W0050487

Additional material from this book can be downloaded from http://extras.springer.com.

ISBN 978-3-642-49455-0 ISBN 978-3-642-49455-0 (eBook) DOI 10.1007/978-3-642-49455-0

Additional material from *Dermatologie,*
ISBN 978-3-642-49455-0, is available at http://extras.springer.com

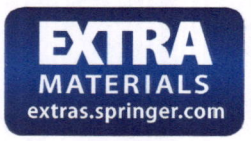

XIII. Congressus Internationalis Dermatologiae

XIII. Congressus Internationalis

Dermatologiae

31.7. – 5. 8. 1967 / München

Editors: W. Jadassohn and C. G. Schirren

Volume 1

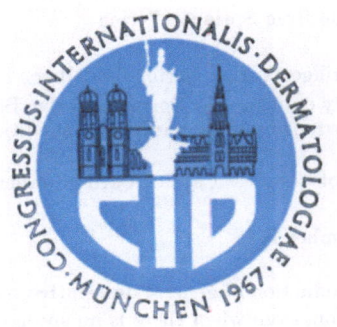

Springer-Verlag Berlin Heidelberg GmbH 1968

Additional material to this book can be downloaded from http://extras.springer.com

ISBN 978-3-642-49455-0   ISBN 978-3-642-49735-3 (eBook)
DOI 10.1007/978-3-642-49735-3

All rights reserved
No part of this book may be translated or reproduced in any form without written
permission from Springer-Verlag

© by Springer-Verlag Berlin Heidelberg 1968
Originally published by Springer-Verlag Berlin-Heidelberg New York in 1968
Softcover reprint of the hardcover 1st edition 1968

Library of Congress Catalog Card Number 68-8552

Title Number 1523

The reproduction of general descriptive names, trade names, trade marks, etc. in this
publication, even when there is no special identification mark, is not to be taken as a sign
that such names, as understood by the Trade Marks and Merchandise Marks Law,
may accordingly be freely used by anyone

Photos: pages *1—128:* L. HEIGL, H. GIESSNER, R. PRÖHL and W. GERSTENBREY

Volume 1

Preface . . . . VII—X

Congressus Internationales Dermatologiae XII

Contents . . . . : . . . . XIII—XXXIX

Organization, Addresses and Course of the Congress . . . . . *1—128*

Main-Theme I—VII . . . . 1—525

Symposium 1—4 . . . . 527—703

Volume 2

Symposium 5—15 . . . . 705—1375

Case Presentations and Fundamentals on Film . . . . 1377—1382

Scientific Exhibition . . . . 1385—1591

Authors Index . . . . 1592—1598

Volume 1

Preface
Congressional Invitation des Begrüssung ....

Contents XIII

Opening Address and Welcome to the Congress ....

Main Theme I ....

Symposium 1 ....

Volume 2

Symposium 1b ....

See Pneumatical and Fundamentals o., Phil ...

Sample Exhibition ....

Author Index ....

Preface

By these volumes, we would like to show how the problems which preoccupy dermatologists were exposed and discussed at the XIII International Congress of Dermatology. Above all, in this preface, we wish to express our joy that the congress has been a success, which is well shown in the scientific parts of these volumes. Worldwide new relations have been established among dermatologists. We owe its success to all participants: to those who have contributed by their scientific works, to those who followed with attention and to those who have helped us so kindly. Our thanks to the International Committee of Dermatology, the Organization Committee and to numerous collaborators, have been expressed in several speeches. Rereading these we notice with much regret that many people who have greatly contributed to the success of the Congress, were not named verbally. We are not going to make a list of them, it would be too long and incomplete. For their work, their constant collaboration, their great kindness, we wish to express to them our gratitude.

The Publishing Firm Springer, with its usual devotion, realized the wishes of the editors, in publishing the present work and printed it in the shortest delay possible.

The Firm Ciba, has generously undertaken, to its own expense, the publication of the patient demonstration by Eidophor.

WERNER JADASSOHN   CARL GEORG SCHIRREN
Genève   München/Marburg (Lahn)

June 15, 1968

Préface

Par le contenu de ces volumes, nous désirons montrer de quelle façon les problèmes qui préoccupent les dermatologues ont été exposés et discutés au XIIIième Congrès International de Dermatologie. Dans cette préface, nous aimerions tout d'abord exprimer notre joie pour la réussite du Congrès, réussite que la partie scientifique de ces volumes montre bien. En outre, de nouveaux liens se sont établis entre les dermatologues du monde entier. Le succès du Congrès, nous le devons à tous les participants: à ceux qui ont contribué par leurs travaux scientifiques, à ceux qui ont pris part aux discussions, à ceux qui ont écouté avec attention et à ceux qui ont aidé avec tant de gentillesse. Les remerciements adressés au Comité International de Dermatologie, au Comité d'Organisation du Congrès et à tous les nombreux collaborateurs ont déjà été exprimés dans plusieurs discours. Relisant ces derniers, nous nous apercevons avec regret que bien des personnes ayant grandement contribué à la réussite du Congrès, n'ont pas été nommées. Nous n'allons pas en donner la liste, car elle serait trop longue et incomplète. Pour leur travail, leur constante collaboration et leur grande amabilité, nous aimerions ici exprimer encore notre gratitude à toutes les collaboratrices et à tous les collaborateurs.

L'impression et la publication du présent ouvrage par la Maison d'Edition Springer, bien connue pour son dévouement, a exaucé les vœux des éditeurs.

La publication de la séance de démonstrations de malades par le procédé Eidophore, a été généreusement offerte par la Maison Ciba.

WERNER JADASSOHN
Genève

CARL GEORG SCHIRREN
München/Marburg (Lahn)

le 15 Juin 1968

Prefacio

Por medio de estos volúmenes, nos es grato demostrar, de que modo, en el XIII Congreso Internacional de Dermatología, fueron expuestos y discutidos aquellos problemas que preocupan a los dermatólogos. En este prefacio, desearíamos, ante todo, proclamar nuestro gozo por el éxito alcanzado por este Congreso. Este triunfo queda bien reflejado en la sección científica contenida en estos volúmenes. Han quedado establecidos nuevos lazos entre los dermatólogos del mundo entero. El éxito del Congreso ha sido debido a la acción conjunta de todos los participantes: los que contribuyeron con sus trabajos científicos; los que tomaron parte en las discusiones; los que escucharon con atención y todos aquellos que nos prestaron su ayuda con tanta gentileza. Las frases de agradecimiento, dirigidas al Comité Internacional de Dermatología, al Comité de Organización y a los innombrables colaboradores, fueron expresadas en muchos discursos. Releyendo estos, nos hemos apercibido que los nombres de un gran número de personas, que contribuyeron grandemente al éxito del Congreso, no fueron citados. Renunciamos a mencionarles, ya que la lista sería demasiado larga y quizás incompleta. Por su trabajo, su constancia y su gran amabilidad, nos satisface expresar aqui nuestra gratitud, a todas las colaboradoras y colaboradores.

La Editorial Springer, con su desinterés acostumbrado, ha impreso y publicado esta obra en muy breve plazo, colmando asi los deseos de los editores.

La Casa Ciba ha tomado, generosamente, a su cargo, la publicación de la sesión en la que fueron presentados enfermos por su sistema Eidophor.

WERNER JADASSOHN   CARL GEORG SCHIRREN
Genève   München/Marburg (Lahn)

15 de Junio de 1968

Vorwort

Die vorliegenden Bände sollen zeigen, wie am XIII. Internationalen Kongreß für Dermatologie die Probleme, die die Dermatologen beschäftigen, abgehandelt und demonstriert wurden. In diesem Vorwort möchten wir unserer Freude darüber Ausdruck geben, daß der Kongreß gelungen ist. Denn er ist gelungen; das zeigt der wissenschaftliche Teil dieser Bände. Das ergibt sich daraus, daß zwischen den Dermatologen der ganzen Welt neue freundschaftliche Bande geknüpft wurden. Wenn der Kongreß gelungen ist, so verdanken wir das allen Teilnehmern, wirklich allen: denen, die wissenschaftliche Beiträge geliefert haben; denen, die diskutiert haben; denen, die interessiert zugehört haben und denen, die uns freundschaftlich entgegengekommen sind. Dem Dank an das Internationale Komitee, an das Organisationskomitee und an alle die vielen Mitarbeiter ist in verschiedenen Reden Ausdruck gegeben worden. Wenn wir jetzt diese Reden wieder lesen, so stellen wir mit Bedauern fest, daß viele, die sich große Verdienste um den Kongreß erworben haben, namentlich nicht erwähnt sind. Wir verzichten auch jetzt darauf, dies nachzuholen, die Liste würde zu lang und trotzdem unvollständig. Aber alle unsere Mitarbeiterinnen und Mitarbeiter sollen hier den Ausdruck unseres Dankes finden für ihre Arbeit, für ihre stetige Hilfsbereitschaft und auch für ihre große Freundlichkeit.

Der Springer-Verlag hat in gewohnter Großzügigkeit die Wünsche der Herausgeber bei der Gestaltung des Verhandlungsberichtes erfüllt und für ein rasches Erscheinen des umfassenden Werkes Sorge getragen.

Die Ciba hat in sehr dankenswerter Weise die Publikation der Eidophordemonstration übernommen.

WERNER JADASSOHN
Genève

CARL GEORG SCHIRREN
München/Marburg (Lahn)

15. Juni 1968

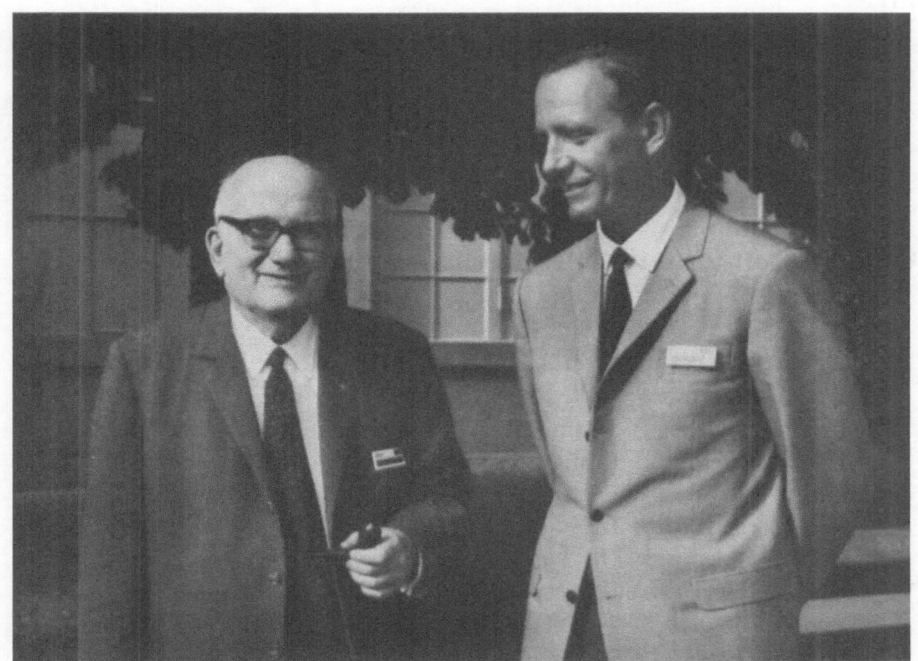

Professor W. JADASSOHN
President of the Congress

Professor C. G. SCHIRREN
Secretary General of the Congress

Congressus Internationales Dermatologiae

	President	*Secretary-General*
I. Paris, 1889	Prof. A. Hardy	
II. Wien, 1892	Prof. Moritz Kaposi	Prof. Gustav Riehl, Sr.
III. London, 1896	Sir Jonathan Hutchinson	Dr. J. J. Pringle
IV. Paris, 1900	Prof. Ernest Besnier	Prof. Georges Thiebierge
V. Berlin, 1904	Prof. E. Lesser	Dr. O. Rosenthal
VI. New York, 1907	Dr. James C. White	Dr. John Fordyce
VII. Roma, 1911	Dr. Tommaso de Amicis	
VIII. København, 1930	Prof. C. Rasch	Prof. Svend Lomholt
IX. Budapest, 1935	Prof. Louis Nékám	Dr. Stephen Rothman
X. London, 1952	Sir Archibald Gray	Dr. G. B. Mitchell-Heggs
XI. Stockholm, 1957	Prof. Sven Hellerström	Dr. Carl Henrik Flodén
XII. Washington, 1962	Prof. Donald M. Pillsbury	Prof. Clarence S. Livingood
XIII. München, 1967	Prof. Werner Jadassohn	Prof. Carl Georg Schirren

Contents Volume 1

	page
Introduction	1
Organization of the Congress	8
Participants Numbers from 1952 to 1967	10
Opening Session — Introduction	13
Opening Addresses	17
Prof. ROBERT DEGOS	17
Dr. h. c. ALFONS GOPPEL	19
Dr. HANS-JOCHEN VOGEL	19
Prof. LUDWIG KOTTER	22
Prof. ALBERT WIEDMANN	22
Prof. WERNER JADASSOHN	23
Prof. CARL GEORG SCHIRREN	27
Medals and Prizes	29
While Sessions	33
Press — Radio — Television	36
Social Program and Ladies' Program	39
Exhibitions — Introduction	53
Technical Exhibition	56
Opening of the Technical Exhibition — Opening Addresses	59
Prof. WERNER JADASSOHN	59
Prof. WILHELM SCHNEIDER	59
Exhibitors	62
The Art Exhibition	65
Film — Introduction	69
Film Program	70
Voyages after the Congress	72
Closing Session — Introduction	74
Concluding Speeches	75
Prof. ROBERT DEGOS	75
Prof. WERNER JADASSOHN	76
Prof. JOSÉ GAY PRIETO	77
Prof. CARL GEORG SCHIRREN	78
Donations	80
List of Donors	81
Members of the Congress	85
International Committee of Dermatology, Meeting of July 30, 1967, Munich	97
Report to the International Committee of Dermatology by SVEN HELLERSTRÖM	102
International League of Dermatological Societies	106
International Committee of Dermatology, Meeting of August 5, 1967, Munich	109
Rules and Regulations of the International League of Dermatological Societies	117

Main Theme I: Cancerous State, Precancerous State and Pseudocancers of the Skin (except Sarcomas and Melanomas)

1. Experimental Studies of the Carcinom Mechanism and Precancerous States

Reports

Electron Microscopic and Histochemical Findings in Basal Cell Epithelioma, Squamous Cell Carcinoma and Some Appendage Tumors. W. F. LEVER and K. HASHIMOTO	3
The Rôle of the Mesoderm in Basaliomas. H. PINKUS	8

page

Interrelation between Structure and Recurrence in Basal-Cell Carcinoma. A. REHÁK 11

Sur les précancéroses cutanées. I. BOSCO 13

Histochemical and Histoenzymological Studies in the Praecancerous Conditions of the Skin. L. SZODORAY and CL. VEZEKENYI-NAGY 16

The Mechanism of Precancerous and Pseudocancerous Conditions. — A Comparative Study. S. JABLONSKA and A. LANGNER 17

Free Communications

The Vascular Pattern of Induced Skin Cancer in Rats. W. A. WELTON 19

Enzymes de la glycolyse et du cycle des pentoses-phosphates dans les épithéliomas. A. RIBUFFO 21

Effect of Prolonged Administration of Testosterone on Normal and X-Ray Radiated Rat Skin. H. S. ZACKHEIM 22

Solar Ultraviolet Radiation and Skin Cancer. F. URBACH and R. E. DAVIES 24

A Clinical and Histological Study of the Evolution of Proliferative Epidermal Lesions of Pitch Workers. G. HODGSON and H. J. WHITELEY 29

Arsenbedingte Präcancerosen und Cancerosen der Haut. W. BRAUN 31

Beitrag zur Beziehung des Traumas zum Hautcarcinom. M. SCHWARZWALD 33

(Prä-)Cancerosen und Elastose. G. NIEBAUER 35

Les nucléases des tumeurs épidermiques. J. DE BERSAQUES and J. PIÉRARD 37

Vergleichende cytophotometrische Untersuchungen an metatypischen Basalzellepitheliomen und Plattenepithelcarcinomen der Haut. G. EHLERS 38

Respiratory Enzymes Activity in Human Skin Neoplasms and Some Praecancerous Lesions. D. CERIMELE, F. SERRI and C. PELFINI 43

Etude histochimique et biochimique comparée de certaines activités enzymatiques dans les cancers de la peau. J. HEWITT, M. GUIGON and J. BOLUBASZ 44

Histologie des lésions précancéreuses de la peau. J. WANET and G. ACHTEN 46

Antigene Wirkung von Tumorgewebe. H. TRITSCH 48

Report

Les dermatoses paranéoplasiques. Y. BUREAU and H. BARRIERE 49

2. Keratoakanthoma

Free Communications

Unusual in Keratoakanthoma. D. V. STEVANOVIĆ 51

Zur Histogenese des Keratoakanthoms. K. W. KALKOFF, H. BERGER and M. HUNDEIKER 53

Unusual Forms of Keratoakanthoma. A. W. KOPF 54

An Ultrastructure Study of the Keratoakanthoma Experimentally Produced. L. PRUTKIN 57

Papilomatosis Florida oral. A. R. DE KAMINSKY, C. A. KAMINSKY, J. ABULAFIA and A. KAMINSKY 58

3. Clinical and Histological Studies

Report

Tumeurs des glandes sudorales. J. CIVATTE and J.-M. MASCARO 61

Free Communications

Das Syndrom der multiplen Basalzellnaevi (Naevobasaliome). W. THIES 63

Xeroderma pigmentosum — ein Modellprozeß der Cancerogenese der Haut. A. KÚTA 67

Clear Celled Epithelial Tumors of the Skin. A. H. MEHREGAN 68

The Pathology of Malignant Angioendothelioma of the Skin. E. WILSON-JONES . . . 70

Importance of Early Recognition of Oculo-cutaneous Metastases in Cancer of the Urinary Bladder. A. HOLLANDER and I. A. GROTS 72

page

Cytologische Untersuchungen der Hautbasaliome in den Ausstrichpräparaten.
K. Lejman and J. Bogdaszewska-Czabanowska 73

Tetracycline Fluorescence in Squamous Cell Carcinoma. H. J. Donsky and G. R.
Mikhail 74

Regional Multiple Carcinoma. G. W. Vavruska and D. S. Kahn 75

A Skin Cancer Consultative Clinic. A. Johnson 76

Corrélations morpho-cliniques dans les récidives des épithéliomas cutanés de la face.
C. Longhin, G. Sandru, R. Dutu and M. Spiridon 78

Neuromyopathy in Skin Cancer. A. K. Afifi, F. S. Farah, A. K. Kurban and F. A.
Sabra 79

Cáncer, precáncer y pseudocáncer cutáneos: Estudio estadistico de la clínica dermatológica de la Universidad de Valencia. J. Calap and J. M. Fortea 81

Electron Microscopic Study of the Morphogenesis of Skin Tumours. J. Sugár 83

Epidermotropic Eccrine Carcinoma. Y. Miura, A. Akano, T. Nakagawa and Y. Kikuchi 84

Considérations sur le potentiel de malignisation des chéilites précancéreuses. Al. Dimitrescu 86

L'influence des radiations artificielles sur la muqueuse des lèvres des trempeurs d'acier.
R. Nicolau, P. Iacob and M. Bichis 87

Erythroplasia of Queyrat: A Precancerous Dermatosis. J. H. Graham and E. B. Helwig 89

Queilitis actínica, glándular y cáncer de labio inferior. P. Parejo and J. Ocaña . . . 91

L'ulcère chronique de la lèvre inférieure. F. Vanbremeersch, B. Duperrat and
J. Y. Noury 92

Squamous Cell Carcinoma in the Nottingham-Derby Combined Tumour Clinic 1959/66.
P. D. C. Kinmont and D. I. McCallum 97

4. Therapy

Reports

The Treatment of Skin Cancer and Pre-Cancer with Topical Cytotoxic Ointments.
J. C. Belisario 99

The Treatment of Skin Cancers with Radiation. H. Goldschmidt 105

Resultado de la radioterapia superficial en los epiteliomas cutáneos. G. Jaqueti and
J. Gay Prieto 107

Free Communications

Experiences with Topical Use of 5-Fluorouracil. A. R. Goddard 110

Therapie des Bowencarcinoms und des Lupuscarcinoms mit konventionellen Röntgenstrahlen. G. Stein 112

Traitement de l'épithélioma cutané par l'exérèse simple avec suture immédiate.
D. Thibaut 113

Tratamiento actual de la enfermedad de Paget del pezon. J. Ocaña Sierra and A. J.
Capilla 117

Tratamiento quirúrgico del cáncer cutáneo-mucoso. F. de Dulanto and J. Sánchez-
Muros 118

Über die Dosisplanung bei der Strahlentherapie der Hauttumoren. K. Balabanov and
P. Pentschev 119

Antimitotica der Podophyllinreihe bei Hautkrebs und seniler Keratose. V. Matanić 120

Chemosurgery for the Microscopically Controlled Excision of Skin Cancer. F. E. Mohs 122

Die Therapie fortgeschrittener Hauttumoren. H. Drepper and F. Ehring 125

Cryosurgery of Cutaneous Carcinoma. S. A. Zacarian 126

Topical 5-Fluorouracil. — An Effective Agent in the Treatment of Multiple Actinic
Keratoses and Some Superficial Malignant Diseases. W. M. Honeycutt, C. J. Dillaha
and G. T. Jansen 128

page

Main Theme II: Corticosteroids in Dermatology

Reports

Corticosteroids in Dermatology. G. Asboe-Hansen 133

Indications de la corticothérapie en dermatologie. S. Longhin 135

The many "Facies" of Iatrogenic Hypercorticism. A. C. Curtis and G. L. Stoker . . 140

Les traitements prolongés par les corticostéroïdes (conduite du traitement). A. Midana,
G. Zina and G. Martina 143

Schädigungen bei lang durchgeführter Steroidtherapie mit besonderer Berücksichtigung
der Hypophyse und Nebennierenrinde. F. Földvári, B. Vértes and J. Masszi . . 145

Topical Corticosteroid Therapy. V. H. Witten 149

Les atrophies cutanées au cours de la corticothérapie générale. R. Touraine, M.
Fournet and S. Belaïch 153

Some Effects of Corticosteroids "in vitro". C. N. D. Cruickshank 156

Free Communications

Long-term Estrogen and Corticosteroid Therapy in Chronic Skin Diseases. A. S. Spangler, S. Sotman and H. N. Antoniades 158

Australian Experiences with the Cortico-steroids. W. W. Lempriere 159

Möglichkeiten der Entwöhnung bzw. Einsparung von Corticoiden in der dermatologischen Therapie. G. Ludwig 160

Indications for and Results of Systemic Corticosteroid Therapy in Dermatology.
J. C. P. Logan and A. Girdwood Fergusson 163

Influencia de los corticosteroides en la queratinización. A. M. Mom 165

Seltene Nebenerscheinungen bei der Therapie mit den Corticosteroiden an der dermatologischen Klinik in Zagreb. D. Karlić and V. Čajkovac 166

Die Insuffizienz der Nebenniere nach Corticoidbehandlung. E. Lacková, J. Rádl and
M. Horáková 168

Corticosteroid-Nebenwirkungen und ihre Behandlung durch klinische Klimatherapie an
der Nordsee. W. Pürschel 169

A Cytotoxic Effect of Fluocinolone Acetonide. A. J. Cox and E. M. Farber 171

Vergleich zwischen der vasoconstrictorischen und antientzündlichen Wirkung verschiedener Corticosteroide. H. Tronnier 172

Penetration Studies with C^{14}-Labelled Fluocinolone Acetonide. M. K. Polano and
L. de Beukelaar 176

Standards for Clinical Evaluation of Topical Steroids. J. R. Scholtz and K. J. Dumas 179

Absorption de l'hydrocortisone par la peau saine. G. Gardenghi and B. Tarquini . . 181

Local Action of Steroids. K. Aso, Y. Tanabe and K. Takenouchi 184

The Penetration of Radiolabeled Hydrocortisone in Human Skin in vivo. R. J. Feldmann and H. I. Maibach. 186

Zur Resorption von Corticoidsalben. K. Winkler 187

Measurement of Percutaneous Absorption of Corticosteroid by Means of an Autoradiography. A. Kukita and T. Matsuzawa 188

Observations concernant l'emploi des corticostéroïdes dans le traitement local de certaines dermatoses. St. Teodorescu and Al. Bădănoiu 192

The Influence of Topical Corticosteroids on Hypothalamic-Pituitary-Adrenal Function.
D. D. Munro, M. Feiwel and V. H. T. James 194

An Evaluation of Intralesional Steroid Therapy in Alopecia Areata. F. O. Meenan . . 197

Effects of Topical Steroids in Normal and Psoriatic Skin. L. Juhlin 198

The Recurrence Rate of Psoriatic Lesions after Topical Treatment with Dithranol and
Corticosteroids under Plastic Dressings. D. Suurmond 200

Effect of Topically Applied 0.1% Betamethasone 17-valerate ("Betnovate") Ointment on
the Adrenal Function of Children. M. Feiwel, D. D. Munro and V. H. T. James 202

Die Ausscheidung der 17-Oxysteroide durch den Harn bei der lokalen Locacorten-
Applikation. M. Horáková and E. Lacková 204

page

Prolongation moyenne de la vie chez les malades de pemphigus vulgaris traités par corticostéroïdes. P. Botzov, T. Pascalev and G. Spirov 205

The Effect of Intraarticular Celestona Chrondose in Rheumatoid Arthritis Associated with Psoriasis. L. Hellgren and A. Björnberg 207

Corticosteroids in the Treatment of Severe Dystrophic Epidermolysis Bullosa. E. J. Moynahan 208

Corticosteroid Therapy in Herpes Zoster. R. W. Carslaw and J. M. Nicolson . . . 209

Avantages thérapeutiques des corticostéroïdes dans un cas de Ainhum. A. Merello 211

The Present Aspect of Corticosteroids. — Therapy of Pemphigus in Japan. K. Ohara 212

Acción tópica de la fluformilona en dermatología. P. A. Viglioglia 213

Main Theme III: Contact Dermatitis (Allergic and Non-Allergic)

Reports

Factors Involved in Contact Non-Allergic Dermatitis. R. R. Suskind 217

Die Epicutanprobe durch wiederholte Benetzung. W. Burckhardt, R. Schmid and P. Schmid 224

Pathogenesis of Sensitization in Allergic Contact Dermatitis in Man. R. L. Baer and M. J. Fellner 226

Chronicity in Allergic Contact Dermatitis. C. D. Calnan 229

Zur Pathogenese der toxischen (ortoergischen) Kontaktdermatitis. H. W. Spier and F. Klaschka 232

Specificity and Cross-Sensitivity in Contact Allergy. V. Pirilä 236

Die Akzentverschiebungen bei den sensibilisierenden Stoffen während der letzten 3 Jahrzehnte. S. Borelli 238

Free Communications

Kontaktekzem und Ekzematoide. Fr. Kogoj and J. Fettich 244

Die passive Übertragung des DNCB-Kontaktekzems beim Meerschweinchen mit Hilfe der kontinuierlichen Austauschtransfusion. F. Schröpl 246

Immunologic Unresponsiveness to Contact Sensitizers. E. D. Lowney 247

The Persistence and Recurrence of Contact Eczema: Clinical Experimental Observations. C. L. Meneghini, F. Rantuccio and G. Cozza 249

Tests épicutanés et épreuve de concentration-dilution. J. Oleffe 252

Experimentelle Untersuchungen über Sensibilisierungen mit chlorierten Imidazolinderivaten. E. Schöpf and K. H. Schulz 254

Problèmes physiochimiques concernant la formation de l'antigène sensibilisant de contact. E. Panconesi 255

The Aetiology of Eczema. J. G. Coburn and J. Reid 257

Cutan-vasculäre Kontaktallergie. — Untersuchungen zur Frage einer Antigen-Antikörperreaktion bei physikalischer Allergie. L. Illig 258

Sur la sensibilisation expérimentale au chrome. V. N. Negulescu 259

Recherches sur la pathogénie de l'eczéma dû aux sels de chrome. A. Sertoli and E. Panconesi 261

Efectos de una substancia antiplasmínica sintética en el eczema. J. M. Gimenez Camarasa 262

Test épicutané et test intradermique au bichromate de potassium. — Etude histopathologique comparative. B. Giannotti and A. Sertoli 265

Aspectos clínicos y pruebas cutáneas de las dermatitis. S. Abeliuk and E. Sylvester 267

The Frequency of Allergic Diseases Among Relatives of Patients with Allergic Eczematous Contact Dermatitis. M. Forsbeck, E. Skog and K. Ytterborn 268

	page
Zunahme von Metallallergien bei Hausfrauen. G. FORCK	270
Hand Dermatitis, a Prospective Study. G. AGRUP	273
Seasonal Variations in the Incidence of Contact Dermatitis. N. HJORTH	275
L'Allergie aux sels d'ammonium quaternaire. — Etat actuel de nos recherches. P. MARTIN, M. MENNECIER, P. AGACHE and CL. HURIEZ	276
Contact Dermatitis due to Plastic Coated Furniture (Tricresyl Phosphate). J. S. PEGUM	279
Study on the Penetration of Mineral Oil into the Human Skin by the Aid of Fluorescence Microscopy. C. SCARPA	280
Vergleichende Untersuchungen verschiedener Testmethoden bei Sensibilisierung gegen Neomycinsulphat (N.). M. NOVÁK and T. BIELICKÝ	282
Photoallergic Reaction in Red Tattoos. Mercury-Cadmium Sensitivity. N. GOLDSTEIN	283
Etude des maladies cutanées provoquées par la Brai de Houille. F.-X. CARTON	286
Dermatitis, verursacht durch das Insekt Simulium erythrocephalum. A. KRSTITSCH and V. ZIVKOVITCH	288
Contact Dermatitis from Static Electricity. H. E. BELLRINGER	289
Les études des facteurs étiologiques chez les dermatites de contact provoquées par le ciment. S. PERIŠIĆ, A. SOFRONIĆ and D. JOVOVIĆ	291
Plants of North America that may Cause Dermatitis Venenata. A. P. ULBRICH	292
Kontaktekzeme in der Landwirtschaft. E. HEGYI	294
L'automatisation dans l'industrie métallurgique élimine la possibilité d'apparition des dermatoses professionnelles de contact (orthoergiques) ? C. C. OANCEA	296

Main Theme IV: Virus Infections of the Skin and Mucosa

Reports

Neuere Entwicklungen dermatologischer Virusforschung. Th. NASEMANN	301
Pox-Viruserkrankungen. G. STÜTTGEN	306
L'étiologie virale des dermatoses bulleuses généralisées (pemphigus et pemphigoïdes). A. CROSTI, F. GIANOTTI, E. HAHN and D. BUBOLA	310
Hand, Foot and Mouth Disease. R. WARIN and E. WADDINGTON	314
Herpès de primo-infection en milieu tropical. A. BASSET and M. ARMENGAUD	316
Survey of 22 Cases of Behçet's Disease. — The Significance of Specific Skin Hyper-Reactivity. I. KATZENELLENBOGEN	321
Contribution à l'étude du rôle des infections rickettsiennes et pararickettsiennes dans l'étiologie de certaines dermatoses à substratum vasculaire. ST. G. NICOLAU, C. SURDAN and G. NOAGHEA	325

Free Communications

Etude histopathologique des lapins et des singes inoculés avec des virus isolés du sang de malades de pemphigus et de pemphigoïdes. F. STROZZI, E. RONCHI and G. CHIAPPINO	326
Caractéristiques physiques, chimiques, biologiques et immunologiques de quatre souches virales isolées de cas de pemphigus, de dermatite de Duhring, d'épidermolyse bulleuse grave et d'érythème polymorphe. G. GIACOMETTI and E. HAHN	327
Etudes immunologiques chez les malades de pemphigus et pemphigoïdes. D. BUBOLA	329
Démonstration de la présence d'immuno-globulines et de la fixation du complément dans les lésions cutanées chez les malades de pemphigus, au moyen de l'immunofluorescence. F. GIANOTTI, M. GOVERNA, B. PERNIS and A. CROSTI	330
Cutaneous Manifestations of Behçet's Disease. M. MONACELLI and P. NAZZARO	331
Untersuchung der Interferenz zwischen den Herpes simplex- und Vacciniaviren. J. ANGYAL and E. BOTTYAN	333

page

Idoxuridine in the Treatment of Cutaneous Herpes Simplex. M. B. CORBETT, CH. M.
SIDELL and M. ZIMMERMAN   334

Studies on "Latent" Motor Palsy Caused by Zoster. K. UEDA, K. IWASHITA and M.
WAKASUGI   335

The Clinical Features of Hand, Foot and Mouth Diseases. E. WADDINGTON and R. P.
WARIN   336

Etude clinique et épidémiologique de la maladie de Nicolas et Favre à Bordeaux.
L. TEXIER, P. LE COULANT, M. GENIAUX and J. M. TAMISIER   338

Observations on Orf in Man. R. D. SWEET   339

Nobecutan-Podophyllin Preparations in Viral Warts. A. BJÖRNBERG and L. HELLGREN   340

Main Theme V: Current Problems in Syphilis

Reports

Syphilis and Human Ecology. T. GUTHE, O. IDSØE and R. R. WILLCOX.   345

Aspects actuels de la syphilis récente. E. LORTAT-JACOB   353

Aktuelle Probleme der Spätsyphilis. A. WIEDMANN   355

Estimation of the Recent Serologic Methods. H. A. NIELSEN   357

Evaluation des renseignements fournis par le T.P.I. et l'immunofluorescence.
G. L. DAGUET   359

Penicillin in the Treatment of Syphilis. W. J. BROWN   360

Autres traitements que la pénicilline. R. DEGOS   363

Free Communications

Epidemiology

Homosexual Transmission of Early Syphilis. N. G. RAUSCH   366

Homosexualité masculine et syphilis. G. MORIAME and P. MEERTS   367

Social Problems of Venereal Disease Among Adolescents and Young Adults in New
York City. W. CURTH   369

General Trend of Syphilis Recenta in Japan in the past 5 Years (1962 to 1966). J. DOHI,
H. MOCHIZUKI, K. AONO and T. KOJIMA   370

Early Infectious Syphilis in Central London. R. D. CATTERALL   372

Clinical, Epidemiological and Therapeutic Aspects of Syphilis in Buenos Aires.
L. M. BALIÑA, J. C. GATTI, J. E. CARDAMA, J. J. AVILA and H. N. CABRERA . . .   373

Syphilis and Japanese Seamen. T. HASEGAWA and R. SHINODA   375

La sífilis en el Uruguay. Tratamiento y profilaxis. R. A. VIGNALE, F. AMOR and C.
RIVEIRO   377

Der diagnostische Wert des Zeichens von Higoumenakis. C. G. HIGOUMENAKIS. . . .   378

Serology and Experimental Syphilis

Some Immunobiological Problems in Experimental Syphilis. K. ITO   380

Serodiagnosis of Syphilis. L. NICHOLAS and H. BEERMAN   381

Zur quantitativen Beurteilung des FTA-Testes. F. FEGELER, S. NOLTING and M. KIFFE   385

Untersuchungen über den Einfluß des Überlebensmediums auf die Sensibilität des
Nelson-Testes. J. LESINSKI, C. WISNIEWSKA and W. ZAJAC   387

The Problem of Recovery from Syphilis. F. FLARER and C. RABITO   389

Biological False-positive Reactors for Syphilis: Studies with the FTA-Absorption Test.
D. L. TUFFANELLI and K. D. WUEPPER   391

Neue diagnostische Methoden bei un- und anbehandelter Frühsyphilis. K. GREGORCZYK   393

Die Aufgabe des Lysozyms bei der experimentellen Syphilis des Kaninchens. L. POSPÍŠIL   395

page

F.T.A. Test quantitatif dans le sérum d'individus non syphilitiques. S. SARTORIS and G. F. STRANI 397

Quantitative FTA Test During Treatment of Recent Syphilis. G. LEIGHEB, G. F. STRANI and S. SARTORIS 398

Modifications du comportement des tréponèmes pales après passages sur des lapins cortisones. P. COLLART, G. POGGI, M. DUNOYER and F. DUNOYER 400

Recherches expérimentales sur la provocation des anticorps fluorescents après administration de spirochète de souche Reiter chez des individus sains et syphilitiques. A. PANTI and S. ULIVI 404

Activité des anticorps fractionnés du serum dans la syphilis. F. OTTOLENGHI and U. SPAGNOLI 405

Activité antigénique des fractions de la protéine purifiée du tréponème de Reiter. U. SPAGNOLI and F. OTTOLENGHI 406

Possible signification du comportement des fractions globuliniques au F.T.A.-test sur le sérum de sujets luétiques. P. PAGNES 408

La stimulation lymphocytaire in vitro en divers stades de la syphilis. G. C. CHIEREGATO and G. FALDARINI 410

Untersuchungen über die Sensibilität und Spezifität des FTA-ABS-Testes. W. LESIŃSKA, J. LESIŃSKI and W. ZAJAC 411

Sérologie de la syphilis chez les sujets de race noire. P. MANY, R. MISSON, J. LAPEYRE, J. TEILLARD, B. BOUTET and F. PAGES 413

Treatment

Traitement de la syphilis. L. CIARROCCHI 415

Long Term Results of Penicillin Therapy of Primary and Secondary Syphilis. J. TOWPIK 416

New Therapeutical Aspects in the Therapy of Syphilis. G. EHRMANN 419

Considérations sur le diagnostic de guérison de la syphilis au moment actuel. U. BONCINELLI 419

Traitement des syphilis récentes par injection unique de 2.400.000 unités de Benzathine-Pénicilline. R. ROLLIER and T. MARKUCH 421

L'effet thérapeutique chez les malades atteints de syphilis traités à la Clinique Universitaire de Dermatovénérologie à Belgrade les 20 dernières années. S. KONSTANTINOVIĆ and S. PERIŠIĆ 423

Stellt die Behandlung der Frühsyphilis heute noch ein Problem dar? J. SÖLTZ-SZÖTS . 425

Main Theme VI: Cutaneous Manifestations of Circulatory Disorders of the Legs

Reports

Die venösen Durchblutungsstörungen der unteren Extremität. W. SCHNEIDER . . . 429

Methoden zur Untersuchung zirkulatorischer Störungen der Beine. H. STORCK and E. STREHLER 438

Arterial Reconstruction in Cutaneous Ischaemic Lesions. G. E. MAVOR and J. M. D. GALLOWAY 441

Medical Treatment of Cutaneous Disorders of Vascular Origin. CL. HURIEZ and F. DESMONS 444

Surgical Treatment of Venous Ulcers and Eczema of the Leg. K. HÆGER 450

Lymphedema of the Lower Extremities. J. BENINSON 452

Hipodermitis nodular subaguda migratiz. J. PIÑOL AGUADÉ 455

An Evaluation of Low Molecular Weight Dextran in Acrocyanosis and Acroscleroderma. E. M. FARBER, H. S. ZACKHEIM and E. ASCHHEIM 458

Free Communications

Oxygénothérapie locale dans les ulcères de jambe. W. RASIEWICZ and B. SZYMCZYK 460

page

Des aspects médico-sociaux et étio-pathogéniques de l'ulcère de jambe. L'importance de l'artério- et de la phlébographie dans l'ulcère dit variqueux. G. NASTASE and G. CHISLEAG 461

Studies on the Healing Time of Leg Ulcers. A Clinical and Statistical Study Based on 200 In-Patients. A. PERDRUP and J. STENE 463

A Mathematical Model for Healing Curves of Leg Ulcers. J. STENE 464

Arterial Occlusions as a Cause of Gangrene and Ischemic Ulcerations of the Legs. R. G. FREEMAN and J. M. KNOX 466

Präventivmaßnahmen bei Rezidiven der Unterschenkelgeschwüre. B. JANOUŠEK, H. DLABALOVÁ and V. ROZSÍVALOVÁ 468

Atrophie blanche. R. SANTLER 469

Stasis Dermatitis and Atrophie Blanche. —A Clinicopathologic and Histochemical Study. A. S. MARQUES, J. H. GRAHAM, W. C. JOHNSON and H. R. GRAY 470

Cutaneous Manifestations of Circulatory Disorders of the Legs. A. BOROTA 474

Neue Gesichtspunkte in der Behandlung venöser Durchblutungsstörungen. H. WEIT-GASSER 474

Angiolopathien und Unterschenkeldermatosen. N. KLÜKEN 476

The Pathogenesis of Nodular Panniculitis of Calves. P. BARTÁK 478

Histopathological Studies on Inflammatory Nodular Diseases in Lower Leg, Especially Concerning on Vascular Change. T. MIYAZAWA and Y. SASAI 479

The Treatment of Tropical Ulcer with an Antibacterial Soap and Topically Applied Sugar. R. A. OSBOURN, B. BENJAMIN and B. E. ELLICKSON 481

Main Theme VII: Regeneration and Transplantation of the Skin

Reports

Regeneration and Transplantation Experiments with Lower Vertebrate Skin as a Guide to Possible Endogenous Sources of Localized Pathogenesis in Man. I. W. WHIMSTER 487

The Cell Turnover of Human Epidermis. A. TOSTI 490

Tissue Banks and Local Therapy for Extensively Burned Patients. G. DOGO 496

Transplantation of Normal Skin to Pathologic Skin. N. ORENTREICH 497

Cultivation and Regeneration of Normal and Psoriatic Cells. B. LAGERHOLM 500

Reactions Between Skin Grafts and Hosts. A. CASTERMANS, G. DEGIOVANNI, A. M. HAENEN-SEVERYNS and G. LEJEUNE 501

Indikationen und Ergebnisse von Transplantationen bei Dermatosen. H. C. FRIEDERICH 503

Free Communications

Electron Microscopic Studies of Epithelial Growth and Keratinization in Cultures of Split-Thickness Adult Human Skin. PH. H. PROSE and A. E. FRIEDMAN-KIEN . . 505

The Management of Extensive Full-thickness Burns by Skin Grafting. T. ANZAI . . 509

Les hétérogreffes animales: Phénomènes de rejet des hétérogreffes répétées et des auto-greffes secondaires. P. LAUGIER, M. VÉRON, J. C. RISOLD and V. ELLENA 510

Transplantation of Epithelial Cell Cultures and the Formation of an Epidermis. M. A. KARASEK 513

Influence of Genetic Relationship on Skin Homotransplantation Survival in Humans. R. CEPPELLINI, M. VISETTI and G. LEIGHEB 514

Über die klinische Anwendung homologer und heterologer Hauttransplantate. W. WITTELS 515

Acid Mucopolysaccharide Synthesis in Scleredema. S. I. LAMBERG 517

La dynamique de la croissance des fibroblastes in vitro à partir des explants de peau humaine. M. GAVRILESCU 518

Biología de las heridas cutáneas. J. SÁNCHEZ-MUROS and F. DE DULANTO 520

page

Electron Microscopy of the Immunologically Competent Cells During Skin Homograft Rejection in the Rhesus Monkey (Macaca mulatta). F. ALLEGRA, M. BELL and L. GIACOMETTI 521

Zur Frage des Ausgangsmaterials der senilen Elastose. — Licht- und elektronenmikroskopische Befunde. H. BERGER 522

Epithelial and Fibroblast Tissue Culture Studies as a Trial to Understand the Action of Asiaticoside as a Healing and as a Fibrolytic Agent. H. EL-HEFNAWI 524

Symposium 1: Genodermatoses

Reports

Classification of Genodermatoses. D. BLOOM 529

Les génodermatoses bulleuses. S. LAPIÈRE 531

Le test gémellaire dans les dermatoses héréditaires. L. GEDDA and R. CAVALIERI . . 534

Epidermolysis bullosa hereditaria. — Klinik, Histologie, Elektronenmikroskopie. U. W. SCHNYDER 539

Le pemphigus familial bénin chronique et les formes bulleuses de la maladie de Darier. J. PIÉRARD and A. KINT 542

The Different Forms of Ichthyosiform Erythrodermia. J. R. SIMPSON 549

Xeroderma pigmentosum. E. HADIDA, F. G. MARILL and J. SAYAG 551

Free Communications

Importance génétique et clinique des altérations atypiques du fond de l'oeil dans le syndrome de Groenblad et Strandberg (pseudo-xanthome élastique et stries angioïdes). A. FRANCESCHETTI 553

The Necessity of Distinguishing Four Types of Acanthosis Nigricans. H. OLLENDORFF CURTH 557

Angiokeratoma Corporis Diffusum Fabry. W. P. DE GROOT 559

Studies on Ichthyosis Vulgaris. Y. IGARASHI, K. UEDA and K. IWASHITA 561

A Genetic Study of X-Linked Ichthyosis in Israel. L. ZIPROWSKI, A. FEINSTEIN, A. ADAM, R. SANGER and R. R. RACE 562

Atrophodermie folliculaire, proliférations baso-cellulaires et hypotrichose. B. CHRISTOL, A. DUPRÉ and A. BAZEX 565

Genetic Analysis of Erythropoietic Protoporphyria (EPP), the Erythrocyte Fluorescence Method. K. D. WUEPPER and J. H. EPSTEIN 566

Erythropoietic Protoporphyria — a Family Study. E. M. DONALDSON, A. D. DONALDSON and C. RIMINGTON 569

Biochemische Untersuchungen bei Porphyria variegata. G. ZIEGLER 570

The Molecular Cause of Albinism. G. F. WILGRAM 571

Zum Mechanismus der Aktivitätsminderung der Phosphoglucose-Isomerase in Erythrocyten von Kranken mit florider Psoriasis vulgaris. H. HOLZMANN and B. MORSCHES 572

Lichtdermatosen mit Hyperaminoacidurien. P. H. CLODI 574

Zur Klinik und Chromosomenanalyse der V. Phakomatose. G. VELTMAN and S. ADARI 575

Incidence of Anti-Nuclear Antibodies Among First-Degree Relatives of Patients with Chronic Discoid Lupus, Systemic Lupus and Normal Subjects. C. MARCH, N. ROTHFIELD and N. PACE 576

Electrocardiographic Abnormalities in a Familiy with Generalized Lentigo. R. J. WALTHER, B. POLANSKY and I. A. GROTS 578

Pachyonychia Congenita. C. B. VIZIAM, R. MATHAI, A. MAMMEN and Z. ISAAC . . . 580

Estudios citogenéticos en dermatología. J. ESTELLER, J. PIÑOL AGUADÉ, A. ALIAGA and E. GIMFERRER 581

Über den Erbgang einiger Formen von palmo-plantarer Keratose in Zusammenhang mit ihrem erbbiologischen und nosologischen Konzept. E. I. BOLOGA 583

page

Disseminated Superficial Actinic Porokeratosis. M. E. CHERNOSKY, R. G. FREEMAN and
D. E. ANDERSON 587
Werner's Syndrome. — Report of a Case with Postmortem Findings. Y. HAMADA . . 588
Unklassifizierte fleckenhafte Atrophie der Haut bei zwei Schwestern (Capillaritis
maculo — keratotica atrophicans familiaris). R. ILEA and M. PAVEL 589

Symposium 2: Pyodermatitis

Reports

The Etiology of Pitted Keratolysis. D. TAPLIN and N. ZAIAS 593
Bacterial Flora. — The Rôle of Local and Environmental Factors. J. M. KNOX, M. E.
MCBRIDE and W. C. DUNCAN 595
Polysaccharidfraktionen von Bakterien in ihrer Bedeutung für die Haut. J. MEYER-ROHN 600
Staphylococcal Strain 502-A in the Treatment of Recurrent Furunculosis. H. I. MAIBACH
and W. G. STRAUSS 602
Some Observations on the Normal Cutaneous Flora of Different Age Groups.
M. J. MARPLES 602

Free Communications

Über die Dynamik der Zusammensetzung der Bakterienflora auf der Haut. A. TODOROV
and P. POPCHRISTOV 605
Keloidal Folliculitis of the Neck in Mongolism. E. KOCSARD, J. E. MOULTON and
F. OFNER 607
Die Auswertung der Einwirkung des Staphylokokken-Anatoxins bei der Therapie und
Diagnostik der Staphylokokken-Hautkrankheiten. J. LAŇCUCKI, J. SAMOS, Z.
JÓZEFCZYK and E. STANOWSKA 609
Die Erysipelfrage. I. Allergologische und immunologische Untersuchungen an Erysipel-
kranken. E. RAJKA, S. KOROSSY, J. BÖSZÖRMÉNYI, J. SZITA and M. GÓZONY 611
Die Erysipelfrage. II. Resultate der Streptococcus-Vaccinetherapie bei rezidivierenden
Erysipelkranken. S. KOROSSY, E. RAJKA, J. BÖSZÖRMÉNYI and M. GÓZONY 611
Bacterial Etiology of Superficial Pyoderma in the Middle East. A. S. DAJANI, F. S. FARAH
and A. K. KURBAN 612
L'influence de l'infection sur la marche du psoriasis. M. ZAJFEN and B. EJMONT-
SKRZYPCZYK 613
Antiovulatorios en el tratamiento del acné juvenil. M. AHUMADA, L. NEUMANN and E.
ORTEGA 615

Symposium 3: Dermatoses, Nervous System and Psychotic Origin

Reports

Haut und Nervensystem in klinischer Sicht. G. W. KORTING 623
Structure des fibres amyéliniques du système nerveux cutané. AD. DUPONT and A.
BOURLOND 626
Dermatologie psychosomatique. P. DE GRACIANSKY and O. DE POLIGNY 628
Alteraciones cutáneas con interacción mental. A. KAMINSKY 630
Rehabilitation in Dermatologic Therapy. H. M. ROBINSON 634
Witchdoctors and their Ways. C. M. ROSS 636

Free Communications

Some Experimental Observations of Psychosomatic Aspects of Allergic Skin Disorders.
K. HIGUCHI 639

page

Psychothérapies et traitements classiques dans les dermatoses psychosomatiques.
P. PICHOT and S. LAMBERGEON 640

Lichen ruber planus und Psyche. R. WEITZ and G. VELTMAN 642

A Controlled Experiment in the Psycho-Therapy of Psoriasis. G. H. V. CLARKE and
P. J. ASHURST 644

Etude psychologique clinique et paraclinique des psoriasiques. M. SOULE, J. M. PIRET,
J. NOEL, G. HUREL and M. BOLGERT 645

Genetic Neurological Disorders of Choreoathetosis and Cerebellar Ataxia with Important
Dermatological Findings. W. B. REED 646

Segmentale Innervation und Hautkrankheiten. W. HAUSER 650

Untersuchungen über den Zustand des vegetativen Nervensystems bei Urticaria-
Kranken. ST. CHLEBAROV 652

Neuropsychiatric Manifestations in Xeroderma Pigmentosum. M. S. ABDEL GAWAD and
H. EL-HEFNAWI 654

Symposium 4: Andrology (Masculine Impotence and Sterility)

Experimental Andrology

Reports

Biochemische Untersuchungen an Spermaplasma unter Berücksichtigung des Prostaglandins und seiner klinischen Bedeutung. R. ELIASSON 659

On the Adrenal Origin of Dehydroepiandrosterone in Human Seminal Plasma.
O. STEENO, C. SCHIRREN, W. HEYNS and P. DE MOOR 660

Oestrogene im menschlichen Sperma. C. SCHIRREN 662

Neue Ergebnisse der Immunologie des Spermaplasma. W. P. HERRMANN 663

Neu re morphologische Untersuchungen an Hodenzellen. H.-J. BANDMANN 665

Free Communications

Basische Proteine in Spermienköpfen fertiler und infertiler Männer. W. MEYHÖFER . . 666

Atomabsorptions-spektrometrische Untersuchungen des Magnesium- und Zinkgehaltes
im Hoden und Prostatagewebe sowie im Ejaculat des Menschen. R. HERRMANN, W.
KNOTH and W. MEYHÖFER 668

Zur Bedeutung der Prostaglandine im humanen Seminalplasma. H.-C. STURDE . . . 670

Vergleichende licht- und elektronenmikroskopische Untersuchungen an Hodenbiopsien
von infertilen Männern. H. SCHMALBRUCH and O. P. HORNSTEIN 672

Clinical and Therapeutical Andrology

Reports

Ursachen der Impotentia coeundi. R. CERNEA 673

Successful Treatment of Azoospermia with Human Gonadotropins. CH. A. JOEL . . 676

Uses and Abuses of Gonadotrophins in the Male. G. HELLINGA 679

Nicht-hormonale Substanzen in der Behandlung der männlichen Infertilität. W. NIKO-
LOWSKI 682

Free Communications

Klinische, histologische und endokrinologische Untersuchungen beim „idiopathischen"
Hyperoestrogenismus. M. F. HOFMANN, G. POZZO and M. CRISTOFOLINI 685

Spermaqualität und Konzeptionsrate. R. KADEN 686

Tératospermie et anomalies évolutives de la grossesse. A. MONTAGNANI and M. DE LUCA 688

Les troubles de l'éjaculation — Observations cliniques. G. SANTORI 690

Impuissance organique par dystrophies spinales congénitales (Spina bifida occulta et
spondylolisthésis). J. SIAGE 691

page

Endocrine Function of the Testes, Gonadotropic Activity and Genetic Sex in Male Infertility. L. ANDREASSI 693

Essais de traitement endocrinien de l'infertilité due à des altérations testiculaires. L. SEMMOLA 694

Die Therapie des Klinefelter-Syndroms. H. NIERMANN 696

Die Gonadotropine menschlicher Herkunft in der Behandlung der männlichen Unfruchtbarkeit. P. CERUTTI and M. DE LUCA 698

Enzymatic Activities on Nucleic Acids and their Derivatives in Human Seminal Plasma. P. SANTOIANNI and G. ARGENZIANO 700

Ein neuer Gesichtspunkt endokriner-normospermatischer Infertilität. ST. ILCA, C. DODICA and Z. IOANOVICI 702

Volume 2

Symposium 5: Malignant Reticuloses and Lymphomas

Reports

Histopathologic and Hematologic Changes in Malignant Lymphomas and Reticuloses. H. MONTGOMERY and R. K. WINKELMANN 707

Zur Nosologie und Einteilung der Reticulosen, Reticulosarkomatosen und verwandter Krankheitsbilder unter Berücksichtigung cytophotometrischer Untersuchungen. W. KNOTH 712

Patología y clínica de los reticulo!infomas óculopalpebrales. P. H. MAGNIN, M. C. MORGENFELD and R. L. CABRINI 714

The Identity and Treatment of the Lymphoma Mycosis fungoides. M. A. LUTZNER . 720

Free Communications

Klinik und Histopathologie der malignen Reticulosen. K. W. MACH 721

Cytological Studies on Lymphoma with Electronmicroscopy. H. FUJITA 724

Cutaneous Lymphoblastoma, Spontaneous Involution of Tumours. D. MAJCAN, D. STEVANOVIĆ and B. LALEVIĆ 725

Blood Vessel Morphology in the Reticuloses. T. J. RYAN 727

Generalized Giant-Cell Reticulohistiocytosis (Lipoid Dermatoarthritis) — Clinical and Histopathological Study of two Cases. P. NAZZARO, U. GRANELLI and A. BIGNAMI . 728

Malignant Development in Mastocytosis. F. SAGHER and Z. EVEN-PAZ 729

Sézary Syndrome. G. L. ROCHA, F. SANTOS, R. AZULAY and A. PETRARCA DE MESQUITA 731

Mycosis Fungoides. — Mode of Presentation of 55 Cases. P. D. SAMMAN 733

Cytological Diagnosis in Mycosis Fungoides. E. BREHMER-ANDERSSON and U. BRUNK 735

Triacetyl 6-Azauridine in Mycosis Fungoides. CH. J. MCDONALD, P. CALABRESI and R. C. DE CONTI 739

Ultrastructure de l'angio-réticulo-sarcomatose cutanée: Maladie de Kaposi. E. CALAS, H. BONNEAU and J. P. CESARINI 741

Zur Entität des sog. Morbus Kaposi. G. OEHLSCHLAEGEL 745

Les localisations cutanées spécifiques de la maladie de Waldenstroem. H. BARRIERE, P. LITOUX and B. BUREAU 747

Esquisse de la physionomie de l'angio-sarcomatose de Kaposi en Algérie (A propos de 25 observations personelles). F. G. MARILL, E. HADIDA and J. SAYAG 748

Intérêt de la lymphographie dans les hématodermies. M. DANA, R. BOURDON, V. BISMUTH and J. P. DESPREZ-CURELY 750

Radiothérapie des hémoréticulopathies malignes. R. BOURDON and M. DANA 752

page

Symposium 6: Cosmetology; Biology and Pathology of the Hair

Cosmetology

Reports

Recherches sur le mécanisme d'action des antiperspirants. R. Brun, N. Hunziker and
P. Evdos 755
Hair Dyes. A. Rostenberg and G. Kass 758

Free Communications

International Dermatology and the World of Cosmetics. E. W. Brauer 761
Hormonal and Microbial Influences on the Sebaceous Follicles in Acne. P. E. Pochi . . 762

Biology and Pathology of the Human Hair

Reports

Development of the Human Hair Follicle. — Biology and Pathology of the Human
Hair. F. Serri 763
Alopecia areata, Basic Notions. G. Moretti, A. Rebora, E. Rampini, F. Crovato and
C. Cipriani 765
Klinik und Therapie der Alopecia areata. R. Schuppli 769
Causes actuelles des alopécies féminines diffuses. E. Sidi †, J. Bourgeois-Spinasse
and J. Arouète 771

Free Communications

Propiedades depilatoria y citotóxica de la seleno-cistationina. F. Kerdel-Vegas. . . 775
Control of Mammalian Hair Growth: Studies with a Cell-Free Protein Synthesizing
System. I. M. Freedberg 776
The Effects of Various Pathologic Conditions of the Scalp upon Hair Melanogenesis and
Hair Growth. W. Kostanecki 780
The Histological Changes in Idiopathic Premature Vertex Baldness in Women.
I. Martin-Scott 781
The Normal Trichogram of People Beyond 50 Years but Apparently not Bald.
J. M. Barman, I. Astore and V. Pecoraro 783
Microscopic Studies of Pili Annulati. V. H. Price, R. S. Thomas and F. T. Jones . . 786
Rate of Hair Growth. M. Saitoh, M. Uzuka, M. Sakamoto and T. Kobori 788
Chronical Female Alopecia. M. Binazzi 791
Le problème des états pseudopeladiques ou pseudopeladoïdes dans le cadre des alopécies
cicatricielles. M. Juon 793
La pelade, maladie psychosomatique. S. Lambergeon 795
Biological Depth Dose Studies in Electron Beam Therapy: Effects on Anagen Mouse
Hairs. L. H. Lanzl and F. D. Malkinson 796
Elektronenmikroskopische Befunde an den peritrichialen Nervenfasern des mensch-
lichen Haarfollikels. C. Orfanos 798
Die Behandlung der Alopecia areata im Kindesalter. J. Tomášková 801
Untersuchungen über die Veränderungen des Haares der Augenbrauen bei endogenem
Ekzem. H. Langhof† and M. Munteanu 803

Symposium 7: Mycoses (Superficial and Deep)

Reports

Untersuchungen über die Zuverlässigkeit eines „in vitro"-Lymphocytentests zwecks
Nachweises einer Dermatophyteninfektion. H. Götz 807
Effects of Human Body Fluids on Candida albicans. V. D. Newcomer, J. W. Landau,
N. Dabrowa and M. L. Fenster 813

page

Histoplasmose Africaine. R. VANBREUSEGHEM 817

Micetomas y actinomicosis. A. GONZÁLEZ OCHOA 819

Pathogenesis of South American Blastomycosis (Lutz's Mycosis). A. PADILHA-GON-
ÇALVES 824

Nouvelles acquisitions sur le mécanisme d'action de la Griséofulvine. P. PINETTI . . 826

Free Communications

Les onychomycoses. G. ACHTEN 828

Aspects particuliers de l'épidermomycose causée par epidermophyton floccosum.
I. ALTERAS and I. COJOCARU 830

Ultraestructura y citoquímica de la Candida albicans. L. F. MONTES and V. S. CON-
STANTINE. 831

Keloidal Blastomycosis (Jorge Lobo's Disease). S. FRAGA and J. LISBÔA MIRANDA . . 831

A Look at Mycetoma in India. B. B. GOKHALE, A. A. PADHYE and M. J. THIRUMALACHAR 833

Esporotricosis, estudio clínico epidemiológico. V. C. JARAMILLO, G. C. VÉLEZ, A. R.
MORENO, I. R. PIZANO and A. C. CORTÉS 835

Favus Infection in Iraq. G. F. RAHIM 837

La macrocheilite de la blastomycose Sud-Américaine. J. RAMOS-SILVA and A. PADILHA-
GONÇALVES 839

Experiencias en cuatro casos de cromoblastomicosis y su tratamiento. F. A. OCAMPO,
R. T. PEREZ and R. V. VICTORIA 841

Quelques aspects de la mycose de Lane-Pedroso (chromoblastomycose ou chromomycose) dans la région Amazonique (Brésil). D. SILVA 842

Survey of the Mycoses in U.A.R. K. EL ZAWAHRY and M. EL ZAWAHRY 847

Main Transmission Routes of Spread of Trichophyton Mentagrophytes var. gran.-
Infection from a Natural Focus to Man in a Foothill Region. L. CHMEL, J. BUCHVALD
and M. VALENTOVÁ 851

Beitrag zum Problem tiefer anorectaler Mykosen. O. MALE 852

Flore dermatomycosique actuelle dans la région d'Athènes et sensibilité des souches isolées à la griséofulvine. C. KANITAKIS, U. MARCELOU-KINTI and CHR. GEORGIADIS . . 854

Biological, Sanitarian and Environmental Factors in Dermatomycoses. D. TRICHO-
POULOS, O. MARSELOU-KINTI and A. POLYCHRONOPOULOU 856

New Experiments on Culture, Immunology and Inoculation. J. DE AZEVEDO CARNEIRO,
R. D. AZULAY and L. M. C. DE ANDRADE 858

Sensibilisations de la peau par les dermatophytes. I. COJOCARU, I. ALTERAS and L.
DULAMITĂ 859

La valeur du milieu Gluzman modifié par Condrea dans la préparation de la trichophytine. V. COSTEA, M. CARNIOL, M. LAZAR and M. ILIES 861

Onychomycose due à alternaria tenuis. J. DELACRÉTAZ and D. GRIGORIOU 863

Fungus-Allergy and its Skin Manifestations. E. FEJÉR 864

The Mycologic Laboratory Specimen. The Collection, Inoculation, and Culture Methods.
H. C. GOLDBERG 866

Tinea Versicolor: The Electron Microscopic Morphology of the Genera Malassezia and
Pityrosporum. F. M. KEDDIE 867

Effect of the Immunosuppressive Agent, Cyclophosphamide, on Experimental Systemic
Coccidioidomycosis. J. W. LANDAU, L. INDIANER and V. D. NEWCOMER 872

Enzyme des Kohlenhydratstoffwechsels bei Dermatophyten. W. MEINHOF and G.
RASSNER 876

Microsporum Nanum as a Cause of Human Infections. J. F. MULLINS and C. J. WILLIS 877

Les dermatophytes du sol en Bulgarie. P. POPCHRISTOV, V. BALABANOFF, T. FILKOV and
P. USUNOV 879

L'ultrastructure des grains dans les maduromycoses provoquée par Monosporium apiospermum. M. STOIAN and A. AVRAM 881

page

On the Mycomimetic Pictures Found in Mycologic Examinations. P. SBERNA 883

Zur fermentativen Leistung von Fadenpilzen. W. ADAM 884

Parenté antigénique et localisation des antigènes dans le genre Candida: Etude par immunofluorescence. P. RIMBAUD, J.-M. BASTIDE, M. BASTIDE and J. ALLEGRINI . 886

Essais de marquage de Candida albicans par radioisotopes. Etude de leur distribution dans l'organisme du lapin. S. ANTONESCU 892

Observations of the Treatment of Superficial Mycosis in South-East Europe with CO_2 Snow (Method Haxthausen). M. BRNIČEVIĆ 893

La contamination staphylococcique des trichophyties suppurées. Résultats d'une thérapie combinée: Griséofulvine, antibiotiques antimicrobiennes et traitement local. I. CAPUSAN, P. BALOSU and N. MAIER 895

Tratamiento de las tiñas on Griseofulvina. M. P. MIGUENS 896

Sporotrichosis Recurrens Cicatrisans (Repeating Self-Healing Sporotrichosis). R. N. MIRANDA 898

Traitement expérimental des mycoses cutanées superficielles par l'Amphotéricine B. D. PERYASSÚ and G. LÖWY 900

Experimentelle Grundlagen der externen antimykotischen Therapie. W. RAAB . . . 901

Über den Einfluß von Moronal (-Nystatin) auf den Zellstoffwechsel von Candida albicans (Autoradiographische Untersuchungen). M. RAHMANN-ESSER and F. FEGELER . . 903

Mechanism of Antifungal Action of Potassium Iodide on Sporotrichosis. H. URABE, T. NAGASHIMA and K. NAKASHIMA 907

Fissured Nipples of Lactating Females and its Relation to Candida Infection. A. M. EL MOFTY, R. MEHAREB, H. M. EL KOMY and C. D. JEFFRIES 908

Symposium 8: Malignant Melanomas

Reports

Melanin Biosynthesis in Melanomas. T. B. FITZPATRICK 913

Mélanoses neurocutanées of Touraine. T. KAWAMURA, S. IKEDA, S. NODA, S. ISHIZU.and T. NAKAJIMA 915

La mélanose circonscrite précancereuse de Hutchinson-Dubreuilh (M.H.D.). B. DUPERRAT and J. M. MASCARO 917

Spontaneous Regression of Malignant Melanoma. L. BOWDEN 918

Elektrometrie zur Früherkennung von malignanten Melanomen. N. MELCZER 925

The Surgical Treatment of Malignant Melanoma. R. W. RAVEN 926

Die Behandlung des malignen Melanoms mit schnellen Elektronen eines 15 MeV-Betatrons. G. F. KLOSTERMANN 928

Histologische Diagnostik der Melanome. J. J. HERZBERG 933

Free Communications

Benign Juvenile Melanoma. — Several Selected Aspects from a Study of 51 Lesions. R. ANDRADE 936

Über das Verhalten der Melanomzellen in vitro. B. ROHDE 938

Production of Melanomas in Hairless Mice with Ultraviolet Light. J. H. EPSTEIN, W. L. EPSTEIN and T. NAKAI 939

Effects of Depigmenting Agents on Melanocytes and Melanogenesis. M. A. PATHAK, G. SZABÓ, E. FRENK, S. S. BLEEHEN, Y. HORI and T. B. FITZPATRICK 941

Dopa in Melanoma. H. RORSMAN 942

Multiple Forms of Tyrosinase from Mammalian Melanoma. J. B. BURNETT and H. SEILER 943

370 Mélanomes malins. — Statistiques et pronostic. J. M. SIMONART 944

A propos de 400 mélanomes malins cutanés. C. DUFOURMENTEL, R. MOULY and J. GLICENSTEIN 946

page

Zur Häufigkeit des malignen Melanoms. Ergebnis einer Umfrage. H. KÄSTNER, P. JORDAN and G. FORCK 948

Lentigo Maligna and Malignant Melanoma. R. JACKSON 949

Un diagnostic différentiel important des mélanomes. L'Angiokératome noir. G. E. GOETSCHEL 951

Les noevocarcinomes de l'enfant. R. MOULY, CL. DUFOURMENTEL and J. GLICENSTEIN 954

Nevus y melanomas malignos. L. A. RUEDA 955

Early Diagnosis of Melanoblastoma with the Aid of Electrometric, Thermo-Differential and ^{32}P Uptake Test. A. GULBERT 957

Histologische Befunde beim transplantierten Melanom des Menschen. H. GARTMANN 958

Veränderungen bei inoculierten Melanocyten. KH. WOEBER and O. GRÜTZ † 960

Macromolecular Differentiation of Melanocytic and Nevocytic Malignant Melanomas. Y. MISHIMA 961

Investigación de células tumorales en sangre periférica en enfermos con melanoma maligno. A. ALIAGA and J. CALAP 968

Some Mechanisms of Pox Virus Oncolysis in Malignant Melanoma. A Review of 50 Cases. G. W. MILTON and M. LANE BROWN 970

Richtlinien und unsere Erfahrungen in der Behandlung des malignen Melanoms. GY. KÁRPÁTI, T. VENKEI, Ö. BIHARI, GY. NÉMETH and A. GULBERT 973

Observations concernant la prophylaxie et le traitement du mélanome malin. E. UJVÁRY and I. KREPSZ 974

Données relatives au problème de la possibilité de dissémination après l'irradiation aux rayons X dans les cas du mélanome malin. T. VENKEI and Ö. BIHARI 975

The Uptake of Radioactively Labelled Compounds by Malignant Melanoma. M. S. BLOIS 976

Sensitization to X-Irradiation of Melanoma Cells Using Alpha-MSH. M. LANE BROWN and G. W. MILTON 978

Symposium 9: Physiology of the Skin

Reports

Enzyme und Physiologie der Haut. G. K. STEIGLEDER 983

Collagen Metabolism in Skin. CH. M. LAPIÈRE 986

Physiological Response of Human Skin to Ultraviolet Light. M. A. EVERETT and R. L. OLSON 988

The Clinical Significance of a Comparative Approach to the Physiology of Hair Growth. A. J. ROOK 993

Physiologie der Hautoberfläche. Die relative Bedeutung verschiedener Befunde. F. HERRMANN 995

Some Remarks on the Barrier Function of the Epidermis. J. HORÁČEK 999

Le pouvoir tampon de la peau. H. THIERS 1002

Free Communications

Studies of Some Glycolytic Pathways in the Skin of Rats Under Experimental Conditions. G. RABBIOSI and A. GIANNETTI 1003

Plasma Kinin Formation and Human Inflammation. H. ZACHARIAE, J. MALMQUIST, J. A. OATES and W. PETTINGER 1006

Synthesis of Unique Proteins in Epidermal Keratinization. I. A. BERNSTEIN 1008

Mechanism of Water Binding in Stratum Corneum. J. D. MIDDLETON 1010

Studies on the Epidermal Keratinization of the Human Fetus in vitro with Special References to the Electron Microscopic and Autoradiographic Observation. K. OKAMURA, K. IWASHITA and K. UEDA 1012

page

The Envelope of Epidermal Horny Cells. A. G. Matoltsy 1014

Follicular Hyperkeratinization Induced in the Rabbit Ear by Human Skin Surface Lipids. A. L. Lorincz, H. Krizek and S. Brown 1016

The Influence of Dimethyl Sulphoxide, Dimethyl Acetamide and Dimethyl Formamide on the Epidermal Barrier to Water. H. Baker 1017

Die hygrometrische Aufzeichnung der Hydromeiose und das Abtrocknen der Horn-schicht als Maß ihrer physiologischen Qualität. J. Rovenský and J. Záhejský . . 1020

Physiologische Antiperspirants. H. P. Fiedler 1022

Sodium Secretion and Reabsorption by the Eccrine Sweat Gland. R. L. Dobson . . 1024

The Insensible Water Loss and Skin Temperature. F. A. J. Thiele and K. G. van Senden 1025

The Fine Structure of the Sebaceous Gland of the Adult Female Rat After Receiving Sexual Hormones. Y. Sato and M. Morohashi 1028

The in vivo Study of Cutaneous Lipogenesis. G. Lipkin and V. R. Wheatley 1029

Physiology of Human Sebaceous Glands-Hormonal Control Mechanisms. J. S. Strauss 1031

Le contrôle hormonal de la glande sébacée chez l'homme. M. Bonelli, E. Alessi, C. Tomasini and S. Piccinini 1033

Der Einfluß des Hautoberflächenmilieus auf Staphylococcus aureus. E. Müller . . . 1036

The pH and the Bacterial Flora of Normal Skin Under Fluocinolone-Plastic Occlusion Treatment. E. A. Knudsen 1038

The Alkali Neutralization Capacity of Human Skin in vivo. K. Schutter 1041

Über ultraviolett-absorbierende Verbindungen im Wasserlöslichen epidermaler Ver-hornungsprodukte. E. Schwarz 1043

Ultraviolettes Licht als Stimulus für Kininbildung in menschlicher Haut. R. K. Winkel-mann, J. Epstein and K. Wolff 1045

Sur la réponse vasculaire biphasique au siège de l'érythème dû aux radiations ultra-violettes. Existe-t-il une réponse plus élémentaire que l'érythème ? G. Zina and A. Benedetto 1047

A Cutaneous Role in the Regulation of the Body's Carbohydrate Milieu. R. M. Fusaro and J. A. Johnson 1048

Research on Sialic Acid in the Human Skin. A. Giannetti and G. Rabbiosi 1050

Mepyramine and Adrenergic Neurone. B. S. Verma and O. D. Gulati 1053

Lysosomes and the Skin. R. L. Olson, R. Nordquist, J. Nordquist and M. A. Eve-rett 1056

Modificaciones clínicas e histológicas de la reacción tuberculínica bajo la acción local del valerato de betametasona en cura oclusiva. A. Casalá, C. Bianchi, O. Bianchi, S. Stringa and O. Roqué 1060

The Significance of Low Serum Iron Levels in the Causation of Itching. I. B. Sneddon and M. Garretts 1061

Comparatively Study on the Effects of Corticosteroids, Resochine and Synopene on the Arthus's Phenomenon in Rabbits. B. Bajdekov, K. Bertchev, B. Bojkov and I. Ismirov 1063

Die Adenosintriphosphatase der normalen menschlichen Haut. C. Ene-Popescu . . 1064

Symposium 10: Effects of Radiation on the Skin

Reports

Radiobiologie cutanée. P. van Caneghem 1069

Strahlenwirkung im Hautbereich in Abhängigkeit von der verwendeten Strahlen-qualität. A. Proppe 1070

Strahlenwirkung im Hautbereich in Abhängigkeit von der verwendeten Strahlen-qualität. F. Wachsmann 1074

page

Indications dermatologiques du traitement ionisant. Traitement ionisant des épithéliomas et des mélanomes malins à l'aide de techniques de radio-sensibilisation nouvelles. E. G. SCOLARI 1078

Indications thérapeutiques des substances radioactives en dermatologie. B. PIERQUIN 1081

Algunos rasgos ultraestructurales de las radiolesiones. J. CABRÉ 1083

Preliminary Investigative Studies of the Laser Treatment of Angiomas. L. GOLDMAN, R. J. ROCKWELL jr. and R. MEYER 1084

Free Communications

The Treatment of Skin Tumours with Radium and Hyperbaric Oxygen. C. VALLECCHI and G. MANTELLASSI 1087

Nouvelle technique de Radiumthérapie en oxygène hyperbaryque. M. NANNELLI and G. MANTELLASSI 1088

Acute Effects of Irradiation on the Skin. — A Histochemical and Chemical Study. A. K. KURBAN and F. S. FARAH. 1090

Biochemische Untersuchungen an Serum und Hauteiweißen von Ratten nach Röntgenbestrahlung. O.-E. RODERMUND 1091

Radiations et tissu élastique cutané. M. LEDOUX-CORBUSIER 1093

Problemas del uso de los rayos grenz en los negros y en los mulatos. M. A. CONTRERAS 1094

Tierexperimentelles zur Röntgenfernbestrahlung der Haut. M. BETETTO 1096

Dermatological Observations in the A-Bomb Survivors of Hiroshima and Nagasaki, Japan. M.-L. T. JOHNSON, T. TAURA and P. B. GREGORY 1097

Studies on Induction, Persistence and Recovery of Radiation Damage in Proliferative (Anagen) and Non-proliferative (Telogen) Rodent Hair Cell Populations. F. D. MALKINSON and M. L. GRIEM 1099

Autoradiographische Untersuchungen zur epidermalen Proliferation unter physiologischen, pathologischen und experimentellen Bedingungen mit Tritium-markierten Nucleosiden. W. BORN 1101

Histochimie des enzymes des follicules irradiés du cobaye. A. KINT and J. DE BERSAQUES 1103

Untersuchungen zur experimentellen Photosensibilisierung mit Sulfanilamid und Phenothiazinen. K. SCHWARZ, J. ROTHENSTEIN and M. SCHWARZ-SPECK 1106

Light is an Aetiological Factor for Certain Dermatoses in U.A.R. M. EL ZAWAHRY . . 1107

Heliotherapie und ihr Einfluß auf die Aktivität mancher Enzyme bei Psoriasiskranken. N. BALEVSKA, J. PETKOV, G. MUSTAKOV, S. JOWEV, N. ZLATKOV and G. TOMOV . . 1110

The Action Spectrum of Erythema Induced by Ultraviolet Radiation. Preliminary Report. D. BERGER, F. URBACH and R. E. DAVIES 1112

The Absorption Spectrum of the Stratum Corneum as the Natural Sunscreen of Human Skin. A. R. H. B. VERHAGEN 1118

Prurigo actínico. F. LONDOÑO 1122

Psoralen Therapy of Vitiligo in the Tropics. T. L. FLEISHER 1124

Zur Kombinationsbehandlung der Mycosis fungoides mit Röntgenstrahlen und Spindelgiften. A. WISKEMANN 1125

Photochemical Movement of Cholesterol in Skin. E. W. RAUSCHKOLB and J. M. KNOX 1126

Symposium 11: Immunology in Dermatology

Reports

Aetiology of Some Autoimmune Diseases. N. R. ROWELL 1131

Aspects immunologiques du lupus érythémateux aigu disséminé. J. THIVOLET . . . 1134

Autoimmunity in Pemphigus. T. CHORZELSKI 1135

Immunology of Acne Vulgaris. Dermal Hypersensitivity and Circulating Antibody Levels to Corynbacterium Acnes. S. M. PUHVEL, T. H. STERNBERG and R. M. REISNER 1136

page

Zur Immunologie in der Dermatologie. J. KIMMIG 1139

The Role of the Basophil in the Immune Response. W. B. SHELLEY 1143

Free Communications

Classes of Immunoglobulins Associated with Skin Sensitizing Properties. M. J. FELLNER
and R. L. BAER 1144

Patterns of Skin Fluorescence in Lupus Erythematosus. R. H. CORMANE 1146

Delayed Hypersensitivity Responses in Immunologic Deficiency States. W. L. EPSTEIN 1148

Antikörpermangelsyndrome und Hautveränderungen. G. BREHM 1149

Zur Frage der Antigenspezifität von 2,4-Dinitrochlorbenzol-Epidermis-Conjugaten im
Meerschweinchenversuch. F. KLASCHKA 1151

Antinuclear Factors in Clinical Dermatology. J. S. BECK, N. R. ROWELL and T. E.
ANDERSON 1153

Vasoactive Substances at Sites of Cutaneous Allergies. TH. M. INDERBITZIN and P. J.
GROB 1154

Application de la technique d'immunofluorescence en dermatologie. Y. MONTET, J.
DUHEILLE and J. BEUREY 1156

Experimental Studies on the Pathogenesis of Acantholysis in Pemphigus. P. J. GROB
and TH. M. INDERBITZIN 1158

Autoantibodies in Pemphigus Foliaceus. T. A. FURTADO, A. O. LIMA, G. O. ANDRADE
and O. SEABRA 1159

L'apport de l'immuno-fluorescence dans la mise en évidence du rôle de l'allergie à
Candida albicans dans certaines dermatoses communes. P. TEMIME, M. BENNE,
M. LEBEUF, J. P. MARCHAND and PH. LATOURELLE 1162

Recherches électrophorétiques et immunophorétiques en moyens gélifiés sur protéines
de muscle strié dans différentes collagénoses d'intérêt dermatologique. G. MARTINA
and A. MIDANA 1168

Immunoelektrophorese der Serumproteine bei akuten und chronischen Formen des
Erythematodes. T. BIELICKÝ, L. MALINA and J. OPPLT 1170

Immunologic Defect of the Skin in Lymphadenopathy. Y. NOGUCHI, K. ISHIWARA,
M. HIGUCHI and S. YOSHIDA 1171

Immunologische Untersuchungen von Lymphocytenkulturen. Eine diagnostische
Methode in der Dermatologie. H. J. HEITMANN 1174

Mechanisms of Anaphylaxis. M. W. GREAVES 1176

The Immunochemical Basis of the Urticarial Reaction. F. S. FARAH and A. K. KURBAN 1176

The Release of Serotonin in Hypersensitivity States. J. S. COMAISH 1179

Réactions sérologiques et terrain d'allergie humorale en dermatologie. CL. MIKOL and
M. RENOUX 1180

Experimentelle Untersuchungen zur Desensibilisierung und Immunotoleranz gegen
niedermolekulare Allergene. K. H. SCHULZ 1181

Experimentelle Sensibilisierung mit drei- und sechswertigem Chrom. M. SCHWARZ-
SPECK 1183

Zur Frage autoallergischer Reaktionen bei der Neurodermitis. B. KOPECKÁ, E. SORKIN,
S. BORELLI and A. FJELDE 1185

Delayed Reactivity to Bacterial, Mold and Viral Allergens in Atopic Dermatitis.
G. RAJKA 1187

Das Shwartzman-Phänomen, eine dem Arthus-Phänomen ähnliche, pseudo-immuno-
logische Reaktion der Haut auf Endotoxin. I. KUNICK and L. ILLIG 1187

Immunological Aspects of the Aldrich's Syndrome. G. IACOVACCI, S. UNGARI and F.
AIUTI 1189

Mise en évidence d'anticorps circulants dans les manifestations cutanées de l'allergie à
la pénicilline. J. PAUPE and CL. MIKOL 1190

Heutige Diagnostik der Penicillinallergie. P. MICHAILOV and N. BEROWA 1191

page

Symposium 12: The Skin and Internal Disease

Reports

Erythropoietic Protoporphyria. I. A. MAGNUS 1195
Xanthomatoses et maladies systémiques. A. BAZEX, A. DUPRÉ and B. CHRISTOL . . 1197
Skin Disorders in Relation to Malabsorption. G. C. WELLS 1200
Further Studies on Acrodermatitis Enteropathica. N. DANBOLT 1202
A New Classification for Lupus Erythematosus. J. R. HASERICK 1204
Angiokeratoma Corporis Diffusum. H. J. WALLACE 1207
Consideration of the Etiology of Pyoderma Gangrenosum. H. O. PERRY and P. DIDIS-
HEIM 1208

Free Communications

A Cutaneous Affection from Malabsorption. A. BACCAREDDA-BOY and F. CROVATO . . 1212
Hauterscheinungen bei Colitis ulcerosa. H. REICH 1214
Crohn's Disease Associated with Cutaneous Lesions. G. A. GRANT PETERKIN 1214
Lung Function in Patients with Cutaneous Vasculitis. M. CATTERALL 1215
Atteinte du rein au cours des allergides nodulaires dermiques de Gougerot. ST. BOULLE
and J. GUILAINE 1217
Therapie der Porphyria cutanea tarda (Ergebnisse in 9 Jahren). H. IPPEN 1218
Hautreaktionen bei rheumatischen Erkrankungen. E. WOHLSTEIN 1219
Studies on Iron Metabolism in the Porphyria Cutanea Tarda (P.C.T.). L. LEVI, C. L.
MENEGHINI, F. SPINELLI-RESSI and C. A. BETTINELLI 1222
Krankhafte Zusammenhänge zwischen Leber und Haut in "Porphyria cutanea tarda".
P. TÎRLEA and I. CĂPUSAN 1222
Schistosomiasis (Bilharziasis) der Haut. C. M. HASSELMANN 1224
Schistosomal Infestation of the Skin. A. M. EL MOFTY 1224
The Hepatitis Associated with Infantile Papular Acrodermatitis. V. A. PUCCINELLI . . 1228
Zum Krankheitsbild des Myxoedema circumscriptum praetibiale. CHR. EBERHARTINGER 1229
Natural Course of Various Types of Scleroderma. A. Follow-up-Study over a Period of
20 Years. Z. STAVA 1230
Preparation and Application of Lesional Casts in the Study of Cutaneous Disease.
D. A. ROE 1231
Perorale Kreatinbelastung bei Haut- und Muskelerkrankungen. H. W. KREYSEL and
M. JÄNNER 1232
Liquen rojo plano de la mucosa bucal. Su asociación con diabetes. Nuevas observaciones.
D. GRINSPAN, J. DÍAZ, L. O. VILLAPOL, J. SCHNEIDERMAN, R. BERDICHESKY, D.
PALESE and J. FAERMAN 1234
Sarcoidosis with Cicatricial Alopecia Resembling Generalized Discoid Lupus Erythema-
tosus. L. S. SAUTER 1235
Dermatological Aspects of Crohn's Disease. D. I. MCCALLUM and P. D. C. KINMONT 1237
A propos du syndrôme de Winterbauer (Syndrôme C.R.S.T.). A. PUISSANT, R. LECLERCQ
and F. VANBREMEERSCH 1238
Acanthosis Nigricans. — A Clinical Manifestation of Internal Disorders. T. YASUDA,
SH. NISHIYAMA and SH. TSUYUKI 1240
Glucorrhoea. Is this Pre-diabetes ? J. R. G. AGIUS 1241
Hormonelle Untersuchungen und Behandlungsmethoden bei Acne vulgaris. F. TÓTH
and L. NÉKÁM 1243
Vorkommen von Paraproteinämie bei Pyoderma gangraenosum. H. RÖCKL 1244
Zur Problematik der Arthropathia psoriatica. F. VLčEK, M. ZBOJANOVA, G. NIEPEL
and Z. SITAY 1246

page

Quelques observations sur l'élimination urinaire des cétostéroïdes dans l'acnée féminine.
R. DUMITRIU, M. HAISUC, L. REITER, M. HONTARU and A. COSER   1248

The Seborrhoic Symptom Complex.— The Expression of a Disturbed Intestinal Malutilization of Vitamin B 12 as Proven by Measuring the Radioactivity after Administration of Co 60 Vitamin B 12. W. A. CASPER   1249

Diabetes and Impetigo Contagiosa (Passage from one Diabetic Family to Another
Diabetic Family Via a Related Cousin Carrier). B. R. HEARST   1251

Dermatitis uraemica Rössle. H. FISCHER   1252

Symposium 13: Bullous Dermatoses

Reports

Zur Klinik bullöser Eruptionen (Exklusive bullöse Genodermatosen). J. TAPPEINER   1257

Herpes Zoster and Nonmalignant Disease. L. H. WINER and E. T. WRIGHT   1259

Producción experimental de ampollas; su correlacción con los cambios estructurales en
las dermatosis ampollosas. D. J. GÓMEZ ORBANEJA   1262

La maladie de Duhring-Brocq à grosses bulles dite «pemphigoïde de Brocq», après la
cinquantaine. P. LE COULANT, L. TEXIER and P. BORAUD   1264

Subcorneal Pustular Dermatosis. A review after 10 years. D. S. WILKINSON   1266

Bullous Lesions in Patients with Internal Disorders. E. SKOG   1267

Corticosteroid Treatment of Pemphigus. C. T. NELSON   1270

Friction Blisters Produced under Controlled Conditions. TH. A. CORTESE jr., T. B.
GRIFFIN and M. B. SULZBERGER   1273

Free Communications

Experimental Investigations on the Acantholysis Induced by Staphylococcus pyogenes.
Comparative Study with the Acantholysis on Pemphigus. B. ZILBERBERG   1275

An Electron Microscopic Study of Cutaneous and Oral Pemphigus Vulgaris. K. HASHI-
MOTO   1278

Localización de gamma globulina IgG y complemento (C'3) en la epidermis de enfermos
de Pénfigo vulgar. S. STRINGA, C. BIANCHI, A. CASALA, C. INGLESINI and O. BIANCHI   1283

Dermatite Bulleuse Mucosynéchante et Atrophiante. A. G. BELLONE, M. F. HOFMANN
and G. CAPUTO   1285

Experimental Friction Blisters: Histological Investigation. K. FUKUYAMA and TH. A.
CORTESE jr.   1288

Etude de la composition protéique du liquide des bulles dans les dermatoses bulleuses.
G. MOULIN and Y. MANUEL   1289

Nouvelles observations sur le phénomène citochémiotatique dans la bulle du pemphigus.
P. SERTOLI   1291

Hepatische Porphyrien: Veränderungen der Serumenzymaktivitäten und hämatologischen Befunde beim Menschen und bei der Ratte. H. PIETSCHMANN and W. RAAB .   1293

Interessante, bei den an bullösen Dermatosen leidenden Kranken erhobene hämatologische und gastroenterologische Befunde. V. ROZSÍVALOVÁ, F. MATĚJA, B. FIXA
and O. KOMÁRKOVÁ   1294

The Treatment of Porphyria Cutanea Tarda by Chelation. G. A. HUNTER and G. F.
DONALD   1296

Toxic Epidermal Necrolysis. M. B. LEWIS   1297

Acute Epidermal Necrolysis (Ritter-Lyell). — The Scalded Skin Syndrome.
P. J. KOBLENZER   1298

The Ultrastructure of Acantholysis in Lichen Planus. L. FRY and F. R. JOHNSON . .   1301

Symposium 14: Mycobacterial Infections of the Skin

Reports

Etude biologique récente dans la lèpre: Analogies antigéniques et séro-diagnostic de la lèpre par immunofluorescence sur bacille de Stefansky. F.-P. MERKLEN and F. COTTENOT 1305

Las formas submicroscópicas del m. leprae. J. GAY PRIETO and G. GABINO 1306

Die gegenwärtige Epidemologie und Bakteriologie der Hauttuberkulose in der Bundesrepublik Deutschland. F. EHRING 1308

Mykobakterienbefunde bei den sog. Tuberkuliden. N. SIMON 1312

Thalidomide in Lepra Reaction and in Hansen's Disease. J. SHESKIN, F. SAGHER, M. DORFMAN and J. CONVIT 1314

Free Communications

Geographical Distribution of Skin Tuberkulosis, Leprosy and Sarcoidosis in Japan. K. KITAMURA 1316

A propos des tuberculoses cutanées — leur classification — leur diagnostic biologique — leur traitement. M. BOLGERT and P. L. DELAIRE 1317

Lupus Vulgaris Gigantea Caused by Mycobacterium Avium. J. V. CHRISTIANSEN . . 1319

Atypical Acid fast Micro-Organisms in Scleroderma. A. R. CANTWELL, E. CRAGGS, J. W. WILSON and F. SWATEK 1320

Nature of the Antigen Responsible for the Kveim Reaction in Sarcoidosis. R. KOOIJ and J. W. VAN WAVEREN HOGERVORST 1322

Present Position of BCG Vaccination against Leprosy. L. M. BECHELLI 1323

Über die pigmentierten Naevi bei lepromatösen Leprakranken. Y. ISHIBASHI and T. KAWAMURA 1325

Mise en évidence du bacille de Hansen dans les lèpres apparemment abacillaires. F. COTTENOT, F.-P. MERKLEN and TRINH THI KIM MONG DON 1326

The Frequency of Intracellular Lipid in the Several Structureal Types of Leprosy. R. D. AZULAY and L. C. DE ANDRADE 1328

Cutaneous Response of Leprosy Patients to Living and Heated Mycobacterium Leprae Cultures on the Olitzki-Gershon Medium. M. DORFMAN, F. SAGHER, J. SHESKIN and A. L. OLITZKI 1329

Serum Immunoglobulin Changes in Leprosy and Tuberculosis. SOO DUK LIM and R. M. FUSARO 1332

Nuevos avances terapéuticos en lepra. J. C. GATTI, J. E. CARDAMA and L. M. BALINA 1334

Double Reversal of the Tuberculin Reaction in Sarcoidosis. S. H. SILVERS and F. S. GLICKMAN 1335

Clinical Applications of Shepard's Mouse Foot Pad Technique. P. FASAL and L. LEVY 1337

Impétigo herpétiforme Hébra Kaposi ou Psoriasis pustuleux généralisé (chez une femme âgée de 22 ans, apparu au cours de 5e mois de sa 2e grossesse). R. SAMII 1339

Symposium 15: Iatrogenic Diseases in Dermatology

Reports

Dermatosis iatrogénicas. Definición, patogénia, clasificación. M. I. QUIROGA 1343

The Aetiology of Toxic Epidermal Necrolysis. A. LYELL 1346

Iatrogenic Disease Due to Physical Treatment. A. N. DOMONKOS 1347

Eruptions du type L. E. et syndromes lupiques provoqués par des médicaments. CH. GRUPPER and G. A. C. MARCEL 1349

Dermatoses des traitements antidiabétiques. J. BEUREY, P. JEANDIDIER and A. BERMONT 1352

Iatrogenic Dyschromies. H. MÖLLER 1355

page

Free Communications

Photosensitive Dermatitis as an Iatrogenic Disease. T. KOBORI and H. ARAKI 1357

Les accidents cutanés de l'allergie humorale médicamenteuse. Intérêt du test de Shelley. J. MALEVILLE, H. BERGOEND and A. BASSET 1359

La thésaurismose cutanée par polyvinylpyrrolidone (PVP). J. M. LACHAPELLE . . . 1362

Mascaras pigmentarias como expresión iatrogénica a dosis altas y prolongadas de feniotiacina y derivados en el control de afecciones psiquiatricas. E. B. MOLINA LEGUIZAMÓN, A. A. CORDERO and E. FOLLMANN 1363

Necrolisis Epidermica Toxica. — Observaciones sobre 12 Casos. A. CORTÉS CORTÉS and V. CÁRDENAS JARAMILLO 1371

Dermatosis por anovulatorios. Y. ORTIZ 1373

Case Presentations and Fundamentals on Film

Second International Film Presentation of the Institute for Dermatologic Communication and Education

Keratosis Follicularis (Darier's Disease). N. KARLTORP and ST. FLODERUS 1379

Congenital Ichthyosiform Erythroderma. K. REHTIJÄRVI, K. KUOKKANEN and P. KARMA 1379

Xeroderma Pigmentosum. H. EL HEFNAWI 1379

Metastasizing Basal Cell Carcinoma. C. CH. THOMAS 1380

The Nevoid Basal Cell Carcinoma Syndrome. J. B. HOWELL and D. E. ANDERSON . . 1380

Gold Leaf Treatment of Cutaneous Ulcers. N. M. KANOF 1380

Diagnosis of Latent Psoriasis. G. HOLTI 1380

Surgical Treatment of Benign Acanthosis Nigricans. H. OLLENDORFF CURTH 1380

Pellagra and other Avitaminoses in the Bantu. M. ROSE 1381

Lupus Erythematosus. D. L. TUFFANELLI and W. B. REED 1381

Lipoid Proteinosis. R. M. CAPLAN 1381

Acrodermatitis Chronica Atrophicans (Herxheimer). F. HERRMANN and O. SCHULTKA . 1381

Granulomatous Dermo-Hypodermitis with Progressive Atrophy. J. CONVIT, FR. KERDEL-VEGAS and M. F. ALLENDE 1381

Report of the Institute for Dermatologic Communication and Education to the International Committee of Dermatology 1382

Scientific Exhibition

Clinical Dermatology

Die spontane Heilungsquote der Blutschwämme und die daraus zu ziehenden Schlüsse für die Prognose und Therapie. G. F. KLOSTERMANN 1387

Spontanverlauf der Säuglingshämangiome. A. PROPPE and H. HAUSS 1387

Laser Surgery of Angiomas with Special Reference to Port-Wine Angiomas. L. GOLD-MAN, E. J. RITTER, R. J. ROCKWELL jr., R. MEYER, B. HENDERSON and K. WM. KITZMILLER 1388

Therapie hypercholesterinämischer Xanthomatosen. N. ZÖLLNER, M. GUDENZI and G. WOLFRAM 1390

Proteolytic Enzyme Treatment of Skin Ulcers. M. C. SPENCER 1393

Chemosurgery for the Microscopically Controlled Excision of Skin Cancer. FR. E. MOHS 1393

Multiple Punch Autografts for the Alopecias. D. B. STOUGH 1394

Evaluation of Parental Methotrexate for Intractable Psoriasis. CH. P. DEFEO, A. ALLYN and S. EISENBERG 1394

Zur Wirkung des hochalpinen Klimas in der atopischen konstitutionellen Neurodermitis. S. BORELLI, H. BRENN, ST. CHLEBAROV, C. ENE-POPESCU, H. GEHRKEN, B. KOPECKA, P. MICHAILOV and H. VOSSIECK. 1395

Klimatherapie von Hautkrankheiten an der Nordsee. W. PÜRSCHEL 1397

page

Die Verbrennung — ein dermatologisches Problem. Komplikationen, Therapie und Prophylaxe. G. WEBER and H. JURSCH 1400

A New Principle in Topical Corticosteroid Treatment. G. HAGERMAN 1406

Casus rari muco-cutanei. A. GREITHER and O. HORNSTEIN 1408

Visualization in Dermatology. K. K. MUSTAKALLIO 1409

Examen radiographique des tissus cutanés et sous-cutanés normaux et pathologiques. CH. GROS, A. BASSET, S. SCHRAUB, J. MALEVILLE, E. GROSSHANS and E. HEID . . 1409

Klassifizierung der Ichthyosen. U. W. SCHNYDER and B. KONRÁD 1411

Andrologie in Klinik und Praxis. C. SCHIRREN and H. GRELL 1413

Papulonecrotic and Acneiform Tuberculids. C. E. SONCK 1413

Exhibit on Genodermatoses. L. ZIPRKOWSKI 1418

A Case of Congenital Erythropoietic Porphyria. K. YAMAMOTO 1420

Contact Allergy in Scandinavia. B. MAGNUSSON, S.-G. BLOHM, S. FREGERT, N. HJORTH, G. HØVDING, V. PIRILÄ and E. SKOG 1421

Klinische Pharmakologie des neuen Histaminblockers Tavegil. L. KERP and H. KASEMIR 1425

Hautveränderungen und Antikörper-Mangelsyndrome. G. BREHM 1426

L'allergie de contact. J. FOUSSEREAU 1429

Chamber Test Method. V. PIRILÄ and L. FÖRSTRÖM 1430

Erythropoietic Protoporphyria. R. M. FUSARO, W. J. RUNGE, E. S. PETERKA. M. O. JAFFE, E. W. GOLTZ and C. J. WATSON 1432

Gegenüberstellung von Angiomatosis Kaposi (Sarcoma idiopathicum haemorrhagicum multiplex) und Stewart-Treves-Syndrom (Sarcoma angioplasticum in elephantiasi). H. TELLER and H. KRÜGER 1435

Une affection liée au sexe: la gérodermie ostéodysplasique. D. KLEIN, F. BAMATTER, A. FRANCESCHETTI, G. BOREUX, J. E. W. BROCHER and P. HOLENSTEIN 1443

Elektronenmikroskopische, histochemische und polarisationsoptische Untersuchungen bei Pemphigus familiaris benignus (Hailey u. Hailey). F. NÜRNBERGER and G. MÜLLER 1444

Pemphigus Benignus Chronicus and Keratosis Palmo-plantaris in a Finnish Family. C. E. SONCK 1444

Shibi-Gatchaki-Syndrome. Y. KATABIRA 1447

Cas Cliniques. A. BASSET 1448

Gnathostomiasis Cutis. Yangtze Edema in China and Similar Migrating Intermittent Swellings of the Skin in Japan, Both Due to Gnathostoma Spinigerum Owen, 1836. K. KITAMURA 1449

Plusieures dermatoses. G. SAKELLARIOU 1450

Seltene Hautkrankheiten. G. HARGITA 1451

Angiokeratoma corporis diffusum Fabry. R. DENK 1459

Die primäre Hautreaktion nach infektiösem Tsetsefliegenstich bei der afrikanischen Schlafkrankheit. H. E. KRAMPITZ 1459

Amoebiasis Skin Manifestations. TH. DOXIADES and J. CAPETANAKIS 1462

Skin Diseases in Arabian Countries: Certain Notes and Comments. M. EL ZAWAHRY . 1464

Die Tumormetastasierung von der Haut und in die Haut. H. DREPPER and F. EHRING 1465

Zur Pathologie cutaner Lymphgefäße. J. TAPPEINER and L. PFLEGER 1467

Neuere Aspekte zur Histopathologie der Alopecia areata. W. THIES and CH. FISCHER 1469

Befund Langerhans-ähnlicher Zellen in den Hauterscheinungen der Reticuloendotheliose von Letterer-Siwe. V. PUCCINELLI, F. GIANOTTI and R. CAPUTO 1472

Tetracycline Fluorescence in Squamous Cell Carcinoma. H. J. DONSKY and G. R. MIKHAIL 1474

Concept of the Molecular Cause of Albinism. G. F. WILGRAM 1475

Xeroderma pigmentosum. H. EL HEFNAWI 1476

Skin Tuberculosis, Leprosy, Cutaneous Leishmanosis, Favus. M. A. MALEKI 1476

page

Experimental Dermatology

A Cutaneous Rôle in the Regulation of the Body's Carbohydrate Milieu. R. M. FUSARO and J. A. JOHNSON 1477

The Interplay of Opposites. Immunological Reactions in the Skin. TH. M. INDERBITZIN and P. J. GROB 1480

Autoradiographic Studies on Psoriatic Epidermis. S. SOTOMATSU, Y. IGARASHI and Y. OOSHIMA 1481

Die Mastzelle. A. SCHAUER 1483

Electronmicroscopy of Merkel's Tastzelle. K. K. MUSTAKALLIO and U. KIISTALA . . . 1493

Bilddemonstration zur mikroskopischen Anatomie des Haarfollikels im Verlauf des Haarcyclus. H.-J. BANDMANN and K. BOSSE 1493

Zur Ultrastruktur des menschlichen Haarfollikels. V. PUCCINELLI and R. CAPUTO . . . 1494

Zur licht- und elektronenoptischen Struktur der Nerven am Haar. E. HAGEN and G. NIEBAUER. 1495

Neuere Entwicklung der dermatologischen Virusforschung. TH. NASEMANN 1499

Recent Observations on Langerhans Cells. K. WOLFF, R. K. WINKELMANN and K. HOLUBAR 1502

Malignant Melanomas: Subcellular Differentiation of Nevocytic and Melanocytic Onto-geny. Y. MISHIMA 1505

Epidermal Melanin Unit. M. A. PATHAK, G. SZABÓ, T. B. FITZPATRICK, Y. HORI, S. S. BLEEHEN, E. FRENK, M. MIYAMOTO, M. SEIJI and A. BREATHNACH 1506

Dermo-Epidermal Separation by Suction. N. KIISTALA and K. K. MUSTAKALLIO . . 1513

Comparative Study with the Acantholysis in Pemphigus. Experimental Investigations on the Acantholysis Induced by the Staphylococcus pyogenes. B. ZILBERBERG . . 1513

Pathophysiologie allergischer Dermatosen. G. STÜTTGEN, I. GIGLI and F. HERRMANN 1514

Das mikrobielle Ekzem. H. RÖCKL, F. SCHRÖPL, E. MÜLLER and G. PETER 1516

Experimental Eczema of the Guinea Pig. N. HUNZIKER 1518

Terpentinöl-Intoxikation bei Arbeitern einer Schuhcreme-Fabrik verursacht durch d-Alpha-Pinen. F. NÜRNBERGER 1522

Enzymaktivitätsmuster im Serum und in Erythrozyten bei verschiedenen Hautkrank-heiten. H. HOLZMANN, B. MORSCHES, G. W. KORTING and R. DENK 1524

Immunofluorescence Studies of the Skin. R. H. CORMANE, E. H. BAART DE LA FAILLE, J. B. VAN DER MEER, A. A. W. TEN HAVE-OPBROEK and W. W. MUIJS VAN DE MOER 1524

Herkunft der mononucleären Entzündungszellen (Makrophagen) bei der unspezifischen Entzündung (Untersuchungen am Rebuck'schen Hautfenster bei der Ratte). M. BEGEMANN 1531

Unspezifische und spezifische Wirkstoffe bei allergischen Reaktionen der Cutis. G. STÜTTGEN, J. GIGLI and F. HERRMANN 1531

Allergens of Quinone Structure. K. H. SCHULZ, P. SCHMIDT and H. GRELL 1531

Methode zur Hornschichtdickenmessung in vivo. F. KLASCHKA and R. A. KRAUSE . . 1533

Dermatological and Immunological Aspects of Cryoglobulinaemia. K. K. MUSTAKALLIO and O. WAGNER 1534

R.U.V., X-Ray and Alpha-particles Micrography of the Skin. A. TOSTI 1535

L'Exploration thermographique en dermatologie. CH. GROS, C. VROUSOS, J. ALT and A. BASSET 1539

The History of the Dermatological Section of the Royal Society of Medicine. T. J. RYAN, Y. M. CLAYTON, E. J. MOYNAHAN, J. F. KENNEDY, P. POLANI and I. A. MAGNUS . . 1541

Zellphysiologische Aspekte der Psoriasis vulgaris. O. BRAUN-FALCO, E. CHRISTOPHERS, S. MARGHESCU, D. PETZOLDT, G. RASSNER and M. RUPEC 1546

Mycology

Mikroskopische Demonstration von Fadenpilzen und Hefen. H. BRAUN and C. SCHÖN-BORN 1550

page

Faserzerstörung durch Dermatophyten und keratinophile Pilze. L. KREMPL-LAMPRECHT   1550

Dermatophyten und ihre Hauptfruchtformen. G. A. DEVRIES and L. KREMPL-LAMPRECHT   1555

Serological Relationship of the Dermatophytes of Emmons-Conant-System. H. PALDROK and K. R. SUNDSTRÖM 1556

Adaptationsphasen der Dermatophyten in Zusammenhang mit ihrer Klassifikation. V. A. BALABANOFF 1556

Epidemiologische Analyse des Vorkommens von Dermatophyten in der Slowakei. L. CHMEL. 1560

Einige biochemische Eigenschaften der Isothiocyanate. A. BOJANOVSKÁ 1560

Trichofytocid Spofa® (5% p-bromphenylisothiocyanat) bei der Behandlung von Trichophytosis. L. CHMEL, M. VALENTOVÁ and J. BUCHVALD 1561

Histopathomorphologische Befunde der Haut nach der Applikation von Trichophytocid. L. CHMEL and A. BOJANOVSKÁ 1561

Chromomycosis Caused by a New Species Chmelia slovaca. L. CHMEL, I. KOCHOVÁ and A. BOJANOVSKÁ 1562

The Third Case of Chromomycosis in the Territory of Czechoslovakia. L. CHMEL, I. KOCHOVÁ, A. BOJANOVSKÁ and B. KONRÁD 1563

Pilzerkrankungen innerer Organe. T. WEGMANN 1563

Survey of Mycoses in U.A.R. M. EL ZAWAHRY 1564

Clinical Diagnosis of Onychotrichophytosis. J. ALKIEWICZ and W. SOWINSKI 1564

Favic Infections in the Surroundings of Göttingen. M. KIRSCH-NIETZKI 1566

Pilzinfektionen im Bereich des Auges. D. H. HOFFMANN 1566

Parasitic Forms of the Causative Fungi in the Cutaneous and Visceral Lesions of Chromoblastomycosis. R. FUKUSHIRO and S. KAGAWA 1568

Chromomycosis (in the World and in Finland). T. PUTKONEN 1570

Relations entre formes cliniques et espèces mycologiques. A. BASSET and M. BASSET . 1570

Dermatomykosen bei Säugetieren. H. KRAFT 1570

Mykosen bei Tieren (Befall durch Aspergillus, verschiedene Dermatophyten und Alternaria). H. KRAFT 1572

Maduromykose beim Pferd. B. SCHIEFER and B. GEDEK 1573

Beitrag zur Mykologie der Systemmykosen: Histoplasmose und Kryptokokkose. H. KARUGA. 1574

Vorkommen von Dermatophyten im Boden und bei Tieren als mögliche Infektionsquellen. D. JANKE 1577

Trichophytie und Blastomykose. Zs. HERPAY 1580

Ultrastructure of Dermatophytes. W. MEINHOF and W. VOGELL 1581

Infektionen durch Candida albicans. J. THURNER 1584

Quantitative Methoden der Antimykotikaprüfung. W. DITTMAR 1586

Enzymhistochemische Untersuchungen an Dermatophyten. K. HOLUBAR and O. MALE 1590

Dermatophyten und Schimmelpilze. B. BRAUN, H. RIETH and C. FINGER 1590

Additional Demonstrations

Kollegheft der Vorlesung von F. VON HEBRA, geschrieben von F. CURTI, zur Verfügung gestellt von O. GRUMBACH unter Vermittlung von O. GANS 1590

Histopathology of Leprosy. M. L. BRUBAKER and P. FASAL 1590

Antibiotics and the Placebo Reaction in Acne. R. C. SAVIN and M. CHANCO-TURNER . 1590

Authors Index   1592

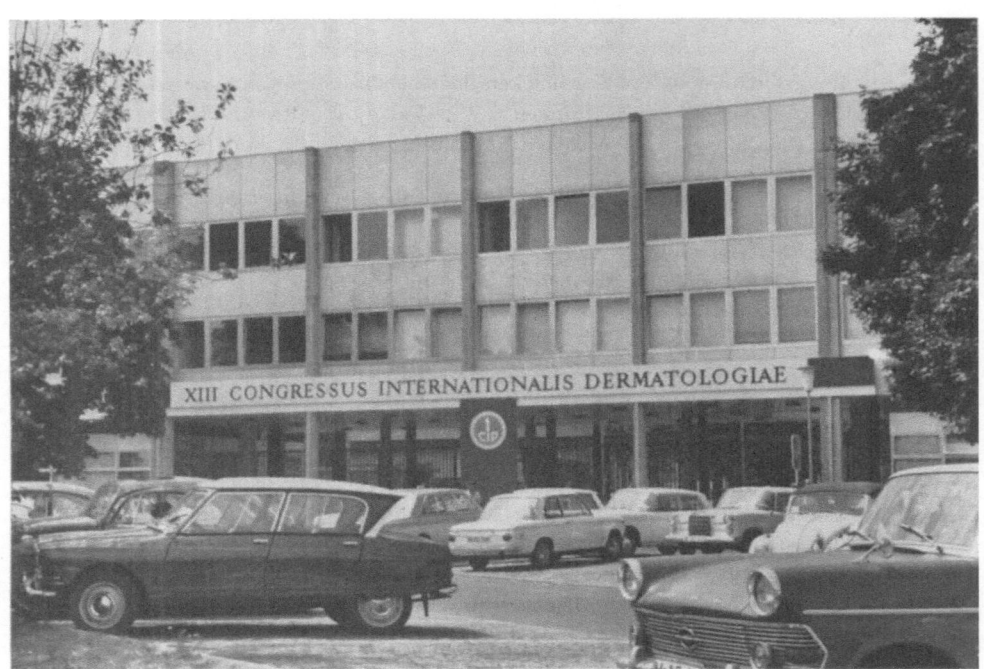

Entrance to the Exhibition Park
on the Theresienhöhe

Entrée du Parc des Expositions
sur la Theresienhöhe

Theresienhöhe, entrada al Parque
de Exposiciones

Eingang zum Kongreßgelände
auf der Münchener Theresienhöhe

XIII International Congress of Dermatology
Munich, 31. 7. to 5. 8. 1967

The International Congress of Dermatology has taken place in Munich from the 31st of July to the 5th of August 1967. 2272 active participants and 824 accompanying persons, from 79 countries, have taken part in it.

At the end of the XII International Congress in Washington, Munich had been chosen as the next congress place and Prof. A. MARCHIONINI had been named president. He died on April 6, 1965 while the International Congress of Munich was under preparation. The Committee of the German Society of Dermatology recommended to the International Committee of Dermatology, Prof. W. JADASSOHN, of Geneva, as the new president of the Congress. During its session of June 1965, the International Committee of Dermatology elected Prof. W. JADASSOHN president of the Congress. He recognized Prof. C. G. SCHIRREN, as General Secretary of the Congress, a position he occupied since 1962. The preparations could thus continue.

The Congress took place in Munich on the territory of congress and exhibition "Theresienhöhe". The various structures consisting of numerous large and small conference rooms, exhibition halls, all kinds of appropriate installations and several restaurants, facilitated the disposition of the whole in a pleasant outline of space and rendered very profitable such a great manifestation. The summer weather throughout the duration of the Congress favored the proceedings and in the same time the voluminous social program.

The International Committee of Dermatology was responsible for the elaboration of the scientific program. With 7 Themes and 15 Symposia, the major present problems concerning dermatology were evoked. The "Bayernhalle" consisting of 4000 seats was the largest conference room. The other rooms consisted of 100 to 850 seats.

The simultaneous translation in the four official languages of the Congress (English, French, Spanish and German) was possible in the three largest rooms.

An exhibition of more than 6000 m² permitted a general view of the pharmaceutical and medical industry concerning our speciality. German participation was the highest compared to foreign enterprises of European and overseas countries.

The Scientific Exhibition had been installed next to the Technical Exhibition. It consisted of 130 divisions. A botanic garden of eczematogenous plants completed this exhibition.

The number of art works of worldwide origin were 170 at the exhibition of the dermatologist-artists. Oil paintings, Indian ink paintings, acquarelles, engravings, sculptures, plastics and others, were the joy of all participants.

The demonstration of patients presenting with important and interesting dermatoses, was rendered possible by color-television. Ciba of Basel, offered its world-wide known Eidophor system. More than 3000 dermatologists and other doctors of the Munich region, followed this demonstration on a 50 m² screen. The session lasted $3^{1}/_{2}$ h and was transmitted directly from the Dermatological University Clinic of Munich. The patients came from different University Clinics and hospital services of the Federal Republic of Germany.

Throughout the duration of the Congress, various films were projected in a 400 seat room. Furthermore a cinematographic session of the "Institute of

Dermatologic Communication and Education" took place one afternoon in the "Bayernhalle".

A wide social program invited the participants and their wifes to know the magnificent sites of the Bavarian alps and gave them a view of artistic life in and around Munich (concerts, opera, museums). History, Folklore as well as fashion were not neglected.

The budget for the Congress was 1,4 million DM. The expenses for each active participant were 610 DM. The participation fee was 240 DM per participant. The remainder of the expenses was completed by different donations which were accepted with gratitude.

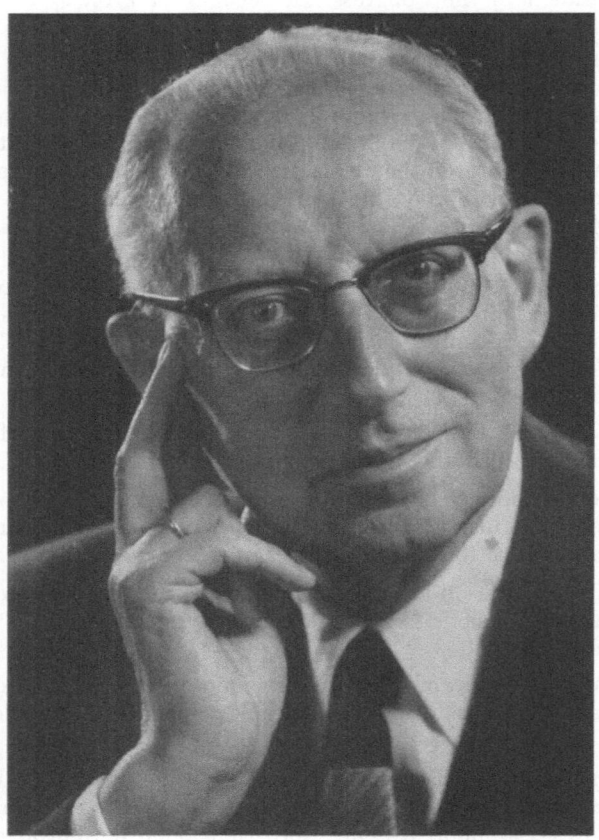

Professor Dr. Dr. h. c. ALFRED MARCHIONINI †

XIIIième Congrès International de Dermatologie
Munich, 31. 7.—5. 8. 1967

Le Congrès International de Dermatologie s'est déroulé à Munich, du 31 juillet au 5 août 1967. 2272 participants actifs et 824 accompagnants officiels, en provenance de 79 pays y ont pris part.

Lors du XIIième Congrès International à Washington la ville de Munich fut désignée pour accueillir le prochain congrès et le Prof. A. MARCHIONINI nommé pour le présider. Malheureusement, le Prof. MARCHIONINI mourut le 6 avril 1965, alors que le Congrès International de Munich était en préparation. Le Comité de la Société Allemande de Dermatologie recommanda au Comité International de Dermatologie, le Prof. W. JADASSOHN pour remplacer le disparu comme nouveau Président du Congrès. Le Comité International de Dermatologie, dans sa réunion du mois de juin 1965, agréa cette recommandation et élut le Prof. W. JADASSOHN nouveau Président. Celui-ci confirma dans son poste le Secrétaire Général du Congrès, le Prof. C. G. SCHIRREN, en fonction depuis 1962. Les préparatifs pour l'organisation du XIIIième Congrès purent ainsi continuer.

A Munich, à la «Theresienhöhe», emplacement réservé à la célébration de congrès et d'expositions, eut lieu le XIIIième Congrès International de Dermatologie. Plusieurs édifices avec de vastes et petites salles de conférences, halles d'expositions, installations appropriées, ainsi que plusieurs restaurants, facilitèrent tout l'aménagement dans un cadre agréable, vaste et verdoyant, et rendirent très accueillante une si grande manifestation.

Le temps estival, qui régna pendant toute la durée du Congrès, en favorisa le déroulement, de même que le programme social très varié.

Le Comité International de Dermatologie eut à sa charge l'élaboration du programme scientifique. Les problèmes majeurs actuels intéressant la Dermatologie, furent évoqués par l'exposé de 7 Thèmes et 15 Symposia. La «Bayernhalle», comprenant 4000 places, fut la plus grande salle de conférences. D'autres salles contenaient entre 850 et 100 places.

La traduction simultanée dans les quatre langues officielles du Congrès, soit l'anglais, le français, l'espagnol et l'allemand, fut possible dans les trois plus grandes salles.

Une exposition d'une superficie de plus de 6000 m², offrit une vue d'ensemble sur l'industrie pharmaceutique et la technique médicale se rapportant à notre spécialité. La très forte participation allemande figurait à côté d'autres exposants européens et d'outre mer.

L'Exposition Scientifique, près de l'Exposition Technique, s'étendait sur 130 cloisons. Un jardin botanique de plantes eczématogènes complétait cette exposition.

Les dermatologues artistes du monde entier, présentèrent 170 œuvres d'art. Des peintures à l'huile, à l'encre de chine, des aquarelles, des gravures, sculptures, plastiques et autres, firent la joie de tous les participants.

Grâce à la Télévision en Couleurs, la démonstration de malades présentant des dermatoses importantes et de haut intérêt, fut possible. La Maison Ciba à Bâle, apporta gracieusement son système Eidophore, mondialement connu. Plus de 3000 dermatologistes ainsi que d'autres médecins de la région munichoise, purent suivre cette démonstration sur un écran géant de 50 m².

La transmission en relais direct de cette séance de la Clinique Universitaire de Dermatologie de Munich, dura 3 heures et demie. Les malades provenaient de plusieurs cliniques universitaires et autres services hospitaliers du pays.

Pendant toute la durée du Congrès fut projeté un grand nombre de films dans une salle de 400 places. En outre, une séance cinématographique de l'«Institute of Dermatologic Communication and Education» eut lieu un après-midi dans la «Bayernhalle».

Un programme social très vaste, dédié aux participants et à leurs épouses, permit de faire la découverte des magnifiques sites des préalpes et alpes bavaroises ainsi que de prendre contact avec la vie artistique munichoise: concerts, opéra, musées. L'histoire, le folklore ainsi que la mode ne furent pas oubliés.

Le budget économique du Congrès s'élevait à 1,4 millions de DM. Les frais pour chaque congressiste actif étaient de 610 DM, tandis que leur participation était de 240 DM. Le surplus des dépenses fut supporté par des dons divers reçu avec reconnaissance.

XIII Congreso Internacional de Dermatología Munich, 31/7 a 5/8/67

El Congreso Internacional de Dermatología se celebró en Munich del 31 de Julio al 5 de Agosto de 1967. Tomaron parte en él, 2272 participantes activos y 824 acompañantes oficiales, llegados de 79 países.

Durante el XII Congreso Internacional de Dermatología, celebrado en Washington, fueron designados la ciudad de Munich, para albergar el próximo Congreso y el Profesor A. MARCHIONINI para presidirlo. Desgraciadamente, el Profesor MARCHIONINI falleció el 6 de Abril de 1965, cuando el Congreso se hallaba en preparación. El Comité de la Sociedad Alemana de Dermatología propuso al Comité Internacional de Dermatología, el nombramiento del Profesor W. JADAS-SOHN de Ginebra, como nuevo Presidente del Congreso. El Comité Internacional de Dermatología, en sesión celebrada en el mes de Junio de 1965, eligió al Profesor JADASSOHN como Presidente del Congreso. Este último, confirmó en su cargo de Secretario General del Congreso al Profesor C. G. SCHIRREN, que lo venía ejerciendo desde 1962. Los preparativos pudieron así continuar.

El Congreso tuvo lugar en Munich, en la zona denominada Theresienhöhe, emplazamiento destinado exclusivamente a Congresos y Exposiciones. Diversos edificios, disponiendo de un gran número de salas de conferencias grandes y pequeñas, pabellones de exhibición, instalaciones adecuadas, así como varios restaurantes, facilitaron la tarea de los organizadores, en un marco de amplios espacios y de vegetación que fueron muy provechosos para una manifestación de esta envergadura. La temperatura estival que se mantuvo durante el desarrollo del Congreso fue propicia al mismo, así como a la celebración de numerosos actos sociales.

El Comité Internacional de Dermatología tuvo a su cargo la elaboración del programa científico. Los mas sobresalientes problemas contemporáneos, relacionados con la dermatología, fueron expuestos y discutidos en 7 temas y 15 simposios. La Bayernhalle, con capacidad para 4.000 personas, fué la mayor sala disponible. Las restantes salas, tenian un aforo comprendido entre 850 y 100 plazas.

Tres de las mayores salas, disponían de un sistema de traducción simultánea en las cuatro lenguas oficiales del Congreso; a saber: inglés, frances, español y alemán.

Una exposición de más de 6.000 m² de superficie, ofrecía una visión de conjunto de la industria farmacéutica y de técnica médica relacionada con nuestra especialidad. La participación alemana, la más importante, figuraba al lado de otros expositores europeos y de ultramar.

La Exposición Científica, cercana a la Exposición Técnica, estaba instalada en 130 parcelas de exposición. Un jardín botánico de plantas eczematógenas completaba esta exposición.

Hubo tambien una Exposición de dermatólogos artistas. Fueron 170 las obras de arte enviadas desde el mundo entero, las expuestas en esta sección. Todos los participantes pudieron admirar pinturas al óleo, a la pluma, acuarelas, grabados, modelajes en plástico, esculturas, etc.

La presentación de enfermos, afectos de importantes dermatosis, de un gran interés, pudo realizarse gracias a la televisión en colores. La Casa Ciba de Basilea participó con su sistema Eidophor, famoso en el mundo entero. Más de 3.000 dermatólogos, junto a otros médicos de la región de Munich, asistieron a esta presentación de enfermos proyectada en una pantalla gigante de 50 m². La sesión, que fué transmitida desde la Clínica Universitaria de Dermatología de Munich, duró tres horas y media. Los enfermos procedían de diversas clínicas universitarias y de los servicios hospitalarios de varios puntos de la República Federal Alemana.

Durante toda la semana en que se desarrolló el Congreso, fueron proyectadas diversas películas en una sala capaz para 400 espectadores. Ademas, "The Institute of Dermatologic Communications and Education", organizó una función cinematográfica en la Bayernhalle en sesión de tarde.

Un programa de actos sociales, muy vasto y variado, dedicado a los participantes y sus esposas, les ofreció la posibilidad de contemplar los magníficos parajes de los Alpes y Prealpes de Baviera asi como de entrar en contacto con los medios artísticos de Munich: música regional, conciertos, funciones de ópera, museos. La historia, el folklore y los desfiles de moda no fueron olvidados.

El presupuesto económico del Congreso se elevó a 1,4 millones de marcos. Los gastos originados por cada congresista fueron del orden de 610 marcos, de los cuales, cada uno de ellos participó con la suma de 240 marcos. El exceso de los gastos fué compensado por diversas donaciones que fueron recibidas con satisfacción y agradecimiento.

XIII. Internationaler Kongreß für Dermatologie
München, 31. 7. bis 5. 8. 1967

Vom 31. Juli bis zum 5. August 1967 fand in München der XIII. Internationale Kongreß für Dermatologie statt. Er wurde von 2272 aktiven Teilnehmern und 824 offiziellen Begleitpersonen aus 79 Ländern besucht.

Am Ende des XII. Internationalen Kongresses in Washington wurde München als Kongreßort bestimmt. Zum Präsidenten war Prof. A. MARCHIONINI gewählt worden. Er starb am 6. April 1965 mitten in den Vorbereitungen zum Münchener Kongreß. Der Ausschuß der Deutschen Dermatologischen Gesellschaft empfahl dem Internationalen Komitee für Dermatologie, Prof. W. JADASSOHN, Genf, zum neuen Kongreßpräsidenten zu ernennen. In seiner Sitzung im Juni 1965 in Paris wählte das Internationale Komitee Prof. JADASSOHN zum neuen Kongreßpräsidenten. Es bestätigte Prof. C. G. SCHIRREN, München, in seinem Amt als Generalsekretär des Kongresses, das er bereits seit 1962 ausgeübt hatte. So konnten die Kongreßvorbereitungen in München fortgesetzt werden.

Der Kongreß fand auf dem Kongreß- und Ausstellungsgelände „Theresienhöhe" der Stadt München statt. Die dort vorhandenen Gebäude mit zahlreichen großen und kleinen Sitzungssälen, die räumlich praktisch unbegrenzten Möglichkeiten für verschiedenste Ausstellungen, das Vorhandensein mehrerer Restaurationsbetriebe sowie die Einbettung des Ganzen in eine aufgelockerte, parkähnliche Grünlandschaft gewährten eine optimale Anpassung an die vielseitigen Bedürfnisse eines so großen Kongresses. Das während der gesamten Kongreßwoche anhaltende hochsommerliche Wetter begünstigte das Geschehen im Kongreßgelände und während des umfangreichen gesellschaftlichen Programms.

Das Internationale Komitee zeichnete für die Zusammenstellung des wissenschaftlichen Programmes verantwortlich. In 7 Hauptthemen und 15 Symposien wurden die meisten die Dermatologie derzeit besonders interessierenden Fragen verhandelt. Der größte Verhandlungssaal, die Bayernhalle, vermochte 4000 Teilnehmer aufzunehmen. Die übrigen Sitzungssäle hatten zwischen 100 und 850 Sitzplätze.

In den drei größten Sälen wurde während der gesamten Kongreßwoche simultan in die vier offiziellen Kongreßsprachen Englisch, Französisch, Spanisch und Deutsch übersetzt.

Eine auf über 6000 qm ausgedehnte Ausstellung vermittelte einen repräsentativen Überblick über die unser Fach betreffende Industrie auf dem pharmazeutischen und medizinisch-technischen Sektor. An ihr hatten sich neben der am stärksten vertretenen deutschen Industrie auch Firmen aus dem übrigen Europa und aus Übersee beteiligt.

Eine in 130 Abteilungen aufgeteilte wissenschaftliche Ausstellung war in räumlicher Nachbarschaft zur Industrieausstellung eingerichtet worden. Ihr zugeordnet war eine botanische Schau häufig hautsensibilisierender Pflanzen.

170 Ausstellungsstücke umfaßte die Kunstausstellung künstlerisch tätiger Dermatologen aus aller Welt. Gemälde in Öl, Aquarell und Tusche, Radierungen, Skulpturen und Plastiken u. a. fanden das besondere Interesse aller Kongreßteilnehmer.

Die Demonstration von Patienten wichtiger und interessanter Dermatosen erfolgte mittels Farbfernsehen. Die Firma Ciba, Basel, hatte ihr weltweit anerkanntes Eidophor zur Verfügung gestellt. Über 3000 Dermatologen und Ärzte aus dem Münchener Raum verfolgten auf einer 50 qm großen Leinwand die 3¹/₂stündige Übertragung aus der Münchener Dermatologischen Universitätsklinik. Die demonstrierten Patienten kamen aus verschiedenen dermatologischen Universitätskliniken und Krankenhäusern des Gastlandes.

In einem 400 Plätze enthaltenden Kinoraum wurden während der ganzen Kongreßdauer sehr verschiedene Filme gezeigt. Ferner wurden an einem Nachmittag in der Bayernhalle die Filme des „Institute for Dermatologic Communication and Education" vorgeführt.

Ein umfangreiches gesellschaftliches Programm sollte den Teilnehmern und ihren Damen die Schönheit der bayerischen Voralpen und des Alpenlandes vermitteln und ihnen Einblick in das Münchener Kunstleben geben (Konzert, Oper und Museen). Historie, Mode und Folkloristik kamen zu ihrem Recht.

Für die wirtschaftliche Fundamentierung des Kongresses mußten 1,4 Millionen DM aufgebracht werden. Umgerechnet auf den einzelnen aktiven Kongreßteilnehmer mußten pro Kopf 610,— DM aufgewendet werden, an denen der Teilnehmer selbst sich durch die Zahlung der Kongreßgebühr in Höhe von 240,— DM beteiligte, während der Rest durch sehr willkommene Spenden und zusätzliche Einnahmen aus der Industrieausstellung usw. gedeckt werden konnte.

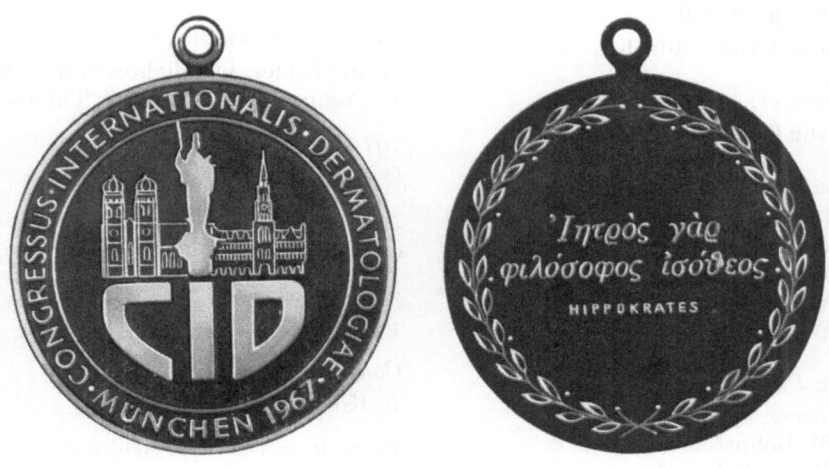

---

* Ἰητρὸς γὰρ φιλόσοφος ἰσόθεος (Der Arzt, der die Weisheit liebt, ist den Göttern ähnlich). — Da Hippokrates den ionischen Dialekt sprach, heißt es Ἰητρὸς und nicht Ἰατρὸς wie im heute geläufigeren attischen Dialekt.

International Committee of Dermatology 1962—1967

President:
R. Degos, France

Secretary General
S. Hellerström, Sweden

Members:

L. A. Brunsting, USA
Fr. Flarer, Italy
J. Gay Prieto, Spain
St. Jablonska, Poland
W. Jadassohn, Switzerland
K. Kitamura, Japan
S. Lapière, Belgium
Cl. Livingood, USA

G. B. Mitchell-Heggs, Great Britain
D. M. Pillsbury, USA
M. J. Quiroga, Argentina
J. Ramos e Silva, Brazil
F. Sagher, Israel
C. G. Schirren, Germany
M. B. Sulzberger, USA

XIII. Congressus Internationalis Dermatologiae

Executive Committee

President:
W. Jadassohn, Genève

Secretary General:
C. G. Schirren, München

Treasurer:
K. von Griesheim, München

Honorary Vice-Presidents:
O. Gans, Comano
H. Gottron, Mainz
J. Kimmig, Hamburg
A. Memmesheimer, Essen
A. Wiedmann, Wien

Vice-Presidents:
H. Aretz, Velbert
R. M. Bohnstedt, Gießen
O. Braun-Falco, München
H. Götz, Essen
F. Herrmann, Frankfurt
K. W. Kalkoff, Freiburg i. Brsg.
G. W. Korting, Mainz
W. Schneider, Tübingen
H. W. Spier, Berlin

Assistant Secretaries:
Th. Nasemann, München
H.-J. Bandmann, München

Scientific Exhibition
(included Scientific Films):
H.-J. Bandmann, in collaboration with
L. Krempl-Lamprecht, München, and
K. Bosse, München

Industrial Exhibition:
W. Schneider, in collaboration with
W. Adam and H. Tronnier, Tübingen

Art Exhibition:
C. E. Sonck, Turku

Itinerary after the Congress:
G. W. Korting, Mainz

Social Program:
Th. Nasemann, München

Congressoffice:
A. Koch, München

Press/Broadcasting/Television
A. Memmesheimer, Essen
H. Götz, Essen
S. Stiel, München

Ladies' Committee
Mrs. K. Jadassohn
Mrs. S. Braun-Falco
Mrs. R. Götz
Mrs. M. Bandmann
Mrs. B. Nasemann
Mrs. L. Schirren

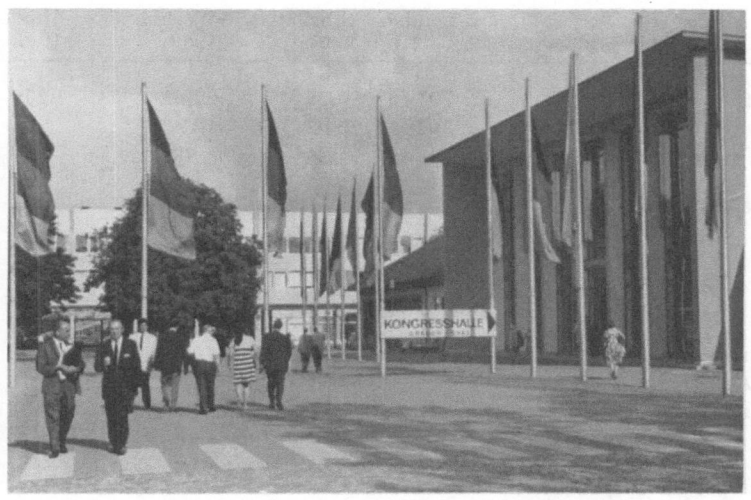

In the Exhibition Park
Dans le Parc des Expositions
En el recinto del Parque de Exposiciones
Im Kongreßgelände

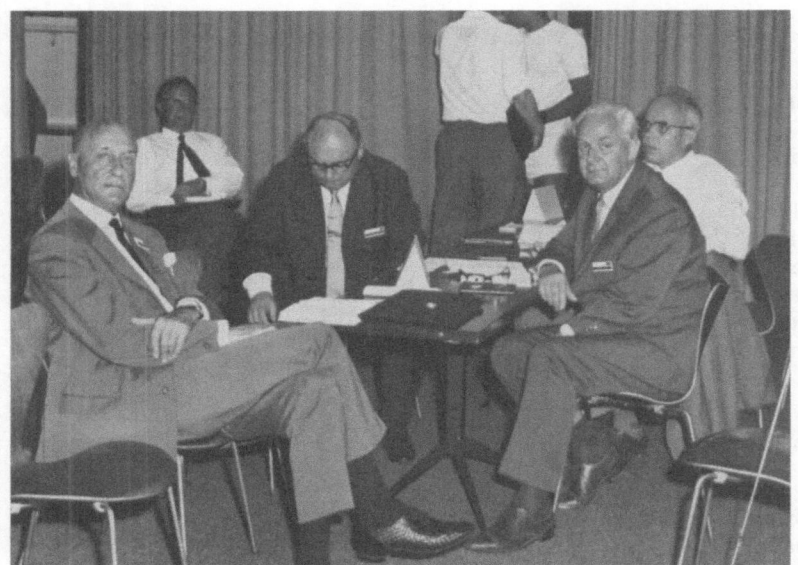

At the Registration   En el local de recepción
A l'Enregistrement   Bei der Anmeldung

→ Prof. LAPIÈRE, Prof. KIMMIG, Prof. TAPPEINER, Prof. PIRILÄ

Comparative Participants Numbers from 1952 to 1967

	London 1952	Stockholm 1957	Washington 1962	Munich 1967
Active participants	707	989	2395	2272
Registered accompanying persons	367	546	1312	824
Number of countries	46	52	66	79
Participants per continent:				
Asia	28	40	67	155
Australia	10	16	12	24
Africa	9	15	17	26
America	236	326	1885	602
North America	210	293	1730	462
Central America	7	11	46	41
South America	19	22	109	99
Europe	424	592	414	1278
Participants per country:				
Algeria		3		1
Argentina	5	6	53	42
Australia	8	12	9	19
Austria	8	12	13	36
Belgium	14	14	11	43
Brazil	6	6	14	19
Bulgaria		3	1	25
Burma			1	
Canada	13	19	81	35
Ceylon				2
Chile			1	2
China		3		1
Columbia	1		11	7
Congo			2	2
Costa Rica		1	1	1
Cuba	3	3	3	3
Czechoslovakia		8		27
Denmark	10	24	13	30
Dominican Republic			2	4
Ecuador			1	2
El Salvador	1		1	1
Ethiopia			1	
Finland	7	21	7	25
France	49	60	48	162
Germany	46	131	106	411
Ghana				1
Greece	5	4	5	16
Great Britain	144	64	51	91
Guatemala				1
Honduras			3	2
Hong-Kong				1
Hungary		8	2	22
Iceland	2	2	1	2
India	8	4	10	6

	London 1952	Stockholm 1957	Washington 1962	Munich 1967
Indonesia	2	1		
Iran		1	5	6
Iraq				2
Ireland	8	3	1	6
Israel	8	16	9	17
Italy	11	34	45	91
Jamaica		1	2	1
Japan	1	6	24	91
Kenya				2
Korea			1	1
Kuwait				1
Lebanon	1	1	2	5
Libya				1
Luxembourg	3	1		2
Madagascar				1
Malaysia	1		1	1
Malta	1		1	1
Mexico	2	6	23	23
Monaco	1	1		
Morocco		2	1	3
Netherlands	42	30	14	44
New Zealand	2	4	3	5
Nicaragua			3	1
Nigeria			1	
Norway	12	16	5	11
Pakistan			1	1
Panama			3	2
Peru	2	4	4	9
Philippines	1		3	3
Poland		10	5	18
Portugal	4	6	6	5
Puerto Rico	1		5	2
S. Rhodesia			1	1
Rumania		4		28
Senegal			1	1
Singapore			1	1
Spain	21	16	16	39
South Africa	3	5	6	8
Sudan				1
Sweden	16	78	40	47
Switzerland	14	22	19	75
Syria				1
Thailand		1	1	3
Turkey	4	7	7	10
United Arab Republic	6	5	4	4
United States of America	197	274	1649	427
Uruguay	4	1	5	3
USSR	2	1	1	
Venezuela	1	5	20	15
S. Vietnam				2
Yugoslavia	6	19	4	21

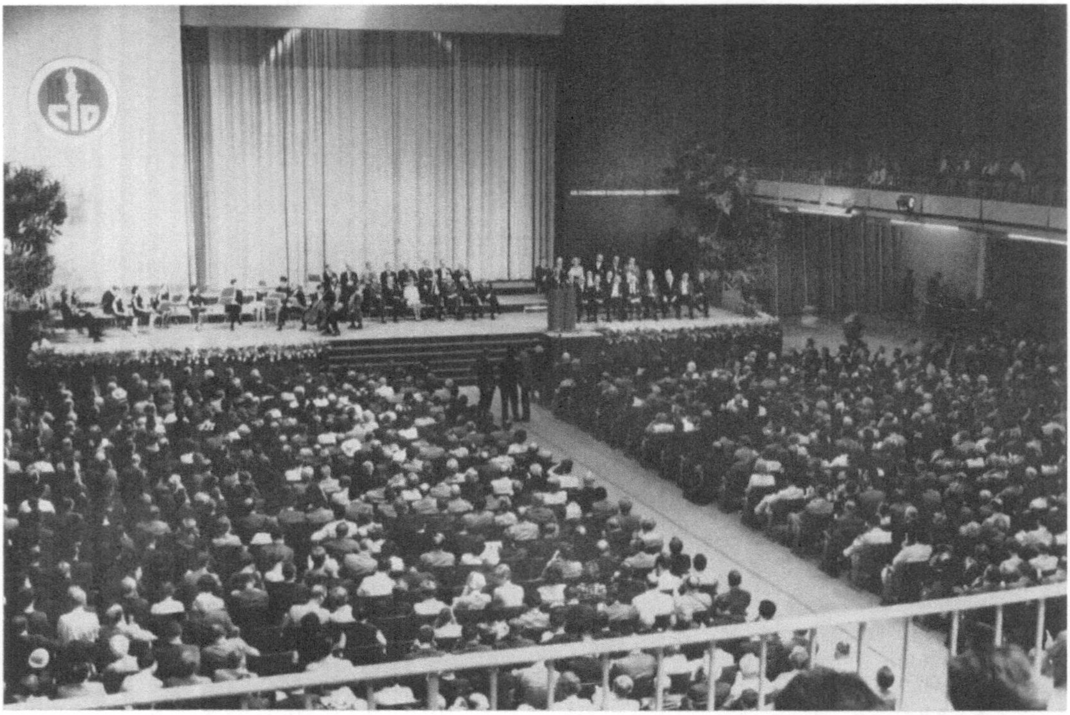

Opening session in the Bayernhalle   Bayernhalle: Ceremonia de inauguración del Congreso

Séance d'ouverture dans la Bayernhalle   Eröffnungssitzung in der Bayernhalle

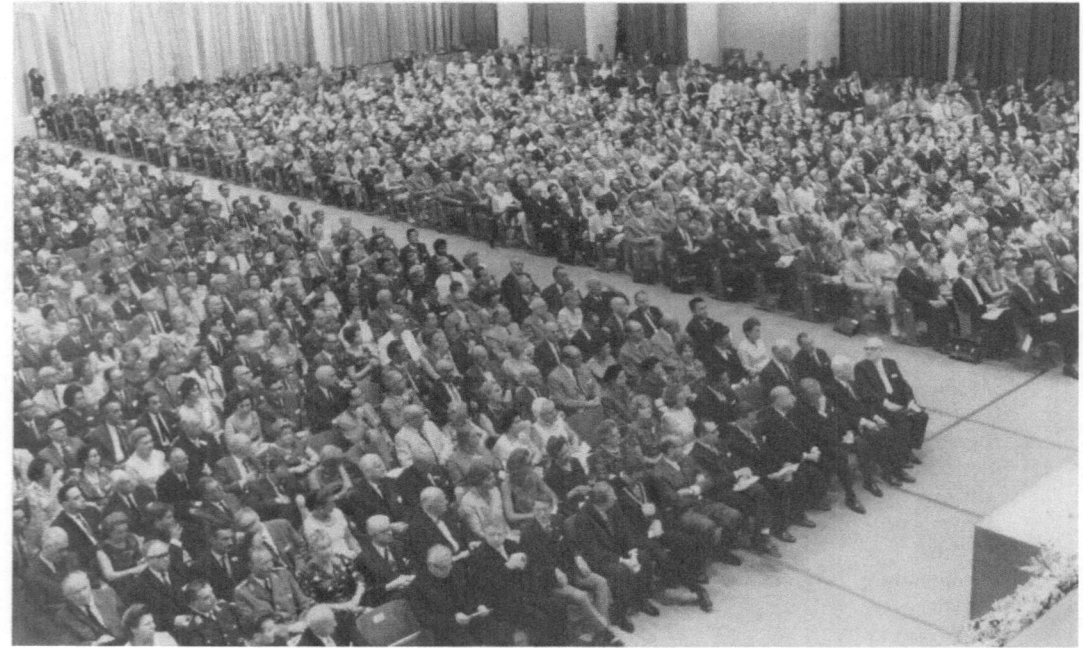

Opening Session

The solemn opening session took place in the "Bayernhalle" on the territory of congress and exhibition "Theresienhöhe" of Munich, on Monday, July 31, 1967, at 9 o'clock.

The "Bayernhalle" consisting of 4000 seats was almost completely packed. Numerous guests of honor assisted, besides the dermatologists of 79 countries and their relatives.

The importance of the Congress was underlined by the presence of the President of the Federal Republic of Germany, Dr. h. c. HEINRICH LÜBKE; the Congress having been realized under his patronage. The presence of the President of the Ministry of the state of Bavaria, Dr. h. c. ALFONS GOPPEL and the Mayor of Munich, Dr. HANS-JOCHEN VOGEL, was remarked. Also were present, the Rector of the University Prof. LUDWIG KOTTER, and the Dean of Medical Faculty of Munich, Prof. MANFRED KIESE.

The participants of the opening session could admire the "Bayernhalle" specially decorated for this occasion. The chamber orchestra of Munich, directed by conductor HANS STADLMAIR, interpreted a concert by J. S. Bach.

To end the session, the Marchionini medal was handed to Prof. W. JADASSOHN, the Marchionini prize to Dr. ST. ANTONESCU, both by Prof. A. WIEDMANN; and finally the Fr. Schaudinn-E. Hoffmann medal was handed to Dr. R. A. NELSON by Prof. A. MEMMESHEIMER.

Séance d'ouverture

La séance solennelle d'ouverture eut lieu le lundi 31 juillet 1967, à 9 heures, dans la «Bayernhalle» à la «Theresienhöhe» de Munich, emplacement réservé aux congrès et expositions de la ville bavaroise.

La «Bayernhalle» d'une capacité de 4000 places, était presque comble. De nombreux invités d'honneur figuraient parmi les dermatologues et leurs proches, venus de 79 pays.

L'importance du Congrès fut mise en relief par la présence du Président de la République Fédérale d'Allemagne, Dr. h. c. HEINRICH LÜBKE. C'est sous son auspice que le Congrès put se célébrer. On remarqua la présence du Ministre Président de Bavière, Dr. h. c. ALFONS GOPPEL, du Maire de la ville de Munich, Dr. HANS-JOCHEN VOGEL. Le Recteur de l'Université, Prof. LUDWIG KOTTER, et le Doyen de la Faculté de Médicine, Prof. MANFRED KIESE, étaient également présents.

Les participants à la séance d'ouverture purent admirer la «Bayernhalle» spécialement décorée à l'occasion de cette cérémonie. L'orchestre de chambre de Munich, sous la direction du chef HANS STADLMAIR, interprèta un concert pour trois violons de J. S. Bach.

Avant la cloture de la séance, le Prof. A. WIEDMANN remit la première médaille Marchionini au Président du Congrès, le Prof. W. JADASSOHN, ainsi que le prix Marchionini au Dr. ST. ANTONESCU. Finalement, le Prof. A. MEMMESHEIMER, remit la médaille Fr. Schaudinn-E. Hoffmann au Dr. R. A. NELSON.

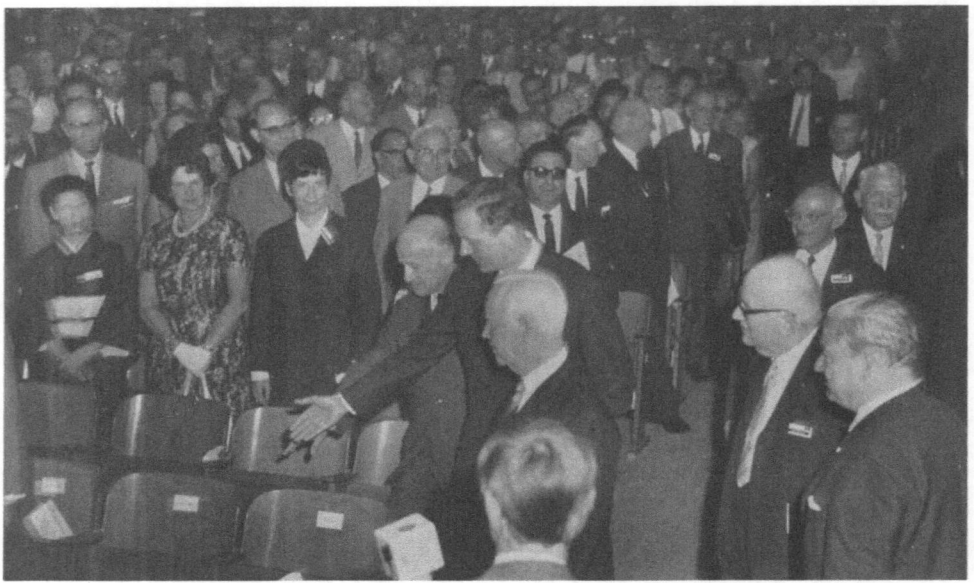

The arrival of the President of the Federal Republic of Germany	Llegada del Presidente de la República Federal Alemana
L'arrivée du Président de la République Fédérale d'Allemagne	Der Präsident der Bundesrepublik Deutschland trifft ein

Sesión de Inauguración

La solemne sesión de inauguración tuvo lugar el lunes 31 de Julio de 1967, a las nueve de la mañana, en la Bayernhalle del Theresienhöhe de Munich, emplazamiento destinado a congresos y exposiciones en la citada ciudad de Baviera.

La Bayernhalle, capaz de albergar hasta 4.000 personas, estaba casi totalmente llena. Numerosas personalidades asistían al acto junto a los dermatólogos y sus familias procedentes de 79 países.

La importancia del Congreso fué realzada con la presencia del Presidente de la República Federal Alemana, Dr. h. c. HEINRICH LÜBKE, bajo cuyos auspicios pudo celebrarse el Congreso. Destacaron, la asistencia del Ministro Presidente de Baviera, Dr. h. c. ALFONS GOPPEL, y la del Alcalde de la ciudad de Munich, Dr. HANS-JOCHEN VOGEL. También hicieron acto de presencia el Rector de la Universidad, Prof. LUDWIG KOTTER, y el Decano de la Facultad de Medicina de Munich, Prof. MANFRED KIESE.

Los asistentes a la sesión de inauguración pudieron admirar la Bayernhalle, especialmente adornada con motivo de esta ceremonia. La orquesta de cámara de Munich, bajo la dirección del maestro HANS STADLMAIR, interpretó el concierto para tres violines de J. S. Bach.

La sesión fue clausurada con la imposición al Presidente del Congreso, Prof. WERNER JADASSOHN, de la primera Medalla Marchionini y la entrega del Premio Marchionini al Dr. ANTONESCU, ambas de la mano del Prof. A. WIEDMANN. Finalmente, el Prof. A. MEMMESHEIMER hizo entrega de la Medalla Fr. Schaudinn-E. Hoffmann al Dr. R. A. NELSON.

Eröffnungssitzung

Die feierliche Eröffnungssitzung fand am Montag, dem 31. Juli 1967, um 9.00 Uhr in der Bayernhalle auf dem Münchener Messe- und Ausstellungsgelände statt.

Die 4000 Sitze fassende Bayernhalle war fast bis auf den letzten Platz besetzt. Neben den Dermatologen aus 79 Ländern und ihren Angehörigen hatten sich zahlreiche Ehrengäste eingefunden.

Die Bedeutung des Kongresses wurde durch die persönliche Anwesenheit des Herrn Bundespräsidenten, Dr. h. c. HEINRICH LÜBKE, unterstrichen, der auch die Schirmherrschaft über diesen Kongreß übernommen hatte. Neben dem Bundespräsidenten waren auch der Ministerpräsident des Freistaates Bayern, Dr. h. c. ALFONS GOPPEL, und der Oberbürgermeister der Stadt München, Dr. HANS-JOCHEN VOGEL, erschienen; ferner der Rektor der Universität München, Prof. LUDWIG KOTTER, der Dekan der Medizinischen Fakultät der Universität München, Prof. MANFRED KIESE, und zahlreiche Ehrengäste.

Die Teilnehmer an der Eröffnungszeremonie fanden in der festlich geschmückten Bayernhalle einen würdigen Rahmen vor. Das Münchener Kammerorchester unter der Leitung von HANS STADLMAIR gab mit dem Konzert für drei Violinen in D-Dur von J. S. Bach die musikalische Umrahmung.

Im Anschluß an die Eröffnungsreden erfolgte die Verleihung der A. Marchionini-Medaille an Prof. WERNER JADASSOHN durch Prof. ALBERT WIEDMANN, die Verleihung des A. Marchionini-Preises an Dr. ST. ANTONESCU durch Prof. ALBERT WIEDMANN sowie die Verleihung der F. R. Schaudinn-E. Hoffmann-Medaille an Dr. R. A. NELSON durch Prof. ALOIS MEMMESHEIMER.

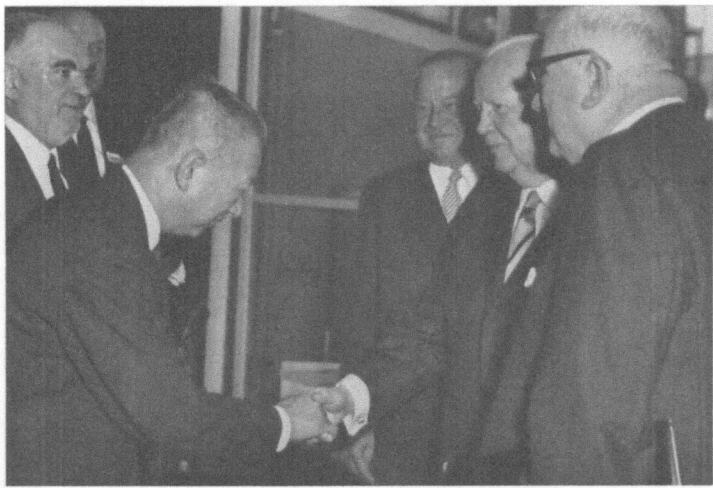

The President of the Federal Republic, Mr. LÜBKE, greets the International Committee of Dermatology

El Presidente de la República Federal Alemana Sr. LÜBKE saludando a los miembros del Comité Internacional de Dermatología

Le Président de la République Fédérale, M. LÜBKE, salue les membres du Comité International de Dermatologie

Bundespräsident LÜBKE bei der Begrüßung des Internationalen Komitees

→ Prof. DEGOS, Prof. LAPIÈRE, Prof. KITAMURA, Ministerpräsident GOPPEL, Bundespräsident LÜBKE, Prof. JADASSOHN

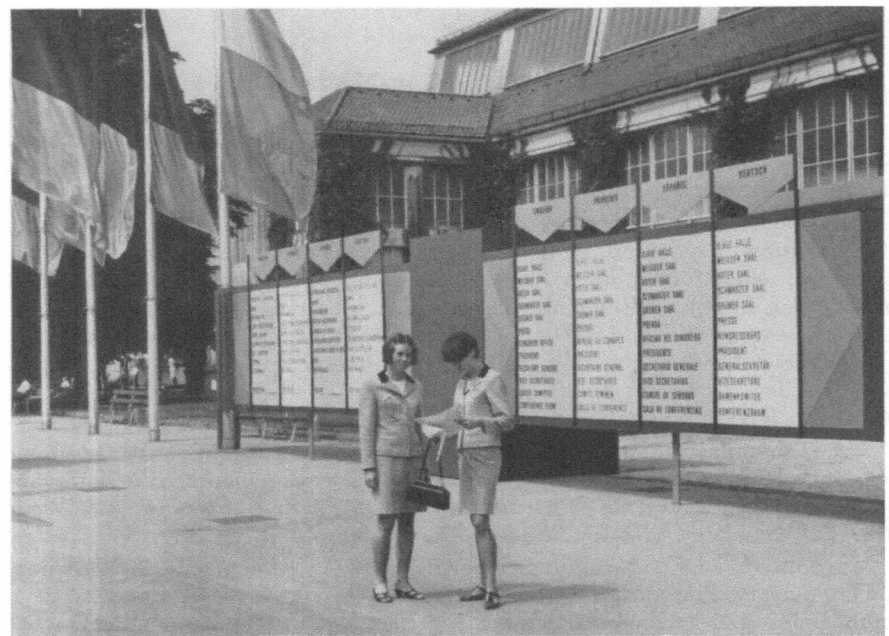

In the Exhibition Park, two hostesses

Dans le Parc des Expositions, deux hôtesses

Parque de Exposiciones, dos señoritas del
servicio de Información

Im Kongreßgelände, zwei Hostessen

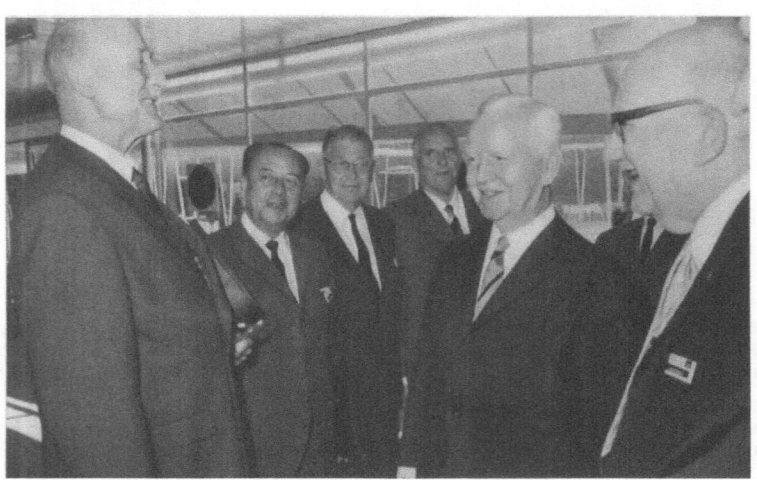

→ Prof. LAPIÈRE, Prof. GAY PRIETO, Prof. PILLSBURY,
   Prof. HELLERSTRÖM, Bundespräsident LÜBKE, Prof. JADASSOHN

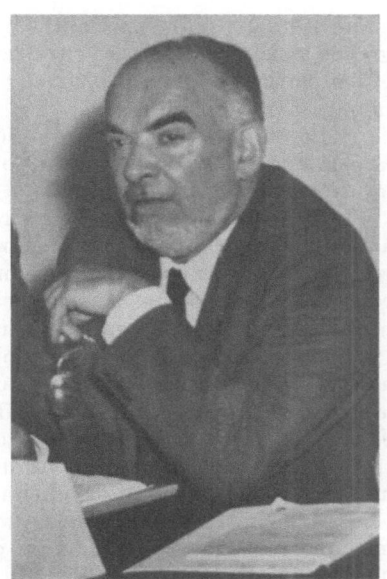

Prof. Robert Degos

Président du Comité International
de Dermatologie et de la Ligue Internationale
des Sociétés Dermatologiques 1962—1967

En tant que Président du Comité International de Dermatologie, j'adresse les remerciements chaleureux des différentes Sociétés Nationales de Dermatologie à la Ville de Munich qui a bien voulu nous recevoir pour y tenir notre XIIIème Congrès International et aux personnalités officielles qui honorent de leur présence cette séance d'ouverture.

Lorsqu'il y a 5 ans, à Washington, nous avons choisi la Bavière comme lieu de nos futures assises, nous étions pleins de joie à la pensée de nous retrouver à Munich, sous la présidence du Prof. Alfred Marchionini. Bien qu'il nous soit très pénible de commencer ce Congrès en évoquant la mémoire de ce grand dermatologiste, je pense que c'est notre devoir de le faire avant toute autre chose. C'est à Marchionini que nous devons d'être ici réunis, c'est lui qui a eu la lourde charge de commencer l'organisation de ce Congrès et je suis sûr qu'en entrant dans cette salle, tous ceux qui l'ont connu ont, comme moi, ressenti très douloureusement le vide immense de son absence parmi nous. Le Comité International, lors de sa réunion à Paris, le 21 juin 1965, avait envoyé une adresse à son incomparable compagne, Tilde Marchionini, dont on ne peut séparer le souvenir de celui auprès duquel elle a lutté toute sa vie pour l'accomplissement d'une œuvre aussi belle sur le plan humain que sur le plan scientifique. Voici cette adresse: «Le Comité International de Dermatologie s'est recueilli pour rendre un hommage ému à la mémoire du Prof. Alfred Marchionini, l'éminent chef de l'Ecole Allemande de Dermatologie, l'homme généreux, épris de liberté et de fraternité humaine — et il communie avec Tilde Marchionini dans le souvenir de celui qui a su acquérir l'estime et l'amitié de tous».

La vie d'Alfred Marchionini, sa personnalité, ses travaux innombrables qui ont tant enrichi la dermatologie mondiale, sa ferveur pour établir un climat de compréhension et d'union entre les peuples, sont trop universellement connus pour qu'il soit besoin de retracer les étapes mouvementées et souvent douloureuses de sa carrière.

D'autres deuils ont, depuis notre dernier Congrès, profondément affecté les différentes Sociétés de Dermatologie. Beaucoup de ces disparus tenaient une place

éminente dans notre spécialité et chacun d'entre nous comptait parmi eux de
grands amis. Je ne puis les citer tant est longue leur liste. Pour tous ces absents
et, en particulier, pour ALFRED et TILDE MARCHIONINI, je vous demanderai une
minute de recueillement. —

Si la tradition veut que le Président du Comité International prenne le premier
la parole, c'est au Président du Congrès que revient l'agréable mission d'adresser
la bienvenue aux Congressistes; je n'usurperai pas ses droits.

Le Comité International s'est réuni à plusieurs reprises — à Munich, à Paris,
à Jérusalem — pour préparer le Congrès. L'atmosphère de véritable amitié qui n'a
cessé de régner au cours de ces réunions a beaucoup facilité notre tâche, et c'est de
cette parfaite entente, de cette confiance mutuelle, que je remercie le plus les
membres du Comité au moment où vont prendre fin mes 5 années de présidence.

La continuité de l'organisation matérielle du Congrès a été heureusement
assurée grâce au Prof. SCHIRREN qui avait été investi des fonctions si difficiles et si
laborieuses de Secrétaire Général du Congrès par MARCHIONINI. Je laisse au Prof.
JADASSOHN le soin de vous dire toutes les qualités d'organisateur de celui qui a
travaillé intensément auprès de lui, mais permettez-moi d'adresser personnellement mes très chaleureuses félicitations au Secrétaire du Congrès.

Par contre, le Prof. JADASSOHN ne pourra faire son propre éloge, et c'est pour
moi une très grande satisfaction que de témoigner notre profonde gratitude et
notre admiration au Président du Congrès. Le décès du Prof. MARCHIONINI, en
pleine organisation de cette Réunion mondiale, avait créé une situation très difficile. Le Comité International a accueilli avec enthousiasme la proposition de la
Société Allemande de Dermatologie de confier la présidence du Congrès au Prof.
JADASSOHN. Le prestige incontesté du Professeur de la Chaire de Genève, ses très
hautes qualités scientifiques et morales, son inlassable capacité de travail, étaient
une garantie qui s'est pleinement justifiée.

Mon cher ami, dans le rôle d'arbitres que nous avons eu parfois à assumer pour
l'établissement final du programme scientifique et pour le choix des présidents des
Thèmes et des Symposia, j'ai pu apprécier votre franchise, votre impartialité, votre
souci de ne froisser aucune susceptibilité individuelle et nationale. Nos rapports ont
été des plus confiants, des plus amicaux et ce fut, pour moi, un véritable plaisir que
de collaborer avec vous et avec le Prof. SCHIRREN, dans des rencontres à Genève et à
Paris et dans des échanges de lettres qui ont été, à certains moments, quotidiens!

Le travail d'un Président de Congrès International est écrasant. Le vôtre le fut
plus encore par le fait que vous ne résidiez pas dans le pays où le Congrès devait
avoir lieu. Que de voyages entre Munich et Genève avez-vous dû accomplir, vous
et le Prof. SCHIRREN! Vous ne serez jamais assez remercié et loué pour avoir accepté
cette tâche surhumaine et pour l'avoir réalisée aussi parfaitement. Avec le Prof.
SCHIRREN et vos équipes de collaborateurs, vous serez justement fier de la magnifique réussite que sera, nous en sommes sûrs, le Congrès International de Munich.

Il me reste une cérémonie à accomplir. Le Prof. SULZBERGER, en prenant la
présidence du Comité International, en 1957, à Stockholm, a généreusement offert
à la Ligue Internationale des Sociétés Dermatologiques un marteau où sont inscrits
les noms des Présidents du Comité International et des Présidents des Congrès
Internationaux de Dermatologie. Cet attribut du pouvoir n'a jusqu'à présent été
qu'un symbole. Aucune table de réunion du Comité ni aucune table de Congrès
n'a retenti de ses coups pour faire taire des indisciplinés. D'autres organisations
internationales pourraient prendre exemple sur nous. Ce marteau m'a été confié à
Washington, en 1962. Je vous le transmets, Monsieur le Président du Congrès, et
que ce viatique vous accompagne dans le déroulement de cette Réunion mondiale
de la dermatologie à laquelle je souhaite le plus éclatant succès.

Dr. h. c. ALFONS GOPPEL

Ministerpräsident des Freistaates Bayern

Hochverehrter Herr Bundespräsident, meine Herren Präsidenten des Bayerischen Landtags und Senates, Magnifizenz, Exzellenzen, meine sehr verehrten Damen und Herren!

Es ist für den Bayerischen Ministerpräsidenten als Vertreter der Bayerischen Staatsregierung eine ebenso große Freude wie Ehre, Sie heute hier in der Landeshauptstadt Bayerns zu Ihrem XIII. Internationalen Kongreß begrüßen zu können und zu dürfen. Daß wir uns auch hier in München freuen, daß Sie, sehr verehrter Herr Bundespräsident, diesen Kongreß durch Ihre Anwesenheit und unser Land mit Ihrem Besuch beehren, brauche ich nicht besonders zu betonen.

Alle Teilnehmer, vor allem auch die zahlreichen Gäste aus dem Ausland, heiße ich herzlich hier in München willkommen. Geben Sie unserem Land die Ehre und besuchen Sie einige der Stätten, die Bayerns Ruf als Land der Kunstfreunde, der Naturfreunde und der Lebensfreude begründen, soweit Ihnen das umfangreiche wissenschaftliche Programm Ihres Kongresses noch Zeit dazu läßt.

Ich darf Sie alle, meine sehr verehrten Damen und Herren, herzlich hier begrüßen!

Dr. HANS-JOCHEN VOGEL

Oberbürgermeister der Bayerischen Landeshauptstadt München

Sehr verehrter Herr Bundespräsident, verehrter Herr Ministerpräsident, meine Herren Präsidenten, Magnifizenz, Exzellenz, meine verehrten Damen und Herren!

Sie haben sich heute hier in München zur feierlichen Eröffnung des XIII. Internationalen Kongresses für Dermatologie versammelt. Als Oberbürgermeister der bayerischen Landeshauptstadt darf ich Sie aus diesem Anlaß im Namen der Münchner Bürgerschaft und des Münchner Stadtrats, aber auch persönlich, auf das herzlichste willkommen heißen. Zugleich möchte ich meiner Freude darüber Ausdruck geben, daß sich zu dieser Veranstaltung so viele hervorragende Persönlichkeiten aus dem In- und Ausland in München eingefunden haben. Allein schon der Teilnehmerzahl nach dürfte es sich damit um einen der bedeutendsten internationalen medizinischen Kongresse handeln, den München bisher gesehen hat, eine Tatsache, die durch Ihre Anwesenheit, sehr verehrter Herr Bundespräsident, noch besonders unterstrichen wird.

Meine sehr verehrten Damen und Herren! Sie haben München 1962 während Ihres Kongresses in Washington als Tagungsort gewählt. Ich bin sicher, daß dafür die Persönlichkeit ALFRED MARCHIONINIS eine ausschlaggebende Rolle gespielt hat. Er war in der Tat der beste Anwalt und Repräsentant, den sich München wünschen konnte. Da ich ihm perönlich bis zu seinem Tode freundschaftlich verbunden war, weiß ich, daß er diesen Kongreß, zu dessen Präsidenten Sie ihn ja bestimmt hatten, als Höhepunkt und Krönung seiner wissenschaftlichen Laufbahn ansah. Das Schicksal hat ihn diesen Tag nicht mehr erleben lassen. Aber sein Andenken lebt fort, unter Ihnen als seinen Berufskollegen ebenso wie in dieser Stadt, der er so sehr zugetan war. Und wenn es eine sinnfällige Verbindung

2*

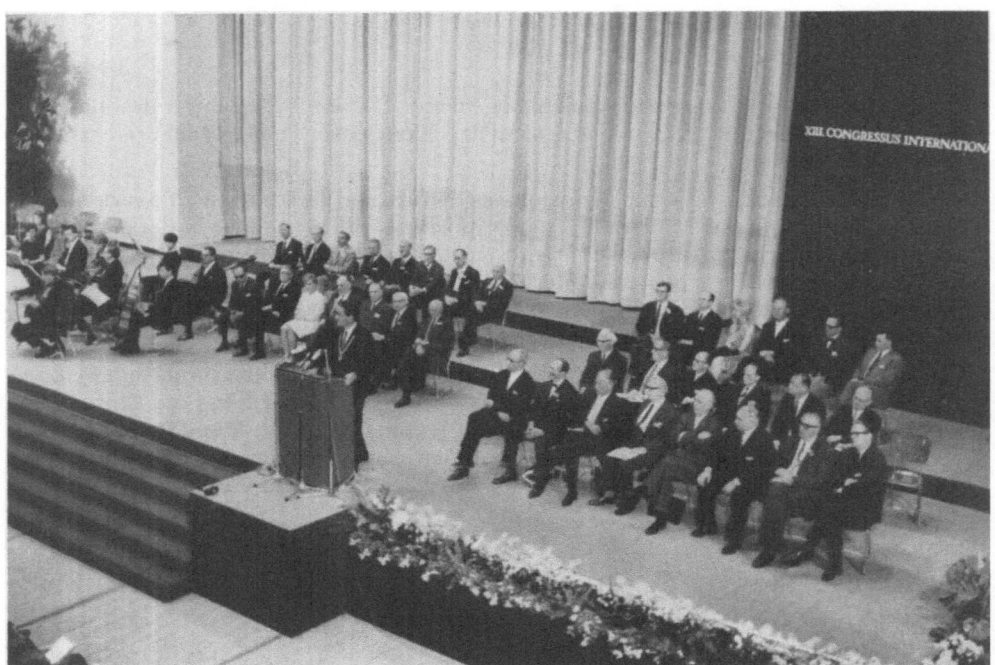

The Mayor of the city of Munich,
Mr. Vogel, at the opening session.
On the podium, on the left, the orchestra;
in the center, the International Committee
of Dermatology; on the right, the
Executive Committee

Le Maire de la ville de Munich, M. Vogel,
lors de la séance d'ouverture. Sur le podium,
à gauche, l'orchestre; au centre, le Comité
International de Dermatologie;
à droite, le Comité Exécutif

El Alcalde de la ciudad de Munich,
Sr. Vogel, durante la ceremonia de la
inauguración. En el estrado: a la izquierda,
la orquesta; en el centro, los miembros del
Comité Internacional de Dermatología;
a la derecha, el Comité Ejecutivo del mismo

Oberbürgermeister Vogel bei der
Begrüßungsansprache.
Auf der Bühne, links das Orchester;
in der Mitte das Internationale Komitee;
rechts das Exekutiv-Komitee

Center, first row: Prof. Gay Prieto, Prof. Pillsbury, Prof. Jablonska, Prof. Degos,
Prof. Hellerström, Prof. Ramos e Silva, Prof. Sulzberger

Center, second row: Prof. Sagher, Prof. Brunsting, Prof. Flarer, Prof. Kitamura,
Prof. Lapière, Prof. Livingood, Dr. Mitchell-Heggs, Prof. Quiroga

Right, first row: Prof. Braun-Falco, Prof. Memmesheimer, Prof. Wiedmann, Prof. Gans,
Prof. Gottron, Prof. Kimmig, Prof. Schneider, Prof. Kalkoff

Right, second row: Dr. Wetzel, Prof. Bohnstedt, Prof. Götz, Prof. Herrmann,
Prof. Korting, Prof. Spier

Right, third row: Doz. Bosse, Prof. Bandmann, Doz. Krempl-Lamprecht,
Prof. Nasemann, Doz. Adam, Doz. Tronnier

zwischen Ihrer Wissenschaft und der Stadt München gibt, dann ist sie in ALFRED MARCHIONINI verkörpert. Er war wahrhaft ein großer, ein ungewöhnlicher Mann — ein Mann, der in kein Schema, in keine Folie unserer so sehr zum Konformismus neigenden Zeit paßt. ALFRED MARCHIONINI war kein Münchner im strengen Sinne — aber er war ein vortrefflicher Bürger dieser Stadt. Er war sicher kein Politiker — aber er war ein eminent politischer Mensch, der sich auch nicht scheute, zu aktuellen Fragen Stellung zu nehmen. Er war weiß Gott kein Nationalist — aber er war vielleicht gerade deshalb ein ebenso wirksamer wie würdiger Repräsentant Deutschlands. ALFRED MARCHIONINI war noch mehr. Er war ein hervorragender Arzt und ein Gelehrter, der weltweites Ansehen genoß. Er war ein begabter und beliebter Lehrer der akademischen Jugend und er war auch ein Diplomat eigener Prägung, der es verstand, Brücken zwischen Institutionen und Körperschaften, aber auch zwischen den Völkern zu schlagen. Ja, diese Vielseitigkeit, diese Universalität, verbunden mit einer seltenen Kontaktfähigkeit und einer Fähigkeit, ja einer Begabung zur Freundschaft — das war eigentlich das Ungewöhnliche, das Besondere an diesem Manne, vor dem sich München in dieser Stunde noch einmal verneigt.

Ohne Zweifel, ich sagte es schon, war MARCHIONINI das stärkste Argument für München. Aber er konnte sich seinerseits auf zwei Umstände berufen, die Ihnen die Wahl erleichtert haben mögen. Darauf nämlich, daß München in Ihrem Fach stets eine gewisse Rolle gespielt und auf Gelehrte, Wissenschaftler und Ärzte immer eine besonders starke Anziehungskraft ausgeübt hat. So geht die Geschichte Ihres Faches in München bis in die erste Hälfte des 19. Jahrhunderts zurück. Schon 1831 wurde eine dermatologische Klinik eingerichtet, und 1863 erhielt München, als erste deutsche Universität überhaupt, eine ordentliche Professur für Dermatologie und Syphilidologie, die dem unvergessenen JOSEF VON LINDWURM übertragen wurde. Die schwierigen Verhandlungen, die dem vorangingen, muten ganz zeitgemäß an. Schrieb doch der Krankenhausinspektor, als er von der Absicht hörte, LINDWURM zunächst als Assistenten zu berufen, warnend an seine vorgesetzte Stelle: „Durch die Vermehrung der Kliniken wird die ärztliche Wissenschaft und Kunst in ihre Elemente aufgelöst und nur das Wissen von Spezialitäten gefördert, was endlich zum Verfall der Wissenschaft selbst führen muß, dem ohnehin schon entgegengestrebt werden muß." Auf LINDWURM folgten später POSSELT, KOPP und, da der Vater Ihres sehr geehrten Herrn Präsidenten, Prof. JOSEPH JADASSOHN, nicht zu gewinnen war, LEO VON ZUMBUSCH. Und aus der kleinen Klinik des Jahres 1831, die originellerweise neben den Betten für die Hautkranken auch die Separatzimmer und die Säle für Kaufleute, Studenten, Hofbeamte und Geisteskranke umfaßte, sind mittlerweile zwei Abteilungen mit 317 Betten geworden. Ein Zeichen dafür, welche Bedeutung wir Ihrem Fach beimessen.

Und was die Anziehungskraft unserer Stadt angeht, so lassen Sie sich bitte durch den äußeren Anschein, durch die Fülle der Baugruben nicht täuschen. In der Sprache Ihres Faches handelt es sich dabei um eine Art „Scabies", bei der ebenfalls die Oberfläche unserer Stadt durch kilometerlange Gänge verunstaltet wird. Kundige Dermatologen werden aber trotz aller dieser passageren Verunzierungen auch gegenwärtig das bestätigt finden, was THOMAS WOLFE vor 40 Jahren über München schrieb: daß nämlich andernorts die Menschen oft davon träumten, sie seien ins Paradies gekommen. In Deutschland, in Bayern hingegen träumten die Menschen davon, sie seien nach München gekommen. Und tatsächlich sei diese Stadt so etwas wie ein großer, ins Leben übersetzter Traum.

Magnifizenz Prof. Ludwig Kotter

Rektor der Ludwig-Maximilians-Universität München

Herr Bundespräsident, Herr Ministerpräsident, meine Herren Präsidenten von Landtag und Senat, Herr Oberbürgermeister, meine Herren Präsidenten, hohe Festversammlung!

Die Universität München freut sich in besonderer Weise, daß der Internationale Kongreß für Dermatologie zum ersten Male in München stattfindet. Im Namen der Ludwig-Maximilians-Universität darf ich die aus 79 Ländern hier versammelten Wissenschaftler und Fachärzte sehr herzlich begrüßen; reflektiert doch der Glanz dieser hohen Versammlung auch auf unsere Medizinische Fakultät, deren Bedeutung dadurch erneut in ein besonderes Licht gerückt wird.

Den Grund für die Auswahl Münchens als Kongreßort der Dermatologen aus aller Welt könnten nur unsere Karikaturisten oder unser Spaziergänger Blasius in der Tatsache suchen, daß die Haut unserer Stadt München derzeit eine Besonderheit darstellt. Ich denke nicht nur an die zahlreichen Ragaden und Aufschürfungen, sondern vor allem an die Riesenmilbe, die derzeit in der Ludwigstraße subcutane Gänge, ja ganze Kavernen bohrt. Dermatologe Vogel hofft, die Haut der Stadt München bis 1972 kuriert zu haben, wobei er allerdings mit diversen Injektionen von Kiesinger-Goppel-Lösung aus den Kanülen von Strauss und Pöhner rechnet.

In Wirklichkeit zur Universität — Herr Präsident Degos hat es bereits deutlich werden lassen: Sie sieht in der Auswahl Münchens als Kongreßort zunächst eine Anerkennung ihres inzwischen verstorbenen Altrektors, des Dermatologen Marchionini, durch dessen Initiative für uns nach dem Kriege zahlreiche internationale Verbindungen neu geknüpft worden sind. Außerdem liegt darin auch eine hohe Ehrung unserer Klinik für Haut- und Geschlechtskrankheiten, deren Oberarzt, Prof. Dr. Schirren, als Generalsekretär die Organisation des Kongresses übernommen hat. Die Dermatologie ist zwar erst verhältnismäßig spät, etwa zu Beginn des 19. Jahrhunderts, wissenschaftlich begründet worden, und erst Anfang des 20. Jahrhunderts wurden an allen Universitäten Deutschlands Hautkliniken und entsprechende Ordinariate errichtet; es wäre jedoch müßig, heute noch ein Wort über die Bedeutung der Dermatologie zu verlieren, sie steht heute mit ihren Forschungen im Dienste der Gesundheit des Menschen in vorderster Front. Dieser Internationale Kongreß wird es erneut deutlich machen.

Auf diesem Wege wieder einen Schritt weiterzukommen, das ist der besondere Wunsch der Universität für den Kongreß und für sich selbst, vor allem aber für die Menschheit.

Prof. Albert Wiedmann

Präsident der Deutschen Dermatologischen Gesellschaft

Meine Damen und Herren!

Es gereicht der Deutschen Dermatologischen Gesellschaft zur außerordentlichen Freude und Ehre, Sie, die Teilnehmer des 13. Internationalen Kongresses für Dermatologie, hier in München begrüßen zu dürfen. Es bedeutet für mich als Vorsitzenden dieser Vereinigung eine große Freude und Genugtuung, diese Grüße Ihnen übermitteln zu dürfen. Es ist uns allen klar, daß Sie München als Tagungsort gewählt haben, um damit ALFRED MARCHIONINI zu ehren. Daß dieser Mann, bevor er selbst hier als Hausherr Sie empfangen durfte, aus dem Leben scheiden mußte, gibt dieser Tagung sicherlich eine gewisse tragische Note. Seine Stelle nimmt ein nicht weniger berühmter Wissenschaftler ein, der ebenso wie MARCHIONINI ein Weltbürger ist. Prof. WERNER JADASSOHN hat nach dem Hinscheiden MARCHIONINIS bereitwillig die mühevolle und schwere Aufgabe übernommen, die Organisation dieser Tagung zu leiten. Ihm zur Seite stand hierbei Prof. SCHIRREN als Generalsekretär. Diesen beiden gebührt unser besonderer Dank dafür, daß sie es ermöglicht haben, daß dieser Kongreß trotz aller Schwierigkeiten nach dem Tode MARCHIONINIS hier stattfinden kann.

Daß dieser Kongreß eine außerordentliche wissenschaftliche Höhe erreicht, dafür bürgt schon der Name WERNER JADASSOHN. Die Deutsche Dermatologische Gesellschaft wünscht aber darüber hinaus, daß Sie sich in diesem Kulturzentrum des deutschen Sprachraumes wohlfühlen mögen und Kontakte finden, welche die Brücke, die ALFRED MARCHIONINI von Volk zu Volk geschlagen hat, weiter stärken.

Prof. WERNER JADASSOHN
Präsident des XIII. Internationalen Kongresses für Dermatologie

„Wir Toten, wir Toten sind größere Heere als ihr auf der Erde, als ihr auf dem Meere, drum ehret die Toten, denn unser sind viele." Der Dichter CONRAD FERDINAND MEYER begründet diese Forderung damit, daß wir auf dem, was die Toten erarbeitet haben, weiter aufbauen konnten. Ein jeder denke an seine verstorbenen Freunde, an seine verstorbenen Lehrer, an diejenigen Menschen, denen er lebenslänglich zu Dank verpflichtet ist, die er verehrt und bewundert hat, und die nicht mehr unter uns weilen. Es besteht heute vielfach die Tendenz, das, was frühere Generationen festgestellt haben, nicht richtig einzuschätzen. Erst kürzlich habe ich einen Vortrag gehört, in dem der Kollege auseinandergesetzt hat, daß in den letzten 30 Jahren mehr Fortschritte in der Medizin gemacht worden seien als in den 300 Jahren vorher. PASTEUR, ROBERT KOCH, RÖNTGEN, VIRCHOW, LISTER, FINSEN, EHRLICH, METSCHNIKOV und viele andere hat er einfach unterschlagen. Wir sind die Zwerge, die auf den Schultern der Riesen sitzen und darum weitersehen können, als es ihnen möglich war. Drum ehret die Toten, denn ihrer sind viele.

Sehr verehrter Herr Bundespräsident!

Es ist eine große Ehre, Sie zum 13. Internationalen Dermatologenkongreß begrüßen zu dürfen. Ihre Anwesenheit beweist uns, daß Sie diesem Kongreß Bedeutung beimessen. Ich spreche hier als Stellvertreter von Prof. MARCHIONINI, der 1962 zum Präsidenten dieses Kongresses gewählt wurde und 1965 gestorben ist. Viel ist über ihn geschrieben worden, über sein erfolgreiches Leben, über seine hervorragenden Eigenschaften als Dermatologe und man darf, glaube ich, das Wort benutzen: als Diplomat. Über zwei Eigenschaften, die mir ausschlaggebend erscheinen, ist wenig gesagt worden: über seinen Optimismus und seine Naivität. Dieser Optimismus und diese Naivität wurden von seiner Frau so in Schranken gehalten, daß alles, was er unternahm, zum guten Ende geführt werden konnte.

Herr Bundespräsident, ich dispensiere Sie vom Anhören der Vorträge, möchte Sie aber höflich einladen, die Ausstellungen zu besuchen. Die Herren Prof. SCHNEI-

DER und BANDMANN, die sie organisiert haben, werden Sie sehr gerne herumführen. Für mich wäre es eine Ehre und Freude, Sie auf diesem Rundgang zu begleiten.

Sehr verehrter Herr Ministerpräsident!

Die dermatologischen Krankheiten haben eine große nationalökonomische Bedeutung. Ich will nur darauf hinweisen, wie viele Arbeitstage durch dermatologische Affektionen verloren gehen und die Geschlechtskrankheiten und die Gewerbedermatosen erwähnen. Ihre Anwesenheit, Herr Ministerpräsident, ist für uns eine große Ehre und ein Beweis dafür, daß Sie uns helfen wollen, prophylaktische Dermatologie zu treiben. Wir danken Ihnen sehr.

Sehr verehrter Herr Oberbürgermeister!

Ich kenne Sie besser als Sie meinen, denn MARCHIONINI hat mir viel von Ihnen erzählt, und ich weiß, wie sehr er Sie schätzte und wie dankbar er Ihnen für sehr vieles gewesen ist. Ich glaube kaum, daß MARCHIONINI München als Kongreßort vorgeschlagen hätte, wenn er nicht gewußt hätte, daß er sich auf den befreundeten Oberbürgermeister voll und ganz verlassen konnte. Wir sind Ihnen sehr dankbar, daß dieser Kongreß in München stattfinden kann.

Es ist ein hohes Ehrenamt, Rektor der berühmten Münchener Universität zu sein, und es ist ein hohes Ehrenamt, Dekan der ausgezeichneten medizinischen Fakultät zu sein. Ehrenämter sind es, aber keine Synekuren. Sie haben, Herr Rektor und Herr Dekan, sicher neben Erfreulichem auch viel Langweiliges und Unangenehmes zu erledigen. Für Ihren Besuch danken wir Ihnen sehr. Sie sind sicher gerne zu dieser Sitzung gekommen, denn schließlich sind wir es, die Ihnen für Ihre Schatzkammer ein neues Schmuckstück geliefert haben, Herrn Prof. BRAUN-FALCO, den neuen Münchener Ordinarius für Dermatologie. Wir wünschen Ihnen, lieber Herr BRAUN-FALCO, von Herzen alles Gute.

Je m'adresse maintenant aux membres du Comité International de Dermatologie:

Chers amis!

C'est vous qui avez pris sur vous l'organisation du programme scientifique. Tous les dermatologues participant à ce congrès et tous ceux qui consulteront plus tard le volume du congrès, vous doivent une très grande reconnaissance. C'était au président du Comité International, le Prof. DEGOS, au Secrétaire Général du congrès, le Prof. SCHIRREN et à moi-même, d'équilibrer ce programme. Je remercierai le Prof. SCHIRREN, les Prof. BRAUN-FALCO et SCHNEIDER, les Prof. NASEMANN et BANDMANN, ainsi que tous les membres du Comité d'Organisation à la fin du congrès. A tous, j'ai une très grande dette de reconnaissance. Mais à vous, mon cher ami DEGOS, je vous dirai aujourd'hui déjà, combien votre collaboration m'a été agréable et utile, combien j'ai apprécié votre gentillesse et vos efforts. Je me contente de vous dire de tout coeur merci.

En ce qui concerne notre programme scientifique, je dois vous avouer, c'était très difficile. Bien que nous soyons dans le pays de Goethe qui a déconseillé de vouloir contenter tout le monde, nous n'avons pas suivi ses conseils; nous avons essayé de contenter autant de collègues que possible, mais: ultra posse nemo obligatur.

Sehr herzlich danken möchte ich auch den Mitgliedern des Ausschusses der Deutschen Dermatologischen Gesellschaft. Unter dem Vorsitz meines Freundes

Prof. WIEDMANN haben sie Herrn Prof. SCHIRREN und mir, in mehreren Sitzungen, immer wieder gezeigt, daß sie uns wohlgesinnt sind, daß sie bereit sind, uns zu helfen, daß sie Vertrauen zu uns haben. Da man nach HEINE nicht Mitleid mit sich selber haben darf, hat uns ihr Mitleid wohlgetan.

I would like to say some words in english, in spite of the fact, that Dr. SULZBERGER once said that, when people like me are speaking in a microphon, it is only the accent which comes out. The accent would like to say: we are very glad that you came to participate on the congress. The international congresses in the english and american speaking countries, in London and in Washington, were wonderfull and all participants will never forget them. You are welcome.

Siento no saber el espanol. Sin embargo, me gustaría desearles una cordial bienvenida a este congreso de dermatología.

Man erwartet, glaube ich, von mir, daß ich hier noch allgemeine Bemerkungen einfüge; ich betone, allgemeine, nicht etwa philosophische Bemerkungen. Ich komme auf etwas zurück, was ich schon gelegentlich betont habe. Die Entwicklung in verschiedenen Ländern, speziell auch bei uns in der Schweiz, hat gezeigt, daß eine Warnung unbedingt wiederholt werden muß. Ich spreche von dem Graben, der immer tiefer ausgehoben wird, zwischen der Klinik einerseits und der Grundlagenforschung andererseits. Ich möchte nicht mißverstanden werden. Ich bin vollständig einverstanden damit, daß dermatologische Grundlagenforschung ohne Rücksicht auf die Klinik getrieben werden muß. Es ist mir klar, daß klinische Untersuchungen (investigations cliniques, clinical investigations) notwendig sind. Aber der Kliniker, der es wünscht (und recht viele sollten es wünschen), muß die Möglichkeit haben, durch die Klinik diktierte Grundlagenprobleme zu bearbeiten, d. h. den oben erwähnten Graben zwischen Klinik und Grundlagenforschung zu überbrücken. Dies immer und immer wieder zu betonen, erscheint mir besonders wichtig, denn es besteht mancherorts die Tendenz, die Kosten dieser Brücken, die, wie ich glaube, in der Dermatologie besonders wichtig sind, in den Budgets zu streichen. Ich bin überzeugt, daß der Kongreßband des 13. Internationalen Kongresses es allen erleichtern wird zu erreichen, daß diese Brücken verbessert, neu erstellt, auf keinen Fall aber abgerissen oder abgesperrt werden dürfen.

Ich möchte hier noch eine Frage erwähnen, über die wir häufig diskutiert haben: Was soll man in den Dermatologievorlesungen oder Demonstrationen den Studenten, die ihr Studium noch nicht abgeschlossen haben, beibringen; was soll man von ihnen im Examen verlangen? Ich bin dagegen, daß man sie mit Raritäten belastet, daß man mit ihnen über die Parapsoriasisformen usw., usw. diskutiert. Sie sollen nur das lernen (das aber gründlich), was sie, wenn sie praktische Ärzte sind, immer und immer wieder in ihrer Praxis werden behandeln müssen: Pyodermien, Carcinome, die verschiedenen Ekzeme und ekzematoiden Dermatosen, die Mykosen, den Erythematodes, die Syphilis, Unterschenkelgeschwüre, Arzneimitteldermatosen usw., usw. Auch so ist das Gebiet noch sehr groß. Sich auf die praktischen Probleme im Unterricht vor dem Arztexamen zu beschränken, erscheint mir richtig, wobei man natürlich nicht darauf verzichten muß, auf theoretisch interessante Fragen kurz hinzuweisen. Häufige Diskussionen mit jungen und alten Kollegen haben mir gezeigt, daß man in diesem Punkte in guten Treuen verschiedener Ansicht sein kann.

Noch einige Worte über ein Kapitel, das mir besonders am Herzen liegt, über die *Prophylaxe*. Aufklärung der Bevölkerung über die Geschlechtskrankheiten ist notwendig, ob sie sehr wirksam ist, erscheint mir zweifelhaft. Das Auffinden der

Infektionsquellen ist eine der wichtigen Aufgaben unserer Sozialassistentinnen. Eine ganz große Bedeutung zum mindesten bei uns in Genf haben die Arzneimitteldermatosen, die ja nicht nur sehr unangenehm sind, sondern oft Spitalbehandlung bedingen und sogar gefährlich werden können. Wenn das Mittel nicht strikt indiziert war, so ist die Erkrankung doppelt peinlich. Wir hatten kürzlich zwei Patientinnen in der Klinik mit schweren Sulfonamidexanthemen. Die eine hatte das Medikament genommen, weil vielleicht ein Schnupfen im Anzug war, der anderen war es verordnet worden, weil beim check-up, mit nicht katheterisiertem Urin, eine positive Bakterienkultur erzielt worden war. Kampf der Tablettensucht, Kampf der Polypragmasie!

Ein besonders wichtiges, aber auch besonders heikles Kapitel ist die Prophylaxe der Berufsdermatosen. Der Wert der Durchführung von Ekzemproben vor der Arbeitsaufnahme, der sog. „prophetic patch test", ist noch umstritten. Der Wert von Hautschutzsalben und anderer Schutzmittel ist intensiv untersucht worden, es bedarf aber hier noch umfassender Arbeit der jungen Generation.

Bei uns ist das wichtigste Kontaktekzem das Zementekzem. Die Häufigkeit dieser Dermatose hängt unzweifelhaft von der Qualität des Zementes ab. Hier könnte in Zusammenarbeit mit den Zementfabriken unter Umständen nützliche Arbeit geleistet werden.

Außer der Prophylaxe im engeren Sinne des Wortes gibt es auch noch eine Prophylaxe der Komplikationen. Man sollte die Hautcarcinome in Behandlung bekommen, bevor das halbe Gesicht weggefressen ist oder Metastasen bestehen. Kleine Unterschenkelgeschwüre werden rascher geheilt als große. Phlebitiden sollten frühzeitig behandelt, meiner Ansicht nach auch mit Röntgen bestrahlt werden, um postphlebitische Ulcera zu vermeiden. Die Acne vulgaris sollte frühzeitig behandelt werden, bevor sich ein Komplex ausgebildet hat, usw., usw.

Die dritte Form von Prophylaxe, von der ich sprechen möchte, betrifft das Vermeiden von Rückfällen. Mit Ekzemproben muß die Ekzemursache festgestellt werden. Dem „geheilten" Neurodermitiker muß eine geeignete Hautpflege verschrieben werden. Der „geheilte" Psoriatiker muß neu auftretende Herde sofort behandeln, usw., usw. Das, was wir als „traitement de maintien" bezeichnen, Dauerbehandlung zur Vermeidung von Rückfällen, spielt für uns eine sehr große Rolle.

Die Wirksamkeit der Prophylaxe hängt sehr stark ab von der Zahl und der Qualität der Sozialassistentinnen. Die kleine Genfer Klinik hat zwei diplomierte „infirmières sociales". Sie suchen die venerischen Infektionsquellen, sie sorgen dafür, daß die geheilten Carcinompatienten zur Kontrolle kommen, sie kontrollieren die geheilten Unterschenkelgeschwüre, sie suchen die ekzemerzeugenden Substanzen am Arbeitsplatz und in der Wohnung, usw., usw.

Ich habe hier auf die Wichtigkeit der Sozialassistentinnen hinweisen wollen, weil ich gedacht habe, diese Ausführungen könnten Klinikleitern nützlich sein, die Gesuche stellen wollen, um solche wichtigen Mitarbeiterinnen zu engagieren.

Comme membre de la Faculté de Médicine de l'Université de la République et Canton de Genève, je terminerai ce discours en français. J'emprunte les phrases de Ricord, qui les a prononcées à Paris, le lundi 5 août 1889, à l'occasion de l'ouverture du premier congrès international de dermatologie: Soyez les bienvenus et permettez-moi de vous présenter cette main qui voudrait serrer toutes les vôtres en vous donnant l'assurance d'une bonne et constante fraternité.

Prof. CARL GEORG SCHIRREN

Generalsekretär des XIII. Internationalen Kongresses für Dermatologie

Herr Bundespräsident, Herr Ministerpräsident, meine sehr verehrten Damen und Herren!

Gestatten Sie mir, daß ich die Ausführungen unseres Präsidenten um einige technische Details ergänze.

Zunächst darf ich namens des Exekutivkomitees unsere Freude darüber zum Ausdruck bringen, mit welch regem Interesse dieser Kongreß von den Dermatologen in aller Welt beachtet worden ist. Bis zur Stunde der feierlichen Eröffnungszeremonie haben sich fast 2100 aktive Kongreßteilnehmer mit über 800 Begleitpersonen registrieren lassen. Bis in die letzten Tage hinein spielte sich ein mit viel Spannung verzeichnetes Kopf-an-Kopf-Rennen zwischen den Teilnehmern des Gastgeberlandes Deutschland und dem wohl mit Dermatologen zahlenmäßig am stärksten besetzten Land, den Vereinigten Staaten von Amerika, ab. Im Augenblick sind unsere amerikanischen Freunde mit 411 aktiven Teilnehmern an die Zahl der Teilnehmer aus Deutschland mit 421 nahe herangekommen. Berücksichtigt man die weite Anreise der amerikanischen Delegation, so kann dieses Ergebnis nur unsere höchste Bewunderung verdienen.

Nach Washington waren 1962 Dermatologen aus 69 Staaten gekommen; 5 Jahre später dürfen wir Gäste aus 79 Staaten in München begrüßen. Nach den bereits genannten beiden Ländern sind im Augenblick in der weiteren Reihenfolge mit beachtlichen Teilnehmerzahlen Frankreich (162), Japan (91), Italien (91), Großbritannien (91), Schweiz (75), Schweden (47), Niederlande (44), Belgien (43), Argentinien (42) vertreten. Ihnen folgen weitere 67 Länder mit Teilnehmerzahlen zwischen 1 und 40.

ALFRED MARCHIONINI hatte noch 1964 eine Reise in die Sowjetunion unternommen, um die Dermatologen dieses Landes persönlich zum Internationalen Kongreß für Dermatologie einzuladen. Sein Verdienst war es, daß eine russische Delegation ihre Teilnahme in Aussicht stellte. 86 sowjetrussische Dermatologen wollten sich mit 32 Vorträgen am Kongreß beteiligen, falls russisch als fünfte Kongreßsprache auch simultan übersetzt werden würde. Das Internationale Komitee hatte zugesagt, bei Teilnahme von mehr als 30 russischen Dermatologen für ein entsprechendes Dolmetscherteam mit russischen Sprachkenntnissen zu sorgen. Dies gelang unter nicht geringen Schwierigkeiten und nur mit erheblichen Geldmitteln. Wenige Wochen vor dem Beginn des Kongresses zog die russische Delegation ihre Zusage zurück. Was der Kongreßleitung blieb, waren die Enttäuschung über diesen Fehlschlag und die Verpflichtung, den bereits unter Vertrag stehenden zwölf russischen Dolmetschern ihr volles Honorar auszuzahlen.

Mit ebenso großem Bedauern verzeichnen wir das Fehlen ostdeutscher Dermatologen. Auch sie hatten zunächst ihr Kommen zugesagt, um dann ebenfalls kurz vor Beginn des Kongresses definitiv ihre Teilnahmezusage zurückzuziehen.

Ein bisher nicht übliches Novum hat dieser XIII. Internationale Kongreß aufzuweisen: Über 40 Kinder von teilnehmenden Dermatologen werden während der Kongreßdauer in einem eigenen dermatologischen Kindergarten im Kongreßgelände betreut und versorgt. Das Jüngste ist gerade 3 Monate alt! Mein Kollege NASEMANN hat sich um die Einrichtung dieses Kindergartens besonders verdient gemacht.

Ein Problem, für das wir eigentlich nicht zuständig sind, hat uns besonders belastet. Als wir Sie alle 1962 nach München einluden, war diese Stadt noch intakt.

Inzwischen hat man begonnen, sie an fast allen bauhistorisch bedeutsamen Stellen aufzureißen, um bis zur Olympiade 1972 eine Untergrundbahn und eine Schnellbahn zu installieren. Sie, Herr Oberbürgermeister Dr. VOGEL, haben vorhin in Ihrer Begrüßungsrede den Vergleich mit der Scabies herangezogen, den wir Dermatologen besonders gut verstehen. Nur ein Unterschied besteht, und darum hinkt dieser Vergleich ein wenig: Therapeutisch wird der Dermatologe heute z. B. mit dem γ-Hexachlorcyclohexan in 2 Tagen mit der Scabies fertig!

Die immensen Kosten eines solchen Kongresses bereiteten uns besondere Sorgen. Ohne die Hilfe der Öffentlichen Hand hätten wir das Finanzierungsproblem nicht lösen können. Die Bundesregierung gab 102000,— DM, der Freistaat Bayern 90000,— DM und die Stadt München 65000,— DM. Die pharmazeutische und medizinisch-technische Industrie unseres Landes und einiger weiterer Länder hat durch ihre großzügige Beteiligung an der Industrieausstellung zur Gestaltung des Kongresses beigetragen. Die Gesamtorganisation dieses wichtigen Kongreßbereichs lag in den Händen von Prof. W. SCHNEIDER aus Tübingen.

Die deutschen Dermatologen haben durch ihre ungewöhnlich große Spendenfreudigkeit, deren Lenkung und Ausrichtung auf den Kongreß durch Prof. H. GÖTZ, Essen, erfolgte, zur Gesamtfinanzierung mit 112000,— DM beigetragen. Einzelne unserer deutschen Dermatologen haben Beträge zwischen drei- und viertausend DM gespendet.

Aber auch Sie, meine verehrten Kollegen und Kongreßteilnehmer, haben uns mit Ihrem offiziellen Kongreßbeitrag in Höhe von 240,— DM in erheblichem Umfang bei der Finanzierung mitgeholfen. Vergessen Sie aber bitte nicht, daß die Teilnahme jedes aktiven Kongreßmitgliedes uns 610,— DM kosten wird, wovon Sie 240,— DM und die Kongreßleitung 370,— DM aufbringen müssen. Und bedenken Sie bitte, daß wir jedem Teilnehmer durch den Vorbericht und durch die Auslieferung des Verhandlungsberichtes, der 2000 Seiten umfassen wird, einen Bücherwert von fast 200,— DM zurückerstatten.

Erlauben Sie mir noch den einen Hinweis, daß das Münchner Exekutivkomitee, in dem ich besonders Prof. TH. NASEMANN und Prof. H.-J. BANDMANN neben vielen anderen nennen möchte, die große Arbeit ohne die aktive Mithilfe der Kliniken für Dermatologie, insbesondere der Univ.-Hautkliniken Deutschlands, nicht hätte leisten können.

Einem Mann fühlen wir uns in dieser Stunde besonders verbunden: Prof. WERNER JADASSOHN aus Genf. Er hat es mit außergewöhnlichem diplomatischen Geschick verstanden, sich in die Situation seines Nachbarlandes hineinzufinden und war nimmermüde an der Kongreßorganisation beteiligt.

Wir haben keine Mühe gescheut, um Ihnen allen eine schöne Kongreßwoche zu bereiten. In unseren Büros in München (A. KOCH) und in Genf (Y. BOSSHARD) haben viele in oft mühseliger, selbstloser Arbeit mitgeholfen. Auch das Wetter hat sich, wenn sie diesen heutigen herrlichen Sonnentag betrachten, auf Ihren Besuch eingestellt. Hoffentlich hält es an!

Möge dieser Kongreß Sie alle bereichern und nach unser aller Wunsch ablaufen: 1. zum Fortschritt der Wissenschaft, 2. zum Nutzen unserer Patienten und 3. zur Festigung von Freundschaften, hinweg über alle Grenzen.

Mögen wir alle an Weisheit zunehmen, auf daß das Wort des Hippokrates, das Sie alle auf der Rückseite Ihrer bronzenen Teilnehmermedaille verzeichnet finden, Wirklichkeit wird: Der Arzt, der die Weisheit liebt, ist den Göttern ähnlich.

Medals and Prizes
Médailles et prix

Medallas y premios
Medaillen und Preise

Rede von Prof. ALBERT WIEDMANN *zur Verleihung der Alfred-Marchionini-Medaille und des Alfred-Marchionini-Preises*

Bevor ich auf den eigentlichen Festakt eingehe, glaube ich im Sinne von Ihnen allen sprechen zu dürfen, wenn ich Herrn KURT HERRMANN den aufrichtigen Dank der Deutschen Dermatologischen Gesellschaft dafür ausspreche, daß er das Andenken an einen der ganz Großen der modernen Dermatologie durch die Stiftung der Alfred-Marchionini-Medaille und des Alfred-Marchionini-Preises geehrt und für die Zukunft fundiert hat.

Gerade die Bestimmung im Statut, daß mit der Verleihung der Alfred-Marchionini-Medaille eine Persönlichkeit ausgezeichnet werden soll, welche nicht nur als Arzt, Lehrer und Forscher, sondern auch im Geiste ALFRED MARCHIONINIS als großer Bürger unserer Zeit zu gelten hat, gibt dieser Ehrung die besondere Note. Dafür möchte ich in Ihrer aller Namen an dieser Stelle Herrn KURT HERRMANN nochmals von Herzen danken.

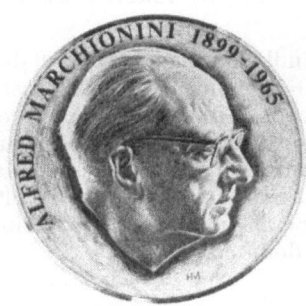

Mein lieber Prof. JADASSOHN!

Es ist eine ständige Redensart, daß der Lebensweg der Söhne großer Männer dadurch erschwert wird, daß die Umwelt immer wieder geneigt erscheint, den Sohn mit dem Vater zu vergleichen. Sicherlich beschattete auch am Beginn Ihrer wissenschaftlichen Laufbahn dieses Vorurteil Ihre Bemühungen, die beschwerliche Straße zum Erfolg zu gehen. Wenn aber in vielen Fällen der Vergleich mit dem Vater zurecht zu Ungunsten des Sohnes ausfällt, wurden hier die Kritiker Lügen gestraft, denn der Sohn JADASSOHN darf heute als der würdige Nachfolger seines Vaters gelten.

Ihr Interesse galt schon von frühester Jugend an der Chemie, einer Wissenschaft, der Sie sich vor allem widmen wollten. Wenn Sie sich später doch gänzlich der Medizin zugewandt haben, so war Ihre Forschungsrichtung durch Ihre Liebe zur Chemie von frühesten Zeiten an bis heute beeinflußt. Dies mag auch einer der Gründe sein, daß der Sohn neben dem großen, dem Trend der Zeit entsprechend vorwiegend morphologisch eingestellten Vater zu gleicher Größe heranwuchs. Ihr Interesse für die morphologische Dermatologie wurde jedoch darüber hinaus nicht nur durch den ständigen Kontakt mit Ihrem Vater, sondern vor allem auch durch Ihren Lehrer BRUNO BLOCH geweckt und gesteigert, der als genialer Meister den jungen aufstrebenden Wissenschaftler maßgeblich beeinflußte.

Den ersten Markstein in Ihrer Gelehrtenlaufbahn bildete die Erteilung der
Venia legendi im Jahre 1928 bei BRUNO BLOCH in Zürich. Den Höhepunkt erreichte Ihre Karriere mit der Berufung auf den Lehrstuhl für Dermatologie an der
Universität Genf im Jahre 1946. Mit dieser Berufung hat Genf eine der ange-
sehensten Kliniken für Hautkrankheiten geschaffen. Daß es nicht gelungen ist, Sie
im Jahre 1957 auf den Hebraschen Lehrstuhl in Wien zu berufen, kann keiner
mehr bedauern als ich selbst, denn im freundschaftlichen Konkurrenzkampf mit
einem der größten Dermatologen der Welt stehen zu dürfen, könnte für jeder-
mann und so auch für mich nur zur besonderen Ehre und Auszeichnung dienen.
Auf die Gründe dieses Mißlingens einzugehen, möchte ich mir versagen. Jedenfalls
hat Ihr wissenschaftliches Oeuvre bewiesen, daß die Synthese der morphologischen
mit der funktionellen Forschung heute der Weg ist, auf dem die Lehre von den
Hautkrankheiten weiterzuschreiten hat.

Wer jedoch über den Gelehrten WERNER JADASSOHN hinaus auch den liebens-
werten Menschen kennt und von ihm mit seiner Freundschaft ausgezeichnet wird,
wird sich ganz besonders glücklich schätzen dürfen. Ihr Humor, der sich nicht nur
in den bestrickenden Tischreden, sondern auch im freundschaftlichen Gespräch
immer wieder zeigt, läßt Sie einem besonders nahe kommen. Daß schließlich zu
Ihnen auch die Pfeife gehört, stellt eine weitere besondere Bindung zwischen Ihnen
und mir dar.

So ist es eine Selbstverständlichkeit gewesen, daß das Kuratorium der Stiftung
für den Alfred-Marchionini-Preis ohne lange Diskussion einhellig den Beschluß
gefaßt hat, Ihnen, Herr Prof. JADASSOHN, die Alfred-Marchionini-Medaille in
Gold zu verleihen, denn keiner könnte würdiger sein, diese Ehrung zu empfangen,
als der wissenschaftlich und menschlich überragende Mann, der im Geiste ALFRED
MARCHIONINIS im wahrsten Sinne des Wortes als Weltbürger bezeichnet werden
kann, was sich letzten Endes auch in der Art, wie Sie in vorbildlicher Weise diesen
Kongreß vorbereitet haben, dokumentiert.

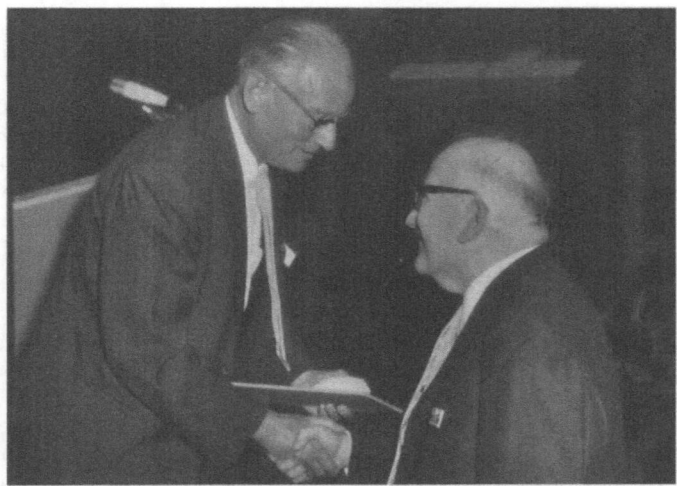

Prof. WIEDMANN hands over the
Marchionini-medal to Prof. JADASSOHN

Le Prof. WIEDMANN remet la médaille
Marchionini au Prof. JADASSOHN

El Prof. WIEDMANN hace entrega de la
Medalla Marchionini al Prof. JADASSOHN

Prof. WIEDMANN überreicht Prof. JADASSOHN
die Marchionini-Medaille

Herr Dr. ANTONESCU!

Sie haben schon in Ihrer Jugend durch die erfolgreiche Ablegung der Konkur-
renzprüfung zur Aufnahme in die medizinische Fakultät der Universität Bukarest
bewiesen und im Jahre 1947 im Rahmen eines Wettbewerbs für die Aufnahme
als Spitalexterner neuerlich unter Beweis gestellt, daß Sie zu den größten Hoffnungen auf wissenschaftlichem Gebiet berechtigen. Die Staatsprüfung legten Sie
im Jahre 1950 mit dem Meritumdiplom ab, wobei Sie als Erster qualifiziert wurden. Schon 5 Jahre später wurden Sie an der von Ihrem Lehrer Prof. LONGHIN
geleiteten dermatologischen Klinik zum Assistenten ernannt und nach weiteren
3 Jahren erhielten Sie die beste Note bei der Assistentenkonkurrenzprüfung.

Ihr besonderes Interesse galt neben der klinischen Tätigkeit der Histopathologie der Hautkrankheiten. Mit ihrer Arbeit über „Untersuchungen über die Hefen
des Genus candida und ihre Rolle in der Pathologie der Haut und Schleimhäute"
haben Sie den Titel eines Doktors der medizinischen Wissenschaften erlangt. Über
120 wissenschaftliche Arbeiten, die Sie unter Leitung Ihres Lehrers Prof. LONGHIN
verfaßten und die sich vor allem mit den Krankheiten, die durch die Candida
hervorgerufen werden und mit der Morphologie der Candida beschäftigen, haben
Sie nicht nur Ihr außerordentliches wissenschaftliches Interesse an den Tag gelegt, sondern auch bewiesen, daß Sie in der Lage sind, wissenschaftliche Probleme
selbständig aufzugreifen und zu lösen und dabei in hervorragender Weise neue
Erkenntnisse zu schöpfen. Sie gehören also sicherlich zu jenen jungen aufstrebenden Wissenschaftlern, die zu den größten Hoffnungen berechtigen.

All diese Erwägungen, Herr Dr. ANTONESCU, waren die Veranlassung, daß das
Kuratorium der Stiftung des Alfred-Marchionini-Preises den Beschluß gefaßt hat,
Ihnen den Alfred-Marchionini-Preis zu verleihen.

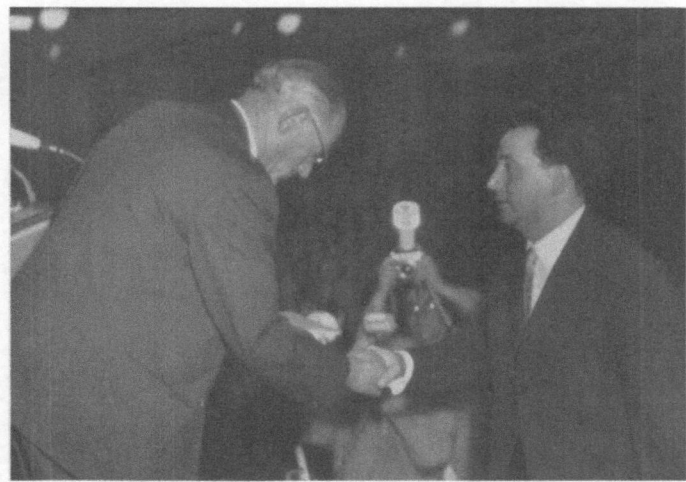

Prof. WIEDMANN hands over the Marchionini-
Prize to Dr. ANTONESCU

Remise du Prix Marchionini par le
Prof. WIEDMANN au Dr. ANTONESCU

El Prof. WIEDMANN hace entrega del
Premio Marchionini al Dr. ANTONESCU

Verleihung des Marchionini-Preises an
Dr. ANTONESCU (rechts) durch
Prof. WIEDMANN

Rede von Prof. ALOIS MEMMESHEIMER *anläßlich der Verleihung
der Fr. Schaudinn-E. Hoffmann-Medaille*

Herr Bundespräsident, Herr Ministerpräsident, Herr Oberbürgermeister, meine
Herren Präsidenten, meine sehr verehrten Damen, meine Herren!

Namens der Deutschen Dermatologischen Gesellschaft habe ich eine weitere
Ehrung mitzuteilen. In Erinnerung an die Entdecker des Erregers der Lustseuche,
FR. SCHAUDINN und ERICH HOFFMANN, hat unsere Gesellschaft eine Plakette geschaffen, die alle 2 bis 3 Jahre einem verdienten Forscher auf diesem Gebiet verliehen wird. Die Kommission hat diesmal einen jungen nordamerikanischen Gelehrten gewählt, ROBERT A. NELSON, der allen Fachleuten durch den Nelson-Test
wohlbekannt ist. Der hervorragende Mikrobiologe der Universität Florida, der
leider nicht selbst kommen konnte, da sein Institut in diesen Tagen von Florida
nach Kalifornien umzieht, der geniale Forscher, hat die Erkennung vor allem alter
und unklarer Erkrankungsfälle und die Feststellung ihrer Heilung durch seinen
Test außerordentlich gefördert. Herr SULZBERGER hat sich bereit erklärt, für den
Gelehrten die Plakette in Empfang zu nehmen und sie ihm demnächst in Kalifornien zu überreichen.

Dankrede von Prof. MARION B. SULZBERGER *anläßlich der Verleihung der Schaudinn-
Hoffmann-Medaille an Dr. R. A.* NELSON

Ich habe die große Ehre, für Herrn Dr. NELSON diese wunderschöne Plakette
zu übernehmen, und ich weiß, wenn Herr Dr. NELSON da sein könnte, würde er
betonen, daß sein Verdienst und seine Forschungen auf einer internationalen Basis
aufgebaut sind, und in diesem Sinne würde er die Auszeichnung annehmen. Im
Namen von Herrn Dr. NELSON besten Dank!

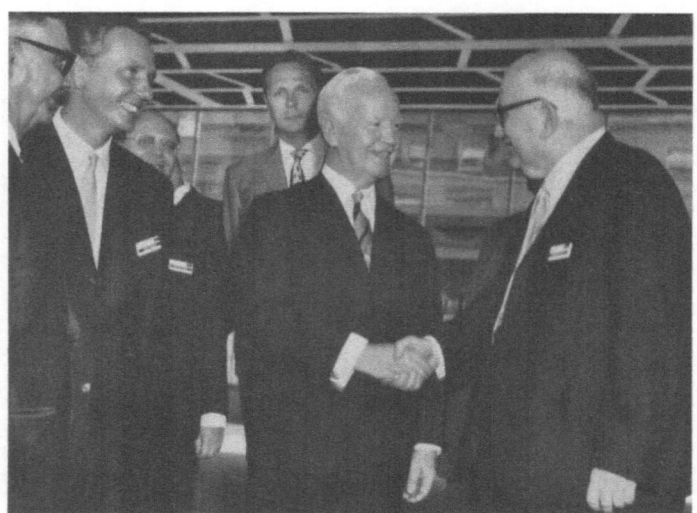

The President of the Federal Republic   El Presidente de la República Federal
of Germany at his departure   Alemana se despide de los congresistas

Le Président de la République Fédérale   Beim Abschied des Bundespräsidenten
d'Allemagne prend congé

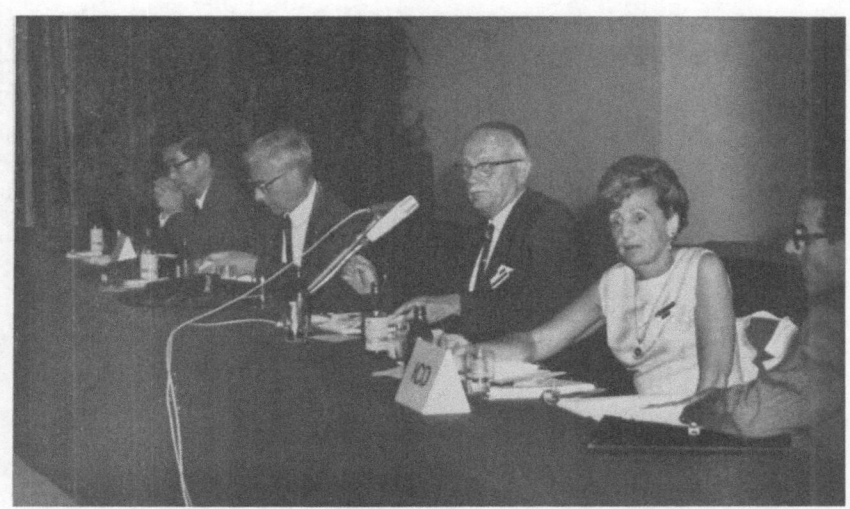

→ Prof. KAWAMURA, Prof. PINKUS, Prof. BELISARIO, Prof. JABLONSKA, Prof. HORNSTEIN

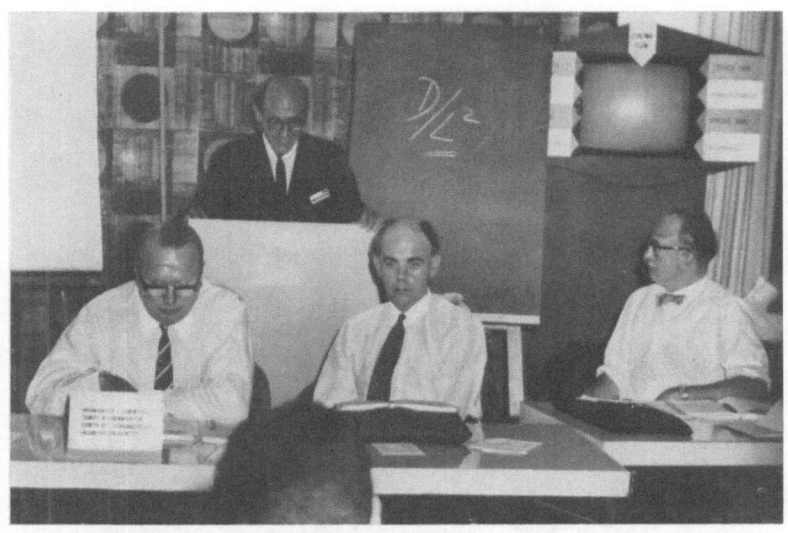

→ Prof. WULF, Dr. ROOK, Dr. MITCHELL HEGGS

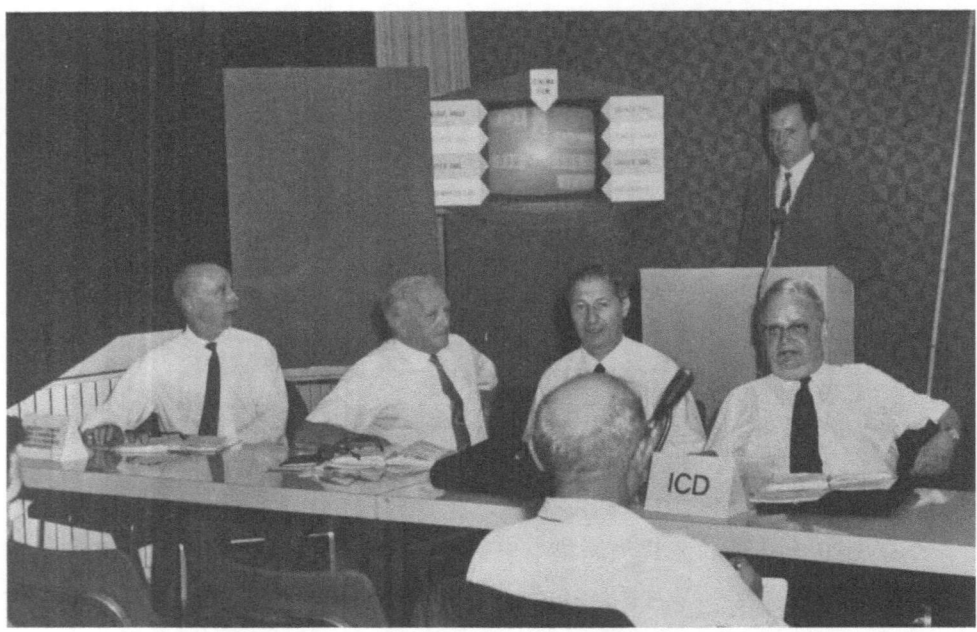

→ Prof. Musger, Prof. Katzenellenbogen, Prof. Sagher, Prof. Montgomery

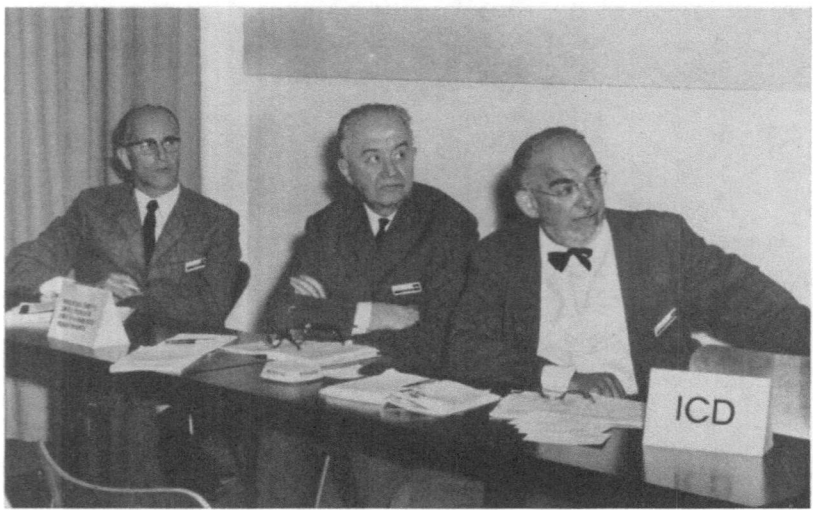

→ Prof. Herzberg, Prof. Longhin, Prof. Degos

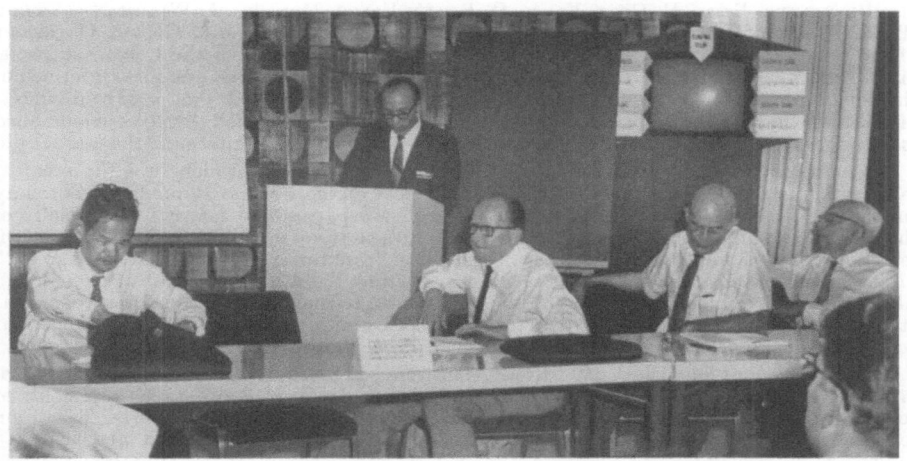

→ Prof. ITO, Prof. LEVER, Prof. GÖTZ, Prof. WILSON, Prof. RAMOS E SILVA

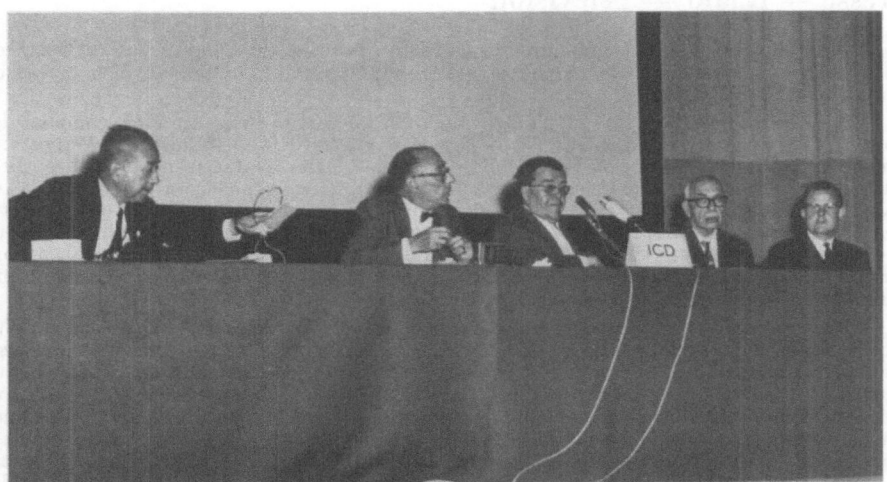

→ Prof. KITAMURA, Prof. LEVER, Prof. DUPERRAT, Prof. BEERMANN, Prof. STEIGLEDER

Press — Radio — Television

A Congress of such an extend as the International Congress of Dermatology, suscites, already before its opening, a great interest in the circle of press, radio and television.

A committee had been formed for the press and information, composed by: Prof. A. MEMMESHEIMER, Essen, H. GÖTZ, Essen, O. BRAUN-FALCO, Munich, A. WIEDMANN, Vienna (President of the Dermatological Society of Germany), W. JADASSOHN, Geneva (President of the Congress), and C. G. SCHIRREN, Munich (General Secretary of the Congress). Profs. MEMMESHEIMER and GÖTZ were chiefly in charge. In this manner, the press was informed of the importance of the conferences before the congress had even started. Two press conferences, of which the first took place before the opening of the congress, informed the press in a detailed and objective way. Mrs. SIGLINDE STIEL of Munich, was in charge of informing the journalists.

Cosmetology is certainly one of the problems of Dermatology which rises the greatest interest of the public. By numerous articles the press of the Federal Republic of Germany supplied ample information on this subject. Many newspapers and magazines, specially of the Federal Republic of Germany, sent their representatives to Munich. The presence of representatives of important dailys, such as: "Die Frankfurter Allgemeine", "Die Welt", "Die Süddeutsche Zeitung", "Die Neue Zürcher Zeitung" and many others, was remarked. All showed a great interest in giving present information to their readers. A medical representative of the press agency of the Federal Republic of Germany, assisted the Congress permanently in order to give information even to small journals of the province.

The dailies alone published 240 articles concerning the Congress, representing a total of 24 million copies. Furthermore, millions of magazine copies, as well as detailed comments of dermatological periodicals must be added. The radio gave almost daily reports. Television commented the event, and many dermatologists were interviewed in radio and television.

Thanks to the aid and comprehension of dermatologists who throughout the Congress placed themselves at the disposal of the press, exact information on a scientific congress could be given.

Presse — Radio — Télévision

Une manifestation d'une envergure aussi vaste que celle du Congrès International de Dermatologie, suscita déjà avant son ouverture, un vif intérêt dans les milieux de la presse, de la radio et de la télévision.

Afin de renseigner la presse et d'autres organes, un comité avait été créé, composé des Profs. A. MEMMESHEIMER (Essen), H. GÖTZ (Essen), O. BRAUN-FALCO (Munich), A. WIEDMANN (Vienne), Président de la Société Allemande de Dermatologie, W. JADASSOHN (Genève), Président du Congrès ainsi que C. G. SCHIRREN (Munich), Secrétaire Général du Congrès. Les Profs. A. MEMMESHEIMER et H. GÖTZ s'étaient spécialement chargés de cette tâche. De cette manière, la presse avait été saisie de l'importance des conférences prévues, avant même que le Congrès n'ait débuté. Deux conférences de presse, dont la première fut donnée avant l'ouverture du Congrès, informèrent la presse d'une façon détaillée et objective. Mme SIGLINDE STIEL (Munich) informait directement les journalistes.

La cosmétologie est certainement un des problèmes de la Dermatologie qui suscite le plus d'intérêt dans le grand public. De nombreux articles parus dans la presse, donnèrent une large information à ce sujet. De nombreux journaux et illustrés, spécialement de la République Fédérale d'Allemagne, envoyèrent leurs représentants à Munich. On nota la présence d'envoyés spéciaux d'importants quotidiens: «Die Frankfurter Allgemeine», «Die Welt», «Die Süddeutsche Zeitung», «Die Neue Zürcher Zeitung» et bien d'autres. Leur vif intérêt donna à leurs lecteurs une intéressante information d'actualité. Un envoyé médical de l'agence de presse allemande, resta en permanence au Congrès, afin d'informer même les journaux locaux à faibles tirages.

Les quotidiens à eux seuls, publièrent 240 articles sur le Congrès, représentant 24 millions d'exemplaires. En outre, il faut ajouter les millions d'exemplaires des journaux illustrés se rapportant au Congrès, ainsi que les commentaires détaillés parus dans des périodiques dermatologiques.

La radio, par de fréquentes émissions spéciales, informa les auditeurs, tandis que la télévision commenta l'événement. Mentionnons encore les interviews radiodiffusées et télévisées de plusieurs dermatologistes.

Grâce à l'aide et la compréhension de quelques dermatologues qui pendant toute la durée du Congrès informèrent volontiers la presse, des commentaires précis et exacts sur cette manifestation scientifique furent donnés.

Prensa — Radio — Televisión

Una manifestación de importancia como este Congreso Internacional de Dermatología, suscitó mucho antes de su inauguración, un vivo interés en el seno de la prensa, la radio y la televisión.

Con objeto de que la prensa y otros órganos similares fueran convenientemente informados se creó un Comité formado por los Profs. MEMMESHEIMER de Essen, H. GÖTZ de Essen, O. BRAUN-FALCO de Munich, A. WIEDMANN de Viena, Presidente del Comité de la Sociedad Alemana de Dermatología, asi como de los Profs. W. JADASSOHN de Ginebra, Presidente del Congreso, y C. G. SCHIRREN de Munich, Secretario General del Congreso. Los Profs. MEMMESHEIMER y GÖTZ se encargaron particularmente de esta misión. De este modo, la prensa tuvo noticias de la gran importancia de las conferencias que deberían celebrarse, incluso con antelación a la inauguración del Congreso. Fueron dadas dos conferencias de prensa, una de ellas antes de la ceremonia de apertura, que permitieron informar a la prensa de manera objetiva y detallada. La Sra. SIGLINDE STIEL, de Munich, fué la encargada de informar personalmente a los periodistas.

La cosmetología es, indudablemente, la rama de la dermatología que más llama la atención de los profanos. Numerosos artículos, publicados en los diarios, informaron ampliamente sobre este tema. Gran número de periódicos y revistas ilustradas, sobretodo de los editados en la República Federal Alemana, estuvieron representados en Munich.

Muchos periódicos importantes enviaron delegados especiales, tales como "Die Frankfurter Allgemeine", "Die Welt", "Die Süddeutsche Zeitung", "Die Neue Zürcher Zeitung" y otros más. El vivo interés que estos redactores testimoniaron al Congreso proporcionó una interesante información de actualidad a sus respectivos lectores. Incluso la Agencia Alemana de Prensa, delegó a un enviado médico especial con caracter permanente a este Congreso, para informar a los mas apartados periódicos de la nación.

Los diarios, por si mismos, publicaron hasta 240 artículos, lo que representa 240 millones de ejemplares, a los que hay que añadir los millones de ejemplares de revistas ilustradas que hicieron mención del Congreso y los comentarios aparecidos en publicaciones médicas destinadas a los dermatólogos.

La radio dedicó al Congreso frecuentes emisiones especiales, informando a sus auditores, al paso que la televisión comentó ampliamente este acontecimiento. Muchos dermatólogos recibieron la visita de los periodistas y sus conversaciones fueron radiodifundidas y televisadas.

Se pudieron facilitar a la prensa, durante todo el desarrollo del Congreso, comunicados precisos y exactos sobre este acontecimiento, todo ello gracias a la ayuda y a la amabilidad de cierto número de dermatólogos que se ofrecieron voluntarios para ello.

Presse — Rundfunk — Fernsehen

Ein Kongreß von der Größenordnung des Dermatologenkongresses findet naturgemäß bereits vor der eigentlichen Eröffnung reges Interesse von seiten der Kommunikationsmittel Presse, Rundfunk und Fernsehen.

Um Presse und Information bekümmerte sich ein spezielles Komitee, bestehend aus den Herren Prof. A. MEMMESHEIMER, Essen, Prof. H. GÖTZ, Essen, Prof. O. BRAUN-FALCO, München, dem Präsidenten der D.D.G. Prof. A. WIEDMANN, Wien, dem Kongreßpräsidenten Prof. W. JADASSOHN, Genf, sowie dem Generalsekretär Prof. C. G. SCHIRREN, München. Die Prof. MEMMESHEIMER und GÖTZ haben sich dieser Aufgabe besonders gewidmet. Auf diese Art und Weise war gewährleistet, daß die Presse bereits vor Beginn des Kongresses auf die Bedeutung der zu erwartenden Verhandlungen aufmerksam gemacht wurde. Zwei Pressekonferenzen, eine bereits vor dem Kongreß, dienten der ausführlichen, sachgemäßen und aktuellen Berichterstattung, die auf journalistischer Seite von Frau SIGLINDE STIEL, München, betreut wurde.

Das Interesse der breiten Öffentlichkeit an den Fragen der Dermatologie wendet sich in erster Linie an das Fachgebiet der Kosmetik. Diesem Interesse des Publikums kamen die deutschen Publikationsorgane durch eingehende Berichterstattung entgegen. So schickten nicht nur Massenblätter wie die Illustrierten ihre Vertreter nach München, sondern auch namhafte Tageszeitungen wie „Die Frankfurter Allgemeine", „Die Welt", „Die Süddeutsche Zeitung", „Die Neue Zürcher Zeitung" und viele andere legten Wert auf eine aktuelle Information ihrer Leser. Ein medizinisch geschulter Korrespondent der Deutschen Presseagentur dpa hielt sich ständig auf dem Kongreßgelände auf, um selbst die kleinsten Provinzblätter mit Nachrichten zu versorgen.

Allein die Tageszeitungen veröffentlichten 240 Berichte über den Kongreß, was einer Auflage von über 24 Millionen Exemplaren gleichkommt. Hinzu kommen die Millionenauflagen der Illustrierten sowie die ausführlichen Kommentare der dermatologischen Fachzeitschriften, in denen die auf dem Kongreß behandelten Probleme zur Sprache kamen. Der Rundfunk gab in mehreren Sendern fast täglich Mitteilungen. Das deutsche Fernsehen nahm das Ereignis in beiden Programmen wahr. Bemerkenswert sind hier die Funk- und Fernsehinterviews, die führende Kongreßteilnehmer gegeben haben.

Die verantwortliche Arbeit der Berichterstattung bei einem wissenschaftlichen Kongreß wurde besonders durch die Hilfsbereitschaft und das Entgegenkommen der einzelnen Professoren gefördert, die während der Kongreßwoche mit der Presse in Berührung kamen. Dank diesem Entgegenkommen lieferten die Pressekonferenzen und Interviews ein für das Publikum befriedigendes Ergebnis.

Im Zusammenhang damit leistete die kongreßeigene Pressestelle dem interessierten Leser einen besonderen Dienst, indem sie es ermöglichte, auch den Laien in verständlicher Darstellung das Wesentliche der wissenschaftlichen Ergebnisse der einzelnen Themen und Symposien zu vermitteln. Gleichzeitig konnten die Wissenschaftler sicher sein, daß keine falsche Information an die Öffentlichkeit gelangte.

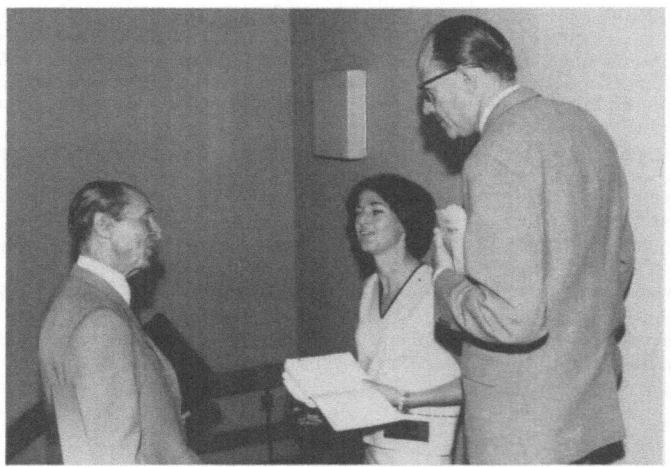

Press-Information   Oficina de la Prensa
Presse-Information   Presse-Information

→ Prof. MEMMESHEIMER, Frau STIEL, Prof. GÖTZ

Das Gesellschafts- und Damenprogramm

Bericht von Prof. THEODOR NASEMANN

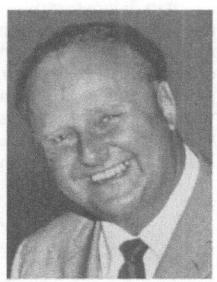

Je größer das Volumen medizinischer Kongresse mit internationaler Beteiligung anwächst, je umfangreicher ihre Vortragsprogramme und je weitläufiger wissenschaftlich-technische wie Industrieausstellungen werden, desto mehr nimmt das Bedürfnis der Teilnehmer zu, persönlichen Kontakt zu finden, Freundschaften zu vertiefen, Erfahrungen auszutauschen und neue, fruchtbare Beziehungen anzuknüpfen. Diesen Wünschen nicht nur entgegenzukommen, sondern sie zwanglos verwirklichen zu helfen, war das Hauptanliegen aller Veranstaltungen des Gesellschafts- und Damenprogramms dieses Münchener Kongresses. Sie wurden so ausgewählt, daß nicht nur verschiedene Geschmacksrichtungen berücksichtigt, sondern auch durch den unterschiedlichen Charakter der Räume Variationen der Stimmungen und der Begegnungsarten erzielt wurden. Schon der von über 2000 Kongressisten mit ihren Damen ungewöhnlich gut besuchte Begrüßungsabend im Kongreßsaal des Deutschen Museums am 30. Juli 1967 auf Einladung der Kongreßleitung war zweifellos ein „Wegbereiter für die aufgeschlossene Atmosphäre der Eröffnungssitzung" am nächsten Vormittag in Gegenwart des deutschen Bundespräsidenten, Dr. h. c. HEINRICH LÜBKE, wie H. W. SPIER, Berlin, es ausgesprochen hat. Der Kongreßsaal war mit Blumenarrangements reich geschmückt und wurde für 3 Std nicht nur Ort für kulinarische Genüsse wahrhaft opulenter kalter Buffets, die durch geschickte Anordnung der langen Tafeln ein Gedränge a priori ausschlossen, sondern auch für zahllose „erste" Begrüßungen und Champagner-beflügelte Gespräche. Es war ein frequentes Hin- und Herwogen, ein bunter Völkerreigen und ein Zusammenklang vieler Sprachen und Dialekte — mithin ein glücklicher Auftakt im Sinne der Kongreßleitung:

„Und wenn Ihr kommt, Ihr sollt willkommen sein!"
und auch des Mottos von Prof. JADASSOHN, des Präsidenten dieses Kongresses:

„Wir wollen sein ein „einzig" Volk von Brüdern!"

(Schiller)

Doch heißt es wohl begründet bei Wilhelm Busch im „Dank" anläßlich seines 70. Geburtstages:

„Fortuna lächelt, doch sie mag
Nur ungern voll beglücken:
Schenkt sie uns einen Sommertag,
So schenkt sie uns auch Mücken."

Hier kamen die „Mücken" in Gestalt einer für die Jahreszeit in München recht ungewöhnlichen, weil anhaltenden schwülen Hitze. Am meisten litten die Gäste aus den nordischen Ländern und die zahlreichen Kongreßbesucher aus den Vereinigten Staaten, die nicht gewohnt waren, auf „Air condition" verzichten zu müssen. Dennoch waren wohl alle froh, daß uns die Sonne lachte und das gute Wetter bis zum Schluß anhielt.

Am Montag, dem 31. Juli 1967, fand das Konzert des Frankfurter Bachorchesters wieder im großen Kongreßsaal des sehr schön auf einer Isarinsel gelegenen und 1903 von OSKAR VON MILLER gegründeten Deutschen Museums statt. Der Blumenschmuck vom Vortage verschaffte wiederum eine wohltemperierte Stimmung und die Darbietungen der Solisten und des Ensembles einen vorzüglichen Kunstgenuß. Wie später eingegangene Briefe bezeugen, wurden diese musikalischen Kostbarkeiten gerade für viele ausländische Teilnehmer zum Parameter Münchner Kunstlebens und bleibende Erinnerung an schöne Environcen eines der Wissenschaft gewidmeten Kongresses. Unter der Leitung von RAINER KOCH, Essen, gelangten folgende Werke zur Aufführung:

Johann Sebastian Bach:
    Suite Nr. 3, D-Dur
Wolfgang Amadeus Mozart:
    Konzert für Flöte und Orchester, D-Dur, KV 314
Georg Friedrich Händel:
    Wassermusik, 1. und 2. Suite — und
Johann Sebastian Bach:
    Brandenburgisches Konzert Nr. 2, F-Dur für Trompete, Flöte, Oboe, Violine und Orchester.

Besonders der Flötist Aurèle Nicotel begeisterte die Zuhörer und riß sie zu anhaltenden Ovationen hin. Aber auch die anderen Solisten, genannt sei noch Adolf Scherbaum, der seine Bach-Trompete virtuos beherrschte, trugen zu dem Gelingen dieser Veranstaltung in hohem Maße bei.

Am Dienstagabend (1. August 1967) folgte eine kunsthistorische Führung durch die bedeutendsten Münchener Kirchen mit eingeschaltetem, kürzerem Orgelkonzert. Die Teilnehmer trafen sich am Hauptportal des spätgotischen Liebfrauendomes, der, 1468 bis 1488 erbaut, noch immer ein Wahrzeichen Münchens darstellt: Die 99 m hohen Doppeltürme grüßen den Besucher der Isarmetropole schon von weitem. Der mächtige dreischiffige Ziegelbau, unweit vom zentral gelegenen Marienplatz, wird vielen Kongressisten mit seinem imponierenden Steildach bei Lektüre dieser Zeilen noch gut vor Augen stehen. Betreut von den sportlich-schick gekleideten Hostessen, Dolmetschern und kunsthistorisch geschulten Führern,

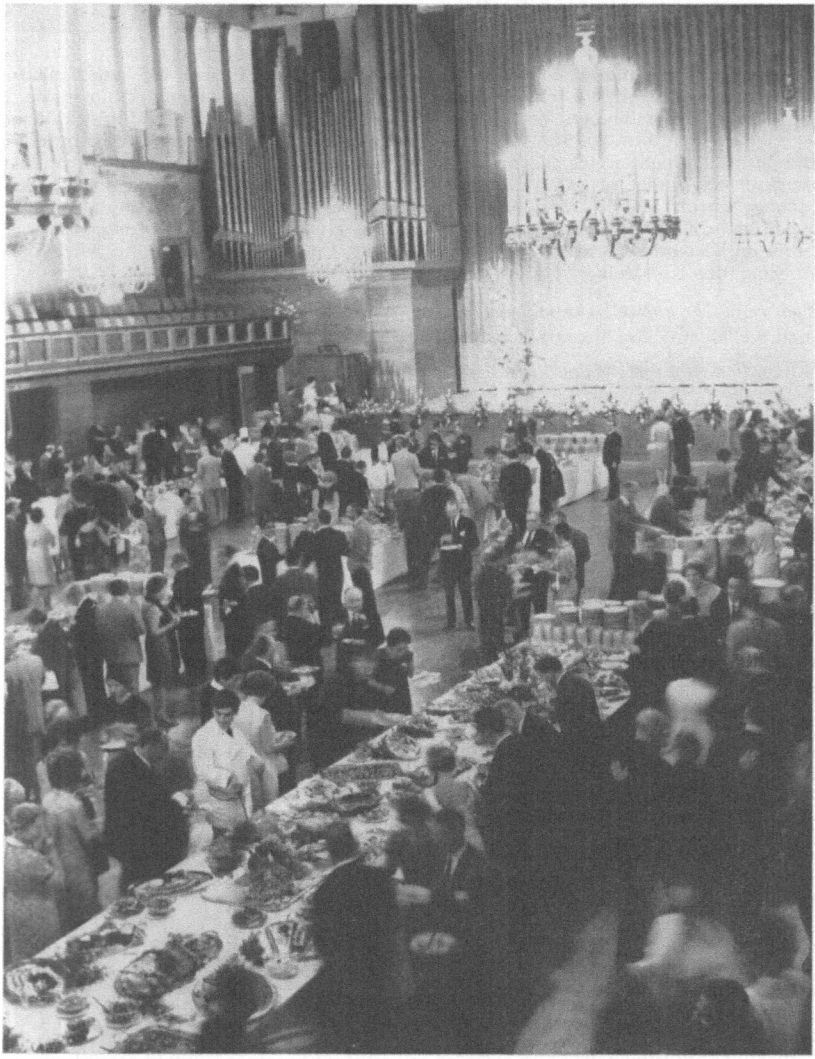

Party for 3,000 persons   Buffet pour 3000 personnes

wurden neben dem Dom die Theatinerkirche, ein stattlicher Barockbau mit wunderschöner, grün-patinierter Kuppel, die Michaeliskirche, die Asamkirche (St. Johann Nepomuk), im Stil des Rokoko erbaut und mit malerischem Portal versehen — sowie die Peterskirche, die im Volksmund „Alter Peter" genannt wird, besichtigt. Für diese Veranstaltung gilt auch an dieser Stelle unser Dank nochmals Herrn Prof. WISMEYER, Herrn Dr. FELLERER, Herrn Domkapitular BAUER und den betreffenden Pfarrämtern.

Am gleichen Abend fand auf Einladung des bayerischen Ministerpräsidenten Dr. h.c. ALFONS GOPPEL im Antiquarium der Münchner Residenz ein Empfang für 400 geladene Gäste statt, in erster Linie für die Mitglieder des Internationalen und des Exekutivkomitees mit ihren Damen sowie für die nationalen Delegierten und die offiziellen Vertreter des Kultusministeriums, der Ludwig-Maximilians-Universität und der Münchner Medizinischen Fakultät. Das Antiquarium, Prunksaal im früheren Sitz des bayerischen Herrscherhauses der Wittelsbacher, gab dieser generösen Rezeption einen würdigen, festlichen Rahmen. Der bayerische Innenminister HECK begrüßte die Gäste im Namen des verhinderten Ministerpräsidenten mit großer Herzlichkeit und Worten, die erkennen ließen, daß auch die Vertreter der Regierung den Anliegen unseres Faches aufgeschlossen gegenüberstehen. Der Präsident, Prof. JADASSOHN, antwortete in seiner stets persönlich gehaltenen und das Wesen treffenden Weise:

„Sehr verehrter Herr Minister,

Wir danken Ihnen sehr für Ihre Einladung. Ich könnte mir vorstellen, daß Sie sich heute abend sagen werden: Ich bin froh, daß ich die Dermatologen hinter mir habe. Vielleicht denken Sie jetzt, da steht der arme Kongreßpräsident und muß eine Dankrede halten. Ich muß Ihnen sagen, daß Sie, falls Sie „armer Kongreßpräsident" gedacht haben, sich geirrt haben. Ich danke gerne für etwas, über das ich mich gefreut habe; und über Ihre Einladung, Herr Minister, haben wir uns alle gefreut, und ich danke Ihnen sehr herzlich im Namen aller Ihrer Gäste. Es war für uns eine große Freude, und wenn Sie es wünschen, kommen wir alle morgen wieder."

Anschließend wurden bayerische „Schmankerl", Sandwichs und allerlei Leckerbissen gereicht, Wein und andere „stärkende" oder erfrischende Getränke ausgeschenkt. Wieder entstand eine fröhliche, aufgeschlossene Atmosphäre. Was erhofft wurde, trat ein: Man traf sich zwanglos zu freundschaftlichen Plaudereien, verabredete Begegnungen für später und diskutierte über gemeinsame Interessen. Abgeschlossen wurde dieser wirklich gelungene Empfang von einer Führung durch die Schatzkammer der Residenz, die durch „hohe Architektur ihres Gehaltes würdig ist", wie NORBERT LIEB es ausdrückte.

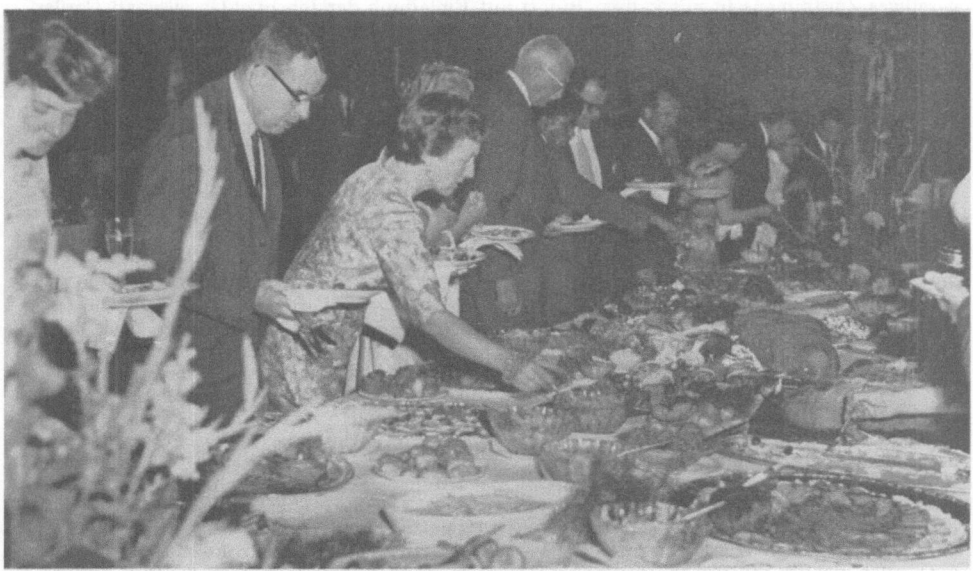

Refectorio para 3.000 comensales   Buffet für 3000 Personen

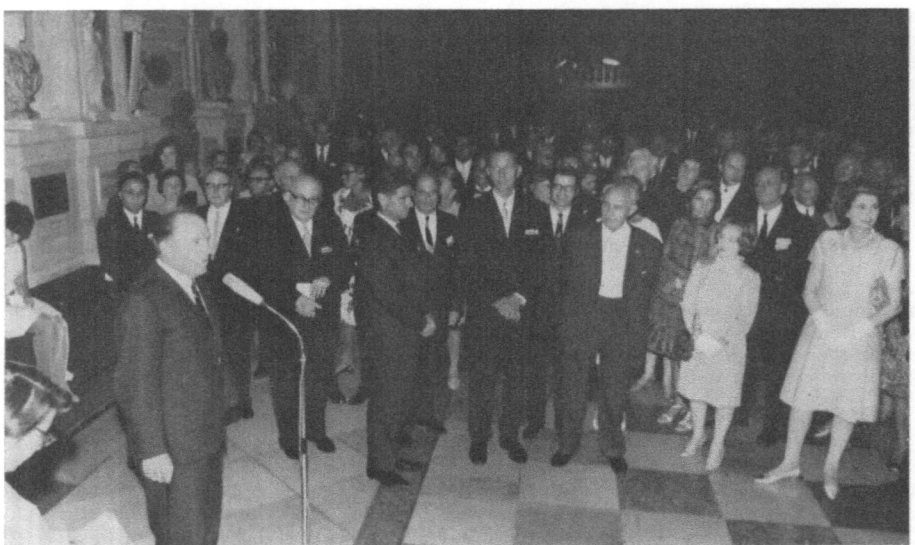

Reception in the Antiquarium by the government of the State of Bavaria. At the microphone, Minister HECK

Réception dans l'Antiquarium par le gouvernement de l'Etat de Bavière. Au microphone, M. le Ministre HECK

Recepción ofrecida por el Gobierno regional de Baviera en el Antiquarium. El Ministro Señor HECK ante el micrófono

Empfang im Antiquarium durch die Bayerische Staatsregierung. Am Mikrophon Minister HECK

Ebenfalls am Abend dieses Tages fand für einen kleineren Kreis der Kongreßteilnehmer ein geselliges Zusammensein mit kaltem Büfett auf Einladung der Ichthyol-Gesellschaft Cordes, Hermanni und Co. im Münchner Künstlerhaus statt. Auch diese Veranstaltung, die sich lang in die warme Sommernacht erstreckte, verlief sehr glücklich. So mancher wird sich gern der angeregten Gespräche unter nächtlichem Himmel auf den oberen Balkonen und Terrassen dieses traditionsreichen Hauses erinnern.

Am Nachmittag und Abend des Dienstages hatten außerdem die bayerischen Kollegen des Verbandes der niedergelassenen Dermatologen Deutschlands mit Unterstützung der „Rhein-Pharma Heidelberg" gleichfalls niedergelassene Praktiker des Auslandes zu einem Treffen eingeladen, das im Restaurant Seehaus am Kleinhesseloher See des Englischen Gartens stattfand. Beabsichtigt war ein Gedankenaustausch über die Probleme des in freier Praxis tätigen Hautfacharztes. Viele persönliche Begegnungen kamen zustande, auch standespolitische Fragen wurden erörtert — und das Temperamente steuerte eine angenehme Bewirtung.

Am Mittwoch, dem 2. August 1967, versprach das Programm zwei besonders schöne Veranstaltungen. Die eine Hälfte der Teilnehmer besuchte eine Festvorstellung des Münchner Nationaltheaters im Rahmen der Opernfestspiele, die andere ein Kammerkonzert im Schloß Herrenchiemsee. Die zweite Gruppe, etwas mehr als 700 Personen, traf sich zur Abfahrt um 14.00 Uhr auf dem Königsplatz. Mit einer langen Autobuskolonne ging es hinaus nach Prien an den Chiemsee. Nach einer Kaffeepause wurde in Schiffen zur Herreninsel übergesetzt, die wahrhaftig ein Paradies genannt werden darf. Im Schloß Herrenchiemsee, dessen schönste Räume herrlich im Lichterglanz zahlloser Kerzen erstrahlten und deren Besichtigung äußerst eindrucksvoll war, fand im großen, prunkvollen Spiegelsaal ein Konzert statt, das den Höhepunkt dieses Ausflugs bildete. Ein Quartett aus Mitgliedern des Mozarteum-Orchesters Salzburg spielte erst das F-Dur Streichquartett von Haydn (Op. 3/5: Serenadenquartett) und dann „Die kleine Nachtmusik" in G-Dur von Mozart (KV 525). Im Schloßhotel wurde anschließend zu Abend gegessen. Hierfür mußten viele Chiemsee-Renken ihr Leben lassen, sie mundeten aber auch denen, die diesen Fisch erstmals aßen, ganz ausgezeichnet. Mit Schiff und Bus ging es dann zurück nach München, „der Stadt des Lebens", wie Hebbel sie nannte. Dem

Chronisten wurde berichtet, daß einige Kongressisten von dieser Fahrt so angeregt zurückkehrten, daß Nachsitzungen in Schwabinger Künstlerlokalen sich wie von selbst ergaben —
etwa im Sinne Goethes, der sagte:

> *Gäste einer solchen Stadt „wandern und weben zwischen ewigen Melodien, der Geist kann nicht*
> *sinken, die Tätigkeit nicht einschlafen, und die Bürger, am gemeinsten Tage, fühlen sich in*
> *einem ideellen Zustand."*

Die andere Gruppe (mehr als 1000 Personen) erlebte im Nationaltheater am Max-Josefs-
Platz die glanzvolle Festaufführung des „Rosenkavaliers" von Richard Strauß. Die 1911 in
Dresden uraufgeführte Oper ist fast schon ein integraler Bestandteil des Münchner Musiklebens geworden, und so war es ein sehnlicher Wunsch ALFRED MARCHIONINIS, der Melodien
von Strauß besonders liebte, gerade diese „Komödie für Musik in drei Aufzügen" auf „seinem
Kongreß" gespielt zu hören. Seine Schüler, die hierum wußten, gedachten an diesem Abend des
Mannes, dem die Erfüllung nicht nur dieses Wunsches versagt blieb.

Am nächsten Tag (3. August 1967) fanden abends zwischen 20.00 und 22.00 Uhr Führungen
durch die bedeutendsten Münchner Museen statt. In vier Partien geteilt, sahen die Kongressisten
Sammlungen des Deutschen Museums, der Alten und Neuen Pinakothek, der neuen Staatsgalerie im Haus der Kunst und der Schatzkammer in der Residenz.

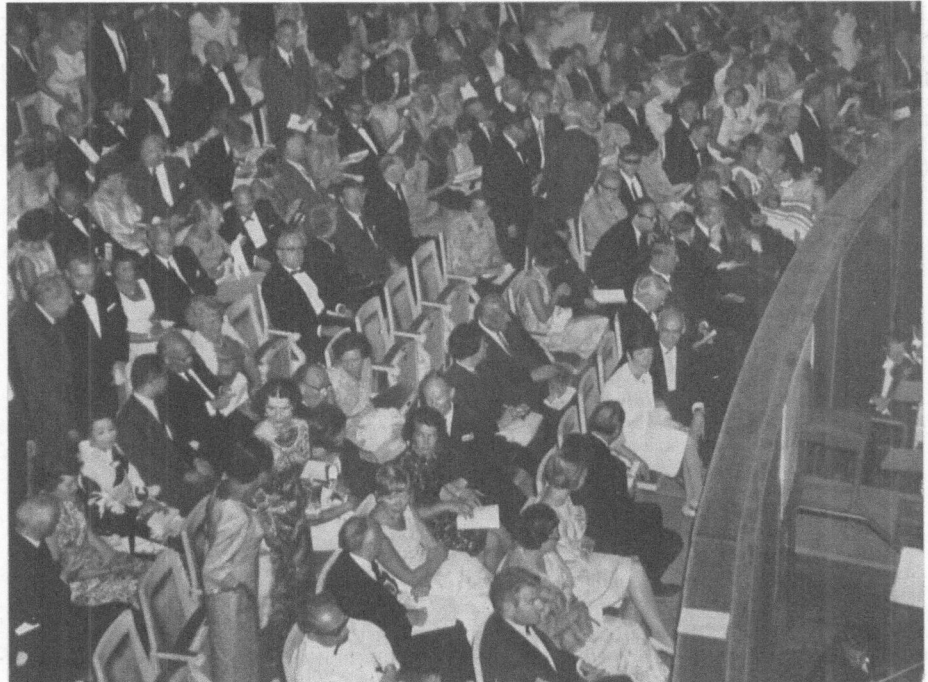

At the gala Opera performance

Au gala de l'Opéra Bavarois

Sesión de gala en el Teatro de la Opera de Baviera

Bei der Festaufführung in der Bayerischen Staatsoper

Ebenfalls am Abend des Donnerstags luden das Präsidium des Kongresses und die Farben-
fabriken Bayer, Leverkusen, etwa 400 Gäste zu einem Empfang in das Kellerrestaurant des
Nationaltheaters ein. Herr Direktor MEYER-UHL sprach sehr herzlich gehaltene Worte der
Begrüßung, auf die der Präsident in launiger Weise wie folgt antwortete:

*„Als die Genfer-Ärztegesellschaft einmal von der Firma Sandoz zum Essen eingeladen war,
hat sich der Präsident versehentlich bei der Firma Hoffmann-La-Roche bedankt. Er hatte
einen außerordentlichen Heiterkeitserfolg. Ich verzichte auf einen solchen Erfolg und danke
der Firma, die unseren Dank verdient, der Firma Bayer, auf das herzlichste. Ich verspreche,
daß ich, obwohl ich die Tablettensucht bekämpfe, gelegentlich eine Aspirin-Tablette nehmen
werde. Sie haben uns, Herr MEYER-UHL, durch die Firma Bayer zu dem heutigen Fest
verholfen. So haben wir nun beides gehabt, einen Münchner Bierabend und ein Fest in diesem
wundervollen Rahmen von Gold und Marmor. Nach Prof. SCHIRREN stammt der Marmor
nicht aus den Bayerischen Alpen. Sie haben mir, Herr MEYER-UHL, bei der Ankunft in
München ein Buch geschenkt, für das ich Ihnen sehr herzlich danke. Darf ich einen Satz
aus dem Buch zitieren: „München, ein liederliches, sittenloses Nest, voll Fanatismus, Grob-
heit, Kellertreiben, voll Heiligenbilder, Knödel, Radiweiber." Der Satz ist von Gottfried Keller.
Ich habe zwar keinerlei Erfahrung mit Radiweibern und Knödel. Ich möchte aber folgendes
feststellen: Die Münchener, die Bayern und die Leute von Bayer sind liebenswürdig, hilfs-
bereit, sympathisch und außerordentlich angenehm. Es lebe München, es lebe Bayern, es
lebe Bayer."*

Auch dieser Gesellschaftsabend mit seiner generösen Bewirtung und einer Auswahl herr-
licher Weine trug sehr zur „physiologisch wirklich notwendigen, komplementären Ergänzung"
des wissenschaftlichen Programms bei, um diese Worte von H. W. SPIER zu zitieren.

Am Freitag, dem 4. August, schloß das Gesellschaftsprogramm mit einem „Bayerischen
Abend" in den Räumen der Mathäser Bierstadt. Spätestens dort werden die Kongressisten
München und die Bayern in ihre Herzen geschlossen haben. Die Stimmung in beiden Fest-
sälen, die wunderschön geschmückt waren — (hierfür gilt auch an dieser Stelle nochmals unser
aller Dank Herrn MINARIK) — erkletterte kaum glaubliche Höhen. An den zahlreichen,
liebevoll gedeckten Tischen saßen mehr als 3000 Gäste, tranken das „süffige" bayrische Bier
aus blumenverzierten Steinkrügen, die zur Erinnerung mitgenommen werden durften. Brat-
hähnchen, würziger Käse, Salat, Rettich und Salzgebäck sorgten für leibliches Wohlbefinden.
Man wurde erinnert an das Gedicht Paul Heyses, der 1910 den Nobelpreis für Literatur
(aber wohl nicht in Ansehung dieser Verse) erhielt:

*„Sei mir gegrüßt, du Held im Schaumgelock,
streitbarer Männer Sieger, edler Bock*!
Nicht graues Zwielicht dampfdurchwölkter Schenken,
den Mittag liebst du und der Gärten Frische.
Hier finden sich auf brüderlichen Bänken
hoch und gering in treulichem Gemische:
Den Knechten nah, die seine Pferde lenken,
der Staatenlenker vom Ministertische,
Pedell, Professor, Famulus, Student —
Du stülpst hinweg die Schranke, die sie trennt.
Es wird von jenem Treviquell berichtet,
daraus man ew'ges Heimweh trinkt nach Rom,
Sehnsucht, die unermüdlich denkt und dichtet,
nur einmal noch zu schauen Sankt Peters Dom.
So hat auf München nie ein Herz verzichtet,
das je hinabgetaucht in deinen Strom.
So rasche Wurzeln hier geschlagen hätt' ich
nie ohne dich und deinen Freund, den Rettich!"*

Für ein musikalisches und folkloristisches Non-stop-Programm sorgte TH. NASEMANN,
dem jetzt in der Rolle des Chronisten erst ganz die Angst um das Gelingen dieses Abends genommen ward. Im bunten Reigen sorgten für die Unterhaltung der Gäste das kleine Berg-
wachtorchester unter Leitung von KARL FODERMAIR, die Turmbläser vom „Alten Peter",
unter Leitung des Kammervirtuosen F. SERTL, die Jodlerin BETTI HORAČEK, das Isar-Trio, die
Bayernlandschrammeln, der Münchner Mandolinenzirkel, die beiden Amateur-Tenore L. HEIGL
(Photograph der Münchner Univ.-Hautklinik) und Herr WERNER (Loewens Pharma) sowie die
Holledauer „Dell'nhauser Musikanten". Der Höhepunkt des Festes wurde zweifellos erreicht,
als Prof. SULZBERGER in Maestro-Manier — hiermit einem Wunsche ALFRED MARCHIONINIS
nachkommend — den bayerischen Defiliermarsch dirigierte, belohnt durch einen Rosenstrauß

---

* Bock, ein besonderes Starkbier.

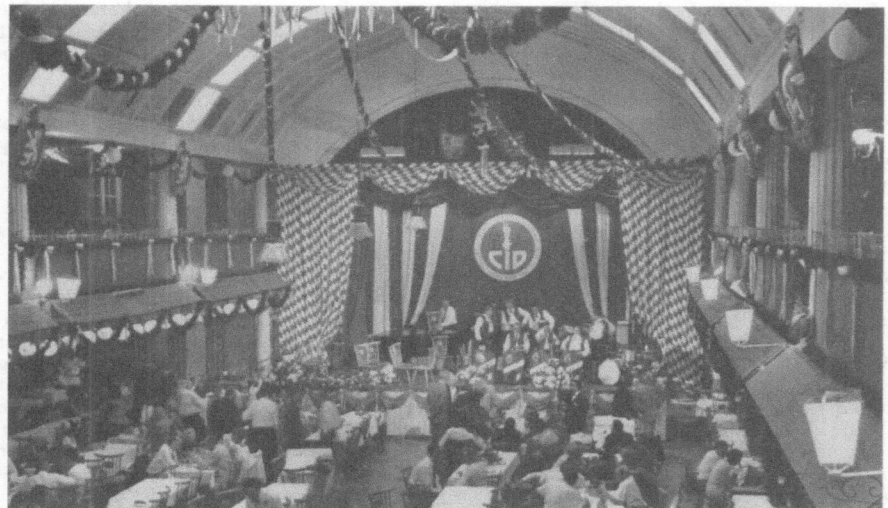

Bavarian folkloric evening   Velada típica bávara
Soirée de folklore Bavarois   Bayerischer Bierabend

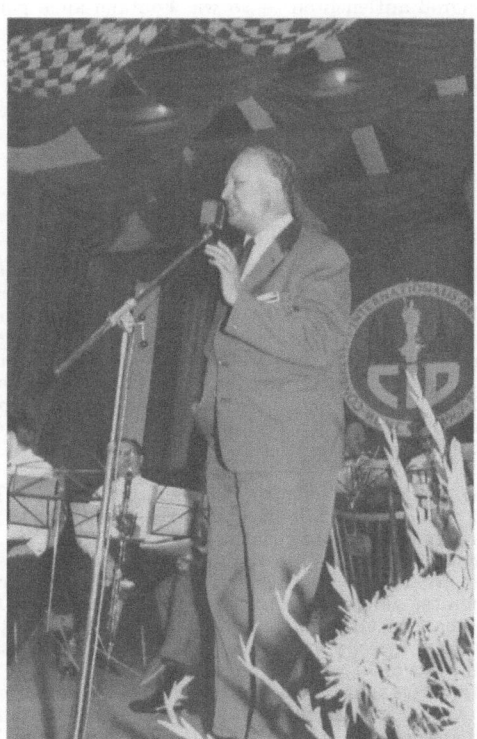

At the microphone Prof. NASEMANN   El Prof. NASEMANN ante el micrófono
Au micro Prof. NASEMANN   Am Mikrophon Prof. NASEMANN

und Kuß einer jungen Verehrerin. Es herrschte froheste Laune, man sang mit, scherzte, lachte und war so recht eine große internationale Dermatologenfamilie. Man kam sich näher — nicht nur beim Tanz zwischen Tischen und Stühlen — sondern im höheren Sinne einer gemeinsamen Zielen zustrebenden Gesellschaft.

Dieses Hauptprogramm wurde umrahmt von vielen weiteren Veranstaltungen des Damen-programms. Stadtrundfahrten am Montag und Dienstag (fast 700 Personen) mit Spaziergang im Englischen Garten und Kaffeepause, Besichtigung von Park und Schloß Nymphenburg (425 Teilnehmerinnen), eine gut besuchte Modenschau mit dem Thema „München macht Mode" im Hotel Bayerischer Hof, dirigiert von der Modezeitschrift „Madame", ein Besuch des Tierparks Hellabrunn, eine Führung durch das Bayerische Nationalmuseum (am Mittwoch, fast 250 Personen) und am Donnerstag Besichtigungen der Alten Pinakothek und des „Hauses der Kunst" waren Stationen dieses Teils der geselligen Veranstaltungen. Am Freitag folgte vor-mittags ein Ausflug der Damen nach dem Kloster Andechs mit Besichtigung der wunder-schönen Barockkirche neben dem Klosterbau, von deren Turm aus man weit über den Ammer-see und das bayerische Voralpenland hinaussehen kann. Hier bot sich anschließend Gelegen-heit zu einem deftigen „ländlichen Frühstück" (in Bayern „Brotzeit" genannt) und einer Probe des köstlichen, von den Mönchen gebrauten Andechser Bieres. Am Freitag-Nachmittag beschloß eine Rundfahrt um den Starnberger See mit Kaffeepause im Undosa-Restaurant Starnbergs das abwechslungsreiche Damenprogramm. Erwähnt sei noch, daß die Firma A. Wolff, Bielefeld, für insgesamt 200 an Fragen der Kosmetik interessierte Teilnehmerinnen (vor allem in der Praxis ihrer Männer mithelfende Ehefrauen) in ihrer in Buch am Ammersee schön gelegenen Kosmetikschule an drei Nachmittagen Kosmetikdemonstrationen mit ge-meinsamer Kaffeetafel und anschließenden regen Diskussionen durchführte. So war das Panorama der neben dem wissenschaftlichen Programm auf gesellschaftlicher Ebene ablau-fenden Folge gegenseitiger Begegnungen und Kontakte in der Tat vielgestaltig und bunt-schillernd wie das Münchner Leben selbst. Als sich am Samstag, dem 5. August 1967, nach beendetem Kongreß das Exekutivkomitee zu einem Abschiedsessen im Restaurant Walterspiel des Hotels „Vier Jahreszeiten" traf, sah man in zwar müden Gesichtern doch Zufriedenheit über den gelungenen Kongreß aufleuchten — so wie Fontane auch gefühlt haben muß, als er schrieb:

„Nur in der Arbeit wohnt der Frieden,
Und in der Mühe wohnt die Ruh!"

Social Program and Ladies' Program

Summary of the Report given by Prof. THEODOR NASEMANN

The increasing of international congresses, the abundance of conferences and the increasing importance of scientific and technical exhibitions, have necessitated personal, friendly and lasting relations among the participants. With this purpose in mind we established a social program as well as a special program for ladies. The congressists, coming from all parts of the world, could choose their pleasure, according to their taste and preference.

At the reception on Sunday evening, July 30th, in the congress hall of the „Deutsches Museum", more than 2000 congressists and their wives were present responding to the cordial invitation offered by the responsibles of the Congress. The hall, generously decorated with flowers, lively conversations, appetizing food and champagne, created a joyful atmosphere during three hours.

On Monday, July 31st, the concert given by the "Bachorchester" of Frankfurt took place. The hall like the previous evening, superbly decorated with flowers, and the exquisite musical interpretation, created an atmosphere of warmth.

Tuesday evening, August 1st, was consecrated to the visit to the most famous and artistic churches followed by brief organ concert. The participants met at the front gate of the "Lieb-frauen" with its Gothic domes, which was built between 1468 and 1488. Being one of the most beautiful religious monuments of Munich, its two 99 m high towers attract the visitor's eye from far distance. Hostesses, interpreters and guides showed the visitors the treasures of the various churches of the town.

The same evening. Mr. A. GOPPEL, President of the State of Bavaria, invited 400 persons to an official reception. Among the assistance the presence of the official delegates of the Ministry of Education, the University and the Faculty of Medicine of Munich, was noticed. The "Antiquarium", anciently parade hall of the Bavarian kings, gave the reception an atmosphere of royal festivity. The Home Secretary, Mr. HECK, greeted the guests in the name of the President of Bavaria, prevented from assisting the reception. He informed us, with

great kindness, of the government's interest in the work of our speciality. The President of the Congress, Prof. W. JADASSOHN, replied in the following very appreciated words:
Mr. Home Secretary.

We thank you for your hospitality. Tonight I could imagine you thinking "I am glad to get rid of the dermatologists" and that even, at present, you say to yourself "Here is this "poor" President of the Congress, supposed to deliver a speech of circumstances". I must bring to your attention that if you thought "poor" President of the Congress, you are mistaken. I thank willingly everything which pleases me. Mr. HOME Secretary, we accepted your invitation with joy, and I express you my gratitude in the name of your guests. Your invitation pleased us very much and we all shall come back tomorrow if you desire.

Then refreshments were offered to the guests who now could continue their friendly conversations and in a cordial atmosphere, establish new relations and engage in long and lively discussions. The reception ended with a visit accros the "Schatzkammer" of the "Residenz".

On Wednesday, August 2nd, two particularly attractive manifestations were on the program. An excursion to "Prien" on "Chiemsee"; where 700 participants were driven by a long column of busses. They crossed the lake on boat to arrive on the "Herreninsel". The castle, illuminated by thousands of candles, enchanted the visitors. The culminating point was, undoubtedly, the concert given in the castle's Hall of Mirrors. A chosen quartett of Salzburg's "Mozart-Orchester" played one of Haydn's masterpieces and Mozart's "Kleine Nachtmusik".

The other great manifestation of the day where more than 1000 persons assisted, was the unforgetable performance of Richard Strauss' "Rosenkavalier" in the grandiose outline of the National Theater of Munich. The much regretted ALFRED MARCHIONINI who was fond of the works of Richard Strauss, would not have missed this musical comedy at the time of "his Congress". That evening, his affected students, thought of the man one of whose wishes had been granted.

The next evening, August 3rd, between 8 and 10 p.m. a visit of the most notable museums of Munich took place. Seperated in four groups, the participants were able to admire the rich collections of "Deutsches Museum", the ancient and new Picture-gallery, the "Staatsgalerie" and the "Schatzkammer" of the "Residenz".

On Thursday evening, upon the joint invitation of the Presidence of the Congress and the Firm Bayer, took place a reception in the National Theatre, where 400 persons participated. Dr. MEYER-UHL greeted the guests cordially. The President of the Congress replied.

On Friday, August 4th, the social program reached its term with an unforgetable bavarian evening in the halls of the "Mathäser Bierstadt". In two well decorated halls, the atmosphere was joyful. 3000 persons were seated around tables decorated with much taste and savoured

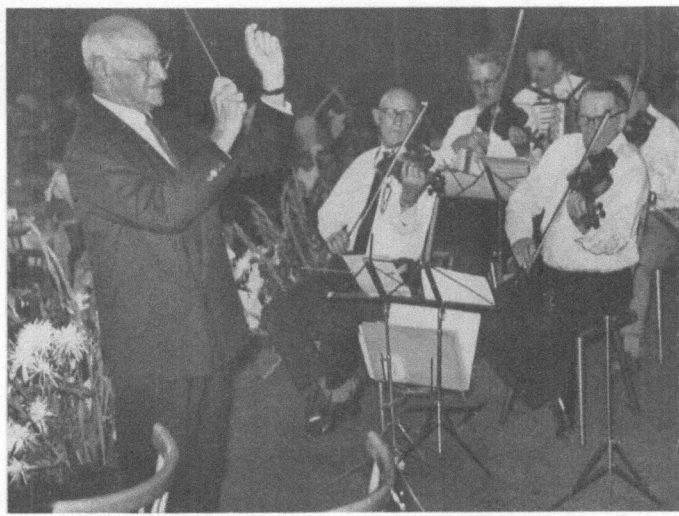

Bavarian Folkloric Evening,
conductor Prof. SULZBERGER

Soirée de folklore Bavarois,
chef d'orchestre Prof. SULZBERGER

Velada típica: el Prof. SULZBERGER,
director de la orquesta

Bayerischer Bierabend: Es dirigiert
Prof. SULZBERGER

the famous bavarian beer, served in special pots, willfully ribboned with flowers, which the participants could take as souvenir. In addition the congressists tasted equisite bavarian specialities. Prof. NASEMANN had organized a session of non-stop folke-lore music. Prof. SULZBERGER distinguished himself as "maestro" directing the bavarian parade march. The joyful atmosphere, the songs, the laughs, the amusements, designed in the best way possible the outline of a bit international family of dermatologists.

To the principal program described above, the various manifestations designed for the ladies must be added. Town visits (approx. 700 persons), excursion to the Park and Castle of Nymphenburg (425 participants), fashion show with the theme "Munich creates fashion", visit of the zoo "Hellabrunn", visit to the Bavarian National Museum (approx. 250 persons) and the "Haus der Kunst" figured among others.

On Friday morning, excursion to the Castle of Andechs and visit to the very beautiful baroque church and its famous cloister. From the top of the towers a magnificent view of the "Ammersee" and the Bavarian prealps is offered to the eye of the visitor. The last event of the ladies' program took place Friday afternoon: excursion around the "Starnberger See". Let us add the demonstration offered by the cosmetic school of the firm A. Wolff Bielefeld in "Buch Ammersee" where 200 ladies participated.

In this manner, at the same time as the Congress and its scientific program, the social program took place showing the treasures and the level of artistic life in Munich.

At the time of the farewell dinner, Saturday, August 5th, the faces of the members of the Organization Committee, even though pale and fatigued, visibly reflected the proudness and joy of a successful Congress.

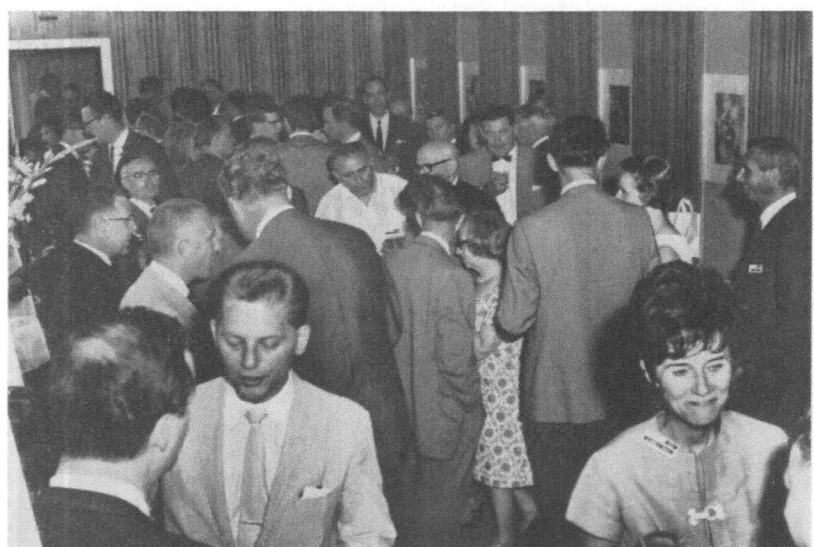

Reception by the Duhring Society   La Sociedad Duhring acoge a los congresistas
Réception offerte par la Société Duhring   Cocktail-Empfang der Duhring Gesellschaft

Programme social et programme des dames

Résumé du rapport du Prof. THEODOR NASEMANN

Le nombre croissant de congrès internationaux, l'ampleur accrue des conférences et l'importance grandissante des expositions scientifiques et techniques s'y rapportant, sont à l'origine, pour les participants, d'un besoin réel de contacts personnels, amicaux et durables. Afin de parvenir à ce but, nous avons établi un programme social et un programme des dames. Nos visiteurs, provenant de tous les coins du monde, purent choisir à leur gré, selon leurs goûts et leurs préférences.

Lors de la soirée d'accueil du dimanche 30 juillet, dans la salle des congrès du «Deutsches Museum», plus de 2000 congressistes et leurs épouses étaient présents, répondant à la cordiale invitation des dirigeants du Congrès. La salle, généreusement décorée de fleurs, des conversations animées, forgèrent une joyeuse ambiance favorisée par des dégustations culinaires sablées au champagne. Et cela trois heures durant.

Le lundi 31 juillet, eut lieu le concert donné par le «Bachorchester» de Francfort. La salle, comme la veille, toujours superbement décorée de fleurs, et l'exquise interprétation musicale, créèrent parmi les auditeurs une chaude ambiance.

Le mardi soir, 1er août, il y eut une visite commentée des églises, les plus fameuses et artistiques, agrémenté d'un bref concert d'orgue. On se donna rendez-vous sous le portail principal aux dômes gothiques de la «Liebfrauen» qui fut érigée entre 1468 et 1488. Toujours un des plus beaux monuments religieux de Munich, elle attire de loin les visiteurs de la hauteur des deux tours de 99 m. Des hôtesses, des interprètes et des guides se succédant, montrèrent aux visiteurs les richesses des diverses églises de la ville.

Le même soir, M. A. GOPPEL, Ministre-Président de l'Etat de Bavière, invita 400 personnes à une réception officielle. Parmi les assistants, on remarqua la présence des délégués officiels du Ministère de l'Education, de l'Université et de la Faculté de Médecine de Munich. L'Antiquarium, anciennement salle de parade des souverains bavarois, donna à cette réception une ambiance de fête royale. Le Ministre de l'Intérieur, M. HECK, salua les invités au nom du Président de la Bavière, empêché d'assister à la réception. Il nous informa, avec beaucoup de gentillesse, de l'intérêt que le gouvernement porte aux travaux de notre spécialité. Le Président du Congrès, le Prof. W. JADASSOHN, lui donna la réplique dans ces termes, qui furent très applaudis:

Monsieur le Ministre,

Nous vous remercions de votre hospitalité. Ce soir, je pourrais m'imaginer que vous pensez «je me réjouis d'être débarrassé des dermatologues» et même, qu'à présent, vous vous dites «voici ce «pauvre» président du Congrès, censé prononcer un discours de circonstances». Je dois vous signaler, que si vous avez pensé «pauvre» Président du Congrès, vous avez fait erreur. Je remercie volontiers pour ce qui me fait plaisir. Monsieur le Ministre-Président, nous avons accepté avec joie votre invitation, et je vous témoigne chaleureusement ma reconnaissance au nom de tous vos hôtes. Votre invitation nous a beaucoup plu et nous reviendrions tous demain si vous le désiriez.

Puis des rafraîchissements furent distribués aux invités; leurs conversations amicales reprirent et dans une ambiance cordiale, les uns établirent de nouvelles relations, tandis que d'autres discutaient longuement. La réception se termina par une visite à travers la «Schatzkammer» de la «Residenz».

Le mercredi 2 août, deux manifestations, particulièrement attrayantes figuraient au programme. Excursion à «Prien au Chiemsee», où une longue colonne d'autocars conduisit les quelques 700 voyageurs. On traversa le lac en bateau pour accoster sur le «Herreninsel». Les salles du château, scintillantes de la lumière de milliers de chandelles, ensorcelèrent les visiteurs. Le point culminant fut, sans doute, le concert donné dans la salle des glaces du château. Un quartett choisi du «Mozarteum-Orchester» de Salzbourg, joua une œuvre de Haydn et la «Kleine Nachtmusik» de Mozart.

L'autre grande manifestation de la journée à laquelle assistaient plus de 1000 personnes, fut l'inoubliable représentation du «Chevalier de la Rose» de Richard Strauß, dans le cadre grandiose du Théâtre National de Munich. Le regretté ALFRED MARCHIONINI qui raffolait des œuvres de Richard Strauß, n'aurait pas manqué cette opéra lors de «son Congrès». Ce soir-là, ses élèves émus, pensèrent à l'homme dont l'un des vœux venait de s'exaucer.

Au lendemain soir, 3 août, entre 20.00 et 22.00 heures eut lieu le parcours des plus notables musées munichois. Divisés en quatre groupes, les participants purent admirer les riches collections du «Deutsches Museum», de l'Ancienne et de la Nouvelle Pinacothèque, la «Staatsgalerie» et la «Schatzkammer» de la «Residenz».

Le jeudi soir, sur l'invitation conjointe de la Présidence du Congrès et de la Maison Bayer, eut lieu une réception au Théâtre National à laquelle participèrent 400 personnes. Le Dr. MEYER-UHL salua cordialement les invités. Le Président du Congrès lui donna la réplique.

Le vendredi 4 août, le programme social arriva à son terme: une inoubliable soirée bavaroise dans les salles de la «Mathäser Bierstadt». Dans deux salles, bien décorées, l'ambiance était joyeuse. 3000 personnes prirent place autour des tables décorées avec beaucoup de goût, dégustèrent la renommée bière bavaroise servie dans de typiques pots de grès enrubannés de fleurs, que l'on emporta en souvenir. Les congressistes se régalèrent, en plus, d'exquises spécialités bavaroises. Le Prof. NASEMANN avait organisé une séance ininterrompue de musique folklorique. Le Prof. SULZBERGER se distingua en «maestro», dirigeant la marche bavaroise de défilé. L'ambiance si joyeuse, les chansons, les rires, les amusements, formèrent le cadre d'une grande famille internationale de dermatologistes.

Au programme principal décrit plus haut, il faut ajouter les diverses manifestations destinées aux dames. Des tours de ville, excursion au Parc et Château de Nymphenbourg, défilé de mode ayant pour thème «Munich crée la mode», visite au Zoo «Hellabrunn», visite au musée National Bavarois et la «Haus der Kunst» figuraient parmi d'autres.

Le vendredi matin, excursion au cloître d'Andechs et visite de la très belle église baroque. Du sommet des tours une vue imprenable de l'«Ammersee» et des préalpes bavaroises s'offre aux yeux des visiteurs. Le dernier acte du programme des dames se déroula dans l'après-midi du vendredi: l'excursion autour du «Starnberger See». Ajoutons la démonstration que l'école de cosmétiques de la firme A. Wolff Bielefeld à «Buch-Ammersee» offrit à quelques 200 dames.

C'est ainsi que, parallèlement au Congrès et à son programme scientifique, se déroula le programme social, ce dernier mettant en relief les richesses et le niveau de la vie artistique munichoise. Lors du déjeuner de clôture du Congrès, le samedi 5 août, les visages des membres du Comité d'Organisation, bien que pâles de fatigue, reflétaient visiblement, la fierté et la joie de la réussite du Congrès.

Programa social y programa destinado a las Señoras

Resúmen del informe del Prof. THEODOR NASEMANN

El creciente número de Congresos Internacionales, la mayor amplitud de las conferencias, la mucha importancia de las exposiciones científicas y técnicas, originan en sus participantes, la necesidad de establecer contactos personales y de anudar amistades duraderas. Este es el fin que nosotros nos propusimos alcanzar estableciendo un programa social y un programa destinado a las Señoras. Ambos programas fueron establecidos teniendo en cuenta las particulares preferencias de nuestros visitantes a los que ofrecimos un sinfín de excursiones, diversiones y gran diversidad de lugares interesantes a visitar.

Los dirigentes del Congreso invitaron a los participantes y a sus esposas a una velada de recepción en la sala de congresos del Deutsches Museum, el día 30 de Julio. Acudieron a este acto más de 2000 personas. La sala estuvo magníficamente adornada con flores. Durante más de tres horas, este bello local fué lugar no solo de degustaciones culinarias sino que también el seno de animadas conversaciones generosamente rociadas de champán.

El lunes, 31 de Julio, tuvo lugar un concierto ejecutado por la "Bachorchester" de Frankfort cuyas interpretaciones entusiasmaron a los asistentes. La sala, siempre soberbiamente adornada de flores, contribuyó al cálido ambiente de esta velada.

En el crepúsculo del martes, 1° de Agosto, tuvo lugar la visita de varias notables iglesias, durante la cual tuvimos la ocasión de escuchar un breve concierto de órgano. El lugar de cita fué el portal principal de la iglesia "Liebfrauen", erigida entre 1468 y 1488 cuyos cimborrios góticos son admirables. Sigue siendo esta iglesia uno de los monumentos mas bellos de Munich. Sus dos torres, de 99 metros de altura, dan de lejos, la bienvenida a los visitantes de la metrópoli del Isar. Intérpretes, guías y simpáticas señoritas acompañaron a los participantes en su recorrido por las diversas iglesias.

El mismo día, el Presidente del Gobierno de Baviera, Sr. A. GOPPEL, dió una recepción a la que asistieron 400 invitados, entre los que figuraban los delegados oficiales del Ministerio de Educación, de la Universidad y de la Facultad de Medicina, los miembros del Comité Internacional de Dermatología y del Comité de Organización, los Delegados Nacionales y las esposas de muchos de ellos. El Antiquarium, antiguamente sala de ceremonias de los soberanos de Baviera, dió a esta recepción un ambiente de fiesta real. El Ministro del Interior, Sr. HECK, saludó a los invitados en nombre del Presidente del Gobierno de Baviera, imposibilitado de asistir a esta recepción. Con gran afabilidad, el Ministro expuso el gran interés que el Gobierno tenía por nuestra especialidad médica. El Presidente del Congreso Internacional de Dermatología, Prof. W. JADASSOHN, le respondió con estas palabras:

Señor Presidente:

Le agradecemos su invitación. Yo podria suponer que esta noche, Vd. pensará "Estoy contento habiéndome desembarazado de los dermatólogos". Tal vez piensa Vd., en este momento "Hé aqui el 'pobre' Presidente del Congreso que debe recitar un discurso de circunstancias". Debo señalarle que si Vd. ha pensado "pobre" Presidente, se ha equivocado. Cualquier cosa que me cause placer la agradezco sinceramente, y en este caso, Sr. Ministro, le estamos reconocidos por su invitación y yo se lo agradezco, muy calurosamente, en nombre de todos. Ha sido de una gran alegria para nosotros y si Vd. lo desea, mañana volveremos de nuevo.

Tras estas alocuciones fueron servidos unos refrescos y se reanimaron las conversaciones, ligándose amistades y entablándose cordiales discusiones. La recepción se terminó con la visita, a través de la Schatzkammer de la Residence.

El miércoles, 2 de Agosto, existia la posibilidad de dos excursiones particularmente atractivas. Una caravana de autocares condujo 700 viajeros a Prien en el Chiemsee. Se cruzó el lago en barco para tomar tierra en el Herreninsel. El castillo, con sus salas iluminadas por miles de bujías, fué el encanto de los visitantes. El punto culminante de la excursión fué el concierto, dado en la Sala de los Espejos, por un escogido cuarteto de la Mozart-orchester de Salzburgo que interpretó una obra de Haydn y la "Kleine Nachtmusik" de Mozart.

El segundo grupo, formado por más de 1000 personas, asistió a la representación extraordinaria de la ópera de Richard Strauss, "El caballero de la rosa" en el Teatro Nacional de la ciudad de Munich. El recordado ALFRED MARCHIONINI, que tanto gustaba de las obras de Richard Strauss hubiera disfrutado escuchando esta bella comedia musical, al tiempo que se desarrollaba "su Congreso". Sus alumnos, tuvieron presente en sus pensamientos, el recuerdo de aquel hombre uno de cuyos deseos estaba realizándose.

La siguiente noche del 3 de Agosto, entre las 20 y las 22 tuvo lugar la visita de los más famosos museos de Munich. Divididos en cuatro grupos, los participantes admiraron las hermosas colecciones del Deutsches museum, de la antigua y la moderna Pinacoteca, de la nueva Staatsgalerie, en la Casa de las Artes y la Schatzkammer de la Residence.

El jueves tuvo lugar una recepción a la que asistieron 400 invitados, de la presidencia del Congreso y de la Casa Bayer, en el marco del Teatro Nacional. El Director, Dr. MEYER UHL saludó cordialmente a los asistentes siendo contestado por el Presidente del Congreso.

El viernes cuatro de agosto llegó a su término el programa social con una fiesta típica bávara en los salones de la "Mathäser Bierstadt". Un auténtico ambiente de fiesta reinó en sus dos amplísimos salones, adornados profusamente. Alrededor de las mesas, adornadas con exquisito gusto, se acomodaron 3000 personas, deleitándose con la famosa cerveza bávara servida en jarros de arcilla adornados con flores, que algunos guardaron como recuerdo de esta fiesta. Fueron servidas exquisitas especialidades culinarias de la región. El Prof. NASEMANN había organizado un programa continuo de música folklórica. El Prof. SULZBERGER dirigió con mano maestra la marcha bávara del desfile. El ambiente fué muy alegre; se cantó, se disfrutó mucho y el regocijo y la camaradería forjaron el molde de una familia internacional de dermatólogos.

Junto al programa social se celebraban muchos actos especialmente dedicados a las Señoras.

Visitas de la ciudad (cerca de 700 personas); visita al Parque y al Castillo de Nymphenburg (425 participantes); un desfile de moda, bajo el lema "Munich crea la moda"; visita al Zoo Hellabrunn; visita al Museo Nacional de Baviera (casi 250 personas) y la visita a la Casa de las Artes formaron parte de este programa.

El viernes por la mañana, excursión al Castillo de Andechs comprendiendo la visita de la bellísima iglesia barroca y su precioso claustro. Desde sus torres la vista se extiende sobre el Ammersee y los Prealpes bávaros. El programa destinado a las Señoras se terminó el viernes con una excursión alrededor del Starnberger See. Debemos añadir que la Casa A. Wolff de Bielefeld invito a unas 200 señoras a la presentación de cosméticos en su escuela de Buch en Ammersee.

Así se desarrollaron ambos programas mostrando a los participantes en ellos la vida artística y pintoresca de Munich, mientras que, paralelamente, se celebraba el programa científico del Congreso.

En la sesión de clausura, del dia sábado 5 de Agosto, los miembros del Comité acusaban la fatiga en sus semblantes pero se sentían satisfechos del triunfo alcanzado por el Congreso.

4*

Number of Participants of the Social and Ladies' Program
Nombre de participants au programme social et au programme des dames
Programas social y dedicado a las Señoras. Número de participantes en los mismos:
Beteiligung an Gesellschaftlichen Veranstaltungen und am Damenprogramm

					persons / personnes / personas / Personen approximately
30. 7.	Reception	Soirée d'accueil	Velada de recepción	Begrüßungsabend	2500
31. 7.	Town sight-seeing	Petit tour de ville	Visita reducida de la ciudad	Kleine Stadtrundfahrt	175
	Nymphenburg Town-visit with coffee break at the English Garden	Nymphenburg Tour de ville avec pause-café au Jardin Anglais	Nymphenburg Visita de la ciudad y merienda en el Jardín Inglés	Nymphenburg Stadtrundfahrt mit Kaffeepause im Englischen Garten	455
					140
	Concert	Concert	Concierto	Konzert	1220
	Grand tour of town	Grand tour de ville	Visita detallada de la ciudad	Große Stadtrundfahrt	470
1. 8.	Fashion show	Défilé de mode	Desfile de moda	Modeschau	355
	Deutsches Museum	Deutsches Museum	Deutsches Museum	Deutsches Museum	35
	Visit of churches	Visite d'églises	Visita a los templos	Kirchenführung	600
	Reception at the Antiquarium	Réception à l'Antiquarium	Recepción en el Antiquarium	Staatsempfang im Antiquarium	350
2. 8.	National Museum	Musée National	Museo Nacional	Nationalmuseum	245
	Zoo	Zoo	Zoo	Tierpark	187
	Chiemsee	Chiemsee	Chiemsee	Chiemsee	900
	Opera	Opéra	Velada de ópera	Oper	1050
3. 8.	Visit of museums	Visite de musées	Visita a los museos	Museenfahrt	245
	Evening-visit of museums	Visite de musées dans le soir	Visita de noche a los museos	Abendbesuch der Museen	800
4. 8.	Andechs	Andechs	Andechs	Andechs	330
	Starnberger See	Starnberger See	Starnberger See	Starnberger See	370
	Bavarian Evening	Soirée Bavaroise	Velada típica regional	Bayer. Abend	2044

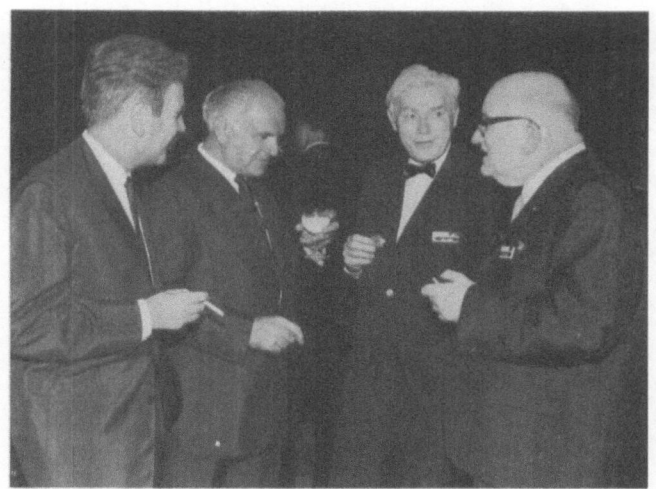

→ Prof. DELACRÉTAZ, Prof. KUSKE, Prof. NELSON, Prof. JADASSOHN

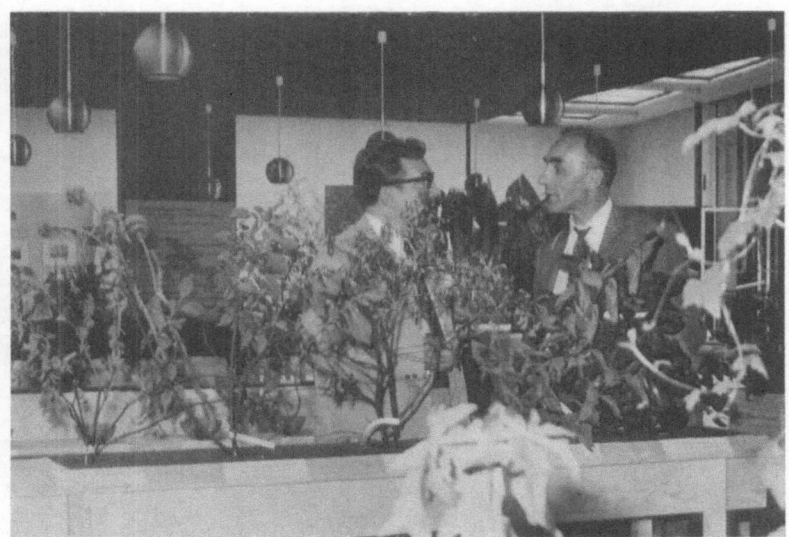

Botanic garden for eczematogenic plants

Jardin botanique de plantes eczématogènes

Jardín Botánico (plantas eczematógenas)

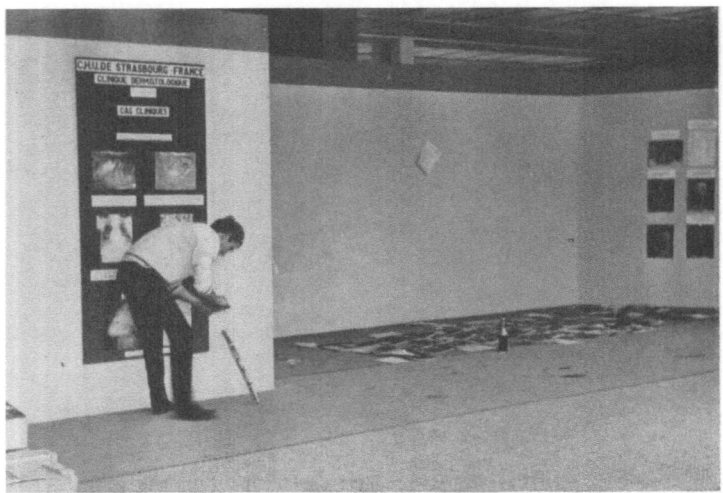

Installation of the Scientific Exhibition
Installation de l'Exposition Scientifique
Instalación de la Exposición Científica
Einrichtung der Wissenschaftlichen Ausstellung

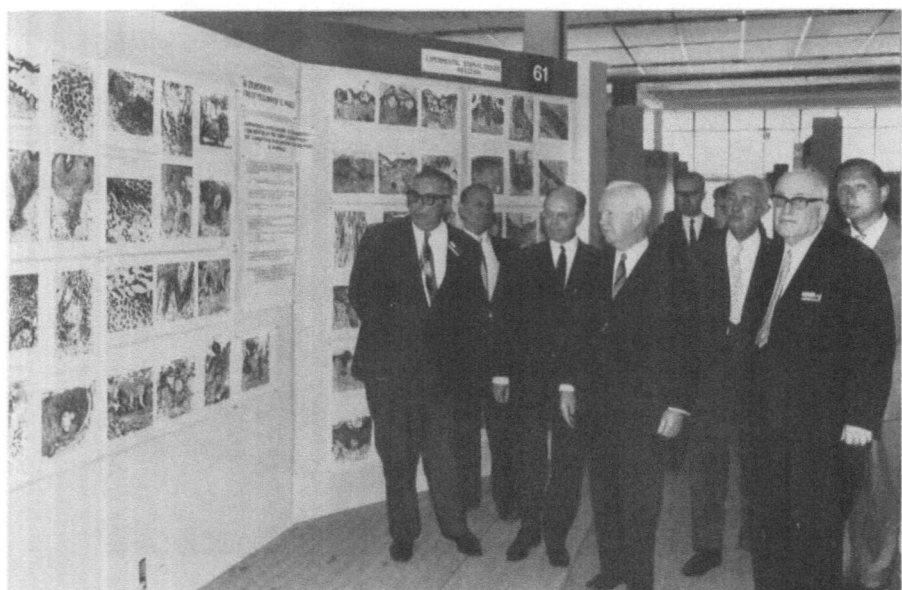

The President of the Federal Republic
goes through the Scientific Exhibition

Le Président de la République Fédérale
visite l'Exposition Scientifique

Visita del Presidente de la República
Federal Alemana a la Exposición Científica

Der Bundespräsident besucht die
Wissenschaftliche Ausstellung

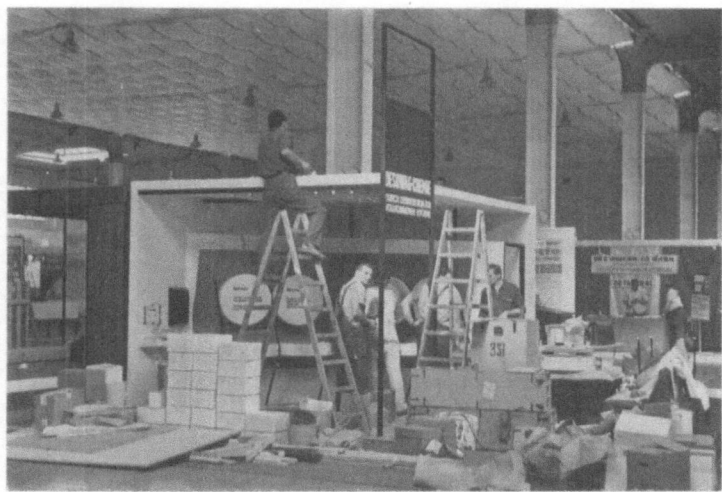

Fitting out of the Technical Exhibition
Derniers préparatifs à l'Exposition Technique
Ultimos preparativos en la Exposición Técnica
Beim Aufbau der Industrieausstellung

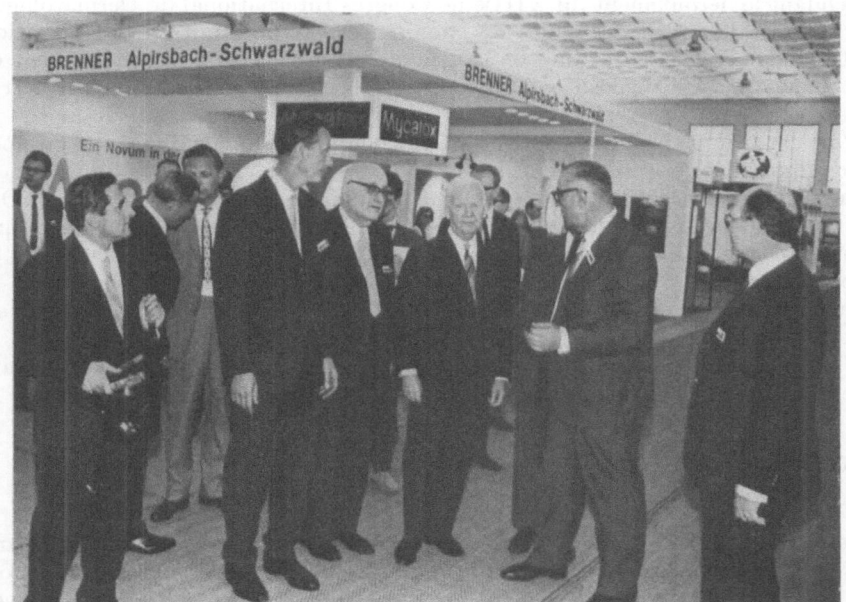

The President of the Federal Republic
goes through the Technical Exhibition

Le Président de la République Fédérale
visite l'Exposition Technique

Visita del Presidente de la República Federal
Alemana a la Exposición Técnica

Der Bundespräsident besucht die
Industrieausstellung

Technical Exhibition
(Prof. WILHELM SCHNEIDER, Tübingen)

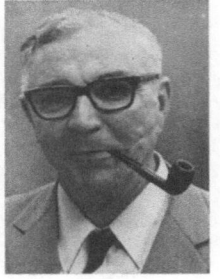

Hall 7, an area of 6000 m², was placed at the disposal of the Technical Exhibition which took place during the International Congress of Dermatology. This site had been chosen, situated in the center of all conference rooms, close to the Scientific Exhibition and not far from the projection room of films; thus facilitating frequent visits.

72 firms exhibited in an area of 2000 m², thus leaving enough space for alleys and seats. Most of the firms represented the pharmaceutical industry. Books and medical reviews were exhibited. The exhibition presented all means of the dermatologists disposal for his medical and scientific activity.

Among the exposants, besides the German, the presence of American, French and Swiss firms was noticed.

The interest of this exhibition suscited among visitors of the Federal Republic of Germany as well as foreign visitors and the press, has been appreciated by the exposants.

Exposition Technique
(Prof. WILHELM SCHNEIDER, Tübingen)

La halle 7, d'une superficie de 6000 m², servit à l'Exposition Technique qui eut lieu pendant le déroulement du XIIIième Congrès International de Dermatologie. Sa situation, au milieu des salles de conférences, sa proximité de l'Exposition Scientifique, et à courte distance de la salle de projection de films, motivèrent ce choix. Grâce à cette disposition, l'Exposition Technique promettait d'être très fréquentée.

72 firmes prirent part à cette exposition. 2000 m² de stands divisés en groupes par de larges allées et groupes de sièges, facilitèrent leur visite.

La plupart des firmes représentaient l'industrie pharmaco-chimique. Des livres et des revues médicales étaient exposés. L'Exposition montrait tout ce que le dermatologue a à sa disposition pour l'exercice de son activité médicale et scientifique.

Parmi les exposants, on notait la présence de firmes allemandes, américaines, françaises et suisses.

L'intérêt que cette exposition suscita parmi les visiteurs nationaux ou étrangers et de la part de la presse, fut très apprécié par les exposants.

Exposición Técnica
(Prof. WILHELM SCHNEIDER, Tübingen)

La nave 7, de 6,000 m² de superficie, fue puesta a la disposición de los organizadores de la Exposición Técnica que tuvo lugar durante la celebración del Congreso Internacional de Dermatología. Fué escogida esta nave por hallarse situada en el centro de todas las salas de conferencias, contigua a las instalaciones de la Exposición Científica y cercana a la destinada a proyección de películas científicas. Gracias a esta situación afortunada la Exposición Técnica estaba llamada a ser muy frecuentada.

72 firmas del ramo, ocupando una superficie de 2,000 m², tomaron parte en esta exposición. La anchura de los pasillos y los espacios reservados a los asientos, facilitaron grandemente, la visita de los pabellones.

Los expositores, en su gran mayoría, pertenecían a la industria médico-química. Libros y revistas médicas ocupaban un lugar importante. En su conjunto, la Exposición Técnica, exhibía todo cuanto el dermatólogo necesita para el ejercicio de sus actividades médica y científica.

Firmas alemanas, americanas, francesas y suizas figuraban entre los expositores.

Estos apreciaron en gran modo el interés suscitado entre los visitantes nacionales y extranjeros. La prensa, por su parte, también se mostró muy interesada por esta Exposición Técnica.

Industrie-Ausstellung
(Prof. WILHELM SCHNEIDER, Tübingen)

Für die Industrieausstellung, die während des XIII. Internationalen Kongresses für Dermatologie abgehalten wurde, stand die Halle 7 des Messegeländes mit rund 6000 m² Fläche zur Verfügung. Dieser Standort wurde vor allem deshalb gewählt, weil er zentral zu allen Vortragssälen, der wissenschaftlichen Ausstellung und dem wissenschaftlichen Filmprojektionsraum lag. Damit war eine bestmögliche Frequenz der Ausstellung schon von ihrer Lage her gewährleistet.

An der Ausstellung beteiligten sich 72 Firmen, die über 2000 m² reine Ausstellungsfläche in Anspruch nahmen, so daß für Gänge und Sitzgelegenheiten genügend Raum zur Verfügung stand.

Unter den Firmen überwog zahlenmäßig die chemisch-pharmazeutische Industrie. Daneben wurden auch Bücher und Fachzeitschriften aufgelegt. Die Ausstellung zeigte, was der Dermatologe bei seiner ärztlichen und wissenschaftlichen Tätigkeit heute benutzen kann.

An der Ausstellung dermatologischer Spezialitäten beteiligten sich außer deutschen Firmen auch Firmen aus den USA, Frankreich und der Schweiz.

Wie bei den einzelnen Ausstellungsständen festgestellt wurde, hat die Ausstellung bei in- und ausländischen Besuchern sowie in der Presse reges Interesse gefunden.

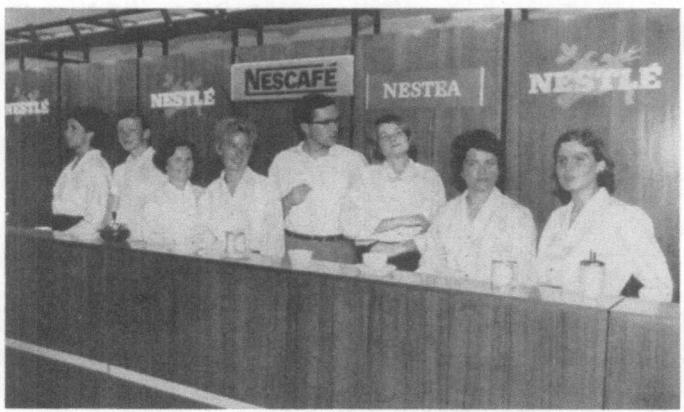

Invited by "Nestlé"   Invitación de la Casa "Nestlé"
Invitation de la «Nestlé»   Zu Gast bei „Nestlé"

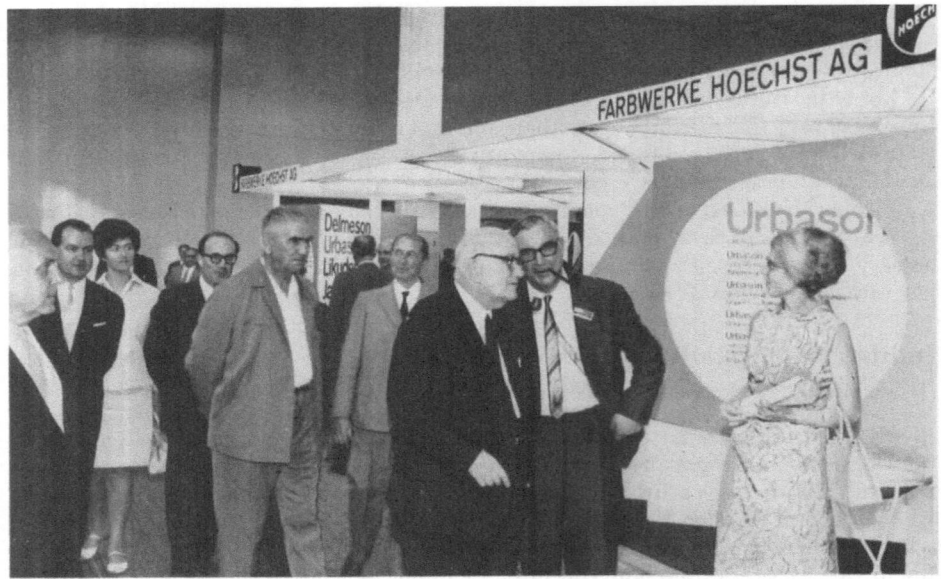

At the Technical Exhibition

A l'Exposition Technique

En la Exposición Técnica

In der Industrieausstellung

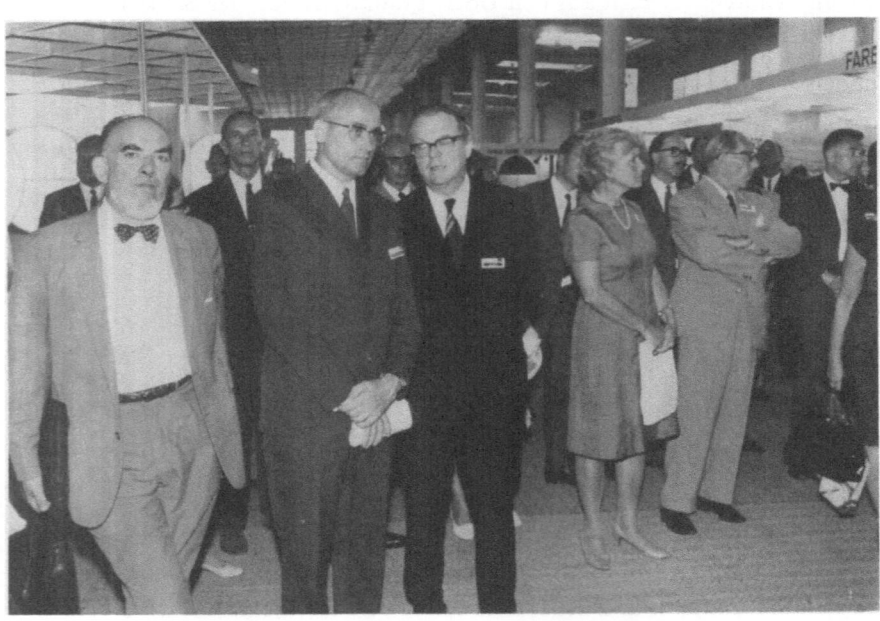

Eröffnung der Industrieausstellung

Prof. Werner Jadassohn

Meine Damen und Herren!

Bevor Herr Prof. SCHNEIDER die industrielle Ausstellung eröffnet, bevor er *seine* Ausstellung eröffnet, seien mir einige Worte gestattet.

Es war ein Glück, daß ich Herrn SCHNEIDER seit Jahren kenne und mit ihm befreundet bin. So wußte ich, daß sich unter seinen zahlreichen Talenten auch eines befindet, das ihn befähigt, eine solche Ausstellung zu organisieren. Wie froh waren wir, daß er die Wahl angenommen hat. Wie ausgezeichnet haben er und seine Mitarbeiter Doz. TRONNIER und Doz. ADAM diese schwierige Aufgabe durchgeführt. Was wäre aus diesem Kongreß geworden, wenn wir diese so wertvollen Mitarbeiter nicht gehabt hätten. Die Herren SCHNEIDER, TRONNIER und ADAM sind dank der an der Ausstellung beteiligten Firmen zu einem ausgezeichneten Resultat gelangt. Den Ausstellern wird Herr Prof. SCHNEIDER im Namen aller Kongreßteilnehmer den Dank aussprechen. Mir fällt die sehr angenehme Aufgabe zu, Herrn Prof. SCHNEIDER und seinen Oberärzten TRONNIER und ADAM sehr herzlich zu gratulieren und ihnen für die große Arbeit, die sie für uns alle geleistet haben, sehr herzlich zu danken.

Ladies and Gentlemen!

Before Prof. SCHNEIDER is opening his exhibition, I would like to say some words. It was a big chance that my friend Prof. SCHNEIDER accepted to organize this exhibition because he is specially gifted to do such a work. He will thank the exhibitors. I want to thank himself and his collaborators Doz. TRONNIER and Doz. ADAM, for the fine work they have done.

Mesdames et Messieurs!

Avant que le Prof. SCHNEIDER inaugure son exposition, j'aimerais dire quelques mots. Je connais mon ami SCHNEIDER depuis bien des années. Je savais qu'il était spécialement doué pour organiser pareille exposition. Je lui laisse le soin de remercier les exposants, mais c'est à moi de le féliciter, lui et ses collaborateurs Doz. TRONNIER et Doz. ADAM pour cette très belle réussite.

Nun wird Herr Prof. SCHNEIDER das Wort ergreifen, sobald sich der Beifall, mit dem sie ihn begrüßen werden, gelegt hat.

Prof. Wilhelm Schneider:

Unser jetziges Zusammentreffen spiegelt die Kräfte wider, die zur Heilung so vieler kranker Menschen am Werke sind. Was wären wir Ärzte ohne die zahlreichen Arzneimittel, die uns — als Ergebnis der industriellen Forschung — in so ausgezeichneter und laufend kontrollierter Güte zur Verfügung gestellt werden, und was wäre die pharmazeutische Industrie ohne die vielfachen Anregungen aus der medizinischen Forschung und die Kontrolle der Arzneiwirkungen und Nebenwirkungen am Kranken selbst? Diese Zusammenarbeit zwischen Industrie und Medizin, hier der Dermatologie, vollzieht sich im Laufe der Jahre in aller Stille durch Austausch von Erfahrungen, durch a) Angebot einerseits und b) kritische Überprüfung andererseits.

Die Industrie hat aber auch durch ihre meist gut ausgebildeten Mitarbeiterstäbe bereits wesentlichen Anteil an der ärztlichen Fortbildung, indem ihre

Vertreter selbst den abgelegensten Landarzt aufsuchen und an Hand sorgfältig ausgearbeiteten Materials unterrichten.

Besondere Freude empfinden wir darüber, daß, wie der Kongreß, so auch die Ausstellung weitgehend internationalen Charakter hat. Wiederum ist dieser ein äußerer Ausdruck der Beiträge, die verschiedene Nationen auf dem Gebiet der Arzneimittel und, das heißt letzten Endes der Therapie, geleistet haben.

Ich denke hier in ungefährer historischer Reihenfolge an das Salvarsan, an das Germanin und die Sulfonamide aus Deutschland, das Penicillin aus England, an die Antihistamine aus Frankreich und schließlich an ACTH-Cortison aus den USA. Das Zusammenspiel der verschiedensten Industrienationen zeigte sich bereits bei der Einführung der Sulfonamide. Das erste deutsche Präparat Prontosil enthielt noch eine AZO-Farbstoffgruppe, während französische Forscher nachweisen konnten, daß diese für den therapeutischen Effekt nicht relevant sei. Auf dem Gebiet der Antibiotica hatte der englische Start weiterführende großartige Entwicklungen in aller Welt, insbesondere in den USA und in Japan zur Folge. Die Tuberculostatica wurden in den USA, in Deutschland und in der Schweiz entwickelt.

Wir wissen aber auch — meine sehr verehrten Vertreter der Industrie — um das Ausmaß der Verantwortlichkeit und des Risikos, das mit Ihrer Entwicklungsforschung und nachfolgender Einführung neuer Präparate verbunden ist. Sie haben einen Grad von Selbstkontrolle erreicht, der durch staatliche Kontrolle (mangels personeller und materieller Ausstattung) schlechterdings nicht zu überbieten wäre.

Schwerwiegende und bedauerliche Nebenwirkungen eines Medikamentes stehen immer noch in aller Welt, insbesondere in Deutschland, im Mittelpunkt des öffentlichen Interesses. Hier trägt die industrielle Forschung besonders schwer an der Verantwortung um das Lebensrisiko in der modernen Industriegesellschaft, wie es sich insbesondere im Straßen- und Luftverkehr ebenfalls bietet. Diese Belastung darf, wie GOTTRON als Präsident der Karlsruher Therapiewoche 1962 betonte, nicht dazu führen, eine wissenschaftliche Entwicklung zu bremsen, die sich für die Menschheit bisher nur segensreich ausgewirkt hat. Hierfür ein paar kurze Daten:

1. Ende des vorigen Jahrhunderts betrug die durchschnittliche Lebenserwartung 35 Jahre, heute beträgt sie 70. Sie hat sich also verdoppelt.

2. Vor der Ära der Sulfonamide und Antibiotica war fast jeder 9. ein Gonorrhoiker und jeder 23. ein Syphilitiker.

3. Die Tuberkulose hat heute in der Seuchenbekämpfung kaum noch eine ernste Bedeutung. Die Entdeckung a) des Streptomycins 1944, b) der Paraaminosalicylsäure 1945, c) des Contebens 1946 sowie d) des Netebens und Rimifons haben zu einer Leerung der Tuberkulose- und der Lupusheilstätten geführt. Heilkurorte für Tuberkulose mußten ob dieser Erfolge umstrukturiert werden wie beispielsweise Davos — ich erinnere in diesem Zusammenhang an den „Zauberberg" von Thomas Mann.

Bis zum Jahre 1921 war der Diabetes mellitus eine Krankheit mit nur begrenzter Lebenserwartung. Durch die Entdeckung und die Einführung des Insulins wurde eine kausale Therapie geschaffen. In letzter Zeit haben sich die Sulfonamide vor allem bei Altersdiabetes besonders bewährt. Gewebefreundliche Desinfektionsmittel und Antibiotica können uns heute von unliebsamen Parasiten befreien. Vor allem haben uns aber die Kontaktinsecticide, wie das DDT von Geigy, in die Lage versetzt, den Vernichtungskampf z. B. gegen die Malaria auf breiter Basis zu führen. Die weltumspannende Vernichtungskampagne gegen die Malaria wird seit Jahren von der WHO energisch und erfolgreich durchgeführt.

Es gäbe noch zahlreiche Beispiele, um zu zeigen, wie segensreich das Zusammenspiel zwischen industrieller und medizinischer Forschung sich für die gesamte Menschheit ausgewirkt hat.

Das sind Tatsachen, meine sehr verehrten Damen und Herren von der pharmazeutischen Industrie, die bekannt sind. Es sollte aber heute und an dieser Stelle nochmals ausdrücklich herausgestellt werden, daß wir um die Bedeutung Ihrer Forschung, Ihrer Produktion und Ihrer gewissenhaften subtilen Selbstkontrolle wissen sowie um die Größe Ihrer Verantwortung. Die Industrie, die sich mit der Herstellung von Bestrahlungsgeräten und anderen medizinischen Apparaten für Diagnostik und Therapie beschäftigt, zeigt ihre neuesten Entwicklungen, wofür wir ihr bestens danken. Das gleiche gilt für die in der Hauttherapie so wichtige Verbandmittel- und Gummistrumpfindustrie. Auch die Körperpflegemittelindustrie ist hier vertreten. Sie steht unter den medizinischen Disziplinen der Dermatologie verständlicherweise am nächsten. Viel des Gesagten trifft auch für sie zu, z. B. im Hinblick auf die Entwicklung und Einführung der Emulsionen, Emulsionslotionen, Lichtschutzmittel und Hautreinigungsmittel. Sie sehen, die Übergänge zur Körperpflege sind fließend. Gute Präparate können zur Prophylaxe, wie z. B. im Lichtschutz, und zur Nachbehandlung eingesetzt werden. An der sog. „dekorativen" Kosmetik sind wir nicht vordergründig interessiert, jedoch gewissermaßen hintergründig ihre Helfer, indem wir Unverträglichkeit bestimmter Produkte oder Komponenten erkennen und gemeinsam mit Ihnen zum Nutzen der Verbraucher ausschalten.

Am Schluß darf ich allen Ausstellern im Namen des Kongresses herzlich danken für die ungewöhnlich große Beteiligung, für den Aufbau dieser schönen und umfassenden Industrieausstellung und für die großzügige und überaus verständnisvolle Mithilfe bei der Gestaltung des Gesamtkongresses. Gedacht und gedankt sei auch einer Reihe von Firmen, die aus bestimmten Gründen nicht ausstellen konnten, dafür aber unser Kongreßvorhaben durch beachtliche Spenden unterstützt haben.

Dank sagen möchte ich weiterhin all denen, die bei der Organisation dieser Ausstellung geholfen haben, d. h. an erster Stelle dem Präsidenten, der überall eifrig die Trommel rührte, mir aber von Anfang an freie Hand ließ, so daß Kompetenzfragen erst gar nicht aufkommen konnten. Entscheidend für das Gelingen war die positive und reibungslose Mitarbeit der Münchner Messegesellschaft, vor allem der Herren SEIFFERT und VOM HÖVEL. Mit dem Letzteren als dem beauftragten Verhandlungspartner der Gesellschaft, hatten wir immer einen erfreulichen persönlichen Kontakt. Der letzte, aber nicht geringste Dank gilt meinen beiden Kongreßsekretären ADAM und TRONNIER, die mit Ausdauer und großem Geschick, wenn auch in aller Stille, zum Gelingen der Ausstellung beitrugen.

Und damit eröffne ich diese Ausstellung als eine weitere Brücke zwischen der Industrie mit ihrer Forschung und der Dermatologie in Klinik und Praxis.

Exhibitors · Exposants · Expositores · Aussteller

Arbeitsgemeinschaft Buchausstellungen
J. F. Lehmann / Otto Spatz
8000 München 15, Schillerstraße 51

Athenstaedt & Redeker KG,
Chem.-Pharm. Fabrik
2800 Bremen 2, Postfach 8660

Dr. Atzinger & Co. KG,
Pharmazeutische Fabrik
8390 Passau, Dr.-Guby-Straße 4—6

Basotherm GmbH
7950 Biberach/Riß, Postfach 130,
Birkendorfer Straße

Johann A. Benckiser GmbH
6700 Ludwigshafen/Rhein 3, Postfach

Georg A. Brenner,
Arzneimittel-Fabrik GmbH
7297 Alpirsbach/Schwarzwald, Postfach 20

Buchler & Co.
3300 Braunschweig, Frankfurter Straße 294

Byk-Essex,
Pharmazeutische Gesellschaft mbH
8000 München 2, Sendlinger-Tor-Platz 1

Chemie Grünenthal GmbH
5190 Stolberg/Rhld., Postfach 129

Ciba AG
7867 Wehr/Baden

Bernd Conzen,
Pharmazeutische GmbH & Co. KG
4000 Düsseldorf-Reisholz, Tönisstraße 27 a

Cooper, Tinsley Lab. Inc.
229 Cleveland Avenue,
Harrison/New Jersey, USA

Ichthyol Gesellschaft,
Cordes, Hermanni & Co.
2000 Hamburg 54
Süderfeldstraße 25, Postfach

Dermik Pharmacal Co.
150 Eileen Way, Syosset / N.Y., USA

Desowag-Chemie GmbH
4000 Düsseldorf 1, Bismarckstraße 83/85

Deutsche Beecham GmbH
7950 Biberach/Riß, Birkendorfer Straße 65

Deutsche Bristol GmbH
8000 München 90, Postfach

Dome Laboratories Division
of Miles Laboratories Inc.
125 West End Avenue,
New York, N.Y. 10 023, USA

Elbeo-Werke, Augsburg—Mannheim
8900 Augsburg, Hofer Straße 10

Dr. med. Josef Ellendorff & Co.
5600 Wuppertal-Barmen, Postfach 124,
Schwarzbach 103

Fabrik Pharmazeutischer Präparate,
Karl Engelhard
6000 Frankfurt/Main,
Sandweg 94, Postfach 3662

Erbe Elektromedizin KG
7400 Tübingen, Ebertstraße 35

Farbenfabriken Bayer AG,
Pharma-Abteilung WG
5090 Leverkusen-Bayerwerk

Arzneimittelwerk Fischer oHG
7580 Bühl/Baden, Hermannstraße 7

Ludwig Frohnhäuser KG
8000 München 15, Lindwurmstraße 1

Ganzoni & Cie. AG
Rittmeyerstraße 15,
CH-9014 St. Gallen, Schweiz

Gilette Roth-Büchner GmbH
1000 Berlin-Tempelhof,
Oberlandstraße 75—84

Glaxo, Pharmazeutika GmbH
4000 Düsseldorf, Volmerswerther Straße 80/84

Grosse Verlag GmbH, Anzeigenabteilung
1000 Berlin-Lichterfelde-West,
Baseler Straße 67

Paul Hartmann AG
7920 Heidenheim/Brenz, Postfach 125

Hefa-Frenon GmbH
4712 Werne a. d. Lippe,
Postfach 220, Capeller Straße 31

Arzneimittelfabrik Hüls, Dr. Albin Hense
4153 Hüls/Krefeld, Wilhelmstraße 39—41

Hermal Chemie, Kurt Herrmann
2057 Reinbek, Danzinger Straße 5

Chemische Fabrik von Heyden AG
8000 München 19, Volkartstraße 83

Farbwerke Hoechst AG,
vormals Meister Lucius & Brüning
6230 Frankfurt/Main-Hoechst, Postfach 70

Kreussler & Co
6202 Wiesbaden-Biebrich, Postfach 9105

Lady Esther, Kosmetik GmbH & Co.
8000 München 90, St. Zenoweg 3

Lederle Arzneimittel,
Abt. der Cyanamid GmbH
8000 München 60, Fritz-Berne-Straße 47

Eli Lilly GmbH, Pharmazeutika
6300 Gießen 2, Postfach 2720, Teichweg 3

Löwens Pharma Düsseldorf GmbH & Co. KG
4000 Düsseldorf 1, Alexanderstraße 28

Lohmann KG
5451 Fahr/Rhein, Postfach

Luitpold-Werk,
Chemisch-pharmazeutische Fabrik
8000 München 25, Zielstattstraße 9—11

Medice, Chemisch-pharmazeutische
Fabrik GmbH
5860 Iserlohn, Postfach 415,
Kuhloweg 37—39

Hädensa Gesellschaft,
Richard Morsch & Co.
1000 Berlin 46, Malteser Straße 136—138

Arznei Müller,
Apotheker Müller GmbH & Co. KG
4800 Bielefeld, Stieghorster Straße 86

Person & Covey
236 South Verdugo Road,
Glendale 5/Calif., USA

Promedica, S.A.
41, rue Camille Pelletan, B. P. 188,
Levallois-Perret (Seine), Frankreich

Protina, Chem. Ges. mbH
8000 München 54, Hofstettenstraße 36

Rhein-Pharma, Arzneimittel GmbH
6900 Heidelberg 1, Postfach 1428

Dr. Rentschler & Co.,
Fabrik chem.-pharm. Präparate Vertrieb
7958 Laupheim, Mittelstraße 16

Dr. Riese & Co
5340 Rhöndorf/Rh., Rhöndorfer Straße 80

Robugen GmbH, Pharm. Fabrik
7300 Eßlingen-Zell, Alleenstraße 22,
Postfach 266

Sandoz AG
8500 Nürnberg, Deutschherrnstraße 15

Dr. Friedrich Sasse,
Pharmazeutische Präparate
1000 Berlin 10, Kaiserin-Augusta-Allee 86,
Postfach 640

Deutsche Milchwerke, Dr. A. Sauer
6144 Zwingenberg/Bergstraße,
Darmstädter Straße 26—36

Schering AG
1000 Berlin 65, Müllerstraße 170/72

A. Schumann, Fabrik für Feinmechanik
4000 Düsseldorf, Poststraße 7

Siegfried GmbH
7880 Säckingen, Postfach 71

Siemens AG
8520 Erlangen, Henkestraße 127

Solco Basel AG
Rührbergstraße 21,
CH-4127 Birsfelden, Schweiz

W. Spitzner, Arzneimittelfabrik GmbH
7505 Ettlingen, Bunsenstraße 6—10

Stiefel Laboratorium GmbH
6050 Offenbach/Main, Postfach 680

Chemische Fabrik Stockhausen & Cie.,
Pharmazeutische Abteilung
4150 Krefeld, Postfach 1238, Bäkerpfad 25

Syntex International Insurgentes
Sur No. 1457, Apartado M-10063,
Mexico 1, D.F.

Dr. E. Uhlhorn & Co. GmbH,
Chem.-Pharm.-Fabrik
6202 Wiesbaden-Biebrich, Postfach 9446,
Am Schloßpark 35—39

Upjohn GmbH
6148 Heppenheim, Graf-von-Galen-Straße 12

Varitex GmbH
4240 Emmerich, Helenenbusch 3

Wilhelm Vogel
6300 Gießen/Lahn, Postfach 119

Dr. August Wolff KG, Chem.-pharm. Fabrik
4800 Bielefeld, Postfach 9540,
Sudbrackstraße 56

Julius Zorn & Co., GmbH
8890 Aichach/Obb., Münchener Straße

Zyma Blaes AG, Arzneimittelfabrik
8000 München 25, Zielstattstraße 34—38

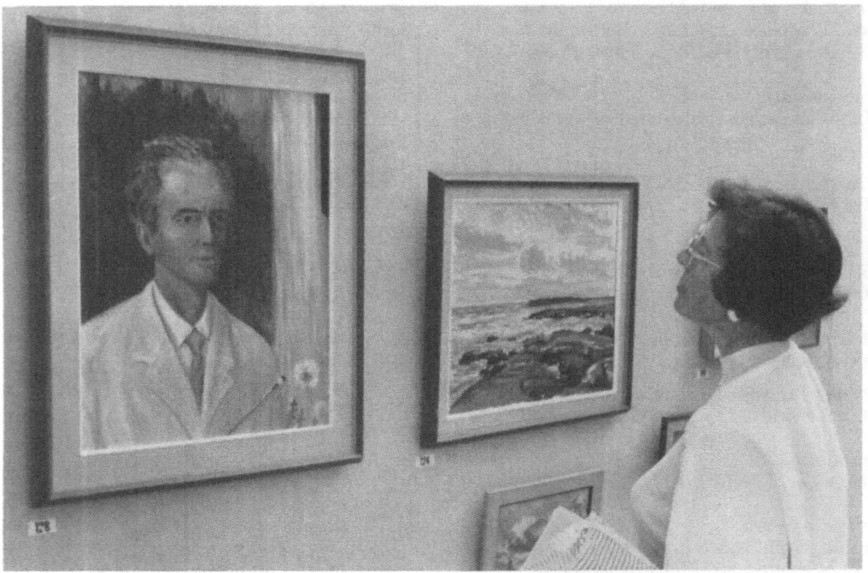

At the Art Exhibition, self-painting by Prof. SONCK

A l'Exposition d'Art, auto-portrait par le Prof. SONCK

Autoretrato del Prof. SONCK en la Exposicíon Artística

In der Kunstausstellung, Selbstbildnis Prof. SONCK

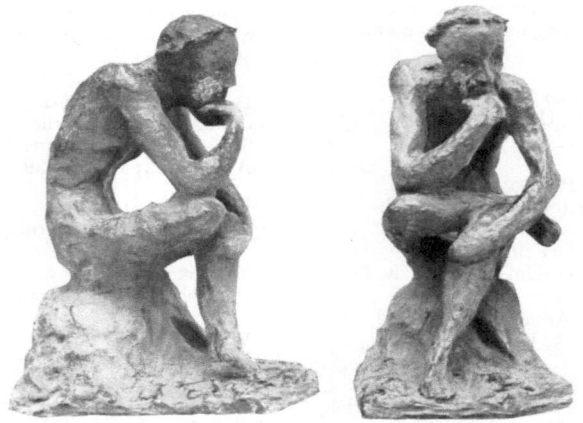

„Philosophe" prophile, enface (R. SABOURAUD)

The Art Exhibition

Summary of the report given by Prof. CARL E. SONCK

In our hectic days, a recreative hobby is of great importance. Whoever has a cherished hobby, may consider himself very happy indeed. Or to quote Alexander Dumas jr.: "L'homme de talent est celui qui sait autre chose que son métier". All through the ages, physicians, especially, have taken an interest in the arts. Besides their work, many of them have been active musicians, singers and even composers. Others have taken interest in sculpture and painting. We can mention, RAYMOND SABOURAUD, the author of the famous work in six volumes "Maladies du cuir chevelu". He was both a well-known dermatologist and an acknowledged sculptor. In a letter to Prof. AXEL CEDERCREUTZ, Sabouraud tells him how he, in his later years, was more and more captivated by his hobby, sculpture. When the last patient left his office Sabouraud produced his tools, covered the floor with a sheet and started to work. In his book "Pêle-mêle" (1933) he says: "Les heures de création sont des heures heureuses". "Toute œuvre d'art est lyrique. Elle comporte une sorte de délire divin où l'artiste, comme la Pythie, parle au nom de son dieu qui la force à parler". "L'œuvre naît au milieu d'une crise. C'est toujours un enfant de la douleur; et souvent son père découragé s'en veut de ne pas l'avoir faite plus belle ...".

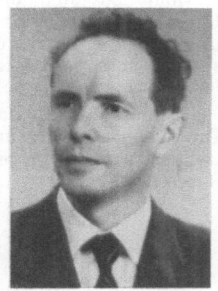

When it was decided that the XIII International Congress of Dermatology was to take place in Munich, the metropolis of arts, I thought that it would be appropriate to have an exhibition of dermatologists' art. In this way, we could also pay a tribute to SABOURAUD.

Exposition artistique

Résumé du rapport du Prof. CARL E. SONCK

De nos jours, un passe-temps, un violon d'Ingres est d'une grande importance. Toute personne ayant un passe-temps, peut se considérer comme vraiment heureux. Citons A. Dumas.: «L'homme de talent est celui qui sait autre chose que son métier». A travers les temps, des médecins ont été attirés par l'art. A côté de leur travail, nombre d'entre eux ont été des musiciens actifs, des chanteurs, des compositeurs même. D'autres se sont intéressés aux arts décoratifs: peinture, sculpture. Citons, par exemple, RAYMOND SABOURAUD, l'auteur des six volumes «Maladies du cuir chevelu». En plus de dermatologue, il était un sculpteur réputé. Lui-même raconte, dans une lettre adressée au Prof. AXEL CEDERCREUTZ, comme il fut, durant ses années de «vieillesse», captivé par son passe-temps, la sculpture. Lorsque le dernier malade quittait son bureau, SABOURAUD sortait ses outils, couvrait le sol d'un drap et se mettait au travail. Dans son livre «Pêle-Mêle» (1933), il écrit «Les heures de création sont des heures heureuses». «Toute œuvre d'art est lyrique. Elle comporte une sorte de délire divin ou l'artiste, comme la Pythie, parle au nom de son dieu qui la force à parler». «L'œuvre naît au milieu d'une crise. C'est toujours un enfant de la douleur, et souvent, son père découragé, s'en veut de ne pas l'avoir faite plus belle ... ».

Munich, capitale des arts, ayant été choisie comme siège du XIIIième Congrès International de Dermatologie, j'ai pensé qu'une exposition d'art, d'œuvres crées par des dermatologistes, serait, elle aussi, le moyen d'honorer la mémoire de RAYMOND SABOURAUD.

La Exposición Artística

Resumén del informe del Prof. CARL E. SONCK

En nuestra época, los pasatiempos tienen una importancia muy grande. Todos aquellos que tienen un pasatiempo preferido pueden considerarse muy felices. Alejandro Dumas decía que "Un hombre de talento es aquel que conoce algo mas que su profesión". Durante todas las épocas, los médicos se han sentido especialmente atraídos por las artes. Independientemente de su profesión, muchos de ellos fueron músicos notables, cantantes, incluso compositores. Otros dieron su preferencia a las artes decorativas, pintura y escultura. Como ejemplo, RAYMOND SABOURAUD, autor de los seis famosos volúmenes "Enfermedades del cuero cabelludo". Por un lado, dermatólogo y escritor bien conocido y por otro, escultor renombrado. En una carta dirigida al Prof. AXEL CEDERCREUTZ, SABOURAUD relata que, a medida que pasaban los años, se sentía, más y más cautivado por su pasatiempo favorito, la escultura. Apenas el último paciente salía de su gabinete Sabouraud, protegiendo el suelo con un lienzo, asía sus cinceles y comenzaba su trabajo. En su libro "Pêle-Mêle" (1933) escribió "Los momentos de creación son momentos felices", "Toda obra de arte es lírica. Como Pythia, forzada por su dios a hablar en su nombre, origina en el artista que la creó una especie de divino delirio". "La obra toma forma durante el desarrollo de una crisis, siendo siempre una criatura fruto del dolor, y a menudo, su progenitor decepcionado se acusa de no haberla creado mas bella...".

Cuando fué tomada la decisión de celebrar en Munich, capital de las artes, el XIII Congreso Internacional de Dermatología, me vino la idea de organizar una exposición de obras de arte creadas por los propios dermatólogos, honrando así, con ella, la memoria de Raymond Sabouraud.

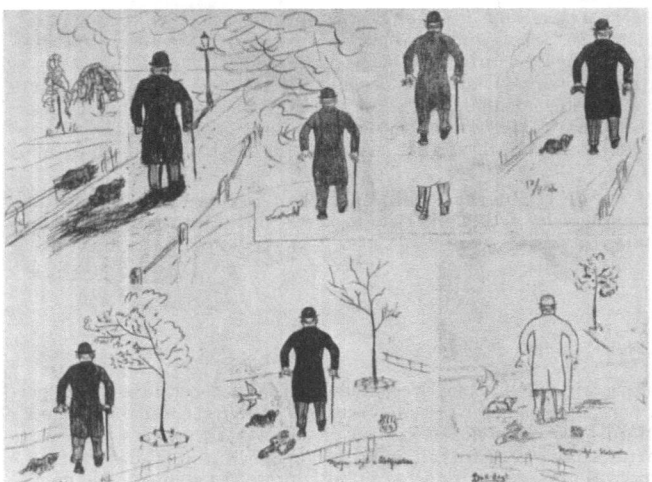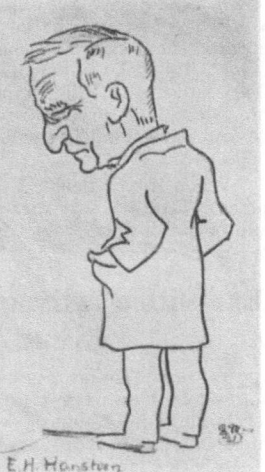

Caricatures: "Morning Walk", "Dr. Hausteen" (Scott Mathiesen)

Kunstausstellung

Bericht von Prof. Carl E. Sonck

Heutzutage ist ein geruhsames Hobby sehr wichtig. Wer solch einen Ausgleich besitzt, kann sich glücklich schätzen. Alexander Dumas sagt: „L'homme de talent est celui qui sait autre chose que son métier". Zu allen Zeiten haben sich die Ärzte mit Kunst beschäftigt. Neben ihrer Berufstätigkeit waren viele aktive Musiker, Sänger und sogar Komponisten. Andere haben sich mit Skulptur und Malerei beschäftigt. Wir erwähnen Raymond Sabouraud, den Autor des berühmten sechsbändigen Werkes „Maladies du cuir chevelu". Als er schon älter war, schrieb er in einem Brief an Axel Cedercreutz, daß er mehr und mehr durch sein Hobby, die Bildhauerei, gefesselt werde. Wenn der letzte Patient sein Ordinationszimmer verlassen hatte, nahm Sabouraud sein Werkzeug hervor, bedeckte den Boden mit einem Leintuch und begann zu arbeiten. In seinem Buch „Pêle-Mêle" (1933) sagt er: "Les heures de création sont des heures heureuses". „Toute œuvre d'art est lyrique. Elle comporte une sorte de délire divin où l'artiste, comme la Pythie, parle au nom de son dieu qui la force à parler". „L'œuvre naît au milieu d'une crise. C'est toujours un enfant de la douleur, et souvent, son père découragé s'en veut de ne pas l'avoir faite plus belle ...".

Als beschlossen worden war, daß der XIII. Internationale Dermatologenkongress in München, der Kunstmetropole Deutschlands, stattfinden sollte, dachte ich, es sei angezeigt, eine Ausstellung dermatologischer Kunst zu organisieren. Auf diese Weise konnten wir auch Sabouraud ehren.

I am indebted also to SABOURAUD's grandson, Dr. OLIVIER SABOURAUD, professor of neurology, who kindly lent the three beautiful bronze statuettes „Manfred", "Philosoph" and "Danseuse" to our exhibition. The art exhibition comprised 186 works in all, by the following 24 "dermatologists-artists":

BYRON H. ARMSTRONG, M. D., Minneapolis, USA. (1 oil, 1 graphic).

V. A. BALABANOFF, Dr. med., Sofia, Bulgaria (3 water colours, 5 groups of caricatures).

LUISE BAUER, Assist. Dr., Rostock, DDR (11 drawings).

JOACHIM BETTERMANN, Dr. med., Dermatologist, Dortmund-Dorstfeld, Germany (13 paintings: 4 in oil, the rest in tempera).

ALF BJÖRNBERG, Dr. med., Gotenburg, Sweden (2 oils).

MINERVA S. BUERK, M. D., Bryn Mawr, Pa.,
   USA (1 water colour).

H. CHATARD, Dermatologist, Grenoble, France
   (1 oil painting).

JAROSLAW DANDA, Dr. med., Docent, Hradec
   Králové, ČSR (6 sculptures).

ADOLPHE DUPONT, Professor, Head of the Department of Dermatology, University of
   Louvain, Belgium (4 oils, 3 water colours).

ÅKE FERNSTRÖM, Dr. med., Stockholm, Sweden
   (3 gouaches).

FRANCO FLARER, Professor, Head of the Department of Dermatology, University of Padova,
   Italy (10 paintings in oil and gouache).

BELLA HEARST, M. D., Chicago, Ill., USA
   (8 graphics: lithographs, dry points and linoleum prints).

D. JANKE, Dr. med., Dermatologist, Fulda,
   Germany (1 oil).

KAZIMIERZ LEJMAN, Professor, Head of the
   Department of Dermatology, University of
   Krakow, Poland (6 graphics).

LUCIEN MARCERON († 1966), Dr. med., Neuilly-
   sur-Seine, France (3 oils, 1 water colour).

SCOTT MATHIESEN († 1963), Dermatologist, Oslo,
   Norway (23 drawings, viz. groups of caricatures, and 3 oil paintings).

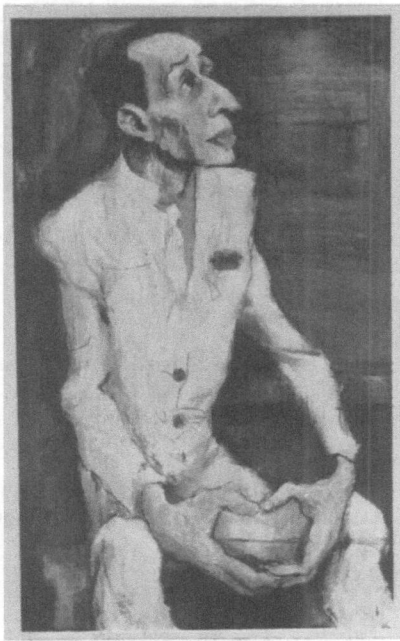

"Dr. Herrmann" (K. STEEN)

THEODOR NASEMANN, Dr. med., Ass. Professor, Munich, Germany (1 diorama).

HANS PFOSI († 1965), Dr. med., Dermatologist, Zürich, Switzerland (6 oils).

RAYMOND JACQUES SABOURAUD († 1938), Dr. med., world-famous Dermatologist and Mycologist, Head of the Laboratory and l'École Lailler at the Hôpital Saint Louis, Paris, France (3 bronze statuettes, 4 photographs of sculptures — Brocq, Darier, Civatte and Jeanselme — signed by SABOURAUD).

JÖRGEN SCHAUMANN († 1953), Dr. med., Professor — well known from his work on sarcoidosis — Stockholm, Sweden (3 oil paintings).

CARL ERIC SONCK, Professor, Head of the Department of Dermatology, University of Turku, Finland (1 group of caricatures, 14 oils).

KLAUS STEEN, Dr. med., Dermatologist, Hamburg-Blankenese, Germany (6 portraits, mixed technique).

HANS STORCK, Professor, Head of the Department of Dermatology, University of Zürich, Switzerland (23 water colours).

HARALD WINTER, Dermatologist, Schwäbisch Gmünd, Germany (6 water colours and 10 ceramics).

5*

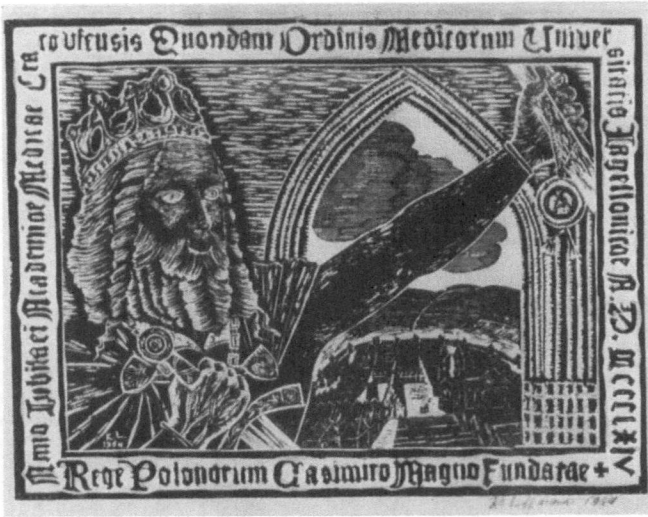

Graphic: "Anno Jubilaei Academiae Medicae
Cracoviensis" (K. LEJMAN)

Only two of the 24 participants (FLARER and WINTER) exhibited non-figurative art.

The exhibition did not comprise works only by living dermatologists, five deceased dermatologists were represented: MARCERON, MATHIESEN, PFOSI, SABOURAUD and SCHAU-MANN. I am indebted to their families, who were kind enough to lend us works for the exhibition.

Unfortunately, the following four "Dermatologists-artists" were unable to send works: SOLANGE LAMBERGEON, Paris; KJELL MOSSIGE and VALD. NYQUIST, Oslo, and ATTILIO ZANCA, Mantova, Italy.

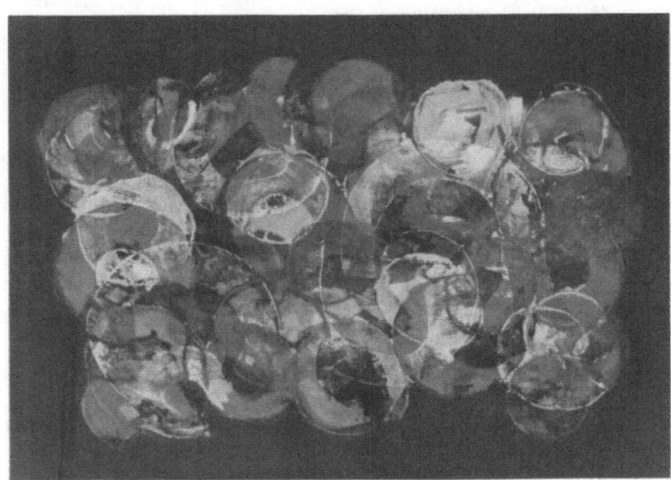

"Structure" (F. FLARER)

Film Program

Throughout the congress, the participants were able to follow two film programs informing them of new techniques, showing them rare ailments, new therapeutical methods etc.

The first program, organized in the context of the Scientific and Technical Exhibition, by Doz. Dr. K. BOSSE, was projected permanently throughout the congress in a 400 seat room.

The second program, prepared by Prof. MARION B. SULZBERGER and Mrs. ROBERTA Z. SULZBERGER, San Francisco, was projected on Friday afternoon, August 4, in the "Bayernhalle" (see page 1377, volume 2).

These two programs were of great interest to most of the visitors.

Projection de films

Pendant la durée du congrès, les participants ont pu suivre deux séries de films les informant sur la pratique de nouvelles techniques, leur montrant des affections rares, les renseignant sur de nouvelles méthodes thérapeutiques etc.

Le programme de la première série, organisé dans le cadre de l'Exposition Scientifique et Technique par le Doz. K. BOSSE, fut projeté en séances permanentes dans une salle de 400 places spécialement aménagée, pendant toute la semaine du congrès.

Le programme de la deuxième série, préparé par le Prof. MARION B. SULZBERGER et Mme. ROBERTA Z. SULZBERGER (San Francisco), fut projeté dans l'après-midi du vendredi 4 août, à la «Bayernhalle» (voir page 1377, volume 2).

Ces deux programmes intéressèrent un grand nombre de visiteurs.

Exhibición de Films

Durante toda la semana en que tuvo lugar el congreso, los participantes pudieron asistir a dos series de películas científicas informándoles sobre la práctica de nuevas técnicas, mostrándoles afecciones raras, dándoles cuenta de nuevos métodos terapéuticos, etc.

El programa de la primera serie, organizado en el cuadro de la Exposición Científica y Técnica por el Doz. Dr. K. BOSSE, fué exhibido en sesión continua, en una sala de 400 plazas, especialmente acondicionada, durante toda la semana de la celebración del congreso.

El programa de la segunda serie, organizado por el Prof. MARION B. SULZBERGER y la Sra. ROBERTA Z. SULZBERGER, de San Francisco, fué proyectado el viernes 4 de Agosto, en sesión de tarde, en la "Bayernhalle" (vease página 1377, volumen 2).

Ambos programas interesaron mucho a un gran número de asistentes a ellos.

Filmprogramme

Während des Kongresses hatten die Teilnehmer Gelegenheit, im Rahmen von zwei voneinander unabhängigen Filmprogrammen sich über neue technische Verfahren, besondere Krankheitsfälle, therapeutische Methoden u. ä. zu informieren.

Das erste Programm, dessen Organisation im Rahmen der wissenschaftlichen und pharmazeutischen Ausstellung durch Dozent Dr. K. BOSSE erfolgte, lief während der gesamten Kongreßwoche in einem Kinoraum mit 400 Sitzplätzen.

Das zweite Programm, das durch Prof. MARION B. SULZBERGER und Frau ROBERTA Z. SULZBERGER, San Francisco, vorbereitet worden war, wurde am Freitag nachmittag, dem 4. August, in der Bayernhalle vorgeführt (s. S. 1377, Band 2).

Das Interesse der Kongreßbesucher an diesen beiden Filmprogrammen war besonders rege.

Film Program — Programme Cinématographique — Películas Científicas — Filmprogramm

presented in the frame of the scientific and pharmaceutical exhibition

organisé dans le cadre de l'exposition scientifique et pharmaceutique

dentro del margen de la exposición científica-farmacéutico

im Rahmen der wissenschaftlichen und pharmazeutischen Ausstellung

(Privatdozent Dr. Dr. KLAUS BOSSE)

Types de mycétomes observés en Roumanie
> Avram, A., Bukarest (Roumanie)

Der heiße Frieden
> Badische Anilin- und Soda-Fabrik AG,
> Ludwigshafen/Rhein (Deutschland)

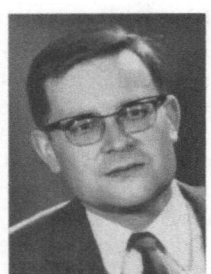

Hochfrequenz — Dermabrasion
Bayer AG, Leverkusen (Deutschland)

UV-Bestrahlung von Zellbestandteilen
Byk-Essex, München (Deutschland)

Psoriasis and its treatment
> Comaish, J. S., G. Holti, and S. Shuster, Newcastle Upon Tyne (Great Britain)

Epizoonosen
> Herrmann, F., und O. Schultka, Frankfurt/Main (Deutschland)

Diabetes
> Hoechst AG, Höchst (Deutschland)

Acanthosis nigricans with Malignancy
> Kleine-Natrop, H. E., Dresden (Deutschland)

Keratoacanthoma
> Kopf, W., New York (USA)

Impetigo herpetiformis
> Leonardi, G., Frankfurt /Main (Deutschland)

Fucidine, Antibioticum
> Löwens Pharma, Düsseldorf (Deutschland)

TG, ein fortschrittliches Verbandmittel, eine moderne Verbandtechnik
> Lohmann KG, Fahr/Rhein (Deutschland)

Der varicöse Symptomenkomplex und seine Behandlung
> Lohmann KG, Fahr/Rhein (Deutschland)

The microcirculation on skin and skin autographs of rat
> Marckmann, A., Copenhagen (Denmark)

The chemosurgical technique for the microscopically controlled excision of cancer in skin
> Mohs, F. E., Madison/Wisc. (USA)

Subläsionale Therapie mit Triamcinolon bei umschriebenen chronischen Dermatosen
> Nasemann, Th., München (Deutschland)

Allergische Dermatosen
Pfizer GmbH, Karlsruhe (Deutschland)

Turban Tumor
Proppe, A., und H. Hauss, Kiel (Deutschland)

Dermatosis cenicienta-Erythema dyschromicum perstans
Ramirez, O., El Salvador (San Salvador) y Convit, J., y F. Kerdel-Vegas, Caracas (Venezuela)

Genetic disorders of interest to dermatologists:
Congenital ectodermal defects Part I
Reed, W. B. (Moderator), and H. McKenzie (Editor), Burbank, Cal. (USA)

Genetic disorders of interest to dermatologists:
Congenital ectodermal defects Part II
Reed, W. B. (Moderator), and H. McKenzie (Editor), Burbank, Cal. (USA)

Genetic disorders of interest to dermatologists:
Neurocutaneous disorders Part I
Reed, W. B. (Moderator), and H. McKenzie (Editor), Burbank, Cal. (USA)

Genetic disorders of interest to dermatologists:
Neurocutaneous disorders Part II
Reed, W. B. (Moderator), and H. McKenzie (Editor), Burbank, Cal. (USA)

Genetic disorders of interest to dermatologists: Chromosomal abnormalities
Reed, W. B. (Moderator), and H. McKenzie (Editor), Burbank, Cal. (USA)

Haltung und Zucht keimfreier Tiere
Rheinpharma, Heidelberg (Deutschland)

Mykosen
Rieth, H., und C. Schirren, Hamburg, und Meinhof, W., München (Deutschland)

Rate of Hairgrowth
Saito, M., Tokyo (Japan)

Zellen im Laser-Strahl
Sandoz AG, Nürnberg (Deutschland)

Mechanismus der Entzündung
Sharp und Dohme, München (Deutschland)

Familial circumscribed Erythrokeratoderma
(Erythrokeratodermia Familiaris Circumscripta)
Sidi, E. †, J. Bourgeois-Spinasse et J. Arouete, Paris (France)

Pustular Psoriasis
Sidi, E. †, J. Bourgeois-Spinasse et J. Arouete, Paris (France)

Le cyto diagnostic
Sidi, E. †, J. Mawas et M. Meignant, Paris (France)

Toxic anhidrosis
Sulzberger, M. B., F. Herrmann, and D. Morrill, L. Mandol, New York (USA)

Dynamic pseudocancerous hyperplasia
Stevanovic, D. W., Belgrad (Yugoslavia)

Erythemosquamous and pustular spongiform eruption — benign variant of pustular psoriasis
Stevanovic, D. W., Belgrad (Yugoslavia)

Voyages after Congress

On the expressed desire of the Congress Organization Committee, a series of voyages were organized, by the German travel agency with its main office in Francfort, for the participants of the XIII Congress of Dermatology. These trips permitted dermatologists who were interested, to visit a certain number of Dermatological clinics, not only in the Federal Republic of Germany, but also in Poland, Hungary, Switzerland, France and Austria.

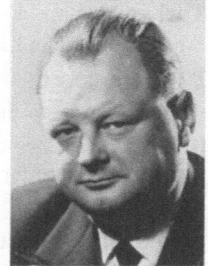

Prof. G. W. KORTING of Mainz, in collaboration with the above named travel agency, arranged five trips. Aside from visits to Dermatological Clinics and discussions with local dermatologists, the participants were able to engage into sight seeing of cities, became familiar with countries and places more or less unknown to them.

Tour 1: Göttingen — Berlin — Hamburg
Tour 2: Mainz — Bonn — Essen
Tour 3: Berlin — Warsaw — Cracow — Danzig
Tour 4: Vienna — Budapest — Debrecen
Tour 5: Zurich — Basel — Paris

Voyages post congrès

L'agence de voyages allemande, siègant à Francfort, organisa, sur demande du Comité d'Organisation, une série de voyages offerts aux participants du XIIIième Congrès International de Dermatologie. Ces voyages permirent aux dermatologistes intéressés de visiter un grand nombre de cliniques de Dermatologie, non seulement en Allemagne, mais également en Pologne, Hongrie, Suisse, France et Autriche.

Le Prof. G. W. KORTING, de Mayence, en collaboration avec cette agence de voyages, mit au point cinq voyages. A part les visites aux cliniques de Dermatologie, les participants eurent le loisir d'admirer de beaux paysages, de visiter des villes, des ports, des fabriques et prendre contact avec des pays parcourus souvent pour la première fois.

Tour 1. Göttingen — Berlin — Hambourg
Tour 2. Mayence — Bonn — Essen
Tour 3. Berlin — Varsovie — Cracovie — Danzig
Tour 4. Vienne — Budapest — Debrecen
Tour 5. Zurich — Bâle — Paris

Viajes post-Congreso

La Agencia Alemana de Viajes, con sede en Frankfort organizó, a petición del Comité de Organización, una serie de viajes destinados a los participantes al Congreso Internacional de Dermatología. Estos viajes ofrecían la posibilidad a los dermatólogos que tomaron parte en ellos, de visitar numerosas clínicas de dermatología, no solamente en Alemania, sino tambien en Polonia, Hungría, Suiza, Francia y Austria.

El Prof. G. W. KORTING de Mayence, en estrecha colaboración con la citada agencia organizó cinco viajes. Junto a las visitas de muchas clínicas dermatológicas y de discusiones animadas con los dermatólogos del lugar, los participantes tuvieron el placer de admirar hermosos paisajes, visitar ciudades, puertos, fábricas, así como de entrar en contacto personal con países que, en general, eran recorridos por vez primera. Los viajes organizados, a satisfacción de todos, fueron los siguientes:

Viaje 1. Göttingen — Berlin — Hamburgo
Viaje 2. Mayence — Bonn — Essen
Viaje 3. Berlin — Varsovia — Cracovia — Danzig
Viaje 4. Viena — Budapest — Debrecen
Viaje 5. Zurich — Basilea — Paris

Nachkongreßreisen

Für die Teilnehmer am XIII. Internationalen Kongreß für Dermatologie hatte das Deutsche Reisebüro in Frankfurt am Main auf Anregung der Kongreßleitung eine Reihe von Reisen zusammengestellt, die den interessierten Dermatologen die Möglichkeit boten, nach Beendigung des Kongresses einen persönlichen Einblick in eine Reihe von Hautkliniken nicht nur in Deutschland, sondern auch in Polen, Ungarn, der Schweiz, Frankreich und Österreich zu bekommen.

Das Deutsche Reisebüro verfügt mit einer eigenen Abteilung für Kongreßreisen über die nötige Erfahrung, um diese spezielle Form von Studienreisen durchführen zu können. In Zusammenarbeit mit dieser Reiseorganisation hatte Prof. G. W. KORTING, Mainz, fünf Rundreisetouren ausgearbeitet. Neben Führungen durch die Kliniken, neben Fachgesprächen mit dort arbeitenden Dermatologen, hatten die Teilnehmer noch ausreichend Gelegenheit, ein Stück Landschaft zu genießen, eine Stadtrundfahrt mit Besichtigung von interessanten Bauten zu unternehmen, Hafen- und Werksgelände zu besichtigen und somit einen abgerundeten Eindruck von den Ländern zu bekommen, die sie oft zum ersten Mal besuchen konnten.

Tour 1: Göttingen — Berlin — Hamburg
Tour 2: Mainz — Bonn — Essen
Tour 3: Berlin — Warschau — Krakau — Danzig
Tour 4: Wien — Budapest — Debrecen
Tour 5: Zürich — Basel — Paris

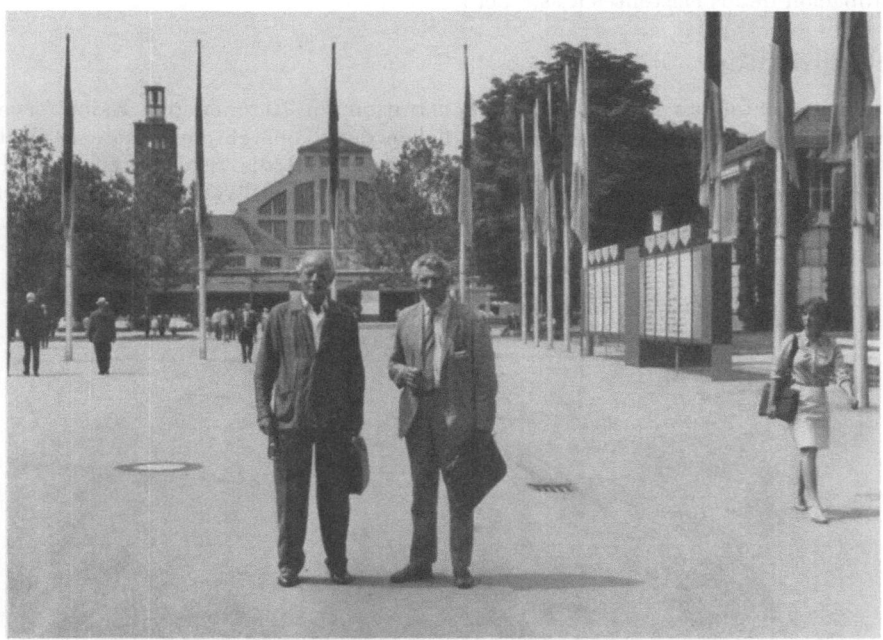

→ Prof. WIEDMANN, Doz. NIEBAUER, Doz. HUNZIKER

Closing Session

The closing session took place in the "Bayernhalle" immediately after the demonstration of patients with the Eidophor system of Ciba, Basle. Congressists as well as other doctors of the Munich area participated. Padua-Venice, chosen as the next congress place, received the approval of the assistance.

Séance de clôture

La séance de clôture eut lieu dans la «Bayernhalle» où venait de se terminer la démonstration de malades par le système Eidophore de la Maison Ciba Bâle. Non seulement des participants au congrès, mais également des médecins munichois y prirent part. Padoue-Venise choisie comme siège du prochain congrès reçut l'approbation de l'assistance.

Sesión de clausura

Tras la presentación televisada de enfermos, gracias al sistema Eidophor de la Casa Ciba de Basilea, en la Bayernhalle, tuvo lugar en esta misma sala la ceremonia de clausura del XIII. Congreso Internacional de Dermatología, a la que asistieron, además de los participantes, buen número de médicos de Munich. Padua-Venecia (Italia), lugar elegido como sede del próximo congreso, recibió la aprobación de los asistentes a este acto.

Schlußsitzung

Im Anschluß an die Krankendemonstration im Rahmen des Eidophorverfahrens der Firma Ciba, Basel, zu der neben den Kongreßteilnehmern auch die Ärzteschaft Münchens eingeladen worden war, fand die Schlußsitzung in der Bayernhalle des Kongreßgeländes statt. Mit großem Beifall verzeichneten die Kongreßteilnehmer die Wahl von Padua/Venedig zum nächsten Kongreßtagungsort.

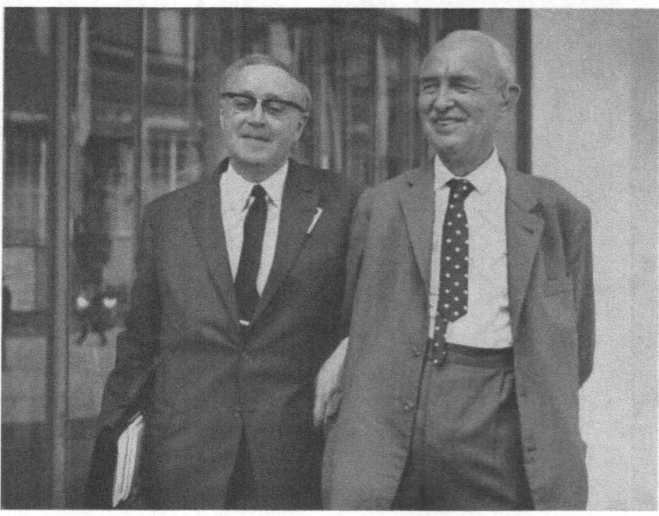

Prof. JORDAN, Prof. GOTTRON

Prof. Robert Degos

Monsieur le Président du Congrès, Mesdames, Messieurs!

Je ne pensais pas qu'il me serait demandé de prendre la parole à la Réunion de Clôture du Congrès. Je le fais avec grand plaisir, car je n'ai à formuler que des remerciements et des éloges.

Les souhaits d'un éclatant succès que je vous avais présentés, Monsieur le Président, à la séance d'ouverture, se sont réalisés sur tous les plans. Un congrès préparé avec autant de soins, et organisé avec autant de maîtrise et de minutie dans ses plus infimes détails, par vous et par le Prof. Schirren, ne pouvait se dérouler que de la façon la plus parfaite. Vous pouvez, tous les deux, être fiers de ce remarquable résultat et je pense qu'à cette joie d'une réussite totale s'ajoute la quiétude justement méritée d'un travail accompli et si bien accompli. Finis les soucis et les appréhensions, la crainte d'un incident de dernière heure: tout s'est merveilleusement passé et vous pouvez maintenant dormir tranquilles!

Vous avez acquis, Monsieur Jadassohn et Monsieur Schirren, la gratitude de la Dermatologie Mondiale pour cette magnifique réalisation qu'a été le XIIIe Congrès International. Grâce à la discipline des organisateurs, des Présidents de séance, des délégués du Comité allemand d'Organisation et des orateurs, le programme scientifique, si chargé, a été exécuté avec un minutage précis, ponctuellement observé, et avec un équilibre horaire permettant la présentation de rapports du plus grand intérêt, l'exposé de toutes les communications inscrites et des discussions fécondes. C'est là un tour de force rarement réalisé et que tous en soient remerciés.

Mais nos remerciements vont également aux femmes des responsables de l'organisation du congrès, aux Dames du Comité d'Accueil, à Madame Jadassohn et à Madame Schirren, en particulier. Elles ont certainement eu la responsabilité de la préparation et de l'exécution du programme social qui fut tout aussi remarquable que le programme scientifique et dont nous avons grandement apprécié les fastes, l'enchantement et l'atmosphère si amicale.

Nos remerciements vont enfin à tous nos hôtes qui nous ont si généreusement et si cordialement reçus. Nous avons été très honorés et très touchés d'être accueillis par le Président de la République Fédérale allemande, par le Ministre Président de l'Etat de Bavière, par le Maire de la ville de Munich et par toutes les hautes personnalités universitaires. Vous voudrez bien, Monsieur le Président et Monsieur le Secrétaire du Congrès, être nos interprètes auprès d'eux pour leur dire notre gratitude.

A vous, Monsieur Jadassohn et Monsieur Schirren, à vos équipes de travail, je vous redis, au nom de tous les congressistes, le plus chaleureux merci.

J'ai le plaisir de vous faire savoir que sur la proposition du Comité International de Dermatologie, l'Assemblée des Délégués de la Ligue Internationale des Sociétés de Dermatologie a nommé le Prof. Gay Prieto, de Madrid, Président du Comité International de Dermatologie pour la période 1967 à 1972.

Je n'ai pas besoin de rappeler la place éminente que le Prof. Gay Prieto occupe dans la dermatologie mondiale. A ce très cher ami, je remets les pouvoirs qui m'avaient été confiés à Washington en 1962, en lui disant mes très affectueuses félicitations.

Le prochain Congrès International aura lieu à Padoue-Venise en 1972. Il sera présidé par le Prof. Flarer que chacun connaissait en tant qu'éminent dermatologiste, mais dont beaucoup viennent de découvrir, à l'Exposition d'Art de ce Congrès, le remarquable talent de peintre.

Prof. WERNER JADASSOHN

Und jetzt wollen wir uns von Ihnen verabschieden. Es hat uns gefreut, daß Sie unsere Gäste waren und wir hoffen, Sie bald wiederzusehen. Danke und auf Wiedersehen.

Et maintenant, nous voulons prendre congé de vous. Nous espérons que ce congrès vous a plût et que nous aurons le plaisir de vous revoir. Merci et à bientôt.

And now we want to say good bye to you. It was a pleasure to have you as our guests and we hope to see you very soon again. Thank you and good bye.

Und jetzt denken Sie sicher, das war kurz und bündig und jetzt geht er weg vom Mikrophon und das Stück ist aus, so habt Ihr was Ihr wollt. Sie irren sich, ich bleibe noch hier, denn ich habe noch Wichtiges zu sagen und ich bedaure, daß ich mich kurz fassen muß.

Dem Präsidenten Herrn DEGOS, dem Generalsekretär Herrn HELLERSTRÖM und den Mitgliedern des Internationalen Komitees habe ich schon gedankt. Ich wiederhole, daß ich ihnen sehr dankbar bin. Ich möchte mich aber bei sehr vielen andern auch noch bedanken, z. B. bei den Mitgliedern des Organisationskomitees, den Kollegen GANS, GÖTZ, MEMMESHEIMER und SIEMENS, die, abgesehen von allem andern was sie getan haben, meine Frau und mich in Genf besucht haben. Herrn WIEDMANN, der mir nie in die Suppe gespuckt hat, trotzdem er das, als Präsident der Deutschen Dermatologischen Gesellschaft, gewiß hätte tun können. Herrn Kollegen GOTTRON danke ich, daß er gekommen ist; man mußte ihm stark zureden. Herrn LINSER, den ich seit Jahrzehnten kenne, und Herrn GERTLER danke ich für ihre freundlichen Briefe. Herrn BRAUN-FALCO habe ich schon gratuliert, jetzt möchte ich ihm und Herrn SCHNEIDER für die so ausgezeichnete Zusammenarbeit danken. Zusammenarbeit, d. h. sie haben gearbeitet und ich habe mich an ihren Resultaten gefreut. Die Herren ARETZ, BOHNSTEDT, HERRMANN, KALKOFF, KIMMIG, KORTING und SPIER haben mich bei den Sitzungen des Ausschusses der Deutschen Dermatologischen Gesellschaft immer unterstützt.

Sehr herzlich danken möchte ich auch noch Herrn Dr. VON GRIESHEIM, der sich um die traurigen Finanzen des Kongresses bemüht hat.

Ganz besonders danken möchte ich Herrn NASEMANN und Herrn BANDMANN. Sie haben nicht nur das Gesellschaftliche Programm respektive die Wissenschaftliche Ausstellung organisiert, sondern mir in schwierigen Situationen immer zur Seite gestanden.

Danken möchte ich, und zwar sehr herzlich, den Mitarbeitern von Herrn SCHNEIDER, Herrn TRONNIER und Herrn ADAM; dem Mitarbeiter von Herrn BANDMANN, Herrn BOSSE.

Danken möchte ich Herrn Kollegen SONCK, der die Kunstausstellung nicht nur durchgeführt, sondern, wenn man so sagen darf, erfunden hat.

Sehr dankbar bin ich Herrn KOCH, Fräulein FREY und ihren Mitarbeitern für ihre Arbeit im Kongreßbüro, die keineswegs leicht war, und meiner Sekretärin, Fräulein BOSSHARD. Ich danke den Kollegenfrauen des Damenkomitees, Frau BANDMANN, Frau BRAUN-FALCO, Frau GÖTZ, Frau NASEMANN und FRAU SCHIRREN; auch meine Frau war Mitglied dieses Komitees. Ich danke, wenn Sie einverstanden sind, in globo, allen Präsidenten der Sitzungen, allen Delegierten des Organisationskomitees, allen Rednern, allen Teilnehmern des Kongresses und allen Ausstellern.

Ich bin noch nicht fertig. Lieber Herr SCHIRREN, lieber Herr Generalsekretär. Man sollte das Sekretär weglassen. Wie ein General, aber wie ein sehr gutmütiger

General, haben Sie die große Arbeit geleistet, und Ihre mir erwiesene Freundschaft während der Kongreßvorbereitung ist für mich etwas sehr Wertvolles gewesen und wird es bleiben.

Meine allerherzlichsten Wünsche dem neuen Präsidenten des Internationalen Komitees, dem neuen Generalsekretär, dem neuen Kongreßpräsidenten, dem neuen Kongreßgeneralsekretär und Ihnen allen, liebe Kolleginnen und Kollegen.

Auf Wiedersehen!

Prof. GAY PRIETO, the newly elected President of the International Committee of Dermatology

Le Prof. GAY PRIETO, nouveau Président du Comité International de Dermatologie

El Prof. GAY PRIETO, nuevo Presidente electo del Comité Internacional de Dermatología

Prof. GAY PRIETO, der neu gewählte Präsident des Internationalen Komitees

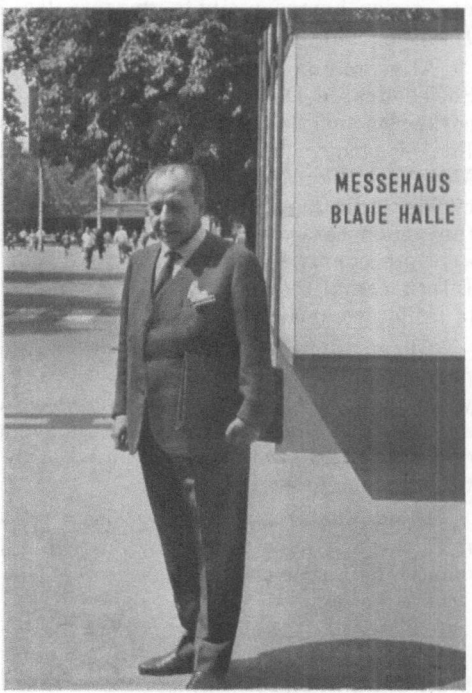

Prof. JOSÉ GAY PRIETO

Señoras y Señores!

Es con profunda emoción que recojo este martillo simbólico, de manos de mi querido y entrañable amigo el Prof. WERNER JADASSOHN.

Estais todos fatigados de 5 días de un Congreso agotador y quiero únicamente pronunciar muy pocas palabras para expresar a todos mi agradecimiento. Vais a perdonarme que abusando de la existencia de la interpretación simultánea hable exclusivamente español, que es 1 de las 4 lenguas oficiales del Congreso. A ello me obliga en primer lugar mi condición de español y el agradecimiento que debo particularmente a todo el grupo hispano-parlante del congreso que con su presencia y con sus votos me ha animado estos años pasados. Ya tuve ocasión de dirigirme a los delegados para agradecerles su elección ayer en los cuatro idiomas oficiales del congreso, hoy el estado emocional me impide hacerlo en cualquier otro, que no sea mi lengua materna.

Debo en primer lugar, resaltar el mérito extraordinario del Presidente del Congreso Prof. JADASSOHN que por el fallecimiento de nuestro llorado amigo el Prof. MARCHIONINI, ha tenido que hacerse cargo de la dirección de un Congreso Internacional de la amplitud del que acaba de terminar, lejos de sus medios habituales de trabajo. Si ha podido llevar a cabo con una perfección no igualada el trabajo extraordinario de organización de este congreso ha sido, y el es, el primero en proclamarlo, gracias a la colaboración desinteresada y abnegada del Secretario General Prof. SCHIRREN, al que me complazco en felicitar, y de todos los colaboradores que han formado el comité local organizador del congreso.

A todos ellos quiero expresar en nombre de todos vosotros el agradecimiento de todos los congresistas, por la perfecta organización del congreso y por las atenciones que todos hemos recibido durante los 5 días inolvidables del XIII. Congreso Internacional de Dermatología.

Al asumir por 5 años el mandato difícil, de presidir la Liga Internacional de Sociedades de Dermatología y el Comité Internacional, no puedo menos de recordar las cualidades de mis predecesores que hacen todavía mas pesada mi carga. Fue el primer Presidente elegido en el congreso de Londres el Prof. GUIDO MIESCHER, figura señera de la dermatología mundial que muchos de vosotros conocisteis y admirásteis; le sucedió una persona de un dinamismo y de una inteligencia tan aguda como el Prof. MARION SULZBERGER de New York y últimamente los 5 años precedentes, la Liga International de Sociedades de Dermatología y el Comité Internacional ha sido regido con singular maestría por el Prof. DEGOS, con toda la brillantez y claridad de su personalidad latina y francesa.

Abrumadora carga es la sucesión de estos tres grandes hombres. Unicamente puedo prometeros el consagrar a este puesto lo mejor de lo que me queda de vida y lo mejor de mis afanes, para intentar (aunque seguramente no podré conseguirlo) que el nuevo Comité Internacional de Dermatología que me cabe la honra de presidir, no desmerezca en su labor de la realizada durante el mandato de mis tres predecesores.

Dando una vez más las gracias a todos por la elección y prometiendo una vez más tratar de hacerme digno de la confianza en mí depositada, digo a todos, hasta dentro de 5 años en Italia.

Prof. CARL GEORG SCHIRREN

Meine sehr verehrten Damen und Herren!

Der XIII. Internationale Kongreß für Dermatologie ist zu Ende. Prof. R. DEGOS und Prof. W. JADASSOHN haben in ihren Vorreden in überaus freundlicher Weise auf meine Verdienste bei der Vorbereitung und Durchführung dieses großen Kongresses hingewiesen. Erlauben Sie mir, daß ich diesen Dank in gleicher Weise wie die Arbeit in den vergangenen Jahren an meine zahlreichen Mitarbeiter delegiere. Ohne ihre Hilfe und ohne ihre Selbstlosigkeit wäre all mein Bemühen nur Stückwerk gewesen.

Ich denke besonders an die Prof. NASEMANN und BANDMANN, an das Kongreßbüro unter Leitung von Herrn A. KOCH mit Fräulein FREY, Fräulein KAHN und Fräulein WALLACH, an die deutschen Dermatologen und Univ.-Hautkliniken, an unser Architektenbüro MINARIK sowie an die 21 Hostessen und 22 technischen Bediensteten, die während des Kongresses tätig waren. Letztere haben ihre Aufgaben während dieser von der Sonne so reich bedachten Kongreßwoche in den zehn Vortragssälen und in den Projektionsräumen unter oft nicht ganz einfachen Bedingungen versehen müssen. Das 25köpfige Dolmetscherteam vom Medizinischen Sprachendienst KLITSCHER hat in den Boxen unserer Verhandlungssäle während eines neunstündigen Arbeitstages fast Übermenschliches geleistet. Ihnen allen gilt heute unser besonderer Dank!

Aber auch Ihnen, meine Damen und Herren, haben wir zu danken, daß Sie eine Woche ausgehalten haben. Sie haben unsere Mühen durch ein ungewöhnlich großes Interesse an den Verhandlungen belohnt. Sie haben darüber hinaus in reichstem Maße an unserem gesellschaftlichen Programm teilgenommen. Der Begrüßungsabend war mit 2500, das Bachkonzert mit 1220, die Oper mit 1050, die Chiemseefahrt mit 900, der Abendbesuch der Museen mit 800 und der Bayerische Abend mit 2044 Teilnehmern erstaunlich gut besucht, um hier nur die wichtigsten der über 20 Veranstaltungen zu nennen.

Wir luden Sie ein unter dem Motto: „Und wenn Ihr kommt, Ihr sollt willkommen sein."

Wir schließen diesen Kongreß mit dem abgewandelten Einladungsmotto: „Und wenn Ihr geht und wart zufrieden, soll's uns willkommen sein."

Auf Wiedersehen 1972 in Padua/Venedig bei Prof. FLARER!

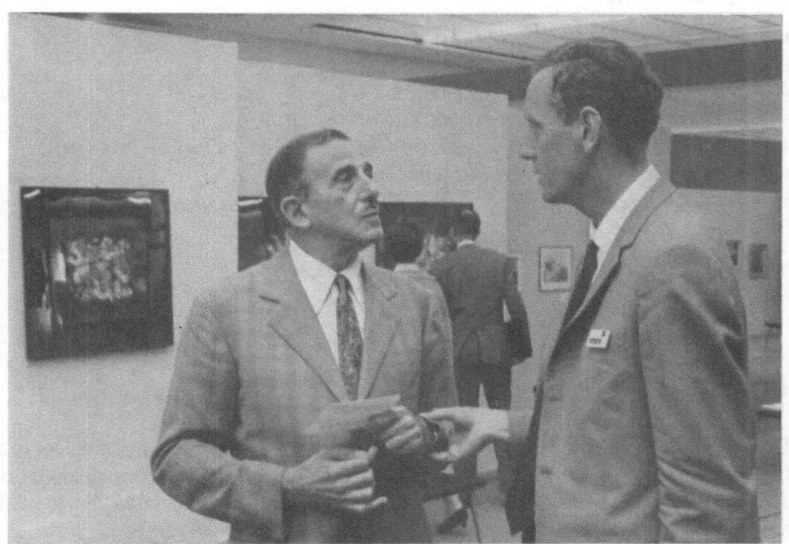

Prof. F. FLARER, President of the XIV. International Congress of Dermatology, Padua/Italy, talking with Prof. C. G. SCHIRREN

Donations

The Organization Committee of the XIIIth International Congress of Dermatology would like to express its gratitude to all those who by their generous donations have contributed to the realization of this great manifestation. We address our thanks especially:

to the *Government of the Federal Republic of Germany*,
to the *Government of the State of Bavaria*,
to the *City of Munich*,
to the *German Academy of Cultural Exchange* as well as,
to the *Pharmaceutical and Medico-Technical Industry*,
to various *Societies of Dermatology*, and,
to the *Dermatologists of the Federal Republic of Germany*.

Dons

Le Comité d'Organisation du XIIIième Congrès International de Dermatologie exprime sa reconnaissance à tous ceux qui, par des dons généreux, ont contribué grandement à la réalisation de cette grande manifestation. Nos remerciements vont tout particulièrement:

au *Gouvernement de la République Fédérale d'Allemagne*,
au *Gouvernement de l'Etat de Bavière*,
à *la ville de Munich*,
à *l'Académie allemande d'échanges culturels*, ainsi,
qu'aux *firmes pharmaceutiques* et de *l'industrie de technique médicale*,
à différentes *sociétés de Dermatologie*, et,
aux *dermatologues de la République Fédérale d'Allemagne*.

Dones

El Comité de Organización del XIII. Congreso Internacional de Dermatología se complace en agradecer todos aquellos, que, por medio de generosos dones, han contribuído a la realización de esta gran manifestación. Nuestro reconocimiento se dirige, muy particularmente, a:

Gobierno de la República Federal Alemana,
Gobierno del Estado de Baviera,
Ciudad de Munich,
Academia alemana del intercambio cultural, asi, como a
las *firmas farmacéuticas* y de la *industria técnica médica*,
a diversos *sociedades de Dermatología*, y
a nuestros *colegas dermatólogos de la República Federal Alemana*.

Spenden

Das Organisationskomitee des XIII. Internationalen Kongresses für Dermatologie möchte an dieser Stelle noch einmal all denen danken, die mit ihrer großzügigen finanziellen Unterstützung diesen Kongreß ermöglicht haben. Unser besonderer Dank gilt:

der *Regierung der Bundesrepublik Deutschland,*
der *Regierung des Freistaates Bayern,*
der *Landeshauptstadt München,*
dem *Deutschen Akademischen Austauschdienst* sowie
den *Firmen der pharmazeutischen und medizinisch-technischen Industrie,*
verschiedenen *dermatologischen Gesellschaften* und
den *deutschen Dermatologen.*

Spenden von Firmen (ausstellende Firmen siehe Seite *62—63*)

P. Beiersdorf und Co. AG, Hamburg
Desitin-Werk Carl Klinke GmbH, Hamburg
Haarmann und Reiner GmbH, Holzminden
Chemische Fabrik von Heyden AG, München
Deutsche Hoffmann-La Roche AG, Grenzach/Baden
Paul Lappe GmbH, Bensberg-Köln
Dr. Madaus und Co., Köln
Pfizer GmbH, Karlsruhe
Röhm und Haas Pharma GmbH, Darmstadt
Dr. K. Thomae, Chem.-pharm. Fabrik, Biberach an der Riss
Chemische Fabrik Carl Wilden, Neu-Isenburg

Spenden von Dermatologischen Gesellschaften

Rheinisch-Westfälische Dermatologische Gesellschaft
Schweizerische Gesellschaft zur Bekämpfung der Geschlechtskrankheiten und
    Dermatologische Klinik der Universität Bern
Verband der Niedergelassenen Dermatologen Deutschlands

Spenden von deutschen Dermatologen

Dr. H. Adae, Stuttgart
Dr. W. Adelung, Singen
Dr. F. Aichinger, Weingarten
Dr. G. Albus, Köln-Brück
Dr. V. Amtmann, Weiden
Dr. R. Anger, Stuttgart
Dr. H. Antz, Mönchengladbach
Dr. H. Aretz, Velbert
Dr. F. Asbeck, Lübeck

Dr. H. Barmeyer, Braunschweig
Dr. H. J. Barnewitz, Witten
Dr. E. Baumann, Freudenstadt
Dr. R. Baumann, Andernach
Dr. F. Beck, Nürnberg
Dr. K. G. Becker, Einbeck
Dr. E. Berg, Hamburg
Dr. F. Betz, Koblenz
Dr. E. Binder, Würzburg
Dr. Th. Blum, Frankfurt a. M.
Dr. Blüthner, Öhringen
Dr. H. D. Bock, Augsburg
Prof. Dr. H. G. Bode, Göttingen
Dr. K. H. Böcker, Walsrode
Dr. C. Böhm, München

Dr. G. Boesmann, Tuttlingen
Prof. Dr. R. M. Bohnstedt, Gießen
Prof. Dr. Dr. S. Borelli, München
Dr. M. Bormann, Hamburg
Dr. A. Brachte, Mainz
Dr. H. Bräuer, Essen
Dr. W. G. Bräuer, Mannheim
Prof. Dr. O. Braun-Falco, Marburg
Dr. M. Brenner-Rheinboldt, Bad Homburg
Dr. E. Breyen, Berlin
Dr. K. Bruder, Fulda
Dr. A. Brun, Wiesbaden
Dr. L. Burgmann, Frankfurt
Dr. H. J. Burmester, Uelzen
Dr. N. Busch, Ulm
Dr. F. Buttermann, Berlin

Prof. Dr. C. Carrié, Dortmund
Dr. M. de La Chaux, Neumünster
Dr. N. Christ, Neuwied
Dr. H. Conzelmann, Bietigheim

Dr. W. Dahlen, Heidenheim
Dr. C. C. Daniels, Bielefeld
Dr. I. Demuth, Pforzheim

Dr. C. Dibowski, Rotenburg
Dr. H. Dittrich, Essen
Dr. K. H. Doerr, Ludwigshafen
Dr. J. Dormann, Freiburg
Dr. A. Drisch, Aachen
Dr. R. Düker, Lüchow
Dr. H. Dürr, Ulm
Dr. G. Dürre, Reutlingen

Dr. A. Edelmann, Bayreuth
Prof. Dr. Ehring, Handorf
Dr. H. Eichert, Koblenz
Dr. U. Ellerbroek, Hamburg
Prof. Dr. W. Engelhardt, Rottweil

Dr. H. Fabry, Bochum
Prof. Dr. F. Fegeler, Münster
Dr. C. Fichtner, München
Dr. M. Fiebig, Köln
Prof. Dr. C. Fischer, Urach
Dr. H. Fischer, Hannover
Dr. H. Fischer, Bad Mergentheim
Dr. H. Fischer, Osnabrück
Dr. R. Fischer, Hamm
Dr. O. Fleischer, Göppingen
Dr. C. Flinsch, Frankfurt
Dr. Fölsch, Bremen
Dr. H. Förster, Paderborn
Prof. Dr. Früwald, Hamburg
Dr. F. Fuchs, Neu-Ulm
Dr. W. Fuchs, Oestrich
Dr. W. Fürste, Berlin
Prof. Dr. C. F. Funk, Regensburg

Prof. Dr. W. Gahlen, Aachen
Dr. G. Gaide, Gelsenkirchen
Prof. Dr. Dr. O. Gans, Frankfurt/Comano
Prof. Dr. H. Gartmann, Köln
Dr. D. Gerke-Mosler, Hannover
Dr. K. Giesing, Krefeld
Dr. W. Gillesberger, München
Dr. G. Giss, Freiburg
Dr. W. Gockell, Bad Dürkheim
Dr. W. Goebel, Minden
Dr. W. Görtz, Hamburg
Prof. Dr. H. Götz, Essen
Dr. Th. Gottron-Killian, Tübingen
Dr. K. Goyert, Traunstein
Dr. H. Graatz, Sulzbach-Rosenberg
Dr. K. Grässner, Lüneburg
Dr. W. Grasreiner, Backnang
Dr. F. Grasser, Volklingen
Dr. J. Gratza, München
Dr. V. Gregorczyk, Kaiserslautern
Prof. Dr. A. Greither, Düsseldorf
Dr. I. Grütz, Siegburg

Dr. F. Haas, Villingen
Dr. O. Habersack, München
Dr. K. Hack, Stuttgart
Dr. H. Hackeloer, Siegen
Dr. R. Hagemann, Bielefeld
Dr. F. Hagen, Dortmund
Dr. H. Hagenburger, Neustadt/Weinstraße
Dr. A. Hamm, Dortmund

Dr. G. Hampel, Aalen
Dr. B. Hanow, Mühlheim
Dr. K. J. Hartmann, Mönchengladbach
Prof. Dr. J. Hartung, Hannover
Dr. L. Hasslinger, Nienburg
Dr. R. Hatton, Günzburg
Prof. Dr. W. Hauser, Bonn
Dr. G. Heilgemeier, Augsburg
Dr. F. Heim, Hildesheim
Dr. L. Heiter-Beier, Nürnberg
Dr. S. Helle, Berlin
Dr. W. Heller, Mülheim
Dr. F. Hennemann, Osnabrück
Dr. H. W. Hennies, Baden-Baden
Dr. Th. Herberhold, Dorsten
Dr. A. Herfeld, Bad Salzuflen
Dr. R. Herger, Langen
Prof. Dr. F. Herrmann, Frankfurt
Dr. W. Hermann, Hamburg
Dr. W. Hertner, Heilbronn
Prof. Dr. J. Herzberg, Bremen
Prof. Dr. P. Hess, Duisburg
Dr. P. Himmel, Wolfsburg
Dr. C. Hövelborn, Bad Cannstatt
Dr. E. Hoffmann, Ludwigsburg
Dr. G. W. Hofmeister, Wiesbaden
Dr. W. Holle, Bielefeld
Dr. K. H. Holtz, Ravensburg
Dr. H. Holzamer, Frankfurt
Prof. Dr. G. Hopf, Hamburg
Dr. W. Hoppe, Stuttgart
Prof. Dr. O. Hornstein, Düsseldorf
Dr. K. H. Huhn, Worms
Dr. B. Huber, München

Prof. Dr. L. Illig, Freiburg
Dr. Immel, Darmstadt
Prof. Dr. H. Ippen, Düsseldorf

Dr. H. Jacobs, Düsseldorf
Dr. M. Jänner, Hamburg
Dr. D. Janke, Fulda
Dr. H. Johne, München
Dr. K. Jonas-Gülden, Neviges
Dr. A. Juncker, Mannheim
Dr. W. Jungfermann, Heidelberg
Dr. W. Junius, Duisburg

Prof. Dr. R. Kaden, Berlin
Dr. L. Kagel, Berlin
Dr. B. Kaiser, Darmstadt
Prof. Dr. K. W. Kalkoff, Freiburg
Dr. K. Kalmus, Wilhelmshaven
Dr. A. Kampa, Heinsberg
Dr. H. Kandler, Frankfurt/M.
Dr. A. Kaul, Berlin
Dr. G. Kauws, Rheine
Dr. W. Keilig, München
Dr. H. Keinath, Stuttgart
Prof. Dr. E. Keining, Mainz
Dr. R. Kersten, Bamberg
Dr. I. Kieferle, Berchtesgaden
Dr. H. Kiermayr, Dortmund
Prof. Dr. J. Kimmig, Hamburg
Dr. Ch. Klärner, Berlin

Dr. H. Klein, Gießen
Dr. H. Kletsch, Kornwestheim
Dr. G. Klostermann, Göttingen
Dr. H. Knapp, Offenbach
Dr. R. C. Knoth, Gießen
Prof. Dr. W. Knoth, Gießen
Dr. F. Knust, Münster
Prof. Dr. H. Koehler, Lübeck
Dr. G. Körfgen, Schwäbisch Gmünd
Dr. W. Kollmeier, Dortmund
Dr. G. Korsukewitz, Berlin
Prof. Dr. G. W. Korting, Mainz
Dr. F. Kortmann, Bielefeld
Dr. W. Korn, Bielefeld
Dr. A. Kowallek, Berlin
Dr. H. Knapp, Offenbach
Dr. H. Krause, Schwäbisch Gmünd
Dr. J. Kremser, Bad Tölz
Dr. M. Kressmann, Nürnberg
Dr. J. Krieg, Düsseldorf
Dr. H. Kriegk, Bremen
Dr. H. Krüger, Berlin
Dr. R. Kurz, Mannheim-Freudenheim
Dr. H. Kutscher, Hamburg

Prof. Dr. E. Landes, Darmstadt
Dr. A. Lauck, München
Dr. U. Laumanns, Duisburg
Dr. R. Ledig, Stuttgart
Dr. H. Lehner, Pirmasens
Prof. Dr. A. Leinbrock, Bonn
Dr. R. Leis, Coburg
Prof. Dr. G. Leonardi, Frankfurt
Dr. Leopold, Gelsenkirchen
Dr. S. Limberger, Stuttgart
Dr. H. Limbourg, Troisdorf
Dr. L. Lindemann, Dieburg
Dr. F. Lippert, Stuttgart
Dr. W. Locher, Ulm
Dr. Lohmann, Rheydt
Dr. K. Lucius, Berlin
Dr. K. H. Lyndian, Limburg

Prof. Dr. A. Marchionini, München
Dr. G. Marhoven, Neuburg/Donau
Dr. M. Marosi, Waldbröl
Dr. H. Martin, Pirmasens
Dr. R. Marx, Wuppertal
Dr. H. H. Mau, Hamburg
Dr. H. K. Mayr, Berlin
Dr. W. Meisterernst, Saarbrücken
Prof. Dr. A. Memmesheimer, Essen
Dr. E. Mendl, Mühldorf
Dr. K. J. Mense, Kassel
Dr. E. Mertin-Ablass, Neustadt
Dr. K. Merzweiler, Freiburg
Dr. G. Meyer-Hamme, Helmstedt
Prof. Dr. J. Meyer-Rohn, Hamburg
Priv. Doz. Dr. W. Meyhöfer, Gießen
Dr. W. Michel, Frankfurt/M.
Dr. K. Miethke, Mettmann
Dr. K. Miso, Augsburg
Dr. B. Mohrmann, Hannover
Dr. J. Morawitz, Brunsbüttelkoog
Dr. F. X. Müller, Rosenheim

Dr. G. Müller, Oberhausen
Dr. J. F. Müller, Recklinghausen
Dr. H. Münzenmaier, Ludwigsburg
Dr. H. Mussler, Emmendingen

Dr. A. Naegele, Speyer
Dr. V. Napp, Duisburg
Dr. M. Nase, Wiedenbrück
Dr. Neidmann, Kamen
Prof. Dr. W. Nikolowski, Neusäss
Dr. E. Niske, Frankfurt
Dr. D. Nitschke, Landshut
Dr. H. Nöhricke, Memmingen
Dr. E. Noske, Frankfurt/M.
Dr. H. Nückel, Oberhausen

Dr. Oberesch, Lippstadt
Prof. Dr. H. Oberste-Lehn, Wuppertal
Dr. Ch. Oehmichen, Urach
Dr. H. Oppermann, Düsseldorf
Dr. H. W. Ortner, Forchheim
Dr. K. M. Ott, Offenbach

Dr. R. Pachur, Hamburg
Dr. U. Pantke, Schwelm
Dr. Th. Papayannis, Frankfurt
Dr. G. Perschmann, Stuttgart
Dr. K. W. Peter, Kassel
Dr. K. Pettker, Verden
Prof. Dr. R. Pfister, Karlsruhe
Prof. Dr. G. Polemann, Krefeld
Dr. E. Prange, Gaggenau-Ottenau
Dr. J. A. von Preyss, Hamburg
Prof. Dr. A. Proppe, Kiel
Dr. W. Pürschel, Nordseebad Norderney
Dr. H. J. Puppel, Braunschweig
Dr. H. Pusch, Kaufbeuren

Dr. R. Reges, Worms
Dr. A. M. Reichel, München
Dr. W. Reipen, Olpe
Dr. P. A. Rentrop, Bonn
Dr. W. Riess, Bamberg
Prof. Dr. H. Röckl, Würzburg
Dr. Rogg, Wilhelmshaven
Dr. R. Rosenkränzer, Essen
Prof. Dr. G. A. Rost, Berlin
Dr. W. Rudolf, Heidelberg
Dr. H. Ruhrmann, Düsseldorf

Dr. W. Sevin, Stuttgart
Dr. C. W. Siewert, Hagen
Dr. K. Sinning, Bad Hersfeld
Dr. J. Sitzberger, Fürth
Dr. H. Smattosch, Ludwigshafen
Dr. M. Söhnchen, Hermülheim
Dr. G. Sparmann, Northeim
Prof. Dr. H. W. Spier, Berlin
Dr. F. Sprenger, Mainz
Dr. Ch. Schäfer, Ansbach
Dr. F. Schandelmaier, Itzehoe
Dr. W. Scharmann, Stuttgart
Dr. B. Schierse, Eschwege
Dr. Schipke, Oberhausen
Prof. Dr. C. G. Schirren, München

6*

Prof. Dr. C. Schirren, Hamburg
Dr. K. Schirren, Kiel
Dr. Schlaeger, Oldenburg
Dr. F. W. Schlockermann, Berlin
Dr. H. Schlote, Krefeld
Prof. Dr. W. Schmidt, Mannheim
Prof. Dr. Schmidt La Baume, Baden-Baden
Prof. Dr. R. Schmitz, Esslingen
Dr. J. Schmitz, Fürth
Prof. Dr. W. Schneider, Tübingen
Prof. Dr. U. Schnyder, Heidelberg
Dr. H. Schöbel, Stuttgart
Dr. K. H. Schölzke, Essen
Dr. H. F. Schrader, Lörrach
Prof. Dr. Th. Schreus, Düsseldorf
Dr. Schrooten, Moers
Dr. W. Schult, Bamberg
Dr. H. Schümmer, Düsseldorf
Dr. R. Schultze, Osnabrück
Dr. F. Schulz, Fulda
Prof. Dr. K. H. Schulz, Hamburg
Dr. W. Schumann, Lübeck
Dr. H. J. Schuppener, Essen
Dr. H. Schuster, Bad Godesberg
Dr. K. Steen, Hamburg
Prof. Dr. G. K. Steigleder, Köln
Dr. H. Stein, Hanau
Dr. R. Steinberg, Bielefeld
Dr. W. Steins, Essen
Dr. W. Stocke, Ludwigshafen
Dr. G. Strocka, Frankfurt
Dr. Dr. F. Sturm, Montabaur
Prof. Dr. G. Stüttgen, Frankfurt

Dr. J. Tangl, Kirchheim
Prof. Dr. H. Teller, Berlin
Dr. G. Thaesler, Radolfszell
Dr. E. Thaler, Regensburg
Dr. K. Thies, Berlin
Dr. K. H. Thies, Celle
Dr. W. Thies, Berlin
Dr. J. Thimm, Essen
Dr. K. Thomae, Biberach
Dr. J. Thomas, Ludwigsburg
Dr. G. Tiedemann, Neu-Ulm
Dr. K. H. Trinczek, Schorndorf
Dr. W. Tschackert, Alsfeld
Dr. B. Tümmers, Ulm

Dr. B. Uedinghoff, Hamm
Dr. W. Uhlmann, Calw
Dr. P. J. Unna, Hamburg

Dr. Vogel, Bremerhaven
Dr. M. Voormann, Berlin
Dr. Fr. Voss, Köln-Riehl
Dr. H. Voss, Hamburg
Dr. K. Walker, Stuttgart
Dr. A. A. Wanger, Heidelberg
Dr. R. Wawersig, Berlin
Prof. Dr. G. Weber, Mainz
Prof. Dr. G. Weger, Stuttgart
Dr. E. Wegner, Hannover
Dr. G. Weigel, Gelsenkirchen
Dr. A. Weigl, Kaiserslautern
Dr. M. Weingärtner, München
Dr. A. Welcker, Wetzlar
Dr. R. Wendt, Heidenheim
Dr. H. Wezel, Fellbach
Dr. A. Wiemers, Frankfurt-Höchst
Dr. L. Wifling, Ansbach
Prof. Dr. H. Wilde, Gelsenkirchen
Dr. H. J. Wilk, Bad Kreuznach
Dr. G. Wilkening, Celle
Dr. H. Willwohl, Mainz
Prof. Dr. K. H. Woeber, Aachen
Prof. Dr. K. Woeber, Verlautenheim
Dr. U. Wolfskehl, Darmstadt
Dr. E. Wollnitza, Schwäbisch Hall
Dr. K. Wolpert, Garmisch
Prof. Dr. K. C. Wulf, Kassel

Dr. K. A. von Zezschwitz, Wangen
Prof. Dr. P. Zierz, Ludwigshafen
Dr. F. Zimmer, Düsseldorf
Dr. A. Zimmermann, Iserlohn
Dr. F. Zimmern, Hamburg
Dr. Zöller, Aschaffenburg

*

Österreich:

Prof. Dr. H. Loos, Innsbruck
Prof. Dr. A. Wiedmann, Wien

USA:

Dr. C. J. S. Herzog, South Norwalk, Conn.

Members of the Congress

This list includes all registrants, some of whom registered before the Congress but due to unforeseen circumstances, were not able to attend the meeting.

Algeria
Marill, François-Georges

Argentina
Acardi, Cesar B.
Ambrosetti, Félix E.
Arditi, Félix
Arguello, Ramón Adrian
Astore, Ignacio
Azar, Abdon
Baliña, Luis Maria
Benzaquen, Iliana
Bianchi, Carlos Albert
Bianchi, Oscar J.
Bianco, Enrique José
Cardama, José Esteban
Casala, Augusto Manuel
Chouela, Alfredo
Daje, Antonio Omar
Duran-Suffern, Luis Alberto
Fuertes, Juan A.
Gatti, Juan Carlos
Grinspan-Bozza, Norberto O.
Grinspan, David
Guillot, Pedro Esteban
Kaminsky, Aaron
Kaminsky, Ana Rosental de
Kaminsky, Carlos Alberto
Kriner, José
Lopez-Gonzales, Gerónimo
Lucena, Carlos Eduardo
Madeo, Vicente
Molina, Eduardo Benito
Mom, Arturo
Nudenberg, Bernardo
Otero, Omar Edmundo
Pecoraro, Vicente
Pierini, Luis E.
Quiroga, Marcial Ignacio
Rechter, Moisés
Sanguinetti, Oscar
Seoane, Manuel
Smith, Gerardo Fr.
Torres, Cortijo
Vallejo-Vallejo, Luis
Viglioglia, Pablo Alberto

Australia
Anderson, Frederick Edwin
Barrack, Bruce Boyle
Belisario, John Colquhoun
Farb, Max
Flaherty, Francis I.
Francis, John Brenton
Hakendorf, Andren John
Hunter, Geoffrey Allan
Johnson, Adrian Mackey
Kocsard, Emery

Lane-Brown, Malcolm M.
Lempriere, William W.
Lewis, Montague B.
Mackie, Bruce Stephen
Macqueen, Ronald
McGeoch, Arthur Hector
Murray-Will, Ewan
O'Loughlin, Michael
White, Walter Barry

Austria
Antoine, Lore
Brunner, Norbert
Eberhartinger, Christoph
Ehrmann, Gertraut
Glöckner, Udo
Gulden, Karl
Hekele, Konrad
Holubar, Karl
Klepsch, Liselotte
Kohler, Josef
Kurzmann, Karl
Lanzl, Lawrence H.
Luger, Anton
Mach, Kurt W.
Male, Otto
Musger, Anton E.
Neuer, Walter
Niebauer, Gustav
Pachinger, Rudolf
Parisot, Herbert
Peter, Helmut
Pfleger, Lilly
Raab, Wolfgang
Santler, Rudolf
Sattler, Alois
Schauer, Ludwig
Söltz-Szöts, Josef
Tappeiner, Josef
Vosicky, Johann
Weitgasser, Hans
Wiedmann, Albert
Wirth, Gerhard
Wittels, Wolf
Wolff, Klaus
Wolfram, Stefan
Zehetner, Hans

Belgium
Achten, Georges
Aupaix, Michel
Baudrez, Eddie
Benekens-Kestelyn,
   Janine G.
Bersaques, Jean de
Bouffioux, Joseph
Bourlond, André
Carpentier, Edmond

Castermans, André
Craps, Lucien Paul
Defresne, Jean H. E.
Delune, Hubert
Dockx, Louis
Duesberg, Jean-Pierre
Dupont, Adolphe
Gillis, Etienne
Hutsebaut, Armand
Haven, E.
Janssens, Jozef P.
Kint, André
Lachapelle, Jean-Marie
Lakaye, Guy
Lamotte, Léon
Lapière, Charles
Lapière, Spartacus
Ledoux-Corbusier,
   Marguérite
Mestdagh, Charles
Moriamé, Gustave
Oleffe, Jacques-Adrien
Piérard, Jean
Pluess, Jacques
Reymen-Bogaert, Alice J.
Seghers, Michel
Sigart, Henri
Simonart, Jean-Marie
Steeno, Omer Pieter
Tanner, Léopold
Thulliez, Michel
Van-Caneghem, Pierre
Van Lierde, Léon J. H.
Vercruysse, André
Vertommen, Jules
Vicca, Eugène-Richard
Wanet, Josette
Wellens, Willy

Brazil
Azulay, Rubem David
Bopp, Clovis
Castelo-Martins, João
Costa, Leopoldo
Costa-Pinto, Wanda
Da-Costa-Araujo-Filho, Fr.
Fraga, Sylvio
Furtado, Tancredo A.
Javor, Zoltan Janos
Lira, Olavo de Andrade
Loisier, Paul
Miranda, Ruy
Padilha-Gonçalves, Antar
Peryassu, Demetrio
Porto Frota de Magalhães,
   Walter
Prado-Sampaio,
   Sebastião A.

Ramos e Silva, João
Rocha, Glyne Leite
Rodrigues-Loivos, José A.
Romiti, Ney
Silva, Domingos
Teixeira-Coelho, Joel
Zilberberg. Benjamin

Bulgaria
Angelov, Nikola
Bajdekov, Belizar
Berowa, Newena
Bojanov, Ljuben
Botzov, Peter Ivanov
Christova, Maria
Filkov, Toma
Georghev, Jordan
Georgiev, Georgi
Grigoroff, J.
Grudov, Totko
Kapuilov, Stoian
Kasandjev, Stoian
Kitova, Lidia
Kutintschev. Michail
Obretenova, Ivanka
Owtscharow, Dimiter
Petrov, Ilia
Popchristov, Petre
Tanev, Nikola
Todorov, Angel
Tonkin, Naderolg
Tscherechev, Petar
Zvetanov, Zvetan

Canada
Albers, Heinrich J.
Bowman, Basil
Buck, Harald William
Clearihue, Joyce G.
Coupe, Robert L.
Donsky, Howard J.
Dumais, Gaston
Ereaux, Lemuel Price
Fekete, Zoltan
Flint, Anna
Forsey, Robert Roy
Freeman, Kenneth
Gallai, Zoltan
Gerstein, William
Getzler, N. A.
Giroux, Jean-Mario
Grandbois, Jean
Gubersky, Victor
Jackson, Robert
Kerbel, Norman
Kinch, Kenneth E.
Leavine, Desta
Maddin, W. Stuart
McLeod, Janey
Panaccio, Victor
Poirier, Paul
Rinne, Herman H.
Scott, Thomas Barrett
Usher, Barney

Vavruska, George W.
Wilkinson, Ralph
Wilson, Arthur P.
Wood, William
Wurm, Karl

Ceylon
Chelvarajah, Thomas
De-Silva, M. J. Pandula

Chile
Klein-Kohn, Oscar
Sylvester, Eduard

Republic of China
Julin-Fan

Columbia
Cardenas, Victor
Cortes C., Alonso
Gutierrz Aldana, Guillermo
Laverde, Alfredo
Londoño, Fabio
Mesa Cock, Jairo
Rueda P., Luis Alfredo

Republic of Congo
Mike-Sovari, Eva
Rossetti, Carlo

Costa Rica
Rosenstock, Noe

Cuba
Diaz-Almeida, José G.
Ruiz-de-Zárate, Serafín
Sagaró-Delgado,
  Bartolomé

Czechoslovakia
Babula, Vaclav
Bartak, Pavel
Bielický, Tibor
Chmel, Ladislav
Hegyi, Eugen
Holan, Vladimír
Horáček, Jaroslav
Horáková, Maruše
Konrad, B.
Kúta, Adolf
Lejhanec, Gustav
Lenart, Wilhelm
Malý, Eugen
Mikolášek, Jiří
Pospíšil, Leopold
Rehák, Alexander
Resl, Vlastimil
Rozsívalová, Věra
Stáva, Zdeněk
Turek, Bohuslav
Uhrík, Július

Vlček, František
Voldánová, Anna
Winter, Valter
Wohlstein, Emanuel
Zabrodsky, Sviatoslav
Zahejsky, Jiri
Zlamal, Josef

Denmark
Asboe-Hansen, Gustav
Auken, Gunnar
Borch-Jorgensen, Birgit
Brodthagen, Holger
Christiansen, Joergen V.
Gadborg, Ejnar
Heilesen, Bjorn
Hjorth, Niels
Knudsen, Erik A.
Kobayasi, Takasi
Konstmann-Meier, Carl H.
Kopp, Heinrich
Lomholt, Gunnar
Ludvigsen, Knud E. D.
Nielsen, Hans Arge
Nielsen, Johannes Peter
Niordson, Ann-Marie
Perdrup, Axel
Reiter, Henry F. H.
Reymann, Flemming
Sasaki, Soichiro
Stoltze, Ruth
Svendsen, Inge Borup
Thomsen, Kristian
Unna, Paul Jacob
Voetmann, Edel
Vosbein, Erich
Wehnert, Robert A.
Winther, Asta
Zachariae, Hugh

Dominican Republic
Coiscou-Weber, Antonio G.
Contreras, Miguel A.
Pimentel, Hernandez Manuel
Pimentel. Imbert M. F.

Ecuador
Murgueytio, Raul
Ollague, Wenceslao

El Salvadore
Oswaldo. Ramirez

Finland
Blomquist, Kirsti
Dammert, Kai Fredrik
Förström, Lars
Helander, Inkeri
Hirvonen, Marsa-Liisa
Hopsu-Havu, Väinö K.
Kauppinen, Kirsti
Kiistala, Urpo

Kilpiö, Olavi
Kuokkanen, Kirsti
Lundell, Eino
Mäkinen, Jiona
Muroma, Ali
Mustakallio, Kimmo K.
Niemi, Kirsti-Maria
Ohela, Kyllikki
Pirilä, Veikko
Putkonen, Tauno
Rehtijärvi, Katri
Salo, Osmo
Siberg, Rauhalea
Siltanen, Inga
Sonck, Carl Eric
Uroma, Eero
Valmari-Kankkunen, Saara

France

Agache, Pierre
Aitken, Georges
Akhoundzadeh, Heydar
Alt, Jean
Araujo, Aides
Aron-Brunetière, Robert
Arouete, Jean
Aubin, Guy M.
Baranger, Jean
Baranger, Henri
Baran, Robert
Barety, Marcel
Barrière, Henri
Basset, André
Bazex, Ande
Belaich, Stéphane
Bénard, Pierre
Benoist, Claude
Bensoussan, Liliane
Bergoend, Henri
Betourné, Michel
Beurey, Jean
Bieber, Philippe
Blez, Francis
Bolgert, Marc
Boulle, Stéphane
Bourdon, René
Bourgeois-Spinasse,
    Jacqueline
Bregevin, Bernard
Bureau, Yves
Burgun, René
Calas, Edmond
Cartier, Jean-Claude
Carton, François-Xavier
Casalis, François
Cauvin, Françoise
Césarini, Jean-Piere
Chambers, William
Charlier, Hector
Chatard, Honoré
Cherif-Cheikh, Jean-Louis
Chichard, André
Christol-Jalby, Bernadette
Civatte, Jean

Collart, Pierre
Cottenot, François
Daguet, Gaston Louis
David, Nathalie
David, Victor
De-Beer, Pierre
Degos, Robert
De-Lestrade, Bernardo
Delort, Joseph
Deltour, Claude
Delzant, Olivier
Deschamps, Pierre
Desmons, François
Desurmont, Michel
Diab, Souheil
Dubois, Philippe
Dufourmentel, Claude
Dugois, Pierre
Duheille, Jean
Duperrat, Bernard
Duverne, Jean
Ellena, Virginio
Fischer, Rosemarie
Friedmann, Elie
Friez, Pierre
Gallet, Philippe
Garelly, Elisabeth
Glasser, René
Goetschel, Eugène
Golé, Laurent
Goudie, Geneviève
Graciansky, Pierre de
Grupper, Charles
Guilaine, Jacques
Gurecki, Henri
Hadida, Elie
Harmel, Louis
Herr, Georges
Hewitt, Jean
Hoffmann-Martinot, Richard
Huriez, Claude
Hy, Robert
Jamain, Claude
Jeandidier, Pierre
Kalis, Bernard
Kohen, Ignace
Labrousse, Claude Jeanne
Lafaurie, Gérard
Lambergeon, Solange
Lapine, Jeanne Marie
Laroche-Navarron,
    Marguerite
Laugier, Paul
Lebeuf, Michel
Lebeurrier, Francine
Leclercq, Robert
Lecoulant, P.
Legoaster, Jacqueline
Lépine, Jacques
Lortat-Jacob, Etienne
Maleville, Jean
Mallet, Pierre
Many, Paul
Marcel, Georges A.
Martin, Pierre

Martinaud, Michel
Mascaro, José M.
Massé, Robert
Merklen, Félix Pierre
Meyer, Jean
Michon, Claude
Mikol, Claude
Monfort, Jean
Montet, Yvette
Moulin, Georges
Mouly, Roger
Navelet, François
Neuman, Arthur
Noury, Jean-Yves
Pailheret, Paul
Parant, Marcel
Payenneville, Henri
Pellerat, Jacques
Peyron, Michel
Pierquin, Bernard Louis
Piret, Jean-Marie
Poisson, Pierre
Pomey, Danièle
Pons, Anuik
Préaux, Jacques
Puissant, Antoine
Renoux, Mario-Louis
Rimbaud, Pierre
Robin, Jean
Roth, Louis
Rousselot, Roland
Schmidl, Serge
Schnitzler, Liliane
Schousboë, Alain
Sirkis, Lucette
Stiegler, Jean-Pierre
Témine, Pierre
Terrier, Henri
Texier, Lucien
Thibaut, David
Thiers, Henri
Thiraud, David
Thivolet, Jean
Touraine, René
Vanbremeersch, François
Vermenouze, Pierre
Vernier, Pierre A.
Vissian, Louis Vincent
Volle, Henri
Weber, Max
Wechsler, Paule
Weille, Raymond
Youénou, Annie
Zéraffa, Jacqueline

Germany

Adam, Wilhelm
Aldick, Wilhelm
Alte, Wolfgang
Amtmann, Valentin
Antz, Heinrich
Aretz, Herbert
Bandmann, Hans-Jürgen
Barkow, Dietrich
Baumann, Rolf

Bause, Eberhard
Bayerl, Peter
Bechter, Elmar
Bender, Elmar
Bentzin, Friedrich
Berger, Hermann
Bergmann, Gertrud
Bergrath, Aristides
Bittar, Elias-Oskar
Blum, Theodor
Boecker, Karl-Heinz
Böhm, Curt
Boesmann, George
Bohnstedt, Rudolf
Borelli, Siegfried
Born, Willi
Bosse, Klaus
Braun, Werner
Braun-Falco, Otto
Brehm, Georg
Breit, Reinhard
Brenske, Eberhard
Bruder, Karl
Brügelmann-Newton, V.
Brun, August
Brune, Regine
Bunge, Ute
Calap, Joaquin
Carrié, Curt
Chlebarov, Stefan
Christ, Klaus
Christahl-Günther, Friderike
Christophers, Enno
Daubach, Emmy
Dehmel, Eva-Maria
Denk, Rolf
Dittmar-Friederichs, Ruth
Dörner, Walter
Drechsler, Wolfgang
Dreiner, Heinz
Drepper, Hubert
Drewes, Irene
Drzezca, Wolfgang
Dürholz, Hans-Hermann
Dürre, Gerhard
Ehlers, Günter
Ehring, Franz
Eichert, Ida Marie
Eichhoff, Dorothee
Engelhardt, Wilhelm
Erdemir, Muammer
Eschler, Wilhelm
Eshelman, Orval M.
Espinoza-Figueroa, Virginia
Fabry, Hermann
Fegeler, Ferdinand
Fichtner, Cläre
Fiebig, Mechthild
Fiedler, Herbert P.
Fischer, Carl
Fischer, Christel
Fischer, Hubert
Fischer, Manfred
Forck, Günther
Frenes, Carl

Friederich, Hugo C.
Fries, Walter
Frydrychowicz, Heinz
Fürste, Waltraut
Funk, Carl Friedrich
Gahlen, Walter
Garhammer, Karl
Garn, Friedrich
Gartmann, Heinz
Gebhardt, Rita
Gefe-Richter, Annemarie
Gent, Werner
Gerke-Mosler, Delia
Giefer, Werner
Giesing, Käte
Gillesberger, Walter
Giss, Gerhard
Gockel, Toni
Gockell, Werner
Goerz, Günter
Götz-Schuster, Ursula
Götz, Hans
Gollnick, Norbert
Gottron, Heinrich Adolf
Graatz, Hans
Gran, Elli
Grasreiner, Werner
Grau, Erich
Gregorczyk, Klaus
Greiner, Gerhard
Greither, Aloys
Greuer, Wilhelm
Griesheim, Kurt von
Grimmer, Heinz
Grobe, Johann-Wilhelm
Grochocki, Franz
Gromzig, Hannelies
Gruber, Elisabeth
Grubmüller, Hanskarl
Grünewald, Hermann
Gündel, Wolfgang
Haas, Franz
Haberl, Lore
Hack, Karl
Hänsch, Rudolf
Hagemann, Rudolf
Hagenburger, Hellmuth
Halbeck, Erich
Halter, Klaus
Hammer, Gerhard
Hampel, Georg
Hanow, Bernhard
Hartmann, Karl Josef
Hasselman, Carl Max
Hartung, Jo
Hasslinger, Ludwig
Hatton, Rudolf
Hauser, Walter
Hauss, Helga
Heim, Franz
Heinke, Ernst
Heintel-Tröster, U.
Heite, Hans-Joachim
Heitmann, Hans Joachim
Helle, Susanne

Hennies, Hermann-Wilhelm
Hermann, Heinz
Hermann, Wolfgang P.
Herrmann, Franz
Hertel, Fritz
Herzberg, Joachim
Hessel, Ludwig
Heusser, Ursula
Himmel, Peter
Höde, Nikolaus
Holzmann, Hans
Hopf, Gustav
Hornstein, Otto
Hornstein, Guido
Huber-Riffeser, Gertraud
Idehen, Humphrey
Illig, Leonhard
Ippen, Margot
Ippen, Helmut
Irisawa, Kaikichi
Iser, Anna
Ishibashi, Yasumasa
Itani, Zouhair
Jacobs, Hermann
Jäger, Gerold
Jänner, Michael
Joel, Günther
Johne, Hans
Jordan, Paul
Juncker, Amelie
Kaden, Rudolf
Kaiser, Bodo
Kalkoff, Karl-Wilhelm
Kampa, Alexander
Kargel, Otto
Karschowsky, Maria
Keilig, Werner
Kemahli, Hasan
Kieferle, Ingeborg
Kiffe, Maria
Kimmig, Josef
Kinoshita, Masako
Kirchesch, Josef
Klabunde, Herta Maria
Klärner, Christoph
Klaschka, Franz
Klempt, Helmut
Klingmüller, Georg
Klostermann, Gerald
Kludas, Martin
Klüken, Norbert
Knierer, Wolfgang
Knoth, Rita
Knoth, Wilhelm
Köhler, Hans
Körte, Carlos
Kohler, Jakob
Korinthenberg, Inge
Korsukewitz, Gottfried
Korting, Günter W.
Krämer, Gisela
Krajewski, Theophil
Krause, Heinrich
Krempl-Lamprecht, Luise
Kremser, Josef

Kreysel, Hans-Wilhelm
Krüger, Arnold
Krüger, Hansgeorg
Kunze, Renate
Landes, Erich
Laumanns, Ulrich
Leinbrock, Arthur
Lemke, Gotthard
Lenger, Josef
Leyh, Frowine
Litschel, Erwin
Locher, Wolfgang
Lucius, Karoline
Ludwig, Gottfried
Lyndian, Karl-Heinz
Mäuser, Bernd
Marghescu, Sandor
Marhoven, Gerhard
Marosi, Marga
Martin, Hans
Mayer, Manfred
Meiers, Hans Günter
Meinhof, Wolf
Memmesheimer, Alois sen.
Memmesheimer, Alois jr.
Mertin-Ablass, Else
Meyer, Wolfgang F.
Meyer-Rohn, Johannes
Meyhöfer, Wolfgang
Milbradt, Rainer
Mönter, Albert
Mooren, Erika
Müller, Eva
Muftic, Mahmud
Nase, Martin
Nasemann, Theodor
Neumann, Leon
Neuner, Yvonne
Niermann, Hans
Nikolowski, Wolfgang
Nödl, Fritz
Nöhricke, Heinz
Noppeney, Georg
Novakovic, Ferdinand
Nückel, Manfred
Nürnberger, Fritz
Nussbaum, Margret
Oberliesen, Christine
Oehlschlaegel, G.
Oehmichen, Christa
Oertel, Hans
Orfanos, Constantin
Ortner, Brigitte
Pabst, Hanni
Paetzold, Otto-Hermann
Pankok, Erich
Pantscharewski, Dimitar
Parisis, Nickolas
Peter, Karl Wilhelm
Peter, Ellen G.
Petzold, Detlef
Pevny, Irmgard
Pfister, Rudolf
Plempel, Manfred
Plöger, H.

Pola, Wolfgang
Polemann, Gerd
Preyss, Johann von
Prinz, Hans Eugen
Pritzsche, Anneliese
Proppe, Albin
Pürschel, Wolfgang
Püschl, Herbert
Pusch, Heinz
Rassner, Gernot
Rauhut, Karl
Reich, Horst
Reich, Anka-Luise
Reichel, A. M.
Reisner, John E.
Rodermund, Otto E.
Röckl, Helmut
Röscher, Wilhelm
Rohde, B.
Rosenberger, Walter
Rosse, Helga
Sakurane, Hirotada
Saueressig, Heinz
Schäfer, Hans
Schalla, Werner
Schaller, Karl-Friedrich
Schandelmaier, Fritz
Schandelmaier, Karin
Scharmann, Willi
Schiedges, Max
Schimpf, Albert
Schirren, Carl
Schirren, Carl Georg
Schirren, Carl Georg, jr.
Schirren, Hermann
Schirren, Karin
Schirren, Michael
Schlaeger, Erich
Schlecht, Karl-Alfred
Schlenger, Theresia
Schlockermann, Fritz-
   Wilhelm
Schlüter, Ilse
Schmid, Otto
Schmidt, Peter
Schmidt-Ehrensberger,
   Marianne
Schmidt-La-Baume,
   Friedrich
Schmidla, Walther
Schneider, Reinhart
Schneider, Wilhelm
Schnyder, Urs Walter
Schöpf, Erwin
Schölzke, Karl Heinz
Schotte, Wolfgang
Schreiber, Reinhard
Schreiner, Hand-Eugen
Schröder, Eckard
Schröpl, Friedrich
Schümmer, Heinrich
Schultze, Rolf
Schulz, Hans-Jürgen
Schulz, Karl-August
Schulz, Karl Heinz

Schuster, Hellmut
Schwark, Edith
Schwarz, Eberhard
Schwarzbauer, Fritz
Schwern, Helga
Schwind, Karl
Sellier, Werner
Seltenreich, Hans
Sevin, Wilhelm
Sicking, Bernhard
Sitzberger-Stählin, Irmgard
Smattosch, Hans
Söhnchen, Max
Spier, Hans Wolfgang
Sprenger, Fritz
Stähle-Klein, Kurt
Steen, Klaus
Steigleder, Gerd Klaus
Stiess, Wolfgang
Strang, David, J.
Strassmann, Horst
Stroux, Bernhard
Stüttgen, Günter
Sturde, Hans
Sturm, Fritz
Stutzer, Gerhard
Sutter, Erika
Swart, B. G.
Teller, Heinrich
Thaesler, Günther
Thaler, E.
Theisen, Hans
Thies, Werner
Thimm, Josef
Throm, Urban
Tiedemann, Günter
Tillmann, Franz
Treeck, Wolfgang
Tritsch, Helmut
Tronnier, Hagen
Tümmers, Burckhart
Ude, Peter
Ulrich, Hermann
Unna, Paul Joachim
Vakilzadeh, Fereydoun
Veltmann, Günther
Vilmar, Traute
Vogt, Hermann
Vollmer, Edmund
Voss, Harald
Wachsmann, Felix
Wagner, Rosemarie
Walker, Kurt
Weber, Gerhard
Webster, Stephen B.
Weidmann, Günter
Weidner, Frank
Weigl, Adolf
Weisenberg, Götz
Welling, Hanneliese
Wenig, Karlhans
Wepner, Heinrich
Werle, Heinz
Wex, Ortrud
Weyer, Hansgeorg

Wezel, Helmut
Wilk, Hans-Joachim
Willwohl, Hans
Winkler, Anton
Winkler, Kurt
Wiskemann, Arthur
Wöber, Karlheinz
Wolfskehl, Ursula
Wolfram, Gottfried
Wollnitza, Ewald
Wolpert, Kurt
Wulf, Karl
Wunsch, Gerhard
Zambal, Zvonimir
Zaun, Hansotto
Zezschwitz, Karl-August
Zierz, Paul
Ziethen, Helene

Germany-East
Naumann, Katharina

Ghana
Mempel, Siegfried

Greece
Belezos, Nickon
Canellis, Panagiotis
Capetanakis, John
Doucas, Christophoros
Doucas, Lydia
Georgiades, Despina
Higoumenakis, Costas
Kanitakis, Constantin
Ktenides, Maria-Anastasia
Marselou-Kinti, Uranie
Photinopoulos, Nick
Polemicos, Antoine
Sakelleariou, Georgios
Stratigos, John
Triantafyllou, Titos
Vlachopoulos, Leontios

Great Britain
Alexander, John
Anderson, Thomas E.
Auckland, Geoffrey
Baker, Harvey
Beck, John Swanson
Bellringer, Hedley E.
Bettley, Francis Ray
Bor, Simon
Brotherton, Janet
Brown, Vernon K. H.
Calnan, Charles
Carslaw, Robert W.
Catterall, Mary
Catterall, Robert D.
Clarke, George H. V.
Coburn, James Garlick
Cohen, Eric Lipman
Comaish, Stanley
Copeman, Peter W. M.

Cram, David L.
Cruickshank, C. N. D.
Dilley, Gordon
Donaldson, Eric Muir
Emslie, Ellen S.
Everall, John Dudley
Feiwel, Michael
Frain-Bell, William
Fry, Lionel
Garretts, Maurice
Greaves, Malcolm
Hall-Smith, Patrick
Hall, Reginald
Hanson, J. Charles Henty
Hellier, Frank
Holti, Gunter
Ingram, John Th.
Johnson, Francis Rea
Kaimis, John
Kinmont, Patrick David
Logan, James C.P.
Lyell, Alan
Lyon, John
Magnus, Ian A.
Marks, Janet Mary
Marsden, Cecil
Martin-Scott, Ian
McCallum, Donald Ian
Meara, Robert Harold
Middleton, John David
Mitchell-Heggs, Gordon B.
Montgomery, Patrick R.
Morgan, John K.
Moynahan, Edmund John
Munro, Dowling D.
Oller, Leonhard
Pegum, Joseph
Peterkin, Georg A.G.
Pettit, John
Philp, Jack McLean
Raffle, Edmund James
Raven, Ronald W.
Robinson, Trevor W.E.
Rook, Arthur
Ross, Alastair A.
Rowell, Neville R.
Ryan, Terence John
Saalfeld, Ulrich
Samman, Peter Derrick
Sanderson, Kenneth V.
Sarkany, Imrich
Scutt, Ronald
Shamy, H. Kamal
Shuster, Sam
Simpson, John R.
Sklarz, Ernst
Smith, Peter
Sneddon, Ian Bruce
Snell, Eric Saxon
Sweet, Robert D.
Szur, Leon
Waddington, Eric
Wallace, Hugh John
Warin, Robert Ph.
Wells, George C.

Whimster, Ian Wesley
Whiteley, Hubert J.
Wilkinson, Darrell Sh.
Willcox, Richard R.
Williams, David
Wilson, Harold
Wilson, Lynley

Guatemala
Galvez-Molina, Luis

Honduras
Corrales, Hernan
Fernandez-Selva, E.

Hong-Kong
Wong, Kwok-Pn

Hungary
Angyal, J.
Balogh, Miklos
Bottyán, Etelka
Fejér, Endre
Földvári, Franz
Frankl, Josef
Fülöp, Eva
Gulbert, Anna
Haraszti, Istvan
Heintz, Elisabeth
Herpay, Zsombor
Károlyi, István
Király, Kálmán
Körössy, Sándor
Melczer, Nikolaus
Nebenführer, László
Rácz, István
Réffy, Franz
Simon, Nikolaus
Szodoray, Ludwig
Török, Ibolya
Venkei, Tibor
Viczián, Mihály

Iceland
Thorarinsson, Hannes
Tryggvason, Olafur

India
Behl, Pran
Gokhale, Balchandra
Majumdar, Taradas
Rebello, Désiré Joseph
Verma, Bhanu B.S.
Viziam, C. Bhakta

Iran
Maleki, Mohamed Ali
Martirossian, Aramais
Mehri, Aazam
Mohaghegh-Yazdi, Hassan
Samii, Rahmatollah
Vaziri, Mansour

Iraq

Akrawi, Fathullah Y.
Rahim, Georgef

Ireland

Barnes, Joseph
Beare, John Artin
Meenan, Francis
Meenan, Livinia
Mitchell, Dorothy
Mitchell, David

Israel

Ellenbogen, Heinrich
Feuerman, Eleasar
Gordon, Josef
Greif, Hersch
Guhrauer, Hans
Haim, Salim
Hernis, Simon
Kanturek, Eduardo
Katzenellenbogen, Isaac
Kochmann, Bruno
Laver, Heinrich
Liquornik, Max
Sagher, Felix
Seligmann, Hans
Sheskin, Jaakov
Spitzer, Rudolf
Ziprkowski, Leo

Italy

Allegra, Fulvio
Andreassi, Lucio
Argenziano, Gabriele
Baccaredda, Boy Aldo
Bazan, Marie Rosaria
Bellone, Angelo
Bergamasco, Arrigo
Binazzi, Maurizio
Boncinelli, Umberto
Bonelli, Mario
Bonu, Giovanni
Bosco, Isidoro
Bruni, Luigi
Buffa, Enrico
Caputo, Ruggero
Cavalieri, Rino
Cerimele, Decio
Cernea, Radu
Cerutti, Pietro
Chieregato, Giancarlo
Ciarrochi, Luigi
Coricciati, Luigi
Cozza, Giovanni
Crosti, Agostino
De-Luca, Massimo
Di-Prima, Guido
Dogo, Giovanni
Donati, Sergid
Ermoli, Guilio
Farris, Guido
Fazzini, Maria Luisa

Flarer, Franco
Gandola, Marco
Gardenghi, Gabriele
Giannotti, Benvenuto
Gianotti, Ferdinando
Gueli, Francesco
Hofmann, Maria Felicitas
Iacovacci, Gianfilippo
Ippolito, Ferdinando
Lancelotti, Mario
Leigheb, Giorgio
Leoni, Aldo
Levi, Luciano
Longhi, Arturo
Lostia, Alberto
Marson, Giambattista
Martina, Giocondo
Meneghini, Carlo
Merello, Andrea
Meringolo, Angelo
Midana, Alberto
Monacelli, Mario
Montagnani, Andrea
Moretti, Guiseppe
Nannelli, Mauro
Nazzaro, Paola
Onorio-Antonio, Carlesimo
Ottolenghi, Franco
Pagnes, Paolo
Panconesi, Emiliano
Panti, Allessandro
Papa, Antonino
Parisi, Paolo
Pezzarosa, Graziano
Pinetti, Pino
Policaro, R. D.
Pozzo, Giorgio
Puccinelli, Vittorio
Rabbiosi, Ciacomo
Ribuffo, Antonio
Rinaldi, Vito
Sabatini, Carlo
Santori, Giacomo
Santoianni, Pietro
Sberna, Paolo
Scarpa, Carmelo
Scolari, Enea Guiseppe
Semmola, Luigi
Serri, Ferdinando
Sertoli, Achille
Sertoli, Paolo
Silvestri, Unita
Simoni, Enrico
Spagnoli, Umberto
Strani, G. Franco
Suchowsky, Giselbert
Tinozzi, Croce C.
Tosti, Antonio
Vaccari, Riccardo
Vallecchi, Carlo
Zina, Guiseppe

Jamaica

Chambers, Henry D.

Japan

Abe, Sadao
Anzai, Takashi
Aono, Kihimide
Arimori, Masanao
Aso, Kazuko
Baba, Masatsugu
Chiba, Keiko
Dohi, Jun-Ichiro
Fujita, Yukio
Fukushiro, Ryoichi
Funabashi, Toshiyuki
Hamada, Yoshiro
Hasegawa, Teruhiko
Hatano, Hitoshi
Hata, Masauji
Hayashi, Yasushi
Higuchi, Kentaro
Hirata, Mitsuo
Honda, Tatsuo
Hosoki, Umeko
Iga, Yukinaka
Ikenaga, Minoru
Ishida, Kei
Ishihara, Fumiyuki
Ishizaki, Hiroshi
Ishizu, Shun
Ito, Kasuke None
Iwashita, Kenzo
Johnson, Marie-Louise
Kageyama, Ryoichi
Kano, Kaichiro
Katabira, Yasuo
Kato, Shiro
Kawada, Akihiro
Kawamura, Taro
Kawamura, Toshimitsu
Kitamura, Seiichi
Kitamura, Kanehiko
Kobayashi, Toshiaki
Kobori, Tatsuji
Kojima, Riichi
Kojima, Takateru
Kukita, Atsushi
Matsuzawa, Tohru
Matsumi, Kazuo
Miura, Yusho
Miyazawa, Teiji
Mochizuki, Hidehiko
Morikawa, Fujio
Mori, Makuso
Mori, Taku
Nagai, Ryukichi
Nagashima, Masaji
Nakagawa, Kiyoshi
Nakahashi, Hisamitsu
Nakajima, Hajime
Nakamura, Iemasa
Nakano, Masao
Nishio, Kazukata
Nishihara, Katsuo
Nishikawa, Takeji
Nobushima, Toku
Nogita, Michio

Noguchi, Yoshikuni
Nonami, Eiichiro
Ohara, Kazue
Oka, Kiyomi
Okuwa, Hiroshi
Otsuko, Sueno
Saito, Masaji
Sakamoto, Kunike None
Sakurai, Jinkichi
Sato, Yoshio
Seiji, Mokoto
Shiratori, Akira
Takada, Hiroshi
Takada, Yoshio
Takeda, Katsuyuki
Tanabe, Kazuko
Tanaka, Hiroshi
Torii, Yuki
Tsukada, Sadao
Ueda, Keiichi
Urabe, Harukuni
Watanabe, Yasushi
Wong Chu-Kwan Wong
Yamamoto, Kazuye
Yamamoto, Masakatsu
Yasuda, Toshiaki
Yukawa, Atsuhiko
Yumino, Isao

Kenya
Patel, Ramanbhai I.
Verhagen, Rudolf H.B.

Korea
Lim Soo Duk

Kuwait
Kanan, Mohammad Wajdi

Lebanon
Afifi, Abdel K.
Dajani, Adnan S.
Farah, Fuad
Johanny, Raymond
Kurban, Amal K.

Libya
Weisz, Adalbert

Luxembourg
Eichhorn, Alfred
Kongs, Albert

Madagascar
Mathurin, Louis

Malaya
Singh-Sachdev, H.

Malta
Agius, John R. G.

Mexico
Ahumada, Miguel Padilla
Arellano-Ocampo,
    Francisco
Atala-Freyat, Assad
Ayala-Uribe, Ma. Guadalupe
Cagigas, Adalid, J.
Estrada-Silos, Concepción
Garza-Toba, Manuel
Gonzalez-Ochoa, Antonio
Guridi-Alatriste, Josefina
Latapi, Fernando
Lavalle, Pedro
Ledesma-Diaz, Virginia
Lepiavka, Arseny
Macotela-Ruiz, Ernesto
Martinez de Escandon, Elena
Novales, Josefa
Ochoa-Mena, Crescensio
Ortiz, Yolanda
Pariser, Hans Georg
Saul, Amado
Trujillo, Valencia Jesus
Valencia de Lao, Jorge
Zermeno-Frias, Carlos

Morocco
Magdelenat, Pierre
Orusco, Marino
Rollier, René

Netherlands
Baes, Hermann G.C.
Beek, C.H.
Beukelaar, Louis de
Bour, D.J.H.
Bruijn, Jacobus H. de
Cormane, R.H.
De-Vries, Hermannus R.
De-Vries, Nikolaas C.T.
Dirksen, Henri Johan
Doeglas, Hendrik
Dragten, Armand
Gieskens, Wilhelmus Nicolas
Groot, Wilhelmus P. de
Grosfeld, J.C.M.
Heijmans, Hans H.
Hermans, Eduard H.
Horst, Pieter
Kooij, Reyer
Kruizinga, Edze Ernst
Mali, J.W.H.
Malten, Klaus E.
Muijs-van-de-Moer,
    Weijer W.
Oswald, Frans H.
Polano, Machiel K.
Renders, Laurentius J.
Reyers, Johan
Ruding, Joseph Rudolph L.
Ruiter, Maximillian
Schutter, Klaas
Siemens, H. W.

Smeenk, G.
Spaas, J. A. J.
Suurmond, Dirk
Thiele, Frederik A. J.
Thoene, A. W.
Tio, T. H.
Van-Aerssen, Robert
Van-der-Meer, Bareld Jan
Van-der-Meer, J. B.
Van-Dooren, M. Hub.
Van-Erp, Ivo, F. R.
Vermeer, Dirk J. H.
Wakkerman, Coenradus
Woerdemann, Martinus J.

New Zealand
Engel, Graham, Bernard
Hill, Brian Henry Rowland
Larnder, Derek
Marples, Mary J.
Muir, Allan D.

Nicaragua
Avalos-Vega, Ernaldo

Norway
Björnstad, Roar Th.
Boe, Einar
Danbolt, Niels
Helle, Gunnar
Kirsentals, Harald
Langeland, Berit
Lium-Strand, Marit
Lunde, Niels Martin
Rokstad, Ingvald
Schanche-Andresen, Solveig
Wennevold, Reidar
Wereide, Knut

Pakistan
Shahidullah, Mohammed

Panama
Carrillo, Lyonel
Merel, Ruben

Peru
Ayaipoma-Vidalón, Marcial
Flores-Cevallos, Luis
González-Pinillos, Víctor
Manrique-Avila, Juán
Manrique-Salas, Aníbal
Navarro-Huaman, Pedro
Rios-Flores, Marcial
Romero-Almeida, Luis
Urrelo-Novoa, Amaro E.

Philippines
Fernandez, Manuel C.
Garcia-Lopez, Milagros
Gutierrez, Guillermo

Poland

Chorzelski, Tadeusz
Golebiowska-Podgórczyk, Irene
Jablonska, Stefanie
Jakubowicz, Kazimierz
Kostanecki, Wojciech
Kozminzka, Anna
Lańcucki, Jan
Langner, Andrzej
Lejman, Kazimierz M,
Lesińska, Wanda
Lesiński, Janusz
Rosner, Julian
Rudowska-Jakubowicz, Irena
Rudzki, Edward
Sokolowski, Franciszek
Sowiński, Witold
Stauber, Marceli
Towpik, Jozeph
Wanic, Aniela
Zalucki, Wojciech

Portugal

Cruz-Sobral, Francisco da
Fonseca, Aureliano
Guimarães, Newton A.
Huffman, Marquis R.
Osswald, Wilhelm

Puerto Rico

Fleisher, Lawrence T.
Torres, Hector R.
Torres-Rodriguez, Victor

Southern Rhodesia

Kingsley, Henry Jack

Rumania

Andermann, I.
Antonescu, Stefan
Bologa, Emil
Chisleag, Gheorghe
Cojocariu, Mihai Ionel D.
Costea, Virgil
Dimitrescu, Alexandru
Ene-Popescu, Constanza-E.
Gavrilescu, Mircea
Iacob, Paul
Ilca, Stefan
Ilea, Romulus
Jonescu, Paul
Kahn, Moise
Longhin, Cornelia
Longhin, Scarlat
Marinescu, Alexander
Munteanu, Mircea
Negulescu, Victor N.
Nicolau, Radu
Noaghea, Gheorghe
Oancea, Constantin

Pintican, Emilia
Schmitzer, Josef
Stoian, Mihai
Tirlea, Petru
Trandafirescu, Maria
Ujváry, Emeric

Senegal

Privat, Yan

Singapore

Chuah Chong Yong

Spain

Aguilera-Maruri, Ceferino
Aliaga-Boniche, Adolfo
Alvarez-Lovell, Luís
Bassas-Grau, Enrique
Cabré, José
Carreras-Verdaguer, Antonio
Carrillo, José M.
Carrillo-Casaux, Diego
Casas, Marin Miguel
Dulanto, Felipe de
El Mehdy, Mohamed
Escartin-Dañobeitia A. J.
Garcia-Perez, Antonio
Esteller, José
Gay-Prieto, José
Gomez-Orbaneja, José
Grimalt, Francisco
Gyoerkoe, Alejandro de
Jaqueti del Pozo, Gerardo
Lecha-Carralero, Eloy
Linarea-de-Mula, Luis
Martin-Gasso, Carlos de
Martinez-Torres, Francisco
Mercadal-Peyri, José
Navarro-Baldeweg, Octavio
Ocaña-Sierra, Juan
Pereiro-Miguens, Manuel
Piñol-Aguadé, Joaquin
Pozueta-Ledo, Antonio
Robledo-Aguilar, Alfredo
Sanchez-Yus, Evaristo
Sans-Mascaro, José
Sanz-Benitez, Huberto
Solla, Laureano
Soto Melo, Joaquin
Telese, Alberto
Terencio-de-las-Aguas, J.
Uruñela-Bernedo, Juan
Vivancos-Gallego, Gines
Zubiri, Antonio

South Africa

Benjamin, Ephraim Sh.
Chitters, Max
Fine, Samuel Harry
Friedlander, Louis
Frootko, Jan
Leeming, John A.L.
Ross, Cyril M.
Stein, Sidney

Sudan

Ahmed, Mohamed

Sweden

Agrup, Gun
Amann, Franz
Bäfverstedt, Jo Erik
Björnberg, Alf
Blumenthal, Börje
Bogg-Berggren, Anna
Brehmer-Anderson, Eva
Brody, Isser
Brogren, Nils
Ekelund, Ann-Greta
Eriksson-Magnusson, G.
Flodén, Carl Henrik
Fredriksson, Torsten
Fregert, Sigfrid
Frithz, Anders
Gip, Lennart Josef
Gisslen, Hakan
Groth, Ove
Grund, Horst
Gudjonsson, Haraldur
Hagerman, Gösta
Heijer, Arne V.
Hellerström, Sven
Hard, Stig
Hellgren, Lars
Juhlin, Lennart A.
Karltorp, Nils
Lagerholm, Björn
Larre, Carl Elis
Liden, Sture
Liden, Sven
Lidmann, Hjördis
Lindgren, Ingemar
Magnusson, Bertil
Martner, Sigbrit
Modee, Jan
Möller, Halvor
Nordqvist, Barbro
Olsson, Karin
Rajka, Georg
Rorsman, Hans R.
Ruhnek-Forsbeck, Margit
Skog, Erik
Swanbeck, Gunnar
Thyresson, Nils
Wahlberg, Jan
Wikström, Kjell

Switzerland

Ahrens, Theodor
Andrial, Milorad
Baumann, Karl
Baumgarner, Paul Rudolf
Bechelli, Luiz Marino
Blum, Gebhard
Börlin, Erich
Bolay, Gustave
Bollag, Raymond
Brand, Paul-Heinrich

Brenn, Hans
Brun, Robert M.
Burckhardt, Walter
Delacrétaz, Jean
Diem, Ernst
Djalali, Amir
Ducel, Georges
Evdos, Peter
Favre, François
Fischer, Emil
Fivaz, Louis
Flüge, Rudolf
Fournet, Monique
Franceschetti, A.
Frenk, Edgar
Gans, Oscar
Garnier, Francis
Gehrken, Hans
Gonzalez, Angel
Grigoriu, Dode
Gutekunst, Jörg A.
Guthe, Thorstein
Huber, Hans Peter
Hunziker, Nicole
Jadassohn, Werner
Jaquier, Jean Jacques
Jeanneret, Jean-Pierre
Jenny, Dieter
Juon, Martin
Kaufmann, Carl E.
Kröpfli, Pierre
Kull, Eugen
Kuske, Hans
Lenggenhager, René
Leu, François
Lilla, Jacques
Löb, Lutz
Loi-Zedda, Prospero
Loretan, Rose Marie
Mäder, Ernst
Muller, Robert
Musso, Emile
Nencki, Leon
Obeid, Vera Maria E.
Paillard, Roger
Paschoud, Jean-Maurice
Pelloni, Enzio
Sachs, Peter
Schaaf, Fritz
Schauwecker, René
Schmid, Ulrich
Schütt, Erich
Schuppli, Rudolf
Schwarz-Speck, Kaspar
Schwersenz, Gerhard
Stierlin-Weber, Soja
Storck, Hans
Suter, Hans
Truffat, Claude
Vidmar-Cvjetanovic.
   Biserka
Walch, Jos.
Weirich, Erich G.
Widmer, Louis
Wilhelmi, Eckehard

Wortmann, Ferdinand

Syria

Siage, Honene

Thailand

Isarabhakdi, Pranpmsri
Suthisomboon, Kalaya
Vejjabul, Pierra

Turkey

Atal, Ali
Cankat, Ilhan
Dogru, Alaeddin
Faruk, Nemlioglu
Gurhan, Necmettin
Kip, Orhan
Kitapci, Baha
Onat, Fuat
Sargin, Cevad
Tat, A. Luetfue
Yemni, Osman

United Arab Republic

El-Mofty, Abdel Monem
El-Zawahry, Mohammed
El-Hefnawi, Hassan
Gawad, Mahmoud Sami A.

United States of America

Aber, Max
Alban, Jan
Anderson, Harold T.
Andrade, Rafael
Andrews, James Claire
Aney, Paul
Armstrong, Byron H.
Baden, Howard P.
Baer, Rudolf L.
Bailey, William
Baird, John W.
Barnes, Gilbert
Barrett, Carey
Barrock, James J.
Bart, Gloria, B.
Bart, Robert S.
Barwasser, Norbert
Becker, Frederic T.
Beerman, Herman
Behling, Ralph
Bembenista, John K.
Beninson, Joseph
Bernstein, I. A.
Berry, Carl Z.
Berke, Meyer
Beyer, Amanda
Bikle, Charles A.
Binkley, George W.
Blankenship, Marshall L.
Blaylock, W. Kenneth
Blaylock, Hoyt C.
Blois, Marsden S.

Bloom, Manuel G.
Bloom, David
Bloom, Robert E.
Boehm, Walter E. F.
Borota, Alexander
Bowden, Lemuel
Brauer, Earle
Brown, William J.
Brown, Martin V.
Brunsting, Henry A.
Brunsting, Louis A.
Buchanan, Robert N.
Buerk, Minerva Smith
Burdick, Kenneth
Burgeon, Carroll
Burnett, Jean B.
Burstein, Rachel
Butler, Milton G.
Butler, John D.
Butterworth, Thomas
Caccamise, Charles W. jr.
Caplan, Richard M.
Carney, Harry
Carson, William E.
Casper, Anne
Casper, Wolfgang
Chargin, Louis
Chernosky, Marvin
Cipollaro, Vincent
Clendenning, William
Clinger, Edwin J.
Cohen, William
Cohen, William B.
Connor, Roger Arthur
Connor, William H.
Constantine, Victor S.
Cook, Thomas
Coon, McIntosh
Corbett, Max B.
Cortese, Thomas A.
Cowan, Leon
Cox, Alvin J.,
Crossland, Paul M.
Cummings, Charles E.
Curth, William
Curth, Helen Ollendorff
Curtis, Arthur Covel
Curtis, John W.
Daly, John F.
Dann, Theod. Alvin
Davenport, Dennies
Davis, Richard Graham
Day, Thomas
Dedehayir, A. Riza
Denton, Cleveland
Dexter, David D.
Dobes, William Lamor
Dobson, Richard L.
Dodge, Billy G.
Domonkos, Anthony N.
Dornbush, Floyd John
Doyle, William H.
d'Avanzo, Charles
d'Urso, John
Ebling, John

Edelstein, Abe James
Ekblad, Gordon
Engel, Marvin F.
Ephraim, Alfred J.
Epstein, William Louis
Everett, Mark Allen
Farber, Eugene M.
Fasal, Paul
Ferguson, Edward
Fischer, Maria
Fishman, Harold, C.
Fitzpatrick, Thomas
Fleisher, Harvey
Flood, James
Fox, Everett
Fox, Jack M.
Freedberg, Irwin M.
Freeman, Robert Glen
Frost, Philip
Fukuyama, Kimie
Fusaro, Ramon
Gant, James
Gaul, L. Edward
Gelber, Anita
German, John Elmer
Gilmore-Brau, Same J.
Goddard, A. Robert
Goldblatt, Marvin
Goldberg, Harry C.
Goldblatt, Samuel
Goldman, Leon
Goldschmidt, Herbert
Goldstein, Norman
Golomb, Herbert
Golubovic, Zivomir
Goodman, J. John
Gould, Arnold H.
Graham, James H.
Griffith, Paul
Grinnell, Ernest Leroy
Grob, Peter, J.
Groel, John T.
Gross, Benjamin A.
Grots, Inta A.
Gudgel, Edward F.
Guthrie, Marschall
Haag, Edgar
Hallet, Joseph
Hambrick, George W.
Hamilton, William
Hamlin, Edwin M.
Hammer, Charles John
Hartson, Mary C.
Haserick, Same J. R.
Hashimoto, Ken
Haynes jr., Harley A.
Hays, Glenn B.
Hearst, Bella
Helfman, Richard J.
Hellreich, Alfred
Helms, Robert W.
Hendren, Owen S.
Hensel, Hilda
Herzog, Carl J. S.
Hicks, John H.

Hidgon, Robert S.
Hitch, Joseph Martin
Hitschmann, Otto
Hollander, Alfred
Holman jr., John Crafford
Honeycutt, W. Mage
Hordinsky, Bohdan Z.
Horvath, Peter N.
Howard, Olga Daiber
Howard, Bruce Godrey
Howell, James B.
Hubler, Winthrope
Hunsicker, Mary
Inderbitzin, Theodor M.
Jacobs, Stanley
James, George W.
Jarecki, Max
Jaross, Robert William
Jennings-Douglass
Jensen, Oswald R.
Jewell, Edward W.
Johnson, Fred
Jones, H. Leon
Jones, Stuart Pannill
Jordon, James Wallace
Juhlin, Einar Axel
Jung, Eduard
Kahn, Guinter
Karasek, Marvin
Keddie, Frances M.
Keiper, Robert James
Keller, Louis
Kersting, David
Keuper, Charles
Kipping, Hans F.
Knoll, George Monroe
Knox, John Marshall
Koblenzer, Peter Johann
Kopf, Alfred W.
Kramer, Jack
Kremer, Ingeborg M.
Kremer, Otto L.
Krugh, Francis J.
Kurtz, Cecilia M.
Kvistberg, Gerald Kent
Lamberg, Stanford
Landau, Joseph W.
Laskas, John J.
Laubenheimer, Roger
Leeper, Roy William
Leland, Carol Margaret
Lessenden, Chester
Lessman, Ellen M.
Lever, Walter F.
Levin, Harold
Levy, S. William
Lewe, Irving A.
Liebmann, Max
Lininger, Thurid B.
Lipkin, George
Livingood, Clarence
Lobitz, Walter C.
Lorincz, Allan L.
Love, William Robert
Lowney, Edmund D.

Lund, Herbert Z.
Lustig, Bernard
Lutzner, Marvin
Lyons, Robert E.
Macdonald, Gordon
Mahood, John
Maibach, Howard
Maksic, Dragutin
Malkinson, Frederick D.
Manson, R. Campbell
March, Cyril H.
Markson, Leonard S.
Marrero, Luis G.
Mathewson, Joseph B.
Matolsty, Alexander
May, Stanton B.
McCusky, John M.
McDaniel, William E.
McDonald, Charles J.
McDonald, Frank
McEleney, Donald A.
McGinley, James
McGrath, Dewis J.
McLean, Lee Davidson
McMullan, Francis H.
Meagher, George B.
Mehregan, Amir H.
Melnikoff, Robert M.
Meltzer, Leonard
Mescon, Herbert
Mihan, Richard
Mihm, Martin Charles
Mikhaul, George R.
Miller, Rolf
Mishima, Yutaka
Miyamoto, Masamitsu
Mohs, Frederic
Molleurus, Couperus
Montagna, William
Montes, Leopold F.
Montgomery, H.
Morginson, William J.
Mortashed, Joan
Mulherin, John
Myers, Cortland
Nelson, Carl Truman
Neuberg, Hans
Newton, Hirma D.
New, William N.
Nicholas, Leslie
Obermayer, Maximilian E.
Oclassen, Charles A.
Olansky, Sidney
Olmstead, Charles B.
Olson, Robert
O'Neill, Charles W.
Orentreich, Norman
Osbourn, Raymond A.
Palmer, Alice
Pathak, Madhukar A.
Payne, Charles Franklin
Perry, Harold Otto
Pfaff, Richard O.
Phillips, Leonard S.
Pillsbury, Donald

Pinkus, Hermann
Pinne, George
Pinski, James Bernard
Pipkin, James L.
Pittelkow, Robert B.
Pochi, Peter E.
Pollard, William Henry
Ponder, Jack Edward
Potts, Kathryn D.
Potts jr., Lew W.
Prager, Paul R.
Price, Vera
Proctor, Wallace Same
Prochazka, J. Fisher
Prose, Philip H.
Prutkin, Lawrence
Puhvel, S. Madli
Quero, Roberto
Quevedo, Walter C., jr.
Quinones, Jesus Maria
Ragsdale, William E., jr.
Ranchoff, John
Rausch, Norbert G.
Rauschkolb, Ruth
Ravits, Harold G.
Reed, Miriam
Reed, William B.
Reisner, Ronals
Reiss, Frederick
Reque, Paul Gerhard
Resnick, Bernard
Richards, Theresa
Riley, Kathleen A.
Robbins, Sidney
Roberton, Joycelin Same
Robins, Perry
Robinson, Harry, jr.
Rodriguez, C.
Roenigk, Hermann H.
Roe, Daphne
Rogachefsky, Hymen
Rogers, George K.
Rogers, John D.
Rosenberg, Eric
Ross, Harold
Rostenberg, Adolph, jr.
Rothman, Sidney
Rubin, Louis
Ruch, Donnald M.
Russo, Joseph
Sanchez, Jose
Saunders, William
Sauter, Lilianna S.
Savin, Ronald C.
Schildkraut, Jacob Max
Schmerold, Wilfried
Schmid, John F.
Schoch, Eugene P.
Schoenfeld, Robert J.
Scholtz, Jud R.
Schröder, Henry
Schwartz, Walter Fr.
Seale, Everett R.

Secrest, James
Sell, Kenneth W.
Senn, Peter
Shapiro, Edward
Shelley, Walter B.
Shields, Thomas L.
Silva, Armando, jr.
Silvers, Seymour H.
Simonson, Louis
Sina, Bahram
Singer, Edward J.
Skinner, Louis C.
Slimp, Thomas E.
Slinger, William N.
Sloughty, Charles A.
Smith, Anna R.
Smith, J. Leslie
Smith, Stuart C.
Sompayrac, Lauren
Spangler, Arthur
Spence, Bart J.
Spencer, Malcolm
Spiller, William F.
Sprowel, Robert Roy
Standish, E. Myles
Stegmaier, Otto
Steiger, Howard P.
Sternberg, Thomas Hunter
Stoker, Gerald Lee
Stolar, Robert
Storkan, Margaret Ann
Strauss, John S.
Strickland, Maurice A.
Sulzberger, Marion B.
Sulzberger, Roberta Z.
Suskind, Raymond R.
Takae, Hirone
Szabo, George
Taplin, David
Thomas, Carmen Chr.
Thompson, Reynolds B.
Thompson, Robert C.
Thomsen, John G.
Tilley, Robert F.
Tobias, Norman
Trice, Ernest R.
Tronstein, Arthur J.
Trunnell, Thomas L.
Tuffanelli, Denny Lee
Ulbrich, Albert Paul
Underwood, Laurence J.
Urbach, Frederick
Vander-Ploeg, Darl Edwin
Vilallonga, Jose M.
Walter, C. Herold
Watt, Thomas
Wecton, William A.
Weinmann, Paul
Weinstein, Gerald
Welton, William A.
Wiggall, Richter H.
Wikiera, Edward S.
Wilgram, George

Wilson, J. Walter
Winer, Louis
Witten, Victor H.
Wolf, Max
Woodburne, Arthur
Wuepper, Kirk D.
Yanowitz, Meyer
Young, James William
Zacarian, Setrag
Zackheim, Herschel S.
Zaffke, Karl Heinz
Zagula-Mally, Zenova

Uruguay

Chiaffitelli, Cezar A.
Montero, Eustaquio D.
Vignale-Peirano, Raul A.

Venezuela

Aguilera, Fernando
Alarcon-Pena, Carlos
Campins, Humberto
Di-Prisco, Juan
Graterol-Rogue, Cruz A.
Hernandez, Jose R.
Homez, Jorge
Kerdel-Vegas, Francisco
Medina, Rafael
Miret, Omar
Moncada, Eleonora
Pedrique-Alvarez, Henry
Rincon, Bratcho Humberto
Scannone, Francisco
Schnidmajer, Ester W.

South Vietnam

Nguyen Van Ut
Trinh Kim Mong Don

Yugoslavia

Adamčič, Milan
Berčič, Maria
Betetto, Milan
Brničevič, Marin
Cajkovac, Vladimir
Fettich, Janez
Jakac, Dušan
Karlić, Djurdjica
Kogoj, Franjo
Konstantinović, Sava
Koražija, Ivo
Kristitsch, Aleksandar
Majcan, Dragan
Matanić, Vladimir
Mravunac, Nikola
Perišić, Slobodan
Premšak, Walter
Radovanovic, Mihajlo
Ruben, Remon
Schwarzwald, Milan
Stevanović, Danilo

International Committee of Dermatology
Meeting of July 30, 1967 (Munich)

Present: DEGOS (President), HELLERSTRÖM (Secretary General), JABLONSKA, RAMOS E SILVA, KITAMURA, QUIROGA, LAPIÈRE, FLARER, BRUNSTING, MITCHELL-HEGGS, GAY PRIETO, SAGHER. Ex officio: SULZBERGER, PILLSBURY, LIVINGOOD, JADASSOHN, SCHIRREN.

The Secretary General, Prof. HELLERSTRÖM, presents his report and informs the Committee that he renounces to his fonctions as Secretary General. The Committee expresses all its gratitude to Prof. HELLERSTRÖM for the 15 years of his fonctions, as Secretary General and Treasurer, perfectly accomplished.

The President opens the discussion in regard to the place of the next International Congress of 1972. Three propositions were officially made:

Australia (Sydney): President Prof. BELISARIO
Italy (Padoua — Venice): President Prof. FLARER
Roumania (Bucarest): President Prof. LONGHIN.

An unofficial, last minute proposition, by Brazil, could not be taken under consideration. Prof. FLARER remarks that Italy's candidature was solicited by the Committee itself.

After secret vote, Italy is chosen in the first place, and Australia in the second. This choice will be communicated to the Assembly of Delegates and will be submitted to its vote.

The President asks the vote of the Committee for the election of the President and the Secretary General-Treasurer of the International Committee for the period 1967 to 1972. By secret vote, Prof. GAY PRIETO is elected President and Prof. SAGHER Secretary General. The Committee decides to submit this double election to the approval of the Assembly of Delegates, even though this procedure is not specified in the present statutes (this procedure had already taken place in Washington).

The President then proceeds to the renewal of one third of the Committee members, according to the modalities specified in chapter two of the statutes. The four outgoing members, according to their age, are: MM. RAMOS e SILVA, KITAMURA, QUIROGA and LAPIÈRE. By secret vote the following are proposed for their replacement: MM. BRAUN-FALCO, BAER, PADILHA-GONÇALVES and CORDERO. This proposition will be submitted to the vote of the Assembly of Delegates.

The Committee was confronted with two propositions of modification of the statutes, one by Prof. DEGOS at the Paris meeting in 1965 and the other by Prof. GAY PRIETO in Jerusalem in 1966. After a unanimous agreement, only one text of modification, associating the points of view of the two proceeding propositions, will be submitted to the vote of the Assembly of Delegates. The Committee confirms the decision, taken in Jerusalem, to propose to the Assembly of the Delegates to establish the contribution of each member of every National Society to $ 1,5 for a period of 5 years.

On the President's proposal, the Committee decided to abolish the Committee of Nomenclature, Classification and Education. Only "The Institute for Dermatologic Communication and Education" will persist. Prof. SULZBERGER drew a statment on the activity of this Institute (see page 1382, Vol. 2).

The relation with the World Health Organization and the Council of International Medical Sciences will be discussed at the next meeting of the Committee which is arranged for August 5.

Comité International de Dermatologie
Réunion du 30 Juillet 1967 (Munich)

Présents: DEGOS (Président), HELLERSTRÖM (Secrétaire Général), JABLONSKA, RAMOS E SILVA, KITAMURA, QUIROGA, LAPIÈRE, FLARER, BRUNSTING, MITCHELL-HEGGS, GAY PRIETO, SAGHER. Ex Officio: SULZBERGER, PILLSBURY, LIVINGOOD, JADASSOHN, SCHIRREN.

Le Secrétaire Général, Prof. HELLERSTRÖM, présente son rapport et fait savoir au Comité qu'il abandonne ses fonctions de Secrétaire Général. Le Comité témoigne au Prof. HELLERSTRÖM toute sa gratitude pour les 15 années où il a si parfaitement rempli ses fonctions de Secrétaire Général et de Trésorier.

Le président met en discussion le lieu où doit se tenir le futur Congrès International en 1972. Trois propositions ont été faites officiellement:

Australie (Sydney): Président Prof. BELISARIO
Italie (Padoue — Venise): Président Prof. FLARER
Roumanie (Bucarest): Président Prof. LONGHIN,

une proposition officieuse, faite en dernière heure, par le Brésil ne pouvant être retenue. Le Prof. FLARER fait remarquer que la candidature de l'Italie a été sollicitée par le Comité lui-même.

Après vote au scrutin secret l'Italie est choisie en premier lieu et l'Australie en deuxième lieu. Ce choix sera communiqué à l'assemblée des Délégués et sera soumis à son vote.

Le Président soumet au vote du Comité l'élection du Président et du Secrétaire Général, Trésorier du Comité International pour la période 1967 à 1972. Au scrutin secret, le Prof. GAY PRIETO est élu Président et le Prof. SAGHER Secrétaire Général. Le Comité décide, dans un esprit démocratique, de soumettre cette double élection à l'approbation de l'assemblée des Délégués bien que cette procédure ne soit pas inscrite dans les statuts actuels (cette procédure a déjà eu lieu à Washington).

Le président fait ensuite procéder au renouvellement du tiers des membres du Comité, suivant les modalités précisées dans le chapitre 2 des statuts. Les quatre membres sortants sont, d'après leur âge: MM RAMOS E SILVA, KITAMURA, QUIROGA et LAPIÈRE. Au scrutin secret, sont proposés pour les remplacer: MM BRAUN-FALCO, BAER, PADILHA-GONÇALVES, CORDERO. Cette proposition sera soumise au vote de l'assemblée des Délégués.

Le Comité a été saisi de deux propositions de modifications des statuts, l'une du Prof. DEGOS à la réunion de Paris en 1965, l'autre du Prof. GAY PRIETO à Jérusalem en 1966. Après un unanime accord, un seul texte de modifications, associant les points de vue des deux propositions précédentes, sera soumis au vote de l'assemblée des Délégués.

Le Comité confirme la décision prise à Jérusalem de proposer à l'assemblée des Délégués, de fixer la contribution de chaque Société Nationale à $ 1.50 pour chacun de ses membres et pour une période de 5 ans.

Sur la proposition du Président, le Comité décide de supprimer les Comités de Nomenclature, de Classification et d'Education. Seul persistera «The Institute for Dermatologic Communication and Education» et le Prof. SULZBERGER fait un exposé sur l'activité de cet Institut (exposé imprimé page 1382, Vol. 2).

Les rapports avec l'O.M.S. et le C.I.O.M.S. seront discutés à la prochaine réunion du Comité qui est fixée au 5 Août.

Comité Internacional de Dermatología
Sesión del 30 de Julio de 1967 (Munich)

Presentes: DEGOS (Presidente), HELLERSTRÖM (Secretario General), JABLONSKA, RAMOS E SILVA, KITAMURA, QUIROGA, LAPIÈRE, FLARER, BRUNSTING, MITCHELL-HEGGS, GAY PRIETO, SAGHER. Ex Officio: SULZBERGER, PILLSBURY, LIVINGOOD, JADASSOHN, SCHIRREN.

El Secretario General, Prof. HELLERSTRÖM, presenta su informe y notifica al Comité que cesa en sus funciones de Secretario General. El Comité expresa al Prof. HELLERSTRÖM toda su gratitud, por los 15 años, en que éste, con tanta competencia, ha ejercido las funciones de Secretario General y Tesorero.

El Presidente somete a discusión el lugar donde, en 1972, deberá celebrarse el próximo Congreso Internacional de Dermatología. Han sido presentadas oficialmente tres propuestas, a saber:

Australia (Sydney): Presidente Prof. BELISARIO
Italia (Padua — Venecia): Presidente Prof. FLARER
Rumania (Bucarest): Presidente Prof. LONGHIN.

Una propuesta oficiosa, presentada por el Brasil en el último momento, no pudo ser tomada en consideración. El Prof. FLARER recuerda que la candidatura en favor de Italia fué presentada por el propio Comité.

Tras voto secreto, Italia obtiene el primer lugar seguida de Australia. Este resultado será comunicado a la Asamblea de los Delegados y sometido a su aprobación.

El Presidente somete al voto del Comité la elección de los cargos de los nuevos Presidente y Secretario General y Tesorero del Comité Internacional durante el período 1967 a 1972. En votación secreta son elegidos, Presidente el Prof. GAY PRIETO, y, Secretario General y Tesorero el Prof. SAGHER. Con espíritu democrático, el Comité decide someter, esta doble elección, a la aprobación de la Asamblea de Delegados, aunque esta formalidad no figure inscrita en los estatutos vigentes. (Un caso similar, sin embargo, tuvo lugar en Washington).

Acto seguido, el Presidente procede a la renovación de un tercio de los miembros del Comité, del modo previsto en el capítulo 2° de los estatutos. Los miembros salientes, por orden de edades, son los Sres. RAMOS E SILVA, KITAMURA, QUIROGA y LAPIÈRE. Son propuestos para reemplazarles los Sres. BRAUN-FALCO, BAER, PADILHA-GONÇALVES y CORDERO. Esta propuesta será sometida al voto de la Asamblea de Delegados.

El Comité delibera, a continuación, sobre dos propuestas de enmienda de los estatutos. Una, presentada por el Prof. DEGOS en la reunión de París de 1965, la otra, por el Prof. GAY PRIETO en Jerusalén en 1966. Por acuerdo unánime, se acepta una sola enmienda que asocia ambas propuestas y que será sometida a la aprobación de la Asamblea de Delegados.

El Comité ratifica su decisión, tomada en Jerusalén, de proponer a la Asamblea de Delegados que establezca la cuota de un dólar cincuenta por cada uno de los miembros de cada Sociedad Nacional y por un período de 5 años.

A propuesta del Presidente, el Comité decide suprimir los comités llamados de Nomenclatura, Clasificación y Educación. Será mantenido, solamente, "The Institute for Dermatologic Communication and Education" sobre cuya actividad presenta un informe el Prof. SULZBERGER (dicho informe se halla impreso página 1382, vol. 2).

Las relaciones con la O.M.S. y el C.I.O.M.S. serán discutidos en la próxima reunión del Comité fijada para el día 5 de Agosto.

Internationales Komitee für Dermatologie
Sitzung vom 30. Juli 1967 (München)

Anwesend: Degos (Präsident), Hellerström (Generalsekretär), Jablonska, Ramos e Silva, Kitamura, Quiroga, Lapière, Flarer, Brunsting, Mitchell-Heggs, Gay Prieto, Sagher. Ex Officio: Sulzberger, Pillsbury, Livingood, Jadassohn, Schirren.

Der Generalsekretär, Prof. Hellerström, verliest seinen Bericht und teilt dem Komitee mit, daß er seine Funktion als Generalsekretär niederlegt. Das Komitee dankt Prof. Hellerström für seine Tätigkeit als Generalsekretär und Quästor, die er 15 Jahre lang zu aller Zufriedenheit ausgeübt hat.

Der Präsident stellt die Frage zur Diskussion, wo der nächste Internationale Kongreß 1972 abgehalten werden soll. Drei Vorschläge wurden offiziell gemacht:

Australien (Sydney): Präsident Prof. Belisario
Italien (Padua — Venedig): Präsident Prof. Flarer
Rumänien (Bukarest): Präsident Prof. Longhin.

Ein nicht offizieller Vorschlag, welcher in letzter Minute von Brasilien eingebracht wurde, konnte nicht mehr berücksichtigt werden. Prof. Flarer betont, daß die Kandidatur Italiens vom Komitee selber gewünscht wurde.

In geheimer Abstimmung wurde in erster Linie Italien bestimmt, in zweiter Linie Australien. Dieses Resultat wird der Versammlung der Delegierten mitgeteilt werden und ihr zur Abstimmung vorgelegt werden.

Der Präsident unterbreitet dem Komitee die Wahl des Präsidenten und des General-sekretär- Quästors des Internationalen Komitees für die Zeitspanne 1967 bis 1972. In geheimer Abstimmung wird Prof. Gay Prieto zum Präsidenten und Prof. Sagher zum Generalsekretär gewählt. Das Komitee entscheidet, um demokratischen Gepflogenheiten gerecht zu werden, diese doppelte Wahl zur Annahme der Versammlung der Delegierten zu unterbreiten, trotzdem dies in den jetzt geltenden Statuten nicht vorgesehen ist (es wurde schon in Washington so vorgegangen). Der Präsident geht dann über zur Neuwahl von vier Mitgliedern des Internationalen Komitees, da die Herren Ramos e Silva, Kitamura, Quiroga und Lapière altershalber zurücktreten. In geheimer Abstimmung werden, um sie zu ersetzen, die Herren Braun-Falco, Baer, Padilha-Gonçalves und Cordero vorgeschlagen. Diese Vorschläge werden zur Abstimmung der Delegiertenversammlung vorgelegt werden.

Danach wurden zwei Änderungsvorschläge in bezug auf die Satzungen zur Diskussion gestellt. Der eine war von Prof. Degos anläßlich der Sitzung des Komitees in Paris 1965, der andere von Prof. Gay Prieto 1966 während der Sitzung in Jerusalem eingebracht worden. Das Komitee beschließt einstimmig, nur einen Änderungstext, der die Punkte beider Vorschläge beinhaltet, der Delegiertenversammlung zur Beschlußfassung vorzulegen.

Das Komitee bestätigt den Beschluß, der in Jerusalem gefaßt wurde, der Delegiertenversammlung vorzuschlagen, für jede nationale Gesellschaft pro Mitglied einen Beitrag von $ 1,5 für 5 Jahre festzusetzen.

Auf Vorschlag des Präsidenten entscheidet das Internationale Komitee, daß die Komitees für Nomenklatur, Klassifikation und Erziehung aufzuheben sind. Nur das „Institute for Dermatologic Communication and Education" soll beibehalten werden, und Prof. Sulzberger gibt einen Bericht über die Aktivität dieses Instituts (siehe Band 2, Seite 1382).

Die Beziehungen zur O.M.S. und der C.I.O.M.S. werden bei der nächsten Sitzung des Komitees diskutiert werden. Die nächste Sitzung wird auf den 5. August festgesetzt.

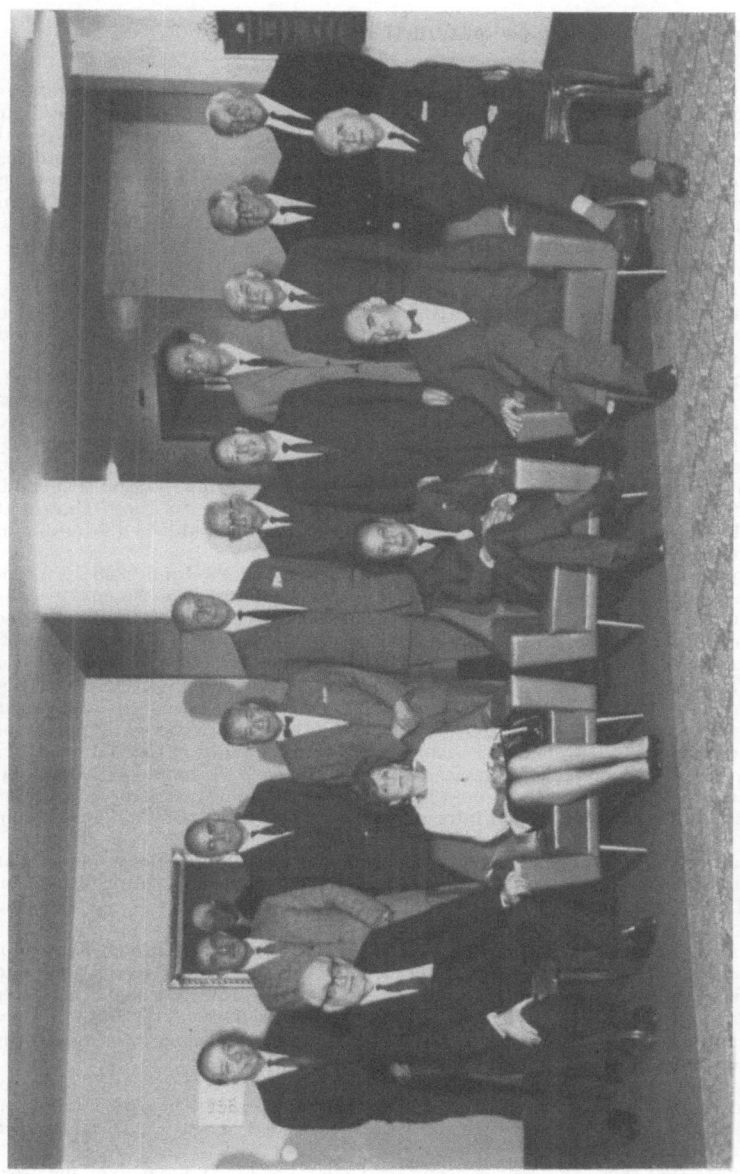

International Committee for Dermatology 1967—1972

First row: Prof. W. Jadassohn/Switzerland, Prof. St. Jablonska/Poland, Prof. J. Gay Prieto/Spain, Prof. R. Degos/France, Prof. S. Hellerström/Sweden

Second row: Prof. R. Baer/USA, Prof. Fr. Flarer/Italy, Prof. O. Braun-Falco/Germany, Prof. K. Kitamura/Japan (guest), Prof. S. Lapière/Belgium, Prof. J. Ramos e Silva/Brazil (guest), Prof. S. Sagher/Israel, Prof. C. G. Schirren/Germany, Prof. M. J. Quiroga/Argentina (guest), Prof. A. Padilha-Gonçalves/Argentina, Prof. M. B. Sulzberger/USA

Report to the International Committee of Dermatology (I.C.D.) at the XIIIth International Congress of Dermatology, Munich (Germany) 1967

by S. HELLERSTRÖM, Secretary-General of the Committee

Since the International Congress of Dermatology in Washington, D.C., 1962 the Secretary-General has continued contact with the different dermatological societies through their presidents and secretaries in order to get delegates nominated to the Assembly of National Delegates and to have a complete list of the members of the above societies. In a few countries having more than one dermatological society there still have been some difficulties in getting the delegates agreed upon and nominated by consultation between the societies as specified in the Rules and Regulations of the International League of Dermatological Societies. Up to now almost 40 countries have nominated their delegates, most of whom will attend the forthcoming congress. A list of delegates is attached to this report.

Prof. S. LAPIÈRE has been the representative of the International Committee of Dermatology in the Council of International Medical Sciences (C.I.O.M.S.). Prof. JOSÉ GAY PRIETO has been the permanent representative of the League in the World Health Organization in Geneva and the official relations with WHO are being continued.

A non-official meeting of the International Committee of Dermatology was held in Munich, 2 to 3 August, 1964, at which the details and organization of the XIIIth International Congress of Dermatology were discussed and accomodation for the Congress was demonstrated by Prof. MARCHIONINI personally. A provisional programme was selected by the committee. Simultaneous translations of the official languages was decided and in addition translation from Russian, providing a sufficiently large number of Russian dermatologists attended. Prof. and Mrs. SULZBERGER indicated that film presentations similar to those shown at Washington 1962 should be arranged. [The protocol of the meeting was published inter alia in the Acta derm.-venereol. Stockholm **45**, 255, (1965).]

A second non-official meeting of I.C.D. was held in Paris, 21 to 22 June 1965 at which Prof. DEGOS paid homage to the memory of Prof. ALFRED MARCHIONINI. The Committee was informed that an invitation had been received from the WHO (through Dr. CANDAU) for the League of Dermatological Societies to be represented at certain Expert Committees. Prof. DEGOS proposed certain modifications of statutes to be put to the vote before the Assembly of Delegates. The I.C.D. unanimously elected Prof. W. JADASSOHN as President of the International Congress in Munich. Prof. JADASSOHN then asked Prof. C. G. SCHIRREN to continue as Secretary-General in Munich. The Organization of the XIIIth International Congress of Dermatology was discussed and preliminary determined as to organizers (consultants) for each theme or symposium. The subjects of themes and symposia, with the names of the responsible organizers, should be published in national journals of dermatology as soon as possible. [The protocol of the meeting was published inter alia in the Acta derm.-venereol. Stockholm **45**, 393 (1965).]

An official statutory meeting of the International Committee of Dermatology was held at Hadassah University Hospital Jerusalem, Israel, May 2 to 3, 1966. At the meeting in Jerusalem the organization of the Scientific session of the Munich Congress was discussed, outlined and special arrangements adopted.

Revisions and amendments of the Rules and Regulations of the International League of Dermatological Societies were also discussed in Jerusalem. An Amendment to Statutes and By-Laws, proposed by Prof. JOSÉ GAY PRIETO, was accepted by the International Committee and will be submitted to the Assembly of Delegates for approval at the XIII International Congress, Munich, August 1967. [The protocol of the meeting was published inter alia in the Acta derm.-venereol. Stockholm **46**, 359 (1966).]

I am sorry to inform you that the finances of the I.C.D. are unsatisfactory with a deficit of 1.674 (onethousandsixhundred and seventyfour) U.S. dollars. The membership contribution of national societies necessarily has to be increased as was decided at the I.C.D. meeting in Jerusalem, 1966.

Finally may I state that these 15 years as Secretary-General of I.C.D. have given me great satisfaction. I wish to thank all the colleagues who have made the work of the Secretary-General interesting, stimulating and pleasant. However I feel that it is about time to withdraw from the Secretary ship. Before doing so I like to underline that the Members of I.C.D. and the representatives of Munich Congress Committee have specially deserved to receive my gratitute for the time passed away. I thank you all most sincerely for the great confidence extended to me during these 15 years.

Comité International de Dermatologie
Rapport présenté au XIIIième Congrès International de Dermatologie, Munich, 1967

par son Secrétaire Général, S. HELLERSTRÖM ·

Dès la fin du XIIième Congrès International de Dermatologie, (Washington, 1962), le Secrétaire Général a maintenu le contact avec les différentes Sociétés Nationales de Dermatologie à travers leurs Présidents et leurs Secrétaires afin de prendre connaissance des noms des Délégués proposés à l'Assemblée des Délégués Nationaux et d'avoir la liste complète de tous les membres des dites Sociétés. Dans les rares pays ayant plus d'une Société Dermatologique, il y a quelques difficultés à ce que les diverses Sociétés se mettent d'accord dans la nomination de leurs Délégués, comme il est prévu dans les statuts et règles de la Ligue Internationale des Sociétés Dermatologiques. Jusqu'à présent, près de 40 pays ont nommé leurs Délégués, la plupart desquels se rendront au prochain Congrès. Une liste des Délégués est annexée au présent rapport.

Le Prof. LAPIÈRE a été le représentant du Comité International de Dermatologie auprès du C.I.O.M.S. (Council of International Medical Sciences). Le Prof. GAY PRIETO a été le représentant permanent de la Ligue auprès de l'OMS à Genève. Nos relations officielles avec ladite Organisation subsistent.

Une réunion officieuse du Comité International de Dermatologie eut lieu à Munich les 2 et 3 août 1964, où furent discutés les préparatifs pour l'organisation du XIIIième Congrès International de Dermatologie. Le Prof. MARCHIONINI lui-même donna des précisions à ce sujet. Un programme provisoire fut rédigé par le Comité.

La traduction simultanée des langues officielles du Congrès fut adoptée, y compris le russe, à condition qu'un nombre suffisant de dermatologistes russes assistent au Congrès. Le Prof. et Mme. SULZBERGER annoncèrent qu'une démonstration de films semblable à celle qui fut faite à Washington serait possible à Munich. [Le Protocole de la réunion fut publié dans Acta derm.-venereol. Stockholm **45**, 255 (1965).]

Une deuxième réunion officieuse du Comité International de Dermatologie eut lieu à Paris, les 21 et 22 juin 1965, où le Prof. DEGOS rendit hommage à la mémoire du Prof. MARCHIONINI. Le Comité fut informé d'une invitation reçue, émanant de l'O.M.S. sollicitant que la Ligue des Sociétés Dermatologiques soit représentée auprès de certains Comités d'Experts de l'OMS.

Le Prof. DEGOS propose quelques amendements aux Statuts qui devront être votés avant la réunion de l'Assemblée des Délégués. Le Comité International de Dermatologie élit le Prof. W. JADASSOHN, à l'unanimité, comme Président du Congrès International de Dermatologie à Munich. Le Prof. W. JADASSOHN demande au Prof. C. G. SCHIRREN de continuer son mandat de Secrétaire Général. On délibère et on désigne, au préalable, les organisateurs (Consultants) de chaque Thème ou Symposium. Les sujets à traiter dans les Thèmes et les Symposia devront être publiés dans les journaux dermatologiques dans le délai le plus bref. [Le protocole de cette réunion fut publié dans Acta derm.-venereol. Stockholm **45**, 393 (1965).]

Une réunion officielle du Comité International de Dermatologie, prévue par les Statuts, eut lieu dans les locaux de l'Hôpital Universitaire Hadassah à Jérusalem, Israel., les 2 et 3 mai 1966. Dans cette réunion fut discutée l'organisation du programme scientifique et celui-ci adopté avec quelques modifications. On discuta aussi à Jérusalem des modifications ou amendements aux Statuts et Règlements de la Ligue Internationale des Sociétés Dermatologiques. Un Amendement présenté par le Prof. GAY PRIETO fut accepté par le C.I.D. et sera soumis à l'approbation de l'Assemblée des Délégués au XIIIième Congrès International de Dermatologie de Munich en 1967. [Le protocole de cette réunion fut publié dans Acta derm.-venereol. Stockholm **46**, 359 (1966).]

Je suis navré de vous informer que les finances du C.I.D. ne sont pas satisfaisantes. Il y a un déficit de 1.674 U.S. dollars. La contribution des membres des Sociétés Nationales devra être augmentée selon décision prise dans la réunion du C.I.D. à Jérusalem en 1966.

Finalement, je déclare la grande satisfaction que j'ai eue pendant les 15 ans où j'ai occupé le poste de Secrétaire Général. J'aimerais remercier tous mes collègues qui ont rendu mon travail de Secrétaire Général intéressant, agréable et encourageant. Néanmoins, je crois qu'il est temps d'abandonner mon poste. Avant mon départ, je dois souligner que les membres du C.I.D. et les représentants du Comité du Congrès de Munich sont, spécialement priés d'accepter ma gratitude pour la période écoulée. Je vous remercie, vous tous, très sincèrement, pour la confiance que vous m'avez témoignée, pendant ces 15 années.

Comité Internacional de Dermatología
Informe presentado en el XIII Congreso Internacional
de Dermatología, Munich, 1967

por S. HELLERSTRÖM, Secretario General del C.I.D.

Tras la clausura del XII Congreso Internacional de Dermatología (Washington, 1962) el Secretario General ha mantenido el contacto con las diversas Sociedades Nacionales de Dermatología a través de sus Presidentes y Secretarios con objeto de inscribir los nombres de los delegados propuestos para formar parte de la Asamblea de Delegados y obtener la lista completa de todos los miembros de cada Sociedad Nacional. En los escasos países, donde existen más de una Sociedad de Dermatología, se han presentado ciertas dificultades en los nombramientos de delegados que deben ser elegidos por acuerdo mutuo entre las diversas Sociedades, según lo estipulan los estatutos de la Liga Internacional de Sociedades de Dermatología. Hasta la fecha, casi 40 paises han nombrado sus delegados, la mayor parte de los cuales acudirán al proximo Congreso. Una lista de los Delegados se adjunta a este informe.

El Prof. LAPIÈRE ha sido el representante del Comité Internacional de Dermatología ante el C.I.O.M.S. (Council of International Medical Sciences). El Prof. GAY PRIETO ha sido el representante permanente de la Liga ante la O.M.S. continuando las relaciones oficiales con dicha Organización.

Una reunión oficiosa del C.I.D. tuvo lugar en Munich los días 2 y 3 de Agosto de 1964, durante la cual, se estudiaron los preparativos necesarios para la buena organización del XIII Congreso Internacional de Dermatología. El Prof. MARCHIONINI comentó aquellos que habian sido adoptados. El C.I.D. preparó un programa provisional.

Se aceptó la traducción simultánea en las lenguas oficiales del Congreso, incluso el ruso, con la condición de que asistan al Congreso un número suficiente de dermatólogos rusos. El Prof. y la Sra. SULZBERGER, declararon, que una serie de películas científicas como las que fueron proyectadas en el Congreso de Washington sería posible en Munich. [El protocolo de esta reunión fué publicado en Acta derm.-venereol. Stockholm **45**, 255 (1965).]

Una segunda reunión oficiosa del C.I.D. tuvo lugar en París, en los días 21 y 22 de Junio de 1965, en la cual, el Prof. DEGOS rindió homenaje a la memoria del Prof. MARCHIONINI. Se informó al C.I.D. de una invitación procedente de la O.M.S. en la cual se solicita que una representación de la Liga Internacional de Sociedades de Dermatología figure en el seno de algunos Comités de Expertos de la O.M.S.

El Prof. DEGOS depositó algunas enmiendas a los estatutos que deberán ser sometidas a votación antes de la reunión de la Asamblea de Delegados. El C.I.D. eligió al Prof. W. JADASSOHN, por unanimidad, Presidente del XIII Congreso Internacional de Dermatología en Munich. El Prof. W. JADASSOHN solicitó del Prof. SCHIRREN su continuación como Secretario General. Se deliberó sobre la organización del XIII Congreso y fueron designados los ponentes de cada tema o simposio. Las materias a tratar en los temas o simposios deberá ser publicada en los periódicos de dermatología en el plazo mas breve posible. [El protocolo de esta reunión se publicó en Acta derm.-venereol. Stockholm **45**, 393 (1965).]

Una reunión estatutaria del Comité Internacional de Dermatología, tuvo lugar en el recinto del Hospital Universitario Hadassah de Jerusalén, los dias 2 y 3 de Mayo de 1966. Se trató en esta reunión de la redacción del programa científico que fué adoptado con ciertas modificaciones. Tambien se trató en Jerusalén de las modificaciones y enmiendas de los estatutos y reglamento de la Liga Internacional de Sociedades de Dermatología. Una enmienda a los mismos fué presentada por el Prof. GAY PRIETO, la cual fué aceptada por el C.I.D. y será sometida a la aprobación de la Asamblea de Delegados del XIII Congreso Internacional de Dermatología de Munich en 1967. [El protocolo de esta reunión fué publicado en Acta derm.-venereol. Stockholm **46**, 359 (1966).]

Siento informarles que la situación financiera del C.I.D. no es nada satisfactoria, y que arroja un déficit de 1.674 dolares. La cuota de los miembros de las Sociedades Dermatológicas debe ser aumentada según se convino en la reunión del C.I.D. en Jerusalén en 1966.

Finalmente, quiero hacer constar la gran satisfacción que he tenido, durante 15 años, en el desempeño de mi cargo de Secretario General. Deseo dar las gracias a todos mis colegas que han facilitado mi misión, haciéndola interesante, agradable y atractiva. Sin embargo, creo que ha llegado el momento de que yo cese de ocuparme de esta Secretaría. Antes de mi partida, designo a los miembros del C.I.D. y del Comité del Congreso Alemán, como recipientarios de mi agradecimiento por el tiempo pasado. Les estoy reconocido, a todos Vds., muy sinceramente, por la confianza que me han otorgado durante estos 15 años.

Bericht für das Internationale Komitee für Dermatologie, vorgelegt am XIII. Internationalen Kongreß für Dermatologie, München, 1967

von S. HELLERSTRÖM, Generalsekretär des Komitees

Seit dem Internationalen Kongreß für Dermatologie 1962 in Washington stand der General-sekretär weiterhin in Kontakt mit den Präsidenten und Sekretären der verschiedenen dermato-logischen Gesellschaften, um vollständige Mitgliederlisten und Nominationen für die Dele-giertenversammlung zu erhalten. In einigen Ländern, die mehr als eine dermatologische Gesellschaft haben, gab es Schwierigkeiten bei der Ernennung der Delegierten, die entspre-chend den Statuten durch Konsultationen der Gesellschaften untereinander erfolgen soll. Bis jetzt haben ungefähr 40 Länder ihre Delegierten ernannt, die fast alle am kommenden Kongreß teilnehmen werden. Eine Liste der Delegierten liegt diesem Bericht bei.

Prof. S. LAPIÈRE vertrat das Internationale Komitee für Dermatologie beim „Council of International Medical Sciences" (Ci.I.O.M.S.). Prof. J. GAY PRIETO war ständiger Vertreter der Liga bei der Weltgesundheits-Organisation (W.H.O.) in Genf. Die offiziellen Beziehungen zur W.H.O. werden fortgesetzt.

Anläßlich einer inoffiziellen Sitzung des Internationalen Komitees für Dermatologie (I.C.D.) am 2. und 3. August 1964 in München wurde die Organisation des XIII. Internationalen Kongresses beraten. Prof. MARCHIONINI demonstrierte persönlich die vorgesehenen Räum-lichkeiten. Das Komitee legte ein vorläufiges Programm fest und beschloß, für die offiziellen Kongreßsprachen Simultanübersetzung einzurichten. Übertragung ins Russische wurde vor-gesehen, falls genügend russische Dermatologen am Kongreß teilnehmen würden. Prof. und Frau SULZBERGER wiesen darauf hin, daß Filmdemonstrationen wie in Washington arrangiert werden sollten (Das Protokoll dieser Sitzung wurde u. a. in den Acta. derm.-venerol., Stock-holm, 45, 255 (1965) publiziert).

Auf einer zweiten inoffiziellen Sitzung des I.C.D. vom 21. bis 22. Juni 1965 in Paris gedachte Prof. DEGOS des verstorbenen Präsidenten, Prof. ALFRED MARCHIONINI. — Dem Komitee wurde mitgeteilt, daß eine Einladung der W.H.O. durch Dr. CANDAU an die Liga der Dermato-logischen Gesellschaften vorlag, Vertreter zu bestimmten Expertenkomitees zu entsenden. Prof. DEGOS schlug einige Statutenänderungen vor, die der Delegiertenversammlung vorge-legt werden sollen. Das Internationale Komitee wählte einstimmig Prof. WERNER JADASSOHN zum neuen Präsidenten des Kongresses. Prof. JADASSOHN bat Prof. C. G. SCHIRREN, weiterhin als Generalsekretär zu fungieren. Das Komitee diskutierte über die Organisation des XIII. Der-matologenkongresses in München und ernannte vorläufig Organisatoren (consultants) für jedes Thema und Symposium. Die Themen und Symposien sowie die Namen der verantwort-lichen Organisatoren sollten in den nationalen Fachzeitschriften so rasch wie möglich publiziert werden [Acta derm.-venereol., Stockholm 45, 393 (1965)].

Gemäß den Statuten fand im Hadassah-Univ.-Krankenhaus von Jerusalem am 2. und 3. Mai 1966 eine offizielle Sitzung des Komitees statt, auf der die Organisation der wissen-schaftlichen Sitzungen beraten und bestimmte Einrichtungen festgelegt wurden.

Außerdem wurde über Änderungen und Ergänzungen der Statuten der Internationalen Liga Dermatologischer Gesellschaften diskutiert. Das Komitee akzeptierte einen Änderungs-vorschlag von Prof. J. GAY PRIETO, der auf dem XIII. Internationalen Kongreß in München der Delegiertenversammlung zur Abstimmung vorgelegt werden wird (Acta derm.-venereol. Stockholm 46, 359 (1966).

Leider muß ich mitteilen, daß die Finanzen des I.C.D. unbefriedigend sind und daß ein Defizit von 1674 U.S. Dollars besteht. Der Mitgliedbeitrag der nationalen Gesellschaften muß erhöht werden, wie es auf der Sitzung des I.C.D. in Jerusalem beschlossen wurde.

Darf ich abschließend versichern, daß mir diese 15 Jahre als Generalsekretär des I.C.D. große Befriedigung verschafft haben. Ich möchte allen Kollegen, die meine Arbeit als General-sekretär interessant und anregend gestaltet haben, danken. Nunmehr ist es an der Zeit, mich von diesem Amt zurückzuziehen. Vorher aber möchte ich unterstreichen, daß die Mitglieder des Internationalen Komitees und die Vertreter des deutschen Organisationskomitees meinen ganz besonderen Dank verdienen. Ich danke Ihnen allen sehr herzlich für das große Vertrauen, das Sie mir in diesen 15 Jahren entgegengebracht haben.

International League of Dermatological Societies

General Assembly of National Delegates, Munich, August 4, 1967 (Presidence: Prof. R. DEGOS)

The President delivers a welcome speech to the National Delegates and reads articles of the Status specifying the number of delegates per National Society and the powers of the Assembly.

The Secretary General, Prof. S. HELLERSTRÖM, proceeds to call the delegates officially appointed by the National Societies (43 nations represented). Then he delivers a moral and financial report which are approved by the Assembly.

The President informs the Assembly of the propositions adopted by the International Committee which are submitted to the vote of the Delegates.

1. Choice of the future place for the International Congress and its President: Italy (Padoua — Venice) being proposed in the first place, Australia in the second. Italy (Padoua — Venice), with Prof. FLARER as the president, obtains by secret vote the majority of voices.

Prof. FLARER thanks the delegates for their vote and assures them that he will do his best to welcome, in the best conditions, a great number of congressists in Padoua in 1972.

2. Designation of the new President and Secretary General of the International Committee of Dermatology. The Committee solicites the vote of the Assembly in order to give a more democratic base to this appointment.

Prof. GAY PRIETO and Prof. SAGHER are elected by secret vote, obtaining the majority of voices, the first as President of the International Committee and the second as Secretary General-Treasurer of the I.C.D.

Prof. GAY PRIETO adresses a short speech to the Assembly thanking for its vote.

3. Election of four new members of the International Committee. Prof. O. BRAUN-FALCO (Republic Federal of Germany), R. BAER (USA), A. PADILHA-GONÇALVES (Brazil) and A. A. CORDERO (Argentina), proposed by the I.C.D. and elected by secret vote.

4. Modifications of status: the propositions of the I.C.D. are voted by show of hands (see page 117).

5. Determination of the financial contributions of National Societies: the Secretary General-Treasurer informs that the league presents a financial deficit and proposes to determine the contribution for every member of the National Societies, to 1,5 $ for a period of 5 years. This amount is voted by show of hands.

6. The President announces the supression of the Committees of Nomenclature, Classification and Education. He specifies that "The Institute for Dermatologic Communication and Education" will continue its activities, one of which the realization of films owed principally to the effects of Mrs. SULZBERGER for which no ample thanks will be expressed.

Prof. SULZBERGER drew up a statement to specify the situation of this Institute.

Ligue Internationale des Sociétés Dermatologiques

Assemblée Générale des Délégués Nationaux, Munich, 4 Août 1697 (Présidence: Prof. R. DEGOS)

Le Président prononce une allocution de bienvenue aux Délégués Nationaux et donne lecture des articles des Statuts précisant le nombre des délégués par Société Nationale et les pouvoirs de l'Assemblée.

Le Secrétaire Général, Prof. S. HELLERSTRÖM, procède à l'appel des délégués officiellement désignés par les Sociétés Nationales (43 nations représentées). Il fait ensuite le rapport moral et le rapport financier qui sont approuvés par l'Assemblée (Rapport à la suite de ce texte).

Le Président communique à l'Assemblée les propositions adoptées par le Comité International et qui sont soumises au vote des délégués:

1. Choix du futur lieu du Congrès International et du Président de ce Congrès: l'Italie (Padoue, Venise) étant proposée en premier lieu, l'Australie en deuxième lieu. L'Italie (Padoue, Venise) avec le Prof. FLARER, comme Président, obtient, au scrutin secret, la majorité des voix

Le Prof. FLARER remercie les délégués de leur vote et les assure qu'il fera tout son possible pour accueillir, dans les meilleures conditions, un grand nombre de Congressistes à Padoue en 1972.

2. Désignation du nouveau Président et du nouveau Secrétaire Général du Comité International de Dermatologie: le Comité sollicite le vote de l'Assemblée pour cette élection afin de donner à celle-ci une base plus démocratique. Au scrutin secret, le Prof. GAY PRIETO et le Prof. SAGHER sont élus, à la majorité des voix, le premier comme Président du C.I.D. et le second comme Secrétaire Général—Trésorier du C.I.D.

Le Prof. GAY PRIETO prononce une courte allocution pour remercier l'Assemblée de son vote.

3. Election des quatre nouveaux membres du C.I.D. Les Prof. O. BRAUN-FALCO (Allemagne), R. BAER (USA), A. PADILHA-GONÇALVES (Brésil) et A. A. CORDERO (Argentine), proposés par le C.I.D., sont élus, au scrutin secret, à la majorité des voix.

4. Modifications des statuts: les propositions du C.I.D. sont votées, à mains levées, à la majorité des voix. (Le nouveau texte des Statuts sera imprimé page *119—122*.)

5. Fixation de la contribution financière des Sociétés Nationales: le Secrétaire Général-Trésorier fait connaître l'état déficitaire des finances de la Ligue et propose de fixer la contribution, pour chaque membre des Sociétés Nationales, à $ 1,50 pour une période de 5 ans. Le chiffre est accepté par vote à mains levées.

6. Le Président annonce la suppression des Comités de Nomenclature, des Classification et d'Education. Il précise que l'«Institute for Dermatologic Communications and Educations» continuera ses activités dont les si heureuses réalisations en matière de films sont dues principalement aux efforts de Madame SULZBERGER qu'on ne saurait trop remercier. Le Prof. SULZBERGER fait un exposé pour préciser la situation de cet Institut.

Liga Internacional de Sociedades Dermatológicas

Asamblea General de Delegados Nacionales, Munich, 4 de Agosto de 1967 (Presidencia: Prof. R. DEGOS)

El Presidente pronuncia una alocución de bienvenida a los Delegados Nacionales y da lectura a los artículos de los estatutos que determinan el número de delegados por cada Asociación Nacional y los poderes de la Asamblea.

El Secretario General, Prof. S. HELLERSTRÖM, pasa lista de los Delegados, designados oficialmente, de cada Asociación Nacional (43 naciones están representadas), presentando, acto seguido, los informes moral y financiero que son aprobados por la Asamblea (estos informes se hallan a continuación de este texto).

El Presidente comunica a la Asamblea las propuestas adoptadas por el Comité Internacional, las cuales son sometidas al voto de los Delegados; a saber,

1. Designación del lugar donde se celebrará el próximo Congreso Internacional y de su Presidente: Padua—Venecia (Italia) es propuesta en primer término; Sydney (Australia), en segundo. Padua—Venecia y el Prof. FLARER en calidad de Presidente alcanzan mayoría de votos en votación secreta.

El Prof. FLARER agradece a los Delegados su voto y les promete que hará cuanto pueda para acoger, en las mejores condiciones posibles, a un gran número de Congresistas en Padua en 1972.

2. Designación de los nuevos Presidente y Secretario General del Comité Internacional de Dermatología. El Comité recaba el voto de la Asamblea a fin de dar a esta elección una base mas democrática. En votación secreta, son elegidos por mayoria de votos, los Prof. GAY PRIETO como Presidente y SAGHER como Secretario General—Tesorero del Comité Internacional de Dermatología.

El Prof. GAY PRIETO pronuncia una corta alocución para agradecer el voto de la Asamblea.

3. Elección de los cuatro nuevos miembros del C.I.D. Por mayoría de votos, en votación secreta, son elegidos los Prof. O. BRAUN-FALCO (Alemania); R. BAER (Estados Unidos de América); A. PADILHA-GONÇALVES (Brasil) y A. A. CORDERO (Argentina).

4. Modificación de los estatutos. Por mayoría de votos, a mano alzada, son aceptadas las propuestas del C.I.D. (Vease página *122* el nuevo texto de los estatutos).

5. Fijar la contribución financiera de cada Asociación Nacional. El Secretario General— Tesorero da cuenta del estado financiero deficitario y propone establecer la cuota de un dólar cincuenta por cada miembro de las diversas Asociaciones Nacionales, durante un período de 5 años. Esta cotización es aceptada mediante votación a mano alzada.

6. El Presidente anuncia la supresión de los Comités de Nomenclatura, de Clasificación y de Enseñanza. En cambio añade, el Instituto de Informaciones y Enseñanzas Dermatológicas proseguirá sus actividades. Gracias a los esfuerzos de la Sra. SULZBERGER, para quien todo elogio es parco, disponemos de magníficas realizaciones en el campo de films científicos. El Prof. SULZBERGER presenta un informe preciso sobre dicho Instituto.

Internationale Liga der Dermatologischen Gesellschaften

Generalversammlung der Nationalen Delegierten, München, 4. August 1967 (Präsident Prof. R. DEGOS)

Der Präsident heißt die nationalen Delegierten willkommen und verliest die Artikel der Statuten, welche die Zahl der Delegierten der einzelnen nationalen Gesellschaften bestimmen und die Kompentenzen der Versammlung regeln.

Der Generalsekretär Prof. HELLERSTRÖM macht Appell bei den offiziellen Delegierten der Nationalen Dermatologischen Gesellschaften (43 Nationen sind vertreten). Anschließend gibt er einen allgemeinen und einen Finanzbericht, die den Beifall der Versammlung finden.

Der Präsident teilt der Versammlung die Vorschläge mit, die vom internationalen Komitee angenommen wurden und die der Abstimmung der Delegierten unterbreitet werden:

1. Wahl des zukünftigen Kongreßortes und des Kongreßpräsidenten: Italien (Padua— Venedig) wird in erster Linie vorgeschlagen, Australien (Sydney) in zweiter Linie. In geheimer Abstimmung wird Italien (Padua—Venedig) bestimmt und als Präsident Prof. FLARER ernannt.

Prof. FLARER dankt den Delegierten für seine Wahl und versichert, daß er sein bestes tun wird, um eine große Anzahl von Kongressisten in Padua 1972 so gut wie möglich zu empfangen.

2. Wahl des neuen Präsidenten und des neuen Generalsekretärs des Internationalen Komitees für Dermatologie. Das Komitee wünscht, daß die Versammlung abstimmt, um diesen Wahlen einen demokratischeren Charakter zu verleihen. In geheimer Abstimmung werden Prof. GAY PRIETO und Prof. SAGHER gewählt, ersterer als Präsident und der zweite als Generalsekretär-Quästor des Internationalen Komitees für Dermatologie.

Prof. GAY PRIETO dankt in einem kurzen Votum für seine Wahl.

3. Wahl von vier neuen Mitgliedern des Internationalen Komitees für Dermatologie: die Prof. O. BRAUN-FALCO (Bundesrepublik Deutschland), R. BAER (U.S.A.), A. PADILHA-GON-ÇALVES (Brasilien) und A. A. CORDERO (Argentinien), die vom Internationalen Komitee vorgeschlagen worden sind, werden in geheimer Abstimmung gewählt.

4. Statutenänderung: Die Vorschläge des Internationalen Komitees werden in offener Abstimmung angenommen (Der neue Text der Statuten findet sich auf Seite *125*).

5. Der Beitrag der nationalen Gesellschaften wird fixiert. Der Generalsekretär-Quästor teilt mit, daß die Finanzen der Liga defizitär sind und schlägt vor, die Beiträge so zu fixieren, daß pro Mitglied jeder nationalen Gesellschaft $ 1,5 in 5 Jahren zu bezahlen sind. In offener Abstimmung wird der Vorschlag angenommen.

6. Der Präsident teilt mit, daß folgende Komitees aufgehoben worden sind: Das Komitee für Nomenklatur, das Komitee für Klassifikation und das Komitee für Erziehung. Er betont, daß das „Institute of Dermatologic Information and Education" seine Tätigkeit fortsetzen wird. Die Filme sind in erster Linie Frau Prof. SULZBERGER zu verdanken, der man für ihre Tätigkeit großen Dank schuldet. Prof. SULZBERGER berichtet über die Situation dieses Instituts.

International Committee of Dermatology
5th August meeting held in Munich, 1967

First part

Present: DEGOS (President), HELLERSTRÖM (Secretary General), JABLONSKA, RAMOS E SILVA, KITAMURA, QUIROGA, LAPIÈRE, FLARER, BRUNSTING, GAY PRIETO, SAGHER. Members of honor: SULZBERGER, JADASSOHN, SCHIRREN. Excused: LIVINGOOD, MITCHELL-HEGGS, PILLSBURY.

Prof. DEGOS announces that Prof. FLARER has been elected as President of the next International Congress of Dermatology. Therefore he may leave his place at the International Committee as a regular member since he will remain a member of the Committee for life. Prof. LAPIÈRE who should have left the International Committee, has therefore remained as regular member.

Three members will leave the International Committee: KITAMURA, QUIROGA and RAMOS E SILVA. Thanks are expressed to them by Prof. DEGOS for all their cooperation.

Prof. RAMOS E SILVA, KITAMURA and QUIROGA express their thanks to the members of the International Committee for their cooperation and friendship.

Prof. DEGOS and HELLERSTRÖM outgoing chairman and Secretary General-treasurer give their power over to the new elected Chairman and the new elected Secretary General-Treasurer, Prof. GAY PRIETO and SAGHER.

Second part

Present: GAY PRIETO (President), SAGHER (Secretary General), JABLONSKA, LAPIÈRE, FLARER, DEGOS, HELLERSTRÖM, BAER, BRAUN-FALCO, PADILHA-GONÇALVES. Members of honor: SULZBERGER, JADASSOHN, SCHIRREN. Excused: BRUNSTING, CORDERO, LIVINGOOD, MITCHELL-HEGGS, PILLSBURY.

Prof. GAY PRIETO welcomes the new members, Prof. BRAUN-FALCO, BAER and PADILHA-GONÇALVES and announces that Prof. CORDERO could not attend because of the conditions in his country. The youth and wisdom of the new members will be of great importance for the Committee. He congratulates Prof. FLARER the new President of the next International Congress, which will be held in Padoua and Venice in 1972. He also expresses his thanks to Prof. JADASSOHN and SCHIRREN, the former President and Secretary General of the Congress in Munich.

Prof. LAPIÈRE expresses his gratefulness for having given him the possibility to continue to be a member of the Committee for further 5 years, and Prof. FLARER was delighted that he could do this for LAPIÈRE, whom he considers a good friend of him.

Prof. PADILHA-GONÇALVES, BRAUN-FALCO and BAER express their thanks and promise to work together for the commun goal.

World Health Organization

The President points out that our relations with the W.H.O. have not changed and are very cordial, and that representatives from the International Committee of Dermatology are invited to the various sessions, such as leprosy, education, etc.

Relations with the Council for International Organizations of Medical Sciences

We are regular member at the C.I.O.M.S. and have to pay $ 250 yearly. The question is raised whether we should become associate member as in this case no dues would have to be paid. The belief is expressed that there is no advantage in remaining a regular member.

HELLERSTRÖM states that we started as associated members but had been voted to become regular members some time ago and that we owe the C.I.O.M.S. already $ 500.

DEGOS expresses his hopes that it will not be necessary to pay the $ 500 should we become an associate member now.

FLARER believes that we could get financial assistance for the next Congress if we apply; therefore one should not change the status immediately.

HELLERSTRÖM points out in that case we would have to pay in addition to the $ 500 which we owe, further 1.250 $ for the next 5 years.

DEGOS states that C.I.O.M.S. is only lending and not giving money, but HELLERSTRÖM could write that we are not in the position to pay but would like to remain associate or regular members.

GAY PRIETO proposes to wait and first speak to the representative of the C.I.O.M.S. in order to find out what the position is in this respect and write only afterwards.

DEGOS remains therefore the representative at C.I.O.M.S. and is charged to discuss this question.

SULZBERGER analyzed the question of large congresses in general. He believes that congresses have changed in spite that they are of great social importance and give a chance to the young colleagues to learn. He thinks that the International Committee should consider also other matters besides congresses every 5 years, and should become more active representatives in dermatology. There are many fields in which this could be done, one of them became clear during the Symposium 6: Dr. BRAUER, an adviser of Revlon pointed out that laws are discussed for the Common Market concerning safety of drugs and cosmetics. No dermatologist is in these committees. He believes that such representatives should be chosen as dermatologists from the International Committee of Dermatology, not only for cosmetics, but also for occupational diseases, venereal diseases and others.

DEGOS knows that dermatologists are representatives in several countries, f.i. DUPERRAT in France.

The President believes that congresses could partly be changed. He proposes that Prof. DEGOS, BRAUN-FALCO and FLARER should find out concerning dermatological representatives at the committees of the Common Market and communicate then their findings to the President or Secretary General.

Mrs. JABLONSKA is in favor to change the congresses. She gives as an example the working session on pemphigus-immunology which was a great success. She would favor such meetings to be held in the time between the congresses. She will send proposals concerning symposia, not at time of the Congresses, under the auspices of the International Committee of Dermatology.

Date of the next International Congress of Dermatology and of the meetings in the next 5 years

It is proposed that the Committee should meet in Padoua next year in order to see the facilities. FLARER is gladly inviting the Committee before the next meeting of the "Association de Dermatologistes et Syphiligraphes de langue française" at Torino and proposes as date of the meeting the 13 to 14 June 1968 in Padoua.

LAPIÈRE is inviting the Committee to meet in Liège in 1969.

The third meeting would be in Madrid in September 1970 according to the invitation of GAY PRIETO.

The fourth meeting for 1971 is not fixed yet.

As date for the next International Congress, May 1972, is proposed.

FLARER proposes Prof. SERRI as Secretary General for the next International Congress.

Financing of meetings

GAY PRIETO asks whether the International Committee is allowed to get financial help for its meetings from industries and other corporations.

HELLERSTRÖM reports that $ 10.000 were spent for the last meeting.

SULZBERGER thinks that members who are obliged to come, should receive the expenses.

DEGOS points out that there is a difference between national and international societies. He does not believe that national societies should accept financial help for their activities, but international societies may do this. He believes that it could be done through people who have connections with firms and is in favor that it should remain up to the President and Secretary General.

A letter from the Netherland Dermatological Society is read concerning a publication "Who is who in Dermatology". It was the consent of the Committee that the President will answer that this is not on our program at the moment and that we are not in the position to take up the question at this time.

Comité International de Dermatologie
Réunion du 5 août 1967 (Munich)

Ière Partie

Présents: DEGOS (Président), HELLERSTRÖM (Secrétaire Général), JABLONSKA, RAMOS E SILVA, KITAMURA, QUIROGA, LAPIÈRE, FLARER, BRUNSTING, GAY PRIETO, SAGHER. Membres d'honneur: SULZBERGER, JADASSOHN, SCHIRREN. Excusés: LIVINGOOD, MITCHELL-HEGGS, PILLSBURY.

Le Prof. DEGOS fait savoir au Comité que le Prof. FLARER ayant été nommé Président du futur Congrès International, a décidé de renoncer à ses fonctions de membre élu du Comité, en faveur du Prof. LAPIÈRE dont l'âge est très proche du sien. Le Prof. FLARER confirme cette décision qui lui a été dictée par son amitié pour le Prof. LAPIÈRE. Le Comité enregistre avec satisfaction l'acte du Prof. FLARER et le Prof. LAPIÈRE remercie le Prof. FLARER en disant sa satisfaction de rester membre du C.I.D.

Le Prof. DEGOS apporte ensuite aux trois membres sortants du C.I.D. les Prof. RAMOS E SILVA, KITAMURA et QUIROGA, l'hommage de gratitude du C.I.D. pour leur si fidèle et si amicale collaboration, et les assure des sentiments de profond regret que leur départ cause à tous leurs collègues du C.I.D. MM. RAMOS E SILVA, KITAMURA et QUIROGA remercient en termes émouvants les membres du C.I.D. avec lesquels ils ont eu tant de plaisir à collaborer.

Les Prof. DEGOS et HELLERSTRÖM, arrivés au terme de leurs fonctions, passent leur pouvoir de Président et de Secrétaire Général-Trésorier aux Prof. GAY PRIETO et SAGHER.

IIème Partie

Présents: GAY PRIETO (Président), SAGHER (Secrétaire Général), JABLONSKA, LAPIÈRE, FLARER, DEGOS, HELLERSTRÖM, BAER, BRAUN-FALCO, PADILHA-GONÇALVES. Membres d'honneur: SULZBERGER, JADASSOHN, SCHIRREN. Excusés: BRUNSTING, CORDERO, LIVINGOOD, MITCHELL-HEGGS, PILLSBURY.

Le Prof. GAY PRIETO, nouveau Président, souhaite la bienvenue aux nouveaux membres du C.I.D., les Prof. BRAUN-FALCO, BAER et PADILHA-GONÇALVES et déclare que le Prof. CORDERO n'a pas pu se déplacer à Munich, à cause de la situation politique de son pays. La jeunesse et la sagesse des nouveaux membres sera de grande importance pour le Comité, ajoute-t-il, félicitant ensuite le Prof. FLARER, Président du prochain Congrès International qui aura lieu à Padoue-Venise en 1972. Finalement, le Prof. GAY PRIETO remercie les Prof. JADASSOHN et SCHIRREN, Président et Secrétaire Général du Congrès de Munich.

Le Prof. LAPIÈRE remercie le Prof. FLARER et se réjouit de pouvoir rester encore 5 ans membre du C.I.D., tandis que le dernier s'en félicite ayant pu être utile à son ami le Prof. LAPIÈRE.

Les Prof. PADILHA-GONÇALVES, BRAUN-FALCO et BAER expriment leurs remerciements et promettent de travailler ensemble dans les objectifs communs.

Organisation Mondiale de la Santé

Le Président fait remarquer que les relations entre l'OMS et le C.I.D. n'ont pas changé, étant toujours très cordiales, comme le prouvent les fréquentes invitations qui lui sont adressées, par exemple à l'occasion des études sur la lèpre, l'éducation, etc.

Relations avec le C.I.O.M.S. (Council for International Organizations of Medical Sciences)

Nous sommes «membre régulier» de cette organisation avec une cotisation annuelle de 250 \$. On se demande s'il ne conviendrait pas de devenir «membre associé», car, dans ce cas, il n'y aurait pas de cotisation à verser. Il semble qu'il n'y a pas de raisons importantes de rester «membre régulier». HELLERSTRÖM rappelle que nous étions dans le passé, «membre associé» et que l'on avait voté pour devenir «membre régulier». D'autre part, il reste une somme de 500 \$ à payer au C.I.O.M.S.

DEGOS espère que si l'on devenait «membre associé», on n'aurait pas à payer cette somme.

FLARER pense que l'on pourrait obtenir une aide financière du C.I.O.M.S. pour le prochain Congrès, si l'on en faisait la demande. Pour le moment, tout changement est à déconseiller.

HELLERSTRÖM souligne que si l'on ne change pas les statuts, qu'en plus des 500 $ dus, 1250 $ seront encore à verser pour les cotisations des 5 années à venir.

DEGOS fait remarquer que le C.I.O.M.S. prête de l'argent mais n'en fait pas cadeau. Cependant, HELLERSTRÖM pourrait écrire à cette association que nous ne sommes pas en mesure d'honorer nos cotisations, mais que nous souhaiterions rester membre «associé» ou «régulier».

GAY PRIETO propose d'attendre et, avant tout, de se mettre en relation avec le représentant du C.I.O.M.S. et le renseigner sur notre situation. Ensuite on écrirait. Notre représentant auprès du C.I.O.M.S., DEGOS, se chargera de cette affaire.

SULZBERGER soulève la question des grands congrès. Il pense qu'il faut les adapter aux besoins, bien qu'ils soient d'une grande importance du point de vue social et qu'ils offrent la possibilité aux jeunes collègues d'approfondir leurs connaissances. SULZBERGER est d'avis que le C.I.D. devrait faire preuve d'une plus grande activité et de ne pas se limiter à l'organisation d'un congrès tous les 5 ans. Plusieurs domaines se prêtent à des modifications; l'un d'eux ayant été exposé au cours du Symposium 6; le Dr. BRAUER de Revlon mettant en relief qu'au sein du Marché Commun, des lois concernant les médicaments et les cosmétiques sont à l'étude. Il n'y a pas de dermatologues parmi les membres des comité qui élaborent des lois. C'est au C.I.D. qu'il appartient de proposer des représentants auprès de ces comités, qui pourraient participer aussi bien dans la branche des cosmétiques que dans le domaine des maladies professionnelles, vénériennes et autres.

DEGOS fait remarquer que dans certains pays, il y a des dermatologues qui sont représentants, par exemple DUPERRAT pour la France.

Le Président croit aussi que les congrès devraient être partiellement modifiés. Il propose que les Prof. DEGOS, BRAUN-FALCO et FLARER se chargent d'étudier la question, de placer des dermatologues dans les comités du Marché Commun, concernant notre spécialité et de présenter un rapport au Président et au Secrétaire Général du C.I.D.

Mme. JABLONSKA partage l'avis de faire quelques additions aux congrès. Elle donne pour exemple, la séance de travail sur le pemphigus et l'immunologie qui a été un grand succès. Elle fera des suggestions concernant les symposia qui pourraient avoir lieu en dehors des périodes de congrès, mais sous les auspices du C.I.D.

Congrès de 1972 et réunions préliminaires. Dates

On propose que le C.I.D. se réunisse à Padoue pour se rendre compte des avantages qu'offre le lieu choisi. FLARER invite cordialement le C.I.D. à se réunir à Padoue les 13 et 14 juin 1968 soit avant la prochaine réunion de la "Association de Dermatologistes et Syphiligraphes de langue française" qui aura lieu à Turin.

LAPIÈRE invite le C.I.D. à se réunir à Liège en 1969.

La troisième réunion serait à célébrer à Madrid en 1970, suite à l'invitation de GAY PRIETO.

La quatrième réunion n'a pas encore été fixée. Il est proposé que le prochain Congrès International de Dermatologie ait lieu en mai 1972.

FLARER propose le Prof. SERRI comme Secrétaire Général du prochain Congrès International.

Financement des réunions

GAY PRIETO demande si le C.I.D. pourrait solliciter des allocations à l'industrie ou d'autres associations.

HELLERSTRÖM informe que lors de la dernière réunion du C.I.D. 10.000 $ ont été dépensés.

SULZBERGER est d'avis que les frais de déplacement des membres au lieu des réunions devraient être remboursés.

DEGOS souligne des nuances entre les Sociétés Nationales et Internationales. Il est d'avis que les Sociétés Nationales ne devraient pas accepter d'aide financière, mais que la question est différente pour les sociétés internationales. Il suggère que les personnes qui ont des liens avec des firmes industrielles, devraient s'occuper de cette affaire et que cette question est du domaine du Président et du Secrétaire Général.

Une lettre de la Société Néerlandaise de Dermatologie au sujet de la publication «Who is who in Dermatology» est lue. On décide que le Président réponde que nous ne sommes pas en mesure, pour le moment, de prendre position dans cette question.

Comité Internacional de Dermatología
Reunión del día 5 de Agosto de 1967. Munich

Parte I

Presentes: DEGOS (Presidente), HELLERSTRÖM (Secretario General), JABLONSKA, RAMOS E SILVA, KITAMURA, QUIROGA, LAPIÈRE, FLARER, BRUNSTING, GAY PRIETO, SAGHER. Miembros de Honor: SULZBERGER, JADASSOHN, SCHIRREN. Excusaron su ausencia: LIVINGOOD, MITCHELL-HEGGS, PILLSBURY.

El Prof. DEGOS comunica al Comité que el Prof. FLARER, habiendo sido nombrado Presidente del futuro Congreso Internacional, ha decidido renunciar a su cargo de miembro electo del Comité, en beneficio del Prof. LAPIÈRE, cuya edad es cercana a la suya. El Prof. FLARER confirma esta decisión que le ha sido dictada por su amistad con el Prof. LAPIÈRE. El Comité toma nota con satisfacción del gesto del Prof. FLARER, mientras que el Prof. LAPIÈRE, expresando su reconocimiento al Prof. FLARER se congratula de poder continuar siendo miembro del Comité Internacional de Dermatología.

El Prof. DEGOS, acto seguido, testimonia su agradecimiento a los tres miembros salientes del C.I.D. los Prof. QUIROGA, RAMOS E SILVA y KITAMURA, por su leal y amistosa colaboración, reiterándoles el profundo sentimiento que su partida causa a todos sus colegas del C.I.D. Los Sres. RAMOS E SILVA, KITAMURA y QUIROGA dan las gracias, con frases emotivas, a todos los miembros del C.I.D. con los cuales se complacieron en colaborar.

Los Prof. DEGOS y HELLERSTRÖM llegados al término de sus mandatos pasan sus poderes respectivos de Presidente y de Secretario General y Tesorero, a los Prof. GAY PRIETO y SAGHER.

Parte II

Presentes: GAY PRIETO (Presidente), SAGHER (Secretario General), JABLONSKA, LAPIÈRE, FLARER, DEGOS, HELLERSTRÖM, BAER, BRAUN-FALCO, PADILHA-GONÇALVES. Miembros de Honor: SULZBERGER, JADASSOHN, SCHIRREN. Excusaron su ausencia: BRUNSTING, CORDERO, LIVINGOOD, MITCHELL-HEGGS, PILLSBURY.

El Prof. GAY PRIETO, nuevo Presidente, da la bienvenida a los nuevos miembros del C.I.D. Prof. BRAUN-FALCO, BAER y PADILHA-GONÇALVES, y comunica que el Prof. CORDERO no ha podido desplazarse a Munich a causa de la situación política de su país. La juventud y la ponderación de los nuevos miembros serán de mucha importancia para el Comité. El Prof. GAY PRIETO felicita al Prof. FLARER, Presidente del próximo Congreso Internacional de Dermatología que tendrá lugar en Padua-Venecia en 1972. Termina dando las gracias a los Prof. JADASSOHN y SCHIRREN, respectivamente Presidente y Secretario General del Congreso de Munich.

El Prof. LAPIÈRE se congratula de su continuidad por 5 años más, como miembro del Comité, mientras que el Prof. FLARER se siente satisfecho de haber ofrecido esta oportunidad a su amigo LAPIÈRE. Los Prof. PADILHA-GONÇALVES, BRAUN-FALCO y BAER exteriorizan su agradecimiento prometiendo aunar sus esfuerzos con vista al objetivo común.

O.M.S. (Organisation Mondiale de la Santé)
El Presidente declara que nuestras relaciones con la O.M.S. en nada han cambiado, siendo muy cordiales, ya que los representantes del C.I.D. son invitados a diversas reuniones, tales que sobre la lepra, la educación, etc.

C.I.O.M.S. (Council for International Organizations of Medical Sciences)
Somos miembros ordinarios de esta Organización a la que abonamos 250 $ al año. La cuestión es la de saber, si no sería preferible, ser miembro asociado, ya que en este último caso no tendríamos que satisfacer cuota alguna. No hay razón de continuar como miembro ordinario.

HELLERSTRÖM recuerda que ya fuimos miembro asociado pero que se acordó, mediante voto, pasar a miembro ordinarío y que ademas debemos al C.I.O.M.S. la suma de 500 $.

DEGOS estima que no habría de satisfacerse esta suma si pasasemos a ser miembro asociado.

FLARER piensa que se podría obtener una ayuda financiera del C.I.O.M.S. para nuestro próximo Congreso si se hiciese la petición. Por esta razón, valdría más no cambiar en nada nuestras relaciones con el C.I.O.M.S.

HELLERSTRÖM advierte que en ese caso tendremos que pagar, además del atraso de 500 $, 1.250 $ más por los 5 años venideros.

DEGOS hace resaltar que el C.I.O.M.S. presta dinero pero no lo regala.

HELLERSTRÖM, sin embargo, podria escribir a dicha asociación, declarando no disponer de fondos para satisfacer las cotizaciones, pero especificando, que nuestro deseo seria de continuar, sea como miembro asociado o como miembro ordinario.

GAY PRIETO propone la espera. Ante todo, ponerse en contacto con el representante del C.I.O.M.S. para aclarar nuestra situación. Más tarde se les escribiría. DEGOS sigue siendo nuestro enlace con el C.I.O.M.S. y puede encargarse de discutir la cuestión.

SULZBERGER hace referencia a los grandes Congresos. Cree que algo debe cambiarse, a pesar de que son de mucha importancia social y que permiten a los jóvenes colegas adquirir nuevos conocimientos. Opina que el C.I.D. debiera ser mas activo y no limitarse solamente a la organización de un Congreso cada 5 años. Deberían hacerse transformaciones en muchos aspectos, uno de los cuales, fué mencionado durante el simposio 6 en el que el Dr. BRAUER de Revlon comunicó que se están preparando leyes sobre medicamentos y cosméticos en el seno del Mercado Común. No hay ningun dermatólogo en esos Comités. Añade que tales representantes deberían ser elegidos por el C.I.D., no solamente en el campo de los cosméticos, sino que tambien en el de las enfermedades profesionales, venéreas y otras.

DEGOS informa que en algunos paises hay dermatólogos que son representantes. En Francia, por ejemplo, DUPERRAT.

El Presidente opina, que, en efecto, los Congresos deberían modificarse en parte. Propone que los Prof. DEGOS, BRAUN-FALCO y FLARER estudien la cuestión concerniente a los representantes de la dermatología en el seno del Comité del Mercado Común y presenten un informe al Presidente y al Secretario General.

La Sra. JABLONSKA tambien cree que deben modificarse los Congresos. Como ejemplo, dijo, la sesión de trabajo sobre el pénfigo y la inmunología que tuvo tanto éxito. La Sra. JABLONSKA presentará proposiciones sobre los simposios que podrían celebrarse en fechas distintas de los Congresos, pero bajo los auspicios del C.I.D.

Determinación de la fecha en que se celebrará el próximo Congreso Internacional de Dermatología y de aquellas otras en que tendrán lugar las reuniones preparatorias en los 5 años venideros.

Se propuso que el C.I.D. se reúna en Padua con el fin de examinar las ventajas que ofrece. FLARER invitó cordialmente al C.I.D. para reunirse en Padua antes de la celebración de la reunión de la "Association de Dermatologistes et Syphiligraphes de langue française" en Turín. Propuso los dias 13 y 14 de Junio de 1968.

LAPIÈRE invitó al C.I.D. a reunirse en Lieja en 1969.

La tercera reunión tendra lugar en Madrid en Septiembre de 1970 por invitación de GAY PRIETO.

La cuarta reunión no fué fijada.

Se propuso que el próximo Congreso Internacional tenga lugar en el mes de Mayo de 1972.

FLARER propone al Prof. SERRI como Secretario General del próximo Congreso Internacional.

Sostén financiero de las reuniones

GAY PRIETO inquiere si el C.I.D. podria solicitar subvenciones de la industria privada o de otras asociaciones.

HELLERSTRÖM informa que se gastaron 10.000 $ en el último certamen.

DEGOS establece un distingo entre las Sociedades Nacionales y las Sociedades Internacionales y opina que las primeras no deberían recabar ayuda financiera para desarrollar sus actividades, pero que la cuestión era distinta para las Sociedades Internacionales. Admite que aquellos que están relacionados con firmas industriales podrían ocuparse de este asunto y sugiere que esta cuestión sea resuelta por el Presidente y el Secretario General.

Se da lectura a una carta de la Sociedad Neerlandesa de Dermatología, referente a la publicación "Who is who in Dermatology ?". Se decide que la respuesta sea dada por el Presidente, ya que esta cuestión no figuraba entre los problemas a estudiar actualmente y no estábamos preparados para darle una solución.

Sitzung des Internationalen Komitees für Dermatologie
München, 5. August 1967

1. Teil

Anwesend: Degos (Präsident), Hellerström (Generalsekretär), Jablonska, Ramos e Silva, Kitamura, Quiroga, Lapière, Flarer, Brunsting, Gay Prieto, Sagher. Ehrenmitglieder: Sulzberger, Jadassohn, Schirren. Entschuldigt: Livingood, Mitchell-Heggs, Pillsbury.

Prof. Degos teilt dem Komitee folgendes mit: Da Prof. Flarer Präsident des nächsten Internationalen Kongresses ist, verzichtet er auf seine Funktion als gewähltes Mitglied des Komitees. Er tut dies zugunsten von Prof. Lapière, der nur wenig älter ist als er. Prof. Flarer bestätigt diesen Entschluß, den er aus Freundschaft zu Prof. Lapière gefaßt hat. Das Komitee nimmt mit Befriedigung Kenntnis vom Beschluß Prof. Flarers. Prof. Lapière dankt Prof. Flarer und gibt seiner Freude Ausdruck, Mitglied des I.C.D. bleiben zu können.

Prof. Degos drückt dann den drei Mitgliedern, die aus dem I.C.D. austreten, den Prof. Ramos e Silva, Kitamura und Quiroga, die Dankbarkeit des I.C.D. aus für ihre treue und freundschaftliche Zusammenarbeit. Er versichert, daß alle Kollegen des I.C.D. ihr Ausscheiden sehr bedauern. Die Herren Ramos e Silva, Kitamura und Quiroga danken herzlich den Mitgliedern des I.C.D., mit denen sie gerne gearbeitet haben.

Die Prof. Degos und Hellerström, die am Ende ihres Mandates angelangt sind, übergeben ihre Ämter als Präsident bzw. Generalsekretär-Quästor an die Prof. Gay Prieto und Sagher.

2. Teil

Anwesend: Gay Prieto (Präsident), Sagher (Generalsekretär), Jablonska, Lapière, Flarer, Degos, Hellerström, Baer, Braun-Falco, Padilha-Gonçalves. Ehrenmitglieder: Sulzberger, Jadassohn, Schirren. Entschuldigt: Brunsting, Cordero. Livingood, Mitchell-Heggs, Pillsbury.

Prof. Gay Prieto, der neue Präsident des I.C.D., heißt die neuen Mitglieder, Prof. Braun-Falco, Prof. Baer und Prof. Padilha-Gonçalves, willkommen und teilt mit, daß Prof. Cordero wegen der politischen Verhältnisse in seiner Heimat nicht nach München kommen konnte. Die Jugend und das Wissen der neuen Mitglieder werden für das Komitee von großer Bedeutung sein. Prof. Gay Prieto gratuliert Prof. Flarer, dem neuen Präsidenten des nächsten internationalen Kongresses, welcher in Padua–Venedig 1972 abgehalten werden wird. Er richtet auch Dankesworte an Prof. Jadassohn und Prof. Schirren, den Präsidenten und den Generalsekretär des Münchener Kongresses.

Prof. Lapière spricht seinen Dank dafür aus, daß es ihm möglich ist, für weitere 5 Jahre ein Mitglied des Komitees zu bleiben. Prof. Flarer war sehr erfreut, auf diese Weise einem guten Freund helfen zu können.

Prof. Padilha-Gonçalves, Braun-Falco und Baer sprachen ihren Dank aus und versichern, mitzuarbeiten für das gemeinsame Ziel.

Weltgesundheitsorganisation

Der Präsident weist darauf hin, daß unsere Beziehungen zur Weltgesundheitsorganisation sich nicht geändert haben und daß sie sehr freundschaftlich sind. Repräsentanten des Internationalen Komitees für Dermatologie waren zu verschiedenen Sitzungen eingeladen, Sitzungen über Lepra, Erziehungsfragen usw.

Beziehungen zum C.I.O.M.S. (Council for International Organizations of Medical Sciences)

Wir sind reguläres Mitglied des C.I.O.M.S. und müssen als solches jährlich $ 250 bezahlen. Es wurde die Frage aufgeworfen, ob wir nicht assoziiertes Mitglied werden sollten, da wir in diesem Fall keine Beiträge bezahlen müßten. Es wurde die Ansicht ausgesprochen, daß es nicht von Vorteil ist, wenn wir reguläres Mitglied bleiben.

Hellerström stellt fest, daß wir als assoziiertes Mitglied begannen, aber es wurde in einer Abstimmung beschlossen, daß wir ein reguläres Mitglied werden sollten. Wir schulden der C.I.O.M.S. bereits $ 500.

Degos hofft, daß es nicht notwendig sein wird, die $ 500 zu bezahlen, wenn wir jetzt assoziiertes Mitglied werden.

8*

FLARER glaubt, daß wir für den nächsten Kongreß finanzielle Beiträge bekommen könnten, wenn wir uns bewerben. Aus diesem Grunde sollten wir den Status quo nicht sofort ändern.

HELLERSTRÖM hebt hervor, daß wir in diesem Fall außer den $ 500, welche wir schuldig sind, noch 1250 $ für die nächsten 5 Jahre bezahlen müssen.

DEGOS macht darauf aufmerksam, daß die C.I.O.M.S. nur Geld ausleiht und kein Geld gibt, aber HELLERSTRÖM möge mitteilen, daß wir nicht in der Lage sind zu bezahlen, daß wir aber gerne assoziiertes oder reguläres Mitglied sein möchten.

GAY PRIETO schlägt vor, abzuwarten und zuerst mit den Repräsentanten des C.I.O.M.S. zu sprechen und erst danach zu schreiben.

DEGOS bleibt also der Repräsentant bei der C.I.O.M.S. und wird beauftragt, diese Frage zu diskutieren.

SULZBERGER analysiert das Problem großer Kongresse im allgemeinen. Er glaubt, daß sich die Kongresse geändert haben, trotzdem sie von großem gesellschaftlichem Interesse sind, und daß sie den jungen Kollegen Gelegenheit geben, zu lernen. Er denkt, daß das internationale Komitee sich auch um andere Dinge kümmern sollte, abgesehen von den alle 5 Jahre stattfindenden Kongressen, und daß das Komitee aktiver die Dermatologie vertreten sollte. Es gebe viele Gelegenheiten, dies zu tun. Eine von diesen zeigte sich während des Symposiums 6: Dr. BRAUER, ein Vertreter von Revlon, wies darauf hin, daß Gesetze für den gemeinsamen Markt diskutiert werden, Gesetze, die die Unschädlichkeit von Medikamenten und kosmctischen Präparaten betreffen. Kein Dermatologe ist in diesen Komitees. SULZBERGER meint, daß Repräsentanten vom Internationalen Komitee für Dermatologie gewählt werden sollten, nicht nur für kosmetische Präparate, sondern auch für Berufskrankheiten, für Geschlechtskrankheiten und anderes mehr.

DEGOS erwidert, daß in verschiedenen Ländern Dermatologen als Repräsentanten vertreten sind, z. B. DUPERRAT in Frankreich.

Der Präsident glaubt, daß die Kongresse teilweise geändert werden können; er schlägt vor, daß Prof. DEGOS, Prof. BRAUN-FALCO und Prof. FLARER sich orientieren sollten über dermatologische Repräsentanten in den Komitees des gemeinsamen Marktes und daß sie dann die Ergebnisse ihrer Ermittlungen dem Präsidenten und dem Generalsekretär des I.C.D. mitteilen sollten.

Frau JABLONSKA ist auch der Ansicht, daß die Kongresse geändert werden sollten. Sie gibt als Beispiel die Sitzung über Pemphigus und Immunologie, die ein großer Erfolg war. Sie möchte solche Sitzungen in der Zeit zwischen den Kongressen abhalten. Sie wird Vorschläge, die solche Symposien betreffen, einreichen. Die Symposien sollten nicht zur Zeit der Kongresse stattfinden, aber unter den Auspizien des internationalen Komitees für Dermatologie.

Daten des nächsten internationalen Dermatologen-Kongresses und der Sitzungen in den nächsten 5 Jahren

Es wurde vorgeschlagen, daß das Komitee nächstes Jahr in Padua tagen sollte, damit man sich über die Möglichkeiten orientieren kann. FLARER freut sich, das Komitee einladen zu können, und zwar vor der Sitzung der „Association de Dermatologistes et Syphiligraphes de langue française", die in Turin stattfindet. Er schlägt als Datum für die Sitzung den 13. und 14. Juni 1968 vor.

LAPIÈRE lädt das Komitee ein, 1969 in Liège zu tagen.

Die dritte Sitzung soll auf Einladung von GAY PRIETO im September 1970 in Madrid stattfinden.

Ort und Zeit der vierten Sitzung wurden noch nicht fixiert.

Als Datum für den nächsten Internationalen Kongreß wird Mai 1972 vorgeschlagen. FLARER beantragt, Prof. SERRI zum Generalsekretär des nächsten Internationalen Kongresses zu ernennen.

Zur Finanzierung von Sitzungen

GAY PRIETO fragt, ob das Internationale Komitee finanzielle Hilfe für seine Sitzungen von der Industrie oder anderen Institutionen annehmen darf.

HELLERSTRÖM teilt mit, daß für die letzte Sitzung des CID 10000 $ ausgegeben wurden.

SULZBERGER meint, daß den Mitgliedern, die an der Sitzung teilnehmen müssen, die Ausgaben bezahlt werden sollten.

DEGOS betont, daß in dieser Beziehung ein Unterschied zwischen nationalen und internationalen Gesellschaften besteht. Nationale Gesellschaften sollten für ihre Tätigkeit keine Unterstützung annehmen. Internationalen Gesellschaften sollte dies erlaubt sein; solche finanziellen Unterstützungen könnten durch Kollegen vermittelt werden, die Beziehungen zur Industrie haben. Er ist der Ansicht, daß man diese Angelegenheit dem Präsidenten und dem Generalsekretär überlassen sollte.

Ein Schreiben der Niederländischen Dermatologischen Gesellschaft wurde verlesen, in dem es um die Publikation von „Who is who in Dermatology?" geht. Das Komitee stimmte überein, daß der Präsident in einem Antwortschreiben mitteilen möge, daß diese Frage zum gegenwärtigen Zeitpunkt nicht behandelt werden kann.

Rules and Regulations of the International League of Dermatological Societies

including the modifications adopted at the XIII. International Congress, Munich, August, 1967.

The aims of the International League of Dermatological Societies are:

to encourage the advancement of dermatology,
to promote personal relations between the dermatologists of the world,
to represent dermatological interest in other international organizations,
to hold international congresses of dermatology.

The component bodies of the league are:

1. The Assembly of National Delegates,
2. The International Committee of Dermatology (I.C.D.),
3. The International Congress of Dermatology,
4. The Organizing Committee responsible for the organization of the Congress in whichever country it is next to be held.

1. *The Assembly of National Delegates*

The delegates are nominated by National Societies of the different countries.

The number of delegates representing each country will be based on the number of regular members in the following proportions:

from 20 to 100 members   1 delegate,
from 100 to 200 members   2 delegates,
more than 200 members   3 delegates,
more than 500 members   4 delegates.

Every member may be replaced by a substitute.

If a country has more than one dermatological society, the delegates are nominated by consultation between the societies.

If a country is already represented on the International Committee of Dermatology, that member or members will automatically be delegates of that country.

The President of each National Dermatological Society will send the names of the delegates to the Secretary-General of the I.C.D. together with the names of those dermatological societies that have supported the appointment, and also a complete list of members.

At the International Congress the Assembly of Delegates holds its sessions under the Chairman of the I.C.D., who is also President of the International League of Dermatological Societies. The Assembly of Delegates is empowered to:

elect, by secret vote, the members of the International Committee of Dermatology, as well as the President and the Secretary General of the I.C.D., on the lists established by the I.C.D.,

to choose the country and city of the next Congress and to elect its President,
to establish the status and regulations for the organization of the International Congress,
to name, if necessary, committees for special purposes,
to determine the membership fee for the next period.

2. *The International Committee of Dermatology (I.C.D.)*

The I.C.D. will be composed of twelve members elected by the Assembly of National Delegates (for their election, personal experience on Congress matters and scientific works will be taken into consideration).

In addition to the elected members, the Presidents and the Secretaries General of the I.C.D., as well as the Presidents and the Secretaries General of the International Congress are named honorary members at the end of their function or at the end of their mandate as elected members of the I.C.D.

The honorary members are named for life. They could assist the meetings of the I.C.D., with the right to vote, but will not receive the displacement indemnities foreseen for one of the I.C.D. meetings.

The President and the Secretary General of the forthcoming Congress officially belong to the I.C.D. and they have the same rights as the elected members.

At the time of each Congress, one third of the members will be renewed, according to age and vacancies due to death or any other valid reason. The new members will be elected by secret vote of the Assembly of Delegates, according to the list proposed by the I.C.D.

At each Congress, the I.C.D., chooses, by secret vote, those of its elected members which will be proposed to the Assembly of Delegates as the new President and Secretary General of the I.C.D. The Assembly of Delegates will then proceed to the election of the President and the Secretary General of the I.C.D. by secret vote. Their functions will begin at the end of the present Congress and continue until the closing session of following Congress.

If the President of the I.C.D. cannot fill his functions, they will be temporarely assured by the Secretary General. A new President will be assigned by the I.C.D. assembled to this purpose by the Secretary General.

If the President of the Congress cannot fill his functions, his place will be taken by the President of the I.C.D. who will consult on this subject, the other members of the Committee. In order to facilitate this nomination, every President of the Congress must, after his election, suggest the name of a substitute to the President and the Secretary General of the I.C.D. At all events, the place of the Congress and its Secretary General cannot be changed if 18 months have elapsed since the preceding Congress. In any other event, a meeting of the I.C.D. must take place as rapidly as possible in order to choose the place and the President of the forthcoming Congress.

The I.C.D. will meet at the time of the Congress, before the meeting of the National Delegates, and at least once in the interval of the Congresses.

The Chairman of the I.C.D. has the power to appoint committees to function between Congresses.

In case of urgency the Chairman may convene an emergency meeting and the decision shall be accepted if a quorum of seven members be present and their vote is unanimous.

The International Committee of Dermatology is empowered:

to deal with all questions regarding dermatological problems of international importance,
to prepare the agenda for the Assembly of National Delegates,
to represent the interests of international Dermatology in relation to other organizations,
to make suggestions to the President of the next Congress regarding the organization of the Congress,
to appoint consultants to collaborate with the Organizing Committee in regard to scientific program, topics and principal speakers at the next International Congress.

Finances of the I.C.D. The members of the I.C.D. are unpaid. To cover the expenses of the Committee (stamps, papers, secretarial work, travel expenses for the members once in the interval between Congresses) every National Society will pay a contribution for each member to cover a period of 5 years (corresponding to the interval between two congresses). The amount of the subscription is fixed by the Assembly of National Delegates.

Countries where there is no Dermatological Organization do not contribute as they have no direct representation in the Assembly of Delegates.

3. *The International Congress of Dermatology*

Object and scope. The International Congress of Dermatology has for its object the development and advancement of dermatology by giving dermatologists of different countries an opportunity for submitting their personal experiences, of exchanging and discussing their ideas and forming personal bonds with their colleagues.

Meeting, membership and regulations. The International Congress of Dermatology shall be held every 5 years, but should it be impossible for a Congress to be held at the time appointed, it will meet at the later date, fixed by the I.C.D. in consultation with the Organizing Committee of the Congress.

All dermatologists of the world may be admitted as members of the Congress on payment of the Congress fee.

The President of the Congress has the right to appoint all the other officers of the International Congress. The President of the Congress may appoint such committees as he feels necessary for the efficient conduct of the Congress.

Consultants shall be appointed by the I.C.D. to work with the Organization Committee of the forthcoming Congress, these consultants do have the power to amend or alter the decisions and arrangements of the Organizing Committee of the Congress in matters relating to the Scientific Program, when in the consultants' opinion these appear to be in conflict with the aims of the International League of Dermatological Societies and of international Dermatology. Disagreements between the consultants appointed by the International Committee and the Organizing Committee of the Congress shall be resolved by appeal to the President of the International League of Dermatological Societies, whose decision shall be final.

The official languages of the Congress are English, French, German and Spanish.

The agenda of each session is drawn up by the Secretary of the Congress.

No report or communication that has previously been printed or read before another learned Society, may be presented in the same form to the Congress.

In the discussion no speech may exceed 5 min in lenght except by authority of the Chairman, based, if necessary, on a majority vote of those present.

The manuscripts of reports, communications and discussions must be handed, before the termination of the Congress! The editorial board may call upon the author to curtail any report or communication which involves more than 1500 words (inclusive of space for schedules, and tables — illustrations are only allowed in exceptional cases at the cost of the author) or to modify or withdraw any report or communication not in keeping with the scientific aim of the Congress. The author may be called upon to contribute towards the cost of the article if it exceeds the specified number of words and cannot reasonably be curtailed.

Any report or communication read before the Congress, but published prior to the appearance of the transactions, can appear therein only in the form of a summary.

The transactions (reports, papers, symposia, discussions) of the Congress shall be published in their original languages.

The subscription of membership of the Congress covers the cost of the transactions. The subscription must be paid at the latest at the beginning of the Congress.

4. Organizing Committee

The President of the Congress and his Organizing Committee are responsible for the organization of the Congress and for the publication of its transactions.

Before the Congress, the Organizing Committee will publish summaries of reports and papers in English, compiled in book form and forwarded to the members of the Congress not later than 6 weeks before the Congress.

The Organizing Committee may make provision for any extra functions at the Congress for films, television, stipends, etc.

Amendments to the Rules. Proposed amendments to those rules must be submitted in writing to the Secretary of the I.C.D. at least 3 months before the meeting of the Assembly of Delegates. The proposal will be circulated to the members of the I.C.D. and then put to the vote before the Assembly of delegates. Adoption requires an affirmative vote of two-thirds of those present and voting.

Statuts et Règlements de la Ligue Internationale des Sociétés Dermatologiques

comportant les modifications adoptées au XIIIième Congrès International de Munich, Août 1967

La Ligue Internationale des Sociétés Dermatologiques a pour objectifs:

de favoriser les progrès de la dermatologie,

de provoquer des contacts personnels entre les dermatologistes du monde entier,

de représenter les intérêts de la dermatologie au sein des autres organisations internationales,

de tenir des congrès internationaux de dermatologie.

Les organes de la Ligue sont:

1. L'Assemblée des Délégués Nationaux.
2. Le Comité International de Dermatologie (C.I.D.).
3. Le Congrès International de Dermatologie.
4. Le Comité d'Organisation responsable de l'organisation du Congrès dans le pays où celui-ci doit avoir lieu.

1. *L'Assemblée des Délégués Nationaux*

Les Délégués sont nommés par les Sociétés Nationales des différents pays.

Le nombre des Délégués, pour chaque pays, sera calculé d'après le nombre des membres titulaires de ces Sociétés, dans les proportions suivantes:

de 20 à 100 membres	1 délégué,
de 100 à 200 membres	2 délégués,
de 200 à 500 membres	3 délégués,
plus de 500 membres	4 délégués.

Chaque membre peut être remplacé par un suppléant.

Si un pays posséde plus d'une Société de Dermatologie, les Délégués seront nommés par accord entre ces Sociétés.

Si un pays est déjà représenté au sein du Comité International de Dermatologie par un ou plusieurs membres, ceux-ci seront automatiquement Délégués Nationaux.

Le Président de chaque Société Nationale communiquera au Secrétaire Général du Comité International de Dermatologie les noms des Délégués, avec une liste des Sociétés de Dermatologie qui ont participé à la nomination des Délégués et la liste complète de leurs membres.

Lors du Congrès International, l'Assemblée des Délégués tient séance sous la présidence du Président du Comité International de Dermatologie qui est aussi le Président de la Ligue Internationale des Sociétés dermatologiques.

L'Assemblée des Délégués a pouvoir:

d'élire au scrutin secret, les membres du Comité International de Dermatologie, ainsi que le Président et le Secrétaire Général du C.I.D. sur des listes établies par le C.I.D.,

de fixer le pays et la ville où se tiendra le prochain Congrès et d'en élire le Président,

de fixer les statuts et règlements pour l'organisation du Congrès International,

de nommer, si nécessaire, des Commissions à des fins spéciales,

de fixer le montant de la cotisation pour la nouvelle période.

2. *Le Comité International de Dermatologie (C.I.D.)*

Le Comité International de Dermatologie sera composé de douze membres élus par l'Assemblée des Délégués Nationaux (il sera tenu compte, pour leur élection, de leur particulière expérience en matière de Congrès et de travaux scientifiques).

En plus des membres élus, les Présidents et les Secrétaires Généraux du C.I.D., ainsi que les Présidents et les Secrétaires généraux des Congrès Internationaux sont nommés *membres d'honneur* à la fin de leurs fonctions ou à la fin de leur mandat de membre élu du C.I.D.

Ces membres d'honneur sont nommés à vie. Ils pourront assister aux réunions du C.I.D. avec droit de vote, mais ne recevront pas l'indemnité de déplacement prévue pour l'une des réunions du C.I.D.

Le Président et le Secrétaire Général du futur Congrès font partie d'office du C.I.D. avec les mêmes droits que les membres élus.

Lors de chaque Congrès, *un tiers* des membres sera renouvelé, en tenant compte de l'âge, des sièges devenus vacants par décès ou par toute autre cause valable. Ces nouveaux membres seront élus, au scrutin secret, par l'Assemblée des Délégués, sur une liste proposée par le C.I.D.

A chaque Congrès, le C.I.D. choisit, par vote au scrutin, ceux de ses membres élus qui seront proposés à l'Assemblée des Délégués comme nouveau Président et nouveau Secrétaire Général du C.I.D. L'Assemblée des Délégués procèdera à l'élection du Président et du Secrétaire Général du C.I.D. par vote à bulletin secret. Leurs fonctions commenceront à la fermeture du Congrès et se poursuivront jusqu'à la fin du Congrès suivant.

Si le Président du C.I.D. ne peut remplir ses fonctions, celles-ci seront assurées provisoirement par le Secrétaire Général. Un nouveau Président sera désigné par le C.I.D. réuni à cet effet par le Secrétaire Général.

Si le Président du Congrès ne peut remplir ses fonctions, son remplacement sera assuré par le Président du C.I.D. qui consultera, à ce sujet, les autres membres du Comité. Pour faciliter cette nomination, chaque Président de Congrès doit, après son élection, suggérer le nom d'un remplaçant au Président et au Secrétaire Général du C.I.D. De toutes façons, le lieu du Congrès et le Secrétaire Général du Congrès ne peuvent être changés si 18 mois se sont écoulés depuis le précédent Congrès. Dans le cas contraire, une réunion du C.I.D. doit avoir lieu aussi rapidement que possible pour décider du lieu et du Président du futur Congrès.

Le C.I.D. se réunira au moment du Congrès, avant la réunion des Délégués Nationaux, et au moins une fois dans l'intervalle des Congrès.

Le Président du C.I.D. est habilité à nommer des commissions dont les fonctions s'exercent entre les Congrès.

En cas d'urgence, le Président peut provoquer une réunion exceptionnelle dont les décisions, pour être valables, exigent un quorum de sept membres et un vote à l'unanimité des présents.

Le C.I.D. est chargé:

de s'occuper de toutes les questions concernant les problèmes dermatologiques d'importance internationale;

de préparer le programme de l'Assemblée des Délégués Nationaux;

de représenter les intérêts de la dermatologie internationale vis-à-vis d'autres organisations;

de présenter des suggestions au Président du prochain Congrès en ce qui concerne l'organisation de ce dernier;

de nommer des conseillers chargés de collaborer avec le Comité d'Organisation en ce qui concerne le programme scientifique, les sujets à traiter et les principaux rapporteurs du prochain congrès international.

Finances du C.I.D. Les membres du C.I.D. ne sont pas rémunérés. Pour couvrir les dépenses du Comité (timbres, papiers, secrétariat, frais de déplacement de ses membres à l'occasion d'une seule des réunions prévues entre les Congrès), chaque Société Nationale versera une cotisation pour chacun de ses membres et pour une période de 5 ans (intervalle entre deux congrès). Le montant de cette cotisation est fixé par l'Assemblée des Délégués.

Les pays qui n'ont pas d'organisation dermatologique n'y participeront pas puisqu'ils n'ont pas de représentation directe à l'Assemblée des Délégués.

3. *Le Congrès International de Dermatologie*

Objet et buts. Le Congrès International de Dermatologie a pour buts le développement et le progrès de la dermatologie en donnant aux dermatologistes de différents pays l'occasion d'exposer leur expérience personnelle, d'échanger et de discuter leurs opinions et de former des liens personnels avec leurs collègues.

Réunions, Elections et Règlements. Le Congrès International de Dermatologie, se tiendra tous les 5 ans. Au cas où il ne pourrait avoir lieu à la date prévue, le congrès se réunirait à une date ultérieure fixée par le C.I.D., en accord avec le Comité d'Organisation du Congrès

Tous les dermatologistes du monde entier ayant acquitté le montant de la cotisation sont admis à participer au Congrès.

Le Président du Congrès a le droit de nommer tous les autres cadres du Congrès International. Le Président du Congrès peut constituer telle Commission qui lui semble nécessaire à la bonne marche du Congrès.

Des conseillers seront désignés par le C.I.D. pour collaborer avec le Comité d'Organisation du Congrès futur; ils auront pouvoir d'amender ou de modifier les décisions et arrangements pris par le Comité d'Organisation du Congrès en ce qui concerne le programme scientifique lorsqu'ils estimeront que ce dernier est en conflit avec les buts de la Ligue Internationale des Sociétés Dermatologiques et de la dermatologie internationale. Les désaccords survenant entre les conseillers nommés par le Comité International et le Comité d'Organisation du Congrès, seront réglés par appel au Président de la Ligue Internationale des Sociétés dermatologiques dont la décision sera définitive.

Les langues officielles du Congrès sont l'anglais, le français, l'espagnol et l'allemand.

Le programme de chaque réunion est préparé par le Secrétaire du Congrès.

Aucun rapport ou communication, déjà imprimé ou exposé a une autre société savante, ne peut être présenté au Congrès sous une forme identique.

Au cours des discussions, aucune intervention ne peut excéder 5 min, sauf sur autorisation du Président, acquise au besoin par un vote majoritaire des congressistes présents à la séance.

Le texte des rapports, communications et discussions doit être remis, avant la fin du Congrès, au Secrétaire du Congrès pour publication dans les comptes-rendus. Le Comité de Rédaction peut demander à un auteur de raccourcir tout rapport ou communication qui dépasse 1500 mots (y compris schémas et tableaux) — les illustrations ne sont admises qu'exceptionnellement et sont imprimées aux frais de l'auteur — ou de modifier ou supprimer tout rapport ou communication qui n'entre pas dans le cadre des buts scientifiques du Congrès. L'auteur peut être invité à contribuer aux frais d'impression d'un article qui dépasse le nombre de mots spécifié et ne peut être raisonnablement raccourci.

Tout rapport ou communication lu devant le Congrès mais publié avant la parution des comptes rendus, ne peut figurer dans ces derniers que sous forme de résumé.

Les comptes rendus du Congrès (rapports, articles, symposia, discussions) seront publiés dans leur langue originale.

La cotisation des membres du Congrès couvre les frais de publication des comptes rendus du Congrès. Cette cotisation doit être versée au plus tard à l'ouverture du Congrès.

4. *Le Comité d'Organisation*

Le Président du Congrès et son Comité d'Organisation sont responsables de l'organisation du Congrès et de la publication des comptes rendus.

Avant le Congrès le Comité d'Organisation publiera des résumés en langue anglaise des rapports et des communications; ces résumés réunis en un volume, seront adressés aux membres du Congrès au moins six semaines avant l'ouverture de celui-ci.

Le Comité d'Organisation du Congrès peut constituer une réserve de fonds destinés à des dépenses de fonctionnement extraordinaires, films, télévision, rénumérations etc.

Amendements aux Règlements. Les propositions d'amendement à ces règles doivent être adressées par écrit au Secrétaire du C.I.D., trois mois au moins avant la Réunion de l'Assemblée des Délégués. Les propositions seront portées à la connaissance des membres du C.I.D., puis soumises au vote de l'Assemblée des Délégués. Leur adoption sera acquise par un vote affirmatif des deux tiers des membres présents et votants.

Estatutos y reglamentos de la Liga Internacional de Sociedades de Dermatología

comprendiendo las enmiendas adoptadas en el XIII C.I.D., Munich, Agosto de 1967

Los objetivos de la Liga Internacional de Dermatología son:
Estimular los adelantos en Dermatología.
Promover relaciones personales entre todos los Dermatólogos del mundo.
Representar los intereses dermatológicos en otras Organizaciones Internacionales.
Organizar los Congresos Internacionales de Dermatología.

Los Organismos que componen la Liga son:
1. La Asamblea de Delegados Nacionales.
2. El Comité Internacional de Dermatología (C.I.D.).
3. Los Congresos Internacionales de Dermatología.
4. El Comité Organizador Local responsable de la Organización del Congreso en cada país en que éste deba tener lugar.

1. *Asamblea de Delegados Nacionales*

Los Delegados son designados por las Sociedades Nacionales de los diferentes países.

El número de Delegados que representa a cada país, se basa en el número de sus socios numerarios con arreglo al siguiente:

de 20 a 100 miembros	1 Delegado,
de 100 a 200 miembros	2 Delegados.
de 200 a 500 miembros	3 Delegados,
superior a 500 miembros	4 Delegados.

Cada miembro puede ser reemplazado por un sustituto.

Si en un país existen más de una Sociedad de Dermatología, sus Delegados serán designados de común acuerdo entre las diversas Sociedades.

Si un país está representado en el Comité Internacional de Dermatología (C.I.D.) este miembro o miembros serán automáticamente Delegados del respectivo país.

El Presidente de cada Sociedad Internacional de Dermatología enviará los nombres de los Delegados al Secretario General del C.I.D., con los nombres de las Sociedades de Dermatología que los han designado así como la lista completa de sus socios.

En cada Congreso Internacional, la Asamblea de Delegados tendrá sus sesiones bajo la presidencia del Presidente del C.I.D., el cual es tambien Presidente de la Liga Internacional de Sociedades de Dermatología.

La Asamblea de Delegados, está capacitada:

Para elegir, en votación secreta, los miembros del C.I.D. así como el Presidente y el Secretario General del C.I.D. de las listas establecidas con este fin por el C.I.D.

Designar el país y el lugar en que deberá celebrarse el próximo Congreso y elegir su Presidente.

Establecer normas y reglamentos para la organización de los Congresos Internacionales.

Designar, si fuere necesario, Comités para objetivos definidos.

Fijar la cuantía de la suscripción para el período siguiente.

2. El Comité Internacional de Dermatologia (C.I.D.)

El C.I.D. está constituido por doce miembros elegidos por la Asamblea de Delegados Nacionales; deben ser considerados en su elección la experiencia en la organización de Congresos y sus trabajos científicos.

Además de los Miembros elegidos, los Presidentes y los Secretarios Generales del C.I.D., así como los Presidentes y los Secretarios Generales de los Congresos Internacionales, son nombrados Miembros de Honor, al término de sus funciones o de sus mandatos de Miembros electos del C.I.D.

Estos Miembros de Honor lo son con caracter vitalicio. Podrán asistir a las reuniones del C.I.D. con derecho a voto, no gozando, sin embargo, de la indemnización de desplazamiento establecida en una precedente reunión del C.I.D.

El Presidente y el Secretario General del futuro Congreso, forman parte, automáticamente, del C.I.D. con los mismos derechos que los Miembros electos.

En cada Congreso, será renovado un tercio de sus Miembros, de acuerdo con su edad; las vacantes ocasionadas por fallecimiento u otras causas deberán ser tenidas en consideración. Los nuevos Miembros serán elegidos por votación de la Asamblea de Delegados de una lista propuesta por el C.I.D.

En cada Congreso, el C.I.D. elegirá por votación, entre sus Miembros electos, aquellos que serán propuestos a la Asamblea de Delegados como nuevos Presidente y Secretario General del C.I.D. La Asamblea de Delegados procederá a la elección del Presidente y del Secretario General del C.I.D. por votación secreta. Sus respectivas funciones se ejercerán desde la clausura del Congreso hasta la terminación del Congreso immediato.

Si el Presidente del C.I.D. se viese incapacitado para ejercer sus funciones, éstas lo serían, con caracter transitorio, por el Secretario General, el cual convocaria el C.I.D. para designar un nuevo Presidente.

Si el Presidente del Congreso no pudiera llenar sus funciones, sería sustituído por el Presidente del C.I.D. el cual llamará a consulta, con este objeto, a los restantes Miembros del Comité. Para facilitar estos nombramientos, cada Presidente de Congreso, deberá, tras su elección, sugerir, al Presidente y al Secretario General del C.I.D. el nombre de un sustituto. De todas formas, la designación del país en que deberá celebrarse el próximo Congreso y la elección de su Presidente no podrán ser revocados si han transcurrido más de 18 meses desde entonces. En caso contrario, tendrá lugar, lo más rápidamente posible, una reunión del C.I.D. con el fin de determinar el país y elegir el Presidente del futuro Congreso.

El C.I.D. deberá reunirse durante el Congreso antes de la reunión de los Delegados Nacionales y cuando menos una vez en el intervalo entre dos Congresos.

El Presidente del Congreso Internacional de Dermatología está facultado para designar Comités que funcionen entre dos Congresos.

En caso de urgencia el Presidente puede convocar reuniones extraordinarias, y su decisión debe ser aceptada si un quorum de siete Miembros presentes, vota de acuerdo.

El Comité Internacional de Dermatología está facultado:

Para ocuparse de cualquier problema dermatológico de importancia internacional.

Para preparar el orden del día de la Asamblea de Delegados Nacionales.

Para representar los intereses de la Dermatología Internacional en otras Organizaciones.

Para hacer sugerencias al Presidente del próximo Congreso, respecto a la organización del mismo.

Para designar Consultantes que colaboren con el Comité Local en la preparación del programa científico, temas y ponentes del próximo Congreso Internacional.

Finanzas del C.I.D. Los Miembros del C.I.D. son honorarios. Para cubrir los gastos del Comité (correo, material de oficina, secretaría, gastos de viaje para sus Miembros una vez en el intervalo de dos Congresos), cada Sociedad Nacional, pagará una contribución por cada uno de sus Miembros, que cubra el periodo de cinco años, correspondiente al intervalo entre dos Congresos. La cuantía de esta contribución será fijada por la Asamblea de Delegados Nacionales. Los países en los que no exista Organización Dermatológica alguna, no contribuirán a estos gastos, pero no tendrán representación en la Asamblea de Delegados.

3. *El Congreso Internacional de Dermatología*

Objetivos: Los Congresos Internacionales de Dermatología, tienen, como misión, el favorecer el desarrollo y progreso de la Dermatología, ofreciendo la oportunidad a los Dermatólogos de diferentes países de dar a conocer sus experiencias personales, intercambiando y discutiendo sus ideas y estableciendo relaciones personales con otros colegas.

Congreso, congresistas y normas: El Congreso Internacional de Dermatología se celebrará cada 5 años. Si fuese imposible celebrarlo en la fecha prevista, se reunirá en una fecha posterior determinada por el C.I.D. de acuerdo con el Comité Local del Congreso.

Todos los Dermatólogos del mundo podrán ser Congresistas previo pago de la cuota del Congreso.

El Presidente del Congreso está facultado para designar todos los otros Miembros del Comité Organizador Local, pudiendo designar todos los Comités que considere necesarios para el eficiente desarrollo del Congreso.

El Comité Internacional de Dermatología designará consultantes para colaborar con el Comité organizador del próximo Congreso autorizados a enmendar o alterar las decisiones y acuerdos del Comité Organizador del Congreso en cuestiones relacionadas con el programa científico, cuando la opinión de los Consultantes esté en conflicto con los fines de la Liga Internacional de Sociedades de Dermatología y de la Dermatología Internacional. Las discrepancias entre los Consultantes designados por el Comité Internacional y el Comité Local de organización del Congreso, se resolverán por el Presidente de la Liga Internacional de Sociedades de Dermatología cuya decisión es inapelable.

Las lenguas oficiales del Congreso son: Alemán, español, francés, inglés e italiano.

El orden del día de cada sesión será establecido por el Secretario del Congreso.

No se admitirá ninguna ponencia o comunicación que haya sido previamente publicada o presentada en otra Sociedad.

El tiempo fijado para la discusión no debe exceder de 5 minutos. El Presidente puede, eventualmente, prolongar este tiempo, si es necesario, con el voto mayoritario de los presentes.

El texto de las ponencias, comunicaciones y discusiones, debe entregarse antes de la terminación del Congreso al Secretario del mismo para su publicación en las actas del Congreso. El Comité editorial puede solicitar del autor de cualquier ponencia o comunicación que exceda de 1500 palabras, que sea acortada (incluido el espacio destinado a gráficos o tablas). Las fotografías serán solamente admitidas en casos excepcionales y por cuenta del autor. Ademas, cualquier ponencia o comunicación en desacuerdo con los objetivos del Congreso podra ser modificada o rechazada. Los autores de artículos que excedan del número de palabras mencionado, que no puedan, razonablemente, ser reducidos, contribuirán al coste de su impresión.

Cualquier ponencia o comunicación presentada al Congreso, pero publicada antes que las actas del mismo, podrá aparecer solamente en forma de resumen.

Las actividades del Congreso (ponencias, comunicaciones, simposio, discusiones) serán publicadas en su lengua original.

La cuota de Miembro del Congreso debe cubrir el coste de las actas. Esta cuota deberá satisfacerse, lo mas tarde, al comenzar el Congreso.

4. *Comité Organizador Local*

El Presidente del Congreso y su Comité Local son responsables de la organización del Congreso y de la publicación de sus actas.

Antes del Congreso el Comité organizador Local publicará resúmenes de las ponencias y comunicaciones, en inglés, en un libro que se enviará a los Miembros del Congreso no más tarde de seis semanas antes de comenzar el Congreso.

El Comité organizador Local deberá disponer de fondos para todas las otras obligaciones del Congreso; películas, televisión, estipendios, etc.

Enmienda de los Reglamentos. Las propuestas de enmiendas a los Reglamentos deberán ser presentadas por escrito al Secretario del C.I.D. por lo menos tres meses antes de la reunión de la Asamblea de Delegados. Las propuestas serán dadas a conocer a todos los Miembros del C.I.D. y sometida al voto de la Asamblea de Delegados. Su adopción requiere el voto favorable de dos tercios de los votantes.

Satzungen und Bestimmungen der Internationalen Liga Dermatologischer Gesellschaften

Die Änderungen, die am XIII. Internationalen Kongreß in München, August 1967, beschlossen wurden, sind einbezogen worden.

Die Ziele der Internationalen Liga der Dermatologischen Gesellschaften sind:

Anregungen zur Weiterbildung in der Dermatologie zu geben,
den persönlichen Kontakt unter den Dermatologen der ganzen Welt zu fördern,
die dermatologischen Interessen bei anderen internationalen Organisationen zu vertreten und internationale dermatologische Kongresse abzuhalten.

Die Liga setzt sich zusammen aus:

1. der Versammlung der Nationalen Delegierten,
2. dem Internationalen Komitee für Dermatologie (I.C.D.),
3. dem Internationalen Kongreß für Dermatologie,
4. dem Komitee, das für die Organisation des nächsten Kongresses verantwortlich ist.

1. *Die Versammlung der Nationalen Delegierten*

Die Delegierten werden von den Nationalen Gesellschaften der einzelnen Länder ernannt.

Die Zahl der Delegierten jedes einzelnen Landes richtet sich nach der Zahl der ordentlichen Mitglieder in dem folgenden Verhältnis:

auf   20 bis 100 Mitglieder   1 Delegierter,
auf 100 bis 200 Mitglieder   2 Delegierte,
auf 200 bis 500 Mitglieder   3 Delegierte,
auf mehr als 500 Mitglieder   4 Delegierte.

Für jeden Delegierten kann ein Ersatzmann eintreten.

Gibt es in einem Land mehr als eine dermatologische Gesellschaft, so werden die Delegierten nach entsprechenden Vereinbarungen zwischen den Gesellschaften nominiert.

Ist ein Land bereits im Internationalen Komitee vertreten, so ist oder sind diese Mitglieder automatisch Delegierte dieses Landes.

Der Präsident jeder Nationalen Dermatologischen Gesellschaft übermittelt die Namen der Delegierten, zusammen mit den Namen der Dermatologischen Gesellschaften, die diese Ernennung durchgeführt haben, und einer vollständigen Mitglieder-Liste an den Generalsekretär des I.C.D.

Beim Internationalen Kongreß hält die Versammlung der Delegierten ihre Sitzung unter der Leitung des Vorsitzenden des I.C.D. ab, welcher zugleich Präsident der Internationalen Liga der Dermatologischen Gesellschaften ist. Die Versammlung der Delegierten ist zu folgendem berechtigt:

Wahl in geheimer Abstimmung der Mitglieder des Internationalen Komitees sowie des Präsidenten und des Generalsekretärs des I.C.D. auf Grund von Listen, die vom I.C.D. vorgelegt werden;

Bestimmung des Landes und des Ortes des nächsten Kongresses sowie die Wahl seines Präsidenten;

Aufstellung von Regeln und Vorschriften über die Organisation des Internationalen Kongresses;

Ernennung von Komitees — falls notwendig — für besondere Zwecke;

Festsetzung der Höhe der Beiträge für die nächste Periode.

2. *Das Internationale Komitee für Dermatologie (I. C. D.)*

Das I.C.D. soll aus zwölf Mitgliedern bestehen, die von der Versammlung der nationalen Delegierten gewählt werden (besondere Erfahrung bezüglich Kongreßangelegenheiten und wissenschaftlicher Arbeit sollen bei der Wahl berücksichtigt werden).

Die Präsidenten und Generalsekretäre des I.C.D. sowie die Präsidenten und Generalsekretäre der Internationalen Kongresse werden zu Ehrenmitgliedern ernannt, entweder wenn sie ihre Funktionen erfüllt haben, oder wenn sie als gewählte Mitglieder des I.C.D. ausscheiden müssen. Die Ehrenmitgliedschaft besteht lebenslänglich. Die Ehrenmitglieder können den Sitzungen des I.C.D. beiwohnen. Sie haben Stimmrecht, erhalten aber keine Reiseentschädigung wie sie für *eine* der Sitzungen des I.C.D. vorgesehen ist. Der Präsident und der Generalsekretär des nächsten Kongresses sind ordentliche Mitglieder des I.C.D. mit den gleichen Rechten wie die gewählten Mitglieder.

Bei jedem Kongreß soll ein Drittel der Mitglieder entsprechend dem Alter ausscheiden, wobei infolge Todes oder aus anderen Gründen frei gewordene Stellen mitgerechnet werden. Neue Mitglieder sollen in geheimer Wahl durch die Delegierten-Versammlung gewählt werden auf Grund einer Vorschlagliste des I.C.D.

Bei jedem Kongreß werden in geheimer Abstimmung vom I.C.D. diejenigen Mitglieder bestimmt, die der Delegiertenversammlung als neuer Präsident und Generalsekretär des I.C.D. vorgeschlagen werden. Die Delegiertenversammlung wählt in geheimer Abstimmung den Präsidenten und den Generalsekretär des I.C.D. Deren Tätigkeit beginnt am Ende des Kongresses und dauert bis zum Abschluß des nächsten Kongresses.

Wenn der Präsident des I.C.D. seine Funktionen nicht versehen kann, so werden sie vorübergehend vom Generalsekretär übernommen. Ein neuer Präsident wird in einer vom Generalsekretär einberufenen Sitzung des I.C.D. gewählt.

Wenn der Kongreßpräsident seine Funktion nicht erfüllen kann, wird der Präsident des I.C.D., nach Konsultation der Komiteemitglieder, für die Nachfolge zu sorgen haben.

Um die Wahl zu erleichtern, soll jeder Kongreßpräsident nach seiner Wahl den Namen eines Stellvertreters dem Präsidenten und Generalsekretär des I.C.D. vorschlagen. Auf keinen Fall dürfen Kongreßort und Generalsekretär des Kongresses 18 Monate nach dem letzten Kongreß noch geändert werden. Ist diese Frist noch nicht verstrichen, so muß so rasch wie möglich eine Sitzung des I.C.D. einberufen werden, um Kongreßpräsident und Kongreßort zu bestimmen.

Das I.C.D. soll zur Zeit des Kongresses einmal vor der Versammlung der Nationalen Delegierten und mindestens einmal im Intervall zwischen den Kongressen eine Sitzung abhalten.

Der Präsident des I.C.D. hat das Recht, Komitees zu ernennen, die in der Zeit zwischen den Kongressen arbeiten sollen.

Bei dringenden Anlässen ist der Präsident berechtigt, eine außerordentliche Sitzung einzuberufen, deren Beschlüsse gültig sind, wenn sie in Anwesenheit von sieben Mitgliedern einstimmig gefaßt werden.

Das Internationale Komitee für Dermatologie ist ermächtigt:

sich mit allen Fragen und Problemen auf dem Gebiete der Dermatologie, die von internationalem Interesse sind, zu beschäftigen;

die Tagesordnung für die Versammlung der Nationalen Delegierten vorzubereiten;

die Interessen der internationalen Dermatologie bei anderen Organisationen zu vertreten;

dem Präsidenten des nächsten Kongresses Vorschläge bezüglich der Organisation des Kongresses zu unterbreiten;

Berater zu ernennen, die mit dem Organisations-Komitee hinsichtlich der Gestaltung des wissenschaftlichen Programms, der Wahl der Themen und der Referenten für den nächsten Internationalen Kongreß zusammenarbeiten.

Finanzen des I.C.D. Die Mitglieder des I.C.D. werden nicht bezahlt. Um die Auslagen des Komitees (Briefmarken, Papier, Arbeiten des Sekretariats, Reisekosten der Mitglieder für eine einmalige Zusammenkunft zwischen den Kongressen) zu decken, wird jede nationale Gesellschaft für jedes ihrer Mitglieder einen Beitrag zahlen, der jeweils eine Periode von 5 Jahren umfaßt (entsprechend dem Intervall zwischen zwei Kongressen). Die Höhe des Beitrags wird von der Versammlung der Nationalen Delegierten festgesetzt.

Länder, in denen keine dermatologische Gesellschaft besteht, haben keinen Beitrag zu zahlen, da sie nicht in der Versammlung der Delegierten vertreten sind.

3. *Der Internationale Kongreß für Dermatologie*

Gegenstand und Ziel. Aufgabe des Internationalen Kongresses ist es, die Entwicklung und den Fortschritt auf dem Gebiet der Dermatologie zu fördern. Er gibt den Dermatologen der verschiedenen Länder die Möglichkeit, persönliche Erfahrungen weiterzureichen, Ideen auszutauschen und zu diskutieren und persönliche Kontakte mit anderen Fachkollegen zu bilden.

Zusammenkünfte, Mitgliedschaft und Regeln. Der Internationale Kongreß für Dermatologie soll alle 5 Jahre abgehalten werden. Sollte die Veranstaltung des Kongresses zum festgesetzten Termin nicht möglich sein, so wird das I.C.D. nach Verständigung mit dem Organisations-Komitee einen neuen Termin festsetzen.

Die Dermatologen der ganzen Welt sind als Mitglieder des Kongresses zugelassen, sofern sie die Kongreßgebühren bezahlen.

Der Präsident des Kongresses hat das Recht, alle anderen für den Kongreß notwendigen Mitarbeiter zu ernennen. Er kann besondere Komitees aufstellen, wenn er sie für einen erfolgreichen Ablauf des Kongresses für notwendig erachtet.

Das I.C.D. soll Berater ernennen, die mit dem Organisations-Komitee für den nächsten Kongreß zusammenarbeiten. Diese Berater haben das Recht, Beschlüsse und Anordnungen des Organisations-Komitees hinsichtlich des wissenschaftlichen Programms zu ändern oder zu ergänzen, wenn sie der Meinung sind, daß diese Beschlüsse im Widerspruch mit den Zielen der Internationalen Liga für Dermatologie und der internationalen Dermatologie stehen. Unstimmigkeiten zwischen den vom I.C.D. bestimmten Beratern und dem Organisations-Komitee des Kongresses sollen dem Präsidenten der Internationalen Liga der Dermatologischen Gesellschaften vorgetragen werden, der dann die endgültige Entscheidung trifft.

Die offiziellen Sprachen des Kongresses sind Deutsch, Englisch, Französisch und Spanisch.

Das Programm jeder Sitzung wird vom Generalsekretär des Kongresses aufgestellt.

Arbeiten oder Mitteilungen, die bereits gedruckt erschienen oder in einer anderen wissenschaftlichen Gesellschaft bekannt gegeben worden sind, dürfen in der gleichen Form auf dem Kongreß nicht vorgetragen werden.

Bei den Diskussionen darf eine Redezeit von 5 min nicht überschritten werden, es sei denn mit Genehmigung des Vorsitzenden und, wenn nötig, in Übereinstimmung mit der Mehrheit der Anwesenden.

Die Manuskripte der Referate, Vorträge und Diskussionen müssen vor Beendigung des Kongresses beim Generalsekretär des Kongresses zur Veröffentlichung im Kongreßbericht abgegeben werden. Das Herausgeberkollegium ist berechtigt, den Autor zur Kürzung aufzufordern, wenn der Bericht mehr als 1500 Worte umfaßt (einschließlich Raum für Tabellen. Abbildungen sind nur in außergewöhnlichen Fällen und auf Kosten des Autors zugelassen). Bei Berichten und Mitteilungen, die nicht dem wissenschaftlichen Ziel des Kongresses entsprechen, sind die Herausgeber berechtigt, den Verfasser zu bitten, den Bericht zu ändern oder zurückzuziehen. Der Autor kann aufgefordert werden, sich an den Kosten für die Veröffentlichung seines Beitrages zu beteiligen, wenn dieser die vereinbarte Zahl von Worten überschreitet und vernünftigerweise nicht gekürzt werden kann.

Berichte oder Mitteilungen, die auf dem Kongreß vorgetragen wurden und vor Erscheinen des Kongreßberichtes andernorts publiziert werden, können in diesem nur als Zusammenfassung erscheinen.

Im Kongreßbericht sollen Referate, Vorträge, Symposien und Diskussionen jeweils in der Originalsprache festgehalten werden.

Im Kongreßbeitrag der Teilnehmer sind die Kosten für den Kongreßbericht inbegriffen. Dieser Kongreßbeitrag muß spätestens bei Beginn des Kongresses bezahlt werden.

4. *Organisations-Komitee*

Der Präsident des Kongresses und sein Organisations-Komitee sind für die Organisation des Kongresses und die Herausgabe des Kongreßberichtes verantwortlich.

Das Organisations-Komitee wird vor dem Kongreß die Zusammenfassungen der Referate und Vorträge in englischer Sprache in Form eines Buches veröffentlichen, welches den Teilnehmern des Kongresses spätestens 6 Wochen vor seinem Beginn zugesandt wird.

Das Organisations-Komitee kann Vorkehrungen für irgendwelche Sonderfunktionen beim Kongreß, wie z. B. für Filme, Fernsehen, Stipendien usw., treffen.

Ergänzungen zu den Regeln. Vorgeschlagene Ergänzungen zu diesen Regeln und Vorschriften müssen mindestens 3 Monate vor der Zusammenkunft der Nationalen Delegierten dem Generalsekretär des I.C.D. schriftlich unterbreitet werden. Die Vorschläge werden unter den Mitgliedern des I.C.D. zirkulieren und danach zur Abstimmung der Versammlung der Nationalen Delegierten vorgelegt.

Zur Annahme ist eine Zweidrittelmehrheit der Anwesenden und ihre Stimme abgebenden Delegierten erforderlich.

XIII. Congressus Internationalis Dermatologiae

XIII. Congressus Internationalis

Dermatologiae

31.7. – 5. 8. 1967 / München

Editors: W. Jadassohn and C. G. Schirren

Volume 2

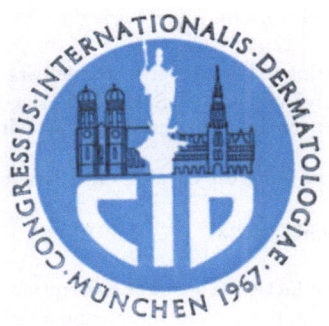

Springer-Verlag Berlin Heidelberg GmbH 1968

Additional material to this book can be downloaded from http://extras.springer.com

ISBN 978-3-642-49455-0   ISBN 978-3-642-49735-3 (eBook)
DOI 10.1007/978-3-642-49735-3

All rights reserved
No part of this book may be translated or reproduced in any form without written
permission from Springer-Verlag

© by Springer-Verlag Berlin Heidelberg 1968
Originally published by Springer-Verlag Berlin-Heidelberg New York in 1968
Softcover reprint of the hardcover 1st edition 1968

Library of Congress Catalog Card Number 68-8552

Title Number 1523

The reproduction of general descriptive names, trade names, trade marks, etc. in this
publication, even when there is no special identification mark, is not to be taken as a sign
that such names, as understood by the Trade Marks and Merchandise Marks Law,
may accordingly be freely used by anyone

Photos: pages *1—128:* L. HEIGL, H. GIESSNER, R. PRÖHL and W. GERSTENBREY

Volume 1

Preface . . . . VII—X

Congressus Internationales Dermatologiae XII

Contents . . . . : . . . . XIII—XXXIX

Organization, Addresses and Course of the Congress . . . . . 1—128

Main-Theme I—VII . . . . 1—525

Symposium 1—4 . . . . 527—703

Volume 2

Symposium 5—15 . . . . 705—1375

Case Presentations and Fundamentals on Film . . . . 1377—1382

Scientific Exhibition . . . . 1385—1591

Authors Index . . . . 1592—1598

Preface

By these volumes, we would like to show how the problems which preoccupy dermatologists were exposed and discussed at the XIII International Congress of Dermatology. Above all, in this preface, we wish to express our joy that the congress has been a success, which is well shown in the scientific parts of these volumes. Worldwide new relations have been established among dermatologists. We owe its success to all participants: to those who have contributed by their scientific works, to those who followed with attention and to those who have helped us so kindly. Our thanks to the International Committee of Dermatology, the Organization Committee and to numerous collaborators, have been expressed in several speeches. Rereading these we notice with much regret that many people who have greatly contributed to the success of the Congress, were not named verbally. We are not going to make a list of them, it would be too long and incomplete. For their work, their constant collaboration, their great kindness, we wish to express to them our gratitude.

The Publishing Firm Springer, with its usual devotion, realized the wishes of the editors, in publishing the present work and printed it in the shortest delay possible.

The Firm Ciba, has generously undertaken, to its own expense, the publication of the patient demonstration by Eidophor.

WERNER JADASSOHN
Genève

CARL GEORG SCHIRREN
München/Marburg (Lahn)

June 15, 1968

Préface

Par le contenu de ces volumes, nous désirons montrer de quelle façon les problèmes qui préoccupent les dermatologues ont été exposés et discutés au XIIIième Congrès International de Dermatologie. Dans cette préface, nous aimerions tout d'abord exprimer notre joie pour la réussite du Congrès, réussite que la partie scientifique de ces volumes montre bien. En outre, de nouveaux liens se sont établis entre les dermatologues du monde entier. Le succès du Congrès, nous le devons à tous les participants: à ceux qui ont contribué par leurs travaux scientifiques, à ceux qui ont pris part aux discussions, à ceux qui ont écouté avec attention et à ceux qui ont aidé avec tant de gentillesse. Les remerciements adressés au Comité International de Dermatologie, au Comité d'Organisation du Congrès et à tous les nombreux collaborateurs ont déjà été exprimés dans plusieurs discours. Relisant ces derniers, nous nous apercevons avec regrêt que bien des personnes ayant grandement contribué à la réussite du Congrès, n'ont pas été nommées. Nous n'allons pas en donner la liste, car elle serait trop longue et incomplète. Pour leur travail, leur constante collaboration et leur grande amabilité, nous aimerions ici exprimer encore notre gratitude à toutes les collaboratrices et à tous les collaborateurs.

L'impression et la publication du présent ouvrage par la Maison d'Edition Springer, bien connue pour son dévouement, a exaucé les vœux des éditeurs.

La publication de la séance de démonstrations de malades par le procédé Eidophore, a été généreusement offerte par la Maison Ciba.

WERNER JADASSOHN
Genève

CARL GEORG SCHIRREN
München/Marburg (Lahn)

le 15 Juin 1968

Prefacio

Por medio de estos volúmenes, nos es grato demostrar, de que modo, en el XIII Congreso Internacional de Dermatología, fueron expuestos y discutidos aquellos problemas que preocupan a los dermatólogos. En este prefacio, desearíamos, ante todo, proclamar nuestro gozo por el éxito alcanzado por este Congreso. Este triunfo queda bien reflejado en la sección científica contenida en estos volúmenes. Han quedado establecidos nuevos lazos entre los dermatólogos del mundo entero. El éxito del Congreso ha sido debido a la acción conjunta de todos los participantes: los que contribuyeron con sus trabajos científicos; los que tomaron parte en las discusiones; los que escucharon con atención y todos aquellos que nos prestaron su ayuda con tanta gentileza. Las frases de agradecimiento, dirigidas al Comité Internacional de Dermatología, al Comité de Organización y a los innombrables colaboradores, fueron expresadas en muchos discursos. Releyendo estos, nos hemos apercibido que los nombres de un gran número de personas, que contribuyeron grandemente al éxito del Congreso, no fueron citados. Renunciamos a mencionarles, ya que la lista sería demasiado larga y quizás incompleta. Por su trabajo, su constancia y su gran amabilidad, nos satisface expresar aquí nuestra gratitud, a todas las colaboradoras y colaboradores.

La Editorial Springer, con su desinterés acostumbrado, ha impreso y publicado esta obra en muy breve plazo, colmando así los deseos de los editores.

La Casa Ciba ha tomado, generosamente, a su cargo, la publicación de la sesión en la que fueron presentados enfermos por su sistema Eidophor.

WERNER JADASSOHN
Genève

CARL GEORG SCHIRREN
München/Marburg (Lahn)

15 de Junio de 1968

X

Vorwort

Die vorliegenden Bände sollen zeigen, wie am XIII. Internationalen Kongreß für Dermatologie die Probleme, die die Dermatologen beschäftigen, abgehandelt und demonstriert wurden. In diesem Vorwort möchten wir unserer Freude darüber Ausdruck geben, daß der Kongreß gelungen ist. Denn er ist gelungen; das zeigt der wissenschaftliche Teil dieser Bände. Das ergibt sich daraus, daß zwischen den Dermatologen der ganzen Welt neue freundschaftliche Bande geknüpft wurden. Wenn der Kongreß gelungen ist, so verdanken wir das allen Teilnehmern, wirklich allen: denen, die wissenschaftliche Beiträge geliefert haben; denen, die diskutiert haben; denen, die interessiert zugehört haben und denen, die uns freundschaftlich entgegengekommen sind. Dem Dank an das Internationale Komitee, an das Organisationskomitee und an alle die vielen Mitarbeiter ist in verschiedenen Reden Ausdruck gegeben worden. Wenn wir jetzt diese Reden wieder lesen, so stellen wir mit Bedauern fest, daß viele, die sich große Verdienste um den Kongreß erworben haben, namentlich nicht erwähnt sind. Wir verzichten auch jetzt darauf, dies nachzuholen, die Liste würde zu lang und trotzdem unvollständig. Aber alle unsere Mitarbeiterinnen und Mitarbeiter sollen hier den Ausdruck unseres Dankes finden für ihre Arbeit, für ihre stetige Hilfsbereitschaft und auch für ihre große Freundlichkeit.

Der Springer-Verlag hat in gewohnter Großzügigkeit die Wünsche der Herausgeber bei der Gestaltung des Verhandlungsberichtes erfüllt und für ein rasches Erscheinen des umfassenden Werkes Sorge getragen.

Die Ciba hat in sehr dankenswerter Weise die Publikation der Eidophordemonstration übernommen.

WERNER JADASSOHN
Genève

CARL GEORG SCHIRREN
München/Marburg (Lahn)

15. Juni 1968

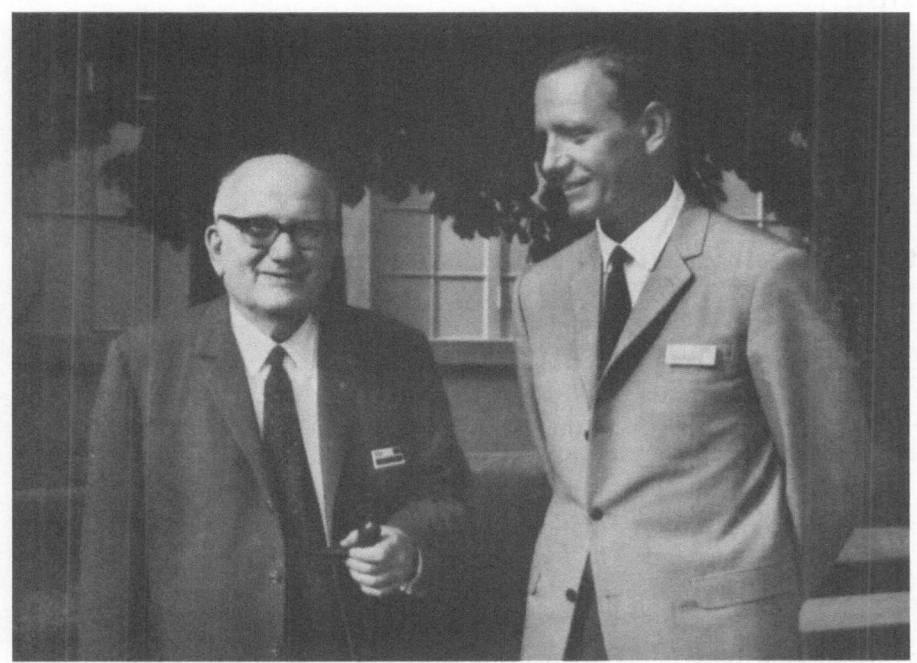

Professor W. JADASSOHN   Professor C. G. SCHIRREN
President of the Congress   Secretary General of the Congress

Congressus Internationales Dermatologiae

	President	*Secretary-General*
I. Paris, 1889	Prof. A. Hardy	
II. Wien, 1892	Prof. Moritz Kaposi	Prof. Gustav Riehl, Sr.
III. London, 1896	Sir Jonathan Hutchinson	Dr. J. J. Pringle
IV. Paris, 1900	Prof. Ernest Besnier	Prof. Georges Thiebierge
V. Berlin, 1904	Prof. E. Lesser	Dr. O. Rosenthal
VI. New York, 1907	Dr. James C. White	Dr. John Fordyce
VII. Roma, 1911	Dr. Tommaso de Amicis	
VIII. København, 1930	Prof. C. Rasch	Prof. Svend Lomholt
IX. Budapest, 1935	Prof. Louis Nékám	Dr. Stephen Rothman
X. London, 1952	Sir Archibald Gray	Dr. G. B. Mitchell-Heggs
XI. Stockholm, 1957	Prof. Sven Hellerström	Dr. Carl Henrik Flodén
XII. Washington, 1962	Prof. Donald M. Pillsbury	Prof. Clarence S. Livingood
XIII. München, 1967	Prof. Werner Jadassohn	Prof. Carl Georg Schirren

Contents Volume 1

	page
Introduction	1
Organization of the Congress	8
Participants Numbers from 1952 to 1967	10
Opening Session — Introduction	13
Opening Addresses	17
Prof. ROBERT DEGOS	17
Dr. h. c. ALFONS GOPPEL	19
Dr. HANS-JOCHEN VOGEL	19
Prof. LUDWIG KOTTER	22
Prof. ALBERT WIEDMANN	22
Prof. WERNER JADASSOHN	23
Prof. CARL GEORG SCHIRREN	27
Medals and Prizes	29
While Sessions	33
Press — Radio — Television	36
Social Program and Ladies' Program	39
Exhibitions — Introduction	53
Technical Exhibition	56
Opening of the Technical Exhibition — Opening Addresses	59
Prof. WERNER JADASSOHN	59
Prof. WILHELM SCHNEIDER	59
Exhibitors	62
The Art Exhibition	65
Film — Introduction	69
Film Program	70
Voyages after the Congress	72
Closing Session — Introduction	74
Concluding Speeches	75
Prof. ROBERT DEGOS	75
Prof. WERNER JADASSOHN	76
Prof. JOSÉ GAY PRIETO	77
Prof. CARL GEORG SCHIRREN	78
Donations	80
List of Donors	81
Members of the Congress	85
International Committee of Dermatology, Meeting of July 30, 1967, Munich	97
Report to the International Committee of Dermatology by SVEN HELLERSTRÖM	102
International League of Dermatological Societies	106
International Committee of Dermatology, Meeting of August 5, 1967, Munich	109
Rules and Regulations of the International League of Dermatological Societies	117

Main Theme I: Cancerous State, Precancerous State and Pseudocancers of the Skin (except Sarcomas and Melanomas)

1. Experimental Studies of the Carcinom Mechanism and Precancerous States

Reports

Electron Microscopic and Histochemical Findings in Basal Cell Epithelioma, Squamous Cell Carcinoma and Some Appendage Tumors. W. F. LEVER and K. HASHIMOTO	3
The Rôle of the Mesoderm in Basaliomas. H. PINKUS	8

page

Interrelation between Structure and Recurrence in Basal-Cell Carcinoma. A. REHÁK   11

Sur les précancéroses cutanées. I. BOSCO   13

Histochemical and Histoenzymological Studies in the Praecancerous Conditions of the
Skin. L. SZODORAY and CL. VEZEKENYI-NAGY   16

The Mechanism of Precancerous and Pseudocancerous Conditions. — A Comparative
Study. S. JABLONSKA and A. LANGNER   17

Free Communications

The Vascular Pattern of Induced Skin Cancer in Rats. W. A. WELTON   19

Enzymes de la glycolyse et du cycle des pentoses-phosphates dans les épithéliomas.
A. RIBUFFO   21

Effect of Prolonged Administration of Testosterone on Normal and X-Ray Radiated
Rat Skin. H. S. ZACKHEIM   22

Solar Ultraviolet Radiation and Skin Cancer. F. URBACH and R. E. DAVIES   24

A Clinical and Histological Study of the Evolution of Proliferative Epidermal Lesions
of Pitch Workers. G. HODGSON and H. J. WHITELEY   29

Arsenbedingte Präcancerosen und Cancerosen der Haut. W. BRAUN   31

Beitrag zur Beziehung des Traumas zum Hautcarcinom. M. SCHWARZWALD   33

(Prä-)Cancerosen und Elastose. G. NIEBAUER   35

Les nucléases des tumeurs épidermiques. J. DE BERSAQUES and J. PIÉRARD   37

Vergleichende cytophotometrische Untersuchungen an metatypischen Basalzellepitheliomen und Plattenepithelcarcinomen der Haut. G. EHLERS   38

Respiratory Enzymes Activity in Human Skin Neoplasms and Some Praecancerous
Lesions. D. CERIMELE, F. SERRI and C. PELFINI   43

Etude histochimique et biochimique comparée de certaines activités enzymatiques dans
les cancers de la peau. J. HEWITT, M. GUIGON and J. BOLUBASZ   44

Histologie des lésions précancéreuses de la peau. J. WANET and G. ACHTEN   46

Antigene Wirkung von Tumorgewebe. H. TRITSCH   48

Report

Les dermatoses paranéoplasiques. Y. BUREAU and H. BARRIERE   49

2. Keratoakanthoma

Free Communications

Unusual in Keratoakanthoma. D. V. STEVANOVIĆ   51

Zur Histogenese des Keratoakanthoms. K. W. KALKOFF, H. BERGER and M. HUNDEIKER   53

Unusual Forms of Keratoakanthoma. A. W. KOPF   54

An Ultrastructure Study of the Keratoakanthoma Experimentally Produced.
L. PRUTKIN   57

Papilomatosis Florida oral. A. R. DE KAMINSKY, C. A. KAMINSKY, J. ABULAFIA and
A. KAMINSKY   58

3. Clinical and Histological Studies

Report

Tumeurs des glandes sudorales. J. CIVATTE and J.-M. MASCARO   61

Free Communications

Das Syndrom der multiplen Basalzellnaevi (Naevobasaliome). W. THIES   63

Xeroderma pigmentosum — ein Modellprozeß der Cancerogenese der Haut. A. KÚTA   67

Clear Celled Epithelial Tumors of the Skin. A. H. MEHREGAN   68

The Pathology of Malignant Angioendothelioma of the Skin. E. WILSON-JONES . . .   70

Importance of Early Recognition of Oculo-cutaneous Metastases in Cancer of the Urinary
Bladder. A. HOLLANDER and I. A. GROTS   72

Cytologische Untersuchungen der Hautbasaliome in den Ausstrichpräparaten.
K. Lejman and J. Bogdaszewska-Czabanowska 73

Tetracycline Fluorescence in Squamous Cell Carcinoma. H. J. Donsky and G. R.
Mikhail 74

Regional Multiple Carcinoma. G. W. Vavruska and D. S. Kahn 75

A Skin Cancer Consultative Clinic. A. Johnson 76

Corrélations morpho-cliniques dans les récidives des épithéliomas cutanés de la face.
C. Longhin, G. Sandru, R. Dutu and M. Spiridon 78

Neuromyopathy in Skin Cancer. A. K. Afifi, F. S. Farah, A. K. Kurban and F. A.
Sabra 79

Cáncer, precáncer y pseudocáncer cutáneos: Estudio estadistico de la clínica dermatológica de la Universidad de Valencia. J. Calap and J. M. Fortea 81

Electron Microscopic Study of the Morphogenesis of Skin Tumours. J. Sugár 83

Epidermotropic Eccrine Carcinoma. Y. Miura, A. Akano, T. Nakagawa and Y. Kikuchi 84

Considérations sur le potentiel de malignisation des chéilites précancéreuses. Al. Dimitrescu 86

L'influence des radiations artificielles sur la muqueuse des lèvres des trempeurs d'acier.
R. Nicolau, P. Iacob and M. Bichis 87

Erythroplasia of Queyrat: A Precancerous Dermatosis. J. H. Graham and E. B. Helwig 89

Queilitis actínica, glándular y cáncer de labio inferior. P. Parejo and J. Ocaña . . . 91

L'ulcère chronique de la lèvre inférieure. F. Vanbremeersch, B. Duferrat and
J. Y. Noury 92

Squamous Cell Carcinoma in the Nottingham-Derby Combined Tumour Clinic 1959/66.
P. D. C. Kinmont and D. I. McCallum 97

4. Therapy

Reports

The Treatment of Skin Cancer and Pre-Cancer with Topical Cytotoxic Ointments.
J. C. Belisario 99

The Treatment of Skin Cancers with Radiation. H. Goldschmidt 105

Resultado de la radioterapia superficial en los epiteliomas cutáneos. G. Jaqueti and
J. Gay Prieto 107

Free Communications

Experiences with Topical Use of 5-Fluorouracil. A. R. Goddard 110

Therapie des Bowencarcinoms und des Lupuscarcinoms mit konventionellen Röntgenstrahlen. G. Stein 112

Traitement de l'épithélioma cutané par l'exérèse simple avec suture immédiate.
D. Thibaut 113

Tratamiento actual de la enfermedad de Paget del pezon. J. Ocaña Sierra and A. J.
Capilla 117

Tratamiento quirúrgico del cáncer cutáneo-mucoso. F. de Dulanto and J. Sánchez-
Muros 118

Über die Dosisplanung bei der Strahlentherapie der Hauttumoren. K. Balabanov and
P. Pentschev 119

Antimitotica der Podophyllinreihe bei Hautkrebs und seniler Keratose. V. Matanić 120

Chemosurgery for the Microscopically Controlled Excision of Skin Cancer. F. E. Mohs 122

Die Therapie fortgeschrittener Hauttumoren. H. Drepper and F. Ehring 125

Cryosurgery of Cutaneous Carcinoma. S. A. Zacarian 126

Topical 5-Fluorouracil. — An Effective Agent in the Treatment of Multiple Actinic
Keratoses and Some Superficial Malignant Diseases. W. M. Honeycutt, C. J. Dillaha
and G. T. Jansen 128

page

Main Theme II: Corticosteroids in Dermatology

Reports

Corticosteroids in Dermatology. G. ASBOE-HANSEN 133
Indications de la corticothérapie en dermatologie. S. LONGHIN 135
The many "Facies" of Iatrogenic Hypercorticism. A. C. CURTIS and G. L. STOKER . . 140
Les traitements prolongés par les corticostéroïdes (conduite du traitement). A. MIDANA,
    G. ZINA and G. MARTINA 143
Schädigungen bei lang durchgeführter Steroidtherapie mit besonderer Berücksichtigung
    der Hypophyse und Nebennierenrinde. F. FÖLDVÁRI, B. VÉRTES and J. MASSZI . . 145
Topical Corticosteroid Therapy. V. H. WITTEN 149
Les atrophies cutanées au cours de la corticothérapie générale. R. TOURAINE, M.
    FOURNET and S. BELAÏCH 153
Some Effects of Corticosteroids "in vitro". C. N. D. CRUICKSHANK 156

Free Communications

Long-term Estrogen and Corticosteroid Therapy in Chronic Skin Diseases. A. S. SPANG-
    LER, S. SOTMAN and H. N. ANTONIADES 158
Australian Experiences with the Cortico-steroids. W. W. LEMPRIERE 159
Möglichkeiten der Entwöhnung bzw. Einsparung von Corticoiden in der dermatologi-
    schen Therapie. G. LUDWIG 160
Indications for and Results of Systemic Corticosteroid Therapy in Dermatology.
    J. C. P. LOGAN and A. GIRDWOOD FERGUSSON 163
Influencia de los corticosteroides en la queratinización. A. M. MOM 165
Seltene Nebenerscheinungen bei der Therapie mit den Corticosteroiden an der dermato-
    logischen Klinik in Zagreb. D. KARLIĆ and V. ČAJKOVAC 166
Die Insuffizienz der Nebenniere nach Corticoidbehandlung. E. LACKOVÁ, J. RÁDL and
    M. HORÁKOVÁ 168
Corticosteroid-Nebenwirkungen und ihre Behandlung durch klinische Klimatherapie an
    der Nordsee. W. PÜRSCHEL 169
A Cytotoxic Effect of Fluocinolone Acetonide. A. J. COX and E. M. FARBER 171
Vergleich zwischen der vasoconstrictorischen und antientzündlichen Wirkung verschie-
    dener Corticosteroide. H. TRONNIER 172
Penetration Studies with C14-Labelled Fluocinolone Acetonide. M. K. POLANO and
    L. DE BEUKELAAR 176
Standards for Clinical Evaluation of Topical Steroids. J. R. SCHOLTZ and K. J. DUMAS 179
Absorption de l'hydrocortisone par la peau saine. G. GARDENGHI and B. TARQUINI . . 181
Local Action of Steroids. K. ASO, Y. TANABE and K. TAKENOUCHI 184
The Penetration of Radiolabeled Hydrocortisone in Human Skin in vivo. R. J. FELD-
    MANN and H. I. MAIBACH. 186
Zur Resorption von Corticoidsalben. K. WINKLER 187
Measurement of Percutaneous Absorption of Corticosteroid by Means of an Autoradio-
    graphy. A. KUKITA and T. MATSUZAWA 188
Observations concernant l'emploi des corticostéroïdes dans le traitement local de cer-
    taines dermatoses. ST. TEODORESCU and AL. BĂDĂNOIU 192
The Influence of Topical Corticosteroids on Hypothalamic-Pituitary-Adrenal Function.
    D. D. MUNRO, M. FEIWEL and V. H. T. JAMES 194
An Evaluation of Intralesional Steroid Therapy in Alopecia Areata. F. O. MEENAN . . 197
Effects of Topical Steroids in Normal and Psoriatic Skin. L. JUHLIN 198
The Recurrence Rate of Psoriatic Lesions after Topical Treatment with Dithranol and
    Corticosteroids under Plastic Dressings. D. SUURMOND 200
Effect of Topically Applied 0.1% Betamethasone 17-valerate ("Betnovate") Ointment on
    the Adrenal Function of Children. M. FEIWEL, D. D. MUNRO and V. H. T. JAMES 202
Die Ausscheidung der 17-Oxysteroide durch den Harn bei der lokalen Locacorten-
    Applikation. M. HORÁKOVÁ and E. LACKOVÁ 204

Prolongation moyenne de la vie chez les malades de pemphigus vulgaris traités par corticostéroïdes. P. Botzov, T. Pascalev and G. Spirov 205

The Effect of Intraarticular Celestona Chrondose in Rheumatoid Arthritis Associated with Psoriasis. L. Hellgren and A. Björnberg 207

Corticosteroids in the Treatment of Severe Dystrophic Epidermolysis Bullosa. E. J. Moynahan 208

Corticosteroid Therapy in Herpes Zoster. R. W. Carslaw and J. M. Nicolson . . . 209

Avantages thérapeutiques des corticostéroïdes dans un cas de Ainhum. A. Merello 211

The Present Aspect of Corticosteroids. — Therapy of Pemphigus in Japan. K. Ohara 212

Acción tópica de la fluformilona en dermatología. P. A. Viglioglia 213

Main Theme III: Contact Dermatitis (Allergic and Non-Allergic)

Reports

Factors Involved in Contact Non-Allergic Dermatitis. R. R. Suskind 217

Die Epicutanprobe durch wiederholte Benetzung. W. Burckhardt, R. Schmid and P. Schmid 224

Pathogenesis of Sensitization in Allergic Contact Dermatitis in Man. R. L. Baer and M. J. Fellner 226

Chronicity in Allergic Contact Dermatitis. C. D. Calnan 229

Zur Pathogenese der toxischen (ortoergischen) Kontaktdermatitis. H. W. Spier and F. Klaschka 232

Specificity and Cross-Sensitivity in Contact Allergy. V. Pirilä 236

Die Akzentverschiebungen bei den sensibilisierenden Stoffen während der letzten 3 Jahrzehnte. S. Borelli. 238

Free Communications

Kontaktekzem und Ekzematoide. Fr. Kogoj and J. Fettich 244

Die passive Übertragung des DNCB-Kontaktekzems beim Meerschweinchen mit Hilfe der kontinuierlichen Austauschtransfusion. F. Schröpl 246

Immunologic Unresponsiveness to Contact Sensitizers. E. D. Lowney 247

The Persistence and Recurrence of Contact Eczema: Clinical Experimental Observations. C. L. Meneghini, F. Rantuccio and G. Cozza 249

Tests épicutanés et épreuve de concentration-dilution. J. Oleffe 252

Experimentelle Untersuchungen über Sensibilisierungen mit chlorierten Imidazolinderivaten. E. Schöpf and K. H. Schulz 254

Problèmes physiochimiques concernant la formation de l'antigène sensibilisant de contact. E. Panconesi 255

The Aetiology of Eczema. J. G. Coburn and J. Reid 257

Cutan-vasculäre Kontaktallergie. — Untersuchungen zur Frage einer Antigen-Antikörperreaktion bei physikalischer Allergie. L. Illig 258

Sur la sensibilisation expérimentale au chrome. V. N. Negulescu 259

Recherches sur la pathogénie de l'eczéma dû aux sels de chrome. A. Sertcli and E. Panconesi 261

Efectos de una substancia antiplasmínica sintética en el eczema. J. M. Gimenez Camarasa 262

Test épicutané et test intradermique au bichromate de potassium. — Etude histopathologique comparative. B. Giannotti and A. Sertoli 265

Aspectos clínicos y pruebas cutáneas de las dermatitis. S. Abeliuk and E. Sylvester 267

The Frequency of Allergic Diseases Among Relatives of Patients with Allergic Eczematous Contact Dermatitis. M. Forsbeck, E. Skog and K. Ytterborn 268

page

Zunahme von Metallallergien bei Hausfrauen. G. FORCK 270

Hand Dermatitis, a Prospective Study. G. AGRUP 273

Seasonal Variations in the Incidence of Contact Dermatitis. N. HJORTH 275

L'Allergie aux sels d'ammonium quaternaire. — Etat actuel de nos recherches. P. MAR-
TIN, M. MENNECIER, P. AGACHE and CL. HURIEZ 276

Contact Dermatitis due to Plastic Coated Furniture (Tricresyl Phosphate). J. S. PEGUM 279

Study on the Penetration of Mineral Oil into the Human Skin by the Aid of Fluorescence
Microscopy. C. SCARPA 280

Vergleichende Untersuchungen verschiedener Testmethoden bei Sensibilisierung gegen
Neomycinsulphat (N.). M. NOVÁK and T. BIELICKÝ 282

Photoallergic Reaction in Red Tattoos. Mercury-Cadmium Sensitivity. N. GOLDSTEIN 283

Etude des maladies cutanées provoquées par la Brai de Houille. F.-X. CARTON . . . 286

Dermatitis, verursacht durch das Insekt Simulium erythrocephalum. A. KRSTITSCH and
V. ZIVKOVITCH 288

Contact Dermatitis from Static Electricity. H. E. BELLRINGER 289

Les études des facteurs étiologiques chez les dermatites de contact provoquées par le
ciment. S. PERIŠIĆ, A. SOFRONIĆ and D. JOVOVIĆ 291

Plants of North America that may Cause Dermatitis Venenata. A. P. ULBRICH . . . 292

Kontaktekzeme in der Landwirtschaft. E. HEGYI 294

L'automatisation dans l'industrie métallurgique élimine la possibilité d'apparition des
dermatoses professionnelles de contact (orthoergiques)? C. C. OANCEA 296

Main Theme IV: Virus Infections of the Skin and Mucosa

Reports

Neuere Entwicklungen dermatologischer Virusforschung. Th. NASEMANN 301

Pox-Viruserkrankungen. G. STÜTTGEN 306

L'étiologie virale des dermatoses bulleuses généralisées (pemphigus et pemphigoïdes).
A. CROSTI, F. GIANOTTI, E. HAHN and D. BUBOLA 310

Hand, Foot and Mouth Disease. R. WARIN and E. WADDINGTON 314

Herpès de primo-infection en milieu tropical. A. BASSET and M. ARMENGAUD 316

Survey of 22 Cases of Behçet's Disease. — The Significance of Specific Skin Hyper-
Reactivity. I. KATZENELLENBOGEN 321

Contribution à l'étude du rôle des infections rickettsiennes et pararickettsiennes dans
l'étiologie de certaines dermatoses à substratum vasculaire. ST. G. NICOLAU, C. SUR-
DAN and G. NOAGHEA 325

Free Communications

Etude histopathologique des lapins et des singes inoculés avec des virus isolés du sang
de malades de pemphigus et de pemphigoïdes. F. STROZZI, E. RONCHI and G. CHIAPPINO 326

Caractéristiques physiques, chimiques, biologiques et immunologiques de quatre souches
virales isolées de cas de pemphigus, de dermatite de Duhring, d'épidermolyse bulleuse
grave et d'érythème polymorphe. G. GIACOMETTI and E. HAHN 327

Etudes immunologiques chez les malades de pemphigus et pemphigoïdes. D. BUBOLA 329

Démonstration de la présence d'immuno-globulines et de la fixation du complément dans
les lésions cutanées chez les malades de pemphigus, au moyen de l'immunofluorescence.
F. GIANOTTI, M. GOVERNA, B. PERNIS and A. CROSTI 330

Cutaneous Manifestations of Behçet's Disease. M. MONACELLI and P. NAZZARO . . . 331

Untersuchung der Interferenz zwischen den Herpes simplex- und Vacciniaviren.
J. ANGYAL and E. BOTTYAN 333

page

Idoxuridine in the Treatment of Cutaneous Herpes Simplex. M. B. CORBETT, CH. M. SIDELL and M. ZIMMERMAN   334

Studies on "Latent" Motor Palsy Caused by Zoster. K. UEDA, K. IWASHITA and M. WAKASUGI   335

The Clinical Features of Hand, Foot and Mouth Diseases. E. WADDINGTON and R. P. WARIN   336

Etude clinique et épidémiologique de la maladie de Nicolas et Favre à Bordeaux. L. TEXIER, P. LE COULANT, M. GENIAUX and J. M. TAMISIER   338

Observations on Orf in Man. R. D. SWEET   339

Nobecutan-Podophyllin Preparations in Viral Warts. A. BJÖRNBERG and L. HELLGREN   340

Main Theme V: Current Problems in Syphilis

Reports

Syphilis and Human Ecology. T. GUTHE, O. IDSØE and R. R. WILLCOX.   345

Aspects actuels de la syphilis récente. E. LORTAT-JACOB   353

Aktuelle Probleme der Spätsyphilis. A. WIEDMANN   355

Estimation of the Recent Serologic Methods. H. A. NIELSEN   357

Evaluation des renseignements fournis par le T.P.I. et l'immunofluorescence. G. L. DAGUET   359

Penicillin in the Treatment of Syphilis. W. J. BROWN   360

Autres traitements que la pénicilline. R. DEGOS   363

Free Communications

Epidemiology

Homosexual Transmission of Early Syphilis. N. G. RAUSCH   366

Homosexualité masculine et syphilis. G. MORIAME and P. MEERTS   367

Social Problems of Venereal Disease Among Adolescents and Young Adults in New York City. W. CURTH   369

General Trend of Syphilis Recenta in Japan in the past 5 Years (1962 to 1966). J. DOHI, H. MOCHIZUKI, K. AONO and T. KOJIMA   370

Early Infectious Syphilis in Central London. R. D. CATTERALL   372

Clinical, Epidemiological and Therapeutic Aspects of Syphilis in Buenos Aires. L. M. BALIÑA, J. C. GATTI, J. E. CARDAMA, J. J. AVILA and H. N. CABRERA . . .   373

Syphilis and Japanese Seamen. T. HASEGAWA and R. SHINODA   375

La sífilis en el Uruguay. Tratamiento y profilaxis. R. A. VIGNALE, F. AMOR and C. RIVEIRO   377

Der diagnostische Wert des Zeichens von Higoumenakis. C. G. HIGOUMENAKIS. . . .   378

Serology and Experimental Syphilis

Some Immunobiological Problems in Experimental Syphilis. K. ITO   380

Serodiagnosis of Syphilis. L. NICHOLAS and H. BEERMAN   381

Zur quantitativen Beurteilung des FTA-Testes. F. FEGELER, S. NOLTING and M. KIFFE   385

Untersuchungen über den Einfluß des Überlebensmediums auf die Sensibilität des Nelson-Testes. J. LESINSKI, C. WISNIEWSKA and W. ZAJAC   387

The Problem of Recovery from Syphilis. F. FLARER and C. RABITO   389

Biological False-positive Reactors for Syphilis: Studies with the FTA-Absorption Test. D. L. TUFFANELLI and K. D. WUEPPER   391

Neue diagnostische Methoden bei un- und anbehandelter Frühsyphilis. K. GREGORCZYK   393

Die Aufgabe des Lysozyms bei der experimentellen Syphilis des Kaninchens. L. POSPÍŠIL   395

page

F.T.A. Test quantitatif dans le sérum d'individus non syphilitiques. S. SARTORIS and G. F. STRANI 397

Quantitative FTA Test During Treatment of Recent Syphilis. G. LEIGHEB, G. F. STRANI and S. SARTORIS 398

Modifications du comportement des tréponèmes pales après passages sur des lapins cortisones. P. COLLART, G. POGGI, M. DUNOYER and F. DUNOYER 400

Recherches expérimentales sur la provocation des anticorps fluorescents après administration de spirochète de souche Reiter chez des individus sains et syphilitiques. A. PANTI and S. ULIVI 404

Activité des anticorps fractionnés du serum dans la syphilis. F. OTTOLENGHI and U. SPAGNOLI 405

Activité antigénique des fractions de la protéine purifiée du tréponème de Reiter. U. SPAGNOLI and F. OTTOLENGHI 406

Possible signification du comportement des fractions globuliniques au F.T.A.-test sur le sérum de sujets luétiques. P. PAGNES 408

La stimulation lymphocytaire in vitro en divers stades de la syphilis. G. C. CHIEREGATO and G. FALDARINI 410

Untersuchungen über die Sensibilität und Spezifität des FTA-ABS-Testes. W. LESIŃSKA, J. LESIŃSKI and W. ZAJAC 411

Sérologie de la syphilis chez les sujets de race noire. P. MANY, R. MISSON, J. LAPEYRE, J. TEILLARD, B. BOUTET and F. PAGES 413

Treatment

Traitement de la syphilis. L. CIARROCCHI 415

Long Term Results of Penicillin Therapy of Primary and Secondary Syphilis. J. TOWPIK 416

New Therapeutical Aspects in the Therapy of Syphilis. G. EHRMANN 419

Considérations sur le diagnostic de guérison de la syphilis au moment actuel. U. BONCINELLI 419

Traitement des syphilis récentes par injection unique de 2.400.000 unités de Benzathine-Pénicilline. R. ROLLIER and T. MARKUCH 421

L'effet thérapeutique chez les malades atteints de syphilis traités à la Clinique Universitaire de Dermatovénérologie à Belgrade les 20 dernières années. S. KONSTANTINOVIĆ and S. PERIŠIĆ 423

Stellt die Behandlung der Frühsyphilis heute noch ein Problem dar? J. SÖLTZ-SZÖTS . 425

Main Theme VI: Cutaneous Manifestations of Circulatory Disorders of the Legs

Reports

Die venösen Durchblutungsstörungen der unteren Extremität. W. SCHNEIDER . . . 429

Methoden zur Untersuchung zirkulatorischer Störungen der Beine. H. STORCK and E. STREHLER 438

Arterial Reconstruction in Cutaneous Ischaemic Lesions. G. E. MAVOR and J. M. D. GALLOWAY 441

Medical Treatment of Cutaneous Disorders of Vascular Origin. CL. HURIEZ and F. DESMONS 444

Surgical Treatment of Venous Ulcers and Eczema of the Leg. K. HÆGER 450

Lymphedema of the Lower Extremities. J. BENINSON 452

Hipodermitis nodular subaguda migratiz. J. PIÑOL AGUADÉ 455

An Evaluation of Low Molecular Weight Dextran in Acrocyanosis and Acroscleroderma. E. M. FARBER, H. S. ZACKHEIM and E. ASCHHEIM 458

Free Communications

Oxygénothérapie locale dans les ulcères de jambe. W. RASIEWICZ and B. SZYMCZYK 460

page

Des aspects médico-sociaux et étio-pathogéniques de l'ulcère de jambe. L'importance de l'artério- et de la phlébographie dans l'ulcère dit variqueux. G. NASTASE and G. CHISLEAG 461

Studies on the Healing Time of Leg Ulcers. A Clinical and Statistical Study Based on 200 In-Patients. A. PERDRUP and J. STENE 463

A Mathematical Model for Healing Curves of Leg Ulcers. J. STENE 464

Arterial Occlusions as a Cause of Gangrene and Ischemic Ulcerations of the Legs. R. G. FREEMAN and J. M. KNOX 466

Präventivmaßnahmen bei Rezidiven der Unterschenkelgeschwüre. B. JANOUŠEK, H. DLABALOVÁ and V. ROZSÍVALOVÁ 468

Atrophie blanche. R. SANTLER 469

Stasis Dermatitis and Atrophie Blanche. —A Clinicopathologic and Histochemical Study. A. S. MARQUES, J. H. GRAHAM, W. C. JOHNSON and H. R. GRAY 470

Cutaneous Manifestations of Circulatory Disorders of the Legs. A. BOROTA 474

Neue Gesichtspunkte in der Behandlung venöser Durchblutungsstörungen. H. WEIT-GASSER 474

Angiolopathien und Unterschenkeldermatosen. N. KLÜKEN 476

The Pathogenesis of Nodular Panniculitis of Calves. P. BARTÁK 478

Histopathological Studies on Inflammatory Nodular Diseases in Lower Leg, Especially Concerning on Vascular Change. T. MIYAZAWA and Y. SASAI 479

The Treatment of Tropical Ulcer with an Antibacterial Soap and Topically Applied Sugar. R. A. OSBOURN, B. BENJAMIN and B. E. ELLICKSON 481

Main Theme VII: Regeneration and Transplantation of the Skin

Reports

Regeneration and Transplantation Experiments with Lower Vertebrate Skin as a Guide to Possible Endogenous Sources of Localized Pathogenesis in Man. I. W. WHIMSTER 487

The Cell Turnover of Human Epidermis. A. TOSTI 490

Tissue Banks and Local Therapy for Extensively Burned Patients. G. DOGC 496

Transplantation of Normal Skin to Pathologic Skin. N. ORENTREICH 497

Cultivation and Regeneration of Normal and Psoriatic Cells. B. LAGERHOLM 500

Reactions Between Skin Grafts and Hosts. A. CASTERMANS, G. DEGIOVANNI, A. M. HAENEN-SEVERYNS and G. LEJEUNE 501

Indikationen und Ergebnisse von Transplantationen bei Dermatosen. H. C. FRIEDERICH 503

Free Communications

Electron Microscopic Studies of Epithelial Growth and Keratinization in Cultures of Split-Thickness Adult Human Skin. PH. H. PROSE and A. E. FRIEDMAN-KIEN . . 505

The Management of Extensive Full-thickness Burns by Skin Grafting. T. ANZAI . . 509

Les hétérogreffes animales: Phénomènes de rejet des hétérogreffes répétées et des auto-greffes secondaires. P. LAUGIER, M. VÉRON, J. C. RISOLD and V. ELLENA 510

Transplantation of Epithelial Cell Cultures and the Formation of an Epidermis. M. A. KARASEK 513

Influence of Genetic Relationship on Skin Homotransplantation Survival in Humans. R. CEPPELLINI, M. VISETTI and G. LEIGHEB 514

Über die klinische Anwendung homologer und heterologer Hauttransplantate. W. WITTELS 515

Acid Mucopolysaccharide Synthesis in Scleredema. S. I. LAMBERG 517

La dynamique de la croissance des fibroblastes in vitro à partir des explants de peau humaine. M. GAVRILESCU 518

Biología de las heridas cutáneas. J. SÁNCHEZ-MUROS and F. DE DULANTO 520

page

Electron Microscopy of the Immunologically Competent Cells During Skin Homograft Rejection in the Rhesus Monkey (Macaca mulatta). F. ALLEGRA, M. BELL and L. GIACOMETTI 521

Zur Frage des Ausgangsmaterials der senilen Elastose. — Licht- und elektronenmikroskopische Befunde. H. BERGER 522

Epithelial and Fibroblast Tissue Culture Studies as a Trial to Understand the Action of Asiaticoside as a Healing and as a Fibrolytic Agent. H. EL-HEFNAWI 524

Symposium 1: Genodermatoses

Reports

Classification of Genodermatoses. D. BLOOM 529

Les génodermatoses bulleuses. S. LAPIÈRE 531

Le test gémellaire dans les dermatoses héréditaires. L. GEDDA and R. CAVALIERI . . 534

Epidermolysis bullosa hereditaria. — Klinik, Histologie, Elektronenmikroskopie. U. W. SCHNYDER 539

Le pemphigus familial bénin chronique et les formes bulleuses de la maladie de Darier. J. PIÉRARD and A. KINT 542

The Different Forms of Ichthyosiform Erythrodermia. J. R. SIMPSON 549

Xeroderma pigmentosum. E. HADIDA, F. G. MARILL and J. SAYAG 551

Free Communications

Importance génétique et clinique des altérations atypiques du fond de l'oeil dans le syndrome de Groenblad et Strandberg (pseudo-xanthome élastique et stries angioïdes). A. FRANCESCHETTI 553

The Necessity of Distinguishing Four Types of Acanthosis Nigricans. H. OLLENDORFF CURTH 557

Angiokeratoma Corporis Diffusum Fabry. W. P. DE GROOT 559

Studies on Ichthyosis Vulgaris. Y. IGARASHI, K. UEDA and K. IWASHITA 561

A Genetic Study of X-Linked Ichthyosis in Israel. L. ZIPROWSKI, A. FEINSTEIN, A. ADAM, R. SANGER and R. R. RACE 562

Atrophodermie folliculaire, proliférations baso-cellulaires et hypotrichose. B. CHRISTOL, A. DUPRÉ and A. BAZEX 565

Genetic Analysis of Erythropoietic Protoporphyria (EPP), the Erythrocyte Fluorescence Method. K. D. WUEPPER and J. H. EPSTEIN 566

Erythropoietic Protoporphyria — a Family Study. E. M. DONALDSON, A. D. DONALDSON and C. RIMINGTON 569

Biochemische Untersuchungen bei Porphyria variegata. G. ZIEGLER 570

The Molecular Cause of Albinism. G. F. WILGRAM 571

Zum Mechanismus der Aktivitätsminderung der Phosphoglucose-Isomerase in Erythrocyten von Kranken mit florider Psoriasis vulgaris. H. HOLZMANN and B. MORSCHES 572

Lichtdermatosen mit Hyperaminoacidurien. P. H. CLODI 574

Zur Klinik und Chromosomenanalyse der V. Phakomatose. G. VELTMAN and S. ADARI 575

Incidence of Anti-Nuclear Antibodies Among First-Degree Relatives of Patients with Chronic Discoid Lupus, Systemic Lupus and Normal Subjects. C. MARCH, N. ROTHFIELD and N. PACE 576

Electrocardiographic Abnormalities in a Familiy with Generalized Lentigo. R. J. WALTHER, B. POLANSKY and I. A. GROTS 578

Pachyonychia Congenita. C. B. VIZIAM, R. MATHAI, A. MAMMEN and Z. ISAAC . . . 580

Estudios citogenéticos en dermatología. J. ESTELLER, J. PIÑOL AGUADÉ, A. ALIAGA and E. GIMFERRER 581

Über den Erbgang einiger Formen von palmo-plantarer Keratose in Zusammenhang mit ihrem erbbiologischen und nosologischen Konzept. E. I. BOLOGA 583

page

Disseminated Superficial Actinic Porokeratosis. M. E. CHERNOSKY, R. G. FREEMAN and D. E. ANDERSON 587

Werner's Syndrome. — Report of a ̃Case with Postmortem Findings. Y. HAMADA . . 588

Unklassifizierte fleckenhafte Atrophie der Haut bei zwei Schwestern (Capillaritis maculo — keratotica atrophicans familiaris). R. ILEA and M. PAVEL 589

Symposium 2: Pyodermatitis

Reports

The Etiology of Pitted Keratolysis. D. TAPLIN and N. ZAIAS 593

Bacterial Flora. — The Rôle of Local and Environmental Factors. J. M. KNOX, M. E. MCBRIDE and W. C. DUNCAN 595

Polysaccharidfraktionen von Bakterien in ihrer Bedeutung für die Haut. J. MEYER-ROHN 600

Staphylococcal Strain 502-A in the Treatment of Recurrent Furunculosis. H. I. MAIBACH and W. G. STRAUSS 602

Some Observations on the Normal Cutaneous Flora of Different Age Groups. M. J. MARPLES 602

Free Communications

Über die Dynamik der Zusammensetzung der Bakterienflora auf der Haut. A. TODOROV and P. POPCHRISTOV 605

Keloidal Folliculitis of the Neck in Mongolism. E. KOCSARD, J. E. MOULTON and F. OFNER 607

Die Auswertung der Einwirkung des Staphylokokken-Anatoxins bei der Therapie und Diagnostik der Staphylokokken-Hautkrankheiten. J. LAŃCUCKI, J. SAMOS, Z. JÓZEFCZYK and E. STANOWSKA 609

Die Erysipelfrage. I. Allergologische und immunologische Untersuchungen an Erysipel-kranken. E. RAJKA, S. KOROSSY, J. BÖSZÖRMÉNYI, J. SZITA and M. GÓZONY 611

Die Erysipelfrage. II. Resultate der Streptococcus-Vaccinetherapie bei rezidivierenden Erysipelkranken. S. KOROSSY, E. RAJKA, J. BÖSZÖRMÉNYI and M. GÓZONY 611

Bacterial Etiology of Superficial Pyoderma in the Middle East. A. S. DAJANI, F. S. FARAH and A. K. KURBAN 612

L'influence de l'infection sur la marche du psoriasis. M. ZAJFEN and B. EJMONT-SKRZYPCZYK 613

Antiovulatorios en el tratamiento del acné juvenil. M. AHUMADA, L. NEUMANN and E. ORTEGA 615

Symposium 3: Dermatoses, Nervous System and Psychotic Origin

Reports

Haut und Nervensystem in klinischer Sicht. G. W. KORTING 623

Structure des fibres amyéliniques du système nerveux cutané. AD. DUPONT and A. BOURLOND 626

Dermatologie psychosomatique. P. DE GRACIANSKY and O. DE POLIGNY 628

Alteraciones cutáneas con interacción mental. A. KAMINSKY 630

Rehabilitation in Dermatologic Therapy. H. M. ROBINSON 634

Witchdoctors and their Ways. C. M. ROSS 636

Free Communications

Some Experimental Observations of Psychosomatic Aspects of Allergic Skin Disorders. K. HIGUCHI 639

page

Psychothérapies et traitements classiques dans les dermatoses psychosomatiques. P. Pichot and S. Lambergeon 640

Lichen ruber planus und Psyche. R. Weitz and G. Veltman 642

A Controlled Experiment in the Psycho-Therapy of Psoriasis. G. H. V. Clarke and P. J. Ashurst 644

Etude psychologique clinique et paraclinique des psoriasiques. M. Soule, J. M. Piret, J. Noel, G. Hurel and M. Bolgert 645

Genetic Neurological Disorders of Choreoathetosis and Cerebellar Ataxia with Important Dermatological Findings. W. B. Reed 646

Segmentale Innervation und Hautkrankheiten. W. Hauser 650

Untersuchungen über den Zustand des vegetativen Nervensystems bei Urticaria-Kranken. St. Chlebarov 652

Neuropsychiatric Manifestations in Xeroderma Pigmentosum. M. S. Abdel Gawad and H. el-Hefnawi 654

Symposium 4: Andrology (Masculine Impotence and Sterility)

Experimental Andrology

Reports

Biochemische Untersuchungen an Spermaplasma unter Berücksichtigung des Prostaglandins und seiner klinischen Bedeutung. R. Eliasson 659

On the Adrenal Origin of Dehydroepiandrosterone in Human Seminal Plasma. O. Steeno, C. Schirren, W. Heyns and P. de Moor 660

Oestrogene im menschlichen Sperma. C. Schirren 662

Neue Ergebnisse der Immunologie des Spermaplasma. W. P. Herrmann 663

Neu re morphologische Untersuchungen an Hodenzellen. H.-J. Bandmann 665

Free Communications

Basische Proteine in Spermienköpfen fertiler und infertiler Männer. W. Meyhöfer . . 666

Atomabsorptions-spektrometrische Untersuchungen des Magnesium- und Zinkgehaltes im Hoden und Prostatagewebe sowie im Ejaculat des Menschen. R. Herrmann, W. Knoth and W. Meyhöfer 668

Zur Bedeutung der Prostaglandine im humanen Seminalplasma. H.-C. Sturde . . . 670

Vergleichende licht- und elektronenmikroskopische Untersuchungen an Hodenbiopsien von infertilen Männern. H. Schmalbruch and O. P. Hornstein 672

Clinical and Therapeutical Andrology

Reports

Ursachen der Impotentia coeundi. R. Cernea 673

Successful Treatment of Azoospermia with Human Gonadotropins. Ch. A. Joel . . 676

Uses and Abuses of Gonadotrophins in the Male. G. Hellinga 679

Nicht-hormonale Substanzen in der Behandlung der männlichen Infertilität. W. Nikolowski 682

Free Communications

Klinische, histologische und endokrinologische Untersuchungen beim „idiopathischen" Hyperoestrogenismus. M. F. Hofmann, G. Pozzo and M. Cristofolini 685

Spermaqualität und Konzeptionsrate. R. Kaden 686

Tératospermie et anomalies évolutives de la grossesse. A. Montagnani and M. de Luca 688

Les troubles de l'éjaculation — Observations cliniques. G. Santori 690

Impuissance organique par dystrophies spinales congénitales (Spina bifida occulta et spondylolisthésis). J. Siage 691

page

Endocrine Function of the Testes, Gonadotropic Activity and Genetic Sex in Male Infertility. L. ANDREASSI 693

Essais de traitement endocrinien de l'infertilité due à des altérations testiculaires. L. SEMMOLA 694

Die Therapie des Klinefelter-Syndroms. H. NIERMANN 696

Die Gonadotropine menschlicher Herkunft in der Behandlung der männlichen Unfruchtbarkeit. P. CERUTTI and M. DE LUCA 698

Enzymatic Activities on Nucleic Acids and their Derivatives in Human Seminal Plasma. P. SANTOIANNI and G. ARGENZIANO 700

Ein neuer Gesichtspunkt endokriner-normospermatischer Infertilität. ST. ILCA, C. DODICA and Z. IOANOVICI 702

Volume 2

Symposium 5: Malignant Reticuloses and Lymphomas

Reports

Histopathologic and Hematologic Changes in Malignant Lymphomas and Reticuloses. H. MONTGOMERY and R. K. WINKELMANN 707

Zur Nosologie und Einteilung der Reticulosen, Reticulosarkomatosen und verwandter Krankheitsbilder unter Berücksichtigung cytophotometrischer Untersuchungen. W. KNOTH 712

Patología y clínica de los reticuloinfomas óculopalpebrales. P. H. MAGNIN, M. C. MORGENFELD and R. L. CABRINI 714

The Identity and Treatment of the Lymphoma Mycosis fungoides. M. A. LUTZNER . 720

Free Communications

Klinik und Histopathologie der malignen Reticulosen. K. W. MACH 721

Cytological Studies on Lymphoma with Electronmicroscopy. H. FUJITA 724

Cutaneous Lymphoblastoma, Spontaneous Involution of Tumours. D. MAJCAN, D. STEVANOVIĆ and B. LALEVIĆ 725

Blood Vessel Morphology in the Reticuloses. T. J. RYAN 727

Generalized Giant-Cell Reticulohistiocytosis (Lipoid Dermatoarthritis) — Clinical and Histopathological Study of two Cases. P. NAZZARO, U. GRANELLI and A. BIGNAMI . 728

Malignant Development in Mastocytosis. F. SAGHER and Z. EVEN-PAZ 729

Sézary Syndrome. G. L. ROCHA, F. SANTOS, R. AZULAY and A. PETRARCA DE MESQUITA 731

Mycosis Fungoides. — Mode of Presentation of 55 Cases. P. D. SAMMAN 733

Cytological Diagnosis in Mycosis Fungoides. E. BREHMER-ANDERSSON and U. BRUNK 735

Triacetyl 6-Azauridine in Mycosis Fungoides. CH. J. MCDONALD, P. CALABRESI and R. C. DE CONTI 739

Ultrastructure de l'angio-réticulo-sarcomatose cutanée: Maladie de Kaposi. E. CALAS, H. BONNEAU and J. P. CESARINI 741

Zur Entität des sog. Morbus Kaposi. G. OEHLSCHLAEGEL 745

Les localisations cutanées spécifiques de la maladie de Waldenstroem. H. BARRIERE, P. LITOUX and B. BUREAU 747

Esquisse de la physionomie de l'angio-sarcomatose de Kaposi en Algérie (A propos de 25 observations personelles). F. G. MARILL, E. HADIDA and J. SAYAG 748

Intérêt de la lymphographie dans les hématodermies. M. DANA, R. BOURDON, V. BISMUTH and J. P. DÉSPREZ-CURELY. 750

Radiothérapie des hémoréticulopathies malignes. R. BOURDON and M. DANA . . . 752

page

Symposium 6: Cosmetology; Biology and Pathology of the Hair

Cosmetology

Reports

Recherches sur le mécanisme d'action des antiperspirants. R. Brun, N. Hunziker and
P. Evdos 755
Hair Dyes. A. Rostenberg and G. Kass 758

Free Communications

International Dermatology and the World of Cosmetics. E. W. Brauer 761
Hormonal and Microbial Influences on the Sebaceous Follicles in Acne. P. E. Pochi . . 762

Biology and Pathology of the Human Hair

Reports

Development of the Human Hair Follicle. — Biology and Pathology of the Human
Hair. F. Serri 763
Alopecia areata, Basic Notions. G. Moretti, A. Rebora, E. Rampini, F. Crovato and
C. Cipriani 765
Klinik und Therapie der Alopecia areata. R. Schuppli 769
Causes actuelles des alopécies féminines diffuses. E. Sidi †, J. Bourgeois-Spinasse
and J. Arouète 771

Free Communications

Propiedades depilatoria y citotóxica de la seleno-cistationina. F. Kerdel-Vegas . . . 775
Control of Mammalian Hair Growth: Studies with a Cell-Free Protein Synthesizing
System. I. M. Freedberg 776
The Effects of Various Pathologic Conditions of the Scalp upon Hair Melanogenesis and
Hair Growth. W. Kostanecki 780
The Histological Changes in Idiopathic Premature Vertex Baldness in Women.
I. Martin-Scott 781
The Normal Trichogram of People Beyond 50 Years but Apparently not Bald.
J. M. Barman, I. Astore and V. Pecoraro 783
Microscopic Studies of Pili Annulati. V. H. Price, R. S. Thomas and F. T. Jones . . 786
Rate of Hair Growth. M. Saitoh, M. Uzuka, M. Sakamoto and T. Kobori 788
Chronical Female Alopecia. M. Binazzi 791
Le problème des états pseudopeladiques ou pseudopeladoïdes dans le cadre des alopécies
cicatricielles. M. Juon 793
La pelade, maladie psychosomatique. S. Lambergeon 795
Biological Depth Dose Studies in Electron Beam Therapy: Effects on Anagen Mouse
Hairs. L. H. Lanzl and F. D. Malkinson 796
Elektronenmikroskopische Befunde an den peritrichialen Nervenfasern des mensch-
lichen Haarfollikels. C. Orfanos 798
Die Behandlung der Alopecia areata im Kindesalter. J. Tomášková 801
Untersuchungen über die Veränderungen des Haares der Augenbrauen bei endogenem
Ekzem. H. Langhof† and M. Munteanu 803

Symposium 7: Mycoses (Superficial and Deep)

Reports

Untersuchungen über die Zuverlässigkeit eines „in vitro"-Lymphocytentests zwecks
Nachweises einer Dermatophyteninfektion. H. Götz 807
Effects of Human Body Fluids on Candida albicans. V. D. Newcomer, J. W. Landau,
N. Dabrowa and M. L. Fenster 813

page

Histoplasmose Africaine. R. VANBREUSEGHEM   817

Micetomas y actinomicosis. A. GONZÁLEZ OCHOA   819

Pathogenesis of South American Blastomycosis (Lutz's Mycosis). A. PADILHA-GON-
ÇALVES   824

Nouvelles acquisitions sur le mécanisme d'action de la Griséofulvine. P. PINETTI . .   826

Free Communications

Les onychomycoses. G. ACHTEN   828

Aspects particuliers de l'épidermomycose causée par epidermophyton floccosum.
I. ALTERAS and I. COJOCARU   830

Ultraestructura y citoquímica de la Candida albicans. L. F. MONTES and V. S. CON-
STANTINE   831

Keloidal Blastomycosis (Jorge Lobo's Disease). S. FRAGA and J. LISBÔA MIRANDA . .   831

A Look at Mycetoma in India. B. B. GOKHALE, A. A. PADHYE and M. J. THIRUMALACHAR   833

Esporotricosis, estudio clínico epidemiológico. V. C. JARAMILLO, G. C. VÉLEZ, A. R.
MORENO, I. R. PIZANO and A. C. CORTÉS   835

Favus Infection in Iraq. G. F. RAHIM   837

La macrocheilite de la blastomycose Sud-Américaine. J. RAMOS-SILVA and A. PADILHA-
GONÇALVES   839

Experiencias en cuatro casos de cromoblastomicosis y su tratamiento. F. A. OCAMPO,
R. T. PEREZ and R. V. VICTORIA   841

Quelques aspects de la mycose de Lane-Pedroso (chromoblastomycose ou chromomycose) dans la région Amazonique (Brésil). D. SILVA   842

Survey of the Mycoses in U.A.R. K. EL ZAWAHRY and M. EL ZAWAHRY   847

Main Transmission Routes of Spread of Trichophyton Mentagrophytes var. gran.-
Infection from a Natural Focus to Man in a Foothill Region. L. CHMEL, J. BUCHVALD
and M. VALENTOVÁ   851

Beitrag zum Problem tiefer anorectaler Mykosen. O. MALE   852

Flore dermatomycosique actuelle dans la région d'Athènes et sensibilité des souches isolées à la griséofulvine. C. KANITAKIS, U. MARCELOU-KINTI and CHR. GEORGIADIS . .   854

Biological, Sanitarian and Environmental Factors in Dermatomycoses. D. TRICHO-
POULOS, O. MARSELOU-KINTI and A. POLYCHRONOPOULOU   856

New Experiments on Culture, Immunology and Inoculation. J. DE AZEVEDO CARNEIRO,
R. D. AZULAY and L. M. C. DE ANDRADE   858

Sensibilisations de la peau par les dermatophytes. I. COJOCARU, I. ALTERAS and L.
DULAMITĂ   859

La valeur du milieu Gluzman modifié par Condrea dans la préparation de la trichophytine. V. COSTEA, M. CARNIOL, M. LAZAR and M. ILIES   861

Onychomycose due à alternaria tenuis. J. DELACRÉTAZ and D. GRIGORIOU   863

Fungus-Allergy and its Skin Manifestations. E. FEJÉR   864

The Mycologic Laboratory Specimen. The Collection, Inoculation, and Culture Methods.
H. C. GOLDBERG   866

Tinea Versicolor: The Electron Microscopic Morphology of the Genera Malassezia and
Pityrosporum. F. M. KEDDIE   867

Effect of the Immunosuppressive Agent, Cyclophosphamide, on Experimental Systemic
Coccidioidomycosis. J. W. LANDAU, L. INDIANER and V. D. NEWCOMER   872

Enzyme des Kohlenhydratstoffwechsels bei Dermatophyten. W. MEINHOF and G.
RASSNER   876

Microsporum Nanum as a Cause of Human Infections. J. F. MULLINS and C. J. WILLIS   877

Les dermatophytes du sol en Bulgarie. P. POPCHRISTOV, V. BALABANOFF, T. FILKOV and
P. USUNOV   879

L'ultrastructure des grains dans les maduromycoses provoquée par Monosporium apiospermum. M. STOIAN and A. AVRAM   881

page

On the Mycomimetic Pictures Found in Mycologic Examinations. P. SBERNA   883

Zur fermentativen Leistung von Fadenpilzen. W. ADAM   884

Parenté antigénique et localisation des antigènes dans le genre Candida: Etude par
immunofluorescence. P. RIMBAUD, J.-M. BASTIDE, M. BASTIDE and J. ALLEGRINI .   886

Essais de marquage de Candida albicans par radioisotopes. Etude de leur distribution
dans l'organisme du lapin. S. ANTONESCU   892

Observations of the Treatment of Superficial Mycosis in South-East Europe with CO_2
Snow (Method Haxthausen). M. BRNIČEVIĆ   893

La contamination staphylococcique des trichophyties suppurées. Résultats d'une thérapie combinée: Griséofulvine, antibiotiques antimicrobiennes et traitement local.
I. CAPUSAN, P. BALOSU and N. MAIER   895

Tratamiento de las tiñas on Griseofulvina. M. P. MIGUENS   896

Sporotrichosis Recurrens Cicatrisans (Repeating Self-Healing Sporotrichosis).
R. N. MIRANDA   898

Traitement expérimental des mycoses cutanées superficielles par l'Amphotéricine B.
D. PERYASSÚ and G. LÖWY   900

Experimentelle Grundlagen der externen antimykotischen Therapie. W. RAAB . . .   901

Über den Einfluß von Moronal (-Nystatin) auf den Zellstoffwechsel von Candida albicans
(Autoradiographische Untersuchungen). M. RAHMANN-ESSER and F. FEGELER . .   903

Mechanism of Antifungal Action of Potassium Iodide on Sporotrichosis. H. URABE,
T. NAGASHIMA and K. NAKASHIMA   907

Fissured Nipples of Lactating Females and its Relation to Candida Infection.
A. M. EL MOFTY, R. MEHAREB, H. M. EL KOMY and C. D. JEFFRIES   908

Symposium 8: Malignant Melanomas

Reports

Melanin Biosynthesis in Melanomas. T. B. FITZPATRICK   913

Mélanoses neurocutanées of Touraine. T. KAWAMURA, S. IKEDA, S. NODA, S. ISHIZU.and
T. NAKAJIMA   915

La mélanose circonscrite précancereuse de Hutchinson-Dubreuilh (M.H.D.).
B. DUPERRAT and J. M. MASCARO   917

Spontaneous Regression of Malignant Melanoma. L. BOWDEN   918

Elektrometrie zur Früherkennung von malignanten Melanomen. N. MELCZER   925

The Surgical Treatment of Malignant Melanoma. R. W. RAVEN   926

Die Behandlung des malignen Melanoms mit schnellen Elektronen eines 15 MeV-
Betatrons. G. F. KLOSTERMANN   928

Histologische Diagnostik der Melanome. J. J. HERZBERG   933

Free Communications

Benign Juvenile Melanoma. — Several Selected Aspects from a Study of 51 Lesions.
R. ANDRADE   936

Über das Verhalten der Melanomzellen in vitro. B. ROHDE   938

Production of Melanomas in Hairless Mice with Ultraviolet Light. J. H. EPSTEIN,
W. L. EPSTEIN and T. NAKAI   939

Effects of Depigmenting Agents on Melanocytes and Melanogenesis. M. A. PATHAK,
G. SZABÓ, E. FRENK, S. S. BLEEHEN, Y. HORI and T. B. FITZPATRICK   941

Dopa in Melanoma. H. RORSMAN   942

Multiple Forms of Tyrosinase from Mammalian Melanoma. J. B. BURNETT and H.
SEILER   943

370 Mélanomes malins. — Statistiques et pronostic. J. M. SIMONART   944

A propos de 400 mélanomes malins cutanés. C. DUFOURMENTEL, R. MOULY and J.
GLICENSTEIN   946

page

Zur Häufigkeit des malignen Melanoms. Ergebnis einer Umfrage. H. KÄSTNER, P.
JORDAN and G. FORCK 948

Lentigo Maligna and Malignant Melanoma. R. JACKSON 949

Un diagnostic différentiel important des mélanomes. L'Angiokératome noi:.
G. E. GOETSCHEL 951

Les noevocarcinomes de l'enfant. R. MOULY, CL. DUFOURMENTEL and J. GLICENSTEIN 954

Nevus y melanomas malignos. L. A. RUEDA 955

Early Diagnosis of Melanoblastoma with the Aid of Electrometric, Thermo-Differential
and ³²P Uptake Test. A. GULBERT 957

Histologische Befunde beim transplantierten Melanom des Menschen. H. GARTMANN 958

Veränderungen bei inoculierten Melanocyten. KH. WOEBER and O. GRÜTZ † 960

Macromolecular Differentiation of Melanocytic and Nevocytic Malignant Melanomas.
Y. MISHIMA 961

Investigación de células tumorales en sangre periférica en enfermos con melanoma
maligno. A. ALIAGA and J. CALAP 968

Some Mechanisms of Pox Virus Oncolysis in Malignant Melanoma. A Review of 50 Cases.
G. W. MILTON and M. LANE BROWN 970

Richtlinien und unsere Erfahrungen in der Behandlung des malignen Melanoms.
GY. KÁRPÁTI, T. VENKEI, Ö. BIHARI, GY. NÉMETH and A. GULBERT 973

Observations concernant la prophylaxie et le traitement du mélanome malin.
E. UJVÁRY and I. KREPSZ 974

Données relatives au problème de la possibilité de dissémination après l'irradiation aux
rayons X dans les cas du mélanome malin. T. VENKEI and Ö. BIHARI 975

The Uptake of Radioactively Labelled Compounds by Malignant Melanoma. M. S. BLOIS 976

Sensitization to X-Irradiation of Melanoma Cells Using Alpha-MSH. M. LANE BROWN
and G. W. MILTON 978

Symposium 9: Physiology of the Skin

Reports

Enzyme und Physiologie der Haut. G. K. STEIGLEDER 983

Collagen Metabolism in Skin. CH. M. LAPIÈRE 986

Physiological Response of Human Skin to Ultraviolet Light. M. A. EVERETT and R. L.
OLSON 988

The Clinical Significance of a Comparative Approach to the Physiology of Hair Growth.
A. J. ROOK 993

Physiologie der Hautoberfläche. Die relative Bedeutung verschiedener Befunde.
F. HERRMANN 995

Some Remarks on the Barrier Function of the Epidermis. J. HORÁČEK 999

Le pouvoir tampon de la peau. H. THIERS 1002

Free Communications

Studies of Some Glycolytic Pathways in the Skin of Rats Under Experimental Conditions. G. RABBIOSI and A. GIANNETTI 1003

Plasma Kinin Formation and Human Inflammation. H. ZACHARIAE, J. MALMQUIST,
J. A. OATES and W. PETTINGER 1006

Synthesis of Unique Proteins in Epidermal Keratinization. I. A. BERNSTEIN 1008

Mechanism of Water Binding in Stratum Corneum. J. D. MIDDLETON 1010

Studies on the Epidermal Keratinization of the Human Fetus in vitro with Special
References to the Electron Microscopic and Autoradiographic Observation.
K. OKAMURA, K. IWASHITA and K. UEDA 1012

page

The Envelope of Epidermal Horny Cells. A. G. Matoltsy 1014

Follicular Hyperkeratinization Induced in the Rabbit Ear by Human Skin Surface Lipids. A. L. Lorincz, H. Krizek and S. Brown 1016

The Influence of Dimethyl Sulphoxide, Dimethyl Acetamide and Dimethyl Formamide on the Epidermal Barrier to Water. H. Baker 1017

Die hygrometrische Aufzeichnung der Hydromeiose und das Abtrocknen der Horn-schicht als Maß ihrer physiologischen Qualität. J. Rovenský and J. Záhejský . . 1020

Physiologische Antiperspirants. H. P. Fiedler 1022

Sodium Secretion and Reabsorption by the Eccrine Sweat Gland. R. L. Dobson . . 1024

The Insensible Water Loss and Skin Temperature. F. A. J. Thiele and K. G. van Senden 1025

The Fine Structure of the Sebaceous Gland of the Adult Female Rat After Receiving Sexual Hormones. Y. Sato and M. Morohashi 1028

The in vivo Study of Cutaneous Lipogenesis. G. Lipkin and V. R. Wheatley 1029

Physiology of Human Sebaceous Glands-Hormonal Control Mechanisms. J. S. Strauss 1031

Le contrôle hormonal de la glande sébacée chez l'homme. M. Bonelli, E. Alessi, C. Tomasini and S. Piccinini 1033

Der Einfluß des Hautoberflächenmilieus auf Staphylococcus aureus. E. Müller . . . 1036

The pH and the Bacterial Flora of Normal Skin Under Fluocinolone-Plastic Occlusion Treatment. E. A. Knudsen 1038

The Alkali Neutralization Capacity of Human Skin in vivo. K. Schutter 1041

Über ultraviolett-absorbierende Verbindungen im Wasserlöslichen epidermaler Ver-hornungsprodukte. E. Schwarz 1043

Ultraviolettes Licht als Stimulus für Kininbildung in menschlicher Haut. R. K. Winkel-mann, J. Epstein and K. Wolff 1045

Sur la réponse vasculaire biphasique au siège de l'érythème dû aux radiations ultra-violettes. Existe-t-il une réponse plus élémentaire que l'érythème ? G. Zina and A. Benedetto 1047

A Cutaneous Role in the Regulation of the Body's Carbohydrate Milieu. R. M. Fusaro and J. A. Johnson 1048

Research on Sialic Acid in the Human Skin. A. Giannetti and G. Rabbiosi 1050

Mepyramine and Adrenergic Neurone. B. S. Verma and O. D. Gulati 1053

Lysosomes and the Skin. R. L. Olson, R. Nordquist, J. Nordquist and M. A. Eve-rett 1056

Modificaciones clínicas e histológicas de la reacción tuberculínica bajo la acción local del valerato de betametasona en cura oclusiva. A. Casalá, C. Bianchi, O. Bianchi, S. Stringa and O. Roqué 1060

The Significance of Low Serum Iron Levels in the Causation of Itching. I. B. Sneddon and M. Garretts 1061

Comparatively Study on the Effects of Corticosteroids, Resochine and Synopene on the Arthus's Phenomenon in Rabbits. B. Bajdekov, K. Bertchev, B. Bojkov and I. Ismirov 1063

Die Adenosintriphosphatase der normalen menschlichen Haut. C. Ene-Popescu . . 1064

Symposium 10: Effects of Radiation on the Skin

Reports

Radiobiologie cutanée. P. van Caneghem 1069

Strahlenwirkung im Hautbereich in Abhängigkeit von der verwendeten Strahlen-qualität. A. Proppe 1070

Strahlenwirkung im Hautbereich in Abhängigkeit von der verwendeten Strahlen-qualität. F. Wachsmann 1074

page

Indications dermatologiques du traitement ionisant. Traitement ionisant des épithéliomas et des mélanomes malins à l'aide de techniques de radio-sensibilisation nouvelles. E. G. Scolari 1078

Indications thérapeutiques des substances radioactives en dermatologie. B. Pierquin 1081

Algunos rasgos ultraestructurales de las radiolesiones. J. Cabré 1083

Preliminary Investigative Studies of the Laser Treatment of Angiomas. L. Goldman, R. J. Rockwell jr. and R. Meyer 1084

Free Communications

The Treatment of Skin Tumours with Radium and Hyperbaric Oxygen. C. Vallecchi and G. Mantellassi 1087

Nouvelle technique de Radiumthérapie en oxygène hyperbaryque. M. Nannelli and G. Mantellassi 1088

Acute Effects of Irradiation on the Skin. — A Histochemical and Chemical Study. A. K. Kurban and F. S. Farah. 1090

Biochemische Untersuchungen an Serum und Hauteiweißen von Ratten nach Röntgenbestrahlung. O.-E. Rodermund 1091

Radiations et tissu élastique cutané. M. Ledoux-Corbusier 1093

Problemas del uso de los rayos grenz en los negros y en los mulatos. M. A. Contreras 1094

Tierexperimentelles zur Röntgenfernbestrahlung der Haut. M. Betetto 1096

Dermatological Observations in the A-Bomb Survivors of Hiroshima and Nagasaki, Japan. M.-L. T. Johnson, T. Taura and P. B. Gregory 1097

Studies on Induction, Persistence and Recovery of Radiation Damage in Proliferative (Anagen) and Non-proliferative (Telogen) Rodent Hair Cell Populations. F. D. Malkinson and M. L. Griem 1099

Autoradiographische Untersuchungen zur epidermalen Proliferation unter physiologischen, pathologischen und experimentellen Bedingungen mit Tritium-markierten Nucleosiden. W. Born 1101

Histochimie des enzymes des follicules irradiés du cobaye. A. Kint and J. de Bersaques 1103

Untersuchungen zur experimentellen Photosensibilisierung mit Sulfanilamid und Phenothiazinen. K. Schwarz, J. Rothenstein and M. Schwarz-Speck 1106

Light is an Aetiological Factor for Certain Dermatoses in U.A.R. M. el Zawahry. . 1107

Heliotherapie und ihr Einfluß auf die Aktivität mancher Enzyme bei Psoriasiskranken. N. Balevska, J. Petkov, G. Mustakov, S. Jowev, N. Zlatkov and G. Tomov . . 1110

The Action Spectrum of Erythema Induced by Ultraviolet Radiation. Preliminary Report. D. Berger, F. Urbach and R. E. Davies 1112

The Absorption Spectrum of the Stratum Corneum as the Natural Sunscreen of Human Skin. A. R. H. B. Verhagen 1118

Prurigo actínico. F. Londoño 1122

Psoralen Therapy of Vitiligo in the Tropics. T. L. Fleisher 1124

Zur Kombinationsbehandlung der Mycosis fungoides mit Röntgenstrahlen und Spindelgiften. A. Wiskemann 1125

Photochemical Movement of Cholesterol in Skin. E. W. Rauschkolb and J. M. Knox 1126

Symposium 11: Immunology in Dermatology

Reports

Aetiology of Some Autoimmune Diseases. N. R. Rowell 1131

Aspects immunologiques du lupus érythémateux aigu disséminé. J. Thivolet . . . 1134

Autoimmunity in Pemphigus. T. Chorzelski 1135

Immunology of Acne Vulgaris. Dermal Hypersensitivity and Circulating Antibody Levels to Corynbacterium Acnes. S. M. Puhvel, T. H. Sternberg and R. M. Reisner 1136

page

Zur Immunologie in der Dermatologie. J. KIMMIG 1139

The Role of the Basophil in the Immune Response. W. B. SHELLEY 1143

Free Communications

Classes of Immunoglobulins Associated with Skin Sensitizing Properties. M. J. FELLNER
and R. L. BAER 1144

Patterns of Skin Fluorescence in Lupus Erythematosus. R. H. CORMANE 1146

Delayed Hypersensitivity Responses in Immunologic Deficiency States. W. L. EPSTEIN 1148

Antikörpermangelsyndrome und Hautveränderungen. G. BREHM 1149

Zur Frage der Antigenspezifität von 2,4-Dinitrochlorbenzol-Epidermis-Conjugaten im
Meerschweinchenversuch. F. KLASCHKA 1151

Antinuclear Factors in Clinical Dermatology. J. S. BECK, N. R. ROWELL and T. E.
ANDERSON 1153

Vasoactive Substances at Sites of Cutaneous Allergies. TH. M. INDERBITZIN and P. J.
GROB 1154

Application de la technique d'immunofluorescence en dermatologie. Y. MONTET, J.
DUHEILLE and J. BEUREY 1156

Experimental Studies on the Pathogenesis of Acantholysis in Pemphigus. P. J. GROB
and TH. M. INDERBITZIN 1158

Autoantibodies in Pemphigus Foliaceus. T. A. FURTADO, A. O. LIMA, G. O. ANDRADE
and O. SEABRA 1159

L'apport de l'immuno-fluorescence dans la mise en évidence du rôle de l'allergie à
Candida albicans dans certaines dermatoses communes. P. TEMIME, M. BENNE,
M. LEBEUF, J. P. MARCHAND and PH. LATOUÆELLE 1162

Recherches électrophorétiques et immunophorétiques en moyens gélifiés sur protéines
de muscle strié dans différentes collagénoses d'intérêt dermatologique. G. MARTINA
and A. MIDANA 1168

Immunoelektrophorese der Serumproteine bei akuten und chronischen Formen des
Erythematodes. T. BIELICKÝ, L. MALINA and J. OPPLT 1170

Immunologic Defect of the Skin in Lymphadenopathy. Y. NOGUCHI, K. ISHIWARA,
M. HIGUCHI and S. YOSHIDA 1171

Immunologische Untersuchungen von Lymphocytenkulturen. Eine diagnostische
Methode in der Dermatologie. H. J. HEITMANN 1174

Mechanisms of Anaphylaxis. M. W. GREAVES 1176

The Immunochemical Basis of the Urticarial Reaction. F. S. FARAH and A. K. KURBAN 1176

The Release of Serotonin in Hypersensitivity States. J. S. COMAISH 1179

Réactions sérologiques et terrain d'allergie humorale en dermatologie. CL. MIKOL and
M. RENOUX 1180

Experimentelle Untersuchungen zur Desensibilisierung und Immunotoleranz gegen
niedermolekulare Allergene. K. H. SCHULZ 1181

Experimentelle Sensibilisierung mit drei- und sechswertigem Chrom. M. SCHWARZ-
SPECK 1183

Zur Frage autoallergischer Reaktionen bei der Neurodermitis. B. KOPECKÁ, E. SORKIN,
S. BORELLI and A. FJELDE 1185

Delayed Reactivity to Bacterial, Mold and Viral Allergens in Atopic Dermatitis.
G. RAJKA 1187

Das Shwartzman-Phänomen, eine dem Arthus-Phänomen ähnliche, pseudo-immuno-
logische Reaktion der Haut auf Endotoxin. I. KUNICK and L. ILLIG 1187

Immunological Aspects of the Aldrich's Syndrome. G. IACOVACCI, S. UNGARI and F.
AIUTI 1189

Mise en évidence d'anticorps circulants dans les manifestations cutanées de l'allergie à
la pénicilline. J. PAUPE and CL. MIKOL 1190

Heutige Diagnostik der Penicillinallergie. P. MICHAILOV and N. BEROWA 1191

Page

Symposium 12: The Skin and Internal Disease

Reports

Erythropoietic Protoporphyria. I. A. MAGNUS 1195
Xanthomatoses et maladies systémiques. A. BAZEX, A. DUPRÉ and B. CHRISTOL . . 1197
Skin Disorders in Relation to Malabsorption. G. C. WELLS 1200
Further Studies on Acrodermatitis Enteropathica. N. DANBOLT 1202
A New Classification for Lupus Erythematosus. J. R. HASERICK 1204
Angiokeratoma Corporis Diffusum. H. J. WALLACE 1207
Consideration of the Etiology of Pyoderma Gangrenosum. H. O. PERRY and P. DIDIS-
HEIM 1208

Free Communications

A Cutaneous Affection from Malabsorption. A. BACCAREDDA-BOY and F. CROVATO . . 1212
Hauterscheinungen bei Colitis ulcerosa. H. REICH 1214
Crohn's Disease Associated with Cutaneous Lesions. G. A. GRANT PETERKIN 1214
Lung Function in Patients with Cutaneous Vasculitis. M. CATTERALL 1215
Atteinte du rein au cours des allergides nodulaires dermiques de Gougerot. ST. BOULLE
and J. GUILAINE 1217
Therapie der Porphyria cutanea tarda (Ergebnisse in 9 Jahren). H. IPPEN 1218
Hautreaktionen bei rheumatischen Erkrankungen. E. WOHLSTEIN 1219
Studies on Iron Metabolism in the Porphyria Cutanea Tarda (P.C.T.). L. LEVI, C. L.
MENEGHINI, F. SPINELLI-RESSI and C. A. BETTINELLI 1222
Krankhafte Zusammenhänge zwischen Leber und Haut in "Porphyria cutanea tarda".
P. TÎRLEA and I. CĂPUSAN 1222
Schistosomiasis (Bilharziasis) der Haut. C. M. HASSELMANN 1224
Schistosomal Infestation of the Skin. A. M. EL MOFTY 1224
The Hepatitis Associated with Infantile Papular Acrodermatitis. V. A. PUCCINELLI . . 1228
Zum Krankheitsbild des Myxoedema circumscriptum praetibiale. CHR. EBERHARTINGER 1229
Natural Course of Various Types of Scleroderma. A. Follow-up-Study over a Period of
20 Years. Z. STAVA 1230
Preparation and Application of Lesional Casts in the Study of Cutaneous Disease.
D. A. ROE 1231
Perorale Kreatinbelastung bei Haut- und Muskelerkrankungen. H. W. KREYSEL and
M. JÄNNER 1232
Liquen rojo plano de la mucosa bucal. Su asociación con diabetes. Nuevas observaciones.
D. GRINSPAN, J. DÍAZ, L. O. VILLAPOL, J. SCHNEIDERMAN, R. BERDICHESKY, D.
PALESE and J. FAERMAN 1234
Sarcoidosis with Cicatricial Alopecia Resembling Generalized Discoid Lupus Erythema-
tosus. L. S. SAUTER 1235
Dermatological Aspects of Crohn's Disease. D. I. MCCALLUM and P. D. C. KINMONT 1237
A propos du syndrôme de Winterbauer (Syndrôme C.R.S.T.). A. PUISSANT, R. LECLERCQ
and F. VANBREMEERSCH 1238
Acanthosis Nigricans. — A Clinical Manifestation of Internal Disorders. T. YASUDA,
SH. NISHIYAMA and SH. TSUYUKI 1240
Glucorrhoea. Is this Pre-diabetes ? J. R. G. AGIUS 1241
Hormonelle Untersuchungen und Behandlungsmethoden bei Acne vulgaris. F. TÓTH
and L. NÉKÁM 1243
Vorkommen von Paraproteinämie bei Pyoderma gangraenosum. H. RÖCKL 1244
Zur Problematik der Arthropathia psoriatica. F. VLČEK, M. ZBOJANOVA, G. NIEPEL
and Z. SITAY 1246

page

Quelques observations sur l'élimination urinaire des cétostéroïdes dans l'acnée féminine.
R. Dumitriu, M. Haisuc, L. Reiter, M. Hontaru and A. Coser   1248

The Seborrhoic Symptom Complex.— The Expression of a Disturbed Intestinal Malutilization of Vitamin B 12 as Proven by Measuring the Radioactivity after Administration of Co 60 Vitamin B 12. W. A. Casper   1249

Diabetes and Impetigo Contagiosa (Passage from one Diabetic Family to Another
Diabetic Family Via a Related Cousin Carrier). B. R. Hearst   1251

Dermatitis uraemica Rössle. H. Fischer   1252

Symposium 13: Bullous Dermatoses

Reports

Zur Klinik bullöser Eruptionen (Exklusive bullöse Genodermatosen). J. Tappeiner   1257

Herpes Zoster and Nonmalignant Disease. L. H. Winer and E. T. Wright   1259

Producción experimental de ampollas; su correlacción con los cambios estructurales en
las dermatosis ampollosas. D. J. Gómez Orbaneja   1262

La maladie de Duhring-Brocq à grosses bulles dite «pemphigoïde de Brocq», après la
cinquantaine. P. le Coulant, L. Texier and P. Boraud   1264

Subcorneal Pustular Dermatosis. A review after 10 years. D. S. Wilkinson   1266

Bullous Lesions in Patients with Internal Disorders. E. Skog   1267

Corticosteroid Treatment of Pemphigus. C. T. Nelson   1270

Friction Blisters Produced under Controlled Conditions. Th. A. Cortese jr., T. B.
Griffin and M. B. Sulzberger   1273

Free Communications

Experimental Investigations on the Acantholysis Induced by Staphylococcus pyogens.
Comparative Study with the Acantholysis on Pemphigus. B. Zilberberg   1275

An Electron Microscopic Study of Cutaneous and Oral Pemphigus Vulgaris. K. Hashimoto   1278

Localización de gamma globulina IgG y complemento (C′3) en la epidermis de enfermos
de Pénfigo vulgar. S. Stringa, C. Bianchi, A. Casala, C. Inglesini and O. Bianchi   1283

Dermatite Bulleuse Mucosynéchante et Atrophiante. A. G. Bellone, M. F. Hofmann
and G. Caputo   1285

Experimental Friction Blisters: Histological Investigation. K. Fukuyama and Th. A.
Cortese jr.   1288

Etude de la composition protéique du liquide des bulles dans les dermatoses bulleuses.
G. Moulin and Y. Manuel   1289

Nouvelles observations sur le phénomène citochémiotatique dans la bulle du pemphigus.
P. Sertoli   1291

Hepatische Porphyrien: Veränderungen der Serumenzymaktivitäten und hämatologischen Befunde beim Menschen und bei der Ratte. H. Pietschmann and W. Raab .   1293

Interessante, bei den an bullösen Dermatosen leidenden Kranken erhobene hämatologische und gastroenterologische Befunde. V. Rozsívalová, F. Matěja, B. Fixa
and O. Komárková   1294

The Treatment of Porphyria Cutanea Tarda by Chelation. G. A. Hunter and G. F.
Donald   1296

Toxic Epidermal Necrolysis. M. B. Lewis   1297

Acute Epidermal Necrolysis (Ritter-Lyell). — The Scalded Skin Syndrome.
P. J. Koblenzer   1298

The Ultrastructure of Acantholysis in Lichen Planus. L. Fry and F. R. Johnson . .   1301

XXXV

page

Symposium 14: Mycobacterial Infections of the Skin

Reports

Etude biologique récente dans la lèpre: Analogies antigéniques et séro-diagnostic de la lèpre par immunofluorescence sur bacille de Stefansky. F.-P. MERKLEN and F. COTTENOT 1305

Las formas submicroscópicas del m. leprae. J. GAY PRIETO and G. GABINO 1306

Die gegenwärtige Epidemologie und Bakteriologie der Hauttuberkulose in der Bundesrepublik Deutschland. F. EHRING 1308

Mykobakterienbefunde bei den sog. Tuberkuliden. N. SIMON 1312

Thalidomide in Lepra Reaction and in Hansen's Disease. J. SHESKIN, F. SAGHER, M. DORFMAN and J. CONVIT 1314

Free Communications

Geographical Distribution of Skin Tuberkulosis, Leprosy and Sarcoidosis in Japan. K. KITAMURA 1316

A propos des tuberculoses cutanées — leur classification — leur diagnostic biologique — leur traitement. M. BOLGERT and P. L. DELAIRE 1317

Lupus Vulgaris Gigantea Caused by Mycobacterium Avium. J. V. CHRISTIANSEN . . 1319

Atypical Acid fast Micro-Organisms in Scleroderma. A. R. CANTWELL, E. CRAGGS, J. W. WILSON and F. SWATEK 1320

Nature of the Antigen Responsible for the Kveim Reaction in Sarcoidosis. R. KOOIJ and J. W. VAN WAVEREN HOGERVORST 1322

Present Position of BCG Vaccination against Leprosy. L. M. BECHELLI 1323

Über die pigmentierten Naevi bei lepromatösen Leprakranken. Y. ISHIBASHI and T. KAWAMURA 1325

Mise en évidence du bacille de Hansen dans les lèpres apparemment abacillaires. F. COTTENOT, F.-P. MERKLEN and TRINH THI KIM MONG DON 1326

The Frequency of Intracellular Lipid in the Several Structureal Types of Leprosy. R. D. AZULAY and L. C. DE ANDRADE 1328

Cutaneous Response of Leprosy Patients to Living and Heated Mycobacterium Leprae Cultures on the Olitzki-Gershon Medium. M. DORFMAN, F. SAGHER, J. SHESKIN and A. L. OLITZKI 1329

Serum Immunoglobulin Changes in Leprosy and Tuberculosis. SOO DUK LIM and R. M. FUSARO 1332

Nuevos avances terapéuticos en lepra. J. C. GATTI, J. E. CARDAMA and L. M. BALINA 1334

Double Reversal of the Tuberculin Reaction in Sarcoidosis. S. H. SILVERS and F. S. GLICKMAN 1335

Clinical Applications of Shepard's Mouse Foot Pad Technique. P. FASAL and L. LEVY 1337

Impétigo herpétiforme Hébra Kaposi ou Psoriasis pustuleux généralisé (chez une femme âgée de 22 ans, apparu au cours de 5e mois de sa 2e grossesse). R. SAMII 1339

Symposium 15: Iatrogenic Diseases in Dermatology

Reports

Dermatosis iatrogénicas. Definición, patogénia, clasificación. M. I. QUIROGA 1343

The Aetiology of Toxic Epidermal Necrolysis. A. LYELL 1346

Iatrogenic Disease Due to Physical Treatment. A. N. DOMONKOS 1347

Eruptions du type L. E. et syndromes lupiques provoqués par des médicaments. CH. GRUPPER and G. A. C. MARCEL 1349

Dermatoses des traitements antidiabétiques. J. BEUREY, P. JEANDIDIER and A. BERMONT 1352

Iatrogenic Dyschromies. H. MÖLLER 1355

III*

page

Free Communications

Photosensitive Dermatitis as an Iatrogenic Disease. T. KOBORI and H. ARAKI 1357

Les accidents cutanés de l'allergie humorale médicamenteuse. Intérêt du test de Shelley. J. MALEVILLE, H. BERGOEND and A. BASSET 1359

La thésaurismose cutanée par polyvinylpyrrolidone (PVP). J. M. LACHAPELLE . . . 1362

Mascaras pigmentarias como expresión iatrogénica a dosis altas y prolongadas de feniotiacina y derivados en el control de afecciones psiquiatricas. E. B. MOLINA LEGUIZAMÓN, A. A. CORDERO and E. FOLLMANN 1363

Necrolisis Epidermica Toxica. — Observaciones sobre 12 Casos. A. CORTÉS CORTÉS and V. CÁRDENAS JARAMILLO 1371

Dermatosis por anovulatorios. Y. ORTIZ 1373

Case Presentations and Fundamentals on Film

Second International Film Presentation of the Institute for Dermatologic Communication and Education

Keratosis Follicularis (Darier's Disease). N. KARLTORP and ST. FLODERUS 1379

Congenital Ichthyosiform Erythroderma. K. REHTIJÄRVI, K. KUOKKANEN and P. KARMA 1379

Xeroderma Pigmentosum. H. EL HEFNAWI 1379

Metastasizing Basal Cell Carcinoma. C. CH. THOMAS 1380

The Nevoid Basal Cell Carcinoma Syndrome. J. B. HOWELL and D. E. ANDERSON . . 1380

Gold Leaf Treatment of Cutaneous Ulcers. N. M. KANOF 1380

Diagnosis of Latent Psoriasis. G. HOLTI 1380

Surgical Treatment of Benign Acanthosis Nigricans. H. OLLENDORFF CURTH 1380

Pellagra and other Avitaminoses in the Bantu. M. ROSE 1381

Lupus Erythematosus. D. L. TUFFANELLI and W. B. REED 1381

Lipoid Proteinosis. R. M. CAPLAN 1381

Acrodermatitis Chronica Atrophicans (Herxheimer). F. HERRMANN and O. SCHULTKA . 1381

Granulomatous Dermo-Hypodermitis with Progressive Atrophy. J. CONVIT, FR. KERDEL-VEGAS and M. F. ALLENDE 1381

Report of the Institute for Dermatologic Communication and Education to the International Committee of Dermatology 1382

Scientific Exhibition

Clinical Dermatology

Die spontane Heilungsquote der Blutschwämme und die daraus zu ziehenden Schlüsse für die Prognose und Therapie. G. F. KLOSTERMANN 1387

Spontanverlauf der Säuglingshämangiome. A. PROPPE and H. HAUSS 1387

Laser Surgery of Angiomas with Special Reference to Port-Wine Angiomas. L. GOLD-MAN, E. J. RITTER, R. J. ROCKWELL jr., R. MEYER, B. HENDERSON and K. WM. KITZMILLER 1388

Therapie hypercholesterinämischer Xanthomatosen. N. ZÖLLNER, M. GUDENZI and G. WOLFRAM 1390

Proteolytic Enzyme Treatment of Skin Ulcers. M. C. SPENCER 1393

Chemosurgery for the Microscopically Controlled Excision of Skin Cancer. FR. E. MOHS 1393

Multiple Punch Autografts for the Alopecias. D. B. STOUGH 1394

Evaluation of Parental Methotrexate for Intractable Psoriasis. CH. P. DEFEO, A. ALLYN and S. EISENBERG 1394

Zur Wirkung des hochalpinen Klimas in der atopischen konstitutionellen Neuro-dermitis. S. BORELLI, H. BRENN, ST. CHLEBAROV, C. ENE-POPESCU, H. GEHRKEN, B. KOPECKA, P. MICHAILOV and H. VOSSIECK. 1395

Klimatherapie von Hautkrankheiten an der Nordsee. W. PÜRSCHEL 1397

page

Die Verbrennung — ein dermatologisches Problem. Komplikationen, Therapie und Prophylaxe. G. WEBER and H. JURSCH 1400

A New Principle in Topical Corticosteroid Treatment. G. HAGERMAN 1406

Casus rari muco-cutanei. A. GREITHER and O. HORNSTEIN 1408

Visualization in Dermatology. K. K. MUSTAKALLIO 1409

Examen radiographique des tissus cutanés et sous-cutanés normaux et pathologiques. CH. GROS, A. BASSET, S. SCHRAUB, J. MALEVILLE, E. GROSSHANS and E. HEID . . 1409

Klassifizierung der Ichthyosen. U. W. SCHNYDER and B. KONRÁD 1411

Andrologie in Klinik und Praxis. C. SCHIRREN and H. GRELL 1413

Papulonecrotic and Acneiform Tuberculids. C. E. SONCK 1413

Exhibit on Genodermatoses. L. ZIPRKOWSKI 1418

A Case of Congenital Erythropoietic Porphyria. K. YAMAMOTO 1420

Contact Allergy in Scandinavia. B. MAGNUSSON, S.-G. BLOHM, S. FREGERT, N. HJORTH, G. HØVDING, V. PIRILÄ and E. SKOG 1421

Klinische Pharmakologie des neuen Histaminblockers Tavegil. L. KERP and H. KASEMIR 1425

Hautveränderungen und Antikörper-Mangelsyndrome. G. BREHM 1426

L'allergie de contact. J. FOUSSEREAU 1429

Chamber Test Method. V. PIRILÄ and L. FÖRSTRÖM 1430

Erythropoietic Protoporphyria. R. M. FUSARO, W. J. RUNGE, E. S. PETERKA. M. O. JAFFE, E. W. GOLTZ and C. J. WATSON 1432

Gegenüberstellung von Angiomatosis Kaposi (Sarcoma idiopathicum haemorrhagicum multiplex) und Stewart-Treves-Syndrom (Sarcoma angioplasticum in elephantiasi). H. TELLER and H. KRÜGER 1435

Une affection liée au sexe: la gérodermie ostéodysplasique. D. KLEIN, F. BAMATTER, A. FRANCESCHETTI, G. BOREUX, J. E. W. BROCHER and P. HOLENSTEIN 1443

Elektronenmikroskopische, histochemische und polarisationsoptische Untersuchungen bei Pemphigus familiaris benignus (Hailey u. Hailey). F. NÜRNBERGER and G. MÜLLER 1444

Pemphigus Benignus Chronicus and Keratosis Palmo-plantaris in a Finnish Family. C. E. SONCK 1444

Shibi-Gatchaki-Syndrome. Y. KATABIRA 1447

Cas Cliniques. A. BASSET 1448

Gnathostomiasis Cutis. Yangtze Edema in China and Similar Migrating Intermittent Swellings of the Skin in Japan, Both Due to Gnathostoma Spinigerum Owen, 1836. K. KITAMURA 1449

Plusieures dermatoses. G. SAKELLARIOU 1450

Seltene Hautkrankheiten. G. HARGITA 1451

Angiokeratoma corporis diffusum Fabry. R. DENK 1459

Die primäre Hautreaktion nach infektiösem Tsetsefliegenstich bei der afrikanischen Schlafkrankheit. H. E. KRAMPITZ 1459

Amoebiasis Skin Manifestations. TH. DOXIADES and J. CAPETANAKIS 1462

Skin Diseases in Arabian Countries: Certain Notes and Comments. M. EL ZAWAHRY . 1464

Die Tumormetastasierung von der Haut und in die Haut. H. DREPPER and F. EHRING 1465

Zur Pathologie cutaner Lymphgefäße. J. TAPPEINER and L. PFLEGER 1467

Neuere Aspekte zur Histopathologie der Alopecia areata. W. THIES and CH. FISCHER 1469

Befund Langerhans-ähnlicher Zellen in den Hauterscheinungen der Reticuloendotheliose von Letterer-Siwe. V. PUCCINELLI, F. GIANOTTI and R. CAPUTO 1472

Tetracycline Fluorescence in Squamous Cell Carcinoma. H. J. DONSKY and G. R. MIKHAIL 1474

Concept of the Molecular Cause of Albinism. G. F. WILGRAM 1475

Xeroderma pigmentosum. H. EL HEFNAWI 1476

Skin Tuberculosis, Leprosy, Cutaneous Leishmanosis, Favus. M. A. MALEKI 1476

page

Experimental Dermatology

A Cutaneous Rôle in the Regulation of the Body's Carbohydrate Milieu. R. M. FUSARO and J. A. JOHNSON 1477

The Interplay of Opposites. Immunological Reactions in the Skin. TH. M. INDERBITZIN and P. J. GROB 1480

Autoradiographic Studies on Psoriatic Epidermis. S. SOTOMATSU, Y. IGARASHI and Y. OOSHIMA 1481

Die Mastzelle. A. SCHAUER 1483

Electronmicroscopy of Merkel's Tastzelle. K. K. MUSTAKALLIO and U. KIISTALA . . . 1493

Bilddemonstration zur mikroskopischen Anatomie des Haarfollikels im Verlauf des Haarcyclus. H.-J. BANDMANN and K. BOSSE 1493

Zur Ultrastruktur des menschlichen Haarfollikels. V. PUCCINELLI and R. CAPUTO . . . 1494

Zur licht- und elektronenoptischen Struktur der Nerven am Haar. E. HAGEN and G. NIEBAUER. 1495

Neuere Entwicklung der dermatologischen Virusforschung. TH. NASEMANN 1499

Recent Observations on Langerhans Cells. K. WOLFF, R. K. WINKELMANN and K. HOLUBAR 1502

Malignant Melanomas: Subcellular Differentiation of Nevocytic and Melanocytic Ontogeny. Y. MISHIMA 1505

Epidermal Melanin Unit. M. A. PATHAK, G. SZABÓ, T. B. FITZPATRICK, Y. HORI, S. S. BLEEHEN, E. FRENK, M. MIYAMOTO, M. SEIJI and A. BREATHNACH 1506

Dermo-Epidermal Separation by Suction. N. KIISTALA and K. K. MUSTAKALLIO . . 1513

Comparative Study with the Acantholysis in Pemphigus. Experimental Investigations on the Acantholysis Induced by the Staphylococcus pyogenes. B. ZILBERBERG . . 1513

Pathophysiologie allergischer Dermatosen. G. STÜTTGEN, I. GIGLI and F. HERRMANN 1514

Das mikrobielle Ekzem. H. RÖCKL, F. SCHRÖPL, E. MÜLLER and G. PETER 1516

Experimental Eczema of the Guinea Pig. N. HUNZIKER 1518

Terpentinöl-Intoxikation bei Arbeitern einer Schuhcreme-Fabrik verursacht durch d-Alpha-Pinen. F. NÜRNBERGER 1522

Enzymaktivitätsmuster im Serum und in Erythrozyten bei verschiedenen Hautkrankheiten. H. HOLZMANN, B. MORSCHES, G. W. KORTING and R. DENK 1524

Immunofluorescence Studies of the Skin. R. H. CORMANE, E. H. BAART DE LA FAILLE, J. B. VAN DER MEER, A. A. W. TEN HAVE-OPBROEK and W. W. MUIJS VAN DE MOER 1524

Herkunft der mononucleären Entzündungszellen (Makrophagen) bei der unspezifischen Entzündung (Untersuchungen am Rebuck'schen Hautfenster bei der Ratte). M. BEGEMANN 1531

Unspezifische und spezifische Wirkstoffe bei allergischen Reaktionen der Cutis. G. STÜTTGEN, J. GIGLI and F. HERRMANN 1531

Allergens of Quinone Structure. K. H. SCHULZ, P. SCHMIDT and H. GRELL 1531

Methode zur Hornschichtdickenmessung in vivo. F. KLASCHKA and R. A. KRAUSE . . 1533

Dermatological and Immunological Aspects of Cryoglobulinaemia. K. K. MUSTAKALLIO and O. WAGNER 1534

R.U.V., X-Ray and Alpha-particles Micrography of the Skin. A. TOSTI 1535

L'Exploration thermographique en dermatologie. CH. GROS, C. VROUSOS, J. ALT and A. BASSET 1539

The History of the Dermatological Section of the Royal Society of Medicine. T. J. RYAN, Y. M. CLAYTON, E. J. MOYNAHAN, J. F. KENNEDY, P. POLANI and I. A. MAGNUS . . 1541

Zellphysiologische Aspekte der Psoriasis vulgaris. O. BRAUN-FALCO, E. CHRISTOPHERS, S. MARGHESCU, D. PETZOLDT, G. RASSNER and M. RUPEC 1546

Mycology

Mikroskopische Demonstration von Fadenpilzen und Hefen. H. BRAUN and C. SCHÖNBORN 1550

page

Faserzerstörung durch Dermatophyten und keratinophile Pilze. L. KREMPL-LAMPRECHT 1550

Dermatophyten und ihre Hauptfruchtformen. G. A. DE VRIES and L. KREMPL-LAMPRECHT 1555

Serological Relationship of the Dermatophytes of Emmons-Conant-System. H. PALDROK and K. R. SUNDSTRÖM 1556

Adaptationsphasen der Dermatophyten in Zusammenhang mit ihrer Klassifikation. V. A. BALABANOFF 1556

Epidemiologische Analyse des Vorkommens von Dermatophyten in der Slowakei. L. CHMEL 1560

Einige biochemische Eigenschaften der Isothiocyanate. A. BOJANOVSKÁ 1560

Trichofytocid Spofa® (5% p-bromphenylisothiocyanat) bei der Behandlung von Trichophytosis. L. CHMEL, M. VALENTOVÁ and J. BUCHVALD 1561

Histopathomorphologische Befunde der Haut nach der Applikation von Trichophytocid. L. CHMEL and A. BOJANOVSKÁ 1561

Chromomycosis Caused by a New Species Chmelia slovaca. L. CHMEL, I. KOCHOVÁ and A. BOJANOVSKÁ 1562

The Third Case of Chromomycosis in the Territory of Czechoslovakia. L. CHMEL, I. KOCHOVÁ, A. BOJANOVSKÁ and B. KONRÁD 1563

Pilzerkrankungen innerer Organe. T. WEGMANN 1563

Survey of Mycoses in U.A.R. M. EL ZAWAHRY 1564

Clinical Diagnosis of Onychotrichophytosis. J. ALKIEWICZ and W. SOWINSKI 1564

Favic Infections in the Surroundings of Göttingen. M. KIRSCH-NIETZKI 1566

Pilzinfektionen im Bereich des Auges. D. H. HOFFMANN 1566

Parasitic Forms of the Causative Fungi in the Cutaneous and Visceral Lesions of Chromoblastomycosis. R. FUKUSHIRO and S. KAGAWA 1568

Chromomycosis (in the World and in Finland). T. PUTKONEN 1570

Relations entre formes cliniques et espèces mycologiques. A. BASSET and M. BASSET . 1570

Dermatomykosen bei Säugetieren. H. KRAFT 1570

Mykosen bei Tieren (Befall durch Aspergillus, verschiedene Dermatophyten und Alternaria). H. KRAFT 1572

Maduromykose beim Pferd. B. SCHIEFER and B. GEDEK 1573

Beitrag zur Mykologie der Systemmykosen: Histoplasmose und Kryptokokkose. H. KARUGA 1574

Vorkommen von Dermatophyten im Boden und bei Tieren als mögliche Infektionsquellen. D. JANKE 1577

Trichophytie und Blastomykose. Zs. HERPAY 1580

Ultrastructure of Dermatophytes. W. MEINHOF and W. VOGELL 1581

Infektionen durch Candida albicans. J. THURNER 1584

Quantitative Methoden der Antimykotikaprüfung. W. DITTMAR 1586

Enzymhistochemische Untersuchungen an Dermatophyten. K. HOLUBAR and O. MALE 1590

Dermatophyten und Schimmelpilze. B. BRAUN, H. RIETH and C. FINGER 1590

Additional Demonstrations

Kollegheft der Vorlesung von F. VON HEBRA, geschrieben von F. CURTI, zur Verfügung gestellt von O. GRUMBACH unter Vermittlung von O. GANS 1590

Histopathology of Leprosy. M. L. BRUBAKER and P. FASAL 1590

Antibiotics and the Placebo Reaction in Acne. R C. SAVIN and M. CHANCO-TURNER . 1590

Authors Index 1592

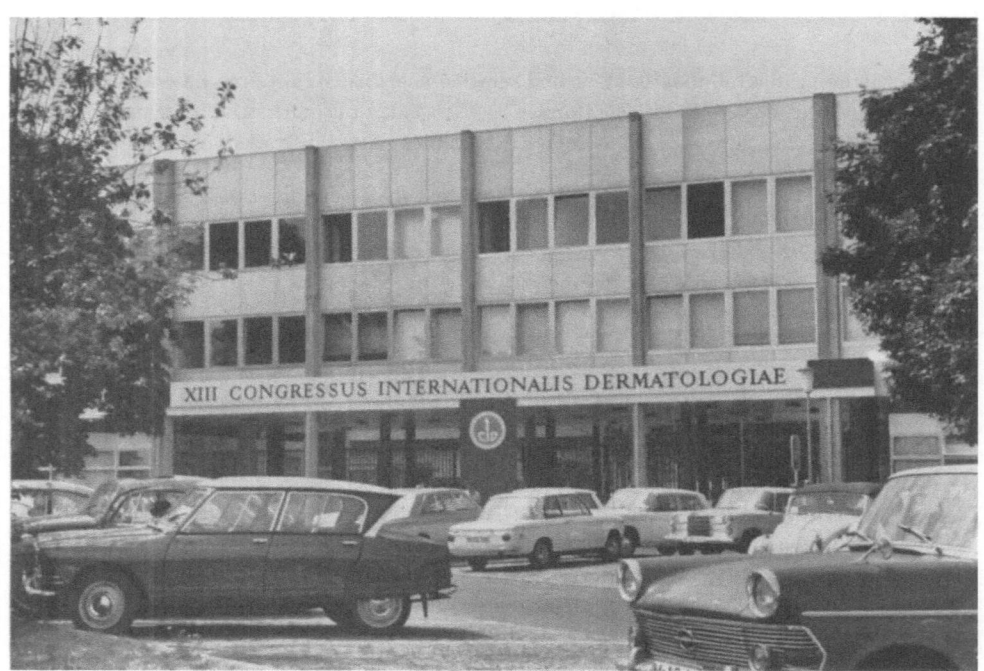

Entrance to the Exhibition Park
on the Theresienhöhe

Entrée du Parc des Expositions
sur la Theresienhöhe

Theresienhöhe, entrada al Parque
de Exposiciones

Eingang zum Kongreßgelände
auf der Münchener Theresienhöhe

Main Theme I   **Cancerous State, Precancerous State and Pseudocancers of the Skin (except Sarcomas and Melanomas)**

Cancers, précancérose et pseudocancérose de la peau (à l'exception des sarcomes et des mélanomes)

Cáncer, precáncer y pseudocáncer de la piel (excepto sarcomas y melanomas)

Cancerosen, Praecancerosen und Pseudocancerosen der Haut (ausschließlich Sarkome und Melanome)

Organizer

St. JABLONSKA, Poland

Presidents

J. C. BELISARIO, Australia

Y. BUREAU, France

T. KAWAMURA, Japan

H. PINKUS, USA

Delegate of the Organization Committee

O. HORNSTEIN, Germany

1. Experimental Studies of the Carcinom Mechanism and Precancerous States

Reports

Electron Microscopic and Histochemical Findings in Basal Cell Epithelioma, Squamous Cell Carcinoma and Some Appendage Tumors

W. F. LEVER and K. HASHIMOTO, Department of Dermatology, Tufts University School of Medicine, Boston, Massachusetts (USA)

Basal Cell Epithelioma. On electron microscopic examination, basal cell epitheliomas showed two types of cells: light cells and dark cells (Fig. 1). Light cells were the predominant type of cells. They were large and rounded, had a light cytoplasm and a large nucleus. Many of the light cells were immature and showed only a few tonofilaments and desmosomes. On higher magnification, most of the immature light cells contained a great number of mitochondria and a fairly well developed endoplasmic reticulum. Some of the immature light cells also contained a moderate amount of glycogen. The immature light cells resembled the immature basal cells of the embryonic epidermis, particularly those of the primary epithelial germ. Embryonic basal cells, like the immature tumor cells, possess large nuclei, are connected with each other by relatively few, poorly developed demosomes, contain only a few tonofilaments but contain a well developed endoplasmic reticulum and a moderate amount of glycogen.

Histochemically, basal cell epitheliomas composed predominantly of immature cells, such as the superficial basal cell epithelioma, contained acid phosphatase, succinic dehydrogenase and amylophosphorylase. These enzymes are present in equivalent amounts in the embryonic epidermis but not in the adult epidermis. This finding further suggests that basal cell, epithelioma and the embryonic epidermis are similar not only structurally but also functionally.

As the cells of the light type matured, many thick bundles of tonofilaments became apparent (Fig. 2). Concomitantly, the number of well developed desmosomes increased. Many of these keratinizing cells also contained dense clumps of homogeneous, dyskeratotic material. In addition, a small number of keratohyaline granules were present. The question whether the keratinization in basal cell epithelioma is of the type occurring in the surface epidermis or of the type occurring in hair cortex cells could not be definitely decided. The presence of small, or even a moderate number of keratohyaline granules does not entirely rule out the theory of the hair type of keratinization, because the Huxley and Henle cells and the cuticular cells of the hair contain trichohyaline granules which are morphologically similar to keratohyaline granules.

As stated at the beginning and shown in the first illustration (Fig. 1), two types of cells were seen in basal cell epithelioma: light cells and dark cells. Cells of the second type, namely dark cells, were few in number. They either lay scattered or in groups. They usually had an elongated shape, a large and very dense nucleus, and a dense cytoplasm containing few or no tonofilaments but usually many ribonucleoprotein particles. The real nature of this type of cell is presently unknown.

The stroma in immediate contact with the tumor islands of basal cell epithelioma had the appearance of a normal subepithelial basement membrane, or basal

1*

lamina, since it consisted of a very thin tropocollagen filaments intermingled with an amorphous substance. In rare instances, such a basement membrane was absent and the basal cells were in direct contact with empty spaces where mucinous material originally had been present. In such instances, the tumor cells showed many pseudopods extending into the spaces.

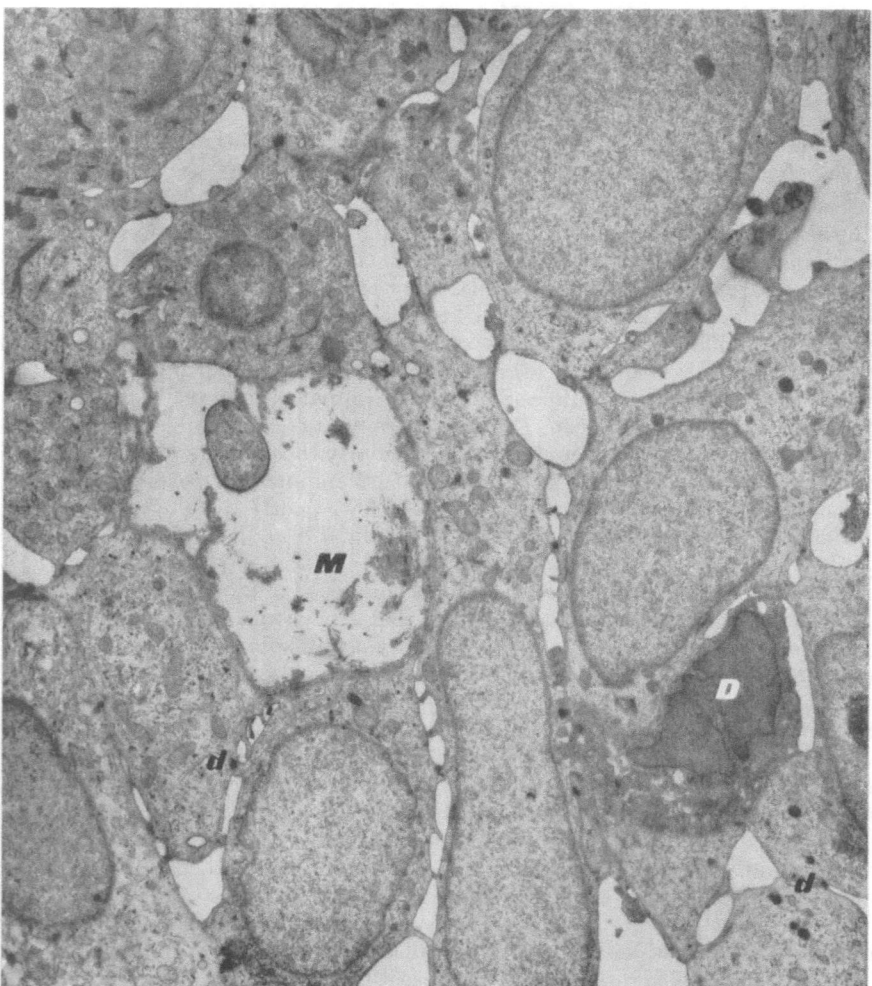

Fig. 1. Basal Cell Epithelioma, Immature Cells. Two types of cells are present: The majority of cells are light cells. One cell (*D*) is a dark cell. Desmosomes (*d*) are inconspicuous. At *M* the stroma has undergone mucinous degeneration. (× 5,750)

Pigmented basal cell epithelioma contained fairly numerous dendritic melano-cytes, mainly at the periphery of the tumor islands. These melanocytes were strongly dopa-positive. Melanophages present in the stroma contained a large amount of melanin granules or melanosomes, enclosed within lysosomes. In addition, also the tumor cells contained quite a few melanosomes (Fig. 3). The melanosomes in the tumor cells were usually located within lysosomes lined by a

membrane, but they were present also outside of lysosomes. Transfer of melanosomes from melanocytes to the adjoining tumor cells thus seemed to take place in a
more or less normal fashion.

Squamous Cell Carcinoma. Squamous cell carcinomas contained only one type
of cell showing varying amounts of tonofilaments and desmosomes. The cells

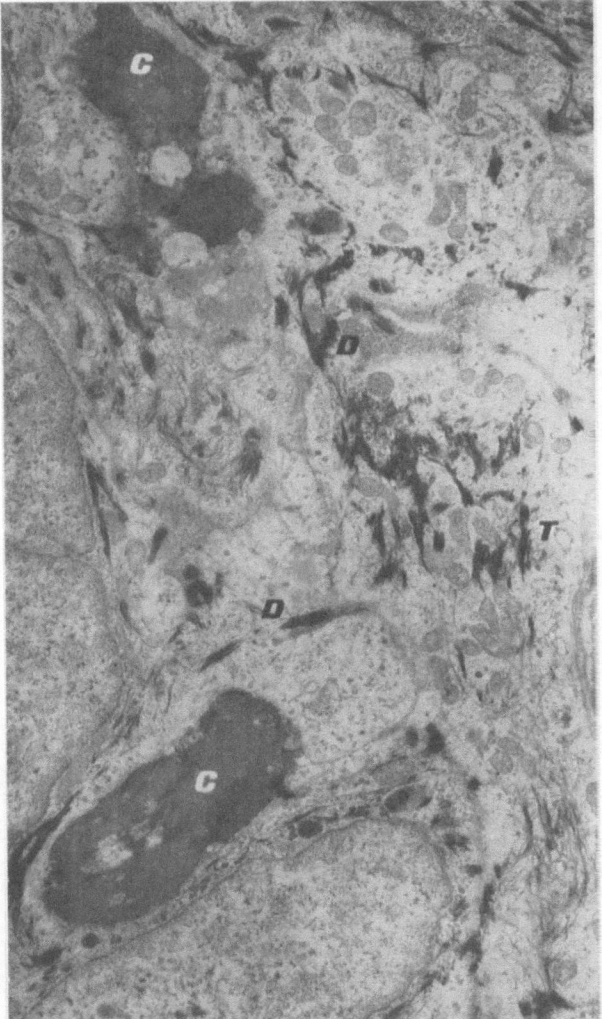

Fig. 2. Basal Cell Epithelioma, Mature Cells. The cells contain aggregates of tonofilaments (*T*).
Some cells also contain clumps of homogeneous, dyskeratotic material (*C*). Desmosomes (*D*) are
well developed. (×14,500)

usually were well developed except in highly malignant carcinomas. The tonofilaments aggregated to keratin in association with keratohyaline granules. The
degree of keratinization varied within the cells of the same tumor so that often
highly keratinized cells lay adjacent to cells showing only little keratinization.
The mechanism of formation of the keratohyaline granules could be easily observed

in most lesions of squamous cell carcinoma. Keratohyaline granules in their earliest stage consisted of small aggregates of dense granules representing ribonucleoprotein particles (Fig. 4, upper portion, arrow). Such aggregates were

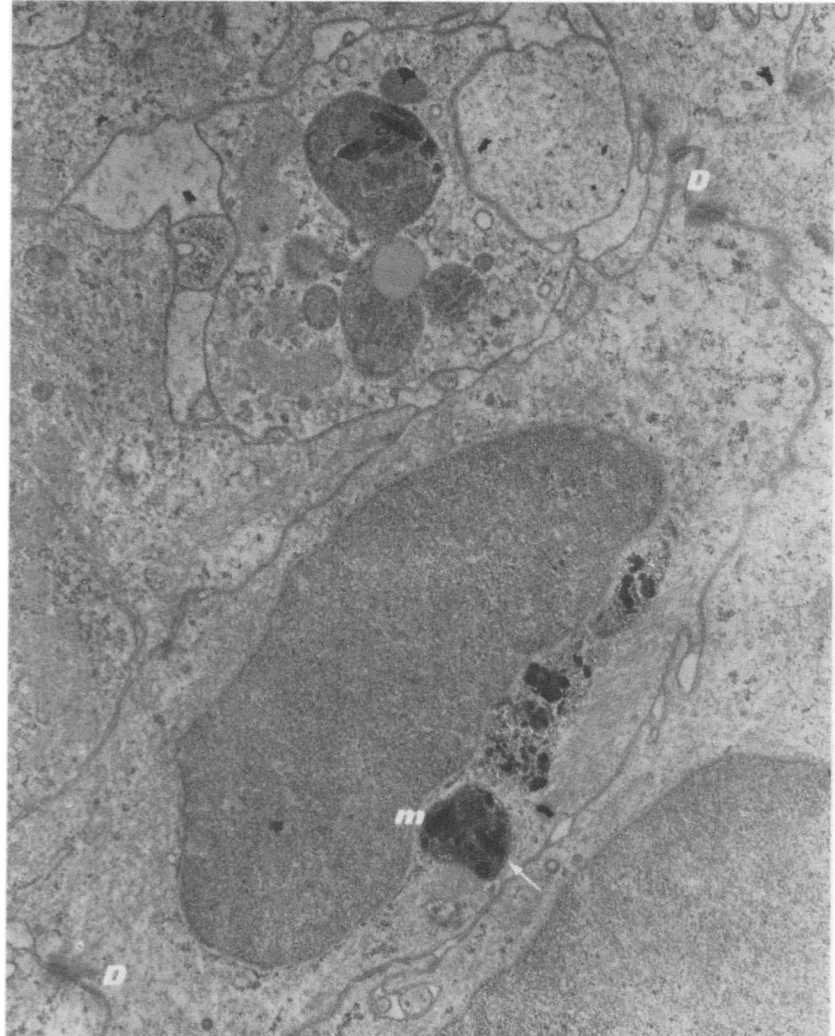

Fig. 3. Pigmented Basal Cell Epithelioma. Melanin (*m*) is present within a membrane-delimited lysosome (arrow). The cell containing the melanin (*m*) is a tumor cell and not a melanocyte because it possesses desmosomes (*D*). (× 20,000)

observed in large numbers in the cytoplasm but occasionally also in the nucleus (Fig. 4, lower portion). In the process of maturation of the keratohyaline granules the individual ribonucleoprotein particles gradually coalesced since these particles produced a dense protein substance. Although this process of formation of keratohyaline granules could be observed also in other keratinizing lesions, it was seen particularly well in squamous cell carcinoma. In squamous cell carcinoma grade III, the basement membrane, or basal lamina, often was disrupted in some areas so that tumor cells lay intermingled with connective tissue components.

Appendage Tumors. As a continuation of Lever's presentation, recent findings on the histogenesis of syringoma and clear cell hidradenoma obtained by the combined technics of histochemistry and electron microscopy will be reported.

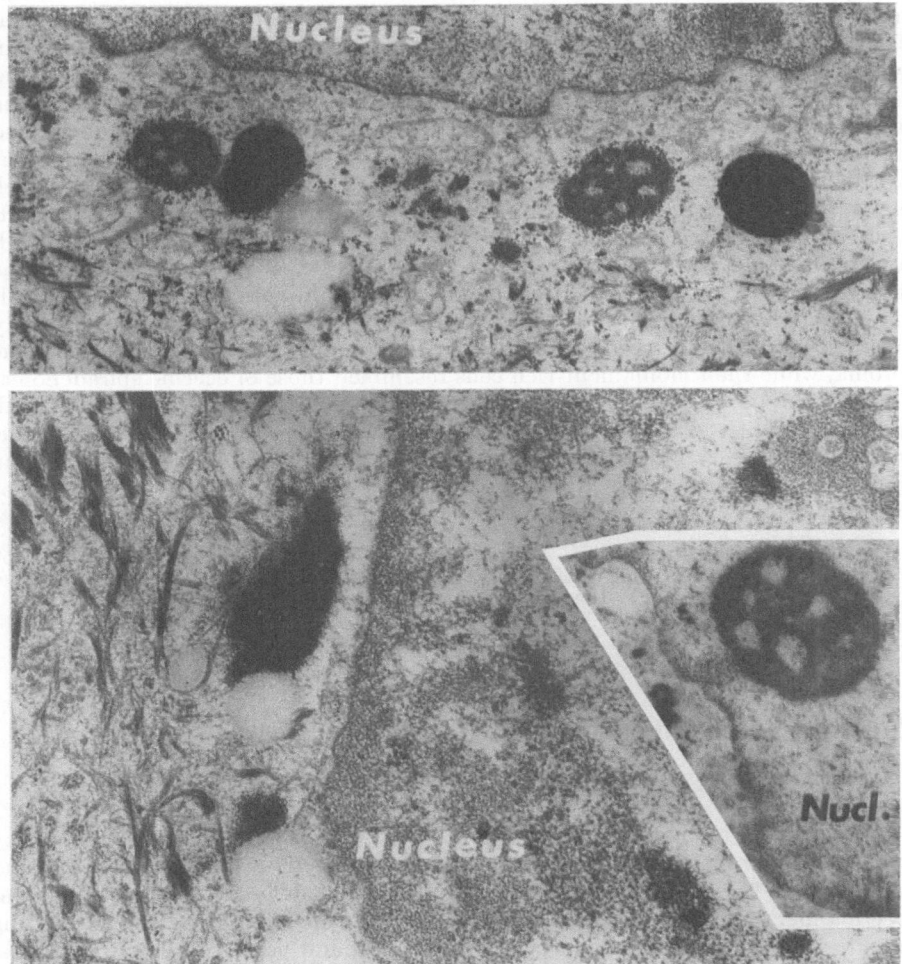

Fig. 4. Squamous Cell Carcinoma. The upper portion shows keratohyaline granules in the cytoplasm of a tumor cell (× 20,000). The lower portion shows the gradual coalescence of ribonucleoprotein particles into keratohyaline granules (× 30,000). The inset in the lower right corner shows a keratohyaline granule within the nucleus of a tumor cell. (× 20,000)

In *syringoma*, enzymes of the eccrine type, such as amylophosphorylase, were very strongly reactive. Amylophosphorylase was found to be strongly positive both in eccrine glands and in the tumor cells of syringoma, whereas it was completely negative in apocrine glands. On the other hand, acid phosphatase and indoxylesterase were strongly reactive in apocrine glands but were negative in eccrine glands and in the tumor cells of syringoma. Thus histochemical evidence strongly suggests that syringoma is an eccrine type of tumor. On electron microscopic examination, the lesion consisted of immature structures greatly resembling the embryonic intraepidermal eccrine sweat duct. The ductal structures in syringoma showed a lumen surrounded by two to four layers of cells. The luminal cells contained four organelles characteristic of cells of the embryonic eccrine intraepidermal duct. They were first, lysosomes; second, keratohyaline granules; third, a periluminal tonofilamentous band; and fourth, short but numerous luminal villi. Since luminal cells of the adult intraepidermal eccrine duct do not contain lysosomes, but only embryonic and regenerating eccrine intraepidermal ductal cells contain them, the presence of lysosomes in the tumor cells of syringoma indicates that the cells are immature cells [1]. Some of the cystic lesions contained several layers of flattened, completely keratinized cells. This keratinization was regarded not as hair type of keratinization but as being equivalent to that which naturally occurs in the upper portion of the intraepidermal eccrine sweat duct unit.

Clear cell hidradenoma, which in the past has also been called clear cell myoepithelioma, was found to contain various types of eccrine enzymes but none of the apocrine type. On electron microscopic examination, some of the cells composing the tumor contained mainly glycogen while others contained mainly tonofilaments. The glycogen-laden cells greatly resembled the tumor cells of eccrine poroma, while the tonofilament-rich cells resembled those of eccrine spiradenoma. Both eccrine poroma and eccrine spiradenoma represent appendage tumors with eccrine differentiation [2, 3]. Thus, both the enzymatic and electron microscopic findings suggest eccrine differentiation in clear cell hidradenoma. Tubular lumina occasionally encountered in this tumor were lined by rather immature ductal or secretory cells.

References. HASHIMOTO, K., B. A. GROSS, and W. F. LEVER: J. invest. Derm. **46**, 150 (1966). — HASHIMOTO, K., and W. F. LEVER: J. invest. Derm. **43**, 237 (1964). — HASHIMOTO, K., R. J. DiBELLA, and W. F. LEVER: Arch. Derm. **96**, 18 (1967).

The Rôle of the Mesoderm in Basaliomas*

H. PINKUS, Wayne State University, Detroit, Michigan (USA)

In epithelial malignancy, relationship of mesoderm to tumor epithelium may take four different forms: 1. the preformed connective tissue is invaded and destroyed, 2. the preformed connective tissue reacts defensively in an inflammatory manner, 3. the medoserm is induced by the tumor to furnish a supporting vascular stroma, 4. the mesoderm interacts with, and possibly induces epithelial growth, it is part of the tumor.

The first of these phenomena, invasion and destruction, is one of the basic signs of cancerous growth and is found in the skin in squamous cell carcinomas and basal cell epitheliomas.

The second phenomenon,defensive reaction, also is pronounced in all cancerous conditions arising in the skin, whether they are invasive or in-situ[1]. It takes the form of a lymphocytic and plasmocytic infiltrate and probably is due to immune mechanisms.

The third phenomenon, production of a vascular supporting stroma under the

* Supported in part by research and training grants from the National Institutes of Health, U. S. Public Health Service.

inductive influence of a cancer, is particularly well known in certain carcinomas of the mamma, where even metastatic deposits of cancerous epithelium may produce a marked proliferation of the connective tissue of the host site.

The fourth phenomenon, organoid interaction between epithelium and native mesoderm, which form a combination tumor, is in my opinion [2] the outstanding and decisive characteristic of cutaneous adnexal tumors, whether we consider them benign adenomas or locally malignant basal cell epitheliomas (basaliomas).

At first glance, there is considerable morphologic similarity between the third and fourth phenomena. In both cases, tumor parenchyma and stroma form a somewhat organoid unit. However, there are deep biologic differences. When a fibroplastic carcinoma metastasizes, it manifests the basic ability of any truly malignant tumor: individual epithelial cells are capable to settle in a new site, to form a colony, and to force the host tissue [3] to supply this epithelial colony with a stroma.

Basal cell epitheliomas, with very few exceptions which will be discussed later, are incapable of single cell metastasis, and even if their epithelial cells are transplanted experimentally, either in the same organism [4, 5], or into suitable foreign hosts [6], they do not grow. The basalioma cells seem to need the support of their native connective tissue to grow locally or to survive after autotransplantation. They behave in this respect like embryonic and adult normal epithelia [7].

Actually, this thought was already expressed in 1903 by Beck and Krompecher [9] in one of their earliest papers. They said that they could not follow Ribbert's ideas about the primary role of connective tissue in carcinogenesis, but they admitted that many basal cell epitheliomas contained much new formed connective tissue and could be considered mixed tumors: carcinoma fibrosum. This idea was later forgotten in the arguments about nature and origin of the epithelial cells, and little attention was paid to the stroma except by a few investigators, e.g. Herzberg [8]. Others, like Nödl [10] and Crossland [11] were more concerned with stromal influences on epithelial morphology and the possible rôle of stromal proliferation in radioresistance of tumors.

About 15 years ago, it had become obvious [12] that the basic biologic difference between the truly malignant and metastasizing squamous cell carcinomas and adenocarcinomas of the skin on the one hand, and the locally destructive, but not metastasizing basal cell epitheliomas on the other hand, could not be found in their site of origin or mode of causation. Carcinogenic rays or chemicals can produce squamous carcinomas and basal cell epitheliomas, and both may be derived from either epidermis or adnexa because the matrix cells of all these structures preserve a certain degree of pluripotentiality. The hypothesis was proposed that the essential biologic difference is to be found in stroma-association and stroma-dependence of the basalioma cells, which can not live and grow if separated from their specific stroma.

Support of this hypothesis has accumulated but slowly [13] because of the difficulty of human experimentation and the unavailability of basaliomas in animals until recently. Swerdlow [14] has supported the view that basalioma oncogenesis recapitulates embryonic development, that the tumor is derived from a basal cell with "locked-in" hair-forming potential, influenced in some way by the dermis, where the potential actually may be "locked". Most of the evidence is indirect and based on experimental embryology [15 to 17].

In that field, it is well established that many epithelia, including those of the skin, need inducing influences, and often continued support, from the mesoderm in order to become differentiated and to maintain polarity and differentiation. The stromal influence in many cases is specific in regard to provenience and age of tissues. An interesting sidelight was HOLTFRETER's report [18] that chemical carcinogens are able to induce normal structures in amphibian embryos, but produce tumors in older larvae.

Experimental embryology also has shown that there may be inter-action between epithelium and mesoderm rather than one-way induction. One of the newest insights in this field is that basement membranes are formed through ectodermal-mesodermal interaction [19], and are not barriers formed by the stroma to mechanically contain the epithelium. The almost constant presence of basement membranes in basal cell epitheliomas [20] thus becomes another point in support of their organoid nature. Basement membranes are usually absent in true carcinomas.

Closer examination of the stroma of basaliomas shows features of specific differentiation similar to those found in benign adnexal tumors. Terms such as mucinous and hyaline degeneration should be replaced by differentiation. The elaboration of elastic fibers [21] or of sulfated mucopolysaccharides [22], histochemically identical with those of the hair papilla, are certainly signs of function rather than degeneration. It is also important to point out that these changes take place in connective tissue newly formed as part of the basalioma, and not in the preformed old tissue which is being replaced. This distinction has not been always recognized [23].

The existence of rare cases of metastasizing basal cell carcinomas does not invalidate the general concept. Our methods of histopathologic examination are crude and can not show biologic differences between similar appearing tumor cells. Besides, a number of those cases reported as metastatic [24] actually resulted from massive implantation of aspirated tumor masses in highly destructive lesions after many years of local growth. These cases rather support the idea that a combination of epithelium and indigenous stroma is needed for autotransplantation of basaliomas.

References. 1. PINKUS, H., M. JALLAD, and A. H. MEHREGAN: J. invest. Derm. **41**, 247 (1963). — 2. PINKUS, H.: In MONTAGNA, W.: Advances in Biology of Skin **7**, 255. Oxford and New York: Pergamon Press 1966. — 3. GULLINO, P. M., and F. H. GRANTHAM: Cancer Res. **23**, 648 (1963). — 4. LYLES, T. W., R. G. FREEMAN, and J. M. KNOX: J. invest. Derm. **34**, 353 (1960). — 5. VAN SCOTT, E. J., and R. P. REINERTSON: J. invest. Derm. **36**, 109 (1961). — 6. GERSTEIN, W.: Arch. Derm. **88**, 834 (1963). — 7. BILLINGHAM, R. E., and W. K. SILVERS: Proc. 12th Internat. Congr. Derm., Washington, D. C. **1**, 257 (1962). — 8. HERZBERG, J. J.: Z. Haut- u. Geschl.-Kr. **16**, 340 (1954). — 9. BECK, C., u. E. KROMPECHER: Dermat. Studien 19; Erg. Heft zu Mh. prakt. Derm. **1903**. — 10. NÖDL, F.: Strahlentherapie **29**, 165 (1953). — 11. CROSSLAND, P. M.: Arch. Derm. **86**, 745 (1962). — 12. PINKUS, H.: Arch. Derm. Syph. (Chic.) **67**, 598 (1953). — 13. VAN SCOTT, E.: Proc. 12th Internat. Congr. Derm., Washington, D. C. **1**, 262 (1962). — 14. SWERDLOW, M.: Arch. Derm. **78**, 563 (1958). — 15. GOETINCK, P. F.: In MOSCONA, A. A., and A. MONROY: Current topics in developmental biology **1**, 253. New York: Academic Press 1966. — 16. JACOBSON, A. G.: Science **152**, 25 (1966). — 17. SENGEL, P.: In MONTAGNA, W., and W. C. LOBITZ JR.: The Epidermis, 15—34. New York: Academic Press 1964. — 18. HOLTFRETER, J.: Science **123**, 674 (1956). — 19. PINKUS, H.: Discussion to CAWLEY, E. P.: The basement membrane in relation to carcinoma of the skin. Arch. Derm. **94**, 715 (1966). — 20. BRAUN-FALCO, O.: Arch. Derm. Syph. (Berl.) **198**, 111 (1964). — 21. RUDNER, E. J., A. H. MEHREGAN, and H. PINKUS: J. invest. Derm. **45**, 70 (1965). — 22. SAMS, jr., W. M., J. G. SMITH jr., and G. R. FINLAYSON: J. invest. Derm. **41**, 457 (1963). — 23. SANDERSON, K. V.: Proc. 12th Internat. Congr. Dermat. **1**, 320 (1962). — 24. COTRAN, R. S.: Cancer (Philad.) **14**, 1036 (1961).

Interrelation between Structure and Recurrence in Basal-Cell Carcinoma

A. Rehák, Children's Hospital, Bratislava (Czechoslovakia)

In our previous studies we have dealt with the morphogenesis of varied structures in basal-cell carcinomas. We have succeeded in distinguishing morphologic patterns which are brought about by histogenetic origin of tumour-tissues and their differentiation from patterns brought about by other random formative factors [1].

The above studies enabled us to divide the structures in basal-cell carcinomas into groups corresponding to the diverse zones of the lanugo-hair follicles. The three main types of these structures are parenchyma analogous to the upper part of the hair sheath, later the so-called hair-matrix type, and at last the rest of several other pilar structures.

Apart from a histogenetic criterion one may choose criteria based on the expansion of the parenchyma itself, closely linked with the behaviour of the mesenchymal tumour-bed. According to the degree of parenchyma fragmentation the foci may appear as solid or cystic ones, later in small strands, and at last pseudoadenoid foci. The connective tissue changes are going mostly side by side with the fragmentation of parenchyma, forming either compressed strands with solid foci, fine laminated fibres with more desintegrated parenchyma or at last myxomatous changes correlated mostly with pseudoadenoid structures of parenchyma.

We have investigated, whether these actual signs may mirror the properties of the tumours namely their malignancy or tendency to recurrence.

Material, Methods. Therefore we selected 181 biopsies of recurring and relapsing tumours and have compaired them with a control group of 238 of non-relapsing tumours. The materials have been divided into groups according to the above criteria.

Results. A statistically significant higher frequency of the matrix type pattern, later of adenoid formations and of myxoid degeneration in the connective tissue, could be seen in the group of relapsing cases in comparison with the control group. The same signs may be present of course in tumours of the control group as well, thus they do not characterize the biological properties of the tumours unequivocally, but only as a certain portentuous symptom [2, 3] (see table).

Discussion. With the aim of verifying the above findings we made advantage of examining the biological properties of basocellular carcinomas in a purely laboratory way: We have studied the nuclear structures and connective tissue damage in an additional group of 100 basocellular carcinomas selected both from among the relapsing and unrelapsing cases. Sections were stained with a series of special simple techniques.

We have correlated the mitotic activity and abnormities in nuclear structures along with their density with the grade of desintegration and damage found in the connective tissue of the tumour-bed. This has been performed by means of separate code-cards for each of the examined tumours. The results of this trial showed that connective tissue damage has been in good correlation with signs of nuclear activity, and the most spectacular symptoms of such an activity were found in the group with the adenoid pattern of parenchyma.

The last attempt to verify the findings was an analysis of clinical data in contrast to the purely laboratory approach to the question. We have studied 783 cases of basal-cell carcinoma with regard to the mode and dosage of therapeutic management, duration, size of the tumours, and their localization, 73 of them being relapsing cases. The analyses failed to show a dependence of relapses on the above conditions [3].

Table

Type	Control group N = 238	Relapsing basal-cell carcinomas	
		Primary tumour N = 41	All biopsies of relapsing tumours N = 181
"Undifferentiated" type	6,3	7,3	8,3
"Matrix" type	38,6	63,4	58,0
Other "pilar" differentiations	86,5	83,0	77,0
Solid and cystic foci	43,3	36,6	33,7
Ribbon-like and little foci	59,0	63,5	66,0
"Pseudoadenoid" structures /total/	28,6	44,0	35,0
"Pseudoadenoid" structures — mucoid inside foci	25,2	34,2	20,4
"Pseudoadenoid" structures—reticular type	8,0	12,2	19,3
Connective tissue — compressed	22,2	14,6	19,3
Connective tissue — subtle laminated	57,2	44,0	46,4
Connective tissue — myxomatous degeneration	39,1	56,0	48,0
Connective tissue — myxomatous degeneration inside foci	29,8	41,5	30,4
Connective tissue — myxomatous degeneration outside the borders of foci	18,5	29,3	36,0

P 0,05;   P 0,01;   P 0,001;

Conclusion. Summing up the materials referred to, we might draw the following conclusions. There is no particular sign which could yield a completely reliable inference on the malignancy in basal-cell carcinoma, nevertheless the so-called matrix pattern and the adenoid pattern of parenchyma are portentuous as signs of a higher activity.

There have been but isolated attempts, as far, to correlate histological findings with clinical properties of the basal-cell carcinomas, the practical importance of such attempts being questioned, at any rate. The ever increasing demands toward a higher standard of the medical service, substantiate such efforts for a more pretentious diagnostical approach with the aim of reducting the relapses as much as possible.

References. 1. REHÁK, A., and J. DRGONEC: Vyd. SAV Bratislava, Czechoslovakia, **1962**, 264. — 2. REHÁK, A., J. LIŠKA, and J. MAŤOŠKA: Neoplasma (Bratisl.) **13**, 2, 169 (1966). — 3. REHÁK, A., J. LIŠKA, and J. MAŤOŠKA: Neoplasma (Bratisl.) **13**, 3, 295 (1966).

Sur les précancéroses cutanées

I. Bosco, Clinica Dermatologica dell' Università di Palermo (Italie)

Je remercie avant tout la Présidence du Symposium et je vous prie de m'excuser si, dans le temps limité qui m'est imparti, il ne m'est pas possible de traiter, fût-ce sommairement, le sujet «Sur les précancéroses cutanées», me limitant au seul énoncé des problèmes variés et complexes inhérents à ce sujet.

Que faut-il entendre par dermatose précancéreuse, par lésions ou états précancéreux? La conception clinico-statistique traditionnelle d'un chapitre sur les dermatoses précancéreuses ne peut pas être maintenue aujourd'hui, par manque d'individualité du chapitre.

Celle de la dermatose précancéreuse est une conception non fondée sur des données pathogénétiques certaines. Même celle de lésion précancéreuse n'aurait pas de signification, sans une corrélation avec la conception biologique du précancer.

On confond encore l'état précancéreux, le cancer « in situ », et la phase prémaligne. Outre que tout en pouvant se référer à la malignité, la question nous entraînerait à un long exposé sur le concept de malignité (malignité clinique, malignité histologique, malignité potentielle, qui coexistent rarement) nous devrons nous en tenir ici, pour ce qui est de la précancérose en question au seul concept de malignité potentielle selon Pentimalli.

Le problème de la précancérose au sens univoque de précancer, est évidemment lié, au sens biologique, au problème biologique du cancer. La dermatologie qui représente un point de rencontre entre la recherche clinique et la recherche biologique expérimentale, ne peut qu'accepter cette orientation univoque, en maintenant par ailleurs la distinction entre cette orientation et: 1. le concept de cancer «in situ» constitué par des entités morbides histo-pathologiquement définies (comme la maladie de Bowen, la maladie de Paget, la maladie de Queirat, la maladie de Jadassohn, la lentigo maligne de Dubreuihl, etc.), 2. les états néoplasitropes, déviations dans de précises directions quantitatives du turnover du tissu, dans l'activité multiplicative différenciative et migratoire qui peuvent constituer un microenvironnement favorable à conditionner l'évolution de la cytomorphose néoplastique (ou le réveil de propriétés aberrantes dans le mécanisme homéostatique) du tissu auquel elle appartient (processus hyperplastiques, productifs, processus atrophiques, processus régréssifs).

Le problème biologique du cancer ne se pose plus aujourd'hui du point de vue étiologique qui trouve une solution dans une étiologie polynomique, mais il réside dans la pathogénèse et dans les schèmes pathogénétiques où il n'a pas encore actuellement une solution univoque certaine.

Le développement de la cellule néoplastique dans un milieu déterminé concerne aussi bien les propriétés intrinsèques de la cellule néoplastique que les propriétés des tissus, de l'organisme hôte où le néoplasme se vérifie.

Les facteurs pathogénétiques

A) La manière dont peut agir dans la pathogénèse ce que l'on appelle le «terrain cancérigène». C'est une question de particulière importance histocytologique, et bien que cette voie de recherche n'ait pas permis d'établir l'existence d'altérations morphologiques absolument spécifiques de la cellule cancéreuse, on a toutefois toujours affirmé l'idée que le problème fondamental réside dans le moment pathogénétique susceptible de déterminer la métamorphose de la cellule, apparemment normale, dans une cellule douée de propriétés progressivement s'égarantes ou malignes.

B) Les systèmes auto-régulateurs dans la prolifération cellulaire homéostatique.

C) Le processus de xénoplasie, dans lequel est important le rapport entre la tumeur et le tissu environnant, qui est caractère nécessaire de la cancérogénèse. Dans les tumeurs cutanées, l'inversion de la polarité de croissance est une marque évidente.

1. Examen de la population des cellules néoplastiques

Le concept de mosaïcisme du tissu néoplastique a gagné du terrain morphologiquement et biochimiquement et actuellement parmi les génétistes qui admettent aussi la difficulté de distinguer rétrospectivement ou par des méthodes indirectes le substratum génétique des variations d'une population cellulaire du tissu. Il n'a pas été possible de démontrer une corrélation dans la constitution chromosomique entre tumeurs classificables du même point de vue histologique. Sur la base de telles observations Hauska soutient que la plus grande partie des tumeurs est constituée par au moins deux clones de cellules néoplastiques.

2. Examen des facteurs cellulaires qui règlent la multiplication

Malheureusement aujourd'hui encore Boulloughs et Laurence affirment que, jusqu'à ce que la nature de l'homéostase du tissu reste obscure, aucune définition satisfaisante du phénomène de la cancérogénèse ne pourra vraisemblablement pas être obtenue. Le même concept avait été exprimé il y a 20 ans par notre Ciaranfi dans ses intéréssantes études sur le problème biologique du cancer « Le problème biologique du cancer, a-t-il dit, est encore en grande partie le problème biologique du non cancer ». Seulement alors ont été commencées les études du métabolisme et de l'enzymologie cellulaire, et c'est depuis peu d'années que quelques essais significatifs ont été accomplis, récemment, à travers le contrôle des gènes (avec l'hypothèse de JACOB et MONOD, avec l'hypothèse de l'homéostase mitotique). Il semble probable que ce dernier mécanisme dépende essentiellement du contrôle exercé par quelques effecteurs sur les gènes qui ne restent pas bloquées pendant la différenciation embryonnaire. Le mécanisme est apte à répondre aux modifications du micro-environnement et spécialement aux modifications de la concentration de l'effecteur tissu-spécifique (dit « Chalon ») qui peut activer le gène du tissu et d'un effecteur non spécifique, peut-être la « retina » de Szent Györgyi qui inactive les gènes des mitoses. La période critique de la vie cellulaire pendant laquelle est réalisé le choix pour la préparation, soit d'une autre mitose successive, soit de l'activité fonctionnelle différenciative cellulaire active est appelé par les auteurs anglo-saxons « dicophase ». Les expériences mentionnées ci-dessus rappellent l'hypothèse du contrôle du gène des effecteurs dans les micro-organismes (MONOD et JACOB et al.) où la production d'un particulier enzyme structural a été appelé « operone ». Le fait qu'un « operone » soit actif ou inactif dépend de la concentration d'un répresseur qui est synthétisé dans une quantité constante correspondant à l'activité du gène régulateur. Un dérangement provoqué par un dé-répresseur change l'orientation biologique du cycle cellulaire. Pour les récents progrès dans l'isolement et la caractérisation du « Chalone » épidermique, il semble que celui-ci puisse être une glycoprotéine basique; il s'agit en effet de substances thermo-labiles non dialysables ni précipitables avec l'alcool. Toutefois ces vues sont acceptables comme hypothèses de travail, mais l'existence de ces schèmes auto-régulateurs n'est pas invraisemblable, non plus que le fait que, dans l'erreur multiplicative des éléments néoplastiques, la prolifération soit contrôlée par de tels facteurs locaux du tissu.

3. *Rôle du tissu connectif dans la prolifération*

Dans la greffe primaire et dans la phase de possibilité d'invasion de développement de la cellule néoplastique, ce rôle s'exerce à travers les phénomènes suivants: la phlogose, la perte de l'inhibition de contact d'Abercombrie, la direction de la cinémathique du processus d'invasions, la réaction du milieu qui influence le mouvement de ce processus. Il est clair que l'un des caractères essentiels de la cancérogénèse réside donc dans la rupture ou la déviation de l'équilibre compensatoire normal entre la valeur de l'activité mitotique et celle des aspects vitaux des cellules du tissu. Le processus de cancérogénèse étant biphasique et distinct dans les deux phase de « l'initiating-process » et du « promoting-process », le préjudice cellulaire fondamental qui est infligé pendant l'initiation est génétique et implique au moins une modification irréversible de l'action du gène. La recherche d'un état de précancer ne peut être destinée qu'à déceler l'aptitude potentielle de la cellule à réaliser un mécanisme génétique erroné de l'homéostase qui peut être cependant latente avant que les conditions cellulaires environnantes ne provoquent cette activité dans la phase de l'initiating-process.

Pour que le mécanisme néoplastique se réalise il faut: 1. une particulière physionomie génomique et par conséquent tissu-spécifique de quelques cellules qui sont aptes à la dégénération néoplastique, non décelables morphologiquement, mais seulement prévisibles potentiellement. 2. une situation microenvironnante qui conditionne le trouble de l'interaction naturelle ou provoquée dans le mécanisme génétique enzimologique, c'est-à-dire qui peut donner lieu à la pathostase néoplastique. Uniquement au point de vue conjectural, en ce qui concerne la précancérose cutanée, il y a dans le xéroderme pigmentaire le syndrome qui permet de prévoir les données nécessaires pour pouvoir y voir la configuration de ce que l'on appelle la maladie précancéreuse, où l'on a comme caractéristique clinique, que l'épithéliome épidermoïde est un véritable apanage de la maladie en elle-même, et par conséquent on présuppose qu'il existe en elle les éléments cellulaires prédisposés et d'une malignité potentielle d'où partiront inévitablement demain les épithéliomes.

Dans le domaine de la cancérogénèse, des précancéroses, des états néoplasitropes, la recherche ne peut être destinée qu'à déceler les variations biophysiques, biochimiques, de la cellule néoplastique ou potentiellement néoplastique, dans son métabolisme cellulaire, avec une étude comparée avec l'homéostase normale du tissu auquel la tumeur appartient. Dans mon Institut j'ai pensé qu'un programme de recherches pouvait consister à suivre les acides aminés les plus importants dans les protéo-synthèses cellulaires, à travers leur marquage avec des isotopes radioactifs. Les substances marquées ont été fournies au tissu « in vivo » dans un essai préliminaire par des injections intramurales dans les épithéliomes, dans le xéroderme et dans les états néoplasitropes.

La même recherche a été d'ailleurs l'object principal d'une étude systematique, à prélèvements périodiques, à rapprocher de celle de l'étude « in vivo » dans la peau normale, dans la peau néoplastique, et dans les états néoplasitropes, suivie sur tissu de survie en culture. C'est pourquoi les divers domaines de recherches ont été confiés à mes collaborateurs (Berna, Grana, Bellafiore, Aricò, etc....) et je me permets ici d'en anticiper seulement quelques résultats globaux pour être bref. D'une comparaison entre le tissu cutané normal et le tissu néoplastique dans les tissus de survie en culture par les recherches d'Aricò, ressort la différence du métabolisme de la méthionine S 35 dans les épithéliomes spinocellulaires en comparaison avec les basaliomes et en rapport avec le tissu épidermique normal. Le cheminement de la méthionine dans un tissu, avec métabolisme nettement plus

accéléré dans les épithéliomes spinocellulaires, qui se montrent riches de la méthionine marquée incorporée pendant le processus de kératinisation concentrique,
contraste avec la rareté du métabolisme de la méthionine S 35 dans les masses
basaliomateuses, même et spécialement en comparaison de l'épiderme normal de
revêtement du même morceau biopsique examiné.

Des résultats très semblables à ceux des épithéliomes épidermoïdes, et par
conséquent significatifs, ont été observés même dans le xéroderme pigmentaire sur
des parties de peau non encore épithéliomateuses.

Histochemical and Histoenzymological Studies in the Praecancerous Conditions of the Skin

L. Szodoray, in collaboration with Cl. Vezekenyi-Nagy, Department of Dermatology, University of Debrecen (Hungary)

It is understandable, that in the possesion of the modern histochemical and
histoenzymological methods the dermatoonkologists are carrying out research work
in order to find characteristic changes in the cells, under malignisation. As early
as 1949 Meyer, Arendt, Doerr and Lüttichen used for this aim the tetrazolium
method and stated that in tumor tissue the formazan-formation is stronger than in
normal tissue (Szodoray, Sóváry).

Newly Wolff and Holubar have made investigations in 95 cases of basalioma, in order to demonstrate their histoenzymologic activity: they found the
Succinodehydrogenase activity variable in each individual case of basalioma and in
the central parts of the tumorcellnests there was an increased acid-phosphatase
activity to be observed. There was no aminopeptidase in the tumorcells, but only
around them in the stroma and likewise there was no alkali-phosphatase activity
in the tumorcells.

In 1954 Braun-Falco published his observations concerning the histochemistry of the skintumors. The basement membrane in basaliomas was always
well developed and gave strong PAS reaction, but in spinaliomas the membrane
was missing or disrupted. It is well known, that in the Spiegler tumors there is a
well defined hyalin formation around the tumornests. In 1967 Sugár and Farago
published their observations concerning the behaviour of the basement membrane
in papillomas and in spinaliomas. The electronmicroscopic pictures showed, that in
spinaliomas the membrane was broken in several places. We have also observed
this phenomenon. Since Fulton's publications several authors dealt with the role
of mastocytes in tumor tissues, but this problem is still unsolved. Many authors
have repeatedly occupied themselves with the role of mucopolysaccharides in
tumor tissue.

It is known since Wenzler that PAS positive mucopolysaccharides can be
demonstrated with appropriate methods relatively often in the tumor tissue.
Quite often in the blood- and lymphatic-capillaries of tumor tissue there is a PAS
positive material to be seen. Elevated serumhexaminases can be observed in
the bloodserum of patients suffering from cancer. My collaborator, E. Török
succeeded in demonstrating pools of PAS positive material around the capillaries
of the tumor tissue: in tar-papillomas of white-mice, caused by dimethylbenzan-
thracen paintings. These observations prove that the mucopolysaccharide formation is a regular phenomenon in carcinogenesis. Gedevanishvili observed,

that during the carcinogenesis the mastocytes-activity diminished in the initial period, but increased later.

During 1966 we investigated the histoenzymologic pattern of skintumors in 67 cases. We made excisions under local anaesthesia from the tumor tissue and then we prepared sections with Kryostat. For the demonstration of succino-dehydrogenase (SD) activity and for the leucinaminopeptidase (LAP) activity and sulfatase (Sulf)activity, we used unfixed sections. For the phosphatase (ac. ph. and alk. ph.) activity we used sections fixed in Ca-formol solution and after washing, treated them for. SD demonstrations with the Pearse-method: for LAP-demonstrations the Glenner-method, for Sulf.-demonstrations the Seligman-method were applied. The ac. ph. and alk. ph. demonstrations were mades by Vadász-method (substrate:naphtol AS-BS and azodye diazo-5-chlor-2-toluidine).

Results: In the examined 27 cases of basalioma the SD-activity appeared to be variable even in the same tumor tissue. Generally in the periferic parts of the nests the activity was the most marked. The SD-activity seemed to be especially intense in the intraepidermic cancer of Bowen-type, and also in the epithelial nests of verruca seborrhoica, condyloma accuminatum, verruca vulgaris and in those of keratoma solare. In the ten cases of examined spinaliom these was a definitely expressed SD-activity and intense ac.ph. activity especially in the central parts of the cellnests. The Sulf-activity was also present. This and the LAP-activity could be demonstrated around the cancer-cellnests in the stroma. The metastases of the carcinoma mammae in the cutis, also showed intense ac. ph. activity. In the tissue of keratoakanthoma and keratoma senile SD-activity and Sulf-activity could be demonstrated. In the keratotic centre there was also ac.ph.-activity present.

In comparing the epithelial tumors with the mesenchymal tumors the latter showed more intense ac. ph-activity and LAP activity (M. Recklinghausen and Dermatofibrosarcoma).

The Mechanism of Precancerous and Pseudocancerous Conditions — A Comparative Study

S. Jablonska and A. Langner, Department of Dermatology, University of Warsaw (Poland)

Material

Diagnosis	Number of cases				
	Total	Electron micro-scopy	Auto-radio-graphy	Histo-chemi-stry	Immuno-fluores-cence
I Epidermodysplasia verruciformis A. Wart E.V.	5	3	3	3	3
B. Proliferative lesion E.V.	5	1	3	3	3
C. Bowen's epithelioma E.V.	4	1	3	3	3
II Keratosis senilis	32	1	6	23	2
III Epithelioma Bowen	13	2	3	5	3
IV Carcinoma spinocellulare	18	1	5	5	7
V Keratoakanthoma	17	2	4	6	5
VI Dyskeratoma	3	—	2	2	1
VII Experimental akanthosis	6	—	6	6	—

Methods

I Electron microscopy	— Ultrasections
	— Negative staining technique
II Autoradiography	— Thymidine — ^{3}H
	— Diisopropyl fluorophosphate /DFP/ — ^{3}H
	— ^{35}S
III Immunofluorescence	— with pemphigus serum
	— with pemphigoid serum
IV Histochemistry	— Lactate dehydrogenase
	— Succinic dehydrogenase
	— Nonspecific esterases
	— Leucinamine peptidase

Thymidine — ^{3}H was used for autoradiography in vitro. Studies in vivo with isotope given intracutaneously and left for one hour were unsatisfactory. In some cases we used also ^{35}S and diisopropyl fluorophosphate (DFP) — ^{3}H, and immunfluorescence with high-titer pemphigus serum for the demonstration of the intercellular substance and pemphigoid serum to show the condition of the basement membrane (T. CHORZELSKI). In electronmicroscopy the instrument Jem 7 was used. Some cases were studied histoenzymatically.

Results

Thymidine — ^{3}H	% normal labelled cells	% atypical labelled cells
Normal epidermis	3,83	—
Akanthotic epidermis	35,60	—
Keratosis senilis	5,90	0,80
Squamous cell carcinoma	6,20	1,10

In senile keratosis the percentage of thymidine-labelled normal cells was raised but little and chiefly in the deeper layers of the epidermis, the percentage of labelled atypical cells was very slight. The same was seen in Bowen's disease and squamous cell carcinoma.

In stripping-induced acanthosis the percentage was five to ten times the normal, depending on proliferation.

Epidermodysplasia verruciformis — Thymidine — ^{3}H	% normal labelled cells	% labelled vacuoles		% atypical labelled cells
		large	small	
Wart E.V.	37,80	12,80	—	—
Transition to Bowen's disease E.V.	30,30	11,50	2,00	—
Bowen's disease E.V.	7,90	—	—	2,10

In e.v. warts labelling was greatly increased and evident also near the surface. Vacuolized cells in warts and proliferating lesions without evident atypia showed DNA synthesis, and in electron-microscopy intranuclear viruses, which in number of capsomers per capside (negative staining technique) corresponded to Papova group viruses, which include also the common wart virus. In another case, histologically similar and with marked vacuolization but without electronmicroscopic evidence of virus, vacuolized cells remained unlabelled near the surface.

In Bowen-like lesions in e.v. labelling was relatively scant, being exceedingly scant among atypical cells; the relatively less atypical cells were synthetizing some DNA.

Viruses were not seen in lesions showing malignancy. In the cells which do not synthetize DNA vacuolization is due to the ergastoplasm's production of and expansion with material containing ribosomes. A keratin-like homogenous substance then collects in the endoplasm cavities, leading to giant vacuoles, depletion of cytoplasm in ultrastructures, and disappearance of nucleus.

In keratoakanthoma there was abundunt thymidine-labelling incorporation of sulphur in the epidermis, fluoroscence with pemphigus serum, which indicates normal intercellular substance and fluorescence with pemphigoid serum, which indicates the presence of immunoglobulins at the basement membrane zone.

The intercellular substance was also present in squamous cell carcinoma, although radiosulphur was scantest over individually keratinizing cells. In dyskeratoma the isotope was absent over dyskeratotic and akantholytic cells. Individual keratinization is shown by electronmicroscopy to involve replacement of about all catoplasm structures by abnormally abundant tonofilaments and separation of cells with disappearance of desmosoms.

These cells became labelled with DFP-^{3}H, its distribution corresponding to that of nonspecific esterases. Labelling is very distinct in squamous cell carcinoma in the cancer pearls, especially their peripheries, and in the inflammatory infiltrates (notably leukocytes and mast cells), which corresponds to leucinamine peptidase activity.

Summarizing, it may be stated, that:

Pseudocarcinomatous conditions differ from the carcinomatous in increased DNA-synthesis, which in atypical cells is usually almost nil.

In epidermodysplasia tending to become malignant (transition to Bowen's disease), no intranuclear virus can be detected, which goes together with the development of morphological features of atypia and failure of DNA-synthesis.

In vacuolized epidermodysplasia cells showing no signs of atypia but containing intranuclear viruses, the synthetized DNA is probably of viral origin.

The behaviour of the intercellular substance can be ascertained with the aid of ^{35}S and immunofluorescence with pemphigus serum.

Individual keratinization and dyskeratosis can be demonstrated with the aid of sulphur 35 and DFP-^{3}H, the latter demonstrating also proteolytic enzymes in inflammatory infiltrates.

Free Communications

The Vascular Pattern of Induced Skin Cancer in Rats

W. A. WELTON, Department of Dermatology, West Virginia University Medical Center, Morgantown, West Virginia (USA)

Introduction. Recent interest in blood vessel relationship to tumor formation [1 to 3] stimulated me to apply a technique of vascular visualization to rat skin exposed to carcinogens.

Method. 50 male albino rats of 3 months of age were used. 25 were painted twice a week with 1% anthramine and 25 with .3% methylcholantrene to the unshaven back (ZACKHEIM, 1949 [4]). — At various intervals they were sacrificed by injecting a cannulated internal carotid artery with potassium dichromate followed by lead acetate. A yellow precipitate of lead chromate occurred in the blood vessels. The skin carcinogen areas on the back were removed and put in cellusolve, then cleared in methyl salicylate (WILLIAMS, 1948 [5]).

2*

— The dermal blood vasculature could be visualized and photographed through the dissecting microscope. Then representative areas and tumors were biopsied and run into paraffin blocks, cut and routinely stained.

Results. Thirteen of the anthramine rats developed tumors in 6 to 10 months.

Diagnosis: Fibrosarcoma   7 (1 metastasized to local node)
          Basal cell carcinoma   8
          Sebaceous carcinoma   4
          Squamous cell carcinoma   1 (metastasized to local node)

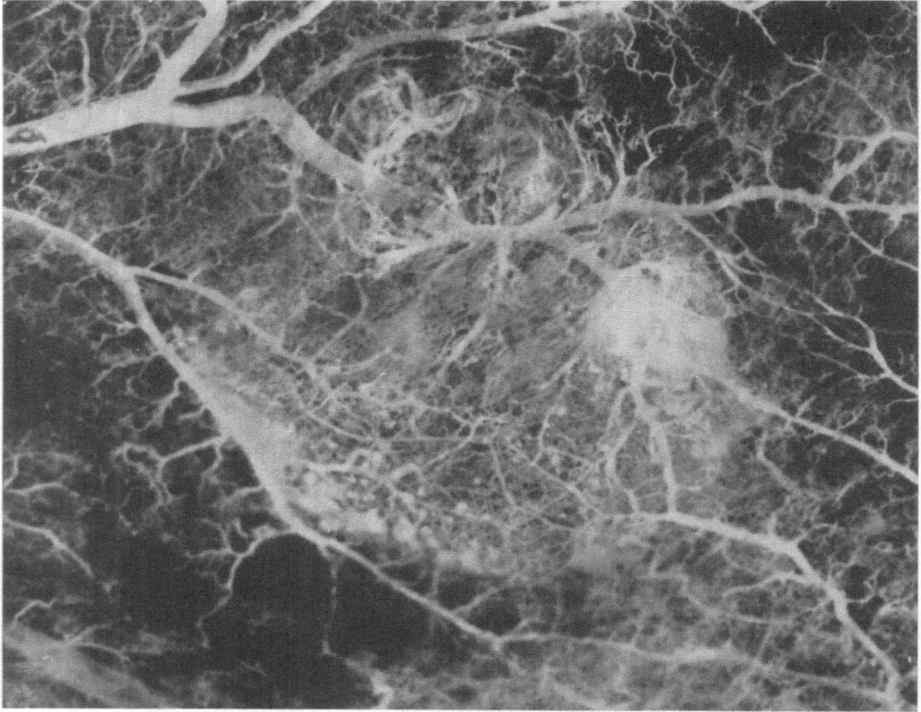

Fig. Vasculature of a well-developed basal cell carcinoma. 8 ×

The two metastatic tumors developed around the mouth persumably from reaching the carcinogen with paws and licking it off. Some rats developed more than one type of tumor. Two had both sarcomas and carcinomas. Several had both basal and sebaceous carcinomas. Nine of the methylcholantrene rats developed tumors in 8 to 11 months.

Diagnosis: Basal cell carcinoma   5
          Sebaceous carcinoma   7
          Sebaceous adenoma   2
          Keratoakanthoma   1

Twelve animals without tumors from the two groups were sacrificed from 1 to 10 months by injecting the precipitate. No definite vessel change was seen.

Nine rats died spontaneously from 1 to 9 months in whom no tumors were found grossly or histologically.

The blood vessels appeared to proliferate and enlarge in relation to the tumor growth. Larger dilated vessels surrounded the base of the tumor sending small branches into it. These surrounding vessels were derived from anastomosis of existing blood supply coming in from different directions. The diagnosis of carcinoma or sarcoma could not be predicted from the vessel pattern.

A method of visualizing tumor blood vessels is presented. It allows for preservation of the gross specimens which can be studied, photographed at low magnifications and then biopsied and microscopic changes observed. A disadvantage is some inconsistency of the lead chromate reaching all the vessels. Before any conclusions can be drawn as to the relationship between vessel change and tumor formation more animals need to be studied at regular intervals prior to tumor formation.

Bibliography. 1. DAY, E. D.: Progr. exp. Tumor Res. (Basel) **4**, 58 (1964). — 2. URBACH, F.: Advanc. biol. Skin. Blood Vessels and Circulation **2**, 123 (Ed. MONTAGNA, W.. and R. A. ELLIS). New York: Pergamon Press 1961. — 3. WARREN, B. A., and P. SHUBIK: Lab. Invest. **15**, 464 (1966). — 4. ZACKHEIM, H. S., W. L. SIMPSON, and L. LANGS: J. invest. Derm. **6**, 385 (1959). — 5. WILLIAMS jr., T. W.: Anat. Rec. **100**, 115 (1948).

Enzymes de la glycolyse et du cycle des pentoses-phosphates dans les épithéliomas

A. RIBUFFO, Institut de Clinique Dermatologique de l'Université de Sassari (Italie)

L'organe le plus convenable pour l'étude biochimique des néoplasies c'est la peau, puisque sa topographie rend facile le prélèvement du tissu.

Malgré cette facilité on a dédié bien peu d'attention à cet argument. Dans ce travail je vais relater sur les résultats du dosage, dans les épithéliomas, de l'activité de quelques enzymes du métabolisme glycidique et précisément d'un parmi ceux du cycle des pentoses-phosphates, la glucose-6-phosphate déhydrogenase et même de deux du cycle glycolytique, l'aldolase et la lactate déhydrogenase. Au même temps j'ai conduit mes recherches sur l'épiderme normal et sur les verrues séborrhéiques afin d'avoir des termes de comparaison. Les résultats obtenus démontrent:

1. que l'activité de la glucose-6-phosphate déhydrogenase a augmenté dans l'épithélioma spinocellulaire, ce qui n'est pas arrivé dans l'épithélioma basocellulaire;

2. que l'activité de l'aldolase a légèrement augmenté dans le seul épithélioma spinocellulaire;

3. que l'activité de la lactate déhydrogenase a remarquablement augmenté dans l'épithélioma basocellulaire et d'une mesure plus petite dans l'épithélioma spinocellulaire.

Pourtant le procédé des enzymes dans les deux types d'épithélioma, soit le spinocellulaire que le basocellulaire c'est tout à fait différent. Tandis que dans le premier l'activité de tous les enzymes considérés a augmenté, particulièrement de la lactate déhydrogenase et de la glucose-6-phosphate déhydrogenase, dans le second l'augmentation est limitée à la seule lactate déhydrogenase.

Tout celà indique que tandis que dans l'épithélioma basocellulaire c'est le cycle glycolytique qui est actif, dans l'épithélioma spinocellulaire au contraire sont efficients soit le cycle des pentoses-phosphates soit la vie glycolytique.

Evidemment les exigences dans les deux types d'épithéliomas sont différentes si dans le premier elles doivent être satisfaites tantôt par celui des pentoses-phosphates et si, dans le second, il suffit la seule vie glycolytique.

Si l'on tient présent que le cycle des pentoses-phosphates c'est l'origine de TPN réduits et de nucléothides et que le cycle glycolytique constitue au contraire une source de seules molécules de ATP, nos données indiquent encore que dans l'épithélioma basocellulaire, à la différence de l'épithélioma spinocellulaire, le cycle des pentoses-phosphates n'est pas fort engagé et ceci c'est le pourquoi, donné son lent accroissement, cette tumeur n'a de remarquables exigences de matériel.

Effect of Prolonged Administration of Testosterone on Normal and X-Ray Radiated Rat Skin

H. S. ZACKHEIM, Department of Dermatology, Stanford University School of Medicine, Palo Alto, California (USA)

The present communication reports the effect of prolonged administration of testosterone on the epidermis and sebaceous glands of female rats, and the effect of testosterone on the induction of pre-cancerous changes in these rats by X-ray.

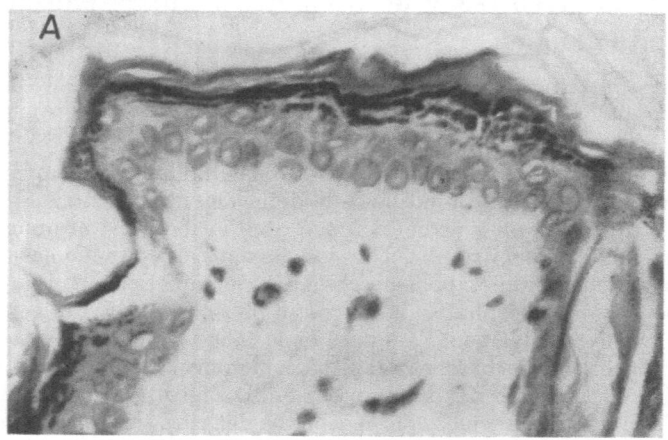

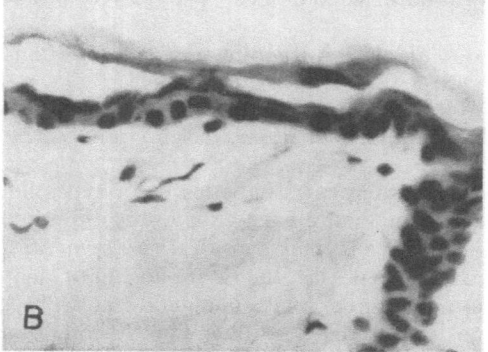

Fig. 1. (A) Epidermis of rat treated with testosterone 2.5 mg 3X/week for 4 weeks. (B) Control rat injected with water for 4 weeks. Both photos taken at 400 X

Procedure. Twelve female albino Sprague-Dawley rats, approximate weight 200 gms, were treated with aqueous testosterone suspension, 2.5 mg, 3 X/week, intra-muscularly for 25 weeks. An equal number of controls were injected with an equal volume of distilled water (0.1 cc). Both the testosterone treated and control rats received weekly X-ray treatments to the mid-back as follows: 500 r at 30 kv (HVL 0.052 mm Al), skin target distance 15 cm, through a 5 cm diameter cone. Biopsies were taken from the unirradiated abdominal skin and from the irradiated region on the mid-back. Since the 50% tissue depth dose of this radiation is only approximately 0.6 mm, the abdominal skin may be regarded as unaffected by the X-ray. This was confirmed by the absence of changes in the abdominal skin of the X-radiated control rats.

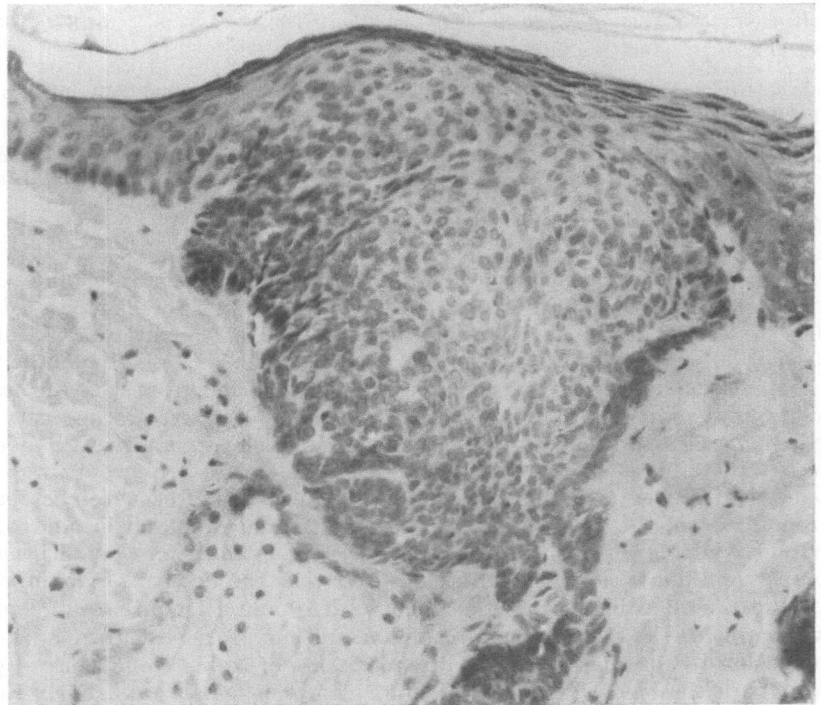

Fig. 2. Early basal cell acrcinoma in rat given 500 r weekly for 25 weeks

Results. I. *Unirradiated abdominal skin.* (1) *Epidermis.* Epidermal thickness is given as the distance from the base of the basal layer to the surface of the stratum granulosum (table). Six measurements were made at approximately equal intervals along the length of each section and then averaged. It can be seen that after 4 weeks of treatment a significant thickening of the epidermis occurs in from 50% to 80% of the testosterone rats. This averaged about a 43% increase in epidermal thickness as compared to the controls. One of the most striking changes was the marked accentuation of the granular cell layer (Fig. 1).

(2) *Sebaceous glands.* The size of the sebaceous glands was estimated by calculating the cross-sectional area of the largest gland in each of 6 high power fields taken at approximately equal distances along the length of the section and then taking their average. No attempt was made to calculate the actual volume of the glands since we were interested in relative values only. The sebaceous glands were consistently and significantly enlarged in all of the rats receiving testosterone (table). All rats receiving testosterone for 8 weeks or longer had sebaceous glands at least 100% larger than the controls.

Table. *Effect of Testosterone on Epidermal and Sebaceous Gland Size*

	0 wk	2 wk	4 wk	8 wk	12 wk	16 wk	20 wk	25 wk
No. rats	12	11	6	12	6	6	6	10
Epid inc[a]	0	1	2	6	4	5	4	7
Test. epid μ[b]	17.2	20.1	20.3	19.8	21.3	29.7	21.1	21.6
Cont. epid μ[c]	16.9	20.2	14.9	15.3	15.3	16.3	18.0	14.9
Seb gld inc[d]	0	7	4	12	6	6	6	10
Test. seb gld[e]	15.5	37.9	38.0	47.5	56.6	53.0	51.8	53.5
Cont. seb gld[f]	14.5	21.8	17.5	16.9	14.5	13.1	17.8	14.2

[a] rats showing a 33% or more increase in epidermal thickness as compared to controls.
[b] epidermal thickness of testosterone rats.
[c] epidermal thickness of control rats.
[d] rats showing a 100% increase or more in sebaceous gland size as compared to controls.
[e] testosterone rats, relative cross-sectional area of sebaceous glands. Multiply by 23 μ^2 for actual value.
[f] control rats, relative cross-sectional area of sebaceous glands.

II. *Radiated skin of back.* One group of 6 testosterone treated rats and 6 water injected controls received 500 r weekly to the mid-back for 25 weeks for a total of 12,500 r. A second group of 6 testosterone rats and 6 controls were similarly radiated for 36 weeks for a total of 18,000. Biopsies taken at 4 and 6 months from the radiated areas revealed that the epidermis was thicker in most of the testosterone rats as compared to the controls. Several of the testosterone rats also showed changes suggesting early stages of squamous cell carcinoma. At 8 months, however, these differences between the testosterone and control groups were less pronounced. However, at 8 months early, but definite, foci of basal cell carcinoma were found in 4 of the 7 surviving testosterone treated rats, and in none of the 6 surviving controls (Fig. 2). No squamous cell carcinomas were found in either group at 8 months. It should be noted however that the bulk of basal and squamous cell carcinomas in the rat appear between 10 and 18 months after weekly X-ray treatments [1] so that these results should not be regarded as conclusive.

Conclusions. Prolonged systemic administration of testosterone causes hyperplasia of both the epidermis and sebaceous glands in female rats. Early results suggest that testosterone stimulates pre-cancerous skin changes in female rats receiving X-radiation.

References. 1. ZACKHEIM, H. S., E. KROBOCK, and L. LANGS: J. invest. Derm. **43.** 519 (1964).

Solar Ultraviolet Radiation and Skin Cancer*

F. URBACH and R. E. DAVIES, Department of Dermatology, Skin and Cancer Hospital, Temple University Health Sciences Center, Philadelphia, Pennsylvania (USA)

As has been shown before (URBACH et al., 1966), there are striking differences between the amounts of ultraviolet radiation to which various parts of the head and neck are exposed. It is quite clear that, under conditions closely simulating natural exposure, the orbital area, the nasolabial fold, the upper lip, the center of

* Supported by The John A. Hartford Foundation.

the chin, the anterior neck and the lower retroauricular area receive little or no radiation unless a very efficient reflector such as sand or snow is present.

In sharp contrast, the rim of the ear and the back of the neck in males and the nose, cheekbones and lower lip in both sexes are the areas of heaviest insolation.

We have made a preliminary study of the prevalence and distribution of squamous cell carcinoma and basal cell carcinoma in these skin areas. The patient material for this evaluation has been obtained from the files of the Skin and Cancer Hospital Tumor Clinic (representing a densely populated urban area), from a splendid report of the experience with skin cancer at the Radiumhemmet in Stockholm (MAGNUSSON, 1935), and from data taken from a series of reports on geographic pathology of skin cancer presented at the 1962 Conference on the Biology of Cutaneous Cancer (URBACH, 1963). Additional information has been kindly contributed by Silverstone of Queensland, Australia (1964), and Sweet of Great Britain (1964). It must be clearly understood that all these data represent highly selected patient groups and cannot even be considered adequate prevalence figures; thus direct comparisons are neither possible nor profitable. We do believe that they represent meaningful trends and are useful for the design of further investigations.

In Tab. 1, the distribution of squamous cell carcinoma and of basal cell carcinoma is compared by sites (experience of the Tumor Clinic of the Skin and Cancer Hospital, 1957 to 1962). It can be seen that 88 per cent of all basal cell carcinomas and 68 per cent of all squamous cell carcinomas occurred on the head and neck. Furthermore, 32 per cent of all basal cell carcinomas occurred in areas relatively protected from ultraviolet light while none of the squamous cell carcinomas arose in such areas.

Table 1. *Prevalence of Basal Cell Carcinoma (BCC) and Squamous Cell Carcinoma (SqCC) by Body Area. (Experience of the Skin and Cancer Hospital Tumor Clinic, 1957 to 1962.) "Protected" Areas Receive less than 20 Per Cent of the Maximum Possible Ultraviolet Radiation*

		Males		Females		Total	
		No.	%	No.	%	No.	%
BCC	Head and neck (unprotected)	159	55 · 3	145	55 · 8	304	55 · 5
	Head and neck (protected)[a]	91	31 · 6	85	32 · 7	176	32 · 2
	Other	38	13 · 1	30	11 · 5	68	12 · 3
	Total	288	100	260	100	548	100
SqCC							
	Head and neck (unprotected)	31	66	10	77	41	68 · 4
	Head and neck (protected)[a]	0	0	0	0	0	0
	Other	16	34	3	23	19	31 · 6
	Total	47	100	13	100	60	100

[a] Protected areas: Upper and lower eyelid, inner and outer canthus, nasolabial fold, post auricular area, upper lip, anterior neck.

Using identical criteria for analysis, it was possible to compare two large series of cases obtained in 1920 to 1935 at the Radiumhemmet (MAGNUSSON, 1935) and in 1957 to 1964 at the Skin and Cancer Hospital of Philadelphia. These data are presented in Tab. 2. Considering only the head and neck area, approximately 38 per cent of all basal cell carcinomas arose in areas of the skin receiving less than 20 per cent of the maximum of ultraviolet radiation, while squamous cell carcinomas occurred only rarely on these sites. (The 6 and 13 per cent incidence, respectively, noted in the table represent 1 and 3 patients only.)

Table 2. *Comparison of Distribution of Basal Cell Carcinoma and Squamous Cell Carcinoma over Protected and Unprotected Areas of the Head and Neck. Experience of the Skin and Cancer Hospital Tumor Clinic, 1957 to 1962, and of the Radiumhemmet* (MAGNUSSON, *1935*)

Area	S and C Hospital			Radiumhemmet		
	Male	Female	Total	Male	Female	Total
	%	%	%	%	%	%
Basal cell carcinoma						
Head and neck (Unshaded)	63 · 3	63 · 0	63 · 2	57 · 1	67 · 3	62 · 2
Head and neck (Shaded)	36 · 7	37 · 0	36 · 8	42 · 9	32 · 7	37 · 8
Squamous cell carcinoma						
Head and neck (Unshaded)	100	88 · 0	94 · 0	84 · 2	90 · 0	86 · 5
Head and neck (Shaded)	0	12 · 0	6 · 0	15 · 8	10 · 0	13 · 5

The correlation between degree of insolation and location of skin cancer is even more strikingly demonstrated by analysis of tumors occurring on and around the external ear. In one large series of cases reported from France (HURIEZ, LEBEURRE and LEPERRE, 1962), 55 per cent of squamous cell carcinomas occurred on the rim of the concha compared to 14 per cent of basal cell carcinomas while 72 per cent of basal cell carcinomas were located in the postauricular, retroauricular and preauricular areas, compared to 26 per cent squamous cell carcinomas.

It thus appears that squamous cell carcinoma of the skin occurs primarily on those skin sites most heavily exposed to ultraviolet radiation. In contrast, about one-third of all basal cell carcinomas appear on areas normally slightly exposed to such radiation. This suggests to us that some factor in addition to ultraviolet radiation plays a significant role in the genesis of basal cell carcinoma, but not in the development of squamous cell carcinoma. If this is the case, it would be expected that the prevalence of squamous cell carcinoma should rise faster than that of basal cell carcinoma with increased exposure, whether because of latitude or occupational and recreational habits. Such data are available to support this hypothesis. Tab. 3 shows squamous cell carcinoma/basal cell carcinoma ratios by occupation in New York State (LEVIN et al., 1960), and Tab. 4 and 5 by latitude and probable exposure. In each case the ratios are greater in those areas and locations which are heavily insolated (i.e. the prevalence of squamous cell carcinoma increases much more rapidly with decreasing latitude and increasing exposure than does the prevalence of basal cell carcinoma). The great and irregular variations in biologically effective ultraviolet radiation reaching the ground in various areas of the world can be seen in the figure.

Table 3. *Comparison of Squamous Cell Carcinoma (SqCC) to Basal Cell Carcinoma (BCC) Ratios by Sites and Probable Exposure. Data of the New York State Cancer Survey* (LEVIN et al., *1960). Note Increase in Ratio (i.e. Relative Greater Frequency of Squamous Cell Carcinomas) with Increased Exposure*

Patients	BCC	SqCC	Ratio
Face			
Urban males	25·9	4·4	0·17
Rural males	22·6	6·8	0·30
Upper extremities			
Urban males	1·3	1·8	1·4
Rural males	0·6	1·4	2·3

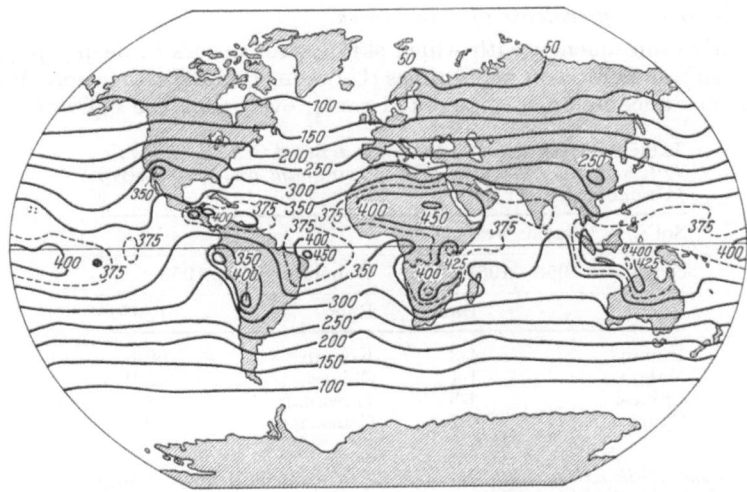

Fig. World distribution of "sunburn" ultraviolet radiation, corrected for latitude, cloud cover and altitude. (Annual values for a 10 mμ wide band of ultraviolet radiation, centered on 307·5 mμ. Calculations and drawing prepared by R. SCHULZE, Hamburg, Germany)

Table 4. *Comparison of Basal Cell Carcinoma (BCC) to Squamous Cell Carcinoma (SqCC) Ratios by Sites and Probable Exposure. Data of the Skin and Cancer Hospital Tumor Clinic (Urban, Low Exposure, Middle Latitude), M. D. Anderson Hospital (Rural, High Exposure, Low Latitude)* (MAC DONALD and BUBENDORF, 1964)*, and Radiumhemmet (Rural, High Exposure, High Latitude)* (MAGNUSSON, 1935)*. Note Rarity of SqCC in Orbital Area, Great Frequency of SqCC on Ear, and Relatively Greater Prevalence of SqCC in Low Latitudes and Rural Areas*

Location	Skin and Cancer 1957—62	M. D. Anderson 1944—61	Radiumhemmet 1916—31
All skin cancers	9·3:1	1·84:1	3·9:1
Head and neck	11·7:1	2·05:1	4·45:1
Body and extr.	3·6:1	1·15:1	1·16:1
Ear	1·9:1	1·1:1	1·2:1
Inner and outher canthus, eyelids	57:0	5·7:1	21:1

Table 5. *Squamous Cell Carcinoma (SqCC)/Basal Cell Carcinoma (BCC) Ratio by Latitude and Probable Exposure. Note Increasing Ratio (i.e. Relatively Greater Increase in Prevalence of SqCC) with Decreasing Latitude and Increasing Exposure. Data of* MAGNUSSON (1935) *(Stockholm),* SWEET (1964) *(Sheffield, Bristol, Plymouth and W. Cornwall),* (LEVIN et al., 1960) *(N. Y. State),* (MAC DONALD and BUBENDORF, 1964) *(Houston) and* TEN SELDAM (1963) *(Perth)*

Origin of data	Latitude	Probable exposure	SqCC/BCC ratio
Stockholm	59°N	Great	0·21
Sheffield	53°25′N	Small	0·07
Bristol	51°30′N	Moderate	0·17
Plymouth	50°20′N	Moderate	0·22
W. Cornwall	50°10′N	Great	0·30
N.Y. State	44°—42′N	Moderate	0·21
Philadelphia	40°N	Small	0·09
Houston	29°30′N	Great	0·55
Perth	32°S	Great	0·50

Ethnic origin and the prevalence of skin cancer

The relative infrequency with which skin cancer occurs in deeply pigmented races has been commented on many times (URBACH, 1963). Furthermore, basal cell carcinomas are uncommon in pigmented races, even near the equator, and the

Table 6. *Squamous Cell Carcinoma/Basal Cell Carcinoma Ratios by Race. Data of Shanmugaratnam and Quisenberry (*URBACH, *1963)*

SqCC/BCC ratios by race

Singapore 1950—1961		Honolulu 1955—1956	
Race	Ratio	Race	Ratio
Indians	4·3	Korean	69·0
Malays	1·4	Chinese	48·0
Chinese	1·3	Hawaiian	1·3
Caucasians	0·2	Caucasians	0·9

Table 7. *Prevalence of Skin Cancer by Ethnic Origin. Experience of the Skin and Cancer Hospital Tumor Clinic, 325 Patients. Expected Percentage Based on "Foreign Born" Category of 1960 Decennial Census for Greater Philadelphia*

Country of origin	% Expected	% Found
Irish	3·45	25·5
Italian	8·3	11·9
German	3·9	9·5
Russian	5·0	7.7
English	4·6	6·9

squamous cell carcinomas reported are most commonly found on the lower extremities and trunk and thus unlikely to be related to ultraviolet radiation (URBACH, 1963) (Tab. 6). Less well known is the apparent frequency of skin cancer in patients of Celtic antecedents (Scots, Irish, Welsh). As can be seen from preliminary data from the Skin and Cancer Hospital (Tab. 7) and Silverstone's (1964) studies in 3 areas of Queensland, Australia (Tab. 8), there appears to be a signifi-

Table 8. *Prevalence of Skin Cancer by Ethnic Origin. Data of* SILVERSTONE *(1964) Obtained by Direct Examination of All Inhabitants of 3 Small Towns in Queensland, Australia. Julia Creek, Located Inland, Latitude 18° S; Tully, Located on Seacoast, Latitude 19° S; Caboolture, Located on Seacoast, Latitude 27° S. Note Greater Prevalence of Skin Cancer in Patients with Celtic Background and Intense Exposure, and Very Low Prevalence in Mediterranean and More Deeply Pigmented Individuals*

Ancestry and incidence of cancers

Ancestry	Percentage with cancers					
	Julia Creek		Tully		Caboolture	
	Males	Females	Males	Females	Males	Females
(A)	32·4	21·9	10·9	6·3	9·3	9·8
(B)	16·4	10·0	29·5	16·4	12·7	6·5
(C)	14·9	8·3	24·4	12·8	7·5	4·3
(D), (E), (F)	0·0	0·0	1·4	1·4	0·0	0·0

(A) = Maternal and paternal ancestry both Scot or Irish.
(B) = One Scot or Irish, the other Australian, North European, etc.
(C) = Both Australian, both North European or one of each.
(D) = One Mediterranean, South American, etc., the other Scot, Irish, Australian or North European.
(E) = One Scot, Irish, Australian, North European, the other Asiatic, Aboriginal or other "pigmented" type. Also, both Mediterranean or South American.
(F) = One Mediterranean or Asiatic, etc., the other Asiatic or Aboriginal.
(G) = Both Aboriginal.

cant excess of skin tumors in Celtic people over that expected based on the distribution of the local population. This phenomenon appears to be due to earlier onset
of skin cancer (by about 10 years) and is probably due to an inherited inability of
Celtic skin to protect itself in the usual fashion against the destructive effects of
ultraviolet radiation.

References. HURIEZ, C., R. LEBEURRE, and B. LEPERRE: Bull. Soc. franç. Derm. Syph.
69, 886 (1962). — LEVIN, M. L., and W. HAENSZEL: J. nat. Cancer Inst. 24, 1243 (1960). —
MACDONALD, E. J., and E. BUBENDORF: Chicago; Year Book Medical Publishers 1964. —
MAGNUSSON, A. H. W.: Acta radiol. (Stockh.) Suppl. 19, 1935. — SILVERSTONE, D.: Pers.
communication. Presented at a conference on ultraviolet light and skin cancer, Airlie House
1964. — SWEET, D.: Pers. communication. Presented at a conference on ultraviolet light and
skin cancer, Airlie House 1964. — TEN SELDAM: In: URBACH, F., ed.: The Biology of Cutaneous
Cancer. Monograph No. 10. J. nat. Cancer Inst. 1963. — URBACH, F.: The Biology of Cutaneous
Cancer. National Cancer Institute Monograph No. 10, U.S. Government Printing Office,
Washington, D.C., USA 1963. — URBACH, F., R. DAVIES, and P. D. FORBES: Ultraviolet
Radiation and Skin Cancer in Man. In Advanc. biology Skin VII: Carcinogenesis. Oxford:
Pergamon Press 1966.

A Clinical and Histological Study of the Evolution
of Proliferative Epidermal Lesions of Pitch Workers

G. HODGSON, Consultant Dermatologist, Cardiff Royal Infirmary (England).
H. J. WHITELEY, Reader in Pathology, Welsh National School of Medicine,
Cardiff (England)

There is a factory in South Wales making patent fuel blocks where coal and
pitch dust are fused together by steam heat. Since 1957 we have had opportunity
to examine the workers referred because of suspicious epithelial proliferative
lesions in all 59 cases have been examined, three with squamous carcinoma, 29 with
active keratoses and 35 with pitchwarts. 17 of those with warts had a history of
previous warts often multiple. In 8 cases exposure was 4 years or less and there
was no difference in incidence between workers with up to 10 years exposure and
those with exposure between 10 to 34 years.

Because the incidence of pitchwarts did not seem to be directly related to
exposure and because certain individuals appeared more susceptible our interest
was stimulated to investigate the evolution of both benign and malignant proliferative epithelial lesions in the total working population; a complete re-examination being carried out after an interval of 2 years. During this time the whole
factory population was and still is under observation. This population has changed
during this time but 70% of those workers seen initially have been reexamined.

All workers at the factory are exposed to pitchdust in varying degree. A total
of 144 at risk being examined. A record of the duration and intensity of exposure
(high medium and low) as estimated by the industry was made. The clinical
examination recorded individual colouring, hair, skin, eyes, the degree of abnormal
pigmentation, together with the type number and distribution of epithelial proliferative lesions, with particular reference to the hair pattern at the site, and
acneform lesions.

Epithelial proliferative lesions were classified into:

A. Benign proliferative lesions, sessile plaque and pedunculated.

B. Premalignant lesion actinic keratoses scars, shagreen skin, chronic tar dermatosis and leucomelanoderma.

C. Malignant squamous lesions.

D. The pitchwart or keratoakanthoma.

Finally acneform keratoses were recorded. Comedones, acne folliculitis and retention cysts.

All pitch warts and suspicious lesions were biopsied.

A control series of 263 persons of the same age group attending outpatient clinics were examined.

A. Benign proliferative lesions occurred in 58% of pitch workers and in 73% of controls. The incidence of these lesions increased with age in both groups. The sessile lesions developing on the hands and forearms in 87% of workers and 95% of controls. These were most common in the fair haired blue eyed workers. B. Actinic keratoses showed an equal distribution of 10 to 12% and 3.5% of workers showed premalignant shagreen skin. C. This was paralled by the development of squamous carcinoma in 2.8% of workers, but only in 0.4% of controls. In one case the carcinoma was scrotal.

Pitchwarts (keratoakanthomas) that were observed in 3.5% of workers at the initial survey compared with 2.7% in controls but over the subsequent 2 years the incidence was 15.7% and only 10.4% of workers were affected, in these over half had multiple lesions. While there was considerable individual variation in the development of pitchwarts there was a definite increase in incidence with prolonged exposure. There was a 4% incidence with 10 to 19 years exposure 20% incidence 20 to 39 years and 75% at 40 to 49 years. It must be recorded however that the one person with over 50 years exposure had not developed a single pitchwart. Those with pitchwarts were all white skinned even though 12.5% of the population at risk were Indian-Negro, but in those developing pitchwarts there was no relationship with hair or eye colour.

Acneform lesions occurred in 93% of the workers and only in 31% of controls. Comedones and acne were three times more common in the workers but folliculitis was ten times more common.

Those workers that developed pitchwarts had a greater tendency to develop other epithelial proliferative lesions, in the benign group 89% as compared with 67% and when the sessile group were assessed the difference was 62% as to 23%. When considering the premalignant lesions the incidence of keratoses was 67% as to 15% and chronic tar dermatoses and pigmentary changes were ten times more frequent in the pitch workers than in the controls. In the malignant proliferative lesions squamous carcinoma was 7.5% as compared to 1.3%, all indicating that the epithelium of the skin and pilosebaceous follicle of certain individuals responds more actively to the stimulus of tar. The site of the lesion was characteristic. 50% of pitchwarts were around the nose, eyes and ears, 28% on the hands and forearms; other sites being scrotum, neck and dorsum of foot. This distribution corresponded with the distribution of the acneform lesions supporting the view that the damaged pilosebaceous follicle may play its part in both lesions.

No histological differences were observed between the lesions of the pitch workers and the control group.

Arsenbedingte Präcancerosen und Cancerosen der Haut*

W. BRAUN, Universitäts-Hautklinik Heidelberg (Deutschland)

Wir wollen über Präcancerosen und Cancerosen als berufsbedingte As-Spätfolgen berichten. Unser Krankengut umfaßt 54 Winzer (Weinbauern) mit gesicherter Arsenexposition durch Umgang mit Insecticiden aus der Zeit von 1921 bis 1942. Alle Kranken hatten die für die Arsenspätintoxikation kennzeichnenden Keratosen der Handteller und Fußsohlen. Von 40 Winzern waren uns die Akten der Berufsgenossenschaft zugänglich. Der Zeitraum zwischen dem wahrscheinlich ersten Kontakt mit arsenhaltigen Insecticiden und der gesetzlich vorgeschriebenen Anzeige der berufsbedingten Arsenfolgen konnte bei 22 Versicherten berechnet werden. Er betrug im Mittel 25 Jahre (3 bis 40 Jahre). Die von uns festgestellten As-Folgen bei 54 Winzern verteilen sich wie folgt (Abb. 1): 54 Kranke mit As-Keratosen, 26 Kranke mit As-Melanosen, 20 Kranke mit malignen Hautveränderungen, 27 Kranke mit chronischer Bronchitis, 22 Kranke mit Bronchialcarcinom, 25 Kranke mit Leberveränderungen (meist Cirrhosen); außerdem bei 8 Kranken Durchblutungsstörungen, 4 Kranken Polyneuritis und bei je einem Kranken ein Dickdarmcarcinom, ein Stimmbandcarcinom, ein Kehlkopfcarcinom, ein Lebersarkom, ein Melanoblastom des Auges.

An *malignen Hautveränderungen* wurden im einzelnen festgestellt: Bei 6 Kranken Basaliome, 12 Kranken Morbus Bowen, 12 Kranken verhornende Plattenepithelcarcinome; bei

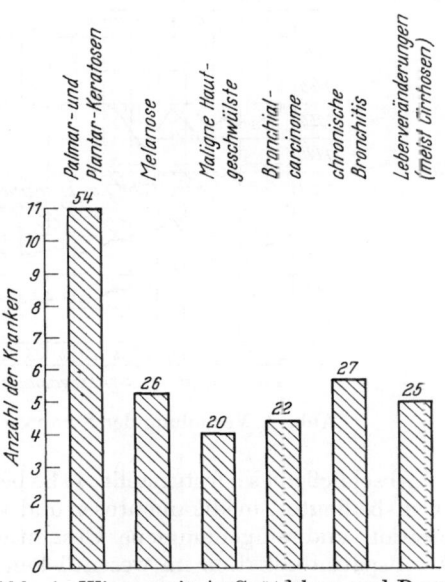

Abb. 1. Winzer mit As-Spätfolgen und Bronchialcarcinom

6 Kranken waren zwei, bei 2 Kranken drei Arten dieser Tumoren gleichzeitig vorhanden. 9 Kranke hatten außerdem ein Bronchialcarcinom. Jeder Typ der Hautgeschwülste kam in der Mehrzahl vor — fast regelmäßig der Morbus Bowen — am meisten am Stamm und an den oberen Extremitäten. Basaliome zeigten gelegentlich die Tendenz zur Verwilderung. In einem Fall war als Besonderheit aus einer Hornwarze an einem Finger ein Cornu cutaneum ohne Übergang in verhornendes Plattenepithelcarcinom, in einem anderen ein Keratoakanthom zu beobachten. Die Keratosen, die auch an Armen und Stamm als kaum erkennbare, flache Tumoren vorhanden sein können [1], sind die Vorstufen für die beobachteten malignen Geschwülste. Die chronische Bronchitis muß bei den ArsenWinzern als Präcancerose gewertet werden und gilt als wichtiges Brückensymptom bei der Entstehung des Lungenkrebses. Die bei ihrer Entdeckung meist inoperablen *Bronchialcarcinome* unserer Patienten führten bei allen 22 Kranken zum Tode. Das Sterbealter betrug im Durchschnitt 57,3 Jahre. Neun Winzer erreichten das 50. Lebensjahr nicht! Die lange Latenzzeit der bösartigen Geschwülste

---

* Die Untersuchungen wurden mit Mitteln der Strebel-Stiftung durchgeführt.

an inneren Organen — unter Bevorzugung der Atemwege — hat dem Arsenspät-
schaden in den letzten 15 Jahren ein neues Gesicht gegeben. ROTH [2] berechnete
1956 für Krebse an inneren Organen der Arsenwinzer (Mosel) 13 bis 22 Jahre. Nach
unserem eigenen Krankengut ist diese Spanne noch größer zu veranschlagen
(Abb. 2). Geht man davon aus, daß die letztmögliche Arsenexposition 1942 bestand (gesetzliches Verbot arsenhaltiger Insecticide im Weinbau), so beträgt bei
unseren Winzern die durchschnittliche Dauer bis zum Tod durch Bronchialcarcinom etwa 15 Jahre (9 bis 24 Jahre). Dieser Zahl muß aber die Dauer der möglichen Arsenexposition hinzugerechnet werden, die 1 bis 21 Jahre betragen haben
kann. (1921 wurden As-haltige Spritzmittel im Weinbau in der hiesigen Gegend
eingeführt.)

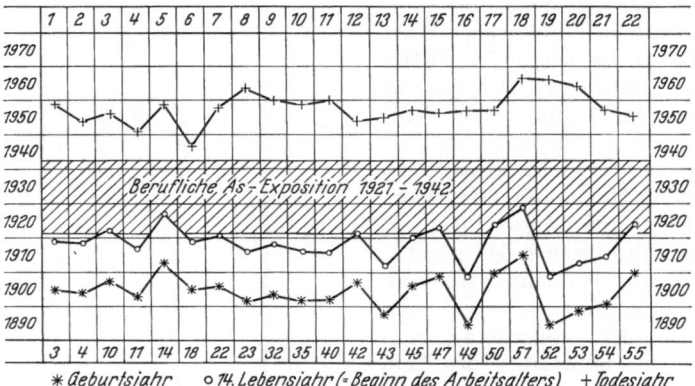

Abb. 2. Verteilung der Symptome bei 54 Winzern mit As-Spätfolgen

Abschließend sei festgestellt: 1. Es besteht prinzipiell *kein* Unterschied zwischen
berufsbedingter, medikamentöser und forensischer Arsenwirkung. Dauer der Ex-
position und aufgenommene Gesamtdosis dürften für den Gesamtverlauf der
Arsenspätintoxikation im wesentlichen verantwortlich sein. — 2. Die Latenzzeit
für die einzelnen Symptome des chronischen Arsenismus ist unterschiedlich:
Melanosen *können* schon nach Wochen, Keratosen nach wenigen Jahren, maligne
Hautgeschwülste nach mehreren Jahren (Minimallatenzzeit nach FIERZ [3]
$3\frac{1}{2}$ Jahre) auftreten. Bei Krebsen an inneren Organen muß die Latenzzeit in
Dekaden angenommen werden, nach unserem Krankengut 15 bis 35 Jahre (nach
SOMMERS und MCMANUS [4]) 13 bis 50 Jahre (Mittel 25 Jahre). — 3. Dem Derma-
tologen kommt durch Erkennung der Arsenspätfolgen und die richtige Beurteilung
des präcancerösen Gesamtzustandes eine wichtige Funktion zu. Es wird seine
Aufgabe sein, Krebsprophylaxe und Therapie auf seinem eigenen Fachgebiet zu
betreiben und die laufende internistische Beobachtung zu veranlassen.

Literatur. 1. BRAUN, W.: Derm. Wschr. **137**, 468 (1958). — 2. ROTH, F.: Z. Krebsforsch.
61, 287 (1956); 468 (1957). — 3. FIERZ, U.: Dermatologica (Basel) **131**, 41 (1965). — 4. SOMMERS,
S. C., u. R. G. MC MANUS: Cancer (Philad.) **6**, 347 (1953).

Beitrag zur Beziehung des Traumas zum Hautcarcinom

M. Schwarzwald, Dermatologische Universitätsklinik Zagreb (Jugoslawien)

Die Pathologen sind im Beurteilen der Beziehungen eines einmaligen Traumas und der Tumorentstehung sehr vorsichtig. Domagk meint, daß auch rein physikalische Ursachen die Entwicklung eines Tumors hervorrufen können und Fischer betont, daß neben dem Trauma auch noch andere Faktoren in Frage kommen.

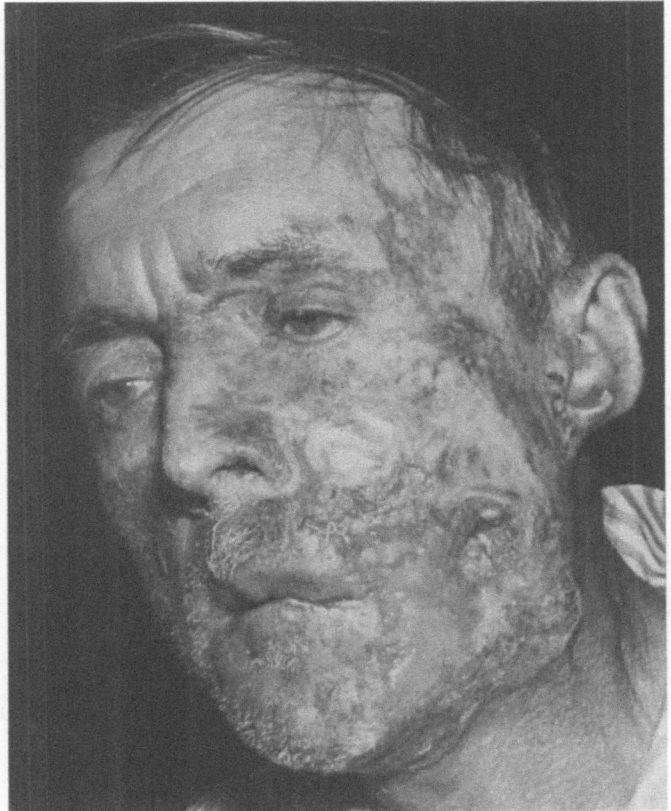

Abb. 1. Posttraumatisches Carcinom auf Lupusnarbe

Aus unserem klinischen Krankengut sollen einige Fälle angeführt werden, wo sich das Carcinom nach einem einmaligen Trauma entwickelte und wo auch die Mitwirkung anderer syncancerogener Faktoren vorausgesetzt werden muß. Ein 63jähriger Patient litt seit seiner Kindheit an Tbc. luposa faciei, die sich auf beide Gesichtsseiten, die Nase und die Ohrmuscheln ausbreitete. Vor einigen Wochen bekam er von einem Pferd auf die linke Seite des Gesichtes einen Hufschlag. Da die traumatische Ulceration keine Heilungstendenz zeigte, wurde der Kranke in die Klinik eingewiesen (Abb. 1). Der histologische Befund ergab ein Carcinoma spinocellulare. Nach Miescher ist die postlupöse Narbe eine Präcancerose im weiteren Sinne. Das einmalige Trauma beschleunigte auf diesem Terrain die Entwicklung des Carcinoms.

Ein 54jähriger Patient arbeitete 7 Jahre als Eisenbahnarbeiter. Beim Tragen einer Schiene entstand eine lineare Verletzung an der linken Seite des Halses. Die Wunde eiterte und vernarbte nie vollständig. Nach 12 Jahren erfolgte Aufnahme in die Klinik. Es bestand ein stellenweise exulceriertes, etwa 12 cm langes, einige Millimeter breites, lineares Infiltrat. Histologisch handelte es sich um ein Basalioma keratoticum. Unterhalb des linearen Infiltrates war die Haut glatt und atrophisch (Druckatrophie), oberhalb war die normale Hautzeichnung erhalten (Abb. 2). Zur Entstehung dieses Carcinoms gab die erste Verletzung, die nie vollkommen verheilte, wahrscheinlich die erste Anregung. Hier haben wir es also mit einem Trauma und einem chronischen Entzündungsprozeß zu tun. Weitere chro-

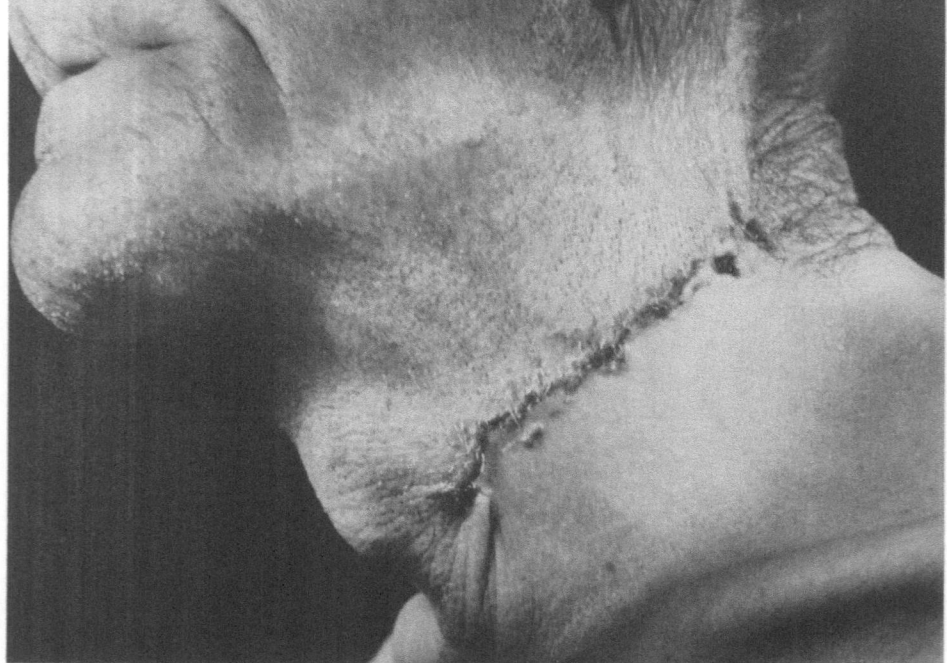

Abb. 2. Posttraumatisches Carcinom

nische Traumata in Form von Dehnung der Haut im Grenzgebiet normaler und atrophischer Haut beim Tragen von Schienen betrachten wir als zusätzliche Ursachen für die Entwicklung dieses Carcinoms.

Nun noch einige Bemerkungen zur Lokalisation des Carcinoms an der Unterlippe. 29 damit behaftete Kranke von insgesamt 216 erinnern sich, daß der Affektion ein Trauma vorausgegangen ist. 16 Kranke führen eine Verbrennung durch eine Zigarette an; einer eine Verbrennung durch Kalk; fünf Verletzungen durch Messer, Rasierklinge oder Biß, die übrigen berichten über einen Schlag mit einem harten Gegenstand. Nur eine Kranke führt eine Verletzung der oberen Lippe mit einem Löffel an. Nach 8 Monaten wurde Spinaliom festgestellt.

Die Unterlippe eines erwachsenen Mannes weist gewöhnlich keine klinischen Veränderungen auf. Darum wird sie unter den Präcancerosen im weiteren oder engeren Sinne meist auch nicht erwähnt. Verschiedenen Statistiken gemäß erscheinen durchschnittlich 95% der Hautcarcinome an photoexponierten Stellen.

Hierher gehört natürlich auch die Unterlippe, was als Beweis für die Bedeutung des Insultes der Sonnen-Irradiation in der Genese des Carcinoms an exponierten Stellen zu werten ist.

Von 1875 Hautcarcinomen, einschließlich der Lippen, fanden wir bei Männern 199 Carcinome der Unterlippe, bei Frauen nur 17. Insgesamt waren an der Unterlippe 216 Carcinome lokalisiert. Die auffallend große Zahl von Männern führt zum Schlusse, daß neben chronischen Reizungen durch Sonnenstrahlung, die nach MIESCHER zur reparatorischen Hyperkompensation führen, auch noch andere Faktoren bestehen, die die Entwicklung des Carcinoms begünstigen. In erster Linie denken wir dabei an die chemische Reizung des durch Speichel erweichten Zigarettentabaks.

Wegen der lange Jahre dauernden Einwirkung der erwähnten zwei Faktoren befindet sich die Schleimhaut der Unterlippe in einer gewissen präcancerosen Bereitschaft, die schließlich zur Entwicklung eines Carcinoms führt. Weitere Traumatisierungen können dann die Realisierung eines Carcinoms beschleunigen. Dies beweist die schnelle Entwicklung des Carcinoms der Unterlippe nach Verbrennung mit der Zigarette. Nach anamnestischen Angaben ist die Verbrennung mit der Zigarette der histologischen Carcinomdiagnose einige Wochen oder Monate vorangegangen. Zwischen der Verbrennung selbst und dem Moment der Diagnosestellung besteht ein gewisses Kontinuum, weil in der Zwischenzeit die Brandwunde nicht verheilt ist. Ebenso hat sich das Carcinom nach dem Hufschlag schnell in eine postlupöse Narbe entwickelt. Bei den übrigen Kranken hat sich das Carcinom in Verbindung mit dem Trauma innerhalb des ersten Jahres entwickelt. Aus unseren Betrachtungen schließen wir, daß die Realisation eines Tumors oft durch eine größere Zahl verschiedener syncancerogener Faktoren beschleunigt wird.

(Prä-)Cancerosen und Elastose

G. NIEBAUER, II. Universitäts-Hautklinik Wien (Österreich)

Die chronische Lichtschädigung der Haut ist ein wesentlicher Faktor für die Carcinomentstehung. Das ist seit den Untersuchungen von DUBREUILH (1907) bekannt, der die Umwandlung seniler Keratosen in Plattenepithelkrebs bei pigmentarmen Menschen häufiger als bei stark pigmentierten Individuen beobachtet hat. Auch die Auswertung des histologisch verifizierten Materials der II. Universitäts-Hautklinik in Wien aus den Jahren 1955 bis 1965, nach Lokalisation und Alter geordnet, beweist das hauptsächliche Auftreten der Carcinome und Präcancerosen in den sog. „exponierten" Regionen bei Menschen älter als 50 Jahre [genauere Angaben s. NIEBAUER und ZENKER (1966)].

	exponierte Region	bedeckte Region	Gesamtzahl
Basaliome	1 963	431	2 394
Spinaliome	329	32	361

	unter 50 Jahre	über 50 Jahre	Gesamtzahl
Basaliome	274	2 120	2 394
Spinaliome	40	321	361

Unter „exponierten" Regionen sind Kopf, Hals, Nacken und Handrücken gemeint. Die 32 Spinaliome in den sog. „bedeckten" Regionen sind meist in Verbrennungsnarben, langdauernden Ulcera, chronischen Röntgenschäden usw.

3*

aufgetreten. In der Gruppe der Basaliome wurde kein Unterschied gemacht zwischen den „einfachen" Basaliomen und den sog. Metatypischen Epitheliomen. In dieser Gruppe sind 431 in den sog. „bedeckten" Regionen aufgetreten. Aber von diesen sind 397 sog. „multizentrische, langsamwachsende Basaliome der Rumpfhaut", die als naevoide Bildungen zu werten und für deren Auftreten daher auch andere Mechanismen verantwortlich zu machen sind. Ein Teil dieser Fälle ist durch Arsen provoziert worden.

In unserem Patientenmaterial (hauptsächlich aus Wien und Umgebung) sind regelmäßig mehr oder weniger stark ausgebildete degenerative Veränderungen des Bindegewebes in den „exponierten" Hautregionen ab dem 40. bis 50. Lebensjahr histologisch nachweisbar.

Das Hauptmerkmal dieser Veränderungen sind einerseits die altersbegünstigte Hypertrophie der elastischen Fasern und andererseits der gleichzeitige Abbau (oder die Auflösung) des kollagenen Fasermaterials. Diese *beiden* zur gleichen Zeit ablaufenden degenerativen Veränderungen des Bindegewebes werden heute als Elastosis senilis sive actinica bezeichnet. Es ist nur eine Frage der histologischen Methode, ob der einen oder anderen Strukturveränderung größere Bedeutung zuerkannt wird. Denn bei den lichtoptischen Untersuchungen (histologische und histochemische Technik) steht die Hyperplasie der elastischen Fasern und die stoffliche und gestaltliche Abänderung ihrer Hüll- und Kittmassen im Vordergrund (FEYRTER und NIEBAUER, 1966), während bei den elektronenoptischen Untersuchungen die Schädigung des kollagenen Fasermaterials, die zum Abbau und zur Auflösung der Fasern führt, der eindrucksvollste Befund ist (NIEBAUER und STOCKINGER, 1965). Daß hier tatsächlich eine Veränderung im Sinne einer degenerativen *Atrophie* vorliegt, beweisen die bei aktinischer Elastose durchgeführten historadiografischen Untersuchungen: in allen Zonen der aktinischen Elastose (auch in ihren Anfangstadien!) ist ein Verlust an Gewebsmasse (d. h. ein relativ geringeres Trockengewicht als in der normalen Cutis) nachweisbar.

Diese bindegewebigen Veränderungen treten immer nur an den freigetragenen Körperstellen auf, und zwar um so stärker und früher, je mehr diese Menschen der Einwirkung des Lichtes ausgesetzt waren und je hellhäutiger (pigmentärmer) sie sind. Die Wellenlänge, die zum UV-Erythem führt und die bei chronischer Applikation auch eine Elastose hervorrufen kann, stimmt mit derjenigen überein, die beim Versuchstier ein Hautcarcinom erzeugt; sie liegt im Bereich von 2900 bis 3200 Å (MACKIE und McGOVERN, 1958).

In unserem Material sind nur eine geringe Zahl von Patienten jünger als 50 Jahre. Von den 40 Spinaliompatienten war keiner jünger als 30 Jahre. In allen Fällen war im Tumorstroma eine Elastose nachweisbar. Bei den 274 Basaliompatienten der jüngeren Altersgruppe handelt es sich entweder um sog. „Naevobasaliome" oder um Tumoren, die ebenfalls durch eine Elastose der Umgebung charakterisiert sind. Somit tritt die überwiegende Mehrzahl von Hautcarcinomen in Regionen auf, wo das Bindegewebe degenerativ, d. h. in Form einer sog. aktinischen Elastose geschädigt ist.

Auf Grund der Erfahrung gilt als sicher, daß diese bindegewebigen Veränderungen der Carcinomentstehung *voraus*gehen. Welche Faktoren letztlich für die Carcinomentstehung verantwortlich sind, ist allerdings nicht bekannt. Zweifellos kommt es im Rahmen der Elastose zur zusätzlichen Schädigung der Epidermis, die sich im weiteren Verlaufe als Atrophie der Epidermis äußert.

In diesem Zusammenhang soll auf Befunde hingewiesen werden, die bisher bei Fragen der Cancerogenese keine Beachtung gefunden haben:

1. In der normalen Epidermis sind regelmäßig suprabasal gelegene Dendritenzellen (Langerhanszellen) nachweisbar. Ihr Verhältnis zur Malpighizelle ist 4 bis

8:1. In der atrophischen Epidermis ist die Zahl der Langerhanszellen stark reduziert. In Fällen weit fortgeschrittener degenerativer Atrophie können sie unter Umständen auch völlig fehlen.

2. Bei Anwendung einer geeigneten Färbung (z. B. der Osmium-Zink-Jodidmethode) lassen sich im gesamten Parenchym der Basaliome und in den Tumorrandzonen der Spinaliome Dendritenzellen ungemein zahlreich nachweisen. Aus elektronenoptischen Befunden geht hervor, daß diese Tumor-Dendritenzellen teilweise identisch sind mit den Langerhanszellen der normalen Haut oder mit den Melanocyten.

3. Die Untersuchungen von WIEDMANN sprechen für eine neurotrophische Funktion der Dendritenzellen. In der geschädigten (atrophischen) Epidermis ist ihre Zahl stark reduziert. Ihr zahlreiches Auftreten in den Hautcarcinomen könnte somit im Sinne einer kompensatorischen Gegenregulation aufgefaßt werden.

Literatur. FEYRTER, F., u. G. NIEBAUER: Derm. Wschr. **152**, 1176 (1966). — NIEBAUER, G., u. L. STOCKINGER: Arch. klin. exp. Derm. **221**, 122 (1965). — NIEBAUER, G., u. F. ZENKER: Przegl. Derm. **53**, 687 (1966).

Les nucléases des tumeurs épidermiques*

J. DE BERSAQUES et J. PIÉRARD, Clinique Dermatologique de l'Université de Gand (Belgique)

L'importance du catabolisme des acides nucléiques dans l'épiderme normal, où ils sont dépolymérisés au moment de la kératinisation, et dans les tumeurs, où certains admettent une altération de leur métabolisme en rapport avec la malignité, nous a incités à doser l'activité de la ribonucléase (RNase) et de la désoxyribonucléase (DNase) dans les épithéliomas cutanés.

Les méthodes utilisées sont des microadaptations (volume final 120 μl) des techniques de précipitation de FIERS (1961) pour la RNase déterminée à pH 7,2 et de SCHNEIDER et HOGEBOOM (1952) pour la DNase II déterminée à pH 5,0. L'activité de la DNase I à pH neutre était chaque fois très minime ou nulle. L'unité d'activité enzymatique correspond à une augmentation de une unité de la densité optique à 260 nm après 1 h d'incubation à 37°. Les dosages ont été effectués sur des fragments obtenus par dissection de coupes lyophilisées. Ils ont porté sur 21 épithéliomas baso-cellulaires, 5 spino-cellulaires et 2 maladies de Bowen; nous les comparerons aux résultats de 12 échantillons d'épiderme normal et de 25 cas de psoriasis.

L'activité de la DNase II était en moyenne de 11,3 (valeurs extrêmes 5,0 à 19,0) unités par mg de poids sec dans les baso-cellulaires, de 7,3 (3,9 à 13,5) unités dans les spino-cellulaires et de 7,9 et 8,9 unités dans les Bowen, contre 2,9 (1,8 à 5,3) unités dans l'épiderme normal et 4,7 (2,3 à 8,6) unités dans l'épiderme psoriasique. L'activité de la RNase était de 65 (28 à 170) unités par mg dans les baso-cellulaires contre 30 (20 à 44) unités dans l'épiderme normal et 52 (19 à 171) unités dans l'épiderme psoriasique.

L'augmentation des activités enzymatiques mesurées dans les baso-cellulaires n'apparaît plus aussi évidente quand on prend comme référence la quantité d'acide désoxyribonucléique (ADN) ou le nombre de noyaux au lieu du poids sec. La quantité d'enzyme par cellule serait à peu près semblable à celle de cellules normales: un peu plus élevée pour la DNase, un peu plus faible pour la RNase.

* Travail réalisé avec le soutien du Fonds de la Recherche Scientifique Médicale.

Nos résultats ne concordent pas avec le travail histochimique de STEIGLEDER et FISCHER (1963) pour qui RNase et DNase sont absentes du parenchyme tumoral, la RNase seule étant présente en quantité appréciable dans le stroma péritumoral.

Le rôle de ces nucléases dans la cellule vivante est encore loin d'être éclairci. On admet que ces enzymes sont en grande partie localisées dans les lysosomes, d'où elles ne seraient libérées qu'au moment de la destruction de la cellule, sous l'effet de certaines agressions ou peut-être à certains moments particuliers de la vie cellulaire. Elles serviraient à un nettoyage préludant à la réutilisation des fragments libérés. Ainsi, sans en comprendre encore le mécanisme exact, a-t-on supposé qu'une forte activité de RNase accompagnait une synthèse active de protéines et que de même la DNase II était en relation avec la synthèse de l'ADN. L'augmentation de l'activité de la DNase précéderait celle de la synthèse de l'ADN: elle servirait à fournir les matériaux nécessaires à cette dernière (LAQUERRIÉRE et LAUMONNIER, 1961; ADAMS, 1963; PRIVAT DE GARILHE, 1964). Cependant, l'activité enzymatique des tumeurs malignes est variable et même souvent abaissée (VORBRODT, 1962; DAOUST et AMANO, 1963; DALE, 1965), ce qui donnerait raison à BRODY et BALIS (1958) qui ont supposé que l'équilibre existant entre la synthèse de l'ADN et les nucléases dans les tissus normaux ou en hyperplasie bénigne, était rompu dans les néoplasmes. Cette hypothèse n'est peut-être pas valable pour les épithéliomas baso-cellulaires, tumeurs dont la malignité est relativement réduite.

Bibliographie. ADAMS, R. L. P.: Biochem. J. **87**, 532 (1963). — BRODY, S., and M. E· BALIS: Nature (Lond.) **182**, 940 (1958). — DALE, R. A.: Clin. chim. Acta **11**, 547 (1965). — DAOUST, R., and H. AMANO: Cancer Res. **23**, 131 (1963). — FIERS, W.: Analyt. Biochem. **2**, 123 (1961). — LAQUERRIÈRE, R., et R. LAUMONNIER: Arch. Biol. (Liège) **74**, 555 (1963). — PRIVAT DE GARILHE, M.: Les nucléases. Paris: Hermann 1964. — SCHNEIDER, W. C., and G. H. HOGEBOOM: J. biol. Chem. **198**, 155 (1952). — STEIGLEDER, G. K., u. I. FISCHER: Arch. klin. exp. Derm. **217**, 553 (1963). — VORBRODT, A.: Acta Un. int. Cancr. **18**, 66 (1962).

Vergleichende cytophotometrische Untersuchungen an metatypischen Basalzellepitheliomen und Plattenepithelcarcinomen der Haut*

G. EHLERS, Universitäts-Hautklinik Gießen (Deutschland)

In den Jahren 1963 bis 1965 haben wir cytophotometrische Untersuchungen über den DNS-Gehalt von Basalzellepitheliomen unterschiedlicher klinischer und histologischer Ausgestaltung durchgeführt. Dabei kamen wir zu folgenden Ergebnissen:

Basalzellepitheliome soliden und adenomatösen Aufbaues weisen ähnlich normalen somatischen Zellen eine Gruppierung der DNS-Werte um das diploide Zentrum auf. Die Streuung in den hypodiploiden und interdiploid-tetraploiden Raum ist gering.

Metatypische Basalzellepitheliome vom Typ des Épithéliome métatypique mixte oder Épithéliome métatypique intermédiaire weichen im DNS-Aufbau von Basalzellepitheliomen typischer Ausgestaltung ab. Eine diploide Gipfelbildung wird vermißt. Dagegen sind Gruppierungen um einen bestimmten DNS-Gehalt in der interdiploid-tetraploiden, tetraploiden sowie hypertetraploiden Phase zu er-

---

* Mit Unterstützung der Deutschen Forschungsgemeinschaft.

kennen. Die Streuung der DNS-Werte ist erheblich und bis in hyperoktoplaide Bereiche zu verfolgen (Abb. 1).

Da sich metatypische Basalzellepitheliome im Hinblick auf klinische, cytologische und cytophotometrische Merkmale echten Carcinomen nähern, dehnten wir unsere Untersuchungen auf Plattenepithelcarcinome der Haut und Übergangsschleimhaut, vergleichsweise auch auf cutane Metastasen von Tumoren innerer Organe aus.

Über DNS-Bestimmungen mittels der Punktmethode an feulgengefärbten Gewebsschnitten von Plattenepithelcarcinomen der Haut berichteten STOWELL; SACCHI; KINT. ATKIN und RICHARDS haben am Ausstrichpräparat den DNS-Gehalt eines Carcinoma spinocellulare der Wangen- und Zungenschleimhaut überprüft. Vergleichende cytophotometrische Untersuchungen zwischen metatypischen Basalzellepitheliomen und Plattenepithelcarcinomen der Haut sind bisher nicht bekannt.

Material und Methodik

Der DNS-Gehalt von je 100 Tumorzellen wurde auf halbquantitativem Wege nach Feulgen-Färbung im sichtbaren Licht bei der Wellenlänge 560 nm am Mikrodensitometer nach DEELEY bestimmt. Zur Ermittlung des diploiden DNS-Gehaltes verwendeten wir menschliche Thymuslymphocyten, die bereits vorher auf demselben Objektträger aufgetragen und somit gleichen histochemischen Bedingungen wie die Tumorzellen unterworfen waren. In entsprechenden Verteilungsdiagrammen wurden in der Abszisse die Arbeitseinheiten AE (AE = Integrationswert der gemessenen Extinktionen), in der Ordinate die Anzahl der gemessenen Zellen (n) aufgetragen.

Zur Untersuchung gelangten folgende Geschwülste:

I. Metatypische Basalzellepitheliome: sieben Fälle, davon

1. Épithéliome métatypique mixte: drei Fälle.

2. Épithéliome métatypique intermédiaire: vier Fälle.

II. Plattenepithelcarcinome der Haut und Übergangsschleimhäute: neun Fälle, davon

1. Plattenepithelcarcinome mit starker Verhornungstendenz: drei Fälle,

2. Plattenepithelcarcinome mit geringer Verhornungstendenz: drei Fälle,

3. Entdifferenzierte Plattenepithelcarcinome (Carcinoma epidermoidale, sog. Bowen-Carcinom): drei Fälle.

III. Cutane Metastasen eines Adeno-Carcinoms: ein Fall.

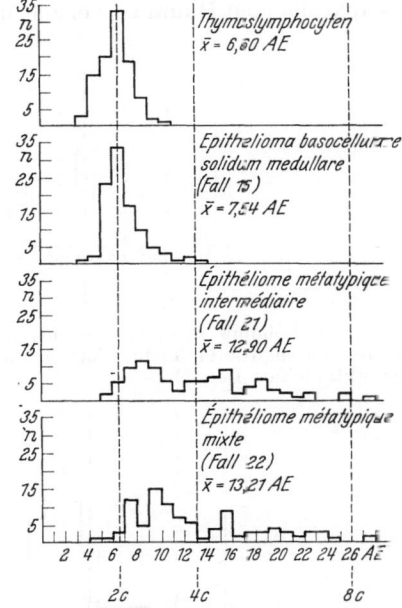

Abb. 1. Cytophotometrische Messung von je 100 Thymuslymphocyten und Zellen unterschiedlicher Basaliomformen im sichtbaren Licht nach Feulgen-Färbung. Identische diploide Gipfelbildung menschlicher Thymuslymphocyten und des Epithelioma basocellulare solidum medullare. Breite Streuung der DNS-Werte mit Gipfelbildung im interdiploid-tetraploiden Raum beim Épithéliome métatypique intermédiaire und Épithéliome metatypique mixte. Zunahme des mittleren DNS-Gehaltes x̄ bei metatypischen Basalzellepitheliomen

Untersuchungsergebnisse

Menschliche Thymuslymphocyten zeigen ein diploides DNS-Verteilungsmuster mit geringer Streuung der Werte in den hypo- und interdiploid-tetraploiden Raum.

Die bisher an metatypischen Basalzellepitheliomen gewonnenen Untersuchungsergebnisse sind reproduzierbar. Diese Geschwülste lassen bei großer Streuung der
DNS-Werte bis in hyperoktoploide Bereiche gewöhnlich in den interdiploid-tetraploiden, selten in den hypertetraploiden Raum verschobene Tumorstammlinien
erkennen. Beim Épithéliome métatypique intermédiaire finden sich DNS-Schwer-
punkte in der hyperdiploiden, tetraploiden oder hypertetraploiden Phase (Abb. 2).
Auch das Épithéliome métatypique mixte ist durch DNS-Gruppierungen in der
hyperdipoliden bzw. hypertetraploiden Phase gekennzeichnet.

Stark verhornende Plattenepithelcarcinome zeigen in allen untersuchten Fällen
eine hypertetraploide Stammlinie. Die Streuung der DNS-Werte ist bis in den
hyperoktoploiden Raum zu verfolgen (Abb. 3).

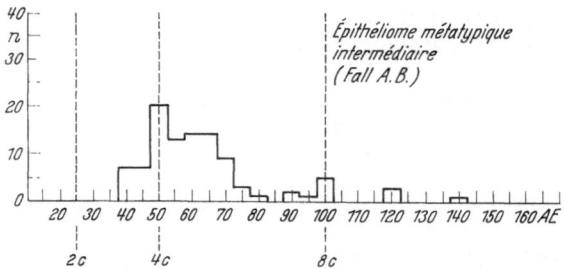

Abb. 2. Épithéliome métatypique intermédiaire. Cytophotometrische Messung des DNS-
Gehaltes im sichtbaren Licht. Tetraploider Gipfel mit Streuung der DNS-Werte bis in den
hyperoktoploiden Bereich

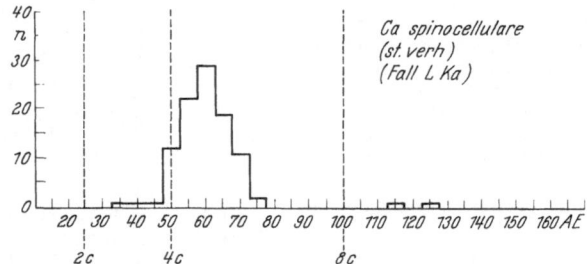

Abb. 3. Plattenepithelcarcinom mit starker Verhornungstendenz. Cytophotometrische Messung des DNS-Gehaltes im sichtbaren Licht. Tumorstammlinie in der hypertetraploiden
Phase mit Streuung der DNS-Werte bis in den hyperoktoploiden Raum

Gering verhornende Plattenepithelcarcinome weisen ebenfalls DNS-Gipfel in
der tetraploiden bzw. hypertetraploiden Phase auf. Die DNS-Streuung reicht bis
in den hyperoktoploiden Bereich.

Bei entdifferenzierten Plattenepithelcarcinomen unter dem Bild des Carcinoma
epidermoidale bzw. des sog. Bowen-Carcinoms liegen bei großer Streuung der
DNS-Werte bis in den hyperoktoploiden Raum die Tumorstammlinien im hypertetraploiden Bereich (Abb. 4).

Im DNS-Verteilungsmuster cutaner Metastasen eines Adenocarcinoms wird
eine Stammlinie vermißt. Eine Gruppierung von Tumorzellen fällt besonders im
hyperoktoploiden Bereich auf. Die erhebliche Streuung der aneuploiden Geschwulstzellen reicht bis 16c (Abb. 5).

Aus dem folgenden Kombinationsdiagramm ist die Verschiebung der Stamm-
linien von Zellen mit diploidem Chromosomensatz bis zu aneuploiden Zellen cuta-

ner Metastasen zu ersehen. Die Gipfelbildung menschlicher Thymuslymphocyten liegt im diploiden Bereich bei 2c, die des Épithéliome métatypique intermédiaire im tetraploiden Raum bei 4c. Plattenepithelcarcinome mit unterschiedlicher Verhornungstendenz und entdifferenzierte Plattenepithelcarcinome lassen die Stammlinie in der hypertetraploiden Phase erkennen. Bei der cutanen Metastase eines Adenocarcinoms wird eine Stammlinie vermißt. Der mittlere DNS-Gehalt $\bar{x}$ zeigt menschlichen Thymuslymphocyten gegenüber beim Épithéliome métatypique intermédiaire, Carcinoma spinocellulare und Carcinoma epidermoidale eine Verdoppelung, bei einer cutanen Carcinom-Metastase eine Verdreifachung (Abb. 6).

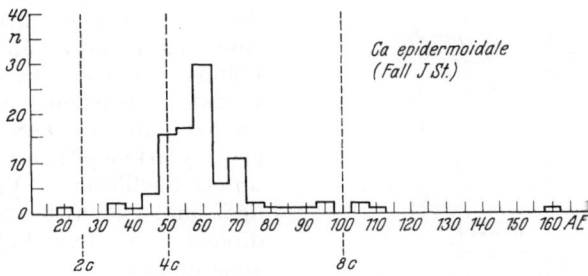

Abb. 4. Entdifferenziertes Plattenepithelcarcinom unter dem Bild des Carcinoma epidermoidale. Cytophotometrische Messung des DNS-Gehaltes im sichtbaren Licht. Ausbildung einer Stammlinie im hypertetraploiden Raum mit Streuung der DNS-Werte bis in die hyperoktoploide Phase.

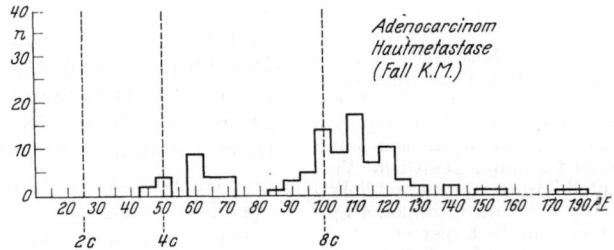

Abb. 5. Cutane Metastase eines Adenocarcinoms. Cytophotometrische Messung des DNS-Gehaltes im sichtbaren Licht. Starke Streuung der DNS-Werte bis in den hyperoktoploiden Bereich mit Gruppierung der DNS-Werte um 110 AE

Fassen wir unsere Untersuchungsergebnisse zusammen, so ergeben sich folgende Befunde:

Metatypische Basalzellepitheliome weisen unterschiedlich stark ausgeprägte und in verschiedenen DNS-Bereichen lokalisierte Tumorstammlinien auf. Diese sind im interdiploid-tetraploiden, tetraploiden oder hypertetraploiden Raum nachweisbar. Die Ausbildung von Gruppierungen um einen bestimmten DNS-Gehalt ist abhängig von der cytologischen Ausgestaltung des Tumors. Gegenüber normalen somatischen Zellen und Basalzellepitheliomen typischen Aufbaues findet sich in der DNS-Verteilung ein deutlicher, gegenüber Plattenepithelcarcinomen der Haut dann ein Unterschied, wenn ihre DNS-Schwerpunktbildungen oder Tumorstammlinien in der interdiploid-tetraploiden Phase gelegen sind. Beiden Geschwulsttypen gemeinsam dagegen ist die große Streubreite der DNS-Werte bis in den hyperoktoploiden Bereich mit Verdoppelung des mittleren DNS-Gehaltes gegenüber normalen somatischen Zellen.

Plattenepithelcarcinome der Haut und Übergangsschleimhäute zeigen im DNS-Verteilungsmuster untereinander nur geringe Unterschiede. Tumorstamm-linien sind in der tetraploiden oder hypertetraploiden Phase zu erkennen. Zellen in verhornenden oder nekrotischen Tumorabschnitten weisen einen niedrigeren DNS-Gehalt auf.

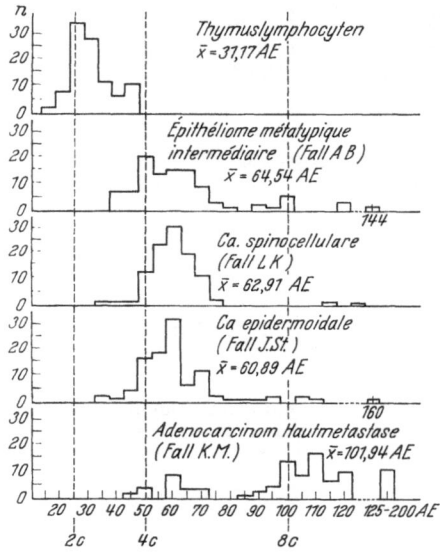

Differenzen in der DNS-Ausstattung zwischen stark verhornenden, gering verhornenden und entdifferenzierten Plattenepithelcarcinomen konnten nicht nachgewiesen werden, da am Ausstrichpräparat die Erfassung von Tumorzellen nach der Einteilung von CASPERSSON und SANDRITTER nicht möglich war. Somit wird die Streuung der DNS-Werte bei einigen Plattenepithelcarcinomen mit unterschiedlicher Verhornungstendenz und Geschwulstnekrosen bis in diploide und hypodiploide Bereiche verständlich.

Aus den angegebenen Gründen lassen sich mit unserer Untersuchungsmethode Rückschlüsse vom DNS-Verteilungsmuster auf den Malignitätsgrad unterschiedlich differenzierter Plattenepithelcarcinome nicht ziehen. Der klinisch malignere Verlauf von Plattenepithelcarcinomen der Übergangsschleimhäute ist cytophotometrisch ebenfalls nicht faßbar.

Abb. 6. Cytophotometrische Messung von je 100 Thymuslymphocyten, Zellen eines metatypischen Basalzellepithelioms, unterschiedlicher Plattenepithelcarcinome und einer cutanen Metastase eines Adenocarcinoms im sichtbaren Licht nach Feulgen-Färbung. Deutliche Verschiebung der Gipfelbildung von menschlichen Thymuslymphocyten bis zum Carcinoma epidermoidale nach rechts in die hypertetraploide Phase, fehlende Stammlinie bei Zellen einer Hautmetastase. Zunahme des mittleren DNS-Gehaltes x̄ bei Tumoren und Metastasen der Haut

Das DNS-Verteilungsmuster cutaner Metastasen eines Adenocarcinoms weicht von dem der metatypischen Basalzellepitheliome und Plattenepithelcarcinome ab. Sowohl das Fehlen der Tumorstammlinie als auch die starke Streuung der DNS-Werte mit weiterer Zunahme des mittleren DNS-Gehaltes lassen auf die erhebliche Verwilderung der Tumorzellen cutaner Metastasen schließen.

Zusammenfassend: Die vergleichenden cytophotometrischen Untersuchungen an Basalzellepitheliomen und Plattenepithelcarcinomen der Haut haben die bereits früher vertretene Ansicht, daß metatypische Basalzellepitheliome auf Grund klinischer und cytologischer Merkmale eine Sonderstellung einnehmen, bestätigt. Auch im Hinblick auf die DNS-Ausstattung nähern sie sich echten Carcinomen der Haut.

Literatur. ATKIN, N. B., and B. M. RICHARDS: Brit. J. Cancer **10**, 769 (1956). — CASPERSSON, T.: Zit. nach SANDRITTER, W. (1952). — EHLERS, G.: Zur Klinik, Histopathologie und Cytologie der Basalzellepitheliome unter besonderer Berücksichtigung cytophotometrischer Untersuchungen im ultravioletten und sichtbaren Licht. Habilitationsschrift, Gießen 1965. — Arch. klin. exp. Derm. **224**, 329, 355 (1966). — Z. Haut- u. Geschl.-Kr. **41**, 261 (1966). — Fortschr. Med. **84**, 463 (1966). — Krebsforschung u. Krebsbekämpfung **6**, 121 (1967). —

KINT, A.: J. Invest. Derm. **40**, 95 (1963). — SACCHI, S.: Atti Soc. ital. Derm. Sif. **1959**, 403. — SANDRITTER, W.: Naturwissenschaften **39**, 46, 47 (1952). — Frankfurt. Z. Path. **63**, 387 (1952). — STOWELL, R. E.: Soc. exp. Biol. **1**, 190 (1947).

Respiratory Enzymes Activity in Human Skin Neoplasms and Some Praecancerous Lesions*

D. CERIMELE, F. SERRI and C. PELFINI, Istituto di Clinica Dermatologica dell'Università, Policlinico S. Matteo, Pavia (Italy)

The relation between respiratory enzyme activity and neoplasms is still doubtful. The leading idea of WARBURG on the shift from aerobic to anaerobic metabolism in neoplasms is not yet settled.

The problem is made still more difficult by many factors: the methods, biochemical or histochemical, the subjects, if humans or animals, the neoplasms, if spontaneous or experimental.

In human squamous cell cancer succinic dehydrogenase activity is low, while lactic and malic dehydrogenase activity is high (MONIS et al., 1959; KAWAKATSU and MORI, 1963). Cytochrome oxidase activity in neoplasms is less high than in stem cells (HANNIBAL et al., 1960). In basal cell epitheliomas succinic dehydrogenase activity is higher than in squamous cell epitheliomas (SERRI, 1955; BRAUN-FALCO and RATHJENS, 1955).

In a previous report on the distribution of respiratory enzymes in human senile skin we observed that in exposed skin lactic dehydrogenase activity was increased, while other enzyme activities were not so well represented (CERIMELE, 1965). As the exposed skin may be considered a praecancerous condition, according to the high frequency of neoplasms observed, we have studied with the same methods many neoplasms of the skin.

Materials and Methods. 29 neoplastic or praecancerous lesions have been studied: among these 16 were basaliomas, 9 were squamous cell epitheliomas, 2 actinic cheilitis and 2 senile hyperkeratosis. The histochemical methods followed have been referred to in a previous paper.

The following enzymes have been studied: succinic and isocitric dehydrogenase, cytochrome oxidase and lactic dehydrogenase: the first two are representative of the Krebs cycle, the cytochrome oxidase is the enzyme to which is owed the reduction of molecular oxygen, lactic dehydrogenase is an enzyme of the glycolitic cycle.

Results. In basaliomas all the enzyme activities were depressed with the exception of succinic dehydrogenase.

In squamous cells epitheliomas isocitric and lactic dehydrogenase activities were highly represented. Succinic dehydrogenase and cytochrome oxidase also were well demonstrable, even if not so outstanding as the aforementioned enzymes.

In some praecancerous lesions studied (actinic cheilitis and senile hyperkeratosis) the hyperplastic epithelium showed high activity of all enzymes studied.

Discussion. The results we have obtained are in agreement with the idea that squamous cells epithelioma and, in lower degree, actinic cheilitis and senile hyperkeratosis, are compound by actively growing epithelium. Namely all the enzymes have been demonstrated very active.

---

* This work was supported in part by C. N. R. GRANT, No. 115.0633.01346.

As to the squamous cells epithelioma we have not been able to get striking results, meaning some peculiar alteration in metabolic pathways of neoplastic cells. The very high activity of lactic dehydrogenase and the relatively moderate activity of succinic dehydrogenase and cytochrome oxidase are not sufficient to state a shift from aerobic to anaerobic pathways, because also isocitric activity is very high: otherwise should be necessary to guess that isocitric dehydrogenase has some metabolic function outside the Krebs cycle.

As to basalioma the very low activity of some enzymes, except succinic dehydrogenase, support the idea that basalioma is not really a malignant tumor, but could be a nevoid tumor (hamartoma) as stated by LEVER (1961). In any case the difference between the enzyme activities in basaliomas and squamous cell epitheliomas is really striking.

References. BRAUN-FALCO, O., u. B. RATHJENS: Arch. klin. exp. Derm. **199**, 152 (1955). — CERIMELE, D.: Boll. Soc. ital. Biol. sper. **XLI**, 19 (1965). — HANNIBAL, M. J., M. M. NACHLAS, and A. M. SELIGMAN: Cancer (Philad.) **13**, 1008 (1960). — KAWAKATSU, K., and M. MORI: Cancer Res. **23**, 539 (1963). — MONIS, B., M. M. NACHLAS, and A. M. SELIGMAN: Cancer (Philad.) **12**, 1238 (1959). — SERRI, F.: Minerva derm. **30**, supl. 12 (1955).

Etude histochimique et biochimique comparée de certaines activités enzymatiques dans les cancers de la peau

J. HEWITT, M. GUIGON et J. BOLUBASZ, Laboratoire de Recherches Dermatologiques, Hôpital Broca, Paris (France)

Ce travail étudie essentiellement l'activité de la glucose-6-phosphate-déshydrogénase dans les épithéliomas cutanés. L'isocitrate-déshydrogénase à NADP n'a été étudiée que dans quelques cas, comparativement à la glucose-6-phosphate-déshydrogénase. Nous avons choisi la glucose-6-phosphate-déshydrogénase pour différentes raisons:

— elle est augmentée dans des cancers de divers organes (COHEN, 1964; MORI, 1964);

— elle intervient dans la kératinisation normale et pathologique, comme nous l'avons montré au Congrès d'Histochimie de Francfort (1964);

— enfin, elle peut s'étudier comparativement sur des portions très voisines de la même tumeur par deux méthodes différentes dans leur principe: la mise en évidence histochimique par la méthode au tétrazolium, sur tissu frais coupé au cryostat, et d'autre part, le dosage biochimique sur l'homogénat de la tumeur, par mesure spectrophotométrique dans l'ultra-violet.

L'isocitrate-déshydrogénase a été choisie comme autre enzyme fonctionnant avec le même coenzyme, le NADP; elle peut être étudiée par les mêmes méthodes. L'étude a porté sur 12 épithéliomas spino-cellulaires et 18 épithéliomas baso-cellulaires.

Résultats

Pour les épithéliomas spino-cellulaires, dans la plupart des cas, les méthodes histochimique et biochimique ont donné des résultats concordants, montrant une forte augmentation de l'activité de la glucose-6-phosphate-déshydrogénase (tableau); dans tous les cas sauf un, il s'agissait d'épithéliomas kératinisants, souvent dyskératosiques. Quelques cas ont montré une discordance relative entre les résultats histochimiques et biochimiques:

Tableau. *Activité de la Glucose-6-phosphate-déshydrogénase dans les épithéliomas cutanés*

Epitheliomas	Nbre de cas	Histochimie	Biochimie[a]
	4	+ + + à + + + +	18 à 26
	3	+ + à + + +	10 à 16
Spino-cellulaires	1	+ + +	32
	1	+ ±	21
	1	+ +	3
	2	±	3 à 5
	13	± à +	0,8 à 7
Baso-cellulaires	3	+ +	7 à 14
	1	+ + +	22
	1	+ +	6,6
Epiderme normal	10	±	3

[a] résultats exprimés en γ de NADPH/10 mg de tissu frais.

— dans un cas, la valeur biochimique comparativement plus élevée que le résultat histochimique peut s'expliquer par l'hypervascularisation de la tumeur et l'augmentation de l'activité par la présence probable de globules rouges dont on connait la richesse en glucose-6-phosphate-déshydrogénase;

— dans un autre cas, la faiblesse relative de la réaction histochimique s'explique peut-être par l'activité particulièrement réduite de la diaphorase de cette tumeur: celle-ci intervient dans la méthode histochimique, mais non dans le dosage biochimique;

— à l'inverse, dans un autre cas, la faible valeur biochimique contrastant avec une réaction histochimique moyenne peut être liée à l'hétérogénéité de la tumeur.

— Enfin, c'est à part qu'il faut signaler 2 cas où les deux méthodes concordent à des niveaux très bas: dans un cas, il s'agissait d'un épithélioma spino-cellulaire en voie de régression spontanée macrophagique, dans l'autre cas, d'un prélèvement très proche de l'ulcération tumorale et de sa nécrose.

Pour les épithéliomas baso-cellulaires, les deux méthodes montrent, dans l'ensemble, une activité enzymatique beaucoup plus faible que celle des épithéliomas spino-cellulaires: dans 13 cas, l'activité est égale ou légèrement supérieure à celle de l'épiderme normal; dans 3 cas, elle est modérément augmentée; dans un cas d'épithélioma baso-cellulaire kératinisant, elle est très fortement accrue, atteignant la valeur obtenue dans les épithéliomas spino-cellulaires. Un seul cas fait apparaître une discordance entre les deux méthodes, que l'on peut attribuer à la structure histologique particulière de la tumeur.

Commentaires et conclusions

Dans l'ensemble, cette étude montre la forte activité en glucose-6-phosphate-déshydrogénase des épithéliomas spino-cellulaires et l'activité beaucoup plus faible des épithéliomas baso-cellulaires. Il semble que l'activité de la glucose-6-phosphate-déshydrogénase soit plus liée à la kératinisation qu'au processus de prolifération cellulaire: elle est en effet très forte dans certains épithéliomas spino-cellulaires dyskératosiques, forte dans un épithélioma baso-cellulaire kératinisant; elle est modérée dans un épithélioma spino-cellulaire non kératinisant type III de Broders. Il semble donc exister, pour les épithéliomas spino-cellulaires, un certain parallèlisme entre le degré de différenciation et l'activité de la glucose-6-phosphate-déshydrogénase; par contre, pour les épithéliomas baso-cellulaires, on ne trouve pas de rapport entre l'activité enzymatique et le type histologique, sauf pour le baso-cellulaire kératinisant; ces résultats rejoignent les observations de WOLFF et HOLUBAR (1965) sur d'autres enzymes.

L'isocitrate-déshydrogénase à NADP n'a pas pu être étudiée par les deux méthodes histochimique et biochimique comparativement à la glucose-6-phosphate-déshydrogénase en raison de la taille souvent réduite des fragments tumoraux. Les résultats obtenus par la méthode histochimique montrent une activité relativement faible de cette enzyme:

— dans les épithéliomas spino-cellulaires, l'activité varie dans le même sens que celle de la glucose-6-phosphate-déshydrogénase, mais à un niveau nettement inférieur;

— dans les épithéliomas baso-cellulaires, l'activité de l'isocitrate-déshydrogénase est très voisine de celle de la glucose-6-phosphate-déshydrogénase. On ne retrouve pas, comme dans le cas de la glucose-6-phosphate-déshydrogénase, une différence d'activité significative entre les deux types d'épithéliomas.

Les résultats biochimiques obtenus sont trop peu nombreux pour que l'on puisse en tirer des conclusions comparatives valables; de toute façon, cette enzyme s'est toujours montrée moins active que la glucose-6-phosphate-déshydrogénase.

En conclusion,

— les deux méthodes histochimique et biochimique d'étude de la glucose-6-phosphate-déshydrogénase dans les cancers de la peau ont montré dans l'ensemble une concordance satisfaisante; les discordances montrent que les insuffisances de chaque méthode peuvent être corrigées ou complétées par l'autre;

— les épithéliomas spino-cellulaires ont une activité beaucoup plus forte, qui parait liée bien plus à la structure kératinisante qu'à l'activité prolifératrice;

— les épithéliomas baso-cellulaires ont une activité beaucoup plus faible.

Histologie des lésions précancéreuses de la peau

J. WANET et G. ACHTEN, Clinique Dermatologique de l'Université de Bruxelles (Belgique)

1. Classification

L'examen microscopique d'un millier de lésions précancéreuses de la peau comprenant les kératoses séniles, leucoplasies, radiodermites, maladies de Bowen et érythroplasies de Queyrat a permis d'adopter pour la peau la classification qu'HINSELMANN a établie pour les précancéroses du col utérin. On peut ainsi distinguer: l'atypie épithéliale simple, l'atypie épithéliale aggravée et l'épithélioma in situ.

a) *L'atypie épithéliale simple* est caractérisée par un épiderme d'épaisseur anormale, soit atrophique, soit hypertrophique. La structure épidermique n'est pas modifiée, la stratification est conservée et les cellules sont normales.

A ce groupe n'appartiennent que des kératoses séniles.

b) *L'atypie épithéliale aggravée* est caractérisée par des anomalies de la structure épidermique: images tourbillonnaires, en moëlle de sureau; globes cornés intra-épidermiques et fentes entre les cellules malpighiennes qui s'isolent par un processus d'acantholyse.

Il n'y a pas d'altérations cellulaires: ni monstruosités ni mitoses anormales. A ce groupe appartiennent des kératoses séniles, quelques leucoplasies et radiodermites.

c) *L'épithélioma in situ* présente en plus des modifications architecturales déjà décrites, de multiples anomalies cellulaires: nombreuses mitoses jusqu'au niveau des couches superficielles, dyskératose, monstruosités nucléaires, anomalies mitotiques dont les métaphases à trois groupes. A cette catégorie appartiennent les kératoses séniles, la maladie de Bowen, l'érythroplasie de Queyrat, quelques leucoplasies et radiodermites.

Statistiquement les mille lésions étudiées se répartissent en:

atypie épithéliale simple	17%
atypie épithéliale aggravée	50%
épithélioma in situ	33%

2. *Étude histochimique*

Elle a porté sur différents constituants cellulaires: glycogène, mucopolysaccharides neutres et acides, acides nucléiques, phosphatase acide. La mise en évidence d'autres enzymes est actuellement en cours.

Nous n'avons pas observé de différences significatives entre l'épiderme normal et les différents types de lésions précancéreuses en ce qui concerne le *glycogène* et les *mucopolysaccharides neutres*. Par contre les *mucopolysaccharides* acides révélés par la métachromasie au bleu de toluidine après fixation au Serra nous sont apparus diminués dans les cellules épidermiques des épithéliomas in situ alors qu'aucune différence importante par rapport à l'épiderme normal n'a été observée dans les atypies épithéliales simples ou aggravées.

C'est au niveau des *acides nucléiques* que s'observent les modifications les plus importantes. L'acide ribonucléique a été étudié par la réaction d'UUNNA-BRACHET sous contrôle de la ribonucléase. Nous n'avons pas observé de modification de la teneur cytoplasmique en RNA dans les atypies épithéliales simples. Par contre la coloration est souvent diminuée dans les atypies épithéliales aggravées sans que ce phénomène ne soit constant. La teneur en RNA apparaît toujours inférieure à la normale dans les épithéliomas in situ. Par ailleurs des colorations des acides nucléiques ont été effectuées au moyen d'un fluorochrome: l'acridine orange et les préparations examinées au microscope à fluorescence. Le complexe acridine orange — RNA donne une fluorescence rouge-orangé tandis que le complexe avec le DNA donne une fluorescence vert-jaune. C'est au niveau de l'épithélioma in situ qu'apparaissent des modifications nettes: le cytoplasme montre une fluorescence rouge orange, très modérée indiquant un contenu faible en RNA alors que les noyaux donnent une fluorescence verte, intense, plus forte qu'au niveau de l'épiderme normal; l'augmentation du DNA est d'autant plus nette que les atypies cellulaires sont plus importantes.

La *basophilie* cytoplasmique des cellules épidermiques est parallèle à leur richesse en RNA lorsque le bleu Alcian est utilisé à un pH inférieur à 5.

Elle apparaît diminuée dans les atypies épithéliales aggravées et les épithéliomas in situ; ceci confirme les observations précédentes portant sur le RNA.

L'étude de la *Phosphatase acide* d'après BURSTONE n'a pas montré de différences significatives entre les kératoses séniles et l'épiderme normal.

Conclusion. A. L'histologie permet de classer les états précancéreux de la peau en atypie épithéliale simple, atypie épithéliale aggravée et épithélioma in situ.

B. L'étude histochimique met essentiellement en évidence des modifications de la teneur en acides nucléiques: ces modifications apparaissent au stade de l'atypie épithéliale aggravée et se précisent à celui de l'épithélioma in situ.

Ces observations confirment les travaux effectués par PIÉRARD et KINT en 1964.

Bibliographie. PIERARD, J., et A. KINT: Arch. belges Derm. **20**, 137 (1964). — VAN DER MEIREN, L., et G. ACHTEN: Arch. belges Derm. **11**, 95 (1955).

Antigene Wirkung von Tumorgewebe

H. TRITSCH, Universitäts-Hautklinik Köln (Deutschland)

Zweck dieser Mitteilung ist es, über Phänomene zu berichten, die bei einem zusätzlichen Behandlungsversuch von Kranken mit malignem Melanom, nach erfolgter konventioneller Therapie, beobachtet wurden. In unserer letzten Mitteilung stellten wir heraus, daß die Aktivierung der körpereigenen Abwehr gegen die Ausbreitung der Geschwulst, wenn überhaupt möglich, eher von der Verabfolgung devitalisierten Auto-Tumorgewebes als von der Tumoraustausch-Homoiotransplantation zu erwarten ist (GARTMANN und TRITSCH).

Wir haben 13 Kranke mit histologisch gesichertem malignem Melanom der Haut ohne Metastasen mit Autotumor-Gewebehomogenat behandelt, nachdem die Geschwulst weit im gesunden Gewebe operativ entfernt worden war. Die theoretischen Überlegungen für dieses Vorgehen basieren im wesentlichen auf Tierversuchen von SCHATTEN. Er fand, daß beim metastasierenden Melanom C 91 der Maus die Entwicklung von Metastasen viel schneller erfolgt, wenn der Primärtumor operativ entfernt worden ist.

Bei unserer Methode wurden die Geschwülste in den Operationspräparaten zur Devitalisierung der Tumorzellen mit 20000 r Röntgenstrahlen (Dermopan, Stufe IV, 50 kV) bestrahlt. Nach exakter Präparation wurde das Tumorgewebe im Homogenisator (50000 r/min) in 40 ml physiologischer Kochsalzlösung zerkleinert. Die Tumorgewebseinwaage lag zwischen 0,7 und 2,0 g. Das Homogenat wurde filtriert, mit 250 mg Reverin versetzt und in vier gleichen Portionen von je etwa 10 ml bei —20° C eingefroren. Jeder Kranke erhielt vier Tumorhomogenat-Injektionen zu je 10 ml. Dabei wurden zweimal 0,1 ml intracutan und der Rest des Homogenates i.m. verabreicht. Die Injektionen erfolgten am 1., 3., 10 und 20. postoperativen Tag.

Bei den Tumorkranken handelte es sich um 6 Männer und 7 Frauen im Alter von 31 bis 70 Jahren. Die histologische Untersuchung der Geschwülste ergab 5 superfiziell und 8 infiltrierend wachsende maligne Melanome, von denen insgesamt 9 aus einer Melanosis praeblastomatosa Dubreilh entstanden waren. Die Entwicklungsdauer der Geschwülste bis zur operativen Entfernung betrug 2 bis 9 Monate. Bei 4 Kranken war die Ausräumung der regionären Lymphknoten und bei einem zusätzlich die Amputation des befallenen Beines vorgenommen worden. Die Nachbeobachtungszeit der 13 Kranken beträgt bis zu 12 Monaten. Keiner bot bislang einen Anhalt für das Vorliegen von Absiedlungen.

Alle Patienten zeigten nach der 1. Homogenatapplikation weder subjektive noch objektive Symptome. Nach der 2. bis 4. Injektion klagten 9 Kranke über Schmerzen an den Injektionsstellen. Bei 6 kam es zu einem kurzfristigen Temperaturanstieg bis auf maximal 38,2 °C.

Klinisch zeigten 3 Patienten keine Reaktionen an den Orten der intracutanen Homogenatinjektionen. 10 Kranke hatten Erscheinungen, die bei einem nach der 2., bei 3 nach der 3. und bei 6 nach der 4. Injektion erstmalig auftraten. Es handelte sich sowohl um Sofort- als auch um Spätreaktionen. Die Sofortreaktion war durch ein frühestens 15 min post injectionem auftretendes rotes Infiltrat gekennzeichnet, das nach etwa 4 Std sein Maximum erreichte. Die Spätreaktion trat etwa 48 bis 72 Std post injectionem auf und war mehrere Tage als bläulich-rotes Knötchen sicht- und tastbar. Von den reagierenden Kranken zeigten 3 eine Sofort- und 2 eine Spätreaktion. Die restlichen 5 Patienten wiesen eine Kombination aus Sofort- und Spätreaktion auf. Bei 4 hatte sich aus der Sofortreaktion die Spätreaktion entwickelt, und nur bei einem war der Sofortreaktion die Spätreaktion insofern vorausgegangen, als daß die letztere sich bereits nach der 2. und 3. Injektion, die erstere sich aber nach der 4. Injektion erst einstellte.

Histologisch konnten die Hautreaktionen von drei Kranken untersucht werden. Beim ersten Kranken erfolgte die Gewebsentnahme 85 min nach Auftreten der Sofortreaktion, aus der sich, wie die Kontrollstelle zeigte, auch eine Spätreaktion entwickelte. Es fand sich das Bild der akuten Vasculitis mit fibrinoiden Gefäßwandveränderungen, Eosinophilen, Granulocyten, Leukocytoklasis, Ödem und nekrobiotischen Erscheinungen im Corium. Die beiden weiteren Untersuchungen betrafen Spätreaktionen (72 Std nach Homogenatinjektion) von zwei Kranken, die sich aus Sofortreaktionen entwickelt hatten. Die Gewebsschnitte zeigten weitgehend übereinstimmende Erscheinungen. Neben hyalinen Gefäßwandveränderungen und Ödem fanden sich im Corium perivasculäre Infiltrate aus Lymphocyten, Histiocyten und einigen Mastzellen.

Die klinischen und histologischen Befunde lassen vermuten, daß ein primär ungiftiger Stoff im Gewebe eine vasculäre, exsudativ-entzündliche Reaktion ausgelöst hat. Die Reaktion gleicht einerseits einem Arthus-Phänomen und läßt nach LETTERER auf eine Antigen-Antikörperreaktion schließen. Andererseits fand sich eine Tuberkulin-ähnliche Hautreaktion, der ebenfalls eine Antigen-Antikörperreaktion zugrunde liegt.

Literatur. GARTMANN, H., u. H. TRITSCH: Hautarzt 17, 529 (1966). — LETTERER, E.: Fortschr. klin. Immunol. 11, 11 (1966). — SCHATTEN, E. W.: Cancer (Philad.) 11, 455 (1958).

Report

Les dermatoses paraneoplasiques

Y. BUREAU et H. BARRIERE, Clinique Dermatologique à la Faculté de Médecine, Nantes (France)

De plus en plus nombreuses sont observées des dermatoses diverses apparaissant au cours de l'évolution de cancers viscéraux, soit ouvrant le cortège et permettant de rechercher ou de dépister ceux-ci, « véritables Dermatoses monitrices du cancer », soit évoluant au cours de ceux-ci, parallèlement avec eux, s'améliorant si la néoplasie viscérale s'améliore, s'aggravant si celle-ci s'aggrave.

Parmi ces Dermatoses, *Certaines ont des rapports indiscutables avec le cancer* Dans ce premier groupe on doit ranger:

L'Acanthosis nigricans dans les formes de l'adulte, bien différente du Pseudo-Acanthosis Nigricans et de l'Acanthosis Juvénile, c'est la plus ancienne connue et la plus indiscutable des dermatoses paranéoplasiques en rapport en général avec des cancers du tube digestif, mais ceci n'est pas exclusif car on a signalé récemment des localisations au poumon, au col utérin, à la vessie.

Les Etats ichtyiosiformes acquis sont en général en relation avec des affections malignes et surtout surviennent au cours de la maladie de HODGKIN, plus rarement peuvent être en rapport avec un cancer pulmonaire.

A côté de ces Ichtyoses, on peut observer les *pseudo-ichtyoses* en taches circulaires de *Ito* et *Tanachra*, et nous pensons que de même pathogénie doivent être certains *Erythemes figures* et en particulier ce très curieux *Erythema gynatum repens* dont les observations se multiplient et qui s'accompagne constamment de cancer profond, le plus souvent broncho-pulmonaire, avec son caractère particulier histologique, présence d'éosinophiles dans l'épiderme et de surchage de mélanine dans le derme.

Les Dermatomyosites sont également un groupe de dermatoses qui doit systématiquement faire rechercher un cancer viscéral qu'on retrouve dans plus de 20% des cas.

On tend à invoquer dans ces cas un mécanisme d'auto-immunisation dû à la présence du néoplasme viscéral. Une observation récente de CHAMBERLAIN et WHITTAKER où s'associent cancer de l'ovaire, Dermatomyosite et Thyroïdite d'Hashimoto permet d'envisager l'hypothèse.

Le Purit sine materia des gens âgés est souvent révélateur de néoplasie viscérale, fait signalé déjà par DARIER il y a de nombreuses années, nous venons d'en observer un certain nombre de cas.

Nous ne ferons que signaler certaines observations rarissimes de *Pachydermoperiostoses et d'Erythemes polymorphes* pouvant accompagner et suivre l'évolution de néoplasies viscérales.

Dans d'autres cas, *Le rapport avec le cancer est plus discutable*. Et tout d'abord, *les Sclerodermies*.

Sans doute se multiplient les observations où la *Sclerodermie* surtout dans ces formes *d'Acrosclerose* s'accompagne de néoplasie en général pulmonaire, mais quand on songe à l'évolution extrêmement longue de ces Acroscléroses il n'est pas étonnant que de temps à autre ces malades présentent des néoplasies, et on peut surtout se demander, puisqu'il s'agit presque toujours de cancer pulmonaire, si la fibrose sclérodermique du poumon ne constitue pas un point d'appel pour le cancer dont elle fait en quelque sorte le lit, car l'on sait l'affinité du cancer pour les tissus de cicatrice.

Les *Amyloidoses* constituent également un chapitre bien particulier soit qu'il s'agisse *d'Amyloidose généralisée* pouvant s'accompagner de cancer, mais plus souvent des formes systématisées type *Lurbach dont les* rapports avec les Myélomes sont si fréquents qu'on peut se demander si l'amyloïdose n'est pas une affection paranéoplasique mais ne constitue pas plutôt dans ces cas un symptôme même de la maladie.

Il en est de même des *Panniculites nodulaires fébriles* (Syndrome de Weber-Christian) oú ainsi que l'observaient récemment LIEVRE et de GRACIANSKI l'affection semble presque toujours en rapport avec une affection pancréatique, le cancer du pancréas restant en général cliniquement muet et n'étant découvert qu'à l'autopsie.

Il s'agit là d'une dermatose bien particulière qui semble liée au cancer puisqu'elle est due à la diffusion d'enzyme lipasique dans l'organisme par voie sanguine et lymphatique. Il ne s'agit donc pas à proprement parler d'un syndrome paranéoplasique.

Les rapports entre la *maladie de Bowen* et les néoplasies profondes semblent de plus en plus fréquents depuis qu'ils ont été signalés pour la première fois en 1959 par GRAHAM et HELWIG. Il semble certain que les malades atteints de Maladie de Bowen ont plus souvent que d'autres des cancers profonds, mais là encore il est peut être difficile de parler d'affection paranéoplasique, mais il s'agirait plutôt d'un terrain particulier sur lequel se développent des cancers multiples.

C'est de la même façon qu'on pourrait interpréter la plus grande fréquence des cancers chez les *malades atteints de Verrues séborrhéiques*, où les cancers viscéraux seraient trois fois plus fréquents que chez les autres individus.

Reste parmi les questions les plus curieuses celle du *Zona* qui est d'une observation tellement fréquente, une maladie tellement répandue, tellement banale, qu'il est difficile de la ranger dans les maladies paranéoplasiques et cependant les statistiques sont formelles les Zonas sont particulièrement fréquents chez les malades porteurs de néoplasie profonde. A signaler également que le Zona apparaît également très fréquemment au cours des affections du tissu réticulé, des leucoses, mais dans ces cas il a une évolution particulièrement grave et d'un très fâcheux pronostic.

Une nouvelle affection paranéoplasique a été signalée récemment par BAZEX et ses collaborateurs qui en ont observé 5 cas, une autre observation a été signalée par HURIEZ et nous-mêmes avons observé un cas comparable.

Il s'agit d'un état particulier pour lequel nous proposons la dénomination d'*Acrokératose paranéoplasique*. Le malade est porteur de lésions érythémato-squameuses et parfois verruqueuses sur le nez, les pommettes, les oreilles et au niveau des mains et des pieds.

L'examen histologique montre dans l'épiderme que certaines cellules Malpighiennes présentent un aspect de dégénérescence cavitaire de type LELOIR qui serait assez caractéristique pour BAZEX.

Ces faits peuvent être rapprochés des *Hyperkeratoses palmaires* que DOPSON et YOUNG PINTO ont décrites récemment. Ces Hyperkératoses sont en général en rapport avec des néoplasies du carrefour pharyngé.

Ce bref rapport ne peut qu'énumérer les différentes dermatoses paranéoplasiques d'un intérêt très grand, puisqu'elles permettent souvent de déceler un cancer profond jusque là méconnu.

2. Keratoakanthoma

Free Communications

Unusual in Keratoakanthoma

D. V. STEVANOVIĆ, Department of Dermatology Belgrade (Yugoslavia)

The time which is allotted to the speaker is too short even to discuss all the unusual features of keratoakanthoma which have been observed by himself. We shall therefore here show only several of them, while the rest is to be presented to this congress in a film.

Similar to man, in hairless mice 2 fundamental types of keratoakanthoma (ka.) can be distinguished viz. superficial and the deep one. With its unusual normal histology characterized by rare hair follicles and deeper in the dermis "hair-cysts", it is clearly seen that the former arises from the hairfollicles and the latter from hair-cysts. Combination of both is also seen.

4*

As the rare site of ka. scalp and beard area can be regarded. They account for less than 1% of all sites. At the same time both clinical and microscopic appearences are slightly altered owing to somehow more numerous cellular architecture of the responsible hairfollicles.

Mucosa, mainly vermilion of the lip, is of particular interest. In all 4 cases observed by us, however, part of the hairy skin below it was also involved. In such a localization, that would suggest its onset also from a hair follicle. Once started, however, tumour grows and spreads quickly along mucosa itself, dissappearing usually after usual time. As the site of origin for ka. the nasal mucosa vibrissae can be surmised.

Among rarer clinical appearences giant and micro, ulcerating, fast spreading and highly pruriginous ka. should be cited. Ulcer in ulcerating type was observed spontaneously or after small dosage of "X" rays; in the highly pruriginous multiple variety it may be speculated on scratching and/or possible virus as the trigger for limited uncontrolled growth of certain hairfollicles.

Talking about the course of ka., a distinction should be made between natural further growth after an inadequate currettage or biopsy in its early phase of evolution, exacerbation — exuberant growth only at the site of biopsy, and recidive — a newgrowth after complete involution of the preceding ka.

Among etiological factors onset on xeroderma pigmentosum and leg ulcer is of considerable interest. These two precancerous conditions here including scars of various origin can be also regarded as prepseudocancerous conditions. Its site among mollusca tumours in an adult may suggest again a nonspecific trigger role of the virus in the onset of ka. The onset on herpes simplex lesions was already signed by us.

With its dyskeratotic and segregating feature ka. has also found its histological counterpart to carcinoma. Thus beside already known similarities in clinical as well as classical histological pictures of ka. and carcinoma, another similarity is presented.

Mucinosis follicularis like picture is more apparent than real. Though the cells of similar stellate-like appearance may be found, histochemical findings on acid mucopolysaccharides remain negative.

We are of the opinion that some cases usually designated as "Vegetating pyoderma" belong to dynamic pseudocancerous hyperplasia.

In some, infection may be incriminated as the trigger. Reinoculation of the pus as well as autotransplantation of the tumorous material together with pus yields negative result. Typical ka. can be also found in some of them.

In another clinical picture and course infection is not present at all. Dynamic pseudocancerous hyperplasia is an accompanying feature of most lesions at the later stage of their evolution, but not necessarily all lesions.

In a distinct dermatose it may appear as an epiphenomenon. It is here also dynamic, and after a spread involutes spontaneously.

Apart from these, certain skin disorders such as Darier's disease, granular cell myoblastoma, verrucous tuberculosis, pyogenic granuloma etc. can also show pseudocarcinomatous hyperplasia which is static and superimposed on the otherwise characteristic histologic picture of the corresponding dermatose. It does not represent the subject of this communication.

During the lecture 42 slides have been shown.

Zur Histogenese des Keratoakanthoms

K. W. Kalkoff, H. Berger und M. Hundeiker, Universitäts-Hautklinik
Freiburg i. Brsg. (Deutschland)

In früheren Publikationen aus unserer Klinik (Kalkoff und Macher, 1961)
wurde die Entstehung des Keratoakanthoms in Bestätigung und Erweiterung der
Untersuchungen von Dupont (1954) und von van der Meiren, Mestdach und
Achten (1956) aus Zellen des supraseboglandulären Bereiches von Haarfollikeln
dargelegt. Dort werden ebenso wie bei Kalkoff (1960) die Arbeiten zitiert, die sich
mit der Histomorphogenese beschäftigt haben. Die von Frau Jablonska gestellte
Aufgabe, im Rahmen dieses Symposions über die Histomorphogenese des Keratoakanthoms zu berichten, habe ich versucht, dadurch zu lösen, daß mit meinen
Mitarbeitern H. Berger und M. Hundeiker 60 Keratoakanthome der Universitäts-Hautklinik Freiburg aus den letzten Jahren auf ihre Entstehung und ihr
Wachstum in Stufenschnitten histologisch verfolgt wurden. Ein Teil des Materials
wurde elektronenmikroskopisch, ein anderer Teil nach Inkubation in ^{3}H-mar-
kierter Thymidin-Lösung autoradiographisch (W. Born) untersucht.

Ergebnisse. In frühen Entwicklungsstadien von Keratoakanthomen ist erkennbar, daß der Proliferationsprozeß seinen Ausgang vom „permanenten" supraseboglandulären Areal der äußeren Haarwurzelscheide nimmt, und zwar einschließlich der besonders bei Lanugohaaren als Hängekragen (Zimmermann) ausgebildeten Talgdrüsenanlage.

Diese Befunde entsprechen auch in ihren Einzelheiten den 1961 von Kalkoff
und Macher publizierten. Autoradiographische Befunde zeigen, daß in Zellen der
Wurzelscheide, und zwar dort, wo das Keratoakanthom auswächst, ein vermehrter
Einbau der radioaktiv markierten Vorstufen der DNS (^{3}H-Thymidin) erfolgt.
In entsprechender Weise ist der Thymidin-Einbau im auswachsenden Kerato-
akanthomzapfen vermehrt.

Die Proliferation erfolgt wohl kaum einmal aus der Wurzelscheide nur *eines*
Haares, sondern in der Regel aus mehreren, vielleicht sogar sämtlichen Haaren
eines umschriebenen Bereiches. Ob die morphologischen Veränderungen des
Keratoakanthoms durch die meist gut erkennbare Hypertrophie und Hyperplasie
des suprabasalen Anteils der äußeren Haarwurzelscheide eingeleitet werden, ist
im zentralen Abschnitt eines Keratoakanthoms nicht zu entscheiden. Ein solcher
Schluß liegt aber nahe, da sich in den Randpartien meist einzelne Follikel finden,
die eine solche Proliferationstendenz der äußeren Wurzelscheide erkennen lassen.
Offenbar klingt die Reaktion der Haarfollikel auf die keratoakanthomauslösende
Noxe zum Tumorrand allmählich ab. Infolgedessen kommt es in der Peripherie zu
beginnenden Veränderungen des Keratoakanthoms, die aber nicht von einer
Tumorzapfenbildung gefolgt sind. Das Steckenbleiben in Anfangsstadien kann
aber auch so gedeutet werden, daß die später in den Krankheitsprozeß einbezogenen peripheren Follikel in der Zwischenzeit wirksam gewordenen immunisatori-
schen Hemmwirkungen ausgesetzt sind.

Die in den Krankheitsprozeß einbezogenen Haare sind in ihrem basalen Fol-
likelteil nicht mehr in Bulbus, Matrix, Haarschaft und Wurzelscheiden gegliedert.
Bisweilen wurde ein undifferenzierter Zellstrang von ähnlicher Art beobachtet,
wie er normalerweise als „Epithelstrang" bei der Kolbenhaarbildung auftritt
(Kalkoff u. Macher). Die Deutung liegt nahe, daß es sich hierbei um Prozesse
handelt, die einer — allerdings pathologischen — Verschiebung der Haarwachs-
tumsphasen entsprechen, wie sie uns als Reaktion auf toxische Reize bekannt ist.

Je nachdem ob die auslösende Noxe an einer Stelle wirksam wird oder an mehreren, dürften streng umschriebene Keratoakanthome entstehen oder aggregierte (SPIER und THIES, 1956). Von der Intensität der Reaktion auf die auslösende Noxe dürfte es abhängen, ob sich typische krateriforme Keratoakanthome oder die seltenen atypischen plattenförmigen Keratoakanthome (KALKOFF, 1960) entwickeln. Auch in fortgeschrittenen Stadien typischer krateriformer Keratoakanthome ist der Tumor zunächst noch völlig von Oberflächenepidermis und einer Coriumlamelle bedeckt. Diese Decke ist ein äußerlich sichtbares, bisher noch nicht recht gewertetes Zeichen für den Ursprung des Keratoakanthoms aus einem unter dem Oberflächenepithel gelegenen Zellmaterial. Mit zunehmendem Wachstum des Keratoakanthoms und entsprechendem Eruptionsdruck gewinnt der zunehmend zentral verhornende Tumor Verbindung zur Oberflächenepidermis, die schließlich zentral schwindet.

Diese charakteristische Überlappung des Tumorrandes durch normale Epidermis bei krateriformen Keratoakanthomen ist ein Rest der ursprünglich kontinuierlichen Decke. Es braucht aber nicht zu einem Schwinden der ursprünglichen Epidermisdecke zu kommen. Dann entstehen plattenförmige Keratoakanthome ohne Krater, von denen ich Ihnen ein eindrucksvolles Beispiel an zwei Diapositiven illustrieren möchte.

Der Verhornungsmodus der Keratoakanthome könnte Rückschlüsse auf ihre Herkunft ermöglichen und ist deshalb für unsere Fragestellung von Interesse. Man trifft nebeneinander ortho- oder auch parakeratotische Hornmassen über einem breiten Stratum granulosum sowie Parakeratose ohne Stratum granulosum. Nur gelegentlich ist auch orthokeratotisches Horn über und zwischen Stachelzellkomplexen ohne Keratohyalingranula, und damit eine abrupte Verhornung, zu beobachten. Somit entspricht der Verhornungsmodus einem pathologisch veränderten Oberflächentyp. Unsere elektronenmikroskopischen Befunde, die einen erheblich gesteigerten Zellstoffwechsel anzeigen, und die typischen Strukturen der lichtmikroskopisch bekannten Glykogenablagerungen haben für unsere Fragestellung nicht weitergeführt. Ein autoradiographischer Befund erscheint uns erwähnenswert: Der ^{3}H-Thymidineinbau beschränkte sich in 3 Fällen auf die peripher gelegenen Zellen. Hierin liegt ein Unterschied zum Carcinoma spinocellulare, bei dem ^{3}H-Thymidin auch im Zentrum der Zapfen in Zellen eingebaut wird, und bei dem sich somit die architektonische Ordnung intermitotischer und postmitotischer Zellen verwischt.

Literatur. BORN, W., u. K. W. KALKOFF: Unveröffentlichte Befunde. — DUPONT, A.: Bull. Soc. franç. Derm. Syph. **67**, 296 (1960). — KALKOFF, K. W.: Strahlentherapie **112**, 133 (1960). — KALKOFF, K. W., u. E. MACHER: Hautarzt **12**, 8 (1961). — SPIER, H. W., u. W. THIES: Hautarzt **7**, 206 (1956). — VAN DER MEIREN, L., CH. MESTDAGH et G. ACHTEN: 9. Cong. Assoc. des Dermatolog. et Syphiligr. de Langue Franç. Lausanne 1956; Kongreßbericht S. 244. — ZIMMERMANN, K. W.: Z. mikr.-anat. Forsch. **38**, 503 (1935).

Unusual Forms of Keratoakanthoma

A. W. KOPF, Department of Dermatology, New York University School of Medicine, New York, N.Y. (USA)

The most common clinical type of keratoakanthoma is the single, hemispheric tumor with a central crater bearing a keratinous plug. Other common anamnestic, clinical and histologic features are: onset usually in later life; rapid growth (usually for 2 to 8 weeks), relatively small maximum size (often under 2 cm in diameter); occurrence on relatively normal or weather-beaten exposed skin; and histologic appearance of hyperkeratinization associated with benign akanthosis or pseudoepitheliomatous hyperplasia of epidermal keratinocytes supported by a stroma of altered dermis.

Keratoakanthomas which deviate from the above "classic" or average type are now becoming recognized as our knowledge of and experience with this variable tumor increase. From variant forms which have come to my personal attention, from formal reports of cases in the literature and from correspondence about cases with colleagues from many lands I distinguish the following:

Peri- and Subungual Keratoakanthomas. This rare type of keratoakanthoma which may be single, but often is multiple was first reported by FISHER under the title "distinctive destructive digital disease". The lesion may affect the deep periungual and subungual tissues as its nodular mass and central keratinous material increases and disrupts the local architecture. Pressure from the expanding tumor may result in painful osteonecrosis of the terminal phalanx. The occurrence of this type of lesion in association with the multiple and eruptive forms is one piece of evidence, among others, of its relation to the common keratoakanthoma. Differentiation from squamous-cell carcinoma is important to recognize because otherwise unnecessary amputations may be performed for this benign disorder. Sometimes, the pain and marked destruction produced by such lesions may necessitate amputation but then it is for sufficient reason despite the recognized non-cancerous nature of the lesion.

Multiple Keratoakanthomas. This uncommon form is characterized by the following features: 1. onset during adolescence or early adult life; 2. preponderance in males; 3. multiplicity of lesions; 4. widespread distribution on unexposed as well as exposed sites; 5. tendency to loss of ability to heal spontaneously; 6. lifelong course with continuous appearance of new lesions; and 7. familial tendency.

While the above is the well-known Ferguson-Smith type of keratoakanthoma, multiple tumors of this type can also appear superimposed upon skin damaged by other dermatoses (vide infra). This form includes the type originally presented by POTH under the appellation "tumor-like keratoses."

Eruptive Keratoakanthomas. In this unusual form the cutaneous surface is studded with 100s or 1000s of keratoakanthomas in all stages of evolution from tiny papules to lesions that may achieve several centimeters in diameter.

Giant Keratoakanthomas. These tumors differ from the ordinary type by their large size (arbitrarily over 3 cm in diameter) and unusual destructiveness. While they have been observed almost everywhere on the skin, those on the face (especially the nose) have presented special therapeutic difficulties and, at times, have led to severe deformity. They serve as a reminder that all keratoakanthomas, though inherently benign, should be respected as potentially mutilating.

Multinodular Keratoakanthomas. These multinodular, often polycyclic, tumefactions develop either by the coalescence of a number of smaller keratoakanthomas or arise as a single lesion which slowly spreads peripherally in the form of a variably shaped continuous or broken row of closely set, nodular masses. Often the typical central crater is missing in the conglomerate although hyperkeratinization remains a constant feature. These multinodular keratoakanthomas have been described under a variety of names like "aggregated keratoakanthoma" (SPIER and THIES), "coralreef keratoakanthoma" (BELISARIO), and "keratoakanthoma centrifugum" (MIEDZINSKI and KOZAKIEWICZ).

Verrucous Keratoakanthoma. Whereas the usual keratoakanthoma has a smooth or slightly scaly periphery surrounding a central keratotic plug, the verrucous type has an entirely or partly irregular surface surmounted by a variable amount of hyperkeratosis that causes clinical confusion with other verrucous conditions such as seborrheic keratosis, nevus verrucosus and verruca vulgaris.

Vegetating Keratoakanthomas. These keratoakanthomas are composed of polypoid excrescences capped by variable amounts of horn. They may resemble granulomas and other vegetating lesions.

Persistent Keratoakanthomas. Although the entire evolution of the "classic" regression the possibility of keratoakanthoma should be suspect in lesions of longer keratoakanthoma requires 2 to 8 months from onset to complete spontaneous duration if other features are compatible. Occasionally, solitary keratoakanthomas have been known to last several years. Giant keratoakanthomas often persist many months more than those of average size and multiple keratoakanthomas seem to lose their tendency for spontaneous involution altogether.

Keratoakanthomas Arising on Pre-existing Dermatoses. While most keratoakanthomas arise on clinically normal skin, or, more commonly, on exposed or weatherbeaten skin, they have also been reported to arise on many other pre-existing dermatoses including the following: psoriasis, discoid lupus erythematosus, radiodermatitis, xeroderma pigmentosum, congenital ichthyosiform erythroderma, arsenical dermatitis, herpes simplex, rosacea, drug eruptions, eczematous conditions, primary irritation caused by mineral oils, pitch tar and other derivatives, erythema multiforme, acne, folliculitis barbae, miliaria, lichen simplex chronicus, burns, seborrheic dermatitis, verrucae vulgares, seborrheic keratoses, atopic dermatitis, and lupus vulgaris.

Keratoakanthomas Arising on Mucous Membranes. Keratoakanthomas have rarely been encountered on oral, laryngeal, nasal, and conjunctival mucous membranes. Lesions situated on mucosae, as well as those which arise on finger pads, palms and soles, indicate that the pilar apparatus is not absolutely essential for the origin of keratoakanthomas.

Keratoakanthomas with Unusual Histologic Features. By means of clinico-pathologic correlation of the histopathologic features of a fusiform biopsy specimen obtained by partial removal of the central portion of the tumor and study of the clinical course of spontaneous involution of the remainder of the lesion, much has been learned about the wide variations of histologic aspects of keratoakanthomas. Virtually all features of primary squamous-cell carcinoma can be seen in selected areas of certain keratoakanthomas. Thus, keratoakanthomas and squamous-cell carcinomas can show similar nuclear aberrations, bizzare mitoses, various cytoplasmic alterations, dyskeratosis, acantholysis, inflammatory response with exocytosis, and invasion by extension into underlying structures such as tendons, bone and perineural tissues. Metastases, of course, are not found.

Recurrent Keratoakanthomas. Regrowth of keratoakanthomas after attempted removal is encountered not infrequently. Less commonly, lesions recur repeatedly even after seemingly complete extirpation. In one patient I know, tumors returned five times in and around an original site. Each recurrence was histologically indubitable keratoakanthoma and each recurrence was treated by thorough surgical excision or electrodesiccation and curettage except the last recurrence which was left undisturbed wherewith it gratifyingly disappeared spontaneously.

Keratoakanthomas Seemingly Arising by Inoculation or as an Isomorphic Effect (KÖBNER). Keratoakanthomas arising at sites of trauma suggest an infectious etiology or Köbner phenomenon. Examples of this are keratoakanthomas arising in sites of donor grafts, at point of puncture of fingers for blood counts, and "kissing" lesions in apposition on oral lips.

Miscellaneous Types of Unusual Keratoakanthomas. To the above variants can be added the following: those keratoakanthomas which have only a very small

opening in the central crater or no opening at all; those which are unusually destructive of neighboring and underlying tissues; those clinically variegate types
(papular, verrucous, papillomatous) which closely resemble acanthomas and
keratoakanthomas induced in experimental animals with carcinogens and electro-
magnetic radiation; those resembling cutaneous horns; those with central ulceration and necrosis, e.g., "kerato-akanthome congestif, necrotique et centrifuge"
(LAPIERE); those of fast spreading and superficially destructive character; those
which are deep seated; and those associated with — but not arising from — other
dermatoses (e.g., acne conglobata, hidradenitis suppurativa, arsenical keratosis,
and squamous-cell carcinoma).

An Ultrastructure Study of the Keratoakanthoma Experimentally Produced

L. PRUTKIN, New York University Medical Center, New York (USA)

In the last few decades, new light has been shed on the whole problem of
experimentally produced cutaneous neoplasms. Investigators in dermatology and
oncology originally thought certain epithelial tumors as early forms of squamous
carcinoma, but now recognize these tumors as keratoakanthoma. This tumor is
clinically benign, rapidly growing and undergoes excessive keratinization and
spontaneous regression. When produced in experimental animals, it is similar in
behavior and morphology to that observed in man.

The keratoakanthoma was studied in the albino male rabbit by applying twice
weekly, for 8 weeks, 1% 7:12 dimethylbenzanthracene (DMBA) in an equal parts
mixture of a lanolin-mineral oil base to the inner surfaces of the ear pinnae of nine
rabbits averaging 1 to 1.25 kg body weight. It was determined by biopsy that the
hair follicles were in the anagen phase of growth. Controls consisted of untreated
animals or animals painted only with the vehicular agent (lanolin-mineral oil in
equal parts). Biopsy material was excised from the earliest stages of tumorigenesis
to the complete regression of the tumor and processed for light and electron
microscopy. Tissue for light microscopy was placed in 10% formalin while tissue
for electron microscopy was fixed in 5% glutaraldehyde and post-fixed in osmium
tetroxide, dehydrated and embedded in Epon 812. The ultrathin sections were cut
on the LKB Ultrotome and stained with uranyl acetate, followed by lead citrate
and examined in the RCA-EMU 2E microscope.

The cells of the upper part of the follicle (above the sebaceous gland) give rise
to the keratoakanthoma and are 3 to 4 cell layers thick in the control sections
with a stratum corneum 6 to 7 cell layers thick. There are numerous free ribonucleoprotein particles, usually in clusters (polysomes) and both sparse rough
surfaced endoplasmic reticulum and Golgi apparatus. In addition, there are tonofibrils in all cell layers while there are stellate keratohyalin granules confined to
one cell layer below the stratum corneum. The stratum spinosum cells contain
membrane-bound inclusions, usually with an internal lamellated structure (membrane-coating granules). Approximately 2 weeks after the initial application of
DMBA, the follicular orifices were prominent due to a hyperkeratosis of the
stratum corneum where it descended into the pilosebaceous orifice. There was also
an increase in the amount of cells of the stratum spinosum and stratum granulosum. However, it was not until the 4th week that tumors developed grossly by

incorporating adjacent hyperplastic follicles. The stratum granulosum enlarged to
6 to 7 cell layers thick, and contained numerous keratohyalin granules. The
granules were usually multifaceted, densely osmiophilic and associated with tonofibrils. The larger granules were closer to the nucleus than the smaller granules.
Tonofibrils, rough surfaced endoplasmic reticulum and membrane coating granules
increased from that seen in the controls. In addition, there were now apparent
between the intact desmosomes of the follicular cells, small intercellular spaces,
a condition not previously seen. Applying DMBA for 6 to 8 weeks to the rabbit
pinna produced the mature stage of the keratoakanthoma. The tumor was superficial and bud-shaped with an average diameter of 0.5 to 1 cm and a central
keratinous plug. Keratinization was excessive in the epithelial elements of the
tumor as evidenced by its horny and brittle condition and the increase in amount
of tonofibrils. The keratohyalin granules were prominent and produced a perinuclear capping. The cells increased their free ribosomes, rough surfaced endoplasmic reticulum, membrane coating granules and intercellular spaces, the latter
producing a "prickle cell" picture. The mature tumor usually existed for 1 to
2 weeks until its central keratinous plug was exfoliated, a period 9 to 10 weeks
after the initial application of DMBA. During regression, the keratinocytes had an
accelerated keratinization, sometimes producing many squamous pearls with their
keratinous whorls. The intercellular spaces increased with a marked decrease of
the cytoplasm of the epithelial cells. Mitochondria underwent degeneration and
there was an increase in the membrane coating granules. As regression continued,
the tumor mass and keratinous whorls decreased. The intercellular spaces were
prominent and within the cytoplasm many cell organelles were observed undergoing autolysis. Intranuclear inclusions were occasionally found and resembled
viral particles. At this stage of the tumor, the keratohyalin granules were markedly
decreased in size and quantity. Complete regression of the keratoakanthoma
usually resulted in scar tissue with a persistent hyperplasia of 5 to 6 cell layers
thick. The tonofibrils were slightly increased from that seen in control sections
while the membrane coating granules returned to the normal quantity.

The keratoakanthoma investigated in these studies has a limited growth and
is well differentiated. The regression of the tumor may be due to a myriad of
factors including a possible immunological mechanism, an inflammatory filtrate,
constant keratinization and the simulation of the growth and regression of the
normal hair follicle. These factors may act independently, or simultaneously with
each other.

Papilomatosis Florida oral

A. R. DE KAMINSKY, C. A. KAMINSKY, J. ABULAFIA y A. KAMINSKY, Servicio
de Clínica Dermatológica del Hospital T. de Alvear, Buenos Aires (Argentina)

Nosotros vamos a relatar nuestra experiencia de un caso de papilomatosis
florida de la mucosa oral, con rasgos histológicos atípicos, que respondió activamente al tratamiento con methotrexate.

Historia clínica

P. M. D. — hombre de 71 años.

Antecedentes personales: úlcera duodenal curada y sífilis a los 21 años bien tratada. Ocho
meses antes comenzó su enfermedad a nivel de la mucosa bucal izquierda, en forma de una

pequeña elevación blanquecina que rápidamente fue aumentando de tamaño para extenderse hasta las vecindades de la encía y gran parte de la mucosa yugal.

Estado actual: mucosa yugal izquierda ocupada por una gran masa vegetante que llega hasta la semimucosa del labio inferior con aspecto de coliflor o de "repollito de Bruselas". La superficie es de color blanco nacarado en franco contraste con el color rosado de la mucosa circundante. Además aislados de la lesión anterior, presenta algunos elementos pequeños, erosivos y elevados en la semimucosa del labio inferior. A la palpación se nota una neta infiltración en la pared de la mucosa yugal sin modificaciones de la piel de la cara. No se palpan adenopatías regionales. Diagnóstico clínico: "Papilomatosis florida oral" o "Carcinoma espino-celular".

Laboratorio: Hemograma: Hematíes por milímetro cúbico 5.060.000; Hb: 15,2 g-%; Relación hematocrita: 47/53; Volumen Corpuscular Medio: 95 micrones cúbicos; Hb Corpuscular Media: 30 microgramos; Concentración Hemoglobínica Media: 33%; Indice de Color: 0,39; Indice de Volumen: 1,04; Indice de saturación; 0,94; Leucocitos por milímetro cúbico: 6.200. Fórmula Leucocitaria: Lobulados: 3% (186 por mm³); Monocitos 6% (3,72 por mm³; Linfocitos 31% (1.922 por mm³). Aspecto de los hematíes: normales. Eritrosedimentación: Indice de Katz: 33.

Histopatología (20-10-1965): La superficie de la lesión es irregular, vellosa y se halla constituída por proyecciones filiformes de un material paraqueratótico sembrado por colonias microbianas. El epitelio mucoso de cubierta ha sido reemplazado por una hiperplasia epiteliomatosa acantótica, con sectores infiltrantes, que invade el corion profundo y muestra una espesísima capa paraqueratótica superficial con leucoedema. Los cordones epiteliales que invaden el corion están constituídos por células espinosas, en sectores de tipo basal, ricas en mitosis, algunas atípicas (tri o tetrapolares), con diferenciación de globos córneos paraqueratóticos. En la zona más profunda, la neoformación muestra sectores desintegrados por la exocitosis de densos acúmulos de polinucleares neutrófilos con eosinófilos. En otras zonas, el tejido conectivo intersticial se presenta edematoso, con vasos dilatados y escasos linfocitos. La submucosa ha sido reemplazada por una fibrosis.

Diagnóstico histopatológico: Proliferación epitelial infiltrante compatible con una papilomatosis florida, con mitosis atípicas.

Tratamiento y evolución: Entre el 21 y el 29 de octubre de 1965 recibió 17 tabletas de Methotrexate, dos por día (5 mg diarios). Al término de esta serie (9 días), la mejoría era realmente importante y la vegetación había perdido aproximadamente un 70% de volumen, reduciéndose la infiltración. En cambio se observaba un buen número de erosiones y ulceraciones, alguna con aspecto aftoide y otras de tipo eritema polimorfo de mucosa tal como sucede en los tratamientos con antagonistas del ácido fólico. La medicación fue suspendida durante 16 días manteniéndose el tratamiento que venía efectuando por vía parenteral con 2500 mcg de ciano-cobalamina y complejo B y pequeñas dosis de antihistamínicos orales El proceso local se mantenía reducido pero se palpaba infiltración geniana.

En este momento (17 días después de iniciado el tratamiento) nuevos exámenes histológicos demostraron:

1. *Zona ulcerada de mucosa yugal izquierda que reemplaza a la lesión tumoral:* Superficie recubierta por espesos exudados fibrino-leucocitarios. En sectores, persisten focos de epitelio necrótico con marcada diferenciación paraqueratótica. El corion se halla invadido por una densa napa de infiltrados inflamatorios subagudos constituídos por linfocitos, plasmocitos y polinucleares neutrófilos. Hay restos epiteliales necróticos en sectores profundos submucosos. Vasos con endotelios tumefactos que muestran intensos fenómenos diapedéticos. *Diagnóstico histopatológico:* Lesión ulcerada con intensos fenómenos inflamatorios subagudos inespecíficos y presencia de restos epiteliales necróticos con acentuada diferenciación paraqueratótica.

2. *Lesión blanquecina de mucosa yugal en zona tumoral:* Cuadro histopatológico similar al de la biopsia anterior, con restos epiteliales paraqueratóticos ubicados en la superficie y en pleno corion. Intensa reacción inflamatoria subaguda inespecífica difusa del corion. *Diagnóstico histopatológico:* Lesión erosiva con restos epiteliales necróticos paraqueratóticos e intensa reacción inflamatoria subaguda inespecífica.

3. *Lesion erosiva de mucosa de labio inferior:* El epitelio se ha necrosado en su totalidad y ha sido reemplazado por una costra fibrino-leucocitaria. Corion con fenómenos inflamatorios subagudos inespecíficos. *Diagnóstico histopatológico:* Necrosis aguda del epitelio mucoso (de tipo eritema polimorfo) con fenómenos inflamatorios subagudos inespecíficos del corion superior.

Un mes después de iniciado el tratamiento, se realizó una segunda serie de Methotrexate (9 tabletas de 2,5 mg) a cuyo término la vegetación se había reducido en un 95%, persistiendo en el centro de la zona una pequeña placa blanquecina y elevada del tamaño de una arveja. Se mantenía un empastamiento inflamatorio geniano perceptible por la palpación. Después de la primer serie la única alteración comprobable consistió en la disminución de los leucocitos a 3.900, con una fórmula relativa conservada, cuya cifra se mantuvo aproximadamente al final de la segunda serie. El 28 de diciembre, (2 meses después de iniciado el tratamiento se

efectuó una tercera serie terapéutica de Methotrexate a razón de 2 tabletas diarias durante
5 días con las que desaparecieron totalmente las lesiones yugales así como la infiltración.
Algunos puntos cremosos superficiales revelaron la presencia de Candida Albicans que
cedieron rápidamente al tratamiento tópico con nistatina.

El estado general, físico y psíquico, se mantuvo con caracteres óptimos durante todo el
tratamiento hasta la actualidad (28-1-1966). En este estado de curación clínica se efectuaron
nuevos exámenes histopatológicos, de mucosa yugal izquierda.

Histopatología (31-1-1966): Epitelio mucoso con crestas interpapilares irregulares que
muestran discreta acantosis. Capa basal normal. No hay atipías celulares ni crecimiento
infiltrativo. El corion superior muestra densos infiltrados inflamatorios plasmolinfocitarios
dispuestos en napas subepitelial. El corion profundo y la submucosa presentan sectores con
acentuada fibro-hialinosis cicatrizal, en cuyo seno se ven vasos con endotelios muy tumefactos;
y pequeños y muy aislados granulomas giganto-celulares de cuerpo extraño que contienen en
su centro restos epiteliales. El músculo esquelético muestra fibras atróficas, algunas con
hipercromatismo de sus núcleos, que son reemplazadas paulatinamente por la fibrosis. Se ven
arteriolas con hiperplasia de la íntima y tendencia a la oclusión de la luz. No hay epitelio
neoplásico en actividad. *Diagnóstico histopatológico:* Fibrosis cicatrizal del corion y de la
submucosa con atrofia de fibras musculares esqueléticas; intensa reacción inflamatoria crónica
subepitelial y presencia de escasos y aislados granulomas giganto-celulares de cuerpo extraño,
alrededor de restos epiteliales.

Histopatología (4-6-1966): Fibrosis Cicatrizal.

Comentario

Los casos de papilomatosis florida se caracterizan por dar lesiones vegetantes,
con aspecto clínico generalmente carcinomatoso, con una histopatología condilo-
matoide y una evolución larga, con crecimiento extensivo o en profundidad de tipo
fistulizante, sin tendencia a dar metástasis. En nuestro caso los rasgos histopatológicos arquitecturales y citológicos de la lesión correspondían a una papilomatosis florida pero con el agregado de francas mitosis atípicas (tri o tetrapolares),
sin aplicaciones previas de podofilino, características de un carcinoma. Basados en
estos aspectos histopatológicos diferentes a los de carcinoma habitual de la mucosa
oral, por la intensa vacuolización de las células superficiales y escasa tendencia
infiltrativa, resolvimos hacer el tratamiento con methotrexate dado el éxito
obtenido (aunque parcialmente) en un paciente anterior. El resultado fue la
curación clínica e histológica con reparación cicatrizal.

Esta experiencia nos hace pensar con MACHACEK y WEAKLEY (1960) que las
papilomatosis floridas tal vez representen una variedad especial de carcinoma,
generalmente con rasgos incompletos para su diagnóstico histopatológico (ausencia
de atipías o de crecimiento infiltrativo) y que biológicamente se comporta de una
manera diferente por no mostrar tendencia a dar metástasis, en ganglios regionales.
Dada la tendencia recidivante de estas lesiones, a los tratamientos radiantes o
quirúrgicos y a la inoperancia del tratamiento local con podofilino, surge que el
tratamiento ideal para las mismas en el momento actual estaría representado por
el methotrexate. Reconocida esta papilomatosis florida por los caracteres clínicos
e histopatológicos, se impone el tratamiento precoz aún en lesiones de escasa
extensión, para evitar fracasos terapéuticos como nos ocurriera en nuestra primera
experiencia.

En nuestro caso la depresión brusca leucocitaria sanguínea originada en la
primera toma de methotrexate, fue de menor importancia en la segunda serie y
prácticamente no repercutió en la tercera serie. El agregado de ADN (800 mg
diarios) a los dos meses de iniciado el tratamiento, elevó bruscamente el nivel de
los glóbulos blancos.

La única complicación observada fué la aparición de lesiones tipo eritema polimorfo en los labios y en la mucosa bucal, después de la primera serie de methotrexate, que repitieron con menor intensidad en las series siguientes. No hubo
enterorragias ni otras manifestaciones digestivas de importancia.

El estudio cromosómico por aplastamiento de un fragmento de tumor de Papilomatosis oral, efectuado por el Dr. JORGE PAULETE-VANRELL, demostró:
1. Escasa apetencia tintorial, lo cual habla de muy discreta aneuploicía;
2. Presencia de muy discreto número de mitosis aptas para el estudio de sus cromosomas; 3. Número cromosómico modal de 47 cromosomas (normal 46); 4. Cariotipo mostrando la presencia de un cromosoma supernumerario de grupo F 19—20 (pequeñas metacéntricos); 5. células con complemento normal, esto es, con 46 cromosomas. Bibliográficamente esto concuerda con lo hallado para tipo de lesiones del tracto digestivo, de tipo papilomatoso, con tendencia a la degeneración maligna en un 25% de los casos y con tendencia metastática mediata o proximal.

Completada la curación clínica e histológica sólo nos resta esperar la curación biológica.

3. Clinical and Histological Studies

Report

Tumeurs des glandes sudorales

J. CIVATTE et J.-M. MASCARO, Clinique des Maladies Cutanées et Syphilitiques et Clinique Dermatologique de la Faculté de Médecine de Paris. Hôpital Saint-Louis, Paris (France)

Il est fort difficile d'établir une classification des tumeurs dérivées des glandes sudorales car les différences entre celles-ci sont souvent tout à fait artificielles. On doit considérer, d'une part, les lésions bénignes, acquises et dysembryoplasiques (naeviques), d'autre part, les épithéliomas sudoripares.

D'une façon très schématique on peut classer ces tumeurs selon le niveau de l'appareil sudoral intéressé ou reproduit par la lésion, en allant de la profondeur vers la superficie et en ne séparant pas les formes eccrines et apocrines.

L'adénome sudoripare (Masson) ou hidradénome nodulaire (Lund) correspond à la prolifération de la partie profonde du peloton sudoripare d'une glande ou d'une ébauche eccrine ou apocrine. Il réalise l'aspect clinique d'un nodule cutané profond, souvent bleuté, ou bien d'une formation globuleuse, mamelonnée et translucide surmontée par des télangiectasies. Presque toujours encapsulé et siégeant dans le derme profond, il est fréquemment kystique au moins partiellement. Il est en général formé de nombreuses digitations ramifiées et anastomosées, séparées par des fentes. Une double assise cellulaire tapisse au moins en partie les végétations. L'aspect peut être plus ou moins modifié par: 1. *une prolifération myo-épithéliale* (myo-épithéliome); 2. un aspect clair des cellules qui sont souvent très riches en glycogène (hidradénome à cellules claires ou myo-épithéliome à cellules claires de Lever); 3. *une métaplasie malpighienne* partielle; 4. *un remaniement du stroma* qui ferait la jonction avec les tumeurs dites mixtes (épithéliomas à stroma remanié, « syringome chondroïde »). Ces différents remaniements peuvent s'associer et réaliser un aspect complexe qui justifie alors le terme d'*hidradénome nodulaire polymorphe*.

Une variété particulière est le *spiradénome eccrine* (KERSTING et HELWIG), tumeur nodulaire douloureuse formant en général une masse arrondie très bien limitée, encapsulée, enchâssée dans le derme, le plus souvent située sur la face antérieure du corps. Ce nodule est composé de plusieurs amas denses séparés les uns des autres par de fines cloisons conjonctives; il est constitué de deux types de cellules, apparemment distinctes par leur taille et leur colorabilité, qui ébauchent parfois des groupements glanduliformes.

Bien qu'il soit habituel de le classer parmi les lésions pré-épithéliomateuses, le *cylindrome* peut en fait être rapproché des hidradénomes nodulaires. L'image clinique la plus suggestive est celle des *tumeurs de Poncet-Spiegler* qui, par leur grand nombre, constituent la *tumeur en turban* (RONCHESE): il s'agit de nodules surtout localisés au cuir chevelu et à la face, pouvant apparaître dès l'adolescence avec un caractère souvent familial et héréditaire, à développement très lent, dont l'exérèse limitée n'empêche pas la récidive in situ, mais qui ne s'ulcèrent qu'exceptionnellement et dont la transformation maligne est assez problématique.

Histologiquement on trouve des lobules épithéliaux situés dans le derme, limités par une rangée de cellules cubiques, disposées en mosaïque, cerclés et séparés les uns des autres par une épaisse gaine hyaline fortement P.A.S. positive. Quelques lobules sont creusés d'une cavité qui, en certains points, est nettement bordée par une double assise cellulaire. Aussi envisage-t-on assez généralement pour ces tumeurs une origine sudoripare, apocrine pour les uns, eccrine (eccrine dermal cylindroma) pour les autres.

L'*hidradénome papillifère de la vulve* résulte de la prolifération de la partie profonde d'une glande apocrine. Cliniquement il se présente comme une formation nodulaire, plus rarement pédiculée ou végétante. L'image histologique est celle d'une cavité kystique arrondie ou anfractueuse, remplie de villosités ramifiées. L'épithélium qui les tapisse ne comporte généralement qu'une assise cellulaire. On voit cependant parfois l'ébauche d'une assise myo-épithéliale.

Les *syringomes* sont des dilatations des canaux sudorifères. Ils se présentent cliniquement sous forme de petites élevures jaunâtres siégeant sur les paupières *(hidradénomes des paupières)* ou sur la face antérieure du tronc *(hidradénomes éruptifs de Darier et Jacquet)*.

L'image histologique est très typique par la présence, dans le derme superficiel et moyen, de cavités souvent kystiques, remplies d'une substance colloïde et parfois bordées par une double assise cellulaire. Des cordons cellulaires pleins sont également visibles. Leur nature apocrine ou eccrine reste discutée.

Les hidrocystomes du visage, dans la génèse desquels interviendrait plus ou moins l'exposition à la chaleur, ont une structure identique. Ils seraient de nature eccrine. La dilatation kystique et la rétention sudorale seraient favorisées par la prolifération des cellules canaliculaires. Mais le nom d'hidrocystome est parfois employé comme synonyme de kyste sudoripare: il s'applique alors à de gros nodules sous-cutanés le plus souvent uniques, de teinte bleutée ou noire, (hidrocystome noir, Monfort; cystadénome apocrine, Mehregan).

L'*hidradénome verruqueux fistulo-végétant* ou *syringo-cystadénome papillifère* est également une lésion du conduit sudorifère, mais accompagnée de phénomènes hyperplasiques de la région où s'abouche le canal excréteur (ostium folliculaire). Assez rare, il est souvent congénital; généralement isolé, il siège sur le cuir chevelu ou la région axillaire et inguinale. Souvent il se développe sur un naevus « sébacé » pré-existant.

Histologiquement la lésion est formée par une cavité profondément invaginée dans le derme, s'abouchant à la surface. La cavité est plus ou moins comblée par des végétations papillaires tapissées par une double assise cellulaire. Le stroma conjonctif contient un infiltrat très dense presque exclusivement plasmocytaire. Sous la cavité on trouve assez souvent des glandes apocrines ectopiques, ce qui confirme la nature apocrine et dysembryoplasique de cette formation.

Récemment a été décrite une autre tumeur n'intéressant que la partie intra-dermique du tube excréteur (*dermal duct tumor*, WINKELMANN et McLEOD).

Le *porome eccrine* (PINKUS, ROGIN et GOLDMAN) correspond à une hyperplasie de la partie intra-épidermique du pore excréteur d'une glande sudoripare eccrine. Cliniquement, il s'agit d'une lésion plantaire ou palmaire, ayant l'aspect d'un bourgeon charnu nettement circonscrit. L'image histologique montre une hyper-plasie épidermique, avec limites latérales parfaitement nettes, faite de cellules foncées, petites, riches en glycogène et munies de ponts d'union. Si la différenciation porale fait totalement défaut, la tumeur mérite alors l'appellation d'*acanthome sudoral intra-épidermique* (hidro-acanthoma simplex, SMITH et COBURN). Un argument diagnostique important est la présence, au sein de la tumeur, de canali-cules à disposition spiralée.

Parfois la tumeur reproduit la structure du pore et de la partie intra-dermique du tube excréteur: on parle alors de *tumeur excréto-sudorale* et certains auteurs utilisent le terme *porosyringome eccrine* (HELWIG).

Enfin il est des cas où la prolifération du pore et celle du canal sont associées à une prolifération adénomateuse sous-jacente, comme si la totalité de l'appareil sudoral était intéressé.

Dans le groupe des *tumeurs sudorales malignes* il faut considérer d'abord les épithéliomas à différenciation sudorale partielle. Cependant, il s'agit en réalité d'épithéliomas baso-cellulaires adénoïdes où cet aspect résulte d'une simple stroma-réaction.

Les *épithéliomas sudoraux fondamentaux*, tumeurs très rares, se présentent sous de multiples aspects histologiques et peuvent être divisés en deux groupes: 1. les *formes « à malignité atténuée »* qui sont, en fait, au moins très proches de certaines tumeurs bénignes (hidradénomes nodulaires) et pourraient presque y être assi-milées; 2. les *formes épithéliomateuses franches* qui présentent des caractères francs de malignité mais dont la nature sudorale est difficile à affirmer.

Free Communications

Das Syndrom der multiplen Basalzellnaevi (Naevobasaliome)

W. THIES, Hautklinik der Freien Universität Berlin (Deutschland)

Der Terminus Basalzellnaevus (BZN) wurde von NOMLAND (1932) eingeführt und die nosologische Selbständigkeit gegenüber dem Epithelioma adenoides cysticum (E.a.c.) (BROOKE) betont anläßlich einer Beobachtung von multiplen basocellulären Epitheliomen (b.E.), die auf dem Boden kongenitaler pigmentierter BZN entstanden waren. HOWELL und CARO (1959) sowie GORLIN und GOLTZ (1960) verdanken wir neben der eingehenden klinischen und histologischen Be-schreibung der bisweilen familiär vorkommenden multiplen BZN und ihrer Neigung zu einer frühzeitigen Umwandlung in ulcerierende Basaliome des Gesichts den Hinweis auf assoziierte Entwicklungsstörungen an der Haut und anderen Organen (Skeletsystem, Zentralnervensystem und innersekretorische Drüsen). Wie komplex das Syndrom der multiplen BZN jedoch sein kann, geht aus der tabellarischen Übersicht von GORLIN u. Mitarb. (1965) hervor, die sich auf mehr als 150 Einzelbeobachtungen des Schrifttums stützt. Sofern der BZN mit neuro-ektodermalen Entwicklungsstörungen oder davon ausgehenden Geschwulst-bildungen verknüpft ist (BINKLEY und JOHNSON, 1951; HERMANS, GROSFELD und

VALK, 1960; HERZBERG und WISKEMANN, 1963), mag es berechtigt sein, das
Syndrom den Phakomatosen im Sinne VAN DER HOEVES zuzuordnen. MUSGER
(1964) rechnet es zu den epitheliomatösen Phakomatosen, wozu als weiterer Vertreter die Brooke-Spieglersche Phakomatose gehört (KNOTH und EHLERS, 1960).

Vom klinischen Standpunkt ist für die BZN kennzeichnend ihr Auftreten in
frühester Kindheit oder in der Pubertät in Form einer mehr oder minder dichten

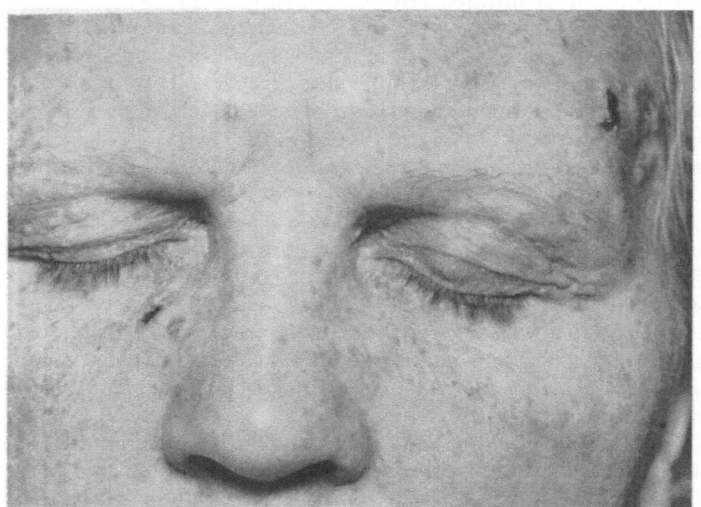

Abb. 1. 45jährige Pat. Multiple stecknadelkopf- bis linsengroße hautfarbene Knötchen auf
Stirn, Lidern und Nasolabialfalten. Knotige, teilweise zentral ulcerierte Basaliome li. Schläfe.
Auffallend breite Nasenwurzel

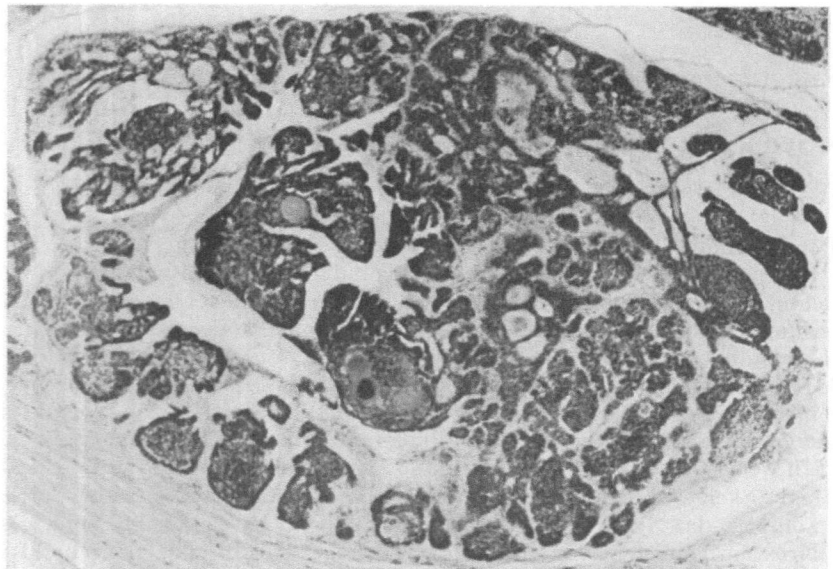

Abb. 2. Erbsgroßer, elastisch-weicher Knoten li. Halsseite. Neben soliden Basalzellkomplexen
mit Knospen und gelegentlich keratotischen Zentren tubuläre Stränge und cystische Hohl-
raumbildungen. H.-E. num. Apertur 0.16

Aussaat meist einzelnstehender, linsen- bis stecknadelkopfgroßer, hautfarbener oder bräunlicher, halbkugeliger oder gestielt aufsitzender, an weiche Naevuszellennaevi oder Neurofibrome erinnernder Knötchen, die vor der Pubertät nur ein ganz begrenztes Wachstum aufweisen, jedoch an Zahl zunehmen können. Prädilektionsstellen sind die mittleren Anteile des Gesichts (Lider, Nasolabialfalten), Stirn, Schläfe, die prä- und retroauriculäre Region, seitliche Halspartie, Nacken, Stamm, Achselhöhle und proximale Extremitätenabschnitte (Abb. 1). Offenbar selten ist eine zosteriforme oder lineare Anordnung (WITTEN und LAZAR, 1952; ANDERSON und BEST, 1962).

Histologisch entsprechen die Knötchen den primordialen Basaliomen mit unterschiedlicher, meist abortiver Differenzierungsrichtung in keratotische,

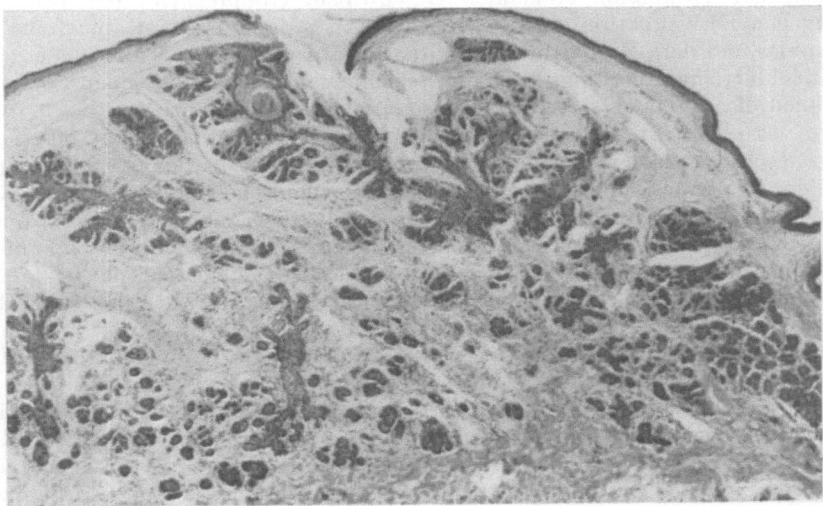

Abb. 3. Stecknadelkopfgroßes Knötchen retroauriculär. Multiple vorwiegend solide, an den primären Epithelkeim erinnernde Knospen basophiler Zellen mit Entfaltung eines faserarmen, fibrocytenreichen Stromas. H.-E. num. Apertur 0.08

adenoide oder cystische Formationen, wobei ohne Kenntnis klinischer Daten eine Abgrenzung vom vulgären Basaliom nicht möglich ist (Abb. 2). Neben multizentrisch vom Oberflächenepithel sich entwickelnden, dem primären Epithelkeim ähnelnden Knospen (Abb. 3) mit und ohne periphere Palisadenstellung der Kerne und zentral wirbelig oder ungeordnet liegenden basalzellähnlichen Formationen findet man auch in den tieferen Cutisschichten knotige, zuweilen glykogenhaltige Zellkomplexe sowie adenoide, an ein Filigrannetzwerk erinnernde Strukturen. Das Stroma ist vielfach ödematös aufgelockert und reich an gewucherten Bindegewebszellen. Bisweilen besteht eine deutliche Metachromasie des eher faserarmen Bindegewebes. Die ausgeprägte korrelierte Stromaentfaltung bildet einen integralen Bestandteil der BZN. Jedoch schwindet der Eindruck eines dynamischen Gleichgewichts zwischen Parenchym und Stroma im Augenblick des Übergangs eines BZN in ein destruierend wachsendes, zentral bisweilen ulceriertes vulgäres Basaliom. Ein Ereignis, das bei dem BZN-Syndrom gar nicht selten bereits im mittleren Lebensalter beobachtet wird (NOMLAND, 1932; NISBET, 1943; BINKLEY und JOHNSON, 1951; HOWELL und CARO, 1959; THIES, DORN und WEISE, 1960; OLIVER, 1960; BAZEX u. Mitarb., 1960; TEMIME und TRAMIER, 1960; JABLONSKA, 1961; HERZBERG und WISKEMANN, 1963). Demgegenüber wird insbesondere von angloamerikanischer Seite der gutartige Verlauf bei dem E.a.c. hervorgehoben, wobei jedoch auch hierbei ausnahmsweise örtliche Destruktionen auftreten können (KNOTH und EHLERS, 1960; Fall 2).

Hinsichtlich der Nomenklatur erscheint der Terminus BZN für diese dysontogenetischen Tumoren weniger geeignet, wenn man sich das von PINKUS (1965) für den Begriff Naevus erhobene Postulat, nämlich Gewebsreife und Stabilität, vor Augen hält. Handelt es sich doch bei den BZN histologisch um unreife, den primordialen Basaliomen ähnliche Strukturen. Dazu kommt vom klinischen Standpunkt die mögliche Wachstumstendenz und ihr häufiger Übergang in ein Ulcus rodens im jugendlichen Alter, weshalb wir der Bezeichnung Naevobasaliom den Vorzug geben, wobei wir mit JABLONSKA (1961) darin übereinstimmen, daß die hier zur Diskussion stehenden Geschwülste entsprechend der bekannten Leverschen Klassifikation eine Übergangsform zwischen dem Hamartoma suborganoides und dem Hamartoma non organomatosum bilden.

Ungeklärt sind allerdings noch die Beziehungen der BZN zu jenen Fällen von multiplen ulcerierenden Basaliomen des Gesichts im höheren Alter (SCOTT, 1952; WADDINGTON, 1952). Theoretisch wäre an eine lange Latenzzeit dysontogenetischer Geschwulstanlagen zu denken, wobei zusätzliche carcinogene Reize (UV-Strahlen, Röntgenstrahlen, Arsen und andere chemische Carcinogene) als Realisationsfaktoren Bedeutung gewinnen. Gehört heute doch zu unserem festen Wissen, daß auch das Basaliom durch cancerogene Noxen hervorgerufen werden kann. Als Geschwulstmatrix wird sowohl die pluripotent bleibende Basalzelle in der Epidermis wie in den vollentwickelten Adnexen erwogen. Im Zuge der beim Haarcyclus sich wiederholenden Regeneration und Degeneration dürfte infolge der Labilität der epithelialen Strukturen mit der Möglichkeit einer geschwulstigen Entartung durch verschiedenste Reize zu rechnen sein.

Mithin ist festzuhalten, daß die b.E. sowohl durch endogene dysontogenetische wie durch exogene Faktoren hervorgerufen werden können. Ersteres wird vor allem bei frühzeitigem Auftreten in Betracht kommen. Ein Musterbeispiel hierfür bietet das Syndrom der multiplen BZN mit dem Auftreten kongenital kurz nach der Geburt oder in der Kindheit, der fakultativen Weiterentwicklung in ulcerierende primordiale Basaliome und der Assoziation mit weiteren Fehlbildungen am ZNS und am Skeletsystem. Die bisher durchgeführten genetischen Untersuchungen (GORLIN u. Mitarb. 1963, 1965) sprechen zugunsten eines autosomal dominanten Erbgangs mit geringer Penetranz.

Literatur. ANDERSON, T. E., and P. V. BEST: Brit. J. Derm. **74**. 20 (1962). — BAZEX, A., A. DUPRÉ, M. PARANT et L. BESSIÈRE: Bull. Soc. franç. Derm. Syph. **67**, 72 (1960). — BINKLEY, G. W., and H. H. JOHNSON: Arch. Derm. Syph. (Chic.) **63**, 73 (1951). — HERMANS, E. H., J. C. M. GROSFELD und L. E. M. VALK: Hautarzt **11**, 160 (1960). — HERZBERG, J. J., u. A. WISKEMANN: Dermatologica (Basel) **126**, 106 (1963). — GORLIN, R. J., and R. W. GOLTZ: New Engl. J. Med. **262**, 908 (1960). — GORLIN, R. J., J. J. YUNIŞ, and N. TUNA: Acta derm.-venereol. (Stockh.) **43**, 39 (1963). — GORLIN, R. J., R. A. VICKERS, E. KELLIN, and J. J. WILLIAMSON: Cancer (Philad.) **18**, 89 (1965). — HOWELL, J. B., and M. R. CARO: Arch. Derm. Syph. (Chic.) **79**, 67 (1959). — JABLONSKA, ST.: Hautarzt **12**, 147 (1961). — KNOTH, W., u. G. EHLERS: Hautarzt **11**, 535 (1960). — MUSGER, A.: Hautarzt **15**, 151 (1964). — NISBET, T. W.: Arch. Derm. Syph. (Chic.) **47**, 373 (1943). — NOMLAND, R.: Arch. Derm. Syph. (Chic.) **25**, 1002 (1932). — OLIVER, R. M.: Arch. Derm. Syph. (Chic.) **81**, 284 (1960). — PINKUS, H.: Hautarzt **16**, 184 (1965). — SCOTT, O. L. S.: Brit. J. Derm. **64**, 342 (1952). — SWERDLOW, M.: Arch. Derm. Syph. (Chic.) **78**, 563 (1958). — TEMIME, P., et G. TRAMIER: Bull. Soc. franç. Derm. Syph. **67**, 99 (1960). — THIES, W., H. DORN und H. J. WEISE: Arch. klin. exp. Derm. **210**, 291 (1960). — WADDINGTON, E.: Brit. J. Derm. **64**, 202 (1952). — WITTEN, Y. H., and M. P. LAZAR: Brit. J. Derm. **64**, 97 (1952).

Xeroderma pigmentosum — ein Modellprozeß der Cancerogenese der Haut

A. Kúta, Hautklinik des Institutes für ärztliche Fortbildung, Krankenanstalten Bulovka, Prag (Tschechoslowakei)

Ich erlaube mir, Ihnen die wesentlichsten Punkte meiner Beobachtung in bezug auf die malignen Hautproliferationen im Terrain von Xeroderma pigmentosum vorzulegen.

In diesen Tagen sind es schon mehr als 10 Jahre, seit wir das heute schon 16jährige Mädchen in klinischer Behandlung haben und 6 Jahre beobachten. Auch ihren nun 10jährigen Bruder behandeln wir. Beide sind von einer drastischen Form von Xeroderma pigmentosum betroffen. In der Familie wird mütterlicherseits ein Fall dieser Erkrankung berichtet.

Beide Kinder werden seit ihrer frühesten Kindheit (5., 4. Lebensjahr), also praktisch seit den ersten klinischen Anzeichen dieser Krankheit in Intervallen von 2 bis 4 Wochen kontrolliert. Somit konnten wir bisher alle Haut-Geschwulsterscheinungen, die sich nach und nach bei diesen Kindern entwickelten, noch in der kleinsten Größe erfassen und auch in der heikelsten Lokalisation beseitigen.

Bis heute excidierten wir nach und nach bei beiden Kindern im ganzen 610 Hautgeschwülste oder als Hautgeschwulst verdächtige Herde. Bei dem Mädchen waren es bisher 359 und bei ihrem Bruder 251. Von der angeführten Gesamtzahl von 610 Excisionen wurde in 555 Fällen eine signifikante carcinomatöse Wucherung histologisch nachgewiesen. Von diesen 555 histologisch verifizierten carcinomatösen Herden handelte es sich in 332 Fällen um Basaliome, in den übrigen 223 um spinocelluläre Carcinome, überwiegend des ersten bis zweiten Grades. In der Topographie dieser beiden Typen war kein signifikanter Unterschied. Über 98% dieser carcinomatosen Proliferationen betrafen Kopf und Hals und 95% nur das Gesicht, und zwar nicht selten an den heikelsten Stellen (Augenlid-Wimperrand, Nasenpyramide-Nasenspitze und Nasenflügel). Ein Spinaliom entwickelte sich sogar auf der Bindehaut des rechten Auges, unmittelbar bei dem Hornhautrand. Einige Basaliome entfalteten sich auch auf den Innenflächen der Ohrmuschel beim Eingang in den Gehörgang.

Unsere Beobachtung dokumentiert also, daß die malignen Proliferationen in dem Terrain des Xeroderma pigmentosum sich praktisch nur in der photogenen Lokalisation entwickeln und zeigt, daß sich in derselben nicht nur spinocelluläre Carcinome sondern ebenfalls, ja sogar noch häufiger, Basaliome entfalten.

Ein bedeutender Teil unseres histologischen Materials von diesen beiden Kindern erfaßt miniature Geschwulstherde bis in die initiale Phase des proliferativen Geschehens. In der begrenzten Zeit kann ich mich nicht mit dieser Problematik befassen. Ich werde sie selbständig bearbeiten. Hier möchte ich nur zusammenfassend erwähnen, daß dieses Material eine auffallende Neubildung von Hautadnexen, insbesondere Follikel, aufweisen. Und gerade aus diesen, sei es aus voll entwickelten oder nur rudimentären, entwickeln sich die meisten Geschwulststrukturen.

An dieser Stelle möchte ich vor allem das Heilverfahren der malignen Hautproliferationen in dem Terrain von Xeroderma pigmentosum betonen, wie es sich bei unseren beiden Patienten bewährte. Daß unsere beiden Kranken — und besonders das heute schon 16jährige Mädchen — auch bei der enormen Häufigkeit oder Frequenz der bösartigen Neubildungen der Haut bisher noch ohne sichtbare Geschwulstveränderungen sind, verdanken wir zweifellos den Tatsachen,

1. daß ihre Hautkrankheit schon seit ihrer frühesten Kindheit fachärztlich kontrolliert und behandelt worden war, und zwar in kurzen Intervallen von 2 bis 4 Wochen, und

2. daß jede noch miniature Hautgeschwulst durch eine ökonomische chirurgische Excision liquidiert wurde und werden konnte.

Eine chirurgische, und zwar ökonomisch durchgeführte Excision erscheint im Lichte dieser und auch anderer unserer Erfahrungen als optimales Heilverfahren in der Therapie der carcinomatösen Hautproliferationen. Das gilt auch und besonders im Terrain von Xeroderma pigmentosum. Die Wunde nach einer glatten und ökonomisch durchgeführten chirurgischen Excision ist gewöhnlich innerhalb von einer Woche geheilt, und außerdem ist es möglich, eine solche auch an den heikelsten Stellen vorzunehmen.

Bei unseren beiden Kranken wurden bisher außer den Hautveränderungen keine wesentlichen Abweichungen von der Norm auch nicht durch Laboruntersuchungen festgestellt, nicht einmal in psychischer Beziehung. Beide Kinder sind von angemessenem Intellekt. Die in der Literatur nicht selten angeführte Debilität dieser Kranken in diesem Lichte gehört nicht zu den primären Teilerscheinungen dieser Krankheit. Sie ist eher erst sekundär und eine Folge davon, daß sie so betroffenen Kinder angesichts ihrer umfangreichen Zerfallserscheinungen und Mutilationen im Gesicht vom Kinderkollektiv und vom psychischen Entwicklungsprozeß überhaupt ausgeschieden sind. Dazu kam es bei diesen unseren Patienten nicht.

Angesichts der Perspektive dieser Kinder ist es bemerkenswert, daß bei dem älteren von ihnen, dem heute 16jährigen Mädchen, in den letzten 2 bis 3 Jahren, also um die Zeit der Pubertät, eine Abnahme in der Frequenz der neuen Geschwulsterscheinungen zu verzeichnen ist. Es läßt sich schwer entscheiden, ob es eine Folge der komplexen hormonalen Faktoren ist, die in der Pubertät in Wirkung treten, oder ob es der Tatsache zuzuschreiben ist, daß ihre ursprüngliche konstitutionell zur Geschwulstwucherung disponierte Haut durch die so viele Excisionen de facto schon beseitigt worden ist. Diese Wirklichkeit gibt die Hoffnung, daß beide Kinder auf diese Weise ohne unbeherrschbare Geschwulstveränderungen erhalten werden; ja — man kann auch optimistisch sagen — bis zu der Zeit, wenn ein tatsächlich wirksames Mittel gegen maligne Geschwulstwucherung bekannt sein wird.

Clear Celled Epithelial Tumors of the Skin*

A. H. Mehregan, Department of Dermatology, Wayne State University, School of Medicine, Detroit, Michigan (USA)

The subject of this presentation is "clear celled epithelial tumors of the skin". With this designation, I eliminate all other varieties of clear celled tumors such as those with melanocytic and connective tissue origin and those which have originated in the internal organs and have invaded the skin secondarily. I will limit my discussion to the clear celled epithelial tumors with epidermal, follicular and sweat glandular differentiations.

This study is based on clinico-pathologic evaluation of 36 cases. Based on structural differentiation and histochemical findings of the tumors these cases may be classified as follows:

* Supported in part by research and training grants from the National Institutes of Health, U. S. Public Health Service.

Epidermal:
{
Benign: Clear cell acanthoma (DEGOS), 3 cases
Anaplastic: Clear celled keratosis senilis, 2 cases
Clear celled Bowen's disease, 2 cases
}

Follicular:
{
Benign: Tricholemmoma (HEADINGTON and FRENCH), 8 cases
Anaplastic: Malignant Tricholemmona, 1 case
}

Sweat glandular: (Eccrine)
{
Benign: Clear cell hidradenoma, 20 cases
Anaplastic: Clear cell hidradenocarcinoma, 1 case
}

Clear cell akanthoma: The growth most commonly appears as a solitary, erythematous, keratotic nodule on the lower extremities of a middle aged person (JONES and WELLS). It is characterized histologically by well defined areas of thickening of the epidermis which consists mainly of large malpighiian cells. These cells possess abundant cytoplasm which appears spongy and edematous. They contain large amounts of glycogen, but no acid mucopolysaccharide (AMPS).

Clear celled keratosis senilis and Bowen's disease: The interfollicular anaplastic epidermis in these precancerous dermatoses may consist entirely of clear epithelial cells (MASCARO). The vesiculated or foamy appearance of the cytoplasm of the anaplastic cells seems to be due to their glycogen content. No AMPS was demonstrated in these cells.

Tricholemmoma: This tumor appears most commonly as a small elevated firm keratotic growth with predilection for face and hairy scalp of middle aged persons. Histologically it is characterized by lobulated tumor masses extending from the epidermis down into the corium. The tumor masses are solid and show no evidence of ductal or cystic transformation. The connection with hair follicle may be observed in an early lesion. The tumor masses are surrounded by a layer of high columnar cells in which the nuclei are displaced toward the inside resembling palisading outer cells of follicular sheath. There is also a thickened PAS positive and diastase resistant basement membrane which resembles the vitreous membrane of the hair follicle. In the central portion of the lobules, there are smaller cells with central nuclei and empty looking cytoplasm. There may be small foci of keratinization by formation of small keratin cysts or squamous eddies. The tumor cells contain varying amounts of glycogen, but no AMPS.

Malignant tricholemmoma: The case reported by BURDICK may be considered as a malignant form of tricholemmoma. The basic structure of the tumor is similar to that of a tricholemmoma, however, extreme variation in the size of tumor cells, presence of cells with atypically large and hyperchromatic nuclei, presence of dyskeratotic cells, abundance of mitotic figures and partial loss of PAS positive basement membrane suggest an anaplastic transformation.

Clear cell hidradenoma: The clinical data of 20 cases in this series may be summarized as follows: Sex: Male 11, Female 9

Age: From 5 to 82 years with an average of 48
Size: Ranging from 5 mm to 30 mm
Duration: From 6 months to 15 years
Location: Head and neck 12
   Extremities   6
   Trunk   2
In one case the lesion was located over the palmar tip of the ring finger.

Histologically, there are lobulated tumor masses in the corium in some cases extending into the subcutaneous fat but showing no attachment to the underlying tissue. Connection with the surface epidermis was noted in more than half of the cases. The tumor masses consist of both solid and cystic areas. The tumor lobules

consist of at least two different type of cells. The clear cells have small hyperchromatic and usually off-center nuclei and abundant empty looking or slightly
foamy cytoplasm. These cells are located mostly toward the center of the lobules
and are surrounded by rows of smaller cells with round central nuclei and slightly
granular cytoplasm. There is gradual transition between these two types of cells.
These two types of cells contain large amount of glycogen but show no AMPS.
However, scattered between the clear cells and lining some of the cystic spaces
are larger clear looking cells containing large amount of PAS positive and diastase
resistant acid mucopolysaccharide which stains deep purplish color by a combination of alcian blue and PAS. It resists digestion with hyaluronidase, it stains
positive with aldehyde fuchsin, colloidal iron, mucicarmine and slightly metachromatic by toluidine blue at pH 2.3. Beside the cystic spaces, there are also
areas of lumina-like cleft formation and a number of duct-like structures. Some of
the duct-like structures and superficial cystic spaces are lined by small cells resembling cells lining eccrine sweat ducts. Occasionally one may see keratinizing
ductal structures as pointed out by KERSTING within the tumor masses. The
tumor lobules are surrounded by a fibrous mesodermal stroma. Close approci-
mation and connection with eccrine glands are present. No connection with
apocrine glands was observed. Prussian blue reaction for iron pigment was negative
in all cases. I believe clear cell hidradenoma is an adnexal tumor with eccrine
type sweat glandular differentiation. Recent study by HASHIMOTO through enzyme
histochemistry and electron microscopy seems to support this hypothesis.

Clear cell hidradenocarcinoma: One case in this series, a 51 year old man, presented
an ulcerated growth on his ear. Histologic sections showed irregular solid tumor
masses growing into the corium. The tumor masses consisted mainly of clear cells
in the center surrounded by rows of smaller cells. There were many mitotic figures.
The PAS positive basement membrane was poorly developed and partially interrupted. There was also some inflammatory reaction in the corium. The tumor is
classified as a clear cell hidradenocarcinoma.

From this presentation I conclude that the clear epithelial cell is not a specific
strain of cells. The cells of various types of epithelial tumors of either epidermal,
follicular or sweat glandular origin may accumulate intracytoplasmic material of
glycogen or AMPS nature which do not stain by the routine hematoxylineosin
stain and will give the cells a clear or vesiculated appearance.

References. BURDICK, C. O., K. P. CLEARKIN, R. K. BROWN, and S. ARAKAKI: Arch.
Derm. Syph. (Chic.) **95**, 73 (1967). — DEGOS, R., J. DELORT, J. CIVATTE et B. POIARES: Ann.
Derm. Syph. (Paris) **89**, 361 (1962). — HASHIMOTO, K., R. J. DiBELLA, and W. F. LEVER: Arch.
Derm. Syph. (Chic.) **96**, 18 (1967). — HEADINGTON, J. T., and J. A. FRENCH: Arch. Derm. Syph.
(Chic.) **86**, 430 (1962). — JONES, W. E., and G. C. WELLS: Arch. Derm. Syph. (Chic.) **98**,
286 (1966). — KERSTING, D. W.: Arch. Derm. Syph. (Chic.) **87**, 323 (1963). — MASCARO, J. D.:
Sem. Hôp. Paris **41**, 473 (1965).

The Pathology of Malignant Angioendothelioma of the Skin

E. WILSON-JONES, Institute of Dermatology, St. John's Hospital for Diseases
of the Skin, London (England)

An earlier report [1] concerning nine primary malignant angioendotheliomas
indicated that these tumours are not exceptionally rare and characteristically
affect the face and scalp of elderly patients. REED et al. [2] have recently published
6 further cases affecting the scalp but preferred the title lymphangiosarcoma

because of the histological similarity to the Stewart and Treves tumour [3, 4, 5], which usually arises as a complication secondary to severe post mastectomy lymphoedema.

This report gives details of 7 further examples of face and scalp angioendotheliomas in the elderly bringing the total of personally studied cases to 16 (3 of the new cases have already been published in meeting records [6, 7, 8]).

The average age of the patients was 75 years (range 60 to 92). Only two have survived, but both with evidence of spreading disease. (Case No. 1 of our original report [1] later died of pneumonia, but with no evidence of local or distant metastases at post mortem; the only example of an apparent cure.) Many of the patients were old and feeble and some of the tumours were merely a contributory cause of death, but evidence of distant metastases was found in 6 patients radiologically or at post mortem. The average duration of the tumours from onset to death was 2 years (range 6 months to $5^1/_2$ years). Characteristically the tumoure spread extensively in the skin to affect large areas of the face, scalp and even the neck. The initial presentation was somewhat variable and usually consisted of a rather diffuse erythematous macules and plaques. In some recurrent haemorrhags or bruise like areas occurred but ulceration tended to be a later manifestation. In one patient diffuse waxy thickening of the skin suggested myxoedema [1] and several of the patients slowly developed chronic bilateral oedema of the eyelids. Another patient presented as a disecting pyoderma of the scalp [8] and another with oedema of the upper lip and bleeding erosions around the nares. The initially affected sites were scalp 5, temple 3, forehead 3, nose 3, upper lip and nares 1, cheek 1. Most of the patients were treated with radiotherapy and although temporary improvement sometimes occurred, in most it did little to check the progress of the disease.

Histological features. Angioendotheliomas are highly characteristic when well differentiated and are not likely to be confused with any other tumour. Anastomosing endothelial lined vascular channels permeate the dermis using the dermal collagen as a scaffolding. The channels are comparatively bloodless, but may contain lymphocytes and shed endothelial cells. The endothelial cells tend to be plump and vary in size and show nuclear hyperchromatism. As the tumour becomes less well differentiated the endothelial cells become heaped up and in places show solid cords of cells with only a slight tendency to cleft or channel formation. These cells are often arranged in a syncytial manner. Sometimes areas occur showing completely undifferentiated tumour closely simulating an anaplastic carcinoma or sarcoma, but usually outlying areas of differentiated angioendothelioma will allow diagnosis.

In addition 4 examples of angioendothelioma of very low grade or borderline malignancy have been studied, three affecting the forearm or wrist (a girl aged 20 [1], a boy aged 16 and a woman aged 57 [9]) and also one example affecting the neck behind the ear of a woman aged 51. Histologically these angioendotheliomas showed vascular clefts lined by plump endothelial cells, but not showing much obvious atypicality. These tumours had slowly developed over the course of several years and they have not recurred after excision.

References. 1. JONES, E. W.: Brit. J. Derm. **76**, 21 (1964). — 2. REED, R. J., F. E. PALOMEQUE, M. A. HAIRSTON, and E. T. KREMENTZ: Arch. Derm. Syph. (Chic.) **94**, 396 (1966). — 3. STEWART, F. W., and N. TREVES: Cancer (Philad.) **1**, 64 (1948). — 4. TASWELL, H. F., E. H. SOULE, and M. B. COVENTRY: J. Bone Jt Surg. **44** A, 277 (1962). — 5. McCONNELL, E. M., and H. R. HARRIS: Brit. J. Surg. **53**, 572 (1966). — 6. McKELVIE, M., and P. J. HARE: Proc. roy. Soc. Med. **58**, 423 (1965). — 7. KINMONT, P. D. C.: Proc. roy. Soc. Med. **58**, 249 (1965). — 8. FORMAN, L.: Trans. St John's Hosp. derm. Soc. (Lond.) **52**, 124 (1966). — 9. LEWIS, R., and H. J. WALLACE: Brit. J. Derm. (In press).

Importance of Early Recognition of Oculo-cutaneous Metastases in Cancer of the Urinary Bladder

A. Hollander and I. A. Grots, Department of Dermatology, Boston University School of Medicine, Boston (USA)

Cutaneous metastases of tumors of the urinary bladder are rare. We found 17 well-documented cases reported in the literature. Cutaneous metastases occurred in predominantly middle-aged males some time after symptoms relating to lower urinary tract disease had led to the diagnosis of malignancy. Oculo-cutaneous metastases of carcinoma of the urinary bladder were observed by us in a 26-year-old man.

In July 1963, about $1/2$ year before the onset of symptoms of urinary tract disease, a verrucous lesion of the frontal part of the scalp was noticed by the patient. He consulted his family physician who excised the lesion on August 11, 1963. Histologic examination was reported as polypoid hidradenoma. The lesion recurred shortly after its removal.

In February 1964 the patient noticed urinary difficulties consisting of frequency of urination, nocturia and urinary incontinence. On March 13, 1964 he was hospitalized by a urologist.

On March 17, 1964, transurethral resection of the bladder neck and the prostate was performed. Deeply invading transitional cell carcinoma (Grade III) of the bladder and the prostatic urethra was found with demonstrable involvement of perineural lymphatics. On March 24, 1964 exploratory laparotomy revealed diffuse metastases of the liver, iliac and inguinal lymph nodes. An ileal segment ureterostomy was carried out to divert the urine. The hospital record does not mention any cutaneous involvement.

In August 1964 new verrucous lesions of the scalp were noticed by the patient. He was referred for dermatologic consultation on October 22, 1964.

Examination revealed 3 light brown verrucous lesions of the scalp; 2 were found in the frontal region of the scalp, close to the hair line, and 1 in the right temporoparietal region of the scalp, measuring 1 to 1.8 cm in diameter. There was another identical growth of the left submandibular angle of the face. The 3 lesions of the scalp were excised on October 24, 1964.

Histologic examination showed a neoplastic process. The epidermis was markedly hyperkeratotic with scattered areas of parakeratosis and foci of crust formation. There was moderate irregular acanthosis; the basal layer appeared intact. The dermis showed well demarcated foci of large oval to cuboidal cells with light staining nuclei and slightly basophilic-staining cytoplasm. There was some variation in the size of these cells, but mitotic figures were rare. Some of these nests of cells were seen to lie within spaces lined by endothelium and therefore presumed to represent intravascular involvement. The surrounding dermis showed areas of fresh hemorrhage and edema of the collagen. There was considerable fragmentation of the connective tissue bundles. Sheets of the above-mentioned tumor cells were also seen in the dermis. There was a chronic inflammatory infiltrate dispersed among the tumor cells. Our histopathologic diagnosis was metastatic carcinoma.

In view of these findings we reviewed the original biopsy of August 11, 1963 and could not concur with the original diagnosis as we found the presence of metastatic malignancy.

On December 19, 1964, 3 new verrucous lesions had developed on a site close to the excision scar of the frontal region of the scalp.

On February 6, 1965, a pea-sized red papillomatous lesion was seen on the medial aspect of the conjunctiva palpebralis of the left upper eyelid, close to the outer margin. Histologic examination of this lesion showed metastatic carcinoma.

The patient consulted us again on November 8, 1965, because 3 new verrucous lesions, measuring 0.5 to 1 cm in diameter, had developed on the scalp. Another lesion had appeared on the outer margin of the skin of the right upper eyelid. The 3 lesions of the scalp were excised. Histologic examination of these tumors also revealed metastatic carcinoma. In April 1965 multiple papular and verrucous lesions were observed on the trunk. From April 28 to May 2, 1965, 5-Fluorouracil, 1 gm daily, was given intravenously. This was repeated from May 6 to May 10, 1965. There was no clinical or histologic change. The patient expired on May 25, 1965. Autopsy was not performed.

Comment. A survey of the pertinent literature shows that skin metastases of carcinoma of the urinary bladder are rare; they are particularly rare in the younger age group. Our case represents several unusual features:

1. At the time of the onset of symptoms the patient's age was 26 years.

2. Cutaneous manifestations in form of a verrucous lesion of the scalp developed about $^1/_2$ year prior to the onset of overt symptoms of urinary tract disease. The skin lesion was misinterpreted and particularly its metastatic nature not recognized.

The recurrence of verrucous tumors of the scalp and the development of additional identical lesions of both scalp, face, and trunk arose our suspicion that we were dealing with malignant cutaneous lesions. Histologic examination revealed metastatic carcinoma.

3. A most unusual finding, previously not recorded, was a mucous membrane metastasis of the conjunction of the left upper eyelid.

4. Cutaneous metastasis from carcinoma of the urinary bladder is considered an indication of early death. Our patient died 26 months after the diagnosis of carcinoma was established and 34 months after the appearance of the first cutaneous metastasis.

Cytologische Untersuchungen der Hautbasaliome in den Ausstrichpräparaten

K. Lejman und J. Bogdaszewska-Czabanowska, Dermatologische Klinik der Medizinischen Akademie Krakau (Polen)

Auf Grund der Untersuchung der von den 76 soliden und 23 adenoiden Hautbasaliomen verfertigten und gefärbten Ausstrichpräparate wurde festgestellt, daß die Krebszellen im Vergleich zu den analogen, in den histologischen Präparaten sichtbaren Zellen, einen deutlicheren Polymorphismus aufweisen. Die Krebsstränge machen einmal den Eindruck eines Syncytiums von großer Dehnbarkeit des Protoplasmas, in den anderen Fällen dagegen und sogar in den soliden Hautbasaliomen sind die Zellgrenzen deutlich sichtbar. Das Stroma der Hautbasaliome weist oft eine beträchtliche Reaktion seitens des fibroblastischen und reticulo-histiocytären Systems auf, die sich nicht nur in der Zellvermehrung, sondern auch in dem Auftreten der hypertrophischen Formen äußert.

In den Ausstrichen von pigmentierten Hautbasaliomen tritt das Melanin in den drei Zellformen auf: erstens in den Melanocyten, die sich durch schaumiges, manchmal die Fortsätze aufweisendes Protoplasma, mit gleichmäßiger Verteilung der Pigmentkörnchen charakterisieren; zweitens in den Makrophagen (Melano-phagen) sowohl im Bereich des Stromas als auch des Krebsparenchyms, welche die typischen Zeichen der freien, phagocytierenden Reticulumzellen aufweisen und in den pigmentierten Basaliomen mit cystischer Umwandlung, im Bereich der Cysten eine ausgesprochene Phagocytose der Pigments vom umgebenden Krebsgewebe, bis zur völligen Überfüllung des Plasmas entwickeln; drittens in den seltenen, Syncytia erinnernden Anhäufungen der Melanocyten.

Die Gewebsmastzellen konnten meistens im Stroma der adenoiden Basaliome, besonders aber beim Schweißdrüsentyp, beobachtet werden; sie treten in zwei Formen auf: erstens als runde, mit gröberen oder feineren Granula gefülltem Plasma und einem durchleuchtenden, helleren Kern; zweitens als spindelige, gleichfalls granulareiche, manchmal zusätzliche Fortsätze aufweisende Zellen. Die Plasmazellen, Lymphocyten und oft zahlreiche, Zelltrümmer enthaltende Makrophagen weisen im Vergleich zu den analogen, in verschiedenen Entzündungszuständen auftretenden Zellen keine wesentliche Unterschiede auf.

Tetracycline Fluorescence in Squamous Cell Carcinoma

H. J. Donsky and G. R. Mikhail, University of Toronto, Toronto General
Hospital, Department of Dermatology, Toronto, Ontario (Canada)

This study was undertaken on 33 patients who had squamous cell carcinoma
or lesions suspected clinically of being squamous cell carcinoma. These patients
were given tetracycline (TC) or demethylchlortetracycline (DMCT) for a three-day
period. Their lesions were examined under Wood's light 48 h after the last
dose for the presence of a canary-yellow fluorescence. Lesions which did not
fluoresce or exhibited a dull yellow colour were considered negative. All lesions
were examined histologically. The presence of squamous cell carcinoma was confirmed in 14 patients. Eleven of these patients were given TC with positive fluorescence in ten instances. All three patients given DMCT showed positive fluorescence.
Of two patients with Bowen's disease, one lesion failed to fluoresce with TC,
while the other showed a "leopard spot" type of fluorescence with DMCT.

Seventeen patients who were clinically suspected of having squamous cell
carcinoma had the following diagnoses on biopsy examination: chronic ulceration
(7), basal cell epthelioma (4), keratoanthoma (1), metastatic adenocarcinoma from
breast (1), syringocystadenoma papilliferum (1), ulcerated periarteritis nodosa (1),
thermal burn ulceration (1), lymphatic hyperplasia (1). Seven of these patients
were given DMCT and none fluoresced. Ten were given TC, and only one fluoresced.

The only false negative result was encountered with TC. This occurred in a
patient who had a scaling erythematous papule on the side of his neck which had
been present for ten months. The pathology report in this case was "Grade I
squamous cell carcinoma". The only false positive result was also observed with TC.
This patient had a chronic ulceration in the pretibial region for 5 years. The
lesion had been enlarging over the $1^{1}/_{2}$ year period before testing. Histology
showed "pseudoepitheliomatous hyperplasia".

Fluorescence, when present, was mainly restricted to the necrotic or granulomatous portions of tumours. The intensity of fluorescence was evenly distributed
in the lesion except in the case of Bowen's disease which showed a "leopard spot"
arrangement.

One of the patients was first given a course of TC without eliciting fluorescence.
At that time he had a granulomatous mass which had gradually developed in the
perianal region for 3 years. The pathology reports in the first seven biopsy
examinations were "pseudoepitheliomatous hyperplasia". The report on the
eighth biopsy specimen was "grade II squamous cell carcinoma". By this time
the lesion had become necrotic and ulcerative. The lesion then showed positive
fluorescence with DMCT. This was the only lesion which demonstrated the "live
coal" fluorescence described by Ronchese. The entire skin was exposed to Woods'
light in all patients, and in no instance was fluorescence observed in any of the
following lesions: nevi, seborrheic and actinic keratoses, psoriasis, seborrhoids, and
xanthelasma palpebrarum.

Many lesions have been reported that fluoresce with ultra violet light. Margarot and Deveze, in 1929, were the first to report fluorescence in naturally occurring
cancers. Ronchese later found that of the various types of skin carcinomata, only
the squamous or epidermoid cell variety is naturally fluorescent. The fluorescence
is restricted to the necrotic ulcerated areas of these lesions. Philips and his group
observed that a thin layer of normal tissue may obscure the fluorescence of an
underlying malignant growth.

RALL and his co-workers induced fluorescence in necrotic animal tumours by administering tetracycline. DUBUY and SHOWACRE demonstrated that tetracycline combined specifically with mitochondria of animal cells. These mitochondria were found to have decreased oxidative phosphorylation, but their oxygen uptake remained normal.

Conclusion: These findings confirm the affinity tetracyclines have for tumour tissue. Their value as an ancillary procedure in the diagnosis of squamous cell carcinoma remains limited by the fact that the tumour must be superficially located in the skin in order to demonstrate positive fluorescence. Demethylchlortetracycline was found to fluorescence more intensely than tetracycline.

Regional Multiple Carcinoma

G. W. VAVRUSKA and D. S. KAHN, St. Mary's Memorial Hospital and the Department of Pathology, McGill University, Montreal (Canada)

Basal cell carcinoma is commonly a single lesion in an older person. Superficial multicentric tumors accur occasionally in adults. Rarely, multiple tumors associated with congenital anomalies (Basal cell nevus syndrome) arise in childhood and continue into adulthood (MONTGOMERY, 1967). Two cases will be presented of multiple, rapidly-growing basal cell carcinomata in adults, that do not appear to belong to the above described types. The tumors developed during a relatively short period and were localized to one region. We suggest as a name for this syndrome, "Regional multiple carcinoma".

Case 1: A 69 year old woman was seen in March 1957 because of recent dermatitis of right retroauricular fold; biopsy showed non-specific changes. Response to therapy (including 500 r Grenz ray) was poor. Second biopsy 6 months later revealed invasive basal cell carcinoma. Chemosurgical excision (MOHS, 1956) showed three independent, closely grouped, invasive basal cell carcinomata: in area of dermatitis, anteriorly, and on the adjacent concha. 3 months later, excision of a new lesion from the upper concha revealed an independent basal cell carcinoma. Another month later, six new independent tumors had become apparent in the region. Excision confirmed carcinomata, three invasive. 15 days later, an infiltrate became apparent in the retroauricular fold, 10 mm below the primary involvement. Chemosurgical excision of the area revealed two new invasive tumors. No further cancers developed in the region. The patient died of carcinoma of the rectum 8 years after the last chemosurgery; 2 years before death, a superficial basal cell carcinoma was excised from the right occipital area (out of the region.).

Case 2: A 63 year old woman was seen in early 1957 with a tumor of the left nasoorbital angle of 2 years' duration, and a recent small tumor on the bridge of the nose, associated with an inflammation that extended to the tip. Biopsies of the two tumors and the tip of the nose all showed invasive basal cell carcinoma. Chemosurgical excision revealed the recent nasal lesion to be the most invasive, out of proportion to the clinically visible cancer. 2-month interval follow-up was instituted. At the sixth visit (1 year after chemosurgery), independent tumors on the upper medial cheek, lower medial cheek and chin, all on the left, were excised. Close follow-up was continued and 1 year later a small infiltrate under the left eye, accompanied by widespread inflammation and blepharitis, occurred. Three of four biopsies of the area contained invasive carcinoma. Chemosurgical excision showed two independent invasive tumors. Post-operatively, the inflammation and blepharitis subsided. There have been no new growths in the region to date. In 1962 a basal cell carcinoma was excised from the right forehead.

Discussion

Both cases developed multiple tumors, many of them rapidly invasive. Case 1 formed eleven tumors during 4 months, and Case 2, eight during 24 months. In each case, the tumors were unilateral and appeared to be limited within one dermatone: right third cervical in Case 1 and left fifth cranial in Case 2. All the carcinomata were successfully excised and no new tumors developed in the region to date (8 and 10 years). In both cases there was marked inflammation, resistant to therapy, which subsided immediately following tumor excision.

Regional multiple carcinoma clearly differs from both superficial multicentric basal cell carcinoma and from the basal cell nevus syndrome. Neither of these is limited to a region, nor do they show rapid growth with invasiveness (MONT-GOMERY). The present cases did not develop in relation to "nevus unius lateris" or other obvious precursor.

To our knowledge, cases of this type have not been reported before. COOPER's case, quoted by BELISARIO (1959), of a locomotive engineer with five basal cell carcinomata on the left cheek, may possibly belong to this syndrome. Also, NÖDL (1953), in discussing peripheral tumor extension after x-ray therapy, suggests that in rare cases this may result from the development of new independent tumors.

LEVER (1961) considers basal cell carcinomata to be nevoid tumors (hamartomas) derived from primary epithelial germ cells. The histopathology of the present tumors was not distinctive; all types of differentiation were found. Numerous small foci of basal cell proliferation occurred in the epithelium between the larger invading tumors, suggesting generalized restlessness of the neoplastic precursor cells in the epithelium of the region.

References. BELISARIO, J. C.: Cancer of the skin. London: Butterworth & Co. 1959. — LEVER, W. F.: Histopathology of the skin, 3rd Edition 1961. Philadelphia and Montreal: J. B. Lippincott Co. 1961. — MOHS, F. E.: Chemosurgery in cancer, gangrene and infections. Springfield: Charles C. Thomas 1956. — MONTGOMERY, H.: Dermatopathology. New York: Hoeber Medical Division, Harper and Row 1967. — NÖDL, F.: Strahlentherapie 90, 265 (1953).

A Skin Cancer Consultative Clinic

A. JOHNSON, University of Sydney (Australia)

The incidence of skin cancer and pre-cancer in Sydney is of the order of 35% of the new cases presenting at a Dermatological Clinic. The latitude of Sydney is 33° S. and the average mean number of sunshine hours to which a population originating mainly from the British Isles is subject is 6.8.

The results of the treatment of skin cancer in competent hands is excellent, no matter whether surgical or radiotherapeutic means are used. It is inevitable that if different methods of treatment are used by workers who do not meet in consultation they tend to see only the failure of the others, and a distorted view ist the result.

Prior to 1960, consultation between the various departments in the Royal Prince Alfred Hospital were haphazard, and it was decided in that year to establish a consultative clinic to which any problem cases could be referred. This Committee meets at monthly intervals in the Belisario Institute of Dermatology, and in consultation the Dermatologist, Radiotherapist and Plastic Surgeon decide at the outset the optimum treatment in each particular case.

It should be explained that in Sydney, treatment with superficial and intermediate radiotherapy is carried out in The Department of Dermatology; the Radiotherapist caring for those patients requiring deep radiotherapy.

The absolute number of cases referred are not great, for the reason mentioned above, and a detailed dissection of the cases, not possible here, is in preparation for publication elsewhere.

As a matter of interest, in the last 179 cases, the method selected for treatment was as follows:

Scalpel Surgery	— 108
Superficial radiotherapy	— 43
Deep radiotherapy	— 18
Radio Cobalt therapy	— 2
Radon Mould	— 1
Local therapy with Cytotoxic Agents —	7

This only reflects, however, the incidence of lesions suitable for such treatment in this particular sample.

The main problems are illustrated by the colour film presented during this communication, and it suffices to say here that they arise with regard to the site of the lesions, the recurrence in previously treated areas, the type of lesion, or, as often happens, with the main aetiological agent still operating, new lesions in or close to previously treated cases. Thus, particular sites — the nasolabial fold, the external ear, particularly if the lesion extends into the auditory canal, the back of the hand in persons engaged in manual labour, are particularly suited to surgery, as are lesions situated below the knee.

Lesions on the lips and eyelids appear to show better cosmetic results when treated with irradiation, except where established ectropion requires surgical correction of itself.

In fact, lesions irradiated by fractional dosage and with varying fields for each fraction extending beyond the minimum area to be treated, and so avoiding a sharp margin, in my view, produced better cosmetic results than surgery, but this is, of course, disputed by surgeons.

The extent of some of these problem cases is shown, where recurrence or new lesions keep ahead of radiotherapy or surgical repair.

Replacement of skin damaged by solar radiation, as a prophylactic procedure, is shown, where a sarcoma occurring in an old burn scar is treated by removal of the whole damaged area, with subsequent grafting.

Morphoeic type basal-celled carcinoma and cicatrizing basal-celled carcinoma, though they are halted by radiotherapy, do not change in appearance and are best treated surgically. Naevoid types are not very radiosensitive, and these too are better treated surgically.

An unusual and extreme case is shown, where a basal-celled carcinoma of the chest wall invades the sternum in a patient who for ten years belonged to a religious sect which forbad the member to consult a doctor.

The final slide presents a patient with Paget's Disease of the scrotum treated with Colcemide Ointment, with apparent cure, but which relapsed within 3 months, and was treated surgically. In this Clinic, we feel that local therapy with cytotoxic drugs, though obviously warranting further investigation, both as a therapeutic agent and as a means of evaluating the effects of these agents on easily accessible malignant cells in situ, is not at this point of time a definitive means of treatment.

Corrélations morpho-cliniques dans les récidives des épithéliomas cutanés de la face

C. LONGHIN, G. SANDRU, R. DUTU et M. SPIRIDON, Institut Oncologique, Bucarest (Roumanie)

Nos considérations seront basées sur l'étude anatomoclinique de 55 cas de récidives de cancer cutané, traités à l'Institut Oncologique de Bucarest, entre 1950 à 1962, et sous contrôle pendant plus de 5 ans.

Sur les 55 récidives, 48 proviennent de tumeurs traitées classiquement par radiothérapie de contact (8000 r) à la base de la tumeur, en doses fractionnées journalières de 500 r auxquelles a été associée, pour les tumeurs bourgeonnantes, l'électrocautérisation comme premier temps [6]. Les 7 cas restants proviennent de tumeurs traitées exclusivement par voie chirurgicale.

La distribution par sexes, présente une fréquence égale à 50%, tandis que par rapport à l'âge, l'incidence maximum après 50 ans est de 87,7%. Les récidives, dans notre lot, ont été localisées exclusivement à la face, avec prédominance nasale (30,30%). Du point de vue anatomo-clinique on a constaté la prédominance de la forme ulcérée (67,25%) suivie par celle bourgeonnante (18,18%) et celle nodulaire (14,57%). En général, une correspondance a été constatée entre les formes anatomo-cliniques des récidives et celles des lésions primaires.

La topographie des récidives quant à la cicatrice primaire post-thérapeutique est comme suit: 95% marginale et 5% seulement dans la zone cicatriciale, ceci pouvant être mis en liaison avec la diminution de la dose à la périphérie du champ d'irradiation et avec la radiorésistance accrue de certaines cellules existantes dans la même tumeur [1].

L'intervalle de temps écoulé depuis la fin du traitement primaire jusqu'à l'apparition des récidives varie entre quelques mois et 12 ans comme suit:

— sous 6 mois   — 7 cas
— entre 7—12 mois   — 6 cas
— entre 13—23 mois   — 14 cas
— entre 24—35 mois   — 8 cas
— entre 36 mois — 10 ans   — 10 cas
— au-dessus de 10 ans   — 5 cas

A remarquer que dans les cas des récidives sous 6 mois (7 cas) la lésion primaire a été traitée exclusivement chirurgical; dans leur majorité ces récidives se sont montrées rebelles au traitement chirurgical répété. Dans le cas des récidives apparues après 5 ans, la lésion primaire a été traitée par irradiation.

La radiothérapie a été moins efficace dans les formes à prédominance infiltrative, dans lesquelles les récidives sont plus fréquentes et apparaissent à des intervalles de temps plus courts.

Au point de vue microscopique, outre le type histologique de la tumeur, ont été étudié par techniques morpho-histo-chimiques appropriées, la distribution du tissu conjonctif, ainsi que la dynamique des éléments cellulaires réactionnels. On a constaté que la forme primitive du processus tumoral a été représentée dans sa plus grande partie par des épithéliomas baso-cellulaires (57,37%) le restant comprenant des formes à différenciation cylindromateuse (24,59%) ou spino-cellulaire (18,03%).

La forme histologique du processus récidivé a toujours reproduit le type histologique de la tumeur primitive.

Les réactions de mise en évidence des muccopolysaccharides et des filets réticuliniques a permis de voir une pseudo-membrane basale qui délimite les îles et les cordons tumoraux, tant dans les formes baso-cellulaires pures que dans celles à évolution cylindromateuse. L'étude du tissu conjonctif ainsi que des cellules réactionnelles de type lympho-plasmocytaire nous a permis de constater des récidives dans les cas dans lesquels ces éléments étaient pratiquement absents ou réduits (30 cas).

Discussion. Le traitement appliqué à l'Institut Oncologique de Bucarest, considère la dose tumoricide à 8000 r et la zone de sûreté péritumorale à 1/4—1/3 du diamètre de la lésion [5, 7], il y a pourtant des récidives dans certains des cas. Cela signifie qu'intervient toute une série de facteurs, à savoir : les données morpho-histo-chimiques mettent en évidence le rôle du tissu conjonctif et de la réaction cellulaire lympho-plasmocytaire dans l'apparition de certaines tumeurs cutanées.

Dans des travaux antérieurs on a établi une relation entre la richesse du tissu conjonctif et l'absence de la possibilité de métastaser [2, 3].

D'autres auteurs ont établi une relation pronostique d'après la distribution du tissu conjonctif, avec un pronostic meilleur, dans le cas des carcinomes délimités par des structures conjonctives [8].

L'état physico-chimique de la substance fondamentale et de la membrane basale ainsi que le rôle de la hialuronidase se trouvent mentionnés dans des travaux récents [4] comme facteurs importants dans le processus d'extension tumorale, la réaction stromale et les modifications histochimiques de la substance fondamentale s'expliquant de cette manière.

En ce qui concerne le processus réactionnel cellulaire lympho-plasmocytaire, il paraîtrait que pour certaines tumeurs au moins, celui-ci serait lié à un pronostic favorable [9].

Bibliografie. 1. BELISARIO, C. J.: Cancer of the skin, p. 169. London: Butterworth & Co. Ltd. 1959. — 2. DUTU, R., and C. LONCHIN: Derm.-Vener. (Buc.) 2, 97 (1959). — 3. DUTU, R., et C. LONGHIN: Folia Histochem. Cytochim 4, 53 (1966). — 4. CAMERON, E.: Hialuronidase and Cancer. London: Pergamon Press 1966. — 5. COSTACHEL, O., et U. BUNESCU: Tratamentul complex al cancerului, p. 246. Bucuresti: Medicală 1965. — 6. LONGHIN, S., AL. DIMITRESCU, and P. TRIFU: Derm.-Vener. (Buc.) 5, 391 (1962). — 7. SPIRIDON, M., C. LONGHIN, and E. IOANID: Eight international cancer congress. Abstr. of papers, p. 369 Moscow: Medghiz 1962. — 8. HEROVICI, C.: Rev. franç. Étud. clin. biol. 8, 1, 59 (1963). — 9. Groupe scientifique de l'OMS sur l'imunothérapie du cancer, Genève 1966.

Neuromyopathy in Skin Cancer*

A. K. AFIFI, F. S. FARAH, A. K. KURBAN and F. A. SABRA, Department of Medicine, Divisions of Neurology and Dermatology, of the American University of Beirut and American University Hospital, Beirut (Lebanon)

During the past two decades, there has been increasing attention to the incidence of neuromuscular disorders in neoplastic disease. The association of dermatomyositis and malignant tumors is well established. The concept of carcinomatous myopathy, introduced in 1954 [1, 2] is being rapidly incorporated into the differential diagnosis of adult myopathies. Although earlier reports referred to a myopathy subsequent studies described a neuropathic component [3] and hence the term carcinomatous neuromyopathy came to be used.

* Supported in part by a grant from the Research Committee of the Faculties of Medical Sciences of the American University of Beirut.

The following table summarizes the incidence of neuromyopathy in cancer of different sites [4].

Table 1. *Incidence of ca neuromyopathy*

Lung	14.2%	Ovary	16.4%
Breast	4.4%	Cervix	2.1%
Stomach	9.0%	Uterus	1.3%
Colon	3.8%	Prostate	6.4%
Rectum	0.5%		

The different neurologic disorders that have been described with carcinoma are:

Myopathy, sensory or motor neuropathy, myelopathy, myasthenia, cerebellar degeneration, motor neuron disease. Of the above, neuromyopathy is the commonest in occurence and accounts for over 50% of the neurologic disorders associated with carcinoma [4]. In the available literature on carcinomatous neuromyopathy no mention is made of an association with skin cancer. This can be interpreted to mean:

1. that carcinomatous neuromyopathy does not occur with skin carcinoma,
2. that it has not been looked for in skin carcinoma.

If the first is true, it may be of significance in elucidating the pathogenesis of this neuromyopathy which todate defies explanation. All patients with biopsy proven carcinoma of skin were screened for any evidence of neurologic disease. The search for neurologic disease was accomplished by

1. a thorough neurologic history and complete neurologic examination,
2. Electrical survey of the neuromuscular system in which

a) motor nerve conduction velocity was measured in two peripheral nerves (Median and Peroneal),

b) needle electromyography was done on a selected group of extremity muscles which included one muscle from each of the arm, forearm, hand, thigh, leg, foot.

Results and Discussion

This study shows that neurological complications do occur in skin cancer. In the 14 patients studied, 8 showed evidence of neuromyopathy. 5 of 10 patients with basal cell carcinoma and 3 of 4 patients with squamous cell carcinoma had neuromyopathy. The apparent preponderance of neuromyopathy in patients with squamous cell carcinoma may represent a false impression because of the small number of patients. Further studies are needed before any final statement could be made.

In four patients, the history and clinical findings were suggestive of neuromyopathy. Electrical studies confirmed the clinical impression in all four. In three patients the neuromyopathy was detected only after electrical studies were done. Only in one case was the diagnosis based on purely clinical grounds. This patient refused electrical studies. The clinical spectrum included complaints of parasthesias, weakness, wasting of muscles, reflex changes and peripheral sensory impairment. The detection of neuromyopathy after electrical studies brings out the necessity of performing such studies before excluding neuromyopathy.

Of the eight cases, six had predominant neuropathy, while two had evidence of neuropathy and myopathy. Only one patient had evidence of cerebellar disease. None of the patients had evidence of cord affection. This relative infrequency of cord and brain manifestations is in agreement with reports in the literature of preponderance of neuromyopathy among the neurological complication of carcinoma (over 50%).

Tab. 2 shows the age distribution of patients with and without neuromyopathy. It is apparent that in every age group except the last (70 to 79) there are control patients with no neuromyopathy. Furthermore, the two youngest patients in the study did have a neuromyopathy.

Table 2. *Age distribution in neuromyopathy*

Age years	No. with neuromyopathy	No. with no neuromyopathy
30—39	1	0
40—49	1	0
50—59	0	3
60—69	4	3
70—79	2	0

While this study helped answer one of the queries raised at the beginning of the presentation, it has failed to answer the more difficult question of why do neuro-myopathies occur in cancer? Everybody agrees that they are not due to metastasis but beyond that, there is a lot of controversy and uncertainty. The metabolic or toxic basis for it is not yet proven. The suggestion that the tumor produces an anti-metabolite against pantothenic acid remains an interesting speculation. The most accepted hypothesis is that of an autoimmune mechanism. Sera of patients w th neuromyopathy contain organ specific complement fixing antibodies against saline extracts of brain [5]. The above has received further support from studies using fluorescent antibody technics [6]. While autoimmunity is an attractive hypothesis, to be finally accepted it has to answer a number of questions, foremost among them is why should fluorescent and complement fixing antibodies be limited to those patients showing sensory neuropathy only.

References. 1. HENSON, R. A., D. S. RUSSELL, and M. WILKINSON: Brain 77, 82 (1954). — 2. HEATHFIELD, K. W. G., and J. R. B. WILLIAMS: Brain 77, 122 (1954). — 3. BRAIN, R., and R. A. HENSON: Lancet 1958, II, 917. — 4. CROFT, P. B. J., and M. WILKINSON: Brain 88, 427 (1965). — 5. WILKINSON, P. C.: Lancet 1964, I, 1301. — 6. WILKINSON, P. C., and J. ZEROMSKI: Brain 88, 529 (1965).

Cancer, precancer y pseudocancer cutaneos: Estudio estadistico de la clinica dermatológica de la Universidad de Valencia

J. CALAP y J. M. FORTEA, Clinica Dermatológica de la Universidad de Valencia (España)

La frecuencia de aparición de algunas dermatosis está intimamente ligada a factores etnológicos y geográficos como demostró MARCHIONINI [1 a 18]. No cabe duda que tambien la aparicion del cancer de piel está influenciada por dichos factores. Demostrativa es la observación de ROTHMAN [19] de que el epitelioma basocelular es casi inexistente en la población Bantú, con excepcion de los bantues albinos, en los que el e.basocelular es muy destructivo.

Para contribuir al capítulo de la dermatologia geográfica y etnográfica aplicado al cancer cutáneo, hemos realizado un estudio en las clinicas dermatológicas de Valencia y Munich. En Valencia de 1944 a 1965 se vieron un total de 31.710 dermatosis de las que se hicieron 4.600 biopsias confirmandose 1.407 epiteliomas: 888 basocelulares y 519 espinocelulares; en las preparaciones en que se precise el tipo de basocelular se encuentra el pagetoide, pigmentado, esclerodermiforme y superficial, por orden decreciente de frecuencia. La media arimetica de los epiteliomas vistos en 22 años es aproximadamente de 40 e. basocelulares y 24 e. espinocelulares por año, cifra relativamente baja si se tiene en cuenta que Valencia tiene una población de mas de 600.000 habitantes. Para comparar la frecuencia y tipo de aparición de los epiteliomas en Valencia con la ciudad de Munich, revisamos los archivos de la clinica dermatologica universitaria de ésta ciudad: en 1965 se diagnosticaron histologicamente en Munich 203 epiteliomas basocelulares y 96 espinocelulares y en 1966; 135 basocelulares y 54 espinocelulares. Si establecemos un cociente benignidad/malignidad en los epiteliomas, vemos que para Munich fue de B/E = 2,11 en 1965 y B/E = 2,50 en 1966, con un cociente global para los dos años de 2,25. En Valencia cifras paralelas nos dan en 1965: 56 basocel. y 48 espinocel. (B/E = 1,16) y en 1966: 68 basocel. y 48 espinocel. (B/E = 1,41). Cociente global 1965 a 1966 = 1,33. Es curioso observar cómo el cociente B/E aumenta en el transcurso del año 1965 a 1966 a favor de la aparición benigna del epitelioma, tanto en Valencia como en Munich. Sin embargo, considerando las cifras globales obtenidas con los datos de 1944 a 1965, obtenemos un B/E = 1,70, lo que no indica una tendencia real hacia las formas benignas del epitelioma, en Valencia, en el transcurso de los ultimos 24 años, evolución que se podria falsamente deducir analizando solo los datos de los dos últimos años.

Formas precancerosas. Predomina en el material de Valencia el queratoma senil, la verruga seborreica y las leucoplasias. El morbus Paget solo lo hemos encontrado en 8 preparaciones (1944 a 1965) lo que da una frecuencia en nuestra clinica, de 1 Paget por cada 3.963 dermatosis. A la frecuencia de aparicion de la enf. de Paget le hemos prestado especial atención por haber estudiado, previamente, esta enfermedad bajo otros aspectos [20, 21].

VILANOVA [22] encontró un caso de Paget de cada 1.900 dermatosis en la clinica universitaria de Barcelona. Esta proporción fue calificada por WIMAN y SKOGH [23] de *exageradamente alta*, por el hecho de encontrar estos autores un Paget de cada 21.000 dermatosis, en Upsala.

La proporción obtenida para' el Paget en Valencia la hemos comparado con un material de Munich abarcando un periodo de 10 años (1956 a 1965): En 1956 se registraron 10.337 nuevos enfermos y en 1965: 15.423 y el total en dichos 10 años: 119.854 enfermos. Ahora bien esta cifra no corresponde al de nuevas dermatosis, pues el sistema de registro de Munich, está hecho de forma que cada enfermo recibe en la historia clinica un nuevo numero a partir del 1 de enero, por ello, para saber el numero total de dermatosis por año hay que ver la historias clinicas aisladamente. El numero real de dermatosis que se vieron en Munich de 1956 a 1965 fue de 102.315, siendo diagnosticados en dicho periodo de tiempo 32 enfermos como enfermedad de Paget, de los cuales en 27 se confirmó histologicamente el diagnostico clínico, en 4 casos se excluyó y en uno fue discutido el diagnostico entre un Paget y un epitelioma intraepidermal. En definitiva, la proporción de Paget/No de dermatosis en Munich es de 1:3.789. Comparando las estadisticas personales con la de VILANOVA y la de WIMAN y SKOGH, tenemos: *Proporcion del Paget según las latitudes:* Upsala: 1/21.000. Munich: 1/3.789. Barcelona: 1/1.900. Valencia: 1/3.963. Vemos cómo los resultados que hemos obtenido en Munich están mas cerca de los de Valencia y los previos de Barcelona (VILANOVA) que de los obtenidos en Upsala (WIMAN y SKOGH). Esta discrepancia de resultados puede ser simplemente debida a la influencia de los factores etnologicos y geograficos en la aparición del cancer.

Pseudocancer. Solo citaremos que en el periodo 1944 a 1965, se establecieron 7 diagnósticos de queratoacantoma en Valencia; teniendo en cuenta que el aislamiento definitivo de este tumor como entidad nosologica se hizo en 1950, vemos que la aparición de este tumor, en nuestra ciudad, es relativamente mayor que la enfermedad de Paget.

Conclusiones: 1. En los dos ultimos años parece haber una tendencia evolutiva a favor de la aparición de formas benignas del epitelioma (Valencia, Munich), afirmación que no se puede hacer observando los valores obtenidos de nuestra estadistica de 22 años (1944 a 1965) (Valencia) comparándolos con los de 1965 a 1966. 2. La discrepancia de resultados de estadísticas realizadas en distintas latitudes, se debe, entre otras cosas, a la influencia que los factores etnologico-geográficos ejercen en la aparición de determinadas dermatosis.

Bibliografía. 1. a 18. MARCHIONINI, A.: Arch. Derm. Syph. (Berl.) **179**, 421 (1931); **181**, 239 (1940); **181**, 127 (1942); **184**, (1942); **185**, 1 (1943); **185**, 363 (1944). — Hautarzt **3**, 109 (1952). — X. Int. Kongr. Derm. London. Proc. Brit. Med. Ass. London 1953. — Hautarzt **4**, 408 (1953); **4**, 455 (1953); **5**, 8 (1954); **5**, 110 (1954); **5**, 205 (1954); **5**, 298 (1954); **5**, 397 (1954); **5**, 504 (1954); **5**, 537 (1954); **6**, 7 (1955). — 19. ROTHMAN, S.: Arch. Derm. Syph. (Chic.) **85**, 311 (1962). — 20. LOZANO, N., y J. CALAP: IV. Congreso Mejicano de Dermatologia, Tampico 1967. — 21. CALAP, J.: VI. Congreso Ibero-Latino Americano de Dermat. Barcelona 1967. — 22. VILANOVA, X., y. F. OLLER: Act. dermo. sifiliogr. (Madr.) **45**, 127 (1953). — 23. WIMAN, L. G., and E. SKOGH: Acta derm.-venereol. (Stockh.) **43**, 32 (1963).

Electron Microscopic Study of the Morphogenesis of Skin Tumours

J. SUGÁR, Research Institute of Oncopathology, Budapest (Hungary)

In the present studies the fine structural changes in relation with the early stage i.e. the beginning of invasive growth were investigated. It has been tried to prove whether cell degeneration and the loosening of the contact, observed in preneoplastic conditions should be of any significance in starting invasive growth.

For these studies methylcholantrene induced skin alterations of mice were used. Preneoplastic hyperplasias, papillomas and carcinomas were embedded for light- and electronmicroscopy. Human skin cancers and precancers were also investigated.

A fundamental structural property of the epithelium undergoing alterations in the course of carcinogenesis was found to be the loosening of cell connections in all layers of the squamous epithelium, including also the basal layer. As a result of the loss of cohesion intercellular spaces were widely enlarged and villiform processes were extruded from the cytoplasm into the intercellular spaces. On account of the considerable dilatation of the intercellular spaces combined with the formation of microvilli and cytoplasmic processes the basement membrane cannot run parallel with the cytoplasmic membrane of the basal cells. In this way spaces are formed between the basement membrane and the cells. These parts of the basement membrane became areas of predilection for gap formation.

The cause of such loosening of the cell contact may be found in cell degeneration which is going on extensively in the epithelial cells and was localized to single cells or to cell groups. That is why intercellular spaces contained varying numbers of ribosomes, remnants of membranes and other cellular debris, referred by us as intercellular exsudate.

In the hyperplastic epithelium electron lucent, light and electron opaque dark cells were alternating.

Invasive growth begins with the breakthrough of the basement membrane. It was observed, however, that in many cases of papillomas, senile keratoma and

6*

keratoacanthomas gaps of 0.05 to 0,1 mμ began to form on basement membranes. Through these gaps cytoplasmic processes of various sizes are protruded into the connective tissue. In these cytoplasmic processes filaments of the epithelial cells can be found. At a site, where the basement membrane in the length of 2 to 3 μ is lacking, a great number of cytoplasmic processes and villi are invading the connective tissue. It may often be observed even in preinvasive or incipient carcinomas that gaps smaller than a cell diameter are found on basement membranes, while frontal breakthrough occurs only at a later stage of invasive growth. Around the non-differentiated epithelial cell rows and bundles of invasive growth, no basement membrane could be detected.

The number of interchromatinic granules in the nucleus of precancer-cells is strikingly high. Parallel with the progress of carcinogenesis chromatin is scattered in the form of crude lumps throughout the nucleoplasm.

The electron microscopic studies of the morphogenesis of squamous cell carcinoma revealed the loosening of the cell contacts in the course of carcinogenesis. Cell degeneration plays a part in the development of the loss of cell cohesion and in starting invasive growth.

Even before the frontal breakthrough of the basement membrane, still in the preneoplastic phase, cytoplasmic processes originating from epithelial cells penetrate into the connective tissue through the gaps of the basement membrane. This phenomenon was referred to as micro-invasion at electron microscopic level.

The fine structure of cell particles containing nucleoproteins i.e. chromatin particles and also interchromatinic granules undergoes considerable modifications in the course of carcinogenesis.

Epidermotropic Eccrine Carcinoma

Y. MIURA, A. AKANO, T. NAKAGAWA and Y. KIKUCHI, University of Hokkaido Medical School, Sapporo, Hokkaido (Japan)

PINKUS and MEHREGAN reported in 1963 a peculiar case with multiple metastatic nodules on all surfaces of the leg and thigh as well as on abdomen and left breast, which showed histologically epidermal involvement with tumor cell nests in Paget's disease-like behavior. A similar case was observed by us.

The patient was a 69-year-old man who was first seen in April, 1963. 12 years previously he had noticed a red, soft papule on the posterior aspect of the right leg, which increased in size slowly to a hen's egg-sized tumor.

Examination showed the right lower extremity lymphedematous and a cauliflower-like tumor, 6 × 5 cm in size, connected to the basis with broad pedicle of about 3 cm in diameter. The surface of the tumor was granulated and eroded with stinking exudates. Right inguinal lymph nodes were enlarged to the size of finger-head.

The tumor was totally resected and the intermediate skin graft was transplanted from the inner site of the right thigh. The right inguinal lymph nodes were enuculated at the same time, and after then irradiation of X-ray was done for the region.

6 months after operation, there appeared keloid-like elevation and multiple verrucous papules on the donor site of the right thigh. After the irradiation of X-ray amounting to 6,000 r, the lesion became flat but eroded. In the following several months, the nodules progressed to involve right leg, left thigh, genitalia

and abdomen up to umbilicus, and began to develop eroded, diffusely indulated and pigmented plaques in some areas. In spite of parenteral administration of antineoplastic drugs, he died with cachexia 8 months after the onset of recurrence. Autopsy revealed wide-spread neoplastic infiltration in the skin of both lower extremities, genitalia and abdomen, which was markedly diffuse and superficial. Metastases were also noticed in the inguinal and periaortic lymph nodes. No other neoplastic lesion was observed at all.

Histopathologic examination of the primary lesion shows papillary proliferation of epidermis, in which nests of tumor cells are present. There are numerous nests of malignant epithelial cells in the corium. Nuclei of these tumor cells tend to be hyperchromatic, of uneven size and shape. The nests vary in size from large masses to small groups, but there are no distinct features of glandular formation.

Tumor cells contain less glycogen, but stain red in Mallory-Heidenhain's azan stained section. On the other hand, one sees dendritic features in the tumor cell nests qualified as melanocytes by Masson-Zimmermann's stain. The tumor cells show no demonstrable tonofibrils. They are often connected with each other by slender cytoplasmic bridges, while in other areas there is a clear space of separation in Unna's waterblue-orcein-eosin-safranin stained section.

Sections from all metastatic nodules show similar characteristics. In the section from recurred lesions on the resected site of the primary tumor, one sees atypical cells in the upper corium in an arrangement suggesting their spread into the lymphatics in the skin. The section from right thigh shows numerous intraepidermal and intradermal nests of tumor cells similar to those of the primary lesion.

The nests in lymph nodes consist of somewhat uneven epithelial cells, which contain a lot of mitotic figures.

From clinical and autopsy findings, it is evident that our case must be a malignant tumor and its diffuse metastases in the skin and in regional lymph nodes, which primarily occurred in the skin. It seems to differ, however, from ordinary malignant epithelial tumors in several points, such as formation of defined intraepidermal cell nests, wide-spread metastases, long course of the disease and clinical features, which resembled Paget's disease in some area.

Various benign and malignant neoplasms of the skin that often or occasionally produce intraepidermal cell nests are divided into three groups by MEHREGAN and PINKUS (1964) as follows:

1. Various benign skin tumors: Seborrheic verruca, Hidroacanthoma simplex, Papillomatous epidermal nevus, Junction nevus.

2. Primary malignant skin tumors: Bowen's precancerous dermatosis, Keratosis senilis, Squamous-cell carcinoma, Basal-cell epithelioma, Malignant melanoma.

3. Secondary invasion of epidermis by foreign neoplastic cells: Epidermotropic carcinoma, Paget's disease.

I shall omit discussion of those forms of benign skin tumors. Bowen's dermatosis, keratosis senilis, squamous-cell carcinoma and malignant melanoma need not to concern us here. There are certain points of similarity between our case and basal-cell epithelioma. One can not see, however, any signs of palisade arrangement of peripheral cell layers in the cell nests, and of distinct connection to basal cell layers of the epidermis. Furthermore, there are diffuse metastatic lesions suggesting spread into the lymphatics, which also show intraepidermal cell nests.

The histologic features of the metastatic lesions remind us of a case described by PINKUS and MEHREGAN (1963) as epidermotropic eccrine carcinoma. Characteristics of tumor cells are completely similar to those of PINKUS' case except for the rather small content of glycogen. If we take into consideration that the histologic picture of the primary lesion provides the characteristics of eccrine poroma, it seems not unreasonable to accept our case as malignant eccrine poroma (or eccrine porocarcinoma suggested by PINKUS, MISHIMA and MORIOKA) and its epidermotropic metastases.

It is interesting that the tumor nests contain symbiotic proliferation of melanocytes, which has been reported by YASUDA et al. (1964) in a case of eccrine poroma of a Japanese patient. As for glycogen, DEGOS et al. (1957) failed to demonstrate glycogen in their specimen of eccrine poroma, and YASUDA et al. (1964) noted it only in a half of the tumor tissue of their case.

Considérations sur le potentiel de malignisation des chéilites précancéreuses

AL. DIMITRESCU, Clinique Dermatologique de Bucarest (Roumanie)

Le sujet de cette étude représente un des aspects et le plus important des chéilites précancéreuses; il a fait de notre part l'objet d'une ample monographie. Dans ce qui suit nous présenterons une synthèse des données qui nous ont été fournies par 343 cas de chéilites chroniques de différents types et origines, étudiées du point de vue clinique, histologique et histochimique. L'objet principal de notre monographie a été justement l'étude de leur degré de cancérisation, ainsi que le mécanisme par lequel elles arrivent à la malignisation; ces deux aspects sont encore sujet à discussions.

1. Concernant les chéilites glandulaires, nous sommes d'avis que:

a) sous leur forme suppurative superficielle et profonde elles possèdent un important potentiel de malignisation, moindre cependant qu'on ne le croit généralement; ce potentiel apparaît encore moins important si l'on tient compte du facteur statistique.

b) Elles ne représentent pas des précancéroses obligatoires, par leur nature glandulaire; la transformation maligne est conditionnée par l'évolution et l'intensité des lésions qui compliquent un petit nombre des chéilites glandulaires simples.

c) Les faits suivants plaident contre la nature et l'origine glandulaire des épithéliomas greffés sur ces chéilites: l'extrême rareté de la transformation maligne de la chéilite glandulaire simple, la rareté des tumeurs malignes et bénignes d'origine glandulaire salivaire, inclusivement des tumeurs mixtes, l'extrême rareté des cas où l'on ne peut surprendre comme point de départ de l'épithélioma de la lèvre, la paroi du canal glandulaire métaplasié.

d) Le mécanisme de la cancérisation des chéilites glandulaires réside essentiellement dans un processus de cocarcinogénèse, dans le cadre duquel les glandes hétérotopiques représentent un simple facteur étiologique prédisposant. Sur ce fond, l'action isolée, mais surtout surajoutée de plusieurs facteurs irritatifs qui agissent en association (le tabac, soleil, tartre dentaire, la paraodontose, certaines prothèses dentaires, des infections microbiennes, des facteurs irritants alimentaires, mécaniques, etc.). Chacun de ces facteurs possède des propriétés leucoplasogènes et cancérigènes, et leur action aboutit à l'aggravation du tableau anatomo-clinique et à la malignisation.

2. En ce qui concerne les chéilites kératosiques qui constituent un groupe relativement hétérogène, mais qui ont comme trait commun l'hyperkératose réactionnelle, nous avons tiré les conclusions suivantes:

a) Le potentiel cancérigène le plus élevé appartient aux chéilites leucoplasiques tabagiques; néanmoins elles sont peu importantes du point de vue statistique.

b) La chéilite actinique chronique a un potentiel de transformation maligne moins élevé, mais elle est la plus importante du point de vue statistique. Dans notre pays elle fournit un très grand taux des épithéliomas de la lèvre (environ 40 à 50%).

c) De même que les chéilites glandulaires, celles kératosiques ne représentent pas des précancéroses à caractère obligatoire. Dans leur stade exfoliatif, ce potentiel est pratiquement nul, n'apparaissant et ne s'accentuant que concomitamment avec l'intensification de l'hyperkératose et des lésions qui peuvent la compliquer. Le point culminant est atteint quand s'installe le tableau anatomo-clinique de la chéilite abrasive ANZILOTTI-MANGANOTTI.

d) Le mécanisme par lequel on arrive à ces complications et à cette malignisation est le même que pour le cas des chéilites glandulaires; rarement intervient un seul facteur étiologique (soleil, tabac). Le plus souvent il s'agit de l'action surajoutée de plusieurs des facteurs irritatifs mentionnés, et en outre de l'hétérotopie des glandes salivaires. Dans ce cadre, l'un des facteurs cocarcinogénétiques exerce une action prépondérante, en imprimant une spécificité étiologique relative (chéilite solaire, tabagique, etc.).

e) Dans le cas des chéilites kératosiques de cause non déterminée, interviennent très probablement des facteurs carentiels de nature alimentaire (troubles digestifs chroniques, alimentation monotone).

3. Quant aux chéilites kératosiques provenant de la localisation labiale de certaines dermatoses, telles que le lupus érythémateux, le lichen plan et le herpes récidivant, le potentiel de leur malignité est discutable. Nous sommes d'avis que les rares cas de malignisation cités dans la littérature, ainsi que ceux que nous avons rencontrés, sont dus à l'intervention de quelques uns des facteurs irritatifs mentionnés, qui ajoutent leur action leucoplasogène et blastogène à l'état leuco-kératosique de l'affection de base.

L'influence des radiations artificielles sur la muqueuse des lèvres des trempeurs d'acier

R. NICOLAU, P. IACOB et M. BICHIS, Section de Dermatologie, Union des Sociétés des Sciences Médicales, Bucarest (Roumanie)

Les cheilites des lèvres inférieures sont des affections provoquées par l'exposition aux radiations naturelles ou artificielles. Elles ont pour cause les actions de la lumière seule ou associée au phototraumatisme. Nous avons étudié cette affection dans un combinat sidérurgique, dans lequel les ouvriers viennent en contact avec diverses radiations ultraviolettes et thermiques.

Des soixante, dix trempeurs d'acier examinés, 58 c'est-à-dire 83% ont été atteints de la cheilite. Les facteurs qui contribuent à l'apparition de cette affection sont d'ordre physique auxquels contribuent le terrain de l'ouvrier et son régime de vie. —

a) Parmi les facteurs physiques citons: la température de l'air, l'humidité et les courants d'air qui existent tous sur le lieu étudié de ce travail. La température de l'air y est constante atteignant 33° — jusqu'à 51 °C. Les déterminations ont été faites à l'aide d'un psychromètre. Les radiations lumineuses émanées des fourneaux ont été mesurées à diverses étapes du travail et à des distances variées atteignant de la 70 lux jusqu'à 5500 lux. La spectroscopie des ultraviolettes faite à l'aide d'un monochromateur Zeiss a montré la présence des rayons ultraviolets compris entre 270 et 400 mμ. Ces radiations sont émises par impulsions qui dépassent la distance d'un mètre de fourneau parfois 600 fois les radiations d'une lampe de mercure mesurées à la même distance. Le manque d'humidité montre les valeurs de 30 à 40% d'humidité relative; les courants d'air ont atteint la vitesse jusqu'à 4,5 msec.

b) L'étude du terrain d'ouvrier a montré en ce qui concerne les gastrites, les ulcères, les fonctions hépatiques et le système nerveux — des données semblables à un autre lieu de travail ce qui nous permet de ne pas attribuer un rôle quelconque au terrain des ouvriers étudiés.

c) Le régime de la vie en ce qui concerne la navette, la qualité de la nourriture, la consommation des médicaments ou l'ingérence de l'alcool n'a pas présenté des données dignes d'être retenues. — Au point de vue clinique, les ouvriers examinés par nous, présentaient un érithème associé des desquamations, fissures et, très rarement d'ailleurs, des croûtes localisées au niveau de la lèvre inférieure qui, en son ensemble, était légèrement oedèmateuse. — On constate par endroits la présence d'une couche blanchâtre ou hyperpigmentée, localisée sur la muqueuse de la lèvre inférieure. — Subjectivement, les ouvriers se plaignaient d'avoir une sensation de sécheresse, brûlure, associée de fourmillement au niveau de la lèvre inférieure. La défense de l'organisme devant les stimules lumineux peut déterminer une réaction congestive au niveau des téguments, une autre pigmentogène et une troisième hyperquératosique.

Nous considérons la réaction pigmentogène comme un moyen de défense de l'organisme. La mélanine a un rôle double de protection optique de même que chimique par le blocage du radical libre des composées toxiques ou cancérogènes. Nous avons considéré la hypérkératose au niveau de la lèvre inférieure aussi comme un moyen de défense.

La couche cornée absorbe les radiations en proportion de 50% à peu près. Parmi les ouvriers examinés par nous, 31% ont présenté la réaction congestive; 68% parmi les ouvriers ont présenté la réaction pigmentogène. Les chéilites associées ou non aux manifestations ci-dessus décrites ont présenté 83% d'ouvriers. Nous insistons que 35% des ouvriers examinés, ont présenté des herpès péribuccaux qui peuvent être attribués à l'association de lumière — infections et qui pourraient avoir un rôle en ce qui concerne la génèse des chéilites.

Les cheilites étaient divisées par nous, en cheilites du premier groupe avec oedème et congestion massive et la forme chronique la seule rencontrée par nous au combinat. L'intensité de l'affection est en rapport avec l'ancienneté dans le travail. — Nous avons rencontré encore des modifications des pavillions auriculaires consistant en télangiectasies, érythèmes, cyanoses et croûtes unilatérales en rapport avec la partie la plus exposée aux radiations. — Les ensemencements pris de la surface de la langue de tous les ouvriers pour identification de candida albicans n'ont montré qu'une positivité de 2,8%.

Ainsi nous avons éliminé la possibilité des affections micotiques de voisinage, qui, soit directement, soit indirectement, par le mécanisme allergique de voisinage ou général, rendraient potentielle l'action des radiations.

Le potentiel cancérogène résulte du grand nombre — 21% des épithélioms des lèvres inférieures, du total — des épithélioms enrégistrés dans cette entreprise.

Du point de vue prophilactique, nous recommandons un contrôle périodique annuel des ouvriers de la section respective, la réduction de l'emploi du tabac par l'ensemble des effets thermiques et chimiques, l'application des onguents pour la protection antiactinique, l'étude des possibilités que la plaque protectrice de verre de cobalt au rôle photoprotecteur, qui préserve à présent les yeux, soit prolongée jusqu'aux lèvres.

Puisque nous n'avons pas trouvé jusqu'à présent la description de cette affection et ayant en vue le grand nombre d'ouvriers malades nous proposons qu'elle soit reconnue comme une maladie professionelle avec toutes les conséquences qui en résultent.

Erythroplasia of Queyrat: A Precancerous Dermatosis*

J. H. GRAHAM, The Skin and Cancer Hospital of Philadelphia, Departments of Dermatology and Pathology, Temple University School of Medicine, Philadelphia, Pennsylvania (USA), and
E. B. HELWIG, The Division of Pathology and Branch of Dermal Pathology, The Armed Forces Institute of Pathology, Washington, D.C. (USA)

Erythroplasia of Queyrat occurs on the glans and prepuce of the penis as a red, velvety plaque, and occasionally is elevated, papillary and ulcerated. The normal epidermis is replaced by atypical hyperplastic epithelial cells and the rete ridges extend into the underlying stroma which is infiltrated with round cells. QUEYRAT [1], in 1911, concluded that erythroplasia of the glans penis represented a precancerous disease. Since then, many similar lesions have been recorded. Furthermore, the concept of erythroplasia has been broadened to include a variety of diseases and sites other than the prepuce and glans such as the glaborous skin, vulva, lips, tongue, and oral mucosa. Because of the striking histologic resemblance, some observers believe that erythroplasia of Queyrat of the glans penis is Bowen's disease of the mucosa. In previous reports [2 to 7], we presented data indicating that erythroplasia of Queyrat was different from Bowen's disease of the skin since there is an apparent significant lack of association with systemic cancer, and patients with the penile lesion fail to show other cutaneous lesions typical of Bowen's disease.

In this report, we shall present clinicopathologic and histochemical observations from 100 adult patients with typical penile lesions of erythroplasia of Queyrat. The group consisted of 90 Caucasians, 9 Negroes, and 1 Oriental. The age range at the time of first biopsy was 20 to 80 years; the median age was 51 years. The duration of the disease from stated onset to biopsy varied from 1 month to 25 years; the median duration was 2 years. The lesions ranged from 2 mm to 3.5 cm; the median size was 1 cm. Information regarding circumcision was available from 87 patients and 84 had not been circumcised before onset of their penile lesion.

Clinical and microscopic evidence of invasion of the underlying stroma as squamous cell carcinoma from lesions of erythroplasia of Queyrat was found in 10 patients. 2 of them had metastasis to the regional lymph nodes and 1 also had distant metastasis. 5 patients had cutaneous premalignant and malignant lesions and these included senile keratosis, senile keratosis with squamous cell carcinoma, squamous cell carcinoma, basal cell carcinoma, adnexal carcinoma, and malignant melanoma. 6 patients had systemic cancer involving sites other than

* This investigation was supported in part by Research Training Grant 2 A-5289 (C_5) from the National Institute of Arthritis and Metabolic Diseases, National Institutes of Health. Public Health Service, Bethesda, Maryland 20014.

the skin. None of the 100 patients showed clinical or microscopic evidence of skin lesions resembling Bowen's disease.

The follow-up period for the 100 patients varied from 1 week to 19 years; the median was 5.2 years. 34 patients were dead after a median period of 3.8 years, and only one death was directly related to erythroplasia of Queyrat. 66 patients are still alive after a median of 6.1 years and follow-up examination indicates that surgical excision is the treatment of choice.

Microscopically, erythroplasia of Queyrat shows a striking histologic resemblance to Bowen's disease. The epidermis is acanthotic with disoriented, atypical cells, vacuolated cells, and mitotic figures at all levels. The upper corium is infiltrated with inflammatory cells. As in Bowen's disease, the adjacent stroma may be invaded by the atypical epithelial proliferation. Histologic differences from Bowen's disease, include hypokeratosis, fewer multinucleated cells and malignant dyskeratotic cells, and usually there is a large number of plasma cells in the inflammatory infiltrate.

Histochemically, some of the atypical vacuolated cells contain glycogen and there are variable amounts of hyaluronic acid in the interstices of the abnormal epidermis and upper corium. Most of the lesions show melanin granules in the atypical epithelial cells and an argyrophilic basement membrane at the dermo-epidermal junction. There is a prominent proliferation of reticular fibers in areas of inflammation and the stroma shows general thinning in the same location. Striking capillary abnormalities occur immediately subjacent to the atypical epithelial changes. Papanicolaou smears show a few atypical individual epithelial cells or clumps of these cells. Chemical analysis of lesions of erythroplasia of Queyrat for arsenic showed lower values than in lesions of Bowen's disease and arsenical keratosis.

Cancer proneness was not prominent in patients with erythroplasia of Queyrat (21%), when compared to that in patients with Bowen's disease (51%). Erythroplasia of Queyrat (10%) is more prone to invade the stroma as carcinoma than Bowen's disease (5%), but for all patients with the respective diseases there is an equal rate of metastasis of 2%. Once invasive carcinoma develops in a Bowen's lesion, metastasis may occur in 37% of the patients unless early adequate treatment is given. Two (20%) of ten patients with erythroplasia of Queyrat showing invasive squamous cell carcinoma had metastasis.

Even though there is a striking histopathologic and histochemical resemblance of erythroplasia of Queyrat to Bowen's disease, the natural history of erythroplasia of Queyrat in our patients indicates that the disease represents a different entity. Factors in the pathogenesis of erythroplasia of Queyrat may be anatomic environmental carcinogens in uncircumcised men.

References. 1. QUEYRAT, L.: Bull. Soc. franç. Derm. Syph. **22**, 378 (1911). — 2. GRAHAM, J. H., and E. B. HELWIG: Arch. Derm. Syph. (Chic.) **80**, 133 (1959). — 3. GRAHAM, J. H., and E. B. HELWIG: Nat. Cancer Inst. Monograph No. 10, p. 323. Washington, D. C., 1963. — 4. HELWIG, E. B., and J. H. GRAHAM: Tumors of the Skin, p. 131. Chicago: Year Book Medical Publishers 1964. — 5. GRAHAM, J. H., and E. B. HELWIG: Tumors of the Skin, p. 209. Chicago: Year Book Medical Publishers 1964. — 6. GRAHAM, J. H., and E. B. HELWIG: Lab. Invest. **13**, 951 (1964). — 7. GRAHAM, J. H., and E. B. HELWIG: Advanc. biology Skin. **VII**, 277 (1966).

Queilitis actinica, glandular y cancer de labio inferior

P. Parejo y J. Ocaña, Universidad de Granada (España)

1. La situación del labio inferior le hace en extremo vulnerable a la acción de las radiaciones actínicas del espectro solar y a los cambios climáticos, experimentando su borde rojo una serie de alteraciones inflamatorias y degenerativas que corresponden a las que se desarrollan en la piel de las zonas descubiertas de los campesinos y marinos. Se atrofia y se retrae progresivamente, tomando un aspecto blanquecino y aparecen unas excrecencias verrugosas que luego se agrietan y ulceran sobreviniendo la cancerización. Es la denominada *queilitis actínica o queratósica*, casi siempre asociada a *leucoplasia*, de patogenia similar, y en la que intervienen, además, otros factores: traumatismos repetidos por piezas dentarias en mal estado, la acción del tabaco y los productos de combustión del papel de fumar y las lesiones producidas por el arrancamiento incesante de la epidermis cuando se lleva adherido el cigarrillo largo tiempo. Contribuye, asimismo, la senilidad prematura, los tratamientos previos con rayos X, alteraciones de la sudoración y metabólicas (diabetes, colesterinosis), existencia de tuberculosis, alcoholismo . . . etc.; estando mas predispuestos los sujetos de piel blanca, cabellos rubios y ojos azules. Al mismo tiempo, la mucosa labial está desprovista de capa córnea, de melanocitos en su epidermis y de glándulas sebaceas, que sabemos dificultan la penetración de los rayos ultravioleta en la superficie cutánea.

Cuando la queilitis actínica y leucoplasia son más o menos difusas la transformación maligna podrá limitarse a una zona, a varias, de modo simultaneo o sucesivo, o afectar la totalidad del borde rojo: es la denominada *"Cancerización en sábana"*.

Histológicamente, la queilitis actínica crónica, presenta en sus etapas iniciales, una hiperplasia epidérmica limitada con hiperqueratosis de tipo paraqueratósico y ligero engrosamiento del cuerpo mucoso de Malpighio. La capa basal prolifera hacia la dermis en forma de prolongaciones tubulares, o rodeando la extremidad de las papilas dérmicas. En estadíos mas avanzados estas características se acentúan aumentando la hiperqueratosis y la acantosis y en el seno del estrato espinoso aparecen células atípicas con nucleos de gran tamaño, hipercromático y de forma irregular, asi como aumento de las mitosis algunas de ellas atípicas. Según Nicolau y Balus la q.a. crónica, no presenta la estructura Bowenoide que caracteriza a la mayoría de las dermatosis precancerosas, pero sí la actividad proliferativa suficiente para considerarla como una dermatosis precancerosa, y aún más, como la base más frecuente del cáncer de labio. En la dermis es patente la presencia de *degeración basófila o elastótica*, señalada hace ya muchos años por los dermatólogos, y que puede ser la causa de los cambios disqueratósicos ocurridos en la epidermis.

2. La *Queilitis Glandular*, está constituida por una inflamación crónica de las glándulas salivales, situadas casi exclusivamente en la mucosa del labio inferior, donde se observan unos orificios pequeños que expulsan gotitas de saliva al presionar el labio. Se han descrito una forma *simple* por Puente y Acevedo, y otra *purulenta* con mayor reacción inflamatoria, bien *superficial* o de Baelz-Unna, y *profunda* de Volkman.

Es posible, pero no cierto, que desempeñe un papel predisponente esta infección crónica de las glándulas salivales, mas abundantes, al parecer en las personas de las regiones meridionales de España, que motivarían una protusión y prognatismo del labio inferior, aumentando la superficie de mucosa que sufriría la acción de la luz solar, desarrollándose entonces una queilitis actínica y queratósica.

Precisa insistir, además, que en estos casos no se trata de glándulas salivales heterotópicas ni de disembrioplasias pues dichas glándulas son normales en la especie humana. Como máximo puede aceptarse que los carcinomas se desarrollan eventualmente, sobre las placas de leucoplasia formada alrededor de los orificios de los conductos excretores.

En un grupo de personas (200 varones y 200 hembras), escogidos al azar entre la población general, con ocupaciones al sol y fuera de él, nos dió el siguiente resultado:

Varones		*Hembras*	
Q. actínica crónica	26%	Q. actínica crónica	14%
Q. glandular simple	4%	Q. glandular simple	6%
Q. actínica y glandular	24%	Q. actínica y glandular	8%

Es bien evidente la mayor frecuencia en nuestros medios, de Q. actínica crónica sola o asociada a Q. glandular simple, que ésta última aisladamente.

Asimismo, el estudio hitológico verificado en 163 pacientes de carcinoma espino-celular, se encontraron en todos los casos alteraciones corresondientes a la Q. actínica y queratósica, muchas veces asociada a leucoplasia, mientras que las glándulas salivales mostraban un aspecto morfológico normal. Solo en cinco casos existia Q. glandular simple y en otro la variedad supurada profunda de VOLKMAN. A pesar del examen detenido de la totalidad de la pieza extirpada no se observaba relación ni continuidad entre las alteraciones histológicas caracteristicas de los carcinomas espinocelulares y los signos inflamatorios a nivel de las glándulas salivales; solo tuvimos oportunidad de estudiar un caso que correspondía a un adenocarcinoma salival ulcerado con zonas epidermoides.

Por tanto, estimamos con BALUS que la queilitis glandular solo excepcional-mente es el punto de partida de un carcinoma espinocelular de labio inferior, y que la mayor parte de los casos publicados representan solo una eventual coincidencia de las dos afecciones; o bien, según nuestra experiencia, por su frecuente asociación con una queilitis actínica y queratósica.

3. Estimando que el sol parece ser el factor más importante en la etiopatogenia del cáncer de labio, al presentar sistematicamente los pacientes una queilitis actínica y lesiones inflamatorias, exfoliación, queratosis, leucoplasia … etc., y a pesar de ser medidas valiosísimas para su profilaxis el empleo de cremas protectoras de la luz solar y grandes sombreros, no llegan nunca a alcanzar el valor y utilidad de la denominada excisión completa del borde rojo labial, incluyendo los planos superficiales del músculo orbicular. Esta técnica ofrece garantías de curación incluso cuando ya existe un carcinoma espinocelular *intraepidérmico*, y permite el examen histológico cuidadoso y detenido de la pieza operatoria mediante cortes seriados que proporcionan datos utilísimos sobre el estado evolutivo de las lesiones, que aconsejarán técnicas mas radicales y extensas: excisión en V-bloque, disección glanglionar terapeútica … etc.

L'ulcère chronique de la lèvre inférieure

F. VANBREMEERSCH, B. DUPERRAT et J. Y. NOURY, Policlinique Alibert, Hôpital Saint-Louis, Paris (France)

Toute ulcération de la lèvre inférieure donne la hantise du cancer quand on ne peut la rattacher d'emblée à une cause précise.

Si le cancer de la lèvre inférieure, même pris à son extrême début, a des signes très évocateurs, il existe, par contre, des lésions ulcéreuses très particulières, qui

ont des caractères cliniques évolutifs et histologiques constants. Ces lésions ulcéreuses ne sont pas exceptionnelles, cependant elles ne sont décrites dans aucun des
Traités de Dermatologie, ni dans aucune des nombreuses publications traitant des
affections des lèvres. Ce sont ces lésions que nous nous permettons de décrire
aujourd'hui, en proposant de les nommer: Ulcère chronique de la lèvre inférieure.

Etiologie

Cette étude est basée sur 10 cas. Il s'agit de 9 hommes et une femme, tous âgés
de plus de 60 ans, vivant et travaillant au grand air, comme agriculteur, horti-
culteur ou comme marin. Tous étaient fumeurs, mais ils avaient cessé de fumer
depuis plusieurs années. Certains d'entre eux avaient des dents en mauvais état,
d'autres portaient une prothèse dentaire
complète depuis plusieurs années. Tous
en excellente santé, aucun d'entre eux ne
prenait de médicaments. La lésion de la
lèvre était unique, isolée, et ne s'accompagnait d'aucune autre altération des
muqueuses buccales ni d'aucune affection
précancéreuse de la peau du visage.

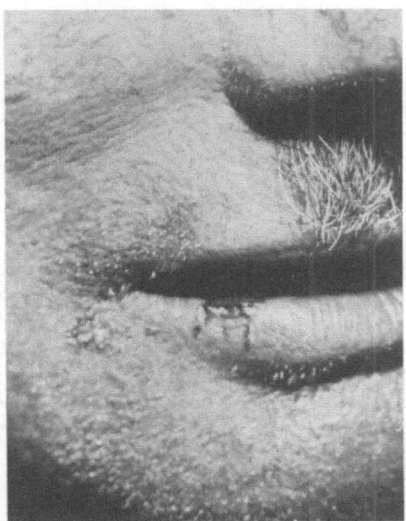

Description

Le mode de début est difficile à préciser chez ces sujets qui ont leur ulcère
depuis des mois. Mais un de nos cas nous
a permis d'assister véritablement au début de la lésion.

C'est un homme de 69 ans, qui a une
lésion ulcéreuse de la lèvre inférieure
depuis 15 jours (Fig. 1). L'ulcération, parfaitement ronde, siège sur la moitié droite
de la lèvre inférieure, dans la zône ver-
millon, proche de la ligne de Kleine. Cette

Fig. 1. Début aigu de l'ulcère de la lèvre

ulcération ronde, rouge vif, saignotante,
est bordée en arrière par un fin liseré blanchâtre, porcelainé, qui fait discuter
un lichen érosif. La palpation est un peu douloureuse mais elle ne montre aucune
induration. Cette ulcération s'est produite spontanément, sans brûlure, sans traumatisme, elle ne succède pas à un herpès, le patient ne fume pas, mais ses dents

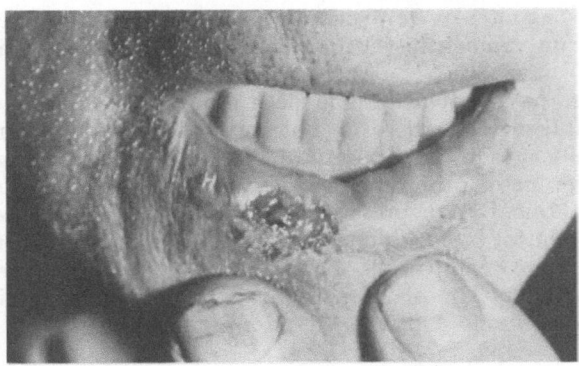

Fig. 2. Ulcère invétéré (2 ans). Noter l'aspect papillomateux, qui est histologiquement bénin,
non tumoral

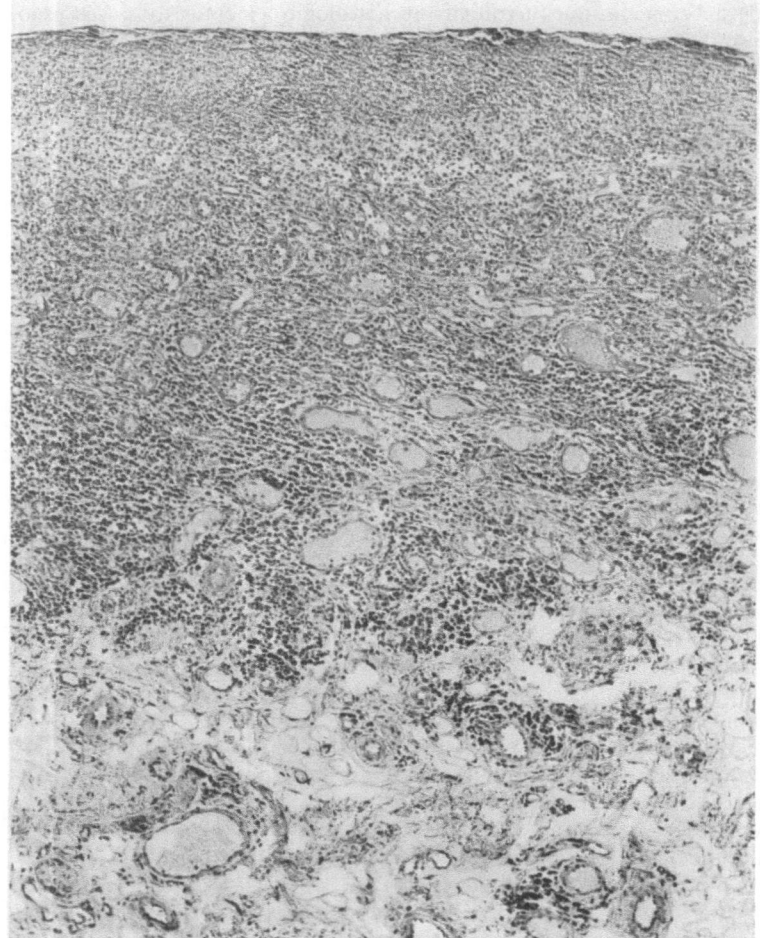

Fig. 3. Aspect typique. Noter, de haut en bas: — la surface horizontale plate — l'infiltrat riche en plasmocytes — le coussin angiomateux. G × 110

et ses gencives sont altérées de pyorrhée. Cette ulcération a été extirpée en bloc pour permettre un examen histologique complet. Et l'aspect microscopique est très particulier.

La muqueuse pavimenteuse est le siège d'une large érosion. L'épiderme est interrompu brutalement au bord de l'ulcération. Cette ulcération repose sur un granulome lymphocytaire qui repose lui-même sur une nappe angiomateuse. Les berges de l'érosion ne montrent aucune altération spécifique si ce n'est des micro-abcès dans l'épiderme. Dans la profondeur, il y a des travées fibreuses qui pénètrent dans le muscle. Un tel tableau donne l'impression d'un trouble trophique brutal et l'ensemble est très comparable à l'aspect de l'ulcère rond de l'estomac, dit «ulcère de Cruveilhier». La plaie opératoire a parfaitement guéri, sans récidive.

Une telle observation est priviligiée qui a permis d'observer le stade initial de l'ulcère.

Le plus souvent, on voit les patients après plusieurs mois d'évolution, et l'aspect clinique est toujours le même. L'ulcère siège toujours sur la lèvre inférieure, franchement latéral, parfois près de la ligne médiane, mais jamais à la commissure. L'ulcère est arrondi ou ovalaire disposé selon le grand axe de la lèvre. Quand il est juxta-médian, il peut être creusé d'une fissure antéro-postérieure douloureuse. Sinon, il n'y a aucune douleur spontanée. Cet ulcère chronique, propre, ne saigne pas sauf s'il est traumatisé. Il n'a aucune induration superficielle ou profonde, tout au plus un léger empâtement inflammatoire s'il y a surinfection passagère.

Cet ulcère chronique persiste inchangé pendant des mois ou des années. Les nombreux topiques antiseptiques, antibiotiques ou antiinflammatoires qui n'ont pas manqué d'être utilisés ne modifient en rien l'évolution. Avec le temps, l'ulcère a tendance à grandir, et tel de nos patients avait un ulcère depuis plus de 2 ans qui mesurait 12 mm (Fig. 2). On remarque, en général, autour de l'ulcère, de petites trainées blanchâtres, dont l'histologie montre qu'il s'agit d'une leucokératose banale, sans la moindre menace de transformation carcinomateuse. Il n'y a jamais aucune tuméfaction ganglionnaire perceptible.

L'examen histologique de tous nos cas montre un aspect uniforme.

Histologie

Nous avons fait de nombreuses coupes des pièces opératoires de nos malades. On constate un ulcère tantôt plan, tantôt déprimé, plus rarement turgescent et saillant. La surface apparait donc, en général, horizontale. Les berges sont tantôt constituées par un amincissement progressif de la muqueuse, tantôt par une coupure brutale. Assez souvent, il existe une papillomatose réactionnelle; celle-ci n'est jamais de type tumoral ni même simplement suspecte.

Sous l'ulcération on observe de haut en bas:

a) un granulome inflammatoire formant une couche continue et compacte. Ce granulome est richement cellulaire avec majorité de plasmocytes,

b) une zône angiomateuse constituée par un lacis capillaire béant,

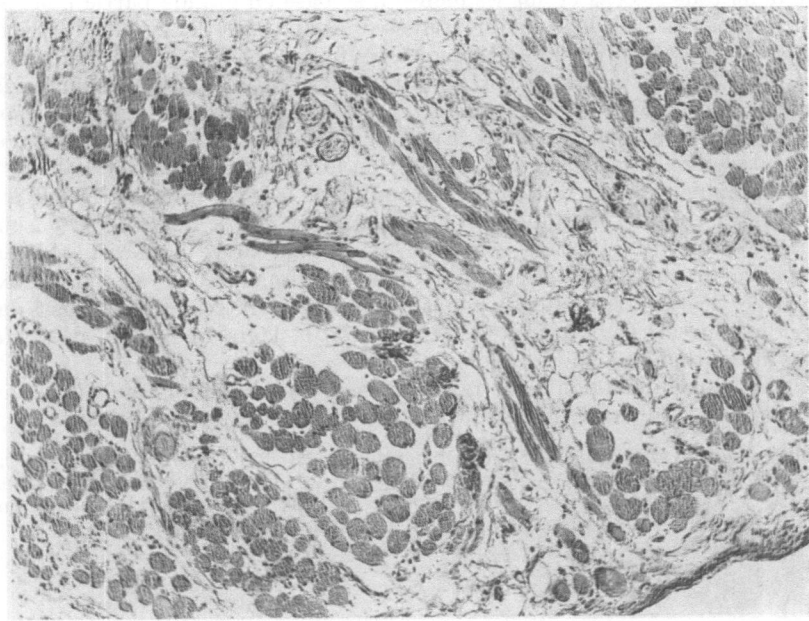

Fig. 4. Noter la sclérose angiomateuse du muscle labial. G × 110

c) une zône de sclérose qui descend jusqu'au muscle labial. Dans les cas invétérés, le muscle apparait morcelé et atrophique. Cette sclérose est également riche en capillaires (Fig. 3 et 4).

Enfin, il faut souligner que les vaisseaux artériels ou veineux qui peuvent être intéressés par l'extirpation chirurgicale sont toujours très altérés. Leur paroi apparait fibreuse, parfois même, il existe un début d'athérome.

Discussion diagnostique et nosologique

Telle est cette lésion que nous proposons de nommer «l'ulcère chronique de la lèvre inférieure». C'est une lésion assez commune, qui semble cependant n'avoir encore jamais été décrite, même dans le travail pourtant si fouillé de SCHUERMANN.

C'est une question d'actualité: tout récemment, à Sydney, MACKIE a décrit les ulcères de la lèvre inférieure provoqués par l'usage de certaines drogues: méthyl-dopa, phénylbutazone, chlorpromazine, ulcères qui guérissent par la simple suppression de la drogue responsable. Nous mêmes, en avons vu un cas dû à la chlorpromazine, chez une femme d'une cinquantaine d'années.

L'ulcère chronique de la lèvre inférieure est distinct, cliniquement et histologiquement, de la leucoplasie verruqueuse ulcérée prénéoplasique, il est différent aussi du lichen érosif et de la maladie de Bowen.

En fait, c'est avec la lésion décrite par ANZILOTTI et MANGANOTTI sous le nom de «chéilite abrasive précancéreuse», que l'ulcère chronique a le plus de similitudes: le siège sur la lèvre inférieure, l'âge déjà avancé des sujets, l'importance des lésions vasculaires. Mais l'évolution est différente: alors que la cheilite abrasive évolue avec des alternances de rémission et de récidive pour aboutir à une érosion permanente qui peut se transformer en cancer, l'ulcère chronique évolue d'une seule tenue, sans aucune rémission et sans transformation. Histologiquement, les différences sont notables. Nous n'avons jamais vu les «perles» épithéliales intra-dermiques décrites par ANZILOTTI, non plus que les cellules dyskératosiques qu'il signale dans tous ses cas et sur lesquelles il se base en grande partie pour établir la nature précancéreuse de la cheilite abrasive. ANZILOTTI et MANGANOTTI décrivent longuement les altérations du collagène et des fibres élastiques, par contre ils n'ont pas vu dans leurs cas cette pénétration du muscle par des travées fibreuses au-dessous du granulome inflammatoire et vasculaire, fibrose qui donne un aspect si particulier à ce que nous décrivons. Et enfin, dans aucun de nos cas, nous n'avons vu un seul élément qui permette de parler de lésion prénéoplasique labiale.

Il semble que le terme d' «Ulcère chronique de la lèvre inférieure» soit justifié. Il s'agit d'un trouble trophique de la lèvre inférieure, à début aigu vasculaire, d'étiologie inconnue. Une fois constitué, il va poursuivre lentement sa carrière avec très peu de modifications cliniques ou histologiques. Et si l'on en fait l'exérèse chirurgicale, c'est parce qu'il n'y a pas d'autre traitement, et c'est aussi dans la crainte où l'on est, devant toute ulcération de la lèvre inférieure, d'assister au début d'un épithélioma spino-cellulaire.

L'ulcère chronique de la lèvre inférieure nous semble donc une entité clinique et histologique, dont la cheilite abrasive n'est peut-être qu'une variante.

Bibliographie. ANZILOTTI, G.: Dermosifilografo **20—21**, 321 (1946). — MANGANOTTI, G.: Arch. ital. Derm. **10**, 25 (1934). — MACKIE, B. S.: Brit. J. Derm. **79**, 106 (1967). — SCHUER-MANN, H., A. GREITHER und O. HORNSTEIN: Krankheiten der Mundschleimhaut und der Lippen. 3. Aufl. S. 289, München-Berlin-Wien: Urban u. Schwarzenberg 1966.

Squamous Cell Carcinoma in the Nottingham-Derby Combined Tumour Clinic 1959/66

P. D. C. KINMONT, Derbyshire Royal Infirmary (England), and D. I. McCALLUM, Nottingham General Hospital (England)

Reports on the incidence of squamous cell carcinoma of the skin made more than 4 years ago, are of little value now because of the diagnostic problems of kerato-acanthoma. This benign self-healing lesion has recently achieved belated recognition, though it was described by DUPONT in 1930. Hitherto it has increased the incidence and improved the cure rate of squamous cancer of the skin by masquerading as a more sinister lesion than can be justified by its behaviour.

Survey: Since 1959, patients suspected of having squamous cell carcinomata of the skin have been referred to a Combined Clinic of dermatologists, radiotherapists, plastic and general surgeons and a histopathologist. During this period of 6 years, 139 such patients with 149 squamous cell carcinomata have been seen. This figure does not include kerato-acanthomata, intra-epidermal carcinomata or premalignant conditions. For comparison, 617 patients with 728 basal cell carcinomata were seen in the same period. The population of the area is 1,115,000. The diagnosis was confirmed by histopathology in every case.

Cytology: For ulcerated lesions cytological examination gives a more rapid answer than biopsy. The result is available in minutes rather than days.

Method. The ulcerated surface is scraped with a thin rounded metal spatula, smears made on microscopic slides, and then fixed in commercial. Iso-propyl alcohol and stained with haematoxylin and eosin.

Cell characteristics: The squamous cells from ulcerated carcinomata are rarely of uniform size. Those from the deeper layers show monstrous or double nuclei, and mitoses may be present. The more superficial dead cells are stratified with elongated nuclei. The cytoplasm is relatively abundant and eosinophilic.

Results

from the 34 ulcerated lesions examined:

Squamous cell carcinoma .. 19
Basal cell carcinoma 4
Seborrhoeic keratosis...... 3
No tumour cells 5
False positive 0
False negative 3

Table 1

Age Group in years	No. of patients			No. of lesions
	Male	Female	Total	
11—20	1	—	1	1
31—40	1	1	1	1
41—50	13	4	17	17
51—60	24	6	30	32
61—70	26	10	36	39
71—80	24	12	36	39
81—90	12	4	16	18
Unknown	1	—	1	1
	102	37	139	149

As expected 124 (82%) of the lesions were situated on exposed areas, but it is noteworthy that 63 (42%) came from relatively circumscribed areas such as pinna, lips and mouth. The peak incidence of carcinoma was in the 5th, 6th and 7th decades and the sex ratio was 3 males to 1 female (b.c.c. 1.2/1).

Duration before Referral: 47% of the lesions had been present for 6 months or less when first seen (b.c.c. 16%) and 65% for less than 1 year (b.c.c. 32%). 20% were ignored for 2 years or more (b.c.c. 50%), yet only five (3.5%) had metastases

when they were first seen. Two were on the lower lip, and the others were on the
lateral buccal sulcus in the mouth, the hand and the shin.

Multiple Lesions: Nine patients had two lesions, and one patient had three.
Nine patients had recurrent lesions after initial treatment when first seen.

Predisposing factors: 89 (60%) of the tumours had some predisposing factor.

Table 2. *Age groups in relation to site*

Years	11/20	31/40	41/50	51/60	61/70	71/80	81/90	Total
Scalp	—	—	1	2	3	7	4	17
Pinna	—	—	2	3	10	13	6	34
Face and Neck	1	—	1	8	6	7	4	26
Lip and Mouth	—	2	7	7	7	6	—	29
Forearm and hand	—	—	2	6	4	4	2	18
Trunk	—	—	2	1	—	—	—	3
Ano-genital	—	—	3	2	4	—	—	9
Leg	—	—	—	3	5	2	2	12
	1	2	18	32	39	39	18	148

Table 3. *Predisposing factors*

Benign Lesions	Premalignant Lesions	Exposures
Lupus Vulgaris	Leukoplakia 5	Sunlight 16
(irradiated 6) 8	Cutaneous horn 4	Radiation 12
Stasis ulcers 2	Bowen's disease 1	Peppermint 1
Cysts 2	Chronic lichen planus	Naphthalene 1
Pigmented mole........ 1	(oral) 1	Tobacco 9
Haemangioma 1	Trauma 2	Oil 3
Lupus erythematosus .. 1	Burns 5	Arsenic 2
		Pitch 2

Results of treatment

Table 4. *Primary*

	No.	Surgery	Radiation	Elect. Dessic	Chemo-therapy	Further Treatment
Satisfactory clear	111	77	23	10	1	16
Unsatisfactory (cosmetic or functional)	6	1	5	—	—	4
Local Recurrence	16	9	4	2	1	13
Metastases	16	9	6	1	—	14
Complications of Treatment	2	1	1	—	—	—
Death — Primary	10	8	1	1	—	8
unrelated	19	13	5	—	—	4
Unknown	2	1	1	—	—	—

Sites of squamous cell carcinomas recurring or metastasizing after primary treatment:

Muco-cutaneous junctions 10	Mouth 6	Lupus vulgaris 5
Irradiated skin.............. 4	Covered skin 4	Exposed skin 3

Follow up: 1 Year 97   Cases discharged after 5 years .. 4
            2 Years 55   Discharged or lost 30
            3 Years 30   Refused treatment 1
            4 Years 20
            5 Years 11

It is too early to compare the merits of surgery and radiotherapy but where
the age and general condition permit, surgery has been the method of choice and
has produced fewer functional and cosmetically unsatisfactory results. Chemotherapy and electrodesiccation have no part to play in the treatment of squamous
cell carcinoma, except in the aged and debilitated patient.

4. Therapy

Reports

The Treatment of Skin Cancer and Pre-Cancer with Topical Cytotoxic Ointments

J. C. BELISARIO, Institute of Dermatology, Royal Prince Alfred Hospital, Sydney (Australia)

Since the first publication by the writer of the results of the topical cytotoxic ointment therapy of skin cancer in 1961, attempts have continued to be made to increase the cure rate by additions to and alterations of the ointment. (BELISARIO, 1961, 1962, 1963, 1964, 1965, 1966, 1967.) The active ingredients have mainly been Colcemid (demecolcine, omaine or N-desacetyl methylcolchicine, Ciba Drug Co.), Methotrexate (4-amino-NlO-methyl pteroglutamic acid, LEDERLE) and Thio-Colciran, R. 261 (N-desacetyl thiocolchicine, Roussel Drug Co.).

At first 0.5% of colcemid was employed in various bases and then methotrexate was added (BELISARIO, 1961) since it had been found to prevent the commencement of cell mitosis, by interfering with the synthesis of desoxyribonucleic acid (SULZBERGER, 1960; VAN SCOTT, 1960). Colcemid on the other hand, inhibits cell mitosis in the metaphase (SCHAER, LOUSTALOT and GROSS, 1954 and others) and the combination of the two was found to exert a synergistic effect.

Colcemid, which comes from the meadow saffron plant, was discovered by SANTAVY and REICHSTEIN, working in conjunction with Ciba Chemists in 1950. Also in the same year MENSHIKOV et al., cited by MUSIN, 1960, dicsovered it independently in Colchicum speciosium and Colchicum vernum.

Then came Thio-colciran, discovered in 1954 by VELLUZ and MÜLLER, which also inhibits mitosis in the metaphase (GRACIANSKY and GRUPPER, 1954; BASSET and MONTFORT, 1955). This drug was found by the writer to exert an additive effect and tended to increase the over-all cure rate which commenced at around 68% for rodent carcinomas and Bowen's disease. The latter being superficial, is almost 100% curable with cytotoxic ointments which are also effective on solar keratoses, leucoplakia and keratoakanthomas. Unfortunately the three drugs mentioned, do not cure squamous carcinomas. They exert a selective, erosive or destructive action on the lesions they affect and the writer is at present employing 0.5% of each, preferably in an ointment base comprised of cetomacrogol emulsifying wax 20 g., soft white paraffin 40 g., and liquid paraffin 200 g. to which is added ephedrine 1,0% and hyaluronidase 80 units per mil. which latter two ingredients increase the efficacy of the cytotoxic drugs (VERMEL, 1963). The ointment is applied twice daily under an occlusive nonadherent dressing (TELFA, BAUER and BLACK, Chicago) for 4 weeks when an antibiotic or antiseptic ointment is applied twice daily for small lesions until healing takes place, usually in 2 or 3 weeks, and up to 4 or 5 weeks for larger ones. The over-all cosmetic effects are better than with other forms of treatment in the great majority of cases. Occasionally the eroded lesion exhibits a hypertrophic appearance and should be lightly curetted at weekly intervals during treatment. At times, there may be some surrounding inflammation, which can be controlled by a zinc paste or steroid ointment. If a lesion is near the eye, conjunctivitis may be caused by the ointment, but can be controlled by 1% hydrocortisone drops or equivalent preparations.

Discomfort caused by the erosion of a lesion is rarely troublesome and can be considerably reduced by the addition of 2% of xylocaine in the ointment. Since 1964 when the over-all cure rate had risen to approximately 85% for ordinary rodent carcinomas (BELISARIO, 1956) the writer has continued to attempt to improve the cure rate by various additions to the ointments employed and by better selection of cases requiring longer treatment or assistance with a cautery and/or curette.

The majority of the lesions which require additional treatment, or recur, are thick nodular fibrous ones or of the superficial cicatricial variety, wich are preventing sufficient penetration of the drugs through the fibrous tissue.

It was thought that incorporation of the cytotoxic drugs in dimethylsulphoxide (DMSO) would overcome this difficulty at least in part. However, to the writer's surprise this was less effective than the ointment base, and of 20 cases treated in this way, only 6 were cured, 12 partly disappeared and 2 were unaffected.

In another attempt to increase the efficiency of the ointment, 5% of griseofulvin was added because of its reputed anti-mitotic effects. However, over a period of 3 years, no obvious increase in the efficiency of the ointment has been noted which could be attributed to griseofulvin.

As the writer has been able to observe treated cases for up to 7 years it appears that the over-all cure rate for cases treated for 4 weeks, observed up to 4 years or longer is still around 85%. For Bowen's disease and the very superficial type of rodent carcinoma however, the cure rate approximates 100%. Of the other 15%, some require a second and even a third course of treatment or assistance with a cautery and/or curette and a few have been removed by surgery, electrochemosurgery or irradiation. Recurrences may appear within a few months, or anytime up to about 3 years. One recurrence appeared after $3^1/_2$ years, but none have been observed after that period of time.

Over the last 12 months, the writer has added chloroquin 5% to the cytotoxic ointments formula because of its reputed fibroblast inhibiting effect and specific deleterious effect on connective tissue (KIMURA et al., 1963; RUIZ-TORRES, 1965). It has also been claimed that chloroquin exerts a synergistic action in combination with cytotoxic agents (KIMURA et al., 1964) in certain malignant conditions.

During this period, 52 rodent carcinomas have been treated in 40 patients with the addition of chloroquin 5% to the ointment. Up to date, all but three cases have been clinically cured following 4 weeks of bi-daily application of the ointment. Eight of the cured lesions were large ones with much nodular fibrosis. Although it will take at least 5 years to evaluate this new combination, it is at least suggestive that an advance has been made in the fact that to date, only three of the 52 cases so treated have required additional treatment in the form of a second course of topical ointment therapy to obtain a clinical cure. Consequently, it seems not unreasonable to hope that the addition of 5% or possibly more of chloroquin to the above mentioned cytotoxic ointment has or will materially increase the overall cure rate.

Trenimon (2,3,5, — triethylene-imino-(1-4)-benzoquinone or Bayer 3231) has also been used by the writer in 0,05% strength in an ointment base. It has produced results more or less similar to those obtained by colcemid, methotrexate and thiocolchicine, before the addition of chloroquin was made, with several variations. These include a greater tendency to cause inflammation of the surrounding skin, the occasional formation of a hard central slough instead of an erosion which causes the lesion to take a week or two longer to heal and an occasional spreading autosensitization of the neighbouring skin to wider areas. It was hoped by the writer (1965) that this sensitization effect might enable the ointment to

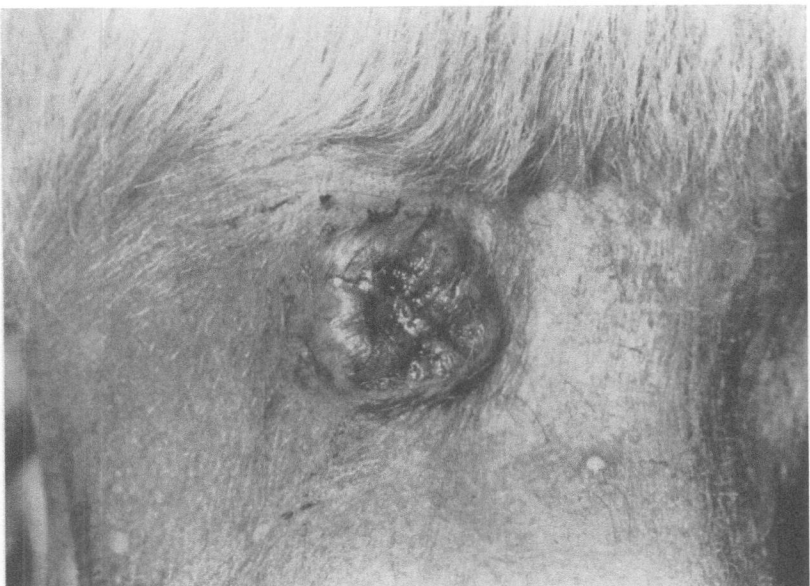

Fig. 1. Large rodent carcinoma on the posterior aspect of the neck

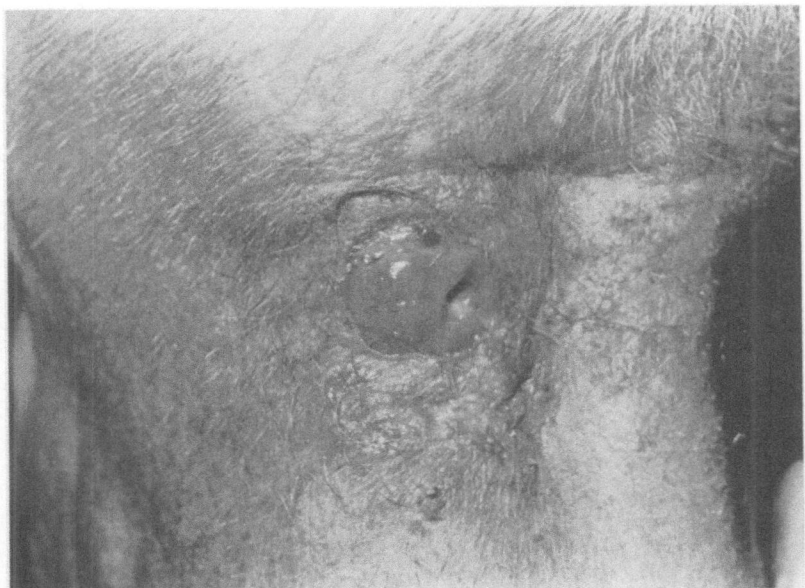

Fig. 2. Same patient as in Fig. 1 showing erosion of the rodent carcinoma after 28 days of bi-daily application of the same ointment

produce a cure of a lesion in a shorter time than usual and thus be developed and utilised for topical treatment generally (see also HELM et al., 1965). However, two cases of the writer's, in whom treatment had been stopped after 2 weeks due to a marked autosensitization eruption (and the lesions disappeared) developed a

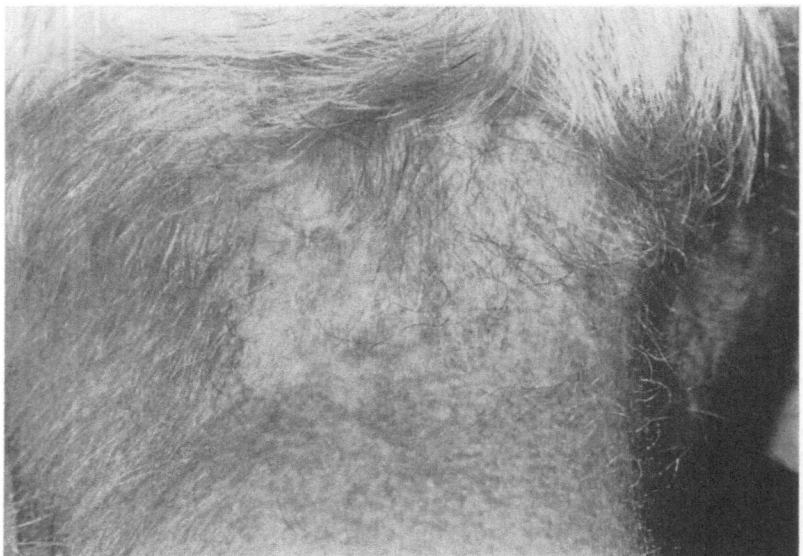

Fig. 3. Same patient as in Figs. 1 and 2, showing disappearance of the rodent carcinoma 5 weeks after the cessation of the cytotoxic ointment

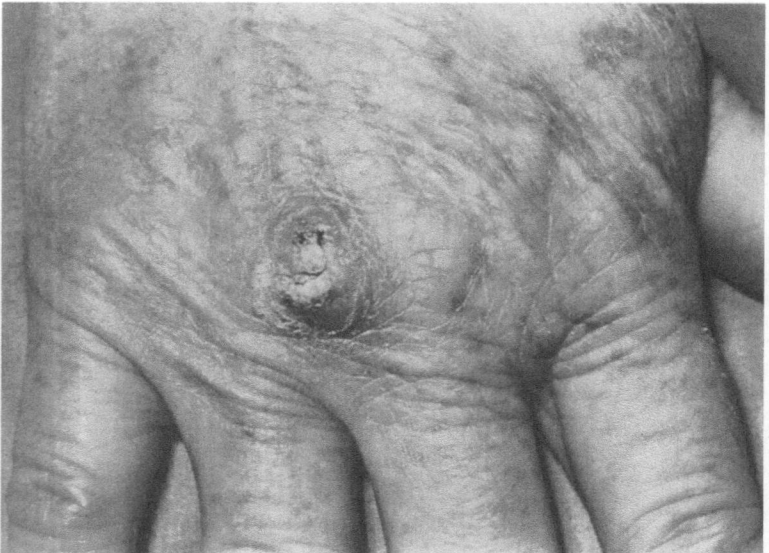

Fig. 4. Keratoakanthoma on the dorsum of the right hand

recurrence in the centre of the treated area after about 3 years of apparent clinical cure.

For some unexplainable reason, three cases of microscopically proven squamous carcinoma have disappeared following the use of trenimon ointment. However, eight other cases were unaffected by this treatment.

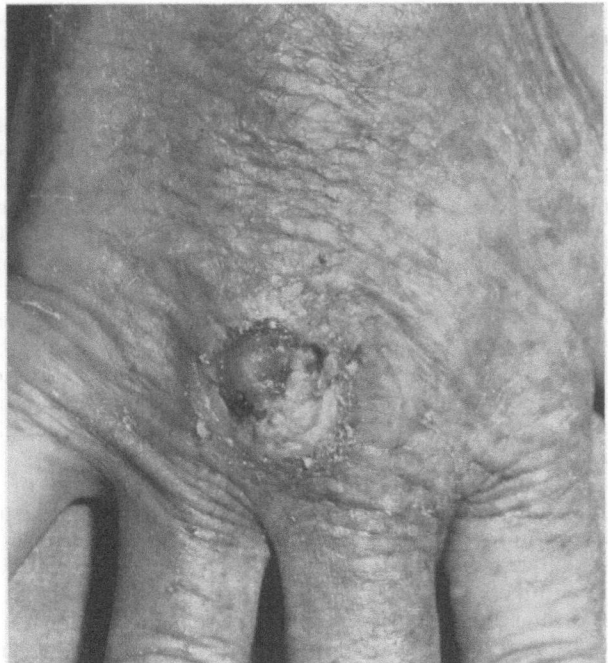

Fig. 5. Same patient as in Fig. 4 showing erosion of the keratoakanthoma (which began within 7 days) after 28 days of bi-daily application of the cytotoxic ointment

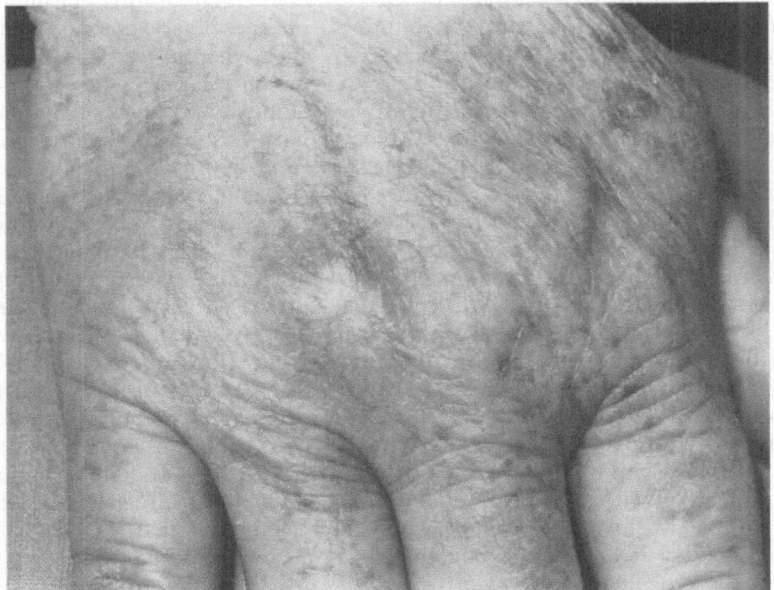

Fig. 6. Same patient as in Figs. 4 and 5 showing disappearance of the keratoakanthoma, 5 weeks after the cessation of the cytotoxic ointment

A further cytotoxic drug which has been employed more recently by Klein et al., 1962; Dillaha, 1963, 1964; Goldman, 1964; Chiaffitelli and Suarez, 1967; is 5-Fluorouracil in 1% to 20% strength. However it has not been found as effective on rodent carcinomas by the writer, Klein et al. (1962) and Dillaha et al. (1963, 1964). It is nevertheless quite effective for solar keratoses and leuco-plakia in 5% strength in polythene glycol, DMSO or an ointment base. Also it is not, in the writer's experience, as effective as the colcemid, methotrexate thio-colciran combination. For these latter conditions, the ointment or lotion has only to be applied twice daily without any occlusive dressing for about 2 weeks, followed by the bi-daily application of 2% of salicylic acid in a steroid ointment base until scaling and erythema have disappeared.

Klein et al. (1962) found topical 5-Fluorouracil ointment effective for some squamous and metastic cutaneous carcinomas. Chiaffitelli and Suarez (1967) have recently found it effective in three cutaneous squamous carcinomas, and the writer has also recently experienced three consecutive clinical cures of these lesions, one of which was a large protruding granulomatous lesion, 3.5 cm in dia-meter and 2 cm above skin level.

Another interesting observation associated with the use of the colcemid combination ointment is the fact that it will (in the writer's experience) invariably erode a keratoakanthoma within 1 to 2 weeks, whereas it does not erode a squa-mous carcinoma. This statement is based on the effects of the topical treatment of 51 keratoakanthomas. The erosion also occurs even with those lesions which exhibit a hypertrophic behaviour, peripheral extension and/or take a long time to heal as in keratoakanthoma centrifugum marginatum (Belisario, 1965). This erosive effect has provided a reasonably reliable method of differential diagnosis between a keratoakanthoma and a low-grade squamous carcinoma, even when the pathologist is in doubt, and in some cases when he has actually favoured the diagnosis of squamous carcinoma (Belisario, 1967).

Since commencing to use topical cytotoxic ointment containing colcemid about 7 years ago, the writer has only encountered one adverse systemic effect. This was in a male aged 83 with four rodent carcinomas, with an average diameter of 2.5 cm, three on the right side of the face and one on the nose.

He was given chloroquin and griseofulvin by mouth and both substances were included in his cytotoxic ointment. His blood count was normal before treatment commenced. 13 days later he became anorexic and generally unwell. His blood haemoglobin had fallen from 13.1 g-% to 11.9 g-%, the white cells from 8700 to 800, 99% of which were lymphocytes, his blood platelets were 160000/cm and his blood urea had risen from 28 mg-% to 121 mg-%. The patient died within 24 h. It was thought at the time, in view of some animal experiments performed by Epstein and Larsen (1961) with colchicine and griseofulvin, that the combina-tion of griseofulvin with colcemid (a derivative of colchicine) might have been responsible for the patient's death. However, complications in two cases following topical colcemid to unusually large lesions were also experienced by Vermel and Kramorenko (1955) in the form of a sharp depression in haemopoiesis. One of them died with signs of agranulocytosis and haemorrhagic diathesis. Kinmont (1967) likewise experienced a fatality in a patient with two large rodent carcinomas on the trunk treated with 1% colcemid ointment, and whose white cell count dropped to 300 per cm and blood platelets to 169000/cm before he died.

Consequently it appears that colcemid alone or in conjunction with metho-trexate and thiocolciran was also responsible in the writer's case, although it is theoretically possible that griseofulvin might have played some additive role. It would seem appropriate here to mention that the writer treated one patient with 0,5% colcemid ointment who had a large rodent carcinoma on his forehead, 9 cm in diameter and another lesion behind one ear 6 cm in diameter. No deleterious effects on this patient's blood count were found at any stage.

However, a strict watch on the blood count should be kept in a patient with large or multiple lesions being treated with cytotoxic ointments. In fact it would appear wise not to treat more than three or four small lesions at any one time and to treat large lesions piecemeal.

References. BELISARIO, J. C.: 12th Ann. Meet. Derm. Assn. Austral., Oct., Sydney. Aust. J. Derm. **6**, 96 (1961). — Proc. XII Internat. Congr. Derm., Washington, D.C., Sept. 1962. — Jap. J. Derm. **72**, 721 (1962). — Ind. J. Derm. Venereol. **29**, 191 (1963). — Skin. **2**, 216 (1963). — Presse méd. **1963**, 71. — Rev. argent. Dermatosif. **48**, 29 (1964). — Acta derm.-venereol. (Stockh.) **44**, Suppl. 56. (1964). — Derm. Digest **4**, 49 (1965). — 84th Ann. Meet. Amer. Derm. Assn., Maui, Hawaii, July. Arch. Derm. **92**, 293 (1965). — Minerva derm. (Torino) **40**, 57 (1965). — Ann. Meet. Derm. Assn. Aust., Aust. J. Derm. **8**, 65 (1965). — Suppl. to Chapter 97, Simon's Handbook of Tropical Dermatology, Vol. II (1953), p. 1551. Elsevier Publ. Co. 1966. — Hautarzt **18**, 66 (1967). — VI-Congreso Ibero-Latino-Americano de Dermatologia, Barcelona, Spain, July 1967. — BASSET, A., et J. MONTFORT: Bull. Soc. franç. Derm. Syph. **3**, 10 (1955). — Xe. Congr. Derm. Syph. de la langue Française (Algier 1959). Paris: Masson et Cie. 1959. — CHIAFFITELLI, C. A.: Montevideo, Pers. communication 1967. — DILLAHA, C. J.: 84th Ann. Meet. Amer. Derm. Assn., Maui, Hawaii, June 1964. — Little Rock, Arkansas. Pers. communication 1964. — DILLAHA, C. J., G. T. JANSON, W. M HONEYCUTT, and A. C. BRADFORD: Arch. Derm. **88**, 63 (1963). — EPSTEIN, W. L., and M. A. LARSEN: J. invest. Derm. **36**, 5 (1961). — GOLDMAN, L.: Cincinatti, Ohio. Pers. communication 1964. — GRACIANSKY, P. DE, et CH. GRUPPER: Bull. Soc. franç. Derm. Syph. **62**, 54 (1955). — HELM, F., E. KLEIN, H. L. TRAENKLE, and E. P. RIVERA: J. invest. Derm. **45**, 152 (1965). — KIMURA, I., H. KAGEYAMA, H. KOTANI, and H. SATO: J. Jap. Soc. intern. Med. **52**, 35 (1963), **53**, 382 (1964). — KINMONT, P. D. C.: Derby, England. Pers. communication 1967. — KLEIN, E., H. MIGROM, F. HELM, J. AMBRUS, and H. L. TRAENKLE: Skin **3**, 81 (1962). — KLEIN, E., F. HELM, H. MIGROM, H. L. STOLL jr., and H. L. TRAENKLE: Skin **1**, 153 (1962). — MUNTONI, S.: Boll. Soc. ital. Biol. sper. **41**, 813 (1965). — MUSIN, N. V.: Vop. Onkol. **6**, 93 (1960). — RUIZ-TORRES, A.: Z. Rheumaforsch. **24**, 320 (1965). — SANTAVY, F., u. F. REICHSTEIN: 12. Mitteilung Helv., Skin Acta **33**, 1606 (1950). — van SCOTT, E. J.: Ann. intern. Med. **59**, 944 (1963). — SHÄR, B., D. LOUSTALOT und F. GROSS: Klin. Wschr. **32**, 49 (1954). — SULZBERGER, M. B., and E. J. van SCOTT: Arch. Derm. **82**, 762 (1960). — VELLUZ, L., et G. MULLER: Bull. Soc. chim. Fr. **6**, (Part 1) 755, **9** (Part 2) 1072 (1954). — VERMEL, E.: Moscow. Pers. communication 1962. — VERMEL, E. M., and I. T. KRAMORENKO: Probl. Onkol. (N Y.) **1**, 69 (1955).

The Treatment of Skin Cancers with Radiation

H. GOLDSCHMIDT, Department of Dermatology, Hospital of the University of Pennsylvania, Philadelphia (USA)

Skin cancers are the most accessible and the most detectable of human malignancies. Yet, in the United States there was a 9% increase in death rate from this cause during the last 10 years. It rose to 2.5% per 100,000 in men and 1.5% in women with a total of 4600 deaths per year. The American Cancer Society has predicted at least 90,000 new skin cancer cases during 1967.

Cutaneous malignancies have been treated with x-rays for over one half century. Newer developments have expanded the indications for x-ray therapy to include certain types of cancer and pre-cancerous conditions which were not amenable to this form of treatment previously, or which gave unsatisfactory results with other forms of radiation.

Changes in this field have been subtle and gradual; no dramatic new developments or breakthroughs can be reported since the last International Congress in

Washington. Progress has been made in the use of radioisotopes in cutaneous malignancies, yet their practical importance outside of medical centers is limited.

Since time does not permit a detailed discussion of various aspects of modern x-ray techniques, this paper will be limited to changing views concerning the selection of x-rays with different penetration. In the past, widely varying suggestions were given by different authors concerning the choice of proper x-ray qualities in skin cancers. It was quite confusing to the inexperienced to see that some authorities recommend Grenz ray qualities (HVL .036 mmAl) in the treatment of basal cell epithelioma, whereas others insist on very penetrating x-rays (HVL 3.0 mmAl).

With few exceptions, agreement has now been reached by most dermatoradiotherapists that the quality of radiation must be correlated to the depth of the tumor. In this connection the most significant recent development has been the gradual change from harder and more penetrating x-rays to softer x-rays. To a large measure, this was inspired and influenced by the excellent scientific contributions on this subject at the XII International Congress, particularly by SCHIRREN, WACHSMANN, PROPPE, ANDREWS and others.

The utilization of softer x-rays (10—50 KV, rarely up to 100 KV) and the elimination of unnecessary deeply penetrating radiation have resulted in better cure rates, less frequent recurrences and superior cosmetic results.

The designation "half value layer" (HVL) has been used for a long time to characterize different qualities of x-rays. The introduction of the new term, "half value depth" (HVD or D 1/2) for the 50% depth dose by JENNINGS has made it easier to formulate practical and logical rules concerning the choice of specific x-ray qualities in relation to the depth of the pathologic process.

As postulated by BELISARIO, a quality or wave length of radiation must be chosen which will exert the maximum deleterious action on abnormal tissues obtainable with the minimal deleterious action on surrounding and underlying normal tissues.

Based on theoretical considerations and practical experience with thousands of skin cancers, these requirements are best fulfilled when the depth of the tumor (measured in millimeters) and the half value depth (measured in millimeters) of the irradiation are equal. Based on the pioneer work of EBBEHOJ, this rule was formulated and defended in many publications by SCHIRREN. Its usefulness and application in benign dermatoses and tumors was discussed by GOLDSCHMIDT.

As an example, a relatively superficial tumor of only 4 mm depth is best treated with x-rays of a half value depth (D 1/2) of 4 mm (= HVL 0.3 mmAl) and not with harder x-rays. Histological measurements of basal cell epitheliomas by POLANO and BURGER et al. have shown that most of these common tumors do not extend beyond 2 or 3 mm tissue depth. On the other hand, a more invasive cutaneous cancer of 12 mm depth should be treated with harder x-rays with a D 1/2 of 12 mm (= HVL 1.0 mm Al) and not with supersoft x-rays. Since biopsies of skin cancers are taken routinely by most dermatologists, the determination of the approximate depth of the tumor does not offer any particular problem.

Most of the newer beryllium windowed x-ray units allow the variation and utilization of softer x-ray qualities. Their wide therapeutic range and high output make them ideal multi-purpose machines for dermatological purposes.

Since the absorption rate in tissue is similar to the absorption in the treatment with radium or the Chaoul (contact) technique, beryllium windowed machines make these older techniques obsolete. They are also more effective, safer and technically easier to use.

Resultado de la radioterapia superficial en los epiteliomas cutaneos

G. Jaqueti, Hospital de San Juan de Dios, Madrid (España), y J. Gay Prieto, Catedrático de Dermatología, Universidad de Madrid, Hospital de San Juan de Dios, Madrid (España)

La acción cancerígena sobre la piel de las radiaciones ultravioletas con longitud de onda comprendida entre los 2.900 Å y 3.100 Å es un hecho admitido desde las investigaciones de Findlay [1] y de Blum [2—3].

El incremento de epiteliomas cutáneos en las zonas no protegidas (cara), en los sujetos de raza blanca que viven y trabajan al aire libre bajo una alta incidencia de radiación solar, es una realidad perfectamente establecida. Belisario [4], nos comunica que en Australia, los epiteliomas cutáneos, representan el 60% de todos los cánceres, incrementándose en las regiones más próximas al ecuador, como en North Queensland, donde alcanza el 75%.

En la meseta central de España donde radica nuestro Hospital (Madrid), las condiciones metereológicas por su altitud sobre el nivel del mar, elevado grado de sequedad atmosférica y alta incidencia solar durante la mayor parte del año, son muy semejantes a las de Australia, y por ello, quizá seamos los dos países con mayor procentaje de epiteliomas cutáneos.

De los 2.200 pacientes que son objeto de revisión, 465 proceden de la provincia de Madrid, siguiendo en orden de frecuencia los de Toledo con 367, Ciudad Real 309, Segovia 212, siendo ya menor el porcentaje para el resto de las provincias menos soleadas.

La profesión guarda relación con la incidencia. De esta forma, han sido los pacientes que trabajan al aire libre los que dan mayor porcentaje; labradores de ambos sexos 1.692 casos, albañiles 126, peones 125, y el resto hasta 2.200 corresponden a empleados, oficinistas, etc.

La edad avanzada con su atrofia epidérmica disminuye la protección frente a laradiación solar y es causa de mayor incidencia. En los grupos de edad de 41 a 50 años tenemos 316 enfermos, que se eleva en los de 51 a 60 años a 560, y en los de 61 a 70 años a 813 enfermos. El sexo no parece guardar influencia ya que el nùmero de varones (1.054) y de hembras (1.146) es equilibrada

En nuestra Clínica del Hospital de San Juan de Dios y Dispensario Martínez Anido han sido asistidos 4.183 enfermos afectos de epiteliomas sobre un total de 85.420 pacientes, de los cuales hemos seleccionado 2.200 para su tratamiento mediante rayos X, el resto ha sido tributario de otras técnicas como la electrocoagulación, extirpación quirúrgica, y radiumterapia.

Desde 1900, fecha en la que Stembeck [5] comunicó el primer caso de cancer-cutáneo curado con rayos X, la radioterapia ha constituído uno de los procedimientos fundamentales empleados por los dermatólogos durante muchos años con éxito.

La multiplicidad de técnicas propuestas plantea una gran dificultad al tratar de esquematizarlas con objeto de dar una idea de conjunto de las mismas. El fin de todas es análogo, la inhibición del desarrollo celular tumoral, pero el método seguido por los diferentes autores varía de unos a atros: la dilución y fraccionamiento de la dosis, su caída en profundidad, la ventaja de dosis masivas o el fraccionamiento, el tamaño del campo a irradiar, la localización, etc. han hecho que sus preconizadores ajusten los factores físicos (kilovoltaje, miliamperaje, filtro y distancia foco-piel) de acuerdo con sus hipótesis de trabajo.

Razones de espacio nos impiden analizar las distintas técnicas y sus resultados que han sido motivo de nuestra atención en otras ocasiones [6—7]. Siguiendo a OTT [8] podemos agruparlas en la siguiente forma: 1° *Extirpación tumoral seguida de dosis masiva única.* 2° *Dosis masiva única.* 3° *Técnicas de radiación fraccionada.* 4° *Método de Chaoul* (irradiación de contacto o proximal).

Técnica personal de radioterapia fraccionada

En publicaciones anteriores [6, 7, 9, 10] hemos realizado análisis periódicos de nuestros resultados pero al cumplirse los veinte años en que iniciamos esta técnica (1946—1966) hemos creído oportuno exponerles lo conseguido sobre un total de 2.200 enfermosafectos de epiteliomas cutáneos.

Al principio tomamos como base el trabajo de nuestro colaborador AZUA DOCHAO [11] realizado en la clínica de Breslau bajo la dirección del Prof. GOTTRON. Intentando adaptar los aparatos de terapia superficial standard a la técnica de Chaoul, determinó la caída de la dosis en profundidad bajo distintas condiciones de voltaje, filtro y distancia foco-piel y llegó a la conclusión de que con 60 Kv, 6 mA (V C H de 0,35 mm de Al) 15 cm foco-piel y sin filtro, las curvas de caida de la dosis en profundidad eran superponibles a las obtenidas por Chaoul. Con dosis diarias de 500 r hasta un total de 10.000 r a 15.000 r consigue un 90% de curaciones definitivas en los cánceres cutáneos. — Desde 1946 modificamos esta técnica en la siguienta forma:

Voltaje. Siendo los epiteliomas cutáneos lesiones superficiales con un lecho tumoral que oscila de 2 mm a 2 ó 3 cm en terminos generales, creemos que las tensiones elevadas son inadmisibles. Utilizamos 30 Kv en los más superficiales; 55 kv en los de profundidad media y 70 Kv para los más penetrantes.

Filtro. — Cuando empleamos tensiones de 30 Kv intercalamos un filtro de 0,30 mm de Al (V C H de 0,2 mm de Al), con 55 kv filtro de 0,78 mm de Al (V C H de 0,75 mm de Al) y con 70 Kv el de 1,25 mm de Al (V C H de 1,25 mm de Al).

Miliamperiaje. — Aun reconociendo la ventaja de la "dilución" utilizamos de 4 a 10 mA ya que intensidades menores alargarían considerablement el tiempo de exposición.

Distancia foco-piel. — Con rayos relativamente blandos la caida de la dosis en profundidad varía poco para distancias foco-piel de 15 cm. En nuestras condiciones de trabajo empleamos distancias de 10 y 15 cm.

Dimensiones del campo. — Es indudable que la extensión de la lesión tiene gran importancia desde el punto de vista pronóstico. Asi, WARREN y LULENSKY [12] tienen un 9% de fracasos en los epiteliomas inferiores a 2 cm, que se eleva al 60% en los superiores a 5 cm. De igual forma, ELLIOT y WELTON [13] encuentran el 50% de fracasos en los epiteliomas que sobrepasan los 5 cm.

El inconveniente que supone las grandes superficies lo evitamos dividiéndolas en pequeñas áreas de 4 cm. que irradiamos sucesivamente. En estas condiciones la radiación es más uniforme y la radiación dispersa menor.

Dosis parciales. — La hemos fijado en 400 r sin tener en cuenta la variedad histológica, forma clínica y localización.

Fraccionamiento. —·La dosis anterior se repite en días alternos hasta alcanzar la dosis necesaria.

Dosis total. — La dosis total que permite la esterilización global de las células cancerosas no se ha podido establecer de una forma exacta. CARTER intentó determinar la "dosis letal carcinoma" en el cancer experimental de la rata, fijándola en 3.000 r.

Prescindiendo de las dosis totales aconsejadas, la tendencia actual (CIPOLLARO, ANDREWS, GORDON, WARD, etc.) es a reducirla entre las 4.000 r y 6.000 r. Estamos por consiguiente lejos de las dosis de 10.000 r y 15.000 r recomendadas hace unos años [14].

Por nuestra parte hemos administrado dosis que oscilan entre las 4.000 r y 5.200 r Hemos de tener en cuenta que en algunos casos, aplanamos las masas vegetantes y destruimos las perlas epiteliales del borde con el bisturí eléctrico, quizá por ello no precisemos de dosis más altas.

Datos clínicos. — En los 2.200 epiteliomas tratados la *distribución topográfica* ha sido lasiguiente:

Cabeza — 2.149

Mejilla	546
Nariz	534
Surco nasogeniano	345
Frontal	356
Preauricular	95
Retroauricular	39
Labio superior	28
Labio inferior	65
Angulo ext. del ojo	36
Angulo int. del ojo	25
Cuero cabelludo	27
Mentón	12
Pabellón auricular	41

Tronco — 28

Torácicos	6
Esternal	1
Lumbar	12
Pene	9

Extremidades — 23

Manos	19
Piernas	4

En cuanto a *variedades clínicas* tratadas se distribuyen en la siguiente forma:

Epitelioma perlado plano	249	Epitelioma terebrante	26
Epitelioma pagetoide	32	Epitelioma ulcerados	553
Epitelioma esclerodermiforme	2	Epitelioma tumoral vegetante	868
Epitelioma ulcus rodens	380	Cuermo cutáneo	90

Respecto a la textura histológica 1.309 casos corresponden a epiteliomas basocelulares, — 842 a epiteliomas espinocelulares y 49 a epiteliomas intermediarios o metatípicos. Aunque la tendencia actual no acepte la existencia de estos últimos, el hecho cierto es, que nos encontramos con este pequeño número de epiteliomas que no podamos incluir en los grupos anteriores.

Resultados. — De los 2.200 enfermos tratados únicamente hemos podido mantener un control superior a los seis meses hasta tres años, en 1.795, habiendo perdido todo contacto con los 405 restantes.

Los resultados que podemos considerar como definitivos son los siguientes:

Curaciones	1.710	(952%,)
Fracasos absolutos	4	(0,2%)
Recidivas	57	(3,1%)
Metástasis post-tratamiento	23	(1,2%)

En cuanto a las recidivas una ha tenido lugar en un adenocantoma sudoríparo que según LENZ [15], TOURAINE, nosotros y recientemente ORBANEJA, constituye-una variedad histológica radioresistente.

En 18 epiteliomas con superficie mayor a 30 cm. hemos podido comprobar la existencia de recidiva o curación incompleta. Otras 5 recidivas han sido comprobadas en epiteliomas terebrantes de nariz y órbita. Finalmente, tenemos 33 recidivas de las que 17 corresponden a epiteliomas basocelulares y 16 a espino-celulares. De los primeros, 5 corresponden a epiteliomas perlados cicatrizales, de cuya resistencia a los rayos X nos ocupamos hace años. El resto de recidivas es difícil de interpretar ya que a nuesto juicio habían recibido una dosis correcta, siendo posible que el campo radiado fuese insuficiente en sus márgenes. Según BAER y KOPF [16] esta es una de las causas más frecuentes de fracasos.

El número de metástasis ganglinares en las regiones tributarias ha sido de 23-(1,2%), todas ellas en espinocelulares. Las más frecuentes (14 casos) son las consecutivas a epiteliomas de localización en pabellones auriculares y regiones pre y retroauriculares por lo que insistimos en que los cánceres de esta localización necesitan de un control cuidadoso y a cortos intervalos después de finalizar el tratamiento.

Bibliografía. 1. FINDLAY, G. M.: Lancet **1928, II**, 1, 070 (1928). — 2. BLUM, H. F.: J. nat. Cancer Inst. **1**, 397 (1940). — 3. BLUM, H. F.: Physiol. Rev. **25**, 483 (1945). — 4. BELISARIO, J. C.: Acta derm.-venereol. (Stockh.) **44**, Supl. 56 (1964). — 5. STEMBECK, T.: Hygiea (Stockh.) **62**, 18 (1900). — 6. JAQUETI, G.: Tesis doctoral. Universidad de Madrid 1949. — 7. GAY PRIETO, G. JAQUETI y J. SOTO: Dermatología (Méx.) **VI**, Fas. 7—8 (1955). — 8. OTT, P.: Strahlentherapie **59**, 189 (1937). — 9. GAY PRIETO, y G. JAQUETI: Medicina Cutánea **1**, 51 (1966). — 10. GAY PRIETO y G. JAQUETI: Archiv. Derm. Syph. **200**, 171 (1955). — 11. AZUA, L.: Tesis doctoral, Zaragoza 1947. — 12. WARREN, and LULENSKY: Arch. Derm. Syph. (Chic.) **44**, 37 (1941). — 13. ELLIOT, and WELTON: Arch. Derm. Syph. (Chic.) **55**, 307 (1946). — 14. CHAOUL, u. ADAM: Strahlentherapie **48**, 31 (1933). — 15. LENZ: Arch. Derm. Syph. (Chic.) **53**, 588 (1946). — 16. BAER, R., and A. KOPF: Year Book Dermat. **1964**.

Free Communications

Experiences with Topical Use of 5-Fluorouracil

A. R. GODDARD, Miami, Florida (USA)

Introduction. Topical 5-Fluorouracil was reported by DILLAHA, JANSEN and HONEYCUTT to be effective for the treatment of actinic keratosis. The therapeutic effect of 5-Fluorouracil is apparently achieved through its ability to block the production of thymine or 5-methyluracil, vital for the synthesis of DNA stopping biological growth at the macromolecular level.

The following is a report on the use of topical 5-Fluorouracil in the treatment of superficial actinic keratoses of 45 caucasians. 82 different anatomical regions were treated with a 10% concentration of topical 5-Fluorouracil.

Method and Materials. Fluorouracil obtained by airdrying the contents of sterile ampules was incorporated into water soluble emulsion bases or propylene glycol.

The patients were instructed to apply the medication with their hands sparingly to the areas treated, rubbing the medication into the skin thoroughly twice each day for a period of 1 month for the face. Treatment in other areas varied from 2 weeks to 2 months.

Five patientscreated the extremeties and upper trunk more than once. Other instructions included avoidan e of exposure to sunlight and contact of the medication with the eyes. All of the patients had been treated in the past for isolated superficial keratoses and each manifested diffuse actinic changes on the areas of their bodies normally exposed to sun.

Results. All of the patients had various degrees of erythema, erosions and edema during the course of treatment. After 1 or 2 weeks of therapy many patches of erythema and erosions in treatment areas were noted that had not been the site of any existing visible changes suggestive of actinic keratosis. Erythema, erosions and edema seemed to uniformly reach a maximum in the 3. to 4. week of treatment when the face was the treatment site. The treated areas seemed to re-epitheliaze in 1 to 2 weeks after cessation of therapy, having a violaceous color which subsided in a few months. The patients all noted burning and soreness of the areas treated at some time during therapy which persisted for 1 or 2 weeks after treatment was stopped. When the antecubital fossae, the sides of the neck and the face of patients having seborrheic dermatitis were treated, erosions and weeping were common.

In 20 patients analgetics, hypnotics and/or both were required. Aggravated response to sunlight, generalized eruption, pyrexia, milia of the face following treatment and hiccups occurred in some patients. In nine patients small non-ulcerated basal cell carcinomas were noted after completing treatment with Fluorouracil. Seborrheic keratoses in treatment sites also appeared to be unaffected by the topical therapy. The post treatment observation period has varied from 1 to 4 years; the majority of subjects being followed longer than 2 years. In four patients isolated keratoses were noted to appear during the 2nd and 3rd year of observation and were treated cryosurgically. Good to excellent results were obtained in all areas treated. No traces of previous keratoses on the face were seen after treatment.

Table 1. *45 Caucasian adults*		Table 2. *82 Treatment sites*		Table 3. *Side effects*	
Females	13/45	Face	32	Pain	20/45
Males	32/45	Arms and fore arms	27	Milia	5/45
Age: Majority in 5th and 6th decade of life		Neck	9	Photo reaction	2/45
		Upper trunk	7	Generalized Eruption	2/45
		Scalp	5	Hiccups	1/45
		Legs	2	Pyrexia	1/45
			82		

Discussion and Conclusions. The favorable results indicate that topical Fluorouracil is the method of choice for the treatment of large areas of exposed surfaces exhibiting "actinic changes".

It appears that deeper lesions such as basal cell and squamous cell carcinomas should be treated differently. The failure to respond to Fluorouracil might aid in the selection of lesions requiring other forms of therapy.

The apparent ability of Fluorouracil to "selectively" pick out early lesions must not be confused with the probable explanation of greater ease of penetration through an altered epidermal barrier at such sites and an unselective cytotoxic effect on all cells in which pyrimidine synthesis is taking place. The erosions seen in the antecubital fossae, sides of the neck, in areas of seborrheic dermatitis, the need to avoid the eyes and the use of propylene glycol as a vehicle to enhance penetration lends credence to this hypothesis. It would appear that any factor that facilitates transport of Fluorouracil to the areas of DNA production in the epidermis such as vehicle, concentration, alteration of epidermal barrier will determine its therapeutic effect. Increasing the treatment time seems to enhance the effect of Fluorouracil.

The generalized eruption, pyrexia and hiccups observed might be an indication that the size of the treatment site at any given time should be limited to reduce absorption and the chance of any systemic toxic side effects.

The aggravated response to sunexposure indicates that Fluorouracil may be phototoxic. In vitro investigations show an absorption spectrum for Fluorouracil that extends into the natural sunlight range. Photohydration and photodimerization may also contribute toward this apparent phototoxic effect.

Therapie des Bowencarcinoms und des Lupuscarcinoms mit konventionellen Röntgenstrahlen

G. Stein, Universitätsklinik für Hautkrankheiten Bonn (Deutschland)

Zwei Hautveränderungen sollen in diesem Referat behandelt werden, deren therapeutische Ergebnisse mit Hilfe konventioneller strahlentherapeutischer Mittel, wie sie der Dermatologie zur Verfügung stehen, nicht befriedigen. Warum gelingt es nicht oder selten, ein Bowen-Carcinom genito-analer Lokalisation oder ein Lupuscarcinom zu heilen? Mit welchen Verfahren sind bessere Ergebnisse zu erwarten?

Beide Veränderungen gehören histologisch zur Gruppe der Plattenepithelcarcinome. Plattenepithelcarcinome der Haut und der Schleimhaut (Unterlippe) sind fast immer heilbar. Das Bowen-Carcinom genito-analer Lokalisation entwickelt sich aus einem Morbus Bowen, einer echten Präcancerose, einer von Beginn an bösartigen Neuentwicklung. Eine eindeutigere Bezeichnung für diese Veränderung ist intraepitheliales Carcinom oder carcinoma in situ. Bereits Beck hat im Jadassohnschen Handbuch auf die Hartnäckigkeit gegenüber Eingriffen hingewiesen. Greither betont ebenfalls, daß der Morbus Bowen der Mundschleimhaut eine schwerwiegende Veränderung darstellt und in der Weiterentwicklung zum Carcinom schnell die Basalzellreihe überschreitet und bei nicht frühzeitiger Erkennung die Erkrankung tödlich verläuft. Auf die Ätiologie der Bowenschen Erkrankung sowie auf die Assoziationen mit visceralen Carcinomen soll nicht eingegangen werden.

Limburg wirft die Frage der erhöhten Strahlenresistenz auf. Der Bowen der Genitalregion wird von zahlreichen Autoren zusammen mit den Vulvacarcinomen abgehandelt, die in der älteren Literatur ebenfalls sehr schlechte Behandlungsergebnisse aufweisen. Liegen dagegen Statistiken mit Stadieneinteilungen vor, sind die Behandlungsergebnisse des Vulvacarcinoms ähnlich den Behandlungsergebnissen der Mammacarcinome oder der weiblichen Beckencarcinome.

Limburg konnte bei 156 primären Vulvacarcinomen sechs Fälle von Morbus Bowen beobachten, die bis auf einen Fall, bei dem nach einem Jahr ein Portiocarcinom entstand, nach ausgiebiger Elektroresektion ausheilten. Weiterhin konnte er unter diesem Kollektiv sechs Bowen-Carcinome beobachten, von denen vier Patienten an Rezidiven und Metastasen trotz ausgedehnter Elektroresektion und Röntgenbestrahlung verstarben. Die Folgerungen aus diesen Ergebnissen bestanden darin, beim Morbus Bowen eine partielle Vulvektomie durchzuführen, beim Bowen-Carcinom die Vulvektomie, Leistenlymphknotenausräumung und eine intensive Strahlenbehandlung durchzuführen, Behandlungsmethoden, die außerhalb der Dermatologie liegen. Die Strahlenbehandlung wurde an einer auswärtigen Strahlenklinik durchgeführt, welche die Möglichkeit der Behandlung mit schnellen Elektronen besitzt. Die Behandlung mit schnellen Elektronen hat nach Aussage des Autors günstigere Behandlungsergebnisse gebracht. Weghaupt hält ebenfalls die Behandlung des Bowen-Carcinoms mit schnellen Elektronen für die Therapie der Wahl.

Wir haben die Ergebnisse von fünf genito-anal gelegenen Bowen-Carcinomen vorliegen. Sie wurden zum Teil mit mehreren Bestrahlungsserien (50 bis 120 kV, pro Serie 6000 ROD) und zusätzlicher Strahlenbehandlung der Lymphabfluß-gebiete (200 kV) behandelt. Da bei vier Patienten mehrmals Rezidive auftraten, wurden bzw. mußten sie operativ behandelt werden. Die Überlebenszeiten betragen 3 bis 8 Jahre. Die Überlebenszeit ist für diese Betrachtung nicht maßgeblich. Die langdauernden, mehrmaligen Bestrahlungen der genito-analen Region stellen nach Eintritt der Strahlenreaktion eine schwere Beeinträchtigung dar. Weiterhin erhebt sich die Frage nach späteren Folgezuständen. Letztlich mußten nach Jahren trotzdem größere operative Eingriffe vorgenommen werden. Diesen Ergebnissen ist zu entnehmen, daß ein Bowen-Carcinom durch 6000 ROD der oben aufgeführten Strahlenqualität nicht vernichtet wird. Unterstellt man dem Bowen-Carcinom eine gewisse Strahlenresistenz, würden vielleicht 10000 R den Tumor vernichten. Eine derartig hohe Strahlenbelastung unter Bedingungen der Oberflächen- oder Halbtiefentherapie in Form von Röntgenstrahlen ist bei der Lokalisation und oftmals größeren Ausdehnung des Tumors nicht vertretbar und zumutbar. Auch wir glauben, daß die Therapie mit schnellen Elektronen günstigere Ergebnisse bringt und überlassen aus diesen Gründen die Behandlung des Bowen-carcinoms der Frauenklinik und der Strahlenklinik.

Das Lupuscarcinom entsteht auf dem Boden einer Narbe, in einem chronisch entzündlichen Gewebe, mit oder ohne äußere Noxen. Auch beim Lupuscarcinom sind die Behandlungsergebnisse mit den konventionellen Methoden schlecht. Die Ursachen hierfür können durch zu kleine Felderwahl, zu niedrige Strahlendosis oder eine Strahlenresistenz des Tumors bedingt sein, obwohl der Tumor wie Plattenepithelcarcinome an sich „dahinschmilzt". In kurzer Zeit entwickeln sich an gleicher Stelle Rezidive. Eine Strahlenresistenz kann durch die herabgesetzte Durchblutung des Narbengewebes (Hypoxämie) gegeben, sein oder das ganze Lupusareal befindet sich im Zustand der Carcinomentwicklung. Günstigere Behandlungsergebnisse sind auch beim Lupuscarcinom durch eine Strahlenqualität, die eine höhere Gesamtdosierung, eine homogenere Durchstrahlung und eine größere Felderwahl erlaubt, oder durch chirurgische Maßnahmen zu erwarten.

Literatur. BECK, S. C.: Handbuch der Haut- und Geschlechtskrankheiten v. J. JADASSOHN. Bd. XII/3, 433. Berlin: Springer 1933. — GREITHER, A.: Dermatologie und Venerologie von GOTTRON, H. A., u. W. SCHÖNFELD, Bd. IV, 656. Stuttgart: Thieme. — GREITHER, A., u. H. TRITSCH: Die Geschwülste der Haut. Stuttgart: Thieme 1957. — SCHUERMANN, H., A. GREITHER und O. HORNSTEIN: Krankheiten der Mundschleimhaut und der Lippen. München: Urban & Schwarzenberg 1966. — LIMBURG, H.: Arch. Gynäk. **196**, 207 (1961). — WEGHAUPT, K.: Wien. klin. Wschr. **1967**, 127. — PETESKA, E. S., F. W. LYNCH, and R. W. GOLTZ: Arch. Derm. (Chic.) **85**, 623 (1961). — DUPERRAT, B., et G. E. GOETSCHEL: Bull. Soc. franç. Derm. Syph. **71**, 301 (1964). — GRIMMER, H.: Z. Haut- u. Geschlecht.-Kr. **38**, XLIX, (1965). — VOLK, R.: Handbuch der Haut- u. Geschlechtskrankheiten von J. JADASSOHN, Bd. X/1, 216. Berlin: Springer 1931. — MICHALOWSKI, R., u. T. KUDEJKO: Derm. Wschr. **151**, 25 (1965). — FRIEDRICH, C. H.: Z. Haut- u. Geschlecht.-Kr. **37**, 163 (1964). — MAGGIORA, A., E. BUZARD und W. JADASSOHN: Derm. Wschr. **147**, 209 (1963). — RIEHL, G., u. O. KÖPF: Die Hauttuberkulose und ihre Therapie. Wien: Wilh. Maudrich 1950. — KALKOFF, K.-W.: Die Tuberkulose der Haut. Tuberkulosebücherei. Stuttgart: Thieme 1950.

Traitement de l'épithélioma cutané par l'exérèse simple avec suture immédiate

D. THIBAUT, Hôpital St. Louis, Paris (France)

D'abord un mot d'histoire. Au cours du XIXe siècle, destruction des cancers cutanés par les caustiques, surtout par le chlorate de Potassium après curetage ou grattage. Des maîtres de la dermatologie tels qu'ALIBERT et BOYER avec DARIER condamnent la chirurgie.

Au seuil du XXe siècle apparaissent les agents physiques: — Electrolyse — Electrocoagulation en France; Radiothérapie, Radiumthérapie en Allemagne. A remarquer que ces diverses techniques sont toujours précédées d'une biopsie. Les lésions dont l'excision entraîne une greffe sont du domaine chirurgical.

Sous l'impulsion de RAVAUT, l'électrocoagulation règne en maîtresse dans tous les services de l'Hôpital St-Louis, sauf dans un: celui de LOUSTE, de 1922 à 1934, puis, après la mort de ce dernier, dans celui de WEISSEMBACH, de 1934 à 1940, l'exérèse simple avec suture immédiate y fut régulièrement pratiquée.

Contre cette technique, existent quelques préjugés: ils sont au nombre de 5.

1. Il est écrit partout que l'excision doit être large; bien que ce ne soit pas précisé, il faut admettre qu'elle doit s'éloigner de la lésion d'au moins 10 m/m. Or, cette règle est fausse absolument. Une marge de sécurité de 5 m/m suffit «largement» et peut même être réduite à 3 ou 4 m/m. Elle doit être admise sans conteste, comme le démontre l'histologie.

Le champ d'action de l'exérèse s'étend donc considérablement et celle-ci peut être employée dans 80% des cas. Le cancer de la peau reste stationnaire pendant des mois au moins, sinon des années, au cours desquels il n'essaime pas. Cette période de latence est celle du bistouri nu.

2. Une autre idée préconçue a fait adopter le bistouri électrique. On en parle avec insistance. Or, il est absolument inutile; il a pour seul effet de rendre plus aléatoire la réunion par première intention et donc de retarder la cicatrisation. Les chirurgiens s'en rendent bien compte puisque après l'électrodissection ils avivent les bords de la plaie opératoire.

3. Un autre reproche est à enregistrer: la possibilité d'une récidive. Outre que celle-ci se produit avec toutes les méthodes, elle est moins à redouter dans l'exérèse. Une deuxième se fera, en effet, en peau saine et non pas dans une peau gravement traumatisée par l'électrocoagulation ou la radiothérapie.

4. Une faute est de compléter l'action de l'exérèse par de la radiothérapie ou par de la chimiothérapie qui agissent souvent sur de la peau saine.

5. Avoir recours à la greffe, lorsque celle-ci n'est pas indispensable, c'est compliquer sans aucune raison valable une intervention particulièrement simple et qui est de la petite chirurgie à la portée du dermatologiste.

Il y a lieu d'éliminer les cancers sur les demi-muqueuses, sur les brûlures, sur les radio ou radiumdermites.

Acte opératoire

Il doit être considéré comme une biopsie «large». Il est indiqué en présence de toute lésion suspecte cutanée sauf si une adénopathie correspondante existe, ou si une induration profonde est constatée.

La biopsie partielle n'est à employer que dans ces deux cas; elle est rejetée pour tous les autres; l'ancien biotome imaginé par PAUTRIER doit être exceptionnellement employé.

D'ailleurs, l'intervention est très simple; elle se fait avec une instrumentation composée d'un bistouri, d'une pince à griffe, d'une paire de ciseaux, d'une aiguille de Reverdin de la plus petite taille — ou d'aiguilles serties — et de crins; une à deux ampoules novocaïne, du coton, des compresses et de l'albuplaste, de l'alcool à 90° sont à prévoir. Catgut et pince à forcipression n'ont jamais été utilisés, car l'hémorragie est facilement arrêtée, soit par pression digitale ou par les crins de la suture.

La durée de l'exérèse ne dépasse pas 15 min et la réunion par première intention est obtenue en 10 jours environ. Elle est suivie d'une ligne cicatricielle qui devient par la suite invisible. Plus belle que celle après l'exérèse d'un lupus. La riche vascularisation de la face explique ces résultats des plus satisfaisants.

Bien que ces divers avantages soient très appréciables, ils s'effacent devant celui d'une importance capitale qui a été pourtant négligé, à savoir: l'examen de

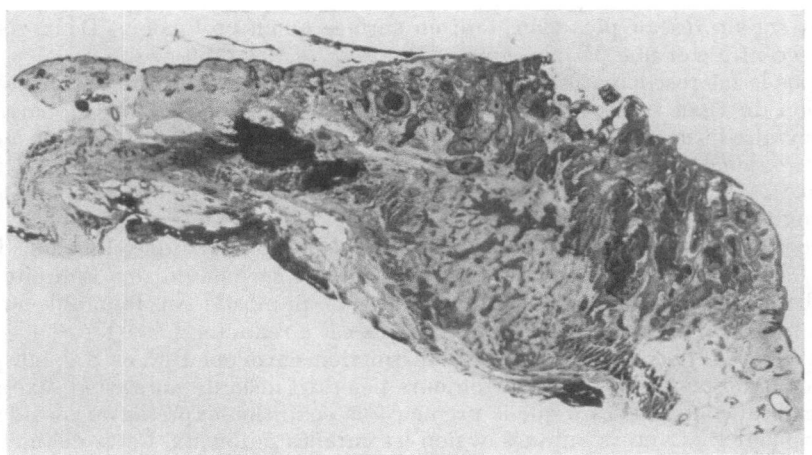

Fig. 1. × 8 — Epithélioma S. C. in the middle normal skin on each side and in depth

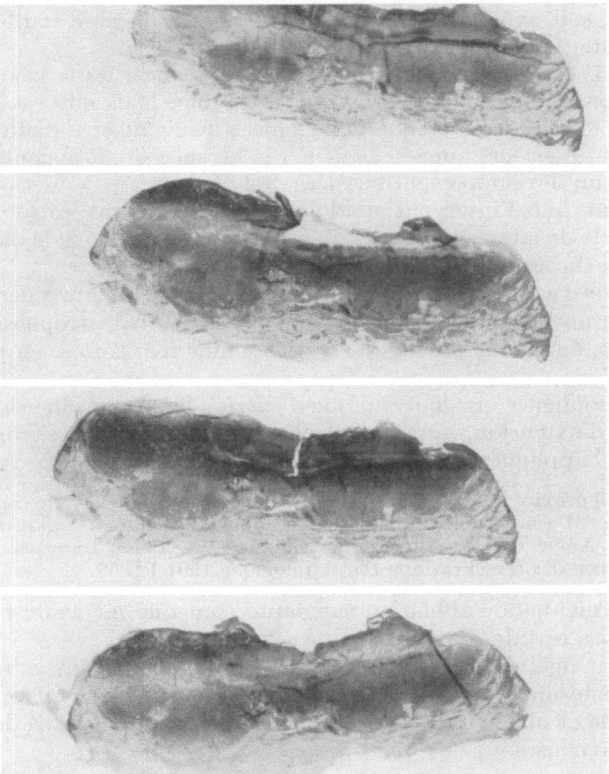

Fig. 2. × 8 — Epithélioma B. C. in the middle normal skin on each side and in depth

la lésion dans «toute son étendue», si toutefois l'exérèse a été correcte. Il peut être exécuté:

1. à l'oeil nu ou à la loupe sur la coupe colorée entre lame et lamelles. Le centre est occupé par un nodule épais opaque ayant pris intensément les colorants et

reposant sur un réseau plus clair, tant en surface qu'en profondeur. Deux zones dont une centrale et une périphérique.

2. Sous le microscope à faible grossissement apparait dans toute sa netteté la séparation du tissu sain et de la néoformation: boyaux épithéliaux et barrière lymphocytaire forment un ensemble cellulaire compact s'opposant à la trame lâche du tissu conjonctif.

Il est très regrettable que cet aspect ne fasse qu'exceptionnellement l'objet de microphotos dans les divers traités.

L'architecture est négligée aux dépens de l'aspect cytologique, lui mille fois répété. La première est cependant d'un gros intérêt car elle dessine la limite de l'épithélioma. Si elle est nettement tranchée, le pronostic est favorable et la récidive improbable. Dans le cas contraire, elle est à redouter.

Il semble, de plus, que la classique distinction entre épi B.C. et S.C. n'a pas une valeur absolue et le caractère toujours péjoratif accordé au second, excessif d'ailleurs beaucoup plus rare que le premier à la condition expresse de considérer exclusivement les Cancers cutanés et non les cutanés muqueux. Cette distinction fondamentale est souvent méconnue.

L'excision révèle les erreurs de diagnostic et évite la confusion, soit avec le noevocarcinome, soit avec les tuberculoses cutanées, soit avec toute lésion chroniqueulcero-croûteuse de la peau.

Conclusions. Il est certain que le traitement du cancer de la peau est dominé par son évolution. La malignité existe incontestable, mais elle est relative, elle reste longtemps locale, de sorte que deux phases peuvent être distinguées: l'une souvent longue — plusieurs années; l'autre, qui lui succède, beaucoup plus rapide, caractérisée par un développement accéléré de la tumeur.

Il est évident que l'intervention doit s'effectuer avant cette accélération, pendant la période de latence; elle sera d'autant plus efficace que le diagnostic sera précoce. Alors le succès est près de 100%.

Le siège au visage (85% des cas) qui inquiète le sujet l'incite à des traitements superficiels, très nocifs, qui conduisent souvent à des catastrophes. Les agents physiques divers, énumérés plus haut, en des mains inexpertes, en sont souvent responsables.

Il faut enfin souligner que la technique d'exérèse longtemps méconnue prendra de plus en plus d'extension, notamment chez les dermatologistes américains qui n'hésitent pas à l'appliquer même dans les noevo-carcinomes.

Bibliographie. THIBAUT, D.: Encyclopédie médico-chirurgicale — Ière Edition 1936 — 12829 P 5. — Anm. Derm. Syph. (Paris), 1948 — Journées Dermatologiques de Marseille-Octobre 1950. — Xème Congrès des Dermatologistes de langue française, Alger 25 à 27 Mai 1959, — DARIER J.: Ière Pratique Dermatologique 1901 PL 59.

«Les inconvénients de l'abblation sanglante sont que mème en taillant largement, on n'est pas certain d'avoir dépassé ces limites.

La mutilation opératoire est souvent énorme pour une tumeur qui paraissait petite. S'il subsiste une parcelle d'épithélioma, comme il arrive trop souvent, la récidive est fatale et oblige à des opérations complémentaires dans des conditions plus ou moins fâcheuses.»

Tratamiento actual de la enfermedad de Paget del pezon

J. Ocaña Sierra y A. J. Capilla, Universidad de Granada (España)

1. Hasta ahora el diagnóstico seguro de cáncer de mama significaba automaticamente una mastectomia radical o incluso super-radical, con todas sus consecuencias. Sin embargo, ciertos conocimientos recientes y los datos aportados por estadisticas amplias y minuciosas, van modificando el criterio clásico en cuanto a las grandes intervenciones muy mutilantes y con elevado índice de mortalidad, para ser sustituidas por los procederes mas conservadores, firmemente complementados con el estudio histológico detenido de la totalidad de la pieza extirpada y la vigilancia estrecha de la paciente. Es decir, en cada caso particular seria necesario un estudio histológico, bioquímico y genético lo mas completo posible, para decidir el método terapeutico más simple y adecuado.

El tratamiento de elección de la enfermedad de Paget del pezon y del cáncer de mama en etapas iniciales continua siendo la cirugia, desde una *simple extirpación del tumor, mastectomia simple o ampliada* con disección de los ganglios linfáticos axilares; intervenciones más conservadoras que el *clásico* Halsted que incluye ademas el musculo pectoral, o bien, las grandes intervenciones, como la *mastectomia radical ampliada* que comprende tambien los ganglios linfaticos de la mamaria interna, o incluso la denominada *super-radical* con liberación, asimismo, de los ganglios linfáticos supra-claviculares; que no han alcanzado mayor porcentaje de supervivencia (Dahl-Iversen, Kaane y Johansen en una serie de 668 pacientes). En este sentido, es interesante la observacion de Temime y cols., en un caso de enfermedad de Paget muy incipiente diagnosticada por dos dermatólogos clínica e histológicamente y que fué intervenida practicandose una mastectomia super-radical, y encontrandose todos los ganglios extirpados, *indemnes histológicamente*.

En el "Symposium" celebrado en Liverpool, abril de 1964, sobre "Cáncer de mama", se ha insistido en que el crecimiento y desarrollo tumoral tiene un curso evolutivo peculiar en cada individuo, no contando todavia con un criterio tanto científico como biológico, suficientemente seguro para justificar el interrumpir, eventualmente, este curso; al estimarse que en ciertos casos ya existian metástasis a través de la corriente sanguínea en una fase muy precoz del proceso, demostrada por la presencia frecuente de células cancerosas circulantes (Cole), asi como la posibilidad de que los ganglios linfáticos actuen frenando la diseminación del proceso neoplásico va adquiriendo cada dia más certeza (Porrit). En tal sentido solo podria influir sobre la diseminación hematógena intentando inhibir el crecimiento de estas células mediante el empleo de la *cirugia endocrina profiláctica* y de los *agentes citotóxicos*.

2. Fundandonos en los datos anteriores, hemos tratado tres casos de la enfermedad de Paget del pezon, en etapas iniciales, localizadas, mediante mastectomia simple, seguido del estudio histológico sistematico de la totalidad del seno extirpado, encontrando una discreta proliferación intra-canalicular en algunos acinis cercanos a su desembocadura, observandose las células de Paget típicas, y en otro de los casos la biopsia reveló un carcinoma de los conductos galactóforos en su porcion terminal con invasión de la epidermis, destruida por el tumor en la zona clínicamente ulcerada.

La herida de la excisión-biopsia cicatrizó normalmente en las tres pacientes. En la actualidad se mantiene la curación clinica y la observación estrecha para practicar una disección ganglionar terapéutica en caso necesario.

3. Las amplias estadísticas recientes de Crile, Porrit y otros, muestran que los resultados del tratamiento del cáncer de mama en etapa I por *mastectomia*

simple, efectuando disección ganglionar axilar posteriormente si aparecen adenopatias, revelan los motivos de la tendencia actual a un tratamiento más conservador sin que ello repercuta en el pronóstico. No hay necesidad, por lo tanto, de exponer por sistema a las enfermas, a la morbilidad y mortalidad de procederes quirúrgicos extensos, y los inconvenientes del linfoedema y fibroedema de la extremidad superior en las disecciones ganglionares axilares.

Fundandonos en los datos anteriores, y contando con la utilidad del citodiagnóstico, mamografia y excisión-biopsia, consideramos que la enfermedad de Paget del pezon, en sus etapas iniciales, localizadas, puede ser tratada con éxito definitivo mediante mastectomia simple y adecuada vigilancia ulterior. En nuestros tres casos se siguió esta directriz satisfactoriamente. El estudio histológico detenido de la totalidad del seno extirpado, en cada caso solo demostro presencia del carcinoma en las zonas inmediatamente adyacentes a las lesiones cutaneas.

Tratamiento quirurgico del cáncer cutaneo-mucoso

F. DE DULANTO y J. SÁNCHEZ-MUROS, Cátedra y Escuela Profesional de Dermatología Médico-Quirúrgica, Universidad de Granada (España)

Con el desarrollo de las técnicas reconstructivas ha desaparecido la principal objeción a la Cirugía para los tumores en zonas descubiertas: la creación de un defecto, dificil de cerrar con resultados estéticos satisfactorios si nó se utilizan. Podemos eliminar el tumor con amplio margen de tejido sano y el examen rápido intraoperatorio mediante cortes por congelación permitirá con frecuencia una garantía de la extirpación completa. "La Cirugía es el más vidente de los métodos o si se quiere el menos ciego." Si se interviene pronto antes que el tumor haya penetrado en estructuras profundas o dado metástasis los problemas a veces insuperables de la excisión radical en otros territorios orgánicos no existen en el cáncer de piel.

La *reparación* de los defectos consecutivos a exéresis, irradiación, (ó quimioterapia) de un cáncer cutáneo-mucoso presenta tres posibilidades fundamentales: 1. la *reparación definitiva inmediata* es el ideal: exéresis-reparación en un tiempo. Es aplicable a la mayoría de los basaliomas y a los carcinomas espinocelulares incipientes. 2. Como *reparación demorada* designamos la que precisa efectuar en tumores avanzados, recidivados, muy irradiados, cuando su exéresis total sea insegura, existan dificultades para la hemostasia o nó puede prolongarse la intervención. La superficie cruenta se cubre provisionalmente con un injerto laminar delgado que nó impide adecuada vigilancia ní el control de recidivas y evita la cicatrización por segunda intención. La reparación definitiva se deja para más adelante, meses o años después, cuando se disponga de razonable certeza de la curación del tumor. 3. Como *reparación definitiva tardia* y de las *secuelas* consideramos el grupo de casos en que el tumor puede considerarse curado después de Cirugía o radiaciones. Nos encontramos frente a mutilaciones de diverse grado, radiodermitis crónica, y sus combinaciones.

Cuando nó es posible la *sutura directa* utilizamos: 1° plastias locales (por deslizamiento, rotación o transposición), 2° Injertos y 3° Colgajos pediculados (planos o tubulares).

El tratamiento de las *adenopatias regionales* hay que contemplarlo siempre que es examen histológico demuestre esta posibilidad. La disección ganglionar es necesaria en muchos carcinomas espinocelulares, melanomas malignos y sarcomas e inútil, habitualmente, en los epiteliomas basocelulares.

En trece años hemos operado personalmente 641 pacientes con predominio de formas avanzadas. Las recidivas alcanzaron, 2% en los epiteliomas basocelulares, 1,9% en los carcinomas espinocelulares y 15% en los melanomas malignos. La cifra de mortalidad global fué de 2,9%. Consideramos la estadística satisfactoria y que aconseja seguir en la orientación expuesta.

Sin duda *la mejor profilaxis del cáncer cutáneo-mucoso es el tratamiento del precáncer.* Insistimos en tres aspectos importantes: 1. La terapeútica de los queratomas actínicos múltiples mediante abrasión rotatoria. 2. El tratamiento de las queilitis queratósicas y leucoplásicas mediante excisión del borde rojo y reconstruccion inmediata desplazando hacia delante la mucosa labial, y 3. La Cirugía reparadora precoz de las radiodermitis.

Demostrada la eficacia de las técnicas quirúrgicas reconstructivas y sus ventajas, permiten a los dermatologos seguir contribuyendo decisivamente al tratamiento y profilaxis del cáncer cutáneo-mucoso. Las técnicas quirúrgicas proporcionan además un amplísimo campo a la Especialidad: deformidades congénitas o consecutivas a accidentes, quemaduras, tumores benignos, alteraciones estéticas, etc. Insistimos en el *concepto integral médico-quirúrgico* de la Dermatología (tegumento, mucosas y forma exterior del organismo), que en España tenemos ya reconocido oficialmente por el Ministerio de Educación y Ciencia.

Über die Dosisplanung bei der Strahlentherapie der Hauttumoren

K. BALABANOV und P. PENTSCHEV, Dermatologische Universitätsklinik und Krebsforschungsinstitut, Sofia (Bulgarien)

Vorbedingung für erfolgreiche Durchführung der Strahlentherapie von Hauttumoren ist die Realisierung einer genügenden Dosis im ganzen Tumor, d. h., auch die am ungünstigsten gelegenen Tumorteile müssen die nötige cancerizide Dosis erhalten. Von der tatsächlichen Höhe der canceriziden Dosis sind unsere Vorstellungen noch ungenau. In der Praxis ist das, was wir Dosis bei den Hauttumoren nennen, die Exposition des Hautniveaus. Die absorbierte Energiemenge, von der ja der biologische Effekt abhängt, zeigt aber in den verschiedenen Tumorteilen bei der Röntgen- und Radiumtherapie erhebliche Unterschiede. In den tiefer gelegenen Tumorteilen ist die Bedeutung der Strahlenempfindlichkeit eines Tumors nach der Exposition der Hautoberfläche aber irreal, ebenso die Angabe der Oberflächenexposition als Dosis, bei der ein Rezidiv aufgetreten ist. Ein solches wird meist in den schwach bestrahlten Anteilen des Tumors beobachtet.

Zur Zeit ist jede Strahlentherapieabteilung, die Ansprüche erhebt, nach modernen Grundsätzen zu arbeiten, bestrebt, bei der Bestrahlung von tief gelegenen Tumoren die genaue Dosisverteilung in den Geweben festzustellen und die minimale Tumordosis genau zu bestimmen. Bei den oberflächlich gelegenen Tumoren, wo das leicht und genau erreichbar ist, ist es falsch und nicht begründet, sich mit der Bestimmung der Oberflächendosis zu begnügen.

Wir haben uns die Aufgabe gestellt, ein zweckmäßigeres und genaueres Verfahren einzuführen, das uns, den heutigen dosimetrischen Möglichkeiten entsprechend, erlaubt:

1. durch Gegenüberstellung der Dosisverteilung im Gewebe bei den verschiedenen Bestrahlungsmethoden die beste Methode für den Einzelfall auszuwählen;

2. die wirklich realisierte Dosis im Tumor festzustellen, indem man den Behandlungseffekt mit der minimalen Tumordosis bezieht;

3. die tatsächliche Behandlungsdosis für die einzelnen Tumoren festzustellen.

Ausgangspunkt bei der Behandlung ist der individuelle Bestrahlungsplan; um ihn anzufertigen, ist es notwendig, die genaue Größe des Tumors zu bestimmen, was für einen erfahrenen Dermatologen oder Röntgenologen keine Schwierigkeit darstellt. Bei der Röntgenkontaktbestrahlung genügt es, transparente Isodosenschablonen für die einzelnen Tubusse [1] auf die maßstäbliche Tumorskizze aufzulegen. Mit dem Ziel der günstigsten Dosisverteilung im Tumor wird der entsprechende Tubus ausgewählt. Nach der Isodose, die die tiefsten Teile des Tumors tangiert, wird die minimale Tumordosis bestimmt. Bei der Radiumtherapie ist es notwendig, für jede Moulage Isodosen zu ermitteln. Zu diesem Zweck benutzen wir die Filmdosimetrie mit den Äquidensitenverfahren [2, 3, 4] und den digitalen Rechenautomaten [5]. Es werden die Möglichkeiten verglichen, die die einzelnen Nahbestrahlungstubusse und die verschiedenen Distanzen und Formen der Moulage ergeben, um eine homogene Tumorbestrahlung ohne große Dosisunterschiede zwischen Oberfläche und Tiefe zu erreichen. Dabei werden auch die Tolerantdosen benachbarter strahlenempfindlicher Gewebe und Organe, z.B. Augenlinse oder darunterliegender Knochen und Knorpel, berücksichtigt.

Unter Berücksichtigung dieser Gesichtspunkte wird die richtige Methodik und Applikationstechnik gewählt und die minimale Dosis bestimmt. In die Krankengeschichte wird eingetragen: 1. die minimale Tumordosis, nach der dann auch das Behandlungsresultat bestimmt wird; 2. die Dosis an der Hautoberfläche, die als Kriterium der Strahlenbelastung dient und erlaubt, die nach der Bestrahlung auftretenden Veränderungen abzulesen, und 3. die Dosis an den kritischen Organen, um eventuelle Veränderungen in ihnen abschätzen zu können. Dieses Verfahren erleichtert die schwere Aufgabe einer eventuellen Rezidivbestrahlung sowohl hinsichtlich der Zweckmäßigkeit einer solchen überhaupt, als auch für die Bestimmung der Dosis und der Methodik.

Literatur. 1. CHAOUL, H., u. F. WACHSMANN: Die Nahbestrahlung. Stuttgart: Thieme 1953. — 2. LAN, E., u. W. KRUG: Äquidensometrie. Grundlagen, Verfahren und Anwendung. Berlin: Akademie Verlag 1957. — 3. RAKOW, A.: Rad. Biol. Ther. **2**, 121 (1962). — 4. SAHATCHIEV, A., and P. PENTSCHEV: Onkologia (Sofia) **2**, 34 (1965). — 5. RICHTER, P. PENTSCHEV und D. SCHIRRMEISTER: Strahlentherapie **132**, 246 (1967).

Antimitotica der Podophyllinreihe bei Hautkrebs und seniler Keratose

V. MATANIĆ, Dermatologische Abteilung des Medizinischen Zentrums, Zadar (Jugoslawien)

Die Zellen der Hautcarcinome und Keratosen zeigen gegenüber Normalzellen viel geringere Unterschiede als die Bakterien. Eine gezielte Wirkung bei Antimitotica, im Vergleich zu Bakteriostatika, kann nie erreicht werden. Man muß also einen Mittelweg suchen, der in der Schonung der sich schnell regenerierenden Gewebe der Haarwurzel und der Basalzellenschicht besteht und doch die Krebszellen angreift.

Ein solches Mittel ist das „Spindelgift" SPG, das ausgesprochen antimitotisch wirkt. Es handelt sich um Podophyllin-D-benzyliden-glucosid der gesamten Podophyllin-glucoside, die mit 70% vertreten sind. Das Medikament blockiert die

Metaphase im Mitosenablauf bzw. desorganisiert die Bildung des Spindelapparates und verhindert die Einordnung der Chromosome in der Äquatorialebene. Es hemmt auf diese Weise die Mitosenbildung der Krebszelle.

Bei verschiedenen Konzentrationen von SPG in Geléeunterlage habe ich versucht, den Wirkungsbereich jeder Konzentration auszuforschen, und welche von denen optimale Auswirkung bei Hautcarcinomen und Keratosis senilis zeigen. Die Versuche wurden bei 466 Patienten eingeleitet.

Die antimitotische Wirkung in der Therapie des Hautkrebses besteht auch hier in der Hemmung womöglichst großer Zellenzahl im pathologisch veränderten Gewebe unter größter Schonung der Normalzellen auf cytotoxischem Weg. Theoretisch besteht hier eine relativ nichttoxische Wirkung. Die Erfolge bei Hautcarcinomen bei lokaler Anwendung der Antimitotica der Podophyllinreihe wurden bei oberflächlig liegenden Hautcarcinomen registriert, weiter bei solchen die inoperabel sind, aber auch als Ergänzung der chirurgischen und radiologischen Bearbeitung.

Konzentration	1%	4%	6%	10%	Total
Anzahl der Fälle	25	55	113	20	213
Erfolgreich	13,3%	21,80%	33,61%	24,40%	

Die Unterschiede in der SPG Konzentrationswirkung auf die Krebszellen sind meiner Meinung nur quantitativ wie in ihrer Wirkung auf die Normalzellen, die gering ist, als auch auf ihre regenerativen Eigenschaften. Die Einwirkungsgrenze ist meines Erachtens in dieser Richtung auf die potenziellen Regenerationseigenschaften der Normalzellen zurückzuführen, deren Grenzen in den normalen Zwischenverhältnissen in der Zelle allein geschaffen sind, abhängig von der Konzentrationshöhe des Antimitoticum in der Einwirkung auf das erkrankte Gewebe. Dabei ist bei SPG die Penetration in die Tiefe langsam und schonend. Deshalb kann auch nicht die Ansprechbarkeit der einzelnen histologisch differenzierten Hautcarcinome die gleiche sein. Man sieht, daß die Basalzellencarcinome gut auf die Therapie anreagieren, die Plattenzellcarcinome und Veruca carcinomatosa bedeutend schwächer. Immerhin gibt es bei einzelnen von diesen Gruppen Versager, trotz der gleichen oder auch erhöhten Konzentration. Meines Erachtens ist der Erfolg zwar von der optimalen Konzentrationsdurchdringung des Mittels abhängig, aber auch von der Beschaffenheit der Haut in dem Krebsgebiet und ihrer Abwehrreaktion. Bei jüngeren Patienten ist eine bessere Ansprechbarkeit zu sehen als bei den älteren Kranken, die schon a priori eine abgenutzte Haut haben. Dazu kommt als bedeutend die Ausbreitung und Tiefe der Geschwulst, ihre Lage und das Konzentrationsvermögen des Antimitoticums. Je oberflächiger in der Haut das Carcinom gelagert ist, desto besser kann SPG einwirken, mit dem Schwerpunkt in der Hemmung der Mitosenbildung der Krebszellen.

Bei *Keratosis senilis* ist SPG auch in den vier Konzentrationen verwendet worden. So sah ich bei:

Konzentration	1%	4%	6%	10%	Total
Anzahl der Fälle	17	85	135	16	253
Erfolgreich	24,20%	58,82%	61,48%	33,5%	

Hier spielt sicherlich eine bedeutende Rolle die Hemmung der Zellverhornung im Stratum corneum. Die Unterschiede gegenüber den Normalzellen sind hier qualitativ im Zellgeschehen wie in der Entstehung als auch in den Rückbildung des Verhornungsprozesses. Das ist nicht nur durch lokales Konzentrationsvermögen des Medikamentes, sondern auch von den optimalen Durchdringungsvermögen abhängig.

Diskussion. KAPLAN hat 1942 die Anwendung von Podophyllinextraten in die Dermatologie wieder eingeführt, nachdem sie seit fast einem Jahrhundert vergessen waren und damals in der Volksmedizin ihre Anwendung bei gewöhnlichen und spitzen Warzen fanden. SULLIVAN und WECHSLER entdeckten 5 Jahre später die Arretierung der Mitose unter der Podophyllum-emmodi-Droge. Durch die Laboruntersuchungen mit markiertem C^{14}-Material bei Ratten zeigte sich, daß die Beimengung von benzyliden Verbindungen der Podophyllum-emmodi-Droge eine deutliche Wirkungssteigerung zur Folge hatte. Das daraus entwickelte SPG übte eine mitotische Wirkung bei Krebszellen aus.

Dies bewog mich, die Versuche mit SPG in Geléeunterlage bei einer großen Anzahl von Hautcarcinomen und Keratosis senilis durchzuführen.

Zusammenfassend kann man sagen, daß SPG zwar auf die Rückbildung der Krebszellen in obengenanntem Sinne einen bestimmten Einfluß auszuwirken vermag, der aber nicht in allen Fällen komplett genügt, diese in ihrem Wachstum ganz zu stoppen und zur kompletten Beseitigung der Hauterscheinungen zu bringen, aber angezeigt ist, um das Leiden auf eine bedeutende Weise anzugreifen und den Kranken eine Hoffnung zu bringen.

Chemosurgery for the Microscopically Controlled Excision of Skin Cancer

F. E. MOHS, University of Wisconsin Medical Center, Madison, Wisconsin (USA)

Because cancers of the skin frequently send out slender strands and thin sheets of cancer cells for a considerable distance beyond the clinically visible and palpable cancerous mass, the cancer therapist must remove or radiate an extra margin of tissue around the grossly visible cancer. However, even with this sacrifice of extra tissue, there is no complete assurance that all of the cancerous outgrowths have been eradicated. To eliminate this uncertainty and also to eliminate the need to remove an extra margin of normal tissues, chemosurgery was developed to provide a means by which cancers of the skin can be excised under complete microscopic control.

The chemosurgical technique consists of three essential steps: first, chemical fixation of the tissues in situ by the application of a zinc chloride fixative paste; second, excision of a layer of fixed tissue; and third, thorough microscopic scanning of the entire undersurface of the excised layer by the systematic use of frozen sections. This process is repeated until a cancer-free plane is reached. Since reapplication of the fixative and reexcision of the tissues are limited to the areas where cancer has been observed microscopically, the "silent" outgrowths may be accurately and selectively followed to their terminations.

For chemical fixation in situ zinc chloride was chosen because it is non-toxic systemically, it produces adequate fixation with good preservation of the microscopic features of the tissues, it is safe to handle because it does not readily penetrate the keratin layer of the skin, it penetrates well through the deeper tissues and its depth of penetration is accurately controlled when it is incorporated in a paste vehicle designed to release the fixative in a predictable manner. Finally, animal experiments and clinical experience show that the chemical has no tendency to increase metastasis.

The chemosurgical technique is illustrated by the following case report. The basal cell carcinoma was of 2 years duration and twice had been treated unsuccessfully by electrodesiccation and curettage (Fig. 1). It was excised in four microscopically controlled stages by the chemosurgical technique. Most of the "silent" extensions were in the dermis at the periphery where the cancer extended at least a centimeter beyond the grossly visible and palpable borders of the neoplasm.

At the completion of chemosurgical treatment the markings on the fixed tissue indicate the sites of origin of the excised specimens (Fig. 2). A map on a pad of paper corresponded to these markings and as the sections were examined microscopically the areas of remaining cancer, had they been present, would have been plotted on the map as a guide to the reapplication of the fixative. The final layer

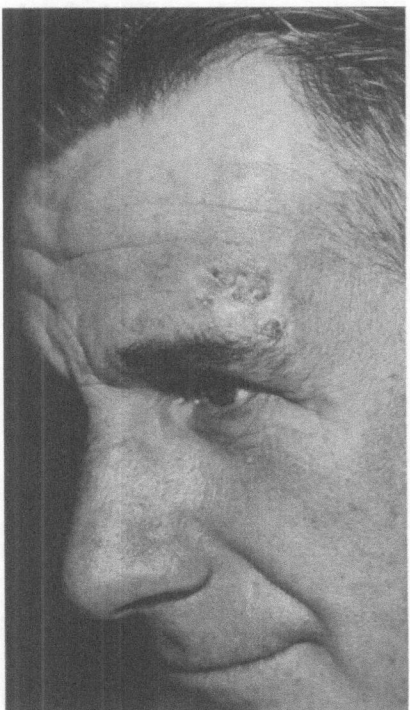

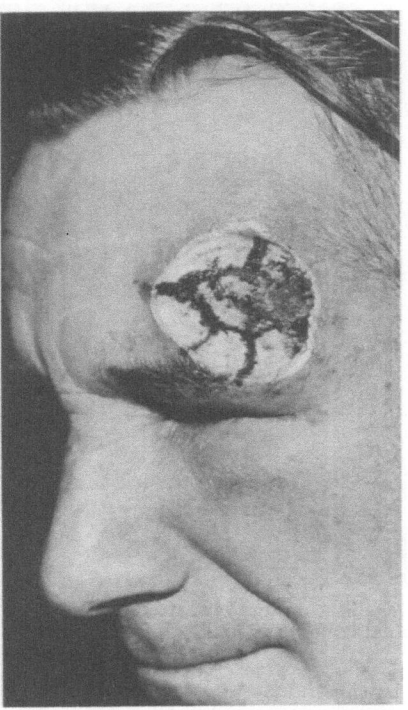

Fig. 1. Basal cell carcinoma, duration 2 years, recurrent after two treatments with electrodesiccation and curettage

Fig. 2. At completion of chemosurgical excision in four microscopically controlled stages

separated 6 days later revealing healthy granulations (Fig. 3). Healing progressed rapidly, and when he returned in 4 months the scar was smooth and pliable (Fig. 4).

In the treatment of cancer of the skin chemosurgery has several advantages. Most important is the unprecedented reliability. In a series of 5423 cases of basal cell carcinoma of the skin, there were 4159 determinate cases with a 5-year cure rate of 99.1%. In a series of 1712 squamous cell carcinomas of the skin there were 1330 determinate cases and the 5-year cure rate was 92.2%. These high rates of cure were attained despite the fact that many of the cancers were extensive and one third of them had recurred after previous radiation or surgical treatment.

The second advantage is the conservatism. Only 1 or 2 mm need be removed beyond the farthest extension of the cancer. Both the conservatism and the reliability are the results of the microscopic control which permits selective removal of the "silent" outgrowths.

A third advantage is the low operative mortality which results from the lack of need for general anesthesia, the lack of trouble with infection, and the conservative approach that can safely be employed.

A fourth advantage is that chemosurgery extends operability to many patients with cancers too extensive for hope of cure with other methods.

Finally, healing is excellent and there are no late complications such as atrophy, ulceration or malignant change.

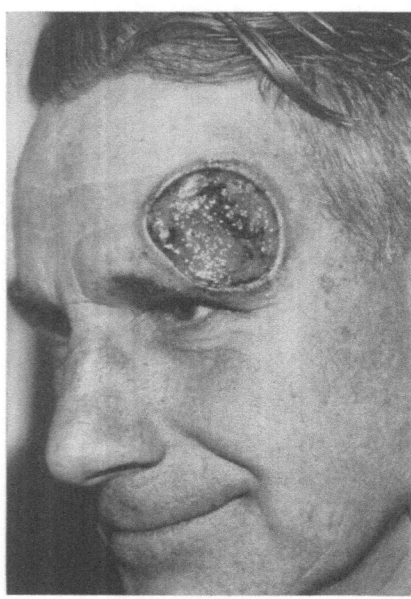
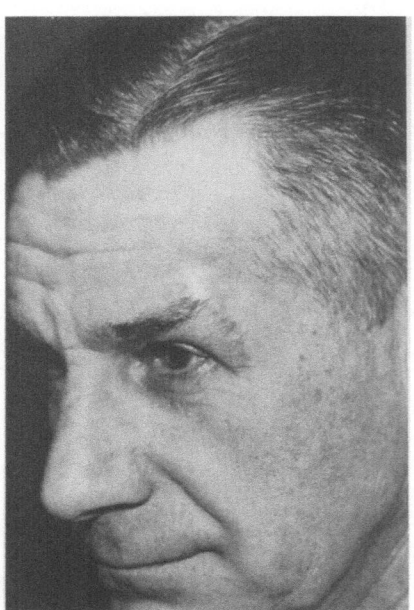

Fig. 3. Granulations after separation of final layer of fixed tissue

Fig. 4. Healed lesion 4 months later

In the treatment of patients with far advanced cancers there may be sufficient pain to require analgesics as potent as morphine, and the process may be time-consuming for the operator. However, since it is in the care of patients with "problem" cancers that chemosurgery is most desperately needed, these disadvantages are not of great significance.

Although the idea of using frozen sections for the complete microscopic guidance of excision is simple in concept, the chemosurgical technique is more complex in practice. Therefore, some training in its use is desirable. Also, the technician who makes the special type of frozen sections should be specially trained.

Chemosurgery is a valuable addition to our armamentarium against cancer of the skin, and the method should be available in every large center of population. More than fifty physicians now are actively using the method, but more are needed.

Die Therapie fortgeschrittener Hauttumoren

H. Drepper und F. Ehring, Fachklinik „Haus Hornheide" des Westfälischen Vereins für Krebs- und Lupusbekämpfung, Handorf über Münster/Westf. (Deutschland)

Unter fortgeschrittenen Hauttumoren verstehen wir in Anlehnung an das TNM-System Geschwülste, die die Unterhaut zur Tiefe überschritten haben oder Metastasen aufweisen. Sie kommen häufiger vor, als vielfach angenommen (Jordan Ehring [8]; Ehling [5]).

Meistens sind diese Tumoren nicht oder nur regional abgrenzbar metastasiert. Eine radikale Behandlung ist relativ aussichtsreich. Allerdings ist es oft schwer, die tatsächliche Tumorausdehnung zu erkennen. Zudem übersteigt die Behandlung und Wiederherstellung vielfach das dermatologische Fachgebiet. Auch Chirurg, Radiologe oder Rhinologe allein sind oft überfordert. Die günstigsten Voraussetzungen bietet die Zusammenarbeit (Teamwork) aller einschlägigen Fachärzte in einer Spezialklinik. Hier kann die Behandlung im ärztlichen Konsilium individuell geplant und durchgeführt werden (Drepper und Ehring [3]).

Die *chirurgische Behandlung* besteht in der en-bloc-Excision — je nach Abgrenzbarkeit des Tumors — 3 bis 30 mm im Gesunden. Leicht implantierbare Tumoren werden möglichst elektrochirurgisch excidiert. Sonst wird das Tumorbett mit einem Cytostatikum, z. B. Trenimon, ausgespült (Spiessl [12]). Anschließend prüfen wir die Vollständigkeit der Excision am Querschnitt, im Zweifelsfall histologisch. In komplizierten Fällen ziehen wir die systematische histologische Schnellschnittkontrolle der Mohsschen chemochirurgischen Methode vor (Drepper [1, 2], Mohs [10, 11]).

Die *radiologische Behandlung* wird durch frühere Bestrahlungen erschwert. Am Schädel liegen oft Tumoranteile hinter Knochen. Hier sind harte Gamma-Strahlen den konventionellen Röntgen-, oft auch den Beta-Strahlen überlegen. Speziell für diese Aufgabe wurde von Ehring, Hellenthal und Schumann sowie der TEM England das ^{60}Co-Kurzdistanztherapiegerät „Cobaltron II" entwickelt. Die Quelle ist hierbei besonders gut abgeschirmt, die Feldbegrenzung sehr scharf. Aufbaueffekt und Knochendurchstrahlung sind wie bei der Telekobalttherapie, der Dosisabfall zur Tiefe aber günstiger, da die GHWT zwischen 3 und 6 cm variierbar ist (Ehring [6]).

Fall 1: 75jährige Hausfrau mit einem 4×4 cm² großen, mit dem Kieferwinkel verbackenen Tumor bei aktiver Tuberculosis luposa, derbe Lymphknotenpakete am Hals, außerdem Diabetes und Herzinsuffizienz. Radiologische Behandlung mit ^{60}Co, INH-Behandlung der Tbc. luposa. Tumor und Tbc. rezidivfrei seit 5 Jahren.

Die *Kombination* von Operation mit Vor- oder Nachbestrahlung verbessert manchmal die Heilungschancen. Technisch inoperable und ausbestrahlte Tumoren sind unter Umständen semiradikal zu entfernen und mit einem 4 bis 6 mm dicken Flap stabil zu decken, so daß sie mit dem Cobaltron II erneut kurativ zu bestrahlen sind (Drepper und Ehring [4]).

Fall 2: 69jähriger Arbeiter mit ausgedehnten, operierten und ausbestrahlten Halslymphknotenmetastasen eines Plattenepithelcarcinoms am li. Mundwinkel. Nach Neck-Dissektion wird der Defekt durch Rotationsplastik gedeckt und fraktioniert mit ^{60}Co (5500 r Oberflächendosis) bestrahlt. Seit 15 Monaten rezidivfrei.

Die *Chemotherapie* hat u. a. bei den Reticulosarkomatosen Erfolgschancen. Aber auch andere Tumoren sind manchmal auf einzelne Cytostatika empfindlich. Aufbauend auf den Erfahrungen von Limburg und Krahe [9] an gynäkologischen

Tumoren testen wir Cytostatika individuell in der Gewebekultur aus. Die ersten Erfahrungen ermutigen zum Ausbau dieser Methode.

Zur *Rehabilitation* muß der Kranke nach Entfernung des Tumors funktionell wie ästhetisch befriedigend wiederhergestellt werden. Die Nachkontrolle darf hierbei nicht behindert werden. Wir decken daher Defekte möglichst mit Vollhauttransplantaten oder provisorisch mit Spalthaut und Epithese und holen die endgültige plastische Wiederherstellung je nach Dauer der Tumoranamnese nach mehrjähriger Beobachtung nach (EHRING [7], DREPPER [2]).

Wie notwendig diese Wartezeit ist, zeige der *Fall 3:* 42jähriger Dreher mit massivem Rezidiv eines mehrfach operierten und plastisch gedeckten Ca. basocellulare terebrans. Radikaloperation, provisorische Spalthautplastik, Gesichtsteilepithese. Der Patient arbeitete wieder. Nach 23 Monaten zeigte sich am Orbitalrand ein Rezidiv, obwohl der Tumor hier 1 cm im Gesunden entfernt war. Bei primär gestielter Plastik wäre dies Rezidiv nicht mehr rechtzeitig entdeckt worden.

Fall 4: 60jährige Angestellte mit einem Ca. basocellulare terebrans des Gesichtes nach Tbc. luposa. Radikaloperation, provisorische Spalthautdeckung. Später wurden Oberlippe, Wange und Nase durch einen akromiopectoralen Rundstiellappen und Rippenknorpelspan wieder aufgebaut. Trotz langjähriger Vereinsamung gelang die volle soziale Rehabilitation. Der Tumor ist 5 Jahre rezidivfrei.

Die endgültige Wiederherstellung ist für den Behandlungserfolg entscheidend. Die Aussicht darauf erleichtert Arzt und Patient den Entschluß zur rechtzeitigen Radikalbehandlung.

Literatur. 1. DREPPER, H.: Hautarzt 14, 420 (1963). — 2. DREPPER, H.: Vortrag 90. Tagung Rhein.-West. Dermatologen, Wuppertal, 15. 11. 1964; ref.: Derm. Wschr. 152, 1032 (1966). — 3. DREPPER, H., u. F. EHRING: Mitteilungsdienst der G.B.K. Nordrhein-Westfalen 4, 595 (1967). — 4. DREPPER, H., u. F. EHRING: Die Tumormetastasierung an der Haut und ihre Behandlung. Krebsforschung und Krebsbekämpfung, Bd. IV. München: Urban u. Schwarzenberg 1967. — 5. EHLING, M.: Inaug. Diss., Münster 1966. — 6. EHRING, F.: Arch. Derm. 219, 504 (1964). — 7. EHRING, F.: Rebahilitative epithetische Medizin. In Rehabilitation. Schriftenreihe der Med. pharm. Studiengesellschaft e.V., Bd. 2/3, Frankfurt am Main: Umschau Verlag 1965. — 8. JORDAN, P., u. F. EHRING: Münch. med. Wschr. 100, 831 (1958). — 9. LIMBURG, H., u. M. KRAHE: Dtsch. med. Wschr. 89, 1938 (1964). — 10. MOHS, F. E.: Proc. Inst. Med. Chic. 21, 134 (1956). — 11. MOHS, F. E.: N. Y. St. J. Med. 56, 3486 (1956). — 12. SPIESSL, B.: Symposon aktueller therapeutischer Probleme 3, 210. Stuttgart: Enke 1961.

Cryosurgery of Cutaneous Carcinoma

S. A. ZACARIAN, Boston University, School of Medicine, Boston, Mass. (USA)

Introduction. Dermatologists were among the pioneers in medicine to utilize liquified gases for medical disorders. As early as 1899, CAMPBELL WHITE [1] used liquid air, with a cotton swab, for the successful treatment of lupus erythematosus, nevi, verrucae, hemangiomas and epitheliomas. By 1907 [2, 3], liquid air and nitrogen were used primarily for benign disorders and precancerous lesions; for it was soon realized that cotton swabs, as applicators were inadequate for eradication of cutaneous carcinomas.

Cotton has a low specific heat. It is a poor conductor and an inferior heat sink, thus lacking tissue penetrability. A substance or material had to be found with a high thermal gradient and conductivity to allow cryogenic temperatures to reach deep into the dermis and subcutaneous tissue, wherein extends malignant epithelioma of the skin. Having found copper to possess the necessary characteristics, solid cylinder discs 1 cm thick with varying diameters and surfaces were designed. The center of the disc is beveled and a plastic handle with a screw tip is readily inserted into it. The copper disc is then immersed into a flask containing liquid nitrogen and within 2 min, the disc assumes equilibrium with its medium. Some copper discs have flat surfaces, while others are concave or convex, and selection is dependent on the morphological surface of the lesion under treatment.

Animal and human temperature studies. In both dogs and guinea pigs, 21 gauge hypodermic needle thermocouples of copper constantan were applied at the cutaneous surface and also inserted at 2, 4 and 5 mm depths. Temperatures were recorded while the chilled copper disc was applied on the cutaneous surface of the animal for over 160 sec [4]. Serial biopsies were obtained on the 1st, 3rd and 5th day following the above temperature studies and varying degrees of cryo-necrosis was noted histologically to extend into the muscular layer of the animals.

To correlate the results of animal experimentation with human experiences may at times be erroneous. A study [5], therefore, was undertaken to obtain in vivo human skin temperatures and to compare the thermal profile between cotton swabs and copper discs. A patient, prepared for mid-thigh amputation for gangrene, was selected for this experiment. A linear incision was made through the skin in the upper thigh and a thermocouple was inserted at the subcutaneous level, exceeding 2 mm depth. Series of temperatures were recorded on a pyrometer following application of cotton swabs saturated with liquid nitrogen and chilled copper discs of varying diameters. Despite *several* applications of cotton swabs for several minutes, temperature gradience varied from +18° to —26 °C. In comparison, with a *single* application of a 1 cm diameter copper cylinder disc, within 15 sec the temperature of the skin at the same depth was recorded at —30 °C and sustained at —44 °C for over 75 sec. With discs of larger diameters, the recorded temperatures were as low as —85 °C. Cryobiologists have established —20 °C as the critical temperature for tissue necrosis. One can readily appreciate the inadequacy of the cotton swab to eradicate malignant neoplasms deep within the integument.

Cryosurgery of skin cancer. In our study, every patient with a skin cancer was biopsied and the neoplasms histologically classified. The appropriate diameter and shaped copper disc is chilled in liquid nitrogen and applied directly onto the lesion. For tumors up to 1.5 cm in diameter, the disc is applied for 120 sec. For larger lesions, 90 sec is adequate. Anesthesia is not required for treatment. The patient feels slight discomfort during the first 10 to 15 sec of freezing and slightly more during the period of thawing, lasting no more than 2 min. There may be a local urticarial reaction at the treatment site within 10 to 15 min, followed with a bullous hemorrhagic reaction within the first 24 h. A necrotic crust follows, with some exudation of serum persisting for several weeks. Within 4 to 5 weeks, the crust sloughs off, leaving a clear wound site. All lesions required a single application and in many instances, multiple lesions were treated with a single sitting.

In the past 2½ years, 250 patients with basal cell and epidermoid carcinomas were cryosurgically treated. The combined total of neoplasms numbered 420. Seven recurrences were noted in 164 patients with a total of 252 tumors during a follow-up period of 1 to 2½ years. This represents a 97.3% cure rate. Recurrences thus far were noted in the earliest patients, where freezing time was between 15 and 60 sec. For the more advanced and larger tumors, a self-pressurizing cryo-surgical instrument has been employed [6]. Liquid nitrogen is directly sprayed onto the larger neoplasms and with thermocouples placed within the tumor mass, temperatures are monitored to assure cryogenic necrosis.

Conclusion. I do not advocate cryosurgery as the single best treatment for cutaneous carcinoma. Each patient and every neoplasm must be evaluated on its own merit. Cryosurgery, however, will offer the cancer therapist another effective modality, with simplicity in technique, least discomfort to the patient and remarkable cosmetic end result.

References. 1. White, A. C.: M. Rec. 56, 109 (1899). — 2. Bowen, J. T., and H. P. Towle: Boston med. surg. J. 157, 561 (1907). — 3. Whitehouse, H. H.: J. Amer. med. Ass. 49, 371 (1907). — 4. Zacarian, S. A., and M. I. Adham: Cryobiology 2, 212 (1966). — 5. Zacarian, S. A., and M. Adham: J. invest. Derm. 48, 7 (1967). — 7. Zacarian, S. A.: Int. J. Surg. 41, (1967).

Topical 5-Fluorouracil — An Effective Agent in the Treatment of Multiple Actinic Keratoses and Some Superficial Malignant Diseases

W. M. Honeycutt, C. J. Dillaha and G. T. Jansen, University of Arkansas Medical Center, Division of Dermatology, Little Rock, Arkansas (USA)

Chronic sun exposure produces many alterations in the skin including actinic keratoses in which early anaplastic and proliferative changes can be seen. When these lesions are distributed over a wide area of the face it is a significant cosmetic defect. More important, however, actinic keratoses have long been associated with progression to a malignant change. The usual means of local destruction for widespread lesions include electrosurgery, cryotherapy and dermabrasive surgery. When scores of lesions are to be treated in an individual, all of these procedures have certain disadvantages. Ideal therapy for such large numbers of lesions would be a treatment which would selectively destroy all of the keratoses in a given area without significant alterations to the normal skin and without undesirable side effects. Our experience with topical 5-fluorouracil (5-FU) leads us to believe that this approach closely approximates such ideal treatment. Other investigators have confirmed this conclusion with reports to us personally.

We previously used 5-FU in 20% and 5% concentrations in a petrolatum vehicle [1, 2], but at the present time a liquid vehicle of propylene glycol is preferred [3]. Its advantages are: 1. greater patient acceptance, 2. a concentration of 1% is effective as opposed to a minimum of 5% in an ointment, 3. a smaller volume of medication is required for a course of therapy, and 4. greater ease of compounding the preparation.

5-FU in a 1% concentration in a vehicle of propylene glycol can be compounded by a pharmacist upon prescription by simply mixing a 10 cc ampule of 5% 5-FU with 40 cc of propylene glycol.

The patient is instructed to apply the medication to his face twice a day, avoiding the eyelids and lips. He may wash and care for his face in the usual way, taking care to have the medication in place most of the time. Selective erythema of the keratoses is expected in 3 to 7 days, which gradually increases until scaling, tenderness, erosion and superficial ulceration occur. Subclinical keratoses, too subtle to detect prior to treatment, will become apparent during this therapy; herein lies one of the major advantages of this treatment.

After a brisk inflammatory reaction has occurred, usually within 7 to 21 days, therapy is discontinued. While the time required to treat the face varies from 7 to 21 days, longer periods of up to 60 days may be required for the hands and forearms.

The erythema subsides in about 2 weeks after discontinuing treatment, and the skin appears smooth and is free of keratoses. There is no alteration in the pigmentation, and no discernable scarring. Thus, the patient's appearance is unaltered except for the absence of the keratoses. A few keratoses may persist and new ones may develop as time passes, but these can be easily handled by conventional means. Retreatment in several years may occasionally be required because of the redevelopment of a large number of keratoses, but this poses no problem and a comparable response can be expected.

A few slides will now be shown to illustrate the effects of topical 5-FU. These demonstrate the appearances of several patients before treatment, at the height of the reaction, and the final result.

The principal undesirable effects are the unsightly appearance of the patient and local discomfort. Sun exposure during the course of therapy may produce a diffuse erythematous phototoxic reaction in actinically damaged areas irrespective of the presence of keratoses. This phototoxic response can be turned to an advantage, however, for it potentiates the selective reaction in the keratoses. We now generally recommend 10 to 15 min of daily sun exposure during treatment.

The topical use of 5-FU as just described is quite safe. No signs or symptoms of systemic toxicity have been noted in hundreds of patients so treated. Experiments in five patients using radioactive 14C-labeled drug indicated that with the 5% ointment, only 6% of the 5-FU was absorbed systemically [2], far below the maximum permissible dosage.

Finally, a word about 5-FU in the treatment of other conditions. Ordinary basal cell and squamous cell carcinomas do not show a predictable response to topical 5-FU and, therefore, it is not recommended in their treatment. However, greater success may be expected in very superficial malignancies such as Bowen's disease, superficial erythematous basal cell epitheliomas and erythroplasia of Queyrat [4].

References. 1. DILLAHA, C. J., G. T. JANSEN, W. M. HONEYCUTT, and A. C. BRADFORD: Arch. Derm. Syph. (Chic.) 88, 247 (1963). — 2. DILLAHA, C. J., G. T. JANSEN, W. M. HONEYCUTT, and G. A. HOLT: Arch. Derm. Syph. (Chic.) 92, 410 (1965). — 3. DILLAHA, C. J., G. T. JANSEN, and W. M. HONEYCUTT: Progr. Dermatol. 1, 1 (1966). — 4. JANSEN, G. T., C. J. DILLAHA, and W. M. HONEYCUTT: Sth. med. J. (Bgham; Ala.) 60, 185 (1967).

Corticosteroids in Dermatology

Les corticostéroïdes en dermatologie

Los corticosteroides en dermatología

Corticosteroide in der Dermatologie

Organizer
G. B. MITCHELL-HEGGS, Great Britain

Presidents
G. ASBOE HANSEN, Denmark
C. NELSON, USA
L. E. PIERINI, Argentina

Delegate of the Organization Committee
J. HÄMEL, Germany

Reports

Corticosteroids in Dermatology

G. Asboe-Hansen, University of Copenhagen, Department of Dermatology, Rigshospital, Copenhagen (Denmark)

The adrenocortical steroids influence most organ functions, because they exert a constant control of the connective tissue as a system. Connective tissues are practically ubiquitous, and they participate in all vital processes of the body. It is impossible to discuss the pathogenesis of any disease without considering the role of the connective-tissue elements.

The skin is a mesenchymal organ covered by the ectodermal epidermis.

It is an almost exciting fact that each component of the skin and the physio-logical processes taking place there is subject to a steady control by various hormones. They may be stimulated or inhibited by administration of hormone preparations produced by the drug industry and placed at disposal of all medical people. These people, while observing favourable effects on a disease, will immediately have to do with side-effects that are untoward but inevitable. This is true because all elements of healthy as well as diseased skin are involved, and because mostly the treatment depends on a pharmacodynamic effect on the tissues rather than substitution therapy of a hormone deficiency.

The *epidermis* has no vessels. It is dependent on nutrition from the underlying connective tissue, the dermis. It is natural only that the epidermis is influenced indirectly by hormones, among others the adrenocortical steroids. This indirect effect is manifested in changes in the growth of hairs and nails, keratinization, pigmentation, function of sebaceous and sweat glands, etc. Very often disorders of connective tissue are reflected in epidermal changes, as in myxedema or sclero-derma. On the other hand, *the dermal and subcutaneous connective tissue connects* the skin organ to all the mesenchymal system. We know skin diseases that simul-taneously involve disorders of joints, eyes, blood, bones, etc.

When the question is of hormone effect on tissue, the cells must be regarded primarily. This is true even of the dermis, that is relatively poor of cells, because the cells are the manufacturers of the extracellular substance that is ample and has an important physiologic and pathophysiologic role. In fibrillar connective tissue there are, as normal inhabitants, fibroblasts, mast cells and histiocytes.

Fibroblasts synthesize collagen. Once laid down in the insoluble form, this substance has a very long biological life-time. It is an almost inert substance. Fibroblasts are influenced by glucocorticoids. Several authors have observed an inhibition of the outgrowth and migration of fibroblasts in tissue culture. Cyto-plasmic vacuoles have been observed, but many have not been able to find changes in the mitotic rate. Collagen synthesis is inhibited by cortisol. Wound healing is restricted as one of the results.

The *mast cells* are responsible for the production of important ground substance components. They synthesize and release the *acid mucopolysaccharides* hyaluronic acid, chondroitin sulfuric acids, and heparin. Besides, they produce histamine.

Glucocorticoids inhibit the synthetic activity of the mast cells. They do not release their granules, or granules may lack entirely. The granules may also form aggregates, or their stainability may change. Acid mucopolysaccharide formation stops or is inhibited, and so is histamine synthesis. These effects are reflected in clinical medicine.

When *histamine* is released, a tissue edema is formed. The increased water content in the tissue brings about degranulation of mast cells with release of acid mucopolysaccharides that bind the extracellular water. This may be a rapid process. The degranulation may also be primary. The acid mucopolysaccharide hyaluronic acid has a strong water-binding capacity. A hydrated gel or a ground substance is formed. Hyaluronic acid has a quick turnover. Within 24 h it is broken down.

If the tissues are under steroid influence, resynthesis of acid mucopolysaccharides is inhibited. It means that an edema disappears. Urticaria or Quincke edema subsides, pemphigus blisters dry, inflammatory swelling in joint capsules or in other locations disappears, wound healing is retarded. One has an explanation of the prompt effect on a disease process. This effect can not be mediated only by a repression of antibody formation.

The activity of tissue *macrophages* is altered. Phagocytosis and intracellular digestion of bacteria are inhibited. After blocking, regeneration of the reticulo-endothelial system is prevented. The concourse of macrophages to an inflammatory area is also restricted.

The effect on lymphocytes, eosinophils, basophils and neutrophils is partially known.

Glucocorticoids increase the *spreading* in skin, and inhibit the spreading activity of hyaluronidase. This effect is complex. Cortisol and similar hormones have a capillary-tightening effect and a vascular constriction comes about. The hyaluronate of the ground substance is changed from a viscous mass to a watery fluid. Particulate matter, bacteria, fluids *e.g.* toxins are allowed to spread easier in the skin. On the other hand, when hyaluronic acid is reduced or depolymerized, the effect of hyaluronidase is logically inhibited.

Similar changes take place in bacterial *infection*. Streptococci and some others produce hyaluronidase, a "spreading factor". Steroids break down the tissue resistance. I am thinking particularly of the viscous ground substance. Invasion is allowed. Simultaneously, however, the attack is weakened. Bacterial, mycotic and viral infection is facilitated, while inflammation, the tissue reaction against infection, is inhibited.

Glucocorticoids display an anti-inflammatory effect. Any change in connective tissue will necessarily change *inflammation* and the balance between the noxious agent and the host. Steroid treatment changes the battle field. This may change the outcome of the battle. Cortisol inhibits exudation and prevents or removes edema. Fibrin becomes less, and the accumulation of phagocytizing granulocytes and macrophages does not come about. Blood flow through the inflamed area is reduced and so is the formation of granulation tissue.

Glucocorticoids exert a distinct effect upon the development and spreading of *tumors* both of which are depending on the present condition of the connective-tissue stroma. It is but natural, therefore, that steroids influence tumors of epidermal as well as dermal origin. Most experimentation has been carried out on animals.

In the dermal connective tissue of precancerous papillomas due to painting of mouse skin with the carcinogenic hydrocarbon 9,10-dimethyl-1,2-benzanthracene a tremendous accumulation of mast cells occurs. Cortisone inhibits the functions and the morphology of mast cells. Cortisone also inhibits the development and growth of papillomas, and cortisol injected in the stroma of the papillomas may bring about a complete regression. Carcinomas also regress, but only for a short time. Thereafter they resume growth and finally kill the animal.

Heterologous and homologous *transplantation* of tumors is facilitated by cortisone treatment of the host. This phenomenon is possibly due to an inhibition of antibody formation, possibly also a direct effect on the tissues, and probably both.

Healing of wounds and bone-fractures are inhibited by steroids. This is immediately understood considering the fact that the healing depends on new-formation of connective tissue, *i.e.* formation of ground substance and fibrils, and epithelization when the conditions of the connective tissue are ideal. Wound healing needs supply of proteins, carbohydrate, ascorbic acid, etc. In man, the inhibition is strongest the first 2 or 3 weeks after start of treatment. However, any clinician knows the Cushing patient or the lupus erythematosus patient on steroids, whose traumatic wounds will not heal.

Keloids will flatten and subside after local injection of cortisol. Contractions and fibroses may loosen or weaken, not because of a break-down of collagen, but because the ground substance becomes less viscous and allows the fibres to move in relation to each other.

What has been mentioned are just examples, of course, examples from daily life. To-day *Cushing's syndrome* is no rarity. In hypercorticism there is deposition of fat at the cost of mucin. All connective tissue is scarce as a result of an anti-anabolic effect. The skin is so thin that the dermal and subcutaneous vessels become visible. Hypertrichosis is possibly produced by an influence of the steroid on the hair sheaths. Striae distensae, often seen on the abdomen, hips and shoulders are due to a reduction of the tensile strength and elasticity of the skin. A similar effect on the connective tissue of the vascular walls produces vascular dilatation, rupture of vessels, and hemorrhage. These hemorrhages may be produced by minor trauma, but also by an accompanying hypertension. Spontaneous fractures are part of the syndrome. Collagen formation is stopped or retarded, and there may be negative calcium-, phosphorus-, and nitrogen balance. Healing of bone fractures is retarded like healing of all wounds. The resistance to infections is broken down. Phagocytosis and antibody-production are inhibited.

Here is the clinical picture of the effect of adrenal cortical steroids on the skin. To-day we recognize a considerable part of the mechanism behind the development of the symptoms.

I have presented the tissue effects. There are, however, other effects, which are quite as interesting and important. It must be clear that the adrenals play an important role in the physiological control of the skin organs as one link in a long chain of regulating effects.

Indications de la corticothérapie en dermatologie

S. LONGHIN, Deuxième Clinique Dermatologique de Bucarest (Roumanie)

Le rapport qui m'a été confié, concernant la corticothérapie en dermatologie, vient remettre en discussion un problème amplement débattu depuis la découverte de la cortisone par HENCH et KENDALL (1949). Ceci surtout par le fait que l'introduction de nouveaux corticoïdes synthétiques, plus puissants mais non dépourvus de risques, posent de nouvelles indications.

La large utilisation des corticoïdes s'explique par le fait que ces produits, intervenant dans les mécanismes physiopathologiques et corrigeant le déséquilibre et les perturbations fonctionnelles, rétablissent les réactions de défense de l'organisme. Ceci explique les effets favorables obtenus dans une série d'affections, les unes assez disparates, et dans lesquelles les médications conventionnelles n'ont pas donné de résultats. Grâce à leur action encore imparfaitement connue, les corticoïdes ont réussi à sauver, ou du moins à prolonger la vie des malades dans toute une série d'affections de cause inconnue. En outre ces produits se sont révélés d'une efficacité exceptionnelle même dans des maladies où la cause initiale était inconnue, mais où, soit qu'il n'y avait pas de traitement spécifique, soit dans les cas où il y en avait un, celui-ci ne parvenait pas à résoudre le problème, à cause du manque de réactivité de l'organisme. Par suite des modifications des réactions de défense de l'organisme, on est arrivé à mettre sur un plan plus important le conflit biologique de la maladie en tant qu'entité, ce qui a fait diminuer l'intérêt concernant l'étiologie.

La corticothérapie garde l'indication d'une thérapie non spécifique, bien entendu la plus importante à l'heure actuelle, car grâce à elle on a réussi à triompher de maladies jadis fatales.

Les indications de la corticothérapie en dermatologie ont été élaborées par de très nombreux auteurs, parmi lesquels nous mentionnons: BAER, BRAUN-FALCO, BRUNNI, CERUTTI, CIAULA, COSTELO, DEGOS, DUPERRAT, DOUGHERTY, E. L. DUBOIS, R. DUMITRIU, FITZPATRICK, GOLDMAN, GOERZ, GRACIANSKY, GREITHER, GRUPPER, JADASSOHN, LEVER, LIVINGOOD, MENKIN, MIDANA, RIMBAUD, SANDERS, SULZBERGER, SOUGHTON, TOURAINE, WEIRICH etc.

Dans le présent exposé, qui est en grande partie en accord avec l'abondante documentation de la littérature, et à la suite de l'expérience personnelle, je montrerai brièvement les indications principales de la corticothérapie en rapport avec leurs effets secondaires, avec leur voie d'administration et avec les indications dermatologiques.

Leur utilisation en thérapeutique est conditionnée par l'action physiologique et par celle pharmacodynamique, en rapport avec l'état morbide, avec la constitution et l'état physiologique du malade, ainsi que par ses contre indications.

Corticostéroïdes par voie buccale

La cortisone est indiquée dans l'insuffisance surrénale lente et aiguë. Dans les états de choc on l'administre par voie parentérale, et quoiqu'elle soit très efficace, on l'utilise moins ces temps-ci. L'Hydrocortisone a les mêmes indications que la cortisone, de plus elle peut être appliquée localement; en outre, elle est mieux tolérée. La Prednisone et la Prednisolone sont quatre fois plus actives que les corticoïdes dont elles sont dérivées. Elles ont les mêmes indications que celles-ci, sauf en cas d'insuffisance surrénale, à cause de la diminution de l'effet de rétention sodique, motif pour lequel elles sont employées dans les états oedémateux et même en cas d'hypertension artérielle. La Méthylprednisolone, 15 à 20 fois plus active que le Prednisolone, ne présente pas d'autres avantages, sauf qu'elle peut être recommandée aux malades déprimés. La Triamcinolone a environ la même action que la Méthylprednisolone; on peut la prescrire en cas d'hypertension artérielle et d'obésité, chez les malades avec troubles gastriques ou excités. Ce produit a une action spéciale dans les syndromes cutanés (SOUGHTON). La Dexaméthasone, qui est six à sept fois plus active que la Prednisone, est prescrite chez les malades mal nourris, chez les diabétiques, mais non chez les personnes âgées. On évitera les doses élevées, parce que ce produit a une grande action de freinage de la production de l'A.C.T.H. La Bétaméthasone, huit fois plus active que la Prednisolone, peut être administrée aux malades hypersensitifs, avec syndromes oedémateux, néphroses ou cirrhoses hépatiques. La Paraméthasone, qui est deux fois et demi moins active que la Prednisone, est indiquée chez les malades avec insuffisance cardiaque, rétention hydrique ou pour cures prolongées. La Fluorprednisolone, trois fois moins active que la Prednisone, ne présente pas d'avantages sur celle-ci. La Fluorcortisone n'est employée que comme traitement supplémentaire à l'Hydrocortisone dans la maladie d'Addison. La Dexaméthasone et la Prednisone, sous forme de combinaisons de corticoïdes oraux, sont très actives et bien tolérées.

Corticostéroïdes injectés par voie intraveineuse

L'Hydrocortisone est le produit le plus indiqué en cas d'insuffisance surrénale, absolue ou relative. Les corticoïdes en injections intraveineuses ou intramusculaires sont indiqués pour leur action rapide. Ainsi nous avons l'Hydrocortisone sodium succinate ou l'Hydrocortisone phosphate. La Prednisolone sodium succinate et la Prednisolone phosphate sont similaires avec l'Hydrocortisone sodium succinate, mais ne sont pas indiquées dans l'insuffisance surrénale; ces produits sont utilisés quand les corticoïdes ne peuvent être pris par voie buccale.

Les corticoïdes pour injections intramusculaires, sont insolubles. Ils sont absorbés et éliminés lentement. La Cortisone acétate en suspension aqueuse est prescrite surtoute dans l'insuffisance de la glande surrénale. La Méthylprednisolone acétate est utilisée comme antiinflammatoire par voie générale.

Les corticoïdes pour emploi local en injections intralésionnelles dont: l'Hydrocortisone acétate, l'Hydrocortisone tertiaire butyl-acétate, la Prednisolone acétate en suspension aqueuse, la Prednisolone butyl tertiaire acétate. Il y a aussi des combinaisons de corticoïdes solubles et insolubles sous forme d'acétate de bétaméthasone et de Bétaméthasone disodium phosphate.

Les corticoïdes pour emploi externe sont des corticoïdes qu'on administre par voie générale (sauf la cortisone), ainsi que les corticoïdes externes spécifiques, qui s'administrent seulement par voie externe, incorporés dans différents véhicules. Ils ont une très grande action antiinflammatoire; cependant les plus actifs sont ceux mono et difluorés. L'ACTH a les mêmes indications que les corticostéroïdes, sauf dans les cas d'insuffisance surrénale.

Indications dermatologiques des corticoïdes administrés par voie générale

Il faut premièrement établir une différence entre les maladies graves, fatales, où le traitement est absolument nécessaire et où il nécessite de longues cures, et les maladies qui ne sont pas fatales, et dans lesquelles l'administration des corticostéroïdes pendant une période plus longue peut provoquer des accidents plus graves que la maladie même pour laquelle on a institué la corticothérapie.

Si dans la première catégorie d'affections la question de la limitation de la corticothérapie ne se pose pas, le problème change d'aspect pour les maladies de la seconde catégorie, où l'administration des corticoïdes doit être faite après avoir attentivement considéré les avantages et les risques.

Dans la catégorie des maladies avec indications absolues, dans lesquelles le traitement doit être intense et continu, nous comprenons: le pemphigus, sous toutes ses formes, le lupus érythémateux systémique aigu et sous-aigu, la dermatomyosite aiguë, la périartérite noueuse, certaines érythrodermies graves, les réticuloses, la mycosis fongoïde.

Nous avons employé d'emblée dans le pemphigus des doses élevées, mais jamais aussi fortes que celles indiquées par LEVER. Si au cours du traitement survenaient de nouvelles poussées, qui n'étaient pas améliorées par une dose augmentée, le produit était changé. Nous avons surtout employé la Triamcinolone, la Bétaméthasone et la Paraméthasone.

Dans le lupus érythémateux systémique aigu avec lésions viscérales, nous avons institué d'emblée un traitement intense, le dosage étant conditionné par les atteintes viscérales, surtout par les lésions rénales. Le corticoïde le plus efficace s'est révélé la Triamcinolone. Quand la symptomatologie s'améliorait, nous ajoutions aussi des antipaludiques de synthèse. Nous avons obtenu des résultats meilleurs avec du chlorhydrate de mépacrine et du phosphate de chloroquine. La Triamcinolone était administrée tous les 2 à 3 jours. Dans l'intervalle, en associant de l'acide acétylsalicylique, on réussissait parfois à maintenir la disparition des phénomènes cliniques et même des signes biologiques, tout en poursuivant le traitement avec les antipaludiques. Les cas avec des lésions rénales avancées et anciennes n'ont pas bénéficié du traitement.

Dans la dermatomyosite, la plupart des auteurs recommandent la cortico-thérapie dans la phase aiguë. Bien souvent nous n'avons pas eu besoin d'y recourir, obtenant de bons résultats avec une autre médication.

Dans la périartérite noueuse, les corticostéroïdes ont modifié les manifestations cliniques de la maladie et la durée moyenne de la vie des malades, étant surtout utiles dans la période où la maladie devient aiguë.

Dans la sclérodermie progressive, les corticostéroïdes peuvent être utiles dans la première phase de la maladie; dans celle tardive, ils peuvent être même nocifs. Dans les formes avancées, nous avons employé des perfusions avec de l'A.C.T.H. naturel ou synthétique, avec de légères améliorations.

Les érythrodermies, soit primitives, telles que celles médicamenteuses ou streptococciques, soit secondaires à d'autres maladies, comme le psoriasis, le lichen plan, etc., bénéficient du traitement avec les corticostéroïdes. La seule recommandation est de ne pas faire des cures prolongées, parce que les récidives sont plus rebelles au traitement. De plus, pour les érythrodermies des femmes enceintes, même si on utilise les corticoïdes, il ne faut pas les administrer pas voie intraveineuse.

Dans le cas des érythrodermies infectieuses, on y associe l'antibiothérapie. Dans le syndrome de Lyell, accompagné de collapse périphérique, on recommande l'administration d'Hydrocortisone par voie intra-veineuse. Dans les formes d'érythrodermies au cours des hématodermies, le traitement corticothérapique favorise l'action des cytostatiques ou de la roentgenthérapie. Dans la maladie de Dühring, une corticothérapie prolongée la rend corticodépendante. C'est pourquoi nous n'y avons eu recours que dans les cas où les autres médicaments ne l'in-fluençaient pas, ou dans la période des poussées accentuées. Dans le lichen plan généralisé, les corticoïdes peuvent être utiles quand l'affection évolue lentement et est très prurigineuse. Dans l'érythème polymorphe Stevens-Johnson, les corticoïdes sont très utiles. Dans le psoriasis, la corticothérapie n'a une action favorable que dans la forme érythrodermique, dans le psoriasis pustuleux et dans la forme arthropatique. Dans cette dernière, l'A.C.T.H. en perfusion peut être efficace. Dans l'eczéma aigu la corticothérapie est recommandable en cures courtes quand celui-ci est exsudatif et étendu. Dans l'eczéma chronique, ainsi que dans la dermatite atopique des adultes, celle-ci n'est indiquée que dans les cas où l'affec-tion devient aiguë, ou quand elle est trop prurigineuse; bien entendu, ces cures doivent être courtes. Dans la dermatite atopique des enfants, la thérapie générale doit être évitée; elle n'y trouve son utilité que dans les formes érythrodermiques. Dans la dermatite actinique, dans les dermatites médicamenteuses, avec des formes plus étendues et plus sévères, les cures courtes peuvent amener des amélio-rations spectaculaires. Dans le choc anaphylactique, traumatique, brûlures, pénicillinique, quand celui-ci est accompagné de collapse périphérique, on préfère l'Hydrocortisone par voie intraveineuse, ou la Bétaméthasone par voie intra-musculaire.

La maladie du sérum répond bien au traitement avec des dérivés stéroïdes. Dans l'urticaire ou dans l'oedème de Quincke, accompagnés de l'oedème de la glotte, les dérivés stéroïdes sont indiqués dans les traitements d'urgence.

Quant à l'urticaire chronique rebelle au traitement, l'ACTH retard administré en trois à quatre injections tous les 4 à 5 jours au cours du traitement de désensibili-sation, peut être utile. Dans la sarcoïdose, les corticostéroïdes sont recommandables sauf la Dexaméthasone. Dans les hématodermies, la maladie de Kaposi, les corticostéroïdes sont d'une aide précieuse.

Les tuberculoses cutanées vraies ou les tuberculides guérissent plus rapidement en les associant aux antibiotiques contre le bacille de Koch. Dans l'oedème chronique streptococcique, la corticothérapie est très utile si on l'ajoute aux traitements antimicrobiens. Dans le zona zoster, quoique certains auteurs s'y opposent, nous l'avons employée avec succès pour calmer les douleurs. Dans le herpès chronique récidivant, il y a des auteurs qui ont signalé des résultats favorables. Nous ne l'avons pas employée. Dans la pelade, on a obtenu la repousse des cheveux, souvent temporaire, mais parfois accompagnée d'accidents sévères, quand on a employé des doses élevées. Nous avons prescrit la Triamcinolone en doses de 4 mg par jour, pour des cures de 20 jours, avec une pause de 20 jours. Nous n'avons pas eu d'accidents, et les guérisons se sont maintenues dans la plupart des cas.

Les indications de la corticothérapie intralésionnelle

Les corticoïdes injectables ont donné des résultats satisfaisants dans les chéloïdes récentes, dans le lichen corneux ou obtus localisé, dans le lupus érythémateux discoïde, dans certaines plaques de psoriasis, dans les névrodermites, les kystes sébacés, l'acné conglobata. Les indurations plastiques des corps caverneux bénéficient rarement de ce traitement. Dans les plaques de pelade, la corticothérapie intralésionnelle peut produire, outre les accidents oculaires, des atrophies cicatricielles; c'est pourquoi nous ne l'appliquons pas.

Les indications de la corticothérapie topique

Outre la cortisone, tous les corticostéroïdes employés par voie générale, nonfluorés ou monofluorés, aussi bien que ceux difluorés (corticoïdes externes spécifiques), ont une action thérapeutique topique dans la majorité des processus inflammatoires, tels que l'eczéma, les névrodermites, le granulome annulaire, l'amyloïdose cutanée, etc. Dans le lupus érythémateux discoïde, dans le psoriasis sont actifs: la Fluorcinolone, la Fluorcortène, la 17 valérate de bétaméthasone, la Fluorméthasone pyvalante, la Fluorométhalone. La Triamcinolone et le phosphate de bétaméthasone sont actifs dans le psoriasis, mais pas dans le lupus érythémateux. La Dexaméthasone, la Prednisone, la Prednisolone et l'hydrocortisone ne sont pas actives dans le psoriasis ou dans le lupus érythémateux. Le succès thérapeutique est dû en grande partie au véhicule adéquat au stade du syndrome inflammatoire. Dans les formes chroniques sèches, le pansement occlusif a permis des résultats supérieurs. Leur association avec des antibiotiques et des antifongiques permet leur emploi dans les dermites microbiennes et mycotiques. La thérapie locale est encore plus efficiente quand on ajoute des substances chimiques actives. La corticothérapie locale est comparable à celle générale du point de vue du progrès du traitement.

Dans ce court exposé je n'ai fait que remettre en question quelques problèmes liés aux indications de la corticothérapie, qui a pris une telle ampleur dans la thérapeutique dermatologique.

Les observations des cliniciens pourront aider les chimistes à synthétiser de nouveaux corticoïdes avec des effets secondaires de plus en plus réduits, par rapport à leur efficacité.

The many "Facies" of Iatrogenic Hypercorticism

A. C. Curtis and G. L. Stoker, Department of Dermatology, University Hospital Ann Arbor, Michigan (USA)

Dermatologists the world over are often criticized by their medical colleagues for their injudicious use of systemic corticosteroids. Many of these instances, however, are related to the short term, or "burst", type therapy in which the risk of complication is minimized. The need for reducing the adverse reactions to prolonged therapy has stimulated investigators to develop new treatment programs. Intermittent regimens have been proposed to provide equal effectiveness but reduced adrenal suppression [1]. Long-lasting intramuscular preparations, as reported by Scher [2], were received with enthusiasm and are currently being used on a universal scale. For the most part, the mode of administration of the steroid relates only to variations in adversity of reaction; namely, time of onset, duration, and severity, rather than to its absence or presence. Therefore, dermatologists need to be acutely aware of the many "facies" of hypercorticism and the treatment trends used by other specialists who employ these agents routinely.

The main groups of natural occurring adrenal corticoids are the glucocorticoids, the mineralocorticoids, and the androgens. The former group of compounds is the one administered in therapeutic dosages for its ability to suppress the immunological mechanisms of defense. Unfortunately, these same compounds may adversely influence protein, carbohydrate, and lipid metabolism, including bone structure. Also they may have a suppressive effect upon the adrenal-pituitary axis. The newer synthetic steroids seem to induce less sodium and water retention and less potassium depletion. Thusly, marked electrolyte imbalance with associated edema, hypotension, cardiac irregularity, etc., is noted less often than with the use of cortisone and cortisol.

Marks et al. [3] investigated the effects of a 5-week course of prednisone therapy in a patient with prostatic carcinoma. They concluded that 20 mgm of prednisone daily for 10 to 14 days was sufficient to moderately reduce the capacity of the adrenal cortex to respond to either ACTH or to the trauma of a surgical procedure. They further evidenced that after 5 weeks of therapy in the same patients, the adrenal output of 17-hydroxy-corticosteroide was negligible even when stimulated with ACTH or by an induced stress. In most individuals the response to stress is restored as the normal pituitary-adrenal mechanism adapts. Evidence of adrenal insufficiency manifested by weakness, malaise, nausea, diarrhea, and hypotension may be noted when the adrenals fail to respond to pituitary stimulation or when steroids directly inhibit the release of ACTH from the pituitary or block the secretion of CRF from the hypothalamus. Complete suppression with cortical atrophy may occur when administration is both prolonged and supraphysiological.

The anti-anabolic action of the glucocorticoids seems predominantly to involve lymphoid, muscular, osseous and connective tissue proteins, leading to a loss of mass of these body constituents. The influence upon lipid metabolism is not well understood but may represent an increased conversion of glucose to fat.

The above metabolic changes may lead to undesirable effects of both minor and major importance. Hypertrichosis, acne, development of striae, atrophy of skin, hemorrhage, redistribution of fat, hypertension, and mental aberrations are reported as evidence of hypercorticism. Menstrual irregularities are commonplace, and patients may complain of alteration and even cessation of flow during periods of steroid usage. Osteoporotic activity may lead to compression fractures of the vertebral column, resulting in back pain and marked loss of stature.

The slow, insidious onset of hip or shoulder pain may be an early sign of degenerative joint disease. No consistent pathogenic relationship has been demonstrated to explain this difficulty, but the association of osseous necrosis and vascular disruption, especially of [4, 5] the femoral head is too frequent to dismiss as purely coincidental.

Hyperglycemia and glycosuria may be noted resulting from a gluconeogenic process. Precipitation of diabetes mellitus or intensification of the diabetic state associated with these changes may require greatly increased amounts of insulin if occurring in types other than maturity-onset diabetes. Glucose tolerance tests which are in the abnormal range can be useful guide lines in directing either treatment or prophylaxis to the latent or the known diabetic-steroid induced or otherwise.

It is often difficult to assess the role of steroids in increasing human susceptibility to infection. Many of the diseases which respond favorably to steroid therapy are related, in themselves, to a higher-than-normal incidence of infection. Much of the early work on the relationship of steroid therapy to infection was done under conditions utilizing high doses of steroids, which often were administered concomitantly with other immuno-suppressive agents.

CASAZZA et al. [6] attempted to establish a relationship between the occurrence of infection and the presence of active lymphomatous disease. They considered the possible influence of radiation therapy, chemotherapy, and corticosteroid therapy on the clinical course of various types of lymphomas. Quarterly case reviews provided tabulated data on the number of infected cases. There was an increased incidence of infection in the terminal stage of disease for all of the lymphomas studied, but the survival curves for infected and non-infected patients were basically the same.

Fungal organisms represent a large portion of the opportunistic invaders. Cases of nocardiosis, aspergillosis, cryptococcosis, mucormycosis, and many others have been reported in increasing numbers. Reactivation of blastomycotic, coccidioidomycotic, and histoplasmotic disease states has been noted and may be related to the depression of a factor responsible for encompassing the infectious process.

Candida albicans has been reported as causing septicemia, endocarditis, perforation of the stomach, formation of renal abscesses, complications in chronic lung disease, and more commonly as producing resistant skin conditions. The dermatophytes, too, are especially difficult to control when found producing disease in patients on high and prolonged steroid schedules.

Bacterial infections are difficult to evaluate in patients on corticosteroids because of the relative frequency of infection in the "non-diseased" population. Reactivation of latent tuberculosis is always feared and can be minimized by obtaining pre-steroid therapy skin tests and chest x-rays. Concomitant use of INH and PAS in persons with positive skin tests is felt by most clinicians to represent the necessary precautionary measures [7]. Septicemia, pneumonitis, enteritis, arthritis, acute glomerulonephritis, etc., have all been reported in association with steroid treated patients, but the exact relationship is difficult to define.

Dissemination of the herpes zoster-varicella virus has been demonstrated by RADO et al. [8] in two cases of a house epidemic involving a total of six patients. ELLIOTT [9], however, used high dosages of prednisone in 15 cases of herpes zoster for a period of 3 weeks to reduce postherpetic neuralgia, and reported no cases of generalized disease. Herpes simplex may become generalized but the incidents reported are largely in persons with an underlying lymphomatous process [10].

CROMPTON and TEARE [11] reported on two cases of acute fatal necrotizing encephalitis which were though to be secondary to the herpes simplex virus and precipitated by the sudden reduction of steroids from a therapeutic to a maintenance dosage.

Abdominal distress related to increased gastric acid and pepsin secretion is well documented. The production and aggravation of peptic ulcer disease has led to fatal hemorrhaging. Acute pancreatitis, which clinically may resemble ulcer disease, also has been reported [12]. Prophylaxis with ulcer bland diets, antacids, and anticholinergic agents has been rewarding.

KLINEBERG and MILLER [13] reported on the possibility of inducing salicylate intoxication in patients receiving both steroids and salicylates. They postulated that the corticosteroids may increase glomerular filtration rate, decrease renal tubular absorption of water, and thus increase the urinary flow and the accompanying salicylate load. In their case, the administration of a constant dosage of salicylates with a tapering dosage of steroids lead to a significant rise in the serum salicylate levels and to intoxication in one instance.

A pseudotumoral syndrome related to intracranial hypertension has been reported in children on prolonged steroid therapy. One or more of the usually ominous signs of headache, ataxia, nausea, vomiting, and the presence of papilledema may occur in cases where steroids are slowly being withdrawn or changed. WALKER and ADAMKIEWICZ [14] related the mechanism of action to that of adrenal cortial suppression because of the similarity of symptoms noted in a few patients with Addison's disease prior to treatment with adrenal corticoids.

There are numerous reports of the association of posterior subcapsular cataracts in patients with rheumatoid arthritis on varying schedules of steroid preparations [15]. Disagreement with the above correlations has been expressed by LEY et al. [16], but further substantiation or denial is forthcoming.

A post-steroid panniculitis presenting with subcutaneous nodules over the cheeks, trunk, and arms has been reported in children undergoing a slow withdrawal of prednisone therapy [17]. Histologically the panniculitis may differ from that of erythema nodosum by the absence of an inflammatory infiltrate about the interlobular septa and veins.

Another difficult management problem is that of a generalized exfoliative psoriasis which may have been triggered by a pre-surgical steroid preparation. We have found methotrexate to be very beneficial in treating these severe psoriatics.

Undoubtedly, numerous other complications arising from prolonged steroid therapy have gone unrecognized. We hope that this presentation will stimulate all clinicians to search for and minimize unnecessary adverse reactions to the oft-used corticosteroids.

References. 1. HARTER, J. G., W. J. REDDY, and G. W. THORN: New Engl. J. Med. 269, 591 (1963). — 2. SCHER, R. K.: J. Amer. Geriat. Soc. 12, 328 (1964). — 3. MARKS, L. J., R. CHUTE, and R. L. SALLADE: New Engl. J. Med. 264, 10 (1961). — 4. SUTTON, R. D., T. G. BENEDECK, and G. A. EDWARDS:: Arch. intern. Med. 112, 594 (1963). — 5. ZOK, S. B. M.: J. Amer. med. Ass. 184, 265 (1963). — 6. CASAZZA, A. R., CH. B. DUVALL, and P. P. CARGONE: J. Amer. med. Ass. 197, 710 (1966). — 7. MEADOR, R. S.: P. Grad. Med. 31, 178 (1962). — 8. RADO, J. P., J. TAKO, L. GEDER, and E. JENEY: Arch. intern. Med. 116, 329 (1965). — 9. ELLIOT, F. A.: Lancet 1964, II, 610. — 10. Editorial J. Amer. med. Ass. 188, 749) 1964). — 11. CROMPTON, M. R., and R. D. TEARE: Lancet 1965, II, 1318. — 12. SCHRIER, R. W., and R. J. BULGER: J. Amer. med. Ass. 194, 564 (1965). — 13. KLINENBERG, J. R., and F. MILLER: J. Amer. med. Ass. 194, 601 (1965). — 14. WALKER. A. E., and J. J. ADAMKIEWICZ: J. Amer. med. Ass. 188, 779 (1964). — 15. GILES, C. L., G. L. MASON, I. E. DUFF, and J. A. McLEAN: J. Amer. med. Ass. 182, 719 (1962). — 16. LEY, A. P., S. BULCANTZ, and C. FALLIERS: J. Amer. med. Ass. 191, 753 (1965). — 17. ROENIGK, jr., H. H., J. R. HASERICK, and F. D. ARUNDELL: Arch. Derm. Syph. (Chic..) 90, 387 (1964).

Les traitements prolongés par les corticostéroïdes (conduite du traitement)

A. Midana, G. Zina et G. Martina, Clinique Dermatologique de l'Université de Turin (Italie)

Il est nécessaire, avant tout, de distinguer les différentes formes morbides où un traitement corticosteroïde prolongé (T.C.P.) peut être envisagé; ces formes peuvent être classées selon le schéma suivant:

a) maladie, où le T.C.P. représente l'unique moyen capable d'arrêter ou de retarder l'évolution mortelle: pemphigus, lupus érythémateux systémique, dermatomyosite, périartérite noueuse.

b) maladie, où le T.C.P. représente un traitement possible, non obligatoire, mais raisonnable, bien que conditionné par l'échec des autres moyens thérapeutiques, dont il peut parfois renforcer l'action ou augmenter la tolérabilité (par ex. antimitotiques, Rx): maladie de Dühring et pemphigoïdes, lupus érythémateux subaigu, érythèmes polymorphes essentiels récidivants, ectodermoses pluriorificielles, érythrodermies chroniques à évolution réticulosique probable, réticuloses et hématodermies, mycosis fongoïdes, etc.

c) maladies, où le traitement T.C.P. est à déconseiller habituellement, souvent dangereux, mais justifié tout de même dans des situations limites particulières, où les doses réduites permettent d'interrompre ou d'éviter de graves conflits ou des frustrations d'ordre psychogène: eczéma diathésique généralisé chez des jeunes gens ou des adultes, psoriasis rebelles avec arthropathies, alopécies en aires malignes, etc.

Dans le premier groupe c'est le pemphigus malin, qui constitue indiscutablement l'indication principale du T.C.P. Dans ces cas il faut entreprendre le traitement, même lorsque de graves contre-indications pathologiques existent (ulcère gastro-duodénal, hypertension, diabète, etc.).

Le choix du corticostéroïde (C) d'attaque n'a aucune importance pratique et la voie d'administration peut être variée en fonction de la situation physiopathologique particulière du malade (nous préférons associer deux ou plusieurs préparations par diverses voies, tout en considérant la voie buccale la plus active et la plus rapide).

La dose d'attaque doit être élevée rapidement, en peu de jours, à des dosages massifs ou héroïques en fonction de la réponse (80 à 200 mg équivalents de δ-cortisone).

L'effet morbistatique — constatable, dans le pemphigus, pour l'arrêt des poussées bulleuses et pour la réparation rapide des lésions cutanées, est atteint le plus tôt possible. Il faut continuer ces doses jusqu'à une stabilisation certaine: dans le pemphigus, à la réparation des lésions muqueuses éventuelles.

La réduction des doses ensuite doit être lente et circonspecte: il ne faut pas se laisser influencer par le décours favorable ni par l'apparition d'effets collatéraux ou de complications même graves. Si la dose de maintien se réalise avec la lenteur nécessaire (dans le pemphigus, même après 5 à 6 mois ou plus), elle peut être faible (5 à 10 mg par jour de δ-cortisone) et peut être continuée indéfiniment.

La réduction précoce du dosage représente un grave danger: les récidives peuvent exiger des doses plus élevées ou même devenir résistantes; il convient, surtout au cours de cette phase, alterner les produits corticoïdes; à ce propos, un choix de corticostéroïde en fonction de la maladie ne nous paraît pas pouvoir être envisagé; ce choix est déterminé plutôt, surtout dans la phase de maintien, en fonction de la sensibilité élective individuelle: soit rapport à l'effet morbistatique, soit rapport aux effets collatéraux. Ni l'emploi de préparations à absorption parentérale ou buccale lente (du type 6 alpha-méthyl-prednisolone, prednilidène), ni l'administration par dose unique à des intervalles de 48 heures ou plus, ne nous semblent offrir d'avantages substantiels en vue de la réduction des effets secondaires. D'ailleurs les données bibliographiques en dermatologie, en allergologie et en rhumatologie confirment une disparité de vues, qui n'est pas rare, soit à propos des indications thérapeutiques électives, soit des effets indésirés.

Il est évident que, dans les formes à décours favorable comme dans les cas du groupe b et c au cours de la phase de maintien à faible dose, l'évaluation de la situation générale du malade pourra guider le choix du corticostéroïde, en tenant compte de ses activités collatérales, caractéristiques et prédominantes.

Dans les maladies du groupe b, la thérapie corticostéroïde est à mettre en route seulement après l'échec des autres tentatives thérapeutiques: dans la dermatite herpétiforme et dans les pemphigoïdes en général, elle peut résoudre des cas rebelles; dans les réticuloses et les mycoses fongoïdes, il faut la limiter aux phases évolutives, résistantes aux antimitotiques et à la radiothérapie.

Elle peut toutefois être utilement employée, à des doses moyennes ou faibles, pour renforcer l'effet des autres moyens. Les doses d'attaque et celles de maintien sont, en général, relativement faibles (20 à 50 mg et 2,5 à 5 mg) équivalents de δ-cortisone, respectivement dans ce groupe comme dans certaines formes du groupe c; de plus, il faut tenir compte du fait que le traitement corticostéroïde peut être alterné — même pendant des périodes relativement longues — avec des préparations à effet cortisonolike, avec des antiréactionnels.

Dans le groupe c dans lequel, à notre avis, à cause de la rareté des succès thérapeutiques, il faut inclure la sclérodermie diffuse progressive, le traitement c est, en principe, à déconseiller.

Des situations limites peuvent toutefois exister, où la dermatose prive pratiquement le patient de toute forme de vie de relation, ce qui provoque parfois de graves conflits psychiques: dans ces cas, une thérapie corticostéroïde prolongée et circonspecte, maintenue à des doses particulièrement faibles, (2,50 à 10 mg de δ-cortisone, par ex.) permet de réaliser un contrôle de la situation objective afin de rompre le cercle vicieux. Le risque d'effets secondaires possibles, limités dans la plupart des cas, est justifié par le nombre assez grand de succès réalisables.

Il est clair que, dans ces formes, le programme thérapeutique est subordonné à l'examen du malade: les graves maladies en cours (diabète, tubercolose, ulcère gastrique) l'empêchent. Il est opportun en outre de considérer l'importance des activités collatérales particulières du stéroïde (par ex. l'action euphorisante du prednisolone et du désaméthasone et l'action déprimante du triancinolone.

En outre la recherche du schéma chronologique d'administration de médicaments, le meilleur qui s'adonne à chaque malade, est indispensable: un malade adroit réussit à trouver, tout seul, le rythme qui lui convient le mieux. Nous répétons, cependant, que dans ces formes l'indication TCP est exceptionnelle.

Traitement collatéral

A part les médicaments spécifiques pour les différentes formes, médicaments qui peuvent s'alterner avec les stéroïdes ou s'y associer par un mécanisme synergique, parfois particulièrement évident, nous pensons que:

l'emploi de l'ACTH d'extraction est, surtout dans le pemphigus, inutile et souvent dangereux, à cause de son action déclenchante sur la symptomatologie clinique; des essais avec l'ACTH de synthèse, au contraire, nous ont fourni, dans les formes du groupe b et surtout c, des résultats encourageants comme traitement de substitution.

L'administration circonspecte d'anabolisants est utile surtout chez les vieux et les malades en mauvaises conditions; de même l'emploi de préparations myo-neurotoniques est utile.

Dans la phase d'attaque de formes particulièrement graves du groupe a et b, nous considérons indispensable le traitement par phléboclyse avec glucose ou, mieux, avec aminoacides associés avec vitamines à doses élevées.

L'antibiose de couverture est à conseiller en théorie. L'antibiose prolongée, jointe au traitement corticostéroïde, peut provoquer avec grande fréquence l'apparition de mucosites systémiques du tube digestif, qui se compliquent facilement de candidose.

Contrôle

Il est clair que le traitement d'attaque et la phase de réduction doivent être pratiqués sous contrôle hospitalier ou, du moins, médical quotidien, qui doit être complété par une série systématique des examens courants en médecine interne pour la thérapie cortisonique (glycémie, équilibre K/Na sérique et endocellulaire, hématocrite, azotémie, cadre protéique, etc.).

Schädigungen bei lang durchgeführter Steroidtherapie mit besonderer Berücksichtigung der Hypophyse und Nebennierenrinde

F. Földvári, B. Vértes und J. Masszi, Universitäts-Hautklinik Budapest (Ungarn)

Eine allgemein anerkannte Tatsache ist, daß längere Zeit hindurch verab-reichte große Dosen von Steroiden (= ACTH + Glucocorticoide) zu einer funktio-nellen Störung des Hypophyse-Nebennierenrindensystems führen können [1]. Die vollständige Restitution des Systems kann mehrere Monate in Anspruch nehmen [4]. Zuerst erhöht sich der Plasmawert des ACTH und übertrifft sogar den gewohnten Blutspiegel. Erst hiernach kommt es zur Normalisierung der Nebennierenrindenfunktion.

Die auf das Hypothalamus-Hypophyse-Nebennierenrindensystem ausgeübte Wirkung der dauernden Glucocorticoidbehandlung wird verschiedenermaßen erklärt. Manche Autoren betonen das In-das-Blut-gelangen des ACTH [9] bzw. die Verminderung des ACTH-Gehaltes der Hypophyse [5], andere verweisen auf die Atrophie der Nebennierenrinde und deren Funktionsverminderung. Histo-pathologische Veränderungen sind sowohl in der Hypophyse, als auch in der Nebennierenrinde zu beobachten [2, 8].

Über das Verhalten des Hypothalamus-Hypophyse-Nebennierenrindensystems ACTH-Dosierung gegenüber herrscht eine viel weniger einheitliche Auffassung. Während manche Autoren [11, 13] schon nach ACTH-Behandlung von einigen Tagen auf Metopironbelastung verminderte Antwort erhielten, beobachteten an-dere [7] normale Werte auch in Fällen von längere Zeit hindurch verabreichtem ACTH. Bei der direkten ACTH-Bestimmung [6] konnte festgestellt werden, daß bei Ratten nach ACTH-Dosierung sowohl die Produktion des ACTH als auch dessen Entleerung aus der Hypophyse behindert war.

Manche Hautkrankheiten erfordern oft eine langdauernde Steroidbehandlung mit recht großer Gesamtdosis, weshalb einige Autoren die Untersuchung der endokrinen Verhältnisse der auf diese Art behandelten Kranken schon früher für notwendig erachteten [15]. Unsere Untersuchungen bezweckten, diesbezüglich weitere Angaben zu ermitteln und durch diese zu therapeutisch verwendbaren Konklusionen zu gelangen.

Untersuchungsmethoden

Mittels Metopironbelastung wünschten wir Aufschluß über den funktionellen Zustand der Hypophyse zu gewinnen. Bekanntlich behindert das Metopiron auf dem Sterangerüst durch Hemmung der elfer Hydroxillation die Cortison-, bzw. Hydrocortisonbildung [15] (Ciba Symp.). Durch den auf diese Weise künstlich zustande gebrachten Glucocorticoidmangel wird die Hypophyse zu erhöhter Funktion angeregt, was bei pathologischen Zuständen nicht der Fall ist. Der funktionelle Zustand der Nebennierenrinden wurde mit der üblichen ACTH-Belastung untersucht.

Die Kranken erhielten 48 Std hindurch keine Steroide. Am 2. Tag der Pause wurden aus dem 24stündigen Urin mit der Zimmermannschen Methode die 17-Ketosteroide und mit dem Norymberskischen Verfahren die Ketogensteroide bestimmt. Am 3. Tag wurde 40 E ACTH verabreicht und gleichzeitig aus dem 24stündigen Urin neuerlich die 17-Keto-, bzw. die Ketogensteroide bestimmt. Nach einer weiteren Pause von 2 Tagen gaben wir am 6. Tag 3 g Metopiron, wonach am 7. Tag im Urin neuerlich die 17-Keto-, bzw. Ketogensteroide bestimmt wurden. Die Wertung der Funktion stützte sich auf die Ketogen-Steroidbestimmungen. Die Funktionsfähigkeit der Nebennieren hielten wir für normal, wenn auf 40 E ACTH die Ketogen-Steroiderhöhung im Urin 5 mg betrug, für die normale Hypophysenfunktion wurde eine Erhöhung auf 7 mg angesehen.

Die in der Tabelle veranschaulichten Resultate umfassen bei Angabe des Geschlechtes, des Alters, der Krankheit und der erfolgten Behandlungen die experimentellen Data der steroidbehandelten Kranken.

Die von uns untersuchten Personen litten an folgenden Krankheiten: 13 an Pemphigus vulgaris, bzw. seborrhoicus, eine an Dermatitis herpetiformis und je eine an Poikilodermie, Erythrodermie bzw. Erythematodes. Wie bereits erwähnt, stützten wir uns bei der Beurteilung der Hypophysenfunktion auf die 17-KGS-Werte. Belastung mit 40 E ACTH bewirkte, daß sich diese Werte von 17 Fällen bei neun erhöhten, bei drei kaum erhöhten und bei fünf verminderten. Nach Metopirondosierung zeigte sich, daß sich die 17-KGS-Werte bei fünf Fällen erhöhten, bei acht verminderten und bei drei unverändert blieben. Die Verminderung, bzw. das Ausbleiben der Erhöhung zeigte sich mit einer Ausnahme (Fall 5) nach hohen Gesamtdosen in drei Fällen über 10000 mg und in sieben Fällen nach Gesamtdosen von 20 bis 70000 mg. Von den fünf Fällen, in denen Erhöhung auftrat, waren zwei Fälle nicht von Pemphigus. Im dritten Kontrollfall, einem Erythematodes systematicus, war der Wert nicht vermindert, aber auch nicht erhöht.

Die Angaben erweisen, daß bei verhältnismäßig kurze Zeit dauernder Behandlung mit kleinen Dosen sowohl die Hypophyse- als auch die Nebennierenfunktion beibehalten ist. Verschieden große Gesamtdosen können bei beibehaltener Nebennierenrindenfunktion zur Schädigung der Hypophyse führen. Bei mehrere Jahre hindurch mit großen Gesamtdosen Behandelten wird sowohl die Hypophyse als auch die Nebennierenfunktion geschädigt. Unter den untersuchten Kranken beobachteten wir in dieser Hinsicht nur eine Ausnahme (Fall 16). Bei einer Kranken (Fall 17) konnte die Metopirondosierung nicht beendet werden. Bereits am steroidlosen Tag klagte sie über schlechtes Allgemeinbefinden, Appetitlosigkeit, nach 1 g Metopiron trat eine weitere Verschlechterung des Allgemeinbefindens mit Übelkeit, Brechreiz, Erbrechen auf und entwickelte sich ein kollapsartiger Zustand. Das Bild entsprach einer Addison-Krise, die sich auf Di-Adreson F. aquosum allmählich löste. In diesem Fall war die Schädigung der Nebennierenrinde so hochgradig, daß wir die weitere Untersuchung unterließen.

Unsere Ergebnisse bekräftigen jene bekannte Feststellung [10], daß durch den infolge der exogenen Steroide dauernd erhöhten Corticoid-Blutspiegel die Bildung

Tabelle. *Schädigung bei Langzeittherapie mit Steroiden*

Zahl der Fälle	Ge-schlecht	Alter	Diagnose	Dauer der Therapie in Monaten	Prednisolon Gesamtdosis mg	Prednisolon Durchschnittliche Tagesdosis mg	ACTH-bewirkte Veränderungen im Urin 17-KS mg	ACTH-bewirkte Veränderungen im Urin 17-KGS mg	Resultate nach ACTH	Veränderungen nach Metopiron 17-KS mg	Veränderungen nach Metopiron 17-KGS mg	Resultate nach Metopiron
1.	♀	63	Poikiloderma	1	500	10	8,1—16,4	5,7—24,6	+	8,1— 2,6	5,7—21,4	+
2.	♀	31	Pemph. vulg.	6	800	40	10,6— 7,0	9,8—55,6	+	10,6— 2,3	9,8—21,4	+
3.	♀	68	Pemph. seb.	5	1 189	10	2,8— 5,2	4,7—47,3	+	2,8— 3,0	4,7—21,4	+
4.	♀	47	Erythroderma	48	4 701	7	5,0— 7,4	4,6—16,0	+	5,0— 5,3	4,6—45,7	+
5.	♀	61	Pemph. vulg.	1	375	5	10,5—12,3	18,5—52,1	+	10,5— 7,4	18,5—11,0	—
6.	♂	39	Pemph. seb.	24	13 000	30	9,8— 8,7	17,0—23,1	+	9,8—16,8	17,0—11,0	—
7.	♂	37	Dermat. herp.	72	30 000	20	25,0—28,0	15,6—29,0	+	25,0— 9,6	15,6—20,4	—
8.	♀	29	Erythemat. syst.	60	13 000	5	14,9—14,2	25,4—50,8	+	14,9—10,6	25,4—27,4	—
9.	♀	53	Pemph. vulg.	72	21 000	15	8,1— 5,8	37,9—18,7	—	8,1— 2,6	37,9— 8,6	—
10.	♂	61	Pemph. vulg.	96	51 687	10	5,3— 5,9	8,7— 8,6	—	5,3— 6,5	8,7— 3,5	—
11.	♂	69	Pemph. vulg.	3	22 655	15	4,5— 5,0	4,7— 0,9	—	4,2— 5,0	4,2— 1,5	—
12.	♀	57	Pemph. vulg.	24	12 000	20	11,4—13,8	8,6—10,2	—	11,4—13,0	8,6— 3,0	—
13.	♀	22	Pemph. vulg.	48	33 000	40	7,3— 9,8	40,1—29,2	—	7,3—10,4	40,1—22,6	—
14.	♀	55	Pemph. vulg.	48	20 000	15	13,0—15,8	31,0—18,4	—	13,0—11,0	31,0— 2,2	—
15.	♂	65	Pemph. vulg.	48	20 500	30	13,0—18,6	18,0—17,0	—	13,0—11,5	18,0—20,0	—
16.	♂	55	Pemph. vulg.	84	40 000	40	21,2— 2,0	19,0—33,4	+	21,2— 8,0	19,0—41,5	+
17.	♀	53	Pemph. vulg.	7	37 610	15	4,5— 6,5	30,5—35,0	—	Die Untersuchung unterbrochen (Zur Addison-Krise ähnlicher Zustand)		—

Bemerkung: + = normale Funktion, — = beschädigte Funktion

10*

bzw. Mobilisation des Corticotropins behindert wird. So kommt es zu einer konsekutiven Schädigung sowohl der Hypophyse als auch der Nebennierenrinde. Im Verlauf längerer Glucocorticoidbehandlung läßt sich das Zustandekommen der Verminderung der Nebennierenfunktion durch die, nach jeden 5 bis 600 mg Mengen, regelmäßig verabreichten 150 bis 200 E ACTH anscheinend nicht abwehren. Dies entspricht den Angaben von LANDON u. Mitarb. [10], die mit wöchentlich 120 E dauernd wirkendem ACTH-Gel die Schädigung der Nebennieren nicht abwenden konnten. Die alleinige und prolongierte ACTH-Behandlung bewirkt eine Dauerschädigung in der Corticotropfunktion der Hypophyse [12, 14]. Am Ende der Steroidbehandlung erscheint ACTH begründet, da bereits eine 4tägige Dosierung die Regeneration der Nebennierenrinde beschleunigt [1], obgleich die Regeneration — mit wenigen Ausnahmen — nach dem endgültigen Einstellen der Steroidbehandlung auch spontan erfolgen kann [1].

Mit der zur Behandlung des Pemphigus verwendeten Steroidtherapie kann in einem großen Teil der Fälle nur mit einer bedeutenden Gesamtmenge ein Resultat erzielt werden. Dies kann selbstverständlich, nebst sonstigen Schädigungen, auch die besprochenen Hypophyse-Nebennierenrindenläsionen nach sich ziehen. Aus diesem Grunde waren wir bestrebt, die Gesamtmengen herabzusetzen oder soweit als möglich die Steroidbehandlung zu vermeiden.

Auf Grund unserer vorhergehenden Untersuchungen der Spinalganglien und auf Grund von diesen folgenden virologischen Untersuchungen begannen wir, bei vier Pemphiguskranken das Sabin-Vaccin anzuwenden. Mit dem Vaccin der Type 2 wurde die Behandlung bisher in vier Fällen angewendet: bei zwei Mund-, einer Alterspemphigus und einer Pemphigus seborrhoicus. Die Vaccination wurde am 21. März des 1. Jahres ausgeführt. Die Tzancksche Probe war vorher bei den zwei Mundpemphigus positiv. Von den zwei Kranken mit Mundpemphigus wurde die eine in 2 Wochen symptomfrei und ist so geblieben; die andere hat sich bedeutend verbessert, doch wurde sie nicht symptomfrei. Nach einer kleinen Menge von Prednisolon (140 mg) wurde sie auch symptomfrei. Der Alterspemphigus wurde innerhalb 3 Wochen symptomfrei und ist seither symptomfrei. Bei dem behandelten Fall mit ausgedehnten Symptomen des Pemphigus seborrhoicus war keine Besserung zu verzeichnen, deshalb wurde er nachträglich mit Prednisolon behandelt. Die tägliche höchste Dosis betrug 35 mg, insgesamt 525 mg, wonach er vollständig symptomfrei wurde. Vorhergehend hatten wir bei der Untersuchung des Poliovirus neutralisierenden Antikörpergehaltes im Blutserum von 16 Pemphiguskranken festgestellt, daß dieser im allgemeinen recht niedrig war. Von den vier behandelten Kranken hatte sich bei den zwei Fällen von Mundpemphigus und in dem Alterspemphigus der Gehalt des Antikörpers nach Verabreichung des Vaccins in großem Maße erhöht, während in dem erwähnten erfolglosen Fall die Erhöhung ganz minimal war. Diese Untersuchungen nahm ich mit meinen Mitarbeitern Dr. FORNOSI und Dr. ANGYAL vor. Natürlich läßt sich auf Grund dieser ersten Erfahrungen der Wert der Behandlung nicht beurteilen, es scheint jedoch die Fortsetzung dieser Untersuchungen wünschenswert und sich mit den anderen zwei Polio-Virustypen zu ergänzen.

Literatur. 1. AMATRUDA, T. T., M. M. HURST, and N. D. D'ESOPO: J. clin. Endocr. **25**, 1207 (1965). — 2. BENETT, W. A.: J. Bone Jt. Surg. **36** A. 867 (1954). — 3. FEKETE, G., and P. GÖRÖG: J. Endocr. **27**, 23 (1963). — 4. GRABER, A. L., R. L. NEY, W. E. NICHOLSON, D. P. ISLAND, and G. W. LIDDLE: J. clin. Endocr. **25**, 11 (1965). — 5. HOLUB, D. A., I. W. JAILER, J. I. KITAY, and G. FRANIZA: J. clin. Endocr. **19**, 1540 (1959). — 6. HOLUB, D. A., J. I. KITAY, and I. W. JAILER: J. clin. Invest. **38**, 291 (1960). — 7. HOLUB, D. A., E. Z. WALLACE, and I. V. JAILER: J. clin. Endocr. **20**, 1294 (1960). — 8. KILBY, R. A., W. A. BENETT, and R. G. SPRAGUE: Ann. J. Path. **33**, 155 (1957). — 9. KYLE, L. H., R. J. MEYER, and I. I. CANARY: New Engl. J. Med. **257**, 57 (1957). — 10. LANDON, I., V. WYNN, V. H. T. JAMES, and I. B.

WOOD: J. clin. Endocr. **25**, 602 (1965). — 11. PLAGER, I. E., and P. CUSHMAN: J. clin. Endocr. **22**, 147 (1962). — 12. RENTSCH, F.: Endocrinologie **48**, 62 (1965). — 13. SOLEM, J. H., and T. BRINCK-JOHNSEN: Acta med. scand. **170**, 89 (1961). — 14. SUSSMAN, L., L. LIBRIK, and G. W. CLAYTON: Metabolism **14**, 583 (1965). — 15. VÉRTES, B., J. MASSZI, and É. TÖRÖK: Börgyógy. Vener. Szemle **1**, 13 (1966).

Topical Corticosteroid Therapy

V. H. WITTEN, Department of Dermatology, University of Miami School of Medicine, Miami, Florida (USA)

It is just 15 years since topical corticosteroids were introduced into dermatologic therapy. In that time they have proven to be, without exception, the most useful and effective of external medicaments. 7 years ago the introduction of thin pliable plastic films as occlusive dressings was another major step in the effective use of these agents, in particular, the fluorinated compounds.

It was apparent immediately that the use of topical corticosteroids had distinct advantages over their systemic administration. For example, topical applications produce: 1. no "lighting" up of latent internal infections; 2. no spreading of superficial cutaneous infections; 3. no acneform eruptions; 4. no retardation of wound healing; 5. no habituation and 6. no clinical manifestations of systemic effects resulting from percutaneous absorption.

The desirable properties of topical corticosteroid preparations include: 1. A high degree of effectiveness in the management of a wide variety of dermatoses; 2. relative ease of use without stain, odor or discomfort; 3. no allergic sensitization or adverse local reactions to the corticosteroid itself; 4. no regular increased resistance; and 5. compatibility with essentially all other commonly used topical medicaments.

The judicious combined use of topical and systemic corticosteroids will, for certain diseases, make it possible to reduce or even discontinue the systemic dose and, in turn, the possibility of undesirable effects.

The adverse side effects of topical corticosteroid preparations have been minimal and consist of the rare occurrence of striae in intertriginous areas and laboratory evidence of absorption with suppressed pituitary and adrenal function. The addition of occlusive pliable plastic dressings accounts for an increasing incidence of complications some of which may be of importance when large body areas are treated. These include: folliculitis, pyoderma and furunculosis; miliaria; apparent thinning of the skin; a disagreeable odor; heat intolerance; and erythema, edema and pruritus. One should also be aware of the possibility of allergic contact dermatitis to and flammability of the plastic.

Numerous techniques have been added for the utilization of topical corticosteroids. It has been found advantageous to remove, wherever possible, crusting and heavy scaling with softening and keratolytic creams and ointments and various abrasives. Modifications of the use of occlusive dressings include the addition of external heat and moist dressings.

The extent to which the suppressed pituitary-adrenal function, which may be demonstrated by careful laboratory examination, should be considered as an adverse response to the use of corticosteroids under occlusive dressings, remains in question. There is scant clinical evidence that this suppression is either harmful or dangerous. Would individuals so affected fail to respond adequately to stress situations or are they likely to be harmed in other ways? It is interesting that the pituitary response, as judged by metyrapone testing, returns to normal within 2 days after discontinuing the occlusive dressings. Further, there is generally a prompt return of plasma cortisol levels and urinary steroid excretion to within normal range after brief periods of topical therapy.

Numerous factors may influence the percutaneous absorption* of corticosteroids and, in turn, their possible systemic effects. Among these are:

1. The compound.

a) In general, acetates are better absorbed than the parent alcohol; phosphates are poorly absorbed and the acetonides of the fluorinated corticosteroids appear to greatly enhance percutaneous absorption.

b) Smaller particle size enhances absorption.

c) Solubility and partition coefficient.

2. Vehicle. Absorption is aided by the addition of agents, e.g. propylene glycol and dimethylsulfoxide.

3. Concentration per gram of vehicle and the total amount applied.

4. Area of body surface treated.

5. Integrity of the epidermal barrier. When absorption takes place it is through skin altered by disease; absorption through normal skin with systemic pituitary-adrenal suppression has not been demonstrated. Increasing the hydration of the stratum corneum apparently increases both the resevoir effect and penetration. The exact role of increased local temperature is not certain.

6. Time of application and duration of therapy.

7. Method of application. Occlusive dressings of impermeable plastic have been shown to markedly enhance percutaneous absorption.

Should not a thorough knowledge of these factors suggest regimens which would enhance therapeutic effectiveness with a reduced incidence of undesirable effects? I am certain that this is so.

In 1955 it was first suggested that there may be a skin depot for the slow release of topically applied corticosteroids. In 1957 the observation was first recorded that hydrocortisone applied to an area of stripped skin caused local vasoconstriction. In 1961 the first publication appeared regarding the use of thin pliable plastic films in conjunction with topical corticosteroids. SULZBERGER and I speculated that the increased effectiveness from this combined therapy was due to: 1. more intimate contact of drug and skin lesions, 2. more ready availability of the therapeutic agent, 3. enhanced percutaneous absorption resulting from maceration of epidermal surface, and 4. increase in vascular flow, temperature, etc.

Numerous studies are available to support the concept of a depot or "resevoir" within the stratum corneum. The phenomenon of local vasoconstriction at the site of application of the corticosteroid has been the major observation used to "prove" the existence of such a resevoir.

The mechanism of the vasoconstriction remains unknown. It has been suggested that it is due to: 1. the effect of the corticosteroid itself or perhaps, 2. the presence of the corticosteroid potentiates the vasoconstrictor action of some normally occurring agents, or increases the sensitivity of the cells to these agents, or inactivates or block enzymes which normally control the action of the vasoconstrictors. I would add that it may be one of the metabolites of the corticosteroid which is responsible.

---

* In all instances the degree of percutaneous absorption has been judged by the extent of the resulting vasoconstriction. However, there is no direct proof that there is any correlation between the vasoconstriction and the anti-inflammatory activity of the corticosteroid or the extent of systematic absorption.

Fig. Transformations of hydrocortisone in human skin

Biochemical studies in our own laboratories at the University of Miami School of Medicine have established the major metabolites resulting from the in vitro incubation of cortisol-4-^{14}C. These transformations are summarized in the figure. The results suggest that oxidation of the 11-β-ol and reduction of a 20-one constitute the two general pathways of metabolism of cortisol in human skin. A third pathway which has been found only in the preputium penis is the formation of allodihydro- and allotetrahydrocortisol.

The metabolism of hydrocortisone was demonstrated for both epidermis and dermis; neither sebaceous glands nor hair follicles are required as shown with skin from the sole.

My own studies utilizing ^{14}C labeled hydrocortisone and triamcinolone acetonide applied to the skin in 95% alcohol suggest that the hydrocortisone, with or without occlusion, is retained within the stratum corneum longer and in larger quantities than triamcinolone acetonide, with or without occlusion. In addition, there is little difference in the amount of radioactivity demonstrable within the stratum corneum as shown by cellophane tape strippings for triamcinolone acetonide, with or without occlusion.

Judging from the results of these studies, there appears to be less of a "reservoir" effect within the stratum corneum for triamcinolone acetonide than for hydrocortisone. This finding is contrary to the concept that hydrocortisone passes through more freely and faster and that triamcinolone acetonide is held longer, thus accounting for the prolonged effect of the latter. According to my findings, it is questionable whether the application of the occlusive plastic alters only the penetration or the "reservoir"; in addition, the conditions created under the occlusive plastic may raise the level of biologic activity within the tissues by increasing the local moisture and heat and, in turn, increase the local metabolic activity and allow for freer passage of the effective compound from the stratum corneum into the underlying tissues.

If this concept is correct, it is not solely the increased absorption of the original compound on the reocclusion which accounts for the reappearance of vaso-constriction, as pointed out by some authors, but rather, there may be increased metabolism on occlusion which provides more of the biologically active agent to produce the vasoconstriction.

One cannot question the fact that impermeable occlusion of topically applied corticosteroids enhances percutaneous absorption; this is evident by the altered pituitary and adrenal gland function. There has been no correlation, however, between such percutaneous absorption, local vasoconstriction and therapeutic benefits. Certainly when reocclusion of previously treated sites results in local vasoconstriction, there is not a repetition of absorption and consequent systemic effects. Nor is there evidence that reocclusion will again bring about therapeutic benefit even when there is vasoconstriction. The mechanism of action of topical corticosteroids remains unknown.

I now quote from the concluding remarks in a paper on "The Corticosteroids in the Management of Diseases of the Skin" which I presented in 1959. I believe these comments are as true today as they were then: "It is evident that, as a group, the corticosteroids have done much to aid in the effective management of many dermatological disorders. This is obviously due to the extraordinary pharmacological and biochemical action of these compounds. However, effective management also results from the accumulation of a vast fund of clinical knowledge concerning these compounds, which aids the practitioner in their safe and success-ful use. Furthermore, understanding the mechanism of action of these products is basic to the understanding of body function in both health and disease. In-vestigations in this field, therefore, by the chemist, biochemist, enzymologist, physiologist, physician, and many others is destined to continue. The discoveries of tomorrow may prove to be as phenomenal as the discovery of cortisone itself. Certainly it is our obligation as practicing physicians to know these compounds well and to use them wisely".

References. BARRETT, C. W., J. W. HADGRAFT, G. A. CARON, and I. SARKANY: Brit. J. Derm. 77, 576 (1965). — HSIA, S. L., and Y. L. HAO: Biochemistry 5, 1469 (1966). — HSIA, S. L., V. H. WITTEN, and Y. L. HAO: J. invest. Derm. 43, 407 (1964). — McKENZIE, A. W.: Arch. Derm. 86, 611 (1962). — McKENZIE, A. W., and R. B. STOUGHTON: Arch. Derm. 86, 608 (1962). — KIRKETERP, M.: Acta derm.-venereol (Stockh.) 44, 54 (1964). — MALKINSON, F. D., and E. H. FERGUSON: J. invest. Derm. 25, 281 (1955). — MARCH, C., T. H. REA jr., and M. J. PORTER: Clin. Pharmacol. Ther. 6, 43 (1965). — SARKANY, I., J. W. HADGRAFT, G. A. CARON, and C. W. BARRETT: Brit. J. Derm. 77, 569 (1965). — SCOGGINS, R. B., and B. KLIMAN: J. invest. Derm. 45, 347 (1965). —STOUGHTON, R. B.: Arch. Derm. 91, 657 (1965). — Arch. environm. Hlth 11, 551 (1965). — SULZBERGER, M. B., and V. H. WITTEN: J. invest. Derm. 19, 101 (1952). — Arch. Derm. 84, 1027 (1961). — VICKERS, C. F. H.: Arch. Derm. 88, 20 (1963). — WELLS, G. C.: Brit. J. Derm. 69, 11 (1957). — WITTEN, V. H.: Ann. N.Y. Acad. Med. 82, 983 (1959).

Les atrophies cutanées au cours de la corticothérapie générale

R. Touraine, M. Fournet et S. Belaïch, Clinique des Maladies Cutanées et Syphilitiques de la Faculté de Médecine de Paris, Hôpital Saint-Louis, Paris (France)

De nombreux travaux ont été consacrés aux atrophies cutanées par cortico-thérapie locale. Mais, peu de publications étudient ou même signalent les divers types d'atrophies cutanées, relativement fréquentes, dues à la corticothérapie générale.

L'examen de 65 malades, fait entre le 3ème mois et la 5ème année après le début de ce traitement, révèle 39 cas d'atrophies cutanées. Cette étude en précise les divers aspects cliniques, envisage les facteurs déclenchants ou favorisants et tente d'en préciser l'origine et le mode de formation.

Description clinique

On peut schématiquement distinguer, dans ce groupe de 39 cas, quatre types d'atrophies cutanées:

— les *atrophies cutanées diffuses* (13 cas), les plus fréquentes. Elles sont aisément décelables, surtout aux avant-bras, sur le dos des mains, sur les jambes, mais sont inconstantes sur le visage. Elles réalisent un amincissement extrême de la peau, véritable «pelure d'oignon», avec nette visibilité du réseau veineux. Cette peau, brillante, rosée, est parsemée de télangiectasies, de pétéchies, et surtout d'ecchymoses provoquées par des traumatismes minimes et entourées de larges zones jaunâtres ou orangées. La pilosité est presque toujours normale. Au palper, la consistance est molle.

— les *atrophies circonscrites isolées* (4 cas) réalisant des plaques de peau amincie, «papier de cigarette», de teinte peu modifiée, laissant nettement voir le réseau veineux. Les ecchymoses sont très rares. On les décèle, par ordre de fréquence, sur le thorax, sur les aisselles, sur les paupières. Ce type ne peut être considéré dans nos cas comme un mode de début ou un stade d'involution de l'atrophie diffuse. Par contre, ces plages peuvent s'associer aux vergetures (5 sur 7 cas de vergetures).

— les *vergetures* (7 cas) ont les caractères de celles décrites dans le syndrome de Cushing, et sont notées, par fréquence décroissante, aux cuisses et aux aines, aux aisselles, sur la région lombaire, l'abdomen et les seins. Les phénomènes hémorragiques sont absents ou minimes.

— les *peaux fines* (15 cas) sont, soit diffuses (6 cas), soit visibles sur le thorax et les membres. La peau est amincie, parfois légèrement ichtyosiforme, sans hémorragies, de couleur quasi-normale. Les cas observés sur des affections cutanées à tendance atrophiante, ainsi que ceux où la différenciation avec une peau sénile étaient difficiles, ont été écartés. Il est impossible de dire actuellement si ces formes évoluent, en cas de continuation du traitement, vers l'atrophie diffuse.

Evolution clinique

Cette étude, faite sur des cas en cours de traitement, ne peut préciser exactement le mode de formation et l'évolution de ces divers types d'atrophies. Il existe des apparitions précoces, dès les premiers mois de la corticothérapie, surtout pour les vergetures. La régression paraît possible, sauf pour les vergetures qui blanchissent. Dans 2 cas, on note une nette régression d'atrophies diffuses, en trois à six mois après arrêt du traitement. Ces faits sont à rapprocher de ceux observés dans les hypercorticismes.

Facteurs étiologiques

1. *Deux facteurs principaux* sont à souligner dans le domaine de la cortico-thérapie:

la *durée* de la corticothérapie (Tableau), sans qu'il soit possible de préciser le temps moyen nécessaire.

Tableau

	nombre total	3 mois	6 mois	9 mois	1 an	2 ans	3 ans	4 ans	5 ans et plus
Atrophies diffuses	13	2		1	1		1	2	6
Atrophies localisées	4		1	1		2			
Vergetures	7				1	1	2		3
Peaux fines	15	2		1	2	1	4	1	4
Peaux normales	26	1	1	5	6	4	3	3	3

La *dose totale* reçue, convertie en delta-cortisone selon les équivalences usuellement admises. Elle paraît avoir un rôle prédominant pour les atrophies diffuses (11 cas sur 13 reçurent des doses totales supérieures à 10 g) ainsi que pour les atrophies localisées et les peaux fines. Par contre, elle apparaît beaucoup moins importante pour les vergetures, ce qui témoignerait d'un terrain individuel.

La *dose d'attaque* est sûrement un facteur favorisant mais non indispensable; elle paraît accélérer l'apparition, comme en témoigne surtout un cas de grande atrophie diffuse apparue au 3ème mois d'un traitement totalisant 8 g.

Ces conclusions sont facilement mises en évidence dans les traitements continus. L'existence de périodes d'arrêt diminue le risque et explique la grande majorité des peaux normales, malgré des traitements prolongés et des doses assez élevées. Ces observations sont également un argument en faveur de la régression possible des modifications cutanées.

Le *type de corticoïde* utilisé ne paraît pas intervenir nettement. Notre statistique semble montrer que les traitements par corticoïde unique sont peut-être moins atrophiants que ceux associant plusieurs dérivés, mais nos chiffres sont insuffisants pour vérifier cette impression.

2. *Autres facteurs*. Le *type de la maladie* ayant nécessité une corticothérapie générale [pemphigus (16), maladie de Duhring (9), lupus érythémateux (8), hématodermies (3), divers (18)] ne semble pas jouer de rôle, sauf dans un cas de syndrome d'Ehlers-Danlos faisant de très nombreuses vergetures au cours d'un traitement de R.A.A.

L'âge et le sexe du patient sont des notions importantes. Les atrophies diffuses sont observées presque uniquement chez la femme âgée de plus de 50 ans (12 cas sur 13). Les atrophies circonscrites et les peaux fines surviennent plus fréquemment chez les sujets après la cinquantaine, sans toujours nécessiter des doses élevées et prolongées. Par contre, les vergetures sont l'apanage du sujet jeune (les 7 cas ont moins de 50 ans), sans influence du sexe.

Les traitements généraux associés à la corticothérapie n'ont pas de rôle particulier dans ce domaine. Un cas avec peau fine a fait une atrophie rapide aux zones de corticothérapie locale associée.

Parmi les antécédents, on ne peut retenir que l'exposition solaire qui a peut-être permis à un sujet jeune de faire une atrophie importante avec une dose totale inférieure à 10 g et qui expliquerait la plus nette visibilité des atrophies des sujets âgés aux bras et aux jambes.

Etio-pathogénie

Il existe une relation évidente entre les atrophies cutanées et les signes témoignant d'un hypercorticisme. Les manifestations habituelles de cet hypercorticisme précèdent les atrophies, puis s'atténuent nettement avec de faibles doses, qui suffisent par contre à entretenir les atrophies.

Dans le groupe des atrophies diffuses, tous les patients avaient ou avaient eu un faciès cushingoïde et un «buffalo-neck», 9 sur 13, une alopécie diffuse due au chevelu, 7 sur 13 un hirsutisme, même en l'absence d'androgènes associés, 6 sur 13 des signes osseux évidents (1 fracture spontanée et 5 ostéoporoses), 6 sur 13 des signes cliniques musculaires, 2 sur 13 une acné, 2 un diabète. Dans le groupe des vergetures, les 7 patients avaient eu, de façon très nette et rapide, le même visage rouge et bouffi. Des signes musculaires sont retrouvés dans 2 cas, une alopécie dans 2 cas, une acné dans 1 cas. Dans le groupe des atrophies circonscrites et des peaux fines, l'interrogatoire retrouvait un faciès caractéristique dans 16 cas, mais ne persistant lors de l'examen que dans 8 cas. Par contre, il ne paraît exister aucune corrélation particulière avec d'autres accidents de la corticothérapie, en particulier digestifs et psychiques.

Des nombreuses études biologiques, on retiendra:

la fréquence de l'hypokaliémie;

l'inconstance, dans le groupe des atrophies diffuses avec ecchymoses, de modifications de la crase sanguine et, en particulier, de fragilité capillaire.

L'étude du fonctionnement des surrénales et de l'hypophyse a été faite par les dosages des 17 C.S., des 17 O.H. et du cortisol plasmatique, et les explorations dynamiques comprenant, dans 20 cas des 5 catégories, un test au synactène (Ciba) avec dosage du cortisol et un test à la métopyrone (S.U. 4885). De ces résultats, on ne peut que signaler la rareté d'une inertie surrénalienne, sans corrélation avec les divers types d'atrophies, et l'absence de facteur hypophysaire associé dans la genèse des atrophies cutanées.

Etude histologique

I. Microscopie optique

66 biopsies cutanées ont été pratiquées chez 55 de nos malades.

a) Les *atrophies diffuses* — 19 biopsies cutanées appartenant aux 13 cas d'atrophie diffuse ont été examinées. Elles furent pratiquées le plus souvent à la face postéro-externe de l'avant-bras.

Les modifications observées furent essentiellement dermiques. Le fait marquant est l'atrophie dermique considérable retrouvée dans pratiquement tous les cas, avec une apparente remontée de l'hypoderme. Cet amincissement est dû à une raréfaction, une véritable fonte des fibres collagènes. En quelques endroits, celles-ci apparaissent fragmentées. La coloration de Hotchkiss-Mac Manus n'a pas montré de modifications importantes. Il n'existe pas de métachromasie au bleu de Toluidine. Les annexes épidermiques ne sont pas modifiées.

Alors que le tissu collagène est nettement raréfié, le tissu élastique est, dans la règle, normal. Dans 3 cas, cependant, de véritables élastomes furent observés dans le derme superficiel. Ils peuvent être rapportés à une élastose solaire ou sénile.

Les lésions vasculaires sont intéressantes à noter. Dans quelques cas, des hémorragies intradermiques sont visibles, bien mises en évidence par la coloration de Turnbull. Sur d'autres coupes, de nombreux capillaires dilatés, mais sans lésions pariétales, sont retrouvés dans le derme superficiel, confirmant l'aspect clinique télangiectasique. Parfois enfin, les vaisseaux sont parfaitement normaux.

L'épiderme est modifié de façon inconstante: atrophie du corps muqueux de Malpighi avec aspect rectiligne de la couche basale et hyperkératose ortho-kératosique.

b) Les *vergetures*. Quatre biopsies de vergetures ont été pratiquées au niveau de l'aisselle, de l'abdomen ou de la hanche. Au-dessous d'un épiderme normal, l'atrophie dermique est considérable, due à une fonte totale du tissu élastique, associée à une diminution des fibres collagènes.

c) Les *atrophies circonscrites*. Cinq biopsies pratiquées chez quatre malades furent examinées. L'épiderme n'est pas modifié. L'amincissement dermique, le plus souvent modéré, est dû à une raréfaction du tissu collagène alors que le réseau élastique est normal. Les parois vasculaires ne sont pas altérées et il n'existe pas d'hémorragies.

d) Les *peaux fines*. 19 biopsies ont été étudiées, appartenant à 14 malades. Dans l'ensemble, les altérations histologiques sont très discrètes. On note un amincissement modéré du derme avec un réseau élastique normal et un épiderme non modifié.

e) Les *peaux normales*. Les 19 biopsies pratiquées sont strictement normales.

II. *Microscopie électronique* (Prof. PIÉRARD et Dr. KINT, Gand)

Huit biopsies cutanées appartenant à huit malades ont été étudiées au microscope électronique (3 atrophies diffuses, 2 atrophies circonscrites, 1 vergeture, 2 peaux fines). Cette étude a porté sur les fibres collagènes, les fibroblastes, les fibres élastiques.

a) Les *atrophie diffuses*. Nous avons pu noter, dans les fibroblastes, une multiplication des fibrilles intra-cytoplasmiques, une disparition des mitochondries. D'autre part, de nombreuses fibrilles entourent le prolongement du fibroblaste avec des fibres collagènes au voisinage de ces fibrilles. Cet aspect fibrillaire représente-il une désintégration des fibres collagènes normales ou une néo-collagénose atypique ? Des structures plus ou moins amorphes ont également été retrouvées; leur signification n'apparaît pas clairement.

Le fait essentiel est que, dans tous les cas, les fibres élastiques sont rigoureusement normales. Le point de départ de l'atrophie cortisonique diffuse n'est donc pas l'atteinte du réseau élastique, mais celle du tissu collagène.

b) Les *atrophies circonscrites*. Dans le fibroblaste, une augmentation du nombre des fibrilles intra-cytoplasmiques a été notée. Les fibres élastiques sont normales.

c) Les *vergetures*. Le tissu collagène n'est pas modifié. Par contre, le tissu élastique est très raréfié et de nombreuses coupes ont été nécessaires pour retrouver l'élastine, de structure d'ailleurs normale.

d) Les *peaux fines*. Leur structure ultra-microscopique est normale.

Some Effects of Corticosteroids "in vitro"

C. N. D. CRUICKSHANK, Medical Research Council, Unit for Research on the Experimental Pathology of the Skin. The Medical School, The University, Birmingham (England)

The use of tissue culture methods to analyse the mechanism of action of drugs on tissues has many advantages. It eliminates indirect effects on cells via the blood and nerve supply, frequently results can be quantitated to form a bio-assay method and usually it represents a saving of time and money.

LAWRENCE and RICKETTS (1957) showed that cortisone could inhibit the uptake of $^{35}SO_4$ by skin "in vitro". This communication, which represents part of the collaborative studies carried out between various members of this Unit and of the Department of Chemistry of Birmingham University, is concerned with the further investigation of this effect and an attempt to use it to compare the potency of corticosteroids.

Initial studies have shown that 60% of $^{35}SO_4$ is incorporated by skin into mucopolysaccharides (BARKER et al., 1964) and more recently the individual $^{35}SO_4$-sulphated mucopolysaccharides have been isolated from rat (BARKER et al., 1965) and human (to be published) epidermis and dermis. One is therefore studying, in effect, the synthesis of mucopolysaccharides.

Methods. The method used was that described by BARKER et al. (1964). In summary, thin slices of human skin obtained at operation were floated for 24 hours at 37 °C on a culture medium containing 0.05 mc Na_2 $^{35}SO_4$. The epidermis was separated from the dermis by subsequent incubation in 0.25% trypsin for approximately 30 min. The two tissues were treated separately and plunged into liquid nitrogen for 30 min. Any excess sulphate was removed by dialysis, followed by rinsing and drying.

Complete destruction of the slices was carried out in 12 N hydrochloric acid at 100 °C and the sulphate was precipitated by addition of 0.1 M sodium sulphate as carrier, followed by 0.1 M barium chloride. Counting was done by the end window method at the calculated infinite thickness.

Experiments were carried out in groups of three with three treated and three control slices.

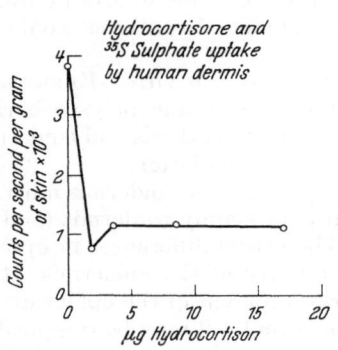
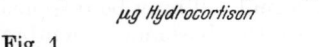

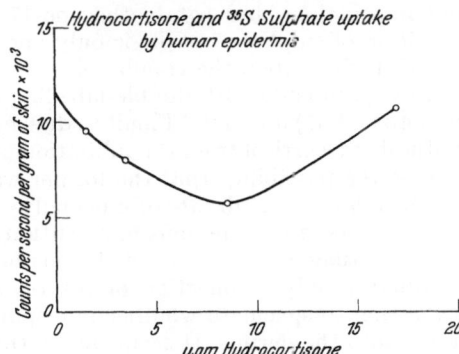

Fig. 1   Fig. 2

Results. The effect of increasing concentrations of hydrocortisone on dermis and epidermis is shown in Figs. 1 and 2. Each point represents the average of three experiments. In the epidermis there is an inhibition which is linear with concentration and which commences with as little as 2 µg/ml hydrocortisone and increases to a maximum of about 46% at 10 µg/ml. In the dermis, a maximum inhibition of 67% occurred at 2 µg/ml and no further increase in the concentration of hydrocortisone caused any further depression.

The table shows the results of a series of experiments comparing the effects of hydrocortisone, fluocinolone and betamethasone-17-valerate. Each experiment with a steroid was accompanied by its own control to allow for the variable $^{35}SO_4$ uptake caused mainly by the variations in slice thickness which were unavoidable. Firstly, it will be seen that the rate of uptake per mg of tissue is considerably

Table. *The effects of hydrocortisone, fluocinolone and betamethasone-17-valerate on $^{35}SO_4$ uptake by human skin "in vitro" (counts/gram/second × 10^3)*

Experiment number	Hydrocortisone		Fluocinolone		Betamethasone-17-valerate	
	C	H/c	C	F	C	BM/v
1. a) Epidermis	8.0[a]	7.8	1.3	0.9	1.8	1.3
b) Dermis	1.6	1.0	1.2	0.7	0.6	0.4
2. a) Epidermis	11.5	11.3	1.8	1.6		
b) Dermis	4.8	2.4	1.4	0.9		

[a] Each figure is the mean of three observations.

higher in the epidermis than in the dermis in all the control slices. However, all the three corticosteroids tested produced about the same degree of depression. In each instance the depression caused in the epidermal slices was of the order of 20 to 30%. Although the actual rate of uptake in the dermis was lower, the depression caused by the steroids was greater.

Discussion. The fact that the inhibition of $^{35}SO_4$ uptakes by hydrocortisone was related to dose seemed to indicate that this method could distinguish the potency of drugs with similar effects. Unfortunately, all three substances inhibited $^{35}SO_4$ uptake to the same extent, whereas clinical experience and skin blanching tests indicate the superiority of the two latter compounds, at least when applied topically. It is unlikely, however, that problems of skin penetration account for the difference between the "in vitro" and "in vivo" results. It seems more likely that fluocinolone and betamethasone-17-valerate have multiple effects of which inhibition of sulphate uptake is only one. The most obvious hypothesis would be a special effect upon the capillaries.

In experiments with double-labelling of chick embryos "in vitro" EBERT and PROCKOP (1967) found it difficult to dissociate the inhibition of mucopolysaccharide synthesis by cortisol from the inhibition of general protein synthesis and could not exclude the possibility that the former was secondary to the latter.

The relatively high rate of mucopolysaccharide synthesis by epidermis must be of interest because, previously, attention has been paid mainly to dermis (and of course cartilage) as a source of these substances. The actual differences in uptake is probably only a reflection of the increased cellularity of the epidermis. It is interesting to speculate whether mucopolysaccharides remain in the epidermis or diffuse into the dermis. It seems likely that the epidermal cell may be responsible for the maintenance of the mucopolysaccharides of the basement membrane. In the dermis the sulphated mucopolysaccharides are associated with the formation of collagen fibres — it is interesting to speculate whether they exercise a similar role in keratin formation.

References. BARKER, S. A., C. N. D. CRUICKSHANK, and T. WEBB: Exp. Cell Res. **35**, 255 (1964). — Carbohydrate Res. **1**, 53 (1965). — EBERT, P. S., and D. J. PROCKOP: Biochim. biophys. Acta. (Amst.) **134**, 45 (1967). — LAWRENCE, J. C., and C. R. RICKETTS: Exp. Cell Res. **12**, 633 (1957).

Free Communications

Long-term Estrogen and Corticosteroid Therapy in Chronic Skin Diseases*

A. S. SPANGLER, Harvard Medical School; S. SOTMAN and H. N. ANTONIADES, Blood Research Institute and Harvard School of Public Health (USA)

Recently NELSON reported the potentiation of the glycosuric effect of hydrocortisone by estrogen therapy. We have investigated the possible potentiation of the anti-inflammatory effect of hydrocortisone by estrogen therapy in certain chronic skin diseases: pemphigus vulgaris, mycosis fungoides, generalized psoriasis, generalized nummular eczema, and chronic erythema nodosum. 13 patients were followed for periods of 1½ to 4 years.

* Supported by USPHS Grant AM-08381 and American Cancer Society (Mass. Division) Inc.

After the minimum maintenance dose of hydrocortisone had been carefully established, estrogen therapy of Chlorotrianisene (TACE) or Diethylstilbesterol (Hexesterol) (in doses approximately equivalent to 100 mg of stilbestrol per day) was added. In each instance the maintenance dose of hydrocortisone could be lowered to 1/3 to 1/10 that previously required. Estrogen therapy alone had little anti-inflammatory effect.

Plasma corticosteroid-binding globulin levels rose from a mean of 12 μg-% to 33 μg-%, and the plasma total unconjugated corticosteroids rose from a mean of 10 μg-% to 24 μg-%, after the addition of estrogen therapy.

It is possible that the prolonged half-life of hydrocortisone observed with estrogen therapy, and the increase in the cortisol-binding globulin-hydrocortisone complex, may provide a depot from which the hydrocortisone can be supplied to the inflamed tissue.

References. NELSON, D. H., H. TANNEY, G. MESTMAN, V. W. GIESCHERN, and L. D. WILSON: J. clin. Endocr. **23**, 261 (1963).

Australian Experiences with the Cortico-steroids

W. W. LEMPRIERE, Melbourne (Australia)

It is only to be expected that Australian experiences with the Cortico-steroids would be largely similar to those in other parts of the civilized world, for Australia is a civilized country, where eleven million inhabitants, mainly of Anglo-saxon origin, are largely concentrated in the bigger cities, and our medical profession is in close touch with world developments, although opportunities for original research are limited. In particular, our dermatologists travel widely to Congresses and exchange ideas with their colleagues throughout the world.

The advances during the past 15 years in the use of Cortico-steroids have been so exciting that many have been tempted to use them unwisely, like a young man with a fast car. The hazards of treatment have been rather slower to emerge. It is said that Knowledge comes but Wisdom lingers.

One restraining factor has been the enormous cost of treatment, also in the earlier years the difffculties of administration. This probably helped to clarify the main indications for the use of Cortico-steroids, namely their life-saving effects in acute emergencies such as pemphigus, exfoliative dermatitis and disseminated lupus erythematosus, also the quick relief of acute contact dermatitis and the suppression of severe atopic eczema. One is justified in calling out the fire brigade to put out the fire. The prolonged use of Cortico-steroids is quite another story.

Naturally, in dermatology the local application of ointments, creams, lotions or sprays predominates, with oral or parenteral administration rightly reserved for emergencies or exceptional cases. Yet the improved formulae, increased potency, wider availability and intense and competitive sales promotion have encouraged the indiscriminate use of these compounds. Their ability to suppress inflammation regardless of its cause leads to a false sense of cure. The patient is loth to come out from under the Cortisone umbrella. He demands some more of that wonderful ointment for his pruritus ani or his eczema.

The temptation to order cortico-steroids for long periods without making a diagnosis is very great, especially in a busy practice, so the cortico-steroid casualties can be said to include both the patient and the doctor.

The commoner complications are well recognised, ranging from disorders of metabolism to effects on intercurrent disorders such as diabetes, gastric ulcer, tuberculosis, psychological upsets, and the masking of infective processes such as perinephric abscesses. The dosage and duration of treatment sufficient to cause serious suppression of natural suprarenal secretions may be quite small, necessitating a prolonged course of a small maintenance dose of cortico-steroids in an apparently healthy patient, with a rapid relapse of his former symptoms if one attempts to stop treatment.

Great interest is being shown at present in the treatment of psoriasis by the fashionable but unpleasant method of inunction of fluorinated cortico-steroids under polythene occlusion. One has to admit that improvement is often rapid, even spectacular, although in hot weather the patient can only endure occlusion for a few hours at a time, at the risk of putrefactive sweat disorders and follicular infections. Apparently the actual maceration of the skin is the important thing, as the same benefits are not obtained by occlusion under Unna's paste.

No doubt to a bad psoriatic, any relief is better than none, but psoriasis is notoriously variable and no one can guarantee a permanent clearance of the lesions. It is not usual for areas cleared by this occlusive technique to remain clear to the same extent as areas treated by superficial X-ray therapy.

One must still be able to treat the patients with the older well-tried remedies, to "trust in God, but keep your gun-powder dry". Again like the young man in the fast car, we should be duly thankful for these wonder-drugs, but keep our eye on the road. ADRIAN JOHNSON of Sydney tells the story of a wise old American at some earlier congress, when everyone had been singing the praises of the cortico-steroids, who sprang up and exclaimed, "Boys, boys, these things aint candy"!

Möglichkeiten der Entwöhnung bzw. Einsparung von Corticoiden in der dermatologischen Therapie

G. LUDWIG, Dermatologische Abteilung der Nordseeklinik Westerland/Sylt (Deutschland)

Die Einsparung von Corticoiden ohne Rückfall der Erkrankung ist zweifellos ebenso erstrebenswert, wie die Corticoidanwendung notwendig sein kann. Inwieweit Corticoidtherapie abgesetzt werden kann, ist gleichsam ein Gradmesser für einen echt kurativen Effekt. Über Corticoideinsparung im Meeresklima berichten auch HARNACK und PÜRSCHEL. — Bei der Durchführung thalassotherapeutischer kurmäßiger Behandlung dermatologischer Patienten unter den Gegebenheiten des Nordsee-Inselklimas konnte an der Nordseeklinik Westerland erneut festgestellt werden, daß in vielen Fällen auf vorangegangene Corticoidtherapie verzichtet werden kann. Im Verlaufe eines knappen Jahres ergaben sich 150 auswertbare Erkrankungsfälle, bei denen eine indizierte, rezente Corticoidanwendung zu eruieren war. Die Diagnosenverteilung, in Gruppen, ist aus der Abbildung ersichtlich.

In 86% der Fälle konnte eine vorangegangene interne Corticoidverabfolgung abgesetzt, in weiteren 5% reduziert werden. Bei den 14%, bei denen auf interne Corticoidtherapie nicht oder nicht ganz verzichtet werden konnte, handelte es sich durchweg um besonders schwere Erkrankungsfälle nach Anamnese, Befund bzw. Diagnose: Erythrodermien, Pemphigus, Mycosis fungoides und besonders schwere Neurodermitis disseminata. Bei allen Schwerkranken, als Gruppe für sich betrachtet, gelang es in der Hälfte dieser Fälle, kurativen Effekt und Corticoidverzicht miteinander zu vereinbaren. — Die Bedeutung dieses Phänomens, auf intern sonst zu verabfolgende Corticoide verzichten oder sie dosismäßig reduzieren zu können, ist angesichts der bekannten Vielfalt und Bedeutsamkeit möglicher Corticoid-Nebenwirkungen offenkundig.

Da ein erreichter Corticoidverzicht aber auch als Kriterium für einen Heilerfolg zu werten ist, interessierte uns die gestellte Frage ebenso im Hinblick auf die Lokalbehandlung, obwohl die Konsequenzen hierbei im allgemeinen nicht so ernst sind und daher meist großzügiger verfahren wird. — Auch bei unseren lokal mit Corticoid vorbehandelten Patienten handelte es sich fast ausschließlich um bis dato trotz intensiver Vorbehandlung unbefriedigend gebliebene Verlaufsformen. Unter zusätzlichem Einsatz thalassotherapeutischer Faktoren konnten in 40% externe Corticoidapplikationen, ohne daß es zu Rezidiven kam, abgesetzt und in 35%

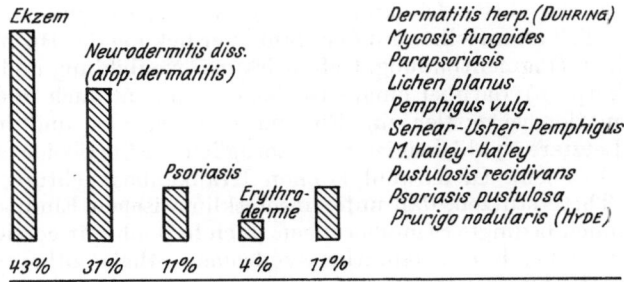

Abb. Diagnosenverteilung der 150 ausgewerteten Erkrankungsfälle

konzentrationsmäßig oder im Hinblick auf die Häufigkeit der Anwendung reduziert werden. Die verbleibenden 25% gliedern sich wie folgt auf: In 8% (der wirkliche Anteil ist sicher noch größer) waren eindeutige Störfaktoren nachweisbar, die nicht irgendeiner Therapie anzulasten sind (z. B. zu spät entdeckte Eigenbehandlung oder nicht ausgeschaltete anderweitige Kontaktnoxen, Renten-Neurosen u. a.), in 6% handelte es sich um besonders schwere Erkrankungsfälle im oben erwähnten Sinne und 11% blieben ohne plausible Erklärung.

Die Gründe für die Möglichkeit der Corticoideinsparung im Meeresklima sind zum Teil bekannt, zum Teil werden sie diskutiert. Es gibt über diese meeresklimatischen Einflüsse Klassifikationen, die ihre Gültigkeit haben. Daraus seien als besonders wichtig zitiert der aktinische und der — besonders von PFLEIDERER erforschte — sog. thermisch-hygrische Wirkungskomplex im weitesten Sinne, die sich ihrerseits wieder aus verschiedenen — zum Teil sehr differenten — Faktoren zusammensetzen (z. B. U.V.-, reine Licht-, Wärmestrahlung, Lufttemperatur, -bewegung, -feuchtigkeit). Diese müssen ärztlicherseits — und wenn dermatologische Probleme es erfordern, dermatologischerseits — gezielt eingesetzt, dosiert und expliziert werden*. Um meeresklimatische Faktoren individuell auszuschöpfen, d. h. auch auszuwählen, auszusortieren, um schädigende (z. B. photosensibilisierende) Einflüsse auszuschalten und schließlich, um parallellaufend geeignete bzw.

---

* Anm. b. d. Korr.: Diese vom Institut für Bioklimatologie und Meeresheilkunde der Universität Kiel seit langem erhobenen Forderungen werden seit einigen Jahren auf dem Therapiegelände dieses Instituts in Westerland bei Freiluft-Sonnenbehandlung von Dermatosen unter Verzicht auf konventionelle Therapie mit gutem Erfolg praktiziert [vgl. H. PFLEIDERER: Internationaler Kongreß für Thalassotherapie Westerland 1966 sowie Z. angew. Bäder- u. Klimaheilk. 8, 38 (1961)].

Auch bei meinen Psoriasispatienten, die dort freundlicherweise behandelt wurden, konnte ich die günstigen Ergebnisse feststellen.

notwendige konventionelle Therapie einsetzen zu können, ist laufende Überwachung der Kranken erforderlich.

Im Optimalfalle geschieht das stationär in unmittelbarer Strandnähe. Dann steht wirklich eine sehr breite Skala einsetzbarer thalassotherapeutischer Einflüsse und gegebenenfalls weiterer physikalischer und balneologischer Therapie zur Verfügung: vom ausgesprochenen „Schongang" der Liegekur unter Behaglichkeitsbedingungen über dosierte Freiluft-Insolationen bis zu stärksten Reizwirkungen beim Brandungsbaden und bei forcierter Bewegungstherapie am Strand: eine Eskalation im Training des Gesamtorganismus wie auch des Integumentes. Eine der wesentlichen Besonderheiten dürfte dabei sein, daß diese Anwendungen, z. B. insbesondere die Heliotherapie mit dem ihr eigentümlichen kontinuierlichen Strahlungsspektrum, einsetzbar sind, ohne daß es zu Hitzestauungen oder Schweißstauungen kommen müßte. Diese werden durch die ständige Luftbewegung verhindert.

Meeresklimatische aktive Direkteinwirkung auf das Integument manifestiert sich zum großen Teil unmittelbar auf der Haut (Verdickung der Hornschicht) oder besser in derselben (Pigmentbildung, Gefäßwirkung, Neubildung und Aktivierung von Sulfhydrilkörpern); darüber hinaus ist das Integument auch in der Thalassotherapie Informationsvermittler zur Einschaltung nervaler und inkretorischer Regulationen. Letztere zu objektivieren, ist bezüglich der Corticoide ein noch nicht völlig gelöstes Problem. Gleichwohl können Krankenbeobachtung und Untersuchungen die These stützen, daß unter meeresklimatischen Einflüssen abgemilderte, stress-ähnlich bedingte Stimulierungen, auch hypophysär-corticotrop, intervenieren. Andererseits gibt es Adaptationssyndrome — thalassotherapeutische auf jeden Fall — auch ohne Intervention der Hypophysen-Nebennieren-„Achse". In Tierversuchen sind Adaptationssyndrome sogar nach operativer Entfernung der Nebennieren bekannt geworden (SELLERS u. Mitarb.).

Zurückkommend auf die Ersetzbarkeit bzw. das Weglassen von Corticoiden durch Einsatz der Thalassotherapie, ist festzustellen, daß hier durch ein Zusammenspiel zahlreicher accessorischer Faktoren Voraussetzungen dafür geschaffen werden, daß auf jeden Fall der Corticoidbedarf absinkt. Darüber hinaus darf als wahrscheinlich gelten, daß zumindest in manchen Fällen auch die körpereigene Produktion stimuliert werden kann.

Die Leistungsfähigkeit der Thalassotherapie ist sicher noch zu steigern, wenn sie weniger als bislang erst als ultima ratio bemüht wird. Sie könnte — und das hat sie interessanterweise mit der Corticoidbehandlung gemeinsam — sogar unter Umständen die Rolle einer echt kausalen Therapie *dann* spielen, wenn es ihr gelingt, einen circulus vitiosus zu durchbrechen.

Literatur. AMELUNG, W., u. A. EVERS: Handbuch der Bäder- und Klimakeilhunde. Stuttgart 1962 (s. hier auch bei JUNGMANN, H., R. LOTZ, W. SCHMIDT-KESSEN und E. G. SCHULTZE). — DAUGHADAY, W. H.: J. clin. Invest. **37**, 51 (1958). — DAUBERT, K., u. F. AICHINGER: In Dermatologie und Venerologie, hrsg. v. GOTTRON, H. A., u. W. SCHÖNFELD, Bd. I, Teil 2. Stuttgart 1962. — HARTUNG, J.: In Dermatologie und Venerologie, hrsg. v. GOTTRON, H. A., u. W. SCHÖNFELD, Bd. II Teil 1. — HARNACK, K.: Derm. Wschr. **151**, 553, 1080 (1965). — HARTUNG, J., u. W. PÜRSCHEL: Kompendium der Klimatherapie von Hautkrankheiten an der Nordsee, hrsg. v. Deutschen Bäderverband E.V., Bonn (Efferen b. Köln, 1964). — JESSEL, U.: Z. angew. Bäder- u. Klimaheilk. **13**, 240 (1966). — LINSER, K.: In Fortschritte der praktischen Dermatologie und Venerologie, Bd. IV. Berlin 1962. — LUDWIG, G.: Internationaler Kongreß für Thalassotherapie Westerland 1966. — MENGER, W., u. W. UNGER: Arch. phys. Ther. (Lpz.) **17**, 225 (1965). — MILCU, S. M., AL. LUNGU, A. TACHE, E. BERLESCU and A. SCHULLER: Z. angew. Bäder- u. Klimaheilk. **14**, 62 (1967). — NELSON, D. H.: Metabolism **11**, 894 (1961). — PFLEIDERER, H.: Z. angew. Bäder- u. Klimaheilk. **8**, 38 (1961). — Arch. phys. Ther. (Lpz.) **17**, 305 (1965). — Stud. gen. (Berl.) **17**, 533 (1964). — Internationaler Kongreß für Thalassotherapie, Westerland 1966. — PÜRSCHEL, W.: Z. Haut- u. Geschl.-Kr. **XXXII**, 199 (1962). — ROBINSON, I. R.: Physiol. Rev. **40**, 112 (1960). — SELLERS, E. A., S. S. YOU, and N. THOMELS: Amer. J. Physiol. **178**, 449 (1951).

Indications for and Results of Systemic Corticosteroid Therapy in Dermatology

J. C. P. LOGAN and A. GIRDWOOD FERGUSSON, Department of Dermatology, Stobhill General Hospital, Glasgow (Scotland)

A clinic concerned as much with prevention as with treatment is surely unique in dermatological practice, yet that is what we have at Stobhill Hospital. When it is added that this clinic is concerned with the control of such killing conditions as the following, it will be clear that it is also a life-saving activity (numbers of cases of each disease are included in parentheses): Early mycosis fungoides (22), acute systemic lupus erythematosus (3), senile dermatitis herpetiformis (10), pemphigus foliaceus (4) and vegetans (1), periarteritis nodosa (3), cranial arteritis (1), nodular vasculitis (1), erythema multiforme with Behçet's (1) and Stevens-Johnson (2) syndromes, urticaria with angioneurotic oedema (1) and lymphadenoma (1) and lymphatic leukaemia (1) both with erythrodermia. Conditions of less urgency comprise psoriasis (28) especially with exfoliation and arthritis, atopic exzema (16), idiopathic exfoliative dermatitis (1), parapsoriasis lichenoides (1), infectious eczematoid dermatitis (1), seborrhoeic eczema (1), dermatitis venenata (1), lichen planus (2), prurigo nodularis (1), aphthous mouth ulcers (3) and relapsing febrile nodular non-suppurative panniculitis (1). Our "Steroid Clinic" has been in operation since 1953.

Material and Methods

107 cases receiving systemic corticosteroid therapy under our care were followed up over the past 10 years. There were 45 females and 62 males whose ages ranged between 9 and 85 years with a mean of 52 years. Various oral preparations were used but we favoured triamcinolone and later betamethasone which we now prescribe most often. Treatment commenced invariably with the patient in hospital on a dose of 8 tablets daily (one tablet is the equivalent of 5 mg of prednisolone), reducing gradually according to response until a recrudescence appeared, after which it was held at the lowest possible maintenance dose. In assessing results the category "excellent or good" signified activity minimal or symptomless on a daily dose of three tablets or less: "fair or poor" signified still active but controlled on a daily maintenance dose of up to three tablets or more.

Results

The favourable effect of corticosteroids in early mycosis fungoides except in one case — a notorious defaulter — is evident in the table. Most of these cases presented as exfoliative dermatitis with adenitis and intense pruritus. A regular feature in the course of therapy was persistent recrudescence of activity whenever the maintenance dose was reduced, but this dose tended in a few to become lower

Table. *Results of corticosteroid therapy in 107 cases*

Diseases	Results		Totals
	Excellent or good	Fair or poor	
Mycosis fungoides	21	1	22
Psoriasis	5	23	28
Atopic eczema	9	7	16
Infective eczema	0	2	2
Bullous conditions	8	10	18
Allergic vascular reactions	5	1	6
Other dermatoses	9	6	15
Totals	57	50	107

through time, allowing even withdrawal of therapy in one case. Histopathology
was seldom typical of the mature reticulosis but revealed generally some abnormality of cells and nuclei. It is our opinion that the satisfactory response in 21 cases
gives promise of being able to control mycosis fungoides indefinitely by this means
if diagnosed at an early stage.

Initial response was good in exfoliative psoriasis and psoriasis with arthritis,
but a high maintenance dose sometimes became necessary thereafter with consequent severity of side-effects requiring gradual withdrawal of therapy. In these
instances no rebound effect was observed. Results recorded in all the other conditions are fairly evenly balanced between the two chosen categories, although
notably good in allergic vascular reactions which included two cases of periarteritis
nodosa in which truly remarkable suppression of active disease was achieved.

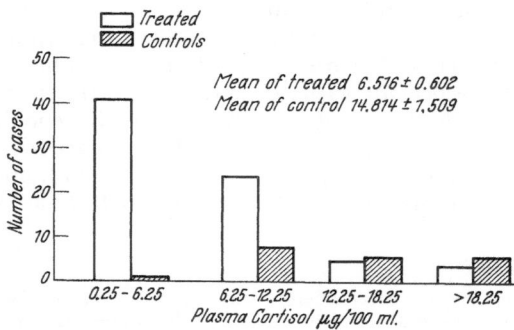

Fig. Reduction in the level of plasma cortisol of 74 treated cases compared with 21 controls

Side-effects. The usual manifestations associated with Cushing's syndrome were
encountered, diminishing since the advent of better oral preparations of the hormone and as our experience increased. The most frequent side-effects were (totals
included in parentheses): infections of the skin (33) with steroid acne (11) and
hypertension of varying degree (24); and the most serious complications were
osteoporosis (3) with vertebral collapse (3), pulmonary tuberculosis supervening (3)
and activated (1), hyperglycaemia (5) with steroid-induced diabetes (3), peptic
ulcer (5) with haemorrhage (1) and perforation (1), and adrenal failure following
septicaemia (1).

Tests of Endocrine Function. The figure shows the level of plasma cortisol in
74 treated cases (open bars) and 21 controls (solid bars). This histogram illustrates
reduction in the level pf plasma cortisol of treated patients. Mean values are
6.516 $\pm$ 0.602 for the treated cases and 14.814 $\pm$ 1.509 for the controls, and they
are significantly different. No correction for skewness was made in the calculation.

The Thirty-minute Synacthen (synthetic corticotrophin) test was carried out
in 19 cases on various doses of corticosteroids and 14 cases showed evidence of
adrenal suppression: 1 of 6 controls was also low. This test was applied to 7 cases
in which corticosteroids had been stopped for varying intervals and the only
2 showing suppression, in one continuing after 3 weeks and in the other up to
4 months, had been on high maintenance doses.

Acknowledgements. We wish to thank Dr. J. K. GRANT of the University Department of
Steroid Biochemistry where the tests of endocrine function were carried out, and Dr. ALEX
BERRIE, also of Glasgow University, for his advice on presentation and statistics, as well as
Mr. P. S. WALDIE of the Medical Photography Department, Stobhill Hospital, Glasgow, for
reproducing the table and the figure.

Influencia de los corticosteroides en la queratinizacion

A. M. Mom, Universidad de Buenos Aires, Hospital Argerich, Buenos Aires (Argentina)

El mecanismo de la queratinización y sus modificaciones por corticosteroides fue estudiado en pacientes con psoriásis, ictiósis y controles. En algunos casos se comparó la actividad diferencial entre corticosteroides y antifólicos.

Este estudio se realizó por medios histológicos e histoquímicos (microscopía óptica y electrónica) y bioquímicos (electroforesis en papel, agar y poliacrilamida).

Ultraestructura de las lesiones: La epidermis psoriásica muestra reducción en cantidad y densidad electrónica de tonofibrillas, disminución progresiva del número y desarrollo de desmosomas, agrandamiento de espacios intercelulares y desaparición del estrato granuloso que es sustituído por un número variable de capas celulares con granos defectuosos de queratohialina.

En los estratos descamantes los desmosomas residuales quedan adheridos a una de las capas córneas. En la psoriásis se dividen por la zona clara media: la perforación de los desmosomas de las capas epidérmicas superiores es etapa previa.

El queratinosoma es el cuarto elemento de la queratinización cuya abundancia y topografía varía en piel normal y psoriásica. Presentes en cuerpo mucoso van disminuyendo en el citoplasma celular hacia la capa córnea y aumentando su relación con la membrana plasmática, como si emigraran hacia el espacio intercelular para colocarse entre los desmosomas. En las capas granulosa y córnea puede verse la alternancia de queratinosomas y desmosomas residuales, perdiendo su aparato fibrilar.

Bajo triamcinolona oral o fluocinolona local se observa: 1. mayor número y densidad de tonofilamentos; 2. disminución en amplitud de espacios intercelulares; 3. aumento de desmosomas con mejor desarrollo filamentoso; 4. secuencia similar a la normal del proceso de queratinización y 5. disminución de células con queratinosomas libres en citoplasma. Estos son mas numerosos en la granulosa y en los espacios intercelulares córneos, que en piel normal.

Bajo metotrexato los cambios son similares, aunque mas lentos. La diferencia estructural más neta se observó en los tonofilamentos. La triamcinolona produce una tendencia notablemente mayor a la disposición en haces y los filamentos son de mayor tamaño y densidad que los inducidos por metotrexato. Los queratinosomas son más abundantes bajo triamcinolona. En síntesis, triamcinolona produce una normalización más rápida y completa de la queratinización que metotrexato.

Histoquímica de las reacciones enzimáticas: Las biopsias se practicaron cada 7 días, durante 6 semanas, en psoriásicos sometidos a triamcinolona oral o metotrexato parenteral. Se estudiaron: fosfatasa alcalina (naftol AS-MX); fosfatasa ácida; adenosintrifosfatasa y esterasa inespecífica.

Bajo metotrexato los resultados fueron:

1. *Esterasas:* La actividad intensamente positiva de la zona queratógena disminuye progresivamente hasta acantonarse en cuerpo granuloso que se reconstituye desde el día 14. En dermis las modificaciones son mucho menos marcadas. La actividad esterásica permanece invariable en las células próximas a los capilares papilares.

2. *Fosfatasa ácida:* La actividad intensa de la zona paraqueratósica declina en forma similar a la de esterasas. Finalmente queda localizada en capa granulosa y parte alta del estrato espinoso. En dermis la gran actividad se atenúa rápidamente, persistiendo pocos elementos celulares con reacción positiva franca en dermis papilar.

3. *ATPasa:* En epidermis sucede lo mismo que con las anteriores, quedando limitada a la capa granulosa. Los pequeños y grandes vasos dérmicos, muestran idéntica y persistente actividad a pesar del tratamiento.

4. *Fosfatasa alcalina:* Esta enzima muestra las modificacione siguientes: disminución del calibre y número de los capilares papilares, rectificación de su trayecto y franca declinación de la reacción durante la actividad antifólica.

Bajo triamcinolona las modificaciones son similares pero se realizan en la mitad del tiempo requerido para el metotrexato. Acantosis y papillomatosis tienden a normalizarse más rápida y netamente con triamcinolona.

Los elementos dérmicos con intensa actividad esterásica y de fosfatasa ácida no sufren influencia aparente por triamcinolona, manteniendo sus reacciones.

En síntesis, salvo para fosfatasa ácida, la influencia de ambas drogas en la queratinización es cualitativamente similar. La velocidad de regresión bajo triamcinolona es el doble de la del metotrexato.

Isoesterasas epidérmicas: El estudio electroforético de enzimas de la epidermis normal, psoriásica, ictiósis y del pénfigo foliáceo así como familiares clínicamente sanos de psoriásis se limita en este análisis a esterasas inespecíficas. Los resultados toman en conjunto las técnicas papel, agar y poliacrilamida.

En los extractos de capa córnea normal se detecta una sola banda esterasa A, inhibida parcialmente por eserina. En *psoriasis* las bandas son 3 (agar-gel y papel, 5 o más en poliacrilamida), A, B_1 y B_2, inhibidas casi totalmente por eserina. Bajo la acción de triamcinolona o de metotrexato las bandas adicionales se atenúan pero no desaparecen totalmente aunque la epidermis aparezca clínicamente normal. En algunos hijos o hermanos de psoriásicos se detectan esterasas B_1 ó B_2 o ambas, poco definidas. En dos oportunidades ambas bandas desaparecieron (agar-gel) después de 8 días de triamcinolona. Dos meses después reaparecieron como originalmente (psoriásis latente?).

En *ictiosis* se detecta a menudo la esterasa B_1, que desaparece con triamcinolona o prednisona aunque por sus respuestas a inhibidores parece de estructura diferente a la de la psoriásis. En *pénfigo foliaceo* se detectan B_1 y B_2 que desaparecen bajo prednisona.

En síntesis, este estudio sugiere la existencia de formas moleculares enzimáticas epidérmicas peculiares, cuya influencia por corticosteroides necesita una detenida investigación.

Seltene Nebenerscheinungen bei der Therapie mit den Corticosteroiden an der dermatologischen Klinik in Zagreb

D. KARLIĆ und V. ČAJKOVAC, Dermatologische Klinik der Medizinischen Fakultät der Universität Zagreb (Jugoslawien)

Lang andauernde Behandlung chronischer Dermatosen mit hohen Dosen von Corticosteroiden, wie z.B. des chronischen vulgären Pemphigus, kann auch unerwünschte Nebenerscheinungen hervorrufen.

Während vor der corticosteroiden Therapie nur 13% der Erkrankten die ersten Anzeichen der Krankheit überlebt haben (RAAB, 1963) und die Mortalität 90% betragen hat, hat sich nach der Einführung der corticosteroiden Therapie die Mortalität auf 30% gesenkt (SÖNNICHSEN, 1964).

Bei unserem an chronischem vulgärem Pemphigus leidenden Kranken kam es im Laufe der lang andauernden Behandlung mit Corticosteroiden neben vielen anderen Begleiterscheinungen zu einer ungewöhnlich starken Wirkung auf das Knochensystem, und deshalb sind wir der Meinung, daß es vom besonderem Interesse ist, dies zu veröffentlichen.

Die durch Corticosteroide hervorgerufene Osteoporose ist der Osteoporese beim Cushing-Syndrom (LICHWITZ, 1961) identisch, und die im Laufe der Medikation mit Corticosteroiden an der Wirbelsäule auftretenden Veränderungen bezeichnete BATZENSCHLAGER (1962) mit dem Namen „vertèbre en poisson", während sie MAURER (1965) „Fischwirbelkrankheit" nennt.

Die Veränderungen kommen am deutlichsten am thorakolumbalen Teil der Wirbelsäule zum Ausdruck, wo es zu sog. Knocheninfarkten kommt, während die gleichzeitige Erscheinung der Osteomalacie nicht vorhanden ist.

Man nimmt an, daß die Corticosteroide primär auf mesenchymale Zellen wirken und so — direkt und indirekt — zur dramatischen Verringerung der Anzahl der für die Bildung des neuen Knochens notwendigen Zentren führen (KLEIN, 1965).

Unter allen Corticosteroiden wird die Osteoporose am häufigsten durch Dexamethason verursacht. BRUNI (1965) analysiert in seiner Arbeit das parallele Vorkommen der Osteoporose und der atrophischen Hautstriae.

An der Dermatovenerologischen Klinik in Zagreb wurden im Laufe der letzten 10 Jahre 49 an chronischem vulgärem Pemphigus leidende Kranke mit verschiedenen Corticosteroiden ärztlich behandelt (Cortison, Prednison, Prednisolon, Dexamethason).

Unser Fall: L. S. 36 Jahre alt, männlich, Landwirt. A. familiae: o.B. A. vitae: außer einem langjährigen Magenkatarrh immer gesund. A. Morbi: im Monat Juli 1960 sind bei ihm an der Schleimhaut der Mundhöhle Blasen in Erscheinung getreten und 7 Monate danach Bullae an der ganzen Haut des Körpers, vorwiegend an der Haut des Rückens, an der inneren Seite der Oberschenkel und perigenital. Rö. der Wirbelsäule, der Rippen und der Oberschenkel- und Oberarmbeine: Hyperlordose der cervicalen Wirbelsäule. Ausgesprochene Kyphoskolose des thorakolumbalen Teiles in Form eines verlängerten S.

Vorhanden ist eine starke Porose der Wirbel mit den sehr durchsichtigen verdünnten und dem Fischschwanz ähnlichen Wirbelcorpora. Auf diese Weise sind Intervertebralräume breiter geworden, was besonders im Lumbalteil zum Ausdruck kommt. Die Spongiose der Wirbel ist völlig reduziert, und die Corticalis, obwohl sie sehr dünn ist, läßt sich doch gut feststellen. Von den erwähnten Veränderungen sind die ersten fünf Halswirbel ausgenommen, die, obwohl osteoporotisch, keine Verkleinerung der Höhe des Rumpfes aufweisen.

Die beiden Oberschenkel und Oberarmbeine haben einen geringeren Kalkgehalt mit ausgesprochener Reduktion der Compacta, vorwiegend in ihrem Mittelteil. Die Dyaphysen der Oberarmbeine unterscheiden sich von der Compacta der Oberschenkelbeine, die nur stellenweise ein wenig reduziert ist, und zwar hauptsächlich in der Mitte des lateralen Teiles der Dyaphyse. Am medialen Rand des distalen Teiles der Dyaphyse des linken Oberschenkelbeines lassen sich geringere längliche Schichten des Periostes feststellen. In der Axillarlinie links sind Deformationen der Rippen, was dem Zustand nach den früheren spontanen Frakturen entspricht.

Orthopädischer Befund: Osteoporosis gradus maioris, Deformatio columnae vertebralis et thoracis, Contracturae, Radiculalgiae, Collapsus vertebrarum multiplicium.

Schlußfolgerungen: Aus dem dargestellten Material geht als Begleiterscheinung corticosteroider Therapie die Wirkung auf die Wirbelsäule selbst und die langen Knochen offensichtlich hervor, was sich durch Verminderung der Körpergröße um 25 cm bemerkbar macht.

Diese Erscheinung läßt sich nur dadurch erklären, daß der Patient durch längere Zeit hohe Dosen steroider Hormone eingenommen hat, obwohl er gleichzeitig mit Anabolika behandelt worden ist.

Durch eine bessere Kenntnis der Pathophysiologie der Corticosteroidwirkung auf das Skelet werden wir vermutlich imstande sein, die Osteoporose und im Zusammenhang damit auch eine eventuelle Verminderung der Körpergröße zu verhindern.

Die Insuffizienz der Nebenniere nach Corticoidbehandlung

E. Lacková, J. Rádl und M. Horáková, I. Kinderklinik, Forschungsinstitut der Entwicklung des Kindes, I. Dermatologische Klinik Prag (Tschechoslowakei)

Wenn auch der Mechanismus der Cortisontherapie bisher nicht ganz aufgeklärt ist, werden die Corticoide sehr oft in der medizinischen Praxis angewendet.

In vielen Fällen ist die Applikation der Corticoide ohne dauernden Effekt auf die Ursache der Krankheit und hat noch dazu viele Nebenwirkungen [1].

Heute wollen wir über einen Patienten mit chronischem Ekzem berichten; das Ekzem wurde mit einer staphylokokken Sepsis kompliziert; die laugdauernde Corticoidtherapie bewirkte eine irreversible Schädigung der Nebenniere, wobei die eigentliche Krankheit ungeheilt blieb.

Bei unserem Patienten, der im Jahre 1956 geboren wurde, begannen die ersten Anzeichen der Erkrankung im 1. Lebensjahr. Er wurde anfangs nur lokal behandelt, später mit Antibiotica, und nach 2 Jahren, als sein Zustand sich nicht besserte, wurden Corticoide verabreicht.

Auch jetzt wurde der Zustand nicht besser; es kam noch eine septische Temperatur dazu. Beim Versuch, die Dosis der Corticoide herabzusetzen oder sie ganz wegzulassen, stellten sich Kopfschmerzen, Schwäche, Erbrechen als Symptome der Insuffizienz der Nebenniere ein.

Im Oktober 1964 wurde das Kind in unsere Klinik aufgenommen. Das Kind war in sehr schlechtem Zustand, die Temperatur bewegte sich zwischen 38 bis 40 °C, die Haut war gerötet, infiltriert, mit vielen nassen Excoriationen. An einigen Stellen erschienen deutliche Desquamationen und papulöse Eruptionen auf erröteter Grundlage.

Nach einige Tage dauernder steriler Behandlung, bei der Applikation von Antibiotica, Plasma und Corticoiden, beruhigte sich die Haut, fiel die Temperatur ab, und der Allgemeinzustand des Patienten wurde besser.

Das führte uns dazu, die Dosis des Prednisons herabzusetzen oder ganz auszulassen. Schon 12 Std nach der Aussetzung des Prednisons stieg die Temperatur auf 39 bis 40 °C an, fingen Kopfschmerzen an, erschien ein Schwächezustand und weitere Anzeichen der Insuffizienz der Nebenniere. Wiederholt versuchten wir Corticoide wenigstens intermittent zu verabreichen, was immer eine schnelle Verschlechterung des Allgemeinzustandes zur Folge hatte. Deshalb waren wir gezwungen, die Corticoidtherapie ohne Unterbrechung fortzusetzen.

Die Haut wurde besser, aber der Knabe hatte ein cushingoides Aussehen. Im Alter von 10 Jahren hatte er eine Größe von 124 cm, eine betonte Osteoporosis und eine um 2 Jahre verspätete Ossifikation.

Von den Laboruntersuchungen führe ich wegen Zeitmangels nur einige Ergebnisse an. Im Blutbild war eine hypochrome Anämie zu sehen, die Antikörper gegen Haut, Leber, Milz waren negativ. Aus der Hämokultur wurde wiederholt pyogener Staphylococcus kultiviert.

Einen sehr interessanten Befund sahen wir bei der immunoelektrophoretischen Untersuchung des Serums. IgD wurde in einer großen Menge (100 mall als normal überschreitend) vorgefunden [2].

Wie wir sehen, hat die langdauernde Behandlung unseres Patienten eine irreversible Schädigung der Nebenniere verursacht. Die Veränderungen in den Immunoglobulinen kann man entweder als primäre (und darum ein so schwerer

Krankheitsverlauf) oder sekundär erklären. Bei der sekundären Auffassung hätte die langdauernde Behandlung mit Antibiotica und Corticoiden eine so ungewöhnliche Veränderung des Eiweißspektrums hervorgerufen.

Literatur. 1. LACKOVA, E., u. J. SVEJCAR: Fortschr. Med. **21**, 875 (1965). — 2. ROWE, D. S., and J. L. FAHEY: J. exp. Med. **121**, 171, 185 (1965).

Corticosteroid-Nebenwirkungen und ihre Behandlung durch klinische Klimatherapie an der Nordsee

W. PÜRSCHEL, Allergie- und Hautklinik Norderney (Deutschland)

In den letzten 10 Jahren wurden 7354 Hautkranke auf der Nordseeinsel Norderney klinischer Klimatherapie unterzogen. Die Kranken, die vorher mit Corticosteroiden behandelt worden waren, wurden nach unerwünschten Corticoid-Nebenwirkungen, wie pro-infektiös, pro-ulcerös, pro-diabetisch, pro-myopathisch, pro-psychotisch usw. untersucht.

Die Untersuchungen bezogen sich auf fast zwei gleich große Patientenkollektive.

Das erste Kollektiv mit 3747 Kranken bestand aus Patienten mit Psoriasis vulgaris bis zur Erythrodermie, mit Parapsoriasis, Mycosis fungoides, Urticaria, Lichen ruber, Ekzemen ohne Neurodermitis, Dermatitis herpetiformis Duhring u. a.

Vor der Klinikaufnahme war eine Corticoidbehandlung in 5% der Fälle (189 von 3747 Patienten) durchgeführt worden. Bei 83% mußte die Corticoidbehandlung schon vorher wegen unerwünschter Nebenwirkungen eingestellt werden. Bei Klinikaufnahme standen 32 Patienten unter einer Langzeitbehandlung, die 81 Nebenwirkungen zur Folge hatte. Vitale Indikation bestand nur bei zwei Pemphiguskranken, hier wurde die Corticoid-Tagesdosis reduziert. Alle anderen wurden von der Dauermedikation befreit und die Nebenwirkungen abgebaut. Entlassung erfolgte in 82% frei von krankhaften Hautveränderungen.

Vom zweiten Kollektiv wurden in 26,3% der Fälle, d. h. bei 950 von 3607 Patienten mit konstitutionellem Ekzem mit/ohne Asthma bronchiale [Synonyma: Neurodermitis (BROCQ), endogenes Ekzem (GOTTRON, KORTING), atopic dermatitis (COCA, SULZBERGER)], vor Klinikaufnahme eine längere Corticoidbehandlung durchgeführt.

Bei der Klinikaufnahme standen 487 Neurodermitiker unter Corticoid-Dauermedikation. Bei 89,5% der Fälle wurden 730 verschiedene Nebenwirkungen festgestellt. 204 Patienten wiesen zwei bzw. drei Nebenwirkungen auf. Corticoid-Abbauversuche waren vorher fehlgeschlagen.

Die Altersverteilung des Kollektivs zeigte, daß besonders die Altersklasse der 20- bis 30jährigen einen deutlichen Unterschied zur Altersverteilung der bundesdeutschen Bevölkerung aufwies.

Die Corticoid-Dauermedikation betrug bei 318 Kranken 6 bis 12 Monate, bei 98 bis 2 Jahre, bei 54 bis 4 Jahre, bei 17 bis 9 Jahre.

Am häufigsten wurde mit 24% das 6-Methyl-Prednisolon und mit 27,1% das Triamcinolon verwendet.

Von den 730 Nebenwirkungen wurden in 26,4% das cushingartige Syndrom mit Gewichtszunahmen bis 20 kg, in 14,6% Pyodermien und Pathomorphosen, in 13,7% allgemeine Resistenzminderung, Adynamie und gehäufte Infekte festgestellt. 89 Patienten, 11,7%, wiesen eine Steigerung der Aktivität bis zur psychomotorischen Unruhe auf, von diesen litten einige unter Suicidgedanken und

zeigten Suchterscheinungen. Herz- und Kreislaufbeschwerden wurden in 10,4%
verifiziert, darunter bedrohliche Kreislaufkollapse auch beim Corticoidabbau.
Gastritische Beschwerden bis zur Magenulcusbildung wurden in 5,7% festgestellt. Zweimal täuschten Röntgenbefunde der Magenschleimhaut ein Malignom
vor.

Weitere Nebenwirkungen waren: Steroid-Striae 4,6%, Menstruationsstörung
in 1,4% und gleich viel Leberschädigungen; Hautblutungen in 0,9% und Provokation einer latenten diabetischen Stoffwechselanomalie in 0,9% mit Blutzucker-
erhöhung von bis zu 500 mg-%. Die Steroidacne wurde in 0,6%, die Corticoid-
myopathien in 0,4% und pathologische Verschiebungen von Natrium, Kalium
und Calcium im Serum in 0,8% beobachtet.

Diese Feststellungen zeigten, daß die durch Corticoid-Dauermedikation gesetzten Schäden in fast allen Fällen größer waren als der therapeutische Nutzen,
daß die sog. Cushing-Schwellendosis keine unbedingte Garantie bietet, um
Schäden zu verhindern, daß ein Individualfaktor beim Auftreten von Schäden
bedeutungsvoll ist und daß vor und während notwendiger Corticoidmedikation
internistische Untersuchungen durchgeführt werden müssen, um Schäden zu verhindern bzw. rechtzeitig zu erkennen. Eine straffe ärztliche Führung ist uner-
läßlich. Dauerbehandelte sollten einen Cortisonpaß besitzen.

Die Corticoid-Dauermedikation und ihre Nebenwirkungen lassen sich klinisch
im Nordseereizklima sehr gut abbauen. Die günstige Nordseeklimawirkung liegt
insbesondere im cyclonalen Westwettergeschehen und führt zur Aktivierung des
Nebennierenrinden-Hypophysensystems und zur Regulierung des vegetativen
Nervensystems. Wichtig ist auch die günstige lokale Einwirkung verschiedener
meteorologischer Elemente und Wirkungskomplexe auf das erkrankte Hautorgan.
Im Nordseereizklima ist der Abbau der Dauermedikation je nach Fall bei Ruhig-
stellung in 2 bis 4 Wochen durchzuführen. Mindestens weitere 4 Wochen Klimabehandlung sind erforderlich, um den Patienten hauterscheinungsfrei zu entlassen.
Insgesamt 3 Monate sollte sich der Kranke nach Corticoidabbau wegen der bekannten Streßanfälligkeit schonen. Von den Nebenwirkungen können die meisten zum
Abklingen gebracht werden. Am längsten halten sich cushingartiges Syndrom und
besonders die Steroidstriae.

Auskunft über die Nordseeklimawirkung gibt unter anderem das Verhalten
absoluter eosinophiler Granulocyten bei konstitutionellen Ekzematikern (7 Wochen
Behandlungszeit). Bei der Klinikaufnahme ist keine Eosinophilie nachweisbar.
Nach Corticoidabbau erfolgt Zunahme der Eosinophilen mit nachfolgender weitgehender Normalisierung. Die Absicherung dieser Ergebnisse hinsichtlich Mittelwert und Streuung erfolgte mit dem R- oder Duncan-Test bzw. der F-Verteilung.
Das Gegenkollektiv ohne Corticoidbehandlung zeigt bei der Aufnahme die Eosinophilie, die sich während klinischer Klimatherapie normalisiert.

Daß sich klinische Klimatherapie bewährt, konnte gezeigt werden; daß sie bei
zu später Einweisung überfordert werden kann, zeigen 2% Mißerfolge. Bei zehn
Kranken konnte die Corticoid-Dauermedikation nicht mehr abgebaut werden, da
sich beim Abbauversuch lebensbedrohliche Krankheitszustände, wie Status
asthmaticus, Kreislaufkollapse je viermal und in zwei Fällen Erythrodermie mit
Kreislaufinsuffizienz einstellten.

A Cytotoxic Effect of Fluocinolone Acetonide

A. J. Cox and E. M. Farber, Department of Dermatology, Stanford University School of Medicine Palo Alto, Calif. (USA)

Much of the success of steroid therapy in dermatology has been attributed to a constricting effect upon hyperemic vessels and to a reduction of inflammatory infiltration. In the past few years it has been found in addition that proliferative processes, such as those of psoriasis and mycosis fungoides, have regressed after topical steroid application [1].

In order to analyze this process, 15 lesions of mycosis fungoides have been studied histologically at intervals up to 2 weeks following the onset of continuous topical therapy with 0.2% fluocinolone acetonide* under a plastic occlusive dressing. Three of the lesions were examined serially by biopsy 3, 6, 12 and 24 h after the onset of therapy. In addition, three chronic plaques from patients with psoriasis were similarly studied from 3 to 48 h after the onset of topical therapy with fluocinolone acetonide.

The lesions of mycosis fungoides selected for this study were plaques that had a typical histological appearance, with well-defined large atypical lymphoid cells both in the dermis and in the thickened epidermis, where they formed Pautrier microabscesses.

By 12 h after the beginning of the steroid treatment the number of infiltrated cells in the superficial dermis had already decreased. This decrease continued rapidly, though a few infiltrated cells remained in the deep dermis even after one week or more.

Changes in the epidermis also appeared early. By 6 h there was a distinct reduction in the number of infiltrated mononuclear cells in the epidermis, with disappearance of all large hyperchromatic nuclei. The loss of infiltrated cells was more pronounced at 12 h, and by 24 h these cells were practically absent from the epidermis.

The epidermal cells were also affected, leading to a rapid decrease in epidermal thickness. In scattered individual epidermal cells in or near the stratum basale, there was evidence of a cytotoxic effect. These cells showed pyknosis and sometimes fragmentation of nuclei. Some of these apparently necrotic cells were in pairs, suggesting that there had been recent division. This focal degenerative change in single epidermal cells, localized to the region of the basal layer, was still present in lesions sampled 1 week after the onset of therapy, but was encountered less frequently after 2 weeks of therapy.

The three similarly treated psoriatic plaques showed comparable changes in epidermal cells, appearing first in the 6 h specimens and. reaching a peak at 24 h. These abnormal cells were still found after several days of continuous treatment, but they were rare after the epidermal thickness had returned to normal.

Whether the remarkably rapid disappearance of infiltrated cells from lesions of mycosis fungoides during topical therapy with 0.2% fluocinolone acetonide resulted from a cytotoxic effect upon the infiltrated cells is not certain, but the appearance at the same time of focal necrosis in epidermal cells suggests that the non-epithelial cells may have received a similar injury which could not be so clearly identified. Apparently certain epidermal cells were particularly susceptible, because the effect was not uniform. The localization of the damaged epidermal

* The fluocinolone acetonide in a cream containing propylene glycol was supplied by Syntex Laboratories, Palo Alto, Calif.

cells almost exclusively to the region of the basal layer, and the presence of pairs
of such cells, suggest that cells in some stage of division may have been the
principal site of injury, although not all phases of the mitotic process are arrested.
This could account for the prominence of regressive changes in the hyperplastic
epidermis of lesions of mycosis fungoides or of psoriasis, while epidermis of normal
thickness is much less modified by topical steroid application.

Inhibitory effects of steroids upon growing cells in culture have been observed,
and fluocinolone acetonide has been shown to have a particularly powerful
inhibitory effect upon cultures of fibroblasts, in which morphological changes
suggest cell injury [2]. Two very recent reports [3, 4] have described growth
inhibition in cultured epidermis in the presence of hydrocortisone. We presume
that such effects are comparable to the cell injury that we have identified in this
in vivo study.

We have concluded that focal cell death plays a role in the involution of
hyperplastic epidermis in lesions of mycosis fungoides and of psoriasis treated by
topical application of concentrated preparations of fluocinolone acetonide. The
appearance is most consistent with a toxic effect that specifically injures dividing
cells.

References. 1. FARBER, E. M., A. J. COX, J. STEINBERG, and R. P. MCCLINTOCK: Cancer
(Philad.) **19**, 237 (1966). — 2. RUHMANN, A. G., and D. L. BERLINER: Endocrinology **76**, 916
(1965). — 3. CARON, G. A.: J. invest. Derm. Submitted for publication. — 4. REAVEN, E. P.,
and A. J. COX: J. invest. Derm. Submitted for publication.

Vergleich zwischen der vasoconstrictorischen und antientzündlichen Wirkung verschiedener Corticosteroide

H. TRONNIER, Universitäts-Hautklinik Tübingen (Deutschland)

Die vergleichende Prüfung der antientzündlichen Wirkung lokal angewendeter
Corticosteroide ist problematisch [3]. Aus den Untersuchungen von MCKENZIE
[4, 5] über die unterschiedliche Vasoconstriction der einzelnen Corticosteroide
wurde später auch auf deren antientzündliche Wirkung geschlossen.

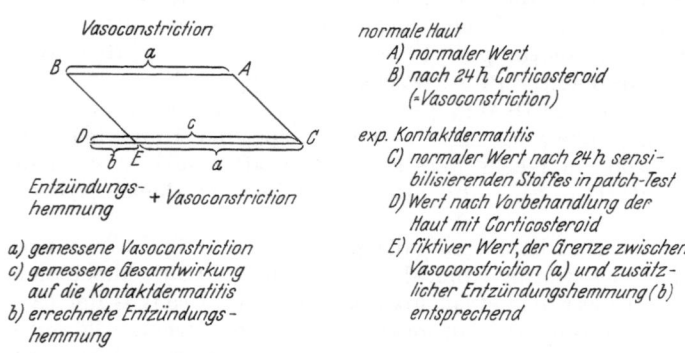

Abb. 1. Schema der Versuchsdurchführung

Unsere Untersuchungen, die ausführlich in zwei Dissertationen dargestellt
sind [1, 2], dienten der Beantwortung der Frage: Ist die Vasoconstriction direkt
ein Maß für die Entzündungshemmung eines Corticosteroids?

Für die Untersuchungen haben wir an der Haut die Temperatur, die modifizierte Wärmeleitfähigkeit [7] und die Farbe [6] gemessen, und zwar zunächst an der normalen Rückenhaut von 35 Versuchspersonen (Abb. 1). Das ergab den Wert A; nach 24stündigem Occlusivverband mit den Corticosteroidsalben ergab sich der Wert B und somit die Strecke a als Maß für die Vasoconstriction. Bei 20 unterschiedlich sensibilisierten Versuchspersonen wurden dann die gleichen Werte für den Epicutantest ohne Behandlung (Punkt C) und nach Vorbehandlung der Haut (2 Std vor Anlage des Patch-Tests) mit Corticosteroiden (Punkt D) bestimmt. Unter der fiktiven Annahme, die Vasoconstriction a_1 sei gleich a, wurde dann b als Entzündungshemmung aus der kombinierten Wirkung c errechnet.

Geprüft wurden insgesamt 32 Präparate mit unterschiedlichen Corticosteroiden und Grundlagen (Abb. 2).

Die Meßwerte a und c sowie die errechneten b-Werte, aufgeschlüsselt für die einzelnen Corticosteroide bei der Temperaturmessung, zeigt die folgende Abb. 3. Niedrige a-Werte entsprechen einer hohen vasoconstrictorischen Wirkung, niedrige c-Werte einem guten kombinierten vasoconstrictorisch-entzündungshemmenden Effekt und hohe, möglichst positive Werte für b zeigen den errechneten Anteil der reinen Entzündungshemmung an.

Günstig liegt also hier Fluocortolon, besonders schlecht mit gerade umgekehrt verlaufender Kurve Dexamethason.

	Creme	Salbe	Lotio (Schaum)	Lösung	Spray
Hydrocortison	1	1	1	—	—
Prednisolon	1	2	—	—	1
Triamcinolon	1	2	1	—	1
Dexamethason	1	2	—	—	—
Methyl-Fluor-Pr.	1	1	1	1	—
Fluocinolon	1	1	1	—	—
Fluorandrenolon	1	1	1	—	—
Beta-methason	1	1	—	—	—
Fluocortolon	—	1	—	—	—
Flumethason	1	1	—	—	—
Fluoprednilyden	—	1	—	—	—
Versuchspräparat	—	1	—	—	—

Abb. 2. Geprüfte Corticosteroidzubereitungen

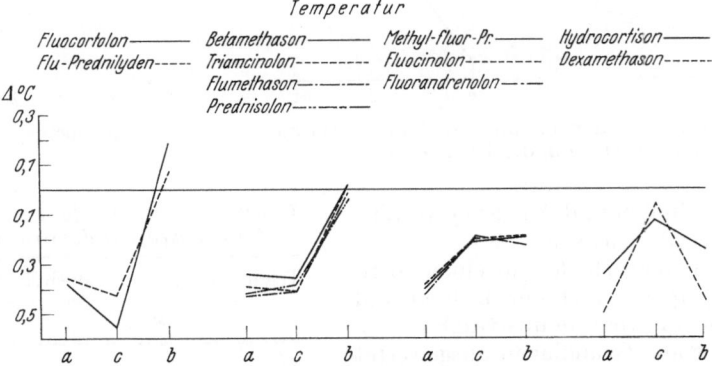

Abb. 3. Vasoconstriction (a) und kombinierte Wirkung (c) sowie errechneter antientzündlicher Wirkungsanteil (b) in der Temperaturmessung

Ähnliche Kurven (Abb. 4) erhält man auch bei der Bestimmung der Wärmeleitfähigkeit; wiederum liegt Fluocortolon besonders günstig, während Dexamethason trotz hohen vasoconstrictorischen Effektes nur eine geringe zusätzliche Entzündungshemmung zeigt. Etwas abweichend sind die Kurven bei der Farbmessung (Abb. 5). Hierbei wird ja die abnehmende Blutfülle, nicht der verringerte Blutdurchfluß erfaßt. Jetzt finden sich die günstigsten Werte für Betamethason

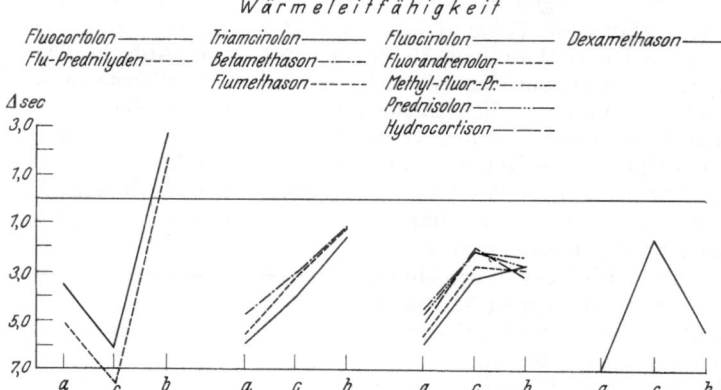

Abb. 4. Vasoconstriction (a) und kombinierte Wirkung (c) sowie errechneter antientzündlicher Wirkungsanteil (b) in der mod. Wärmeleitfähigkeitsmessung

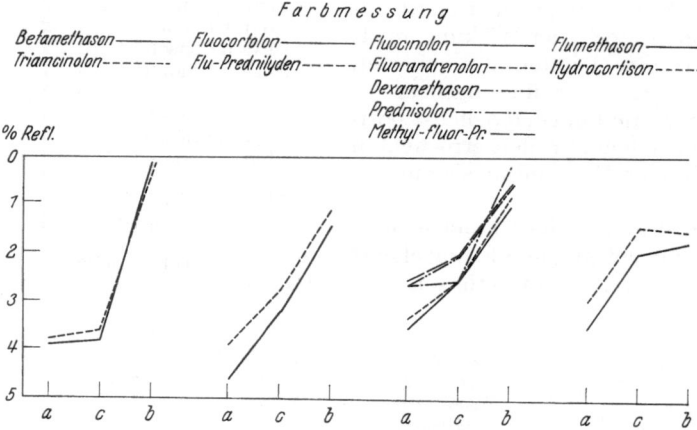

Abb. 5. Vasoconstriction (a) und kombinierte Wirkung (c) sowie errechneter antientzündlicher Wirkungsanteil (b) in der Farbmessung

und Triamcinolon und die geringste Wirkung für Hydrocortison.

Diese Mittelwerte der einzelnen Corti-
costeroidgruppen sind nur bedingt auf
die einzelnen Präparate übertragbar, weil
hier immer alle Grundlagen ausgewertet
wurden und, wie die Tab. 1 zeigt, Salben und Cremes meist wirksamer als die
anderen Formen sind. Da die einzelnen
Werte der drei Tests untereinander nicht
direkt vergleichbar sind, wurde für die
weitere Auswertung immer der Platz der
einzelnen Präparate der Serien zugrunde
gelegt und jeweils die Summe der Plätze
für die drei Tests (Sp) aufgeführt.

Tabelle 1. *Unterschiedliche Wirkung (c)*
in Abhängigkeit von der Grundlage

Triamcinolon		Methyl-Fluor-Prednisolon	
	$S_{p\ (c)}$		$S_{p\ (c)}$
Creme	11	Creme	56
Salbe	14	Salbe	59
Lotio	31	Lösung	62
Spray	78	Schaum	80

Schlüsselt man in gleicher Weise die einzelnen Präparate auf, und zwar einmal
nach der kombinierten Wirkung (c), zum
anderen nach der reinen Vasoconstriction
(a), so erhält man für die jeweils acht
wirksamsten die folgenden Werte (Tab. 2).

Es ist zu sehen, daß keines der Präparate gleichzeitig in beiden Gruppen vorkommt. In der ersten finden sich Triamcinolon, Betamethason und Fluocortolon, in der zweiten u. a. Dexamethason. Für den Volon-A-Spray liegen offenbar besondere Resorptionsverhältnisse vor, auf die hier nicht eingegangen werden kann.

Tabelle 2. *Zusammenstellung der acht Präparate A. mit der besten kombinierten Wirkung (c) B. dem stärksten vasoconstrictorischen Effekt (a)*

Präparat	Wirkstoff	$S_{p\,(c)}$	$S_{p\,(a)}$
A. Volon-A-Creme	Triamcinolon	11	42
Ultralan-Salbe	Fluocortolon	11	53
Volon-A-Salbe	Triamcinolon	14	49
Celestan-Salbe	Betamethason	16	65
Delphicort-Salbe	Triamcinolon	19	44
Decoderm	Fluoprednilyden	19	57
Volon-A-Lotio	Triamcinolon	31	48
Celstan-Creme	Betamethason	32	45
B. Fortecortin-Creme	Dexamethason	79	25
Jellin-Creme	Fluocinolon	33	31
Volon-A-Spray	Triamcinolon	78	31
Sermaka-Creme	Fluorandrenolon	56	33
Decortin-Creme	Prednisolon	73	34
Delmeson-Creme	Methyl-Fluor-Pr.	56	36
Millicorten-V-Cr.	Dexamethason	43	40
Jellin-Lotio	Fluocinolon	44	40

Bestimmt man nun noch die Differenz zwischen Vasoconstriction (a) und kombinierter Wirkung (c), so kann man wieder zwei Gruppen bilden: A. mit einer gegenüber der Vasoconstriction besonders guten kombinierten Wirkung, B. einer zwar relativ guten vasoconstrictorischen, aber vergleichsweise geringen kombinierten Wirkung (Tab. 3).

Tabelle 3. *Differenz zwischen $S_{p\,(a)}$ und $S_{p\,(c)}$, A. $S_{p\,(c)}$ besser als $S_{p\,(a)}$, B. $S_{p\,(a)}$ besser als $S_{p\,(c)}$*

Präparat	Wirkstoff	$S_{p\,(a)} - S_{p\,(c)}$
A. Celestan-Salbe	Beta-Methason	+ 49
Ultralan-Salbe	Fluocortolon	+ 42
Versuchspräp. 1106	—	+ 38
Volon-A-Salbe	Triamcinolon	+ 35
Voloh-A-Creme	Triamcinolon	+ 31
B. Volon-A-Spray	Triamcinolon	— 47
Eucortyl-Salbe	Dexamethason	— 45
Fortecortin-Creme	Dexamethason	— 44
Decortin-Creme	Prednisolon	— 39
Cohortan-Salbe	Hydrocortison	— 27

Aus den Ergebnissen der Gruppe B ist jetzt noch deutlicher abzulesen, daß Dexamethason zwar eine gute Vasoconstriction zeigt, aber bezüglich der Entzündungshemmung besonders ungünstig liegt.

Daß die Grundlagen eine wesentliche Rolle spielen, ist wieder am Volon-A-Spray in dieser Gruppe zu erkennen. Sie sind es wohl auch, die für die unterschiedlichen Ergebnisse in Abhängigkeit von dem verwendeten Allergen verantwortlich sind. Diese Abhängigkeit, auf die hier nicht näher eingegangen werden kann, sei an einer letzten Tabelle (Tab. 4) dargestellt, in der die acht wirksamsten Präparate mit ihren Plätzen bei zwei unterschiedlichen Allergenen aufgeführt sind.

Tabelle 4. *Verteilung der Plätze für die Hauttemperaturmessung für die acht insgesamt wirksamsten Präparate bei zwei unterschiedlichen Allergenen*

Präparat	Allergen	
	K-Dichromat $S_{p(c)}$ temp.	Terpentin $S_{p(c)}$ temp.
Volon-A-Creme	14	7
Ultralan-Salbe	4	4
Volon-A-Salbe	16	16
Celestan-Salbe	8	17
Delphicort-Salbe	1	1
Decoderm	32 (!)	3
Volon-A-Lotio	5	25 (!)
Celestan-Creme	2	27 (!)

Zusammenfassend ergaben die Versuche:

1. Triamcinolon, Betamethason und Fluocortolon sind in dieser Versuchsanordnung am wirksamsten.

2. Dexamethason und Hydrocortison sind am wenigsten wirksam, obwohl die Vasoconstriction beim Dexamethason besonders deutlich ist.

3. Salben und Cremes sind in der Regel wirksamer als Lotio, Lösung und Spray.

4. Der vasoconstrictorische Effekt der Corticosteroide geht nicht mit einer Entzündungshemmung parallel.

Literatur. 1. KOHLER, H. G.: Methodische Untersuchungen zur getrennten Erfassung von Vasoconstriction und Entzündungshemmung bei externen Corticoidsteroidzubereitungen unter Berücksichtigung der Grundlage. Inaug. Dissertation, Tübingen 1967. — 2. HEINECKE, F.: Prüfung verschiedener Corticosteroide im Hinblick auf ihre Vasoconstriction und Entzündungshemmung an der menschlichen Haut. Inaug. Dissertation, Tübingen 1967. — 3. HEITE. H.-J., K. W. KALKOFF und H. KOHLER: Hautarzt 14, 222 (1960). — 4. McKENZIE, A. W.: Arch. Derm. Syph. (Chic.) 86, 611 (1962). — 5. McKENZIE, A. W., and R. B. STOUGHTON: Arch. Derm. Syph. (Chic.) 86, 608 (1962). — 6. TRONNIER, H.: Strahlentherapie 121, 392 (1963). — 7. TRONNIER, H., u. G. HOPPE-SEYLER: Aesth. Med. 14, 254 (1965).

Penetration Studies with C^{14}-Labelled Fluocinolone Acetonide

M. K. POLANO and L. DE BEUKELAAR, Department of Dermatology, University Hospital, Leiden (Holland)

Let me begin to state that erroneously the program attributes this paper to me alone. It is a joint effort of DE BEUKELAAR and me, we planned together, but he did most of the work. Secondly I must remark that when we promised in November 1965 to read a paper on the penetration of corticosteroids into the skin, we hoped to be able to tell you now, in August 1967, about the results of experiments then being carried out. This turned out to be an error too.

We started from the fact that although fluocorticosteroids have no effect on psoriasislesions after simple inunction, they have a marked effect after inunction plus plastic occlusion. We considered it important to establish, by using isotope-labelled fluocinolone acetonide, the differences in the penetration of corticosteroids into the skin with and without plastic occlusion. We hoped that this might provide us with a clue about the point of impact of the drug, as well as provide information on drug penetration generally. We used fluocinolone acetonide cream (0.025% 6.4 microcurie/gr) in our ointments. 50 mg of this cream was evenly distributed over a circular spot with a diameter of 4 cm on the thigh of volunteers. We wanted to establish first two things:

1. whether with this concentration of isotope-labelled substance the skin would take up enough radioactive material to permit autoradiographic observations, and

2. whether the radioactivity would disappear from the skin sufficiently rapidly to safeguard the patients from undesirable radiation consequences.

Punch-biopsysamples (5 mm diameter) were made 1, 4 and 16 days after application of the ointment and the radioactivity of the sample was determined in a liquid photoscintillator. The results in five persons were:

Table. *Results of radioactivity measurements in a liquid photo-scintillator of punch-biop-sysamples determined at various intervals after inunction with C^{14}-labelled fluocinolone acetonide*

Interval	24 h	4 days	16 days
T 3	33 560 C/50 min	10 520 C/50 min	7 605 C/50 min
T 4	21 817 C/50 min	11 952 C/50 min	3 740 C/50 min
T 5	36 620 C/50 min	1 835 C/50 min	3 270 C/50 min
T 6	30 370 C/50 min	9 215 C/50 min	1 210 C/50 min /14th. day
T 7	23 565 C/50 min	2 347 C/50 min	662 C/50 min

This table shows: 1. after 24 h enough radioactivity is still present to make it probable that positive autoradiographs can be obtained and 2. that the biological half life of the radioactive material in the skin was sufficiently within the limits of safety to make the method acceptable.

In our first series of experiments also a second biopsy was made 24 h after application of the ointment. Deepfrozen cryostate sections were "sanwiched" between a slide and dental X-ray film and exposed for 80 to 100 days. In most cases a clearly visible black line became apparent after the film was developed. To our disappointment, here on the contrary no photographic grains were found with the stripping technique, in which the section is covered with a photosensitive emulsion that is floated upon water.

We supposed that in spite of the fact that fluocinolone acetonide is only 1:10000 soluble in water, the radioactive material is washed out from the section during the time that the slide carrying the sections is manipulated in water to catch the floating emulsion. To check this, we covered a section with water, which was later pipetted of and transferred to the liquid photoscintillator. The number of the counts was within the range that could be expected from the content of radioactive material of the section.

Our next step was to treat a new series of volunteers. On the assumption that the transport of the radioactive material through the skin during the first 24 h would be the most interesting, we performed biopsies at 2, 4, 8 and 24 h. The sections were worked up with the sandwich technique so that the exposed film could be re-aligned on the section responsible for the print on the dental X-ray film. To make this re-alignment possible, marks were made with tritium-labelled ink around the sections that registered on the film. A total of 4 biopsies were performed in each of 6 volunteers. Generally speaking we saw two types of photographic prints: one consisting of black dots on a line corresponding to depressions in the surface of the epidermis and the other consisting of more regular black lines (Figs. 1 and 2). As far as could be judged from the re-aligned films, this black zone lay either just above the stratum corneum or in its upper layer. This

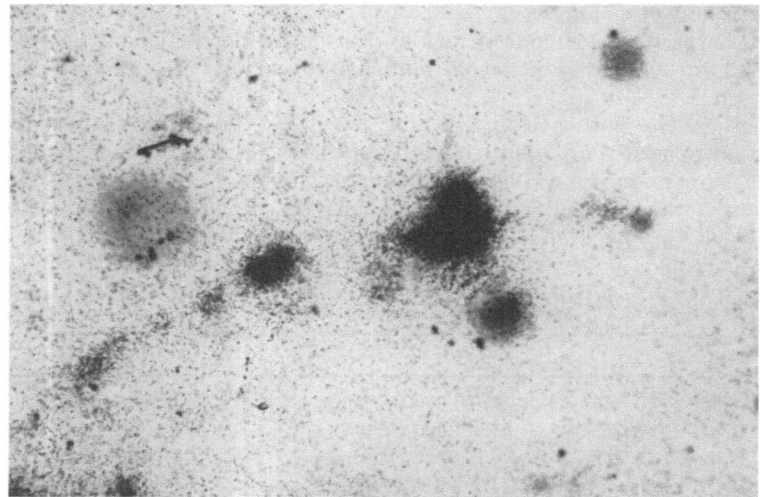

Fig. 1. Black dots, corresponding to depressions in the epidermal surface (dental X-ray, sandwich technique)

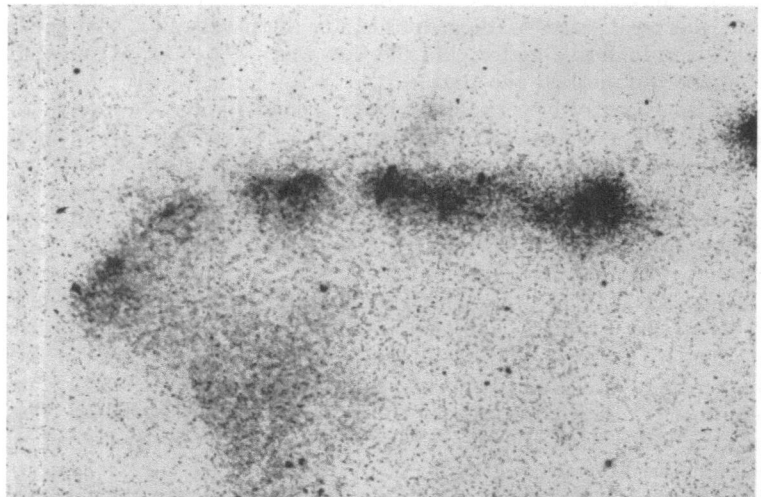

Fig. 2. Blackening as a regular black line (dental X-ray sandwich technique)

localization seemed the more likely because in slides on which, during the handling of the section, the stratum corneum had become partly detached from the epidermis, it had taken the black line with it (Fig. 3). No specific pattern could be observed in the distribution of these two phenomena, dots or lines, between the earlier and the later biopsy samples.

In this study, the following facts were established:

1. After 24 h and even after 96 h, appreciable quantities of the ointment are still present. This is proven by the number of counts in the liquid photoscintillator. Presumably this ointment is present, not only in the epidermis but also on it. It is more likely that the loss between 24 h and 96 h is due to rubbing off than to penetration. This assumption is based on comparisons between the results obtained after 2 and 24 h and on the fact that MALKINSON found signs of radioactivety in the urine only in the first 16 h after inunction of radioactive ointment.

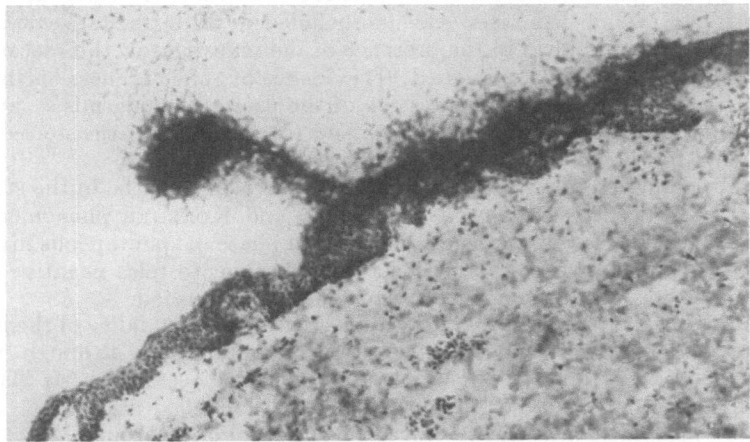

Fig. 3. The stratum corneum is partly detached and has moved radioactive material upwards

2. A considerable proportion of the radioactive material applied is still on the stratum corneum 24 h after application. This is in accordance with the fact that most authors suppose that only a small proportion of the applicated drug penetrates through the epidermis*.

This report is more an account of the many technical difficulties, which were partially overcome, than a enumeration of results. We hope that we are not too rash in promising more results for the XIVth international congress.

Acknowledgement: The authors are greatly indebted to Miss K. POSTEMA for her expert technical assistance.

References. MALKINSON, F. D., E. H. FERGUSON, and M. C. WANG: J. invest. Derm. 28, 211 (1957).

Standards for Clinical Evaluation of Topical Steroids

J. R. SCHOLTZ, School of Medicine, University of Southern California, Los Angeles, California (USA) and
K. J. DUMAS, Institute of Clinical Medicine, Syntex Research, Palo Alto, California (USA)

A semi-quantitative, objective, clinical assay of efficacy of topical corticosteroids has been used by one of us (J.R.S.) for the past 3 years. This method was designed to identify formulations of adrenal corticoids which would consistently

---

* During the congress papers are presented which suggest that under various conditions the resorption might be more important.

12*

produce significant therapeutic results in clinical therapy. Although numerous
methods for in vivo and in vitro assay have been developed, a satisfactory clinical
method in humans has not been available. Numerous new compounds reported as
statistically validated have failed to perform and survive in clinical therapeutics.
This subject has recently been comprehensively reviewed [1].

The method here presented has the following features: (a) naturally occuring
inflammation in humans (chronic stable psoriasis) is the test subject; (b) measured
amounts of medication are applied to measured areas of lesion; (c) final formulations of medication can be used; (d) positive (fluocinolone acetonide 0.025%)
and negative (placebo) "controls" can be included in all tests; (e) sealed plastic
film dressings [2] are applied in the presence of the investigator, thus ascertaining
that treatment is executed as designed; (f) evidence of "effectiveness" is indicated
by nothing less than complete suppression of the psoriatic epidermis — an essentially objective, "all or none", end point; and (g) systemic corticosteroid effects
are precluded by the small amounts of drug required.

Proper selection of patients is essential. The psoriasis must be in the stabilized
phase, lesions static, no new lesions appearing, and KOEBNER phenomenon not
elicited by adhesive used in dressings. Psoriasis in phase of spontaneous involution
will lead to false positive results, and in exacerbation, to false negative results.
All systemic therapy is discontinued during the testing period.

"Reading" of the therapeutic end result is critical to the validity of the method.
When the epidermis is normal to inspection and palpation, although residual
erythema may be present, this is a clear-cut positive result, and is classed as
"effective". Anything less than this response has been called negative.

In the double blind study here described, fluocinolone acetonide in its regular
commercial base was prepared in concentrations of 0.0, 0.0001, 0.00025, 0.001,
0.0025, 0.005, 0.025, and 0.1 per cent. Each concentration appeared twelve times in
the total of 96 coded tubes. Tubes were marked in groups of three, e.g. 1-A, 1-B,
1-C, in a total of 32 groups. Selection of the three concentrations in any group was
based on a balanced incomplete block design [3].

96 sites in 8 patients were treated, usually 3 or 6 in one patient at one time, with
one minim cream per 4 sq. cm of lesion under occlusive "surface depot" dressings
[2] on days 1, 4, 7, 10, and reading of results on days 4, 7, 10, 14. Results were
recorded as "0" (no response), "1" (improved), and "2" (complete involution except
residual erythema). Final data are tabulated on basis of results at 14th day, and
only results rated "2" are accepted as "effective". Results are shown in the table.

Table. *Results with fluocinolone acetonide with occlusive (surface
depot) dressings in chronic psoriasis*

Conc. %	Mcg./sq.cm./ 14 days[a]	No. "effective" /No. tested	Per cent "effective"
0.0	0	0/12	0
0.0001	0.064	0/12	0
0.00025	0.160	0/12	0
0.001	0.66	6/12	50
0.0025	1.60	10/12	83
0.005	3.30	9/12	75
0.025	16.5	12/12	100
0.10	70.0	10/12	83

[a] Absolute amount of corticoid — total of 4 applications.

Noteworthy points include: (a) Placebo creams showed no signs of treatment
effect. (b) The 0.025% concentration proved 100% effective in this group. This

agrees with past experience (J.R.S.) that this concentration consistently induces (at least temporary) involution of the epidermal component of chronic psoriasis, and therefore can be included in studies of this type as a "positive control." (c) With concentrations below 0.0005%, there were no positives out of 36 trials, while concentrations above 0.0005% produced 47 positives out of 60 possibles. (d) The clinically significant threshold concentration ("effective" in 50% of the trials) was 0.001%. This is in close agreement with E.C.[50] reported for fluocinolone acetonide in several other forms of assay in lower animals and man [4, 5, 6]. In our study, the 0.0005% concentration was not tested, but it may well be the significant threshold. (e) From 0.001% to 0.025%, there is a direct dose-response relationship. (f) At high concentration (0.1%), there is some decreased effectiveness, possibly the result of difficulty in keeping higher concentrations in solution. (g) The absolute amounts of drug necessary to produce good results is remarkably small; e.g., at 0.001% concentration, 0.66 mcg. per sq. cm per 14 days. See table.

Limitations and sources of error. 1. Availability of suitable patients. 2. Change in status of patient — onset of exacerbation or remission. 3. Inaccurate measurement of treatment site. 4. Air bubbles in dispensing syringe. 5. Defects in dressings: (a) failure of sealing, allowing drying; (b) loose dressing not in apposition to skin. 6. Loose dressings, allowing admixing in adjacent sites. 7. Bias in reading end point in agents with borderline effectiveness. 8. Confusion in identification of treatment sites on succeeding application. 9. Method not applicable with oily, greasy, or liquid vehicles which would loosen dressings.

References. 1. SCHLAGEL, C. A.: J. pharm. Sci. **54**, 335 (1965). — 2. SCHOLTZ, J. R., L. GOLDMAN, and H. M. ROBINSON: Proc. of XII. Int. Cong. of Derm., Vol. II, p. 1642. — 3. COCHRAN, W. G., and G. M. Cox: Experimental Designs, 2nd Edition. New York: John Wiley & Sons 1957. — 4. SCOTT, A. I.: Brit. J. Derm. **77**, 586 (1965). — 5 BAKER, H., and A. M. KLIGMAN: Human Assay of Topical Activity of Anti-Inflammatory Corticosteroids. To be published. — 6. McKENZIE, A. W., and R. B. STOUGHTON: Arch. Derm. **86**, 608 (1962).

Absorption de l'hydrocortisone par la peau saine

G. GARDENGHI et B. TARQUINI, Clinique Dermatologique et Clinique Médicale Florence (Italie)

Pour étudier la possibilité d'une absorption cutanée de l'hydrocortisone, nous avons pratiqué le dosage de corticoïdes plasmatiques libres. Nous l'avons réalisé selon une technique simple et relativement spécifique, la méthode fluorimétrique.

On a appliqué à cinq sujets sur la face antérieure des membres supérieurs 40 g d'une crème à l'hydrocortisone 2,5% (= 1 g d'hydrocortisone) avec une médication simple ou occlusive. On a observé un net accroissement dans la concentration plasmatique du cortisol qui commence plutôt précocement (après ½ h) et tend rapidement à s'épuiser dans le 4 h successives. Cependant la variabilité individuelle et la décroissance physiologique pendant la journée du niveau hématique du cortisol endogène ne nous a pas permis de standardiser les résultats. Il a toutefois été démontré récemment que l'administration à minuit, par voie orale ou intraveineuse, de 0,5 à 1 mg de déxaméthasone, ou d'une dose équivalente d'un autre corticostéroïde de synthèse, produit une suppression de l'activité surrénale qui persiste pendant 30 h. Nous avons donc pensé à utiliser cette méthode pour étudier avec une plus grande clarté l'importance et la durée de l'absorption de l'hydrocortisone.

Les recherches ont été effectuées chez 18 sujets de sexe masculin, d'âge compris entre 15 et 40 ans, dans de bonnes conditions de santé, avec une peau saine, tous

Table 1. Hydrocortisone acétate en médication normale et occlusive 17-OH-CS plasmatiques libres. Valeurs moyennes en µg/100 ml (± E.S.)

Groupe	N° des subjects	Type de médication	Hydrocorti- sone acétate	Temps en minutes après l'application						
				0	30'	60'	120'	180'	240'	300'
A	5	N	0,125	2,8 (±0,5)	2,5 (±0,4)	2,8 (±0,4)	2,4 (±0,2)	2,7 (±0,5)	2,5 (±0,3)	2,9 (±0,4)
B	5	O	0,125	2,1 (±0,3)	2,4 (±0,2)	2,4 (±0,5)	2,9 (±0,2)	2,8 (±0,3)	2,8 (±0,2)	2,7 (±0,2)
C	4	N	1,000	4,9 (±0,5)	14,3 (±0,7)	11,4 (±0,1)	8,6 (±0,5)	6,9 (±0,5)	4,5 (±0,4)	4,3 (±0,4)
D	4	O	1,000	4,3 (±0,8)	21,3 (±1,3)	15,2 (±0,6)	9,4 (±0,3)	7,8 (±1,1)	5,0 (±1,1)	4,6 (±0,1)

heure d'application: 7 a.m. — N = normale, O = occlusive

hospitalisés et pourtant dans les conditions idéales pour être suivis à l'abri de toute influence extérieure. A ces sujets on a administré, par voie orale, à 24 h du jour précédent la médication, 1 mg de déxaméthasone. Les prélèvements du sang ont été effectués avec une seringue héparinisée. Il faut remarquer qu'avec la technique suivie, n'est pas relevée la déxaméthasone, qui n'est pas douée de fluorescence.

Nous avons avant tout observé que, pour relever des variation dans le taux cortisolique plasmatique, il faut faire usage des quantités d'hydrocortisone sensiblement supérieures à celles qui sont utilisées dans la pratique quotidienne.

Avec 5 g de crème (correspondant à 125 mg d'hydrocortisone) nous n'avons pas observé de variations (voir Tab. 1, groupes A et B). En revanche avec 40 g (correspondant à 1 g d'hydrocortisone), 30 min après à peine, on peut observer un accroissement sensible du cortisol plasmatique. Celui-ci est notablement plus élevé à la suite d'une médication occlusive que d'une médication simple, mais sa durée, à parité de doses de médicament et de surface cutanée utilisée, apparaît indépendante du type de médication: en effet, au bout de 4 h, on peut observer un retour aux niveaux initiaux dans les deux types de médication (voir Tab. 1, groupes C et D).

La récente démonstration d'un rythme circadien de la réactivité cutanée nous a conduits à considérer la possibilité d'une variation circadienne même dans le cas de l'absorption des stéroïdes. Nous avons donc étudié cette absorption à différentes heures de la journée. Aux sujets pris en examen, on a administré 1 mg de déxaméthasone à 24 h du jour qui a précédé l'expérimentation, et l'on a par la suite appliqué une médication non occlusive avec 40 g de crème à l'hydrocortisone 2,5 % à différentes heures de la journée: à 7 h pour un premier groupe, à 16 h pour un second et à 22 h 30 pour un troisième.

Les résultats observés (Tab. 2) ne permettent pas de relever des différences sensibles entre les différents groupes. Il faut toutefois remarquer un fait d'un certain intérêt: lorsque le stéroïde était appliqué à 22 h 30, on observait dans trois cas sur cinq (Tab. 2, cas numéros 9, 10, 12), un prolongement du blocage de la sécrétion surrénale du même type que celui réalisé par l'administration de déxaméthasone par voie orale à la même heure, lorsque l'action de la déxaméthasone administrée 24 h avant, était déjà epuisée.

Table 2. *Hydrocortisone acétate (g 1) en médication normale 17-OH-CS plasmatiques libres µg/100 ml*

N.	Heure d'application	Heures 8[a]	7	8	9	10	11	12	8[b]
1	7.00	14,4	4,0	11,4	8,3	7,0	4,3	4,6	14,4
2		16,0	3,9	12,0	9,2	8,0	5,5	3,3	16,0
3		23,5	7,8	10,4	7,5	6,6	3,5	5,0	18,0
4		15,1	4,2	11,8	9,3	6,0	4,6	3,4	15,8
Valeurs moyennes		17,2 (±2,1)	4,9 (±0,5)	11,4 (±0,1)	8,6 (±0,5)	6,9 (±0,5)	4,5 (±0,4)	4,1 (±0,4)	16,0 (±0,9)

N.	Heure d'application	8[a]	16	17	18	19	20	24	8[b]
5	16,00	15,2	5,2	13,4	8,3	5,0	3,5	2,7	17,6
6		16,5	3,2	4,7	4,7	5,5	2,6	2,6	16,5
7		18,0	1,8	9,3	—	5,5	1,8	2,5	18,0
8		15,8	1,8	6,2	6,5	6,0	2,6	2,2	15,9
Valeurs moyennes		16,4 (±0,6)	3,0 (±0,6)	8,4 (±1,9)	6,5 (±0,7)	5,5 (±0,2)	2,6 (±0,4)	2,5 (±0,1)	17,0 (±0,4)

N.	Heure d'application	8[a]	22,30	24	8	12	17	24	8[b]
9	22,30	15,8	4,8	12,5	5,6	5,6	3,3	2,5	14,1
10		14,4	3,0	10,0	5,6	4,5	7,5	2,2	—
11		16,0	4,2	11,4	14,0	11,2	9,4	2,7	10,9
12		18,0	5,1	13,6	7,5	6,0	5,0	2,4	16,7
13[c]		16,0	2,8	9,8	12,5	9,2	7,0	2,9	16,2

[a] Valeurs des 17-OH-CS plasmatiques libres trois jours avant la recherche.
[b] Valeurs des 17-OH-CS plasmatiques libres après la recherche.
[c] On a renoncé pour ce groupe à donner des valeurs moyennes car le résultats n'ont pas montré de modifications constantes.

Local Action of Steroids

K. Aso, Y. Tanabe and K. Takenouchi, Department of Dermatology, School of Medicine Chiba University, Chiba (Japan)

The external application of steroids suppressed the respiration of the skin, that is so-called "local activity" of steroids different from that when administered systematically. The local inhibitory effect of the steroids on the energy formation of the inflamed skin is seemingly explained as one of the anti-inflammatory activities.

Materials and Methods

Oxygen uptake of the skin was measured manometrically by the Criesemer method [1], whereas esterified P^{32} of the rat skin slice was estimated by the procedure of Decker [2], while oxidation of NADH as well as reduction of cytochrome C was estimated spectrophotometrically. Rat liver mitochondria was prepared to estimate the effect of steroids upon the respiratory chain and coupled ATP formation. The cell membrane of the rat liver was prepared after Emmelot's [3] method. Autoradiogram with C^{14}-cortisol denoted the way of percutaneous absorption.

Results

1. *Inhibition of skin respiration by steroids:* Respiration of the inflamed rat skin induced by xenon lamp irradiation, reached highest on the 4th day of inflammation with $QO_2:0.80$, while $QO_2:0.45$ of the normal skin substrate being

Table. *Inhibition of the skin respiration by C-21 steroids Warburg manometric method air 37 °C*

steroids	conc. mM	no. of cases examined	% of inhibition
1. None		10	0
2. Cortisol	0.0001	8	0.3
	0.001	4	29.9
	0.001	7	32.3
	0.1	5	28.0
3. Prednisolone	0.1	4	26.8
4. Dexamethasone	0.0001	4	0
	0.001	4	24.2
	0.01	4	25.0
	1.0	4	42.4
5. Corticosterone	0.0001	4	0
	0.001	4	12.2
	0.01	4	19.3
	0.1	4	29.6
6. DOC	0.001	4	22.0
	0.01	4	49.4
	0.1	4	51.5
7. Progesterone	0.001	4	29.6
	0.01	4	33.3
	0.1	4	50.0
8. THF	0.1	4	0

succinate. The accelerated respiration was suppressed by the external application of steroids as is shown in the table, steroids that are not active systematically inhibited the respiration of skin slice. Inhibitory activity on the respiration of skin by those steroids is correlated reasonably with Glenn's [4] study that steroids such as progesterone, desoxycorticosterone show in fact very active local anti-inflammatory activity. These steroids inhibited oxidation of NADH and reduction of cytochrome C of rat liver mitochondria. It is considered that the site of the steroids in the respiratory chain lies between the flavo-protein and cytochrome C, agreed with JENSEN's [5] result.

2. *Effects of steroids upon ATP formation:* It was proved that esterified P^{32} formation was decreased when the skin slice was incubated with inorganic P^{32} and cortisol together, the concentration 10^{-4} M. To ascertain the effect on the formation of ATP, oxymetric investigation of rat liver mitochondria was performed. In the well prepared mitochondria, respiratory control, that is, ATP formation is remarkable when Pi, substrate, and ADP are added. This state of oxygen uptake is called as step 3. Less ATP formation was observed when the steroids are incu-

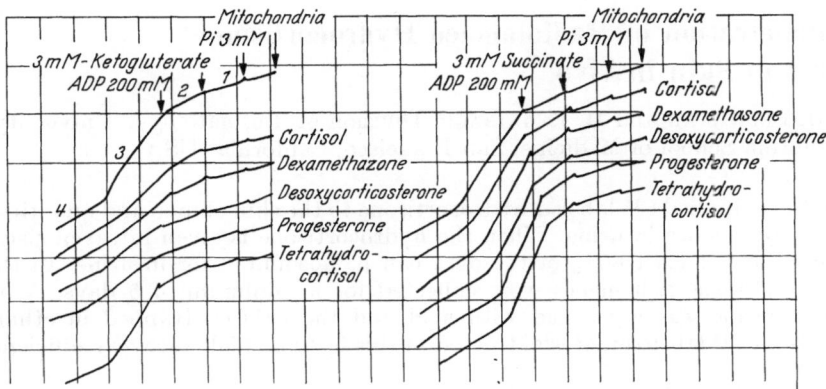

Fig. Oxymetric observation of the suppressed ATP formation of rat liver mitochondria by C-21 steroids when electron pass through NADH linked path way

1: step 1 reaction mixture: sucrose 200 mM, KCl 20 mM, EDTA 0.1 mM,
2: step 2   MgCl$_2$ 3 mM, tris-HCl pH 7.4 10 mM and steroids 10^{-4}M
3: step 3

bated, the concentration ranged between 10^{-5} and 10^{-6} M as shown in the figure. It was also ascertained that steroids inhibit respiratory chain and coupled ATP formation by interferring NADH linked respiratory chain whereas inhibitory effect was not observed when the substrate was succinate.

3. *Effects on the cell membrane electron transport system by cortisol and corticosterone:* Cortisol absorbed transepidermally from the inflamed skin as if passed through intercellular space of epidermis, influencing some effects on the cell membrane. Cell membrane of rat liver has NADH linked electron transport system. The epidermal cell is considered to have the same system. To observe whether steroids exert any effects upon the cell membrane system, cortisol and corticosterone were incubated to the rat liver cell membrane and cytochrome C reductase was estimated. Among both of them, cortisol was more inhibitory, the concentration being 10^{-4} M.

Discussion

Though it is still unclear, the mode of action of steroids to the inflammation has been explained by several workers, such as the inhibitory effect of glucose utilization [6], glycolysis pathway [4] and the formation of kinin [7]. WEISSMANN [8] reported on the stabilizing effect of cortisol on the lysosomal membrane, liberation of the inflammatory agents was thus inhibited. Inhibition of the respiration of the skin, particulary that of inflamed skin by local application of steroids, might be share another explanation to the mode of steroids activity.

Literatur. 1. Griesemer, R. D., and E. Gould: J. invest. Derm. **22**, 299 (1954). — 2. Decker, R. H., and R. L. Anderson: J. invest. Derm. **45**, 168 (1965). — 3. Emmelot, P., C. J. Bos, and E. L. Benedetti: Biochim. biophys. Acta (Amst.) **90**, 126 (1964). — 4. Glenn, E. M., W. L. Miller, and C. A. Schlagel: Recent Progr. Hormone. Res. **19**, 107 (1963). — 5. Jensen, P. K.: Nature (Lond.) **4664**, 451 (1959). — 6. Overell, B. G., S. E. Condon, and V. Petrow: J. Pharm. Pharmacol. **12**, 150 (1960). — 7. Cline, J. M., and K. L. Melmon: Science **153**, 1135 (1966). — 8. Weissmann, G., and L. Thomas: Recent Progr. Hormone Res. **10**, 215 (1964).

The Penetration of Radiolabeled Hydrocortisone in Human Skin in vivo

R. J. Feldmann and H. I. Maibach, Division of Dermatology, University of California School of Medicine, San Francisco, California (USA)

We have applied C^{14} labeled hydrocortisone to the skin of man and quantitated it by its appearance in urine. When the hydrocortisone is given intravenously or intradermally, at least 80% of the dose can be accounted for in urine. In these metabolic studies 24 h urines were collected for a minimum of 5 days. A 5 ml aliquot of urine was wet-ashed with acid and the $C^{14} CO_2$ trapped in ethanolamine. With C^{14} labeled material treated in this fashion, high recovery efficiencies were found.

In 20 individuals we found that approximately 1% of hydrocortisone penetrates the forearm when applied in acetone to a 13 sq cm area at a concentration of approximately $1/_4$%. This figure represents an average; there is considerable variation between people. The variation is between the individuals and not the method, as replicate determinations on the same individual tend to be similar.

It previously has been thought that the stripping of the stratum corneum removes its barrier to foreign compounds. In our experiments stripping only doubles penetration and obviously does not remove the barrier. Occlusion is a far more potent method of increasing penetration. The application of plastic film occlusion increases penetration ten-fold. When stripping and occlusion are done together, penetration increases additively with about a twenty-fold rise.

Certain bases influence the penetration of hydrocortisone but none nearly so much as a change in the parent molecule to other steroids. Mineral oil, propylene glycol and dimethyl acetamide were found not to influence penetration, but dimethyl formamide and dimethyl sulfoxide increase penetration two- and four-fold. None were nearly as effective as occlusion.

Slight modifications of the chemical configuration of the steroid allow for much greater changes in penetration than altering bases. For instance testosterone penetrates under similar conditions to approximately 12%.

There is considerable variation in various anatomical sites. Previously it had been thought that the palm was impenetrable to most chemicals thus accounting for the rarity of allergic contact dermatitis in this area. Much to our surprise, 4/5 as much hydrocortisone penetrated the palm as the forearm. The scrotum had almost no barrier to penetration and approximately 40% of the applied dose penetrated. In areas in which there were increased numbers of hair follicles, such as the forehead, scalp and beard, there was as much as a ten-fold increase in penetration compared to the forearm. This is not to state that the presence of the hair follicle itself accounted for this increase but only that certain peculiarities of the anatomy in this area are related to this increase.

These findings are being extended to other steroids and to benzene ring derivatives.

Zur Resorption von Corticoidsalben

K. WINKLER, Dermatologische Abteilung des Städtischen Krankenhauses Berlin-Britz, Berlin (Deutschland)

Es stehen im wesentlichen zwei Methoden zur Verfügung, mit denen man etwas über die Resorption von Corticoidsalben aussagen kann:

1. die Bestimmung des Plasmacortisolspiegels und der 17-Hydroxycorticoide und 17-Ketosteroide im Harn;

2. die Anwendung markierter Substanzen.

Wenn bei der äußerlichen Behandlung größere Corticoidmengen in aktiver Form resorbiert werden, so sind Rückwirkungen auf den Plasmacortisolspiegel sowie auf die Steroidwerte im Harn zu erwarten. Hierbei ist zu berücksichtigen, daß der Plasmacortisolspiegel ein wesentlich empfindlicherer Indikator für eine abgeschwächte Nebennierenrindenfunktion ist als die Corticoidwerte im Harn. Denn verschiedene Faktoren können die Corticoidausscheidungen im Harn verändern, ohne daß die NNR-Funktion selbst beeinträchtigt ist. So bedingen Urinmengen von 400 ml und weniger pro Tag scheinbar erniedrigte Werte für die 17-Hydroxycorticoide. Außerdem ist die Ausscheidung der Corticosteroide von der Funktion der Leber und verschiedener endokriner Drüsen abhängig. Eine weitere Schwierigkeit ist, daß die Patienten die gesamte Tagesharnmenge sammeln müssen. Deshalb haben wir besonderen Wert auf die Bestimmung des Cortisolspiegels im Plasma gelegt.

Da der Plasmacortisolspiegel innerhalb eines Tages große Schwankungen aufweist, wurden die Blutabnahmen immer um 8.30 Uhr morgens durchgeführt. Auch wenn man die Blutentnahme immer zur selben Zeit macht, muß man mit spontanen Schwankungen rechnen und das bei der Beurteilung der Werte berücksichtigen. Zu bedenken ist ferner, daß auch andere Arzneimittel den Cortisolspiegel beeinflussen können.

Wir haben seit 3 Jahren bei 62 Patienten den Plasmacortisolspiegel und die Steroidwerte im Harn bestimmt, und zwar vor, während und nach der Behandlung mit verschiedenen Corticoidsalben.

Das Ergebnis der Untersuchung ist, daß selbst große Mengen hochprozentiger Corticoidsalben, z. B. 60 g einer 0,5%igen Fluocortolonsalbe, die täglich auf die Haut aufgetragen oder in die Haut eingerieben werden, den Cortisolspiegel und die Hormonausscheidung nicht verändern. Auch bei Anwendung großer Salbenmengen ist also keine Rückwirkung auf das NNR-Hypophysensystem infolge von Corticoidresorption aus der Salbe zu befürchten.

Wesentlich genauer kann man etwas über die Resorption aus Salben aussagen, wenn man markierte Substanzen verwendet. Wir gebrauchten eine Salbe, die zu gleichen Teilen Fluocortolon und Fluocortoloncapronat enthielt. Fluocortolon wurde mit Tritium, Fluocortoloncapronat mit C 14 markiert. Die Salbe wurde in die erkrankten Hautpartien von Ekzematikern und Psoriatikern kräftig eingerieben. Zum Vergleich wurde die Salbe auch in die Haut von Gesunden einmassiert.

An den Tagen, die dieser Behandlung folgten, haben wir die Radioaktivität im Blut, im Harn und im Stuhl gemessen und die wiedergefundene Menge der markierten Substanzen bestimmt.

Bei Ekzematikern wurden mehr als 50% der angewandten Fluocortolondosis im Stuhl und Harn wiedergefunden. Dagegen war die wiedergefundene Menge des Fluocortoloncapronats wesentlich geringer. Daraus folgt, daß der Ester viel weniger resorbiert wird als der freie Alkohol. Bei Psoriatikern war die wiedergefundene Menge an Corticoiden geringer als bei Ekzematikern. Bei Patienten mit gesunder Haut waren die ausgeschiedenen Corticoidmengen am geringsten.

Trotzdem die Corticoide also von der Ekzemhaut sehr gut resorbiert werden, sieht man keine Rückwirkungen auf den Plasmacortisolspiegel und auch bei langdauernder Anwendung keine Nebenerscheinungen. Es ist deshalb wohl anzunehmen, daß das resorbierte Corticoid im Organismus — vielleicht durch Bindung an Eiweiß — nicht aktiv werden kann.

Measurement of Percutaneous Absorption of Corticosteroid by Means of an Autoradiography*

A. Kukita and T. Matsuzawa, Department of Dermatology, Sapporo Medical College, Sapporo (Japan)

Topical application of corticosteroid has been widely used for the treatment of certain dermatoses. Since the occlusive dressing therapy (O.D.T.) has been developed, topical corticosteroid therapy has much advanced. It is generally believed that absorption of the drug into the skin is enhanced by the use of O.D.T. and the problems of possible systemic corticosteroid effects have been repeatedly discussed [1, 2].

In Malkinson and his co-workers' studies [3 to 6] on percutaneous absorption of C-14 labeled corticosteroids applied on the skin surface, the absorption of the compounds used has been proved by the demonstration of radioactivity in the urine specimens and remaining radioactivity on the skin surface in the normal, stripped or inflamed skin. Using radioactive triamcinolone acetonide cream [7], they have found about 50% of the steroid was absorbed over 4 to 6 h period on the stripped skin. On the normal skin, 1.5 to 2% of the steroid applied on the skin surface was absorbed, similar to their earlier observations for cortisone and hydrocortisone.

Our autoradiographic studies have been carried out to investigate the following three major subjects: the pathway of percutaneous absorption of corticosteroid, percutaneous absorption of corticosteroid of skin site to which corticosteroid had been applied previously and the site of steroid depot of the skin after the application under plastic film using fluocinolone acetonide labeled with C-14 in the acetonide group. Kukita and Fitzpatrick [8] have developed the autoradiographic histochemical method using C-14 labeled tyrosine for demonstrating tyrosinase activity in human melanocytes. For this study, this modified technic was employed.

* This study was supported in part by a grant from the Far East Basic Research Fund of Sears, Roebuck and Co. Inc. Chicago, Ill. USA.

C-14 labeled fluocinolone acetonide cream was kindly supplied from Syntex Laboratories, Inc. Palo Alto, Calif. USA through Tanabe Pharmaceutical Co. Osaka, Japan.

Materials and Methods

Human axillary skins, skin of the palm and scar tissue of the scalp were used for this study. 0.025% C-14 fluocinolone acetonide cream (specific activity, 1.23 ci per Gm.) was applied under plastic film. After the application, cream was removed, then excision biopsy was performed. In order to prevent the displacement of the radioactive substances, the excised skin specimens were not fixed in any fixatives. Then the unfixed skin specimens were frozen at 20 °C below zero. Then the specimens were cut 10 microns thick in a cryostat freezing microtome. For preparing autoradiography, the frozen specimens cut were directly mounted on Nuclear Track Plate NTB-3 (Eastman Kodak) in dark room. They were exposed for 2 weeks at 4 °C, then were developed in Kodak D-19 developer for 25 min and were fixed on 20% hypo solution for 10 min. And they were washed in running water for 30 min, stained with cold lithium carmine, counterstained with picric acid in 100% alcohol and were mounted in synthetic resin.

Results

Radioactive substances were demonstrated in all autoradiographs. Dense silver grains were noted in the horny layer of the epidermis, hair follicles and lumina of apocrine gland in 4 h after the topical application under plastic film in the axillary skin (Fig. 1 and 2). The distribution of the radioactive substances was sharply defined, therefore, this findings indicate that there is no or little artificial displacement of the substances during the experimental procedures.

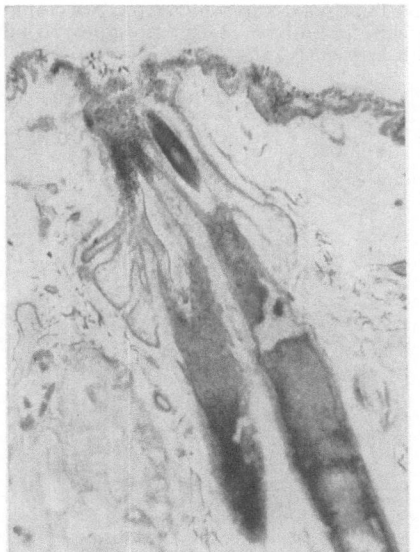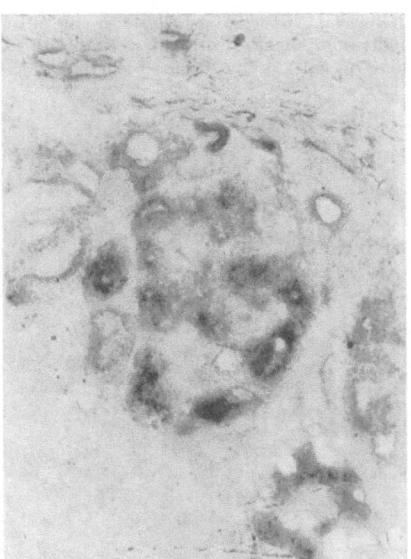

1   2

Fig. 1 and 2. Autoradiographs in 4 h after the topical application under plastic film in the human axillary skin. Radioactive substances were present in the horny layer of the epidermis, hair follicles and lumina of apocrine gland

As compared with the experiments of radioactive corticosteroid cream was topically applied under plastic film to the axillary skin for 16 h to which non-radioactive same steroid had been applied for 8 h previously and cream base alone applied for 8 h previously, the localization of radioactive substances on autoradiographs was different. In these studies, the slow absorption of radioactive substances into the skin has been proved in the former experiment. It is assumed that this inhibitory effect on percutaneous absorption of corticosteroid may be due to

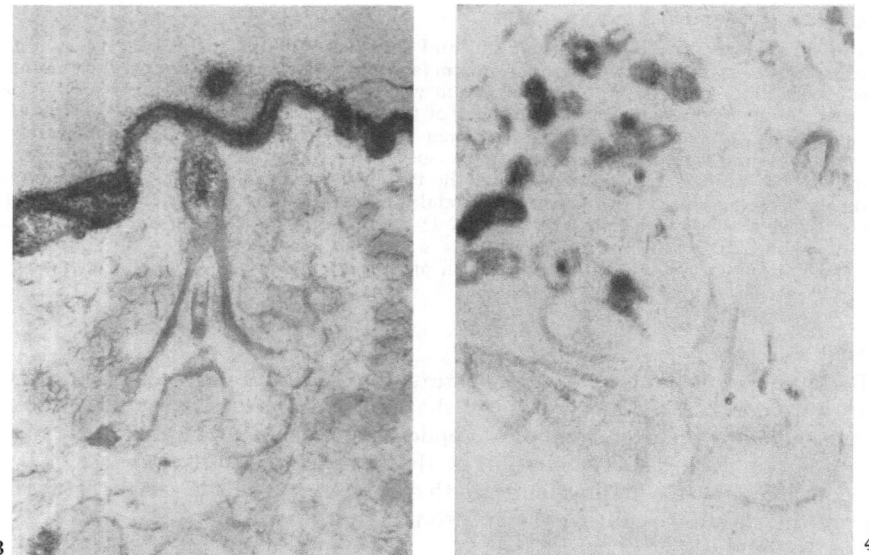

Fig. 3 and 4. Autoradiographs showing radioactive fluocinolone acetonide cream was topically applied under plastic film to the human axillary skin for 16 h to which non-radioactive fluocinolone acetonide cream had been applied for 8 h previously

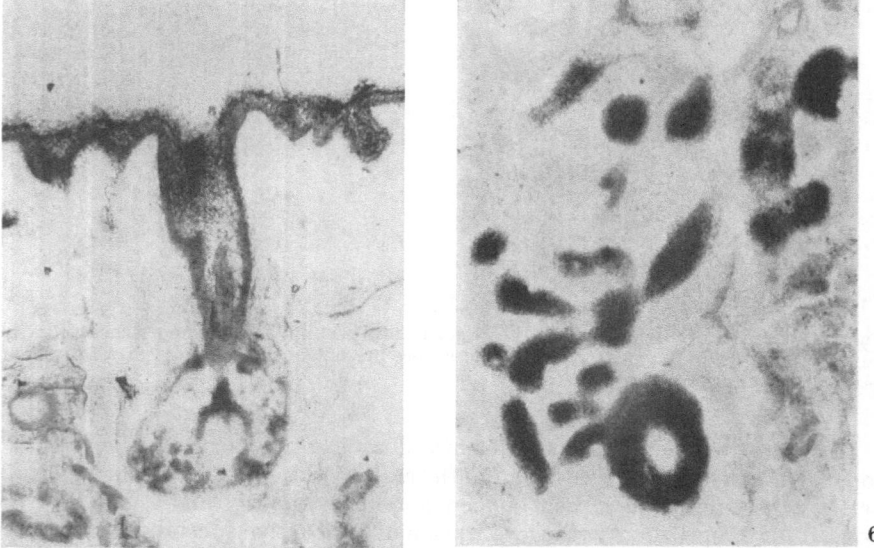

Fig. 5 and 6. Autoradiographs showing radioactive fluocinolone acetonide cream was topically applied under plastic film to the human axillary skin to which cream base alone had been applied for 8 h previously

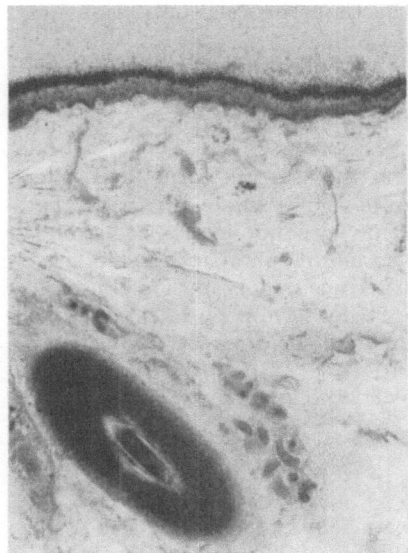

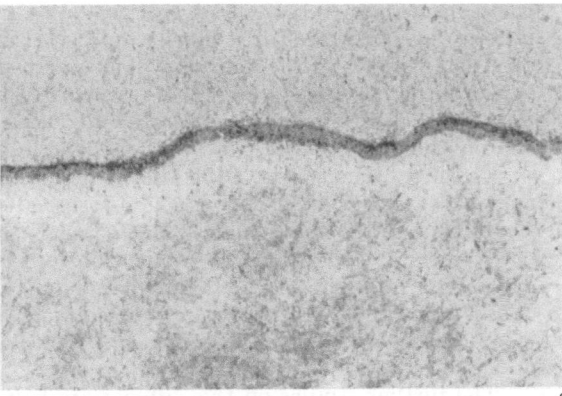

8

Fig. 7 and 8. Autoradiographs, Radioactive fluocinolone acetonide cream was applied locally on the
non-stripped skin of scar tissue of the scalp (Fig. 7)
and stripped skin (Fig. 8) for 24 h

7

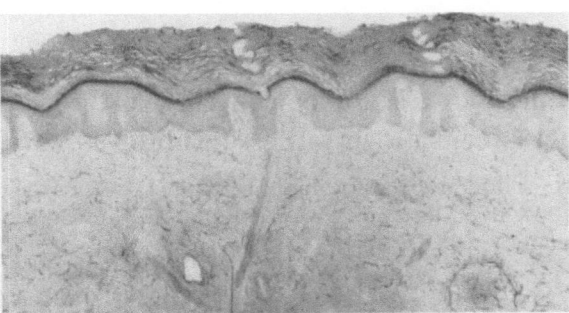

9

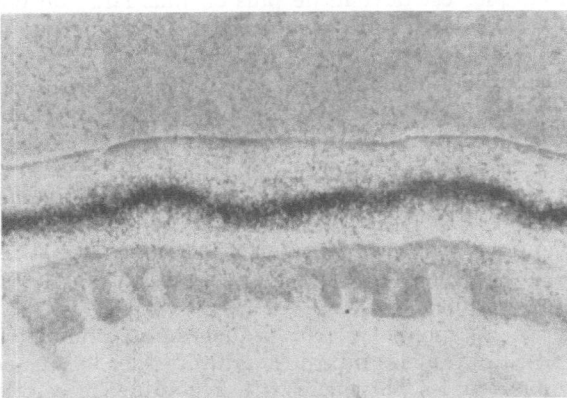

10

Fig. 9 and 10. Skin of the palm (Fig. 9, hematoxylin-eosin Staining). Autoradiograph: In 24 h
after the application under plastic film of radioactive fluocinolone acetonide cream in skin of
the palm (Fig. 10)

the concentration gradient of corticosteroid in the tissue or vasocontriction induced by corticosteroid previously applied (Fig. 3 to 6).

The existence in the skin of a depot for topically applied substances has been suggested in the past years. This reservoir of the substances has been proved by the clinical observation, such as vasocontriction after topical application of corticosteroid and the experimental findings using radioisotope.

VICKERS [9] suggested the site of depots lay in the stratum corneum of the epidermis. In our experiment of non-stripped skin of scar tissue of the scalp, the site of steroid depots was demonstrated in the stratum corneum and the remaining hair follicle in 24 h after the application under plastic film. In stripped skin site, autoradiographs showed no definite radioactive substance depots in the epidermis (Fig. 7 and 8). In the palm skin, dense band-like radioactive zone in the middle layer of the thick horny layer was demonstrated in 24 h after the application under plastic film (Fig. 9 and 10).

The further studies on this subject are being carried out.

References. 1. SCOGGINS, R. B.: J. invest. Derm. **39**, 473 (1962). — 2. SCOGGINS, R. B., and B. KLIMAN: J. invest. Derm. **45**, 347 (1965). — 3. MALKINSON, F. D., and E. H. FERGUSON: J. invest. Derm. **25**, 281 (1955). — 4. MALKINSON, F. D., E. H. FERGUSON, and M. C. WANG: J. invest. Derm. **28**, 211 (1957). — 5. MALKINSON, F. D.: J. invest. Derm. **31**, 19 (1958). — 6. MALKINSON, F. D.: J. Soc. Cosm. Chem. 11, 146 (1960). — 7. MALKINSON, F. D., and M. B. KIRSCHENBAUM: Arch. (Chic.) 88, 427 (1963). — 8. KUKITA, A., and T. B. FITZPATRICK: Science 121, 893 (1955). — 9. VICKERS, C. F. H.: Arch. (Chic.) 88, 20 (1963).

Observations concernant l'emploi des corticostéroïdes dans le traitement local de certaines dermatoses

ST. TEODORESCU, Clinique Dermatologique, Hôpital Colentina Bucarest, et AL. BĂDĂNOIU, Centre dermato-vénérologique du Ministère de la Santé, Bucarest (Roumanie)

Depuis 1952, lorsque SULZBERGER et WITTEN ont signalé des résultats bénéfiques obtenus par l'application locale d'une pommade à cortisone, l'emploi des topiques corticostéroïdiques est devenu de plus en plus large de telle façon qu'il peut être considéré actuellement — à juste raison — comme une thérapeutique dermatologique usuelle.

Par suite de la découverte de nouveaux corticoïdes, nous possédons à présent toute une série de produits cortisoniques destinés au traitement local de différentes affections cutanées, l'expérience des dermatologistes s'étant enrichie, de ce fait, de nouvelles connaissances.

A ce sujet, nous désirons présenter ici nos observations personnelles en liaison avec 638 cas traités, par voie locale, à l'aide de différentes substances corticostéroïdiques. Etant donné l'espace restreint dont nous disposons, nous nous limiterons d'exposer brièvement dans cette communication, les faits les plus significatifs qui en ressortent.

En ce qui concerne les modalités par lesquelles fut administrée la corticothérapie locale, on a utilisé tant les mixtures agitantes, les lotions et les produits écumeux, que les crèmes et les pommades. Chez nombre de cas, les pommades cortisoniques ont été appliquées sous pansements occlusifs à feuilles de plastique. Ajoutons que, par rapport à la nature des affections traitées, le topique employé contenait suivant les cas, à part le corticoïde, aussi d'autres substances actives, à savoir: antibiotiques (tétracyclines, cloramphénicol, néomycine), réducteurs, kératolytiques ou antiacnéiques (soufre, résorcine).

Parmi les dermatoses que nous avons soumises au traitement cortisonique local se trouvaient: l'eczéma avec ses différentes formes cliniques, eczématides et neurodermites récentes, des prurigos, des angiodermites des jambes, des impetigos strépto- ou staphylococciques, l'acnée vulgaire; le traitement intralésionnel a été réservé aux neurodermites invétérées, au lichen plan corné, lichen amyloïde, aux formes fixes du lupus érythémateux chronique, aux pélades en plaques circonscrites et, enfin, à l'induration plastique du pénis.

Quant au type des corticoïdes, il s'agissait de l'hydrocortisone 1%; delta-hydrocortisone 0,5%, triamcinolone 0,1%, fluorométolone 0,025%; flumétasone 0,02%; fluocinolone 0,025%; bétamétasone valérianée 0,1%.

D'autre part, pour le traitement intralésionnel ont été utilisées seulement l'hydrocortisone, la delta-hydrocortisone et la 6-métil-prednisolone, injectées sous la forme d'une suspension microcristaline.

Comme suite des traitements cortisoniques locaux, on a enregistré une proportion globale de 80% résultats favorables. En effet, quelques jours après les applications en question, s'amendaient tant les lésions cutanées — et plus spécialement la congestion locale — que les symptômes subjectifs, à savoir le prurit. Disons, à cette occasion, que le délai de l'amélioration des neurodermites se prolongeait jusqu'à une dizaine de jours. Ajoutons encore que les eczémas, les intertrigos de même que d'autres états cutanés congestifs ont mieux réagi aux médications en question. En effet, en contrôlant histologiquement, à l'aide des biopsies périodiques, l'évolution des cas traités, nous avons remarqué dans le derme la diminution graduelle de l'oedème, de la congestion vasculaire et des infiltrations périvasculaires, et la disparition de la spongiose et de la vésiculation dans l'épiderme.

Quant aux injections corticostéroïdiques intralésionnelles, il faut mentionner l'influence bénéfique qu'elles ont exercée, sur les neurodermites invétérées, le lichen plan corné et le lichen amyloïde, à condition que le traitement soit poursuivi une durée plus longue, tandis que dans l'induration plastique du pénis la médication en question ne donne que des résultats partiaux. Enfin, dans les plaques péladiques, on a vu que l'injection de corticoïdes détermine l'accroissement temporaire des poils.

Selon leur efficacité locale, les corticoïdes employées par nous, se rangeaient dans l'ordre suivante: un premier groupe, englobant la fluocinolone et la bétamétazone valérianée, s'est montré le plus actif; ce groupe est suivi d'un autre incluant la flumétasone, la fluorométalone et la triamcinolone, en troisième ligne se plaçant la delta-hydrocortisone et l'hydrocortisone.

Une autre question que nous voulons souligner ici se rapporte à l'inocuité des traitements locaux cortisoniques. En effet, sur 638 cas traités nous n'avons observé que seulement chez deux d'entre eux l'apparition tardive d'une atrophie dermique, comme suite des injections intralésionnelles. En ce qui concerne l'eventuelle résorbtion des corticoïdes dans l'économie générale, risque qui surviendrait — selon certains auteurs — surtout après les applications occlusives, sur les lésions multiples et de longue durée, nous n'avons remarqué aucune signe clinique ou bien biologique pouvant être invoqué dans ce sens. En effet, ni le nombre des lymphocytes ou des éosinophiles sanguines, ni le taux des 17-kétostéroïdes urinaires n'étaient pas influencés par la médication locale en question.

Tels étant les résultats de nos observations, il ressort que le traitement cortisonique local offre bien d'avantages qui justifient son large emploi dans la thérapeutique dermatologique.

The Influence of Topical Corticosteroids
on Hypothalamic-Pituitary-Adrenal Function

D. D. MUNRO M. FEIWEL and V. H. T. JAMES, Departments of Dermatology and Chemical Pathology, St. Mary's Hospital, London (England)

Introduction. The intact stratum corneum forms an efficient barrier to absorption of chemicals applied to its surface, but damage results in penetration of topical therapeutic agents. Depression of adrenal activity may follow the use of corticosteroid ointments (SCOGGINS and KLIMAN, 1965; MARCH and KERBEL, 1962; KIRKETERP, 1964).

The purpose of this paper is to document more fully than previously, the function of the hypothalamic-pituitary-adrenal axis in adult patients treated with corticosteroid ointments for 2 weeks.

Methods and Materials

The patients suffered from eczema or acute psoriasis, and had over 60% of their skin involved. Throughout the investigation blood samples were taken at 9.0 a.m. each day for plasma cortisol estimation (MATTINGLY, 1962) and each 24-h urine sample was collected and 17-oxogenic steroid (17-OGS) determined (JAMES and CAIE, 1964).

A "pretreatment period" of 3 or 4 days was used to obtain baseline estimations of plasma cortisols, urinary 17-OGS and response to insulin stress test (I.S.T.). During this period 30 g of inert ointment base was applied to the skin daily, and a polythene suit was worn for 20 h each day.

During the 14 day "treatment period", 30 g of the steroid ointment was applied daily and a polythene suit worn. The ointments investigated were "Locorten" (flumethasone pivalate 0.02%), "Betnovate" (betamethasone 17 valerate 0.1%) and "Ultralanum Plain" (flucortolone 0.25% with flucortolone caproate 0.25%).

In the "post treatment period" the I.S.T. was repeated on the second or third day after stopping steroid ointments and a metyrapone test performed the next day.

Insulin stress tests were conducted as described by LANDON et al. (1963), in which soluble insulin 0.15 units/kg body weight, was injected intravenously and serial estimations made of the plasma cortisol and blood sugar response. In control subjects, this procedure produces a rise in plasma cortisol of 8 μg/100 ml over the resting level, to a value above 20 μg/100 ml.

The metyrapone test consisted of six oral doses of 750 mg of metyrapone at four hourly intervals with collection of urine during that day and the following day. The urinary 17-OGS were estimated and a normal response was taken as a rise greater than 10 mg/24 h above the resting level.

Results

The results are shown in the table, divided into patients treated with "Locorten", "Betnovate" and "Ultralanum Plain" ointments. The resting levels of urinary 17-OGS and plasma cortisols are the mean levels during the pre-treatment, treatment and post-treatment periods, and are represented graphically in Figs. 1, 2 and 3.

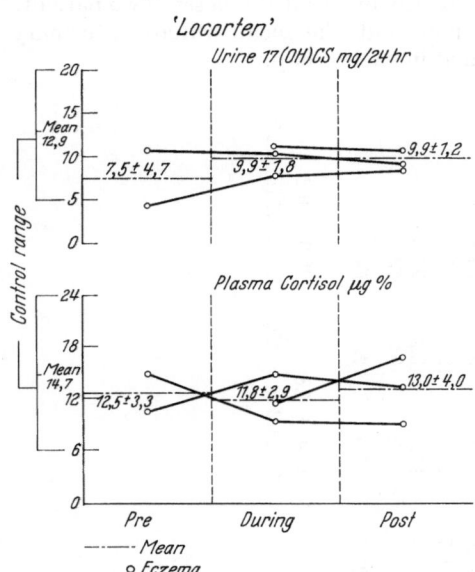

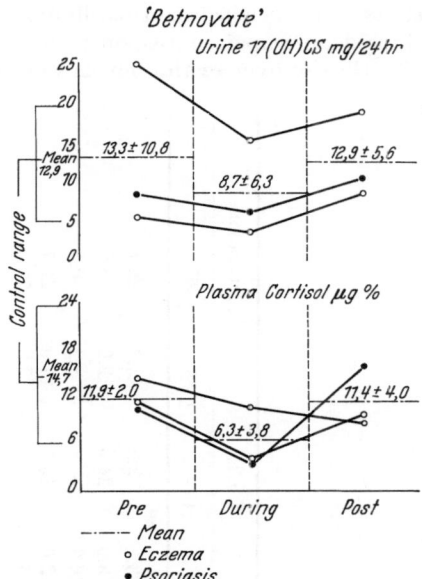

Fig. 1. Urinary 17 oxogenic steroids and plasma cortisol levels before, during and after treatment with Locorten

Fig. 2. Urinary 17 oxogenic steroids and plasma cortisol levels before, during and after treatment with Betnovate

In the three patients treated with "Locorten" mean levels for urinary 17-OGS are, throughout the investigation, a little lower than the control values, but there is no depression of the values during treatment. Similarly the plasma cortisol levels are minimally below the control values but are not significantly altered during steroid ointment therapy.

In three patients treated with "Betnovate" ointment the urinary 17-OGS are normal before and after treatment, while during treatment the levels are depressed but not to a statistically significant degree. The mean plasma cortisol levels are similar before and after treatment. During treatment they are significantly lowered (P < 0.05).

One patient treated with "Ultralanum Plain" ointment had normal urinary 17-OGS readings before and after treatment, while there was reduction in the values during therapy but not to significant degree. Highly significant depression of plasma cortisol levels (P < 0.001) was seen during treatment, when compared with pre and post treatment levels.

Plasma cortisol elevation in the insulin

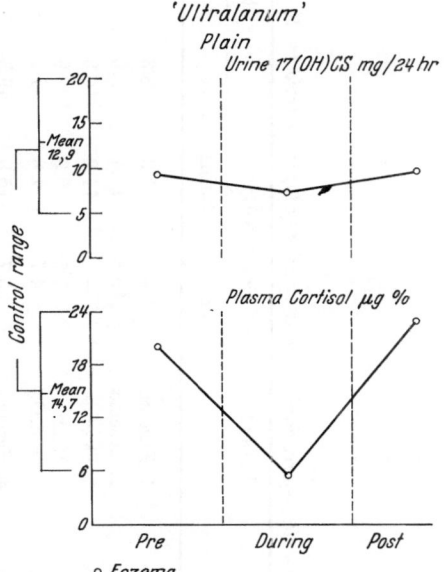

Fig. 3. Urinary 17 oxogenic steroids and plasma cortisol levels before, during and after treatment with Ultralanum

13*

stress test was within normal limits after treatment in all the cases. Two patients showed an impaired response to metyrapone but the mean values of urinary 17-OGS rise over resting levels were normal in each group.

Table. Results before, during and after 14 day topical steroid treatment

Steroid	Patient	Urine 17-OGS[a]			Plasma cortisol[b]			I.S.T.[c]		Metyrapone[d]
		Pre	During	Post	Pre	During	Post	Pre	Post	Post
Locorten	1. Eczema	4.2	7.9	8.3	10.1	14.9	13.1	3.3	23.2	26.1
	2. Eczema	10.8	10.4	9.0	14.9	9.1	9.0	24.0	19.6	8.6
	3. Eczema	—	11.2	10.8	—	11.4	16.9	—	8.2	30.5
	Mean	7.5	9.9	9.9	12.5	11.8	13.0	13.7	17.0	21.7
	± S.D.	± 4.7	± 1.8	± 1.2	± 3.3	± 2.9	± 4.0	±14.6	± 7.8	±11.6
Betnovate	4. Eczema	25.7	15.8	19.3	14.2	10.6	8.5	23.3	13.8	35.9
	5. Psoriasis	8.5	6.3	10.7	10.4	3.4	16.0	14.4	13.7	38.8
	6. Eczema	5.7	3.9	8.7	11.2	4.9	9.7	14.1	12.2	6.1
	Mean	13.3	8.7	12.9	11.9	6.3	11.4	17.3	13.2	26.9
	± S.D.	±10.8	± 6.3	± 5.6	± 2.0	± 3.8	± 4.0	± 5.2	± 0.9	±18.1
Ultralanum	7. Eczema	9.2	7.1	9.8	20.0	5.5	23.0	7.0	12.0	54.8
Control	Mean	12.9±2.8			14.7 ± 4.0			15.4 ± 4.8		23.9 ± 8.2
	± S.D.									
	Range	5—20 (n = 16)			6—24 (n = 66)			7.7—24.2 (n = 29)		10.8—37.6 (n = 29)

a Urine 17 oxogenic steroids mg/24 h.
b Resting levels plasma cortisol μg/100 ml.
c Insulin stress test: plasma cortisol rise above resting level μg/100 ml.
d Urine 17 oxogenic steroid rise above resting level mg/24 h.

Discussion

Short term depression of the hypothalamic-pituitary-adrenal axis is probably not important. Long term mild depression of function from prolonged use of steroid ointments may give rise to impaired cortisol output at times of stress, and may interfere with normal tissue physiology.

Under the conditions of this investigation, significant depression of cortisol levels was demonstrated in patients treated with "Betnovate" and "Ultralanum Plain" ointments whereas "Locorten" ointment did not give this depression. When treatment stopped no significant depression of hypothalamic-pituitary-adrenal function could be detected in any group.

The response of the patients' dermatoses to treatment was most marked with "Betnovate", and less with "Ultralanum Plain" and "Locorten". It would appear that efficiency of the preparation in terms of skin healing correlated with the potency of the steroid and its effect on adrenal function.

We acknowledge research grants from Glaxo Laboratories Ltd., England, and CIBA Laboratories Ltd., England. MERCK, SHARP and DOHME, Pennsylvania, USA kindly made a personal grant to D.D.M.

References. James, V. H. T., and E. CAIE: J. clin. Endocr. **24**, 180 (1964). — KIRKETERP, M.: Acta derm-venerol. (Stockh.) **44**, 54 (1964). — LANDON, J., V. WYNN, and V. H. T. JAMES: J. Endocr. **27**, 183 (1963). — MATTINGLY, D.: J. clin. Path. **15**, 374 (1962). — MARCH, C., and G. KERBEL: J. Amer. med. Ass. **187**, 676 (1964). — SCOGGINS, R. B., and B. KLIMAN: New Engl. J. Med. **273**, 831 (1965).

An Evaluation of Intralesional Steroid Therapy in Alopecia Areata

F. O. MEENAN, Department of Medicine and Therapeutics, University College, "Woodview", Dublin (Ireland)

A steroid suspension was injected locally into the affected areas of 100 patients with alopecia areata of the scalp. There were 61 females and 39 males, ranging in age from 2 to 65 years, the average age being 25. 36 had one patch of alopecia areata while 58 had multiple patches. 6 patients had alopecia totalis.

The steroids used were 2.5% suspension prednisolone acetate in 10 cases, 2.5% triamcinolone diacetate in 10 cases, and 1% triamcinolone diacetate in 80 cases. The injections varied in amount from 0.1 to 0.2 cc. In smaller patches, the injection was given into the centre; in larger patches several injections were given; on an average the distance between the injections was 1/2 inch. The patient returned at intervals of 4 weeks for further injections, if necessary. The depths of the injection were sub-lesional and superficially sub-cutaneous. There were no side effects; in some cases there was slight atrophy at the site of injection, but this disappeared after about 6 months.

In 87 cases approximately 4 to 6 weeks after an injection, there was a definite tuft of hair growing at the site of injection. The colour of this hair was the normal colour of the patient's hair. Simultaneously, or within the next few weeks, fine non-pigmented hair appeared in the untreated areas around the injection site, and also in other affected areas of the scalp that had not been treated. There were two types of hair, thus, filling in a patch of treated alopecia areata: the tufts of steroid-induced hair which were of normal colour and which appeared only at the site of injection, and spontaneous non-pigmented hair which grew in non-injected areas. The spontaneous hair gradually assumed the normal hair colour. In the other 13 cases which included the six cases of alopecia totalis, there was either no hair growth at the site of injection, or else a weak growth which was not sustained and which quickly fell out. Spontaneous hair behaved in a similar manner. If there was a weak and unsustained growth of steroid hair, there migth also be a weak growth of spontaneous hair, but it soon fell out. The six cases of alopecia totalis were observed over 2 to 3 years. During this time periodic waves of weak but definite activity could be detected in the hair follicles. Injections were given at intervals of several months. Sometimes there was no steroid response, and no spontaneous hair grew either. Occasionally, there would be a weak response of steroid hair accompanied by slight spontaneous growth. This might continue for a few weeks. Then the steroid hair fell out, and was followed inevitably by a fall of spontaneous hair. There was no difference between the various strengths of steroid suspension used. Injections into the edge of a spreading patch did not check spread.

It would appear from these results that this therapy does not alter the prognosis in alopecia areata. Judging from the 87 cases whenever steroid hair grew, spontaneous hair grew as well. In the other 13 cases the growth of steroid hair waxed and waned with the growth of spontaneous hair. Treatment with steroid injections does not correct the basic fault which causes alopecia areata. However, in reviewing these 100 cases, it would be unwise to dismiss completely this therapy. It has two virtues. Firstly, if it is accepted that psychological factors play a part in the occurrence of the condition, this form of therapy is attractive, as the patient can see that something positive is being done for his condition. To see a tuft of hair growing at the site of injection helps to keep up the patient's morale, and he can be assured that the hair follicles are not dead. Secondly, it can also be used as a test for prognosis. If there is a sustained hair growth at the site of injection, it means that the outlook for subsequent hair regrowth is good. If there is no growth or a weak and unsustained growth of steroid hair, the immediate prognosis is poor. This test is especially useful in alopecia totalis.

Effects of Topical Steroids in Normal and Psoriatic Skin

L. JUHLIN, Department of Dermatology, University Hospital,
Uppsala (Sweden)

We have in a double-blind investigation studied the effects of corticosteroids applied topically for 4 to 6 weeks without occlusion on psoriatic lesions [1]. The best effect was obtained with 0.025% fluocinolone acetonide ointment. Complete healing was noted on the arms in 43% and on the legs in 34% of the patients. The effect was better if the ointments were applied three instead of two times daily. The amount of steroids applied daily varied between 0.3 to 3.0 gm/dm². There was no correlation between the effect and the amount of ointment used. Relapses were seen within 3 to 28 days in 90% of the patients. After combined therapy with dithranol paste, tar bath and ultraviolet light only 13 to 26% of the patients are reported to relapse after 1 month [2, 3]. Although the skin after both treatments appears normal, it is uncertain if it really has healed and minor histological changes around the vessels might persist for month. No histological differences are seen between steroid and dithranol-treated skin [4]. Histological examinations seem therefore to be of little value to predict relapses.

Lesions of psoriasis are anhidrotic and may show an absence of sweating for a long time after they have cleared clinically. Halter found that anhidrosis preceded the eruption of psoriasis [5]. Searching for a functional measure of healing which might help to predict relapses, we have compared the sweat response before and after treatment with fluocinolone and our conventional therapy. We stained the sweat pores with 5% ortophthaldialdehyde in xylene after stimulation of sweating with metacholine and epinephrine. In psoriatic lesions we saw a few comma-shaped sweat pores [6]. After 3 to 4 weeks treatment with dithranol, tar bath and ultraviolet light as described by INGRAM the number of sweat pores usually became normal. This rarely happened after treatment with fluocinolone. The sweat response could, however, not be used to predict the relapses which were common after fluocinolone. The number of sweat pores in fluocinolone-treated healthy skin was normal.

Histamine has earlier been considered as a stimulator for cell growth during fetal life and early childhood. KAHLSON has postulated a connection between a high rate of histamine formation and rapid tissue growth [7]. Since the cell growth is increased in psoriais we have studied the amount and localisation of histamine in affected and fluocinolone-treated psoriatic skin. Freeze dried histological sections were stained selectively for histamine with the orthopthaldialdehyde method [8, 9]. Histamine was determined in small biopsies and histological sections with a combined electrophoretic and fluorometric method [10]. A marked yellow fluorescense indicating histamine is seen in the tortuous capillaries and in mast cells. The amount of histamine in patients with psoriasis was usually within normal limits in psoriatic lesions, fluocinolone-treated areas and normal appearing skin (Tab. 1). Hyperkeratotic and acanthotic cells without histamine explain the

Table 1

Diagnosis	No. of subjects	Histamine base $\mu g/g$ fresh skin
Healthy	15	3.9 ± 0.4
Psoriasis		
non-treated lesions	15	5.9 ± 0.8
fluocinolone-treated lesions	10	5.0 ± 0.9
normal appearing skin	15	4.8 ± 0.5

Table 2

Material	No. of subjects	Histamine base $\mu g/g$ dry weight		
		Normal	Psoriasis	
			Non treated	Fluocinolone-treated
Stratum corneum and granulosum	8	0	0	0
Basal cell layer and papillae	8	18 ± 2	31 ± 3	19 ± 3
Dermis	7	10 ± 1	11 ± 1	9 ± 2

normal histamine values in total biopsy determinations. We have therefore made sections parallel with the skin surface. An increase of histamine is now found in the sections containing basal cell layer and papillae. The histamine increase is normalized in fluocinolone-treated areas. In normal appearing skin treated with fluocinolone the amount and distribution of histamine remained unchanged. The dermis shows normal histamine values (Tab. 2). Histamine is a physiological vaso-dilator in the skin. Its increase in psoriatic lesions might explain the dilated vessels and it might probably also be involved in the increased growth-rate of the basal cells. Our results with a normalisation of the histamine content after corticosteroid treatment might indicate a pathway for their effect on psoriatic lesions.

References. 1. GROTH, O., L. JUHLIN, G. MICHAËLSSON, and S. ÖHMAN: Acta derm.-venereol. (Stockh.) **47**, 216 (1967). — 2. CHURCH, R.: Brit. J. Derm. **70**, 139 (1958). — 3. PRAKKEN, J. R.: Dermatologica (Basel) **117**, 379 (1958). — 4. SUURMOND, D.: Dermatologica (Basel) **131**, 357 (1965). — 5. HALTER, K.: Arch. Derm. Syph. (Berl.) **191**, 134 (1950). — 6. JUHLIN, L.: Acta derm.-venerol. (Stockh.) **47**, 98 (1967). — 7. KAHLSON, G.: Proc. Int. Union. Physiol. Sciences **1**, 856 (1962). — 8. JUHLIN, L., and W. B. SHELLEY: J. Histochem. Cytochem. **14**, 525 (1966). — 9. JUHLIN, L.: Acta derm.-venerol. (Stockh.) **47**, 383 (1967). — 10. JUHLIN, L.: Acta physiol. scand. **71**, 30 (1967).

The Recurrence Rate of Psoriatic Lesions after Topical Treatment with Dithranol and Corticosteroids under Plastic Dressings

D. SUURMOND, Department of Dermatology, University Hospital, Leiden (The Netherlands)

It is common knowledge that psoriatic lesions improve more rapidly when treated with fluorcorticosteroid creams applied under plastic dressings than when dithranol pastes are used. However, some investigators emphasize, that cortico-steroid-treated lesions tend to relapse sooner (e.g. VERHAGEN, ALEXANDER). This phenomenon is attributed to the fact that many corticosteroid-treated lesions do not disappear completely (according to BRAUN-FALCO and others); persistent residual erythemas and minor histological changes are indeed frequently found in association with these lesions.

In view of the great practical importance of this problem, we have continued our comparative studies (SUURMOND, 1965, 1966) in an attempt to answer two questions:

1. Does the rate of recurrence of corticosteroid-treated lesions and dithranol-treated lesions differ significantly?

2. Are relapses more severe in cases treated with corticosteroids under plastic occlusion than in cases in which dithranol treatment is applied?

Methods and Material

To give an answer to these questions 33 patients with generalized and symmetrically-distributed psoriatic lesions were treated simultaneously with 0.1% triamcinolon acetonide in an O/W emulsion under plastic occlusion on one arm or leg and with dithranol in a zinc paste on the opposite extremity. All patients concerned in this paired comparison trial were admitted to the hospital. Most of the case-histories revealed a strong tendency to rapid recurrences after previous hospital treatments.

Dithranol was employed in gradually increasing concentrations from 0.1 to 1%. Triam-cinolon acetonide cream was applied under thin tubular plastic films for 14 h daily. During the remaining 10 h the cream was applied without plastic occlusion. The favourable effect of this intermittent occlusive therapy appeared to be equal to that of two successive 12-h applications; however, the former has the advantage, that complications due to occlusion occur less frequently.

When the patient was discharged from the hospital, the lesions concerned in this trial had either cleared up completely or showed a slight persistent residual erythema. The latter was observed in ten of the corticosteroid-treated extremities.

Both kinds of treatment were discontinued at the time of discharge and were replaced by application of 20% liquor carbonis detergens (coal tar solution NF) in an O/W emulsion. This weak antipsoriatic after-treatment was given mainly for psychological reasons. The patients were then seen once a week until a relapse was observed, at which the time and the severity of the relapse were recorded.

Results

The comparative treatment had to be discontinued in 11 out of the 33 patients before both sides had cleared up. This was due in five cases to repeated complications caused by the plastic dressing (skin irritation, pustular reactions, and candida infections); in two cases to insufficient improvement of the lesions under occlusive therapy; and in four cases to skin irritations or insufficient improvement under dithranol treatment.

The mean duration of the hospital treatment in the remaining 22 cases was 5½ weeks (varying from 3 to 8 weeks). The duration of the follow-up varied from 2 to 8 weeks in 20 cases, and was 28 and 36 weeks in the two cases which showed no relapse.

The results were as follows:

1. *Worse with corticosteroid treatment* than with dithranol: *6 cases.* Five of these cases showed an earlier relapse and in the sixth case the relapse was more severe than on the dithranol side.

2. *Better with corticosteroid treatment: 5 cases.* In four of these cases the relapses started later than on the dithranol sides and in one case the relapse was less severe than on the opposite side.

3. *No difference* was found in: *9 cases.* In these cases the recurrence rate and the clinical aspect of the relapses were the same for both sides.

4. *No recurrence* on either side was noted in: *2 cases.*

The mean recurrence time for the corticosteroid treatment was 2.9 weeks, for dithranol 3 weeks (varying between 1 and 8 weeks). Very marked differences between the severity of the relapses in individual cases occurred only occasionally.

Conclusions. From the results obtained in this study it may be concluded that no significant differences between the two kinds of treatment were detected with respect to the incidence, the rate and the severity of the relapses. The chance that such differences would be found if the same trial were performed in a larger number of patients can considered slight on the basis of these results.

In a previous study published in Dermatologica (SUURMOND, 1965, 1966), we described the presence of residual histological and enzyme histochemical changes in lesions showing clinical signs of a persistent slight erythema after occlusive corticosteroid therapy. The findings obtained in a small number of cases led us to assume that such lesions generally relapse sooner than completely cleared-up lesions. In the present study, comprising 22 cases, a residual erythema was found in ten patients for the corticosteroid treatment. In five of these cases the erythema faded away during the after-treatment with the liquor carbonis detergens cream, whereas in the other five cases the erythema remained unaltered until the relapse was noted. The rate of recurrence in these lesions did not differ significantly from the rate in lesions which had completely disappeared. This is an unexpected and interesting phenomenon warranting further study.

References. ALEXANDER, S.: Brit. J. Derm. 77, 162 (1965). — SUURMOND, D.: Dermatologica (Basel) **131**, 357 (1965). — Dermatologica (Basel) **132**, 237 (1966). — VERHAGEN, A. R. H. B.: Ned. T. Geneesk. **108**, 1404 (1964).

Effect of Topically Applied 0.1% Betamethasone 17-valerate ("Betnovate") Ointment on the Adrenal Function of Children

M. Feiwel, D. D. Munro and V. H. T. James, Dermatological and Chemical Pathology Departments, St. Mary's Hospital, London (England)

Introduction. In results presented to this Congress (Munro, Feiwel and James, 1967) it has been shown that 30 gm of Betnovate ointment, applied daily under polythene occlusion to adult patients with widespread skin disease impairs hypothalamic-pituitary-adrenal function, but that this is usually associated with rapid recovery on cessation of treatment. Previous investigations with other potent topical corticosteroids (e.g. Scoggins, 1962; Strange and Hjorth, 1965) had also demonstrated some of these effects. The possible consequences of percutaneous absorption in children do not, however, appear to have been studied.

We have investigated nine young children. Selection of cases was not restricted to those most severely or acutely affected, amounts of ointment applied were not very large and the children were not occluded with polythene. In this way we sought to make the study representative of cases not uncommonly seen in dermatological practice and to use treatment a general practitioner might prescribe.

Table. *Clinical Features in the nine Children*

Case	Age Sex Nationality	Diagnosis	Description	Degree of surface involvement	Estimate of severity
1	4 F Jamaican	Atopic dermatitis	dry lichenified	2/3	Moderately severe
2	4 M Indian	Atopic dermatitis	partly exudative	2/3	severe
3	5 M Indian	Atopic dermatitis	partly exudative	2/3	moderately severe
4	6 M Jamaican	Atopic dermatitis	lichenified	1/2	moderately severe
5	$1^1/_2$ M Jamaican	Atopic dermatitis	partly exudative	1/2	moderately severe
6	4 M English	Atopic dermatitis	lichenified excoriated	1/2	severe
7	2 M English	Atopic dermatitis	exudative infected	2/3	severe
8	3 M English	Atopic dermatitis	exudative infected	2/3	severe
9	4 M English	Psoriasis	widespread erythema	1/2	severe

Patients and Methods. The clinical features in the nine children are shown in the table. The children were admitted to hospital but not confined to bed. On the day of admission each child was treated by two applications of ointment base, the affected parts being dressed with stockinette secured with strapping. Gloves were worn if the hands were involved. A bath containing emulsifying ointment preceeded the morning treatment and oral trimeprazine ("Vallergan") was prescribed if irritation was severe. At 9.00 a.m. on the second day a blood-sample was taken by venesection for estimation of the plasma cortisol (method of Mattingly, 1962). Betnovate ointment was then substituted for the inert base but otherwise the same treatment schedule was continued. 7.5 gm of ointment was usually applied in one dressing. If more was required multiples of 7.5 gm were, if possible, used and the total noted. Blood-samples for plasma cortisol estimations were taken twice weekly until the end of active treatment, indicated by complete or near-complete resolution of the skin condition. Application of Betnovate ointment was then stopped. 2 days later a "Synacthen" stimulation test

(WOOD, FRANKLAND, JAMES and LANDON, 1965) was performed, 125 μgm of Synacthen being administered by intramuscular injection and samples for cortisol being taken before injection and 30 min later. The mean period of treatment was 14 days, ranging in individual cases from 6 to 29 days.

Results. The plasma cortisol levels are given in Fig. 1. They are expressed as mean values with the standard error. Results of the Synacthen stimulation test are recorded in Fig. 2.

Discussion. Application of Betnovate ointment in young children with skin disease produced a fall in plasma cortisol levels. In only one case was adrenal function unaffected and this child differed from the rest by having widespread lichenification but minimal acute eczema. In the children, we had chosen conditions less favourable to percutaneous absorption than in the adults (less average

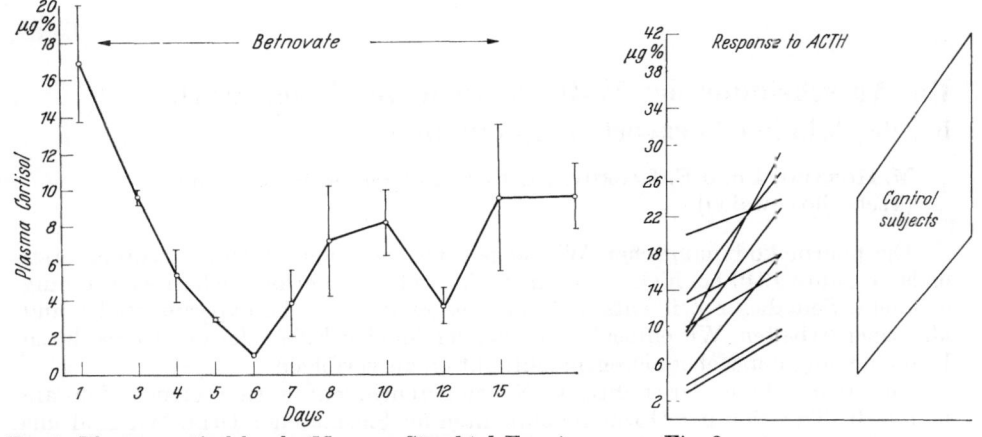

Fig. 1. Plasma cortisol levels (Mean ± Standard Error)   Fig. 2
in nine children treated with 0.1% Betnovate ointment

Fig. 2. Response to ACTH (Synacthen) in children immediately after treatment with Betnovate ointment. Results in adult control subjects are shown for comparison

body-surface involvement, less erythema and exudation, and no polythene occlusion) so these results were somewhat unexpected. Furthermore, eight of the nine children had atopic dermatitis and while most had some exudative areas much of their affected skin was dry and lichenified. Also, five of the nine children were of West Indian or Indian stock (we have many immigrant patients) and these may have a somewhat thicker epidermis than Caucasian children. The finding that low plasma cortisol levels tended to rise again towards the end of the treatment period when, because of clinical resolution, the barrier to cutaneous penetration was being restored, indicated that the observed fall in cortisol levels had not resulted from inadvertent ingestion of Betnovate ointment. Percutaneous absorption thus appears to occur rather readily in children and this finding is important.

Our experience of the Synacthen stimulation test in children is limited but the results show that at the end of treatment eight children had diminution of their adrenal reserve. It should be emphasised, however, that this conclusion is drawn using the criteria in adult patients, and three of the children failed only marginally to achieve these criteria. Results in the remaining five patients were more markedly abnormal and would seem to justify the conclusion that they had an impaired response.

The clinical benefits of potent corticosteroids like Betnovate ointment need no emphasis. However, if the type of the disorder and the treatment approximates that of the children in our series, then the consequences of systemic absorption should be borne in mind especially under ambulant conditions when progress may be slower than in hospital. The case should be managed as if a small dose of oral corticosteroid were being administered.

Acknowledgements. We are indebted to Glaxo Laboratories Ltd. England, and CIBA Laboratories Ltd., England for grants towards our Research Funds. MERCK, SHARP and DOHME, Pennsylvania, USA kindly made a personal grants to one of us (D.D.M.).

References. MUNRO, D. D., M. FEIWEL, and V. H. T. JAMES: Proc. XIIIth Int. Cong. Dermat. 1968, P. 194. — MATTINGLY, D.: J. clin. Path. **15**, 374 (1962). — SCOGGINS, R. B.: J. invest. Derm. **39**, 473 (1962). — STRANGE, H. A., and B. HJORTH: 17th Meeting of Scandinavian Dermat. Soc. Copenhagen 1965. — WOOD, J. B., A. W. FRANKLAND, V. H. T. JAMES, and J. LANDON: Lancet **1965**, I, 243.

Die Ausscheidung der 17-Oxysteroide durch den Harn bei der lokalen Locacorten-Applikation

M. HORÁKOVÁ und E. LACKOVÁ, I. Dermatologische Klinik Prag (Tschechoslowakei)

Die pharmakodynamischen Wirkungen der corticalen Hormone wurden erstmals im Jahre 1949 bei nichtendokrinen Erkrankungen erfolgreich in Anwendung gebracht. Seit dieser Zeit entstand eine unabsehbare Reihe experimenteller und klinischer Arbeiten. Wir entschlossen uns, den lokalen Effekt der Corticoide durch Untersuchung der Nebennierenrindenfunktion zu verfolgen.

Zur Beurteilung der richtigen Nebennierenrindenfunktion eignet sich am besten die Titration der Hormonmetaboliten im Plasma oder Urin. Wir sind uns dessen bewußt, daß auch diese Bewertung nur eine approximative ist, daß sie uns z. B. die Funktion der Mineralcorticoide nicht näher beleuchtet. Aber es ist dies bislang die präziseste Methode zur Beurteilung der richtigen oder alterierten Funktion. Wir ermittelten also die Ausscheidung der 17-OHCS im Urin, denn diese sind die Repräsentanten der für das Leben unerläßlichen Hormonmetaboliten, und zwar Hydrocortison, Corticosteron und Cortison.

Methodik. Wir behandelten zehn Patienten im Alter von 13 bis 84 Jahren mit der Diagnose Psoriasis vulgaris (vier) und Eczema atopicum und chronicum (sechs Patienten). Für sämtliche Ekzematiker verwendeten wir zur Therapie das Präparat Locacorten Creme (Ciba) und für Psoriatiker Locacorten Tar (Ciba). Beide Präparate enthalten 0,02% Flumethason-Pivalat, Locacorten Tar außerdem noch 1,5% Pix lithantrax und 1,0% Acidum salicylicum. Locacorten applizierten wir auf die krankhafte Fläche zweimal täglich und legten für die Nacht durchweg einen luftdichten Verband an. Die Tagesdosis von Locacorten Creme betrug 2,65 bis 10,0 g und Locacorten Tar 4,2 bis 7,0 g.

Wir sammelten den Harn der Kranken innerhalb von 24 Std, und zwar 3 Tage vor Beginn der Therapie mit Corticoiden, 14 Tage während der Behandlung und 3 Tage nach Beendigung der Kur. Die Bestimmung der 17-Oxysteroide im Harn führten wir mittels der von KANDRÁČ modifizierten Methode [1] nach PORTER-SILBER [2] durch. Zur Hydrolyse verwendeten wir die Beta-Glucuronidase aus dem Magensaft der Gartenschnecke (Helix pomatica).

Ergebnisse. Bei unseren zehn Kranken trat während der 14tägigen Locacorten-Applikation keine Veränderung in der 17-Oxysteroidausscheidung zutage, aus der man auf eine Beeinflussung der Nebennierenrindenfunktion durch Resorption des Corticoids schließen könnte. Die Werte der ausgeschiedenen Hormone bei den einzelnen Kranken bewegten sich in den Grenzen der Norm und sind annähernd identisch vor der Einleitung der Therapie, im Verlauf der Behandlung sowie nach

Absetzen der lokalen Therapie. (Zum Beispiel beim Patienten K.O. bewegten sich die Werte der ausgeschiedenen 17-Oxysteroide im Mittel vor der Therapie 3,7 mg/24 Std, während der Behandlung 3,7 mg/24 Std und nach der Therapie 3,7 mg/24 Std. Beim Patienten Z. M. betrugen die Werte vor der Therapie 5,7 mg/ 24 Std, während der Behandlung 5,9 mg/24 Std und nach der Therapie 8,0 mg/ 24 Std.) Wir konnten also weder im Verlauf der Therapie, noch nach Absetzen der lokalen Behandlung einen wertbaren Abfall der corticalen Hormone wahrnehmen.

Diskussion. Aus unseren Ergebnissen können wir urteilen, daß die lokale Applikation von Locacorten (Ciba) die eigene Elimination der 17-Oxysteroide im Urin nicht beeinflußt, und daß auch nach Absetzen der lokalen Applikation ihr Abfall nicht eintritt, der bei der allgemeinen Therapie mit Corticoiden so auffallend ist. Wir können also abschließend sagen, daß bei kurzfristiger lokaler Applikation keine Störung der Nebennierenrindenfunktion droht. Bei der langzeitigen, einige Monate dauernden lokalen Verabreichung der Corticoide, empfehlen wir, auch trotz unserer positiven Ergebnisse, eine intermittierende Therapie [3, 4, 5].

Schlußfolgerung. Nach der kurzfristigen lokalen Locacorten-Applikation trat keine Beeinflussung der durch den Harn ausgeschiedenen 17-OHCS in Erscheinung. Daraus geht hervor, daß die in dieser Form applizierten Hormone keine Nebenwirkungen hervorrufen und daß die lokale Applikation mit keinem Risiko wie bei der allgemeinen Applikation verbunden ist.

Literatur. 1. KANDRÁČ, M. Š.: Steroide Diagnostik. Bratislava; SAC 1955. — 2. PORTER, C. C., and R. H. SILBER: J. biol. Chem. **185**, 201 (1950). — 3. KRACHT, J.: Endokrinologie **39**, 80 (1960). — 4. LACKOVÁ, E., J. POKORNÁ, J. RÁDL, and J. MASOPUST: Čs. Pediat. **22**, 1 (1967). — 5. LACKOVÁ, E., u. J. ŠVEJCAR: Fortschr. Med. **83**, 21, 857 (1950).

Prolongation moyenne de la vie chez les malades de pemphigus vulgaris traités par corticosteroïdes

P. BOTZOV, T. PASCALEV et G. SPIROV, Clinique Derm. Vener. Sofia (Bulgarie)

Pour évaluer la prolongation moyenne de la vie des malades de pemphigus vulgaris (P. V.), nous avons utilisé la méthode d'élaboration de tables de léthalité et de survie (Life tables) appliquées chez des malades soumis à un traitement déterminé.

Tous les malades de P.V. en Bulgarie sont hospitalisés, enregistrés, observés et soignés gratuitement et systématiquement par l'établissement dermatologique le plus proche à leur domicile. Pendant la période 1946 à 1954 nous avons observé 77 malades soignés par les anciennes méthodes, dont le nombre des survivants à la fin de l'année initiale (O) était 51, de la première — 14, de la deuxième — 2 et après la deuxième — pas un seul. Nous avons évalué pour chaque année légale la probabilité de survic pour les malades traités. Cet indice, appellé P_x représente le rapport entre le nombre des malades restés vivants jusqu'au début de l'année légale suivante et le nombre des malades, qui ont été vivants vers le début de l'année précédente. La probabilité de survie pour l'année initiale est $P_o = 0,6623$, pour la première année légale — $P_1 = 0,2916$, pour la deuxième — $P_2 = 0,1538$ et pour la troisième — $P_3 = 0$.

Pour évaluer la probabilité de morbidité, nous avons formé l'équation $P_x + Q_x = 1$. Il en résulte que la probabilité de morbidité (Q) pour les années correspondantes est $Q = 1—P_x$.

La méthode exige qu'on prenne un chiffre arbitraire rond, par exemple 10000 malades, pour faciliter l'évaluation. A l'aide de l'indice d_x (nombre des malades morts dans l'intervalle de x à x + 1 années), nous avons calculé la léthalité des personnes soignées de P. V. par les anciennes méthodes, qui a été 33,77% pendant l'année initiale (0), 80,69% entre la première et la deuxième année, 97,03%-entre la deuxième et la troisième, la période entre la troisième et la quatrième année ayant été fatale pour tous les malades.

En utilisant les valeurs de P_x, Q_x et d_x, nous avons évalué l'indice de la durée moyenne de la vie (e_x^0) des malades, en admettant l'hypothèse, que les cas morbides ont été rhythmiques pendant l'année correspondante, ce qui conditionne que chaque malade mort a vécu dans l'année de sa mort 0,5 année. Pendant l'année initiale (0) les 3377 morts (des 10000 malades) ayant une durée moyenne de la vie de 0,5 année ont survécu au total — 1688,5 années; les 4692 morts entre la première et la deuxième année, ayant une vie moyenne de 1,5 années ont survécu générale-ment 7038 années etc. La somme totale des années vécues par tous les malades morts est 13,851. Etant donné, que pas un seul des malades observés n'a survécu, le chiffre indiqué exprime les années vécues par tous les malades. En divisant le nombre des années vécues par tous les malades soignés au nombre initial des malades, c'est à dire à 10000, on obtient le nombre 1,38. Par conséquent, la durée moyenne de la vie des malades de pemphigus vulgaris soignés par les méthodes anciennes dans la période 1946 à 1954 a été une année et 5 mois.

Dans la période 1955 à 1956 le traitement des malades de P.V. en Bulgarie a été combiné — par les moyens anciens et seulement pour quelques malades — par les corticosteroïdes. Voila pourquoi, nous avons éliminé cette période du spectre d'observation.

Un traitement réalisé exclusivement par des cortisones et par ACTH des malades de P.V. chez nous s'applique depuis 1957. Nous avons observé 132 malades jusqu'au début de l'année 66, desquels ont survécu 68,1% dans cette période de neuf années, tandis qu'à la fin de la troisième année (délai dans lequel mouraient tous les malades soignés par les méthodes anciennes), ont été vivants 74,1% de ce groupe. L'élaboration des données pour ce groupe a été effectuée par la méthode indiquée déjà. Il est indispensable de noter, qu'en calculant à e_x^0 au nombre total des années vécues par les malades morts (8947,5) nous avons ajouté les années vécues (61281) des 6809 malades restés vivants, chacun d'eux ayant vécu 9 années en moyenne jusqu'a la fin de l'observation. Le nombre total des années vécues de tous les malades étant 70228,5, la durée moyenne de la vie des malades de P.V. soignés par les corticosteroïdes dans la période 1957 à 1965 a été 7,02.

La comparaison des données des deux groupes a montré le suivant:

1. La léthalité des malades de P.V. soignés par les méthodes anciennes à la fin de la troisième année a atteint 100%, tandis que pour la même période (trois années) les malades soignés par les corticosteroïdes meurent seulement dans 25,9% des cas.

2. Pour une période d'observation de 9 années sur les malades de P.V. soignés par les corticostéroïdes restent vivant 68,1% du nombre initial des malades.

3. La durée moyenne de la vie des malades de P.V. après l'application des nouvelles méthodes de traitement (corticostéroïdes et ACTH) monte à 7,02 années, tandis que pour ceux traités par les anciennes méthodes, la durée moyenne de la vie est 1,38 années.

Cela signifie que par les nouvelles méthodes de traitement, la vie des malades de P.V. a été prolongée par 5 années et 7 mois.

The Effect of Intraarticular Celestona Chrondose in Rheumatoid Arthritis Associated with Psoriasis

L. HELLGREN and A. BJÖRNBERG, Dept. of Dermatology, University Hospital, Gothenburg (Sweden)

In a total population in Sweden about 10% of the patients with psoriasis have classical, definite or probable rheumatoid arthritis, which is about four to five times higher than for persons without psoriasis in the general population. The clinical picture may be arthritis psoriatica or rheumatoid arthritis. The disease is progressive and may result in deformities if special treatment to the joints is not given. Rheumatoid arthritis in connection with psoriasis cannot usually be treated with antimalarials as the rheumatoid arthritis without the skin disease since exfoliative dermatitis may appear. Also gold salts may lead to exacerbations of the psoriasis.

The symptoms of inflammation in the joints may be reduced in two ways locally, by surgery or by injections of corticosteroids. These are usually rapidly resorbed and need for a longacting effect special preparation as prednisolone in tert. butylacetate, which has a depot action in the joints for weeks or months. During this period the joint symptoms are often lessened subjectively and objectively, normal function of the joints is restored, the pain disappear and deformities can be prevented.

On the skin lesions in psoriasis prednisolone in ointments has very little effect in contrast to the potent betamethasone-17-valerate ointment. To find out if this difference also applies to the arthritis of rheumatoid type associated with psoriasis, betamethasone in a depot preparation (Chrondose, Schering Corp.) was compared with the effect of prednisolone tert. butylacetat.

A double blind technique was used in the investigation. Each patient served as his own control and symmetrical joints affected were chosen for the test. All the joints had typical capsular swelling, exsudate and were painful on motion. The clinical diagnose in all was definite rheumatoid arthritis.

The study was performed in 26 patients. In two symmetrical joints of the same clinical picture one was injected with prednisolone, the other with betamethasone preparation. In smaller joints, i.e. metacarpophalangeal joints and interphalangeal joints 0,3 to 0,4 ml were injected with a fine needle. The effect was judged after 2 weeks and then after 2 to 3 months. Before the injection and in reading the results a sum index was calculated for small indices concerning the different objective and subjective symptoms: Capsular swelling: 0 to 3: exsudate: 0 to 3: pain on active and passive motion: 0 to 3: degree of motion 0 to 3. Null means normal conditions, one means slight symptoms, two moderate symptoms, three extensive symptoms.

It could be demonstrated that betamethasone after 2 weeks had a better effect in 15 of the 26 patients, prednisolone in five.

In six there were no difference in effect between the drugs.

In two respects the betamethasone preparation had disadvantages as compared with the prednisolone preparation. It gave more pain after injections lasting for a period of one or two hours, and was also more turbide.

In conclusion it can be stated that betamethasone in a depot preparation is a valuable steroid for treatment with injections in joint lesions in rheumatoid arthritis associated with psoriasis.

Corticosteroids in the Treatment of Severe Dystrophic Epidermolysis Bullosa

E. J. Moynahan, Hospital for Sick Children and Guy's Hospital, London (England)

Reports of the use of corticosteroids for the treatment of Epidermolysis Bullosa, especially the severe dystrophic and 'letalis' forms continue to be disappointing on the whole. However few authors appear to have treated a significant number of patients and in many the dosage of the corticosteroids was inadequate. The purpose of this communication is to give a brief account of our experience with these drugs in the management of upwards of 20 cases of severe dystrophic epidermolysis bullosa and six of 'letalis' variant at the H.S.C. during the period 1960 to 1967. All other forms of Epidermolysis are excluded and it should be emphasized at the onset, that not only the dosage but the need for steroid therapy was assessed by the clinical severity of the disease and its response to treatment. It did not take long to establish that corticosteroids *when administered in sufficient doses* will control and even suppress blistering in the severest cases and to establish that they are life saving. They will relieve dysphagia and obviate the need for mechanical dilation of the oesophagus or gastrostomy; furthermore, they make it possible for the plastic surgeons to restore useful function to crippled hands, which may be reduced virtually to a barely mobile stump.

It will be convenient to group cases together on clinical grounds, and thus avoid the vexed question of their aetiology and taxonomy, although it does seem likely that each clinico-genetic variant will be shown to be an independent entity. Prednisolone is the steroid of choice though others have been used.

Severe Epidermolysis in the Newborn. Treatment should begin as soon as the diagnosis is established. An initial dose of 60 mg/diem is usually sufficient to prevent fresh blistering in the newborn, but if this is not obtained in 24 to 48 h, the dose should be increased by 50% and if this, too, is inadequate by 100% or more. When satisfactory control is obtained, the dose can be reduced step wise, the rate and amount by which the dosage is reduced being determined by the number and size of new blisters that may appear.

Careful microbiological monitoring of the flora of the skin, mouth and pharynx is essential if serious sepsis is to be avoided. Moniliasis of mouth, pharynx and occasionally the skin is common, and should not be mistaken for fresh blistering; control with Nystatin or Amphotericin is usually easy. Daily bathing using Ung. Emulsificans or similar emollient instead of soap is helpful. Careful toilet of the blistered skin, removing the roof and tattered edges aseptically with scissors also helps to reduce the risk of sepsis. The infant should be nursed naked on parachute silk sheeting — no diaper is worn. Premature infants will require an incubator and should be fed through a nasal tube. Blood transfusions are sometimes required. Careful physiotherapy will prevent contractures when these are threatened.

Complications of Infection in Newborn. Infection is the most serious risk and was responsible for three out of four deaths in the present series. Steroid cardiomyopathy leading to failure is not infrequent in the small infant on high doses, but will respond to appropriate measures — the clinician should not reduce the dose of steroids because of this.

Corticosteroids in the Treatment of Dysphagia. Blistering of the mucosae of the mouth, pharynx and oesophagus invariably occurs in severe cases, whether of the lethal or dystrophic from. Tube feeding may be necessary in the newborn or small infants, until blistering is controlled. Painful dysphagia is a frequent complaint in untreated older patients, in some of whom it may be severe enough to demand mechanical dilation of the gullet or even gastrostomy, if nutrition is to be maintained. *Oesophagoscopy* in these cases has shown that despite radiological findings, there is no organic structure present, but the oesophagus is denuded of much of its epithelial surfaces, which may hang in shreds. Some of these may form synechial bars or ribbons which impede deglutition. Mucosal lesions repond quickly as a rule, to corticosteroids with dramatic improvement in swallowing. This followed in two siblings who required dilation at fortnightly intervals and a grossly affected boy who was sent to us with a view to gastrostomy.

Corticosteroids and the Correction of Deformities in the hands. Many patients with severe involvement develop syndactyly and later lose the use of their digits, as their hands become reduced to a stump covered by thin fragile epidermis beneath which lie clenched and buried their atrophied digits. My colleagues Mr. DAVID MATTHEWS and Mr. IVOR BROOMHEAD have now been successful in restoring useful function to five patients, with severely crippled hands, thanks to the blister-suppressing properties of the steroids. Mutilation will be prevented in earlier cases by careful dosage and suitable physiotherapy designed to prevent contractures and atrophy.

Corticosteroid Therapy in Herpes Zoster

R. W. CARSLAW and J. M. NICOLSON, Victoria Infirmary, Glasgow (Scotland)

The need for a therapeutic method to control post herpetic pain is clear. The management of a case of herpes zoster is still symptomatic in nature. No regime has as yet been suggested that can abort the course of the disease. Many therapeutic measures have been suggested but none have stood the test of controlled trial. In a survey of 916 patients DE MORAGAS and KIERLAND (1957) found that different forms of treatment used during the acute and chronic phase of the process did not modify substantially the natural course of the disease. JORDA, LENFIELD and ROTHSCHILD (1957) found emetine hydrochloride effective in preventing post herpetic neuralgia in a series of 40 cases, whereas pain occurred in 32.5% of controls. They considered that this was due to the antiinflammatory effect of emetine hydrochloride.

Corticosteroid therapy to control or prevent the inflammatory reaction may be considered justifiable in the management of herpes zoster in the adult. This is based on the assumption that post herpetic neuralgia may be due to post inflammatory fibrosis in the root ganglia or sensory roots. ELLIOT (1964) in a series of 16 cases had no incidence of post herpetic neuralgia using prednisolone in high dosage as the antiinflammatory agent.

At the present time simple analgesics are the routine, coupled with local measures to control or prevent sepsis. The course is self limiting. In the young subject there is surprisingly little symptomatic effect and normally no sequelae. In the older patient, however, symptoms may be severe. Pre-herpetic pain, pain and discomfort with the herpetic eruption and post herpetic neuralgia are found. This sequel of post herpetic neuralgia, a sequel to the acute inflammatory stage of the disease, may persist for years. It can result in prolonged and severe disablement.

An investigation of consecutive cases of herpes zoster seen at a major teaching hospital was carried out. 32 cases were included in the investigation. 12 cases received analgesics only; 8 cases received emetine hydrochloride; 4 cases received

emetine hydrochloride and later cortisone acetate; 4 cases received Prednisolone
and 4 Betamethasone.

Table 1. *Distribution of cases by age*

	Total	Post Herpetic Neuralgia	%
Under 40 years	4	1	25
40 to 70 years	21	4	20
Over 70 years	7	3	42

Table 2. *Distribution of cases by site*

	Total	Post Herpetic Neuralgia	%
Cerebral	15	3	20
Cervical	3	—	—
Thoracic	8	4	50
Lumbar	6	1	16.6

Table 3. *Therapy related to post herpetic neuralgia*

Treatment	Total	Post Herpetic Neuralgia	%
Analgesics	12	3	25
Emetine Hydrochl.	8	2	25
Emetine and Cortisone	4	3	75
Prednisolone	4	—	—
Betamethasone	4	—	—

The poor result with the combined Emetine and Cortisone Acetate was
probably due to the fact that the Cortisone Acetate was given after Emetine had
appeared to be ineffective and so was given late in the course of the disease. It is
probable that it was also given in insufficient dosage.

It is our belief that the corticosteroids, by controlling the acute inflammatory
reaction, both give much needed relief to the patient in the acute stage and lessen
the possibility of post herpetic neuralgia.

This survey of 32 consecutive cases of herpes zoster has shown an overall
figure of 25% with the sequela of post herpetic neuralgia. This is the experience
of other authors (CARTER and ROYDS, 1957). The age distribution is again that
which is generally accepted. Pain was a symptom of the acute phase in 29 cases
and was absent in only three cases aged 10, 27 and 72.

Cortisone acetate was given in a daily dose of 100 mg to 4 cases, in all at a
late stage, and 3 had the sequela of post herpetic neuralgia. The therapy was given
too late and the dosage was too low. But in 4 cases receiving Prednisolone 20 mg
daily and 4 receiving Betamethasone 3 mg daily all escaped this sequela. These
8 cases had pain during the acute phase and in all there was also pre-herpetic
pain. In all but 2 cases the corticosteroid was given during the first week. The
segment involved was cerebral 5, thoracic 1 and lumbar 2 cases. The average age
was 63, the youngest 54 and the oldest 74.

The eight cases on Prednisolone or Betamethasone had rapid relief from the
acute symptoms although the course of the disease was probably unaffected.

It is suggested that it is justifiable to take such measures as we can to control
the inflammatory phase of the disease as this will, we believe, lessen the risk of the
disabling sequela of post herpetic neuralgia. No case of spread of the viral infection
was found. However, it is considered that this form of therapy should not be given
to the young patient. The young patient suffers little discomfort and the risk of
post herpetic neuralgia is very slight.

References. CARTER, A. B., and J. E. ROYDS: Brit. med. J. **2**, 746 (1957). — ELLIOTT, F. A.:
Lancet **2**, 610 (1964). — DE MORAGAS, J. M., and R. R. KIERLAND: Arch. Derm. **75**, 193 (1957).
— JORDA, V., J. LENFIELD, and L. ROTHSCHILD: Čs. Derm. **32**, 309 (1957).

Avantages thérapeutiques des corticostéroïdes dans un cas de Ainhum

A. MERELLO, Aiuto Inc. Reparto Dermatologico Ospedale San Carlo di Genova Voltri (Italie)

P. EDA agée de 42 ans. Le grand-père paternel affecté de chératodermie paume-plantaire a eu une fille avec cataracte congénitale. La p. affectée de chératodermie paume-plantaire avec cataracte zonulaire congénitale bilatérale a eu une fille affectée de cararacte congénitale. De touts les membres de la dite famille, seule la p. a commencé depuis quelque temps à remarquer des étranglements annulaires symétriques aux petits orteils des pieds en correspondance de l'interligne articulaire entre la seconde et la troisième phalange sans altérations des ongles.

Les sillons annulaires se sont toujours plus approfondis avec l'apparition de phénomène ulcératif, cause d'intenses douleurs spontanées et provoquées par la déambulation.

La p. est en outre une poliartrosique avec une colicistite calculeuse et une colite spastique. Elle a un métabolisme de base $+ 19$. Modiquement anémique elle a une discrète augmentation de l'indice de Katz avec iperglobulinémie. Elle a des périodes de petite fièvre. Rien d'autre de particulier ne révèlent tous les plus variés examens de laboratoire. On pose le diagnostic d'une forme d'étranglement

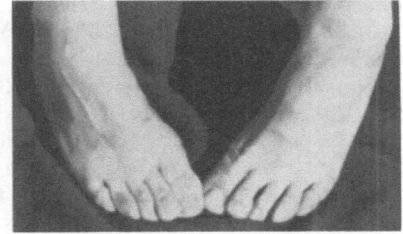

annulaire simile-Ainhum avec chératodermie paume-plantaire sur base disgénique ecto-mésodermique, en artrosique, colélitiasique et disthyroïde. Le cas rappelle ceux de MIANI et RASPONI et D'ACTON, HYDE MONTGOMERY, PARDO-CASTELLO et DE MESTRE. On a commencé un traitement polivalent, antidisréactif, polivitaminique, antibiotique et symptomatique.

La situation pathologique des orteils, cependant, ne s'améliore pas. On obtient une amélioration décisive, subjective, et objective avec des infiltrations locales d'une solution de bétamétasone (Célestone) en dose d'un mgr. par orteil à jours alternés pour un ensemble de 15 piqûres. La p. a ainsi pu éviter de subir une amputation et elle est remise en de bonnes conditions. Contrôlée à périodes elle est soumise à quelques piqûres locales pour maintenir les résultats obtenus.

Bibliographie. BECKER, W., and M. E. OBERMAYER: Modern Dermatology and Syphilology, 2 ed. London: Lippincot 1947. — CAVALIERI, R.: Cronache dell'I.D.I. **6**, 403 (1961). — EHRMANN, S., u. R. BRUNAUER: Handbuch der Haut- u. Geschl.-Kr., Bd. VIII/2. Berlin: Springer 1931. — MIANI, G., e L. RASPONI: Arch. ital. Derm. **XXV**, (I) (1952). — ORMSBY, S. O., and H. MONTGOMERY: Diseases of the Skin, 8 ed. London: Kimpton 1954. — RIVA, P. C.: Arch. ital. Derm. **XXXI**, (V) 281. — SIMONS, PH., PERIS, and GONZALES: Ainhum or dactylolysis spontanea Handbook of Tropical Dermatology and Medical Mycology. Amsterdam: Elsevier Publ. Company 1953. — ZUCCARINI, N.: Dermatologia (Napoli) **13**, 34 (1962).

The Present Aspect of Corticosteroids — Therapy of Pemphigus in Japan

K. OHARA, Dept. of Dermatology, Kansai Medical School, Osaka (Japan)

The purpose of this study is to realize the present aspect of corticosteroids therapy and the prognosis of pemphigus in Japan in comparison with other countries.

The data of 240 cases collected from 103 hospitals throughout Japan have been analyzed.

The advent of corticotropin and various synthetic corticosteroids for the treatment of pemphigus resulted in a marked improvement in the prognosis of the disease. The mortality in the presteroid era ranged from 43.6 to 100% in countries other than Japan. In Japan, it was between 35.0 and 60.4%. The mortality in the poststeroid era is from 4.0 to 44% in non-Japanese series. Statistically, it revealed 22.5% on an average of 185 deaths among 823 cases in 27 reports from Austria, Brazil, Canada, England, Germany, Holland, Hungary, India, USA and USSR.

In Japan, it was 10 to 25% by YAMASAKI et al., and in my present series, it revealed 20.1%.

Results of corticoid therapy in 73 living patients with pemphigus in Japan. 33 of these patients were free of lesions without treatment for 4 to 80 months, 16 of them were found with a few lesions without treatment and 15 with a few lesions with maintenance doses, the remaining 9 being in an exacerbation.

Among 232 living patients from ten non-Japanese reports including NELSON, MATTER, SANDERS et al., STEVENSON, WITTELS, LINTON et al., PEL et al., LEVER, SÖNNICHSEN and KÜRNER, 75 were clear without treatment, 103 were clear with maintenance doses, 34 were found with a few lesions with maintenance doses, one was in an exacerbation and the remaining 19 were unknown.

An analysis was made of various factors related to the mortality, such as the age of onset, known duration, severity of the disease and laboratory findings. Regarding the mortality by the age of onset in 168 pemphigus cases in Japan, the younger and older age groups show a higher mortality than the middle age group. The same tendency is seen in 50 American cases reported by SANDERS et al. in 1960. Next, mortality was studied related to the known duration in 106 Japanese pemphigus vulgaris cases. Almost all fatal cases were those with less than a 3-year known duration.

Regarding the total protein level and A/G ratio, the fatal cases are found with less total protein and lower A/G ratio. It is to be noted that there is no difference in mortality irrespective of the presence or absence of oral lesions in our series.

Initial daily doses used in Japan are as follows: less than 4 tablets 41%, 4 to 8 tablets 44.7%, 8 to 12 tablets 8.7%, 12 to 16 tablets 1.9%, more than 16 Tablets 3.7%. That is to say, in Japan, most of the patients were treated by rather small doses, i.e., less than 12 tablets. These doses were about a half or one third of those of western countries. The mortality in reference to initial, maintenance and average daily doses of corticosteroids was discussed.

Next, causes of death were analyzed. It is noticed that Japanese cases showed more deaths due to pemphigus and less deaths due to corticoid therapy than cases in the non-Japanese literature (Tab. 1). 17 fatal Japanese cases due to or probably due to corticoid therapy consisted of 10 cases (58.5%) of bacterial or monilial infections, 5 cases (29.4%) of peptic ulcer and 2 cases (11.8%) of others; the non-Japanese counterpart revealed 44.4, 28.9 and 6.7%, respectively, with 20% thromboembolism. Japanese fatal cases due to corticoid therapy were more

attributable to infections and less to thromboembolism than non-Japanese cases
(Tab. 2).

Table 1. *Cause of Death*

	Deaths of Pemphigus	Deaths from Therapy	Deaths of Incidental Diseases	Unknown	Total Deaths
Japanese Cases	22 (48.9%)	17 (37.8%)	6 (13.3%)	0	45
Non-Japanese Cases	35 (26.1%)	66 (49.3%)	29 (21.6%)	4 (3%)	134

Table 2. *Analysis of Deaths Attributable to Therapy*

	Infection	Peptic Ulcer	Thrombosis or Embolism	Others	Total Deaths Attr. to Therapy
Japanese Cases	10 (58.8%)	5 (29.4%)	0	2 (11.8%)	17
Non-Japanese Cases	20 (44,4%)	13 (28.9%)	9 (20%)	3 (6.7%)	45

Table 3. *Summarized Data*

	Death Rate	Deaths due to Pemphigus / Total Deaths	Deaths attributable to Therapy / Total Deaths	Deaths due to Infections / Deaths attributable to Therapy	Dosage of Corticoids
Japanese Cases	20.1%	48,9%	37.8%	58.8%	low
Non-Japanese Cases	22.5%	26.1%	49.3%	44.4%	high

The summarized data are shown in the Tab. 3. It seems safe to interpret
that more deaths due to corticoid therapy of non-Japanese cases are probably
attributable to a higher dosage, and more deaths due to pemphigus of the Japanese
series are probably attributable to a lower dosage. As COSTELLO, SANDERS and
LEVER have stated, early and vigorous treatment with rather a high initial dosage
is preferable. It is suggested that a little higher dosage would be reasonably recommended in the treatment of pemphigus in Japan.

Accion topica de la fluformilona en dermatologia

P. A. VIGLIOGLIA, Universidad de Buenos Aires (Argentina)

Los córticosteroides representan la medicación tópica mas ampliamente empleada en el tratamiento de las dermopatías. La fluformilona es un nuevo esteroide
anti-inflamatorio, de acción fundamentalmente tópica, dotado de intensa actividad
antiflogística y antirreaccional.

Con este nuevo compuesto hemos sometido a tratamiento local a un numeroso
grupo de pacientes con la finalidad de establecer: su actividad tópica; y posibilidad
de efectos sistémicos por absorción percutánea eventual.

Empleamos el esteroide a la concentración de 0,025%, en vehículo hidrosoluble y oleaginoso. Se siguió el procedimiento "doble ciego", utilizando alternativamente excipiente solo y preparación completa conteniendo el esteroide.

Se efectuaron además estudios comparativos con preparados de hidrocortisona, alcohol libre (al 1%), de fluorandrenolona (al 0,05%) y de fluocinolona (al 0,025%), estableciéndose las indicaciones preferenciales de ungüento, crema y cura oclusiva.

El método "doble ciego" se experimentó en dermopatías simétricas y el oclusivo en procesos crónicos, empleándolo con ritmo intermitente de 48 h para evitar complicaciones (piodermitis, miliar roja, estrías atróficas) y nunca en más de la cuarta parte del cuerpo (25 grs.) para eludir posibles riesgos de absorción percutánea.

Al justipreciar los resultados se tuvieron en cuenta las respuestas objetivas y subjetivas; como criterios de mejoría se consideraron: reducción de los síntomas (en especial prurito); disminución del edema, eritema y/o descamación; atenuación o desaparición de la lesión. El ensayo se efectuó en un grupo de 217 pacientes que comprendió: Dermatitis atópica (37), Psoriasis (26), Dermatitis de estasis (24), Eczema del lactante (23), Dermatitis seborreica (18), Dermatitis de contacto (14), Prurito vulvar (12), Dishidrosis (12), Neurodermitis circunscripta (9), Prurito anal (8), Otitis externa (8), Eritema solar (8), Picadura de insecto (6), Eczema numular (5), Toxicodermia (4) y Liquen rojo plano (3).

La aplicación del medicamento se llevó a cabo en pacientes vírgenes de tratamiento o en aquellos que venían recibiendo terapéutica general, después de haberlo interrumpido durante 15 días.

En 25 pacientes con cura oclusiva, se controló la eliminación de los 17-cetosteroides urinarios para descartar absorción percutánea. En el 80% de los casos tratados con aplicaciones tópicas de fluformilona, los resultados obtenidos fueron satisfactorios y las diferencias con los placebos resultaron netas. No hubo evidencias de sensibilización alérgica a la medicación, ni signos o síntomas que hicieran presumir fenómenos por absorción percutánea.

Los estudios comparativos demostraron que la fluformilona al 0,025% posee una eficacia superior a la hidrocortisona alcohol libre al 1%; y similar a la fluorandrenolona al 0,05% y a la fluocinolona al 0,025% (considerada hasta ahora como el esteroide local más activo). Las bajas concentraciones medicamentosas (0,025%) reducen el costo y permiten emplear los esteroides en áreas mas extensas de la piel.

En períodos evolutivos o en zonas donde se impone lubricación, la base oleosa fué preferida a la hidrosoluble.

La cura oclusiva es preferible a la infiltración local con esteroides anti-inflamatorios porque no causa dolor, hemorragia ni atrofia; puede repetirse a voluntad; puede aplicarla el propio paciente y el riesgo de absorción sistémica es menor.

En las curas oclusivas y tomando las precauciones ya mencionadas, no hemos observado fenómenos humorales atribuíbles a absorción sistémica. El tratamiento oclusivo se halla especialmente indicado en dermopatías crónicas.

Recomendamos la cura oclusiva con fluformilona en psoriasis, neurodermitis circunscripta, dermatitis atópica, dermatitis de estasis y en el lupus eritematoso crónico.

En resumen, la fluformilona representa un nuevo esteroide, con neta disociación entre efectos locales y sistémicos, que demuestra una eficacia antiflogística y antirreaccional prácticamente superior a la de los esteroides de acción Tópica más activa.

Main Theme III

**Contact Dermatitis
(Allergic and Non-Allergic)**

**Dermatitis de contact
(allergiques et non-allergiques)**

**Dermatitis por contacto
(Alérgicas y no alérgicas)**

**Kontaktdermatitis
(allergische und nicht-allergische)**

Organizer

S. LAPIÈRE, Belgium

Presidents

CL. HURIEZ, France
M. A. MALEKI, Iran
V. PIRILÄ, Finland
J. TAPPEINER, Austria

Delegate of the Organization Committee

J. KIMMIG, Germany

Reports

Factors Involved in Contact Non-Allergic Dermatitis*

R. R. SUSKIND, Divisions of Environmental Medicine and Dermatology, University of Oregon Medical School (USA)

Any comprehensive discussion of critical factors which determine the responsiveness of the skin in contact dermatitis should include: 1. The nature of the substance and its inherent capacity to damage; 2. the degree of exposure i.e., concentration, duration of contact and size of the area exposed; 3. the vulnerability of the skin as determined by genetic considerations or presence of prior existing skin disease; 4. the vulnerability of the skin as determined by environmental factors such as ambient humidity, wetting, ambient temperature and prior exposure to chemical agents; 5. the habits of the patient.

We have been impressed with the clinical observation that non-allergic contact dermatitis is in many instances provoked by repeated exposure to marginal irritants and that the clinical reactions are clearly influenced by environmental factors such as wetting, ambient humidity and temperature, as well as prior or concomitant exposure to chemical agents. All of these environmental factors have a measurable influence on percutaneous absorption and render the skin more vulnerable to specific penetrants.

The best examples are the cases which occur in so-called "wet work", among machine tool operators, housewives, restaurant workers, loggers and wood-pulp workers in which the common factor is frequent exposure to water.

This report is concerned primarily with the influence of wetting on reactivity to marginal irritants and on the penetration of a series of nicotinates as it may be measured experimentally. The questions which we have attempted to answer are: 1. Will water produce identifiable structural injury in mammalian skin? 2. If barrier characteristics are altered by water, can such alterations be measured in terms of intensified responses to low-level irritants such as edible oils, and pharmacologic agents? 3. How long after removal from the water does it take for the penetration characteristics to return to their normal pre-wetted state? 4. Does repeated immersion result in cumulative change penetration characteristics? 5. Can the degree of permeability change induced by hydration be correlated with the duration and/or frequency of exposure? 6. How does water effect the penetration of substances with widely different water/ether partition coefficients?

A. Water Immersion Vulnerability to "Innocuous" Chemical Agents

1. Guinea Pig Reactions. It was observed that when shaved albino guinea pigs were immersed in tap water at 37 °C as frequently as one hour four times daily for as long as 4 weeks, no gross or histological injury was detected (Fig. 1). No changes were observed when biopsy material was stained with H and E, PAS, sulfhydryl and disulfide localization methods, Sudan Black and acid hematin (Fig. 1). No changes in localization or intensity of epidermal enzymes were observed when the water-exposed animals were compared with non-immersed controls. The enzymes studied histochemically included cytochrome oxidase, acid phosphatase, lactic dehydrogenase, leucine aminopeptidase, alpha-naphthol esterase, glucose-6-phosphatase, glucose-6-phosphate dehydrogenase, succinic dehydrogenase, and Tween esterases.

---

* These studies were supported in part by research grant OH 00137 National Institutes of Health U.S.P.H.S.

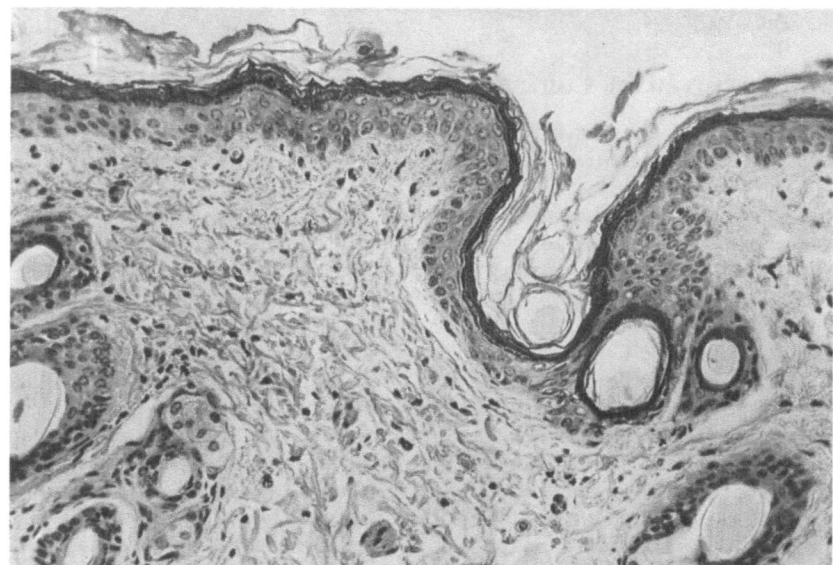

Fig. 1. Section of guinea pig skin from animal immersed in water at 37 °C, 2 h daily for 3 weeks (hematoxylin and eosin; X 180)

When measured amounts (0.05 ml) of edible oils, such as cottonseed and corn oil, were applied daily for 3 weeks to shaved guinea pigs, mild reactions were seen in a limited number of animals. Edible oils were chosen initially because they are common contactants for those involved in kitchen work among whom the incidence of irritant hand dermatitis is high. 80% of the animals failed to show any gross change in 3 weeks. When the same number of animals were immersed in water for 1 h daily, or longer, and the oils applied 30 min after removal from the water bath, moderate-to-severe inflammatory reactions resulted within 2 to 5 days, varying with the specific oil (Fig. 2). The inflammatory responses in wetted animals differed from the non-wetted animals in that they were of much greater intensity, developed in a much shorter period of time, and a larger number of animals were affected (Fig. 2).

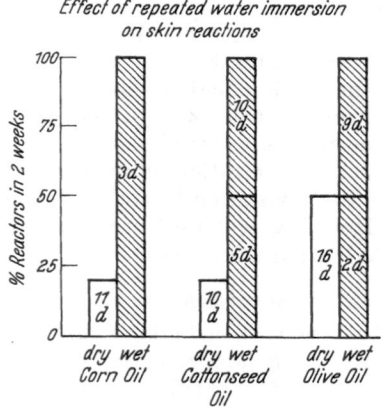

Effect of repeated water immersion on skin reactions

Fig. 2. Percentage of guinea pigs reacting within 2 weeks of exposure to measured amounts of edible oils: nonimmersed compared to water-immersed animals (d indicates maximum number of days required to produce reactions)

Striking histological differences are observed when the skin of the non-immersed, oil-exposed animals is compared with the water-immersed oil-exposed groups (Fig. 3 to 5). The oils alone produce some epidermal hyperplasia and minimal dermal reaction in the non-wetted skin. The normal guinea pig epidermis, which is 1 to 2 cell layers in thickness may increase to 3 to 5 cells in thickness and a slight increase in inflammatory cells is noted. By contrast the reaction of repeatedly-immersed skin to the edible oils is

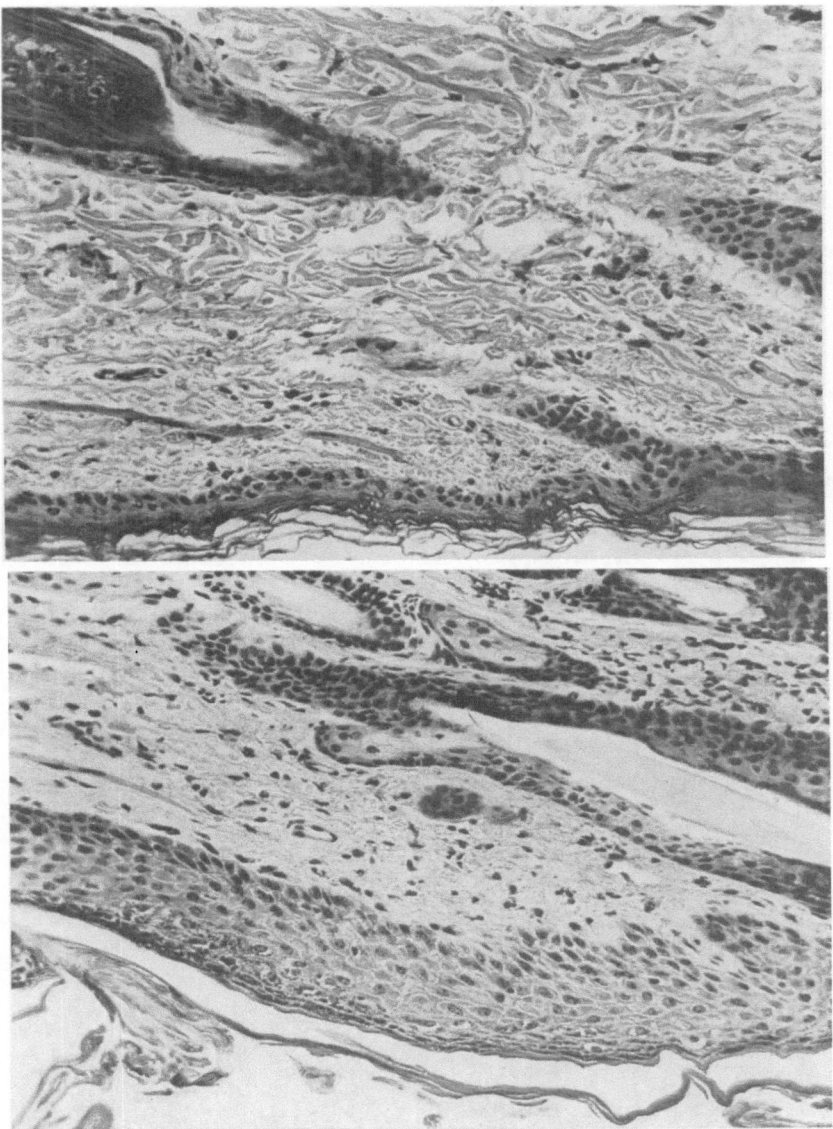

Fig. 3. Reaction of guinea pig skin to daily application of cottonseed oil for 3 weeks in the nonimmersed animal (top) compared with untreated side of same animal (bottom) (hematoxylin and eosin; X 180)

characterized by intense acanthosis (7 to 15 cells in thickness), spongiosis, and a significant inflammatory infiltrate. The hyperplastic response may extend to the follicular epithelium as well. The results of applying some simple straight-chain aliphatic acids and alcohols in subthreshold irritant concentrations to the skin of non-immersed, as compared with immersed is shown in Fig. 6.

   2. Human Skin Reactions. Measured amounts (0.2 ml) of a series of common edible oils and their significant fatty acid components were applied daily to the

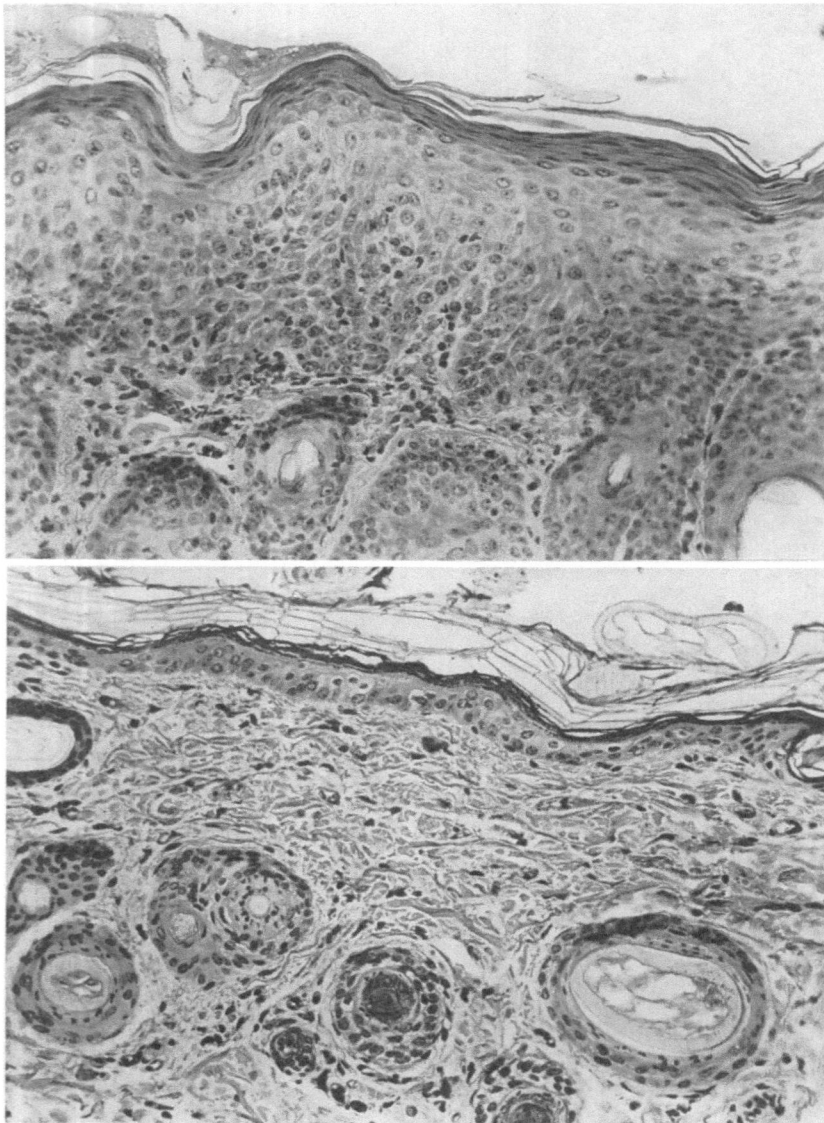

Fig. 4. Reaction of guinea pig skin to daily application of cottonseed oil for 3 weeks in the water-immersed animal (top) as compared to the untreated side of the same animal (bottom) (hematoxylin and eosin; X 180)

forearms of human subjects for 3 weeks. A greater number of reactions were observed on the forearm previously immersed in water for 1 h than on the non-immersed forearm and in a shorter period of time. The table below summarizes the result of one of several typical experiments using 15 subjects. Octyl alcohol was the positive control. The materials were undiluted and both the oleic and linoleic acids were of commercial grade and in liquid state.

The major fatty acid components of the corn oil used were 53% linoleic acid

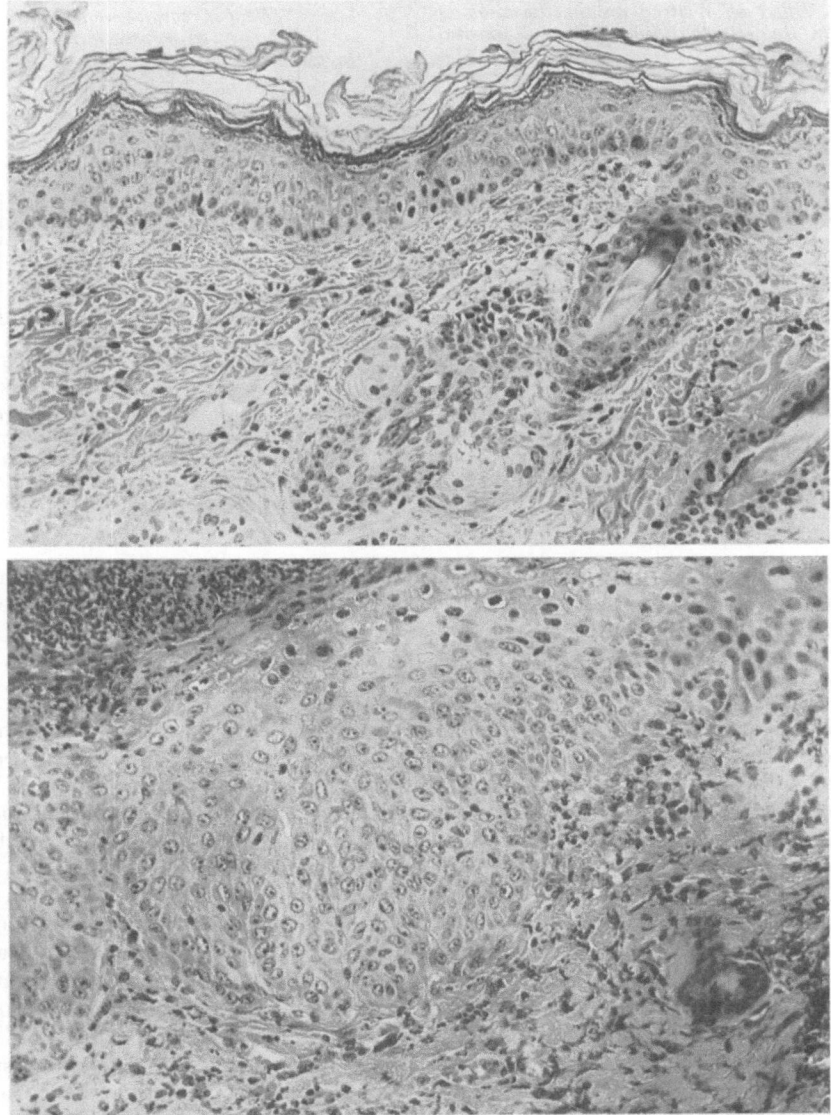

Fig. 5. Reaction of guinea pig skin to daily application of olive oil for 3 weeks in the non-immersed animal (top) as compared with reaction in the immersed animal (bottom); (hematoxylin and eosin; X 180)

and 29% oleic acid; olive oil contained 74% oleic acid and 8% linoleic acid. It appears from these results that the irritant effect in human skin of corn oil is probably from the linoleic acid rather than from the oleic acid, since olive oil evoked no clinical damage in either non-wetted or wetted skin while corn oil with its higher concentration of linoleic acid produced responses in 20% of the subjects on the immersed side. More than 50% of the subjects were frankly irritated by linoleic acid on the immersed side as compared with 13% on the non-immersed side. Histological examination revealed much more intense epidermal and dermal

Table. *Effect of Wetting on the Reaction of Human Subjects to Edible Oils and unsaturated Fatty Acids*

Material	Percentage of Subjects Reacting	
	Immersed forearm %	Dry forearm %
corn oil	20	0
soybean oil	7	0
olive oil	0	0
oleic acid	20	7
linoleic acid	53	13
triolein	0	0
mineral oil	20	0
octyl alcohol	100	80

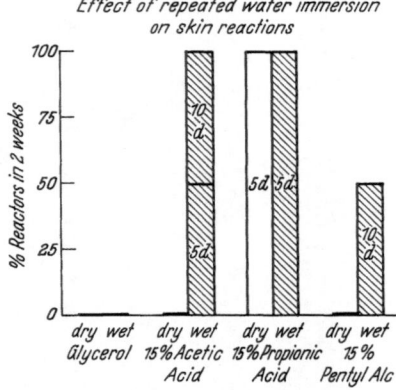

Fig. 6. Percentage of guinea pigs reacting within 2 weeks of exposure to organic compounds: nonimmersed compared to water-immersed animals (*d* indicates maximum days required to produce reactions)

responses on the wetted forearm to which the materials were applied than on the non-wetted side. These histological observations paralleled very closely those described for the guinea pigs.

B. Effect of Wetting on Absorption of a Homologous Series of Nicotinates

Using a modified technique described by STOUGHTON et al. [2], we demonstrated that the penetration of methyl nicotinate in guinea pig skin was measurably altered by whole body immersion in water at 37 °C and by ambient humidity [1]. The skin was tested with a series of concentrations prior to and at intervals after wetting to determine the minimal concentration which would induce a reaction. The data indicated that the degree of change in penetrability as well as the persistence and reversibility of such change can be correlated with the duration and frequency of water immersion and with the duration and level of relative humidity. Cumulative effects were observed with immersion of 2 h/day or greater after 2 weeks of such exposure [1]. Similar experiments were conducted with human subjects using two different techniques of wetting: 1. whole forearm immersion in water at 37 °C in which reactions before and after immersion were determined and compared with reactions in the non-immersed forearm and, 2. a series of small areas on one side of the forearm was kept moist by filter paper squares measuring 1 cm² saturated with water at 37 °C for specified periods of time. Wetted areas were tested with a series of concentrations of each nicotinate to determine the threshold concentration which would produce a reaction. These were compared with adjacent non-wetted areas of the same forearm before and at stated intervals after the water exposure had been terminated.

In experiments using whole forearm immersion and methyl nicotinate as the indicator, the skin reactivity was increased almost six times immediately following the immersion; 30 min following immersion the reactivity was still altered by a factor of 3 X and the skin of most of the subjects returned to their pre-immersion levels at the end of 1 h.

Using the more sensitive filter paper technique, 1 h of wetting resulted in an 18-fold increase in reactivity when tested with methyl nicotinate immediately after wetting; there was still a three-fold increase within ½ h after wetting. The reactivity returned to the level of the non-wetted sites within 1 h after the termination of the wetting.

8 Subjects					H_2O at 37 °C
30 min immersion		1 h immersion			
Tested Post Immersion	15 min	Immed.	15 min	30 min	1 h
Reactivity Factor Average	3.4	5.6	3.8	3.0	1.0

Fig. 7. Effect of water immersion on skin reactivity to methyl nicotinate

1 h filter paper wetting

Post Wetting Test	Immed.			10 min		
Reagent	B	M	Ac	B	M	Ac
Reaction factor average	14	18	1.5	12	9	1.5

20 min			30 min			1 h			2 h		
B	M	Ac	B	M	Ac	B	M	Ac	B	M	Ac
11	4	1	4	3	1	1	2	1	1	1	1

B = Butyl nicotinate; M = Methyl nicotinate; Ac = Nicotinic acid

Fig. 8. Effect of wetting on nicotinate penetration and skin reactions

The nicotinic acid esters: methyl and butyl nicotinate and nicotinic acid, provides a small homologous series of compounds which differ in their water solubilities and their H_2O/ether partition coefficient as well as in their individual ability to form hydrogen bonds. There is a dramatic difference in the effect of water on methyl and butyl nicotinate, e.g. 14 to 18 times, immediately after water exposure. The skin response returns to the level of the non-wetted site at the same rate within 1 h. By contrast, prior wetting of the skin has *no effect* on the activity of the much more water soluble nicotinic acid. The H_2O/ether partition coefficient of nicotinic acid is 9.25 as contrasted with methyl and butyl nicotinate which have coefficients of 0.373 and 0.028 respectively [3]. The increased activity of the more lipid soluble esters in previously wetted skin is a reflection of the enhanced penetration by hydration of the barrier. A plausible but intriguing explanation is that water alters the non-polar pathways utilized by the lipid soluble esters but has no apparent effect on the polar or aqueous pathway utilized by the nicotinic acid. This idea is further supported by the observation that the penetration of heavy white mineral oil (the water solubility of which approaches zero) is also enhanced by wetting.

We wish to acknowledge with gratitude the efforts of Dr. M. Ishihara, Dr. H. Nitto, and Dr. T. Ryan; Mrs. G. Christian and Miss J. C. Hopkins all of whom made substantial contributions to these investigations.

References. 1. Suskind, R., R. and M. Ishihara: Arch. environm. Hlth 11, 529 (1965). — 2. Stoughton, R., W. E. Clendenning, and D. Kruse: J. invest. Derm. 35, 337 (1960). — 3. Stoughton, R.: Some In-Vivo- and In-Vitro-Methods for Measuring Percutaneous Absorption. In: Progress in the Biological Sciences in Relation to Dermatology, p. 263. Cambridge: Univ. Press 1964.

Die Epicutanprobe durch wiederholte Benetzung

W. Burckhardt, R. Schmid und P. Schmid, Städt. Dermat. Poliklinik, Zürich (Schweiz)

Die 1896 von J. Jadassohn eingeführte Läppchenprobe ist noch immer die Standardmethode zur Abklärung des Kontaktekzems. Es gibt jedoch Situationen, bei welchen die Applikation eines einzigen Tropfens der Noxe unter einem Okklusivverband mit einer Expositionszeit von 24 Std nicht die adäquate, der tatsächlichen Exposition am nächsten kommende, Testform ist. Insbesondere für die Prüfung der Empfindlichkeit der Haut gegenüber Flüssigkeiten, die wiederholt und massiv im Berufe mit der Haut in Berührung kommen, kann die Testung eines einzigen Tropfens ein falsches Resultat geben, da die Chemie der Hautoberfläche diese kleine Menge der Noxe verändern kann, so daß die Hornhautbarriere nicht mehr durchdrungen wird. Es gibt zahlreiche Arbeitssituationen, bei welchen die Haut wiederholt mit Flüssigkeiten — Detergentien, Lösungsmittel, Kühlwasser, Bohrwasser, Zementaufschwemmungen — in Berührung kommt, wobei offenbar die Zahl und die Dauer der Arbeitskontakte eine wesentliche Rolle spielen, indem diese Flüssigkeiten zunächst die Oberflächenchemie der Haut verändern, um dadurch andere Permeabilitätsverhältnisse zu schaffen, so daß spätere Kontakte zu Reaktionen führen, welche durch den ersten Kontakt nicht hervorgerufen werden konnten.

An der Städtischen Poliklinik für Hautkrankheiten in Zürich haben wir deshalb seit einigen Jahren die Epicutanprobe durch wiederholte Benetzung durchgeführt. Eine mit einem Gentianaviolett-Kreis markierte, handtellergroße Hautpartie — meistens am Oberarm — wird mit einem Wattestäbchen wiederholt benetzt. Der Patient kann diese Benetzung selbst durchführen. Pro Minute werden zwei Benetzungen vorgenommen. Am 1. Tag der Prüfung werden im allgemeinen 30 Benetzungen in 15 min appliziert, nur ausnahmsweise weniger. Die Hautreaktion wird sofort und nach 24 Std beurteilt. Entscheidend ist eine noch nach 24 Std sichtbare, ekzematoide Reaktion. Tritt nach 30 Benetzungen keine Reaktion auf, und zeigt die Anamnese einen täglichen, mindestens 30maligen Kontakt mit der Noxe, so wird am 2. Tage auf der gleichen Hautstelle eine erneute Prüfung mit 30 bis eventuell 60 Benetzungen in 15 oder 30 min vorgenommen. Ausnahmsweise wird auch am 3. Tage die Probe noch einmal auf der gleichen Hautstelle mit 30 bis 60 Benetzungen wiederholt. Dies jedoch nur dann, wenn ein täglicher, massiver Kontakt mit der Noxe im Berufe stattfindet.

Als positives Resultat betrachten wir eine mehrere Tage dauernde sichtbare ekzematoide Reaktion. So entstand z. B. nach 30maligem Benetzen mit Bohrwasser eine ausgedehnte Rötung und Schwellung, Knötchenbildung der Haut mit deutlichem ekzematoidem Charakter, welche erst nach mehreren Tagen abheilte. In einem anderen Fall bei einer Wäscherin entstand durch 60maliges Benetzen mit 10%igem PER, einem Waschmittel, eine erosiv-ekzematoide Reaktion mit Rötung und Schwellung.

In einzelnen Fällen haben wir histologische Untersuchungen vorgenommen und das klassische Bild einer intra-epithelialen lymphocytären Spongiose gefunden.

Die Konzentration der zu prüfenden Flüssigkeiten soll so gewählt werden, daß eine normale Haut die 30, 60 oder eventuell häufigeren Benetzungen ohne Reaktion erträgt. Wir haben deshalb speziell zu Beginn unserer Untersuchungen, parallel mit den Benetzungen, an unseren Patienten die entsprechende Zahl von Benetzungen an jeweils drei hautgesunden Kontrollpersonen vorgenommen, die immer negativ ausfielen. Wenn neue, noch unbekannte Noxen zu prüfen sind, sollten solche Kontrolluntersuchungen immer vorgenommen werden.

Von 100 Patienten mit Gewerbeekzem, bei welchen die klassischen Läppchen-proben keine eindeutige Reaktion ergaben, konnten wir bei 67 mit der Methode der wiederholten Benetzung eine ezkematoide Reaktion erzielen.

Tabelle

Noxe	Zahl der Fälle	Benetzungs-konzentration	Zahl der Benetzungen	Min
Detergentien	30	2—10%	30—60	15—30
Organische Lösungsmittel, Xylol, Benzin, Petrol, Sangaiol	20	100%	6—140 (60)	3—70 (30)
Bohrwasser, Kühlwasser	7	2—4%	30—60	15—30
Zement	10	20—40%	60	20—30

Aus der Tabelle ist zu sehen, daß es sich 30mal um Ekzeme durch Detergentien handelte. Meistens waren es Waschmittel, Reinigungsmittel, Abwaschmittel, welche aus alkalischen oder neutralen Detergentien bestanden. Die größere Anzahl dieser Fälle waren Frauen, welche täglich, manchmal stundenlang, Geschirr spülen mußten.

Detergentien wurden in einer Konzentration von 2 bis 10% geprüft. Es kommt immer wieder vor, daß entgegen den Vorschriften mit zu hoch konzentrierten Detergentien gearbeitet wird. Wir führten je 30 bis 60 Benetzungen in 15 bis 30 min durch. Einzelheiten über die Art der Detergentien können in den Arbeiten von René Schmid und Peter Schmid nachgelesen werden.

Eine zweite Gruppe von 20 Fällen betrifft Gewerbeekzeme durch organische Lösungsmittel wie Xylol, Benzin, Petrol, Sangaiol. Es handelte sich vorwiegend um männliche Arbeiter aus mechanischen Werkstätten oder aus dem grafischen Ge-werbe, welche Maschinenbestandteile oder ganze Maschinen täglich oder mehrmals wöchentlich mit diesen Lösungsmitteln reinigen, so daß ihre Hände wiederholt während ½ bis 1 Std von diesen Lösungsmitteln benetzt wurden. Da diese Lö-sungsmittel während der Arbeit immer unverdünnt angewandt werden, werden auch die Benetzungsproben unverdünnt vorgenommen.

Fanden die Benetzungen bei der Arbeit nur selten statt, so haben wir auch nur sechs Benetzungen in 3 min durchgeführt. In der Regel wurden 60 Benetzungen in 30 min vorgenommen, nur ausnahmsweise mehr. Insbesondere bei den Lösungs-mitteln waren wir froh, von der hier besonders unzuverlässigen Läppchenprobe losgekommen zu sein, rufen doch diese Lösungsmittel bei der Läppchenprobe Blasen hervor, fast unabhängig von der individuellen Empfindlichkeit des Pa-tienten.

Ein weiteres Kapitel sind die Bohr- und Kühlwasser-Ekzeme. Die Bohr- und Kühlwasser sind Mischungen von Wasser mit Emulgatoren, die oft den Charakter von Detergentien haben. Manchmal sind auch Antioxydantien oder Rohöle oder Pflanzenöle als Rostschutzmittel beigegeben. An vielen Arbeitsplätzen in der Maschinenindustrie wird die Haut beständig von diesen Bohrölen benetzt. In sieben Fällen, in welchen die Läppchenproben versagten, konnten wir durch 30- bis 60maliges Benetzen in 15 bis 30 min ekzematoide Reaktionen erzielen.

Beim Maurerekzem durch Zement gibt es besonders beim ersten Ekzemschub Fälle, bei welchen man noch keine deutliche, positive Kaliumbichromatprobe erhält, obwohl der Zusammenhang in bezug auf Anamnese und klinisches Bild eindeutig ist. Durch die Benetzungsprobe mit 20- bis 40%igem Zement bei 30 bis 60 Benetzungen konnten wir in zehn Fällen eine deutlich ekzematoide Reaktion erzielen.

Zur Abklärung der Biologie der Benetzungsprobe haben wir eine Anzahl von Untersuchungen durchgeführt. Zunächst wurde der pH-Wert der Hautoberfläche in 19 Fällen gemessen. Er erhöhte sich insbesondere nach Verwendung alkalischer Detergentien und Bohrwasser und durch Zement um zwei bis drei Punkte. Den Aminosäuregehalt der Hautoberfläche kontrollierten wir mit Hilfe der Ninhydrin-Reaktion und fanden dabei in neun von elf Fällen eine Verminderung des Aminosäurengehaltes der Hautoberfläche nach der Benetzung insbesondere mit Detergentien und Bohrwasser. Die Alkaliresistenz war in allen 13 kontrollierten Fällen auf der wiederholt benetzten Haut deutlich vermindert. Diese Versuche zeigen, in welchem Sinne eine Benetzungsprobe den Oberflächenfilm der Haut verändert und die Widerstandskraft gegen chemische Noxen herabsetzt, so daß gegen Ende der Benetzungsprobe andere Verhältnisse vorliegen als zu ihrem Beginn. Diese ermöglichten ein besseres Eindringen der Noxe in die Haut.

Zusammenfassend ist die Benetzungsprobe eine weitere Möglichkeit der epicutanen Testung insbesondere mit Flüssigkeiten. Sie ahmt den Arbeitskontakt weitgehend nach und kann deshalb in vielen Fällen in Ergänzung der üblichen Läppchenproben den Zusammenhang von Arbeit und Ekzem beweisen, in welchen andere Methoden versagt haben.

Literatur. BURCKHARDT, W., u. R. SCHMID: Hautarzt 15, 555 (1964). — SCHMID, P.: Med. Diss., Zürich 1967. Dermatologica (Basel) 1968 (Im Druck). — SCHMID, R.: Die Erfahrungen mit einer Epicutanprobe durch wiederholte Benetzung beim Kontaktekzem. Med. Diss., Zürich 1963.

Pathogenesis of Sensitization in Allergic Contact Dermatitis in Man*

R. L. BAER and M. J. FELLNER, Department of Dermatology, New York University School of Medicine, New York, N.Y. (USA)

The conventional concept holds that in order to induce allergic eczematous contact sensitivity, low molecular weight allergens such as dinitrochlorobenzene, paraphenylenediamine, nickel, penicillin, etc., must first combine irreversibly, i.e., covalently, with skin proteins to form the complete antigen. It is generally assumed that covalent conjugates of hapten and protein are also required for elicitation of allergic contact reactions in previously sensitized individuals.

Since some substances which are known to engender contact sensitization in man do not react covalently with proteins, their allergenicity must involve additional factors. In many instances such substances may be considered precursors of haptens, i.e., a metabolite or degradation product of the parent allergen is formed in the skin or elsewhere and it is this compound which is the actual hapten. The classical example for this are compounds of quinone structure derived from paraphenylenediamine [1]. It is reasonable then to assume that at times more than a single haptenic compound may be formed from the application to the skin of a single allergen. Indeed in experimentally induced contact dermatitis in guinea pigs due to penicillin it has been shown [2] that several haptenic groups are formed which are capable of eliciting contact allergy. Also, some contact allergens, among them common contact allergens such as nickel and chromium, do not bind co-

* This work was supported in part by grant AI 07728 from the United States Public Health Service.

valently with proteins. Rather, it appears likely that they form relatively stable, although not irreversible, combinations with proteins by chelation. The dermal collagen which affords many closely spaced polar groups is more suitable for such chelation than are the epidermal fibrous proteins such as keratins and keratin precursors.

Ordinarily, the hapten gains access to cutaneous proteins by crossing the barrier zone and via the adnexal structures. In exceptional cases, however, contact sensitization may be engendered by administration of the hapten by other than topical routes including the oral and parenteral routes.

Even though conjugation with protein is required to induce and elicit allergic contact responses, sensitization is most easily produced by contact with the simple chemical alone rather than in conjugated form. This is attributed to the important role of the carrier proteins in determining the specificity of the reaction to the hapten-protein conjugate.

It also appears possible for haptens to form conjugates with more than a single protein after topical application to the skin. If one considers the fact that more than one haptenic compound can be derived from a single contact allergen and that each hapten in turn may conjugate with one or more carrier proteins, then one is forced to conclude that multiple hapten-protein-conjugates may well be involved in some instances of allergic contact dermatitis.

Among the important unresolved problems with respect to the mechanism of allergic contact sensitization is whether delayed hypersensitivity is mediated, as has been assumed now for about 25 years by immunologically competent cells containing or having at their surface so-called cellbound antibodies or whether it is mediated by circulating antibodies.

In 1962, it was proposed [3] that delayed hypersensitivity reactions are mediated by freely circulating antibodies with extremely high binding affinity, but that these antibodies are present in such low concentrations so as not to be detectable by conventional methods. This explanation was based on the known heterogeneity in antibody response. Since that time some experimental evidence has been reported which supports the hypothesis that delayed hypersensitivity reactions are mediated by circulating antibodies. For example it was shown [4] that insoluble antigen-antibody complexes prepared from high affinity circulating antibodies against dinitrophenyl-guinea pig albumin were able to elicit delayed reactions in sensitized animals. This indicates that delayed antibodies can compete successfully for antigen with conventional antibodies. It was also shown that desensitization by injection of minute doses of antigen results in moderate specific desensitization of delayed sensitivity without affecting Arthus reactivity to the same antigenic determinant [4].

In another experiment [5] comparisons were made of the capacity of two homologous conjugates of different average molecular sizes of dinitrophenyl groups lightly coupled with poly-L-lysine for elicitation of delayed sensitivity in previously sensitized animals. It was found that equal weight concentrations of the two conjugates elicited equally intense Arthus and delayed sensitivity reactions while equimolar concentrations did not. These results suggest that delayed sensitivity reactions are initiated by the reaction of antigen with antibody molecules in true solution, and not by simple antigen bridging of antibody molecules fixed to the surface of cell membranes. This would mean that antibody molecules are freely movable in the extracellular fluid. Most recently, successful passive transfer of delayed sensitivity in guinea pigs has been claimed with serum [6, 7]. If these findings, which are in conflict with previous reports, are confirmed they would also support the hypothesis that antibody of conventional type rather than cell-bound

15*

factor is involved in delayed hypersensitivity. However, if delayed hypersensitivity antibody exists "free" in the serum, complete desensitization of delayed hypersensitivity should be possible with very small doses of antigen and passive transfer should be feasible with large amounts of anti-serum [8]. Attempts to prove these points habe failed.

The lymphocyte which formerly was thought to be an "end" cell, in recent years has been shown to be capable of further transformation [9]. Lymphocytes stimulated with phytohemagglutinin, an extract of the kidney bean, phaseolus vulgaris, elaborate gamma-globulin; so do lymphocytes cultured in a medium containing the specific antigen or allergen to which the donor of the lymphocytes is allergic. More recently it has been demonstrated also that specific antibody is produced by lymphocytes from patients sensitive to penicillin [10].

Recent studies suggest that antigenic material before it initiates immunologic changes in the lymphoid system is first taken up by macrophages [11]. The immunogenic part of the antigen molecule is complexed with RNA in macrophages and it is thought that it is this RNA-antigen complex which then acts on lymph node cells (presumably lymphocytes) to initiate antibody formation. These findings have been confirmed in a bacteriophage T 2 system [12] in which the actual antigens were demonstrated in the antigen-RNA complexes isolated from macrophages. An important unresolved question at the present time is whether macrophages are involved only in preparing antigen-RNA complexes or whether they serve other functions in the immunologic system.

The earliest change in the ultrastructure of the contact response of the skin of guinea pigs sensitized to DNCB is a diffuse increase in the number of mononuclear cells in the upper dermis at 6 h, and a gradual increase in the number of these cells in the epidermis [13]. In regions adjacent to these mononuclear cells, an appreciable extracellular space appeared between epidermal cells and there was loss of desmosomes. Other studies in delayed sensitivity have shown close apposition of macrophages to lymphocytes [14], supporting the possibility that some immunologically important material may be passed from macrophages to lymphocytes or that material be exchanged between these cells.

The currently available evidence then suggests that the contact allergen or its haptenic derivatives form hapten-protein conjugates by combining with keratin or keratin precursors (e.g. tonofilaments) in the epidermis or with collagen and collagen precursors in the dermis. It is possible that serum proteins, particularly globulins, and mucopolysaccharides also serve as carriers. These conjugates are recognized as "foreign", or non-self material, and are engulfed by tissue macrophages in the dermis. Within the macrophages part of the antigenic hapten-protein conjugate is complexed with RNA. Either the entire complex or some part or replica of the complex is released to lymph node cells, probably lymphocytes, which are instructed to make cellbound factor or antibody.

After reexposure in the sensitized individual the antigen interacts with "antibody" furnished by such immunocompetent lymphoid cells or with circulating antibodies released in very low concentrations. This produces "toxic" antigen-antibody complexes many of them probably at the surface of epidermal cells. In the epidermis, the primary damage involves tonofilaments and desmosomes thus producing the pathologic picture of spongiosis. This type of mechanism has been described as a cytotoxic response [15] in which the antibody, either multivalent or less usually incomplete, reacts with an antigenic component of a tissue cell or with an antigen which has become intimately associated with a tissue cell. To this extent, the cytotoxic response can be considered an autoimmune phenomenon.

Photoallergic contact dermatitis (PA CD) is a variety of allergic contact dermatitis (ACD) which has attracted much attention in recent years. Its clinical manifestations are erythematous and papulovesicular and thus are similar to those of ACD. Since the lesions of PA CD are usually limited to the light exposed regions, the most common differential diagnostic possibility is contact dermatitis due to airborne allergens. The histologic changes of PA CD also have shown to be indistinguishable from ACD. The causal agents thus far reported all have been small molecular compounds. The difference between PA CD and ACD lies in the fact that in order to induce sensitization and to elicit a reaction in the sensitized individual exposure to specific wavelengths of light is required in addition to exposure to the simple chemical compound. Thus, substances which cause PA CD must have the capacity to capture photons of light. The energy supplied by these photons causes the photoactive compound to be transformed into another compound which has haptenic properties and to conjugate with carrier protein to form a complete antigen.

Many years ago the characteristic clinical features of an allergic sensitization were demonstrated in photosensitization engendered by certain small molecular compounds such as sulfonamides [16]. At that time, the differentiation between phototoxic and photoallergic reactions was suggested. Experimental induction of photocontact allergic sensitization in guinea pigs was reported with sulfanilmide [17], and with 3, 3', 4', 5 tetrachlorosalicylanilide [18]. Recently we have reported induction of PA CD in guinea pigs with 3, 3', 4', 5 tetrachlorosalicylanilide and, 3, 4', 5 tribromosalicylanilide and related compounds [19] as well as preliminary findings on passive transfer of photoallergic contact sensitivity to TCSA in guinea pigs. The procedure involved the use of large numbers of mononuclear cells obtained from the peritoneal cavity of strongly TCSA photoallergic animals injected intraperitoneally into previously nonsensitive animals.

The demonstration of passive transfer of photocontact sensitivity adds immunologic proof of an allergic mechanism to the previously available clinical and experimental evidence favoring the concept of photoallergic contact sensitization to small molecular compounds.

References. 1. MAYER, R. L.: Arch. Derm. Syph. (Berl.) 156, 312 (1928). — 2. LEVINE, B. B.: J. exp. Med. 112, 1131 (1960). — 3. KARUSH, F., and H. N. EISEN: Science 136, 428 (1962). — 4. LEVINE, B. B.: J. exp. Med. 121, 873 (1965). — 5. LEVINE, B. B.: Science 149, 3680 (1965). — 6. ROTHMAN, U., and S. LIDEN: Acta derm.-venereol. (Stockh.) 47, 1 (1967). — 7. KOCHAN, I., and W. BENDEL: J. Allergy 37, 284 (1966). — 8. UHR, J. W.: Physiol. Rev. 46, 359 (1966). — 9. HIRSCHHORN, K.: Science 142, 1185 (1963). — 10. FELLNER, M. J., C. S. RIPPS, K. HIRSCHHORN, and R. L. BAER: Nature (Lond.). In press. — 11. FISHMAN, M.: Nature (Lond.) 198, 549 (1963). — 12. FRIEDMAN, H. P.: Science 149, 1106 (1965). — 13. FLAX, M. H., and J. B. CAULFIELD: Amer. J. Path. 43, 1031 (1963). — 14. WIENER, J.: Amer. J. Path. 47, 723 (1965). — 15. GELL, P. G. H., and R. R. A. COOMBS (editors): Clinical Aspects of Immunology. Philadelphia: F. A. Davis and Co. 1963. — 16. EPSTEIN, S.: J. invest. Derm. 2, 43 (1939). — 17. SCHWARZ-SPECK, M.: Dermatologica (Basel) 114, 232 (1957). — 18. VINSON, L. J., and V. F. BERSELLI: J. Soc. Comet. Chem. 17, 123 (1966). — 19. HARBER, L. C., S. E. TARGOVNIK, and R. L. BAER: Arch. Derm. (In press).

Chronicity in Allergic Contact Dermatitis

C. D. CALNAN, Institute of Dermatology, University of London (England)

All discussion of allergic contact dermatitis presupposes accurate diagnosis. But all investigators in this field soon appreciate that such accuracy is not easily achieved, mainly because it rests on the patch test which is subject to all the variations of biological material. The problem is well illustrated by the failure of WARSHAW and HERMANN (1951) to decide whether propylene glycol was an allergen or not after carrying out hundreds of tests. The causes of false positive re- actions are numerous and cannot be discussed here. But even when a positive patch test is accepted as evidence of allergy, its precise relationship to a patient's dermatitis must be established. The choice is threefold: the allergy may be (1) the cause of, (2) an effect of, or (3) unrelated to the dermatitis. Strong aller- gens are often irritants also, and hence when they initiate a toxic dermatitis, sensitization is likely to follow.

Allergic contact dermatitis may be primary and uncomplicated by other fac- tors, or secondary to another pattern of dermatitis such as atopic, varicose or seborrhoeic. The aetiology of allergic contact dermatitis may be unifactorial or multifactorial. With very strong allergens nothing except exposure to the agent appears to be required since virtually 100% of those exposed are sensitized. But with weak allergens which sensitize only a small number of those exposed, some precipitating factor is thought to exist, whether it be genetic predisposition, psychic trauma, physical or chemical injury to the skin, or something else.

There are seven main causes of chronicity in allergic contact dermatitis. These are:

1. The primary cause is still acting.

2. Adverse reactions to treatment.

3. Secondary factors such as an additional pattern of eczema, or secondary allergens.

4. The inherent character of eczema.

5. The nature of the allergen.

6. The skin sites affected.

7. Constitutional factors.

Much interest in recent years has been focussed on the first cause, namely, that chronicity could be attributable to the primary cause persisting in an occult form. This could occur in several ways. One is the presence of micro amounts of allergen in the patient's environment; examples of this are (a) chromate in cement and its products, matches, welding fumes, oils and anticorrosive fluids; (b) impurities such as cobalt in nickel salts; (c) nickel in detergents; and (d) the constituents of balsam of Peru. Another is chemical cross reaction to other allergens via group sensitiza- tion, examples of which are now very numerous. And a third way is by exposure to light in cases of contact photosensitization; in some patients, although the allergen is avoided, exposure to sunlight or artificial light alone is enough to elicit the reaction.

Adverse reactions to treatment may be responsible for the persistence of an allergic dermatitis. This may be the result of the physical charactersistics of a topical application whether it be an ointment, cream, paste or a type of dressing which proves unsuitable in an individual case. It is more evident, however, when allergy occurs to a drug, a preservative or a constituent of the base. In such cases the degree of sensitization may be so low as not to induce an acute reaction but merely to retard recovery. This occurs especially with neomycin derivatives, lanolin, parahydroxybenzoates, chlorocresol and so on (HJORTH and TROLLE- LASSEN, 1965). These are chemically unrelated secondary allergens. In fact, any additionally acquired allergic sensitivity may result in chronicity of the primary dermatitis.

Perhaps the most important causes of chronicity are the secondary eczema factors. Most eczemas are multifactorial (PILLSBURY, 1952), and many cases of allergic contact eczema are either at the outset or later complicated by an element of atopic, seborrhoeic, varicose, nummular or other pattern of eczema. MALTEN has called these "eczema hybrids". Failure to recognise them can be an important cause of misunderstanding. Eczema is a pathological state in the skin, rather akin to cirrhosis or nephritis, and will not necessarily be dependant on a single causal factor.

Many cases of eczema show what appears to be an inherent tendency to spread, often irrespective of their apparent origin or pattern. This is usually least evident in allergic contact eczema, but is more likely to appear after repeated attacks or if the dermatitis is severe and extensive. Generalised dermatitis is the most likely to persist. In such circumstances complete removal from the allergen does not always result in cure; the eczema process appears to adopt a momentum of its own and not to be readily reversible. Such an event may occur after a single or repeated attacks.

The nature of the allergen itself certainly has some relevance to chronicity. Contactants which frequently induce chronicity are chromate, nickel, formalin and turpentine. All of them are both irritants and allergens. They have no special chemical or biological characteristics. They are, however, widely dispersed in an industrialised community. But dyes, drugs, plants, timbers and cosmetics do not usually induce chronicity.

The site of an allergic contact dermatitis is also relevant. Chronicity is more prone to occur when the hands, feet, or lower legs are affected. But chronicity in these areas is also a feature of other patterns of eczema. The reasons for it are quite obscure.

Psychogenic factors are frequently regarded as a cause of chronicity, particularly when financial compensation is involved in medicolegal cases. There is little or no evidence to support this. BENTLEY PHILLIPS (1954) found that the majority of patients with chronic dermatitis before legal settlement continued to have it afterwards, but he did not strictly separate allergic from irritant cases. My own experience is similar. In a psychiatric study of twelve patients with allergic and twelve with toxic contact dermatitis no difference was found in the mental background and attitudes.

Two other factors are sometimes regarded as relevant, namely bacterial infection and liver insufficiency. I have not specifically studied them, but have not been impressed that either were relevant to chronicity. Nor are the histological changes any different in chronic allergic contact dermatitis from those of a non-allergic one. Yet another factor cited is occult ingestion of the allergen. Its relevance is debatable. Nickel was used in the manufacture of margarine, chromate may be present in rhubarb, and azo dyes are used in foodstuffs. There is no doubt that oral feeding of an allergen can aggravate a dermatitis, but the dosage normally has to be large. Feeding of nickel salts (in acceptable amounts) does not alter nickel dermatitis (WHITTLE, personal communication), but small amounts of chromate by mouth may aggravate a chromate dermatitis (FREGERT, personal communication). No evidence has been adduced to prove that azo dyes in foodstuffs have been responsible for inducing or aggravating dermatitis.

References. BENTLEY PHILLIPS, B.: Practitioner 172, 531 (1954). — HJORTH, N., and C. TROLLE-LASSEN: Trans. St John's Hosp. derm. Soc. (Lond.) 1963. 49, 127 (1965). — PILLSBURY, D. M.: Proc. X Int. Cong. Derm. 1952. London: 58 (1953). — WARSHAW, T., and F. HERMANN: J. invest. Derm. 19, 423 (1951).

Zur Pathogenese der toxischen (orthoergischen) Kontaktdermatitis

H. W. Spier und F. Klaschka, Hautklinik der Freien Universität Berlin (Deutschland)

Das in Deutschland meist nach Schreus sog. *degenerative Ekzem* (deg. E.) spielt eine bedeutende Rolle bei den Berufsdermatosen. Wie das allergische Kontaktekzem befolgt auch das deg. E. die Regel: cessante causa, cessat effectus (Schreus, 1957). Klinisch zeigt es Ekzempolymorphie mit Betonung fissuriert-hyperkeratotischer und Zurücktreten papulo-vesiculöser Morphen.

Zur Nomenklatur: degeneratives Ekzem (Schreus, 1939); Abnutzungsdermatose (Bering, 1939); toxogenes Ekzem (Miescher, 1945); unspecific contact eczema (Becker u. Obermayer, 1947); orthoergische Dermatitis (Sézary); Eczema detritivum (Kogoj, 1955); traumiteratives Ekzem (Hagerman, 1957).

Eigene Untersuchungen

Zum Studium der Morphodynamik des deg. E. Modell-Expositionsserie an vier hautgesunden Probanden:

Eintauchen jeweils des linken Unterarmes in drei Cylinder, je 4 l Aceton + Benzin 9:1, für 60″, 30′, 30′, anschließend in Aq. dest. für 60″ unter gleichmäßigen Bewegungen. An Stelle Wasser späterhin KOH n/100, abschließend KOH n/60 (Abb. 1). — Durchführung dieser kombinierten, fakultativ subtoxischen Eluierungen von Lipiden und wasserlöslichen Bestandteilen der Hornschicht täglich hintereinander bis viermal — individuell etwas unterschiedlich —, gegebenenfalls in Verbindung mit Laurylsulfat-Bürstenbädern, mit dem Ziel, die individuelle toxische Schwelle zu erreichen, aber nicht zu überschreiten.

Trotz täglich neu angepaßter Exposition zeigte nur eine Probe (D) ein Eczema craquelée am 8. bis 12. Tag, die anderen lediglich Brennen, leichte Rötung, sehr diskrete Schuppung und allenfalls — mit Hilfe der Nitrazingelbprobe (Burckhardt und Locher) — demonstrierbare punktförmige Erosionen. — 19 3 mm-Stanzenbiopsien (Abb. 1).

Histologische Untersuchungen: a) Unter dem Einfluß der aggressiven Bäder Anstieg des *Durchmessers des Zellepithels* von vier bis sechs auf etwa zehn bis elf Zellagen, meist mit Zurücktreten des Wellenmusters der Papillarepithelleisten zugunsten mehr block- oder bandartiger numerischer Hyperplasie, unabhängig vom klinischen Effekt.

b) Ähnlich unabhängig verhielt sich der *Mitosequotient* (M. Qu.). Es wurden strikt nur sichere Meta-, Ana- und Telophasen (Abb. 2) berücksichtigt (d. h. realer Mitosequotient > 0,8 bis 5,5⁰/₀₀-). Von Pinkus, Brophy und Lobitz sowie Williams und Hunter wurden nach Abrissen maximale M. Qu. von 20⁰/₀₀- (bis über 50⁰/₀₀-) ausgezählt! — Leider bedingt die zeitraubende M.-Zählung an humaner Epidermis noch viele Lücken unserer Kenntnisse. — Die interkurrente Senkung des M. Qu. auf Werte normaler Regeneration bei Probe C und D kann vielleicht als Ausdruck eines synchronisierten, wellenartigen Verlaufes der Mitosendichte gedeutet werden, muß es aber nicht zwingend; die Stanzen konnten nicht in dichterer Aufeinanderfolge entnommen werden.

c) Eine Histometrie der *Hornschichtdicke* war wegen Ablösung meist nicht möglich. Immerhin: die Stanze des 12. Tages zeigte beim Prob. A als Zeichen einer Aktivierung der Differenzierung eine lucidum-ähnliche gußartige, die des Prob. C bereits am 10. Tage eine kreppgummiartige Hyperkeratose. UV-Schwellenwerte (Prob. C) (30. Tag) bei 17 min li., 10 min re. Unterarm; beim Prob. D (15. Tag) li. 8,5 min, re. 7 min nach Erst-Exposition.

d) Selbst beim Probanden D mit seinem anlaufenden polymorphen Reaktionsbild konnte das erwartete Phänomen einer ekzemspezifischen erhöhten

Contact Dermatitis (allergic and non-allergic) 233

räumlichen Inhomogenität der Mitosedichte nicht genügend verifiziert werden. —
Hier half die Auszählung von 110 Einzelgesichtsfeldern einer Stanze eines Patienten
mit *genuinem subakutem* Unterarm-deg.-E.* (Abb. 3) weiter. Bei allgemein

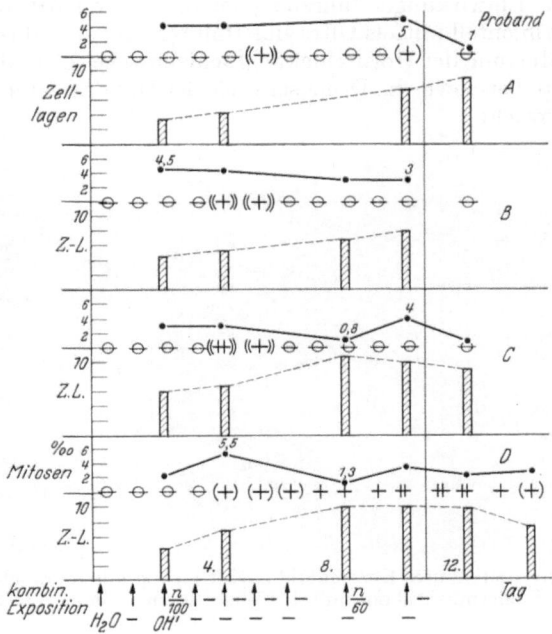

Abb. 1. Expositionsserie. Übersicht. Klinische Reaktionsstärken jeweils in Feldmitte

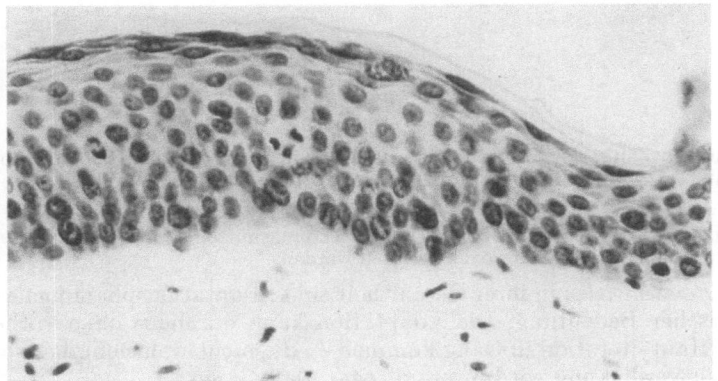

Abb. 2. Drei Mitosen: li Ana-, Mitte Telo-, re. Meta-Phase. (Proband D — Stanze am 5. Tag.
Carnoy-Gallocyanin)

erhöhtem M. Qu. von 9⁰/₀₀, d. h. etwa dem Zehnfachen der orthologen Maus-
erungsquote, konnte im Detail eine glaubhaft überdurchschnittliche Variabilität
der Mitosedichte ermittelt werden (Abb. 4).

* Durchgeführt von Frau Dipl. biol. SPATA und Dipl. biol. LIPP.

Diese Analyse — gewiß die eines Zufallquerschnittes — sei der Aufhänger für eine Zusammenfassung unserer Auffassung der Pathogenese, d. h. der Mikro- und Makro-Morphodynamik des deg. E.

1. Die Epidermis ist bekanntlich ein Wechsel- oder Dauer-Mausergewebe.

2. Physikalische Einwirkungen führen zu der bereits von MIESCHER vor 30 und mehr Jahren experimentell mittels Ultravioletteinwirkungen induzierten homogenen reaktiven Verdickung der Hornschicht („Lichtschwiele"), der die Hornschichtverdickung nach Reiben sowie die Druckschwiele der Handarbeiter, die Fußsohlenschwiele usw. entspricht.

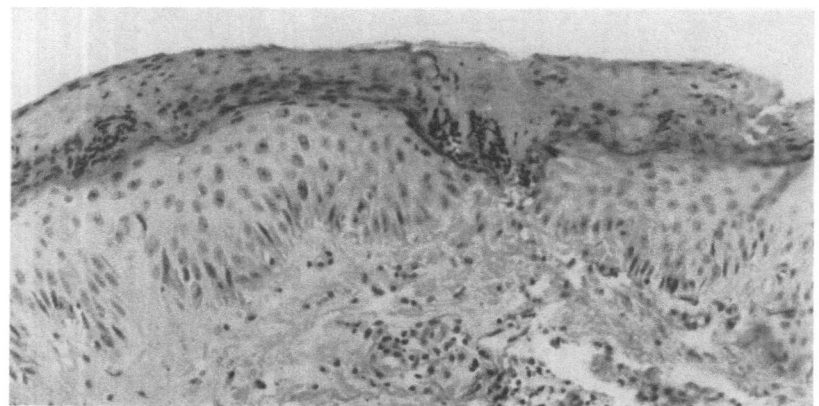

Abb. 3. Traumiteratives subakutes Ekzematoid nach Umgang mit gebrauchten Autoölen und Benzin. Schlotartige Epidermis-Diskontinuität. Keine Bläschen. (Pat. C.L. Unterarm, 626/67, Formol-H.E.)

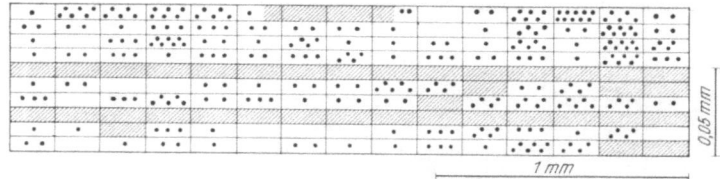

Abb. 4. Inhomogenität der Mitosendichte in der Epidermis. Pat. der Abb. 3. „Aufsicht" auf 110 Gesichtsfelder von acht (von zehn) Einzelschnitten. Ein Punkt = eine Mitose

Auch nach atoxischen Einwirkungen von Lösungsmitteln konnte von uns mit SPATA reaktive Hornschichtverdickung nachgewiesen werden.

Diese *Reizschwielen* in ihrer Gesamtheit sind Adaptationsphänomene von größter praktischer Bedeutung. Die Adaptation kann durchaus ohne vorhergehende sichtbare Hautalteration in Gang kommen — die nicht wahrnehmbare adaptative Hornschichtverdickung wird in praxi sogar überwiegen.

3. Mitogene Reize kommen erst nach 2 bis 3 Tagen zur Auswirkung. Da Mitosesteigerung zunächst zu numerischer Epithelhyperplasie führt, läuft erst nach einer zweiten, zeitlich unscharfen Latenz die reaktive Hyperkerose an. Das Ingangkommen der Adaptation braucht demnach Zeit, andererseits hält die Hornschichtverdickung mehrere Wochen an.

4. Insbesondere aggressive Lösungsmittel, Laugen usw. sind oft ambivalent wirkende Reize: Bis zu einem gewissen Maximum besteht eine positive Korrelation (oder Rückkoppelung) zwischen effektiver Reizstärke und Mitoseaktivierung, bei

weiterer Steigerung der effektiven Reizstärke dagegen eine Depression der Mitose-aktivität, d. h. eine negative Korrelation (oder Rückkoppelung), offenbar als Folge direkter toxischer Schädigung der Epithelzellen.

Die Effektivität der Wirkung eines exogenen Reizagens auf den Mitosequotien-ten ist davon abhängig, was die Hornschicht jeweils durchläßt. Im Bereich all-fälliger subklinischer Hornschichtläsionen oder relativ dünner Hornschicht kann ein bestimmtes aggressives Lösungsmittel usw. in das Zellepithel eindringen und zur Mitosedepression führen, während in der Sphäre unversehrter abwehrtüchtiger Hornschicht in der Nachbarschaft eine mehr oder weniger deutliche Aktivierung der Mitosentätigkeit erfolgt. Bei iterativer, d. h. wiederholter Reizexposition wird sich diese *Disproportionierung der Geschwindigkeit der Keratogenese* immer mehr verstärken, gegebenen Falles bis zur klinischen Polymorphie, bevorzugt in Form von Erosionen und Hyperkeratosen.

5. Ob die Haut auf iterative Exposition gegenüber fakultativ toxischen Chemi-kalien mit Adaptation oder mit Dysregeneration reagiert, ist oft schon vor Auf-nahme der betreffenden Berufsexposition entschieden. Eine klinisch gesunde, aber mit relativ dünner Hornschicht versehene Haut ist dazu prädestiniert, in der kritischen Initialphase der Exposition überfordert zu werden: Die Entwicklung der Adaptationshyperkeratose braucht Zeit; zunächst muß die Hornschicht, so wie sie ist, abwehren.

6. In der Praxis kommt allerdings diese Adaptation nicht selten nach bzw. trotz einer dermatitischen Phase mit oft nur kurzfristiger oder fehlender Unter-brechung der Arbeitsfähigkeit in Gang. Dieses bekannte *Härtungsphänomen* sollte nicht mit dem seltsamen Phänomen der temporären Ekzemdesensibilisierung bei Allergendauerkontakt verwechselt werden.

7. Der positive Läppchentest beim *allergischen* Kontaktekzem ist ein echtes allergisches Ekzem. Für das hier zu diskutierende *orthoergische* Ekzem gibt es nur allgemeine Resistenz- und Permeabilitätsproben, aber weder spezielle diagno-stische Tests noch wirklich befriedigend reproduzierbare, für spezielle Berufs-schädigungen relevante Modellexpositionen: Es gehen zu viele Einzelfaktoren in die Gleichung ein, z. B. auch Milieutemperatur, Reibe- und Reinigungsmodi, Art der Arbeitspausen, Freizeitbeschäftigung.

Hinsichtlich der *Abgrenzung* sowie der *Nomenklatur* der hier zu besprechenden Ekzemform besteht leider keine Einigkeit. Selbstunterhalt wie Streuphänomene sind ihr wesensfremd. Persistenz nach Expositionsabbruch wird meist auf Über-gang in ein mikrobielles Ekzem hinweisen, oft kenntlich an figurierten Morphen.

Beispiel: primär toxisches, sekundär chromat-allergisches, tertiär so oft mikrobielles Maurer-Ekzem (Huriez — Stockholm).

Es erscheint bedenklich, die Dermatose als *Ekzem* zu bezeichnen: Wohl kom-men fakultativ subcorneal oder subgranulär Vesikeln und Vesicopusteln vor, da-gegen keine primär basalständigen Spongiovesikeln.

Diese orthoergische Reaktionsform mag daher in Anbetracht ihrer Polymorphie einerseits, dem Fehlen von eigentlichen Ekzembläschen zum anderen, den *Ek-zematoiden* zugeordnet werden. Ferner: *Traumiteration* ist die unbedingte Voraus-setzung ihrer Entstehung. Um die Nomenklatur nicht mit einem neuen Term (etwa „*dysregeneratorisches Ekzematoid*") noch mehr zu verwirren, sollte dem Hagermanschen Vorschlag zum Teil gefolgt und von einem *traumiterativen Ekzematoid* gesprochen werden.

Specificity and Cross-Sensitivity in Contact Allergy

V. Pirilä, Institute of Occupational Health, Helsinki (Finland)

The specificity and cross-sensitivity in contact sensitization have during the past 30 years been dealt with by many authors [e.g. 1, 8, 10, 15, 17, 21]. However, the development of chemical industry has brought with it new problems and, on the other hand, the advanced scientific methods have given new possibilities to study these problems and the old unsolved ones more thoroughly than earlier. Therefore, the significance of these phenomena can be regarded to be still increasing.

The eczematous sensitization is highly specific. The specificity is, as a rule, obvious when sensitization to a certain element or a simple molecule is concerned. In such a case exposure to the same substance only or possibly to a compound containing it will elicit a hypersensitivity reaction. The situation is more complicated in case of a complex compound, such as aromatic amines or neomycin. Perhaps the only difference, however, may be that this kind of molecule is composed of different biologically active fragments or atom groupings which often occur in other compounds as well. Therefore, in a case of sensitization, exposure not only to the primary allergen but also to a new immunochemically related secondary allergen may cause an allergic reaction. Thus the law of specificity is also valid for cross-sensitivity.

The extreme variety of individual sensitivity patterns in patients sensitized to paraphenylenediamine or other nitrogeneous aromatic compounds [1, 4, 10, 18] is confusing. Since the number of those compounds, more or less related to each other, is almost unrestricted, it is often impossible to decide to which of them the patients have previously been exposed and to know which are the metabolites. Hence differentiation of the reactions into multiple primary sensitizations and/or those due to true cross-sensitivity renders difficulties. Therefore the phenomena of specificity and cross-sensitivity may be more clearly illustrated by combined sensitivity to other groups of substances, such as cobalt and nickel and the neomycin group of antibiotics.

The nonexistence of true cross-sensitivity between chromate, cobalt and nickel has not yet been accepted by all dermatologists. This disagreement applies mainly to combined sensitivity to cobalt and nickel. However, the results of most authors speak for independent coincidental sensitizations, as do ours [for the literature see 2, 5, 9, 11].

We performed patch tests with both cobalt and nickel during a 16-year period ranging from 1949 to 1964 in 180 cases of sensitization to nickel acquired in nickel plating or due to suspender buckles [11]. It was found that combined sensitivity to cobalt and nickel was astonishingly more common in patients with eczema due to suspenders than in nickel platers. Furthermore, an obvious decrease in the incidence of the combined sensitivity during the 16-year period could be observed. These discrepancies are explained by a change in the nickel plating technique until the mid 1950s in Finland.

In order to obtain a highly lustrous surface, a large number of agents have been added to nickel baths as brighteners. More than 12 years ago the addition of cobalt salts in a ratio of approx. 1 to 20 to the nickel solutions for the bright-nickel-process used to be a rather common practice. This method, however, is not only expensive but the resulting coating also less resistant to corrosion than that obtained without the addition of cobalt. Therefore, organic brighteners have largely replaced cobalt. Furthermore, the nickel salts for electroplating produced by modern methods are very pure, containing, as a rule, not more than 0.04% cobalt. Thus whereas about 12 years ago nickel platers were still often exposed to cobalt such exposure to this metal in connection with nickel plating is today almost negligible. Hence it can be understood that most cases of combined sensitivity to cobalt and nickel among nickel platers occurred during the earlier 8-year period. Since 1956 only two such patients were seen. Both had exceptionally been exposed to cobalt at the time they acquired eczema. Therefore, I think it reasonable to conclude that sensitivity to cobalt never — or very seldom — occurs as a result of nickel plating, provided that the nickel solutions contain no more than minute amounts of cobalt. This leads further to the conclusion that there is no true cross-sensitivity between cobalt and nickel, but that the once very common combined sensitivity to cobalt and nickel has to be regarded as due to two independent highly specific primary sensitizations. In agreement with this view VANDENBERG and EPSTEIN [22] in tests on eight subjects experimentally sensitized to nickel found no reactions to cobalt, chromate or copper.

Cross-sensitization to the neomycin group of antibiotics and coincidental sensitization to bacitracin are suitable for studying the laws of specificity and cross-sensitivity for several reasons: Firstly, these sensitivities did not occur in Finland before the introduction of these antibiotics and have thus been induced primarily by themselves, as suggested by the steady rise of the incidences of sensitization starting from zero and going parallel with the increase of consumption of ointments containing neomycin and bacitracin [12]. Secondly, sensitization has been induced by neomycin and bacitracin almost exclusively, since the topical use of the related antibiotics has been negligible in Finland. Thirdly, the variety of cross-reacting antibiotics is still small.

SIDI et al. have reported cross-sensitivity between neomycin and streptomycin [19, 20]. However, although positive reactions to streptomycin have been found in some cases of neomycin sensitivity by other authors also [3, 12], true cross-sensitivity has not been confirmed. Thus positive reactions to streptomycin were obtained in only 3% out of more than 200 neomycin-sensitive patients tested by us and in most of them a previous exposure to streptomycin was discovered [12].

We have investigated the cross-sensitivity between neomycin, framycetin, kanamycin, paromomycin and gentamicin, for instance by testing sensitized patients with several related compounds, including some rubber chemicals and various fragments of neomycin and paromomycin obtained by degradation. From the results, which have been published elsewhere [14], it can be concluded that neomycin obviously contains at least two different chemical groupings possessing sensitizing capacity. This gives rise to different patterns of cross-sensitivity, as yet not very complicated.

However, our recent observation that gentamicin, a new antibiotic, the chemical structure of which is known to be close to that of kanamycin [16], causes positive reactions in only a part of the kanamycin-sensitive patients [12, 13] suggests that the pattern of cross-sensitivity is more complicated than has hitherto been apparent. Furthermore, there is no doubt that in patients with primary sensitization to the other related antibiotics other types of patterns are to be expected.

Obviously, however, the patterns will never reach the great variety of the cross-sensitivity between "para compounds" which has led BAER to compare it with the well-known variety in finger-print patterns [1]. According to FISHER et al. the spectrum of this cross-sensitivity appears to be related to an individual "host" factor and to be established early on in life [6].

This kind of individual susceptibility and different types of exposure could be responsible for the exceptionally common coincidental sensitization to some substances, such as cobalt and nickel, as well as neomycin and bacitracin in Denmark [7] and Finland or neomycin and streptomycin in France. Some individuals would more likely become sensitized to the neomycin group of antibiotics and bacitracin, for instance, others to cobalt and nickel and possibly to chromate as well. This idea is further supported by our observation that in painters combined sensitivity to oil of turpentine and cobalt is not equally common, although both substances are potent sensitizers and patients have certainly been exposed to both of them. If this hypothesis is correct, it may in the future of an already acquired sensitivity to some extent to be predictable to which types of allergens the individual can be expected to become sensitized in case of adequate exposure.

References. 1. BAER, R. L.: Cross-sensitization phenomena. In Mac Kenna: Modern trends of dermatology, 2. Ser., p. 232. London: Butterworth & Co. 1954. — 2. BANDMANN, H.-J., and G. FUCHS: Hautarzt 14, 207 (1963). — 3. CALNAN, C. D., and I. SARKANY: Brit. J. Derm. 70, 435 (1958). — 4. DÜNGEMANN, H., and S. BORELLI: Berufsdermatosen 14, 281 (1966). — 5. FISHER, A. A.: Contact dermatitis. Philadelphia: Lea & Febiger 1967. — 6. FISHER, A. A., A. PELZIG, and N. B. KANOF: J. invest. Derm. 30, 9 (1958). — 7. HJORTH, N.: Ugeskr. Laeg. 120, 1323 (1958). — 8. JADASSOHN, W.: Arch. klin. exp. Derm. 211, 230 (1958).— 9. MARCUSSEN, P. V.: Acta allerg. (Kbh.) 17, 311 (1962). — 10. MAYER, R. L.: Kallós' Progress in allergy, 4, 79 Basel/New York: S. Karger 1954. — 11. PIRILÄ, V., and L. FÖRSTRÖM: Acta derm.-venereol. (Stockh.) 46, 40 (1966). — 12. PIRILÄ, V., L. FÖRSTRÖM, and S. ROUHUNKOSKI: Acta derm.-venereol. (Stockh.) 47, 419 (1967). — 13. PIRILÄ, V., M.-L. HIRVONEN, and S. ROUHUNKOSKI: Dermatologica (Basel) (In press). — 14. PIRILÄ, V., and L. PIRILÄ: Acta derm.-venereol. (Stockh.) 46, 489 (1966). — 15. ROSTENBERG, A., and N. M. KANOF: J. invest. Derm. 6, 201 (1945). — 16. SCHAFFNER, C. P., and H. MAEHR: 149th Meet. Am. Chem. Soc. p. 17. Detroit 1965. — 17. SCHULZ, K. H.: Chemische Struktur und allergene Wirkung unter besonderer Berücksichtigune von Kontaktallergenen. Berufsdermatosen 4, Monogr. Aulendorf i. Württ.: Editio Cantor K.G. 1962. — 18. SIDI, E., and S. DOBKEVITCH-MORRILL: J. invest. Derm. 16, 299 (1951). — 19. SIDI, E., A. GERVAIS, and P. GERVAIS: Acta allerg. (Kbh.) 17, 529 (1962). — 20. SIDI, E., M. HINCKY, and R. LONGUEVILLE: J. invest. Derm. 30, 225 (1958). — 21. SULZBERGER, M. B., and R. L. BAER: J. invest. Derm. 1, 45 (1938). — 22. VANDENBERG, J. J., and W. L. EPSTEIN: J. invest. Derm. 41, 413 (1963).

Die Akzentverschiebungen bei den sensibilisierenden Stoffen während der letzten 3 Jahrzehnte

S. BORELLI, Dermatol. Klinik und Poliklinik der Univ. München (Deutschland)

Der Akzent und der Akzentwandel dermatologischer Kontaktnoxen differiert je nach der statistischen Fragestellung. Ein maßgeblicher Spiegel des späteren allgemeinen Trends in der Sensibilisierung der Bevölkerung ist grundsätzlich dem Akzentwandel gewerbedermatologischer Kontaktekzematogene zu entnehmen, so daß wir unsere — natürlich nur aphoristischen — Folgerungen aus den Berufsbereichen ableiten können.

1. a) In der *Landwirtschaft* dominierten in den 30er Jahren die Kontaktnoxen Kunstdünger, z. B. durch Kalkammonsalpeter, Ammonsulfat, ferner Pflanzenschutzmittel mit Quecksilberzusatz. Heute sind es ebenfalls noch die Kunstdünger, viele neue Insektizide und Fungizide und neue Pflanzenschutzmittel, z. B. Thiocarbamidsäurederivate (Anticryptogam), das 1-, 2-, 3-, 4-, 5-, 6-Hexachlorcyclohexan. Melkfette und Eutersalben, heute z. B. mit quaternären Ammoniumbasen, reizen mitunter. Jetzt und für die Zukunft bedeutungsvoll sind Viehfutternoxen, z. B. durch Kobalt im Mineralfutter, durch Antibiotica im Mastfutter, weiter Chromverbindungen, Kaliumbichromat, durch Beimischung als Konservierungsmittel für Milchproben. Zunehmend sind Gummi- und Gummibestandteil-, sowie

Maschinen-bedingte Noxen, wie sie in der Metallindustrie vorkommen, durch die Motorisierung und Automatisierung der Landwirtschaft.

1. b) *Gärtner* hatten früher vorzugsweise mit Pflanzenallergien, z. B. Primel- oder Giftefeuekzemen zu tun. Heute sind auch in diesem Bereich die Pflanzen- schutzmittel, die Gumminoxen und Maschinennoxen bedeutungsvoll.

1. c) In der von der Landwirtschaft und vom Gartenbau abhängenden *Nah- rungsmittelindustrie* kannte man früher z. B. Reaktionen auf Spargel und Citrusöle. Diese Möglichkeiten bestehen auch heute weiter, haben sich jedoch durch Pflanzen- schutzmittel- und Haltbarkeitsmittel-bedingte Noxen vermehrt.

2. In den *Bauberufen* beschuldigte man früher Kalk und Zementbestandteile (Calciumoxyd, Calciumhydroxyd und dergleichen). Heute stellen Sensibilisierun- gen durch Chrom-, Kobalt-, Nickelverbindungen, Terpentin und Lösungsmittel, Anilinabkömmlinge, die bedeutendsten Irritantien dar, unter denen das Chrom dominiert. Der Akzent verlagert sich weiter auf Spezialgipse, Spezialzemente und für die Zukunft wahrscheinlich Kunstharzprodukte, wie zur Zeit bereits Phenol- formaldehyd-Harzkitte, -Verputze und dergleichen.

3. *Maler, Anstreicher und Lackierer* kannten Sensibilisierungen durch Lacke, Lösungsmittel, Farben, auch schon Kunstharzbausteine, Phenol und Formalin. Terpentin spielt heute zwar noch eine große Rolle, ist im Akzent jedoch um 50% weniger bedeutungsvoll (Abfall der Registrierung positiver Terpentintestungen von früher 10 bis 20 bis 30% auf 5 bis 10% des Probandengutes). Paragruppenver- wandte Sensibilisierungen, solche durch Metallionen (insbesondere Chrom, ferner Nickel, Kobalt), auf Nitrolacke, gehören weiter zum Üblichen. Terpentinnachfolge- stoffe, Formalin-haltige Kunststoffe, Leime, Leimfarben, Kunststofflösungsmittel lassen sich für die Zukunft als zunehmend bedeutende Irritantien voraussetzen.

4. Im Sektor *Metallindustrie*, Mechaniker, Dreher und dergleichen, wurden Chromverbindungen sowie Produkte technischer Öle und Fette als Kontaktnoxen in den 30er Jahren zum Teil selbst, zum Teil deren Additive, wie Phenol, Kresol, Napthol, Teerabkömmlinge, angeschuldet. — Chromallergien sind in diesem Be- reich heute ebenso geläufig wie die mit ihnen gekoppelt aber auch isoliert vorkom- menden Irritationen durch Nickel, Kobalt, mitunter Kadmium, Beryllium. Als seltenere Agentien wurden neben dem Kaliumbichromat das Chromylchlorid und das Manganchlorid identifiziert. Terpentin und Lösungsmittel, ebenso Anilin- und Anilinderivatreizungen sind bekannt. Von den technischen Ölen und Fetten weiß man heute, daß sie selbst weitaus weniger gefährlich sind als — insbesondere im Übermaß zugegebene und alkalische — Additive, wie Merkaptobenzothiazol, ferner Triacine, wahrscheinlich aber letztlich weiterhin Formalin und Phenol. Die relative Neuerung, statt der früher zum Löten benutzten Salzsäure heute Hydra- cinhydrobromid anzuwenden, hatte Überempfindlichkeitsreaktionen zur Folge. Weiterhin erwies sich unter den Reinigungsmitteln als irritierend Trichloräthylen. Bedeutend in den Vordergrund getreten sind Bestandteile der Kunststoffe, Kunst- harze, insbesondere aus Halbfertigfabrikaten dieser Art, Kunstharzklebstoffe, z. B. Formaldehydharze wie Paratertiärbutylphenolformaldehydharz, Araldid- kleber und dergleichen. Auch in Zukunft sind auf diesem Sektor noch viele Irrita- tionen zu erwarten. — Bei Arbeitern in Atomkraftwerken wird das Auftreten von allergischen Ekzemen als Folge von Sensibilisierungen gegenüber *Natrium-* und *Calciumuranaten* angenommen.

5. In der *Galvanikindustrie* sind es früher wie heute Sensibilisierungen gegen- über Metallionen, Nickel (-Sulfat, -Chlorit), Chrom-, Kobalt-, Kupfer-, sehr selten Eisen-, Goldverbindungen, auch Terpentin. Das klassische Ekzem des Galvani- seurs, das Nickelekzem, hat seine frühere zentrale Bedeutung aber doch weitgehend eingebüßt (Automation!).

6. Im *Bergbau* kommen alle industriellen Noxen der Maurer, Metallarbeiter vor.

7. Im Bereich der *Elektroindustrie*, bei Elektrikern, wurden vor 30 Jahren mitunter Formaldehyd und Phenol als Sensibilisatoren nach Erhitzen von Kunstharzschaltern und dergleichen eliminiert. Diese Entwicklung hat sich bis heute mit dem Vormarsch der Kunststoffe und -harze, auch im Elektrobereich (Epoxydharze, -Äthoxylinharze, -Triäthylentetraminhärter, Phenoloxypropenoxyd [= Chlorparaffin], z. B. als Kabelmantelmasse) weiter akzentuiert.

8. Der Raum der *chemischen Industrie* bereitet besondere Schwierigkeiten infolge der Vielzahl dort in Frage kommender Noxen. Viel wurde früher und wird heute über Chrom-, Nickel-, Terpentin-, Anilinderivate-, Nitro-, Phenacin-, Diphenylamin-, Triphenylmethan-, (-Farben)-Unverträglichkeiten, wie Benzol-, Toluol-, Dinitrochlorbenzol-, Anisolirritationen und dergleichen berichtet. Inzwischen ist allerdings der Begriff der Paragruppenverbindungen und gekreuzten Sensibilisierung bekannt geworden. Sensibilisierungen durch Phenol, Formalin, Epoxyde sind heute und in Zukunft im Rahmen der Akzentverschiedung besonders zu erwähnen!

9. In der *Gummiindustrie* haben die altbekannten Gummilösungsmittel Benzin, Tetra, Benzol, die Acceleratoren (Hexamethylentetramin), dann aromatische Nitroverbindungen, Benzolabkömmlinge, Farbstoffe, Schwefelmonochlorid heute noch ihre Bedeutung. In den Vordergrund getreten sind die Vulkanisationsbeschleuniger wie Merkaptobenzothiazole, Dithiocarbaminsäurederivate, Guanidinderivate (z. B. Diphenylguanidin), Formalinderivate, ferner die Alterungsschutzmittel, z. B. vom Typ des n-Phenyl-cyclohexyl-p-phenylendiamin (4010), des Phenyl-Beta-Napthylamin (PBN), des 4,4-dioxyddiphenol (DOD), des Aldol-Alpha-Napthylamin (Aldolharz), Stabilisatoren wie PVC, Chlorparaffine, die unter Umständen mit Phenoxypropenoxyd stabilisiert sind. Immer ist zu denken an die Möglichkeit von Reaktionen auf Terpentin- und Paragruppenverbindungen. Mitunter spielen auch zugesetzte Antimycotica (z. B. Thiram) eine Rolle. Bei der zu erwartenden weiteren Verschmelzung der Echtgummi und Kunststoffgummi bzw. kunstharzgummiartigen Produkte herstellenden Industrie ist natürlich in diesem Bereich für die Zukunft eine breite Verschiebung in Richtung Kunstharzbestandteilallergien zu erwarten.

10. Eine *Kunstharz-herstellende Industrie* kannte man vor 3 Jahrzehnten mit Phenol und Formalin als Sensibilisatoren auch bereits, allerdings nicht den Breiteneffekt der Jetztzeit in dieser Hinsicht. Es läßt sich sagen: auf Grund der immer größeren Vielfalt der Chemieprodukte steigt, abgesehen von der Verursachung durch die üblichen Noxen, die Zahl der Hauterkrankungen — vor allem durch die Kunstharze — insbesondere bei Chemiewerkern außerordentlich rapid. Hervorzuheben sind dabei die Epoxydharze (Dian, Epichlorhydrin) und die Phenol-formaldehyd-Harze. Diese finden außerdem überall, z. B. als Veredelungsmittel in der Textilindustrie, als Klebstoffe der lederverarbeitenden Industrie, in zugehörigen Gewerben, bei den Tischlern, in der Säurebautechnik, ein immer größeres Verwendungsgebiet, so daß die Zahl der Sensibilisierungen und Irritationen hier eine massive Akzentverschiebung erkennen läßt.

11. In der *Bodenbeläge-herstellenden Industrie* kannte man in den 30er Jahren nur außerordentlich wenig Schäden, in Anbetracht der weitgehend maschinellen Produktion, durch Leinöl, Terpentinverbindungen, Harze (Colophonium) und Farben, z. B. aus der Reihe der Anilinderivate. Heute, soweit Sensibilisierungen vorkommen, dominieren hier ebenfalls die Schäden der Kunstharzindustrie.

12. *Holzverarbeitende und -bearbeitende Berufszweige* und Einflußgebiete hatten um 1930 mit Sensibilisierungen durch Leime, Lösungsmittel (Terpentine usw.), Beizen, Haltbarkeitslösungen, z. B. Chromunverträglichkeiten, durch Lacke, Po-

liermittel (Pyridin) sowie Benzolabkömmlinge zu rechnen. Bekannt waren Überempfindlichkeiten gegenüber verschiedensten Hölzern, deren Harze, Alkaloide,
man vor allem anschuldigte. Formalindämpfe, Basilit (Fluornatrium, Arsen, Bichromat, Dinitrophenol), Pyridin wurden genannt. Die heute beobachteten Noxen
sind ähnlich. Aber die Phenol- und Formalinallergien sind erheblich vermehrt.
Zugenommen haben auch die Chromallergien (Chrombeizen!) und die Sensibilisierungen durch eine Vielzahl von Hölzern, insbesondere die neuerdings mehr verwendeten exotischen Hölzer bzw. in ihnen enthaltenen Harze, Balsame, Terpene,
Alkaloide, Saponine, Kardiotonica, Glykoside, Farbstoffe, Chinone usw. Die neuerliche Aufklärung dieser ekzematogenen Strukturen gibt den sensibilisierenden
Faktoren einen neuen Akzent.

13. Formalin-haltige Kleister, Farbstoffe, Paragruppenderivate, Lumpen- und
Hadernbestandteile, Holzbestandteile, Metallionen, fanden sich vor 30 Jahren
ebenso wie heute in der *Papier-herstellenden und verarbeitenden Industrie*. Größer
geworden ist z. B. sowohl in der Herstellung wie in der Anwendung der Sektor
Glaspapier bzw. filmbeschichtetes Papier (Noxe z. B. Metol oder 1-Diäthylamino-
4-diazobenzen) bzw. imprägniertes Kopierpapier (z. B. Noxe Aminophenyldiazon).

14. Waren es im *fotografischen Gewerbe* vor 3 Jahrzehnten die Entwickler Metol
(Aminophenolderivate, Monomethyl-p-aminophenol), Amidol, Rodinal, Pyrogallol,
Hydrochinon (die letzten vier relativ selten), ferner Fixiersalze, insbesondere Ammoniumpersulfat, Tönungsmittel, insbesondere Chromverbindungen, wie Kaliumbichromat, Verstärker, wie Quecksilberverbindungen, z. B. Hg-chlorid-Sublimat,
so kommen diese heute ebenso als Irritantien in Betracht. Durch die anderweitige
erhebliche Verbreitung von Paragruppenverbindungen dürften diese etwas häufiger als Sensibilisatoren beobachtet werden, ebenso spielt Chrom eine sichtbare
Rolle. Akzentverschiebungen ergeben sich im übrigen durch Intensivierung des
Lichtpausgeschäftes, z. B. durch Diazoäthylanilinchlorid, sowie des Farbfilmgeschäftes, z. B. Farbentwickler CD-2 (3-methyl-4-amino-N-diäthyl-anilin-monohydrochlorid), TSS (4-amino-N-diäthylanilinsulfat), also substituierte p-Phenyldiamine! Hinzu kommen Veränderungen in der Herstellung von Härtern, z. B. als
Noxe Hexahydrotriacin, oder von Stabilisatoren, in denen den Kontaktpersonen
wieder Formalin begegnet. Die Möglichkeit, mit Fotokopierpapier-Aktivatoren in
Berührung zu kommen, gehört heute zu den Alltäglichkeiten.

15. Das *Graphische Gewerbe* (Drucker, Lithographen) hatte mit Terpentin, Terpentinersatzstoffen (Kienöl, Xylol), mit technischen Ölen und Fetten, bei denen
die Additive meist noch nicht als Noxen genannt wurden bzw. in den Vordergrund
gerückt waren, mit Chromverbindungen und Anilinabkömmlingen zu tun. Formalin spielt neben den genannten Substanzen auch heute noch eine größere Rolle in
diesem Sektor. Außerdem hat man Kobalt-, Nickelverbindungen ein größeres
Augenmerk geschenkt, seitdem die häufig beobachtete Koppelung mit Chromallergien bekannt ist. In diesem Bereich wird es sich jedoch um Direktsensibilisierungen durch Kontakt mit Kobalt- und Nickelverbindungen in der Druckerschwärze handeln.

16. Farbstoffe der Anilinreihe liegen in der *Textilindustrie* als Sensibilisatoren
nahe, ferner früher Mottenschutzmittel, Antiseptica, Appreturen, in den beiden
letzteren Formalin, bei den Antiseptica auch Lysol, Phenol, Kresol und dergleichen.
Terpentin- und Chromallergien dürften insgesamt auch heute von einer gewissen
Bedeutung sein. Die Sensibilisierungsmöglichkeit durch Paragruppenverbindungen
ist auch hier hervorzuheben und desgleichen die Kobalt- und Nickelsensibilisierung, die durch Quecksilber in Appreturen selten vorkommende Quecksilberüberempfindlichkeit und naturgemäß die allseits erhöhte Zahl von Formalinallergikern.
Vernetzer und Arbeitslösungen der Spinnerei, Farbstoffe der Baumwollindustrie

(z. B. Eisrot TR) sind zu nennen. Die Anzahl der Personen, die auf Kleiderfarben und Formaldehydharz enthaltende Stoffe reagieren, ist auffallend hoch, ebenso das vermehrte Auftreten der Nickel- und überhaupt der Metallionendermatosen in der Gesamtbevölkerung durch die häufige Verwendung im Bekleidungssektor.

17. In der *Hutfabrikation* der 30er Jahre kennt man Chrom-, ferner Farbstoff-, darunter Anilinderivat- und schließlich Lösungsmittelallergien. In den 50er Jahren kommt die Lorbeerölallergie als erkannte Noxe hinzu, die heute ebenso ihre Rolle spielt.

18. In der *Leder- und Schuhherstellung* kommen 1930 Allergien durch Chromverbindungen (insbesondere im Gerbprozeß), bei den Schuhmachern durch Klebstoffe, Gummilösungen, Benzinverbindungen, Benzolverbindungen, chlorierte Kohlenwasserstoffe, Harze, Harzlösungsmittel, Terpentinverbindungen, Terpentinersatz, Anilinabkömmlinge, Naturharz- und Kunstharzlacke vor. Inzwischen werden die Azo- und Antrachinonverbindungen vermehrt Paragruppenreaktionen genannt. Insbesondere aber hat sich der Akzent gewandelt, indem auch hier vermehrt Formalinunverträglichkeiten (einmal durch Anwendung in Gerbmitteln), berichtet werden, und alle bekannten Kunststoff- und Kunstharzbestandteile eine intensive und immer stärker werdende Anwendung in den verschiedensten Branchen der Leder- und Schuhwarenverarbeitung gefunden haben. In Zukunft wird man auf diese Noxen noch weitaus größere Aufmerksamkeit verwenden müssen.

19. Die *Zündholzindustrie* im Jahr 1930 nannte Phosphorabkömmlinge, wie Phosphorsesquichlorid, Phosphortrisulfid, Phosphorsaures Ammoniak, ferner Schwefelantimon, Farbstoffe (Rosin), später Chromabkömmlinge, die für die sog. Streichholzschachteldermatitis verantwortlich zu machen waren.

20. Im *Bäckergewerbe* hat sich ein maßgeblicher Akzentwandel vollzogen. Die früher primären Allergene Mehlaufheller Ammoniumpersulfat, Kaliumpersulfat, Calciumpersulfat, Kaliumbromat (in Deutschland), sekundär reine Mehlstauballergie, sind seit 1957 (dem Verbot der Aufheller in der Bundesrepublik) praktisch ausgeschaltet. Neben den genannten Noxen sind Farbstoffe, z. B. der Azogruppe (z. B. der Azofarbstoff Ponceaurot 6 R) und Aromastoffe, heute also mehr die Backhilfsmittel, als Kontaktnoxen zu nennen. Letzthin haben Antioxydantien der Margarine von sich reden gemacht, z. B. Laurylgallat, Propylgallat, Octylgallat, Dodecylgallat. In Zukunft könnten derartige Substanzen an Bedeutung gewinnen, da die Anwendung von natürlichen Produkten in der Lebensmittelindustrie im allgemeinen und somit auch im Bäckergewerbe zurückgeht.

21. In der *Tabakindustrie* kannte man früher das Tabaksaftekzem, das heute infolge der fast völlig maschinellen und automatisierten Herstellung, jedenfalls in der Zigarettenindustrie, praktisch kaum mehr vorkommt.

22. Im *Friseurbereich* der 30er Jahre kannte man als Kontaktallergen Chinin, Quecksilber, selten Resorcin, oft Haarfarben, insbesondere das deswegen verbotene Ursol und seine Abkömmlinge. Heute ist die Möglichkeit einer Sensibilisierung gegen Paragruppenabkömmlinge weitaus größer, auch gegen Haarfarben und Farbstoffgrundsubstanzen, die eigentlich als verträglich gegolten haben. Metallionenallergien, wie im hauswirtschaftlichen Bereich, gegen Chrom-, Kobaltverbindungen aus Waschmitteln, sind zu beobachten. Fixiermittel der Dauerwellen, z. B. Bromate, Kaliumbromat, sind nennenswert, insbesondere aber ist die Gruppe der Kaltwelldauerwellenentwicklerlösungen als früher nicht bekannte bzw. gar nicht existente Kontaktnoxe aufgetreten (Thioglykolsäurehydracide, Thioglycerine, Ammoniumthioglykolate usw.). Im Friseurbereich werden heute außerordentlich viel Hautunverträglichkeiten beobachtet. Da zugleich auch die Präparate der dekorativen Kosmetik von der Gesamtpopulation, insbesondere der weiblichen, in einem früher nicht geahnten Ausmaß in ihren Konsum einbezogen worden sind,

ist auch hier eine Vermehrung der Kontaktreaktionen erfolgt und weiter zu erwarten.

23. a) Im *medizinischen Bereich* kannte man als Sensibilisatoren vor 3 Jahrzehnten Quecksilber, Desinfizientien, insbesondere Formalin-, Phenolverbindungen (Lysol, Kresol), Anaesthetica (der Begriff der Paragruppenverbindungen war damals noch nicht geläufig), insbesondere Alypin, Anaesthesin, Prokain, ferner Gummihandschuhnoxen wie in der Gummiindustrie. Hier hat sich der Akzent heute verlagert auf früher nicht existierende Antibiotica, z. B. Streptomycin, Penicillin u. a., auf die Phenothiacine (Chlorpromacin), sowie auf eine Vielzahl von neueren Paragruppenverbindungen, nämlich die Sulfonamide, die zu den Anästhetica hinzugetreten sind. Insofern ist auch die Gesamtpopulation mehr Paragruppenallergisch als früher, da diese Kontaktstoffe sich zahlenmäßig vervielfacht haben.

23. b) Im *zahnärztlichen* Sektor sprach man weitgehend nur von Überempfindlichkeiten gegenüber ätherischen Ölen, z. B. Nelkenöl (Eugenol). Nach Einführung der Harze und Kunstharze in die zahnärztliche Prothetik sind auch hier diese Stoffe, insbesondere Methylmetacrylat, Benzylperoxyd, ferner Hydrochinon, Farbstoffe, zu Irritantien geworden.

23. c) Bei den *Apothekern und der pharmazeutischen Industrie* waren früher in erster Linie nur Irritantien die Quecksilberverbindungen, Chininstaub und Radix-Ipecacuanhae (Emetin), ferner Alkaloide, Atropinmutterlaugen, seltener Resochin, ferner Formalin-Lysophorm. Heute findet sich vom Erzeuger bis zum Verbraucher ein ganz breites zusätzliches Spektrum von Stoffen. Die Chininüberempfindlichkeiten wurden bedeutungslos gegenüber den neu hinzugekommenen Medikamenten, in erster Linie den Paragruppenverbindungen, d. h. Sulfonamiden, dann den Antibiotica, insbesondere Streptomycin, Penicillin, Chloramphenicol, Neomycin, Framycetin, Bacitracin, Kanamycin, Nipagin (mit Zwischenprodukten wie p-Nitroaminoacetophenon, p-Nitroacetamidohydroxypropiophenon), dann den Phenothiacinen, Antihistaminen (Bromadryl, Benzhydrilgruppe!), Vitamin K_3 (Menadion), Vitamin K_4 (Menadiol), Vitamin B_1, Vitamin B_6 (Pyridinderivaten), sowie mitunter Hydracinen, Resochin, Äthylendiamin, Piperazinderivaten, Rizinin des Rizinus und dem Formalin als Stoff, der allgemein von größerer Bedeutung geworden ist.

24. Im *häuslichen Bereich*, auch in Hauswirtschaftsberufen und -Tätigkeiten, lag der Schwerpunkt in den 30er Jahren auf Sidol, Sil, Persil, insbesondere Terpentin (in Bohnerwachs und Schuhcremes), Farbstoffen, z. B. Anilinderivaten, Nigrosin, Echtgelb (in Schuhcremes), Harzen, Wachsen, sowie auf Bleichmitteln, z. B. dem Kaliumhypochlorit (KClO im Eau de Javel). Der Akzent ruht heute auf Terpentin und Lösungsmitteln, Metallionen, z. B. Chrom, aber auch Kobalt- und Nickelverbindungen, die in Waschmitteln vorkommen, Paragruppenverbindungen, mancherlei chemischen Substanzen, z. B. Fleckentfernern (hydracinhaltigen), Bakteriostatica (z. B. Tetrachlorsalicylanilid, TCSA), wie sie Putzmitteln zugesetzt werden, und optischen Aufhellern in Waschmitteln. Die Beobachtungen der letzten Jahre in bezug auf die Kontaktsensibilisierung bei Hausfrauen und Hausangestellten beziehen sich vor allem auf die Schädigung durch die neuen synthetischen Waschmittel, Reinigungsmittel, Netzmittel, Fußbodenpflegemittel. Die Gummiekzeme durch Tragen von Gummischuhen und -handschuhen nehmen einerseits zu, während bei Nichttragen derselben die Reaktionen auf den direkten Kontakt mit Einwirkungsstoffen sich vermehren.

Zusammenfassend kann man sagen, daß im gesamten hauswirtschaftlichen Bereich eine erhebliche Akzentänderung an Kontaktstoffen vor sich gegangen ist. Die Zahl der Kontaktstoffe hat sich massiv vermehrt, zugleich die Zahl der Stoffe, die als Netzmittel im Sinne von Schlitten reizende Noxen intensiv mit dem

Hautorgan in Berührung zu bringen vermögen. Damit konform gehend hat auch die Zahl der Unverträglichkeitsreaktionen extrem zugenommen. Was das Terpentin betrifft, so wurde diese Substanz heute weitgehend durch andere organische Lösungsmittel ersetzt und ist dadurch im Gegensatz zu früher in einem etwas geringerem Maße als Allergen beteiligt. Eine Ausnahme machen hier die hauswirtschaftlichen Bereiche und dementsprechend der nichtberufliche Sensibilisierungsgang gegen Terpentine, da die dort tätigen Personen, d. h. die Allgemeinpopulation, weiterhin gehäuft mit Terpentin-haltigen Bohnerwachsen und Schuhcremes in Berührung kommt.

Noch einige Worte zur allgemeinen Situation: Greifen wir noch einige wenige Beobachtungen heraus!

Die drei meist reagierenden Kontaktallergene (MAGNUSSON, BLOHM, FREGERT, HJORTH, HOVDING, PIRILÄ und SKOG) bei Männern (Skandinavien) waren 1965 Chromverbindungen, Perubalsam, Kobaltverbindungen, bei Frauen Nickelverbindungen, Perubalsam, p-Phenylendiamin, also Paragruppenverbindungen.

In den USA (BAER, New York) fiel im Vergleich zwischen 1937 und 1962 auf, daß das Vorkommen von Nickel- und Chromunverträglichkeiten relativ gleich häufig war. Dagegen reagierten Quecksilberverbindungen (um 180%), Paragruppenstoffe, p-Phenylendiamin (um 140%) und Formaldehyd (um 290%) häufiger!

Ein Überblick über die 12000 bis 13000 Personen umfassende Klientel der Dermatologischen Klinik und Poliklinik der Universität München in vier verschiedenen Jahren erbringt, daß als hauptsächlichste berufliche Kontaktallergene neben technischen Fetten und Ölen die Farben, Zemente, Chromverbindungen und deren vielfältige Möglichkeiten vorkommen.

An der Spitze liegen in 4 Vergleichsjahren Terpentine, Wasch- und Reinigungsmittel bzw. -tinkturen, Friseurbedarfsstoffe, Öle und p-Gruppenverbindungen. Im Gegensatz zu 1952/53 liegen 1962/63 Terpentin, Terpentinersatz, Schmieröle, Spezialgipse und -zemente an der Spitze. Berufsstoffe, die 1952 nicht oder kaum auffällig waren, bzw. nicht ermittelt wurden, sind bestimmte Kaliumbichromat enthaltende Farben, ferner Hölzer, Hopfen, Retuschierlösungen, Antibiotica, Nipagin und Nipasol, Xanthocillin und Gummibedarfsstoffe wie TMTD usw. 1962/63 ist gegenüber früher die Zahl der Allergien auf Spezialbaustoffe, Spezialgipse, Spezialhärter und -zemente angestiegen. Allergien auf Kohlenwasserstoffe, technische Bleich-, Wasch- und Reinigungsmittel sowie Leime und Farbstoffe nahmen neben anderen Stoffen stetig zu.

Free Communications

Kontaktekzem und Ekzematoide

FR. KOGOJ und J. FETTICH, Dermatologische Klinik Ljubljana (Jugoslawien)

Das vulgäre Ekzem ist in der Regel ein an das Kontaktgebiet gebundenes, nur relativ selten sich generalisierendes, akut ablaufendes, allergisches Hautgeschehen. Für den Übergang in eine chronische Hautalteration sind nach Ausschaltung des Primärantigens andere Faktoren verantwortlich. Die eventuelle Ausbreitung des ursprünglich auf kleinere Hautareale beschränkten Ekzems auf größere Gebiete oder gar seine universelle Ausbreitung sind auf dieselben Mechanismen zurückzuführen, denen die Erstveränderungen ihr Entstehen verdanken. Das periphere Fortschreiten erfolgt sowohl auf exogenem als auch auf endogenem Wege, wobei das Allergen unseres Erachtens nicht nur hämatogen oder lymphogen, sondern auch von Zellkomplex zu Zellkomplex verschleppt werden kann.

Er gibt ekzemähnliche Hautmanifestationen, die ebenfalls hämatogen, lymphogen oder auf dem Gewebeweg entstehen und im Anschluß an ein vulgäres Ekzem oder an eine pyodermische oder pyodermisierte Affektion auftreten. Wir nennen diese Veränderungen Ekzematoide. Von 7341 Neueingängen diagnostizierten wir 192mal (2,61%) ein nummuläres oder papulovesiculöses Ekzematoid und 244mal (3,05%) ein vulgäres Kontaktekzem. Die mikrobiellen Dermoepidermitiden und das reine mikrobielle Ekzem bilden nur einen Teil der Ekzematoide, zu welchen auch das sog. papulo-vesiculöse Ekzem von BROCQ und das sog. nummuläre Ekzem von DEVERGIE gehören. Diese verdanken ihr Erscheinen der hämatogenen Aussaat des kausalen Agens aus einem Herd. Sie sind also Fokalosen. Ist der Herd ein vulgäres Ekzem, erscheinen die Ekzematoide nicht in den ersten Tagen nach dem Auftreten des Ekzems, sondern etwas später, sehr oft zu einer Zeit, wo das Ekzematogen schon durch eine längere Zeitspanne nicht mehr an die Haut herangebracht wurde. Zwischen nummulärem und papulo-vesiculösem Ekzematoid bestehen Kombinationen und Übergänge. Bemerkenswert ist die bei den Ekzematoiden bestehende lokale Therapieresistenz.

Die Frage, ob die auf dem Blutweg im Anschluß an ein Eczema vulgare entstandenen Ekzematoide auf die Wirkung des ursprünglichen Ekzematogens zurückzuführen sind oder es sich um „Ide" anderer Genese, z. B. Mikrobide handelt, wurde schon oft untersucht (MIESCHER, ROBERT, STORCK, RAJKA u. Mitarb., die Schule von MARCHIONINI, insbesondere RÖCKL, MEYER-ROHN u. a.). Eigene (K.) Versuche (1964) zeigten, daß es in fünf von zwölf Ekzematoidfällen gelungen ist, aus dem Blut hämolytische Staphylokokken herauszuzüchten, ein Befund, der im Einzelfalle vielleicht anfechtbar ist, als Kollektivergebnis jedoch seine Bedeutung besitzt. Auch das vom vulgären Ekzem abweichende, makrovisuelle Bild der Ekzematoide weist auf ein, vom ursprünglichen Ekzematogen abweichendes, pathogenes Agens hin. Der histologische Befund zeigte beim nummulären Ekzematoid neben eventuell gleichzeitig bestehender Spongiose und oberflächlichen nekrobiotischen Veränderungen (vgl. MIESCHER, RÖCKL) in der Papillar- und Subpapillarschicht kleine lymphocytäre Elemente, die zusammen mit einer größeren oder kleineren Anzahl gelapptkerniger Leukocyten stellenweise in die Epidermis einwandern (Mikrodia). Sehr oft sahen wir als auffallendes Merkmal lang ausgezogene Papillen mit entsprechender digitiformer Akanthose, ein Befund, der beim Eczema vulgare in dieser Form kaum beschrieben worden ist (Mikrodia).

Manches, ganz besonders aber die positive Hämokultur und die Sterilität der frischen Ekzematoidbläschen weisen in Richtung eines Mikrobides, wobei wir die antigene Rolle nicht den Pyokokken als solchen zuschreiben, es aber dahingestellt bleiben soll, ob metabolische Produkte der Staphylokokken oder ihre Toxine als Allergen wirken.

Es gibt Gründe, die Zweifel darüber berechtigt erscheinen lassen, ob mit dieser Erklärung die Pathogenese der mit dem Ekzemherd verbundenen Ekzematoide ausgeschöpft ist. Das ist vor allem die Erkenntnis, daß überall dort, wo der pathologische Prozeß zu einer Zell- und Gewebsdesintegration führt, mit der Bildung von körpereigenem, autoantigenem Material zu rechnen ist. Wir erinnern dabei nur an WHITFIELDS Autosensibilisierung, die Autoekzematisation von CORMIA und ESPLIN und zum Teil an die Versuche von RÖCKL, der bei mikrobiellem Ekzem mit Ekzemherddetritus positive Epicutanreaktionen erhielt.

Obwohl uns klar war, daß im Tierexperiment die Verhältnisse, wie sie beim Zustandekommen der Ekzematoide vorhanden sind, nicht reproduzierbar sind, versuchten wir an Meerschweinchen einen indirekten Einblick in den Ablauf der

Geschehnisse dabei zu gewinnen. Aus der Haut mit DNCB sensibilisierter und nichtsensibilisierter Meerschweinchen wurde je ein wäßriger und ein Etanol-extrakt hergestellt. Nach 6 bis 9 Wochen injizierten wir die einzelnen Extrakte der Reihenfolge nach in die Zitze. In keinem Falle erzielten wir ein positives Resultat, was natürlich nicht als Beweis für die Nichtbeteiligung autoallergischer Vorgänge bei den hämatogenen Ekzematoiden gewertet werden kann. Jedenfalls ist ihre Entstehung einem anderen Allergen zu verdanken als dem, der das Erscheinen des vulgären Ekzems zur Folge hatte. Dieses Zweitantigen ist wahrscheinlich entstanden durch Interferenz mikrobieller und dermogener Komponenten bzw. Einwirkungen. Deshalb wäre die Bezeichnung Ekzematide irreführend. Mit dem Worte „Ekzematoid" soll zweierlei zum Ausdruck gebracht werden: die Ekzemähnlichkeit und die fokale Allergengenese. Wenn das Ekzem ein primäres allergisches Hautphänomen ist, dann können wir die Ekzematoide als sekundär allergische Hautphänomene auffassen.

Die passive Übertragung des DNCB-Kontaktekzems beim Meerschweinchen mit Hilfe der kontinuierlichen Austauschtransfusion

F. SCHRÖPL, Dermatologische Klinik und Poliklinik der Universität Würzburg (Deutschland)

Das tierexperimentelle Kontaktekzem war zuerst von HAXTHAUSEN durch *Parabiose* übertragen worden, was später von KALKOFF und SKOG bestätigt wurde. Die verwendete Technik war einfach: Zwei Tiere wurden mit Peritoneum und/oder Haut zusammengenäht. Der Zeitpunkt des Eintritts von Kreislaufanastomosen war dabei nicht exakt festzulegen.

Unseren eigenen Parabioseversuchen liegt die Technik der kontinuierlichen Austauschtransfusion zugrunde, die auf MÜLLER-RUCHHOLZ und PFEIFFER zurückgeht und von uns für das Meerschweinchen modifiziert wurde.

Wir gehen dabei folgendermaßen vor: Von einem Halsschnitt aus werden 1 mm starke Kunststoffkatheter durch einen Subcutantunnel zum Nacken geführt und dort herausgeleitet. Bild 1 zeigt die Katheter mit dem Ansatz der Halterung, dunkel die blutführenden Schläuche, hell ein zusätzlicher Subcutankatheter. Die Schläuche werden am Hals in die Arteria carotis und Vena jugularis eingeführt und fixiert. Die Tiere erhalten laufend Depotheparin, wozu der auf der ersten Abbildung gezeigte Subcutankatheter dient.

Nach Versorgung der Wunden werden die blutführenden Schläuche mit einem Zwischenstück miteinander verbunden, so daß ein extracorporaler Kreislauf entsteht. Eine von uns konstruierte Spezialhalterung erlaubt den Tieren relativ viel Bewegungsfreiheit. Zwei dermaßen operierte Tiere sind leicht in kontinuierlichen Blutaustausch zu bringen.

Die Arterie des einen Tieres wird jeweils mit der Vene des anderen Tieres verbunden und umgekehrt. Bei dieser Parabiosemethode sind Beginn und Dauer des Blutaustauschs exakt definiert, ebenso die ausgetauschte Blutmenge, die 2,5 bis 5 l pro Tag beträgt. Der Blutaustausch gelingt ohne Schwierigkeiten über 24 Std und länger.

Mit dieser Versuchsanordnung war es uns möglich, das experimentelle DNCB-Ekzem des Meerschweinchens passiv zu übertragen. Wir koppelten dabei stark sensibilisierte Spendertiere mit unbehandelten Empfängern. Die Auslösung der Reaktion erfolgte unmittelbar im Anschluß an den Beginn des Blutaustausches. Zur Auslösung der Tests wurde die nichttoxische DNCB-Konzentration von 15 γ/cm² verwendet. Mit dieser Methode erzielten wir bei 8 von 15 Empfängern eine passive Übertragung. Alle Testreaktionen wurden histologisch kontrolliert und nur solche als positiv bewertet, bei denen eine typische Spongiose vorhanden war. Kontrollversuche mit unbehandelten Tieren verliefen negativ.

Die von uns operierten Einzeltiere lassen sich darüber hinaus als Herz-Lungen-Maschine verwenden, da sie über einen gut funktionierenden extracorporalen Kreislauf verfügen. Es mußte daher möglich sein, eine Versuchsanordnung auszuarbeiten, bei der Haut überlebend gehalten und von einem solchen Tier durchblutet werden konnte. Nach langwierigen Vorversuchen gelang es uns, eine derartige Methodik zu entwickeln.

Wir exstirpieren hierzu die Vorderpfote eines Meerschweinchens und führen in die Arteria und Vena axillaris Katheter ein. Diese werden mit einem in der oben angegebenen Weise voroperierten Spender verbunden, wobei die Zwischenschaltung eines Pumpsystems erforderlich ist. Es war uns bereits möglich, auf diesem Wege auf der überlebenden Haut unspezifische entzündliche Reaktionen auszulösen. Bei der gezeigten Abbildung handelt es sich um eine 21-Std-Reaktion einer Crotonöldermatitis auf der Haut eines solchen Explantates. Entsprechende Kontrollversuche wurden selbstverständlich durchgeführt. Diese Versuchsanordnung wird es unseres Erachtens ermöglichen, die Frage der Hautständigkeit des Antikörpers beim Ekzem exakt zu beantworten. Wir versuchen hierzu gegenwärtig, die Extremitäten sensibilisierter Tiere von nicht sensibilisierten Spendern aus am Leben zu erhalten und darauf die ekzematöse Kontaktreaktion auszulösen. Unsere diesbezüglichen Versuche, die mit beträchtlichen methodischen Schwierigkeiten verbunden sind, sind noch nicht abgeschlossen. Wir werden an anderer Stelle darüber berichten.

Literatur. HAXTHAUSEN, H.: Acta derm.-venereol. (Stockh.) **24**, 286 (1944). — MÜLLER-RUCHHOLZ, W., W. DETTWYLER und E. F. PFEIFFER: Z. ges. exp. Med. **135**, 368 (1962). — SCHRÖPL, F., u. P. RIPPMANN: Arch. klin. exp. Derm. **229**, 331 (1967). — SKOG, E.: Acta derm.-venereol. (Stockh.) **35**, 264 (1955).

Immunologic Unresponsiveness to Contact Sensitizers

E. D. LOWNEY, Medical College of Virginia, Richmond, Virginia (USA)

I am going to describe briefly the results of our studies of immunologic unresponsiveness to contact sensitizers. Because some of this work has already appeared in print, and because time is short, we will not go into the methodology in detail.

When a contact sensitizer, such as paranitrosodimethylaniline (NDMA), is put on the skin of a guinea pig, two things are seen to happen. First, as a result of the topical application of the sensitizing compound, the animal becomes sensitized to a moderate degree, so that a skin test with the sensitizer will be mildly positive 10 days later. The second, and more interesting thing that happens is that the animal becomes unresponsive to the compound, so that we cannot raise the level of sensitivity to a higher level.

Experiments on unresponsiveness always have three parts: First, a suppressing exposure to the compound is given and, as a result of this exposure, the animal fails to respond, or is unresponsive, to a second procedure which would normally cause an increase in sensitivity. The third step is a set of skin tests, to measure the degree of sensitivity produced in response to the second step.

In our experiments the previous exposure was given by the topical route. Since topical exposure itself causes mild sensitivity, we had to use a highly sensitizing exposure, such as the injection of 50 γ NDMA mixed with FREUND's complete adjuvant into the foot-pad, in an attempt to elicit a measurable increase in sensitivity.

We have shown [1] that when as much as 175 γ NDMA is put on the skin of the guinea pig 4 weeks before the sensitizing injection, there is no response to the injection at all. In the figure, the bottom animal is a control animal, he received the sensitizing injection only with no previous exposure, and he responded normally to it, with strongly positive reaction to skin tests applied 10 days later. The upper animal, on the other hand, was made unresponsive by topical application of NDMA 4 weeks before the injection. He shows a very mild reaction, which represents residual sensitivity from the topical exposure itself, but he shows no evidence of response to the injection of NDMA in complete adjuvant.

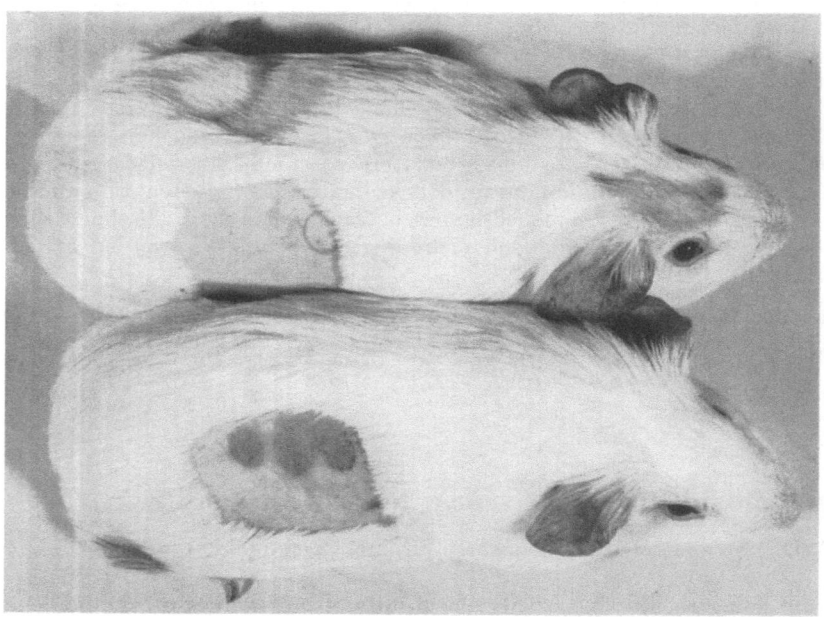

Fig. Both animals were given a strongly sensitizing foot-pad injection of 50 γ NDMA in FREUND's complete adjuvant 10 days before these tests were applied. The upper animal had been rendered unresponsive to this injection by topical application of 175 γ NDMA 30 days previously. The lower, control, animals shows strongly positive epicutaneous test reactions, which is the normal response to the injection

We have found that the degree of unresponsiveness induced by topical exposure to a contact sensitizer is related to the amount of sensitizer applied. In the case of NDMA, application of as much as 175 γ induces virtually complete unresponsiveness, while response is only partially impaired by a topical dose of 25 γ [2].

Unresponsiveness does not appear at once after topical application of a sensitizer, but develops gradually over a 2 to 3 week period [3]. Thus, after the sensitizer is put on the skin, unresponsiveness and sensitivity develop simultaneously over the same period of time, and may represent two semantically different aspects of the same phenomenon.

Can such unresponsiveness be demonstrated to occur in man ? We have shown that human subjects who are very slowly sensitized by a series of exposures to minute amounts of a contact sensitizer develop a weak, attenuated sensitivity. This is in contrast to a higher degree of sensitivity seen in subjects who are rapidly sensitized by massive exposures to the chemical [4]. Preliminary evidence indicates that human subjects in whom such a weak sensitivity has been induced do not respond to efforts to induce a strong sensitivity by application of larger sensitizing doses. If these preliminary studies are confirmed, then, we will have demonstrated unresponsiveness in man as well as in the guinea pig.

References. LOWNEY, E. D.: J. Immunol. **95**, 397 (1965). — J. invest. Derm. **45**, 378 (1965). — J. invest. Derm. **48**, 391 (1967). — Attenuation of contact sensitivity in man. J. invest. Derm. (In press). — Many excellent papers by other authors are referred to in the cited papers.

The Persistence and Recurrence of Contact Eczema: Clinical Experimental Observations

C. L. MENEGHINI, F. RANTUCCIO and G. COZZA, Dermatology Department, University of Bari (Italy)

The chief pathogenetic factors in the recurrence and persistence of contact eczema are:

1. persistence of the allergen,
2. subsequent sensitisation to other substances, including cross sensitisation,
3. sensitisation to pyogens and mycetes,
4. aspecific agents: mechanical, physical, etc.,
5. individual neurogenic or dysmetabolic factors or factors arising out of other diseases,
6. autosensitisation.

This note is concerned with the first three factors:

1. The persistence of the contact is an important factor in hypersensitivity to chromium, turpentine and aniline substances, which are ubiquitous. Chromium may even be found in drinking water, especially if it comes from wells in industrial areas. In the Milan area, for example, hexavalent chromium is present in water in traces or as much as 50 γ/l.

It is also found in soaps and detergents, products used daily by many persons [1].

Turpentine is still used extensively in Italy and hence contact with it is frequent. Terpenes of the same type but of different provenance can give rise to reactions. As a matter of fact, it has been shown that some persons who are hypersensitive to turpentine have positive reactions to orange essence.

Aniline-containing compounds are also widely used. And so repeated contact with the above substances occurs frequently, without people being aware of it.

The following findings bear out this point: of 343 patients hospitalised from 2 to 10 times for clinically-ascertained contact eczema over the past 8 years the majority were hypersensitive to these allergens (Tab. 1), whereas patients hypersensitive to substances not widely used were less prone to recurrence, once the contact had been removed.

Experimental data point in the same direction (Tab. 2). Of 139 subjects experimentally sensitised to DNCB over half desensitised spontaneously during the

observation period of 3 to 6 years, whereas subjects sensitised to dimethylpara-
nitrosoaniline during the same period showed greater persistence of hypersensi-
vity [2].

2. Another important factor is sensitisation to other substances. In our experience drugs applied to eczematous lesions induced further hypersensitivity in
5% of 4500 cases of contact eczema.

Evidence of polyhypersensitivity to other allergens was present in 10% of
the cases.

3. With regard to the role of microbial agents, pyogens and mycetes, as infective or allergenic agents, the following investigations were conducted on subjects with recurrent or persistent contact eczema.

a) infectivity tests: staphylococci, streptococci and Candida albicans, active
and isolated from the skin of eczematous subjects and concentrated by culturing
were applied to the skin for 24 h; tests were conducted with autologous or homologous mixed or differentiated bacteria;

b) tests of cutaneous allergic reactivity to inactivated pyogens and Candida
and to their antigens;

c) serologic tests (autologous complement deviation to microbial antigens in
the same eczematous subjects).

Table 1. *343 patients hospitalised 2 to 10 times over a period
of 8 years for relapsing eczematous contact-type dermatitis:
incidence of the allergens responsible*

N° patients	allergens
118	chromium
21	chromium + turpentine
20	chromium + cobalt
3	chromium + nickel
49	turpentine
3	turpentine + aniline
2	turpentine + cobalt
15	aniline
22	aniline + other substances of the "para" group
14	sulfanilamide
11	antihistaminics
16	other substances
49	allergens not determined

Table 2. *Persistence of eczematous hypersensitivity induced experimentally with dinitrochloro-
benzol 2.5 to 30% in 139 subjects checked up 3 to 6 years later*

No. subjects	Positive	Negative
139	53	86

*Persistence of eczematous hypersensitivity induced experimentally withd imethyl-paranitrosoaniline
in 19 subjects checked up 3 to 6 years later*

No. subjects	Positive	Negative
19	14	5

For details of the methods used the reader is referred to a previous note on the
subject [3]. Further type tests (in addition to hemolytic and coagulase activity
tests) were performed (fermentation and phosphatase activity tests).

The microorganisms taken from the healthy and diseases skin of eczematous
subjects and cultured on plates of agar-broth, agar-broth-blood and gelatin were

in the main saprophytic micrococci and pyogenic staphylococci (aureus, citreus and albus); pyogenyc streptococci and, occasionally, Candida albicans, were among the other bacteria found.

The results taken as a whole (Tab. 3) broadly bear out the observations made in preliminary studies. The application of a film of autologous and homologous staphylococci or streptococci to healthy skin was not followed by a significant response indicating direct infection or delayed hypersensitivity. Candida albicans gave rise to vescicopustulation in one case and to erythema in others. The same pyogens on skin altered by stripping gave rise to abraded erythematous reactions, even more impetiginoid because of the streptococcus in more than half of the cases; but in most cases the skin responses, evident at 24/36 h, receded in the days that followed.

Table 3. *Contact eczema: infectivity tests*

Type of skin reaction	Cases n.	Evolution after exposure			
		24 h	48 h	96 h	192 h
A. Staphylococcus pyogenes		cases n. 102			
Erythema at site of contact	39	++	+	—	—
Eryth., edema, weak exudation at site of contact	28	+++	++	+—	—
Eryth., vesiculation (beyond area of contact)	—				
No reaction	35				
B. Streptococcus pyogenes		cases n. 82			
Erythema at site of contact	12	++	+	—	—
Eryth., edema, weak exudation at site of contact	9	++	+	—	—
Eryth., vesiculation (beyond area of contact)	—				
Eryth., vesiculo-pustular lesion	16	++	++	+	—
No reaction	45				
C. Candida albicans		cases n. 102			
Erythema at site of contact	17	++	+—	—	—
Eryth., edema, weak exudation at site of contact	5	++	+	—	—
Eryth., vesiculation (beyond area of contact)	11	+	++	+++	++
Eryth., vesiculo-pustular lesion	33	++	+++·	++	+—
No reaction	36				

The application of mixed bacteria from broth cultures to eczematous lesions did not rekindle the cutaneous reactions either at the site or at distance from it.

Tests for cutaneous reactivity to inactivated microorganisms, toxoids or anatoxins elicited no responses of the allergic eczematous erythematovesicular type, except in the case of Candida albicans suspensions.

The search for serologic antibodies to pyogens and to Candida albicans showed that high antistaphylococcus concentrations were frequently present in eczematous subject.

According to the findings reported here, surface pyogens do not seem to take part in the pathogenesis of the continuity of contact eczema by inducing a specific allergy, though perhaps we have not yet got a reliable immunologic model for this. Pyogens probably play a more important role through their infective and lympho-angioitic action, which further upsets the immunologic mechanisms that are already altered in eczematous subjects.

References. 1. QUINONES, P. A., et G. M. GARCIA MUNOZ: Ann. Derm. Syph. (Paris) 92, 383 (1965). — 2. MENEGHINI, C. L., F. RANTUCCIO, A. RIBOLDI und M. F. HOFMANN: Berufs-dermatosen 15, 103 (1967). — 3. MENEGHINI, C. L., I. VIVARELLI e G. COZZA: G. ital. Derm. Sif. 107, 899 (1966).

Tests épicutanés et épreuve de concentration-dilution

J. OLEFFE, Clinique dermatologique de l'Université de Bruxelles (Belgique)

1. Orthoergie et allergie

Pour le dermatologue comme pour le médecin du travail il est extrêmement important de faire la distinction entre l'eczéma orthoergique (par irritation primaire) et l'eczéma allergique. Dans le premier cas, les contacts avec le produit nocif doivent être supprimés pour l'ensemble des travailleurs exposés; dans le second cas, c'est le travailleur devenu allergique qui devra le plus souvent être écarté de ses occupations professionnelles. Par la pratique des tests épicutanés il n'est pas toujours possible d'établir par quel mécanisme, orthoergique ou allergique, une substance déterminée a pu déclencher l'apparition d'un eczéma. En fait on qualifie trop souvent d'allergique une réaction cutanée à une substance caustique diluée.

2. Histologie des tests épicutanés

L'étude histologique des tests épicutanés met en évidence des images assez caractéristiques correspondant aux réactions orthoergique et allergique. Dans le cas d'un «test orthoergique» on observe selon la concentration utilisée:

une nécrose totale ou partielle de l'épiderme,

la formation de grandes vésicules ou de petites vésicules, généralement superficielles,

la libération des cellules épidermiques par un phénomène comparable à l'acantholyse.

dans le derme s'observe un infiltrat composé de lymphocytes et de poly-nucléaires, pouvant dissocier l'épiderme et les zones vésiculeuses.

Le «test allergique» présente l'image de l'eczéma: spongiose des cellules malpighiennes avec éventuellement formation de vésicules, infiltrat dermique lymphocytaire qui vient persiller la face profonde de l'épiderme. Ces deux types d'images ne sont cependant pas toujours bien tranchés: des études expérimentales effectuées par VAN DER MEIREN et ACHTEN avec de l'acide sulfurique et de la potasse caustique dilués montrent qu'entre les images histologiques de l'orthoergie et de l'allergie existent des phénomènes de zone. En fait, il n'est pas toujours possible par l'examen histologique seul de faire la distinction entre allergie et orthoergie.

3. Épreuve de concentration-dilution

C'est pourquoi nous estimons qu'une révision des taux de dilution habituels des réactogènes professionnels devrait se faire sur la base de l'application de l'épreuve de concentration-dilution.

Cette épreuve s'adresse à la fois à des sujets allergiques et non allergiques. Elle consiste à pratiquer des tests épicutanés à l'aide de la substance étudiée, à des concentrations progressivement croissantes et décroissantes au départ du taux de dilution mentionné dans les listes de dilution usuelles.

Nos premiers résultats basés sur l'aspect clinique des réactions cutanées ainsi que sur leur étude histologique nous ont paru encourageants et doivent à notre avis permettre de déterminer avec plus de précision le seuil de l'allergie et celui de l'irritation primaire.

Nous relaterons brièvement les conclusions des épreuves de concentration-dilution appliquées au bichromate de potassium et à la térébenthine.

A. Bichromate de potassium. Chez des sujets sensibilisés, le bichromate de potassium à la concentration de 0,5% à 1% (taux de dilution couramment admis) donne une réaction cliniquement et histologiquement allergique. De 10 à 20% l'image est celle d'une réaction toxique qui s'observe aussi chez des sujets non sensibilisés. Chez des sujets sensibilisés, le bichromate de potassium à la concentration de 0,01 à 0,001% donne une image histologique allergique alors que la réaction clinique est négative.

B. Térébenthine. Nos travaux actuellement en cours envisagent l'étude comparative de plusieurs lots de térébenthine de provenance géographique et d'origine botanique différentes. Nos résultats actuels concernent deux variétés de térébenthine du commerce (correspondant à des mélanges). Chez des sujets sensibilisés, toutes deux donnent des images allergiques quelle que soit la concentration utilisée de 5 à 50%. A une dilution plus poussée (0,5%) on met en évidence une image allergique, en l'absence de réaction clinique.

Chez des sujets non sensibilisés, une de ces deux térébenthines ne nous a jamais donné de tests positifs jusqu'à la concentration de 75%, tandis que la seconde provoquait à cette même concentration de 75%, une réaction orthoergique dans 41% des cas.

Nous basant sur les travaux de PIRILÄ et collab. ainsi que de HELLERSTRÖM et RAJKA nous avons également appliqué l'épreuve de concentration-dilution à l'étude des divers constituants de la térébenthine et notamment du Δ-3-carène. Nos premières conclusions au sujet de ce produit rejoignent celles des auteurs précités, à savoir que le Δ-3-carène fraîchement distillé ne donnerait lieu à des réactions d'irritation cutanée que pour des concentrations égales ou supérieures à 75%.

Par l'application de l'épreuve de concentration-dilution nous espérons pouvoir faciliter la différenciation entre orthoergie et allergie et permettre de ranger les réactogènes professionnels dans une classification que nous avons esquissée précédemment et qui comprendrait des substances caustiques, toxiques et allergiques.

Bibliographie. (La bibliographie détaillée peut être consultée dans). — ACHTEN, G., et J. OLEFFE: Tests épicutanés et dermatoses professionnelles. Bull. Soc. franç. Derm. Syph. **73**, 49 (1966). — HELLERSTRÖM, S., and G. RAJKA: Turpentine Allergy: Artificial sensitization. Dermatologica (Basel) **130**, 287 (1965). — PIRILÄ, V., E. SILTANEN, and L. PIRILÄ: On the chemical nature of the eczematogenic agent in oil of turpentine. Dermatologica (Basel) **128**, 16 (1964). —

Experimentelle Untersuchungen über Sensibilisierungen mit chlorierten Imidazolinderivaten

E. Schöpf und K. H. Schulz, Universitäts-Hautklinik Hamburg (Deutschland)

Nach der Beschreibung des 2-Benzylimidazolins im Jahre 1939 durch Meyer und Schnetz als stark sympathicolytisch wirksame Substanz — bekannt unter dem Handelsnamen Priscol —, sind eine Vielzahl von Derivaten des Imidazolins als Pharmaka mit vorwiegend antihistaminem Effekt in Gebrauch, wie z. B. Antazolin, Naphazolin, Xylometazolin, Clemizol u. a. Über die sensibilisierenden Eigenschaften eines chlorierten Imidazolinderivates, das bei der Synthese von pharmakologisch wirksamen Imidazolinderivaten eine Rolle spielt, soll im folgenden berichtet werden.

Bei zwei Chemielaboranten eines pharmazeutischen Betriebes konnten wir innerhalb von 6 Monaten Kontaktekzeme der Hände beobachten. Die Ekzeme wiesen Verlaufsabhängigkeit von der Labortätigkeit auf, die in der Entwicklung neuer Derivate des Imidazolins bestand. Nach Abheilung der Hauterscheinungen vorgenommene epicutane Testuntersuchungen mit verschiedenen infrage kommenden Imidazolinabkömmlingen ergaben noch mit 0,001 molaren (= 0,0158%) wäßrigen Lösungen von Chlormethylimidazolinhydrochlorid positive Reaktionen. Toxicitätskontrollen waren bis zu einer 0,1 (= 1,58%) molaren Konzentration negativ. Aus den vorliegenden Befunden ergab sich, daß Chlormethylimidazolin das führende Allergen darstellt. Bei einem mit der Synthese dieser Verbindung beschäftigten Chemiestudenten konnte eine Sensibilisierung gegenüber Chlormethylimidazolin außer durch positive Epicutanteste auch durch einen positiven Lymphocytentransformationstest nachgewiesen werden. Dabei wurden die Blutlymphocyten des sensibilisierten Spenders für 120 Std bei 37 °C mit einer wäßrigen Lösung von Chlormethylimidazolin (Endkonzentration 0,0001 molar) zu einem Kulturmedium inkubiert. Anschließend wurden die Prozentsätze der sog. transformierten Lymphocyten und der Mitosen im Vergleich zu einem Kontrollansatz ohne Haptenzusatz bestimmt. Chlormethylimidazolin war in der Lage, 18% der Blutlymphocyten des Chlormethylimidazolinallergikers zu Transformation und 0,4% zu Mitose zu stimulieren. Im Kontrollansatz waren Transformationen und Mitosen nicht nachweisbar.

Zur Untersuchung der Sensibilisierungsfähigkeit von Chlormethylimidazolin wurden darüber hinaus Experimente an Meerschweinchen durchgeführt. Die toxische Reizschwelle von Chlormethylimidazolin lag nach epicutaner Applikation bei einer Konzentration von etwa 0,3 molar. Als Lösungsmittel diente für alle epicutanen Versuche ein Gemisch von Äthanol 45%, Methylcellosolve 45% und Tween 80 10%. Die Sensibilisierungsversuche wurden in folgender Weise durchgeführt: Eine Gruppe von zehn Meerschweinchen wurde durch zweimalige s.c.-Injektion einer 0,01 molaren Lösung von Chlormethylimidazolin unter Zusatz von Freundschem Adjuvans sensibilisiert. Bei einer zweiten Gruppe von zehn Meerschweinchen wurde eine 0,5 molare Lösung von Chlormethylimidazolin an 3 aufeinanderfolgenden Tagen epicutan appliziert. 8 Tage nach Beginn der Sensibilisierung durchgeführte Epicutanteste zeigten bei allen Tieren beider Gruppen eine Sensibilisierung gegenüber Chlormethylimidazolin. Es waren noch eindeutig positive Reaktionen bei einer Konzentration von 0,002 molar zu beobachten. Auch auf Grund histologischer Kriterien war die Reaktion als allergisch zu betrachten.

In einer weiteren Versuchsreihe wurde die Sensibilisierungsfähigkeit von Chlormethylimidazolin mit der von Dinitrochlorbenzol (DNCB) verglichen. Unter gleichen Bedingungen wurden zwei Gruppen von Meerschweinchen mit 0,5 molaren Lösungen von Chlormethylimidazolin bzw. DNCB sensibilisiert. Dabei zeigte sich, daß die 0,5 molare DNCB-Lösung stärkere toxische Reaktionen verursachte als die gleich konzentrierte Chlormethylimidazolinlösung. Im Gegensatz hierzu waren allergische Reaktionen mit DNCB nur bis zu 0,01 molaren, mit Chlormethylimidazolin aber bis zu 0,002 molaren Konzentrationen nachweisbar. Diese Befunde sprechen für eine im Vergleich zu DNCB geringere Toxizität, aber stärkere Sensibilisierungsfähigkeit von Chlormethylimidazolin unter diesen Bedingungen.

Gegenstand weiterer Untersuchungen waren die Beziehungen zwischen chemischer Struktur und allergener Wirkung von Imidazolinderivaten. Wir untersuchten die folgenden Imidazolinabkömmlinge auf etwaige gruppenallergische Reaktionen an sensibilisierten Meerschweinchen und den Patienten, die eine Kontaktallergie gegenüber Chlormethylimidazolin aufwiesen. Sämtliche getesteten Imidazolinabkömmlinge ohne Cl-Atom an der Methylgruppe bewirkten keine Reaktionen. So waren z. B. die Teste auf Imidazolinderivate, bei denen das Cl-Atom durch eine Diäthylamino- bzw. Hydroxylgruppe ersetzt war, negativ. Aus diesen Befunden ist zu schließen, daß die Reaktionsfähigkeit des Chlormethylimidazolins an die Chlormethylgruppe gebunden ist. Durch das labile, leicht abspaltbare Cl-Atom wird das C-Atom der Methylgruppe aktiviert und zur Bindung an Aminogruppen von Proteinen befähigt, wodurch eine Komplettierung zum Vollantigen erfolgt.

Zusammenfassend möchten wir feststellen, daß Chlormethylimidazolinhydrochlorid auf Grund seiner hervorragenden Wasserlöslichkeit und seiner dem DNCB überlegenen Sensibilisierungsfähigkeit ein für experimentelle Untersuchungen der Spätreaktionsallergie geeignetes Allergen darstellt.

Problèmes physiochimiques concernant la formation de l'antigène sensibilisant de contact

E. Panconesi, Clinique Dermatologique de l'Université Florence (Italie)

Nous nous intéressons depuis quelque temps aux problèmes de la pathogénie de l'eczéma de contact du point de vue de la chimie physique [1, 2], en nous référant à une vision générale de ces problèmes de ce même point de vue et aux méthodes utilisables pour leur solution. Nous n'aborderons dans cette communication que deux nouveaux groupes de recherches concernant la formation de l'antigène de contact, en omettant de rappeler nos expériences précédentes et le plan général de nos études. Ces dernières recherches ont été faites en collaboration avec A. Sertoli et G. Sgaragli de la Clinique Dermatologique et G. Gabrielli, A. Ficalbi de l'Institut de Chimie Physique de l'Université de Florence.

1. La manifestation cutanée la plus significative pour un jugement sur l'affinité d'un haptène vis-à-vis des protéines cutanées d'un sujet sensibilisé à ce même haptène semble être l'apparition d'un érythème, premier stade de la réaction allergique complète (érythème, oedème et vésiculation). A ce sujet, dans le cadre d'une étude cinétique de la réaction allergique de contact, on a pris en considération, pour une évaluation adéquate du temps d'apparition de ce premier stade, 50 sujets sensibilisés: au Cr, à la térébenthine, au Ni et au Co. L'observation effectuée toutes les 6 h a permis de relever au préalable une distribution casuistique dans le temps qui nous a permis de mettre en évidence avec une crédibilité suffisante la valeur du temps moyen d'apparition de l'érythème. Cette

valeur doit être entendue comme *le temps le plus probable* (Tp) correspondant c'est à dire à celui pendant lequel le plus grand nombre de cas réagit par érythème. On peut synthétiser les résultats de la façon suivante: le Ni^{++} et le Co^{+++} se comportent de manière analogue de ce point de vue c'est à dire que la valeur du Tp s'avère de 24 h pour tous deux; alors que l'on a pareillement pour les haptènes Cr et térébenthine un comportement analogue avec un Tp de 6 h pour tous deux. Il est significatif de relever que ce dernier couple d'haptènes a un Tp de $^1/_4$ de la valeur du premier couple. On sait que le bichromate de K (Cr^{+6}) subit une réduction à Cr^{+3}, qui devient le véritable haptène, sous l'action de substances diverses, même intrinsèques de la peau [3]. De même il semble qu'on puisse admettre que l'activité sensibilisante de la térébenthine est attribuable à

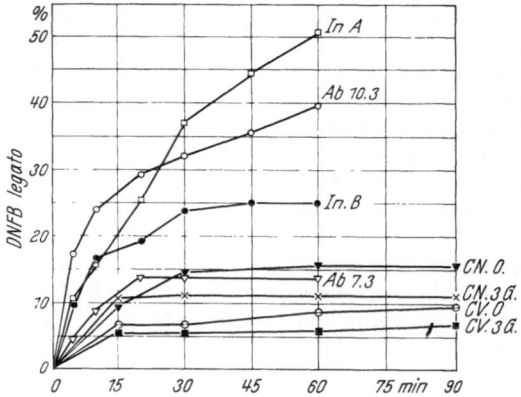

Fig. Quantité de DNFB (valeur en pour cent par rapport à la quantité devant réagir) qui se sont unies respectivement à: *En A* insuline de Eli Lilly Italia S.p.a. (master lot 47), pH du produit de réaction 10,3. *En B* insuline de Eli Lilly Italia S.p.a. (master lot 52), pH du produit de réaction 10,3. *Ab 10,3* albumine de sérum de boeuf cristallisée Calbiochem, pH du produit de réaction 10,3. *Ab 7,3* albumine de sérum de boeuf cristallisée Calbiochem. pH du produit de réaction 7,3. *CN 0* protéines hydrosolubles de peau de lapin, pH du produit de réaction 7,6. *CN 3* idem 3 jours après la préparation. *CV 0* protéines hydrosolubles de peau de cobaye, pH du produit de réaction 7,6. *CV 3* idem 3 jours après la préparation

quelques composants qui sont sujets à des processus d'oxydo-réduction qui engendrent vraisemblablement le véritable haptène final qui s'unit aux protéines. Dans ce tableau hypothétique, on visualise une justification pour nos résultats. Les substances dont nous supposons qu'elles donnent lieu à des haptènes à la suite d'un processus d'oxydo-réduction seraient individualisables par une valeur de Tp qui s'avère être $^1/_4$ de la valeur de Tp des haptènes non sujets, d'après nos connaissances, à des processus d'oxydo-réduction. D'un point de vue de la chimie-physique, la justification de ceci doit être recherchée dans la plus grande stabilité du complexe haptène-protéine pour le second couple (Cr et térébenthine) par rapport au premier (Ni et Co). A la plus grande stabilité correspond en effet une plus grande rapidité de réaction globale. D'un point de vue simplement énergétique la plus grande stabilité semblerait confirmée d'une manière suggestive même par les valeurs de diminution d'énergie libre (ΔG) se rapportant aux processus d'oxydo-réduction pour le Cr et la térébenthine et à ceux qui se rapportent à la formation d'associés pour le Co et le Ni. En effet on a calculé (G. GABRIELLI), en première approximation, pour le Cr une valeur de ΔG de 89.950 cal., pour la térébenthine de 62.794 tandis que pour le Co ($\Delta G = 22.452$) et pour le Ni ($\Delta G = 15.930$) on a des valeurs nettement inférieures. On doit souligner en outre que même les Tp concernant les autres stades de la manifestation allergique (œdème et vésiculation) se sont avérés à peu près dans le même rapport pour les deux couples.

2. La réaction allergique cutanée au DNFB présuppose une véritable réaction chimique entre ce composé et les protéines cutanées, avec formation d'un DNB-dérivé. Il nous a semblé d'un grand intérêt d'étudier la réactivité du DNFB avec les protéines cutanées hydrosolubles de cobaye et de lapin. Nous avons d'abord étudié par la méthode spectrophotométrique la réactivité du DNFB avec deux protéines hydrosolubles purifiées du commerce (albumine de sérum de bœuf et insuline), et ensuite avec les protéines de la fraction soluble d'un homogéné de peau de cobaye et de lapin.

Les résultats obtenus jusqu'à présent (voir figure) sont les suivants: A. Albumine: la réactivité varie en fonction du pH; B. insuline: la réactivité varie selon l'échantillon utilisé; C. protéines hydrosolubles de peau de cobaye et de peau de lapin: il n'y a pas de différences appréciables de réactivité entre les deux groupes de protéines, il y a peut-être une plus grande réactivité des protéines extraites de la peau de lapin; avec le vieillissement de la solution protéique la réactivité diminue.

Bibliographie. 1. SCOLARI, E. G., E. PANCONESI e A. SERTOLI: Comunic. V Congr. Internaz. Allergologia, Madrid ottobre 1964. — 2. PANCONESI, E.: XLVII. Congr. Naz. della S.I.D.E.S. (Siena, 29—31 ottobre 1965). Minerva derm. (Torino) **40**, 6 (1965). — 3. SGARAGLI, G., e. E. PANCONESI: Minerva derm. (Torino) **40**, 359 (1965).

The Aetiology of Eczema

J. G. COBURN and J. REID, Manchester and Salford Hospital for Skin Diseases, Manchester (England)

Introduction. The clinical manifestations of eczema occur in the skin, but this paper suggests a hypothesis indicating that the disease has its primary origin in the central nervous system. Both skin and nervous tissue arise from the ectoderm and thus have natural affinities in their development. Apart from specialised nerve endings the epidermis is well supplied with non-medullated fibres which ramify freely around the cells of the basal layer and at higher levels among the Malphigian and granular layers. The sensation of itching is conveyed to the thalamic nuclei and cortex by pain fibres, the particular quality of the sensation being determined by its intensity and duration. In addition to itching sensations passing to the cortex, there exists a spinal cord reflex which causes surrounding skin to become hypersensitive. When the free fibres in the epidermis are stimulated, acetylcholine is produced with consequent rise in the total acetylcholine in the epidermis. This increase has been shown to take place by biological assay on many occasions and acetylcholine has been assumed to be there for the purpose of conveying the sensory impulse and also to transmit antidromic impulses concerned with axon reflexes in response to physical and mechanical stimuli. In our view it is there for an entirely different reason.

Mechanism of the production of eczema. We agree that acetylcholine is the chemical primarily concerned in eczema, and in doing so would emphasise that it is also primarily concerned in the activities of the autonomic nervous system. Acting on the epidermal cells (possibly with noradrenaline as an intermediary) it produces spongiosis and local vascular dilatation. Enzyme interaction with specific cholinesterase results in vesicle formation. The action of Cortisone is to abolish the enzyme activity and suppress the eczema. The atropine-like drugs would have to be given in huge doses to produce the same effect. Acetylcholine is usually assumed to be mainly concerned with the activation of the sweat apparatus; the existence of this apparatus is fundamental to our hypothesis, as we suggest that many of the non-medullated fibres in the epidermis are supplied with motor nerves in preparation for the innervation of sweat glands which never develop. The eccrine sweat gland is a late development in evolution, coming from the follicle in the first place as an apocrine gland and later achieving a more refined function. If the nerve supply to a sweat gland is stimulated acetylcholine produces sweat secretion. If the same nerve is stimulated in the absence of a gland, acetyl-choline is liberated into the epidermis with the production of eczema.

Such stimulation may be produced through the autonomic nervous system by:

1. Emotional stress from the cortex and hypothalamus via the white rami.
2. Trauma — locally by spinal reflex.
3. By contact antigen-antibody dermatitis — the so-called eczematoid dermatitis.
4. By inflammation of bacterial origin.

Combinations of these factors increase the likelihood of eczema and there is a familial tendency to this type of activity.

Cutan-vasculäre Kontaktallergie
Untersuchungen zur Frage einer Antigen-Antikörperreaktion bei physikalischer Allergie*

L. ILLIG, Universitäts-Hautklinik Freiburg im Breisgau (Deutschland)

Wenn von „Kontaktallergie" der Haut die Rede ist, denken wir unwillkürlich an eine *epidermale* Sensibilisierung bzw. an eine Kontaktdermatitis. Tatsächlich ist eine Sensibilisierung in Form einer chemischen Kontakt-*Urticaria* — z. B. auf Citrusfrüchte — extrem selten. Nicht so selten sehen wir dagegen eine *physikalische* Kontakt-*Urticaria*; nur hat man bis in letzter Zeit immer wieder gezweifelt, ob in diesem Fall tatsächlich eine Antigen-Antikörperreaktion zugrunde liegt. Zwar ist schon lange bekannt, daß die sog. physikalische Allergie gegen Kälte, Wärme und Licht mit dem Patientenserum im Prausnitz-Küstner-Versuch passiv übertragen werden kann. Nur hat man in diesen Fällen immer wieder eingewandt, es müsse sich bei dem übertragbaren Serumfaktor nicht unbedingt um einen Antikörper handeln, sondern es könne auch ein unspezifischer Entzündungsmediator sein (CALNAN, 1964). Andererseits kann nicht bestritten werden, daß der Prausnitz-Küstner-Versuch keineswegs in jedem Fall physikalischer Urticaria gelingt.

Zur Abklärung dieser Frage haben wir uns bei zwei Fällen von Lichturticaria und bei einem Fall cholinergischer Urticaria eingehender mit der Prausnitz-Küstner-Reaktion beschäftigt. Dabei konnten wir einen echten Antikörper als übertragbaren Serumfaktor sehr wahrscheinlich machen. Würde die passive Über-tragbarkeit einer physikalischen Urticaria auf einem Entzündungsmediator im Serum beruhen, so dürfte dieser eigentlich nur direkt nach experimenteller Aus-lösung *vorübergehend* im Blut erscheinen. Zumindestens müßte er im Urticaria-anfall viel stärker angereichert sein als im Intervall. Dies ist aber nach unseren Beobachtungen nicht der Fall. Wir konnten keine gesetzmäßige Abhängigkeit der

---

* Mit Unterstützung der Deutschen Forschungsgemeinschaft.

Serumaktivität im Prausnitz-Küstner-Test von der physikalischen Exposition feststellen; sie war stets auch im erscheinungsfreien Intervall nachweisbar. Bei der Lichturticaria erwies sich der fragliche Serumfaktor als thermolabil und nicht-dialysierbar. Wochenlanges Einfrieren des Serums in der Tiefkühltruhe verminderte seine Wirksamkeit nicht; in die Haut injiziert blieb er bei der Lichturticaria bis 48 Tage lang aktiv, was mit der Annahme eines Mediators schwer vereinbar ist, für das Verhalten eines Antikörpers dagegen als typisch angesehen werden muß. In gleicher Richtung liegt die Beobachtung, daß die Prausnitz-Küstner-Reaktionen bei einer cholinergischen Urticaria innerhalb von 12 Tagen oftmals erneut wieder aufflammten. Das Patientenserum blieb also in der präparierten Haut erstaunlich lange wirksam. Außerdem boten die Reaktionen bei mehreren Versuchspersonen das für die cholinergische Urticaria typische morphologische Bild von gruppierten Quaddeln follikulären Typs. Schließlich konnte die Prausnitz-Küstner-Reaktion in diesem Fall durch Cholinomimetica anstelle der sonst üblichen Wärmeexposition ausgelöst und durch Atropin gehemmt werden, was im Falle eines Entzündungsmediators unverständlich wäre.

Wir kommen daher zu dem Schluß, daß die physikalische Urticaria zumindestens in denjenigen Fällen auf einer Antigen-Antikörperreaktion beruht, bei welchen der Prausnitz-Küstner-Versuch eindeutig positiv ausfällt; sehr wahrscheinlich gilt dies aber auch für gleichartige Fälle mit negativer Reaktion. Nur bei der mechanogenen Urticaria (auf Dermographie und Druck) ist eine passive Übertragung bisher nicht in allgemein anerkannter Form gelungen.

Man kann also der *epidermalen* Kontaktallergie das gar nicht so seltene, eigenartige Krankheitsbild der Kälte-Wärme- und Lichturticaria als Beispiel einer „*cutan-vasculären* Kontaktallergie" zur Seite stellen. Nur stellt der Kontaktreiz — die physikalische Einwirkung — in diesem Fall nicht das Allergen selbst dar, sondern nur einen Trigger bzw. Provokator. Das Allergen muß in einer körpereigenen, physiologischen, reizspezifischen Substanz gesucht werden, die in *jeder* Haut nach entsprechenden physikalischen Einwirkungen gebildet wird. Im Gegensatz zur Kontaktdermatitis handelt es sich bei der physikalischen Urticaria natürlich um eine Allergie vom Soforttyp. Histologische Untersuchungen haben uns gezeigt, daß der Schwerpunkt der Reaktion nicht — wie man erwarten könnte — im Papillarkörper an den *Capillaren* gelegen ist, sondern im Bereich des subpapillären Gefäßplexus bzw. sogar im *mittleren* Corium. Das perivasculäre Zellinfiltrat besteht vornehmlich aus Granulocyten und reichlich Eosinophilen. Es stellt offenbar — im Gegensatz zum Rundzellinfiltrat der Kontaktdermatitis — nur einen *sekundären*, reaktiven Vorgang dar. Seine Unterdrückung mit Cortison beeinträchtigt das urticarielle Exanthem bemerkenswerterweise *nicht*.

Literatur. ILLIG, L.: Arch. klin. exp. Derm. **217**, 82 (1963). — ILLIG, L., u. W. BORN: Arch. klin. exp. Derm. **220**, 19 (1964). — ILLIG, L., u. A. HEINICKE: Arch. klin. exp. Derm. **229**, 360 (1967). — ILLIG, L., u. A. HEINICKE: Arch. klin. exp. Derm. 1967 V. Mitt. (Im Druck).

Sur la sensibilisation expérimentale au chrome

V. N. NEGULESCU, Centre Dermatovénéréologique Bucarest (Roumanie)

Jusqu'à présent, quoique l'existence de l'allergie au chrome soit reconnue à l'unanimité, les opinions sur l'antigénicité de ses sels sont encore divisées. En vérité, si la majorité des auteurs admettent cette qualité seulement pour les sels hexavalents, d'autres comme MORRIS, BOCKENDAHL, DA FONSECA, COHEN, MALI,

17*

VAN NEER, VAN KOOTEN, FREGERT, RORSMAN etc. sont les partisans de l'anti-génicité des sels trivalents.

La même controverse s'est fait remarquée aussi parmi les résultats des sensi-bilisations expérimentales publiées par NIELZEN, HUNZIKER et SCHINAS, WIKSTRÖM, COHEN, SAMITZ, FREGERT et RORSMAN, PENDERS, WAHLBERG et SKOG etc., tandis que beaucoup d'autres comme CHARPY, CIVATTE, SULZBERGER, EPSTEIN, MIE-SCHER, TZANCK, HUNZIKER, SCHINAS, JADASSOHN, KLASCHKA, GROTH, DE GRACI-ANSKI et collab. etc. discutent sur la valeur des études histologiques des lésions provoquées aux animaux d'expérience.

Matériel et méthode. Dans nos recherches appliquées sur les cobayes, nous avons utilisé en guise d'allergène le bichromate de potassium en solution hyperalcaline (pour des applications percutanées) ou incorporé dans les adjuvants de FREUND (pour des inoculations intracutanées ou intramusculaires).

Par les mêmes voies d'autres cobayes ont reçu des solutions similaires d'alun de chrome (sel trivalent).

La sensibilisation des animaux a été estimée par l'aspect des lésions et aussi par le résultat des tests épicutanés et intradermiques, vérifiés à leur tour par des biopsies.

Conclusions. Nos recherches nous ont fourni les constatations suivantes:

1. Les sensibilisations au chrome ont réussi seulement avec les composés hexa-valents mais d'une manière moins régulière que celles obtenues avec le DNCB. Les résultats favorables avec le chrome trivalent, publiés par certains auteurs sur les cobayes ou les lapins, sont probablement dus à l'utilisation dans leurs expériences, de certains échantillons contenant, en plus, des traces de chrome hexa-valent. Tout comme ZINA et BONU, nous avons décelé nous mêmes dans quelques solutions de sulphate basique de chrome (trivalent) provenant de diverses tan-neries, l'existence de petites quantités de chrome hexavalent. Cette impureté nous a expliqué l'apparition des tests positifs au sulphate basique de chrome dans quelques cas hypersensibilisés au bichromate.

2. La voie intracutanée s'est avérée plus sûre que la voie percutanée, à condi-tion que le bichromate soit incorporé dans les adjuvants de FREUND; en échange l'inoculation intramusculaire s'est montrée inefficace.

3. La sensibilisation expérimentale au bichromate semble être favorisée par l'hyperalcalinisation de la solution antigénique — effet similaire avec celui produit par le ciment hyperalcalin dans l'apparition des eczémas des maçons.

4. Pour confirmer les états allergiques provoqués, il faut appliquer la méthode des tests cutanés. Mais les résultats des ceux-ci doivent être à leur tour vérifiés au microscope, étant donné leur aspect macroscopique, souvent douteux. Les tests épicutanés se sont avérés plus fidèles que les intradermoréactions.

5. Sur les sections seriées — aussi dans les cas de dermites que dans les tests positifs — nous avons observé une structure histologique de type eczémateux, caractérisé par: hyperacanthose, spongiose insulaire avec exosérose et exocitose, jusqu'à former même des microvésicules surbasales dans l'intérieur desquelles nageaient quelques lymphocytes et polynucléaires; dans le derme superficiel on distinguait un œdème avec infiltrat mononucléaire (surtout lymphocytaire), massé le plus souvent autour des follicules pilleux, dont les cellules présentaient sur cer-taines sections une tendance à la spongiose jusqu'à former même de petites vésicules.

Les tests épicutanés positifs au bichromat, caractérisés cliniquement par éry-thème et papulo-vésicules, présentaient les mêmes modifications histologiques mais d'une moindre intensité.

Les ganglions satellites appartenant aux zones inoculées étaient volumineux, avec une remarquable réaction lymphoréticulaire qui suggérait le rôle important joué par le système lymphatique dans la sensibilisation.

Recherches sur la pathogénie de l'eczéma dû aux sels de chrome

A. Sertoli et E. Panconesi, Clinique Dermatologique de l'Université Florence (Italie)

Les problèmes théoriques concernant l'étiopathogénie de l'eczéma allergique de contact au ciment (chrome) ont été exposés dans le récent rapport de Scolari et collab. [1]. On a consacré à ces problèmes, déjà au centre de nos précédentes recherches [2 à 5], deux groupes d'expériences dont nous rapportons les résultats.

1. Nous avons cherché, en collaboration avec le Dr. Giannetti, chimiste, à vérifier l'union du chrome aux amino-acides, aux polypeptides et aux protéines «in vivo» et «in vitro» et de contrôler la présence de ce métal dans la peau et dans le sang de sujets allergiques au chrome.

On a incubé durant 48 h à 37° des solutions de 18 levo-amino-acides avec du potassium bichromate (Cr^{+6}) et avec le radioisotope Cr 51 (mélange de Cr^{+6} et de Cr^{+3}). On a effectué la chromatographie sur couche mince monodimensionelle de chacune des solutions contenant l'amino-acide et le chrome. Sur les taches du chromatogramme se rapportant au seul amino-acide, au Cr^{+6} et au Cr^{+3} on a effectué une détermination qualitative et quantitative du chrome par la méthode spectrophotométrique et autoradiographique. Cette vérification est possible parce qu'à la phase utilisée, le Cr^{+3} se sépare nettement du Cr^{+6}. On a constaté: 1. la réduction du Cr^{+6} au Cr^{+3}; 2. l'absence de chrome dans les taches correspondant à chaque amino-acide; 3. l'apparition dans les solutions de tyrosine traitées au chrome de deux fractions dépourvues de chrome mais que l'on peut distinguer au moyen de la chromatographie tandis qu'avec la solution d'amino-acide pure on a une fraction unique. On conclu que dans les limites des conditions que nous avons réalisées dans notre expérience, la réduction du chrome ne se concilie pas avec l'union aux amino-acides. D'autres expériences ont été faites «in vivo» consistant à traiter le cobaye au chrome 51 par voie épidermique et intradermique. La peau a été enlevée au bout de 24 h. On a séparé par homogénéisation et par centrifuga-tion les protéines solubles dont on a obtenu des amino-acides et des polypeptides par hydrolyse acide à courant d'azote et par hydrolyse triptyque. On a effectué une chromatographie mono- et bidimensionnelle sur couche mince avec l'homo-génisé superflottant (protéines solubles plus chrome 51) et avec les hydrolysés (amino-acides et polypeptides plus chrome 51). L'évaluation qualitative et quanti-tative du chrome 51 a été faite par la méthode radiométrique et autoradio-graphique. On a constaté encore: 1. la réduction du Cr^{+6} au Cr^{+3}; 2. l'absence de chrome dans les taches correspondant au matériel organique. Une partie des pro-téines solubles, hydrolysées et non hydrolisées, a été soumise à la dialyse. On a constaté la progressive évidente diminution de la radioactivité du matériel or-ganique au profit du dialysé. On peut conclure que dans nos conditions expéri-mentales, nous n'avons pu démontrer l'union du chrome aux protéines solubles, aux amino-acides et aux polypeptides qui en dérivent par hydrolyse. Nous avions déjà pratiqué le dosage polarographique du chrome [4] sur des fragments de peau atteinte d'eczéma, provenant de cinq sujets. Les résultats avaient semblé indicatifs de la présence du chrome en quantité supérieure à celle que nous avions relevée chez les sujets de contrôle. Le dosage spectrophotométrique du chrome hématique chez 25 sujets pris par l'eczéma dû au chrome n'a pas donné par contre de valeurs différentes de celles que nous avons relevées chez dix sujets normaux.

2. Le second groupe d'expériences a été fait pour établir si quelques substances peuvent diminuer ou bloquer la réaction du chrome contenu dans le ciment avec la peau. Nous avons démontré que la réactivité vis-à-vis: a) des solutions de

potassium bichromate, b) des suspensions de ciment dans de l'eau bidistillée, c) des suspensions de ciment dans des solutions de sulfate de soude (activation du chrome selon BRUN) est diminuée ou bloquée quand le matériel est traité avant l'exécution des tests, au baryum hydroxyde ou en plomb acétate qui précipitent le chrome sous forme de sels insolubles (chromate de baryum). En outre, on a démontré que sodium hyposulfite et sodium ascorbate réduisent le chrome hexavalent du ciment, précédemment activé par du sulfate de sodium, à la forme trivalente (qui est moins active et qui peut être facilement bloquée par différents chélateurs).

Bibliographie. 1. SCOLARI, E. G.: LXVII Congresso Nazionale SIDES (Siena, ott. 1965). Minerva derm. (Torino) 40, 1 (1965). — 2. SERTOLI, A., e E. PANCONESI: Rass. Derm. Sif. 19, 333 (1966). — 3. SGARAGLI, G., e E. PANCONESI: Minerva derm. (Torino) 40, 395 (1965). — 4. MACCHI, G., A. SERTOLI, C. VALLECCHI e E. PANCONESI: Minerva derm. (Torino) 40, 369 (1965). — 5. GIANNOTTI, B., e. A. SERTOLI: Rass. Derm. Sif. 17, 323 (1964).

Efectos de una substancia antiplasmínica sintética en el eczema

J. M. GIMENEZ CAMARASA, Dermatólogo del Estado Barcelona (España)

Introduccion

Actualmente se admite como lo más verosímil que los fenómenos alérgicos son debidos a un cambio coloidal, causado por una reacción antígeno-anticuerpo. Ello motivaría cambios enzimáticos que liberando determinadas substancias, condicionarían toda la fenomenología subsiguiente.

Una de las enzimas activadas por la reacción antígeno-anticuerpo es la plasmina o fibrinolisina, la cual ataca a diversas proteinas plasmáticas y celulares [1]. De esta agresión se liberan las substancias inductoras de la reacción alérgica. Según UNGAR [5], la actividad de esta enzima está en equilibrio con la de otra, presente en la fracción albúmina, denominada antiplasmina. OKAMOTO [2] la halló también en la fracción euglobulina. Estudios sobre la posibilidad de inhibición de la actividad de aquel fermento llevaron al empleo en clínica del ácido épsilon-aminocaproico, primer compuesto sintético utilizado con este objeto.

Aunque este fenómeno de la fibrinolisis se conoce desde antiguo [3, 4], el concepto de que el sistema enzimático fibrinolítico participe en ciertas formas de la reacción alérgica es de reciente adquisición [5, 6]. OKAMOTO [7] demostró cómo aquella substancia de síntesis era capaz de inhibir los fenómenos anafilácticos a la vez que corregir la fibrinolisis. Por tanto, parecía lógico admitir que la reacción antígeno-anticuerpo corria paralela a una exacerbación del sistema enzimático fibrinolítico.

KITAMURA [8], SUZUKI [9], AOKI [10], HAKUGAWA [11] y otros autores, han demostrado que el sistema enzimático de la fibrinolisis se halla activado en el eczema agudo, eczema crónico, eczema por contacto, eritema polimorfo, eritema nudoso, urticaria, en las toxicodermias, quemaduras, enfermedad de Gibert, acné y en la forunculosis. CORMIA y cols. [12], y DOUGHERTY y cols. [13] lo han observado en el prurito *sine materia* y en el pénfigo vulgar. NILSSON y cols. [14] han constatado el mismo fenómeno en el sarcoide de Boeck.

El ácido épsilon-aminocaproico es una substancia sintética prácticamente atóxica que tiene, tanto *in vitro* como *in vivo*, un gran poder de inhibición de la activación del plasminógeno, así como de la acción de la plasmina. Su gran poder antiexudativo ha permitido a varios autores usarlo con éxito en la terapia del eczema [8 a 18], [1, 23]. BERTELLI y cols. [19], WORINGER [21], LAUGIER [22] y otros investigadores, lo emplean con éxito en la urticaria *a frigore*. Por último, SOTTY y GILLOT [20] constatan su eficacia en las respuestas de intolerancia o alergia frente a alimentos y medicamentos.

Estas y otras publicaciones nos han llevado a verificar los posibles efectos de esta nueva substancia sintética en un grupo de enfermos con eczema.

Este trabajo constituye el primer estudio realizado en nuestro país y por nosotros conocido, sobre la acción medicamentosa del ácido épsilon-aminocaproico en dermatología.

Material y metodos

El estudio se ha realizado en 40 enfermos sin seleccionar. Entre ellos, se encontraban casos con eczema por contacto, eczema seborreico, eczema atópico, dermatitis por álcalis, dishidrosis y urticaria. Las dermatitis por contacto se dividieron provisionalmente en agudas y crónicas, para distinguir las más exudativas con menos de quince días de evolución, de las más secas y con más tiempo evolutivo. En la tabla siguiente se resumen todos los casos tratados.

A cada sujeto se le administraron de 3 a 4 ampollas ingeribles de 10 ml al día, conteniendo ácido épsilon-aminocaproico en solución acuosa al 40%. Dicha posología se mantuvo en cada paciente durante 1 semana. Ningún enfermo fué controlado después de los 8 días. Ninguno de los pacientes recibió otro tipo de medicación general o tópica.

El efecto de la medicación fué valorado en

afección	casos
eczema agudo por contacto	20
eczema crónico por contacto	10
eczema atópico	3
eczema seborreico diseminado	2
eczema por álcalis	2
urticaria	2
dishidrosis	1
Total	40

varios aspectos: 1°) rapidez de aparición y características del supuesto efecto beneficioso; 2°) estado general de la dermatitis a la semana de la medicación, y 3°) intolerancias.

Resultados

En quince enfermos con eczema agudo por contacto, muy exudativo y vesiculoso, se obtuvieron resultados que pueden considerarse como excelentes. La mejoría se refiere sobre todo al prurito, que llega a desaparecer al tercero o cuarto día de la medicación. Igualmente, en este espacio de tiempo la vesiculación, la exudación y el edema se reducen de modo rápido secándose las lesiones. Ambos efectos aparecen al segundo o tercer día de iniciado el tratamiento, y se prolongan mientras dura el mismo. No obstante, la extensión de las lesiones al octavo día permaneció poco modificada, si bien seca, descamativa, mucho menos eritematosa y sin o escasísimo prurito. En los cinco enfermos restantes se obtuvieron los mismos efectos beneficiosos pero en menor cuantía, de manera que el prurito y la exudación, habiendo remitido considerablemente, persistían con mayor o menor intensidad, según los casos. Ambos efectos pueden considerarse como muy aceptables, dada la ausencia de medicación tópica no empleada en ningún caso, y que supone una eficaz ayuda en esta clase de enfermos.

En ocho casos de eczema crónico se obtuvieron excelentes resultados en la sedación del prurito y en la regresión del eczema. La aparición del efecto fue más tardía (4° a 5° días). En dos enfermos no se obtuvo mejoría alguna.

No se consiguió ningún éxito en tres pacientes afectados de neurodermatitis difusa (atopía tardía), localizada en la cara y en la superficie de flexión de codos, brazos y rodillas. Ni el prurito intenso, ni la mayor o menor liquenificación de las lesiones se beneficiaron durante la semana que duró el tratamiento.

Ningún éxito se obtuvo bajo ningún aspecto, en dos casos tratados de urticaria crónica o de urticaria enfermedad.

El efecto sedativo del prurito fué asimismo rápido y evidente en dos enfermos con dermatitis seborreica diseminada. También este efecto fué brillante en dos enfermas con dermatitis causada por álcalis, y en un caso de eczema dishidrósico, en el cual el efecto sedante y antiexudativo de la medicación fue de rápida y drástica aparición entre el segundo y tercer día de tratamiento.

En dos casos, los enfermo notaron en el primer día del tratamiento náuseas con o sin vómitos, que cedieron al proseguir la medicación al día siguiente. En otro caso el paciente acusó cierto desasosiego e intranquilidad nerviosa. Otro enfermo se quejó de escalofríos. Por último, un sujeto refería que se le presentó somnolencia desacostumbrada al beber vino, mientras duró la medicación. Estas intolerancias, que siempre aparecieron en las primeras dosis, cedieron posteriormente y no motivaron en ningún caso el cese de la medicación. En los treinta y cinco casos restantes (87,5%) la tolerancia fue total. En las dos tablas siguientes se resumen todos los casos tratados y la mejoría sintomática obtenida.

Tabla

afección	efecto medicamentoso			
	casos	muy bueno	bueno	nulo
eczema contacto agudo	20	15	5	0
eczema contacto crónico	10	8	2	0
eczema por álcalis	2	0	2	0
eczema seborreico	2	0	2	0
eczema atópico	3	0	0	3
dishidrosis	1	1	0	0
urticaria	2	0	0	2
Total	40	24	11	5

afección	mejoría sintomática			
	prurito	vesiculación	edema	extensión lesiones
eczema contacto agudo	20	20	20	12
eczema contacto crónico	8	8	0	0
eczema por álcalis	2	0	0	0
eczema seborreico	2	0	0	0
eczema atópico	0	0	0	0
dishidrosis	1	1	1	1
urticaria	0	0	0	0
Total	33	29	21	13

Resumen y conclusiones

Este es un estudio previo acerca de la capacidad curativa del ácido épsilon-aminocaproico en el eczema. Sus resultados permiten analizar con una mayor casuística, la acción de este fármaco en el mismo eczema, y en todas aquellas dermatitis de índole alérgica o no, y en las que pudiera estar incriminada una alteración de los mecanismos del sistema enzimático fibrinolítico. Dicho fármaco actúa de modo evidente como un eficaz resolutivo de los fenómenos de exudación y vesiculación, tan importantes en la clínica del eczema. Esta peculiaridad permite asegurar cierta preferencia por los estados agudos, en comparación con los eczemas más cronicos y más secos. Tal vez por la misma acción, o por otro mecanismo desconocido, dicho fármaco actúa como un buen sedante del prurito y del escozor que acompaña a estos fenómenos agudos.

Su eficacia está limitada en lo que se refiere a modificar, reducir o aclarar la extensión de las lesiones. Si bien en algún caso la curación ha sido total, no es lo frecuente. Es muy posible que su eficacia pueda ser multiplicada con la ayuda de una medicación local adecuada e incrementando el tiempo de tratamiento.

Si bien el número de enfermos examinados es muy pequeño y por lo tanto no puede generalizarse, llama la atención la ineficacia del fármaco frente a los casos de urticaria enfermedad y de dermatitis atópica.

En ningún caso se han observado intolerancias que motivaran el abandono del tratamiento.

Nombre genérico y registrado de la droga: ácido épsilon-aminocaproico (Caproamin Fides).

Bibliografía. 1. NAKANE, S.: Clin. Rep. Ipsilon **1**, 124 (1962). — 2. OKAMOTO, A.: Jap. J. clin. Med. **17**, 2182 (1959). — 3. DASTRE, A.: Arch. Physiol. Norm. Pathol. **6**, 464 (1894). — 4. NOLF, P.: Arch. intern. Physiol. **3**, 1 (1905). — 5. UNGAR, G., and H. HAYASHI: Ann. Allergy **16**, 542 (1958). — 6. ROCHA e SILVA, M., and R. M. TEIXEIRA: Proc. Soc. exp. Biol. Med. **61**, 376 (1946). — 7. OKAMOTO, A., and Y. TSUKADA: Keio J. Med. **28**, 295 (1951). — 8. KITAMURA, S.: Jap. J. Allergy **3**, 361 (1955). — 9. SUZUKI, S., T. KAWASHIMA, and E. MIKAMI: Jap. J. Dermat. **66**, 561 (1956). — 10. AOKI, Y.: Jap. J. Dermat. **68**, 100 (1958). — 11. HAKUGAWA, S.: Jap. J. Dermat. **69**, 1753 (1959). — 12. CORMIA, F. E., J. W. DOUGHERTY, and S. A. UNRAU: J. invest. Derm. **28**, 425 (1957); **30**, 21 (1958). — 13. DOUGHERTY, J. W., F. E. CORMIA, and S. A. UNRAU: Arch. Derm. **77**, 281 (1958). — 14. NILSSON, I. M., H. SKANSE, and K. GYDELL: Acta med. scand. **159**, 463 (1957). — 15. KITAMURA, S., T. YAMURA, and S. NISHIDA: Derm. Urol. **9**, 111 (1955). — 16. IZAKI, M., S. KUROSAWA, I. MAYAMA, S. KON, Y. UEHARA, and R. MURAKAMI: Clin. Rep. Ipsilon **1**, 107 (1962). — 17. HATANO, H., M. OGAWA, N. KONO, Y. YAMAMOTO, and T. HORIUCHI: Derm. Urol. **14**, 882 (1960). — 18. SAKUMA, G.: Derm. Urol. **23**, 51 (1961). — 19. BERTELLI, A., L. DONATI, S. FERRI e I. GALATULAS: Atti Accad. Med. lombarda **20**, 391 (1965). — 20. SOTTY, M., et C. GILLOT: Presse méd. **74**, 1943 (1966). — 21. WORINGER, F., J.-F. LEVY, H. BERGOEND et E. GROSHANS: Bull. Soc. franç. Derm. Syph. **71**, 224 (1964). — 22. LAUGIER, P.: Rev. Inform. Cps. Med. **3**, 70 (1965). — 23. YOKOYAMA, K., and H. HATANO: Keio J. Med. **8**, 303 (1959).

Test épicutané et test intradermique au bichromate de potassium Etude histopathologique comparative

B. GIANNOTTI et A. SERTOLI, Clinique Dermatologique de l'Université Florence (Italie)

Chez la Clinique Dermatologique de l'Université de Florence, nous nous dédions depuis quelques années à l'étude des aspects histopathologiques de l'eczéma professionnel de contact, des tests épicutanés, et de l'eczéma expérimental du cobaye [1, 2, 3, 4, 5].

Au cours de notre dernière recherche nous avons procédé à l'examen histologique de la peau soumise au test épicutané et au test intradermique au bichromate de potassium sur un groupe de maçons atteints d'eczéma professionnel allergique de contact. L'évolution de la réaction allergique a été suivie de la 1ère à la 24ème h. On a pratiqué sur le dos de chaque sujet deux tests épicutanés et deux tests intradermiques. Par la suite, à différents intervalles chez les divers individus, on a pratiqué la biopsie en même temps dans le siège du test épicutané et dans le siège du test intradermique. Les fragments ont été fixés en Carnoy et colorés à l'hématoxyline-éosinee. M. LO BRUTTO a collaboré à cette première partie de notre recherche.

De la comparaison entre les deux tableaux histopathologiques des tests épicutanés et intradermiques chez le même individu, il ressort qu'en général l'un et l'autre test provoquent dans la peau les mêmes modifications, et que celles-ci apparaissent et évoluent dans les deux sièges avec des différences chronologiques de faible importance. Les altérations deviennent évidentes à la 6ème - 7ème h : des zones de spongiose apparaissent dans l'épiderme, pendant que dans le derme se constitue un infiltrat périvasculaire de cellules mononuclées qui se répandent vers le haut, s'insinuant au-dessus de la jonction dermo-épidermique entre les cellules épidermiques. Au cours des heures suivantes, on voit une augmentation de la spongiose jusqu'à ce que vers la 15ème h apparaissent les premiers vésicules ; les cellules mononuclées de l'infiltrat dermique augmentent progressivement en nombre. Les altérations acquièrent souvent une évidence particulière dans la portion distale des glandes sudoripares eccrines ; on observe autour des follicules pileux et des glandes sébacées une accentuation de l'infiltration cellulaire. De la 15ème à la 24ème h les altérations acquièrent de plus en plus d'évidence. Dans cette uniformité fondamentale de nos observations, quelques différences ne font cependant pas défaut : en effet, dans le test intradermique l'infiltrat dermique est généralement plus considérable, et quelquefois les altérations épidermiques aussi sont plus prononcées, ou même plus précoces, par rapport au test épicutané.

L'infiltrat cellulaire dermique, disposé le plus souvent en manchons périvasculaires, est constitué presque exclusivement de cellules mononuclées. Celles-ci apparaissent pour la plupart de forme arrondie ou polyédrique, avec un noyau sombre ; le cytoplasme, limité à un mince halo ou même invisible dans les éléments de petites dimensions, est bien évident dans les cellules de dimensions supérieures.

Quelques fragments de peau soumise au test intradermique, prélevés à la 4ème, 8ème, 11ème, 13ème, 16ème h, ont été examinés au microscope électronique pour une observation plus approfondie des cellules de l'infiltrat. Dans les manchons périvasculaires, on reconnaît facilement les fibroblastes, les fibrocytes, les mastocytes, les macrophages, les péricytes. La grande majorité des cellules est cependant représentée par des lymphocytes typiques et par des cellules mononuclées que nous définirons, en raison de leurs caractéristiques morphologiques, « lymphocyte-like ».

Les lymphocytes sont reconnaissables à leurs petites dimensions, à leur noyau sombre avec chromatine disposée en blocs irréguliers et condensée à la périphérie, à leur cytoplasme très mince, riche en ribosomes mais pratiquement dépourvu d'organites exception faite de quelques mitochondries.

Les cellules que nous avons définies « lymphocyte-like » ont fréquemment des dimensions à peine supérieures à celles des éléments typiquement lymphocytaires, et se différencient de ceux-ci par quelques détails de structure. Le noyau présente souvent une irrégularité de son contour. Le cytoplasme est abondant, et on peut y reconnaître : un nombre remarquable de mitochondries, qui ont souvent des dimensions considérables, une forme grossièrement sphérique, une matrice claire et des crêtes disposées irrégulièrement ; des membranes de réticulum endoplasmique, auxquelles s'associent souvent des ribosomes ; enfin, chez un léger pourcentage de cellules seulement, quelques « microbodies » et lysosomes. Ces cellules semblent correspondre aux mononucléaires qui ont été décrits dans la sensibilisation retardée expérimentale à la tuberculine ou aux protéines, définis par quelques auteurs « moyens ou grands lymphocytes », par d'autres « jeunes macrophages ». L'observation des caractéristiques morphologiques ne nous fournit pas d'éléments sûrs ni pour évaluer le siège d'où dérivent les cellules du type lymphocytaire qui composent l'infiltrat dermique, ni pour évaluer le rôle qu'elles jouent dans la réaction allergique du type retardé.

Le microscope électronique nous a montré en outre un aspect morphologique tout à fait particulier des éléments lymphocytaires. Ces cellules présentent, surtout quand elles se trouvent isolées dans le derme papillaire, une nette irrégularité de leur contour nucléaire et un grand nombre d'expansions cytoplasmiques en forme de pseudopodes, qui semblent souligner leur mouvement de migration vers l'épiderme, attesté par la présence de cellules du type lymphocytaire dans l'épithélium.

Bibliographie. 1. GIANNOTTI, B.: XLVII Congresso Nazionale della S.I.D.E.S., Siena 29—31 ottobre 1965. Minerva derm. (Torino) **40**, 50 (1965). — 2. GIANNOTTI, B., C. VALLECCHI e E. PANCONESI: Minerva derm. (Torino) **40**, suppl. 8, 357 (1965). — 3. GIANNOTTI, B., e C. VALLECCHI: Folia allerg. (Roma) **13**, 1 (1966). — 4. GIANNOTTI, B., e A. SERTOLI: Rass. Derm. Sif. **19**, 81 (1966). — 5. GIANNOTTI, B., A. SERTOLI e M. LO BRUTTO: Rass. Derm. Sif. **19**, 297 (1966).

Aspectos clinicos y pruebas cutaneas de las dermatitis

S. ABELIUK, Servicio de Dermatología del Hospital del Salvador; Servicio Nacional de Salud, Santiago de Chile, y
E. SYLVESTER, Departamento de Alergia del Servicio de Dermatología y del Hospital del Salvador

Este trabajo se refiere al estudio de 102 enfermos realizado en el Departamento de Alergia del Servicio de Dermatología del Hospital del Salvador, en Santiago de Chile.

Los pacientes fueron sometidos a un examen dermatológico y clínico médico detallado. Se practicó una anamnesis completa en relación especialmente a antecedentes alérgicos personales y familiares, intolerancias medicamentosas, alimenticias y de contacto. Se exploró lo concerniente al ambiente profesional, ocupacional y habitacional.

A cada uno de los pacientes se le practicó una serie de 20 pruebas epicutáneos y 20 intradermoreacciones, iguales para todos. El objeto primordial es conocer el valor del procedimiento como método diferencial diagnóstico en la clasificación alergológica de las dermatitis.

En las pruebas epicutáneos se usaron las substancias corrientemente aplicadas en este caso y los extractos de la intradermo-reacción corresponden todos, excepto uno, a alimentos que se consideran comunmente alergizantes. Como elemento de control y excepción se incluyó el extracto de Litre (Litrea caústica o venenosa) muy conocida en nuestro país y causante de frecuentes dermatitis.

Nuestros enfermos fueron tomados sin selección y comprenden 71 casos de dermatitis o eczemas de los diferentes tipos, repartidos en 59 con dermatitis tópica o de contacto, 9 de dermatitis atópica y 3 de eczema seborreico.

Los otros 31 casos corresponden a otras dermatosis y sirvieron de control. Se observó una frecuencia en la mujer doble a la del hombre, de alergia cutánea tópica y atópica, explicable por diversas circunstancias, fuera de mayor susceptibilidad. La dermatitis tópica aparece con mayor frecuencia en la edad adulta.

La dermatitis atópica frecuente en la primera infancia tendería a desaparecer con la edad. En las dermatitis tópicas se clasifican 22 casos profesionales y 37 no profesionales. Los agentes causales más frecuentes en las profesionales fueron los productos químicos, luz solar, lana y cemento. En las no profesionales predominaron los detergentes caseros, cosméticos, lanas, luz solar y el nylon.

La localización más frecuente tanto de las dermatitis tópicas profesionales como de las no profesionales fueron las extremidades y la cara. Hay relación clara entre localización y agente irritante en las dermatitis no profesionales; en las profesionales esta relación no es tan aparente.

Los antecedentes personales y familiares predominan en general en las dermatitis atópicas y caracteriza especialmente este tipo de dermatitis. La intolerancia
a las drogas es más o menos el doble en la atopia que en la tópica y no alérgicas
de control. Existe predominio de pruebas epicutáns positivas en las dermatitis
tópicas y predominio de intradermoreacciones positivas en las dermatitis atópicas.
Resultó que en 59 casos de dermatitis tópicas detectados:

> 43% fueron con predominio positivo al parche prueba
> 32% fueron con predominio positivo a intradermoreacciones
> 25% Sin predominio
>
> En los casos de atopia:
>
> 22% fueron con predominio positivo al parche prueba
> 50% fueron con predominio positivo a intradermoreacciones
> 22% Sin predominio

Como agentes que arrojan mayor positividad en los parches pruebas resaltan:

Pomada salicílica benzoica	18%
Formalina	16%
Jabón neutro	14%
Intradermoreacciones:	
Litre	43%
Cacao	14%
Pescado y mariscos	8%

(Los demás agentes que dieron reacciones positivas con menos frecuencia, completan el saldo
al 100%)

Desgraciadamente no hay posibilidad de proyectar junto con este resúmen.
Los numerosos cuadros y tablas contenidos en el trabajo in extenso. Se hace
notar:

1. El valor diagnóstico y pronóstico que en el examen del paciente tienen, el
reconocimiento anamnésico y clínico, en alergia cutánea especialmente.

2. El valor diagnóstico diferencial entre atopia y topia por medio de las
pruebas cutáneas de parches e intradermoreacciones; al respecto no se debe
olvidar que con frecuencia hay una superposición de diferentes tipos de dermatitis,
especialmente en los casos crónicos.

The Frequency of Allergic Diseases Among Relatives of Patients with Allergic Eczematous Contact Dermatitis

M. FORSBECK, E. SKOG and K. YTTERBORN, Department of Dermatology,
Department of Occupational Dermatoses, Karolinska sjukhuset and Institute
of Genetics, University of Stockholm (Sweden)

This investigation has been made for the purpose of finding out whether
hereditary constitution is of any importance in the development of allergic
contact dermatitis, and if there is a connection between this delayed type allergy
and atopy [1].

Materials and Methods. 54 probands (42 men and 12 women) suffering from allergic
contact dermatitis, were selected at random from consecutive patients admitted to the skin
clinic at Karolinska Hospital, in Stockholm. The diagnosis was based upon the history of the
disease and the results of the patch test. The patient's relatives, including parents, wives or
husbands, siblings and children older than 10 years, were questioned about past or current
atopic diseases (atopic dermatitis, asthma and hay fever) and examined for the presence of
allergic eczematous contact dermatitis. Patch testing was performed with substances known

to be the most common contact allergens in Sweden [3, 4, 5]. They include metals, chemicals in rubber, locally used antibiotics, perfumes and plant leaves. The test substances were applied to the skin on the patient's back with circular occlusive patches. These were removed after 48 h and the readings were made 24 h later [6].

Table 1. *Probands*

Contact allergens	Male Age 26—70	Female Age 10—60
Chromium	27	1
Turpentine	5	
Formaldehyde	2	4
Cobalt	2	
Chemicals in rubber	3	2
Nickel	1	3
Primrose		1
Colour-developers	2	1
	42	12

Table 2. *Results of patch test in relatives of the probands*

Relatives tested	Pos. patch test and allergic dermatitis	Pos. patch test only	Neg. patch test
Number	%	%	%
281	13.5	8.5	78.0

Results and Conclusions. Tab. 1 shows the sex of the probands and the causing agents. Only what was thought to be the main allergen has been included. 23 probands reacted to more than one allergen. The dominating allergen in men was chromium and in women, formalin and nickel.

The results of the patch tests of 281 relatives of the probands are recorded in Tab. 2. 22% reacted positively to the patch tests. About two thirds of these positive reactors had a previous or current allergic contact dermatitis, while the rest had only positive tests indicating a latent sensitivity. These figures are much higher than found in the literature where the prevalence has been estimated from 1 to 3% in a normal population, but there are only few investigations reported [2].

Table 3. *Comparison of the frequencies of positive patch tests between males and females*

Relatives	Number	Pos. patch test %	Corrected chi square
Sons	39	8	
Daughters	32	31	5.04[a]
Fathers	22	9	
Mothers	22	36	3.24[b]

Comparison of the frequencies of positive patch tests between males and females

[a] $0.025 > p > 0.01$. — [b] $0.10 > p > 0.05$.

Table 4. *The occurrence of atopic diseases among the relatives and probands*

	Patch test	Number	Atopy %
Relatives	Pos.	62	19.4
	Neg.	219	16.4
Probands	Pos.	54	7.4
Total	Pos.	116	13.8

The incidence of positive reactions was higher amongst women than amongst men. Since there were more male than female probands there was expected to be a higher number of positive reactors among the female siblings, if one assumes the morbidity rate of both sexes to be the same.

As is shown in Tab. 3 however there was also a higher number of positive reactions among the mothers and the daughters than among the male relatives. The high incidence of positive reactors among the relatives of the probands in the present investigation may indicate that the genetic constitution is of importance for the manifestation of contact dermatitis.

The occurrence of atopy among the probands and patch tested relatives is shown in tab. 4. A noticibly high incidence of atopy was however found among the children of the probands, 27% had or had had atopic diseases. Because of this high frequency of atopic diseases among the children of the probands it seems possible that the allergic contact dermatitis and the atopy may have some hereditary link. We intend to further investigate more female probands and their relatives.

References. 1. FORSBECK, M., E. SKOG, and K. H. YTTERBORN: Acta derm.-venereol. (Stockh.) **46**, 149 (1966). — 2. HELLGREN, L.: An epidemiological survey of skin diseases, tattooing and rheumatic diseases. Uppsala: Almqvist and Wiksell 1967. — 3. MAGNUSSON, B., S.-G. BLOHM, S. FREGERT, N. HJORT, G. HOVDING, V. PIRILÄ, and E. SKOG: Acta derm.-venereol. (Stockh.) **46**, 153 (1966). — 4. MAGNUSSON, B., S.-G. BLOHM, S. FREGERT, N. HJORT, G. HOVDING, V. PIRILÄ, and E. SKOG: Acta derm.-venereol. (Stockh.) **46**, 396 (1966). — 5. MAGNUSSON, B., S.-G. BLOHM, S. FREGERT, N. HJORT, G. HOVDING, V. PIRILÄ, and E. SKOG: Acta derm.-venereol. (Stockh.) (In press). — 6. SKOG, E.: Arch. Derm. **92**, 276 (1960).

Zunahme von Metallallergien bei Hausfrauen

G. FORCK, Hautklinik der Westfälischen Wilhelms-Universität Münster (Deutschland)

Im Krankengut vieler Hautkliniken nimmt unter den Berufserkrankungen die Anzahl der Patienten mit Kontaktekzemen — insbesondere verursacht durch eine beruflich erworbene Allergie gegen Metalle und Metallsalze — eine Spitzenstellung ein.

Zu den häufigsten Kontaktallergenen gehören ohne Zweifel die *Chromate*, denen in der sechswertigen Form eine besonders hohe Allergiepotenz zukommt. In Deutschland stammt der überwiegende Teil aller Patienten mit beruflich erworbenen Chromatallergien aus der Bau- und Metallindustrie.

Die beruflich erworbenen *Nickel*allergien sind dagegen viel seltener und stammen meist aus Galvanisierabteilungen. *Kobalt*allergien sind gewerbedermatologisch bei der Metallgewinnung aus Erz sowie in der Glas- und Keramikindustrie von Bedeutung, während das beruflich bedingte Auftreten von Allergien gegen andere Metalle (Eisen, Kupfer, Edelmetalle, Beryllium usw.) sehr selten ist und eigentlich nur dann gelegentlich an Bedeutung gewinnt, wenn entsprechende Gewerbebetriebe benachbart sind.

Auf Grund der in Deutschland bestehenden Berufskrankheitenverordnung werden alle Patienten mit beruflich bedingten Metallallergien erfaßt, so daß über deren Häufigkeit verhältnismäßig genaue Vorstellungen bestehen. Nicht unter diese Gesetzgebung fallen die Hausfrauen, da die Tätigkeit einer Hausfrau nicht als Beruf anerkannt und daher auch versicherungsfrei ist. Um so mehr dürften Untersuchungen über die Art und die Häufigkeit von Metallallergien bei Hausfrauen von Interesse sein.

In Übereinstimmung mit anderen Untersuchern konnte in den letzten Jahren auch innerhalb des dermatologischen Krankengutes der Münsteraner Klinik eine Zunahme der Metallallergien festgestellt werden. Diese Beobachtung bezieht sich sowohl auf die männlichen wie auf die weiblichen Patienten. Bei einer ungefähr gleichbleibenden Patientenfrequenz von etwa 11 bis 12000 Patienten pro Jahr und einer konstanten Testkonzentration von 0,25%igem Kaliumbichromat (im Standardtest der Klinik enthalten) zeigt die Tab. 1 die Häufigkeit der Chromatallergien, aufgeschlüsselt in männliche und weibliche Patienten.

Tabelle 1. *Häufigkeit der Chromatallergien im Patientengut der Univ.-Hautklinik Münster*

Jahr	♂	♀	insgesamt
1960	101	15	116
1961	65	17	82
1962	80	24	104
1963	99	34	133
1964	96	42	138
1965	132	36	168
1966	140	57	197
total	713	225	938

Da in diesen Zahlen auch die Anzahl der Gutachtenpatienten enthalten ist, die der Klinik aus versicherungsrechtlichen Gründen zugeschickt worden sind, wird in der Tab. 2 eine Aufteilung der Chromatallergien in Gutachtenpatienten und Nichtgutachtenpatienten vorgenommen.

Tabelle 2. *Aufteilung der Chromatallergiker in Begutachtungs- und Nichtbegutachtungspatienten*

Jahr	Chromat positiv	Gutachten-Patienten	Nicht-gutachten-Patienten
1960	116	74	42
1961	82	39	43
1962	104	45	59
1963	133	46	87
1964	138	42	96
1965	168	59	109
1966	197	56	141
total	938	361	577

Aus der letzten Spalte ist jetzt sehr deutlich ersichtlich, daß innerhalb einer Zeitspanne von 7 Jahren eine Zunahme der Chromatallergien um das $3^1/_2$fache eingetreten ist.

In der Tab. 3 wird eine Differenzierung aller Chromatallergiker nach Berufen vorgenommen. Hierbei ergibt sich nun die sehr interessante Tatsache, daß unter den Chromatallergikern die Hausfrauen nach den Maurer- und Bauberufen an zweiter Stelle stehen, und daß die Zahl der Patienten pro Jahr sich innerhalb eines Zeitraumes von 7 Jahren versiebenfacht hat.

Die Tab. 4 führt den jeweiligen Beruf des Ehemannes bei Hausfrauen mit Chromatallergien auf.

Diese Tabelle zeigt, daß 71% der Hausfrauen mit Chromatallergien mit Männern verheiratet sind, die nur diesen sechs Berufsgruppen angehören.

Von weiterem Interesse ist die Feststellung, daß die Männer von 45% der Hausfrauen mit Chromatallergien zwar nur fünf verschiedenen Berufsgruppen angehören (Maurer, Metallarbeiter, Büroangestellte, Maler, Hilfsarbeiter), ihrerseits aber 61% aller männlichen Chromatallergiker stellen (Tab. 5).

Tabelle 3. *Berufliche Differenzierung der Chromatallergiker*

Beruf	1960	1961	1962	1963	1964	1965	1966	insgesamt
Maurer, Fliesenleger, Bauarbeiter	58	31	43	43	33	80	69	357[a]
Hausfrauen	5	7	16	19	24	22	35	128
Metallarbeiter u. a.	8	14	7	15	21	13	16	94[a]
Büroangestellte, Kaufleute, Verkäufer ♂	3	6	5	7	8	9	10	48 ⎫ 70
♀	1	1	3	4	4	2	7	22 ⎭
Raumpflegerinnen, Küchenhilfen	4	3	0	5	3	7	2	24
Maler, Anstreicher	6	1	3	6	2	3	2	23
Schneider, Näherin, Textilarbeiter	2	1	1	2	2	7	7	22
Färbereiarbeiter u. a.	8	2	2	1	7	1	0	21
Tischler, Schreiner	3	0	1	2	1	5	5	17
Gärtner, Landarbeiter	1	3	1	4	3	0	5	17
Kopierer, Chemiearbeiter	2	1	1	3	3	3	3	16
Post-Bahnbeamte, Soldaten	3	2	5	1	3	0	2	16
Elektriker	1	2	1	3	3	1	3	14
Bäcker	1	1	0	4	3	3	2	14
Kraftfahrer, Fahrzeugführer	1	1	3	4	1	2	1	13
Pflegepersonal	2	4	1	1	1	0	1	10
Lokführer	1	0	3	0	0	2	2	8
Schulkinder, Studenten	1	1	0	2	1	1	1	7
Lederarbeiter, Schuhmacher	1	0	0	1	1	1	3	7
Friseure	1	0	0	0	3	0	1	5
Hilfsarbeiter	1	1	4	5	7	1	9	28
Andere Berufe	2	0	4	1	4	5	11	27
total	116	82	104	133	138	168	197	938

[a] einschl. Gutachtenpatienten.

Tabelle 4. *Beruf der Ehemänner bei Hausfrauen mit Chromatallergien*

Büroangestellte, Kaufleute, Verkäufer	20 = 19.0%
Metallarbeiter u. a.	13 = 12.4%
Maurer, Fliesenleger, Bauarbeiter	11 = 10.5%
Gärtner, Landarbeiter	11 = 10.5%
Hilfsarbeiter	11 = 10.5%
Kraftfahrer, Fahrzeugführer	9 = 8.6%
insgesamt	75 = 71.5%

Tabelle 5. *Beziehung zwischen chromatallergischen Hausfrauen/Beruf des Ehemannes und Verteilung der Chromatallergien bei fünf Berufsgruppen*

	chromatallergische männl. Berufstätige	chromatallergische Hausfrauen
Maurer, Fliesenleger, Bauarbeiter	239	11
Metallarbeiter u. a.	94	13
Büroangestellte, Kaufleute, Verkäufer	48	20
Maler, Anstreicher	23	3
Hilfsarbeiter	28	11
insgesamt	432	58
Entspricht einem Anteil an der Gesamtzahl von	61%	45%

Es besteht daher der dringende Verdacht, daß der Beruf des Ehemannes bei der Sensibilisierung der Ehefrau gegen Chromate zumindest mittelbar von Bedeutung sein könnte. Zu denken wäre hier beispielsweise an das Waschen der Berufskleidung. Sollte sich dieser Verdacht weiterhin festigen, so könnte man die Chromatallergie bei Hausfrauen bis zu einem gewissen Grade als sekundäre Berufskrankheit auffassen. Aber auch der Kontakt mit (chromathaltigen?) Waschmitteln selbst könnte von Bedeutung sein, zumal der relativ größte Anteil chromatallergischer Hausfrauen von Ehefrauen gestellt wird, die mit Büroangestellten, Kaufleuten oder Verkäufern verheiratet sind; einer Berufsgruppe also, deren Wäsche erfahrungsgemäß öfter gereinigt wird (z. B. tägliche Wäsche von Synthetic-Hemden und -Socken).

Während außerberuflich erworbene *Kobalt*allergien bei Hausfrauen in unserem Krankengut recht selten nachgewiesen worden sind, ist bei den Nickelallergien — wie bei den Chromatallergien — eine Zunahme innerhalb des Berichtszeitraumes festzustellen. Die Allergie wurde jeweils durch das im Standardtest enthaltene Nickelsulfat 5%ig nachgewiesen. In der weit überwiegenden Zahl der Fälle wurde die Nickelallergie durch unmittelbaren (scheuernden) Kontakt mit vernickelten Gegenständen (Strumpfbandschnallen, Reißverschlüssen usw.) hervorgerufen, gelegentlich auch durch Nickelanteile bei Schmuck und Armbanduhren. Nach der Untersuchung von KROEPFLI und SCHUPPLI können gelegentlich auch (nickelhaltige) Waschmittel einer Sensibilisierung Vorschub leisten. Die Tab. 6 zeigt die Zunahme der Nickelallergien bei weiblichen Patienten; innerhalb von 7 Jahren konnte somit in unserem Krankengut mehr als eine Verdoppelung der nichtberuflich bedingten Nickelallergien bei weiblichen Patienten, insbesondere Hausfrauen, festgestellt werden.

Tabelle 6. *Patientinnen mit nicht-berufsbedingten Nickelallergien*

Jahr	Patientinnen
1960	27
1961	19
1962	52
1963	42
1964	43
1965	48
1966	68
total	299

Zusammenfassend kann somit gesagt werden, daß die Allergie gegen Chromate und Nickel bei Hausfrauen und anderen weiblichen Patienten offenbar deutlich zunimmt. Schlecht abheilende, eventuell rezidivierende Ekzeme bei weiblichen Patienten sollten daher den behandelnden Arzt auch daran denken lassen, daß es sich um Kontaktekzeme bei Allergie gegen Chromate und Nickel handeln könnte.

Hand Dermatitis, a Prospective Study

G. AGRUP, University of Lund (Sweden)

The dermatologic investigation to be presented was performed in patients who took part in a health survey in Malmöhus county, Sweden.

The reason for our participation in the health survey was that we wanted to know the prevalence of hand dermatoses in the county because a section for occupational dermatology is just under development at the University hospital in Lund. As it is known that hand dermatoses are mainly responsible for the occupational dermatoses our attention was only directed to the occurrence of lesions on the hands. — Patients who had given a positive answer to a question with regard to hand dermatosis were asked to come to the department of dermatology in Lund for an examination. This examination was without any costs for the patients and the travel costs were also covered by the county authorities.

2.3% out of 107,000 persons answered positively to the question on hand dermatosis. 65% of those with a positive answer came for dermatologic examination at our department. In all 1600 patients came for dermatologic examination. 75% of the patients were from towns with chemical and mechanical factories and with shipping and 25% were from the rural area. All patients were over 10 years old. 56% were females and 44% males.

As our department has been especially interested in contact allergy, attention was paid to the occurrence and type of contact dermatitis. For treatment of the data obtained at the examinations we used IBM punch cards. In these were registered relevant clinical data and the results of laboratory test examinations. In the history special attention was paid to their occupational activities, how long time the patients had been away from their work, their earlier visits to physicians because of skin trouble, the treatments given, earlier investigations performed, with special regard to earlier contact allergy test examinations.

In all these patients patch tests were performed with 20 different substances used in the routine screening tests at the department.

Out of the 739 patients tested 398 were found to have one or several positive patch tests. The most common positive patch tests were any of the *balsams*. Examples of compounds belonging to this group are different spices, perfumes, and pharmaceutical products, cosmetics, detergents, etc. Furthermore, our common Swedish trees, spruce and pine, are responsible for a big proportion of the balsams giving positive tests in this group. Other common allergens were *metals*. Here chromium, nickel, and cobalt allergies were the most frequent. Another common allergen was *rubber*. Here the antioxidants and accelerating substances are responsible for the allergies. Thus these compounds often gave rise to hand dermatitis in house-wives and factory workers wearing rubber gloves. The common *flowers* were important causes of hand dermatitis. The most common one in Sweden is the primula. Another important group of contact allergens were the *topical treatment substances* which had earlier been used by the patients. The sensitizing agents were antibiotics like neomycin, aromatic esters used as conservating agents like p-hydroxy benzoic acid esters, and different brands of wool-fat.

Plastic products formed another group of contact allergens. The formaldehyde resins were of special importance. The epoxy resins were also found to be responsible agents in some cases. As these resins are innoxious in cured form it was most surprising that we had a great number of dermatitis due to epoxy resins. However, it has been described that uncured epoxy resins may be used as softening agents in polyvinyl chloride products and this type of plastic is so commonly used that it is probable that we get many epoxy contacts in this way.

The hand dermatites in the house-wives were seldom induced by contact allergy to the commonly used *detergents*. In a few cases the perfumes added to the detergents were of importance as allergens.

This type of investigation seems to give us a good basis for the planning of the occupational dermatology in the region.

We have now been reinvestigating the patients with diagnosed contact dermatitis. In this reinvestigation it is analysed to what extent it has been of value to change details in the occupational activity. Protective measures are also evaluated. Special attention is paid to the large group of house-wives with hand dermatitis. They are patients who often had not reached the specialist and who often got a chronic dermatitis.

Routine patch testing was found to be of great value in the investigation of hand dermatitis. Many of the contact allergens causing chronic dermatitis were diagnosed where history alone was found to be insufficient.

The other side of the medal is, however, the sensitization caused by the routine patch test. Thus the retesting demonstrated a high number of reactions to some allergens namely diaminodifenylmetane, azo dye, parafenylendiamine and primula extract.

Seasonal Variations in the Incidence of Contact Dermatitis

N. Hjorth, Department of Dermatology, Finsen Institute, Copenhagen (Denmark)

Between 1935 and 1961, a total of 48.000 patients with dermatitis have been examined with a uniform series of 21 standard patch tests. We have tabulated this material according to the months of examination. And in order to estimate any seasonal variations we calculated the average per month of the patients tested and the positive reactions obtained. These averages were used as base-lines, and the number of patients examined in each individual month was then calculated as percentage deviations from the monthly average. Positive reactions were calculated in the same way.

In Denmark the number of patients referred for contact dermatitis is low during summer. During winter it is correspondingly higher. In January, for example, the incidence of contact dermatitis is 122% of the monthly average.

Positive reactions to the series of patch tests, however, are relatively common during summer. In other words, the percentage of patients examined showing positive reactions to one or several patch tests is·higher in summer than in winter.

Dark shading used on this and the following graphs indicates that positive reactions are relatively frequent. Light shading that they are relatively rare in a particular season.

Positive reactions are common during summer, but this is because *Primula obconica* is included in the standard series. Without this, positive reactions might occur with a uniform percentage throughout the year.

Sensitivity to rubber chemicals is comparatively common in late summer. It should be noted that rubber sensitivity in our clinic is a consumer's allergy. Occupational rubber dermatitis may show a different trend. The consumer's goods most likely to give rubber dermatitis in late summer are shoes.

Nickel makes a striking contrast to rubber. This curve includes women with suspender dermatitis and women with nickel dermatitis of the hands as a sequel to the primary suspender sensitisation. Suspenders are constantly worn from September to June but the incidence of nickel dermatitis varies. The peaks of the curves coincide with the periods when dermatitis of the hands is most likely to start.

In the late summer we have an influx of patients referred for chromate dermatitis. Dermatitis from cement is the most likely reason for chromate dermatitis at this season. The few persons suffering from shoe dermatitis due to chromate could hardly influence the total incidence of chromate dermatitis.

The major sources of sensitisation to formaldehyde are textiles and anti-perspirants. These allergens may give rise to the peak observed in September. But why should positive reactions be relatively rare in summer and common in winter? A possible explanation is that false positive reactions mainly occur during winter. Mercury has similar seasonal variations, and likewise this is a primary irritant substance.

18*

L'Allergie aux sels d'ammonium quaternaire
Etat actuel de nos recherches

P. MARTIN, M. MENNECIER, P. AGACHE et CL. HURIEZ, Clinique Dermatologique, Centre Hospitalier Régional de Lille (France)

Comme STÜPEL et SZAKALL [1], WAHLBERG [2], nous avons constaté, ces dernières années, l'apparition d'allergies de contact aux sels d'ammonium quaternaire chez des malades porteurs d'ulcères de jambes, d'eczémas ou d'infections cutanées traités par des topiques qui en contenaient. Nous avions essayé précédemment [3 à 5] de préciser l'importance de ces faits que cette note actualise. La formule générale des ammoniums quaternaires est la suivante:

$$R-\overset{+}{N}\overset{\diagup R_1}{\underset{\diagdown R_3}{-R_2}} \quad X^- .$$

R représente une longue chaîne hydrocarbonée de 8 à 18 atomes de carbone (le plus souvent en C_{12} lauryl-, ou en C_{16} cétyl-), R_1, R_2, R_3 représentant des groupes organiques de faible poids moléculaire (méthyl-, éthyl-, benzyl- ou cyclohexanol-, etc.) et X un anion tel que Cl, Br ou SO_4CH_3, etc. L'azote peut également faire partie d'un hétérocycle tel que la pyridine. Ils possèdent des propriétés bactéricides, bactériostatiques et mouillantes utilisées contre les infections cutanées. Sont notamment employés (Tab. 1):

Tableau 1

Dénomination commune Française	Formules développées	Noms des spécialités pharmaceutiques
Céthexonium (bromure)	$C_{16}H_{33} - \overset{+}{N} \overset{\diagup CH_3}{\underset{\diagdown}{-CH_3}}$ (cyclohexyl, H, HO) Br^-	Biocidan Stamycil
Cétrimonium (bromure)	$C_{16}H_{33} - \overset{+}{N} \overset{\diagup CH_3}{\underset{\diagdown CH_3}{-CH_3}}$ Br^-	Cétavlon
Dodécyl-Diméthyl-Carbéthoxyméthylamm. (bromure)	$C_{12}H_{25} - \overset{+}{N} \overset{\diagup CH_3}{\underset{\diagdown CH_3}{-CH_2-COO-C_2H_5}}$ Br^-	Fongeryl
Benzalkonium (chlorure)	$R - \overset{+}{N} \overset{\diagup CH_3}{\underset{\diagdown CH_2-C_6H_5}{-CH_3}}$ Cl^- $R = C_8$ à C_{18}	Benzalkonium
Benzododécinium (chlorure ou bromure)	$C_{12}H_{25} - \overset{+}{N} \overset{\diagup CH_3}{\underset{\diagdown CH_2-C_6H_5}{-CH_3}}$ Cl^- ou Br^-	Benzododécinium

inspiré de LECHAT [6] et BALATRE [7].

le *céthexonium* ou bromure de cétyl-diméthyl (hydroxy-2-cyclohexyl) ammonium;

le *cétrimonium* ou bromure de cétyl-triméthyl ammonium;

le *bromure de dodécyl-diméthyl-carbéthoxy-méthylammonium*. Une préparation pharmaceutique fréquemment utilisée contient en outre un dérivé du dichloro-crésol.

L'allergie a été recherchée par patch-tests, parfois en scratch. Les topiques étaient appliqués tels quels, puis des tests étaient effectués avec les ammoniums quaternaires correspondants. Pour faciliter l'interrogatoire, nous présentions aux malades les diverses préparations sur un «banc des aveux».

Seules furent retenues comme positives les réactions $\geq$ ++.

Nous avons testé au *céthexonium* (solution à $0,1\%$ dans l'eau distillée) 201 malades susceptibles de s'y être sensibilisés. 34 malades y étaient allergiques, soit $16,9\%$ des cas. Par ailleurs, nous n'avons trouvé que 10 allergiques chez 440 eczémateux n'ayant jamais utilisé ce corps: soit $2,3\%$. Entre ces deux populations le test X^2 est hautement significatif: $p \leq 0,001$.

Pour 126 malades traités par le *carbéthoxyméthylammonium*, 18 réagirent positivement: soit $14,2\%$. 195 témoins testés dans les mêmes conditions (solution à $1,5\%$) donnaient $7,6\%$ de réactions positives (15 épreuves positives). Ce pourcentage ne se trouve pas modifié par 45 autres témoins (3 réponses positives) testés à une dilution de $0,1\%$.

Avec le *cétrimonium* 130 malades donnèrent $9,2\%$ de positivité (12 malades allergiques). Pour 240 témoins, il y eut 14 réactions positives: $5,8\%$ (solution de cétrimonium à $0,5\%$).

Nos résultats confirment l'allergie au céthexonium. Ils sont moins significatifs pour les deux autres corps; pourtant, les réactions étaient parfois vésiculeuses, attestant de la réalité de phénomènes allergiques. Mais *les ammoniums quaternaires donnent des réactions cytotoxiques qui gênent la lecture des tests.* D'après THIERS [8], certains peuvent fournir pas décomposition des mono- ou diméthylamines caustiques. Ils ont aussi des propriétés histaminolibératrices. *Le pouvoir sensibilisant de certains ammoniums quaternaires est difficilement dissociable de leurs propriétés irritantes, et certaines intolérances cutanées réputées allergiques relèvent peut-être exclusivement de ces dernières.* Avec SIDI et HINCKY [9] nous dirons que le problème de leur utilisation en dermatologie devrait être revu sous l'angle des concentrations minima actives pour limiter le nombre des intolérances. Il est en tous cas prudent de s'abstenir de les appliquer sur les dermatoses irritables.

Les pommades contenant des ammoniums quaternaires peuvent donner des réactions positives par allergie aux composants des excipients. Les remarques de DE GRACIANSKY et TAIEB [10] sont confirmées chez 23 malades sensibilisés à la pommade au céthexonium-hydrocortisone:

teinture de benjoin	16 épreuves positives
céthexonium	13 épreuves positives
gallate de lauryle	7 épreuves positives
huile de maïs estérifiée	2 épreuves positives

Les firmes pharmaceutiques devraient éliminer de leurs préparations des composants tels que le benjoin ou l'essence de lavande.

Les problèmes soulevés s'étendent à de plus vastes horizons (Tab. 2):

1. Ces corps sont employés pour la désinfection des mains et des champs opératoires. Nous avons récemment observé une allergie professionnelle au cétrimonium et au céthexonium chez une infirmière d'un bloc opératoire. SCHULZ [11] les mentionne dans ses listes d'allergènes professionnels.

2. Ils ont des propriétés antispasmodiques, hypotensives, etc. utilisées en thérapeutique interne. SIDI [12] a rapporté l'existence de sensibilisations très violentes chez les chimistes mettant au point la fabrication des ganglioplégiques.

3. Ils sont employés dans de nombreux domaines : excipients modernes, shampooings cationiques, désinfectants, colorants, teintures, huiles solubles, liquides de flottation, liants pour peintures, etc. Il est bon d'y penser dans les enquêtes allergologiques.

4. Des cosensibilisations peuvent se rencontrer à plusieurs ammoniums quaternaires, ainsi que nous l'avons constaté chez 48 malades sur 127 (Tab. 3). Nous ne pouvons toutefois rien en déduire sur la fréquence exacte de tel type de cosensibilisation, tous nos malades n'ayant pas été testés avec l'ensemble des corps.

Tableau 2

Thérapeutiques générales	*Industrie chimique, industrie pharmaceutique*
Hypotenseurs	Chimie des ammoniums quaternaires
Ganglioplégiques	Fabrication des dérivés cationiques
Antispasmodiques	Chimie des colorants
Analgésiques centraux	Fabrication des médicaments
Antitussifs	
	Industrie textile, industrie des teintures
	Traitement des fibres textiles/Teintures
	Imperméabilisation, etc.
Thérapeutiques locales	*Métallurgie*
Excipients modernes du type huile dans eau	Certaines huiles solubles
Conservateurs pour excipients classiques	Certaines graisses
(cold-cream,...) et pour collyres	*Exploitations minières*
Crèmes, pommades, solutions,	Liquides de flottation
poudres antiseptiques et antifungiques	*Peintures*
	Liants pour peintures
Hygiène et cosmétologie	*Agriculture*
Shampooings cationiques	Stérilisation des équipements et des
Crèmes de beauté	étables
Dentifrices	Désinfection des champignonnières
Talcs, produits hygiéniques	Traitements vétérinaires
Crèmes antisudorales	*Industrie alimentaire*
Stérilisation du linge et des langes	Désinfection des appareils, équipements et
Désodorisants d'hôpital	ustensiles
Désinfectants pour salles et véhicules	Industrie sucrière, conserverie, etc.
publiques	
Algaecides pour piscines	

Professions médicales
Manipulation des produits pharmaceutiques
Désinfection des salles, des masques, instruments, langes.
Désinfection des mains
Chirurgie, obstétrique, gynécologie
Dermatologie

Tableau 3

Consensibilisations	Ammoniums quaternaires	Nombre de cas
5 Composés	céthexonium, carbéthoxy-méthylamm., cétrimonium, sulfométhylate de méthylphényl-dodécyl-triméthyl-amm., chlorure de benzalkonium	1
4 Composés	les quatre premiers ci-dessus	9
3 Composés	les trois premiers = 14 cas autres associations = 6 cas	20
2 Composés	les deux premiers = 12 cas autres associations = 6 cas	18

Nous remercions sincèrement MM. DEQUIDT, LESPAGNOL, MARCHAND et MERVILLE † pour leurs conseils et la documentation qu'ils nous ont aimablement fournie.

Bibliographie. 1. STÜPEL, H., u. A. SZAKALL: Die Wirkung von Waschmitteln auf die Haut. Heidelberg: A. HUTHIG 1957. — 2. WAHLBERG, J. E.: Acta derm.-venereol. (Stockh.) 42, 230 (1962). — 3. HURIEZ, CL., P. AGACHE, P. MARTIN, G. VANDAMME et J. MENNECIER: Rev. franç. Allerg. 3, 134 (1965). — 4. Sem. Hôp. Paris 1965, 2301. — 5. HURIEZ, CL., P. MARTIN, M. VANOVERSCHELDE et J. MENNECIER: Bull. Soc. franç. Derm. Syph. 73, 260 (1966). — 6. LECHAT, P.: Thérapie 1954, 835. — 7. BALATRE, P.: Bull. Soc. Pharm. Lille. 2, 111 (1955). — 8. THIERS, H.: Manuel d'allergologie. Paris: Masson et Cie. 1964. — 9. SIDI, E., et M. HINCKY: Gaz. Hôp (Paris) 7, 301 (1965). — 10. DE GRACIANSKY, P., et M. TAIEB: Discussion de la communication de HURIEZ, CL. et coll. Bull. Soc. franç. Derm. Syph. 72, (2), 106 (1965). — 11. SCHULZ, K. H.: Berufsdermatosen: In Dermatologie und Venerologie von GOTTRON, H. A., u. W. SCHONFELD, V/I. Stuttgart: Thieme 1963. — 12. SIDI, E.: Syndromes cutanés. In: SCHÖNFELD, Traité des maladies allergiques par PASTEUR VALLERY-RADOT, WOLFROMM, R., J. CHARPIN et B. N. HALPERN, p. 443. Paris: Flammarion 1963.

Contact Dermatitis due to Plastic Coated Furniture (Tricresyl Phosphate)

J. S. PEGUM, The London Hospital, London (England)

A patient with eczema gave a strongly positive reaction to the adhesive tape used in applying patch tests. The tape was made of polyvinyl chloride (PVC) plasticized with tricresyl phosphate (TCP). It was the TCP to which she was allergic. It was found that furniture in her house was upholstered with PVC and the kitchen floor tiles were of the same material. She also reacted to her spectacle frames, made of cellulose acetate, plasticized with triphenyl phosphate (TPP) which is chemically related to TCP and to a plastic kitchen spoon and beater. The eczema improved following withdrawal from contact with most of these things.

Polyvinyl chloride is used very widely as car and furniture upholstery; for gloves and shoes and handbags; as wall covering; for simulated wood veneer in furniture; for baby chairs, carry cots and prams. For rainwear and clothing. For brush handles, tablecloths, table mats. For toys, wallets and electric cable covering. For adhesive tape, oxygen tents and waterproof sheets.

Cellulose acetate is widely used for spectacle frames, tooth brushes, pencils, ball point pens, lamp shades, record sleeves, magnetic tape, wine lists and office equipment.

In spite of the widespread distribution of TCP and TPP containing plastic there is no evidence that dermatitis from this cause is at present common, and there are few reports of the matter in the literature. The earliest is BERKOFF's (1938) about spectacle dermatitis and one of the most interesting is HJORTH's (1964), whose patient reacted to cellulose acetate objects containing TPP and to non-smudge carbon paper, containing TCP. Recently CALNAN and LEWIS discovered a patient with spectacle dermatitis who reacted to TCP and TPP (1967).

References. BERKOFF, H. S.: Arch. Derm. Syph. (Chic.) 38, 746 (1938). — CALNAN, C. D., and R. LEWIS: Pers. communication 1967. — HJORTH, N.: Berufsdermatosen 12, 86 (1964).

Study on the Penetration of Mineral Oil into the Human Skin by the Aid of Fluorescence Microscopy

C. Scarpa, Clinica Dermatologica-Policlinico Umberto I, Rome (Italy)

Normal primary fluorescence of human skin is mainly limited, as already known, to elastic fibers, keratin and granules belonging to sweat glands. We planned to study the eventual increase of fluorescence of human skin after local

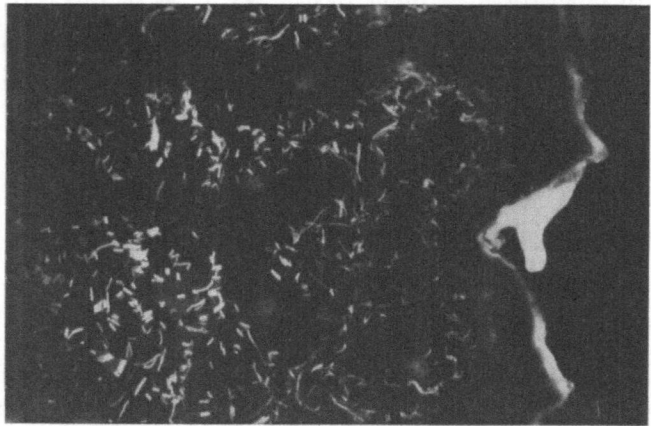

Fig. 1. Control skin

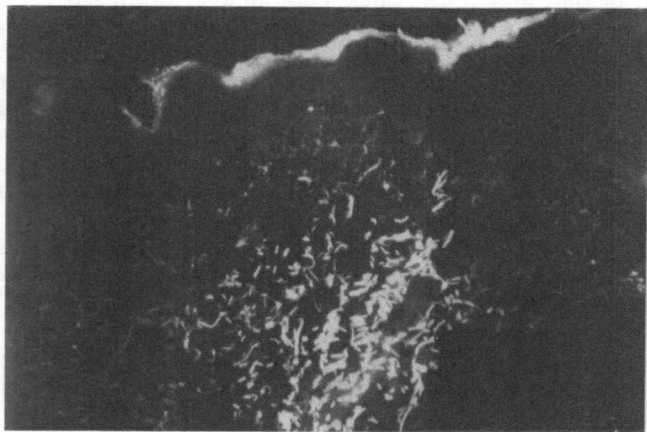

Fig. 2. Control skin

application of mineral oil with additives. This oil is supposed to penetrate in a certain quantity into the impregnated skin. Unfixed biopsy specimens were sectioned directly by cryostat (sections of 10 microns), then were examined at the fluorescence microscope (Zeiss-Optar GFL) in dark field (primary filters BG 12/4 and BG 3/4; secondary filters 53/47).

In a first series of experiments we stated that the fluorescence of impregnated skin and control skin, was almost equal. The skin was impregnated for 48 h with paraffinic oil SAE 30, additivated by calcium alkylsalycilate 5% and primarily fluorescent. We then turned to a new technique which, in our intention, should render easier the scope of ascertaining the limits of penetration of oil into the skin. We mixed beforehand the oil with acridine orange 1% in water, by means of vaseline oil (liquid petrolatum) and propyleneglycol as vehicles, emulsified by Tinovetin NR (alkylarylpolyglycolether) and Cetiol. We applied the emulsion under a closed patch on a skin area of the shoulders. By this procedure the difference of impregnation between oil with fluorochrome and unstained oil, in the same indivi-

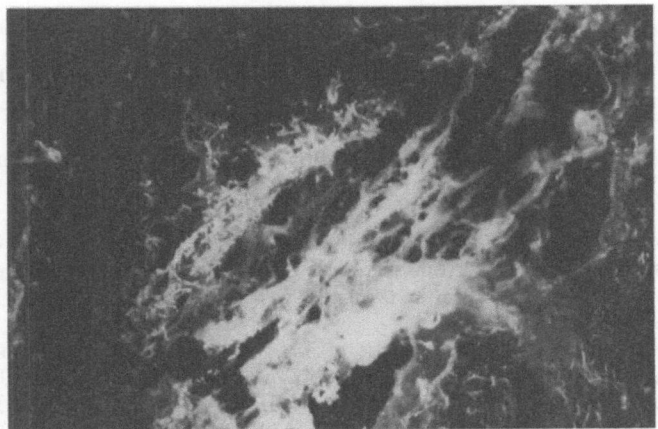

Fig. 3. With fluorochrome oil treated skin

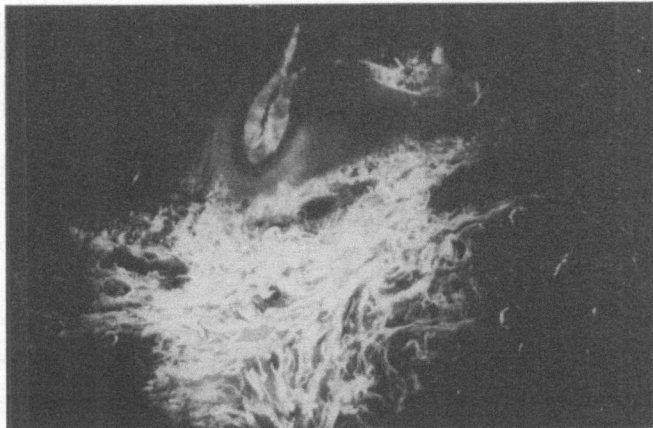

Fig. 4. With fluorochrome oil treated skin

dual, is rather clearcut. We point out that the fluorochrome is well emulsified with the mineral oil.

On careful examination, in two specimens among eight, elastic fibers appear as more fluorescent than normally and more crowded in the subpapillary layer, where they use to be scanty. The general greenish hue of fluorescence, which is due also to clumps of collagen, is found increased in the subpapillary and perifollicular areas. Surface keratin fluoresces in a deeper green-yellowish hue than are fluorescing control sections (Fig. 1 to 4).

In the other six biopsy specimens the oil fluorescence was not found increased employing oil + fluorochrome.

The mineral oil which was selected by us, seems to seldom penetrate human skin after 48 h impregnation. It seems to do so probably as an effect of the additive content, and to enter mainly through the sweat pores. This oil was sometimes recognizable in the skin by emulsifying it with fluorochrome and subsequently observing skin sections at the fluorescence microscope by dark field.

Vergleichende Untersuchungen verschiedener Testmethoden bei Sensibilisierung gegen Neomycinsulphat (N.)

M. NOVÁK und T. BIELICKÝ, Dermatologische Klinik der Medizinisch-Hygienischen Fakultät der Karls-Universität in Prag (Tschechoslowakei)

Bei der Sensibilisierung gegen N. bestehen über die Art der Testmethoden und über die Konzentration von N. Meinungsverschiedenheiten. Es werden folgende Testmethoden empfohlen: ET mit 0,5 bis 50% N., IKT, AT, SKT und NaLST mit 1 bis 10% N.

Da die Penetration des N. durch die intakte Haut ungenügend ist, sind die ET oft falsch negativ. Darum versuchten wir mit quantitativ abgestuften ET und mit anderen Testmethoden die optimale Art und die niedrigste wirksame Konzentration bei N.-Testen festzustellen. Zur Erhöhung der Penetration von N. durch die Haut bedienten wir uns des SKT, NaLST, AT und des IT. Die Reaktionen wurden über 7 Tage verfolgt.

Vorläufige Untersuchungen zeigten, daß etwa 34% aller hospitalisierten getesteten Ekzematiker gegen N. sensibilisiert sind. Am häufigsten sind es Kranke mit Unterschenkelekzemen und Unterschenkelgeschwüren.

61 gegen N. sensibilisierte Patienten untersuchten wir in drei Gruppen. In der ersten Orientierungsgruppe verglichen wir ET mit 1% und 50% N. in Salbengrundlage, 20% N.-Lösung und den 1% SKT. Der 1% SKT und die 20% und 50% ET waren bei allen Patienten positiv. Falsch negative Reaktionen wurden nach 1% N. bei vier (23%) und fragliche bei zwei Kranken (11%) beobachtet. Die Reaktionen nach 50% N. waren oft sehr stark. Diese Untersuchung zeigt, daß die 1%-Konzentration für ET zu niedrig und die 50% zu hoch ist.

Tabelle. *Numerische Wertung der Reaktionsintensitäten bei den einzelnen Testmethoden bei 30 Patienten/+++ = 3, ++ = 2, + = 1, + = 0,5/*

	+++ = 3	++ = 2	+ = 1	+ — = 0,5	0	S
ET	2	5	18	4	1	36
AT	2	12	12	3	1	43,5
SKT	4	15	10	—	1	52
NaLST	8	13	8	—	1	58
IT	12	12	6	—	—	66

Abkürzungen: ET = Epicutantest, AT = Abrißtest, SKT = Skarifikationsepicutantest, NaLST = Natriumlaurylsulphat-Provokationstest (KLIGMAN), IT = Iontophoresetest, IKT = Intracutantest.

Zur Feststellung der niedrigsten wirksamen Konzentration untersuchten wir 14 Kranke mit 2%-, 4%-, 10%- und 20%-Lösungen epicutan und mit 2%-Lösung im SKT. Die 10% und 20% ET waren in allen Fällen positiv. Die 2% und 4%

waren in fünf bzw. drei Fällen falsch negativ. In dieser Gruppe erfaßte der 10% ET alle sensibilisierten Personen.

Bei einer weiteren Gruppe von 30 Kranken wurden der 10% ET, die 1% SKT, AT, NaLST und IT verglichen. Nur der IT war in allen 30 Fällen positiv. Je eine falsch negative Reaktion wurde beim SKT und NaLST beobachtet, beim ET und AT je eine falsch negative und drei bzw. vier fragliche Reaktionen. Die Reaktions-intensitäten numerisch ausgedrückt zeigen diese Reihenfolge (Tabelle): 1. IT, 2. NaLST, 3. SKT, 4. AT und 5. ET. Der NaLST gibt zwar starke Reaktionen, die doch durch Summation der Reizwirkung von NaLST und der allergischen Reaktion entstehen. Die Reaktionen waren meistens verzögert, in einigen Fällen 5 bis 6 Tage.

Vorläufig können wir zusammenfassend schließen, daß der empfindlichste der IT ist. Die Durchführung in der Praxis ist doch schwierig. Die ET in niedrigeren als 10%-Konzentrationen geben häufig falsch negative Reaktionen. Aber auch nach 10% N. können falsch negative Reaktionen entstehen. Für die Praxis empfehlen wir darum den 20% ET und den 1% SKT, da sie leicht durchführbar sind. Für wissenschaftliche Zwecke und bei fraglichen Reaktionen ist der 1% IT der empfindlichste. Die Reaktionen muß man 7 Tage verfolgen, da sie oft ver-zögert erscheinen.

Photoallergic Reaction in Red Tattoos
Mercury-Cadmium Sensitivity

N. GOLDSTEIN, Dermatology Department, The Medical Group, Honolulu, Hawaii (USA)

Allergic reactions in tattoos are rare, but have been documented; the most frequent being red, which is usually mercuric sulfide. BROSE [1], in 1927, was first to describe an irritative phenomenon in red tattoo sites. In 1954, BEERMAN and LANES review [2] uncovered a total of 18 case reports of mercurial sensitivity in tattoos. Since then, BONNELL [3], RAVITS [4] and WEIDMAN et al. [5] have each reported single cases. LAMB et al. [6] described two cases and BJORNBERG [7] reported four men with reactions in red pigmented sites. The author has investi-gated twelve cases of allergic reactions in red tattoo sites from 1965 to 1967. The subjects were all military personnel stationed in Hawaii. Each noted pruritic, nodular or verrucous lesions develop only in the red tattoo sites after exposure to sunshine. The duration of the tattoos prior to the development of symptoms ranged from 2 weeks to 17 years! (Fig. 1 to 3)

Pathologic. Pathologic examinations were performed in eight patients. Two biopsies revealed a mild perivascular lymphocytic infiltration. Two demonstrated massive pseudoepitheliomatous hyperplasia, hyperkeratosis and parakeratosis as well as a perivascular lymphocytic infiltration. Four biopsies revealed a sarcoid-*like* granuloma. (Fig. 4)

Etiology. Various explanations have been proposed concerning the prolonged delay of symptoms. Exposure to mercurial solutions, ointments and diuretics [6], and trace amounts of mercurial preservatives in Asian influenza vaccine [8] have been postulated. LAMB et al. [6] suggest a histamine-like chemical elaborated by sunlight in a rare case of solar urticaria in red tattoo sites.

Actinic radiation does indeed play a role in each subject of this report. Each noted symptoms in the red tattoo sites only after exposure to the sunshine in

Hawaii. None of the subjects had received mercurial diuretics, and none had been given mercury-containing ointments.

Relationship to Immunizations? In 1959, SULZBERGER and TOLMACH [8] described a patient who had symptoms in red tattoo sites after receiving trace

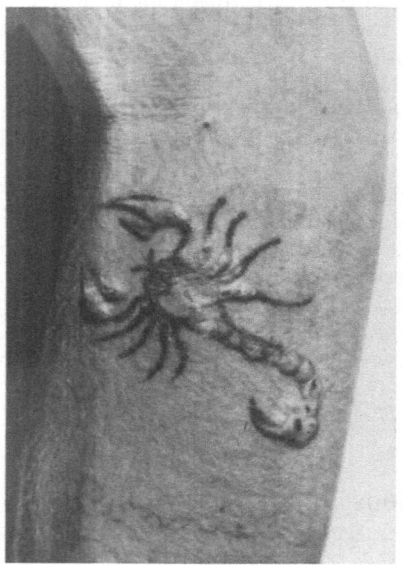

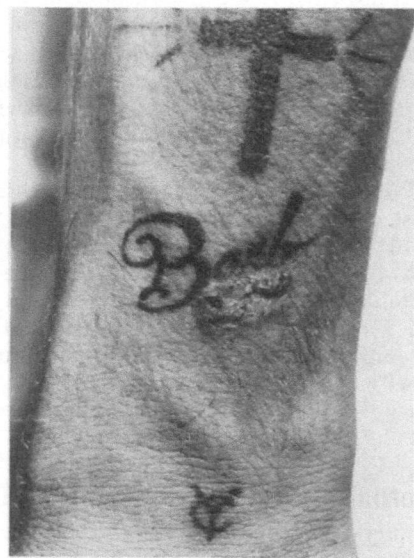

Fig. 1   Fig. 2

Fig. 1—3. Granulomatous reactions in red tattoo sites after sun exposure

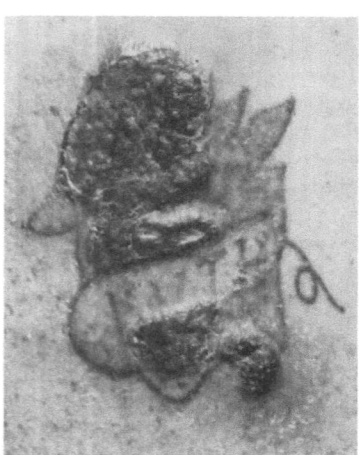

Fig. 3

amounts of a mercurial preservative in an influenza vaccine. Vaccines and antigens frequently used in the Military were reviewed for mercurial preservatives. Typhus and influenza vaccines as well as blastomycin, coccidioidin and histoplasmin antigens do indeed contain 1:10,000 thimerosal (merthiolate). Immunization records were reviewed. In only three was there any *possible* relationship of receiving these immunizations and the onset of symptoms.

Sarcoidosis? LUBECK and EPSTEIN [9] described a man with sarcoidosis who developed a "raised, scaly dermatitis" in tatto sites. The biopsy was "probably sarcoid". The reports of POST [10], BONNELL [3] and WEIDMAN et al. [5] as well as four of the eight skin biopsies in this study, represent a sarcoid-*like* granuloma rather than true cutaneous sarcoidosis. All of the subjects were in good health and had neither signs nor symptoms of sarcoidosis. Chest roentgenograms were all normal.

Patch Testing. Subjects were patch tester to various mercurial preparations. While most had negative or mild reactions, the two cases with verrucous responses

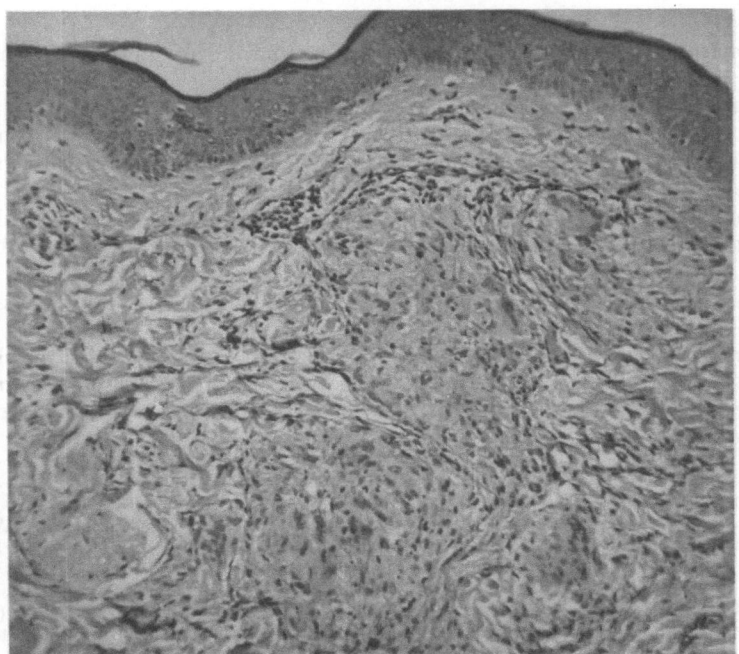

Fig. 4. Sarcoid-like granuloma in red tattoo site — Human (H & E x 60)

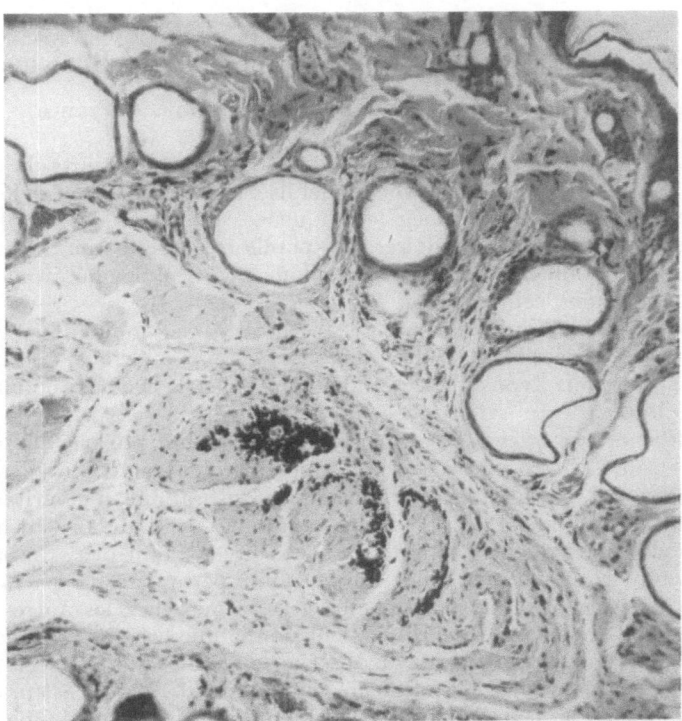

Fig. 5. Sarcoid-like granuloma in hairless mouse tattooed with "Red" pigment and exposed to sunshine (H & E x 60)

in red tattoo sites had strong reactions to bichloride of mercury, ammoniated mercury and aqueous and tincture of Merthiolate (thimerosal, Lilly).

Therapy. The only topical preparation that relieved the symptoms in some patients was a sunscreen cream. One patient noted complete resolution of the pruritic nodules by the use of this sunscreen preparation. Dermabrasions were performed in nine subjects.

Animal Studies. Reproduction of the clinical lesion and a sarcoid-like granuloma was accomplished in hairless mice tattooed with a commercial "red" tattoo pigment followed by sun exposure, but not in control sites [11] (Fig. 5).

Chemical Analysis. Analysis of biopsies revealed mercuric sulfide as well as trace amounts of cadmium sulfide.

Comment. Samples of Commercial Red Tattoo pigment were also shown to contain trace amounts of cadmium sulfide. This light sensitive substance induces a photoallergic reaction in red tattoo sites. The granulomatous response is unrelated to sarcoidosis.

References. 1. BROSE: Derm. Wschr. **84**, 461 (1927). — 2. BEERMAN, H., and R. A. G. LANE: Amer. J. med. Sci. **227**, 444 (1954). — 3. BONNELL, J. A., and B. RUSSELL: Proc. roy Soc. Med. **49**, 823 (1956). — 4. RAVITS. H. G.: Arch. Derm. **86**, 287 (1962). — 5. WEIDMAN, A. I., R. ANDRADE, and A. G. FRANKS: Arch. Derm. **94**, 320 (1966). — 6. LAMB, J. H.: Arch. Derm. **83**, 568 (1961). — 7. BJORNBERG, A.: Arch. Derm. **88**, 267 (1963). — 8. SULZBERGER, M. B., u. J. A. TOLMACH: Hautarzt **10**, 110 (1959). — 9. LUBECK, G., and E. EPSTEIN: Calif. Med. **76**, 83 (1952). — 10. POST, C. F.: Arch. Derm. Syph. (Chic.) **66**, 762 (1952). — 11. GOLDSTEIN, N.: Bumps and Lumps in the Sun. Clinical Investigation Session, 48th Annual Session of the American College of Physicians, April 10, 1967, San Francisco, California.

Etude des maladies cutanées provoquées par la Brai de Houille

F.-X. CARTON, Centre Hospitalier Universitaire Amiens (France)

Nous avons pu observer plusieurs dizaines d'ouvriers atteints de dermatoses provoquées par le brai de houille avec lequel ils étaient ou avaient été en contact. Leurs lésions cutanées sont d'inégale fréquence. Ce sont: des érythèmes, des pigmentations, des lésions folliculaires, des papillomes vérruqueux, des kératoses, des épithéliomas papillaires cornés ou papillomes cornés, des kérato-acanthomes, des épithéliomas spino-cellulaires.

Trois ordres de lésions: érythèmes, pigmentations, folliculites, des parties découvertes ont été décrites de nombreuses fois. Nous voudrions, à la lumière des observations que nous avons faites, étudier plutôt les lésions exubérantes provoquées par le brai.

Les papillomes verruqueux sont extrêmement fréquents, plus de 30% de malades observés. Ils peuvent être très petits, filiformes. Le plus souvent d'ailleurs ils sont vus très tôt, car les ouvriers qui travaillent près du brai ont une véritable hantise des lésions cutanées. Dans d'autres cas, les papillomes verruqueux sont un peu plus volumineux. Ils surviennent à tout âge et sont souvent multiples. En fait ils n'ont aucun caractère clinique particulier qui puissent permettre de les rattacher au brai. Seules leur fréquence beaucoup plus grande que chez les autres individus, et leur répétition en des endroits divers leur donne une certaine autonomie.

Outre les papillomes verruqueux on observe des *kératoses*. Là aussi la distinction avec les kératoses séniles est très difficile. Cliniquement l'aspect est pratiquement le même, mis à part les cas où leur association à d'autres lésions donne l'aspect de «peau de chagrin». Ces kératoses sont uniques ou multiples: elles siègent essentiellement sur le visage et sur les membres supérieurs, en particulier le dos des mains. Elles n'apparaissent qu'après un délai d'exposition au brai d'une dizaine d'années mais peuvent survenir longtemps après la cessation du contact avec le brai. En fait les malades que nous avons vus atteints de kératoses étaient âgés de 55 à 68 ans, si bien que beaucoup d'entre eux ne travaillaient plus depuis longtemps. Il est extrêmement difficile chez une personne de 50 ans de savoir s'il s'agit d'une kératose sénile ou d'une kératose du brai. Y a-t-il d'ailleurs une différence entre elles ? Cela est bien difficile à dire puisque les kératoses séniles surviennent plus fréquemment chez des personnes qui ont eu pendant leur vie une exposition prolongée au soleil. Or les ouvriers qui travaillent au brai ont eu cette exposition solaire prolongée, aggravée souvent par des érythèmes provoqués par le brai. Ils font donc plus fréquemment que d'autres des kératoses qui peuvent évidemment dégénérer en épithéliomas spino-cellulaires.

Il était habituel depuis de très nombreuses années de distinguer parmi les lésions provoquées par le brai, ce que l'on a appelé «le bouton de brai», ou «papillome du brai»: tumeur arrondie, à tête cornée, de couleur brun grisâtre, et dont le volume pouvait varier d'une grosse tête d'épingle à celui d'une noisette, évoluant soit vers l'épithélioma spinocellulaire, soit vers la guérison. A la suite de l'observation d'un certain nombre d'ouvriers travaillant au brai, nous pouvons dire que nous n'avons jamais vu de lésion cutanée particulière, que l'on aurait pu appeler «bouton de brai», car toutes pouvaient cliniquement être rangées dans le cadre des papillomes cornés ou des kérato-acanthomes. Notre diagnostic clinique a été confirmé ou précisé par un diagnostic histologique fait par le Professeur DUPERRAT.

Nous avons observé des *papillomes cornés*, assez rarement en réalité. Nous savons combien il est difficile et souvent impossible de les distinguer cliniquement des épithéliomas spino-cellulaires débutants. L'évolution vers l'épithélioma que l'on a dit être celle d'un certain nombre de boutons de brai était en réalité celle des papillomes cornés.

Mais la définition du bouton de brai correspond surtout à la description du *kérato-acanthome*, et ceci est admis depuis un certain temps. Les études de ROOK et WHIMSTER en 1950, celles de BINKLEY et JOHNSON en 1955 signalaient l'idendité vraisemblable du K. A. avec des tumeurs des ouvriers des cokeries et les carcinoïdes du goudron. Ceci était repris dans le rapport de ROOK au Congrès des Dermatologistes de Langue Française à Lausanne en 1956. Dans une communication à ce même congrès, MM. HURIEZ et coll. trouvent dans la moitié des K. A. qu'ils ont observés un contact avec le brai et ils évoquent l'analogie avec le carcinome du brai. Les K. A. que nous avons observés chez les ouvriers du brai ont les mêmes caractères cliniques et évolutifs que tout K. A. Mais leur fréquence est grande: près de 20% des lésions observées. Uniques ou multiples, ils ont guéri spontanément; parfois, mais rarement, ils ont récidivé. Cette évolution vers la guérison décrite dans le bouton de brai, correspond à l'évolution habituelle du K. A. Nous n'avons observé aucun K. A. qui ait évolué vers l'épithélioma spino-cellulaire.

Les épithéliomas provoqués par le brai sont toujours spino-cellulaires. Ils revêtent les aspects cliniques de cette catégorie de tumeur, mais parfois peuvent être vus à leur début sous l'aspect clinique d'un papillome corné, d'une kératose épaissie, ou même d'une tumeur ressemblant au K. A. Ces épithéliomas siègent souvent sur le visage, parfois sur le dos des mains. Nous en avons observé un du scrotum et un autre du nez. Ils sont assez rares: 2,5% des malades que nous avons observés.

Dermatitis, verursacht durch das Insekt
Simulium erythrocephalum

A. Krstitsch, Dermato-venerologische Abteilung, Allgemeines Krankenhaus in Zemun-Beograd und
V. Zivkovitch, Parasitologische Abteilung, Institut für medizinische Forschungen, Beograd (Jugoslawien)

Im Laufe der Monate Juni und Juli 1965 hatten wir öfters Gelegenheit, bei unseren Patienten der Purpura ähnliche Veränderungen auf der Haut zu beobachten, die aber bei allen anderen Merkmalen ein ziemlich gleichmäßiges Bild ergaben. Bei allen Fällen handelte es sich um die Veränderungen, die durch die Stiche einer Kriebelmückenart — Simulium erythrocephalum DE GEER 1776 (Diptera, Simuliidae) verursacht werden. Zweite Hälfte Juni, Anfang Juli 1965, kam es zu einer Invasion dieser Insekten auf dem Gebiet der Vojvodina (nordöstliches Jugoslawien). Diese Kriebelmücke hat in Schwärmen die Menschen und Haustiere angegriffen und gestochen. Am meisten hat sie in frühen Morgenstunden und vor dem Sonnenuntergang angegriffen. Bei schwülem Wetter und vor dem Regen sind diese Simulie angriffslustig gewesen. An einigen Tagen waren die Mücken so zahlreich und aggressiv, daß sie die Feldarbeiten erschwert und sogar unmöglich gemacht haben.

Um die Brutstätten der S. erythrocephalum in dem Invasionsgebiet von Vojvodina festzustellen, wurden die Donau auf mehreren Lokalitäten (in der Länge von 393 km) sowie zwei ihrer Nebenflüsse — die Drau (in der Länge von 12 km) und die Karasica — im Sommer 1965 untersucht. In allen diesen fließenden Gewässern wurden Eier, Larven und Puppen von S. erythrocephalum gefunden. Die reichsten Brutstätten hat man in der Karasica entdeckt.

Wir haben insgesamt 37 Patienten mit Veränderungen auf der Haut als Folge der Stiche von S. erythrocephalum behandelt. Die Mehrzahl dieser Patienten meldete sich im Monat Juli. Dem Geschlecht nach waren es 22 weibliche und 15 männliche Personen im Alter von 3 bis 62 Jahren. Die Veränderungen waren am häufigsten auf die unteren Gliedmaßen lokalisiert, seltener auf die oberen, im Gesicht, in der Hals- und Ohrengegend. Bei einem Patienten bestanden auch Veränderungen auf dem Rumpf. Die Einstichstellen wiesen hämorrhagische Veränderungen in Form von klar umgrenzten, unregelmäßigen Petechien und Eckhymosen (Durchmesser 1 bis 3 cm) auf. Auf diesen Stellen befanden sich öfters Bläschen mit serohämorrhagischem Inhalt. Nach dem Aufgehen der Bläschen bleiben bräunliche Krusten und Erosien mit nekrotischem Grund, die auch beim Ausbleiben sekundärer Infektion schwer verheilten. Sehr oft kam es zu Ödemen der ergriffenen Hautpartien, aber ohne Inflammationszeichen. Außer zwei Patienten, die Schüttelfrost und Schwächeanfälle hatten, gab es keine anderen allgemeinen Symptome. Am häufigsten spürten die Patienten nur ein leichtes Brennen und Jucken an der betroffenen Stelle. Bei einem Fall bestanden Zeichen einer Lymphangitis und inguinaler Lymphadenitis. Die Behandlung der Patienten bestand aus Zink-Talkum-Mixtur und antibiotischen Salben. Außer einer Patientin, bei der die Veränderungen fast 30 Tage erkennbar waren, verschwanden sie bei den übrigen Patienten im Laufe von 5 bis 15 Tagen mit restitutio ad integrum, leichte Pigmentation hinterlassend. Bei der hospitalisierten Patientin wurden keine Veränderungen im Blutbild, Sedimentation und Urin festgestellt.

Beim Aufstellen der Differentialdiagnose kann man die oben erwähnten Veränderungen mit der akuten Purpura verwechseln. Die Anamnese dagegen, weiterhin das saisonbedingte Auftreten, gewöhnlich kleinere Anzahl der hämorrhagischen Veränderungen sowie die übrigen erwähnten Merkmale weisen auf die parasitäre Ätiologie hin. Von den übrigen parasitären Dermatosen, verursacht durch verschiedene Arthropoden, unterscheiden sich die Hautveränderungen bei unseren Fällen durch ausgesprochene und ständig ausgeprägte hämorrhagische Komponenten, ohne exudative Papeln. Bei der Dermatitis ex insectis (Paederus), die in Jugoslawien von FANINGER und VUKOV beschrieben wurde, ist die erythemato-oedematöse Veränderung mit eigentümlich verteilten und ineinander übergehenden Pusteln charakteristisch für die Hautveränderungen.

Die allergologische Untersuchung bei unseren Patienten haben wir mit dem Antigen von toten Weibchen des S. erythrocephalum in einer Lösung 1:10000 in Form von intradermalen Proben angestellt. Von insgesamt 19 Fällen waren nur bei drei die Reaktionen stark positiv, wogegen bei anderen die Reaktionen negativ ausliefen*.

Um das Agens festzustellen, das durch Stiche des S. erythrocephalum verursachte Veränderungen auf der Haut bewirkt, haben wir mehrere Versuche angestellt. Zu diesem Zweck hat man dieselben Methoden angewandt, wie bei Untersuchungen der Toxine des Simulium colombaschense FABRICIUS 1787. Sowohl bei dieser Art als auch bei S. erythrocephalum stellte man im Extrakt der Köpfe und Thorax von Weibchen kein Toxin fest, sondern nur eine Protease. Nachdem proteolytische Fermente nach neueren Auffassungen eine wichtige Rolle spielen können, nicht nur bei dem Entstehen der allergischen Hautreaktionen, sondern durch ihren proteolytischen Mechanismus durch Polipeptiden auch bei inflammatorischen Prozessen, so nehmen wir an, daß diese Protease auf der Einstichstelle des S. erythrocephalum die beschriebenen Veränderungen der Haut verursacht. Dabei kommt es wahrscheinlich durch direkte Wirkung dieser Protease oder durch proteolytische Zerfallprodukte zur Permeabilitätssteigerung bei Capillaren, zur Gefäßerweiterung, Capillaritis und Entzündungsreaktionen der Haut.

---

* Experimentelle Arbeiten und Gewinnung des Antigens verdanken wir der Mitarbeit von Dr. M. LAZAREVITCH.

Contact Dermatitis from Static Electricity

H. E. BELLRINGER, Central Medical Establishment, Royal Air Force, London (England)

Following the discovery of an irritating dermatitis affecting parachute packers, an investigation was undertaken to determine the cause, during the summer of 1963. Out of a total work force of 27, 15 exhibited the dermatitis. Four males; eleven females; but approximately two females were employed for each male packer. The men worked in collarless shirts, with sleeves rolled up; while the women wore an open-necked blouse with short sleeves.

The parachutes were cleaned and dried in a room kept at a temperature of 80 ° to 85 °F (27 ° to 29 °C) with a 50% humidity, while a separate packing room was kept between 55 ° to 65 °F (13 ° to 18 °C) and also with 50% humidity.

Symptoms arose in the packing room only. Suspicion was centred on the nylon parachute cords, when it was seen that the cords were flicked on the ventral surface of the outstretched arm lying palm upwards on the long table. This enabled the cords to be held neatly together. This was precisely the area where eight of the patients claimed their rash first appeared.

Initially almost all the packers noticed a sense of "pins and needles" which eventually became more severe in those who developed the rash. This was a faint, reticulate, or blotchy erythema, deepening in places, with a tight cluster of minute vesicles where it was most intense. At times serous oozing was noticed, while the severest cases showed a number of small, superficial ulcers.

The rash appeared over one, or both forearms, and often extended to the other exposed areas, particularly the forehead, the sides of the cheeks and neck, across the shoulders and the top of the breasts. Itching could be sufficiently intense to interfere with sleep.

Both the symptoms and the rash waxed and waned erratically. They had been present, at intervals for periods ranging from a few weeks to more than a year. All noticed that discomfort was greatest towards the end of each week and that the rash disappeared after 3 or 4 days rest from work.

Subsequently one male and three females were found with the dermatitis at other parachute packing centres.

It was then noticed that quite a large amount of static electricity was generated, as shown by movement of hairs and fine particles, when the cords were passed over the arms. Subsequent observation confirmed that aggravation of the dermatitis always accompanied thundery weather.

Debris picked up from the ground as a cause of the dermatitis was eliminated by the careful cleaning prior to drying. As a small quantity of hydrochloric acid forms when nylon is exposed to sunlight, old cords were frayed and used as material for patch tests. No primary or secondary reaction occurred. Neither preservatives, bleaches nor dyes were used in the manufacture of the cords.

Enquiries were then made to the manufacturers of the parachutes and their components. The major supplier revealed that workers commonly complain of a prickling sensation when handling nylon cordage. Some show the characteristic rash from time to time. It is accepted as a minor work hazard, and very few need to seek alternative work.

Alerted by this experience, 16 women have been found with a similar, but less severe, dermatitis, confined to the lower legs. All noticed an association with some, but not all, brands of nylon stockings. The faint, erratically variable, blotchy erythema is quite unlike the nylon dye dermatitis described by CALNAN et al. (1958).

A further three women have presented with a much more severe erythema restricted sharply to the bare areas of the thighs between pants and the tops of nylon stockings. All were affected only when wearing a particular brush-nylon petticoat, but not on every exposure. Careful patch tests, using the garments and the colouring dyes have proved negative.

It seems reasonable to postulate that both of the last two groups of patients have also suffered from a skin reaction to static electricity generated and conducted by fine nylon fibre threads.

References. CALNAN, C. D., R. H. MARTEN, and H. T. H. WILSON: Brit. med. J. 11, 544 (1958).

Les études des facteurs étiologiques chez les dermatites de contact provoquées par le ciment

S. Perišić, A. Sofronić et D. Jovović, Clinique Dermatologique de l'Université de Belgrade (Yougoslavie)

Les études des facteurs étiologiques des manifestations eczématiques chez les ouvriers qui sont, au cours du processus de travail, dans le contact permanent avec le ciment sec ou humide, représentent un problème qui attire de plus en plus un grand intérêt. L'importance de ce problème résulte des conséquences qui se reflètent sur l'activité professionnelle ultérieure.

On sait que cet eczéma est une conséquence de l'action des différents facteurs: mécaniques, rhagades, érosions, macérations de la peau pendant le travail, de l'alcalinité du ciment — surtout humide, ainsi que la sensibilisation des sels métalliques, spécialement du chrome, qui se trouvent dans tous les ciments en quantités minimums.

Différents auteurs (Jaeger, Meneghini, Gianotti, Calnan, Fregert, Geiser et d'autres) ont trouvé un haut degré de sensibilité envers les sels de chrome, un degré plus petit pour les sels de cobalt et de nickel chez les malades avec l'eczéma des cimentiers. Le but de nos études était le suivant:

déterminer la fréquence des eczémas chez les cimentiers;

déterminer la fréquence des manifestations chez les cimentiers qui travaillent avec le ciment humide, ainsi que chez ceux qui travaillent avec le ciment sec;

déterminer le pourcentage de l'allergie latente chez les personnes qui travaillent avec le ciment.

Nous avons testé 193 ouvriers parmi ceux qui ont travaillé avec le ciment sec, d'autres qui ont travaillé avec le ciment humide.

Les testes epicutanés sont effectués avec bichromate de potassium 0,5%, avec l'oxyde pur de cobalt, aqua calcis 25%, sulfate de nickel 10%, avec le ciment sec et humide de deux usines yougoslaves: Beočin et Popovac. Du nombre mentionné des ouvriers, 18 ont présenté eczéma vulgaire, c'est à dire l'eczéma s'est manifesté dans 9,38% des cas. Ces ouvriers ont travaillé entre 3 et 30 ans avec le ciment.

Dans les groupes de contrôle il y avait 30 personnes qui n'ont pas eu de contact avec le ciment. De ceux-ci 23 personnes n'ont manifesté aucune dermatite de contact, tandis que sept ont eu des eczéma d'autre étyologie. Toutes les personnes testées ont été partagées en quatre groupes:

1. groupe: ceux qui ont la dermatite de contact et travaillent avec le ciment (35);

2. groupe: les personnes qui ont la dermatite de contact, mais ne travaillent pas avec le ciment (7);

3. groupe: les personnes sans manifestation cutanée (158);

4. groupe: les personnes qui ont une autre dermatose, mais n'ont pas de contact avec le ciment.

Les résultats des tests épicutanés sont présentés dans les Tab. 1 et 2.

A la base des résultats obtenus on peut constater:

que le pourcentage des eczéma des cimentiers chez les ouvriers qui sont en contact permanent avec le ciment est assez élevé (9,38%);

chez les ouvriers malades le nombre de l'eczéma est beaucoup plus grand chez les ouvriers qui travaillent avec le ciment humide (93,7%);

le pourcentage de l'allergie latente est également relativement grand (9,88%) — plus grand avec le ciment humide;

influence allergique des sels de chrome est la plus grande parmi tous les constituants de ciment;

19*

Tableau 1

Les groupes avec eczéma		patch test	Cr	Co	Ni	A. calcis	le cim. sec	le cim. hum.
1. person. 35	avec eczéma (18)	+	12	2	—	1	—	3
		—	7	17	18	16	18	15
	avec la dermatite non aller. (17)	+	1	—	—	—	—	—
		—	16	17	17	17	17	17
3. person. 158	travaille avec le cim. humide (103)	+	10	3	2	—	2	—
		—	93	100	101	—	101	—
	travaille avec. le cim. sec (55)	+	3	1	—	—	—	—
		—	52	54	55	55	55	55

Tableau 2

Les groupes	patch test.	Cr	Co	Ni	a. calcis	le ciment sec	le ciment hum.
2.	+	4	—	1	1	—	—
7 person.	—	3	7	6	6	7	7
4.	+	—	—	—	—	—	—
23 person.	—	23	23	23	23	23	23

Dans le Tab. 3 se trouvent les résultats des tests épicutanés positifs chez 16 ouvriers malades de l'eczéma de cimentiers spécifiés d'après l'allergent.

Tableau 3

Cr	Ni	C o	le ciment humide	no. des personnes testées
+	+	+	—	1
+	+	+	—	1
+	—	—	+	3
+	—	—	—	10
—	—	+	—	1
totalité des personnes sensibilisées				16

il n'y a pas de sensibilisation croisée, mais on peut constater une sensibilisation parallèles envers chrome, nickel et cobalt;

les facteurs favorisants ont un rôle important dans le mécanisme de sensibilisation.

Plants of North America that may Cause Dermatitis Venenata

A. P. ULBRICH, Detroit, Michigan (USA)

In North Central United States the most common plant causing dermatitis venenata is rhus radicans or poison ivy [1]. The variations of this plant range from the original germinating leaf of three leaflets to large woody vines 15 cm or more in diameter. The seed or drupe is readily eaten by birds and is a winter food for some 60 species [2]. The exterior is digested, but the hard seed or pit remains viable after passing through the birds digestive tract. A cross section of the stem shows an abundance of veins that contain the antigen. Following any trauma the veins fracture and the sap containing the antigen bleeds to the surface. The ability of the plant to extrude this material is phenomenal. While insects are not commonly found on the leaves, the leaves frequently show insect damage. A one-meter section of vine of rhus radicans was cut in late September. 3 months later both ends were cut off to remove the original exudate, and 10 h later it had again extruded potential antigen to a height of 12 mm. The leaf structure on cross section also shows the potential of antigen to any fracturing of its brittle surface. The plant, as it burns, disperses microparticles of toxin in smoke, combustion is incomplete. These particles may precipitate on patients or fomites. Another means of transmission are animal fomites. Often pets carry antigen on their fur causing dermatitis venenata. Patients exposed to fomites have a more diffuse dermatitis than when contacting the toxin from the plant direct.

The root is just as potent a source. A patient had transplanted a common shrub. She did not recognize that the shrub also had rhus radicans entwined through it. She fractured the roots and had been exposed.

The sap of rhus vernix or poison sumac [3] is as antigenic, but the plant is not as common and grows only in moist areas of high acidity. The shrub is 2 to 5 m tall with a compound leaf from 7 to 13 leaflets. Because of the height of the plant, the site of reaction occurs most often on the upper extremities, the head and neck. The reaction time is the same as rhus radicans, 6 h to 12 days. The leaf loses its chlorophyll early in the fall and becomes a brilliant red. The seed hangs down. The wood of both plants is soft, but may be made into furniture. The thouroughly dry woods do not transmit the antigen.

Euphorbia cyparissias has established itself well in its adopted land. It grows profusely along some roads. It also has been adapted to gardens and trimmed. A patient had her husband bring in the plant as she developed a dermatitis each time she pulled it as a weed from her flower garden.

Another euphorbia that is grown in flower gardens is euphorbia marginata. Fortunately, it is not often used as a table flower. One text [4] claims the juice of this plant can be used to brand cattle. I made one unsuccessful attempt to do this.

Podophyllum peltatum, the source of podophyllin resin, has the common name of May apple. The white flower is beneath its leaf. The fruit in autumn may be eaten, but the podophyllin resin is in the rhizomes and would be contacted by gardeners or those clearing wooded land. The leaf may affect some patients.

The cypripedium family of orchids have four species: reginae, calceolus, acaule and candidum. The seedpods may be antigenic. The first three favor a moist area of peat bogs and shade, the areas where rhus vernix is commonly found. Only the candidum [5] favors well drained areas of open sunlight.

Asmina triloba with the common name of Paw Paw has a fruit that may be made into jam or marmalade. The fruit is the more common source of antigen.

The ranunculus or buttercup family [6, 7] have numerous species in North America. When the plant is injured an unsaturated lactone, protoanemonin, is formed by the breakdown of a glucoside. This is contained in the leaves and stem and may cause blistering of the skin.

Arisaema atrorubens — Jack-in-the-Pulpit, is a plant readily grown in wild flower gardens. The leaf contains oxalic acid, but it is the seed or the bulb that would give more reaction. This grows in moist areas and here too patients who would dig this would potentially be exposed to rhus radicans roots. I had one patient who claimed her dermatitis was from Jack-in-the-Pulpit, but when I went over the site with her, I identified the broken roots leading to rhus radicans or poison ivy.

Lobelia cardinalis attracts people by its brilliance, fortunately it grows only in moist areas along streams and meadows so it is a rare cause of dermatitis.

References. 1. ULBRICH, A. P.: J. Amer. O. Ass. **64**, 10 (1965). — 2. PETRIDES, G. A.: A. Field Guide To Trees and Shrubs, 81. Boston/Massachusetts: Houghton-Mifflin Co., Riverside Press 1958. — 3. BILLINGTON, C.: Shrubs of Michigan, Cranbrook Institute of Science, 197. Bulletin 22nd Edition. Michigan: Bloomfield Hills 1949. — 4. KINGSBURY, J. M.: Poisonous Plants of the United States and Canada. Englewood Cliffs/New Jersey: Prentice-Hall. Inc. 1964. — 5. SMITH, H. V.: Michigan Wild Flowers, Cranbrook Institute of Science, Bulletin 12. Michigan: Bloomfield Hills 1961. — 6. FISHER, A. A.: Contact Dermatitis, 70. Philadelphia/Pennsylvania: Lea & Febiger. 1967. — 7. BURBACH, J.: Ned T. Geneesk **107**, 1128 (1963).

Kontaktekzeme in der Landwirtschaft

E. HEGYI, Univ.-Hautklinik der Komenský-Universität, Bratislava (Tschechoslowakei)

Die Palette der Ekzemnoxen in der Landwirtschaft verliert immer mehr ihre frühere Charakteristik und nähert sich der Fülle der Allergene in der Industrie. Die Ekzemnoxen in der Landwirtschaft sind charakterisiert durch ihre Zugehörigkeit einerseits zu den pflanzlichen und tierischen Allergenen, andererseits zu den chemischen Noxen, unter denen besonders die Gruppe der Agrochemikalien und Zement bedeutsam sind.

Die Kontaktdermatitis nimmt zwar in der Landwirtschaft neben den Berufsinfektionen einen bescheidenen Platz ein, ihrer Incidenz gehört aber in den Jahren 1958 bis 1960 unter den Berufsabteilungen der sechste Platz, in den letzten Jahren — inklusiv der Fälle in der Agrochemikalienproduktion — schon der fünfte.

Das Sensibilisationspotential der pflanzlichen Allergene ist steigend, z. B. Kamillenextrakt erwies sich in den letzten Jahren als ein Allergen von 6% Vorkommen und wurde deshalb in die Routineserie eingeführt.

Sehr interessant ist die Spezifität der phytogenen Allergie, die aber nicht verallgemeinert werden kann. Bei Tabakekzem reagierten manche Patienten nur auf eine bestimmte Tabaksorte. Die Spezifität und die Gruppenallergie war bei der Sensibilisation auf die Pflanze *Inula Britannica L.* durch phylogenetische Zusammenhänge bestimmt, da die Reaktion auf *Inula salicina, I. enzifolia, I. hirta* und *I. conyza* negativ, aber auf *I. Germanica*, die phylogenetisch *I. Britannica* am nächsten steht, positiv war.

Bei der Überempfindlichkeit auf technisches Hexachlorcyclohexan war es gelungen, das eigentliche Allergen, Delta-Heptachlorcyclohexan, aufzufinden und eine Gruppenallergie festzustellen, die einerseits sterisch determiniert (Gruppenüberempfindlichkeit auf die Stellungsisomere der Heptachlorcyclohexane oder auf Epsilon-Hexachlorcyclohexan-Ähnlichkeit der Konformationen), andererseits durch die chemische Reaktivität gegeben sein kann (Tab. 1, 2).

Auch Allergene wie Zement sind in den landwirtschaftlichen Betrieben häufiger geworden. Hier gelang es, signifikante Unterschiede zwischen den einzelnen Zementsorten festzustellen (Tab. 3) und im Falle der Zementart mit dem größten Chromgehalt, diesen Unterschied durch den unterschiedlichen Chromgehalt der Kalksteine aufzuklären (Tab. 4). Diese Befunde ermöglichten, den Kalksteinbruch mit dem hohen Chromgehalt zu eliminieren und so den Gesamtchromgehalt dieser Zemente zu reduzieren.

Tabelle 1. *Die Resultate der Epicutanproben bei gegenüber technischem Hexachlorcyclohexan sensibilisierten Patienten*

Geprüfte Substanzen	Patienten					
	1	2	3	4	5	6
Hexachlorcyclohexan (Rohmaterial)	+++	+++	+++	+++	+	++++
Alpha-Hexachlorcyclohexan	+	—	—	—	—	—
Beta-Hexachlorcyclohexan	—	—	—	—	—	—
Gamma-Hexachlorcyclohexan	—	—	—	—	—	—
Delta-Hexachlorcyclohexan	—	—	—	—	—	—
Epsilon-Hexachlorcyclohexan	—	—	++	—	—	—
Alpha-Heptachlorcyclohexan	+	—	—	+	—	+++
Gamma-Heptachlorcyclohexan	+++	—	—	—	—	+++
Delta-Heptachlorcyclohexan	++++	++++	+++	++++	+++	++++
Epsilon-Heptachlorcyclohexan	—	—	—	—	—	++
Alpha-Oktachlorcyclohexan	—	—	—	—	—	+++
Beta-Oktachlorcyclohexan	—	—	—	—	—	
Alpha-Pentachlorcyclohexen (1)	—	—	—	—	—	++
Delta-Pentachlorcyclohexen(1)	+++	+++	+++	+++	—	+++

Tabelle 2. *Die Ähnlichkeit der Konformationen zwischen Delta-Heptachlorcyclohexan und Epsilon-Hexachlorcyclohexan*

Delta-Heptachlorcyclohexan

e a a e e /a c/ $\rightleftharpoons$ a e e a a /e a/

e a a e a a $\rightleftharpoons$ a e e a e c

Epsilon-Hexachlorcyclohexan
e = equatorial; a = axial

Tabelle 3. *Chromgehalt der Zemente in vier Betrieben*

Betrieb	mg Cr^{VI}/kg Zement
A	14,94 ± 1,31
B	3,20 ± 0,24
C	5,06 ± 0,41
D	8,00

Tabelle 4. *Der Gesamtchromgehalt der Kalksteine aus fünf Kalksteinbrüchen des Betriebes A*

Kalksteinbruch	mg Cr^{VI}/kg Kalkstein
1.	0 (oder weniger als 0,5)
2.	etwa 0,5
3.	0 (oder weniger als 0,5)
4.	0 (oder weniger als 0,5)
5.	47

Die Entwicklung der landwirtschaftlichen Produktion und die technologischen Neuerungen erfordern weitere Aufmerksamkeit für die dermatologische Problematik in der Landwirtschaft.

L'automatisation dans l'industrie métallurgique élimine la possibilité d'apparition des dermatoses professionnelles de contact (orthoergiques)?

C. C. Oancea, Brasov (Roumanie)

En cadre d'une dissertation avec le sujet: «Les dermatoses professionnelles dans une grande entreprise métallurgique constructrice de machines», on a discuté l'automatisation, entre autres sous l'aspect si cette automatisation élimine la possibilité d'apparition des dermatoses professionnelles orthoergiques, notamment l'acnée professionnelle, parce que cette dermatose professionnelle est la plus fréquente dans les entreprises métallurgiques.

En général à cause de l'acnée professionnelle l'activité n'est pas interrompue, mais l'affection est inesthétique et par les complications que'elle peut présenter, constitue un important problème, dans le chapitre des dermatoses professionnelles.

Sur un nombres de approximativement 10.000 d'ouvriers d'une usine métallurgique, constructrice des machines, l'acnée professionnelle a constitué non seulement la dermatose professionnelle, mais encore, en général la maladie professionnelle la plus fréquente, en pourcentage de 80%, rapportée à toutes les autres maladies professionnelles.

On avait fait des recherches pour voir où se trouve plus fréquente la dermatose professionnelle orthoergique, aux ouvriers qui travaillent avec des machines automatisées, ou à ceux qui travaillent avec des machines sans automatisation (universelles).

En 1962 on constate que 18% d'ouvriers qui travaillent avec des machines automatisées ont présenté l'acnée professionnelle, devant 19% d'ouvriers qui travaillent avec des machines sans automatisation (universelles).

En 1963 le pourcentage des cas d'acnée professionnelle est de 8,66 aux ouvriers qui travaillent avec des machines automatisées, devant 8% des cas d'acnée professionnelle aux ouvriers qui travaillent avec des machines sans automatisation.

En 1964 le pourcentage d'acnée professionnelle est de 3,33% aux ouvriers qui travaillent avec des machines automatisées, devant 3,5% cas d'acnée professionnelle aux ouvriers qui travaillent avec des machines sans automatisation.

Comme on voit, la proportion est approximativement égale en ce qui concerne la fréquence d'acnée professionnelle aux ouvriers qui travaillent avec des machines automatisées et à ceux qui travaillent avec des machines sans automatisation.

En 1963 nous observons une fréquence plus grande d'acnée professionnelle: 19% aux ouvriers qui travaillent avec les machines automatisées, devant 8% acnée professionnelle aux ouvriers qui travaillent avec des machines sans automatisation (universelles).

Comment s'explique cette situation?

Les ouvriers qui travaillent avec des machines sans automatisation (universelles), peuvent remplacer l'huile minérale, dans le processus technologique de fabrication (la coupe et le refroidissement)avec d'eau et savon, chose qu'on ne peut faire aux machines automatisées, ou l'huile minérale n'est pas possible remplacer dans le processus technologique d'emploi de cette sorte de machine, tant en ce qui concerne le refroidissement et le graissage de la machine dans la perfection du processus de la coupe.

Si la quantité de coupeaux, dans l'unité du temps, croît, certainement la consomation d'énergie et de la chaleur croît aussi, s'impose donc l'emploi d'un liquide pour graissage et refroidisement, qui éloigne un pourcentage le plus grand possible de chaleur développée et en même temps réduit le frottement au minimum possible.

L'huile minérale offre aussi encore des avantages qui pour le moment ne peuvent être remplacés dans le processus technologique, comme sont : 1. une consommation réduite d'énergie de la machine, 2. la suppresion presque complète des vibrations entre la pièce travailleuse et l'outil coupeur, s'obtient ainsi une face plus uniforme des superfices coupées, 3. enfin la conservation en temps prolongé des outils coupeurs. Resulte d'ici que, bien que la machine soit automatisée, la main d'ouvrier, qui dessert cette machine, ou plusieurs machines automatisées, car un seul ouvrier peut travailler, avec plusieurs machines automatisées, en même temps, vient en contact direct avec l'huile minérale en différentes phases du processus technologique : au changement des machines, au contrôle des pièces pendant le processus du fonctionement, au contrôle des machines au cas ou celles-ci s'arrètent et enfin la réception du matériel fini.

Ainsi s'explique pourquoi la proportion entre la fréquence d'acnée professionnelle est approximativement égale aux ouvriers qui travaillent avec les machines automatisées et à ceux qui travaillent avec les machines sans automatisation (universelles). L'automatisation n'éloigne pas le contact direct entre la main d'ouvrier et l'huile minérale, indispensable justement à cette sorte de machines ; en conséquence l'acnée professionelle peut apparaître.

Le médecin dermatologique de l'entreprise métallurgique est obligé d'accorder toute l'attention aussi aux ouvriers qui travaillent avec les machines automatisées. Donc l'automatisation dans l'industrie métallurgique n'élimine pas la possibilité d'apparition des dermatoses professionnelles de contact (orthoergiques)!

Bibliographie. La thèse de doctorat pour obtenir le titre de Docteur en Sciences Médicales du Dr. CONSTANTIN C. OANCEA, Romania-Brasov, p. 23, 31, 41, 74.

Virus Infections of the Skin and Mucosa

Maladies virales cutanéo-muqueuses

Afecciones, por virus, de la piel y de las mucosas

Virusinfektionen der Haut und der Schleimhaut

Organizer

J. GAY PRIETO, Spain

Presidents

R. D. AZULAY, Brazil

A. CROSTI, Italy

A. C. CURTIS, USA

M. MONACELLI, Italy

Delegate of the Organization Committee:

A. GREITHER, Germany

Reports

Neuere Entwicklungen dermatologischer Virusforschung

Th. Nasemann, Dermatologische Klinik der Universität München (Deutschland)

In dieser Einführung zum 4. Hauptthema des Kongresses, das die dermatologische Virusforschung zum Gegenstand hat, soll versucht werden, nicht nur die neueren Entwicklungen experimenteller Virologie in ihrer Bedeutung für unser Fach aufzuzeigen, sondern auch auf Ergebnisse hinzuweisen, die für Praxis und Klinik wichtig sind und in den Vordergrund des Interesses rückten. Der Organisator dieses Themenkreises Gay Prieto hat in glücklicher Weise den Rahmen weit gesteckt. So reicht das Spektrum dieses Vormittags vom kleinsten dermotropen Virus, dem Erreger der Maul- und Klauenseuche (hierüber berichtet das Referat von Warin), bis zu den Rickettsienarten, durch deren Befall auch Hauterscheinungen bedingt werden. Hierüber wird später Nicolau vortragen. Im folgenden gilt es weniger auf Erreichtes zurückzublicken — das ist Aufgabe der Handbücher! — sondern vielmehr die gegenwärtigen Tendenzen und ihre Ziele darzustellen. Dies soll in fünf Abschnitten geschehen, wobei die Kürze der Zeit nur eine subjektive Auswahl zuläßt.

I. *Wie wird heute methodisch vorgegangen, um bei einer Krankheit mit noch unbekannter Ätiologie, für die eine Virusgenese vermutet wird, den Virusnachweis zu erbringen?*

Nicht alle Veröffentlichungen der letzten Jahre auf diesem Sektor brachten jeder Kritik standhaltende Beweise bei. Noch immer — das sollte nicht vergessen werden! — gelten hier die von Henle und Koch aufgestellten Postulate. Die entscheidenden Kriterien sind also: *Nachweis, Isolierung* und *Charakterisierung* des Erregers. So wichtig mikromorphologische Befunde nach Einführung der Elektronenmikroskopie für die Virologie auch geworden sind, sie allein reichen nicht aus. Dies sei an einem Beispiel demonstriert. Zelickson (1961/62) fand bei seinen schönen Dünnschnittuntersuchungen beim Keratoakanthom im Zellkern der Epithelien Spiralkörper von gut Rickettsiengröße. Schon von anderer Seite war die mögliche Virusätiologie dieser Tumoren diskutiert worden. Was lag also näher, diese Einschlüsse für den ursächlichen „Viruserreger" zu halten?! Diese aus mehreren Lamellen aufgebauten intranucleären Spiralkörper sind aber sicher keine Viruselemente, noch sind sie überhaupt spezifische Bildungen. Sie kommen u. a. bei der Sarkoidose, bei spitzen Kondylomen, bei der Psoriasis vulgaris, beim Lichen ruber und vulgären Warzen vor. Sie sind möglicherweise nur Ausdruck einer Änderung des Stoffwechsels. Auch Bellone und Caputo (1966) faßten diese Inklusionen als unspezifische Bildungen auf, desgleichen Bierwolf und Thormann (1965). Morphologisch gleichen die von Forck, Fromme und Jordan beschriebenen Strukturen in Keratoakanthomschnitten viel eher Viruselementarkörpern. Caputo und Bellone zeigten kürzlich in Ultraschnitten vom benignen Schleimhautpemphigus andere Kerneinschlüsse, die zahlreiche 200 Å große Granula enthalten und insgesamt von einer Membran umschlossen werden. Kürzlich konnten wir analoge Gebilde elektronenoptisch in Sarkoidoseschnitten auffinden, und zwar im Zellkern von Epitheloidzellen. Wenn gleiche Gebilde in ganz verschiedenen Substraten gefunden werden, so spricht dies nicht für ihre Spezifität. Aus dem Arbeitskreis von Crosti werden wir nachher Details zu diesem Problem hören, vor allem aber den letzten Stand der Ätiologieaufklärung bei den blasenbildenden Dermatosen erfahren. Für mögliche Viruskrankheiten der Haut gaben

BLANK und RAKE (1955) die Direktiven ätiologischer Beweisführung an. Sie forderten die Erfüllung von sechs Kriterien, die hier nicht ausführlich aufgezählt werden können. Im wesentlichen aber sind es: 1. Induktion einer analogen Krankheit mit dem isolierten Virus bei einem Zwischenwirt; 2. Rückübertragung auch nach zahlreichen Passagen in Zwischenwirten auf freiwillige Versuchspersonen, Menschenaffen oder höhere Säugetiere; 3. immunologische Evidenz (beweisender Antikörper-Titeranstieg im Serum des Kranken); 4. cytologische Resultate (z. B. Einschlußkörper); 5. Darstellung der Viruselemente im Elektronenmikroskop und 6. epidemiologische Hinweise auf die Infektiosität der Erkrankung. Die alleinige Isolierung einer Virusart in einem Laboratoriumstier oder in der Gewebekultur besitzt keine ausreichende Beweiskraft.

   II. Im zweiten Teil dieses Referates sollen einige *ausgewählte Fortschritte der Virusdiagnostik* erörtert werden.

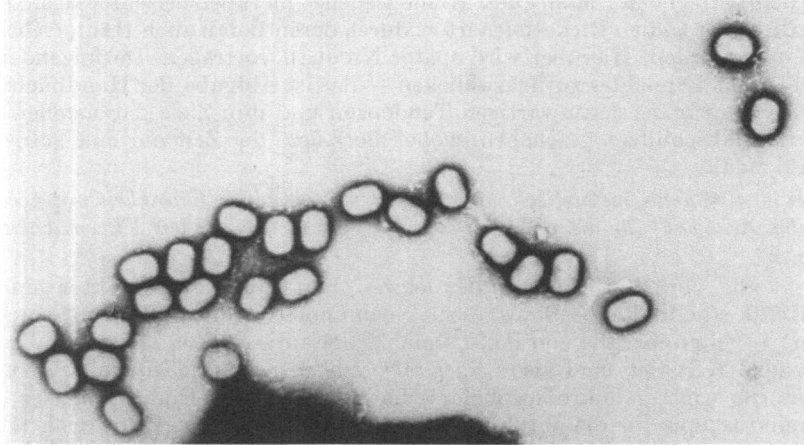

Abb. 1. Molluscum contagiosum-Virus, Negativkontrastierung mit Phosphor-Wolframsäure. Elektronenopt. Vergr. 28000mal

   Hier hat die *Elektronenmikroskopie* in der Tat revolutionierend gewirkt. Wir werden von STÜTTGEN hören, daß die elektronenoptische Präparation eine Schnelldiagnose der Pocken (Variola vera) erlaubt. Die Technik ist denkbar einfach — und das Ergebnis kann schon in wenigen Stunden vorliegen. Dies gelingt sowohl mit der direkten Präparation als auch mit der *negativen Kontrastierungstechnik* durch Phosphorwolframsäurebehandlung (negative staining technique). Dieses Verfahren ist auch zum Nachweis des Vaccinevirus (z. B. bei einem Fall von Eczema vaccinatum), des Molluscum contagiosum- und Melkerknoten-Virus (s. Abb. 1) geeignet, ebenfalls — wie SÖLTZ-SZÖTS (1967) zeigen konnte — zur Darstellung des Zostervirus. Die Präparationen brauchen nicht einmal extrem sauber zu sein. Selbst in Eiweißniederschlägen leuchten die Elementarkörper hell auf und machen so ihre Erkennung möglich. Die kleinen Viren der Herpesgruppe sind dieser Methode auch zugänglich und jede moderne Hautklinik, in der elektronenmikroskopisch gearbeitet werden kann, ist ohne weiteres in der Lage, Virusdiagnostik durch Negativkontrastierung zu betreiben. Noch genauere Aussage über die Feinstruktur der Viren erlaubt die elektronenoptische Analyse ultradünner Schnitte. Die *Ultramikrotomie* hat in den letzten Jahren bedeutende Fortschritte gemacht. Dies sei an einigen Dünnschnitten von Molluscum contagiosum, Herpes simplex und Warzen demonstriert (s. Abb. 2 bis 4!). Auch von BLANK werden wir

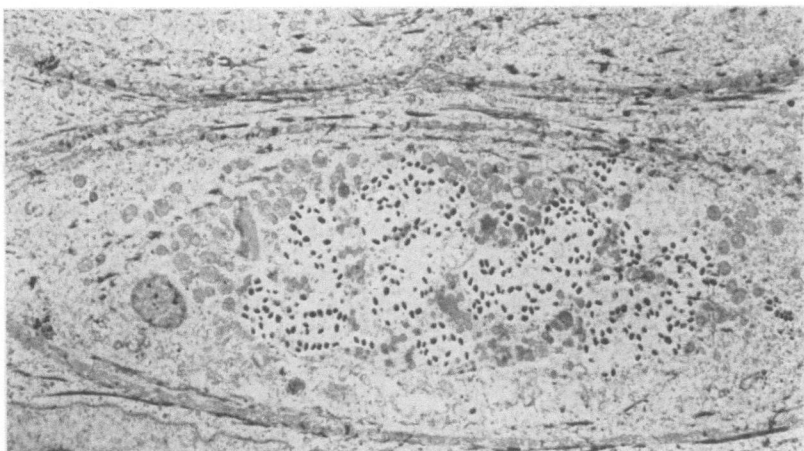

Abb. 2. Molluscum contagiosum, Ultraschnitt. Spinalzelle mit zahlreichen Elementarkörpern im Cytoplasma, darum herum Wall aus Mitochondrien. Elektronenopt. Vergr. 6000mal

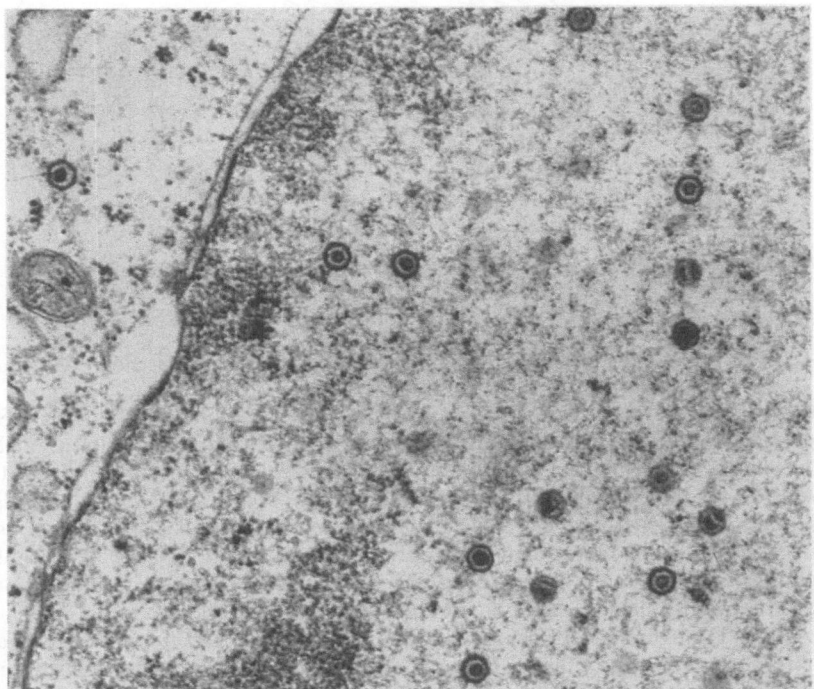

Abb. 3. Herpes simplex-Virus in HeLa-Zelle. Elementarkörper vorwiegend im Zellkern Ultraschnitt. Elektronenopt. Vergr. 70000mal

nachher sicher schöne Schnittbilder gezeigt bekommen. Weiteres Bildmaterial ist in der wissenschaftlichen Ausstellung zu sehen!

Die Methode der Isolierung von Viren in *Zellkulturen* findet immer mehr Berücksichtigung in der dermatologischen Forschung. Erwähnt sei hier nur, daß es

1961 MENDELSON und KLIGMAN gelang, das Warzenvirus in Zellkulturen aus Affen-
nierenepithel zu züchten. Neben der Zellkultur eignet sich die elektronenoptische
Untersuchung von Dünnschnitten vorzüglich zur Analyse von *Virustumoren der
Haut,* über die uns SOHIER berichten wird.

III. Der dritte Abschnitt soll *klinischen Fragen* gewidmet sein. Der zeitlichen
Begrenzung wegen können nur zwei Krankheiten berücksichtigt werden: Die
Verrucosis generalisata und die *Herpessepsis des Neugeborenen.*

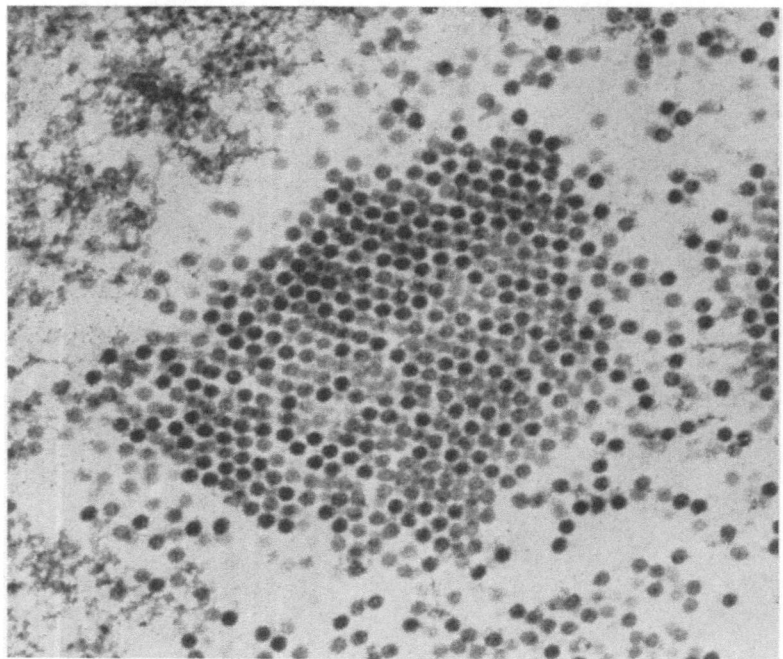

Abb. 4. Warzenvirusaggregat im Zellkern. Ultraschnitt. Elektronenopt. Vergr. 70000mal

Oft beginnt die *generalisierte Verrucosis* schon vor dem 7. Lebensjahr. Sie ist
zunächst an Hand- und Fußrücken sowie im Gesicht lokalisiert und kann nach und
nach große Teile der Körperhaut befallen, eventuell fast die gesamte Hautoberfläche. Die Läsionen gleichen überwiegend den planen, zum Teil auch den vulgären
Warzen. Auch das histologische Bild gleicht mehr dem der planen Warzen, jedoch
ist die Zahl der vergrößerten vacuolisierten Zellen besonders groß. Die Zellkerne
der letzteren zeigen eine ausgesprochene Pyknose und Fragmentierung. Spontane
Rückbildung eines Teiles oder des gesamten Krankheitsbildes wurde bisher nicht
beobachtet. Die Aussichten für eine erfolgreiche Therapie sind schlecht. Maligne
Entartung ist selten und kommt fast nur bei Kranken aus konsanguinen Ehen vor.
Hinsichtlich der Ätiologie des Leidens entwickelte sich bekanntlich ein Streit, ob
eine echte Genodermatose oder eine generalisierte Warzenform bei Vorhandensein
einer besonderen Disposition vorliegt. Durch Untersuchungen des Arbeitskreises
von JABLONSKA mittels gelungener Auto- und Heteroinoculationen unter Verwendung des Gewebsbreies der Läsionen wurde die Frage zugunsten der letzteren
Hypothese entschieden.

Die Herpessepsis des Neugeborenen wurde erst in den letzten 15 Jahren genauer
untersucht. Bisher sind etwa 60 Fälle in der Literatur beschrieben worden. Man

kann aber schon jetzt zwei Formen mit unterschiedlicher Prognose unterscheiden: 1. die meist bei Frühgeburten auftretende herpetische Sepsis mit schlechter Prognose, die in der Regel bereits einige Tage nach der Geburt beginnt, und 2. die Herpessepsis des Kleinkindes mit desto besserer Prognose, je älter die Kinder sind. Die Häufigkeit des Krankheitsbeginnes weist hier einen Gipfel zwischen der 10. Lebenswoche und dem 24. Lebensmonat auf. — Prädisponierend für den Erwerb einer Herpessepsis können verschiedene Faktoren sein, z. B. Toxämie und Hypertension bei der Mutter, Kaiserschnitt und Zangengeburt, Zwillingsgeburt, Unreife der Kinder und niedriges Geburtsgewicht, Cyanose am 1. Lebenstag und Cortisontherapie. MICHELS (1963) fand in der Literatur, daß unter 24 Neugeborenen mit Herpessepsis zwölf Frühgeburten und zwei operativ entbundene Kinder waren. Als Gründe für den bevorzugten Befall von Neugeborenen gelten physiologische Unreife der Leber und damit verbundene Unfähigkeit, Antikörper zu bilden. Auch das Knochenmark ist unreif und ist daher mitverantwortlich am Gamma-Globulinmangel. Da die mütterliche Leihimmunität erst in den letzten Wochen vor dem normalen Geburtstermin den Kindern verliehen wird, bedingt dies, daß Frühgeburten eventuell völlig ungeschützt bleiben. — Eine wirklich erfolgversprechende Therapie der Herpessepsis gibt es noch nicht, da alle Maßnahmen in der Regel zu spät kommen. Theoretisch ließe sich ein prophylaktischer Effekt nur von Gamma-Globulinen erwarten, wenn sie gleich nach der Geburt appliziert würden. Dies käme wohl nur dann in Betracht, wenn eine Infektionsquelle a priori angenommen werden muß, z. B. wenn die Mutter zum Geburtstermin eine primäre Vulvitis herpetica aufweist. Bei so gelegenen Fällen sollten sowohl vorher der Mutter als auch nachher dem Neugeborenen wiederholt Gamma-Globuline zugeführt werden. Außerdem sollten bei der Mutter die Haut- und Schleimhautareale mit Herpeseruption unter der Geburt sorgfältig abgedeckt werden. Schwestern mit floridem Lippenherpes gehören nicht auf Neugeborenenstationen. Übrigens werden nachher BASSET und ARMANGAUD über spezielle Fragen der herpetischen Primärinfektion vortragen.

IV. Hiermit wird schon der 4. Teil des Referates berührt, die *Virustherapie*, die nur kurz gestreift werden kann. Es darf daher auf die kürzlich erschienene Arbeit von ROHDE und HELLMIG (1967) verwiesen werden. Gegenwärtig ragen aus den vielen experimentell geprüften Substanzen zwei heraus: das bei Pocken und Vaccinia wirksame *Marboran*, um das es aber schon ruhiger wird, und das 5-Jod-2'-Desoxyuridin (IDU), das vor allem bei der frischen, oberflächlichen Keratitis herpetica gute Behandlungsresultate zeigte. Das IDU wirkt kaum noch bei der tiefen Keratitis disciformis, die eine kräftige Stromareaktion aufweist. Auch der Herpes der Halbschleimhäute (Herpes labialis, Herpes genitalis) spricht nur bei frühzeitiger Anwendung von IDU-Salben an. Experimentell fanden wir hierfür eine interessante Parallele. In der HeLa-Zellkultur hemmen schon 1 bis 2,5 γ/cm^3 Kulturmedium die Vermehrung des Herpes simplex-Virus. Mit vergleichbaren Konzentrationen wird aber in der Eikultur keine Virustase erzielt. Die Chorionallantois ist reich vascularisiert. Die Cornea aber ist ein gefäßloses Gewebe und kann im Aufbau eher mit einer Gewebekultur verglichen werden als die Allantois. Die etwa gleichgute Wirkung des IDU in Zellkultur und auf der Cornea hat also eine morphologische Entsprechung. Wahrscheinlich wird bei Gefäßbeteiligung das IDU rasch verstoffwechselt. Dies erklärt vielleicht die geringe Wirkung beim Herpes der Haut. Für eine interne Anwendung ist das IDU zu toxisch.

V. Der letzte Abschnitt ist der *Prophylaxe* gewidmet. Hier wurden in den vergangenen Jahren große Fortschritte erzielt. Erinnert sei nur an die Polioimpfung mit der Salk-Vaccine. In unserem Fach wurden von verschiedener Seite zur Behandlung des rekurrierenden Herpes simplex Impfungen mit einem inaktivierten

Herpesimpfstoff, dem sog. Herpin, durchgeführt. Die Tab. 1 orientiert über die Ergebnisse verschiedener Autoren.

Tabelle 1. *Ergebnisse der Vaccinationsbehandlung mit Herpin*

Arbeit von	Patienten-zahl	Besserung Anzahl	%	erfolglos Anzahl	%
BIBERSTEIN u. JESSNER	24	20	83,4	4	16,6
SÖLTZ-SZÖTS	74	~ 54	72,3	20	27,7
DEGOS u. TOURAINE	50	42	84,0	8	16,0
Münchener Dermato-logische Klinik	63	57	90,48	6	9,52

Tabelle 2. *Intracutantest mit Herpesantigenen*

Antigen	Mittlere Erythemfläche bei je 30 getesteten Patienten
Herpin Behring 66/24	45 cm²
Herpin H	30 cm²
Herpin G	15 cm²
Vacciniaantigen Behring	43 cm²
Leerantigen (Eimembran)	0
physiol. Kochsalzlösung	0

Wir fanden nun gemeinsam mit CALAP, daß bei intracutaner Einspritzung verschiedener Herpesantigene die Erythemflächen im Bereich der Impfstellen unterschiedlich groß waren.

Hieraus darf abgeleitet werden, daß ein universeller Herpesimpfstoff aus möglichst vielen Herpesstämmen hergestellt werden sollte. Wenn ein Patient auf die Impfungen überhaupt nicht anspricht, muß der spezifische Herpesstamm isoliert und zur Impfstoffgewinnung herangezogen werden. Wir erwarten uns noch bessere Resultate durch einen Hühnereiweiß-freien und durch Ultrazentrifugation angereicherten Herpesimpfstoff, der in etwa mit dem Grippeimpfstoff der Behringwerke zu vergleichen wäre. Mit diesem Ausblick in die Zukunft möchte ich dies Referat, das zu den folgenden Vorträgen überleiten sollte und nur wenige Details herausstellen konnte, schließen.

Pox-Viruserkrankungen

G. STÜTTGEN, Universitäts-Hautklinik Frankfurt a. M. (Deutschland)

Die Erreger der Pox-Virusgruppe gehören insgesamt zu den Quaderviren. Während Variola major, Variola minor und Vaccinia (Vaccinationen, Kuhpockeninfektion) durch Gemeinsamkeiten in der Entwicklung überkreuzter relativer Immunität gekennzeichnet sind, weisen Molluscum contagiosum und Melkerknoten als Paravaccine (NASEMANN) derartige Merkmale nicht auf (Abb. 1).

Die Infektion bei Variola vera und Variola minor erfolgt in über 90% als Tröpfcheninfektion über den Respirationstrakt. Es entwickelt sich eine cyclische Infektionskrankheit mit charakteristischen Stadien der Virämie, Initiatsyndromen und Hautsymptomen. Unter der Voraussetzung mangelnder Immunität kann sich auch bei cutaner Inoculation mit Vaccine- (selten) und Variolaviren kurzfristig eine Generalisierung der Hauteruptionen entwickeln, die gegenüber der Tröpfcheninfektion bei Variola eine Raffung der Entwicklungsstadien aufweist.

Ich möchte meine Ausführungen aus zeitlichen Gründen im wesentlichen auf die Variola vera beschränken, die durch die heutigen vielfältigen Kontaktmöglichkeiten mit den Weltpockenreservoiren (Indien, Afrika) und bereits erfolgten Infektionen in Europa in den Vordergrund getreten ist. Unabhängig von der

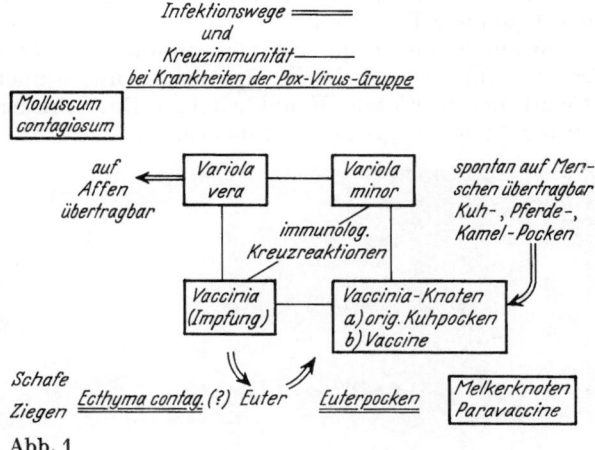

Abb. 1

praktischen Aufgabe des Dermatologen bei der Differentialdiagnose, ist die Verlaufsform der Pocken ein Beispiel für die Beziehung zwischen Morphokinetik und immunologischer Besonderheit. Die Prognose einer Pockenerkrankung entwickelt sich im Initialstadium bei Einsetzen des zweiten Virämieschubes vor dem Nachweis von Antikörpern [Hämagglutinationshemmtest (HAH), Komplementbindungsreaktion (KB), Virusneutralisationstest (VN)] und eruptivem Aufschießen

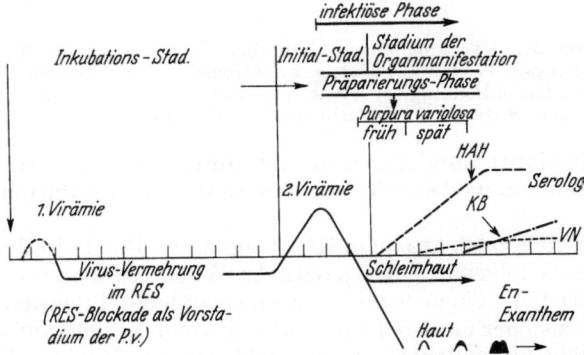

Abb. 2. Verlauf der Variola-vera-Erkrankung unter besonderer Berücksichtigung der einzelnen Stadien, der Serologie, des Exanthems und der „Präparierungsphase" für die Purpura variolosa (s. HERRLICH, 1967)

der Hauteffloreszenzen, deren Charakteristika Aufschluß über die voraussichtliche Entwicklung des Krankheitsbildes geben (Abb. 2). Je mehr das exanthematische Bild zur konfluierenden, schlaffen, flächigen Blasenbildung hinneigt, je mehr eine hämorrhagische Komponente sich in den Vordergrund spielt, um so dubiöser wird die Prognose (Abb. 3).

Während bei Vorliegen einer hämorrhagischen Diathese sich sekundär eine hämorrhagische Pustel entwickeln kann, entsteht die Purpura variolosa (P. v.)

spontan aus einer immunopathologischen Situation heraus, die arbeitshypothetisch einmal der Purpura anaphylakt., zum anderen dem Typ des Shwartzmann-Sanarelli-Phänomens (SSP) zugeordnet werden kann. Geimpfte und Nichtgeimpfte können an dieser Form der Variola erkranken. (Geimpfte: Nichtgeimpfte = 1,5:1 Männer: Frauen: Gravide: 2:3:5). Damit verdient diese Krankheitsform aus mehreren Gründen besondere Beachtung.

Die P. v. ist sowohl in der Frühform (subconjunctivale Blutung vor dem papulo-vesiculösen Schub) als auch in der Spätform (subconjunctivale Blutung nach dem Exanthem) ein sicher letales Krankheitsbild. Das Schicksal der Kranken ist mit Auftreten der hämorrhagischen Veränderungen in 24 Std besiegelt. Der

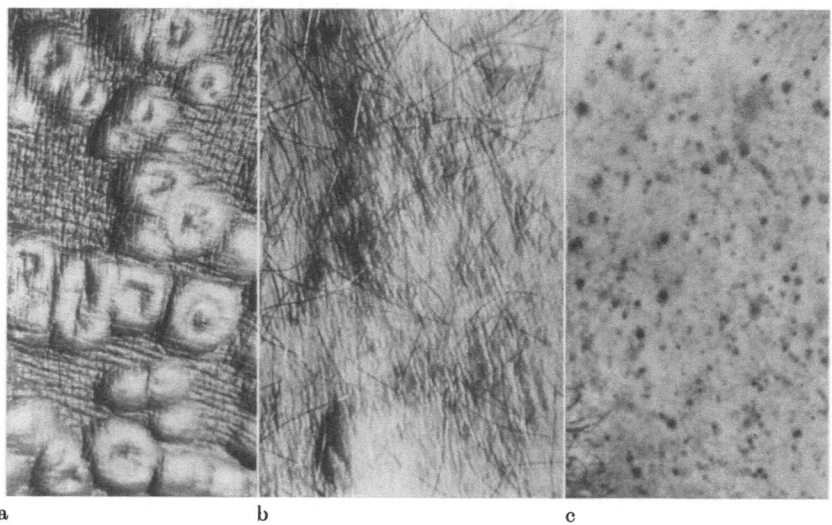

a   b   c

Abb. 3. Variationen der Exanthementwicklung bei Variola vera. a) Ausgeprägte Pustelbildung 7. Exanthemtag, 11. Krankheitstag. b) Hämorrhagische Blasenbildung konfluierend 4. Exanthemtag, 8. Krankheitstag. c) Kleine papulo-vesiculöse, petechiale Hämorrhagie bei Purpura variolosa vom Spättyp. 2. Exanthemtag, 6. Krankheitstag

P. v. geht im Initialstadium ein Ödem mit diffuser Rötung oder eine Urticaria mit Hämorrhagien voraus. Diese Vorstadien werden bei der Purpura fulmians vermißt (Abb. 4).

Eigene Untersuchungen an einem Krankengut von P.v. in Indien, Pakistan und Deutschland lassen folgende pathogenetische Wege diskutabel erscheinen:

1. Die Variola trifft einen bereits mit einer anderen Infektionskrankheit infizierten Organismus oder ein Infekt pfropft sich einer Variola auf (eine Gravidität ist einer Infektion äquivalent) bzw. die früheren Stadien der Variola sind die Präparierungsphasen, nach denen der zweite Variola-Virämieschub im Initialstadium das Blutungsübel auslöst. Bedeutungsvoll für die Entwicklung eines SSP (zumindest im Tierexperiment) ist der kurze Zeitabstand zwischen der Präparierungs- und Auslösungsphase.

2. Unter der Virämie ist eine Endothel-Antigen(Virus)-Komplexbildung erfolgt, die zum allergisch-anaphylaktoiden Zusammenbruch des Gefäßsystems unter den Zeichen einer Verbrauchscoagulopathie bei Thromboplastinfreisetzung führt. Es liegen Hinweise dafür vor, daß sich bei diesem Typ der Hämorrhagie ein Komplementverbrauch entwickelt, der die Neutralisation der Variolaviren verhindert und die außergewöhnlich hohe Virämie beim P.v. erklären könnte.

Untersuchungen der physiologischen Gerinnungszeiten im lyophilisierten Plasma akuter hämorrhagischer Purpuraformen der Variola zeigten einen etwa 50%igen Abfall des Fibrinogen (FI), des Prothrombin (FII), des Accellerin (FV) und des antihämophilen Globulin-A (FV) (BRÜSTER, DESAI, RICHTER und STÜTTGEN 1965). Verbunden mit einem hochgradigen Thrombocytenschwund geben diese gerinnungsphysiologischen Daten einen Hinweis für eine Verbrauchscoagulopathie.

Der Erfolg täglicher Infusionen von 200 ml Vaccine-Rekonvaleszentenserum über 8 Tage im Frühstadium akuter hämorrhagischer Variola vom Spättyp — noch ohne subconjunctivale Blutungen — (Bombay 1965) scheinen darauf hinzu-

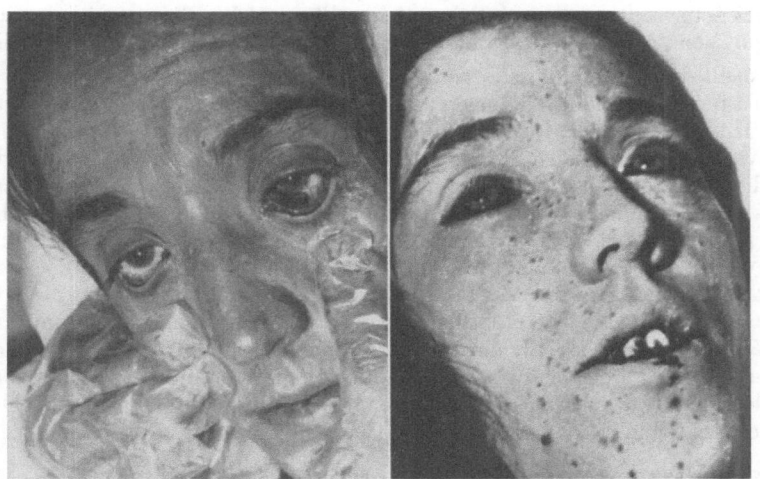

a   b

Abb. 4. Purpura variolosa vom Spättyp. a) Subconjunctivale Blutung, 2. Exanthemtag, 5. Krankheitstag. b) Weitere Entwicklung am 3. Exanthemtag, 6. Krankheitstag. Ante exitus

weisen, daß das Blutungsübel mit der Entwicklung der Variolainfektion verbunden ist, und daß bei Überstehen der hämorrhagischen Phase durch die obengenannte Therapie der cyclische Verlauf der Infektion mit Entwicklung diskreter Pusteln ohne Hämorrhagie seinen Fortgang nimmt.

Anaphylaktische Purpuraformen sind nach Vaccination selten beschrieben worden. Infektionsallergische Prozesse im weiten Sinne, gegebenenfalls kombiniert mit Unverträglichkeiten der Chemotherapie, sind Komplikationen der Infektionskrankheiten im allgemeinen einschließlich der Variola. Eine Abschirmung möglicher sekundärer Infektionen mit Antibiotica sollte erst zum Zeitpunkt der Pustelbildung erfolgen. Eine Prophylaxe der Variola mit viruciden Substanzen empfiehlt sich zur Zeit nur bei Kontaktpersonen im Frühstadium. Bei ausgebrochener Erkrankung steht nach unseren Erfahrungen die Verabreichung spezifischer heparinisierter Immunseren im Vordergrund.

Literatur. BRAS, G.: Docum. Med. geogr. trop. (Amst.) **4**, 303 (1952). — BRÜSTER, H., SH. DESAI, K. H. RICHTER und G. STÜTTGEN: Unveröffentlicht, Bombay 1965. — DIXON, C. W.: Smallpox, London: J. u. A. Churchill 1962. — HERRLICH, A.: Die Pocken. Stuttgart: Thieme 1967. — Handbuch der Schutzimpfungen. Berlin-Heidelberg-New York: Springer 1965. — KRECKE, H.-J.: Zum generalisierten Shwartzman-Phänomen. Stuttgart: Fischer 1964. — MARCHIONINI, A., u. TH. NASEMANN: Die Viruskrankheiten der Haut. In Handbuch der Haut- und Geschlechtskrankheiten, Ergänzungsband IV/2, Berlin-Göttingen-Heidelberg: Springer 1961. — STÜTTGEN, G.: Pox-Virus-Krankheiten in Infektionskrankheiten, hrsg. von GSELL, O., u. W. MOHR. Berlin-Heidelberg-New York: Springer 1967.

L'étiologie virale des dermatoses bulleuses généralisées (pemphigus et pemphigoïdes)

A. Crosti, F. Gianotti, E. Hahn et D. Bubola, Clinique Dermatologique de l'Université de Milan (Italie)

Ce n'est qu'au cours de ces dernières années que, grâce au progrès des recherches virologiques, la question dont nous nous occupons ici semble s'orienter vers d'intéressantes acquisitions.

Pendant ce dernier demi-siècle, périodiquement, les recherches expérimentales ont polarisé l'attention des chercheurs sur l'hypothèse d'une origine virale du pemphigus, sans que cette orientation ait pu avoir l'appui d'autres confirmations.

Les résultats obtenus dans le pemphigus par des cultures cellulaires et publiés par nous à partir de 1959 — nous en avons donné communication, entre autres, au Congrès International de Dermatologie tenu à Washington en 1962 — semblent avoir ouvert la voie à une série plus heureuse de recherches sur l'étiologie virale de la maladie considérée. En effet, depuis 1964, plusieurs groupes de chercheurs ont confirmé d'une façon ou d'une autre la possibilité d'isoler des virus pathogènes dans le pemphigus et dans la dermatite de Duhring (Kisljakova, Tseraidis, Zhdanov et Bogdanova, Földvari et Angyal, Studnitchine, Akopjan, Avakjian et Danilova, Gay-Prieto et coll., Schetscherbakow etc.) Ces recherches ont été par la suite étendues par nous du pemphigus chronique vrai et de ses variétés (végétant, de Senear Usher, foliacé, brésilien, oculomucosynéchant) aux trois autres groupes éruptifs bulleux à étiologie inconnue susceptibles de constituer des formes de passage aboutissant au pemphigus (dermatites de Duhring, épidermolyses congénitales graves et érythèmes exsudatifs multiformes.).

Notre expérience nous permet d'exposer les constatations suivantes:

1. Isolement des virus

Il est plus facile sur la souche cellulaire KB dérivant de l'individu humain ou la souche BS-C-1 dérivée de cellules rénales de cercopithèque, l'une et l'autre libres de toute infection virale spontanée.

2. Caractéristiques des cultures

L'effet cytopathogène est initialement modique et il faut avoir une certaine expérience pour pouvoir l'apprécier; il est plus évident dans les subcultures et permet le passage des virus à d'autres souches cellulaires et à l'embryon de poulet. Les altérations cellulaires, du type à foyer, provoquent la formation de masses syncitiales, plus aidées à observer en cas de souches isolées de l'épidermolyse bulleuse congénitale que si l'on a affaire au pemphigus ou à la dermatite de Duhring. Les virus isolés d'érythèmes polymorphes procurent une souffrance cellulaire légèrement différente et leur croissance est moins rapide. Dans les oeufs embryonnés, ces virus peuvent provoquer des fissures pseudo-bulleuses.

3. Titre infectieux

Ce titre, exprimé en TCID 50/cc — dose virale infectant le 50% des cultures tissulaires — est ordinairement inférieur à l'unité; il s'élève ensuite à la $10^e - 15^e$ culture et se stabilise ensuite aux environs de $10^5 - 10^6$ (Tab. 1). Le passage des virus dans différentes cultures cellulaires diminue le taux d'infectiosité.

Tableau 1. *Titre infectieux*

Souche virale isolée de	Sub-culture N°	Titre TCID$_{50}$/ 0.5 ml	Souche virale isolée de	Sub-culture N°	Titre TCID$_{50}$/ml
Pemphigus vulgaire	1	0,37	Epidermolyse	4	2,42
	7	4,8	Bulleuse congen.	12	4,27
	16	6,34	Type herpétiforme		
	25	6,4	(du sang)		
Pemphigus vulgaire	2	2,23	Epid. bull. cong.	1	0,56
	10	6,63	Grave mortelle	7	3,44
	20	6,58	(du sang)	16	6,54
				30	6,60
				38	6,15
Pemphigus séborrhéique	2	0,81			
	8	3,0			
	11	5,15	Epid. Bull. cong.	6	3,81
			Type dystrophique	14	5,50
			(du liquide de bulle)		
Pemphigus séborrhéique	3	1,21			
	6	2,67			
	11	5,69	Epid. bull. cong.	5	2,17
			Type herpétiforme	10	4,41
			(du liquide de bulle)		
Pemphigoïde	3	1,5			
	7	3,15			
	12	6,3			
Dermatite	3	1,5			
Muco-synéchante	5	2,49			
	10	5,85			

4. Matériel d'isolement

Les virus ont été isolés:

de l'organisme des malades (sérum de sang, liquide de bulle, liquide céphalo-rachidien, fragments de lésions cutanées et muqueuses);

de cadavres récents d'individus décédés des suites de pemphigus (cerveau, moelle épinière);

d'animaux inoculés (avec du sérum de sang, ou du liquide de bulle ou des filtrats de cultures infectées) et tués (sang, moelle épinière, cerveau, etc.).

5. Séro-neutralisation de l'effet cytopathogène viral

Elle a été effectuée moyennant sérums hyper-immunisés de lapin infectés par des souches isolées de cas de *pemphigus vulgaris*, de dermatite de Duhring, d'épidermolyse bulleuse généralisée et de pemphigus brésilien, avec les résultats suivants:

L'action cytopathogène est neutralisée par le sérum hyper-immunisé homologue à titre élevé (jusqu'à 1:512 pour IOO TCID 50); par contre, le sérum hétérologue hyperimmunisé ne provoque pas la neutralisation, ou ne la détermine qu'à des titres très faibles (Tab. 2).

Tableau 2. *Neutralisation croisée entre les souches virales isolées et leurs sérums hyperimmunisés*

		Sérums hyperimmunisés (lapin)			
		Pemphigus	D. Duhring	Epiderm. bull.	P. brésil.
Souches virales (= 100 TCID$_{50}$/ 0,5 cc)	Pemphigus	1:128	1:16	1:16	1:16
	D. Duhring	1:4	1:512	1:64	1:14
	Epidermol. bulleuse	1:4	1:32	1:512	1:4
	P. brésil.	1:16	1:4	1:4	1:160

Les souches isolées de cas cliniques différents semblent avoir une base antigène de groupe, mais chacune a une constitution antigène autonome; la séro-neutralisation croisée avec 10 souches isolées de l'organisme de malades de pemphigus appartenant à différents types cliniques et 11 souches dérivant d'érythème polymorphe a permis en effet de relever des différences immunologiques en pareil sens. Par contre, 5 souches isolées de cas de pemphigus foliacé brésilien et 5 autres isolées de cas d'epidermolyse bulleuse congénitale se sont avérées immunologiquement identiques (Cf. Bubola).

6. Séro-neutralisation avec sérums hyper-immunisés d'affections virales connues

Elle s'est avérée négative. Les sérums immunés d'herpes simplex, des trois types de poliomyélite, d'aphte épizootique A, de virus syncitial respiratoire, de rougeole et de parotite épidémique, n'exercent aucun effect neutralisant sur l'action cytopathogène des souches isolées de nos maladies bulleuses; un effet tout aussi négatif a été constaté pour les sérums hyper-immunisés de nos souches sur les pouvoirs pathogènes des virus cités, sur l'adénovirus 7 et sur le virus de Newcastle.

7. Typisation des souches virales

Une série de recherches plus vastes d'ordre physique, chimique, biologique et immunologique ont été effectuées sur quatre souches isolées de cas de pemphigus, de dermatite de Duhring, d'épidermolyse bulleuse grave et d'érythème polymorphe, en vue d'en effectuer la classification (Cf. GIACOMETTI et HAHN). Des recherches précédentes, effectuées également par le Dr. HAYFLICK de l'Institut Wistar de Philadelphie, avaient affirmé l'impossibilité d'identifier ces agents pathogènes avec les PPLO. Un rapport étroit a été maintenant confirmé entre les souches isolées du pemphigus, de Duhring et de l'épidermolyse bulleuse: il s'agit de virus RNA présentant des caractéristiques susceptibles de motiver leur classement parmi les Myxovirus. Le virus isolé de l'érythème polymorphe se différencie des autres: c'est un virus DNA présentant les caractéristiques des PaPoVa.-virus.

8. Expérimentation sur l'animal

Il a été procédé à l'inoculation intraveineuse, intrathalamique et médullaire de virus chez le lapin et le singe. Aucune des souches inoculées n'a donné épreuve d'une virulence spéciale: symptômes cliniques légers et transitoires, à part quelques parésies de l'arrière-train et quelques dystrophies graves parmi les lapins. Les animaux, sacrifiés à des distances de 2 à 12 mois, ont toujours présenté cependant (GIANOTTI et RONCHI) des dégénérations parcellaires nucléocytoplasmatiques des neurones corticaux, de la corne d'Ammon et des moto-neurones spinaux; les altérations les plus graves ont été constatées dans les ganglions spinaux postérieurs, qui présentaient les symptômes de la dégénération macrovacuolaire décrite par FOLDVARI et BALO chez les malades décédés des suites de pemphigus, dans l'organisme desquels ces mêmes Auteurs on pu prélever et isoler un virus.

9. Recherches au microscope électronique

Bien que nous les ayons effectuées à plusieurs reprises, ces recherches n'ont pu aboutir à aucune identification de virus sur le matériel humain ou sur l'animal inoculé.

10. Observations cliniques

a) *fréquence d'isolement:* l'isolement du virus du sang est relativement aisé chez le malade en phase active. Dès le premier prélèvement, le pourcentage de positivité dépasse le 50% des cas; il augmente encore avec l'intensification des recherches chez le même malade ainsi que dans le sang et les tissus malades. La fréquence varie également selon le type clinique examiné.

Nos recherches virologiques se sont étendues à un total de 300 malades: 100 cas de pemphigus vrai, 61 du groupe de la dermatite de Duhring, 79 du groupe des érythèmes polymorphes, 16 d'épidermolyse bulleuse congénitale, 23 de dermatites bulleuses mucosynéchantes ou de pemphigoïdes bulleux, 15 de pemphigus brésilien, 6 d'*Herpes gestationis* (Tab. 3, 4 et 5).

Tableau 3. *Pemphigus*

	Nombre de cas	Sérum pos.	Sérum nég.	Liquide de bulle pos.	Liquide de bulle nég	Liquor pos.	Liquor nég.	Encéphale pos.	Encéphale nég.	Moelle épinière pos.	Moelle épinière nég.
Pemphigus vulgaire Subaigu et chronique	70	40	30	15	7	4	1	7		4	
Pemphigus séborrhéique de Senear-Usher	19	14	5	3	1	1					
Pemphigus végétant	9		9	3	3		1				
Pemphigus foliacé	2		2	2							
Pemphigus foliacé Brésilien	15	15									
Guéris de pemphigus	12		12								

Tableau 4. *Pemphigoïdes*

	Nombre de cas	Sérum pos.	Sérum nég.	Liquide de bulle pos.	Liquide de bulle nég.	Liquor pos.	Liquor nég.	Encéphale pos.	Encéphale nég.
Dermatite de Duhring et pemphigoïdes	69	42	27	17	9	1	1	1	
Dermatite bulleuse Muco-synéchante (Pemphigus oculaire)	15	10	5	3	1	1			
Herpes gestationis	6	3	3	2	2				
Guéris de la dermatite de Duhring ou pemphigoïde	9		9						

Tableau 5. *Epidermolyse bulleuse congénitale grave*

	Nombre de cas	Sérum pos.	Sérum nég.	Liquide de bulle pos.	Liquide de bulle nég.
Epidermolyse bulleuse congénitale grave	16	14	2	6	2
Parents de ces enfants	14		14		

Tableau 6. *Erythème polymorphe vésiculo-bulleux*

	Nombre de cas	Sérum pos.	Sérum nég.	Liquide de bulle pos.	Liquide de bulle nég.
Erythème polymorphe	79	42	37	8	6

Le sang a été trouvé négatif dans le pemphigus végétant, positif dans dix cas sur 15 pour le pemphigus oculaire, entièrement positif dans les 15 cas de pemphigus brésilien. Les sujets guéris de leur pemphigus (11 cas) ont toujours donné des résultats hématologiques négatifs.

b) *enquêtes séro-immunologiques:* ces recherches se heurtent, chez le malade, à des difficultés considérables (antigènes anti-complémentaires, présence réduite d'anticorps dans le pemphigus actif); seule la séro-neutralisation de l'effet cytopathogène nous a donné des informations intéressantes qui nous permettent d'affirmer ce qui suit:

Le sang inactivé du malade n'exerce aucune inhibition sur cette action;

le sang des malades guéris de leur pemphigus (absence de manifestations depuis une période allant d'un an à 20 ans) neutralise l'action pathogène des souches de pemphigus et non celle des autres affections bulleuses considérées.

c) *cutiréactivité des malades:* l'intradermoréaction pratiquée avec les antigènes viraux a prouvé que les malades ne présentent aucune réactivité du type retardé; la réactivité devient positive dans les phases de régression de la maladie ou après guérison. Cette hypersensibilité est également présente chez les mères qui, après avoir eu des enfants atteints d'épidermolyse bulleuse dès la naissance, ont accouché d'enfants sains.

d) *interférence d'infections virales:* nous avons remarqué que la manifestation de la rougeole résout l'évolution des dermatites de Duhring graves et récidivantes de l'enfance.

Les interférences de quelques virus connus sur l'action cytopathogène du virus pemphigus dans les cultures cellulaires ont été particulièrement actives dans le cas du poliovirus 1.

Conclusions. Toutes ces données cliniques et expérimentales suggèrent de grouper pemphigus et pemphigoïdes, ainsi que les autres affections bulleuses à étiologie inconnue examinées ici, en un seul chapitre pathologique qui semble trouver son étiologie dans une infection virale. Des virus différents à activité principalement neuro-dermotrope et des conditions pathogénétiques différentes détermineraient les divers tableaux cliniques.

Les auto-anticorps anticutanés constatés dans le pemphigus et dans les pemphigoïdes par BEUTNER et JORDAN, et confirmés par nos recherches en tant que réaction liée au complément humain, ont une signification jusqu'ici obscure. Les virus isolés par nous pourraient déterminer la dénaturation des tissus, avec formation d'antigènes susceptibles d'évoquer des réactions autoimmunes. Il a été, en effet, récemment signalé (ISACSON, 1967) que les myxovirus — dont feraient également partie les virus étudiés par nous — agissent par l'intermédiaire de réactions auto-immunes.

Hand, Foot and Mouth Disease

R. WARIN and E. WADDINGTON, Departments of Dermatology, United Bristol Hospitals and Cardiff Royal Infirmary (England)

Historical. Hand Foot and Mouth Disease is an infection due to a Coxsackie A virus with characteristic lesions in the mouth, on the hands and feet and occasionally the buttocks and limbs. Outbreaks have been reported in 1957 in Toronto and New Zealand, 1959 in California, 1963 in Arizona and 1964-5 in Copenhagen. In the United Kingdom, the first outbreak was reported from Birmingham in

1959. In 1961 a few cases were seen in Bristol and Birmingham, and in 1963-4 there were reports of cases scattered over the whole of England. In 1964, the largest outbreak reported occurred in South Wales, and involved about 800 cases.

Epidemiology. The outbreaks have been explosive and often involved schools. In one school in South Wales 123 out of 374 pupils, and six out of eleven teachers developed the disease. In a follow-up study of the forty-two affected families one in six of the adults and one in eight of the children under 5 years became infected. Isolated pockets of infection have occurred in the regions involved. Apart from the outbreaks, occasional cases have been seen throughout the last 6 years. Because this is usually a mild illness many cases are probably not recognised. The seasonal incidence varies, but most cases have been reported in mid Summer and Autumn. The highest incidence occurred between the ages of 3 and 9 years and few adults are affected.

In most outbreaks cases have occurred with lesions confined to the mouth and Meadow (1965) considered that in these patients the lesions were slightly different from those seen in association with the rash elsewhere. However in the South Wales epidemic no such distinction could be made and the same virus was isolated from cases with lesions confined to the mouth. It has been demonstrated (HIGGINS et al., 1965) that mothers, brothers and sisters of the affected children commonly excrete the virus, although they may be free of symptoms.

Virology. A Coxsachie A virus has been isolated in all the outbreaks chiefly from the stools but also from vesicle fluid. The recovery rate from stool specimens varies but in the Bristol cases the virus was isolated from 20 out of 27 specimens examined. In all the large outbreaks the sero type of the virus has been A 16 but in the more limited outbreaks and in sporadic cases, A 5 and A 6 and A 10 have all been isolated from typical cases. The virus often remains in the stools for a period of 3 to 4 weeks (HIGGINS et al., 1965) and has been demonstrated for a period up to 40 days.

Clinical. The incubation period is generally between 3 to 6 days. Prodromal symptoms have consisted of headache and malaise, but in the South Wales outbreak most of the patients had abdominal pain and mild diorrhoea and two infants had a morbilliform erythema of the face and trunk for 4 days before the characteristic eruption developed. Constitutional upset in most cases is mild and lasts 2 to 3 days. In a few the temperature has been up to 39 °C and general symptoms have lasted 1 to 2 weeks. Although usually a mild illness, serious complications associated with Coxsachie A 16 infection have been described, including two cases of meningo-encephalitis, one of whom died, and fatal myocarditis in another child (WRIGHT et al, 1963; GOLDBERG and McADAMS, 1963; GOHD and FAIGEL, 1966).

Appearance of Mouth Lesions and Eruption discussed in the following paper page 336.

References. ALSOP, J., T. H. FLEWETT, and J. R. FOSTER: Brit. med. J. **1960**, 1708. — CLARKE, S. K. R., T. MORLEY, and R. P. WARIN: Brit. med. J. **1964**, 58. — FLEWETT, T. H., R. P. WARIN, and S. K. R. CLARKE: J. clin. Path. **16**, 53 (1963). — GOHD. R. S., and H. C. FAIGEL: Pediatrics **37**, 644 (1966). — GOLDBERG, M. F., F. MORTON, and A. J. McADAMS: J. Pediat. **62**, 762 (1963). — HIGGINS, P. G., E. M. ELLIS, D. G. BOSTON, and W. L. CALNAN: Mth. Bull. Minist. Hlth. Lab. Serv. **24**, 38 (1965). — HJORTH, N., u. H. KOPP: Hautarzt **12**, 533 (1966). — MAGOFFIN, R. L., E. W. JACKSON, and E. H. LENNETTE: J. Amer. med. Ass. **175**, 441 (1961). — MEADOW, S. R.: Arch. Dis. Childh. **40**, 560 (1965). — RICHARDSON, H. B., and A. LEIBOVITZ: J. Pediat. **67**, 6 (1965). — ROBINSON, C. R., F. W. DOANE, and A. J. RHODES: Canad. med. Ass. J. (1958). — SEDDON, J. H.: Research. Newsletter No. 2. Research Committee of New Zealand. Council, College of General Practitioners 1961. — WRIGHT, H. T., B. H. LANDING, E. H. LENNETTE, and R. M. McALLISTER: New Engl. J. Med. **268**, 1041 (1963).

Herpès de primo-infection en milieu tropical

A. BASSET et M. ARMENGAUD, Clinique des Maladies Cutanées de l'Université
Strasbourg (France)

Dès notre arrivée à DAKAR en 1956, nous avions été frappés par la fréquence
de lésions chéilobuccales au décours de la rougeole chez les petits Africains. Ces
accidents évoquaient la primo-infection herpétique; mais nous n'avions pas l'expérience clinique de cette forme, exceptionnelle en Europe; et ce n'est qu'après
plusieurs années que nous avons pu affirmer avec certitude la nature de ces
accidents bulleux.

Fréquence et gravité

La primo-infection herpétique est féquente en milieu Africain: 244 cas observés
de juin 1960 à janvier 1963 dans le service des maladies infectieuses de DAKAR,
soit 5% des hospitalisés. Elle est grave en Afrique: 10% de mortalité.

Facteurs étiologiques

1. *Le jeune âge des sujets* en moyenne de 1 à 4 ans, le plus jeune avait 8 mois,
le plus âgé 8 ans.

2. *L'association à une maladie intercurrente*, presque exclusivement la rougeole,
plus rarement une entéro-virose, la coqueluche ou la diphtérie. L'association avec
la rougeole explique le caractère saisonnier de la primo-infection herpétique; c'est
entre janvier et juillet, saison sèche au Sénégal, que sévit habituellement l'endo-
épidémie morbilleuse.

3. *Le facteur nutritionnel* n'est retrouvé que dans un cas sur deux (habituellement syndrome de malnutrition fruste, deux fois seulement un Kwashiorkor
évident); chez les autres enfants le taux de protéinémie est supérieur ou égal
à 60%.

4. *Le terrain*, les auteurs sud Africains (HANSEN, BECKER, McKENZIE) ont
constaté comme nous que la primo-infection herpétique est beaucoup plus fréquente en Afrique qu'en Europe, ils attribuent cette prédominance uniquement
aux troubles nutritionnels. Dans nos observations ce facteur est inconstant et
comme ces primo-infections se rencontrent presque uniquement chez des enfants
de race Noire il est logique d'incriminer le terrain de l'enfant Africain conditionné
par le mode de vie des Noirs en Afrique.

Symptomatologie

Il est caractérisé par un ensemble de signes muqueux, cutanés et généraux et
ne réalise jamais le bouquet d'herpès de l'adulte.

1. *Début*. Les premiers symptomes apparaissent entre le 5e et le 9e jour après
le début de l'éruption d'une rougeole.

2. *Signes muqueux et cutanés.*

a) les lésions chéilobuccales sont les plus fréquentes et résument parfois à elles
seules toute la symptomatologie. Elles siègent sur les lèvres, la face interne des
joues et la langue. Ce sont des lésions bulleuses de 5 à 10 mm de diamètre plus ou
moins confluantes, elles s'ulcèrent rapidement, saignent au moindre contact et
sont douloureuses. Elles réalisent un tableau de stomatite aphteuse. La gingivite
n'est pas majeure ni constante.

b) *atteinte cutanée*, peut aller de quelques bulles péribuccales, à l'envahissement
de tout le pourtour des orifices naturels de la face.

c) *formes bipolaires* accompagnées de manifestations bulleuses dans les régions anales et génitales. Dans certains cas, la primo-infection herpétique réalise un véritable syndrome d'ectodermose pluriorificielle.

d) *formes extensives* avec atteinte du pharynx, larynx et même de la trachée. Toutes les lésions cutanéo-muqueuses guérissent en général sans laisser de cicatrices.

3. *Signes généraux*. Leur intensité constitue un facteur de gravité. La dysphagie due aux ulcérations bucco-pharyngées aggrave la dénutrition et favorise la deshydratation.

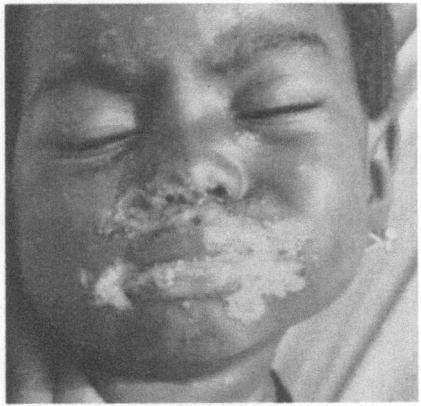

Fig. 1. Lésions cheilobuccales

a) la fièvre qui peut manquer dans les formes bénignes, se traduit par une courbe oscillante entre 38° et 40° dont l'acmé correspond à l'efflorescence des éléments cutanéo-muqueux. Elle se prolonge pendant une ou deux semaines; elle précède, accompagne, et suit l'apparition des aphtes.

b) *atteintes viscérales et nerveuses* hépatomégalie et encéphalite sont les témoins d'une véritable maladie herpétique généralisée.

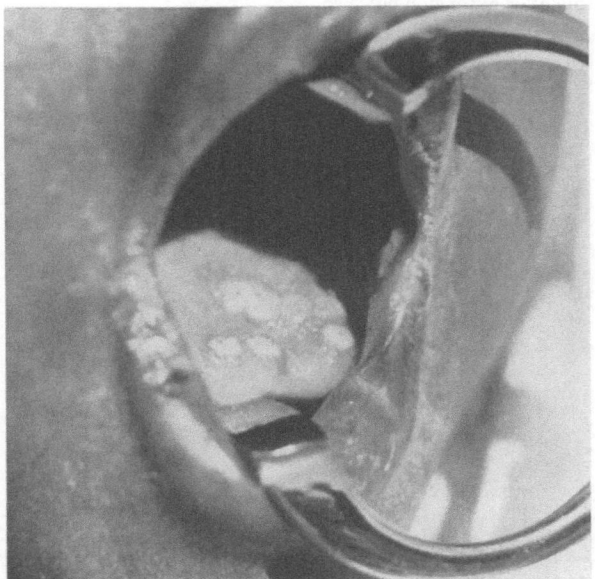

Fig. 2. Primo infection herpétique

Etude Virologique

La nature herpétique a pu être démontrée dans 42 observations.

1. *par la recherche des anticorps déviant le complément*. Faite à différentes périodes, elle montre que le taux des anticorps nul au moment de l'apparition des premiers aphtes croit jusqu'au 15e jour et persiste pendant plus de 2 mois.

2. *par les inoculations* — à des cellules de la souche K. B. — au souriceau nouveau né — à la membrane chorioallantoïde de l'oeuf — à la cornée du lapin.

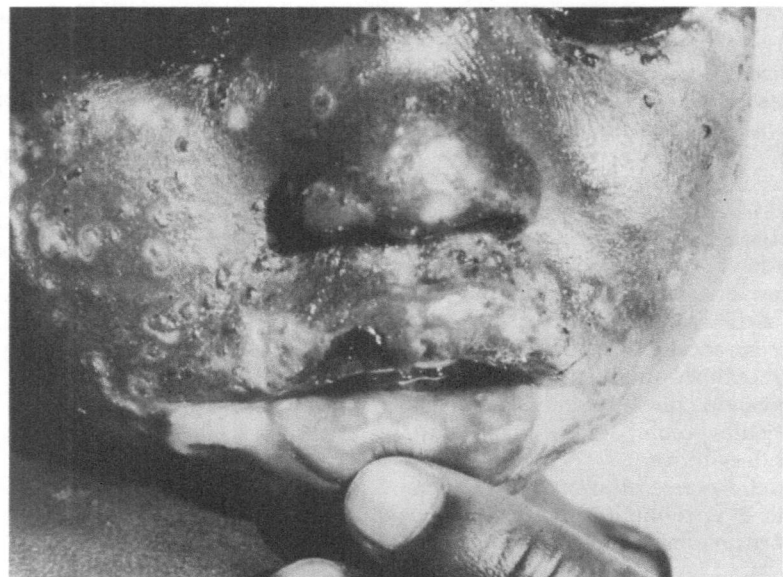

Fig. 3. Forme avec extension cutanée

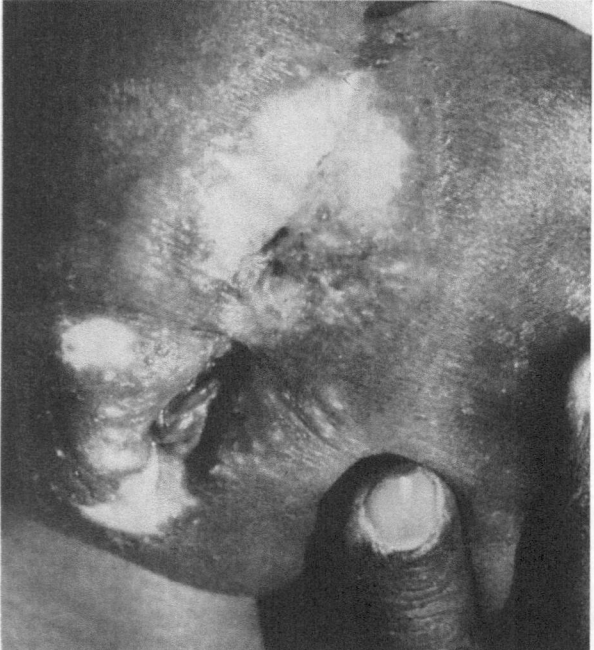

Fig. 4. Atteinte périano-génitale

Etude Anatomopathologique

Pratiquée chez onze malades, l'anatomie pathologique montre des lésions caractéristiques.

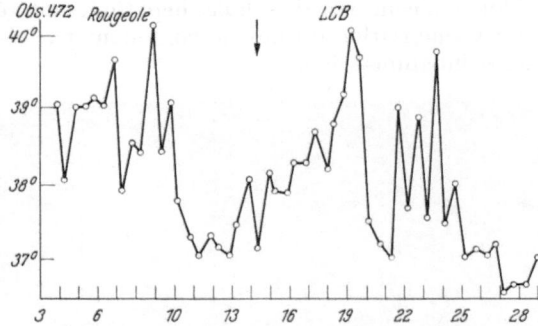

Fig. 5. Courbe de température. La flèche marque le
début de la primo-infection herpétique au décours de
la rougeole

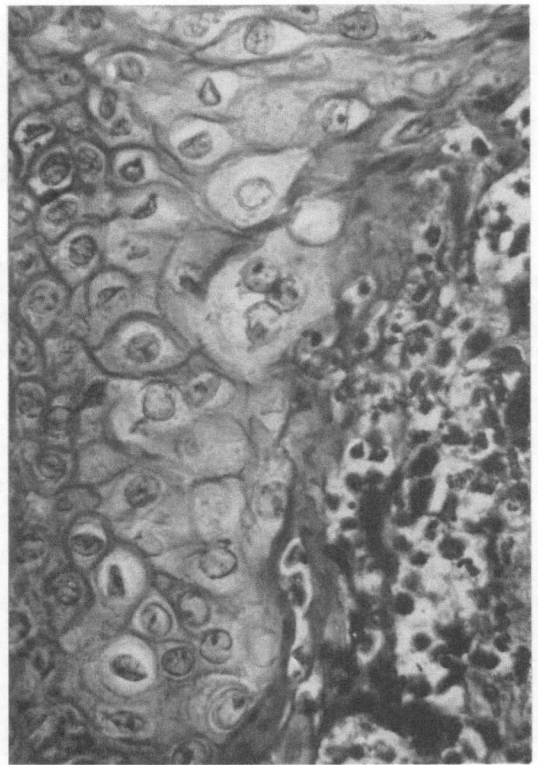

Fig. 6. Histopathologie de la langue, ballonisation des
cellules épithéliales

1. *au niveau des muqueuses* (buccales, pharyngées et même trachéales) —
nécrose — dégénérescence ballonisante de la couche de Malpighi (caractère pathognomonique).

2. *au niveau du foie*, hépatomégalie parsemée de foyers nécrotiques blancs
grisâtres de la grosseur d'une tête d'épingle, Microscopiquement autour de ces

foyers de nécrose acidophile, couronne de cellules hépatiques altérées (multinucléa-tions condensation ou vacuolisation du noyau, contenant parfois des inclusions), absence de phénomènes inflammatoires.

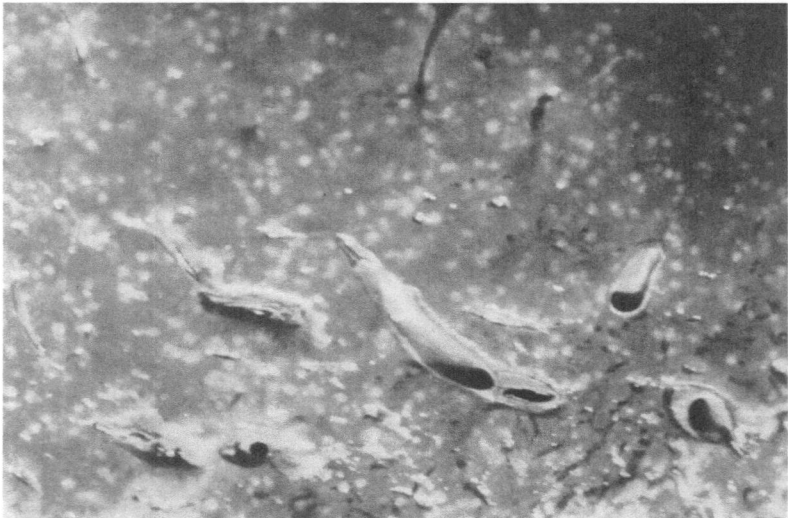

Fig. 7. Hépatite herpétique

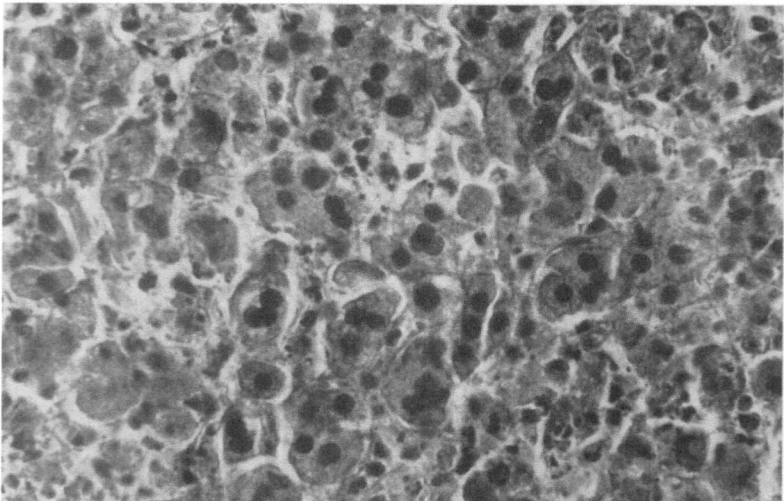

Fig. 8. Hépatite lésions microscopiques

3. des lésions herpétiques ont été retrouvées au *niveau d'autres organes:* (sur-rénales, système nerveux). Trois points méritent d'être soulignés — les lésions des muqueuses sont caractéristiques de l'herpès — les lésions hépatiques sont patho-gnominiques. Elles permettent de faire retrospectivement le diagnostic d'herpès généralisé — les broyats d'organes des enfants décédés ont permis d'isoler le virus herpétique par inoculation.

Diagnostic

Il repose sur l'identification du virus herpétique et l'ascension du taux des anticorps déviant le complément. Sans cette preuve biologique le diagnostic n'était pas facile à porter en milieu Africain.

D'une part, il existe de nombreuses autres étiologies : stomatites microbiennes, et moniliasiques : syphilis endémique ; avitaminose. D'autre part, on doit discuter le rôle de la primo-infection herpétique dans les syndromes de Stevens-Johnson, syndromes d'étiologie complexes souvent observés au cours des toxidermies.

Pronostic et traitement

Le pronostic dépend : 1. de la maladie herpétique elle-même ; les cas mortels sont le fait de formes généralisées. 2. de l'état nutritionnel bien que dans certaines formes léthales on n'ait pas trouvé la stéatose hépatique habituellement rencontrée dans les malnutritions de l'enfant africain. Le traitement consiste en réanimation, réhydratation et lutte contre les surinfections notamment moniliasiques. A cette époque, nous n'avions pas à notre disposition la vaccination qui aurait peut-être donné des résultats satisfaisants (R. Touraine).

Conclusion

La primo-infection herpétique en milieu tropical tire son originalité de — sa fréquence — sa gravité — sa localisation chéilobuccale réalisant le tableau de la stomatite aphteuse — de l'âge du sujet qu'elle atteint (dans les trois premières années de la vie).

Elle est semblable dans la grande majorité des cas à la stomatite herpétique de primo-infection exceptionnellement observée en Europe chez le jeune enfant.

Elle peut être à cet âge, bien que plus rarement, assez semblable à la maladie herpétique généralisée que l'on observe en Europe chez les seuls prématurés et nouveau-nés. Elle s'observe communément au décours de la rougeole.

Survey of 22 Cases of Behçet's Disease
The Significance of Specific Skin Hyper-Reactivity

I. Katzenellenbogen, Tel-Aviv University Medical School, Department of Dermatology, Beilinson Hospital (Israel)

It is by now will recognized that Behçet's disease is a protean disorder with a wide spectrum of clinical manifestations. As more and more specialities are concerned in the research into this disease, more and more laboratory methods are involved the more the differences in the findings and evaluation of the syndrome. In a disease often extending over many years the three phases of activity do not always occur. The outstanding feature of Behçet's disease is the non-specific skin and mucosa hypersensitivity. Diagnosis is possible with two major symptoms if this "pathergy" is present.

In 18 cases seen by us, cutaneo-mucosal signs preceded the eye symptoms by 2 or 3 years. During the course of the disease our patient's sensitivity changed. At the height of an attack it was more evident, while during a remission it often disappeared. In two women with Lipschutz-like ulcerations in the vulva and mild aphthous stomatitis, the non-specific skin sensitivity preceded the eye symptoms by 3 years.

Table

Case	1	2	3	4	5	6	7	8	9	10	11
Sex	M	M	M	M	M	M	M	M	M	M	M
Origin	Syria	Palest.	Leban.	Turkey	Turkey	Turkey	Irak	Irak	Poland	Poland	Russia
Age	24	41	25	40	30	40	22	33	48	36	26
Age at onset	20	31	21	20	21	25	19	23	44	28	19
Family history	X	X	–	–	–	–	–	–	–	–	–
First lesions	Eye	Oral	Genit Oral	Genit.	Eyes	Eyes	Genit. oral	Genit. oral	Eyes	Genit. oral	Oral
Eye lesions	X	X	X	X	X	X	X	X	X	X	X
Oral lesions	X	X	X	X	X	X	X	X	X	X	X
Genital lesions	X	X	X	X	X	X	X	X	X	X	X
Cutaneous les.	X	X	X	X	–	X	X	X	X	X	X
Thrombophleb.	–	–	–	X	–	X	–	–	X	–	X
Erythema nod.	XX	XX	XX	–	XX	–	X	XX	XX	X	–
Headaches	X	–	–	X	X	–	X	X	X	–	X
Remittant fever	X	–	–	–	–	–	–	XX	–	–	–
Neurolog. compl.	–	–	–	–	–	–	–	–	–	–	–
E. S. R.	XX	XXX	XX	XX	XX	XX	XXX	XXX	XX	X	XXX
Rheumat. symp.	X	X	–	X	X	X	X	X	X	X	–
Dysproteinemia	?	?	?	?	?	?	no	no	no	no	–
Pathergy	XXX	XXX	XXX	XXX	XXX	XXXX	XX	XXX	XXX	X	X
Relapsing Epid.	XX	XX	–	XX	–	–	XX	–	–	–	–
Urethritis	–	–	–	XX	–	–	XX	–	–	–	–

The table summarizes the data concerning the patients seen by us in the years 1943 to 1967. 22 patients were treated, 18 males and 4 females. 19 were natives of the Middle East, 3 were born in Europe. The earliest age at onset was 13, the latest 44. The great majority started in the twenties. In four cases there was a family history of oral lesions. 16 patients showed eye lesions, such as

Table (continued)

	12 M Egypt.	13 M Irak	14 F Maroc.	15 M Maroc.	16 M Yemen	17 F Yemen	18 F Maroc	19 F Persia	20 M Persia	21 M Persia	22 M Israel
Age	33	29	37	38	19	17	30	37	33	36	35
Age at onset	20	18	13	37	17	16	27	36	24	33	34
Family History	—	X	X	—	—	—	—	—	—	—	—
First lesions	Oral Genit	Oral	Oral	Oral	Oral	Genit	Genit	Genit	Oral	Oral	Oral Genit
Eye lesions	X	—	X	—	—	—	X	X	—	X	X
Oral lesions	X	X	X	X	X	X	X	X	X	X	X
Genital lesions	X	X	X	X	X	X	X	X	X	X	X
Cutaneous les.	X	X	X	X	X	X	—	—	X	X	X
Thrombophleb.	X	X	X	X	—	—	X	—	X	—	X
Erythema nod.	X	X	X	—	X	X	—	—	X	—	X
Headaches	X	X	XXX	X	X	—	—	—	—	—	—
Remittant fever	X	X	—	—	—	X	—	X	—	—	—
Neurolog. compl.	—	—	—	—	—	—	—	—	—	—	—
E.S.R.	XX	XXXX	XX	XXX	XX	XXXX	XX	XX	X	—	X
Rheumat. symp.	X	—	X	—	—	—	—	X	X	—	—
Dyoprotoinemia	X	X	—	XX	X	X	X	X	—	—	—
Pathergy	X	XXX	XXX	X	XXX	X	XX	XXX	XXX	XXX	XXX
Relapsing Epid.	—	—	—	—	—	—	—	—	—	—	—
Urethritis	—	—	—	—	—	—	—	—	—	—	—

recurrent iridocyclitis with an hypopyon, retinal and vitreous haemorrhages, retinopathy, conjunctivitis and episcleritis. All cases showed oral and genital signs. In addition to other signs, 18 cases had cutaneous lesions. In 11 cases thrombophlebitis was observed and in 11 cases erythema nodosum. 14 patients complained of headaches and 12 suffered from remittent fever. 2 patients had severe neurological complications. 7 complained of arthralgia. In 4 cases recurrent epididymitis was observed; in 2 urethritis was observed.

The outstanding feature in all our cases was the hyperreactivity of the skin and mucosa to any intracutaneous injection or needle prick. Within 24 h papules, nodules or pustules appeared on the skin and aphthous lesions on the oral mucosa. However, this hyper-reactivity, specific for Behcet's disease, was not stable and alternated in the course of the disease. It was manifested at the height of the outbreaks and faded away at the time of periodic remissions. This applied to Behçetin as well as to physiological saline. In a patient who displayed a "complete" Behçet syndrome with recurrent epididymitis, arthralgic pains and erythema nodosum, Behçetin test at time of remission was negative while positive with other solutions at the period of activity. The pathergy test was used to find out the state of the patient; often a positive test preceded the new outbreak. In one case we found a long delay before the test became positive.

R. M. female, married, age 28, born in Irak. In 1964 patient was seen with a large deep ulcer on the left labium vulvae and numerous oral aphthous lesions, including the tongue and with a superficial ulcer on the leg. Laboratory test: E.S.R. — 33/59, W.B.C. 7900, inversion of the A/G ration 3.40/4.30 but no increase of the α_2 and gamma-globulin. Pathergy tests were negative. 1967: Numerous oral lesions, no genital signs at time of examination, erythema nodosum-like lesions on the left leg, arthritis of the left knee and beginning of eye troubles; conjunctivitis and episcleritis. Laboratory test: E.S.R. 42/76, W.B.C. 8400, inversion of the A/G ration 3.8/4.5, increase of the α_2 and gamma-globulins and a strong positive pathergy reaction of the skin and the oral mucosa.

In this case the appearance of the positive skin tests 3 years later coincided with the clinical appearance of eye signs, monoarthritis and erythema nodosum-like nodules of the skin. Incidentally there was now an increase of the α_2- and gamma-globulins in the serum.

Control tests of skin hyper-reactivity in 20 cases with aphthous stomatitis of the recurrent type and in five patients with S.L.E. all proved negative.

Histological examination of early papules produced by Behçetin or physiological saline has revealed in both oedema in the dermis with diffuse inflammatory infiltrates. These infiltrates often perivascular, were composed of lymphocytes and a large number of polymorphnuclear leucocytes and eosinophiles. In biopsies taken after 48 h in addition the epithelium became necrotic as in aphthous lesions.

Treatment

Steroids in the treatment of Behçet's Disease have changed the prognosis of the disease and are helping the wellbeing of the patients. Comparing the fate of my first patients in the pre-steroid period with those treated later by steroids, the significant change in the prognosis becomes obvious. No patient treated in the post-steroid period has lost his eyesight, while in the first group 4 out of 5 became blind. Diamino-diphenyl sulfone preparations (DDS) were useful in some cases but could not be substituted for steroids at times of severe attacks. The question of the etiology of Behçet's disease is so far not definitely settled. My own investigations and those by more competent authorities have failed to verify the claims for a virus etiology. The auto-immune hypothesis is the only one to give some explanation of the hyper-reactivity of the skin and mucosa in periods of attack and lack in periods of remission. The spectacular morbidistatic effect of corticosteroids on Behçet's disease also suggests an auto-immune disease.

Contribution à l'étude du rôle des infections rickettsiennes et pararickettsiennes dans l'étiologie de certaines dermatoses à substratum vasculaire

St. G. Nicolau, C. Surdan et G. Noaghea, Central Dermato-Venerologie al MSPS et Inst. Inframicrobiologie al Academie, Bucarest (Roumanie)

Etant donnée la faculté dont les rickettsies et les pararickettsies jouissent de persister dans l'organisme, à état latent, un temps souvent indéfini après l'infection première et le tropisme spécial que leurs toxines affectent pour le système vasculaire et spécialement pour les capillaires, ainsi que la faculté qu'ils ont d'agir parfois par un mécanisme allergique, on a été amené à se demander, à juste raison, si les germes en question n'interviendraient-ils pas dans l'étiopathogénie de certaines dermatoses au substratum angiopate.

Les premiers résultats confirmatifs dans ce domaine ont été publiés en France, dans le courant des dernières années, par Bazex et par Degos. A notre tour, nous avons d'abord abordé l'étude de ce problème par l'examen de 112 cas de dermatoses à étiologie obscure (erythème migrans, erythème polymorphe, pitiriasis Gibert, pustuloses amicrobiennes, maladie de Behçet etc.), les résultats positifs obtenus dans chacune de ces catégories de cas ayant déjà fait l'objet de publications antérieures.

Dans la présente communication, pressés par le temps qui nous est accordé, nous sommes obligés donc de nous limiter à l'exposition des résultats obtenus dans le dernier temps, chez 40 malades, appartenant aux trois catégories éruptives suivantes: a) capillarites accompagnées de purpures anhémopathiques; b) ulcérations cutanées nécrotiques récidivantes et c) hypodermites nodulaires des jambes.

Comme moyen diagnostique de base nous avons utilisé la réaction sérologique de microagglutination sur lame, de Giroud, pratiquée à tour de rôle, dans chaque cas, avec quatre antigènes rickettsiens: r. prowazecki, r. moseri, r. conori et r. burneti, ainsi qu'avec deux antigènes pararickettsiens du type Q_{18} et T_{13}, ces produits provenant tous de l'Institut Pasteur de Paris. Nous n'avons retenu comme valable que les réactions, dont le titre minimum d'agglutination était de 1/820 pour r. prowazecki, de 1/160 pour r. mooseri et conori et de 1/20 pour r. burneti et les pararickettsioses. Dernièrement nous avons également utilisé, dans un nombre de cas, des intradermoréactions, pratiquées avec l'antigène s'étant montré positif dans le cas respectif, mais la technique et les résultats de ces recherches feront l'objet d'une publication ultérieure.

Le temps nous empêchant d'exposer les observations de nos malades appartenant aux trois groupes dermatologiques mentionnés, nous nous contenterons d'indiquer seulement numériquement les cas positifs découverts parmi eux.

I. Le groupe de dermatoses purpuriques était représenté par 16 cas, dont un revêtait l'aspect d'un purpura nécrotisant et les 15 autres celui d'eczématides purpuriques. Ajoutons que dans tous ces cas il s'agissait de purpuras liés strictement à des lésions vasculaires pariétales et indépendantes de toute modification de la crasse sanguine, ou des organes hématopoïetiques. Parmi ces 16 malades en question, 7 d'entre eux montraient une forte puissance agglutinatrice en présence des espèces rickettsiennes suivantes: 4 pour prowazecki, 3 pour mooseri et 1 pour les deux à la fois. Chez un huitième de nos malades, l'épreuve sérologique n'était que faiblement positive à une pararickettsie du groupe T_{13}, mais en échange l'intradermoréaction était fortement positive à l'antigène en question. Chez nos huit autres malades les réactions sérologiques étaient franchement négatives.

II. Le groupe des vascularites nécrotiques était représenté par 13 malades, dont cinq présentaient une réaction sérologique Giroud fortement positive aux anti-gènes suivants: 1 pour prowazecki, 2 pour conori, 1 à celui de la psitacose et 1 à celui du typhus murin. Dans ce dernier cas, atteint d'une ulcération du scrotum et de la cuisse, nous avons réussi d'isoler la souche rickettsienne en cause, par l'ensemencement du sang et de la moelle osseuse du malade dans le poumon de la souris, et dans un autre cas, atteint d'ulcérations du gland et ayant réagi au conori, nous avons pu mettre en évidence les corpuscules rickettsiens sur les coupes histologiques.

III. Groupe des hypodermites nodulaires. Six de nos 19 cas, dans lesquels on ne pouvait invoquer aucune autre étiologie, ont montré tous une microagglutination franchement positive, 3 d'entre eux au r. conori, 1 au prowazecki, un autre au mooseri et 1 dernier à 1 pararickettsiose du type T_{13}.

En conclusion, nous devons convenir que malgré les résultats confirmatifs ob-tenus jusqu'à présent, le problème des rickettsioses se trouve encore dans sa phase d'exploration et que nous ne devons nous y avancer qu'avec prudence. En effet, en tenant compte du fait que la majorité des moyens de diagnostic couramment employés aujourd'hui sont d'ordre indirect et, en attendant que ces moyens s'enrichissent d'autres plus probatoires, nous croyons pour l'instant, devoir for-muler, les critériums suivants qui représenteraient pour nous, dans leur ensemble, un minimum d'exigences nécessaires à l'affirmation d'un diagnostic de rickettsiose cutanée, sinon de certitude, au moins de très grande probabilité: a) une micro-agglutination GIROUD à un titre élevé; b) augmentation du titre initial de l'agglu-tination sous l'influence des tétracyclines, l'intervention du traitement en question mettant en liberté les produits solubles des germes détruits, et sa diminution ultérieure traduisant l'épuisement de ces produits; c) l'existence de données anamnestiques révélatrices d'une infection rickettsienne antérieure (critérium re-latif, car au cours de grandes épidémies, bien de cas évoluent d'une façon asympto-matique); d) l'épreuve thérapeutique aux tétracyclines, qui guérissent, parfois d'une façon spectaculaire, des lésions en question, chroniques et récidivantes depuis des années et, enfin e) l'exclusion de tout autre facteur étiologique possible.

En nous conformant à la discipline énoncée, nous croyons avoir pu établir dans certains cas de diagnostics de certitude et dans d'autres de très grande probabilité, de rickettsioses, dans un nombre notable de dermatoses à étiologie obscure jusqu'à présent.

Free Communications

Etude histopathologique des lapins et des singes inoculés avec des virus isolés du sang de malades de pemphigus et de pemphigoïdes

F. STROZZI, E. RONCHI et G. CHIAPPINO, Clinique Dermatologique de l'Uni-versité de Milan (Italie)

Nos programmes d'étude de l'étiopathogénie des affections pemphigo-pemphi-goïdes ont inclu une enquête sur la transmissibilité de la maladie à un certain nombre d'animaux, et précisément, dans notre cas, à 47 lapins et à 30 singes (Rhésus ou Cymolgus), moyennant inoculation intraveineuse et/ou intracérébrale ou intraspinale, des agents viraux cytopathogènes isolés du sang de malades atteints de pemphigus proprement dit, de dermatite herpétiforme, de pemphi-goïdes et d'épidermolyse bulleuse congénitale.

33 lapins ont été inoculés par voie intraveineuse avec des liquides de subculture de cellules KB infectées. L'inoculation a été effectuée avec 5 cc de liquide sur des cultures cellulaires (centrifugées à 1000 tours pendant 30') et ayant un titre infectieux compris entre 10^{-4} et 10^{-6}, tous les 5 jours, à dix reprises. Sur les quatorze lapins restants, l'inoculation a eu lieu par voie intracérébrale, avec emploi de 0,25 cc de liquide de subculture de cellules KB ou BS-C-1-infectées. Les animaux ont été sacrifiés à 60 jours de distance.

Les singes ont été inoculés, avec du liquide de subcultures infectées, par voie intrathalamique (0,5 cc dans chaque thalamus), ou par voie intraspinale lombaire (0,1 cc) et sacrifiés à un intervalle de temps allant de 2 à 12 mois.

Alors que ces inoculations n'ont déterminé que des symptômes cliniques très peu marqués — à part une parésie de l'arrière-train et une dystrophie grave chez quelques-uns des lapins traités, par contre l'enquête histopathologique effectuée sur les différents organes a révélé des lésions significatives.

Nous rapporterons, en résumé, les aspects histopathologiques constatés chez ces animaux, sans préciser les différences éventuellement attribuables aux différents types de virus et à l'intervalle de temps plus ou moins prolongé entre l'inoculation et le sacrifice de l'animal.

Les lapins présentaient des pathoses viscérales plus ou moins accentuées, mais c'est dans le système nerveux que les lésions les plus significatives ont été constatées.

Les lapins inoculés par voie intracérébrale ont présenté, dans l'encéphale, des signes de dégénération parcellaire nucléo-cytoplasmatique des neurones corticaux et des lamelles de la corne d'Ammon, ainsi qu'une dégénération grave des moto-neurones dans la moelle épinière.

Les singes inoculés par voie intrathalamique, ou dans la moelle lombaire, et les lapins simplement injectés par voie veineuse ont uniquement accusé une chromato-lyse centrale de quelques neurones moteurs, avec colliquation des amas tigroïdes.

Chez tous les animaux traités, indépendamment du siège d'inoculation choisi, on a constaté de graves altérations nucléo-cytoplasmatiques des ganglions spinaux postérieurs avec dégénération macrovacuolaire des cellules somato-sensitives. Autour des gros vacuoles contenant quelques rares résidus protoplasmatiques, les cellules capsulaires étaient aplaties, tandis qu'elles s'avéraient hyperplasiques et polystratifiées autour des cellules en état de dégénération.

La coloration de KLÜVER, pratiquée sur les singes, a révélé une démyélinisation du nerf efférent du ganglion spinal postérieur.

Cette pathologie correspond à celle qui caractérise — comme il a été donné de le reconnaître de façon certaine — les cas mortels de pemphigus chez l'homme; elle peut indiquer de façon significative la responsabilité casuelle des virus étudiés et de la pathogénèse de la maladie.

Caractéristiques physiques, chimiques, biologiques et immunologiques de quatre souches virales isolées de cas de pemphigus, de dermatite de Duhring, d'épidermolyse bulleuse grave et d'érythème polymorphe

G. GIACOMETTI et E. HAHN, Istituto Sieroterapico Milanese «S. Belfanti»
Clinique Dermatologique de l'Université de Milan (Italie)

Il a été procédé à l'étude des propriétés physiques, chimiques, biologiques et immunologiques les plus importantes et les plus significatives de quatre souches

Tableau. *Some properties of isolated viruses (log $TCID_{50}$/1 ml)*

Virus isolated from	IDUR ♀ 10^-4 M		pH 3, 2 h at 25 °C		Chloroform 5% for 10'		Temperature 1 h at			Guanidine HCL 50 γ/ml		Trypsin DIFCO 0.2% 2 h at 37 °C		Hemo-agglutination	Hem-ad-sorption
	n. tr.	tr.	n. tr.	tr.	n. tr.	tr.	25 °C	60 °C −MgCl$_2$	60 °C +MgCl$_2$	n. tr.	tr.	n. tr.	tr.		
Pemphigus	7.1	6.9	6.6	4.7	7.3	<1	6.4	3.2	2.9	7.0	6.9	7.3	6.9	+++	+++
Cong. bullous epidermolysis	6.9	6.8	6.2	4.5	6.9	<1	6.5	2.7	2.4	7.1	7.0	6.8	7.0		
Duhring's dermatitis	7.3	7.2	6.7	5.2	7.2	<1	6.8	3.9	3.5	7.2	7.0	7.1	6.9		
Erythema multiforme	5.2	<1	4.8	4.2	5.3	5	4.7	3.5	3.3	4.9	4.6	5.1	4.7		
Reference viruses															
Polio 1	7.8	7.6	7.2	7.3	7.9	7.8	7.6	2.1	5.9	7.7	3.9	7.6	7.5		
N.D.V.	6.8	6.8	6.5	1.9	6.5	<1									
Herpes S.	5.6	<1					5.8	<1	<1						
F.M.D. A												6.8	2.3		

n. tr. = non treated   tr. = treated

virales isolées sur des cultures de cellules KB provenant du sang de malades de pemphigus vulgaire (PV), de dermatite de Duhring (DD), d'épidermolyse bulleuse congénitale (CEB) et d'érythème polymorphe (EP) afin d'en effectuer le classement. Nos recherches et celles du Dr. HAYFLICK (de l'Institut Wistar de Philadelphie) ont exclu toute possibilité d'identifier ces agents viraux avec les PPLO.

Les souches virales PV, DD et CEB possèdent des propriétés analogues l'une à l'autre, mais différant de façon assez sensible de celles de la souche EP. Ce sont des RNA-virus, la 5-iododésoxyuridine n'exerçant aucune inhibition sur eux; leur composition comprend des lipides essentiels, leur pouvoir infectieux disparaissant à la suite du traitement par le chloroforme; la labilité de leur pH est assez réduite; leur thermo-résistance n'est aucunement influencée par la présence de chlorure de magnésium; la guanidine n'exerce à leur égard aucune inhibition, ni la trypsine aucune inactivation; elles agglutinent, enfin, les érythrocytes humains comme les érythrocytes de poussin et déterminent une hémoabsorption dans les cultures cellulaires infectées.

Ces souches traversent des filtres millipores à pores de 100 mμ de diamètre, en y perdant cependant une partie considérable de leur titre infectieux; par contre, elles ne peuvent traverser les filtres à pores de 50 mμ.

La séro-neutralisation croisée a permis d'identifier un rapport antigénique étroit entre les souches PV, DD et CEB; par contre, la souche EP s'avère nettement différente.

A notre avis, toutefois, les souches PV, DD et CEB sont différentes, ou constituent peut-être des sous-types d'une même souche caractérisés par un comportement différent en milieu de culture cellulaire: A) leurs courbes d'accroissement différent légèrement les unes des autres; B) la souche CEB est la seule à former régulièrement des syncyces; C) la souche DD — contrairement aux autres — ne se développe pas sur les cultures de rein de porc.

Le virus EP est un virus DNA (inhibition complète par la 5-désoxyuridine); son pH est peu stable; il résiste au chloroforme (absence d'inhibition par la guanidine, et de modification par la trypsine); il ne provoque aucune hémo-agglutination ni aucune hémo-absorption dans les cultures cellulaires infectées. Le virus EP a un cycle lent de croissance, il est considérablement thermo-résistant et sa stabilité ne semble pas devoir subir l'influence des cathions bivalents. Il passe au travers des filtres millipores à pores de 100 mμ de diamètre avec réduction peu marquée du titre infectieux et ne traverse pas les filtres à pores de 50 mμ.

Ces souches, inoculées par voie sous-cutanée à des souris et à des hamsters nouveau-nés, n'ont donné lieu à aucun signe clinique après 8 mois d'observation.

Les caractéristiques citées nous permettent d'affirmer, pour conclure, que les souches virales PV, DD et CEB appartiennent au groupe des myxovirus, tandis que la souche virale EP appartient à celui des PaPoVa-virus.

Etudes immunologiques chez les malades de pemphigus et pemphigoïdes

D. Bubola, Clinique Dermatologique de l'Université de Milan (Italie)

L'étude de l'agent causal et celle des aspects immunologiques s'avèrent également importantes dans le domaine de l'étiopathogénie du pemphigus et des pemphigoïdes.

Au cours de nos recherches précédentes, nous avons vu que les souches virales isolées des différents cas cliniques de pemphigus vrai, de dermatite herpétiforme de Duhring, de pemphigoïde bulleux, d'érythème polymorphe vésico-bulleux et d'épidermolyse bulleuse dystrophique grave appartiennent à des types antigéniques différents, même à identité de variété clinique, en dépit de l'existence d'une certaine corrélation antigénique fondamentale.

Les enquêtes effectuées sur dix souches virales, isolées du sérum de sang et du liquide de bulle d'un certain nombre de malades atteints de pemphigus vrai en phase active, se sont révélées en effet nettement significatives. La séroneutralisation croisée, effectuée au moyen de sérums autoimmunisés obtenus à partir d'un certain nombre de lapins, a permis de distinguer trois types différents de virus. Onze souches virales, prélevées de cas d'érythème polymorphe bulleux muco-cutané, nous ont permis de différencier quatre types antigéniques différents. Par contre, les cinq souches de virus isolées du sang d'enfants atteints d'épidermolyse bulleuse congénitale appartenaient à un type unique; un virus unique a été également isolé, d'autre part, de cinq cas de pemphigus foliacé brésilien.

La technique de la séro-neutralisation nous a encore permis de remarquer que le sérum de ces malades est presque dépourvu ou même totalement dépourvu d'anticorps neutralisant les virus homologues ou hétérologues; en effet, sur un total de 50 malades atteints de ces dermatites bulleuses, peu de sérums ont neutralisé (au titre de 1:4 à 1:8) les trois souches virales de pemphigus, alors que tous les autres se sont avérés dépourvus d'anticorps neutralisants. Par contre, les sérums de sang de douze individus guéris de leur pemphigus ont neutralisé 100 TCID$_{50}$ des trois types de virus de pemphigus, à un titre variant de 1:4 à 1:80, et les sérums de six individus guéris de leur dermatite de Duhring ont neutralisé le virus homologue à un titre de 1:8 à 1:32, sans neutraliser par ailleurs (sauf à faible titre) les souches virales isolées de cas de pemphigus. Signalons, à ce sujet, que nous entendons par «individus guéris» ceux dont les manifestations cliniques ont cessé depuis un an au moins, sans l'aide d'aucun traitement pendant cette période de temps; bien entendu, le sang de ces sujets a toujours été trouvé dépourvu d'effet cytopathique.

Nous avons cherché en outre à évaluer la capacité défensive aspécifique de ces malades moyennant dosage de la properdine effectué sur 37 sujets (12 cas de pemphigus vrai, 10 de dermatite de Duhring, 6 de pemphigoïde, 9 d'érythème polymorphe bulleux). Le système properdinique, évalué moyennant neutralisation du bactériophage selon la méthode de BARLOW et coll. modifiée par PERNIS et TURRI, a donné pour nos malades des valeurs de 2 à 23 PhN/50, avec une moyenne de 11,5 (valeurs normales moyennes de 8,7). Le taux constaté ne nous a semblé avoir aucune corrélation ni avec le type de l'affection, ni avec sa gravité; par contre, chez les sept sujets guéris de leur pemphigus ou de leur dermatite de Duhring, la properdinémie a accusé une augmentation (valeurs comprises entre 13 et 30 PhN/50, avec une moyenne de 25). L'évaluation de l'hypersensibilité du type retardé a été effectuée par nous moyennant intradermoréaction avec emploi d'antigènes viraux obtenus à partir de cultures de tissu infecté. L'hypersensibilisation a été toujours absente pendant la phase active de la maladie, alors que sa présence s'est manifestée pendant la phase de régression et celle de guérison. Cette hyper-réactivité a été également constatée par nous chez les mères ayant accouché d'enfants normaux après avoir mis au monde des enfants atteints d'épidermolyse bulleuse.

Démonstration de la présence d'immuno-globulines et de la fixation du complément dans les lésions cutanées chez les malades de pemphigus, au moyen de l'immunofluorescence

F. GIANOTTI, M. GOVERNA, B. PERNIS et A. CROSTI, Laboratoire de Pathologie Expérimentale de la Clinique du Travail de l'Université de Gênes, Clinique Dermatologique de l'Université de Milan (Italie)

L'examen des lésions cutanées présentées par les malades de *pemphigus vulgaris*, pratiqué moyennant immuno-fluorescence sur des coupes histologiques obtenues au cryostat et colorées par des anti-sérums anti-IgG, anti-IgM et anti-B_1C conjugués à la fluorescéine, nous a permis de déceler la présence des immuno-globulines dans la couche filamenteuse de l'épiderme de ces malades.

Les observations en question confirment les données précédemment obtenues par BEUTNER et coll. (1965) et par WALDORF et coll. (1966). Les immuno-globulines identifiées appartiennent aux classes IgG et IgM. Nous avons constaté en outre, au cours de nos recherches, que ces amas d'immuno-globulines sont sièges de fixation du complément.

Cette immuno-fluorescence est spécifique: en effet, la coloration n'a pas lieu dans les coupes cutanées de sujet normal, ou dans les coupes cutanées des cas de pemphigus pré-traitées par les mêmes fractions de globuline non marquée ou par des fractions de globuline marquée de sérum non immunisé.

L'interprétation la plus plausible de ces accumulations d'immuno-globulines, c'est celle d'une interaction locale antigène-anticorps.

La démonstration du fait que ces immuno-globulines ne sont pas constituées par toutes les classes, mais uniquement par les IgG et les IgM, et la présence, en outre, d'une fixation du complément rendent plus vraisemblable l'hypothèse identifiant le siège de l'immuno-fluorescence à l'endroit de l'immunoréaction.

Nous avons également vu que le sérum des malades atteints de *pemphigus vulgaris* contiennent des anticorps anti-épiderme, comme signalé précédemment par d'autres chercheurs (BEUTNER et JORDON, 1964; BEUTNER et coll., 1965) WALDORF et coll., 1966; BEUTNER et coll., 1967). Cette immuno-fluorescence est spécifique; elle ne se produit aucunement lorsqu'on procède à un pré-traitement par les mêmes fractions globuliniques non marquées, ou par des fractions globuliniques marquées de sérums non immunes.

Il n'a pas encore été exactement précisé si les faibles titres de réactivité de ces sérums ont une signification biologique. L'origine et la signification de cette immuno-réaction ne sont pas encore claires. Chez le malade de pemphigus, la production d'anticorps anti-épiderme pourrait bien être l'évènement pathogène principal, mais ces anticorps pourraient être même produits par une réaction secondaire déterminée par d'autres agents dans les cellules altérées (WRIGHT et coll., 1966). Cela permettrait de comprendre le rôle des agents viraux (du groupe des myxovirus) isolés depuis 1959 par CROSTI, GIANOTTI, HAHN et BUBOLA du sang des malades de pemphigus.

L'infection virale cutanée pourrait donner lieu à des antigènes, soit directement produits par le virus, soit dérivant indirectement de la déformation provoquée par le virus sur la synthèse protéique des cellules infectées (LURIA, 1959); elle pourrait déterminer également la mise en liberté de certains antigènes autologues précédemment dissimulés, comme l'affirme ISACSON (1967) pour les myxovirus.

Cutaneous Manifestations of Behçet's Disease

M. MONACELLI, Dermatological Clinic, University of Rome, and
P. NAZZARO, Institute of Dermatology "S. Gallicano Hospital", Rome (Italy)

To the triple symptom complex (recurrent iritis with hypopion and aphthous lesions of the oral and genital mucous membranes) first described by ULUSHI BEHÇET in 1937, have been added, as a result of extended observations, a number of manifestations affecting various organs and systems. Even though the early descriptions of the disease frequently mentioned nodular and pustular skin manifestations, only recently has the attention of authors been focused on skin lesions.

In the past decade we studied 20 cases of Behçet's disease. Cutaneous lesions were found in almost all our patients. In four cases they constituted the initial symptoms of the disease and the patients were for a long time thought to be suffering from pyogenic dermatitis and from recurrent erythema nodosum. In four cases skin manifestations were quite relevant and became prominent among the other manifestations of the disease.

The cutaneous lesions include various morphological elements: *Papulopustular manifestations* (85% of our cases). — The lesions are most frequently localized in the limbs, in the scalp and in the face, where they generally assume the aspect of acne. They usually appear as papular lesions which in 24 to 48 h become pustular. On the thighs, in the gluteal regions, on the penis and scrotum the lesions frequently ulcers and assumes the aspect of "skin aphtha".

Papulo-nodular manifestations: These lesions were observed by us in the four cases with preeminently cutaneous symptoms. They are larger than the papulopustular lesions, bright red, more or less prominent on the surface of the skin and very painful. They are typically transient and regress rapidly within a few days leaving no trace. They do not evolve into ulcers or pustules. In our cases they were observed on the back of the hands and on the lateral surface of the fingers.

Dermo-hypodermitis of Behçet's disease (80% of our cases) — Nodular manifestations appear acutely as rounded or ovoidal dermo-hypodermic nodules, varying in size from that of a hazelnut to that of a walnut, bright red in color, tender, slightly painful. Occasionally these elements are larger in size and may coalesce to form sizable indurations at times localized along the course of a vein, most often along the internal saphena. The number of nodules varies with each attack; though usually small it may reach 20 elements. The lesions occur in the lower limbs, particularly on the legs, but may also be seen on the thighs, on the forearms or on the trunck. The latter localizations are seldom mentioned in the literature, but were present in three of our patients.

Spontaneous regression occurs within 10 to 15 days without ulceration and usually without residual lesions. Occasionally small sclerotic areas are left after the regression of the lesions; atrophy is never seen. The chromatic variations of erythema nodosum are lacking.

Non-specific skin sensitivity. Patients with Behçet's disease present a peculiary condition of non-specific skin sensitivity. A needle-prick, particularly in the active stage of the disease, can produce lesions altogether similar to those wich occur spontaneously. This reactive condition involves not only the skin but also the oral and genital mucous membranes, as we proved by provoking lesions which were both clinically and histologically similar to spontaneous aphthous lesions. Non-specific skin sensitivity has a great diagnostic significance in the initial and incomplete forms of Behçet's disease.

Histopathological findings: In the aphthous lesions of the mucous membranes our investigations constantly showed a condition of inflammation with pronounced involvement of the blood vessels followed by necrosis of the superficial dermis and of the epithelium. The vessels show swelling of endothelial cells resulting in partial obliteration of the lumen. Endothelial proliferation, typical of proliferating and obliterating vasculitis can be noted in some of the small arteries. Vascular walls are thickened and it is often possible to observe homogeneization and dissociation of the media. A perivascular infiltration with lymphomonocytes, polynuclear leukocytes, some in karyorrhexis and some plasmacells is also observed. The aphthae are consequent upon an acute necrotizing angiitis.

The same findings show superficial papulo-pustular cutaneous lesions and papulo-nodular manifestations. Nodular manifestations present perivascular, and, exceptionally, periadnexial foci of infiltration, localized in the middle and deep dermis and involving the surrounding adipose tissue. No giant-cells, not hystiocytic granulomata, typical of eythema nodosum, are observed. In this case the venous and arterial vessels of the dermis and of the hypodermis are involved. In one case a thrombotic panarteriitis was observed in a hypodermal artery. In two cases we were able to note extensive area of connective tissue degeneration surrounded by cellular infiltrate chiefly consisting of lymphocytes and histiocytes. The lesions are similar to granuloma anulare.

On the basis of our histopathological observations, it can be held that the various manifestations have a common histopathogenesis and that blood vessels are mainly affected. The histopathological aspects of these alterations can in fact be referred to a vasculitis involving the capillaries and venous vessels of the dermis and hypodermis. The histological alterations, the clinical course and the association in some cases of migrating phlebitis, are suggestive of an allergic vasculitis consequent upon sensitization towards various antigens (bacterial or possibly viral).

Untersuchung der Interferenz zwischen den Herpes simplex- und Vacciniaviren

J. Angyal und E. Bottyan, Staatsinstitut für Dermato-Venerologie, Klinik für Haut- und Geschlechtskrankheiten der Medizinischen Universität Budapest (Ungarn)

Schon Jenner beobachtete im Jahre 1804, daß das Bestehen der Herpes simplex-Infektion das Keimen der Pockenschutzimpfung behindert. Für diese Erscheinung, die von Jenner nicht erklärt wurde, gibt es zwei Möglichkeiten:

a) Antigenverwandtschaft, Gruppenimmunität;

b) Virusinterferenz.

Da die Gruppenimmunität durch Kreuzneutralisation-Hemagglutinationbehinderung und -Präcipitation in vitro nicht bewiesen werden konnte, haben wir Versuche bezüglich der Interferenz angestellt.

Methode. Die Untersuchung erfolgte in HeLa Zellkultur, mit je zwei Herpes- und Vaccinia Virusstämmen. Zuerst wurde der Herpes- und der Vacciniavirus simultan auf dieselbe Gewebekultur geimpft. Im weiteren wurde 24 bis 48 Std nach vorheriger Impfung des Herpesvirus die HeLa Zellkultur mit Vaccinia infiziert (Tab. 1), sodann impften wir umgekehrt 24 bis 48 Std nach vorheriger Vacciniainfektion den Herpes virus auf die Gewebekultur (Tab. 2). Die Anwesenheit des Vacciniavirus versuchten wir, teils mit Hahnerythrocyten-Hemagglutination, teils nach mit Herpes Immunserum erfolgender Inkubation von Nährflüssigkeit der Gewebekultur das Auftreten etwaiger cytopathogenen Wirkung nachzuweisen

Tabelle 1

Beimpfter Virus	Zahl der vergangenen Tage				
	1	2	3	4	5
Herpes C^a	—	—	++++	++++	++++
H^b			0	0	0
Herpes + Vaccinia	—	—	+	++	++++
			0	1:9	0
Herpes + nach 24 Std Vaccinia	—	—	++	++++	++++
			0	0	0
Herpes + nach 48 Std Vaccinia	—	—	++	++++	++++
			0	0	0
Vaccinia	—	—	+	++++	++++
			0	1:9	1:27
Ungeimpfte HeLa	—	—	—	—	—

C^a = cytopathogene Wirkung — H^b = Hemagglutinationstiter

Ergebnisse. Tab. 1 veranschaulicht, daß der Herpesvirus nach 3 und der Vacciniavirus nach 4 Tagen eine vollständige Zerstörung der Gewebekultur bewirkte. Wenn der Herpes- und der Vacciniavirus in gleichem Verhältnis gemischt auf die HeLa-Zellkultur geimpft wurden, so konnte am 3. Tag noch kaum cytopathogener Effekt beobachtet werden. Auf die Vermehrung der Vaccinia deutet der am 4. Tag beobachtete Hemagglutinationstiter von 1:9. Am 5. Tag erfolgte die Zerstörung der Gewebekultur, Hemagglutination wurde nicht mehr beobachtet. Auch bei der nach der Inkubation des Supernatans mit Herpesimmunserum vorgenommenen Impfung wurde keine cytopathogene Wirkung beobachtet. Demnach hatte sich der Vacciniavirus nicht vermehrt. Wurde 24 bis 48 Std nach der Impfung des Herpesvirus mit Vaccinia infiziert, so konnte bereits am 3. Tag — der Kontrolle ähnlich — eine schwere cytopathogene Wirkung beobachtet werden. Der

Vacciniavirus war weder mit Hemagglutination noch nach Neutralisation mit Herpesimmunserum nachweisbar.

Bei der 24 bis 48 Std nach der Vacciniaimpfung erfolgenden Herpesinfektion (Tab. 2) sind am 3. bzw. 5. Tag keine lebenden Vacciniaviren mehr in der Nährflüssigkeit zu finden.

Tabelle 2

Beimpfter Virus	Zahl der vergangenen Tage				
	1	2	3	4	5
Vaccinia Cᵃ	—	+	++	++++	++++
Hᵇ		1:3	1:9	1:9	1:27
Vaccinia + nach 24 Std Herpes	—	+ / 1:3	+++ / 0	++++ / 0	++++ / 0
Vaccinia + nach 48 Std Herpes	—	+ / 1:3	++ / 1:9	+++ / 1:9	++++ / 0
Ungeimpfte HeLa	—	—	—	—	—

Cᵃ = cytopathogene Wirkung — Hᵇ = Hemagglutinationstiter

Zusammenfassend läßt sich feststellen, daß die Herpesviren die Vermehrung der Vaccinia verhindern. Auf Grund von Modellversuchen läßt sich JENNERs Beobachtung erklären. Bei den Herpeskranken erfolgte wahrscheinlich deshalb nicht die Keimung der Pockenschutzimpfung, weil die gegenwärtigen aktiven Herpesviren die Vermehrung der Vaccinia verhindern. Unsere weiteren Untersuchungen sprechen dafür, daß dieser Effekt mit Produktion des Interferons zusammenhängt.

Idoxuridine in the Treatment of Cutaneous Herpes Simplex

M. B. CORBETT, CH. M. SIDELL and M. ZIMMERMAN, University of Southern California, Pasadena (USA)

The antiviral activity of 5-iodo 2′deoxyuridine was first demonstrated in vitro by HERRMANN [1], in 1961; 1 year later, KAUFMAN [2] proved its effectiveness in vivo in the treatment of herpes simplex keratitis. The rationale for this treatment rested on the fact that idoxuridine imitated the chemical structure of thymidine used in the build up of deoxyribonucleic acid (DNA).

The herpes infected cell, using idoxuridine in place of thymidine to replicate new virus, constructs faulty virus with a false or weak link in the viral DNA. The virus is unable to replicate itself hence does not infect other cells.

Where does this fit in the chain of events? At 0 h the capsid is engulfed and absorbed by the cell. In 2 to 4 h the capsid of the virus is stripped resulting in release of viral DNA. Between the absorption and eclipse stage is the time interferon can be effective. The synthesis of DNA occurs from the 4. to the 14. h. It is during this period that idoxuridine and cytosine arabinoside have their action.

From the 14. to the 18. h the assembly of the capsid protein occurs. This step can be blocked by the use of isatin p thyosemicarbozone. During the 18. to 24. h in the cycle the virus is released. Following the release of the virus and before it is engulfed, antibodies or amantidine can interrupt the cycle.

It seemed reasonable that idoxuridine would be effective in the treatment of cutaneous herpes simplex. In designing a test program, the following variables were taken into account:

1. Herpes simplex is self-limited. Average duration of an attack is 2 weeks, but varies from 4 to 30 days.

2. Herpes simplex is recurrent. Intervals of recurrence are completely variable.

3. Herpes simplex has numerous precipitating factors such as sunlight, menses, physical trauma, psychic stress, fever and many others.

4. The manifestations of a given herpetic attack are erratic. Marked variation is characteristic of attacks in different persons and in recurrences in the same person.

5. There is marked psychic overlay in herpes simplex. It has long been known that herpes can be provoked by hypnosis or by psychic stress [3].

6. Idoxuridine can inhibit mammalian cells replication as well as viral cells.

We have learned from HARVEY BLANK that in the 1. day the herpetic vesicle fluid grows to contain 1 million virus particles/cu mm. This number drops rapidly on the 2. day to 100 organisms/cu mm of vesicle fluid. By introducing idoxuridine in the 4. to 10. h of its cycle we should be able to depress the number of developing organisms. This would reflect in a minimal clinical reaction or an abortive lesion.

Patients were instructed to apply idoxuridine with the first prodromal symptom every 5 min for the 1. h, then every hour for 12 h, then every 2 h for a total of 48 h. Discontinuing the drug at the end of 48 h allowed normal tissue repair to take place. Patients frequently had well developed late herpes when first seen. They were told it was too late in the course of their existing infection for them to derive any benefit from the medication.

A total of 111 patients were treated for recurrent herpes simplex lesions. Idoxuridine treated lesions showed a mean healing time of 5.7 days as compared to a mean healing time of 12.5 days for untreated lesions. Other evaluations of idoxuridine in treatment of cutaneous herpes simplex has varied from highly effected to completely negative [5 to 11].

Our results also varied depending upon variation in treatment schedule, time at which treatment was started, time at which treatment was stopped, concentration of idoxuridine, and the vehicle used. With proper selection of all these factors, we found idoxuridine was effective in treating cutaneous herpes simplex.

References. 1. KAUFMAN, H. E., E. C. MARTOLA, and E. H. DOHLMAN: Arch Ophthal. 68, 235 (1962). — 2. ROIZMAN, B., L. AURELIAN, and P. R. ROANE jr.: Virology 21, 482 (1963). — 3. BLACK, H., and M. W. BRODY: Psychosom. Med. 12, 254 (1950). — 4. HALL-SMITH, S. P., M. J. CORRIGAN, and M. J. GILKES: Brit. med. J. 1962, II, 1515. — 5. SCHOFIELD, C. B. S.: Brit. J. Derm. 76, 465 (1964). — 6. Man Turns Tide Against the Virus, Med. World News 4, 37 (1963). — 7. JACKSON, N.: J. Irish. med. Ass. 52, 156 (1963). — 8. BURNETT, J. W., and S. L. KATZ: J. invest. Derm. 40, 7 (1963). — 9. JUEL-JENSEN, B. E., and F. O. MacCALLUM: Brit. med. J. 1964, II, 987, — 10. IVE, F. A.: Brit. J. Derm. 76, 463 (1964). — 11. JUEL-JENSEN, B. E., and F. O. MacCALLUM: Brit. med. J. 1965, I, 901.

Studies on "Latent" Motor Palsy Caused by Zoster

K. UEDA, K. IWASHITA and M. WAKASUGI, Department of Dermatology, Kyoto Prefectural University of Medicine, Kyoto (Japan)

The clinically manifested motor palsy in zoster has been reported in many papers, e.g. an oculomotor palsy in ophthalmic zoster and a facial palsy in aural zoster. But there are no reports in literature about the clinically "latent" motor palsy caused by zoster. During the past several years 92 cases of zoster were studied electromyographically to find the latent motor palsy caused by zoster.

Results: The latent motor palsy was found in 10 cases compared 6 cases of the manifested one out of 28 cases involving cranial nerves, and the latent in 6 cases compared 6 cases of the manifest out of 64 cases involving spinal nerves. In our series, both of the manifest and latent motor palsy in cases involving spinal nerves were observed in patients with rash over the trunk and the lower extremities, but not in patients with eruption over the occipital region and the upper extremities. Thus, if specifically examined the motor palsy including the latent occurs fairly frequently in zoster.

The motor palsy was always of a peripheral and flaccid paresis in either manifest or latent cases in our series.

The manifest motor palsy was confirmed in the muscles of the region corresponded approximately to the distribution of rash, i.e. frontal muscle, orbicularis oculi muscle and zygomaticus major muscle (facial nerve) and masseter (the third branch of trigeminal nerve) in cases involving cranial nerves, and intercostal muscle (D_2—$_6$), rectus abdominis muscle (D_9—$_{11}$), vastus lateralis muscle ($L_3, _4$) and rectus femoris muscle (L_2—$_6$) in cases involving spinal nerves. They began 5 to 21 days after the appearance of skin lesion in almost all cases and persisted for 1 to 8 months showing various severities.

However, following the manifest motor palsy the latent one could be detected electromyographically in the same muscles in all cases and lasted for 1 week to 6 months, shorter than the manifested period.

The latent motor palsy not preceded by the manifest motor palsy was found in 10 cases involving cranial nerves: frontal muscle in 6 cases, frontal muscle and orbicularis oculi muscle in 2 cases and masseter in 2 cases; in 6 cases involving spinal nerves: sternomastoid muscle ($C_2, _3$) and trapezius muscle (C_2—$_4$) in 1 case, intercostal muscle (D_2—$_7$) in 4 cases and tibialis anterior muscle (L_4) in 1 case.

Although the muscle of the region corresponded approximately to the distribution of rash were also here impaired, it was noticeable that the impaired muscles were less in number than those of the manifest motor palsy in cases involving cranial nerves. Further this latent palsy began 2 to 10 days after the onset of eruption and lasted for 10 to 24 days in most of cases. In general, it was detectable on the earlier stage of disease and persisted in the shorter period than those of the manifest. But it might be not overlooked that in a few cases the latent motor palsy began as late as 21 to 30 days after the onset of skin lesion, consequently after the disappearance of rash, and persisted as long as 1 to 4 months.

The motor palsy found electromyographically was ordinarily of slight degree, having nothing to do with the severity of the rash as well as the neuralgic pain.

The relation of either manifest or latent motor palsy to the sensory disturbance couldn't be exactly found, because the latter is primarily variable in this disease. Furthermore, the cerebrospinal fluid showed a slight increase of pressure, a slight pleocytosis and a positive Pandy's test, either alone or combined, in 28 out of 62 cases examined, but they were nothing significant related to the motor palsy in the present work.

The Clinical Features of Hand, Foot and Mouth Diseases

E. WADDINGTON and R. P. WARIN, Departments of Dermatology, Cardiff Royal Infirmary and United Bristol Hospitals (England)

The Mouth

The lesions affect the gingivolabial grooves, the floor of the mouth, the tongue, buccal mucosae and palate. They begin as bright red macules 2 to 8 mm in diameter which are occasionally associated with petechiae. They later form thin walled flaccid oval grey vesicles with a surrounding zone of erythema. Vesicles on the tongue and buccal mucosae rupture early leaving shallow ulcers with a yellow base and hyperaemic margin. On the palate the vesicles are often arranged in groups and resolve without ulceration.

The Skin

Most children have a sparse eruption of 10 to 30 vesicles restricted to the hands and feet but particularly in children under 5 years of age the buttocks, upper thighs, and extensor aspects of the joints are often affected. The vesicles develop on the flexor aspects of the fingers and toes, on the terminal phalanges below the distal end of the nails and on the borders of the palms and heels. The grey colour and shape of the vesicles is characteristic. They are oval, linear or crescentic and run parallel to the skin lines. The lesions resolve within 10 days leaving pigmented macules.

There are three types of eruption on the buttocks, the most common consists of erythematous macules and papules which do not form vesicles but resolve within 2 weeks. In the second type, vesicles identical to those on the hands and feet affect the perianal area where friction and maceration produce early rupture. The third type is rare and consists of lichenoid papules scattered over the buttocks and posterior aspects of the thighs. Papular lesions also occur on the limbs and often resolve without forming vesicles.

Chronic Infection

A woman aged 84 years has had a unique chronic infection for 3 years. She had always been healthy apart from an attack of Herpes Zoster at the age of 72 years. In June, 1964, during the outbreak of Hand, Foot and Mouth disease in South Wales, she developed a febrile illness with diarrhoea. 3 days later vesicles and ulcers appeared in the mouth. She recovered in 3 weeks. In September, 1964, there was a recurrence of the oral vesicles which were associated with a vesicular rash on the abdomen, vulva and legs. The lesions began as a small group of vesicles which gradually enlarged to form a ring of flaccid haemorrhagic bullae. She was admitted to hospital for investigation.

On examination: She was afebrile. Small vesicles were present on the inner aspect of the lower lip. On the lower abdomen, vulva, groins, upper thighs and popliteal fossae, there were several circular patches 2 to 6 cm in diameter. In the centre the skin was macerated at the site of the collapsed vesicles. The margin was crenated due to the coalescence of flaccid vesicles, some of which were haemorrhagic. In the popliteal fossae the skin was lichenified with numerous vesicles at the edges of the thickened skin. There were pigmented patches on the legs at the site of healed lesions. There were no lesions on the hands or feet and no abnormality was detected in the other systems.

Investigations: Coxsackie A 16 virus was isolated on six separate occasions over the course of several months from both faeces and vesicle fluid. Neutralisation tests on the serum had titres of up to 1/250 against 100 L.D. 50 of virus. Antibody to Herpes Simplex virus was not detected by complement fixation. Histological examination showed an intraepidermal bullae containing eosinophils. There was reticular degeneration and "ballooning" of the malpighian cells with the formation of a multilocular vesicle. Blood examination was normal. Quantitative studies showed no defect in gammaglobulin.

Course: 2 weeks after her admission the dermatologist looking after her developed typical lesions of hand foot and mouth disease from which the same subtype of Coxsackie A 16 virus was isolated. He recovered within 10 days. The patient continued to develop crops of vesicles in the mouth, on the lower abdomen, vulva and legs during the following year, but in the last 2 years she has had occasional remissions, followed by relapses which have been provoked by intercurrent infection. The course of the disease has been uninfluenced by Dapsone, Sulphapyridine and 5-iodo-2-desoxyuridine.

We have not found any report of chronic infection with Coxsackie A 16 virus.

The pathogenesis of the infection in this patient is difficult to explain. She has no evidence of a defect in gammaglobulin formation. During the first year the eruption persisted without remission but recently the disease has resembled Herpes Simplex in that both conditions have periods of remission followed by vesicle production in the presence of antibody and relapses have been provoked by intercurrent infection.

References see previous paper page 314.

Etude clinique et épidémiologique de la maladie de Nicolas et Favre à Bordeaux

L. Texier, P. le Coulant, M. Geniaux et J. M. Tamisier, Centre Hospitalier et Universitaire de Bordeaux, Hôpital Saint-André (France)

On constate actuellement que la maladie de Nicolas et Favre a pratiquement disparu de l'Europe Occidentale, alors qu'elle existe encore à l'état endémique dans certaines régions tropicales. Mais par sa position géographique, Bordeaux reste une des villes de notre continent où sévit encore cette maladie. C'est ainsi que nous avons pu en détecter 48 cas, de 1942 à 1966, parmi lesquels 35% d'autochtones. A titre de comparaison, nous avons retrouvé 73 cas dans les archives de la Clinique Dermatologique, de 1920 à 1939, dont 71% d'autochtones: l'endémie régionale a certes régressé, mais elle n'est pas encore éteinte; elle ne gagne plus cependant l'arrière-pays.

L'âge de nos 48 malades, 44 hommes et 4 femmes, s'échelonne de 19 à 52 ans. Le lieu de la contamination a pu être précisé dans 45 cas: Europe Nord 1; Europe Sud 2; Afrique du Nord 2; Afrique Noire 8; Afrique du Sud 2; Madagascar 2; Extrême-Orient 3; Amérique du Nord 2; Antilles 6; Bordeaux 17. Parmi les hommes, on trouve 22 marins (contaminations extramétropolitaines), chez les 4 femmes, 3 étaient des cas autochtones (dont 2 prostituées).

Sur le plan clinique, il faut mettre à part trois localisations anorectales, dont deux très évoluées chez des hommes (stade chirurgical), une décelée précocement chez une femme, ainsi qu'une forme asymptomatique (révélée simplement par les examens biologiques) chez une jeune femme (couple Nord-Américain). Tous les autres cas correspondaient à la forme classique.

L'incubation a pu être précisée dans 30 cas. Elle s'est montrée très variable: 5 jours, en moyenne, dans 10 cas, 10 jours dans 6, 18 jours dans 6, 1 mois dans 8.

Le chancre d'inoculation a été retrouvé 23 fois, toujours de petites dimensions, souvent balanopréputial: 6 nodulaires, 4 chancrelliformes, 5 syphiloïdes, 2 herpétiformes, 6 mal définis. Chez un jeune homme de 22 ans, l'affection a débuté par une uréthrite amicrobienne suivie d'une polyadénopathie classique (nous n'avons pas retenu ici les uréthrites virales pures, malgré une étiologie lymphogranulomateuse possible, mais difficile à prouver).

L'adénite inguinale se caractérisait chez 44 malades par une polyadénopathie à large prédominance unilatérale, avec atteinte constante des ganglions rétrocruraux. Sur le plan évolutif, on pouvait distinguer: 10 simples polyadénopathies, 19 périadénites avec prise en masse des ganglions, 10 adhérences à la peau avec ramollissement, 4 fistulisations uni- ou plurifocales, 1 éléphantiasis. Dans 14 cas, on a décelé une adénite iliaque interne et dans 10 cas, une splénomégalie, avec fièvre, céphalées et asthénie.

Sur le plan biologique, la classique leucocytose n'a été constatée que cinq fois. Une biopsie ganglionnaire pratiquée quatre fois. L'intradermoréaction de FREI a confirmé toute sa valeur (Institut Pasteur et Lygranum ST Squibb). Nous ne l'avons trouvée défaillante que dans quatre cas (retard de virage ?).

Le diagnostic biologique doit être complété actuellement par les réactions de déviation du complément au Lygranum CF Squibb, ou à l'antigène ornithosique de l'Institut Pasteur. Elles sont comparables au FREI, par leur sensibilité, mais plus précoces et permettent de suivre l'élimination des anticorps, après traitement. Mais ces «réactions de groupe» ne permettent pas le diagnostic différentiel avec d'autres viroses «sœurs», la lymphoréticulose bénigne d'inoculation en particulier (maladie des griffes du chat). C'est donc à la clinique, à l'enquête épidémiologique, et à la réaction de FREI qu'il faut encore recourir pour trancher les cas litigieux.

Sur le plan thérapeutique, l'Auréomycine (2 gr par jour) nous a donné des guérisons définitives chez 36 malades traités, en 2 à 6 semaines. On peut y adjoindre la corticothérapie dans les formes anciennes évoluant vers la fibrose.

Observations on Orf in Man

R. D. SWEET, Department of Dermatology, Plymouth General Hospital (England)

Orf is the farmer's name for a virus disease of sheep and goats found in all parts of the British Isles and usually referred to by Veterinary Surgeons as "Contagious pustular dermatitis". In some areas it is endemic and of sufficient economic importance to warrant routine vaccination of flocks. The virus belongs to the Pox group of DNA containing viruses and was first grown from human lesions in tissue culture and isolated by NAGINGTON and his colleagues in Cambridge in 1961 [1]. Human infections are not uncommon in country districts in Great Britain and I saw six cases in the South West of England in the spring and early summer of 1966. Nonetheless case reports are rare in the world literature: for instance, only five papers are mentioned in 20 years in the Year Book of Dermatology (Chicago), three of them from England and two from the USA [1 to 5]. Clinical descriptions are limited to the classical painless nodule on a finger which so characteristically attracts the Surgeon's knife and is found to be solid, that this in itself is strongly suggestive of the correct diagnosis. In fact it is usually some other aspect of the disease that brings it to the notice of a Dermatologist because country people accustomed to handling sheep are more familiar with it than are their physicians.

Records of 16 cases have been reviewed, six male and ten female. Most occurred in the spring and early summer, either from handling infected lambs, usually when bottle feeding, or from shearing. Three infections definitely followed shearing, ewes in particular being infected, mainly on the belly or around the vulva. One of the three cases in which the human lesion was not on hand or fore-arm was on the face of a woman who spent a week-end on her daughter's farm. She had no contact with animals at all but her husband tried his hand at shearing and must have infected his wife. The incubation period in this case was 14 days and virus was demonstrated by electron-microscopy in a biopsy [6]. The other two were in an ear and on the shaft of the penis, both in boys caring for pet lambs. The latter, appearing about 2 weeks after an alleged abrasion in a privy, was accompanied by erythema multiforme which was bullous on the thighs — it might otherwise have closely resembled a primary chancre. In two patients there were multiple primary lesions — one man had two on the same hand and one woman four on hands and fore-arms.

Histologically there is the usual explosive ballooning of epidermal cells seen in virus infections, but no actual vesiculation. There is a dense subepidermal inflammatory reaction which in older cases invades and almost replaces the remains of the epidermis.

Only two patients complained of any pain and in one of these there was obvious secondary bacterial infection. Nevertheless, in three other patients there was clinical lymphangiitis and there were enlarged regional lymph glands in 10 of the 16 cases. Healing took place in between 4 and 6 weeks and seemed quite uninfluenced by treatment. Virus was cultured from two and observed microscopically in two more.

There is one major complication of human orf about which little, if anything, has been published. This is a rather distinct form of bullous erythema multiforme which may occur at any time from 3 or 4 days to 3 weeks after the appearance of the primary lesion. It was the occurrence of erythema multiforme that determined the reference of half of my cases to Hospital. The eruption affected all four limbs in each case, and the trunk in the boy with the penile lesion and in one other. In two there was mild but definite involvement of mouth and eyes. In all but one the erythema multiforme lesions were bullous in the vicinity of the actual infection and to a lesser extent on the other hand also. In several the bullae were haemorrhagic. Lesions elsewhere were usually small and typical. In these very acute reactions there was fever and severe discomfort and the patient had to retire to bed. In one case only, with infection of a finger, the bullae were generalised and this was the only one in which repeated crops were seen, or in which the erythema multiforme lasted more than 10 days. Most subsided in about a week. Virus was not isolated from the blister fluid in two cases where this was attempted.

It is well known that herpes simplex infections may be followed by erythema multiforme and it has also been described in association with Milker's Nodes, lesions indistinguishable from orf, which can be acquired from cattle infected by an almost identical virus [7, 8].

References. 1. NAGINGTON, J., and C. H. WHITTLE: Brit. med. J. 1961, II, 1324. — 2. BLAKEMORE, F., M. ABDUSSALAM, and W. N. GOLDSMITH: Brit. J. Derm. 60, 404 (1948). — 3. LLOYD, G. M., A. MAC DONALD, and E. R. GLOVER: Lancet 1951, I, 720. — 4. WHEELER, C. E., E. P. CAWLEY, and J. H. JOHNSON: Arch. Derm. 71, 481 (1955). — 5. FARMER, J. L., and H. O. PERRY: Minn. Med. 43, 818 (1960). — 6. NAGINGTON, J.: Brit. med. J. 1964, II, 1499. — 7. SONCK, C. E.: Acta allerg. (Kbh.) 4, 251 (1951). — 8. SEDLACEK, V.: čs. Derm. 29, 32 (1955).

Nobecutan-Podophyllin Preparations in Viral Warts

A. BJÖRNBERG and L. HELLGREN, Department of Dermatology, Sahlgrenska Sjukhuset, University of Gothenburg (Sweden)

This paper is presented as a methodological and clinical study to evaluate the effect of topical treatment of virus warts, in this case Nobecutan solutions. Because of the great tendency of selfhealing of warts it is difficult to judge the efficiency of the treatment without knowing the spontaneous cure rate in a comparable material. In these investigation such factors have less importance as the patients were their own controls, the warts being treated in the same individual. The variances between individuals were reduced and a relatively smaller series of patients was needed for a reliable conclusion.

A plastic base, Nobecutan, manufactured by Bofors Company in Sweden, had in an English study in 1965 been shown to have a good effect in itself in plantar warts. In the study performed by us Nobecutan base was compared to Nobecutan with 20% podophyllotoxin and with 20% podophyllotoxin and 10% salicylic acid (the compositions suggested by SVEN HAMMARSKJÖLD). The three plastic solutions were dispensed in exactly similar small bottles with code marks. One third of each solution was randomly coloured red, one third brown and one third green. Each patient got one of each colour in such way that he also got all the three compositions. As the colour was randomly chosen neither he nor the doctor could identify the contents of the bottles.

For the treatment 40 patients were chosen who were considered to be reliable and who had at least three warts (or three groups of warts) of about the same duration and size on the feet *or* on the hands. On these three skin lesions the three coloured plastic solutions were applied each evening, after cleaning of the surface with acetone. Macerated parts of the warts were cautiously removed by cutting. Every week it was controlled that the treatment was properly performed which was easy by because of the colouring of the warts by the dyes in the plastics.

The judgement of the results of treatment was made according to an index scale defined as a numerical expression for the morphological picture of the warts, the highest number, five, meaning a fully developed wart without any signs of regressive changes, the lowest, 0, no visible verrucous changes. The morphology was registrated definitely after 4 weeks independently by two doctors and the means of their judgements were used in the statistical evaluation of the results with the Kendall's concordance test. The significance level was 95%.

It was found that the solutions containing podophyllotoxin and salicylic acid had a statistically significant better clinical effect than the Nobecutan solution itself and than Nobecutan-podophyllotoxin. In a later study on 25 other patients it was also demonstrated that a 20% podophyllotoxin + 10% salicylic acid-Nobecutan solution had better effect than a 10% salicylic acid-Nobecutan solution. The reactions to the podophyllin preparations varied much individually and some patients got painful reactions for some time.

The described method used in the evaluation of the effect of topical treatment of virus warts is valuable when patients are chosen who are reliable and who have comparable warts of the same duration, size and localization.

Main Theme V	**Current Problems in Syphilis**
	Problèmes actuels de la syphilis
	Problemas actuales de la sífilis
	Aktuelle Probleme der Syphilis

Organizer

R. Degos, France

Presidents

G. Hagerman, Sweden

A. King, Great Britain

S. Longhin, Rumania

S. Olansky, USA

Delegate of the Organization Committee

J. Herzberg, Germany

Reports

Syphilis and Human Ecology

T. GUTHE, O. IDSØE and R. R. WILLCOX, Division of Communicable Diseases, World Health Organization, Geneva (Switzerland)

More than in most other conditions the transmission of venereal disease relates to fundamental human behaviour, regulated by facilitating and restraining forces in the environment, forces of a broad educational, social and economic nature. The intensity of the epidemiological process concerned in the spread of venereal disease depends on a somewhat precarious balance between these ecological forces and the nature and extent of case-finding, diagnostic and treatment facilities in individual countries, and in an international context.

1. Incidence trends and wars

Wars are classically known to influence the frequency of venereal infections. Information on incidence in armed forces is often available before similar information concerning civilian populations. Data from the United Kingdom and France

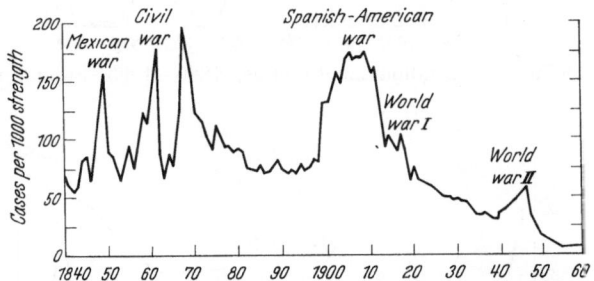

Fig. 1. Venereal disease trends in United States Army, 1840—1960. Annual rates per 1000 strength (adapted from MOORE, J. E. 1943)

show a marked general incidence recession in the last 100 years, interrupted by periodic recurrences associated in time with wars or war-like conditions at home or abroad. This pattern has perhaps best been documented in the USA (Fig. 1) where the annual VD rate per 1000 strength from 1840 to 1960 showed epidemic peaks at the time of the Mexican war, the Civil war, the Spanish-American war and the two World Wars. The general long-term recession is nevertheless evident. This graphic presentation included US-Forces at home and abroad and did not show the very high VD rates in disturbed areas in the Far East in recent years. Information released [1] indicates that in 1951/52 the VD rate in Korea was 150/200 new cases annually per 1000 men and that it has been some 280/300 new cases annually per 1000 men in the recent Viet Nam conflict.

In the civilian population trends similar to those in the military can be discerned in the latter part of the last and the early part of the present century. Thus the incidence of acquired syphilis from 1880 to 1965 in the capitals of the Nordic countries (Fig. 2) shows the outbreaks of wars reflected in periodic recurrences in the civilian populations — whether the countries were neutral (as in the first World War) or were actually occupied (as were Norway and Denmark in the second World War). Other peaks are probably associated with overseas wars (e.g. the Russo-Turkish war in the 1880's and the Russo-Japanese war at the turn of the century) where Scandinavian shipping was deeply involved and where import of disease to the home countries was frequent. The general recession of disease incidence over a period of time is nevertheless evident. This decline in civilian morbidity in the Nordic countries — and elsewhere — was also reflected

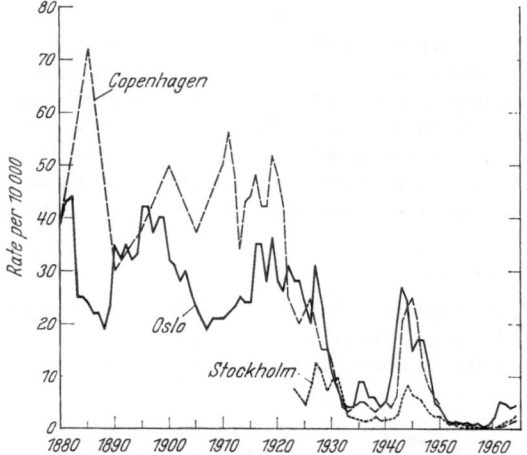

Fig. 2. Acquired syphilis in Scandinavian Capitals, 1880—1965, annual rates per 10000 population

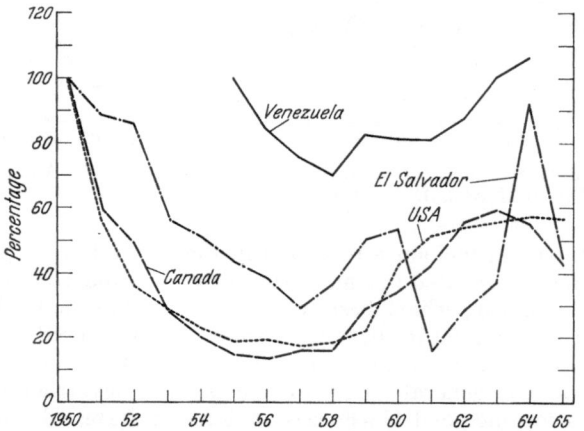

Fig. 3. Reported primary/secondary, cases of syphilis in four countries in the Americas, 1950 to 1965. Yearly percentage variations of incidence rates using 1950 as reference (100%)

by a decline in late and latent syphilis, although the rates were several times that of the early infection, picturing the prevalence of untreated syphilis in the population 5 to 20 years earlier as well as the effectiveness of treatment at that time.

The recurrence of early syphilis associated with the Second World War was followed by an unprecedented fall in incidence to an all time low by the mid 1950's. The subsequent recrudescence (still continuing in many countries) aroused considerable interest in developing and developed countries alike. This fall and rise have taken place on a global scale and have been marked in some regions, less marked in others, as far as can be appraised on the basis of data from countries where continuous information is available over the 15 to 20 years. Fig. 3 shows in four countries in the Americas the percentage annual variation in incidence rates

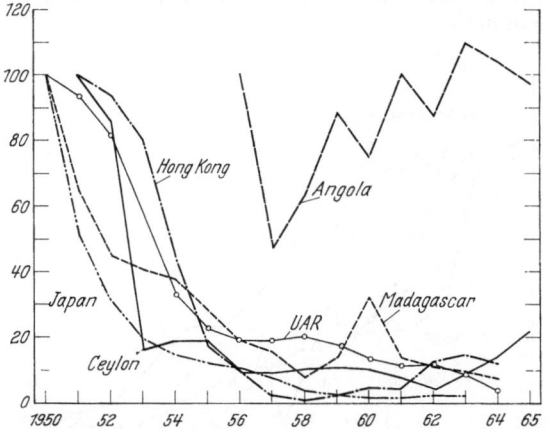

Fig. 4. Reported primary/secondary cases of syphilis in six African and Asian countries, 1950—1965. Yearly percentage variations of incidence rates using 1950 as reference (100%)

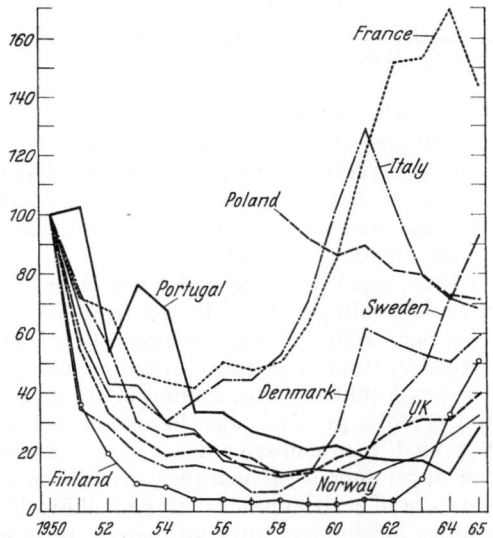

Fig. 5. Reported primary/secondary cases of syphilis in nine european countries, 1950—1965. Yearly percentage variations of incidence rates using 1950 as reference (100%)

of early syphilis 1950 to 1965, using reported cases in 1950 as a 100% reference point. Fig. 4 shows similar data from six countries of Asia and Africa. Fig. 5 shows the perspective in nine European countries. The recrudescence began in most countries around 1956/58 and has continued, with individual variations. It is obvious that the data are not always directly comparable owing to differences in the nature and completeness of morbidity reporting in time and in place — the reasons for which are well known. Nevertheless such information does give an indication of long-term incidence trends of early syphilis. The same applies to data on congenital syphilis, as shown in Fig. 6. Although a remarkable fall has taken place in the incidence of congenital disease since around 1950 it has levelled off since 1960, and congenital syphilis has remained a maternal and child health problem in some countries.

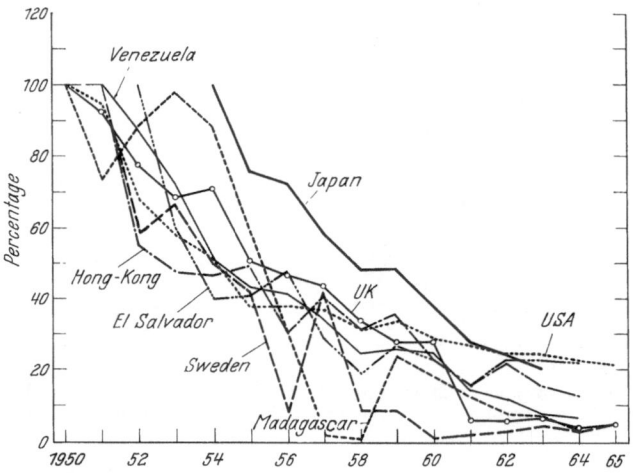

Fig. 6. Reported congenital syphilis in eight countries, 1950—1965. Yearly percentage variations of incidence rates using 1950 as reference (100%)

2. Medical and Public Health Aspects

a) The introduction of *penicillin therapy* was certainly a causative factor in the sharp decline of infectious syphilis after the second World War [2]. This development, however, could not prevent the recurrence which has taken place since 1956 1957, although there is no evidence that the treponemicidal power of penicillin in individual therapy has decreased [3, 4].

b) FINGER [5], in 1920, suggested that following "mass-infection" of syphilis, acquired immunity would again be "lost" in the next generation, and that this *change in the volume of susceptibles* played a major role in cyclic variations of the disease. This basic consideration — also observed in many other infections — is in accord with subsequent evidence that immunity towards reinfection generally develops in untreated syphilis [6]. It is also in accord with subsequent evidence that metal therapy applied in subcurative doses over a prolonged period did not substantially obstruct development of such protective immunity [7]. In contrast to this, adequate treatment of early syphilis with penicillin will obviate a prolonged stimulus of the immunity mechanism, preventing long-term resistance to reinfection [8]. Actually, in population groups with high exposure rates, reinfections after penicillin treatment have emerged as an epidemiological problem ("repeaters" and "ping-pong" syphilis).

There is also the public health implication of the changed immunological picture demonstrated by the World Health Organization in developing countries following mass penicillin campaigns against the non-venereal endemic treponematoses of childhood, particularly yaws. Such campaigns have been undertaken in the last 10 to 15 years in 45 countries where some 150 million people were examined and some 45 million clinical cases, latent cases and contacts were treated with longacting penicillin. In such areas, veneral syphilis was previously exceedingly rare; but the relative cross-immunity from yaws possessed by the previous generation against venereal syphilis is now present to a much lower extent in the new generation. Only 5 to 10% are now sero-reactive (FTA, TPI) at puberty, as contrasted to 60 to 70% in some areas 15 to 20 years ago. It is, however, too early to appraise how far this new immunological situation may — in conjunction with a whole set of other ecological changes — favour spread of syphilis in the future.

c) It has been suggested that the wide use of penicillin for other conditions than syphilis during the first 15 to 20 years of the penicillin era may have had a general *"happenstance" preventive effect* on syphilis in exposed persons among the population at large [9, 10]. This may have contributed to the observed sharp decline in early syphilis after 1948—1950. Conversely the diminishing of this preventive effect may have been one of the causes of the recrudescence of syphilis in recent years. In fact it has been shown that the penicillin doses resulting in such happenstance effect would suffice to abort most cases during the incubation period [11].

d) Since the end of the last and at the beginning of the present century, *public health laws* in many countries (e.g. the Nordic countries, Great Britain, USA) provided for special activities against venereal diseases, including free examination and treatment facilities [12]. The International Union against the Venereal Diseases and the Treponematoses (IUVDT) was instrumental in obtaining introduction of such measures.

Public health activities affected the frequency of venereal disease in many countries at about the same time, regardless of the differences of methods used [13]. Subsequently the high venereal disease incidence during and immediately after the second World War led to some further strengthening of public health control measures and their modernisation (e.g. the Rapid Treatment Centre programme in the USA).

The impressive early therapeutic achievements of penicillin apparently lured health administrations as well as the public into indifference to control measures [14]. It is only recently that some reorientation in the public health aspects of syphilis control has become discernable in some countries, where the rise in early syphilis has reactivated health administrations. It is reasonable to suggest that, for example, the incidence fall in 1965 in France — which continued also in 1966 — and the levelling off in the incidence rise in the United States and the United Kingdom, may be ascribed to intensification of anti-venereal disease activities [15 to 17].

e) In many countries ambulatory syphilis treatment with penicillin has been to a great extent taken over by *private practitioners* [18, 19] who cannot easily manage complicated and time-consuming modern control activities (and the paperwork that goes with them). In the opinion of many, failure of epidemiological cooperation between private doctors and public health authorities has in some countries become a significant cause for the upsurge of syphilis since the mid-fifties.

3. Economic, social and behavioural changes

a) We have already indicated the association between wars and periodic recurrence of early syphilis. Causal links between periods of *expanding economy* and spread of syphilis have also been pointed out, particularly by HAUSTEIN in the 1920's [20] and in more recent years by GJESSING [21]. There is no contradiction between these aspects, since a war economy is usually of an inflationary nature leading to temporary economic affluence and easy money spending. On the other hand the global incidence rise of early syphilis since 1956—1957 has taken place in peace-time, and the post-war cycle of fall and rise has covered an almost un-broken period of economic expansion. It is logical — and notable — that during the first part of the post-war period individual and collective investments of money in most parts of the world were used for resettlement, reconstruction and rehabili-tation needs. In recent years funds have increasingly been used for "living stand-ard" goods combined to an amazing extent with travel, tourism and entertain-ment, of importance in the epidemiology of syphilis. But obviously, in addition to the economic forces, other factors also influence the treponeme-host balance in man.

b) *Changing ethical, moral and behavioural codes* of the post-war years have been associated with increased promiscuous sexual activity [22, 23]. But we must re-member that so-called morality has undergone great variations also in the past. Today, however, due to rapid social, economic and technical progress such changes infiltrate society almost explosively. Several aspects in this context must be con-sidered:

i) *There is first the changing pattern of prostitution:* Following the improvement in recent years of socioeconomic conditions, industrialization, female emancipation, expanding civil rights, etc., the general pattern of prostitution has changed in developed countries. Traffic in women and children and legalised controlled pros-titution have in principle been abolished by international action at the United Nations level (1956) [24], and legalised prostitution and brothels have since almost ceased to be reported as major sources of venereal infection [25]. During the post-war reconstruction period prostitution continued to be viewed optimistically as of minor epidemiological importance. There is, however, evidence that the problem of prostitution has reappeared in modified form with the economic affluence of recent years. But, it is now striking that women in developed countries are rarely driven into sale of sex to obtain the basic necessities of life — as was previously often the case. They are rather driven by urges to obtain the extra luxuries and consumer goods considered essential in today's modern life, stimulated by a sex-conscious advertising industry — articles often beyond their social and economic possibilities [25]. There is a trend towards an increasing role of prostitutes in this sense as sources of infection, although "bread and butter" prostitution remains in developing countries. Furthermore, mental deviations, hereditary factors, ethnic and group minority traits, inadequate family, social and educational background, alcohol and drug addiction [26 to 28] result to a larger extent than before in maladjustment to society and failure to overcome the complexities of modern life. Prosmicuous behaviour patterns are frequent in these groups.

ii) *The second aspect of importance in the spread of syphilis relates to male homosexuals:* In the mid-twenties homosexual practices were considered subordi-nate as a source of syphilis infection [29]. During recent years, however, attention has been called to the increasing role of male homosexuals in the epidemiology of venereal diseases. Homosexual contacts have been reported to range from about ten to more than 90%. Also the problem is particularly one of big cities, where young homosexual male prostitutes congregate [30, 31]. Frequently they have heterosexual contacts also [32], a fact which adds to their significant role in the spread of infection.

iii) *The third aspect of importance for the spread of infection relates to syphilis (and gonorrhoea) among young people* [23]: For example, in the USA the rate of primary and secondary syphilis in this group increased from 10.1 in 1956 to 24.2 per 100.000 population in 1965, compared with a rate of 11.6 for all age groups [33]. A similar trend has been reported from several countries, including Canada [34], Western Germany [35], the Netherlands [36], Italy [37], and the Nordic Countries [38 to 40].

4. Population Movements

The international aspects of venereal disease control have been emphasized in relation to population movements by many investigators.

a) Several investigations have been undertaken in regard to the potential spread of venereal diseases by *migrant* and *immigrant labourers*. The pattern in the United Kingdom concerning the West Indians has been well documented in British Cooperative Clinical Group Studies and otherwise [41 to 43]. In West Germany and Switzerland there are extensive foreign labour forces (respectively 1.2 and 0.7 millions) who have by and large been found not to contribute to the importation and spread of disease in the guest countries [44, 45]; (thus the sero-reactivity rate 1957—1963 in the foreign labour force of West Germany was 0.22% compared to 0.20% in home populations, and in Switzerland in 1963 it was 0.09% in foreign labourers as against 0.03—0.04% among blood donors in the general population). In France the rate among foreign labourers increased, however, from 1.4% in 1958 to 2.9% in 1965 owing to the influx of labour from North African countries [15]. Measures have been taken which may be responsible for an apparent downward trend in reported early syphilis in France in 1965 and which has continued in 1966.

b) There is evidence that in recent years the incidence of syphilis and other genital infections in areas of *urbanisation and industrialization* has increased in many countries [46]. While 6% of the population of the USA lived in cities in 1880 some 70% of the population was urban in 1960 [47]. In 1966, 59 cities, comprising 21.8% of the population in the USA, accounted for 53.8% of the total reported primary and secondary syphilis cases [33]. Epidemic outbreaks of venereal infections have been reported in several countries in relation to implantation of large industrial complexes into rural areas, e.g. in Odense in Denmark [48]. On the other hand, the venereal disease problem of rapidly growing industrial settlements can be checked when adequate environmental, health and education programmes are set up from the beginning. This has been shown in Poland [49] where the infectious syphilis rate per 1.000 fell from 1.70 to 0.38 in the Nova Hota area during the first 10 years despite a significant population increase.

c) The present floating population in overseas trade is estimated not to exceed a million *seafarers*. While European countries account for the bulk of the 100% increase in the world's merchant fleet between 1945 and 1963, an impressive growth has taken place also in African and Asian countries, indicating that a more comprehensive and modernised international co-operation in maritime health services and venereal disease control is required than exists at present. The increasing importance of veneral disease in seafarers has been documented in recent years by several investigators in European and other countries [51]. In Finland in 1961 more than half of the seafarers infected with venereal disease had acquired their infections abroad [52]. The same applied to Danish seafarers in Copenhagen [53]. In an English seaport 60% of the seafarers treated had acquired their disease in eleven different countries of the world [54]. Among 4.066 infected sailors of 30 nationalities treated in French ports (1960—1964), 64.5% had acquired their disease in non-French ports [55].

d) The combination of economic affluence and peace-time *tourism* for the masses has to a large extent replaced the epidemiological element previously represented by movements of armed forces. The year 1967 has been declared "International Year of Tourism" and a further rise must be expected in this very great industry of modern times. The enormous increase in the tourist industry in recent years is illustrated in the table on page 352 — leaving to our imagination the epidemiological potential for exchange of venereal contagion between countries.

Only sporadic direct documentation is available on the prevalence and spread of infection among tourists and travellers. But, in Sweden, 24% of total patients with early syphilis acquired their infection abroad; for those in the U.K. it was

Table. *Extent of International Tourism from 1958 to 1966*
Arrivals of tourists in 26 countries and estimated economic value

Year	Arrivals	Indices	Receipts ($ million)	Indices
1958	55,250,000	100	5,449	100
1959	63,000,000	114	5,847	107
1960	71,138,674	129	6,842	126
1961	75,281,000	136	7,284	134
1962	81,406,000	147	8,027	147
1963	93,756,000	170	8,834	162
1964	107,744,447	195	10,159.1	186
1965	115,892,595	210	11,633.5	213
1966	127,990,000	232	12,997.0	239

Source: International Bureau of Tourism, Geneva, 1967.

estimated that 40% of infected males acquired the infection during visits outside the country [41]. Moreover, examples from Ceylon [56] and Western Germany [57] illustrate the rôle in the spread of venereal infections of gatherings of people during exhibitions and fairs arranged on a regional or world basis.

5. Population Control

In addition to the problems arising from aggregations of existing populations we finally have the even greater problems arising from the increasing populations of the future. Millions of women utilise anticonceptional devices and pills in the present-day orientation towards population control. Their use is reported to increase sexual activity and multiply sexual contacts. While conception may well be prevented by gestogens and intrauterine loops, the transmission of venereal disease will not. On the contrary, this new element in our rapidly changing environment may well become of epidemiological importance in the spread of genital infections in the future. The time may have come for a more integrated approach between the groups working in the population control field and the communicable disease groups concerned with genital infections, and it would seem logical that case finding activities for genital infections be associated with anticonceptional programmes.

Conclusion. In summing up this introduction to theme V of the XIIIth International Congress of Dermatology on syphilis and human ecology, it may be said that most of what can reasonably be expected from individual therapy has been reached by penicillin in the treatment of syphilis; and new treponemicidal agents cannot improve considerably the present situation. But even if complete perfection of therapy could be attained in all stages of the disease the multitude of human ecological factors concerned in our times in the spread of disease — and beyond the influence of antibiotics — suggest that true control or elimination of syphilis can hardly be attained in society as a whole with present epidemiological methods.

Bibliography. 1. Navy Times: Washington, D. C., 8 March 1967. — 2. MALGRAS, J.: Proph. sanit. morale **39**, 37 (1967). — 3. COLLART, P., L. J. BOREL et P. DUREL: Ann. Inst. Pasteur **102**, 596 (1962). — 4. YOBS, A. R., S. OLANSKY, D. H. ROCKWELL, and J. W. CLARK: Arch. Derm. Syph. (Chic.) **91**, 379 (1965). — 5. Cited by HAUSTEIN, H.: In JADASSOHN, J. (Ed.) Handbuch der Haut- und Geschlechtskrankheiten, **22.** Berlin: Springer 1927. — 6. CHESNEY, A. M.: Immunity in syphilis. Baltimore: Williams & Wilkins 1927. — 7. EAGLE,

H., H. J. Magnuson, and R. Fleischman: J. exp. Med. **85**, 423 (1947). — 8. Thomas, E. W.: Syphilis, its course and management. New York: Macmillan Company 1949. — 9. Schamberg, I. L.: Brit. J. vener. Dis. **39**, 87 (1963). — 10. Danehower, W. F., and I. L. Schamberg: Arch. Derm. Syph. (Chic.) **88**, 930 (1963). — 11. Magnusson, H. J., H. Eagle, and R. Fleischman: Amer. J. Syph. **32**, 1 (1948). — 12. Royal Commission on Venereal Diseases Final Report of the Commissioners. London: H. M. Stationary Office 1916. — 13. Willcox, R. R.: A Textbook of Venereal Diseases and Treponematoses, 2nd edition. London: William Heinemann Medical Books Ltd. 1964. — 14. King, A.: Lancet **I**, 651, (1958). — 15. Vernier, A.: Prcph. sanit. morale **37**, 219 (1965). — 16. Eradication of Syphilis. A task force report to the Surgeon General, US Dept. of Health, Education and Welfare, Public Health Service, Publication No. 918 (1963). — 17. King, A.: Discussion at meeting of the Medical Society for the Study of Venereal Diseases (MSSVD) London, April 1967. — 18. Curtis, C.: J. Amer. med. Ass. 186, 46 (1963). — 19. Degos, R., et O. Delzant: Vie méd. **44**, 330 (1963). — 20. Haustein, H.: In Jadassohn, J. (Ed.) Handbuch der Haut- und Geschlechtskrankheiten **22**, Berlin: Springer 1927. — 21. Gjessing, H. C.: Brit. J. vener. Dis. **32**, 86 (1956). — 22. Time **83**, No. 4, 42 (1964). — 23. British Medical Association: Venereal disease and Young People, London 1964. — 24. Study on Traffic in Persons and Prostitution. United Nations, New York, ST/SOA/SD/8 (1959). — 25. French, E.: Brit. J. vener. Dis. **31**, 113 (1955). — 26. Ducrey, C.: Sem. Hôp. Paris **36**, 1 (1960). — 27. Mayer, H.: Pers. communication to WHO 1962. — 28. Brandao, F. N., F. da Cruz Sobral, and A. da Fonseca: Proceedings of the XXIVth General Assembly and Technical Meeting of the International Union against the Venereal Disease and the Treponematoses, Lisbon, 197 (1965). — 29. Hecht, H.: In Jadassohn, J. (Ed.) Handbuch der Haut- und Geschlechtskrankheiten **22**, Berlin: Springer 1927. — 30. Hooker, E.: Male Homosexual life styles and venereal disease, Los Ángeles: University of California 1962. — 31. Tarr, J. D.: Gen. Pract. **25**, 91 (1962). — 32. Eck, M.: Sodome: Essai sur l'homosexualité, p. 189. Paris: Libraire Arthème Fayard 1966. — 33. Today's VD Control Problem. The American Social Health Association, New York 1967. — 34. Venereal Disease in Canada. Annual Report. Ottawa, Dept. of National Health & Welfare, Epidemiological Division 1965. — 35. Communication from Bundesministerium für Gesundheitswesen, Federal Republic of Germany, 18. 2. 1965. — 36. Staatsgezicht op de Volksgezondheid, Luesenquete 1963, Ghi Bulletin, The Hague 1966. — 37. Coffari, V.: Proceedings of the XXIVth General Assembly and Technical Meeting of the International Union against the Venereal Diseases and the Treponematoses, Lisbon 189 (1965). — 38. Danbolt, N.: Medicinsk årbog. Copenhagen: Munksgaards Forlag 1966. — 39. Ekstrøm, K.: Acta psychiat. scand. Suppl. **180**, 241 (1964). — 40. Hellerstrøm, S., M. Ruhnek-Forsbeck, B. Hederstedt, and C. Palme: Svenska Läk.-Tidn. **61**, 3585 (1964). — 41. British Co-operative clinical group. Brit. J. vener. Dis. **36**, 233 (1960). — 42. British Co-operative clinical group. Brit. J. vener. Dis. **41**, 251 (1965). — 43. Willcox, R. R.: Brit. J. vener. Dis. **39**, 214 (1963). — 44. Lundt, P. V.: WHO unpublished working document EURO-240/9.2 (1963). — 45. Communication from Eidgenössisches Gesundheitsamt, Berne (Switzerland). 18. 8. 1966. — 46. Degos, R.: Bull. Soc. Méd. Hôp. Paris **76**, 362 (1960). — 47. Revelle, R.: J. Amer. med. Ass. **197**, 638 (1966). — 48. Perdrup, A.: Pers. communication 1966. — 49. Capinski, T. Z.: WHO unpublished working document WHO/VDT/66.337/WHO/HE.66.1 (1966). — 50. Wld. Hlth. Org. techn. Rep. Ser. **190**, 4 (1960) — 51. Idsøe, O., and T. Guthe: Bull. Wld. Hlth. Org. **29**, 773 (1963). — 52. Härö, A. S., and R. Pätiäla: Bull. Wld Hlth Org. **24**, 394 (1961). — 53. Hartmann, G.: In Maritime venereal-disease control, WHO unpublished working document WHO/EURO, 111 (1956) — 54. Schofield, C. B. S.: Bull. Wld Hlth Org. **33**, 867 (1965). — 55. Communication to WHO from the French Ministry of Foreign Affairs (1967). — 56. Annual Administration Report, Anti-VD Campaign 1946—1965, Colombo, Ceylon. — 57. Memmesheimer, A. R.: Dtsch. med. Wschr. **89**, 2021 (1964).

Aspects actuels de la syphilis récente

E. Lortat-Jacob, Hôpital Saint-Louis, Paris (France)

En relisant les auteurs classiques, on s'aperçoit qu'il n'y a aucune modification à apporter aux descriptions anciennes de la syphilis récente. Fournier les a toutes décrites, même celles qui nous paraissent actuellement moins conformes aux descriptions classiques. Ceci signifie que nous avons oublié l'enseignement de nos maîtres.

La seule modification notable à apporter est celle dûe à l'incidence d'une anti-biothérapie dangereusement insuffisante, qui peut décapiter, masquer ou modifier l'évolution d'une syphilis récente. Il nous paraît donc utile de réaffirmer certaines descriptions classiques, connues, mais oubliées, conformes à nos observations actuelles.

Une seule question se pose : Ces aspects cliniques qui s'avéraient rares autrefois sont-ils plus fréquents actuellement ?

Période préchancreuse

L'incubation de la syphilis reste de 15 à 20 jours, en moyenne, parfois raccourcie dans le cas de lésion pré-existante (herpès, balanite de Follmann). L'incubation prolongée mérite de retenir notre attention. C'est le cas des incubations retardées, allongées, par une antibiothérapie locale ou générale. Une antibiothérapie adminis-trée pour une infection intermittente (blennorragie) entraine non seulement un allongement de l'incubation, quelquefois une atypie du chancre, parfois une ab-sence de tréponèmes sur les prélèvements, sans parler du retard du virage séro-logique. Ce sont là des faits nouveaux, d'où la règle d'instituer une surveillance sérologique pendant 6 mois, dans ces cas particuliers.

Accident primaire

Dans la majorité des cas le chancre garde ses caractères classiques : « la plus insignifiante des érosions, une écorchure, une égratignure, un rien, reposant sur une base épaissie » (FOURNIER). Tous les aspects classiques se voient : chancres nains, de grande taille, plus ou moins indurés, chancres gangréneux etc., mais, actuellement, il nous semble que deux aspects, bien que classiques, apparaissent avec une plus grande fréquence :
— les chancres ulcéreux,
— les chancres d'aspect inflammatoire.

Le chancre ulcéreux, fréquent surtout chez les Nord-Africains (50%) est une ulcération ronde, régulière à fond sanieux ou cruenté. Mais parfois, cette ulcération est irrégulière, purulente, peu indurée qui fait hésiter à porter le diagnostie d'acci-dent primitif. Lorsque le siège n'est pas génital, le diagnostic est rendu délicat.

Le chancre d'aspect inflammatoire, bien que classique, nous paraît plus fréquent. Le chancre perd ses caractères d'*aphlegmasie* et d'*indolence*. Il s'agit, le plus souvent, de chancre ulcéreux, purulent, entouré d'une réaction oedémateuse, rouge, douloureuse spontanément et à la palpation. Ce caractère inflammatoire (peut-être dû à une surinfection par des cocci banaux) ne doit pas être confondu avec le *syphilome primaire* classique caractérisé soit par une zone rouge sombre, quelquefois squameuse qui entoure le chancre et engaine parfois le fourreau ou le gland, soit par une simple infiltration rouge dure, squameuse, sans ulcération. L'indolence qui caractérise classiquement le chancre syphilitique ne peut donc plus être retenue comme signe majeur pour affirmer le chancre syphilitique ou le con-sidérer comme un chancre mixte.

L'adénopathie peut également prendre une allure inflammatoire. Déjà signalée par FOURNIER dans 1,2% des cas, nos statistiques montrent une discrète augmen-tation de fréquence, puisque nous la retrouvons dans 3% des cas de syphilis primaire. La pléiade de RICORD, aphlegmasique, dure, indolente, polyganglionnaire peut perdre ses caractères classiques : les ganglions se groupent, deviennent cohérents et semblent se fondre en une seule masse. Il se forme une tumeur unique, c'est un *bubon conglo méré*. D'autre fois le bubon déroge à ses habitudes d'aphleg-masie et d'indolence pour prendre les caractères d'une adénite subaigue. Les ganglions deviennent douloureux, la peau rosit. On a l'impression qu'une suppuration s'installe, mais la ponction ne ramène ni pus, ni germes. Beaucoup plus rarement, le bubon évolue vers un abcès sous forme «d'abcès puriforme aseptique». En général, ce n'est qu'une menace d'abcès, un feu de paille qui tombe aussitôt. L'évolution vers la fistulisation est tout à fait exceptionnelle Degos, De Graciansky ne l'ont observé chacun que dans deux cas. Par la fistule, le pus aseptique s'évacue, puis se ferme. Elle ne donne jamais lieu à une suppuration prolongée avec persistance de trajets fistuleux. «Rien d'autre, rien de plus ne se manifeste» (Fournier). Depuis toujours ces bubons inflammatoires ont posé le problème de la possibilité pour le tréponème de provoquer une adénite aigue. Autrefois, l'association du tréponème au bacille de Ducrey ou au virus de la maladie de Nicolas-Favre pouvaient expliquer ces aspects cliniques. Mais, à l'heure actuelle où le chancre simple, où la maladie de Nicolas-Favre ont pratiquement disparu, cette explication ne peut être retenue. Les auto-inoculations, les recherches bactériologiques s'avèrent toujours et constamment négatives. La surinfection du chancre par des germes banaux pourrait être en cause, mais comment expliquer la constante stérilité des cultures de ponctions pratiquées dans les adénites inflammatoires?

La localisation des chancres ne présente aucune particularité nouvelle, sauf pourtant la plus grande fréquence des chancres pubiens chez les Nords-Africains. Cette localisation s'explique-t-elle par une balistique particulière de la race africaine, ou par la pratique du rasage du pubis des Arabes? Les chancres multiples sont surtout l'apanage de chancres génitaux (18%).

La syphilis modifiée par l'antibiothérapie constitue les faits nouveaux de la syphilis récente. La syphilis sans chancre est connue de longue date. «Syphilis décapitées», dues soit à des chancres inapparents, soit à une inoculation au-dessous d'une «dose seuil» (Levaditi-Gastinel). Mais la plus grande part revient actuellement à une antibiothérapie administrée pendant la période d'incubation à dose insuffisante, soit à l'occasion d'une infection intercurrente, soit à titre préventif et qui ne suffit pas à stériliser l'organisme, mais permet encore l'éclosion de manifestations syphilitiques retardées sans chancre apparent (Hollander, Turner). C'est peut être là le principal danger d'un traitement pénicillé préventif.

Syphilis secondaire

Tous les aspects de la syphilis secondaire se rencontrent toujours et d'autant plus que les «internistes» ont oublié la syphilis aux dépens de l'allergie ou de l'hépatisme. Certaines syphilis évoluent plusieurs mois avant d'être reconnues. C'est ainsi que les *syphilides florides* réapparaissent chez des malades traités pendant plusieurs semaines pour «allergie» ou «troubles hépatiques». Celles-ci ne trompent pas un oeil averti. Par contre, certaines formes discrètes, beaucoup plus rarement observées, méritent de retenir notre attention ainsi que le prouvent ces dernières photographies que nous vous présentons. Elles permettent de nous rappeler que la «grande simulatrice» continue à se manifester sous les aspects les plus variés. Retenons cependant que toutes ces formes qualifiées d'atypiques ont toutes été magistralement décrites par A. Fournier.

Aktuelle Probleme der Spätsyphilis

A. Wiedmann, II. Univ.-Hautklinik Wien (Österreich)

Die Einteilung in Früh- und Spätsyphilis ist zweckmäßiger als die bisher übliche Unterteilung in drei Stadien. Dies auch deshalb, weil durch die moderne Therapie und Diagnostik die Erkrankung einen anderen Aspekt bekommen hat.

In diesem Zusammenhang muß auf die modernen Erkenntnisse bei der endemischen Syphilis hingewiesen werden. Die Ursache für die Zunahme der luischen Infektionen muß besonders berücksichtigt werden. In Österreich haben die Meldungen von frischen Luesfällen vom Jahr 1959 bis zum Jahr 1966 von 194 auf 1123 zugenommen. Aus einer Zusammenstellung eines russischen Autopsiegutes geht hervor, daß die Mortalität an Organlues von 1933 bis 1957 von 1,3% auf 0,2% zurückgegangen ist.

Unsere Ansichten über die Heilung der Syphilis haben durch die Einführung des TPI-Tests einen einschneidenden Wandel erfahren. Die Zahl der Fälle von spätlatenter Syphilis hat in den letzten Jahren zugenommen, woraus sich ein soziales wie ein wirtschaftliches Problem ergibt. Dies kann zum großen Teil auf die unterschwellige Penicillinbehandlung zurückgeführt werden, vor allem auf die indikationslose Anwendung des Antibioticums. Die Erscheinungen der Frühsyphilis sind dadurch flüchtiger und uncharakteristischer geworden.

Als besonders bedeutungsvoll hat sich der TPI-Test zur Unterscheidung der alten latenten Lues von den falsch positiven Reaginereaktionen erwiesen. Besonders interessant ist die Frage nach der Allergie und Immunität im Verlaufe der syphilitischen Erkrankung. Insbesondere muß darauf hingewiesen werden, daß Intradermoreaktionen mit Luetin nur mit großer Vorsicht beurteilt werden dürfen. Vor allem das aus Kaninchenhoden hergestellte Organluetin birgt eine große Reihe von Fehlerquellen in sich; es eignet sich aber sicherlich ausgezeichnet zur Provokation negativer Reaginereaktionen. Schlüsse aus solchen Beobachtungen zu ziehen, birgt die Gefahr in sich, daß sie zu spekulativen Überlegungen verleiten.

Auch die Frage Schanker redux, Neuinfektion oder Superinfektion bedarf der Klärung, und es sollte derselben größere Aufmerksamkeit zugewandt werden. Die Forderung, welche RUDOLF MÜLLER vor fast 50 Jahren aufgestellt hat, ein zweites schankerähnliches Geschwür, welches im Lymphbereich des ersten Geschwürs auftritt, nicht unbedingt als Neuinfektion zu betrachten, ist wohl durch die antibiotische Behandlung erschüttert worden, geklärt ist die Frage aber noch nicht. Vor allem muß in diesen Fällen unbedingt gefordert werden, daß eine histologische Untersuchung des neuerlichen Geschwürs vorgenommen wird.

Aus diesen Überlegungen ergibt sich die weitere Frage, inwieweit wir bei Fällen von alter latenter Syphilis die Möglichkeit haben, die Anwesenheit von Treponemen im Organismus noch nachzuweisen, ohne daß klinische Erscheinungen bestehen. Gibt uns diesbezüglich der TPI-Test bindende Aufschlüsse? Ich glaube, daß ein positiver TPI-Test einen Hinweis für das Vorhandensein von Treponemen im Organismus darstellt. Es ist uns gelungen, bei Kranken mit alter latenter Lues und positivem TPI-Test durch eine Behandlung mit Cortison und hohen Penicillindosen die Immobilisine zu beseitigen, das heißt, den TPI-Test dauernd zu negativieren. Daraus kann der weitere Schluß gezogen werden, daß, ähnlich wie das Cortison, jeder entsprechende zur ACTH-Ausschüttung führende Stress eine ähnliche Virulenzsteigerung der Treponemen nach sich ziehen kann. Wir konnten weiterhin beobachten, daß bei Fällen mit schwach positivem TPI-Test durch die Verabreichung von Cortison die Reaktion bis zur vollkommenen Positivität provoziert werden kann. So sehen wir in der Provokation des TPI-Tests mit Cortison bei der alten Syphilis eine Möglichkeit, der Feststellung einer biologischen Heilung der Erkrankung näher zu kommen.

Estimation of the Recent Serologic Methods

H. A. NIELSEN, Statens Seruminstitut Copenhagen (Denmark)

As an introduction I just want to remind you that studies on circulating anti-bodies produced during infections have demonstrated that the more important circulating antibodies can be separated into two groups: the first group having smaller molecules (7 S proteins) is called IgG, and the second group having heavier molecules (19 S proteins) is called IgM.

It is well known that the IgM appear before the IgG; for a shorter or longer time the two groups of antibodies will be present together, but then it seems from some observations that IgG is maintained longer than IgM, other observations give, however, quite the opposite information. Sometimes we have sera containing antibodies which have not been produced against an infecting organism but are appearing during collagen or auto-immune diseases, such antibodies are sometimes exclusively of the IgM group, but IgG are often present simultaneously.

If the latter molecular type of antibodies does react with the antigen we use in syphilis serology we will have a serum showing biologically false reactivity or better non-treponematic reactivity.

Now, if we had information on which group of antibodies is reacting in the various serological tests for syphilis, we could from a theoretical point of view be able to some extent to predict what sensitivity the various tests would have for early syphilis and at the same time we could deduce upon the specificity. The character of the antigens is of course very important in this connection.

In my department in Copenhagen Dr. E. HOLST has performed some studies — not yet published — in order to get information on the group of antibodies which reacts in the various tests. The main results from his studies are: The im-mobilizing antibodies reacting in the treponema pallidum immobilization test (TPI) are in the first line IgG antibodies, but IgM might occasionally show immo-bilizing activity. This explains why the TPI test as a rule is negative in primary syphilis whereas tests which are able to react with IgM will give reactive results.

The fluorescent treponemal antibody test (FTA) seems also to react with the IgG. In many papers it has been stressed that FTA is earlier reactive in fresh syphilis than the TPI test. I think all authors can agree in this. Whether it is exactly the same antibodies which are active in the two tests is not definitely decided, but the antibodies do belong to the same group, namely IgG, in accordance at least to our experiments. However, MATUHASI et al. [1] have found that IgM antibodies do react in the FTA test.

Also from papers published it is evident that the FTA test is less specific than the TPI test if the sera tested in the FTA test have not been diluted f. inst. 1:200 or absorbed. This is easier to understand if IgG as well as IgM are able to react in FTA. In the TPI test such measures are not needed, it is a real specific test.

The recent modification of the FTA test, the absorption technique [2], seems to have increased the specificity without having reduced the sensitivity signifi-cantly. In this connection I would like to make the following remarks: The absorb-ing substance is prepared from the Reiter organism. Perhaps the active substance is the Reiter protein, but I have not seen any publication telling us the real chemi-cal nature of the absorbing substance. Now, the sorbent should bind all reacting non-treponematic related substance from the sera under examination, and it is strange to say that the same substance which here is used to remove the non-specific reacting substance in the Reiter protein complement fixation test (RPCF) should be able to give specific results; again I refer to several publications con-cerning the use and value of RPCF.

It is correct that the TPI test is time consuming and demands much technical skill, but it is in fact a very simple and elegant test with a so far unsurpassed specificity. The test is non-reactive in early cases, but this is — as already said — to some extent explained through its ability to react mainly with IgG [3]. If IgM were able to immobilize T. pallidum the TPI test could be reactive earlier, but at the same time the high specificity of the TPI test might disappear.

The FTA test is technically more simple, but the readings are even more subjective than the readings of the TPI test. If the FTA readings could be done by a spectrophotometric arrangement, handy and quick in use, it would be a big advantage by the elimination of some sources for deviating results between laboratories.

Concerning the RPCF test I refer to a WHO document [4] in which BEKKER, DE BRUIJN and MILLER stress that it is important to employ the correct RPCF technique, and even in that case they point out that the RPCF will give about 1% reactive results in non-treponematic cases — compared to 0.1% in an examination with cardiolipin antigen.

The number of laboratories performing the complement fixation test with cardiolipin antigen has reduced considerably in the recent years, the reason is that laboratories find the test too difficult and time consuming. It has in a wider scale beem replaced by the slide microflocculation test mostly the VDRL test. The results of these two tests are rather similar, both can be performed sensitive enough to serve as screen tests. Now it is possible that the CF test will meet a "renaissance period", because some laboratories have with success automatized the CF test.

The well known microflocculation slide test has been modified in the recent years, f. inst. the rapid plasma reagin card test [6]. This test is very simple to perform, it can in fact be done on any spot, because the whole laboratory is a real "pocket-lab.". Cardiolipin antigen is used. If the technique is correctly performed and the readings are made by a qualified person, the sensitivity is high enough to point out all suspicious cases, but otherwise the test is not adequate in itself, but needs a supporting verification test. There is one point in this test which I consider very advantageous namely the use of plasma. In a personal communication Dr. JOSEPH PORTNOY mentioned that it might be better in the serology as far as possible to use plasma in stead of serum and I agree in this point with Dr. PORTNOY. The technical performance of some of the tests mentioned so far have in recent years been simplified in order to meet extraordinary situations. For inst. does OVCHINNIKOV's [7] simplification of the TPI test enable laboratories to avoid difficulties with the special gas mixture, and VAISMAN et al. [8] rondelle technique in the FTA test has made it easier to collect and ship blood from a team working under field conditions to a remote laboratory. In my opinion these modifications will not enter a well equipped routine laboratory.

At last I want to call your attention to a very recent procedure, a passive hemagglutination test for syphilis worked out by Dr. RATHLEV in my department in Copenhagen. A paper describing this test including preliminary results will appear in British Journal of Veneral Diseases in a few months.

References. 1. MATUHASI, T., K. MIZUOKA, and USUI MITSUKO: Bull. Wld. Hlth Org. **34**, 466 (1966). — 2. HUNTER, ELIZABETH F., W. E. DEACON, and PATRICIA E. MEYER: Pub. Hlth Rep. (Wash.) **79**, 410 (1964). — 3. TRINGALI, G., C. DEL CARPIO, and N. GIAMMANCO: WHO/VDT/RES/66.103 (1966). — 4. BEKKER, J. H., J. H. DE BRUIJN, and N. MILLER: Brit. J. vener. Dis. **42**, 42 (1966). — 5. PUGH, V. W., and W. T. GAZE: Brit. J. vener. Dis. **41**, 221 (1965). — 6. PORTNOY, J., JOHN H. BREWER, and AD. HARRIS: Pub. Hlth Rep. (Wash.) **77**, 645 (1962). — 7. OVCHINNIKOV, N. M.: Methodological Letters. 16. March 1962. — 8. VAISMAN, A., A. HAMELIN, and T. GUTHE: Bull. Wld Hlth Org. **29**, 1 (1963).

Evaluation des renseignements fournis par le T.P.I. et l'immunofluorescence

G. L. DAGUET, Laboratoire de Bactériologie-Virologie, Faculté de Médecine, C. H. U. Saint-Antoine, Paris (France)

Les tests d'immobilisation et d'immunofluorescence faisant appel à des antigènes constitués par des tréponèmes pathogènes sont actuellement considérés comme plus spécifiques et plus sensibles que les réactions cardiolipidiques.

Toutefois, nous devons souligner que dans notre expérience, poursuivie à Paris depuis 1952, les réactions cardiolipidiques s'avèrent très bien adaptées pour résoudre les problèmes courants posés par le diagnostic de la syphilis et la surveillance de l'infection après traitement. D'après nos observations, les défauts de spécificité ou de sensibilité des réactions cardiolipidiques concernent environ 2 pour 100 des sérums examinés en routine.

Depuis 15 ans, le TPI a acquis une situation privilégiée : il est considéré comme la réaction la plus spécifique des tréponématoses et, de ce fait, joue le rôle de test de référence pour clarifier les problèmes difficiles. L'apparition tardive de l'anticorps immobilisant au début de l'infection tréponémique lui enlève cependant toute valeur pour le diagnostic précoce. Par contre, la persistance indéfinie de cet anticorps, lors des phases latentes et tardives de la syphilis, confère au TPI une grande valeur dans les cas d'infection cliniquement muette ou discutable. L'étude de la courbe, reflétant l'évolution des titres en anticorps immobilisant chez les sujets traités aux phases latentes et tardives, s'avère de peu d'intérêt pronostic. La disparition de l'anticorps immobilisant chez les sujets traités ne représente pas un test rigoureux de guérison : des examens répétés plusieurs années après traitement peuvent démontrer la réapparition temporaire de petites quantités d'anticorps. De plus, l'anticorps immobilisant peut être absent chez des malades porteurs de manifestations de syphilis tardive typique, notamment le tabès.

Depuis quelques années différentes tentatives ont été entreprises pour simplifier la technique originale de Nelson dont les difficultés sont bien connues. D'autre part, un accroissement de la sensibilité de TPI a été proposé et réalisé dans une certaine mesure par addition de lysozyme ou par prolongation de la durée d'incubation. Or, toutes les modifications apportées à la technique de Nelson sont capables de perturber, dans des proportions variables, la spécificité et la sensibilité de la réaction. Le TPI ne peut jouer son rôle de test de référence que lorsqu'il est exécuté selon une technique directement dérivée de la méthode originale de Nelson. Ses indications doivent être réservées aux cas litigieux. Il faut reconnaître que le TPI est parfois positif chez des sujets exempts de tout antécédent et de tout signe clinique de syphilis.

Depuis 1957, l'application de l'immunofluorescence à la syphilis a été largement étudiée. D'importantes améliorations techniques ont été apportées. Celles-ci concernent :

1. les équipements des microscopes à fluorescence ;

2. la sélection des suspensions de tréponèmes (encore que beaucoup d'antigènes commercialisés soient de médiocre qualité) ;

3. la préparation de sérum antigammaglobuline humaine de titre élevé, marqué dans des proportions optima par l'isothiocyanate de fluorescéine ;

4. la dilution initiale des sérums à examiner à 1:200 (FTA 200) ;

5. L'absorption des sérums par un ultra-sonnat de tréponèmes de Reiter (FTA ABS) permettant un examen qualitatif après dilution à 1:5 ou 1:50.

Sur la base de notre expérience, portant sur un millier de sérums posant des problèmes, le FTA 200 est en accord avec le TPI dans 90 pour 100 des cas: sa spécificité est défaillante dans 5 pour 100 des cas; sa sensibilité est inférieure à celle du TPI dans 5 pour 100 des cas. Ces constatations sont conformes à celles observées par de nombreux expérimentateurs. Le FTA 200 ne peut ni remplacer les réactions cardiolipidiques dans les examens de dépistage, ni remplacer le TPI dans l'étude des cas litigieux.

Le FTA ABS avec dilution du sérum à 1:5 dans l'ultra-sonnat de Reiter (préparé par PILLOT à l'Institut Pasteur) est en accord avec le TPI dans près de 95 pour 100 des cas; sa spécificité est inférieure à celle du TPI dans 3 pour 100 des cas, sa sensibilité est supérieure dans 2 pour 100 des cas.

Le FTA ABS représente un progrès par rapport au FTA 200. Cependant, des variations de réactivité sont observées selon les préparations d'ultra-sonnat utilisées. De plus, la dilution du sérum à 1:5 dans l'ultra-sonnat ne peut être considérée comme obligatoirement optima pour un examen qualitatif applicable au dépistage.

La standardisation des réactifs et des modalités techniques de l'immunofluorescence appliquée à la syphilis n'est pas encore atteinte. Aussi est-il impossible de considérer actuellement le FTA comme une méthode de référence susceptible de remplacer le TPI, ou comme une méthode de dépistage à la place des réactions cardiolipidiques.

Des recherches doivent être poursuivies aussi bien pour isoler et préparer des antigènes rigoureusement spécifiques des tréponèmes pathogènes que pour analyser les immunoglobulines correspondantes.

Enfin, il faut tenir compte du fait que les syphilitiques subissent des examens sérologiques répétés pendant plusieurs années: toute modification technique ou toute technique nouvelle pose de difficiles problèmes d'interprétation aux cliniciens surveillant ces malades, d'autant qu'aucune réaction biologique ne peut être considérée comme valable dans 100 pour 100 des cas.

Penicillin in the Treatment of Syphilis

W. J. BROWN, Venereal Disease Program, National Communicable Disease Center, Atlanta, Georgia (USA)

In October 1943, Dr. JOHN F. MAHONEY, Director of the United States Public Health Service Venereal Disease Research Laboratory, cautiously reported on the apparently successful treatment of four cases of primary syphilis with penicillin. Dr. MAHONEY had undertaken this study only after limited animal experimentation indicated that penicillin possessed spirocheticidal activity. These preliminary animal studies indicated that exhaustive studies of the time-dose relationship would be necessary to establish maximally effective schedules since he had already noted that minimal amounts of penicillin given for brief time periods failed to sterilize experimentally infected animals. In December of that year a preliminary report detailing the treatment schedule clinical response in the four patients was published [1].

MAHONEY's treatment consisted of an intramuscular injection of 25,000 Oxford units of amorphous penicillin at 4 h intervals, day and night, for 8 days. This totalled 48 injections and 1,200,000 units. Mild Herxheimer reactions were noted within the first 8 h and repeated darkfield examinations were negative after 16 h. These reports clearly marked the beginning of a new epoch in syphilotherapy.

Regardless of future developments it is unlikely that such a revolutionary advance in the treatment of this infection will again occur.

Supplies of penicillin were both very limited and of widely varying purity, potency and constitution. Of the four natural penicillins, G, K, F, and X, occurring in amorphous penicillin, penicillin G was later established as by far the most active [2, 3].

Because of the exigencies of wartime it was essential that the value of penicillin be established quickly. This was accomplished by a nation-wide cooperative program of studies sponsored by the United States Government, in which the medical departments of the Army and Navy, many university hospitals, and the rapid treatment centers of the Public Health Service were active participants.

In these early years the great advantage of penicillin over arsenic and bismuth in the treatment of syphilis was its almost non-existent toxicity. Massive intravenous infusion arsenotherapy was actually being accomplished in a shorter period (5 days) than comparable effective penicillin schedules which required up to 80 injections and 10 or more days. However, massive arsenotherapy entailed a high incidence of serious reactions and approximately one patient in 200 died prior to the advent of Dimercaprol (British Anti-Lewisite) in 1945 which provided a method of reducing this mortality [4].

In the decade that followed MAHONEY's discovery, most of the problems of penicillin syphilotherapy were solved. Treatment schedules were rapidly devised not only for early syphilis, but also for syphilis in pregnancy, congenital syphilis, latent syphilis, late gummatous syphilis, cardiovascular and neurosyphilis [5]. By 1947 penicillin was firmly established as the treatment of choice in early syphilis and many of the schedules studied during that decade have remained essentially unchanged to the present day.

The problem of avoiding the frequent injections that were necessary to maintain treponemocidal blood levels was eventually solved by the development of repository preparations. ROMANSKY [6] introduced penicillin G in oil and beeswax (POB), in 1944, which permitted treatment with only a single daily injection. Subsequently, procaine penicillin G and procaine penicillin G in oil with 2% aluminium monostearate (PAM) were introduced. Injections of the latter preparation resulted in extension of the interval between injections to twice a week instead of daily. The apparent ultimate in repository preparations, benzathine penicillin G was introduced in 1954 [7]. A single injection of 2.4 million units of this preparation, which can produce detectable blood levels for up to 30 days, was shown to produce results equivalent to those obtained with more protracted schedules in the cure of early syphilis. The single dose therapy of primary and secondary syphilis is now firmly established as the treatment of choice in venereal disease clinics in the United States. Latent and late syphilis is treated with 6 to 9 million units of benzathine penicillin G given 30 million units per session at 7-day intervals. Thus, EHRLICH's goal of a single curative dose of antisyphilitic drug has been very nearly realized, for all forms of the disease. The results of proper penicillin treatment of syphilis are most satisfactory and excel those obtained in the pre-penicillin era.

Many studies after the discovery of the effectiveness of penicillin in syphilis employed the adjuvant agents of arsenic, bismuth, and fever in various combinations. These studies were carried out not only because penicillin was then both relatively scarce and expensive, but with the hope of shortening treatment or further reducing the number of treatment failures. Although, as might be expected, the clinical results showed some variance, the vast majority of investigators believed that such adjuvant therapy provided no definite advantage over penicillin alone, but only added inconvenience and distinct hazard to the patients.

The advent of penicillin radically changed the public health aspects of syphilis control in the United States. Treatment was reduced from months and years to days, hours and finally minutes. This brevity has undoubtedly hampered the education of patients and necessitated the development of new and improved epidemiologic techniques for contact tracing. Therapy has become so simple and rapid that reinfection has become commonplace. Indeed, reinfection, which was a relatively rare phenomenon following long term heavy metal therapy, now constitutes one of the serious problems of syphilis control. It is an interesting footnote to history that one of MAHONEY's original four patients subsequently became infected [8].

As penicillin became plentiful and cheap, the need for the specialized management of syphilis disappeared and treatment became the providence of the general practitioner rather than the syphilologist. Indeed it appeared that in the late 1940's and early 1950's that the reservoir of early infectious syphilis was drying up and the disease might be entirely eliminated. The dramatic decline in the number of newly reported cases of infectious syphilis witnessed throughout the world in that period has never been fully explained. However, it would seem a logical conclusion, since penicillin was being very widely employed during this period, that hundreds of thousands of undiagnosed and incubating syphilitics received penicillin for various unrelated conditions and were coincidentally cured.

By the mid 1950's the hazards of parenteral penicillin therapy were receiving considerable publicity and penicillin was beginning once again to be used only when more rational indications existed. During this same period broad spectrum antibiotics were coming into use and the indications for these drugs were frequently such as to be used in place of penicillin. While effective in syphilotherapy in the proper prolonged dosage, broad spectrum antibiotics cannot be compared with penicillin in treponemocidal activity and in only rare instances would patients receive sufficient quantities to produce inadvertant cure as was formerly undoubtedly commonplace with penicillin.

While the reasons invoked are conjectural, it is undeniable that a startling recurrence of infections occurred not only in the United States but in many other areas of the world during the late 1950's and early 1960's. Increases in incidence of the magnitude of 50% per year were recorded and once again the mechanisms of syphilis control were re-established and new control measures developed. Among the most effective new measures invoked has been the prophylactic penicillin treatment of known sexual contacts to infectious syphilis. Prophylactic treatment is proving to be an indispensible part of our program [9, 10].

One of the truly fortunate things in the penicillin therapy of syphilis has been the failure of the treponeme to develop resistance to penicillin. During the more than two decades of widespread clinical usage, many formerly highly susceptible organisms have gradually developed resistance to penicillin.

Since it would be exceedingly important to know whether the treponema is also following this pattern, the Venereal Disease Program began in 1965 a re-evaluation of those penicillin schedules that had been established for many years to affirm their continuing efficiency. While the number of patients studied has been small, compared with the numbers originally treated with these same schedules over 15 years ago, a preliminary analysis of the data gives absolutely no indication that any clinically evident resistance to penicillin has developed.

In this study three penicillin G schedules: 1. aqueous procaine, 600,000 units daily for 8 days; 2. benzathine, 2,400,000 units in a single injection and; 3. procaine in oil (PAM), 2,400,000 units followed at 3-day intervals by two further injections of 1,200,000 units are under evaluation in early syphilis. The cumulative retreatment rate after 9 months of observation has been 6.7, 5.3, and 8.0% respectively. In almost every case where retreatment has been necessary, available epidemiological and clinical evidence has indicated reinfection rather than treatment failure or relapse.

We currently feel that oral erythromycin or tetracycline in doses of 30 to 40 g given over a 10 to 15 day period are the alternate antibiotics of choice in treating infectious syphilis in penicillin sensitive patients. In latent or late syphilis the total dosage of broad spectrum antibiotics should be doubled. Unfortunately, these schedules are somewhat less dependable than parenteral penicillin because of their variable absorption, the necessary reliance upon the patient to take his medication, and the significant number of side effects, particularly gastrointestinal, which may limit their administration. Also, treatment with alternate antibiotics must be accompanied by close follow-up of the syphilitic patient since none of these drugs have had adequate evaluation in all stages of syphilis.

What penicillin has accomplished in the therapy of syphilis has been little short of miraculous. The vast majority of syphilitics have now been treated and spared the ravages of late syphilis and premature death. The treatment of infectious patients remains swift and certain. The extension of the benefits of penicillin, in the form of prophylactic or preventive therapy, to persons exposed to infectious syphilis is but a further logical step in syphilis control. We firmly believe that this step is the key to eventual syphilis eradication.

References. 1. MAHONEY, J. F., R. C. ARNOLD, and AD. HARRIS: J. vener. Dis. Inform. **24**, 355 (1943). — 2. OLANSKY, S., and L. E. PUTNAM: J. vener. Dis. Inform. **27**, 178 (1946). — 3. TURNER, T. B., M. C. CUMBERLAND, and H.-Y. LI: Am. J. Syph. **31**, 276 (1947). — 4. EAGLE, H., and H. J. MAGNUSON: Am. J. Syph. **30**, 420 (1946). — 5. Syphilis Treatment Schedules Based on Statement issued December 1, 1947 by Syphilis Study Section, National Institutes of Health, to Council on Pharmacy and Chemistry, American Medical Association. — 6. ROMANSKY, M. J., and G. R. RITTMAN: Bul. U.S. Army Med. Department Carlisle Barracks 81, 43 (1944). — 7. SMITH, C. A., J. F. O'BRIEN, W. G. SIMPSON, F. W. HARB, and J. K. SHAFER: Amer. J Syph. **38**, 136 (1954). — 8. MAHONEY, J. F., R. C. ARNOLD, and AD. HARRIS: J. vener. Dis. Inform. **30**, 350 (1949). — 9. ALLISON, jr., J. R.: J. S. C. med. Ass. **6**, 239 (1965). — 10. Epidemiologic Treatment of Syphilis-Editorial J. Amer. med. Ass. **188**, 820 (1964).

Autres traitements que la pénicilline

R. DEGOS, Hôpital Saint-Louis, Paris (France)

Parler d'autres médicaments antisyphilitiques que la pénicilline peut sembler anachronique. Dans beaucoup de pays, la pénicilline est devenue la seule thérapeutique utilisée dans le traitement des syphilis récentes et tardives, sauf cas d'intolérance à cet antibiotique. Cependant, si la pénicillinothérapie a une place prééminente incontestée, elle n'exclut pas d'autres médications.

Les *cyclines* ont une action tréponémicide qui apparaît équivalente à celle de la pénicilline. Dans les cas de sensibilisation à la pénicilline, la tétracycline et la terramycine permettent d'appliquer une antibiothérapie très valable, dont nous avons constaté l'efficacité. Mais, il serait dangereux de diffuser l'emploi d'une thérapeutique orale dont la facilité conduirait à des traitements sans contrôle médical.

Les arsénobenzols et autres arsénicaux ont été abandonnés par la plupart des syphiligraphes et nous n'y avons plus jamais recours. Par contre, les sels de *bismuth*, surtout oléosolubles, sont encore employés de façon courante dans certains pays, en particulier en France. Le mercure sous forme de *cyanure* de mercure, garde quelques indications.

Dans le traitement des *Syphilis récentes*, l'opportunité ou l'inutilité de faire suivre la cure pénicillinée initiale par des cures bismuthiques ou pénicillino-bismuthiques est discutable.

Nous avons revu 1981 dossiers de syphilis primaire et secondaire, traitées dans notre service, soit par une à trois cures de pénicilline, soit par un traitement pénicillino-bismuthique prolongé.

Dans les syphilis primaires, les résultats sont identiques. Dans les syphilis secondaires, les pourcentages de négativation de la sérologie de réagines sont plus élevés avec le traitement pénicillino-bismuthique, et la différence est surtout marquée lorsque le malade est traité plus de 3 mois après la contamination. Nous avons, en outre, éliminé de notre statistique les malades soumis à un traitement pénicilliné et qui ont été retraités par le bismuth du fait d'une séro-positivité persistante, ce qui diminue encore le pourcentage réel de négativation sérologique après pénicillinothérapie isolée.

Quel que soit le traitement, les pourcentages de négativation sérologique sont faibles lorsque la syphilis est traitée plus de 6 mois après la contamination, surtout si l'on déduit de ces chiffres les TPI positifs avec sérologie classique négative.

Tableau 1. *Syphilis primaire et secondaire pourcentage de négativation sérologique après traitement*

	S^1 présérologique	S^1 sérologique	S^2 précoce	S^2 3 à 6 mois après contamination	S^2 tardive
	198 cas	783 cas	316 cas	491 cas	193 cas
Pénicilline Seule	93%	88%	68%	55%	43%
Pénicilline + Bismuth	91%	86%	78%	73%	54%

Les pourcentages de négativation sérologique (sérologie de réagines) ont été calculés en éliminant les malades perdus après le traitement initial.

Pourcentages des T P I positifs isolés (sérologie classique négative) chez les malades traités

S^1 présérologique	S^1 sérologique	S^2 précoce	S^2 3 à 6 mois après contamination	S^2 tardive
8%	18%	45%	55%	80%

En faveur du traitement pénicillino-bismuthique, il faut aussi noter que le nombre de malades ayant échappé à notre surveillance est moins élevé avec un traitement prolongé.

Tableau 2. *Pourcentage de malades perdus pendant la première année*

	S^1 présérologique	S^1 serologique	S^2 précoce	S^2 3 à 6 mois après contamination	S^2 tardive
Malades perdus dans la 1ère année de traitement:					
après Pénicilline	44%	49%	53%	56%	50%
après Pénicilline- + Bismuth ..	32%	35%	30%	31%	25%

La valeur de cette statistique comparative est très relative, comme l'est celle de toute statistique qui concerne le traitement des syphilis récentes. Cependant, nos résultats incitent à appliquer un traitement complémentaire bismuthique ou pénicillino-bismuthique lorsque la contamination remonte à plus de 4 mois et lorsque le genre de vie du sujet crée des risques importants de dissémination de la maladie. Nous poursuivons ce traitement pendant un à quatre ans suivant l'ancienneté de la contamination et l'évolution de la sérologie, avec des repos de 1 à 2 mois entre les cures. Ce traitement prolongé est d'autant plus justifié en France que nos malades redoutent l'inefficacité des traitements courts et qu'ils sont par la suite fréquemment traités de façon anarchique pendant de très nombreuses années.

Les *syphilis demeurant séro-positives* plus d'un an après une cure pénicillinén unique et isolée commandent, pour la plupart des syphiligraphes, la reprise d'ue traitement énergique, bien que la séro-négativité puisse apparaître dans des délais plus prolongés. Ces séro-positivités persistantes posent le problème de la pénicillino-résistance. Aussi, nous semble-t-il logique, dans ces reprises de traitement, d'adjoindre le bismuth à la pénicilline dans des cures alternées et répétées. Mais, ce traitement tardif, même prolongé, négative beaucoup plus difficilement la sérologie, ce qui peut être un argument contre les traitements initiaux de courte durée.

Dans ces cas, comme dans ceux où la syphilis reste séro-positive après un traitement prolongé, aucun élément ne nous permet de fixer la durée du traitement. Après 4 ans de cures régulières bismuthiques et pénicillino-bismuthiques, nous laissons le malade sous simple surveillance annuelle.

Les *Syphilis sérologiques* découvertes fortuitement ou celles qui se rapportent à une *contamination très ancienne*, gardent habituellement une sérologie toujours positive ou dissociée, malgré tous les traitements. Les mêmes constatations ont été faites dans la syphilis expérimentale. Est-il utile, dans ces conditions, d'instituer un traitement ? Si l'on admet le fait biologique que la présence des anticorps sériques traduit la persistance de tréponèmes vivants dans l'organisme, la prudence oblige à faire un traitement énergique, en prévenant le malade que sa sérologie restera positive. Cependant, les recherches de P. COLLART et d'autres auteurs montrent bien que, chez l'animal et chez l'homme atteints de syphilis tardive, la thérapeutique ne parvient pas à obtenir une stérilisation bactériologique, des tréponèmes — peut-être avirulents — étant retrouvés dans les ganglions, dans différents organes et dans le liquide céphalo-rachidien. Malgré l'absence de donnée scientifique pour juger de l'opportunité du traitement, de ses modalités et de sa durée, nous conseillons un traitement bismuthique, puis pénicillino-bismuthique de 4 ans.

De toutes façons, il nous paraît dangereux d'attaquer d'emblée par la pénicilline des syphilis anciennes qui n'ont jamais été traitées, ou qui ont été laissées depuis longtemps sans traitement. Le risque d'une réactivation de lésions latentes, surtout nerveuses et sensorielles, pouvant amener à la cécité et à la surdité, nous fait pratiquer deux à trois cures bismuthiques avant de recourir à la pénicillino-thérapie.

Dans les *Syphilis viscérales* authentifiées, ce risque de réactivation par la pénicilline est encore plus grand. Une corticothérapie concomitante ne met pas toujours à l'abri de ces complications et les expériences de McLEOD et MAGNUSON, et celles plus récentes de COLLART, font craindre une reprise de virulence des tréponèmes sous l'effet des corticostéroïdes.

Malgré ces réserves, la pénicilline reste, pour beaucoup de syphiligraphes et de cardiologues, le seul médicament qui mérite d'être retenu dans les *aortites syphilitiques:* la pénicilline peut cependant réveiller des crises angineuses et même provoquer des anévrysmes aortiques d'évolution rapide. Comme nous l'avions signalé il y a plus de 30 ans, le bismuth a une action dépressive sur le myocarde. Sans partager l'opinion de ceux qui excluent formellement le bismuth dans toute syphilis cardioaortique, nous avons recours à ce métalloïde lorsque l'aortite n'a pas retenti sur le myocarde et ne s'accompagne pas d'atteinte rénale. Les longues séries de 150 injections de cyanure de mercure, telles que nous les avions préconisées dès 1943, ont un effet souvent remarquable sur les douleurs angineuses et peuvent améliorer l'insuffisance cardiaque. Ce traitement mercuriel prolongé est parfois le seul qui puisse être conseillé dans les aortites syphilitiques avec angor et défaillance cardiaque.

Dans la *paralysie générale*, les médications autres que la pénicilline sont inefficaces, en dehors de l'acétarsol (stovarsol), peu employé actuellement. Le seul problème est celui de l'indication de la malariathérapie qui peut être envisagée, ainsi que la pyrétothérapie, après échec de la pénicilline.

Pour le tabès et pour les autres formes de syphilis nerveuse, nous sommes beaucoup plus éclectiques. Si la pénicilline à doses progressives prudentes constitue la médication de choix, le bismuth peut être bénéfique et le cyanure de mercure garde des indications surtout dans les syphilis oculaires et auditives. Nous commençons habituellement par des cures de cyanure et de bismuth avant de recourir à la pénicilline. Ce sont les effets comparatifs, favorables ou aggravants, de chacun de ces médicaments sur les signes fonctionnels qui dictent notre conduite thérapeutique ultérieure. Parfois, nous conseillons l'abstention de toute médication anti-syphilitique, chaque essai de médicament étant suivi d'une recrudescence des symptômes, en provoquant une congestion des lésions cicatricielles ou dégénératives du tissu nerveux.

Nous n'avons pas à envisager le traitement préventif de la *Syphilis congénitale*, la pénicillinothérapie pendant la grossesse de la mère garantissant complètement l'enfant. Notre expérience du traitement de la syphilis congénitale précoce est très réduite, mais le danger d'activation des lésions polyviscérales fait conseiller, par certains, des frictions mercurielles avant les premières injections de pénicilline. La syphilis congénitale tardive requiert le même traitement que la syphilis acquise tardive, et nous utilisons des cures alternées de bismuth et de pénicilline pendant 4 ans, la kératite interstitielle commandant une corticothérapie locale.

Free Communications

Epidemiology

Homosexual Transmission of Early Syphilis

N. G. Rausch, Erie County Health Dept. V. D. Clinic, Buffalo, N.Y. (USA)

Syphilis can be eradicated completely through a combination of education and epidemiology, or epidemic control. The latter depends for the most part on the results of securing a complete list of contacts from the patient during the incubation and/or infectious stages of his disease. A well trained interviewer knows that there are many males of all social strata who have sexual relations with not just one or several but even 100 of females! He does an excellent job of eliciting the names of female contacts. Not so well understood is the fact that many of these same patients have homosexual contacts as well. The purpose of this communication is to call attention to this problem.

Homosexual relations during and since "Old Testament" times both in the Jewish and later in the Christian culture have emphasized the fact that they are immoral and abnormal. Modern western society condems severly one who has homosexual relations. Consequently it is difficult for the interviewer to have the person so questioned admit such exposures. Tact and patience on the part of the questioner is essential for a thorough and complete list of both heterosexual and homosexual contacts.

KINSEY [1] insists that only 50% of the population is exclusively heterosexual after adolescence and since only 4% of the population is exclusively homosexual, 46% or nearly half then are "bisexual". These latter individuals engage in both heterosexual and homosexual activities and react to persons of both sexes in the course of their adult lives. There is no specific evidence that an individual's choice of a sexual partner is affected by some basic anatomic and/or physiologic capacity. It should be pointed out that only an infinitesimal number of these persons have abnormal gentalia or other secondary sex characteristics. KINSEY states further that "The homosexual has been a significant part of human sexual activity ever since the dawn of history, primarily because it is an expression of capacities that are basic in the human animal".

During a recent 2 year period careful interviewing technique at the Buffalo-Erie County New York Health Department revealed that 61 or about 33% out of a total of 185 male patients with early (less than 1 year in duration) syphilis, gave a history of homosexual exposure during the incubation period of their infection. This figure is even more impressive in the white males where our statistics show such a homosexual history was elicited in 45% of this group. The figure for the non-white males who admitted homosexual exposure was about 25%. The 20 to 24 year old age group yielded the greatest number of such patients, as one might expect, since the incidence of early syphilis was greatest in this area also.

There were 55 females who had early syphilis during this 2 year study period, but no female homosexuals or lesbians were discovered during the patient contact interviews. Our past experience has shown that the transmission of veneral disease is practically nil in this latter group.

It should be noted that in two instances only were homosexual exposures admitted exclusively. The great majority listed both female and male contacts. These individuals were then "bisexual" as KINSEY states are 46% of the male population.

To summarize then, knowledge of the possibility of both hetero and homosexual transmission of syphilis is of paramount importance. The facts listed above should be comprehended and remembered by clinicians, public health officials and para-medical personell in order to insure the eradication of syphilis as promptly as possible.

Rerefence. 1. KINSEY, A. C., W. B. POMEROY, and C. E. MARTIN: Sexual Behavior in the Human Male, p. 656. Philadelphia: W. B. Saunders Company 1948.

Homosexualité masculine et syphilis

G. MORIAME et P. MEERTS, Clinique Dermatologique de l'Université de Bruxelles (Belgique)

Depuis une dizaine d'années, de nombreux auteurs ont attiré l'attention sur l'importance croissante prise, un peu partout dans le monde, par les faits d'homosexualité masculine dans la propagation de l'endémie syphilitique (THIERS, 1959; GOODMAN, 1960; SCHUPPLI, 1962; HERMANS, 1963; DEGOS, 1964).

En ce qui concerne Bruxelles, les statistiques du Service Universitaire de Dermato-Syphiligraphie révèlent que l'homosexualité masculine a été la principale responsable du maintien de l'endémie syphilitique de 1958 à 1962, c'est-à-dire pendant les années «creuses». Pendant cette période en effet, les pédérastes ont représenté 60 à 100% des cas de syphilis récente dépistés chaque année. Les homosexuels participent également dans la proportion de 10% environ, au raz-de-marée tréponémique qui, depuis 1964, a plus que quintuplé le nombre des cas de syphilis contagieuse enregistrés annuellement à Bruxelles.

L'interrogatoire approfondi de nos patients, ainsi que de leurs partenaires indemnes, nous a permis de constater que:

1. Tous, sans exception, acceptent leur déviation comme une chose naturelle; ils n'en souffrent guère et s'y adonnent sans aucune retenue. Ce sont des amoraux et des pervers au sens psychiatrique du terme.

2. L'activité sexuelle des invertis se caractérise toujours par son extraordinaire intensité. Toujours inassouvis, non seulement ils multiplient les contacts sexuels mais sont perpétuellement à la recherche de partenaires nouveaux.

3. Tous ignorent la menace vénérienne ou pensent qu'elle ne concerne que les hommes ayant des rapports hétérosexuels.

Hypergénitalisme, promiscuité sexuelle et ignorance de la menace vénérienne sont trois faits capitaux qu'il convient de souligner. Ils expliquent en effet le rôle particulièrement néfaste que les milieux homosexuels sont susceptibles de jouer dans la dissémination du tréponème. Ces constatations rejoignent en tous points celles de nombreux auteurs et notamment de TOURAINE (1960). Diverses enquêtes menées, entr'autres, auprès des milieux judiciaires et policiers de notre capitale, nous ont fourni un certain nombre de données intéressantes. Le nombre des homosexuels est en augmentation constante depuis 1945 et on assiste en Belgique, comme dans de nombreux autres pays, à une véritable «démocratisation» de la pédérastie. La prostitution masculine, d'apparition relativement récente à Bruxelles, tend à s'accroître et à s'organiser. L'homosexualité se fait de plus en plus voyante et ses adeptes se livrent, notamment auprès de la jeunesse, à un prosélytisme aussi dangereux qu'actif. Comme tels, les faits d'homosexualité ne sont pas punissables. Ils ne le deviennent que pour autant qu'ils aient été commis sur des mineurs de moins de 16 ans ou en infraction aux articles de la loi pénale relatifs à la protection de la pudeur. En matière d'homosexualité, la protection des mineurs jusqu'à l'âge de 16 ans apparaît comme insuffisante et devrait être, de l'avis des juristes, étendue à tous les jeunes de moins de 21 ans (MASSION-VERNIORY et CHARLES, 1957).

Mesures thérapeutiques et prophylactiques

1. Thérapeutique de l'homosexualité. Tous les patients que nous avons examinés acceptent leur déviation et se considèrent comme parfaitement normaux. Il n'est donc pas surprenant qu'aucun d'entr'eux n'ait accepté de se soumettre à une thérapeutique quelconque. Il ne nous paraît donc pas exagéré de dire qu'il est pratiquement impossible de guérir un homosexuel avéré.

2. Prophylaxie de l'homosexualité. Il est admis que le milieu familial de l'enfant ainsi que les premières expériences sexuelles de l'adolescent jouent un rôle important dans l'orientation de la sexualité. De ce point de vue le prosélytisme et le proxénétisme auxquels nous assistons actuellement contribuent certainement à l'accroissement de l'homosexualité. Il convient par des mesures éducatives pour les jeunes, coercitives si nécessaire pour les autres, de pallier à cet état de fait.

3. Prophylaxie antivénérienne. «Tout homosexuel est un syphilitique en puissance». Il est donc indispensable, quel que soit le motif de sa consultation, de lui faire subir un examen clinique complet, ainsi que des examens sérologiques.

D'autre part, un dépistage systématique s'impose dans les milieux homosexuels. Dans la mesure du possible, ce dépistage devrait être réalisé avec la
collaboration des intéressés et notamment par l'intermédiaire de leurs associations.

A défaut de dépistage librement consenti, il y aurait peut-être lieu de prendre
des mesures légales visant au même but.

Bibliographie. La bibliographie complète peut être consultée dans: MEERTS, P.: Homosexualité masculine et syphilis. Rev. Méd. Pharm. **21**, 559, 599 (1965).

Social Problems of Venereal Disease Among Adolescents and Young Adults in New York City

W. CURTH, Division of Social Hygiene, Department of Health, City of New
York, New York (USA)

The treatment of venereal disease among negro or Puerto Rican adolescents and
young adults in New York City is complicated by the problems of housing and
drug addiction, which perhaps are not unique to the United States but are found
in New York City on an unprecedented scale. Most of the central parts of the larger
American cities were built during the last century. The houses are now obsolete,
kept in bad repair, and are lacking in bathroom and toilet facilities. As a consequence, the more prosperous white classes have moved to surburbs leaving the core
of the town to the poor.

Most of these are Negroes from the Southern States, who were displaced by the
increasing mechanization of agriculture, then there are Puerto Ricans from the
Carribean Island, which is heavily overpopulated, or Mexicans, who are also
seeking a better life in the United States. In New York City alone, there are
500,000 people living on public support. Because these people cannot pay the usual
rents, two or three families have moved together into an old, unsanitary apart-
ment. There are, of course, not enough playgrounds or parks for the children or
young adolescents. The public schools face an almost impossible task to teach the
children even the fundamentals of learning. The result is that as adolescents they
are ill-prepared for almost any job. With no work awaiting them and too much
free time on theirs hands, it is not surprising that pregnancies and prostitution
among the females and homosexuality among the males have become rampant.
The rate of venereal disease is high among both. The hopelessness of their way of
life has driven many young people into addiction to heroin or other drugs. There
are 30,000 drug addicts in New York City alone. The drugs are so expensive that
the user cannot earn the money by honest work, which he cannot obtain anyhow,
and so he or she has to resort to crime or prostitution. The family life among the
Negroes does not offer refuge from the harrowing influences of the street. The
mother rules in the house but her supervision is limited. Moral or ethical values
get scant attention. Quite often the children's fathers have disappeared. They do
not pay alimony or support the children. They cannot be found because registration of addresses is unknown in the United States.

As a Chief of a Venereal Clinic of the City of New York in the Negro district of
Harlem for the past 30 years, I have noted that the age of our patients has steadily
become lower. Gonorrhea and syphilis among children of 13 or 14 is not at all rare.
Boys of all ages try to obtain money by stealing or offering themselves for pay to
homosexuals, who are frequently infected with venereal disease. 40% of cases of
fresh syphilis in the City Clinics occur among homosexuals. To give you an

example: a 12 year old boy with syphilitic condylomata ad anum was infected by a 17 year old self-appointed youth leader, who infected 14 other young boys. He was supposed to take them into playgrounds. Through case finding by federal investigators assigned to practically every Venereal Disease Clinic in the USA we located a together 26 infected males or females in connection with this incident. — Usually we are able to bring three to four contact cases into the clinic per case of infectious syphilis.

The sero reaction among heroin addicts frequently gives a false positive result. It, therefore, becomes necessary to use TPI or FTA tests to determine the significance of the result of the blood test. Treatment of syphilis with the various penicillins presents no special problems; we usually give a total of 6,000,000 units. In case of allergy to penicillin, we hand out to the patient enough capsules of tetracycline for 4 to 7 days only then he has to return for another supply; the total amount is 50 g. One problem has arisen: the increasing resistance of gonorrhea to penicillin or even streptomycin; again we may have to resort to orally given tetracycline in such cases. Complications of gonorrhea such as epididymitis, prostatitis, and arthritis are rarely seen.

The late cutaneous manifestations of syphilis have practically disappeared; systemic lesions such as aortitis or cerebro-spinal syphilis are very rare. The dermatologist in private practice rarely sees cases of fresh syphilis. The government of the United States has undertaken a big program to improve the status of the poor. Let us hope that with a restoration of economic health there will be a betterment of mental and physical well-being and as a consequence a lessening of venereal disease.

General Trend of Syphilis Recenta in Japan in the past 5 Years (1962 to 1966)

J. Dohi, H. Mochizuki, K. Aono and T. Kojima, Tokyo Jikeikai University, School of Medicine Tokyo (Japan)

The incidence of syphilis recenta increased throughout the world immediately after World War II, but later declined for a time. In recent years, however, there has been a marked world-wide rise again in this disease.

According to the statistics of foreign countries, complied by the Ministry of Health and Welfare, the incidence of syphilis recenta generally followed a downward curve from 1950, hitting bottom from 1956 to 1958 before rising again in recent years. However, much of data collected by this speaker and others in Japan shows that the ebb before the fresh rise came around 1961 or 3 to 5 years later than it occurred in other countries.

This is a report on the trend of syphilis recenta in Japan for the 5 years beginning 1962, based on a survey conducted by this speaker and associates.

Method of Survey

In Japan, a compulsory system is in force of reporting all cases of venereal disease to the public health authorities. But regrettably, this system is not necessarily strictly observed, making it impossible to obtain accurate figures on the incidence of veneral diseases in our country. Therefore, we focused our survey on patients with syphilis recenta visiting the dermatological departments of hospitals attached to universities and doctors of the Japan Dermatological Society. Though unable to gain accurate figures covering all patients throughout the country, we could clarify the general tendency of syphilis recenta in Japan for the past 5 years.

Data

Covered by the survey were 1,128 patients visiting the dermatological department of 46 universities and 8,853 patients visiting at hospitals and clinics operated by 458 members of the Japan Dermatological Society. Their total came to 9,981.

Increase and Decrease in Number of Patients for the past 5 Years

The index of the number of patients on the basis of 100 for 1962 rose sharply to 144 in 1963 and to 222 in 1964, but it dropped to 123 in 1965 and to 125 in 1966.

Geographical Distribution

If Japan is divided into northern and southern halves, an interesting phenomenon was observed in the geographical distribution of syphilis recenta. That is, in the period under review, the most rapid and marked rise in the incidence of this disease was noted in the southern half. The average annual number of patients visiting the dermatological department of each university hospital or each hospital or clinic of a dermatologist, which stood at 5.3 in 1962, gradually increased in 1963 and 1964. From 1965, however, it showed a downward trend.

By contrast, the average number of patients per hospital or clinic in the northern half of Japan stood at only 0.4 in 1962, or far less than that in the southern half, but continued on the upgrade in subsequent years, reaching 4.4 in 1966.

These facts indicate that the rising trend of syphilis recenta in Japan has been shifting from warm areas in the south to cold districts in the north. And a closer analysis naturally shows the fastest and clearest increase in those areas which are advanced in industry, pelagic fishing and marine transport for international trade.

Distribution by Age

One of the recent characteristics of syphilis recenta in foreign countries is said to be a sharp increase in the incidence of the disease among juveniles. In stark contrast, however, patients aged 19 or less accounted for 7.4% of the total number of patients with syphilis recenta in Japan, on the annual average, in the 1962 to 1966 period. This represented only about half of the annual average up to 1954. Nevertheless, it is noteworthy that when analysed on a year-to-year basis, the proportion of 19-year-old or younger patients showed a marked rise, reaching 9.4% in 1966 or about four times as high as the 2.5% of 1962. By contrast, the percentage of patients in their 20 declined from 54.9 in 1962 to 45.5 in 1966.

Symptoms

Significant differences are seen between patients up to 1954 and those since 1962. That is, a notable increase has been observed in psoriasis syphilitica and alopecia syphilitica, while condylomata lata has shown a sharp decline. These facts are confirmed by many reports in Japan. Meanwhile, the eruption of tertiary syphilis has scarcely been reported in Japan since 1962.

Source of Infection

It was impossible to trace the sources of the infection in the social conditions in which Japan now finds itself.

24*

Early Infectious Syphilis in Central London

R. D. Catterall, The Middlesex Hospital, London (England)

In May, 1965, a new department of venereology was opened at the Middlesex Hospital in London, close to the Soho district, famous for its restaurants, night clubs and coffee bars. During the 2 year period between May, 1965, and May, 1967, 10,627 new patients attended the department and 214 were found to have early infectious syphilis.

There were 183 men, of whom 85 had primary syphilis, 68 secondary syphilis and 30 early latent syphilis of less than 1 year's duration. Only 31 women were found to have infectious syphilis. 9 had primary syphilis, 8 secondary syphilis and 14 early latent syphilis.

Homosexual intercourse was the commonest source of infection amongst the men and was responsible for 116 infections (63%). There were 40 homosexual men with primary syphilis, 54 with secondary syphilis and 22 with early latent syphilis. 96 (83%) of the men stated that their exposures were both casual and promiscuous. 85 (73%) said that they were both active and passive, 21 (18%) were always passive and 10 (9%) were always active. The primary chancres were anal in 22 (55%), penile in 12 (30%), rectal in 4 (10%) and buccal in 2 (5%). There were no homosexual women.

A number of atypical non-indurated lesions occurred in the anal area but lymphadenopathy was a marked feature of the majority of cases. It was present in 76 (89%) of the 85 men and in 8 (81%) of the 9 women with primary syphilis and in 67 (88%) of the 76 cases of secondary syphilis. The commonest skin lesions were papular and were found in 43 (56%), but macular and squamous lesions were also frequently observed. Mucous patches were present in the mouth in 30, on the penis in 20 and in the rectum in 11 patients. Palmar and plantar lesions were found in 26 men and 4 women.

Herxheimer reactions occurred in 118 men (64%) and 15 women (48%). They were most frequent in patients with seropositive primary syphilis and early secondary syphilis.

The majority of the patients were treated with procaine penicillin 600,000 units intramuscularly daily for 10 days. Eight patients stated that they were sensitive to penicillin and were treated with erythromycin orally to a total dose of 30 g. There were 7 (3%) treatment failures with penicillin, 4 having serological relapses and 3 having abnormalities of the cerebrospinal fluid 1 year after treatment.

Contact tracing was successful in 36 (40%) of the 85 men with primary syphilis, 36 (53%) of the 68 men with secondary syphilis and in 13 (43%) of the 30 men with early latent syphilis. The contacts of 8 (88%) of the 9 women with primary syphilis, 4 (50%) of the 8 women with secondary syphilis and 7 (50%) of the 14 women with early latent syphilis were traced and treated. Failure of contact tracing was usually due to the casual nature of the contact, language difficulties, especially with Pakistanis, Indians and Cypriots, and to lack of cooperation from some patients.

Reinfection with syphilis during the period of observation occurred in 14 men (8%), 13 of whom were homosexuals. Only one of the women was reinfected. Multiple infections were common in many of the patients. 68 other sexually transmitted diseases were found amongst the 183 men. The commonest conditions were rectal and urethral gonorrhoea, non-specific urethritis, scabies and pediculosis pubis. Amongst the 31 women, 28 other diseases were diagnosed, the most frequent being gonorrhoea, trichomoniasis and vaginal candidosis.

At a new clinic in central London over half of the cases of early infectious syphilis were in homosexual men. Despite a number of atypical anal lesions, lymphadenopathy was found to be a valuable physical sign. Reinfection with syphilis was a problem amongst homosexual men and multiple infections with sexually transmitted diseases occurred frequently in both sexes. Contact tracing was often unsuccessful owing to the casual nature of the relationships, intense promiscuity amongst homosexuals, language difficulties and lack of cooperation from some of the patients.

Clinical, Epidemiological and Therapeutic Aspects of Syphilis in Buenos Aires

L. M. Baliña, J. C. Gatti and J. E. Cardama, Universidad del Salvador, Facultad de Medicina, Departamento de Dermatología, Buenos Aires (Argentina), and J. J. Avila and H. N. Cabrera, Municipalidad de Buenos Aires-Hospital Francisco J. Muñiz, Servicio de Piel (Argentina)

331 syphilitic patients were studied. This constitutes 2.87% of a total of 11,513 patients examined during the last 4 years at the Skin Diseases ward Muñiz Hospital.

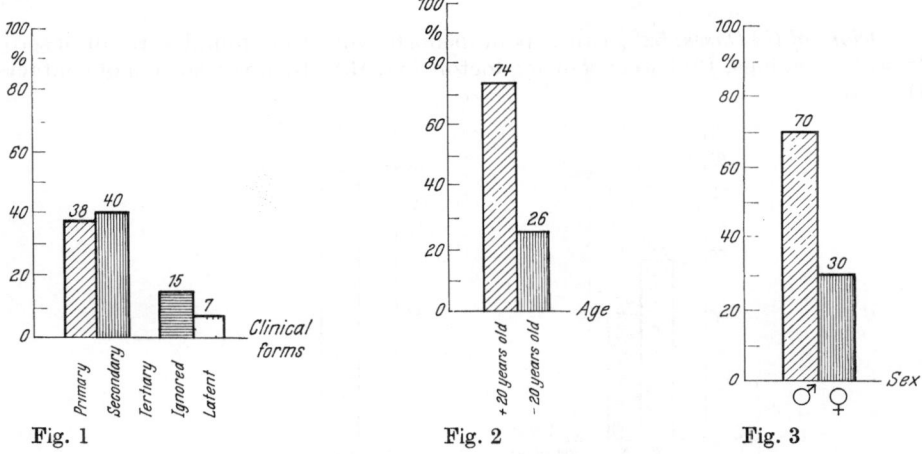

Fig. 1   Fig. 2   Fig. 3

Clinical Manifestations: The most frequent form was secondary syphilis (40%) followed by primary syphilis (38%) no case in the tertiary stage was observed, in 15% of the cases the disease was ignored, and in 7% it was latent (Fig. 1). In the primary stage, apart from the typical primary lesion, that was seen almost exclusivly in men (only once in a woman) we recorded manifold, herpetic and ulcerous cases and Follman's balanitis.

Age: 26% were less than 20 years old, 74% over that age (Fig. 2).

Sex: The majority (70%) were men as compared with 30% among women (Fig. 3).

Epidemiology: The likely source of contagion was: boy-girl friend relationship 29%; wives and husband 26%; homosexuals 16%; prostitutes 13%; promiscuous women 7%; parents 3%; engaged couples 3%; permanent extramarital relationships 3%.

The high incidence of homosexuals as compared with prostitutes is remarkable ; the same can be said of that of wives as compared with that of permanent extra- marital relationships (Fig. 4).

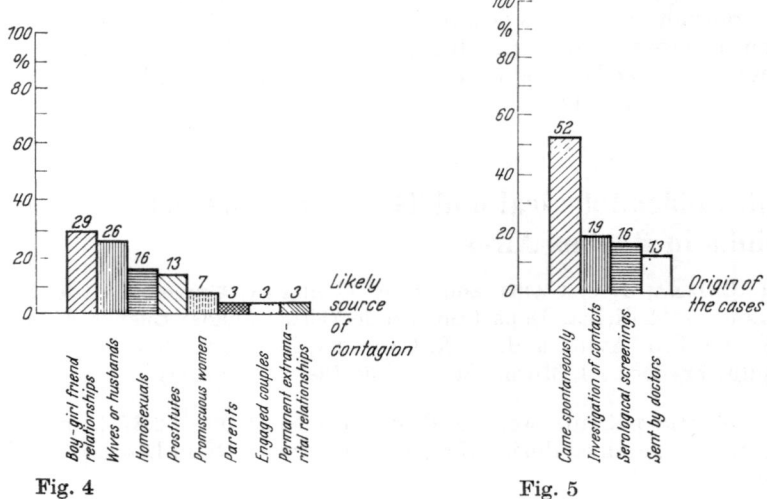

Fig. 4   Fig. 5

Origin of the Cases: 52% came spontaneously, 16% were found as result of sero- logical screenings, 13% were sent by doctors and 19% by investigation of contacts (Fig. 5).

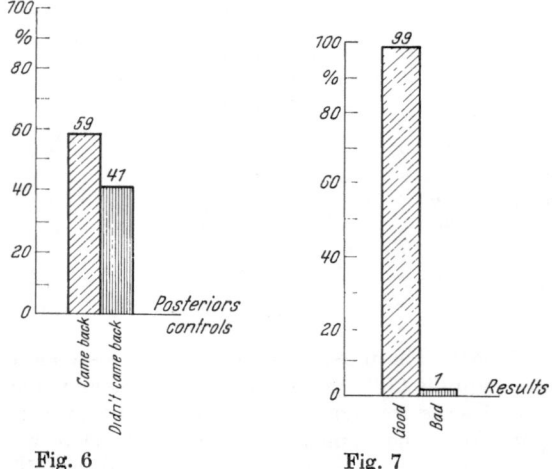

Fig. 6   Fig. 7

Therapeutics: 90% of the patients received benzatine penicillin in 4 weekly doses of 2,400,000 units each Crystalline penicillin 1,000,000 units daily up to a total of 10 to 20,000,000 units was tried only as an exception. In one patient who was allergic to penicillin tetracyclines were used. Only 50% of the patients returned tobe followed up, in those treatment was 99% effective (Fig. 6 and 7).

Sensitation. In 25 patients, before treatment intradermal and pathological studies were performed on the injection site after the injection of a 1% solution of sodium G-penicillin. There was one case of penicillin intolerance (nettle rash and dizzines). Histological studies of injection sites revealed lesions in papillary and subpappillary capillaries, with endothelial swelling surrounded by neutrophilic and lymphocitic cells with kariorexis, that recalls allergic vasculitis (GOU-GEROT-RUITER). This was seen in half of the cases studied with penicillin; almost all the patients showed symptoms of Herxheimer phenomenon 3 to 8 h after injection.

Prophylaxis: We have edited a booklet on sexual and antiveneral education for doctors, teachers and parents. It points out that sex is a gift and has to be faced in an absolutely positive way. The education has to be progressive, objective and straightforward and must inspire respect. Appeals to feelings of moral and decency are more effective than warnings or prohibitions. Any assistance demands a helpfull and comprehensive attitude on a part of the instructor. Sexual information usually reaches the young in the street or because they have heard adults speaking about it in an undesirable way.

What must and what must not be done in the case of a genital lesion is pointed out.

It is stated that preventive or epidemiological treatment can be applied in suspicious cases provided the treatment is completed.

A profounder study of skin and venereal diseases in the pregraduate levels, is recommended. A world wide statistical study by WEBSTER and BRANIGIN supported by the WHO showed that in 437 medicals schools which answered an average of 25,5 h were devoted to venerology as combined subject. For this reason "intensification in the activities in this field is recommended in view of the significant increase in veneral infections".

Public Health and epidemiological studies seemed to receive minimum attention. Epidemiological treatment of all contacts must be encouraged, because the benefits for the comunity overcame the individual risks of penicillin.

Localization of contacts, epidemiological inquires

Emphasis must be laid upon the need for Social Services and on the adequate motivation of social assistant and auxiliary staff specialized in veneral diseases to give them a clear notion of the social importance of contacts localization.

Leading serological centers; to set norms for serological; treponemal and fluorescent reactions; serological screenings every 3 years specially before marriage, in workers, schools and military establisment.

Syphilis and Japanese Seamen

T. HASEGAWA and R. SHINODA Kyoto (Japan)

The recent resurgence of syphilis has become a world-wide problem, and Japan which is now the one of the foremost maritime nation is no exception. Sailors have been held responsible for carrying syphilis from one port to another since the days of Columbus.

In an attempt to obtain new information about syphilis among seamen, questionaires were sent to 95 hospitals and clinics in Japanese ports, and to several shipping companies. 46 replies (48.4%) were received from hospitals and clinics.

The survey covered the 3 years from 1964 through 1966. An average of 207 seamen with syphilis were treated in each port clinic each year. The incidence of syphilis was higher in the Tokyo-Yokohama, the Nagoya-Shimizu, and the Kobe-Osaka port areas. Replies from the companies showed much lower incidence of syphilis, presumably since sailors do not tell the truth about venereal disease to the health services of their companies. The 1966 statistics of venereal disease in Kobe and Kyoto revealed that the highest incidence of syphilis was among white collar workers and those in heavy labor and that it was lower among sailors.

However, the statistics of dermatology clinic of the Tokyo-Seamen's-Insurance-Hospital indicated a higher incidence of syphilis than in the general out-patient population. 2.76% of the total number of out-patients were sailors with syphilis. 1% of all the out-patients seen in the dermatology clinic of the Kobe-Ekisaikai-Hospital, and 0.5% of those in the Nagoya-Pier-Ekisaikai-Clinic were seamen with syphilis. The number of registered seamen in Japan is 180,665. Thus the incidence of syphilis among seamen is not so high as among white collar workers and laborers working on the land.

The incidence of syphilis among young people has increased in many countries. Our survey also showed that the incidence of infection was highest in the sex-active 20-agers. 459 seamen with syphilis, 159 (42.6%) were between 20 and 30 years age. Replies from shipping companies also indicated a higher incidence among young seafarers. Similar results were obtained in the general population in Kyoto and Kobe. The incidence of syphilis among teen-age sailors was the same as in the general teen-age population. Probably sexual behaviour of young seafarers does not differ from that of the general population.

An increased incidence of primary and secondary syphilis was noted. Alopecia was a frequent symptom of secondary syphilis.

One of the most important problems is the source of infection. Replies from hospitals indicated that 80% of the seamen were infected in Japan. In contrast to this, replies from shipping companies indicated that 62% caught syphilis in foreign countries. This discrepancy can be attributed to the difference between the ocean-going and the coasted seamen.

The treatment of syphilis has been done by penicillin alone, penicillin and metals, penicillin plus other antibiotics, or other antibiotics alone. The first choice antibiotic is still penicillin. In general, 12 million units of penicillin were given in the treatment of secondary syphilis. The new synthesized penicillins were also used. In one clinic, metals, metals combined with other antibiotics were preferred. Common antibiotics other than penicillin used in the therapy of syphilis were erythromycin, tetracycline and chloramphenicol.

30% of the infected seamen were seen in the clinic within 3 months of infection, and 36% after 3 to 6 months. Most of them were not treated continuously. Some of them were treated by the ship's surgeon or responsible officer dealing with health on board ship.

In most cases, treatment was paid for by Seamen's Insurance, and very few by private fees. In one company, the health statistics of 1966 indicated that 35.6% of all diseases were gastrointestinal disorders, and 4.4% venereal diseases. In this company, the average age at the time of marriage was 27.9 years for officers and 27.0 years for sailors.

The different attitudes towards sexual behaviour and the different religions in each country make the solution of the problem of prostitution difficult. Venereal disease is basically a separate problem from that of extramarital intercourse, I think. Among seafarers, syphilis is still an occupational hazard.

However, maritime traffic is now changing rapidly. Remote control ships, submarine tankers, giant tankers, containerization are examples of recent innovation, which may soon change the nature and the problem of the seamen themselves.

La sifilis en Uruguay. Tratamiento y profilaxis*

R. A. VIGNALE, Clínica Dermosifilopática de la Facultad de Medicina de Montevideo (Uruguay), F. AMOR y C. RIVEIRO, Ministerio de Salud Pública, Montevideo (Uruguay)

La sífilis constituye en Uruguay un problema sanitario importante, con un aumento de la morbilidad paralelo al observado en la mayoría de los países.

Clinica. No creemos que haya variado la patobiología del treponema es decir, no hay formas clínicas nuevas ni atípicas de las ya clásicamente conocidas. No observamos DUCREY, pero sí NICOLAS y FAVRE. La asociación sífilo-poradénica explicaría en parte, las formas atípicas clínicas y serológicas, en especial las inflamatorias. También el tratamiento insuficiente enmascara y desfigura las lesiones. Las reinfecciones son cada vez más frecuentes, debido a la eficacia del tratamiento. Con sífilis I y II, se obtuvieron los siguientes porcentajes: 1960, 1.02%; 1961, 1.65%; 1962, 1.88%; 1963, 2.50%; 1964, 3.47%; 1965, 4.60%; 1966, 4.94%.

Factores epidemiologicos: 1. *Médico:* disminución de la enseñanza de la Dermatología y de la venerología, uso indiscriminado de los antibióticos, especialmente en el tratamiento de la blenorragia; automedicación y tratamiento por idóneos, abandono de las medidas de profilaxis, uso de anticonceptivos orales. 2. *Higiénicosanitarios:* falta de educación sanitaria en la población, escasez de personal técnico. 3. *Socio-económico-morales:* auge de la prostitución reglamentada y clandestina, incremento del homosexualismo y proxenetismo, disminución del temor a las enfermedades, pobreza y promiscuidad en las zonas marginales de las ciudades, relajamiento de las costumbres con aumento de las relaciones sexuales en los adolescentes, debilitamiento y desintegración del núcleo familiar, independencia económica de la mujer, rapidez de las comunicaciones nacionales e internacionales, aparición de la llamada "nueva moral". — El homosexualismo se presenta en forma similar a la de los otros países. Es un problema de orden psiquiátrico con múltiples factores en juego. La frecuencia de chancros anales ha ido en aumento: 1957, 0.5%; 1961, 1% y 1967, 5%. Además de los prostíbulos masculinos clandestinos, existe la prostitución callejera, en hoteles y en ambientes socio-culturales y artísticos.

Prostitución. De acuerdo con la Ley Orgánica del Ministerio de Salud Pública, el sistema legal es el *abolicionismo* pero en la práctica rige el *reglamentarismo:* ejercicio en prostíbulos, casas de "huéspedes", revisión médica periódica, inscripción en registros, etc.

Profilaxis. a) *Sobre el reservorio:* Efectuar la búsqueda y tratamiento de los enfermos; localización de la fuente de contagio; tratamiento integral de la prostituta, contralor del ambiente "para prostitución" proxenetismo y trata de blancas; mejorar el medio socioeconómico de los aledaños de las ciudades; creación de Servicios Sanitarios especializados; realizar catastros serológicos en la población de todo el país. b) *Vias de trasmisión:* educación sexual, en especial de la juventud, cierre de prostíbulos y lugares afines.

Montevideo, la capital, concentra el 80% de los casos y debe ser el objeto inmediato de la orientación profiláctica.

Tratamiento. Empleamos *exclusivamente* la penicilina para todo tipo de sífilis. Importa no solamente la dosis sino el tiempo de administración, que no debe ser menor de 30 días. La penicilina es siempre de gran eficacia. No hemos observado hasta el momento actual, sífilis III, cutáneas o viscerales, *clínicamente activas,* en

* Trabajo de la Sección Asistencia y Profilaxis Venérea del Ministerio de Salud Pública, Montevideo, Uruguay. Colaboración del Departamento de Biofísica de la Facultad de Medicina, Montevideo, Uruguay.

enfermos que hayan sido bien tratados con penicilina, a pesar de la persistencia de una serología y un Nelson positivos. Preferimos la penicilina de acción retardada en especial la benzatínica, excepto en embarazadas, lactantes y en las viscerales que iniciamos con la cristalina para evitar el Herxheimer. En casos de intolerancia empleamos la penicilina por vía oral, eritromicina o tetraciclinas.

Plan de tratamiento. No usamos dosis mínimas hemos observado serologías positivas en sífilis recientes en enfermos que abandonaron el tratamiento luego de una o dos inyecciones de benzatínica; serologías persistentemente positivas durante muchos años. En sífilis recientes, latentes y terciarias cutáneas en dosis semanales de 2.400.000 U de benzatínica con un total de 4 inyecciones. En terciarias viscerales y en embarazadas, cristalina en suero fisiológico diarias, en dosis crecientes por 10 días continuando con la benzatínica al igual que en las anteriores. En el lactante, 40 o 50.000 U de cristalina por kilo de peso, repartidas en los 10 primeros días, siguiendo con un millón, hasta completar un mes de tratamiento. También se puede terminar con benzatínica 600.000 U según la edad. En casos de empleo de penicilina oral, indicamos la fenoximetilpenicilina: 1.200.000 U por día, tres dosis diarias durante 25 a 30 días. Si se indica la tetraciclina o eritromicina, 2 gr diarios durante un período de 25 a 30 días. La repetición de las series de penicilina benzatínica, en casos de serologías y Nelson persistentemente positivos, se hará de acuerdo con el criterio evolutivo del enfermo. En general no somos partidarios de la reiteración de los tratamientos.

En Sintesis. La sífilis no constituye un problema de orden médico sino sanitario y social. La penicilina ha solucionado el tratamiento. Si logramos ajustar el contralor de la prostitución y si empleamos las modernas técnicas de educación sanitaria en todo su vasto plan, podremos disminuir la morbilidad de esta enfermedad.

Der diagnostische Wert des Zeichens von Higoumenakis

C. G. HIGOUMENAKIS, Universitätsklinik „A. SYNGROU" für dermatologische und venerische Krankheiten, Athen (Griechenland)

Die Diagnose der *erworbenen* Syphilis erfolgt, wie bekannt, einerseits an Hand der klinischen Erscheinungen während des ersten, zweiten und dritten Stadiums und andererseits laboratorisch an Hand der Untersuchungen des syphilitischen Treponema auf kontagiöse syphilitische Erscheinungen hin während des ersten und zweiten Stadiums sowie auch auf Grund der Wassermannschen Reaktion.

Die *angeborene* (konnatale) Syphilis dagegen wird auf Grund der permanenten sicheren und unsicheren Zeichen, die sich auf die Nachkommen des an Syphilis Leidenden übertragen, festgestellt.

Zu den sicheren Zeichen der *angeborenen* Syphilis zählt seit 1936 das von meinem Vater entdeckte, beschriebene und interpretierte Zeichen, das in der internationalen Bibliographie unter dem Namen „Hyperostosis Claviculae Signum Higoumenakis" bekannt ist. Dieses Zeichen — die Schwellung am sternalen Ende der Schlüsselbeine — ist klinisch leicht feststellbar und tritt durchwegs bei *allen* an angeborener Syphilis Leidenden auf; eine Tatsache, die ihm seinen besonderen diagnostischen Wert verleiht.

Personen, die an *erworbener* Syphilis leiden sowie jene, die absolut gesund sind, weisen dieses Zeichen niemals auf.

Zur Begründung dieser Behauptung, daß die Schwellung am sternalen Ende der Schlüsselbeine ein sicheres Zeichen für die Diagnose der angeborenen Syphilis ist, hat mein Vater auch röntgenologische Beweise erbracht. Die Röntgenaufnahme hat aber auch einen praktischen Wert, da sie die Diagnose des sicheren Zeichens bei korpulenten Personen ermöglicht, bei denen es wegen des Fettansatzes meist äußerst schwer ist, das Zeichen von Higoumenakis klinisch festzustellen. Histologisch wurde die durch die Spirochäten verursachte syphilitische Schwellung der sternalen Schlüsselbeinenden von TOURAINE, RIBADEAU, DUMAS und BERMON bestätigt.

Die Tatsache, daß das Zeichen von Higoumenakis bei allen an *angeborener* Syphilis Leidenden vorhanden ist, beruht auf anatomischer, biologischer und mechanischer Basis.

Aus der *Anatomie* ist uns bekannt, daß die Osteose des inneren Drittels des Schlüsselbeins, des sternalen Endes, aus dem späteren Kern erfolgt, und zwar zwischen dem 18. und 20. Lebensjahr; die Osteose des Schulterblattendes und des Clavikels dagegen erfolgt bereits zwischen dem 30. und 35. Tag des intrauterinen Lebens. Die Osteose des Schlüsselbeins unterscheidet sich von der Osteose der übrigen Knochen insofern, als hier die Kerne der Osteose unmittelbar auf dem Bindegewebe erscheinen. Der Knochen bildet sich also direkt aus dem Bindegewebe; die Wandlung des Bindegewebes zu Knorpel wird hier übergangen.

Biologisch gesehen: Das syphilitische Treponema, das ein ausgesprochener Parasit der Lymphen und des Bindegewebes ist, wird bereits während des intrauterinen Lebens von der Mutter dem Embryo durch das Blut zugeführt. Es setzt sich während der Ausstreuung in allen Organen und Geweben des Embryo sowie am sternalen Ende beider Schlüsselbeine, die aus dem Bindegewebe gebildet werden, fest.

Mechanisch gesehen: Die wichtigste Aufgabe des Schlüsselbeins besteht darin, die Zuführung des Akromium zur Mittellinie des Körpers zu verhindern. Folglich stoßen sich die sternalen Enden der Schlüsselbeine am Sternum. Hierdurch wird eine leichte Verletzung verursacht, besonders am sternalen Ende des rechten Schlüsselbeins, da die rechte Hand am meisten gebraucht wird. Das syphilitische Treponema, das sich nun als Parasit des Bindegewebes am sternalen Ende der Schlüsselbeine festgesetzt hat, bleibt hier so lange verborgen, bis es, gereizt durch die andauernden Anstoßungen des sternalen Endes des Schlüsselbeins am Sternum, erwacht und durch seine Toxine einen chronischen Reiz verursacht, der schließlich eine Schwellung des sternalen Endes, besonders am rechten Schlüsselbein, bewirkt. Diese Schwellung ist die Folge einer Bindegewebehyperplasie und der traumatischen Osteitis. Die Schwellung bleibt für immer und ist *das* wertvolle Zeichen, an Hand dessen die angeborene Syphilis klinisch festgestellt werden kann.

Daß man die Schwellung am sternalen Ende des rechten Schlüsselbeins deutlicher feststellen kann, ist darauf zurückzuführen, daß die Mehrheit der Menschen die rechte Hand mehr gebraucht. Die Schwellung kann jedoch auch am sternalen Ende des linken Schlüsselbeins deutlicher auftreten; eine Erscheinung, die bei Personen auftritt, die bei ihrer Arbeit mehr die linke als die rechte Hand gebrauchen. Auch bei einer Agenesie der rechten Hand tritt die Schwellung linksseitig deutlicher auf.

Abschließend zeige ich drei Krankheitsfälle angeborener Syphilis, die außer dem Zeichen von Higoumenakis auch unsichere Zeichen der konnatalen Syphilis aufweisen:

1. Fall: Zeichen von Higoumenakis. Vitiligo. Totale Alopecie der Kopfhaut. Zeichen von Dubois. Wassermannsche Reaktion negativ.

2. Fall: Zeichen von Higoumenakis. Zeichen von Dubois. Totale Alopecie. Wassermannsche Reaktion negativ.

3. Fall: Zeichen von Higoumenakis. Zeichen von Dubois. Totale Alopecie Areata. Unbegründete Schwerhörigkeit. Wassermannsche Reaktion negativ.

Die Diagnose der angeborenen Syphilis war in diesen Fällen also nur an Hand des Zeichens von Higoumenakis möglich, da es das *einzige* sichere Zeichen ist, das bei *jedem* an angeborener Syphilis Leidenden vorhanden ist. (Das Zeichen der Trias von HUTCHINSON tritt nur bei 20 bis 25% der an angeborener Syphilis Leidenden auf; die Wassermannsche Reaktion ist nur in 10 bis 40% der Fälle positiv.)

Serology and Experimental Syphilis

Some Immunobiological Problems in Experimental Syphilis

K. ITO, University Skin Clinic Gifu (Japan)

Even though it is 62 years since SHAUDINN-HOFFMAN discovered T. p. there are still many problems concerning syphilis yet to be solved. Recently, the inadequate treatment of syphilis has become a big problem. Needless to say, such subject bears some relation to the immunity of syphilis. Here I present our permal data obtained from some immunobiological research in experimental rabbit syphilis, together with that from various methods of staining T. p.

1. The Long Endurance of Stained Specimens of Treponema pallidum

Concerning the long endurance of stained specimens of T. p. we have attempted various staining methods and re-studied more than 2000 T. p. smear samples which have been stored for more than 33 years at our laboratory. Regarding positive staining of T. p., we used 15 kinds of fixatives and solvents, and we observed specimens stained by 31 kinds of dyes. The fixatives and solvents which were comparatively better than others were potassium permanganate etc. Some dyes gave good results as shown. Regarding negative staining we used 63 different kinds of dyes. 25 dyes out of these dyes gave good results. Several dyes are listed.

2. Staining of Treponema pallidum in Tissue

Here we are dealing with a new simple method of the staining of T. p. in the tissue.

Method: Section is soaked in the 1st solution (uranylnitrate and surfactants) for 5 min, the 2nd solution (silvernitrate and surfactants) for 5 min and the 3rd solution (hydroquinon, acetone, pyridine, sodiumbisulphate and surfactants) for 5 min. This method has the following points to recommend it. (1) Simple and rapid staining. (2) A clear picture. (3) Stable for a long time. (4) So stable that the specimen can be subjected to double staining.

3. Reinduration, Corymbiform Syphilid and Gumma-like Eruption

Following an intracutaneous inoculation with T. p. suspension on the dorsum, syphilitic papule was produced in that area. Following inadequate treatment with Penicillin (25 mg/kg 1 to 2 times) the papule disappeared leaving only a scar, but within about a week there was recurrence of the papule in the scar-area. Apparently the new papule was the same kind of papule as the old one. However, histopathologically there was the presence of T. p. in collagenous tissue and the lumina of dilatated lymphvessel. This papule gradually increased in size. Around it there were many corymbiform eruptions. These became bigger and amalgamated to form an ulcer. Histopathologically a dense infiltration of plasma cells and severe vasculitis were observed. Partial portion of this ulcer healed leaving a scar, it resembled a gumma-like eruption.

4. The Problem of Reinfection

a) Treatment (thought to be adequate) given to rabbits infected with T. p. S.T.S. (Wassermann, Reiter, F. T. A. etc.) showed a negative result. These rabbits were divided into two groups. One group was reinoculated at a relatively early stage lent no syphilitic reaction was produced. The other group was reinoculated after a relatively long time and the syphilitic reaction was produced.

b) No treatment given to rabbits infected with T. p. Reinoculation was immediately given to a group of those rabbits which showed a positive S. T. S. result. This group of rabbits showed no further syphilitic eruption. However, in the case of a S. T. S. positive group, reinoculation was made after a long time lapse. Sometimes a slight syphilitic eruption was observed.

The above results suggest that local immunity is an important condition in success of reinoculation with Treponema Pallidum.

5. Local immunity and immunity

First. Healthy rabbits were inoculated intravenously with T. p.-suspension. About 4 or 5 weeks afterwards even before the S. T. S. revealed the disease, syphilitic papule and orchitis broke out. Histopathologically, T. p. was shown to be present in these papule and orchitis. Material from these papule and orchitis were excised and pressed in a mortar. Then, using tissue fluid thus obtained, the S. T. S. showed positive.

Secondly. The skin and the testicle were inoculated with T. p.-suspension. Syphilitic papule and orchitis broke out. While the S. T. S. still gave a negative result, fluid pressed from papule and orchitis tissue when subjected to S. T. S. provoked a positive reaction.

These two experiments suggest that local immunity precedes immunity in case of hematogenous inoculation with T. p.

Serodiagnosis of Syphilis

L. NICHOLAS, Hahnemann Medical College and Hospital, Philadelphia (USA), and H. BEERMAN, School of Medicine, University of Pennsylvania, Philadelphia (USA)

Since 1906 when AUGUST VON WASSERMANN applied the then recently described complement fixation reaction to the diagnosis of syphilis, the significance of the serologic reactions has been challenged many times. In fact, today the meaning of a reactive serologic test for syphilis is still being questioned. Therefore, a large number of serologic tests were devised which aimed for a higher degree of specificity and/or sensitivity. In the final analysis, each test detected reagin, a non-specific globulin complex of high molecular weight. Since many other diseases produced reactivity to these tests, a large number of false positive results were observed.

One of the biggest steps in recent years was the utilization of treponemes as the antigen in newly-devised procedures. The era of treponemal testing began in 1949 when NELSON and MAYER described the immobilization of treponemes by syphilitic serum in the presence of complement. Then, in less than 15 years, a host of tests were developed, some of academic and research interest only, and some of proved clinical value. At best, treponemal tests likewise suffer from definite limitations. They do no more than inform of the immunologic status of the patient and do not answer the question of whether or not he has syphilis.

The first fluorescent treponemal antibody (FTA) test was introduced by
DEACON, FALCONE and HARRIS in 1957. The original test utilized a 1:5 dilution of
the patient's serum, at which dilution 25% of normal serums gave low-titred false
positive reactions. These were due to reaction of the treponemal antigen with a
group antibody which was shown by DEACON and HUNTER to react with such non-
pathogenic treponemes as the Reiter treponeme and T. microdentium, as well as
with T. pallidum. The titer of serums containing nonspecific group antibody
ranged from 1:5 to 1:100. In 1960, DEACON, FREEMAN and HARRIS introduced a
modification called the FTA-200 test, utilizing a 1:200 dilution of patient's serum.
Thus, the group antitreponemal antibody was diluted beyond its reactive titer and
no longer interfered with the test. However, by testing with such high dilution of
serum, the sensitivity of the test was decreased. After DEACON and HUNTER

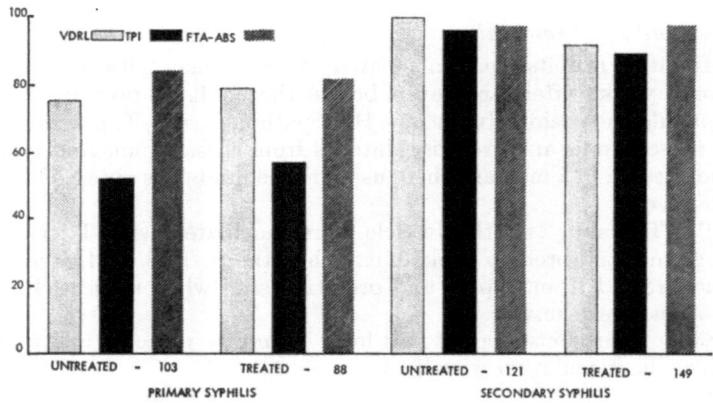

Fig. 1. Comparative reactivity of VDRL, TPI, and FTA-ABS tests in primary and secondary
syphilis based on 2,252 specimens; this test is reactive in a higher percentage of instances
than the TPI or VDRL in all diagnostic categories except untreated secondary syphilis

showed that the group antibody could be eliminated from test serums by absorption with intact Reiter treponemes, the serums so treated and subsequently
examined resulted in a increase specificity and sensitivity of test results. The use
of sonic-disrupted Reiter treponemes in place of intact organisms for absorption
was described in 1964 by HUNTER, DEACON and MEYER as the FTA-ABS test.
Now, in place of the sonicate, the FTA-Sorbent is a standardized water-soluble
extract of the non-pathogenic Reiter treponeme, which is used in place of buffered
saline in making the 1:5 dilution of the patient's serum.

DEACON, LUCAS and PRICE reported an evaluation of the FTA-ABS test based
on 2,252 specimens and studied through the cooperation of two academic institutions (Baylor University and University of Michigan), two State laboratories
(Tennessee and Florida) and one City laboratory (St. Louis, Missouri). We will
briefly summarize a few of their data by presenting two of their charts. Fig. 1
shows the FTA-ABS test is reactive in a higher percentage of cases than the TPI
or VDRL in all diagnostic categories except untreated secondary syphilis, where
all tests approach reactivity of 100%. Fig. 2 includes a comparison of the tests in
other syphilitic categories and again in all phases the FTA-ABS test shows the
highest reactivity rate.

According to DEACON, LUCAS and PRICE, the differences in these results are
attributable primarily to the greater sensitivity of the FTA-ABS test, particularly

in very early syphilis and in syphilis of long duration. There is no evidence that the FTA-ABS test is any less specific than the TPI test.

DEACON, LUCAS and PRICE state in their summary that "repeat testing of 215 specimens with discrepancies between the FTA-ABS and TPI tests suggests that if the FTA-ABS test gives a positive reaction and the TPI test a negative reaction, the difference is due to the greater sensitivity of the FTA-ABS test; if the TPI gives a positive reaction and the FTA-ABS a negative reaction, testing is at fault".

These conclusions are not universally accepted. WILKINSON and RAYNER studied the relationship between immobilizing antibody and the antibodies detected

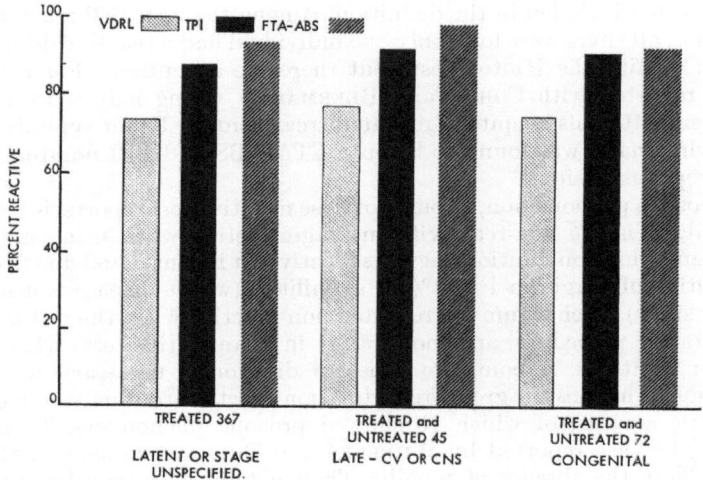

Fig. 2. Comparative reactivity of VDRL, TPI, and FTA-ABS tests in latent and late acquired syphilis and in congenital syphilis; in all phases FTA-ABS shows the highest reactivity rate

by the fluorescent tests. To these English investigators, the discrepancies between TPI titer and absorbed FTA titers suggest "a difference between the two antibodies rather than a difference in the sensitivity level of the two tests".

There are four special situations which may cause an etiologic diagnostic problem. These are first, the case of early syphilis; second, the biologic false reactor; third, the prozone phenomenon; and lastly, sero-nonreactive late syphilis, usually ocular or neurologic.

Following infection by Treponema pallidum, formation of various antibodies ensues. Suffice to say that the rate of reagin production is such that its detection by the VDRL slide test is usually delayed about 30 days, that is, 7 to 10 days after the chancre appears. In addition to reagin, these are at least two separate treponemal antibodies. One, reacting with the Reiter treponeme as well as with T. pallidum, unites with the shared or group antigen common to these and other treponemes; the other is apparently specific for T. pallidum itself. Except in some cases of early syphilis, the group component of the antibody predominates. This justifies to some clinicians the use of the Reiter treponeme in place of T. pallidum as antigen. Referring again to DEACON et al., of their 25 cases of sero-negative primary syphilis (that is, non-reactive to the VDRL slide test), 16 or 64% were reactive to the FTA-ABS test. Thus, the FTA-ABS test may detect syphilis earlier than the VDRL. This should be remembered in trying to make a diagnosis in a VDRL non-reactive person with a lesion which is either negative on darkfield examination or inaccessible for either direct or indirect darkfield examination.

The entire subject of biologic false reactivity is getting more attention now. The old oft-repeated lists of the percentage of BFPs in various diseases must be revamped because so many of the figures are based on tests performed with the old, crude tissue extract antigens rather than with cardiolipin described by PANGBORN in 1941. In HOAGLAND's study of 300 cases of infectious mononucleosis, only three patients had reactive STS, one of which was proved to have syphilis, while the other two were biologic false reactors. This reported incidence of 0.66% BFP in infectious mononucleosis is far from the commonly cited 20 to 30% figure.

The BFP is usually considered to be of low titer. In fact, this weakness of reaction is often included in the definition. Among the 200 BFP reactors reported by FIUMARA, all titers were low; only one individual had a reactive dilution titer as high as 1:16 with the Hinton test. But there are exceptions. For example, the patient I reported with COHEN and BEERMAN, a young lady with a persistent VDRL titer of 100 dils in spite of repeated treatment for latent syphilis (5 times in 8 years) who finally was found to be both FTA-ABS and TPI non-reactive, while her LE prep was positive.

The prozone phenomenon, a source of false negative test reports, is incompletely understood, It is the non-reactivity in reagin testing when using more concentrated serum, which on dilution becomes reactive. It is considered due to exaggerated production of reagin in 1 to 2% of syphilitics (whose diaease is usually in the secondary stage). Such serum are reported non-reactive when the test is performed as a qualitative procedure, and more rarely in quantitative tests when limited to 3 or fewer dilutions. A complete series of dilution is necessary to detect this phenomenon. The Boston group reported non-reactive routine serollogic tests in 24 syphilitic serums, of which 16 showed prozone phenomena. To add to the confusion, the case reported by WUEPPER and TUFFANELLI showed the prozone phenomenon in the absence of syphilis. Their patient with lymphosarcoma was a biologic false reactor whose VDRL was reactive at 1:256, but both the TPI and FTA-ABS tests were non-reactive. Fortunately, in these treponemal tests nothing resembling a prozone phenomenon has been observed.

Again, a false negative reagin test may occur in late syphilis when it is not unusual for the reagin level to dip below the line of detection. A non-reactive routine STS is to be expected in 10% of late benign (mucocutaneous, osseous and visceral) syphilis, in 20% of cardiovascular syphilis, and in 33% of tabes dorsalis. However, doubt of the etiologic agent in these cases is dispelled by performing the proper treponemal test. SMITH and others in a survey of patients with ocular syphilis and neurosyphilis, studied 175 serums which were reactive to the FTA-ABS test and/or the TPI test; 65% reacted to both treponemal tests; 28% reacted to the FTA-ABS, but not the TPI; and 6.3% were TPI reactive, but were missed by the FTA-ABS test; most significant was their finding of a reactive or weakly reactive VDRL test in only 81% of the 175 serums. Hence, about 20% of their cases of late syphilis were sero-negative with the routine reagin test. Therefore, to avoid this source of error in determining the etiologic diagnosis when the reagin tests are non-reactive, these investigators list the following definite indications for ordering specific serologic tests (preferably the FTA-ABS test): (1) any abnormal pupil; (2) dislocated lenses (except frank Marfan's syndrone); (3) chronic uveitis; (4) retinitis pigmentosa-like fundi; and (5) optic atrophy.

With these repeated encomiums for the treponemal tests, one might ask why the reagin tests are continued. There are several reasons. The value of the reagin test is almost undisputed in the following situations: (1) Because of their economy and relative ease of perforance, they are invaluable as screening tests. (2) When correlated with history and clinical evidence of syphilis, a reactive reagin test is confirmatory. (3) When used in conjunction with epidemiological investigations, a reactive reagin test in a contact, suspect or associate is highly significant. (4) When reactive in high or rapidly increasing titer, a reactive test is almost diagnostic of syphilis, though occasionally false positive reactions occur in high titer as previously noted. (5) When used to follow babies suspected of congenital syphilis, a good quantitative reagin test is an excellent diagnostic tool. (6) Finally, the serologic response following treatment should be observed by repeated quantitative determinations with tests that measure reagin rather than tests that measure treponemal antibodies, because the latter do not change substantially following therapy.

On the other hand, treponemal testing has found its greatest value in the three following areas:

(1) to help distinguish between biologic false reactive and a true reactive reagin tests for syphilis;

(2) to help establish a correct diagnosis in patients who have clinical evidence of syphilis, particularly late syphilis, but who have non-reactive blood and spinal fluid reagin tests, and

(3) to assist in the diagnosis in patients who epidemiologically should have the disease, but who have non-reactive clinical serological evidence (such as a marital partner or an apparently normal parent of a congenitally syphilitic child).

In closing, we must answer a question which many of you are asking yourselves. "What about the Reiter tests — call it RPCF or KRP — you failed to mention them?" Yes, that is true because we consider these tests obsolete. The antigen employed in performing the RPCF or KRP tests is essentially the material used to absorb the non-specific group antibodies from the serum in the FTA-ABS test. In other words, the tests employing Reiter protein detect the non-specific or group antibodies rather than the antibodies specific for the treponema pallidum.

The only factors which stand in the way of world wide acceptance of the FTA-ABS test are: (1) the special ultra-violet microscope which is required. Fortunately, fluorescence is a factor in so many tests now, most up to date laboratories are buying such scopes. (2) Visual fatigue of the technician is a limiting factor. Somewhere between 30 and 60 tests per day is the upper limit for a technician. (3) Automation of the test has been completed by a company which is now working out many factors needed prior to production. If as and when automation is commercially available, the machine will cost about $ 15,000, and it will require technicians with much less training than do the tests now; the machine will be able to do 600 tests a day which will permit its use as a screening test.

Zur quantitativen Beurteilung des FTA-Testes

F. Fegeler, S. Nolting und M. Kiffe, Universitäts-Hautklinik Münster (Deutschland)

Aus der anwachsenden Zahl spezifischer Seroreaktionen haben bisher zwei ihren festen Platz behaupten können, und zwar der TPI-Nelson-Test und der FTA-(Fluoreszenz-Treponemen-Antikörper)Test. Die Schwierigkeit der technischen Durchführung, vor allem des Nelson-Testes, schließt bei nahezu absoluter Spezifität Fehlermöglichkeiten und daher falsch positive Ergebnisse nicht aus. Es erscheint daher zweckmäßig, auch in der spezifischen Luesserologie mehrere

Seroreaktionen durchzuführen, wie es für die klassische Serologie schon seit langem gefordert wird.

Mehr als der TPI-Test ist der FTA-Test bei der Beurteilung subjektiven Einflüssen unterworfen. Es erhebt sich oft die Frage, ob bei bestimmten Serumkonzentrationen eine gerade noch wahrnehmbare Fluorescenz als positiv anzusehen ist, ganz abgesehen davon, daß eine derartige Beurteilung manchem Untersucher visuell Schwierigkeiten bereitet. Bei den eigenen Untersuchungen wurden für die Beurteilung Serumverdünnungen von 1:10, 1:50, 1:100, 1:200 und 1:500 gewählt.

Insgesamt wurden an 604 Seren entsprechende Untersuchungen durchgeführt und das Ergebnis mit dem TPI-Test und den klassischen Seroreaktionen verglichen. Der TPI-Test war hierbei in 195 Fällen positiv, 18mal zweifelhaft und 29mal wies er einen Grenzwert auf. Die Bezeichnung Grenzwert wurde von uns eingeführt für eine spezifische Immobilisation von 50 bis 75%. Wir sind der Meinung, daß alle Untersuchungen mit einer spezifischen Immobilisation von 25 bis 75% wiederholt werden sollten, um Fehlermöglichkeiten weitestgehend auszuschalten.

Vergleicht man die Ergebnisse des FTA-Testes mit dem TPI-Test, so fällt auf, daß die größte Übereinstimmung mit den positiven TPI-Testergebnissen bei einer Verdünnung des Serums von 1:50 bis 1:100 liegt, während die größte Übereinstimmung mit den negativen Seren bei einer Verdünnung zwischen 1:10 und 1:50 zu beobachten ist. Teilt man die zweifelhaften Ergebnisse auf die positiven und negativen Reaktionsausfälle auf, so liegt die größte Übereinstimmung bei einer Serumverdünnung von 1:50 sowohl für die positiven als auch für die negativen Reaktionen. Die klassischen Seroreaktionen zeigen in dem vorliegenden Kollektiv eine erhebliche Abweichung von den spezifischen Seroreaktionen. Dies kommt daher, weil es sich fast ausschließlich um ein Krankengut handelt, bei dem Zweifel an der Diagnose Syphilis bestanden.

Bei zunehmender Verdünnung wird die Reaktivität des FTA-Testes unterschiedlich. Bei 195 im TPI-Test positiven Seren lag bei einer Serumverdünnung von 1:10 eine Übereinstimmung von 97% vor, während bei einer Verdünnung von 1:500 lediglich noch eine Übereinstimmung von 46,1% vorhanden war. Demgegenüber zeigte die Serumverdünnung von 1:10 die höchste Abweichung vom negativen TPI-Test. Die Untersuchung von zehn im TPI-Test positiven Liquores ergab in einer Verdünnung von 1:10 bei neun Fällen eine Übereinstimmung.

Aus den vorliegenden Beobachtungen ergibt sich die Frage, in welcher Verdünnung der FTA-Test durchgeführt werden soll. Die Beantwortung hängt von der Funktion ab, die man dem FTA-Test im Rahmen der Luesserologie zuerkennen will, d. h. soll er als Ergänzung der klassischen Luesserologie dienen oder soll er die spezifische Serologie ergänzen.

Zweifellos stellt er in beiden Fällen eine erhebliche Bereicherung der diagnostischen Möglichkeiten dar. Im ersten Fall sollte eine Verdünnung von 1:10 und 1:100 gewählt werden, um Empfindlichkeit und Spezifität möglichst weitgehend zu gewährleisten. Im zweiten Fall würde unseres Erachtens eine Verdünnung von 1:50 ausreichen, da der TPI-Test eine Kontrollfunktion ausübt.

Von den klassischen Seroreaktionen differierende Ergebnisse sollten unbedingt Veranlassung sein, eine TPI-Testuntersuchung durchzuführen, soweit nicht klinische Symptome den Ausfall des TFA-Testes einwandfrei bestätigen. Ergebnisse, die mit dem TPI-Test nicht übereinstimmen, bedürfen der Kontrolle. Inwieweit der FTA-Test sich für die Beurteilung der Wirksamkeit einer antiluischen Behandlung bewährt, müßten weitere Untersuchungen zeigen. Mit Sicherheit weiß man bisher, daß der FTA-Test im Gegensatz zum TPI-Test auch dann noch negativ werden kann, wenn die Behandlung im späteren Stadium der Lues begonnen wird.

Untersuchungen über den Einfluß des Überlebensmediums auf die Sensibilität des Nelson-Testes

J. LESINSKI, C. WISNIEWSKA und W. ZAJAC, Dermatologische Klinik der Medizinischen Akademie Bialystok (Polen)

Dem Nelson-Test wird heute, dank seiner absoluten Spezifität und hohen Empfindlichkeit, eine entscheidende Bedeutung in der Luesserodiagnostik beigemessen. Doch ein zweifelloser Mangel dieser Methode ist ihre unbefriedigende Reproduzierbarkeit.

Die Sensibilitätsschwankungen des Testes sind vor allem mit dem unstandarisierbaren Antigen, welches lebendige und bewegliche Treponemen bilden, verbunden. In dem bisherigen Schrifttum wurde zu wenig Aufmerksamkeit dem Einfluß des Basalmediums und seiner Modifikationen auf die Sensibilität und Reproduzierbarkeit des Testes geschenkt.

Tabelle 1. *Zusammensetzung der sechs untersuchten Basalmedien*

Stoff	Modifikationen des Basalmedien					
	Lysozym ml	Albumin ml	Gelatin ml	Dextran	Periston ml	nach BOAK ml
5% Rindalbuminlösung[a]	50	50	—	—	—	—
0,2% Gelatinlösung[b]	—	—	50	—	—	—
3% Dextranlösung[a]	—	—	—	100	—	—
Kaninchenserum	—	—	—	—	—	50
NaCl	—	—	—	0,3 g	—	—
Phosphatpuffer pH 7[a]	15,7	15,7	15,7	1,68 Na$_2$ HPO$_4$ 0,96gKH$_2$PO$_4$	17,8	—
1,5% Na-Thioglykolatlösung[b]	12	12	12	—	16,7	—
0,63% Cystein-Hydrochlorid-lösung[b]	3,2	3,2	3,2	0,1 g	3,6	—
1,23% Glutathionlösung[b]	6,3	6,3	6,3	—	3,6	—
1% Na-Pyruvatlösung[b]	1,5	1,5	1,5	—	1,75	—
1,26% Na-Bicarbonatlösung[a]	5,6	5,6	5,6	0,45 g	6,45	—
0,85% Kochsalzlösung	5,7	5,7	5,7	—	—	50
Periston N	—	—	—	—	50	—
Fructose	—	—	—	0,5 g	—	—
Lysozym	2 mg	—	—	—	—	—

[a] Wasserlösung
[b] Kochsalzlösung

Die vorliegende Mitteilung umfaßt Untersuchungen über sechs Modifikationen des Nelsonschen Basalmediums, die in der Praxis am meisten benutzt werden. Tab. 1 zeigt die Zusammensetzung der untersuchten Medien. Es sind: das Albuminmedium nach NELSON und DIESENDRUCK in der Modifikation des WHO-Labors in Kopenhagen, das Gelatinmedium nach HARDY, das Peristonmedium nach BERLINGHOFF, das Dextranmedium nach RIETSCHEL, ein Medium mit Kaninchenserum nach BOAK sowie ein Medium mit Lysozymzusatz in der Modifikation von FRIBOURG-BLANC.

In unseren Untersuchungen wurde das Überlebensvermögen der Spirochaeten untersucht. Die Ergebnisse zeigt die Tab. 2. Die besten Überlebensmöglichkeiten bot das Albuminmedium nach NELSON und DIESENDRUCK. Diesem folgen der Reihe nach: das Gelatin-medium nach HARDY, das Peristonmedium und das

Dextranmedium. Die schlechtesten Überlebensmöglichkeiten bietet das Boaksche Medium.

In den weiteren Untersuchungen wurde der Einfluß der Zusammensetzung des Basalmediums auf die Spezifität des Nelson-Testes geprüft. Die Untersuchungsergebnisse von 300 nichtluetischen Seren zeigen eine absolute, von der angewandten Modifikation unabhängige Spezifität des Nelson-Testes.

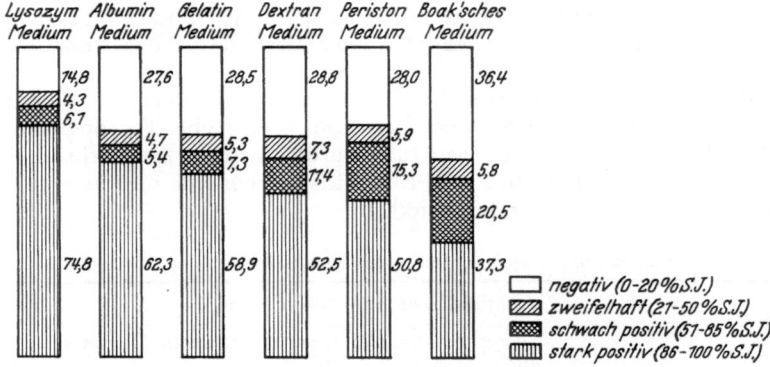

Abb. Vergleich der mit 6 Nelson-Test-Modifikationen erzielten Resultate bei 700 luetischen Seren

Tabelle 2. *Die Überlebensrate der Treponema pallidum in sechs untersuchten Medien nach 18, 24, 32, 36 und 40 Inkubationsstunden*

Medium	Durchschnittsprozent[a] der Überlebensrate der Treponema pallidum nach				
	18 Std %	24 Std %	32 Std %	36 Std %	40 Std %
Albumin	96	92	84	80	80
Gelatin	88	88	72	64	52
Periston	88	84	72	64	52
Dextran	84	80	64	56	32
nach BOAK	80	64	49	28	0

[a] Der Durchschnittsprozentsatz der Überlebensrate der Treponema pallidum wurde an Hand von fünfmal wiederholten Bestimmungen berechnet.

Das Hauptziel unserer Untersuchungen war aber die Prüfung der Abhängigkeit der Sensibilität des Nelson-Testes von der Zusammensetzung des Basalmediums. Die Ergebnisse zeigt das Diagramm. Insgesamt wurden 700 luetische Seren untersucht, die teilweise von den behandelten Kranken stammten. Der Nelson-Test wurde gleichzeitig mit allen sechs untersuchten Modifikationen angesetzt. Mit der Lysozymmodifikation aber wurde nur die Hälfte der Untersuchungen durchgeführt. Wie es aus dem Diagramm hervorgeht, ist die Sensibilität der Lysozymmodifikation die höchste. Die nächsthöchste Empfindlichkeit weist unter den anderen Medien das Albuminmedium nach NELSON und DIESENDRUCK vor. Unbedeutend steht ihm das Gelatinmedium nach. Eine wesentlich geringere Sensibilität weisen das Peristonmedium nach BERLINGHOFF und das Dextranmedium nach RIETSCHEL vor. Ein charakteristisches Merkmal der erwähnten Modifikationen des Nelsontestes ist ein verhältnismäßig bedeutender Prozentsatz zweifelhafter und schwach positiver Resultate. Diese Ergebnisse, die oft Interpretationsschwierigkeiten ergaben, werden in 19% der mit Hilfe des Dextranmediums und sogar bei 21% der mit Hilfe des Berlinghoffschen Mediums durchgeführten Untersuchungen festgestellt. Die Sensibilität des Nelson-Testes in der Boakschen Modifikation hat sich als gering und diagnostisch ungenügend erwiesen.

Die auf dem Diagramm vorgestellten qualitativen Untersuchungsresultate zeigen sich als vollkommen übereinstimmend mit den quantitativen Untersuchungsergebnissen, die hier aus Raummangel nicht im Detail besprochen werden. Unsere Untersuchungen haben den Mechanismus der Einwirkung des Basalmediums auf die Sensibilität des Testes nicht völlig geklärt.

Die Bestimmung des Restkomplementes zeigt keine antikomplementäre Wirkung keines der untersuchten Basalmedien in einem auf die Sensibilität einwirkenden Grade.

Die erhöhte Sensibilität der Modifikation mit Lysozymzusatz ist laut METZGER mit der Wirkung dieses Enzyms auf die nichtantigene Hülle der Treponemen verbunden. Hinsichtlich der anderen untersuchten Modifikationen haben wir einen Zusammenhang zwischen den Überlebensbedingungen der Treponemen und der Sensibilität der Reaktion festgestellt. Je bessere Überlebensmöglichkeiten das untersuchte Medium bot, desto höher war die Sensibilität des Nelson-Testes. Dieses Phänomen könnte besagen, daß die Treponemen im ungünstigen Milieu weniger empfindlich auf die Wirkung der Antikörper werden. Diese Beobachtungen sind übereinstimmend mit den experimentellen Untersuchungen von COLLART u. Mitarb.

Unsere Untersuchungen ergeben folgende praktische Schlußfolgerungen. Wir haben bedeutende Sensibilitätsschwankungen des Nelson-Testes in Abhängigkeit von der Zusammensetzung des Basalmediums festgestellt. Diese Unterschiede könnten die Ursache einer schlechten Reproduzierbarkeit und wesentlicher Diagnoseschwierigkeiten sein. Die Einführung immer neuer Modifikationen des Mediums in die serologische Praxis führt zu wesentlichen Mißverständnissen zwischen dem Serologen und Klinizisten und untergräbt das Vertrauen der Kranken zum Arzt.

Aus unseren Untersuchungen ergibt sich die Notwendigkeit einer Standardisierung der Nelson-Technik, und der erste Schritt in dieser Richtung wäre die Standardisierung des Basalmediums.

The Problem of Recovery from Syphilis

F. FLARER and C. RABITO, Dermatologic Clinic of the University of Padua (Italy)

It is possible to recover from a luetic infection, rarely spontaneously, more often by adequate treatment. We can assert this in consequence of the observation of very numerous men and women who had contracted the infection and recovered many years ago and today after all this time have either died from some other disease or, if still alive, have shown no clinical serological sign of the proceeding illness and may have given birth to children perfectly healthy and normal, as well as from the observation of a certain number of subjects who had contracted the infection twice or three times again, that was seen to be a new initial syphilis.

The luetic infection may also remain uncured in spite of adequate treatment. We can assert this on the basis of the observation of subjects in whom, after treatment considered apt to cure the disease and that had actually produced the disappearance of clinical and serological manifestations, after a more or less prolonged interval of time, presumably not due to reinfection, belated manifestations or re-positivation of the serologic manifestations showed up; also on the basis of subjects in whom the diagnosis of lues had been made only on the hand of sero-positivity (with the absence of clinical manifestations; latent lues) together with incurability of this symptom in spite of treatment.

These two assertions, valid in general for luetic infection, depend also on the single patient, so that one may say, one may recover and the other not. But in pratice when can we say that an individual has recovered ? When he hasn't re-covered ? When he can recover and when he cannot ?

These four questions, that in the last analysis make up the pith of the problem of the recovery criterium of syphilis, do not allow an easy answer in an absolute sense, even if in some cases there may be greater probability of validity and cer-tainty. Without making an analysis of the possible answers that case by case may be given to each question, anyone who has even slight familiarity with the problem can at once see the vast series of factors, from the clinical form to the treatments carried out, the serologic behaviour, the time that has elapsed, the constitution etc. that must be taken into consideration and be statistically appraised in order to try to find rules and suitable results to answer these questions in single cases.

Practically, with the aim of reaching a more and more reliable answer as regards the necessary individual appraisal of recovery and of the eventual real meaning of the so-called latency (postivity eventually persisting without clinical manifestations) I have considered the following three main directive lines necessary:

1. A statistic analysis made on the hand of the variables that come into play in the determinism of the criterium of recovery, an analysis that, given the con-siderable number of variables, can only be carried out with the modern methods of electronic calculations and by means of the compilation of index-card allowing these calculations. We are examining an index-card that will permit anyone to gather data according to the index-card itself and avail himself of the progra-mation worked out, in order to reach results comparable one with the other and valid for the above mentioned ends.

2. A comparative study of the various types of penicillin and of the modality of their action, given the necessity of clearing up the still obscure motivations of the disappointing use of penicillin in cases of latent syphilis.

3. The recourse to researches in the field of serology and of immunologic reactivity of the tissues in luetic infection which may enlighten us as to the real meaning of positivity and of the persistence of serological positivity in so-called latent syphilis. And in fact it is necessary to establish or differentiate the eventual modalities of the serological mechanism or of the immunitary tissue response between the positivity of the actual disease and the positivity persisting in spite of treatment.

Or the factors that must be taken into consideration for a judgment of re-covery from syphilis, those that at first sight appear and are perhaps the most significant are the therapeutic treatment and the serologic behaviour.

As regards the treatment, a problem that in my opinion is particularly inter-esting is the way in which a drug-like penicillin, atoxic, so that one can increase the dose ad libitum reaching a very high percentage in clinically active cases of luetic infection so as to obtain the disappearance of the clinical symptoms and the negativization of the non-positivisation of the serologic reactions always very active in vitro on spirochetes, in some cases is seen to be clinically inefficacious at least from the point of view of serologic negativisation. The problem might be faced, besides from the point of view of the actual study of cases of particular individuals in which the phenomenon is verified, and has been done in my Clinic by RABITO and cow. with the individualization of a factor protecting the spirochetes from penicillin, also with a more thorough study of the mechanism of action pertaining to the antibiotic.

As regards the serologic factor, if we can all agree as to the meaning of the negativity of the serologic reactions in the luetic patient and of T.P.I. after treatment, persistent negativity for a certain period of time may be discussed as to their meaning of persistent positivity in spite of treatment. It may be a consequence of the desirable preparation of new serologic reactions or of new modalities used in the carrying out of those already in use, so as to put into evidence eventual differences between positivity as a symptom of the persistence of the infection and persistent positivity in spite of actual recovery.

I think that following these three main lines it will be possible to reach an appraisal of the criterium of individual recovery on the hand of methods that are scientifically more suitable and therefore clinically more satisfactory.

Biological False-positive Reactors for Syphilis: Studies with the FTA-Absorption Test

D. L. TUFFANELLI and K. D. WUEPPER, Division of Dermatology, San Francisco Medical Center, University of California (USA)

The association of systemic diseases, particularly diseases of immunologic aberration on patients with chronic false-positive nontreponemal tests for syphilis, has repeatedly been stressed. Newer treponemal tests, particularly those employing fluorescent-antibody methods, are modifying previous diagnostic tenets and changing concepts of the false-positive reaction. The *Treponema pallidum* immobilization test (TPI) is less sensitive than the fluorescent treponemal-antibody absorption test (FTA-ABS) in primary, secondary and late syphilis.

A number of patients, considered to have false-positive reactions on the basis of a nonreactive TPI test, have been found to have reactive TFA-ABS tests. Because of the disparity in results we have restudied our patients with a previous diagnosis of false-positive reaction. In this report these patients are reclassified by their response to the newer treponemal tests. In addition, the incidence and serologic evidence of immunologic disease in these patients is determined.

Study Groups and Methods

100 and 76 of 347 diagnosed BFP reactors responded to an inquiry and were interviewed and re-examined, and serum specimens were obtained for laboratory studies. *TPI-Tests* were performed as in the usual procedure.

TPI-Tests were performed as in the usual procedure.

FTA-ABS-Tests were performed as described by HUNTER et al.

LE-Cell-Tests. L.E.-cell preparations, latex nucleoprotein slide test, antinuclear antibodies, and Tiselius paper electrophoresis was done on all serum specimens.

Results

On the basis of the results of nontreponemal and treponemal tests for syphilis the 176 patients studied serologically could be divided into four groups.

Transient Reactions. 211 had acute or transient reactions according to the history. All had reactive reagin tests of less than 6 month's duration and nonreactive TPI tests on one or two occasions. The majority of these patients had only a single reactive VDRL followed by two nonreactive VDRL tests, and many may have represented technical errors. 76 of the 211 were re-examined. All had nonreactive VDRL, TPI, FTA-200 and FTA-ABS tests at the time of re-examination.

Chronic Reactions. 136 patients had persistently reactive reagin tests of more than 6 months' duration and one or more nonreactive TPI tests when originally studied. 100 were re-examined in this study. The results of repeated treponemal testing allowed these patients to be grouped as having syphilis, "indeterminate" reaction or chronic false-positive reaction.

Syphilis. 12 patients, when restudied had reactive TPI and FTA-ABS tests though an initial TPI test had been negative. All of these were re-diagnosed as having syphilis.

"Indeterminate" reaction. 38 patients initially diagnosed as having false-positive reactions on the basis of a nonreactive TPI test had repeatedly nonreactive TPI tests but reactive FTA-ABS tests on repeat testing. These were termed "indeterminate" reactions. The TPI test was nonreactive in 61 of 63 determinations. The FTA-ABS test gave repeatedly reactive results (a total of 63 determinations in 38 patients). 7 had clinical evidence of late syphilis when reexamined.

Chronic false-positive reaction. 50 of the 100 patients initially diagnosed as having chronic false-positive reactions for syphilis had repeatedly reactive reagin tests of more than 6 months' duration and nonreactive TPI and FTA-ABS tests. These were true chronic false-positive reactions. In 5 patients the titer was higher than eight dilutions; the highest titer obtained (from a narcotic addict) was 64 dilutions. 24 had diseases considered to be immunologic in nature. 39 of the 50 had serious systemic illnesses.

Other serologic tests. The incidence of serologic abnormalities in patients with transient reactions was not remarkable, nor was it abnormal in the indeterminate and syphilitic groups. However, of those with chronic false-positive reactions, 25% had antinuclear antibodies, 27.6% rheumatoid factor, 11.1% L.E. cells, and 27.2% hyper-gamma-globulinemia.

Discussion

Reagin (Wassermann antibody) is an ubiquitous serum protein that may indicate syphilis or a predisposition to a disease of immunologic aberration. Patients with serum reagin and nonreactive treponemal-antibody tests have classically been considered to have "biologic" false-positive seroreactions.

Most studies of false-positive reactions have employed the *T. pallidum* immobilization test as the definitive diagnostic procedure, and previous studies depend upon its validity. Recently, however, fluorescent treponemal-antibody (FTA) studies utilizing absorption technics to remove "group" treponemal antibodies have resulted in the FTA-ABS test with an improvement in sensitivity. Sensitivity of the TPI in late syphilis is approximately 90%. The FTA-ABS is 8 to 10% more sensitive than the TPI in late syphilis. It is quite likely that this group forms a fair proportion of cases previously reported as chronic false-positive reactions.

In our study 50% of 100 patients previously diagnosed as having chronic false-positive reactions on the basis of a nonreactive TPI had reactive FTA-ABS tests. Repeated serologic and clinical evaluations confirmed syphilis in 19 patients (38%). On the basis of the findings described above, the treponemal tests necessary to establish false-positive reactions should include the FTA-ABS test. At present in our clinic the presence of repeatedly reactive reagin tests, a nonreactive TPI and a nonreactive FTA-ABS test is required. Previous reports of false-positive reactions may have included patients with syphilis. The transient presence of reagin is of little importance. Clinically and serologically, the patients do not appear to be different from normal controls.

The finding of 50 patients with reactive FTA-ABS tests in our original series of 100 chronic false-positive reactions was unsuspected and of value in increasing our understanding of such false-positive reactions. Treponemal-antibody tests were repeated several times in this group. Twelve subsequently gave reactive TPI tests, and seven others had clinical evidence of late syphilis. Thus, the original diagnosis based on single nonreactive TPI was in error. The 38 patients with nonreactive TPI tests and reactive FTA-ABS tests cannot all be given diagnoses at present on the basis of clinical evidence of late syphilis. For the reasons noted above, 19 to 50% of the patients with previous diagnoses of chronic false-positive reactions on the basis of a single nonreactive TPI test may actually have had syphilis.

Of the patients with persistent false-positive reactions 39 of 50 had serious systemic disease. This incidence is greater than that of previous reports, possibly because patients with latent syphilis and a nonreactive TPI test were excluded. The prevalence of serologic abnormalities such as antinuclear antibodies, rheumatoid factor and hyper-gamma-globulinemia in patients with persistent false-positive reactions is elevated and usually reflects an underlying immunologic disorder.

Neue diagnostische Methoden bei un- und anbehandelter Frühsyphilis

K. GREGORCZYK, Städt. Krankenhaus Kaiserslautern (Deutschland)

Für die in den letzten Jahren berichtete und vielfach auch statistisch gesicherte erneute Zunahme der syphilitischen Infektionen werden zahlreiche Ursachen diskutiert: Vermehrte Promiskuität und Homosexualität, eine verstärkte Bevölkerungsfluktuation und eine dadurch erschwerte oder ohnehin nachlässig gehandhabte Infektionsquellenerfassung dürften nicht allein verantwortlich sein.

Die nach GREITHER schleichende und daher besonders gefährliche Ausbreitung der Frühsyphilis ist zumindest in gleichem Maße auf nicht oder nicht frühzeitig erfolgende Erkennung zurückzuführen. Die Gründe hierfür mögen zum Teil in einer vorübergehend vernachlässigten Aus- und Fortbildung auf venerologischem Gebiet wie auch in einem durch zeitweisen Morbiditätsrückgang bedingten Unterlassen entsprechender differentialdiagnostischer Erwägung zu suchen sein.

Im Vordergrund dürfte jedoch die mit dem Wiederanstieg der Infektionszahlen beobachtete Zunahme diagnostischer Schwierigkeiten auch für erfahrene Venerologen stehen: Der fast allgemein registrierte Gestaltwandel der Syphilis aller Stadien mit klinisch— und nach eigenen Beobachtungen auch serologisch — symptomarmen bzw. symptomfrei erscheinenden Formen wird begleitet von einer Erschwerung des Erregernachweises als Folge oraler, parenteraler oder lokaler An- oder Mitbehandlung.

Aus dieser Situation ist es verständlich, daß eine höchstempfindliche und in ihrer Spezifität an den TPI-Test heranreichende serodiagnostische Methode wie der FTA-Test von zahlreichen Klinikern und Serologen und auch in eigenen mehrjährigen tierexperimentellen und klinisch-serologischen Untersuchungen auf seine Aussagekraft besonders bei der Frühsyphilis überprüft wurde. Diese Untersuchungen hatten in weitgehender Übereinstimmung gezeigt, daß die mit der Fluorescenzmethode erfaßten, gegen das Treponema pallidum gerichteten Antikörper nicht mit den Immobilisinen identisch sind, unabhängig von ihnen und bis zu 10 Tagen vor den selbst mit höchstempfindlichen Reaktionen nachgewiesenen Reaginen auftreten und einen von Immobilisinen und Reaginen unabhängigen Titerverlauf aufweisen. Andererseits zeigte sich, daß durch die von DEACON, FREEMAN und HARRIS empfohlene Anwendung einer Serumverdünnung von 1:200 die bei der Primärsyphilis gelegentlich geringen Antikörpermengen nicht immer ein eindeutiges Resultat ergaben; geringere Verdünnungen wiederum bedingten unspezifische Reaktionsausfälle, und das FTA-Absorptionsverfahren führte bei quantitativer Auswertung gelegentlich zu niedrigen Titern, wie sie auch nach frühzeitiger Behandlung isoliert im FTA-Test noch längere Zeit nachweisbar sind.

Beim eigenen serologischen Untersuchungsgut, das jetzt vorwiegend von auswärtigen, nur zum Teil venerologisch erfahrenen Einsendern unter Hinweis auf das Fehlen eindeutiger klinischer und serologischer Symptome sowie ausreichender anamnestischer Angaben eingesandt wird, ergeben sich daher insbesondere bei isoliert positivem Resultat des FTA-Tests folgende Fragen: Handelt es sich hier um

a) eine Primärsyphilis mit bereits positivem FTA-Test bei noch nicht nachweisbaren Reaginen,

b) eine bereits energisch, wenn auch unbewußt behandelte Frühsyphilis mit nur noch positivem FTA-Test,

c) eine serologisch sich gleichartig verhaltende Lues latens,

d) eine — ohne Wissen des Einsenders — lediglich anbehandelte Frühsyphilis oder

e) einen Patienten mit gegebenenfalls genital oder perigenital lokalisierten nichtsyphilitischen Haut- oder Schleimhautveränderungen und unspezifischpositivem Resultat im FTA-Test oder auch in einer oder mehreren der klassischen Seroreaktionen ?

Unter Berücksichtigung der bisherigen eigenen Erfahrungen mit dem FTA-Test bei über 8000 Serumuntersuchungen (davon über 7000 mit gleichzeitiger Untersuchung im TPI-Test und in den klassischen Lues-Seroreaktionen) und bei jetzt mehr als 200 Sera unbehandelter und behandelter Patienten mit einer Primärsyphilis wird daher bei diesem in Betracht zu ziehenden Patientenkreis folgende diagnostische Methodik für erforderlich gehalten:

1. Der FTA-Test wird grundsätzlich quantitativ und gleichzeitig mit den klassischen Seroreaktionen durchgeführt. Dem Einsender werden bei isoliert positivem Resultat des FTA-Tests dringend Wiederholungsuntersuchungen angeraten, da bei einer Primärsyphilis (auch bei lokaler Anbehandlung) der Titer des hochempfindlichen FTA-Tests in wenigen Tagen deutlich, bei sonstiger Anbehandlung ebenfalls, jedoch verzögert ansteigt, und gegebenenfalls die klassischen Lues-Seroreaktionen ein reaktives Verhalten aufzuweisen beginnen.

2. Bei gleichbleibendem oder auch absinkendem, insbesondere niedrigem Titer ist zur Klärung der Frage, ob lediglich gruppen-, jedoch nicht erregerspezifische Antikörper das positive Reagieren auslösen, zumindest zusätzlich das von HUNTER, DEACON und MAYER angegebene Absorptionsverfahren anzuwenden. Eine schon kurzfristig mögliche Wiederholung wird bei Vorliegen einer Primärsyphilis auch hier einen deutlichen Anstieg des Absorptionstiters ergeben. Bei Ausbleiben eines Titeranstiegs oder -abfalls bis zur Negativität muß durch Untersuchung im TPI-Test geklärt werden, ob eine in den klassischen Lues-Seroreaktionen nicht oder nur schwach reaktive Resultate auslösende Lues latens vorliegt.

3. Dem Einsender wird zusammen mit der Aufforderung zur wiederholten Serumeinsendung empfohlen, die weitere, unbedingt erforderliche Beobachtung des Patienten durch mehrfach zu wiederholende Versuche des Erregernachweises durch ihn oder einen anderen Untersucher auch bei nicht klassisch ausgeprägten Effloreszenzen zu ergänzen. Bei fehlender mikroskopischer Ausrüstung, unzureichender Erfahrung in der Differenzierung pathogener Treponemata pallida oder mangelnder Bereitschaft des Patienten zur Überweisung an einen anderen

Untersucher wird dem Serumeinsender empfohlen, ein von ihm gewonnenes Reiz-serum auf Objektträgern ausgestrichen und luftgetrocknet einzusenden. In An-lehnung an die von KELLOG und DEACON angeregte Methodik können dann durch Beschickung mit einem jedoch durch Absorption von Gruppen-Antikörpern weit-gehend befreiten, erregerspezifischen Antiserum und nachfolgender Fluorescein-markierung die fixierten und sogar morphologisch veränderten Treponemata pallida nachgewiesen bzw. von apathogenen Spirochaetales differenziert werden.

Zusammenfassend ist zu sagen, daß die selbst bei Anwendung neuester diagno-stischer Verfahren sich ergebenden Probleme bei klinisch Untersuchten und dort fortlaufend beobachteten Patienten ohne Zweifel leichter zu lösen sind. Wir müssen jedoch die Tatsache zur Kenntnis nehmen, daß heute eine große Zahl von Syphilitikern nicht in dermatologische Kliniken oder Abteilungen und auch nicht zum freipraktizierenden Dermatologen kommt. In diesen Fällen ist daher die Forderung nach gegebenenfalls mehrmaliger und vor allem quantitativer Wieder-holung des FTA-Tests unabweisbar und schon aus technischen Gründen leichter als die nach einer — leider vielfach unterbleibenden — Wiederholung des TPI-Tests zu stellen.

Die Aufgabe des Lysozyms bei der experimentellen Syphilis des Kaninchens

L. POSPÍŠIL, Mikrobiologisches Laboratorium der dermatologischen und venerologischen Universitätsklinik Brno (Tschechoslowakei)

Dem Lysozym, 1922 von FLEMING entdeckt, wird in den letzten Jahren eine erhöhte Aufmerksamkeit gewidmet. Das gilt sowohl für die Grundforschung als auch für die Möglichkeiten der praktischen Anwendung in der Diagnostik und Therapie. Die Frage über die Aufgabe des Lysozyms in der syphilitischen Infektion wurde aktuell, als von METZGER, HARDY und NELL (1961) beobachtet wurde, daß das Lysozym die notwendige Zeit für die spezifische Immobilisation der Tre-ponemen wesentlich verkürzt. Wie bekannt ist, gibt es bei Tr. pallidum aus frischen syphilitischen Läsionen einen Zustand der immunologischen Nichtreaktivität, deren Dauer durch Zugabe von Lysozym verkürzt werden kann. Die durch Zugabe von Lysozym verursachte Beschleunigung der Reaktion wird durch die Destruk-tion der hypothetischen Mucopeptidschicht von Tr. pallidum, deren Beweis jedoch bis heute nicht erbracht wurde, erklärt. Wir haben unsere Aufmerksamkeit folgenden Fragen gewidmet:

1. Wie groß ist die Lysozymaktivität unter den Bedingungen der experimen-tellen syphilitischen Infektion, und können diese Quanten eine immunologische Rolle spielen (Lysozymspiegel im Serum und Lysozymspiegel in dem mit Trepo-nemen infizierten Hodengewebe)?

2. Gibt es einen Zusammenhang zwischen dem Serumlysozym und den Leuko-cyten?

3. Wird die Ultrastruktur der Treponemen durch Lysozym verändert?

Material und Methodik. Die Lysozymaktivität wurde spektrophotometrisch nach der Lysis von Micrococcus lysodeikticus gemessen (POSPÍŠIL und JAKUBOWSKI, 1966) und auf 1 ml Serum bzw. 1 g Hodengewebe umgerechnet. Die Zählung der Leukocyten geschah in der Bürkerschen Kammer. Die elektronoptischen Präparate wurden in der von ADAMIKER u. Mitarb. (1965) beschriebenen Modifikation zubereitet und mit dem Elektronenmikroskop Tesla BS 242 A untersucht (Prof. Dr. Z. O. NEČAS).

Resultate. Die Werte der einzelnen Messungen (ausgeglichene Mittelwerte) und deren graphische Darstellung sind in den Abb. 1 bis 5 veranschaulicht. Die Abb. 1 zeigt, daß es nach einem anfänglichen Sinken der Lysozymaktivität bis zum 7. Tage

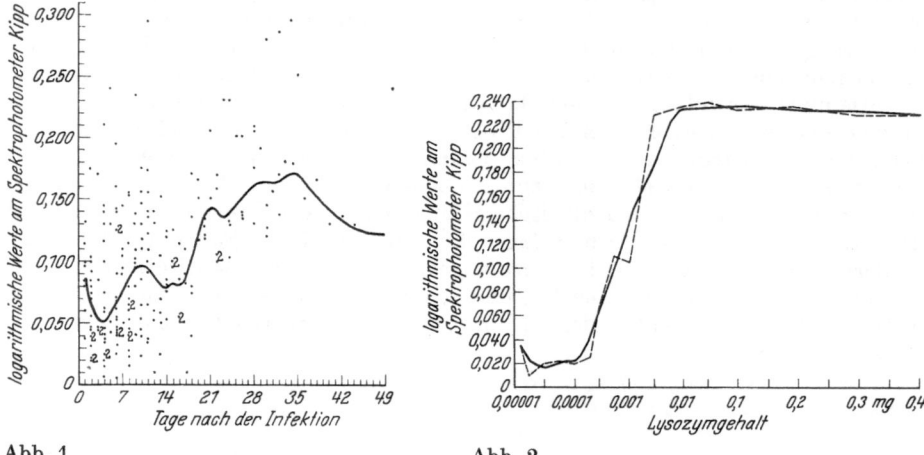

Abb. 1

Abb. 2

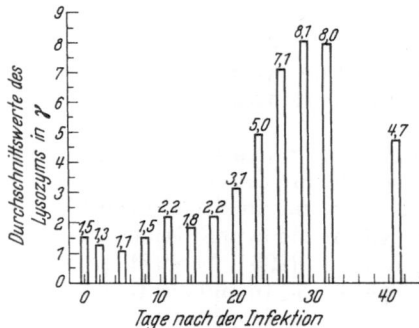

Abb. 3

zu einem deutlichen Anstieg über den Normalwert kommt. Zum Zweck der quantitativen Auswertung wurde eine Kalibrierungskurve mit bekannten Mengen eines kristallinen Lysozyms hergestellt (Abb. 2). Die nach dieser Kurve umgerechneten Lysozymmengen sind in der Abb. 3 dargestellt. Es ergibt sich, daß der Durchschnittswert des Lysozyms im Serum von gesunden Kaninchen 1,5 γ/ml beträgt. Bei der experimentellen Kaninchensyphilis kommt es zunächst zu einem Abfall auf 1,1 γ/ml und dann zu einem

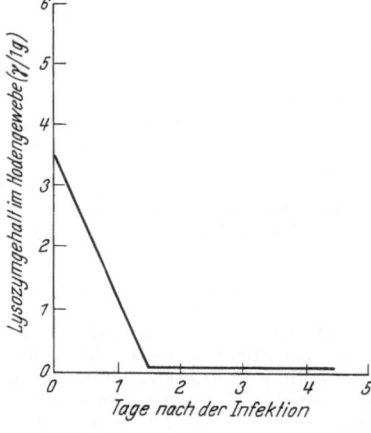

Abb. 4

Abb. 5

Aufstieg am 28. bis 30. Tage nach der Infektion auf 8,1 γ/ml. Der Verlauf der aus den Medianwerten der Leukocytenzahlen zusammengesetzten Kurve hat einen ähnlichen Charakter (Abb. 4). Was den Lysozymgehalt in dem infizierten Hoden-gewebe betrifft, haben wir folgendes festgestellt: Der Normalwert von Lysozym beträgt 3,45 γ/g. Nach der Infizierung mit Tr. pallidum kommt es zu einem raschen Sinken des Lysozyms, so daß nach 48 Std keine Spur nachzuweisen ist (Abb. 5). Mit Hilfe des Elektronenmikroskops ist es nicht gelungen, den Beweis zu bringen, daß das Lysozym die Treponema-Ultrastruktur verändert.

Besprechung. Im Verlaufe der experimentellen Syphilis des Kaninchens kommt es zu wesentlichen Veränderungen der Lysozymquanten im Serum und im infi-zierten Hodengewebe. Der Verlauf der Lysozymveränderungen im Serum ent-spricht den Veränderungen der Leukocyten. Da die Leukocyten das Lysozym in riesigen Mengen enthalten (bis 10000 γ/ml), ist es sehr wahrscheinlich, daß die Veränderungen des Serumlysozyms eng mit den Veränderungen der Leukocyten-zahl zusammenhängen. Die schon nach 48stündiger Infektion festgestellte Ab-wesenheit des Lysozyms im Hodengewebe kann die Ursache der erwähnten an-fänglichen immunologischen Nichtreaktivität der Treponemen aus frischen Läsionen sein. Vorläufig ist es uns nicht gelungen, die hypothetische empfindliche Schicht der Treponemen, die durch das Lysozym attackiert werden kann, zu be-weisen.

Literatur. ADAMIKER, D., G. BREITFELLNER und R. NEUHOLD: Mikroskopie **20**, 201 (1965). — FLEMING, A.: Proc. roy. Soc. B. **93**, 306 (1922). — METZGER, M., P. H. HARDY jr., and E. E. NELL: Amer. J. Hyg. **73**, 236 (1961). — POSPÍŠIL, L., u. A. JAKUBOWSKI: Z. Immun.-Forsch. **131**, 444 (1966).

F.T.A. Test quantitatif dans le sérum d'individus non syphilitiques

S. SARTORIS et G. F. STRANI, Clinique Dermatologique de l'Université de Turin (Italie)

Il est bien connu que l'inconvénient le plus important, et presque le seul, de l'Immunofluorescence (I.F.) appliquée au diagnostic de la syphilis est son défaut de spécificité aux très faibles dilutions. Cette remarque déjà a été faite par DUREL, BOREL, FRIBOURG-BLANC et NIEL, lesquels ont observé que les sérums non dilués d'individus normaux au contact de l'antigène tréponémique résultent fréquemment positifs, probablement à cause de la présence d'anticorps inconnus, en tout cas non tréponémiques. Ces auteurs rapportent que le 2 à 3% des sérums d'individus non syphilitiques peut atteindre un titre de 1/150 et, exceptionnelle-ment, même de 1/300. Cette spécificité non absolue impose donc la recherche d'une dilution standard des sérums dans le but d'éliminer cet inconvénient sans perte des faibles positivités d'origine sûrement spécifique.

Se basant sur une très vaste expérience, FRIBOURG-BLANC et coll. ont proposé une dilution standard de 1/150 que nous avons adoptée dans notre routine. Sur la base de ces données, nous avons déterminé le titre des sérums d'individus sûrement non atteints d'infection syphilitique; à ce but nous avons effectué l'I.F. sur 200 sérums selon la méthode quantitative (FRIBOURG-BLANC et coll.; SARTORIS, STRANI, LEIGHEB G.) aux dilutions suivantes: 1/1 (sérum non dilué), 1/5, 1/10, 1/20, 1/50, 1/150. On a répété ensuite l'I.F. sur chaque sérum après inactivation à

56 °C pendant 30 min. Les résultats de notre recherche sont exposés dans le tableau suivant:

Tableau

Dilution des sérums	négatifs	titre (+)
1/1	38%	
1/1		20%
1/5		12%
1/10		14%
1/20		13,5%
1/50		2%
1/150		0,5%

L'examen des données démontre que:

1. seulement le 38% des sérums normaux non dilués est négatif,

2. à la dilution de 1/5 le pourcentage des sérums négatifs est de 58%,

3. la fréquence des positivités non spécifiques aux dilutions successives se réduit rapidement: le 2% à la dilution de 1/50,

4. un seul sérum est résulté faiblement positif à la dilution de 1/150 (0,5 %).

Il faut encore signaler que l'inactivation des sérums à 56 °C pendant 30 min ne provoque pas de variation significative du titre.

Sur la base de ces observations nous pouvons confirmer les conclusions de FRIBOURG-BLANC et coll., selon lesquels la dilution standard de 1/150 peut être considérée comme optimale pour le dépistage systématique avec l'I.F. Cette dilution permet de réduire au minimum les positivités non spécifiques et de mettre en évidence en même temps les faibles positivités vraiment spécifiques dans les sérums de sujets syphilitiques.

Quantitative FTA Test During Treatment of Recent Syphilis

G. LEIGHEB, G. F. STRANI and S. SARTORIS, Department of Dermatology, University of Turin (Italy)

The behaviour of the quantitative FTA. test was studied in 20 cases of primary syphilis (5 to 30 day-old syphilomas) and in 20 cases of syphilodermas. The study was conducted during a standard treatment (one vial of bismuth, a mixed cycle — 12 million Vi benzathine penicillin and ten vials of 0.20 g basic salicylate of bismuth) followed by a month's break and a second mixed cycle. Control samples were taken before therapy, after one vial of bismuth, after 6 million penicillin, after 12 million, after ten vials of bismuth, before the IInd cycle, at the end of the IInd cycle and before the IIIrd cycle. The Wassermann reaction with protein treponemic antigen and the VDRL test were done at the same time as the FTA test.

In the cases of syphilomas of a few days standing, in preserological period, the VDRL was negative or weakly positive and the FTA test showed a titre of $\leq$ 150 rising to a maximum of 300 after reactivation. It then fell progressively to 100 before the IInd cycle and to 0 after the second. The variations of the FTA titre observed during therapy are shown in the graph where the downward curves represent some cases of recent syphilomas. In more long-standing cases, with positive WR and VDRL, the initial FTA titre varied from 300 to 2500 and in the primary-secondary forms was as high as 4000.

The curves at the top show the strange behaviour of the FTA serum titre in some cases of 15 to 30 day-old syphilomas. These show that peaks may occur in various phases of treatment due to serological Herxheimer phenomena. The contrast between cases where antibodies fall sharply after only 6 to 12 million penicillin and others with later, sometimes considerable increases in antibodies at the end of the Ist cycle is noteworthy. These increases are presumably related to the destruction of treponemic foci by therapy.

The curves tend to fall in correspondence with the break in therapy because of the lack of fresh therapeutic stimulus and the consequent fall in antibody production. The continuation of the gradual decrease in antibody level, documented by comparing titres before and after completion of the IInd cycle, suggests that there are no new phases of increase in the course of this treatment. At the very most such phases are slight and very short-lived, as shown by the almost total negativization observed at the end of the cycle. RW nad VDRL became negative before the FTA test when the latter was still positive 1:300, 1:1350.

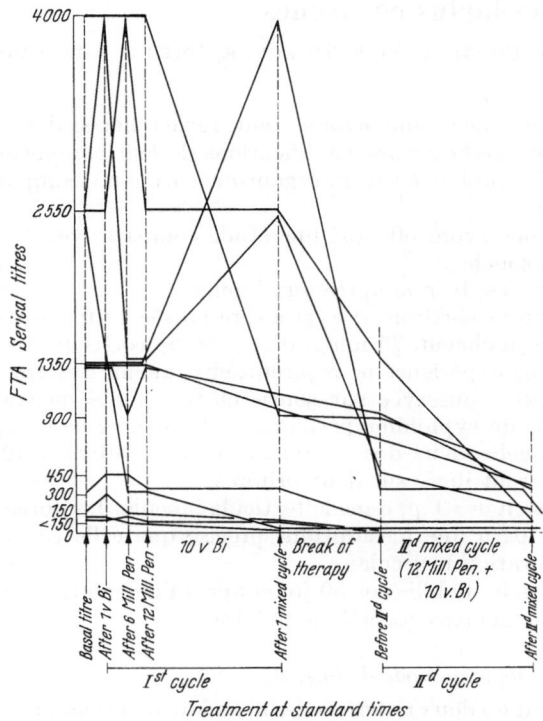

Fig. Behaviour of FTA-titre during treatment in primary syphilis

In florid secondary syphilis, titres varied from 2500 to 24,000 without very high serological Herxheimer activity and titres were observed, on average, after 6 million penicillin. There was a progressive fall in antibodies both after the penicillin and after the bismuth cycles. Upon completion of the second cycle, titres of 1:300, 1:900, indicating successful therapy, were often reached.

However, this behaviour was not the rule: alongside subjects with low serum titres after two cycles, others demonstrated a slow but steady fall in antibodies.

To conclude: 1. The therapeutic effect is more pronounced the earlier the treatment begins. 2. In more long-standing primary forms, serological Herxheimer activity is more evident. This may occur at various stages of the initial treatment. 3. Considerable falls in serum curves are evident after the very first penicillin cycle and last throughout the break because of the lack of therapeutic stimulus and the probable extinction of most treponemic foci. 4. The curve then falls slowly during the IInd cycle and in this phase, the FTA is possibly the result of persistent stimuli (related to destruction of residual active treponemic foci) or solely of serological inertia with slow return to negativity. 5. In secondary syphilis, the very high initial titres decrease greatly and progressively during the first cycle. Later, however, they show a slower return to negativity with respect to cases of primary syphilis.

Modifications du comportement des tréponèmes pales après passages sur des lapins cortisones

P. Collart, G. Poggi, M. et F. Dunoyer, Institut Alfred Fournier, Paris (France)

Dans cette expérience, nous avons voulu rechercher si des T.p. de la souche Nichols pouvaient présenter des modifications de leur comportement habituel à la suite d'un contact prolongé sur un organisme cortisoné, comparativement à des T.p. d'autre origine.

Dans ce but, nous avons effectué une étude comparative, sur des bases statistiques, avec trois souches:

La souche Nichols, bien adaptée aux lapins.

La souche Nichols cortisonée: c'est à dire passée 13 fois consécutivement sur des lapins ayant reçu chacun 75 mmg. d'acétate de cortisone en 6 jours. Mais les lapins entrant dans l'expérience ne reçurent, eux, aucun traitement hormonal.

La souche Gand, conservée sur souris et transférée successivement sur six lapins pour obtenir un syphilome permettant de réaliser une suspension calibrée.

Pour chaque souche, deux doses furent utilisées: 100000 et 10000 tréponèmes.

Les résultats furent jugés sur deux critères:

1. La réapparition des T.p. dans le testicule inoculé. La durée de cette période de latence nous a paru une mesure plus précise que celle consistant à juger les résultats sur l'induration testiculaire.

2. Le dosage des immobilisines 50 jours après l'inoculation. Tous ces résultats furent l'objet d'une analyse statistique précise.

A. Au point de vue de la période de latence

1. En comparant les deux richesses des inoculats pour chaque souche, l'influence très nette de ce facteur sur la durée de cette phase pour les deux souches à multiplication accélérée (souche Nichols cortisonée et Nichols habituelle). Par contre, pour la souche Gand, à végétabilité réduite, nous n'observons aucune dissemblance.

2. En comparant les résultats des trois souches entre elles, pour chaque inoculum, on constate une inégalité marquée, significative avec une probabilité de un pour mille. Donc, le délai de réappariton des T.p. après l'inoculation est fonction, dans une certaine mesure, de la richesse de l'inoculum mais surtout de la qualité des germes utilisés.

3. Toutes ces injections intratesticulaires furent faites unilatéralement; or, ultérieurement, nous avons observé une bilatéralité des lésions six fois sur dix avec la souche cortisonée, cinq fois sur huit avec la souche habituelle; mais une fois sur neuf avec la souche Gand.

B. Au point de vue des résultats sérologiques au 50ème jour après l'inoculation virulente

1. Selon le nombre de T.p. injectés, les différences obtenues sont significatives pour les deux souches à pouvoir de multiplication accélérée, mais nulles pour la souche Gand.

Tableau 1. *Résultats de l'injection intratesticulaire à des lapins de deux séries de suspension calibrées en T.p. provenant de trois souches différentes*

	Souche Nichols cortisonée				Souche Nichols				Souche Gand			
	N° des lapins	Période de latence en jours	T.I.T. au 50° j %	F.T.A. au 50° j	N° des lapins	Période de latence en jours	T.I.T. au 50° j %	F.T.A. au 50° j	N° des lapins	Période de latence en jours	T.I.T. au 50° j %	F.T.A. au 50° j
100 000	1	5	100	4+	17	13	80	3+	32	29	5	1+
	2	6	60	3+	18	6	52	3+	33	47	2	1+
	3	6	100	3+	19	19	60	3+	34	26	4	1+
T.p.	4	6	75	4+	20	16	70	4+	35	58	2	1+
	5	6	80	3+	21	19	Mort		36	32	8	1+
Moyenne		5,6	83			14,6	65,4			38,4	4,2	
10 000	6	13	65	3+	22	Mort			37	40	4	3+
	7	12	70	3+	23	33	32	3+	38	32	16	1+
	8	12	25	3+	24	20	4	1+	39	32	4	1+
T.p.	9	12	12	3+	25	26	16	2+	40	Mort		
	10	15	25	3+	26	Echec[a]			41	41	4%	3+
Moyenne		12,8	39,4			26,3	17,3			36,3	7	

[a] Cette inoculation n'a été suivie d'aucun effet.

Tableau 2. *Résultats thérapeutiques obtenus avec 200 000 U.O. de benz. péni. par kg. chez des lapins infectés depuis 130 jours avec des inoculats calibres provenant de trois souches de T. p. différentes*

	N° des lapins	Nb. de Tp Inoc.	Incubation en jours	T.I.T. au 100° j	F.T.A au 100° j	traitement au 130° j	Sérologie		Post-Thérapeutique		
							40 j	90 j	200 j	250 j	330 j
Souche	2	100 000	6	100% tt 300	4000	546 000 U.O. de Péni.	TIT = 37% FTA = 2+	TIT = 92% FTA = 2+	TIT = 100% FTA = 1+	TIT = 80% tt = 20 FTA = 450	TIT = 84% FTA = 300
Nichols	9	10 000	12	100% tt 1 200	4 000	688 000 U.O. de Péni.	TIT = 50% FTA = 1+	TIT = 46% FTA = 2+	TIT = 100% FTA =	TIT = 50% tt = 10 FTA = 450	TIT = 75% FTA = 450
Cortisone	10	10 000	15	100% tt 4 000	8 000	588 000 U.O. de Péni.	TIT = 100% FTA = 1+	TIT = 93% FTA = 3+	TIT = 100% FTA =	TIT = 100% tt = 150 FTA = 300	TIT = 100% tt = 50 FTA = 150
Souche	18	100 000	6	100% tt 900	4 000	693 000 U.O. de Péni.	TIT = 100% FTA = 2+	TIT = 89% FTA = 2+	TIT = 100% FTA = 3+	TIT = 100% FTA = 450	Mort
Nichols	23	10 000	33	100% tt 1 500	4 000	756 000 U.O. de Péni.	TIT = 100% FTA = 1+	TIT = 97% FTA = 2+	TIT = 100% FTA = 3+	TIT = 96% tt = 30 FTA = 450	TIT = 75% FTA = 300
	28	1 000	36	100% tt 300	1 350	651 000 U.O. de Péni.	TIT = 87% FTA = 1+	TIT = 100% FTA = 2+	TIT = 100% FTA = 3+	TIT = 100% FTA = 150	TIT = 98% FTA = 150
Souche	32	100 000	29	100% tt 2 000	4 000	525 000 U.O. de Péni.	TIT = 80% FTA = 1+	TIT = 26% FTA = 2+	TIT = 100% FTA = 3+	TIT = 100% tt = 90 FTA = 900	TIT = 100% tt = 70 FTA = 150
Gand	33	100 000	47	100% tt 900	1 350	672 000 U.O. de Péni.	TIT = 0% FTA = 1+	TIT = 0% FTA = 1+	TIT = 2% FTA =	TIT = 0% FTA = 0	TIT = 4% FTA = 0
	37	10 000	40	100% tt 150	1 350	630 000 U.O. de Péni.	TIT = 75% FTA = 1+	TIT = 0% FTA = 1+	Mort.		

2. Selon les souches utilisées: que ce soit avec 100000 ou 10000 T.p., nous observons une différence significative dans la rapidité d'apparition des immobilisines.

3. Même constation pour le test F.T.A.: presque toutes les réponses sont positives pour les deux premières souches et toutes négatives, hormis deux, pour la souche GAND. Mais ces épreuves effectuées non quantitativement, n'ont pas été évaluées statistiquement. Il résulte que l'immobilisation spécifique au 50 ème jour de l'inoculation varie avec la qualité de la souche avec une probabilité de un pour mille et en fonction de la richesse de l'inoculum avec une probabilité de un 1%.

4. Par contre, 100 jours après l'injection virulente, ni la richesse initiale de l'inoculum, ni la qualité des germes, ni l'extension des lésions au côté opposé, ne paraissent jouer un rôle influant dans l'induction du taux des immobilisines, non plus que des titres F.T.A..

Le Tab. 2 montre les résultats sérologiques obtenus après un traitement de 200000 U.O. de benzathine pénicilline par kg effectué au 130ème jour de l'infection.

En dépit d'oscillations transitoires et de quelques résultats discordants, la souche GAND, à période de latence prolongée, s'est montrée plus sensible à l'action de l'antibiotique (deux résultats négatifs sur trois) que les deux autres souches dont les T.I.T. étaient encore positifs au bout d'un an. Toutefois, les passages ganglionnaires étaient encore tous négatifs mais après trois mois d'observation.

Discussion

1. En ce qui concerne la période de latence: Si l'on admet avec le Pf. TURNER que les T.p. se multiplient toutes les 30 à 33 heures et que les lésions cliniquement reconnaissables débutent lorsque le nombre de T.p. atteint localement 10 millions, il faut reconnaitre que cette multiplication, à échelle logarithmique, n'apparaît qu'à la fin de cette période de latence, à la phase de croissance exponentielle qui précède de peu l'apparition des lésions et non pas dès l'inoculation.

2. En ce qui concerne l'action de la cortisone: Les épreuves statistiques montrent que des T.p. en contact prolongé avec un organisme cortisoné, présentent une réduction notable de cette phase de latence, ce qui expliquerait les phénomènes de réactivation rapportés par CH. MCLEOD et MAGNUSON, de même que ceux que nous avons publiés.

3. En ce qui concerne la sérologie: Si avant le 50 ème jour, l'apparition des Ac. paraît être fonction de la rapidité du pouvoir de multiplication des T.p. il n'en est plus de même après le 100ème jour. Aussi, semble-t-il difficile d'attribuer à un titre d'anticorps, pris isolément, une valeur précise; seule l'étude de ces variations, pour chaque sujet, pourrait apporter des renseignements sur l'évolution ultérieure de l'infection.

Conclusion. Tout ceci montre bien la variabilité du comportement biologique des T.p. qu'il n'est pas possible de schématiser d'une façon uniforme par comparaison avec une souche, modifiée par 20 ans de passages accélérés sur une seule et même espèce.

Bibliographie. 1. COLLART, P., L. J. BOREL, P. DUREL M. et F. DUNOYER: Ann. Inst. Pasteur **102**, 596, 693 (1962). — 2. MCLEOD, CH., and H. J. MAGNUSON: J. Immunol **76**, 373 (1956). — 3. TURNER, TH. B., and D. H. HOLLANDER: Biology of Treponematoses 1959; O.M.S.

Recherches expérimentales sur la provocation des anticorps fluorescents après administration de spirochète de souche Reiter chez des individus sains et syphilitiques

A. PANTI et S. ULIVI, Florence (Italie)

Il est connu que l'introduction endoveineuse d'une suspension de tréponème Reiter provoque, dans le sérum de l'individu sain et du syphilitique, l'apparition d'anticorps antitréponémiques et parfois, chez les syphilitiques, paraît aussi l'antilipoide, phénomène qui ne se vérifie jamais chez les sains.

Nos précédentes expérimentations ont fait remarquer qu'en changeant la voie d'introduction, c'est à dire en recourant à l'intramusculaire, on provoque toujours chez le syphilitique, l'apparition de l'anticorps antitréponémique, mais jamais celui antilipoïde, tandis que chez l'individu sain jamais aucun des deux anticorps ne paraît.

Le but de notre travail a été de voir si l'introduction intramusculaire de tréponèmes Reiter provoque chez le syphilitique, outre l'apparition des anticorps antitréponémiques, aussi l'apparition des anticorps responsables de l'immunofluorescence, et si ces derniers pouvaient être évacués même dans les sains. Nos essais ont été faits sur 20 individus, dont 15 syphilitiques et 5 sains. La casuistique des syphilitiques comprend des individus contaminés soit depuis nombre d'années, soit plus récemment, et tous assez régulièrement soignés.

Nous nous sommes assurés, avant de commencer nos expériences, qu'il y avait négativité des réactions classiques et du test d'immunofluorescence.

A chaque sujet on injectait par voie intra-musculaire, à jours alternés et pour un total de huit injections, une suspension de tréponèmes non pathogènes, commençant par un $^1/_2$ cm³ jusqu'à un maximum de 2 cm sans avoir jamais vu paraître des phénomènes d'intolérance soit locale soit générale. Les prélèvements pour les réaction se faisaient à partir du 4è jour après la dernière injection et successivement tous les 3 jours pour les 2 premières semaines, et toutes les semaines au cours des 2 mois suivants.

Exposé des résultats

a) non syphilitiques: l'anticorps antilipoïde et celui antitréponémique n'ont jamais été mis en évidence. L'immuno-fluorescence s'est toujours révélée négative;

b) syphilitiques:

1. chez quatre malades syphilitiques très anciens on a remarqué l'apparition (précoce et persistante) de l'anticorps antitréponémique, mais jamais de l'antilipoïde; phénomène qui a été constant dans toute notre casuistique. L'F.T.A. est devenu positif en deux cas, et cette positivité s'est avérée plus tardivement que les réactions classiques et avec une persistance plus ou moins prolongée;

2. chez neuf syphilitiques plus récents on a remarqué: dans un cas, où le traitement eut son début dans une phase secondaire, l'anticorps antitréponémique est apparu précocement et aussi précoce a été la positivité de l'immuno-fluorescence, positivité qui a persisté pendant toute la durée de nos expérimentations. Dans les autres cas, où le traitement eut son début dans la phase primaire, on a constaté que tandis que l'anticorps antitréponémique a paru dans tous les malades avec précocité et persistance, la positivité de l'immuno-fluorescence ne s'est révélée qu'en trois cas et telle positivité s'est avérée toujours plus tardivement que celle de la déviation du complément;

3. chez deux syphilitiques, malades depuis un peu plus d'un an et soignés dans la phase primaire l'F.T.A. est résulté positif en un seul cas.

Pour provoquer une réactivation on a même tenté l'introduction de spirochète Reiter, et GRÜNEBERG qui le premier se servit de cette méthode, pensa que la réactivation pourrait se réaliser parce que les spirochètes, à travers une réaction de foyer, agissaient sur le processus syphilitique latent.

OLIVETTI s'aperçut que l'introduction endoveineuse faisait paraître des anticorps antitréponémiques soit chez l'individu sain soit chez le malade, enlevant ainsi toute valeur pratique à l'apparition de ces anticorps, tandis que l'évocation de la réagine antilipoïdée, possible seulement chez les syphilitiques, pouvait avoir plus de valeur parce qu'elle pouvait être interprêtée comme une réaction de foyer par la présence d'un état pathologique encore actif.

Nous avions précédemment constaté que l'introduction intramusculaire ne fait pas paraître chez l'individu sain des anticorps spécifiques (de même qu'il arrive avec «l'organoluétine» qui, par voie intramusculaire provoque des anticorps seulement chez les syphilitiques, et par voie endoveineuse chez les syphilitiques et les individus sains), par conséquent la diversité de la voie d'introduction peut avoir de l'importance dans le déterminisme de la provocation des anticorps.

Actuellement nous avons reconfirmé ces expérimentations en outre nous avons vu que chez l'individu sain il ne se provoque jamais de positivité de l'F.T.A. tandis que chez le syphilitique cela arrive assez fréquemment.

Les phénomènes que l'on a observés peuvent être interprétés ou comme une réaction anamnestique type BIELING (réveil d'une fonction présente dans l'organisme, mais assoupie) ou par rapport à une provocation d'anticorps à la suite d'une réaction de foyer.

On pourrait incliner pour la seconde hypothèse puisque la positivité de l'F.T.A. ne se provoque pas chez tous les syphilitiques, mais se vérifie plus facilement dans les cas où la cure a commencé plus tardivement ou n'a pas été très régulière, et aussi parce que cette positivité est toujours plus tardive que l'apparition des anticorps antitréponémiques.

Activité des anticorps fractionnés du sérum dans la syphilis

F. OTTOLENGHI et U. SPAGNOLI, Clinique Dermatologique de l'Université de Sienne (Italie)

L'étude du comportement sérologique des fractions protéiques du sérum séparées par fluxophorèse, dosées spectrophotométriquement et successivement lyophilisées, a démontré que pendant le cours de la syphilis primaire de l'homme, les anticorps flocculants et déviants paraissent d'abord dans les fractions gamma-globuliniques douées d'une moyenne vitesse électrophorétique. Cependant, avec le temps, le patrimoine d'anticorps s'étend à des fractions gamma-globuliniques toujours nouvelles, surtout dans le sens de la direction du flux électrophorétique, de sorte que, la période secondaire approchant, il est possible de démontrer la présence de réagines même dans les sous-fractions bêta-globuliniques plus lentes. Cela vaut, en particulier, pour les anticorps déviants, et non pour les anticorps flocculants, que l'on retrouve dans les fractions bêta-globuliniques dans une phase plus avancée de la période secondaire, avec une dissociation de comportement qui vient s'ajouter aux autres preuves déposant en faveur de l'individualité des anticorps antilipoïdiques déviants et flocculants.

Se servant des quantitatifs maximums de $1000\,\gamma$ de fraction protidique et effectuant pour les réactions de déviation du complément la Microwassermann selon VAN DER VEEN et, pour les réactions de flocculation, la V.D.R.L., il a été possible de constater que, chez l'homme, la positivité paraît environ 20 jours après la pénétration du tréponème dans l'organisme. Les premiers à paraître sont les anticorps déviants avec l'antigène tréponémique, suivis, à quelque distance de temps, par les anticorps déviants avec l'antigène cardiolipinique et par les anticorps flocculants avec la V.D.R.L.

Avec le temps ces quantitatifs se réduisent progressivement de sorte que, 35 jours après le contact infectieux, 200 et 100 γ de gamma-globulines sont en général suffisantes pour dévier le complément et provoquer une flocculation.

Dans le lapin infecté de syphilis se répètent, en principe, les phénomènes décrits chez l'homme, mais le rongeur s'est révélé un producteur d'anticorps plus vigoureux, car, 8 jours seulement après l'inoculation du tréponème, nous avons pu obtenir parfois des réactions positives avec 250 γ de gamma-globulines d'une moyenne vitesse électrophorétique, quantitatif qui dans l'homme résultait suffisant seulement 4 semaines après la pénétration du tréponème dans l'organisme.

Cette différence de comportement entre l'homme et le lapin à notre avis, est rapportable plutôt à l'espèce qu'à la modalité de l'infection syphilitique ou à la souche tréponémique en jeu.

D'après nos études, conduites dans 16 sujets, les bêtalipoprotéines peuvent être vectrices d'anticorps flocculants et déviants antilipoïdiques et antitréponémiques, mais surtout d'anticorps antilipoïdiques: il est ressorti que, en moyenne, 285 γ et 592 γ de bêtalipoprotéines étaient suffisantes pour dévier le complément en présence de cardiolipine ou de Tréponine, tandis que le sérum privé du composant lipoprotéique perd d'une façon sensible la capacité de dévier le complément en présence de cardiolipine. Les bêtalipoprotéines peuvent, dans la syphilis primaire très récente, être dépourvues d'anticorps, même antilipoïdiques qui paraissent dans les bêtalipoprotéines dans une période primaire plus avancée. En employant la méthode de COOMBS et en se servant d'antigène de ROEMER et SCHLIPKOETER pour la réaction d'agglutination, nous n'avons pas retrouvé dans le sérum du sang du syphilitique des anticorps incomplets.

En introduisant dans la veine de lapins sains et syphilisés 6,3 mg d'antigène tréponémique protidique de Reiter purifié conjugué avec 0,255 mg de isothiocyanate de fluorescéine et en tuant les rongeurs 4 h après injection et en recherchant à fluorescence sur fond noir des frottis de foie, moelle, rate, glandes lymphatiques et sang, nous avons constaté l'absence de fluorescence chez lapin sain, tandis qu'on a retrouvé la présence de fluorescence dans les splénocytes et dans les lymphocytes des glandes lymphatiques. Les glandes lymphatiques et la rate sont, en effet, sans doute, les sièges de production d'anticorps antiluétiques. Au contraire, il ne semble pas que les cellules de sections de moelle, foie et sang soient des producteurs actifs d'anticorps. Nos recherches histologiques qui vont paraître dans un prochain travail nous permetteront de mieux examiner les structures histologiques d'organes et de compléter et perfectionner les résultats.

Activité antigénique des fractions de la protéine purifiée du tréponème de Reiter

U. SPAGNOLI et F. OTTOLENGHI, Clinique Dermatologique de l'Université de Sienne (Italie)

L'importance du composant protéique du tréponème, élevé par SACHS à la dignité d'antigène complet, a été démontrée par l'école de D'Alessandro. On sait, en outre, que le complexe protéique du tréponème de Reiter occupe dans le germe une position profonde, toutefois, pour une activité antigénique plus marquée, il faut des procédés d'extraction et de purification.

Mais, bien que l'on sache beaucoup à propos de cet antigène, il continue à intéresser les nombreux expérimentateurs à cause des questions non résolues qui encore affrontent le problème de l'infection syphilitique. Par l'électrophorèse inidirectionnelle on met en évidence dans l'antigène protéique purifié du tréponème de Reiter deux bandes de migration, l'une plus lente, mais quantitativement dominante, l'autre plus rapide, mais moins abondante.

Toutefois nos recherches ont démontré que la protéine du tréponème de Reiter est électrophorétiquement un peu plus complexe.

En effet, en soumettant l'extrait protéique purifié à l'électrophorèse continuelle, méthode de recherche particulièrement convenable pour l'étude de complexes protéiques, nous avons obtenu toute une série de fractions dont on a étudié soit le comportement dans le champ électrique, soit la réactivité de chaque fraction avec les sérums d'hommes syphilitiques et les sérums de lapins inoculés avec des tréponèmes de la souche de Reiter. Dans le champ électrique fluxophorétique et dans nos conditions de travail, nous avons obtenu neuf bandes, dont cinq sont distribuées dans la zone négative et quatre dans la zone positive. Les quantitatives protéiques de la tréponine purifiée de la zone négative du champ (54,76%) dépassent celles de la zone positive (45,24%). Pour la valutation de l'activité du sérum, après avoir déterminé la concentration protéique on a soumis les fractions à la lyophilisation ce qui nous a permis de travailler avec des dilutions antigéniques que l'on peut comparer quantitativement. Nous avons ainsi pu constater que toutes les fractions ne sont pas de la même valeur pour ce qui concerne l'activité du sérum et à côté de fractions qui ont beaucoup d'activité antigénique, 6,5 et 2γ desquelles sont respectivement capables de dévier le complément, il y en a d'autres apparemment dépourvues d'activité sérologique. Les fractions actives dominent sur celles inactives et sont également réactives soit avec du sérum de l'homme syphilitique soit avec du sérum anti-Reiter de lapin. De nos recherches vient un jugement particulièrement favorable pour l'antigène purifié, tandis qu'un contrôle de l'activité de la suspension protéique après la filtration en membranes «Millipores» nous a permis de constater que des filtres avec les pores au-dessous du diamètre de 0,1 micron, arrêtent les micelles et privent la suspension de toute activité du sérum. Donc ça vient à démontrer que l'antigène purifié n'est pas en dispersion moléculaire.

L'inhomogénéité de l'antigène qui vient par l'électrophorèse continuelle et par la filtration en «Millipores» nous dit que la dénomination de purifiée par l'antigène protéique de Reiter a une signification plus sérologique que physico-chimique.

Toutefois, en acceptant la valeur immunologique de l'antigène protéique de la souche de Reiter, confirmée par la méthode d'immunoprécipitation d'Oudin, nous avons utilisé la protéine purifiée pour la recherche des centres anticorpo-génétiques. Et en effet la protéine purifiée du tréponème de Reiter, conjuguée avec de l'isothiocyanate de fluorescéine et injectée dans des lapins syphilisés, s'est révélée un moyen utile aussi pour l'étude des centres anticorpo-génétiques luétiques, comme l'on trouve expliqué dans la communication du Professeur OTTO-LENGHI.

Possible signification du comportement des fractions globuliniques au F.T.A.-test sur le sérum de sujets luétiques

P. Pagnes, Clinique Dermatologique de l'Université de Padoue (Italie)

L'organisme humain parasité par le tréponéma pallidum, peut présenter des cadres cliniques polimorphes et caractéristiques et des cadres sérologiques qui coïncident ou qui sont indépendants de ceux là. Ils apparaissent comme le résultat d'une réponse organique à l'agression de l'agent pathogène et ils comprennent même son action comme élément étranger et éthérogène. Les nombreuses et variables expressions morbides se développent dans le temps parallèlement à l'évolution de l'état immunitaire lequel peut être apprécié et évalué technique- ment mais non défini dans son essence et dans sa véritable signification.

Les anticorps évoqués par le mosaïque antigénique du tréponéma pallidum, peuvent être mis en évidence par différentes méthodes et classés comme réagines non protectives ou comme vrais anticorps à caractère défensif. Et dans le temps, même indépendamment de toute thérapeutique adéquate, on peut observer, parallèlement, une évolution immunitaire polimorphe au sens large. Ces facteurs, qui dans leur complexité caractérisent l'expression morbide individuelle, sont le résultat de la possible variabilité agressive dans le temps de l'agent parasitaire et de la variabilité quantitative et qualitative de la réactivité immunitaire organique. L'infection tréponémique provoque donc, même pour la réactivité fonctionelle conséquant à l'introduction de matériel étranger et éthérogène à l'organisme, une production anticorpale, spécifique, expression d'une modification dans la synthèse des séroglobulines naturelles.

A la lumière des recherches et théories les plus récentes, la cellule productrice d'anticorps ne répondrait pas passivement au stimulus antigénique: la théorie «informative» selon laquelle la portion stéréospécifique de la molécule anticorpale est construite sur le moule fourni par l'antigène, est dépassée par celle «élective». Les moules anticorpaux sont préexistants, et parmi ceux-ci, sont mobilisés ceux à structure moléculaire spécifique pour l'antigène stimulateur. On admet, ainsi, l'existence de gènes structuraux dont l'ADN, après message de l'ARN, informe les ribosomes siège de la synthèse anticorpale. Il existe en effet des groupes sériques génétiquement déterminés qui conditionnent donc, un polimorphisme héréditaire dans les immunoglobulines. Si on ajoute encore qu'à chaque type immunoglobulinique correspond une classe cellulaire prédisposée à sa synthèse, on peut en déduire combien la réponse immunitaire sera spécifique pour chaque individu ou groupe particulier d'individus soit du point de vue quantitatif que qualitatif.

Le problème de l'identification dans le spectre protidémique des anticorps à type immunitaire et réaginique chez le luétique, leur dynamique évolutive et involutive, a été déjà affronté par de nombreux auteurs étrangers et italiens selon les méthodes les plus diverses et raffinées. Magistrales sont les contributions apportées par Cerutti, Boncinelli, Bonelli, D'Alessandro, Ottolenghi-Lodigiani, Puccinelli, Spagnoli, Deacon, Cannefox, Garson, Harris, Hunter, Laurell, Magnuson, Mathasi, Portnoy, Vaisman, et par d'autres encore.

Recherche actuelle: III sérums ont été testés, dont 20 de syphilis primaire, 23 de syphilis secondaire, 30 de syphilis secondaire en traitement, 17 de syphilis latente, 1 de syphilis congénitale, 8 de syphilis congénitale latente, 7 à F.P.B., Le reste comme contrôle.

Pour chaque échantillon on a pratiqué la R.B.W. par les antigènes C. et T., V.D.R.L., et le T.P.I. Ensuite le FTA-test/200 selon la technique de Deacon-

FALCONE-HARRIS, utilisant des sérums anti-fractions protéiques humaines conjugués à F.I.T.C. selon la méthode de COONS-KAPLAN-NAIRN. De chaque sérum on a
évalué la réactivité à côté des antifractions suivantes : globulines totales ; gamma A ;
gamma G ; gamma M ; C/3 — C/4 ; transferrine ; alfa 2 M ; alfa 2 L ; aptoglobine ;
Gc ; albumine. Dans les Figs. 1 et 2, sont reportées les valeurs moyennes de réactivité pour chaque fraction, aux différents moments luétiques pris en considération. Une complète aréactivité est résultée pour : albumine ; Gc ; transferrine ;

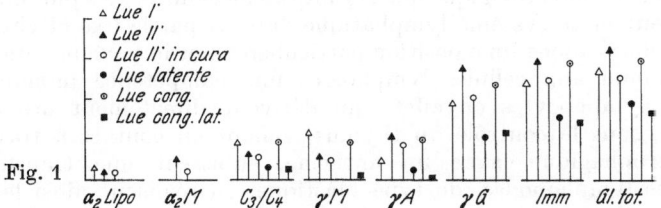

Fig. 1

aptoglobine. En quelques cas de syphilis primaire et secondaire actuelle et
en traitement, une réactivité a été dé
celée pour alfa 2 M et alfa 2 L. La plus
grande réactivité a été obtenue avec
les globulines totales et les immuno-
globulines ; les indications les plus
précises sont dérivées de l'observation
du comportement de chaque fraction
immunoglobulinique caractéristique
dans son développement évolutif et
involutif. De plus, on a remarqué une

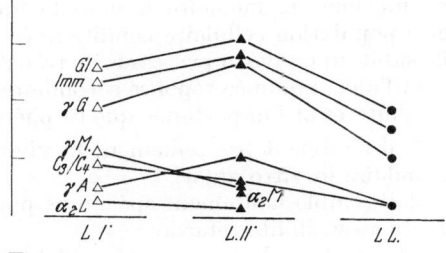

Fig. 2

réactivité C/3 à C/4 avec décroissance, de la syphilis primaire à la syphilis latente. Il faut maintenant rappeler que pas tous les échantillons testés pour chaque
moment luétique, correspondent au résultat final de groupe soit du point de vue
qualitatif que du point de vue quantitatif.

Cette recherche met en évidence une certaine caractérisation des diverses
périodes luétiques considérées. Elle nous semble encore insuffisante pour ce qui
concerne le but final de cette recherche. En rappelant l'hypothèse initiale de
l'individualité quantitative et qualitative de la réponse immunitaire sur la base de
sa prédisposition génétique, l'intérêt global de la recherche sérologique, devra
dépasser son but immédiat diagnostique, et se projeter dans la recherche d'une
possible «typisation» sérologique. C'est à dire, de l'ensemble des résultats obtenus
de l'évaluation des anticorps réaginiques et immunitaires, peut dériver la possibilité de construire pour chaque individu ou groupe particulier d'individus, un
«schéma réactif» lequel nous donne l'indication de l'état réactif actuel et, en
même temps, de son possibilisme évolutif. C'est à dire, qu'il ait cette valeur
prognostique, même en fonction de la thérapie, obligatoirement requise pour cette
phase mal définie, appelée «syphilis latente».

La stimulation lymphocytaire in vitro en divers stades de la syphilis

G. C. Chieregato et G. Faldarini, Clinique Dermatologique de l'Université de Padoue (Italie)

L'évaluation des réponses immunologiques tend à considérer même pour la syphilis soit la recherche sérologique que l'étude des mécanismes les plus intimes des tissus. Parmi ceux-ci, le système lymphatique dans sa partie fixe et circulante a pris, depuis quelques années une position particulièrement importante étant donné que l'on a reconnu aux cellules lymphoïdes une compétence immunologique spécifique. Les lymphocytes en effet, qui dérivent directement des éléments mésenchymaux, sous le contrôle du thymus, venant en contact à travers l'information macrophagique, avec un antigène, subissent une transformation surtout dans les lymphonodes, de type blastique, en réalisant ainsi la réponse primaire. De ces éléments prennent origine, en peu de temps, de petits lymphocytes morphologiquement semblables à ceux qui sont «vierges» mais dans lesquels est imprimée la mémoire immunologique de l'antigène conditionnant. Lorsque cette population cellulaire conditionnée rencontre de nouveau le même antigène, elle subit un nouveau processus de transformation blastique, manifestant, de cette façon l'ainsi nommée réponse secondaire.

L'intérêt et l'importance que ce phénomène a pris, consistent dans le fait que:

1. il n'advient pas seulement in vivo mais il est reproduisible comme réponse secondaire in vitro aussi;

2. il semble hautement spécifique pour l'antigène responsable surtout dans les procès à sensibilité retardée;

3. dans les cellules qui ont subi la transformation blastique on reconnaîtrait des facteurs gamma-globulines de probable nature et fonction anticorpale. Ce processus permettrait donc, non seulement d'identifier mais même de pouvoir mieux préciser le rôle de certains antigènes ou partigènes vis-à-vis de la manifestation et de l'évolution de certains cadres morbides.

Avec l'expérience acquise, appliquant la culture «in vitro» des lymphocytes dans le domaine des dermatoses à sensibilisation retardée et dans les procès d'autosensibilisation, nous avons depuis quelque temps mis en contact in vitro les lymphocytes de malades luétiques en divers stades avec des spirochètes lysés, de souche Nichols, Reiter, cardiolipine et tréponime à plusieurs concentrations et avec des modalités techniques précisées ailleurs (Chieregato—Faldarini).

Pour le moment nous rapportons les données obtenues avec les spirochètes souche Nichols car les résultats obtenus avec les autres antigènes n'ont pas été univoques et ils exigent des recherches et des évaluations plutôt complexes que nous nous réservons de faire le plus tôt possible.

La documentation sur laquelle a été conduite l'expérience est représentée par: 5 cas de syphilis Ière avec R.B.W. partiellement positive et T.P.I. négatif; 10 cas de syphilis II avec R.B.W. et T.P.I. positifs; 10 cas de syphilis latente dont 5 à R.B.W. et T.P.I. positifs et 5 avec R.B.W. négativisée et T.P.I. encore positif; 10 cas de malades précédemment atteints de syphilis mais cliniquement guéris et avec R.B.W. et T.P.I. complètement négativisés; et comme contrôle 20 malades atteints de dermatoses diverses à anamnèse et clinique pour ce qui concerne la syphilis, R.B.W. et T.P.I. négatifs.

D'après l'expérience de centaines d'épreuves que nous avons exécutées, nous avons fixé la limité de positivité dans un pourcentage de transformation blastique supérieur à 5%, classifiant comme négatifs même les cas avec une faible présence de blastes mais inférieure à cette limite.

Le test a donné les résultats suivants : réponse constamment négative outre que dans les 20 contrôles même dans les cinq cas de syphilis Ière, résultat toujours positif dans les dix malades atteints de syphilis II avec de hauts pourcentages de transformation blastique (de 15 à 30%); toujours positif dans tous les dix cas de syphilis latente mais des pourcentages oscillant de 15 à 20% dans les cinq cas avec R.B.W. et T.P.I. positifs et de huit à 14% dans les cinq cas avec seulement T.P.I. positif. Dans le groupe des dix malades cliniquement guéris et sérologiquement négativisés nous avons obtenu neuf cas négatifs tandis que un cas a donné une réponse sûrement positive avec transformation blastique de 15%.

Dans le but de documenter si, dans le procès de transformation blastique, il était possible de mettre en évidence la présence de globulines, nous avons traité les éléments lymphocytaires, à la fin de la culture, avec des antiglobulines totales conjuguées avec de l'isotyocianate de fluorescéine et des fractions anti-gamma A.G. et M conjuguées avec la méthode de COONS et KAPLAN.

On a pu observer une fluorescence positive, surtout dans les cas de syphilis II active, non seulement pour les globulines totales mais aussi pour les trois fractions avec une particulière intensité pour les gamma G.

Pour conclure rapidement d'après les données exposées, nous pouvons observer comment la transformation blastique obtenue avec l'agent spécifique dans la syphilis suit en principe le cours du test de Nelson-Mayer; alors qu'elle se dissocie partiellement de la réaction de Bordet-Wassermann en apparaissant et en disparaissant plus tardivement vis-à-vis de la phase de positivisation et de négativisation de l'épreuve sérologique :

La perte de la mémoire immunologique des lymphocytes dans les individues guéris de syphilis confirme les caractéristiques clinico-évolutives allergisantes mais non immunisantes que l'on vérifie dans cette maladie.

En conclusion la stimulation lymphocytaire in vitro apparaît, même pour la syphilis, non seulement une preuve diagnostique hautement spécifique mais promet, en l'adaptant de façon particulière de préciser ultérieurement quelques procès immunobiologiques tissulaires dans une maladie exquisement «sérologique».

Untersuchungen über die Sensibilität und Spezifität des FTA-ABS-Testes

W. LESIŃSKA, J. LESIŃSKI und W. ZAJAC, Bialystok (Polen)

Der 1957 von DEACON beschriebene Fluorescenz-Treponemen-Antikörpertest (FTA) findet immer breitere Anwendung in der Lues-Serodiagnostik. Er zeichnet sich durch eine außerordentlich hohe Sensibilität aus, doch ist seine Spezifität im Vergleich zum Nelson-Test unbefriedigend. Die Untersuchungen von DEACON und HUNTER sowie vieler anderer Verfasser haben gezeigt, daß im FTA-Test neben den für die pathogenen Treponemen spezifischen Antikörpern auch Antikörper nachgewiesen werden, die gegen saprophytische und Kulturspirochaeten gerichtet sind. DEACON und HUNTER sind der Meinung, daß die unspezifisch, positiven Ergebnisse des FTA durch eine immunologische Antwort auf saprophytierende Mundschleimhaut-Spirochaeten hervorgerufen werden. Unsere eigenen, durch spätere Untersuchungen von KIRALY bestätigten Beobachtungen scheinen nachweisen zu können, daß auch die Borellia refringens für die unspezifischen FTA-Ergebnisse verantwortlich seien.

Im Jahre 1963 arbeiteten DEACON und HUNTER eine Methode aus, welche auf einer Vorabsorption des untersuchten Serums mit Reiter-Spirochaeten beruht. Diese Modifikation, FTA-ABS genannt, ist jetzt Gegenstand zahlreicher Forschungen, die auch von uns schon seit 2 Jahren geführt werden.

In der vorliegenden Mitteilung werden an Hand von 2500 untersuchten Seren die Sensibilität und Spezifität und der diagnostische Wert des FTA-ABS-Testes eingeschätzt. Mit allen Seren wurden der FTA, FTA-ABS und Nelson-Test durchgeführt. Der FTA-Originaltest wurde nach der von uns früher beschriebenen quantitativen Technik durchgeführt, wobei wir uns einer 1:150 betragenden Verdünnung des zu untersuchenden Serums bedienten.

Tabelle 1. *Quantitative Resultate des FTA-ABS und FTA-Testes*

FTA-ABS Titer	FTA-Titer							Zusammen
	50	150	450	1350	4000	12000	36000	
10		2						2
50		17	3					20
150		42	74					116
450			79	40	1			120
1350				109	33			142
4000					68	12		80
12000					1	14	4	19
36000							1	1
Zusammen	—	61	156	149	103	26	5	500

Tab. 1 zeigt die quantitativen Resultate des FTA-ABS im Vergleich zu den Ergebnissen des FTA-Testes. Die Untersuchungen wurden an 500 luetischen Seren durchgeführt. Der quantitative Titer war bei fast zwei Drittel der Untersuchten in beiden Testen gleich. Beim Rest ist der FTA-ABS-Titer um eine Verdünnung niedriger als der FTA-Titer. Die Ergebnisse der Tab. 1 zeigen demnach, daß die Anwendung einer Vorabsorption mit Reiter-Spirochaeten-Ultrasonal die ausgezeichnete Sensibilität des FTA-Testes fast nicht vermindert.

In der Tab. 2 werden die Resultate der mit sog. Problemseren durchgeführten FTA-, FTA-ABS- und Nelson-Teste vorgestellt. Zu dieser Gruppe wurden 2000 Seren gezählt. Ein Teil dieser waren Seren, die uns zur Verifikation der klassischen

Tabelle 2. *Ergebnisse des FTA-ABS und FTA-Testes im Vergleich mit dem Nelson-Test bei 2000 „Problemseren"*

Nelson-Test	Zahl der Fälle	FTA-ABS		FTA 1/150		KS	
		positiv	negativ	positiv	negativ	positiv	negativ
positiv	578	578		578		518	60
zweifelhaft	61	53	8	53	8	35	26
negativ	1361	38	1323	351	1010	117	1244

Seroreaktionen überwiesen wurden. Den weiteren Teil bildeten FTA-positive Seren, bei denen eine unspezifische Fluorescenz vermutet wurde. Diese stammten aus serologischen Reihenuntersuchungen, die von uns in den letzten Jahren mit Hilfe des FTA-Testes durchgeführt wurden. Die Untersuchungen umfaßten etwa 80000 Personen.

Die Nelson-positiven Seren gaben immer, auch in den beiden Fluorescenztesten, positive Ergebnisse. Besonders wesentlich sind für die Beurteilung des diagnostischen Wertes des FTA-ABS die Ergebnisse von 1351 Nelson-negativen Seren.

In dieser Gruppe war der FTA-Test bei 351 Seren positiv, der FTA-ABS-Test demgegenüber aber nur bei 38 Fällen. Eine genaue Analyse der anamnestischen und epidemiologischen Daten sowie eine wiederholte serologische Untersuchung erlaubten, die Diagnose Lues latens der connata in 15 von den 38 erwähnten Fällen zu stellen. In einem großen Teil der weiteren Fälle darf ebenfalls mit einer alten, spontan negativierenden Lues gerechnet werden, wo die Restantikörper noch mit dem FTA-ABS nachweisbar blieben. Dagegen war die wiederholte Untersuchung im FTA-ABS bei vier Fällen negativ, was dafür zeugen könnte, daß in der ersten Untersuchung es nicht gelungen ist, die unspezifischen Antikörper gänzlich herauszuabsorbieren. Dieses kann mit einer unterschiedlichen immunologischen Verwandtschaft zwischen den saprophytischen Stämmen und den Reiter-Spirochaeten verbunden sein, was beweist, daß die Spezifität des FTA-ABS in einer 1:10 Verdünnung nicht absolut ist.

Tabelle 3. *Ergebnisse der quantitativen Untersuchung der 982 FTA-positiven „Problemseren"*

Ausfall	FTA-Titer						Zu-
FTA-ABS	150	450	1350	4000	12000	> 12000	sammen
positiv	20	54	165	255	139	36	669
negativ	153	124	35	1	—	—	313
Zusammen	173	178	200	256	139	36	982

Tab. 3 zeigt eine quantitative Analyse von 982 FTA-positiven Problemseren. Wie es aus der Tabelle hervorgeht, hat die bedeutende Mehrheit der FTA-positiven Ergebnisse mit den Titerwerten 150 bis 450 unspezifischen Charakter. Es muß aber hervorgehoben werden, daß die in Tab. 3 demonstrierten Ergebnisse Problemseren betreffen, die a priori um eine unspezifische Fluorescenz verdächtigt gewesen sind und die aus 80000 FTA-Proben herausselektioniert gewesen sind. Im Durchschnittsmaterial ist der Prozentsatz unspezifischer Ergebnisse selbstverständlich bedeutend geringer.

Die Resultate der vorgestellten Untersuchungen zeigen, daß der FTA-ABS eine Methode von großem diagnostischen Wert ist, welche durch eine ausgezeichnete Sensibilität und hohe Spezifität gekennzeichnet ist. Die Spezifität des FTA-ABS nähert sich praktisch der des Nelson-Testes, besitzt aber keinen absoluten Charakter, da in Ausnahmefällen die Absorption der unspezifischen Antikörper auf Schwierigkeiten stößt.

Weitere Forschungen zur Entwicklung und Standardisierung der Technik dieser wertvollen Methode sind zu empfehlen.

Sérologie de la syphilis chez les sujets de race noire

P. Many, R. Misson, J. Lapeyre, J. Teillard, B. Boutet et F. Pages,
Hôpital du Val de Grâce, Paris (France)

Depuis une vingtaine d'années la pratique des examens sérologiques systématiques a attiré l'attention sur la fréquence des réactions de réagine positives chez des sujets de race noire ne présentant ni signes cliniques ni antécédents de syphilis.

Diverses hypothèses ont été avancées pour expliquer ce fait: mauvaise qualité d'examens effectués outre mer dans des conditions techniques défectueuses, choix de réactions pêchant par excès de sensibilité, particularités immunologiques déterminées par des facteurs ethniques ou nutritionnels, fréquence sous les tropiques d'affections capables de provoquer des «fausses réactions biologiques»: paludisme, lèpre, parasitoses, etc. Tous ces arguments ont longtemps pesé sur l'interprétation des réactions sérologiques classiques de la syphilis chez les noirs et ont conduit maints esprits à leur dénier toute valeur.

Heureusement le test d'immobilisation tréponémique de NELSON et MAYER nous permet maintenant de contrôler la spécificité du résultat des réactions de réagine dans tous les cas sujets à caution. C'est ce qui a été systématiquement fait pour tous les éléments de la statistique que nous vous présentons.

Il s'agit de 217 sujets (200 hommes et 17 femmes) de race noire, pure ou métissée, originaires des états d'Afrique noire francophone, des départements ou des territoires français d'Outre mer (Antilles en particulier) que nous avons eu l'occasion d'examiner à Paris dans les meilleures conditions techniques en raison d'anomalies sérologiques, découvertes lors d'examens systématiques, et non confirmées par la clinique ou les anamnestiques. Nous avons donc éliminé de notre statistique tous les sujets présentant des antécédents certains de syphilis, ou qui avaient déjà reçu un traitement par antibiotiques susceptible de modifier l'état sérologique antérieur. Par contre 23 hommes avaient présenté un pian, certain dans dix cas, probable dans 13 cas.

Les résultats du test de NELSON et MAYER pour les 200 hommes sont les suivants: Positif dans 191 cas. Douteux dans un cas. Négatif dans huit cas.

Le cas douteux (42%) concerne un sujet ayant présenté un pian dans l'enfance. Il n'existe donc que huit cas soit une proportion faible de 4%, où les résultats de la sérologie de réagine apparaissent comme faussement positifs. Nous avons recherché une cause éventuelle à ces réactions faussement positives. Dans quatre cas il s'agit d'africains: 1 présente une bilharziose vésicale, 1 est porteur d'une ankylostomiase, 1 est atteint d'une névrite optique d'étiologie indéterminée. L'enquête est négative pour le quatrième.

Quatre cas concernent des mélanésiens faisant partie d'un petit groupe de sujets originaires des iles WALLIS et FUTUNA. Outre une éosinophilie sanguine respectivement à 2, 4, 13 et 20%, tous ont une importante augmentation de 27 à 36% du taux de leur gamma-globulines sériques. Cette hyper-gamma-globulinémie n'a reçu aucune explication.

Pour 17 femmes nous avons douze tests de NELSON positifs et cinq négatifs. La proportion de réactions de réagine faussement positives: cinq cas sur 17, est donc plus importante que pour les hommes. Mais parmi ces cinq femmes quatre étaient enceintes et l'état de grossesse est une cause classique des réactions de réagines faussement positives.

Ces chiffres permettent de conclure à la spécificité de la sérologie de réagine chez les noirs, spécificité qui nous parait équivalente à celle communément admise pour les blancs. Les travaux du Professeur BASSET et de l'Ecole de Dakar corroborent d'ailleurs cette opinion. A notre avis le pourcentage élevé des réactions de réagines positives chez les noirs ne peut s'expliquer par l'influence des multiples causes de réaction pseudo-syphilitiques.

Familiers de la syphilis vénérienne, seule tréponématose pratiquement connue en Europe occidentale, nous n'avons cependant pas le droit d'ignorer les autres tréponématoses humaines (ou les divers aspects de la tréponématose si nous admettons la théorie uniciste d'Hudson) qui fleurissent électivement dans les régions chaudes, humides ou sèches, de notre globe.

Depuis la fin de la II° guerre mondiale le gigantesque effort de prospection et d'éradication mené grâce aux initiatives de l'OMS nous a même fait connaître la syphilis endémique et la pinta; il nous a appris l'importance numérique de l'extension géographique du pian. Toutes ces tréponématoses ont avec la syphilis vénérienne d'étroites affinités biologiques et leurs réponses immunologiques, qu'il s'agisse de la sérologie classique ou des tests tréponémiques, sont jusqu ici communes.

Chez un sujet présentant un test de Nelson positif, en l'absence d'éléments décisifs permettant une différenciation certaine, nous ne pouvons raisonnablement poser qu'un diagnostic: celui de *tréponématose*.

Treatment

Traitement de la syphilis

L. Ciarrocchi, Rome (Italie)

L'observation d'un certain nombre de patients atteints de syphilis récente m'induit à faire des importantes considérations sur le traitement de la lues. Quelques-uns de ces sujets ont été soignés exclusivement avec la pénicilline, pendant une année; d'autres à thérapeutique plurimédicamenteuse pendant 24—36 mois et tous suivis pendant un long période de temps.

En 1946, au XXXVième Congrès S.I.D.E.S., dans une communication relative à des syphilitiques qui présentaient une persistance d'infection après un court traitement de pénicilline, je conclus: «Il me semble plus probable, dès ce moment, que la valeur de la pénicilline doit se référer plus à la possibilité de remplacer un, eu plusieurs des médicaments existants, à la probable augmentation d'activité réciproque et à la conséquente réduction du long période de temps nécessaire pour considérer que le mal a été vaincu, qu'à une action résolutive, rapide, exclusive».

En 1951, au XXXVIIIième Congrés S.I.D.E.S., après avoir illustré un cas de manifestation luétique tertaire qui avait paru après une cure prolongée, basée exclusivement sur la pénicilline, (manifestation qui confirmait que la pénicilline ne pouvait réussir toute seule à guérir la syphilis), je redis que le syphilographe avait le devoir de ne pas mettre en oubli les vieux médiquements antiluétiques, puisqu'ils conservaient leur valeur même après la découverte de la médecine miraculeuse.

A ce propos, j'ai précisé encore d'avoir soigné avec les antiluétiques traditionnels pendant 4 ou 5 ans, un considérable nombre de syphilitiques premier-secondaires: que je les ai suivis pendant 20 ans environ, après la suspension du traitement, avec des contrôles cliniques et sérologiques (y compris la Nelson), contrôles que j'ai étendus à leurs femmes et à leurs fils, sans rencontrer une rechute clinique ou sérologique; ou bien la trasmission de l'infection à leurs parents. Ce traitement qui démontrait d'avoir obtenu une guérison clinique et biologique, posait cette question: les vieux médicaments antiluétiques sont ils inférieurs à la pénicilline dans les cures d'attaque ou de consolidement? Je crois pouvoir confirmer aujourd'hui la même réponse négative de ce temps-la, sur la base aussi d'ultérieures observations de patients de syphilis récente et traités avec la pénicilline seulement.

Colbert et coll. par leurs recherches, ont pu démontrer que dans des lapins infectés et traités avec des prises élévés de pénicilline et dans douze cas humains de syphilis tardive, soignés longuement, mais encore TIT positifs, on pouvait mettre en évidence dans les ganglions lymphatiques et dans le liquor, = un an après le traitement =, des éléments spiraux pareils au tréponème pallidum. Parmi les

recherches de contrôle confirmant les données françaises (YOBS-OLANSKI), celles de
Boncinelli (1965) méritent une particulière mention pour avoir obtenu des reperts
bactérioscopiques positifs dans les ganglions lymphatiques d'un sur huit sujets,
traités pour syphilis récente, tous avec test de NELSON positifs et tous séronégatifs.

L'association des vieux antiluétiques à la pénicilline, = dont on connaît
l'avantage d'une considérable tolérance et de la simple provision =, doit être considérée indispensable aujourd'hui, même en considération de récentes recherches
expérimentales, selon lesquelles le mécanisme d'action de la pénicilline sur le
tréponème serait différent en comparaison de celui des métalloïdes, car ceux-ci
l'expliqueraient en toutes les phases du cycle biologique, tandis que l'antibiotique
le ferait seulement dans la phase multiplicative.

Je retiens également indispensable une cure prolongée pour 2 ans, au moins
dans les cas où elle a été commencée dans le premier période, ou au commencement
du secondaire et de 3 ans au moins, si elle a été entreprise plus tardivement, à
condition que ce soit rapide la disparition des manifestations cliniques et de la
positivité de la sérologie classique: cette négativité clinique et sérologique doit
s'accompagner à celle du test de NELSON, qui doit demeurer négatif pendant les
3 années qui suivent la fin du traitement.

Enfin le vieux syphilographe —, specialiste depuis 40 ans —, comme il retient
absurde la limitation de la cure antiluétique à quelques cycles de pénicilline,
autant il juge imprudent de ne vouloir considérer la positivité de la NELSON —,
même après un traitement à propos prolongé —, comme un indice très probable de
persistante infection et de la nécessité d'ultérieure cure.

On sait que, dans un certain pour cent de luétiques cliniquement indemnes, il
n'est pas possible d'obtenir le virage de la positivité à la négativité du test de
NELSON, avec une ultérieure thérapeutique, — la durée de la quelle doit être
établie selon les cas et non prolongée indéfinement —: cependant il ne semble que
ce motif doit porter à exclure la susdite nécessité, comme beaucoup de AA sou-
tiennent. On aura, en quelque manière, l'avantage de pouvoir retenir plus probable
que la positivité soit liée à des reliquats cliniques microbiques.

L'avenir seulement, — et non les données acquises jusqu'à présent —, pourra
nous dire si la pénicilline est capable de déterminer toute seule la guérison clinique
et étiologique de la syphilis et la durée de provision.

Long Term Results of Penicillin Therapy of Primary and Secondary Syphilis

J. TOWPIK, Klinika Dermatologiczna Warsaw (Poland)

In the course of 20 years (1947 to 1966) 5875 cases of early syphilis were
treated in the Clinic. Several experimental and routine schedules of treatment
were applied. Prior to ending of observation special attention was given to the
possibility of changes in the central nervous system and the cardiovascular
system. In a smaller group of patients the TPI test at the end of the period of
observation was performed. Because part of the investigation was presented at the
XII. Congres of Dermatology, this paper will deal with only two other methods of
treatment. This means:

Method A. 4.2 MU of Procain Penicillin (0.3 MU daily for period of 14 days) +
one to four courses of metalo-therapy (As + Bi depending on the stage of the
disease. This method was applied during the years 1954 to 1956.

Table 1 to 4. *Results of Long Term Observation*

Treatment method: A

Period of observation (in months)	Primary syphilis					Secondary syphilis				
	N. of patients observed	Clinical relapse (early)	Serological relapse	Late systemic syphilis	Reinfection	N. of patients observed	Clinical relapse (early)	Serological relapse	Late systemic syphilis	Re-infection
	Table 1					**Table 2**				
0—12	112		1		2	236				
13—24	84					172		2		
25—36	72					146				2
37—48	70					130		2		
49—60	62				4	118				
61—84	38					102		2	2	
85—120	4					34				

Treatment method: B

Period of observation (in months)	Primary syphilis					Secondary syphilis				
	N. of patients observed	Clinical relapse (early)	Serological relapse	Late systemic syphilis	Reinfection	N. of patients observed	Clinical relapse (early)	Serological relapse	Late systemic syphilis	Re-infection
	Table 3					**Table 4**				
0—12	265	1			6	219	1	9		4
12—24	187		1		1	147		3		3
25—36	134	1				111	1			3
37—48	41					70				1
49—60	12				1	35				
61—84	3				1	5			1	

Table 5 to 6. *Results of T.P.I. Test in Patients Whose Clinical and Serological Follow up was Satisfactory*

Table 5

In primary syphilis

Period of observation (in months)	N. of patients observed	N. of TPI test performed	Results of TPI test			
			−	+/−	+	++
0—12	455	2	2			
13—24	325	10	10			
25—36	257	19	15	3		1
37—48	150	26	21	4		1
49—60	108	12	9	1	2	
61—84	75	25	21	2	2	
85—120	26	16	14	1		1
121—180						
Total %		110 100	92 83,7	11 10	4 3,62	3 2,7

Table 6

In secondary syphilis

Period of observation (in months)	N. of patients observed	N. of TPI test performed	Results of TPI test			
			−	+/−	+	++
0—12	360					
13—24	235	5	4			1
25—36	180	7	5			2
37—48	132	18	14	2	1	1
49—60	92	16	9	2	1	4
61—84	59	16	12	1	1	2
85—120	33	18	11	2	2	3
121—180	11	9	5	2	1	1
Total %		89 100	60 67,5	9 10,1	6 6,7	14 15,7

Method B (a) 6.0 to 12.0 to 18.0 MU of Procain Penicillin or B (b) 4.8 to 7.2 to 9.6 MU of Benzathin Penicillin depending on the stage of syphilis (Benzathin Penicillin was injected in doses 1.2 MU every fifth day). This method was used during the years 1960 to 1963. Results obtained with method A are shown in the Tabs. 1 and 2.

Out of 112 patients suffering from primary syphilis only one case of treatment failure occured. Apart from this three cases of reinfection were confirmed (Tab. 1).

Out of 236 patients suffering from secondary syphilis eight cases of treatment failures occured. Among these in the 10. year of observation two cases of early neurosyphilis were discovered (Tab. 2). Results obtained with method B are shown in Tabs. 3 and 4.

Taking into acount that results achieved with method B (a) and B (b) both in primary and secondary syphilis (respectively) were very similar, they were considered inclusively. In primary syphilis out of 265 cases treated three were two cases of clinical relapse and one case of serological relapse. Apart from this there were ten cases of reinfection (Tab. 3). In secondary syphilis out of 219 cases treated, there were three cases of clinical failures, twelve cases of serological failures and eleven cases of reinfection.

Conclusions

1. In general the results achieved using treatment method A are slightly better than when method B is used. On the other hand, irrespective of which method is used, there is a significant difference between results obtained in the treatment of primary and secondary syphilis. In cases of secondary syphilis, especially in cases of secondary relapsing syphilis, in spite of intensive treatment, the possibility of a relapse does exist.

2. In cases where a 2 to 3 year follow up after treatment was satisfactory the late systemic changes were rather rare.

3. After treatment with penicillin alone the risk of reinfection was much higher than in cases treated with penicillin + metalotherapy. In a significant number of cases, where penicillin + metalotherapy was used, the course of treatment was not completed.

In seven cases the treatment was interrupted because of the sideeffects of the metalotherapy. Long term observation has revealed (Tabs. 5 and 6) that the TPI test as a criterium of complete cure plays a certain part in primary syphilis whereas, in sencodary syphilis, in spite of adequate treatment and satisfactory clinical results, it may remain positive for period of several years.

New Therapeutical Aspects in the Therapy of Syphilis

G. EHRMANN, II. Universitäts-Hautklinik Wien (Österreich)

There are no therapeutical problems if treatment is started before the onset of the "critical point". After this point, the treponemas, by a sublethal antibody-effect, are no longer virulent, antigen active and sensitive against antisyphilitic treatment. But this state is theoretically reversible by unknown factors. — There is the problem to restore the sensitivity of these dangerous latent treponemas artificially and to start immediately afterwards with massive penicillin — or other antibiotic-treatment. — To increase the sensitivity of the treponemas we can restore the virulence by a cortisone-effect or erode the surface by lysozymes. The investigations and the results are reported and discussed.

Considérations sur le diagnostic de guérison de la syphilis au moment actuel

U. BONCINELLI, Clinica Dermatologica Modena (Italie)

Le mot «guérison» de la syphilis est ici employé dans son sens classique et indique cette condition par laquelle «le syphilitique a perdu tout pouvoir de transmission, il échappe à toute suite morbide et peut arriver à un âge avancé sans plus montrer aucun signe clinique et sérologique de la maladie» (J. CAPPELLI).

Les critères de guérison dont nous disposons sont différentes par leur nature: cliniques, sérologiques, statistiques.

L'absence de signes cliniques (et radiologiques) reste évidemment d'ordre fondamental par rapport à un diagnostic de guérison, même si l'on tient compte qu'un complet silence du point de vue clinique peut caractériser des périodes même tres longues de la syphilis, surtout dans les phases les plus avancées. Il est encore à remarquer que tous les signes cliniques ne constituent pas toujours une preuve certaine d'infection active. On accepte de plus en plus l'idée qu'il existe quelques manifestations, surtout dans le domaine du système nerveux et du système cardiovasculaire, qui peuvent représenter — lorsque toutes les réactions sérologiques, classiques et modernes, sont complètement absentes — les *signes* indiquant les traces d'une infection désormais éteinte.

Le critère sérologique de guérison doit être considéré dans ses justes limites. Les réactions sérologiques classiques ont une grande importance dans la façon dont on pose le problème individuel de la guérison, mais leur valeur est diminuée de beaucoup par un fait bien connu: dans les phases avancées de la maladie les activités cliniques et sérologiques tendent à se dissocier et en quelques cas les réactions sérologiques classiques deviennent négatives même sans traitement, ce qui n'exclut point du tout le risque de complications tardives.

Les tests sérologiques modernes (TPI et FTA, mais spécialement le premier) sont considérés par plusieurs auteurs comme un critère indispensable de guérison. Le motif de cette opinion — surtout en ce qui concerne le TPI — consiste tout d'abord dans les qualités que possède le test et précisément une très haute spécificité et une grande sensibilité. Alors que les réactions sérologiques classiques peuvent être négatives dans les phases latentes, surtout dans les phases tardives, le test de NELSON les révèle toujours. En outre la négativité du TPI — lorsqu'elle est complète et contrôlée pendant une certaine période (trois tests négatifs en 3 ans) — apparaît stable dans le temps, de même qu'il résulte aussi par nos observations systématiques. Toutefois *la positivité du test de Nelson n'exclut point la guérison considérée comme inactivité permanente d'une infection qui d'ailleurs persiste*. Cela est démontré par les recherches sur le groupe d'Oslo (ENG et WEREIDE, 1962).

On doit encore considérer que la valeur des réactions sérologiques — entendues dans le sens le plus large du mot — n'est probablement pas la même et cela suivant les anticorps amenés par l'infection syphilitique n'ont pas le même sens, surtout dans les phases tardives latentes. Quelques anticorps révèlent probablement la seule *infection* (persistance de tréponèmes inactifs, sans *maladie*), d'autres sont considérés peut-être comme anticorps résiduels, soit comme réponse à la lente élimination de partigènes tréponémiques, soit comme un produit de l'activité particulière des organes formateurs des anticorps, activité indépendante de l'antigène et conservée à travers l'expérience morbide antérieure. Il est logique de supposer que la formation des anticorps résiduels est réduite du point de vue de la quantité à l'égard de la formation des anticorps des phases actives et que, par conséquent, les tests quantitatifs nous offrent la possibilité de distinguer — compte tenu des variations individuelles — les phases d'une *latence active*, préparatoires de futures complications, d'avec les phases d'une latence véritable lesquelles peuvent coincider avec l'inactivité durable de l'infection, c'est-à-dire avec la guérison clinique. De cette façon les termes de *latence active* et *inactive* pourraient être utilement introduits à côté des termes classiques de latence clinique, sérologique et totale.

Le *critère statistique* représente une aide précieuse pour évaluer les possibilités de guérison de sujets convenablement traités dans les différents stades de la maladie syphilitique. Les statistiques enseignent que, lorsque le traitement a commencé dans les phases précoces, le pourcentage des complications tardives sérieuses, pendant une période d'observation jusqu'à 20 à 30 ans (JORDON et DOLCE, BOHNSTEDT, LANCELLOTTI) ne dépasse pars le 4%. Même si ces chiffres se rapportent à des sujets traités suivant la thérapie classique, il est juste de supposer que l'introduction de la pénicilline a probablement réduit ce pourcentage. Ces données confirment que *la syphilis est une maladie dont on peut sûrement guérir, puisque la plupart des sujets convenablement traités en phase récente peuvent échapper pour toujours à toute complication tardive*, même s'il se trouve encore dans l'organisme quelques foyers de tréponémés en état d'activité pathogène.

Il paraît que les directives de la recherche future par rapport au problème de la guérison se développent dans une triple direction: bactériologique, immunologique et sérologique.

Bactérologique: en vue de possibles futures complications, éclarcir l'importance des données lymphoglandulaires de tréponèmes chez des sujets traités tardivement.

Immunologique: possibilités et limites d'une synthèse des anticorps indépendante de la présence de l'antigène.

Sérologique: affinement de la sérologie quantitative, dans le but d'établir s'il existe, dans les cas avec persistance sérologique positive, une formule sérologique de latence inactive, coincidente avec la guérison, et une formule sérologique d'activité asymptômatique ou subclinique (latence active) admonitive de futures complications.

Bibliographie. Boncinelli, U., R. Vaccari, L. Pincelli e M. Lancellotti: La guarigione della sifilide — Relazione al 48 Congr. S.I.D.E.S. Merano, 5—9 ottobre 1966 (in corso di stampa).

Traitement des syphilis récentes par injection unique de 2.400.000 unités de Benzathine-Pénicilline

R. Rollier et T. Markuch, Service Jeanselme Hôpital Averroës, Casablanca (Maroc)

Dans le cadre de la lutte antisyphilitique menée par le Ministère de la Santé Publique, il nous fallait, en prévision d'une campagne de masse, déterminer les résultats, incidents et accidents éventuels de la thérapeutique par injection unique de 2.400.000 u. de Benzathine-Pénicilline. Nous avons donc, depuis plus de 3 ans, traité de la sorte 1472 Syphilis primo-secondaires, dont la répartition par tranches d'ages et par type est résumée dans le tableau ci-joint.

Epidémiologie: nous constatons que les femmes n'interviennent que pour 10% des cas de SI, alors que le pourcentage de S. II est sensiblement le même dans les deux sexes.

Technique: a/L'injection de Benzathine-Pénicilline était en principe pratiquée lors des premières heures de la matinée et les malades laissés sous surveillance jusqu'à 18 heures, hospitalisés à la demande en cas de réaction fébrile et systématiquement s'il s'agissait de mineurs ou de femmes enceintes.

b/La dose administrée était de 2.400.000 u pour tous les sujets de plus de 15 ans, dose réduite en fonction de l'age jusqu'à 800.000 u pour un enfant de 5 ans. 10% des patients nous signalèrent avoir reçu au préaable une ou deux injections de Pénicilline ordinaire, pratiquées par un infirmier ou un préparateur en Pharmacie.

c/La tolérance à l'injection fut bonne: phénomènes douloureux à minima, quelques lipothymies chez des sujets pusillanimes; nous n'avons enrégistré aucune réaction allergique contrairement à notre collègue Orusco de Rabat qui en a signalé quelques rares cas.

Réaction d'Herxheimer: Il ne se produisit aucune réaction dans 20% des cas. La température fut inférieure à 38°5 chez 64% de nos patients, à 40° chez 12%, et supérieure à 40° chez 4% d'entre eux. Cette hyperthermie débutait en règle entre les 4ème et 6ème heures, le retour à la normale s'effectuant en 24 heures. Les réactions focales furent pratiquement nulles chez 32% des malades, discrètes chez 47%, moyennes chez 16%, très marquées chez 5% seulement. Les céphalées furent absentes chez 73% des sujets, supportables chez 18%, violentes chez 9%. Leur durée suivait la courbe de température. Les P.L. pratiquées après l'épisode hyperthermique furent toujours normales. L'on observa enfin quatre Ictères Syphilitiques, le retour à

Tableau. *Répartition des cas en fonction de l'age*

Age		0—9	10—14	15—19	20—24	25—39	+ de 40	Total
$\sum 1$	Hommes	12	19	92	264	468	80	935
	Femmes	8	12	32	24	16	4	96
$\sum 2$	Hommes	7	4	37	83	72	9	212
	Femmes	12	15	61	63	69	9	229
	Total	39	50	222	434	625	102	1472

la normale des tests hépatiques s'effectua en 3 mois. Les femmes enceintes de plus 4 de mois ainsi traitées ne présentèrent pas de troubles importants: seules survinrent quelques colliques utérines. Huit enfants examinés à leur naissance étaient normaux; quatre revus après le sixième mois avaient une sérologie négative. En ce qui concerne la Syphilis Congénitale, l'injection de 2.400.000 u de Benzathine-Pénicilline chez la mère allaitant a déclenché une réaction fébrile à plus de 40° chez le nourrisson, rapidement jugulée par l'administration de 100.000 à 200.000 u par jour de Pénicilline G.

Cicatrisation des lésions: les chancres cicatrisèrent entre les 8 ème et 15 ème jours, les Syphilides secondaires en 8 jours.

Evolution sérologique: HECHT, Kline, VDRL quantitatif et KOHLER furent pratiqués systématiquement. Moins de 5% des sérologies des S.I étaient négatives, et dans ces cas la recherche des Tréponèmes était positive dans les lésions. Les contrôles sérologiques devaient être pratiqués après 1, 3, 6, 12, 18 et 24 mois. 80% des patients se présentèrent entre les 8 ème et 15 ème jours; 30% des malades se présentèrent après un mois; moins de 20% ont satisfait au contrôles ultérieurs bien que tous les patients fussent convoqués régulièrement par lettre personnelle. Si l'on en juge par les malades revus, la sérologie se négative entre les Ier et 8 ème mois pour les S I, entre les 6 ème et 24 ème mois pour les S II.

Réinfections: 28 cas observés dont 15 de «Ping-Pong Syphilis»: le mari traité est recontaminé par son épouse; celle-ci nous est alors amenée en période secondaire, le mari étant à nouveau en période primaire. Six homosexuels de moins de 20 ans sept sujets non mariés. Aucune femme ne fut revue victime d'une réinfection. Il est à remarquer toutefois que les femmes revues à la consultation étaient une minorité. Tous les cas revus étaient porteurs d'accidents primaires de localisation différente des lésions notées lors de leur premier examen. Quatre d'entre eux en étaient à leurs troisième et quatrième recontaminations. Deux avaient été pris en traitement avec une Syphilis secondaire.

Récidives: dans quatre cas de reprise sérologique, nous avons constaté la réascension du VDRL quantitatif; tous ces patients avouaient avoir eu de nombreux rapports avec des prostituées clandestines.

Conclusions: Nous étant placés dans les conditions expérimentales du traitement de masse nous pouvons déduire:

1. l'absolue inocuïté et la parfait etolérance de la Benzathine-Pénicilline en suspension huileuse préférable à la préparation aqueuse du produit;

2. l'absence de Procaïne évite de façon presque complète les manifestations allergiques, d'où progrès par rapport à la PAM;

3. la longue activité -retard de la drogue limite les risques d'élimination rapide parfois rencontrés avec la PAM.

4. Absence totale d'accidents et même d'incidents chez les femmes enceintes; tous les enfants examinés dès leur naissance étaient sains; en revanche, le nourrisson porteur d'une Syphilis congénitale précoce, allaité par sa mère encourt le risque d'une réaction d'Herxheimer grave, ce qui doit inciter à la prudence.

5. L'injection unique de 2.400.000 u de Benzathine-Pénicilline semble assurer la guérison si nous en jugeons par les sérologies et TIT négatifs et le caractère quasi-expérimental des recontaminations et des «Ping-Pong Syphilis».

7. Appliquée à près de 1000 Syphilis latentes cette thérapeutique n'a suscité ni incident ni accident imputable à la Syphilis, ni réaction allergique.

8. L'inconnue demeure l'application de la méthode aux Syphilis Cardio-Vasculaires et Nerveuses.

Nous retenons donc l'injection unique de Benzathine-Pénicilline comme le traitement de choix dans les Syphilis récentes, pour les pays où la carence d'état-civil, de législation, d'éducation sanitaire et d'assistantes sociales fait obstacle à une éducation suffisante et à des contrôles rigoureux du syphilitique et de ses contacts. Toute autre technique peut sembler scholastiquement plus séduisante: elle risque d'être prophylactiquement plus dangereuse.

L'effet thérapeutique chez les malades atteints de syphilis traités à la Clinique Universitaire de Dermatovénérologie à Belgrade les 20 dernières années

S. KONSTANTINOVIĆ et S. PERIŠIĆ, Clinique de Dermatologie à la Faculté de Médecine, Belgrade (Jougoslavie)

Durant la période 1947 à 1967 ont été hospitalisés et traités 3258 malades atteints de la syphilis. Le Tab. 1 nous montre le nombre des malades hospitalisés de 1947 à 1967, pour chaque année de cette période.

Le nombre de cas de la syphilis avait augmenté de l'année 1947 à 1950. A partir de cette année le nombre de cas diminue jusqu'à l'année 1958. De 1958 augmente de nouveau jusqu'à 1964, et depuis cette année diminue de nouveau. Ont été analysés 1.106 dossiers de malades mis en traitement de janvier 1955 à décembre 1965, donc avec un recul actuel de 12 à 2 ans. Le Tab. 2 présente la répartition de ces 1.106 cas.

Tableau 1

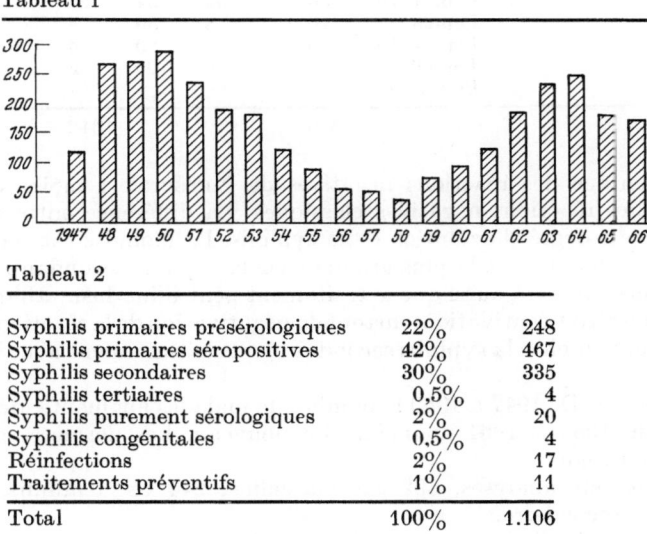

Tableau 2

Syphilis primaires présérologiques	22%	248
Syphilis primaires séropositives	42%	467
Syphilis secondaires	30%	335
Syphilis tertiaires	0,5%	4
Syphilis purement sérologiques	2%	20
Syphilis congénitales	0,5%	4
Réinfections	2%	17
Traitements préventifs	1%	11
Total	100%	1.106

Nous avons vu que nos malades en général sont atteints de la syphilis primo-secondaire. Le traitement antisyphilitique de 1947 à 1955 se faisait par l'application de salvarsan, de bismuth et de la pénicilline. De 1955 à 1961 à tous les malades avait été appliqué un traitement pénicillino-bismuthique.

Depuis 1961 nous avons traité la syphilis primo-secondaire avec de la pénicilline seule. Autres formes de la syphilis ont été traitées par la pénicilline et bismuth. Jusqu'à présent sous notre surveillance sérologique nous avons 566 cas syphilitiques traités. La sérologie de réagine a été suivie régulièrment (KOLMER, KAHN et MEINICKE). Les résultats de sérologie de réagine nous avons comparés à la réaction de NELSON chez 312 malades. Nous présentons les résultats obtenus chez ces malades au Tab. 3.

On voit que chez tous nos malades atteints de la syphilis primaire présérologique les réactions classiques étaient régulièrement négatives. Cependant chez nos malades atteints de la syphilis primaire séropositive, traités par la pénicilline seule, la séronégativation se manifeste en 97% de cas, tandis que chez les malades traités par l'association pénicilline — bismuth en 98% de cas. Chez les malades atteints de la syphilis secondaire la séronégativation se présentait en 90 à 94% des cas seulement. L'évolution sérologique des réinfections a été moins satisfaisante que celle des sujets infectés pour la première fois. De 15 cas de réinfection la séronégativation s'est présentée chez 12 cas (80%) seulement. La séronégativation des cas traités préventivement était de 100%.

Tableau 3

	Traités par	Cas traités	Sérologie de réagine neg. %	Cas traités	Réactions de Nelson neg. %
Syphilis primaires	Penicil.	121	121 100	62	58 93
présérologiques	Pen. + Bi.	21	21 100	13	13 100
Syphilis primaires	Penicill.	172	167 97	81	66 81
séropositives	Pen. + Bi.	57	56 98	36	33 92
Syphilis	Penicil.	135	121 90	80	44 55
secondaires	Pen. + Bi.	36	34 94	25	18 72
Réinfections	Penicil.	10	8 80	8	5 63
	Pen. + Bi.	5	4 80	4	2 50
Traitements	Penicil.	9	9 100	3	3 100
préventifs	Pen.+Bi.	—	—	—	—
Total		566		312	

Le pourcentage des réactions négatives de NELSON est moins élevé que le pourcentage des réactions négatives classiques. La différence entre ces pourcentages dépend du degré d'évolution de la syphilis. La moindre est chez la syphilis primaire présérologique, et la plus grande chez la syphilis secondaire.

Nous avons constaté aussi que le traitement pénicillino-bismuthique donne un pourcentage de séro-négativation, surtout de négativation de la réaction de NELSON, plus grand (surtout chez la syphilis secondaire) que le traitement avec la pénicilline seule.

Conclusions. 1. De 1947 à 1950 le nombre de malades augmente, de 1950 à 1958 diminue et de 1958 à 1964 augmente de nouveau. Les dernières deux années diminue de nouveau.

2. 1106 dossiers analysés, 862 cas masculins, 244 cas féminins, 94% de la syphilis primo-secondaire.

3. 566 de cas régulièrement controlés jusqu'à présent.

4. Syphilis primaire présérologique: les réactions classique négatives.

5. Syphilis primaire séropositive: la séronégativation dans 97 à 98%.

6. Syphilis secondaire: séronégativation dans 90 à 94% de cas.

7. Réinfections: l'évolution sérologique moins satisfaisante que celle des sujets infectés pour la première fois.

8. Le pourcentage des réactions négatives de NELSON est moins élevé que le pourcentage des réactions négatives classiques.

9. Chez la syphilis secondaire un pourcentage de séronégativation plus grand s'obtient par traitement pénicillino-bismuthique, que par un traitement par la pénicilline seule.

Stellt die Behandlung der Frühsyphilis heute noch ein Problem dar?

J. Söltz-Szöts, II. Universitäts-Hautklinik Wien (Österreich)

Therapeutisch hat sich bei der Lues das Penicillin ausgezeichnet bewährt. Bis jetzt wurde keine Abnahme der Empfindlichkeit der Spirochaeten gegenüber dem Penicillin beobachtet.

In der Therapie der Frühsyphilis (Manifestation der Lues zwischen dem Zeitpunkt der Ansteckung und etwa Ende des 2. Jahres post infectionem) wurde in den letzten Jahren fast auf der ganzen Welt die sog. Kurzzeitbehandlung angewandt. Bei dieser muß ein Blutspiegel von 0,03 E Penicillin/ml für die Dauer von 2 Wochen erhalten werden. Die dabei gegebenen Penicillindosen sind abhängig von der Menge und der Depotwirkung des verwendeten Präparates sowie auch von Schwankungen in Resorption und Ausscheidung. Die mit dieser Behandlung erzielten Resultate sind, wie den Literaturberichten übereinstimmend zu entnehmen ist, ausgezeichnet. Die von uns gewonnenen Ergebnisse können dies nur bestätigen. Da einzelne Autoren bereits auf eine fast 25jährige Nachbeobachtungszeit ihrer Patienten zurückblicken können, muß diese Behandlung als optimal angesehen werden. Auch die Kinder von so behandelten Frauen, die sich während einer späteren Gravidität keiner weiteren Behandlung unterzogen haben, waren durchwegs gesund und zeigten auch in einer 3jährigen Nachbeobachtungszeit keine Symptome einer Lues congenita. Trotz dieser guten Ergebnisse soll jedoch weder auf mehrjährige quantitative serologische Nachkontrollen, noch bei Graviden mit positiv gebliebenem TPI-Test auf eine Präventivbehandlung verzichtet werden.

Eine Gefahr für den Patienten besteht bei dieser Behandlung nicht, da Herxheimer-Reaktionen bei der Frühsyphilis, bei ansonst gesunden Individuen, niemals einen bedrohlichen Verlauf nehmen und durch vorherige Wismut-Gaben oder durch gleichzeitig mit der ersten Penicillininjektion verabreichte Corticosteroide gemildert werden können.

Die in den letzten Jahren zunehmenden allergischen Reaktionen auf Penicillin stellen sicher ein nicht zu unterschätzendes Problem dar, jedoch sind dadurch bedingte Todesfälle äußerst selten. Außerdem kann bei bestehender Penicillinallergie die Behandlung mit Breitbandantibiotica durchgeführt werden.

Wenn man bedenkt, daß damit bereits sämtliche, durch das Penicillin hervorgerufene Schäden aufgezählt sind, kann man im Vergleich zu den früher gegebenen Arsenobenzolen und Schwermetallen die Penicillintherapie als ungefährlich bezeichnen.

Die Verkürzung der Behandlungszeit wie deren Vereinfachung brachten es mit sich, daß eine luetische Infektion, besonders bei der jungen Generation, nicht mehr ernst genommen wird. Dies führt dazu, daß einerseits die Behandlung vom Patienten willkürlich abgebrochen wird und damit ihre Wirksamkeit einbüßt, andererseits wiederholte Neuerkrankungen, besonders bei Jugendlichen, in kurzen zeitlichen Abständen keine Seltenheit darstellen. Bei diesen Jugendlichen findet sich fast immer eine abgeschlossene körperliche Entwicklung, jedoch in vielen Fällen ein Mangel an geistiger Reife.

Die Lues und ihre Therapie wird jedoch nicht nur vielfach vom Patienten, sondern leider auch in Einzelfällen von den behandelnden Ärzten bagatellisiert. Dies führt nicht nur zu einer Vernachlässigung der Infektionsquellenforschung wie auch der unumgänglich notwendigen Nachtkontrollen, sondern es kommt auch immer wieder zu einer Behandlungsunterbrechung (etwa an Wochenenden), ohne daß für diese Zeitspanne ein entsprechendes lange wirksames Depotpräparat gegeben wird.

Zwei weitere Faktoren sind bei der Erkennung und Behandlung der Frühsyphilis von Bedeutung. Die ausgedehnte Anwendung der Antibiotica in nicht-venerologischen Indikationen kann dazu führen, daß in manchen Fällen die Infektion durch die Verlängerung der Inkubation einen anderen Verlauf nimmt.

Das nahezu völlige Verschwinden frischer luetischer Infektionen in den 50er Jahren führte dazu, daß viele Ärzte, auch Dermatologen nicht ausgenommen, die luetische Genese einer Erkrankung kaum mehr in Erwägung zogen, wodurch luetische Manifestationen in manchen Fällen verkannt und erst verspätet einer spezifischen Therapie zugeführt wurden. In diesem Zusammenhang soll auch nicht unerwähnt bleiben, daß die zunehmende Verbreitung von Geschlechtskrankheiten unter den Homosexuellen es mit sich brachte, daß die Frühsymptome der Lues bei diesen, oft außerhalb des Genitalbereiches, in Erscheinung treten (Anus, Wangenschleimhaut) und vom Patienten wie auch vom Arzt längere Zeit übersehen werden. Dazu kommt noch, daß solche Personen, da Homosexualität noch in vielen Staaten unter Strafe steht, sich keiner ärztlichen Behandlung unterziehen.

Die Behandlung der Frühsyphilis stellt heute kein therapeutisches, wohl aber noch immer oder mehr denn je ein soziales Problem dar. Eine Penicillinbehandlung, die einen Blutspiegel von 0,03 E/ml über 14 Tage gewährleistet, ist als ausreichend anzusehen. Die einzige Nebenwirkung von Bedeutung ist die Penicillinallergie. Aber selbst in solchen Fällen kann mit Hilfe der Breitbandantibiotica eine verläßliche und wirksame Syphilistherapie durchgeführt werden.

Die Lösung der sozialen Probleme, die sich aus der Kürze der Behandlung wie aus der Änderung im Sexualverhalten in den letzten Jahren ergeben haben, verlangt nicht nur eine verstärkte Aufklärung bei der Bevölkerung, eine verantwortungsvolle Einstellung der Ärzte, sondern auch eine Gesetzgebung, die den sozialen medizinischen Problemen der Venerologie mehr als bisher Rechnung trägt.

Main Theme VI

Cutaneous Manifestations of Circulatory Disorders of the Legs

Les manifestations cutanées des désordres circulatoires des jambes

Afecciones cutàneas por alteraciones vasculares en las piernas

Gefäßbedingte Unterschenkeldermatosen

Organizer

D. M. PILLSBURY, USA

Presidents

C. D. CALNAN, Great Britain

E. FARBER, USA

G. LECLERC, Canada

J. PINOL AGUADÉ, Spain

Delegate of the Organization Committee

H. KOEHLER, Germany

Reports

Die venösen Durchblutungsstörungen der unteren Extremität

W. Schneider, Universitäts-Hautklinik Tübingen (Deutschland)

Die Pathophysiologie der Durchblutungsstörungen der Beine wird dadurch geprägt, daß einem zuführenden System, dem arteriellen, zwei ableitende, nämlich das Venen- und das Lymphsystem, gegenüberstehen, wobei die Venen als Teil des Niederdrucksystems eine doppelte Aufgabe, d. h. Blutspeicherung und -transport zu erfüllen haben. Das Blut wird aus den tiefen Arterien, die am Unterschenkel in den Fascienlogen verlaufen, über zahlreiche kleine Muskeläste der Haut zugeführt. Diese besitzt also keine größeren eigenen arteriellen Versorgungsstämme. Muskel- und Hautdurchblutung verlaufen meist gegensinnig.

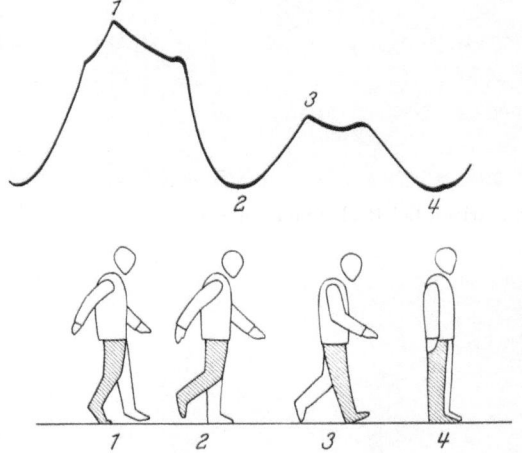

Abb. 1. Schwankungen des Venendruckes im Laufe eines Schrittes (n. Fegan)

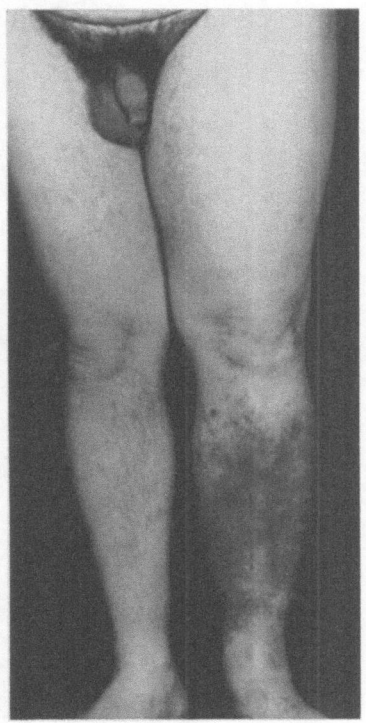

Abb. 2. Stauungsödem des ganzen Beines bei Beckenvenensperre

Der Blutabstrom erfolgt aus der Muskulatur durch die Begleitvenen der tiefen Arterien intrafascial. Das extrafasciale Geflecht sammelt dagegen das Hautblut in einem weit verzweigten, untereinander anastomosierenden Netzwerk mit den beiden Saphenae als den großen Leitvenen. Aus diesen gelangt das Hautblut von Etage zu Etage durch die jeweiligen Venae perforantes in die Tiefe. Die Einmündungen der beiden Saphenae können somit funktionell als letzte und oberste Venae perforantes angesehen werden. Ein Abstrom in die Tiefe kann jedoch nur dann erfolgen, wenn ein negativer Druckgradient besteht. Dieser wird durch die Muskelpumpe in den tiefen Leitvenen erzeugt. Abb. 1 zeigt die venösen Druckschwankungen im Laufe eines einzigen Schrittes nach Fegan.

Bei primärer Varicose mit erhöhtem Druck in den extrafascialen Venen, jedoch intakten Verbindungen zur Tiefe, kommt es eher zu einem vermehrten Abstrom in das intrafasciale Stromgebiet und daher nicht zu Stauungsödem und

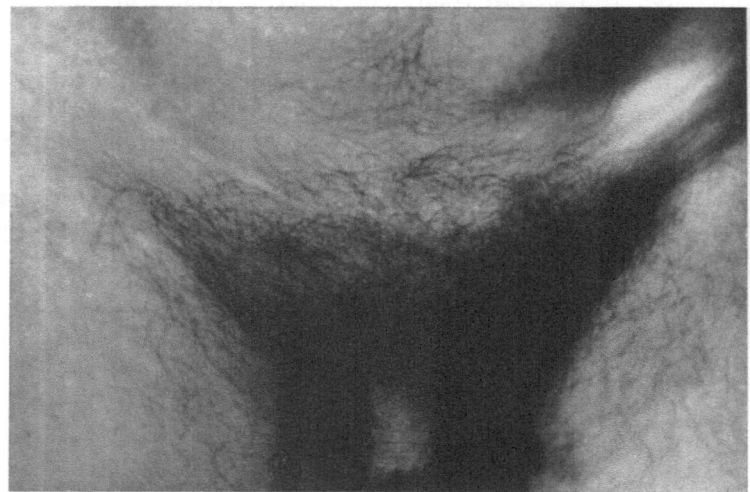

Abb. 3. Suprapubische Kollateralvaricen bei Beckenvenensperre

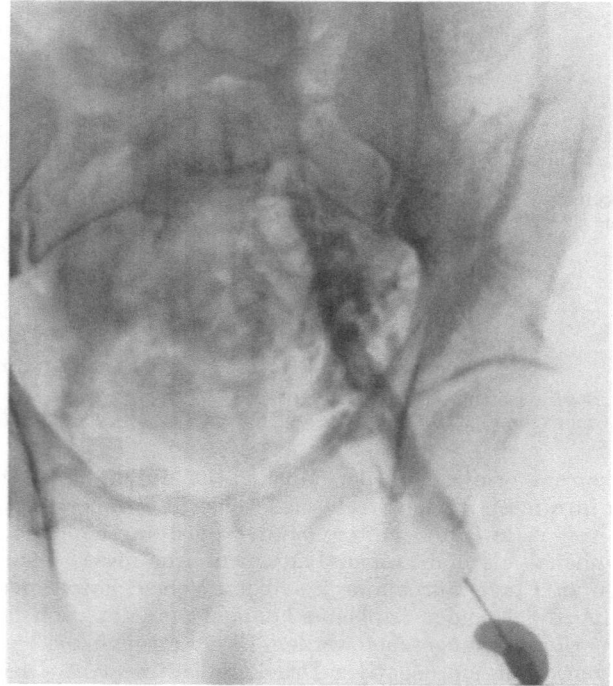

Abb. 4. Kollateralkreislauf zur kontralateralen Seite und durch die V. epigastrica

Ulceration. Im Gegensatz hierzu führt ein Verschluß der tiefen Leitvenen einerseits, aber auch der Perforantes andererseits, zwangsläufig zum Ödem und damit zu Beschwerden und unter Umständen zum Ulcus. Die Lokalisation des Verschlusses ist bestimmend für die Entwicklung des Kollateralkreislaufes und die Ausbreitung des Ödems.

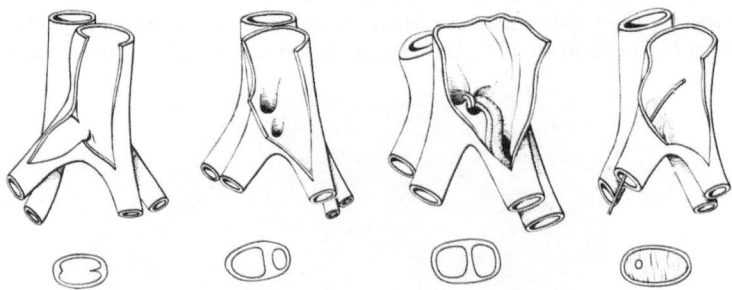

Abb. 5. Bifurkationssyndrom (n. MAY und THURNER)

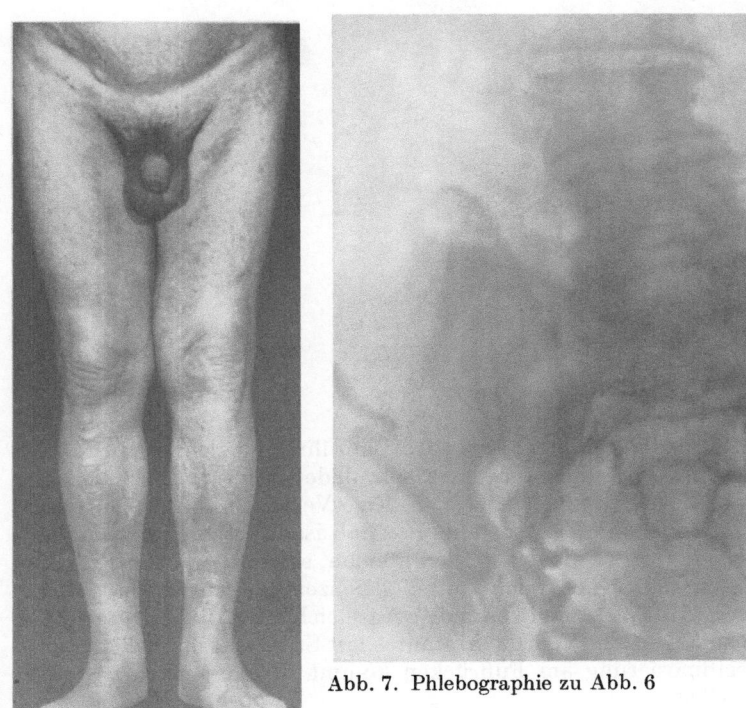

Abb. 7. Phlebographie zu Abb. 6

Abb. 6. Doppelseitiges Beinödem mit Kollateralvaricen beider Vv. epigastricae bei Verlegung der V. cava caudalis

Bei Beckenvenensperre ist das gesamte Bein ödematös (Abb. 2) mit sichtbaren Kollateralen in der Inguinalbeuge und suprapubisch (Abb. 3). Die Femoralisphlebographie (Abb. 4) zeigt die schweren postthrombotischen Veränderungen der Beckenvenen und die Kollateralen zur kontralateralen Seite. Beim Bifurkationssyndrom

(WANKE, GUMRICH), wie hier im Schema (Abb. 5), und beim Cavaverschluß (Abb. 6) können beide Beine betroffen sein mit kompensatorischer Erweiterung der Venae epigastricae (deren Verödung unseres Erachtens nicht in Frage kommt). Phlebographisch erkennt man (Abb. 7) deutlich die Kollateralvenen, während die Beckenvenen und die Vena Cava nicht gefüllt sind. Die Lymphographie (Abb. 8) zeigt das vikariierende Einspringen der Lymphgefäße.

Am Unterschenkel sind die Verhältnisse besonders kompliziert, schon allein durch die sowohl horizontale als auch vertikale Gliederung. Die vertikale wird von

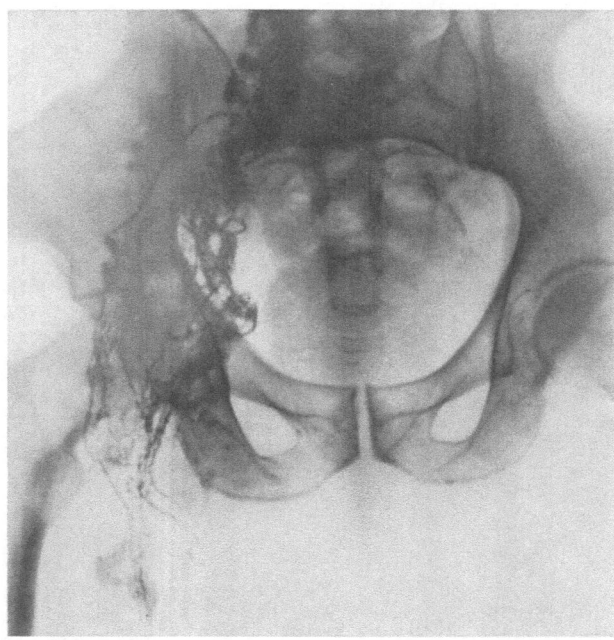

Abb. 8. Lymphographie zu Abb. 6

den drei großen Fascienlogen gebildet (Abb. 9), die mit ihren Muskeln und Gefäßen in sich selbständige Funktionseinheiten darstellen. Jeder Arterie (Tib. ant., Tib. post., Peronaea) entsprechen zwei Begleitvenen. Eine Verbindung der drei Gefäßstränge kommt erst wieder am Fuß zustande, so daß isolierte Strömungshindernisse nicht untereinander ausgeglichen werden können, sondern zu einer Stauung führen, die bis in den Fußrücken reicht unter gleichzeitiger Entwicklung einer Corona phlebectatica (Abb. 10). Ein eventueller Ausgleich über die extrafascialen Venen setzt eine Insuffizienz der Venae perforantes mit Strömungsumkehr voraus. Ob der guten Anastomosierung am Fußrücken kommt es hier — trotz acraler Lage — nicht zum Ulcus.

Entscheidend für die horizontale Gliederung sind die Muskeln mit ihrer Pumpfunktion (Abb. 11). Bei der Kontraktion der Wadenmuskeln werden die tiefen Leitvenen im mittleren Drittel des Unterschenkels durch den Muskelbauch komprimiert. Da sich der Muskel aber auch verkürzt, werden die proximalen und distalen Venenabschnitte, deren Wand in den Muskelzwickeln (intermuskuläres Bindegewebe) fest verankert ist, nunmehr erweitert (Abb. 12), so daß ein negativer Druck entsteht und gleichzeitig Raum für das aus den Fuß- und Wadenmuskeln ausgepreßte Blut geschaffen wird (Abb. 11). Das Umgekehrte tritt bei der

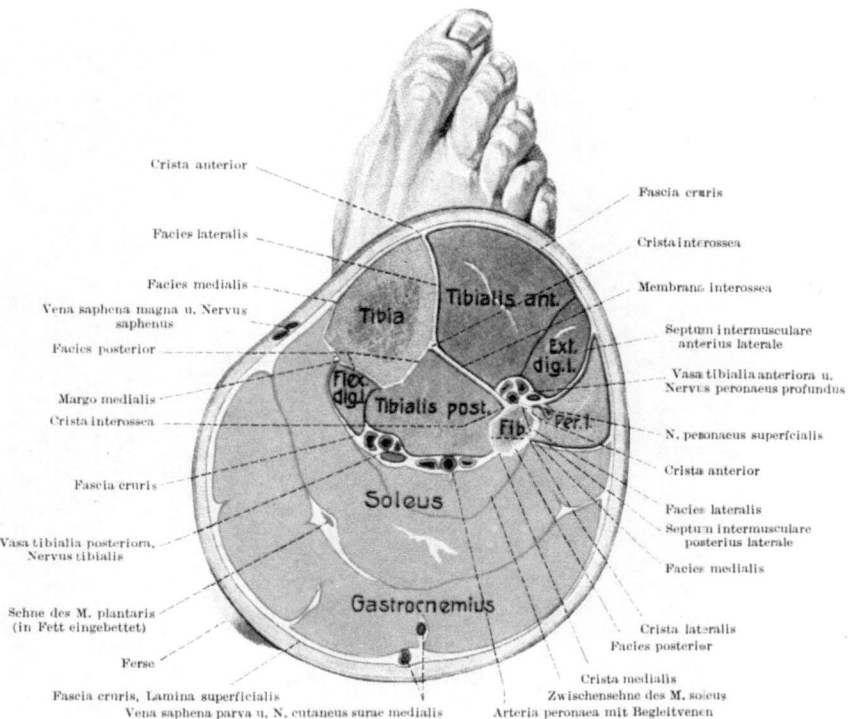

Abb. 9. Muskel- und Fasciculogen
des Unterschenkels (n. Braus)

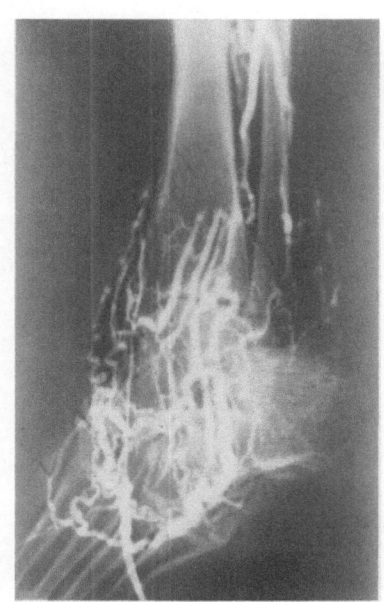

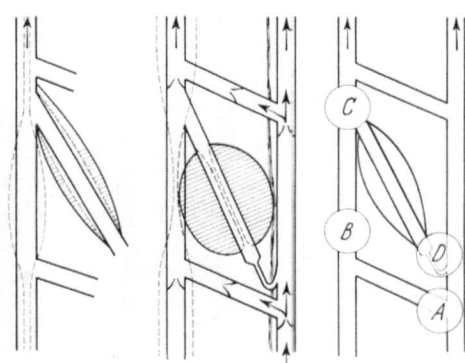

Abb. 11. Schema der Muskelvenenpumpe

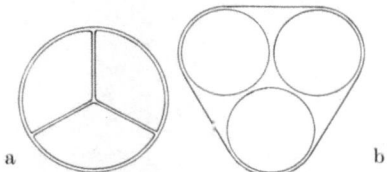

Abb. 12. Erweiterung der bindegewebigen Mus-
kelzwickel bei der Muskelkontraktion (n. Krug
und Schlicher

Abb. 10. Corona phlebectatica

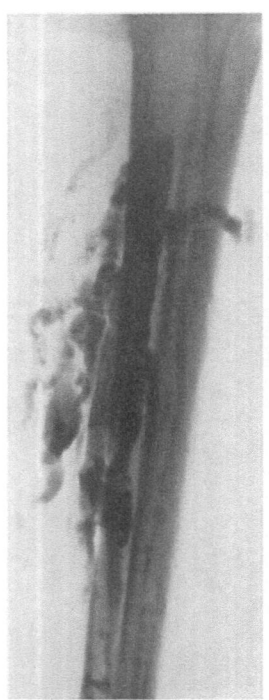

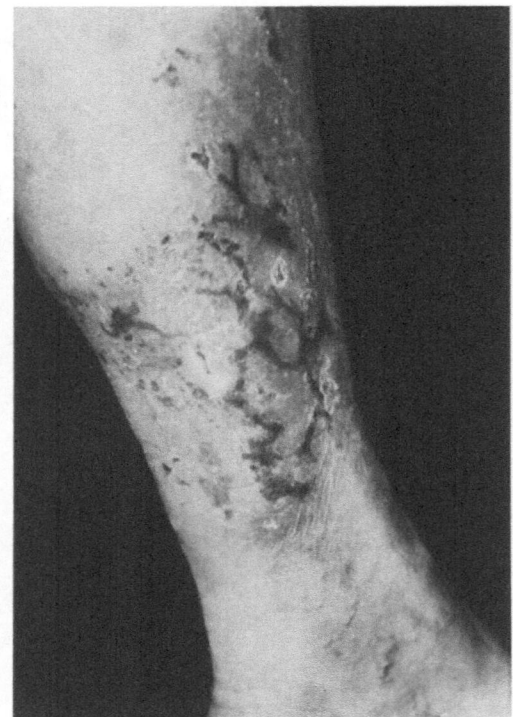

Abb. 13. Erweiterte
Soleusmuskelvene

Abb. 14. Durchtrittspunkte insuffizienter Muskel-
veneneinflußschleifen

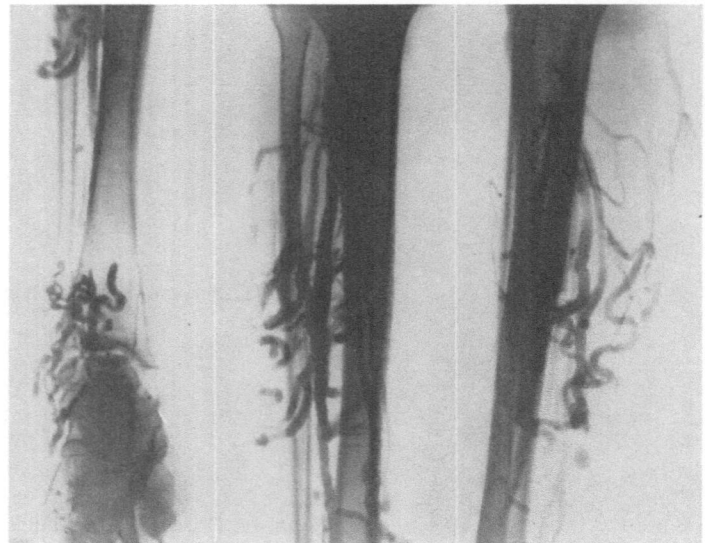

Abb. 15. Phlebographie zu Abb. 14

Muskelerschlaffung ein: Das Blut wird vom distalen ins mittlere Drittel verschoben und vom proximalen in die Vena poplitea. Die Klappen bestimmen die *Richtung* der Strömung. Entscheidend ist, daß die Muskelpumpe nicht im Haupt-, sondern im Nebenschluß liegt (Schema).

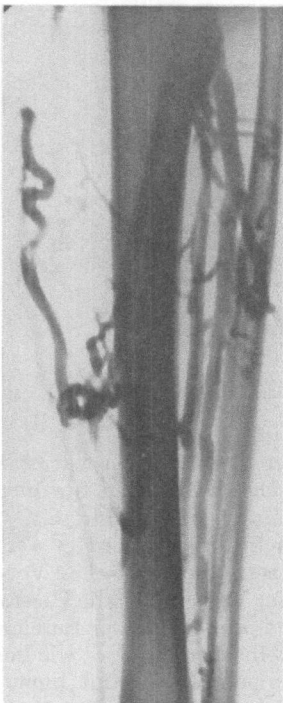

Am Fußrücken fließt die Hauptmasse des arteriellen Blutes in die Haut und wird im suprafascialen Netz wieder gesammelt. Es gelangt erst wieder in Höhe der Fußgelenke in die Tiefe, um intrafascial abgeführt zu werden. Ein Verschluß an dieser Stelle (A) bedingt eine Umleitung über das extrafasciale Netz (Saphena) und — was entscheidend ist — einen Ausfall der Muskelpumpe für den Fuß, dessen tiefes Venennetz nur ganz spärlich ausgebildet ist. Der Verschluß einer tiefen Vene im unteren Drittel (B) muß ebenfalls eine Umleitung über das extrafasciale Netz zur Folge haben, wiederum unter Wegfall der Muskelpumpe.

Ein Verschluß im oberen Drittel (C) muß sich besonders schwer auswirken, weil dann die gesamte Kraft der Muskelpumpe zu einer erheblichen Drucksteigerung im vorgeschalteten peripheren tiefen Netz führt, vergleichbar einer am Oberarm angelegten Stauung bei der Cubitalvenenpunktion. Ohne Stauung führt Faustschluß nur zur Strömungsbeschleunigung ohne wesentlichen Druckanstieg. Unter Stauung sind Druckanstiege bis 80 mm Hg möglich. Dasselbe gilt für einen Verschluß der Muskelausflußbahn. Deshalb sind Thrombosen der Muskelvenen auch so besonders folgenschwer. Das Muskelblut findet dann nur noch einen Ausweg nach außen über die Einflußschleife (D), deren Insuffizienz ein Leck in der Pumpe bedeutet. Zunächst

Abb. 16.
Muskelveneneinflußschleife

zeige ich Ihnen eine Muskelvarice mit noch suffizienter Einflußschleife, d. h. ohne Leck, da die zugehörige

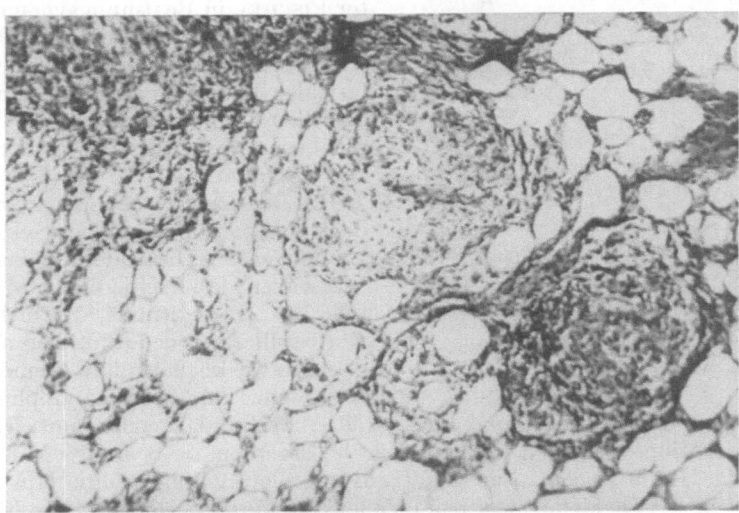

Abb. 17. Epitheloidzellige Aufräumgranulome bei tiefer Vasculitis

28*

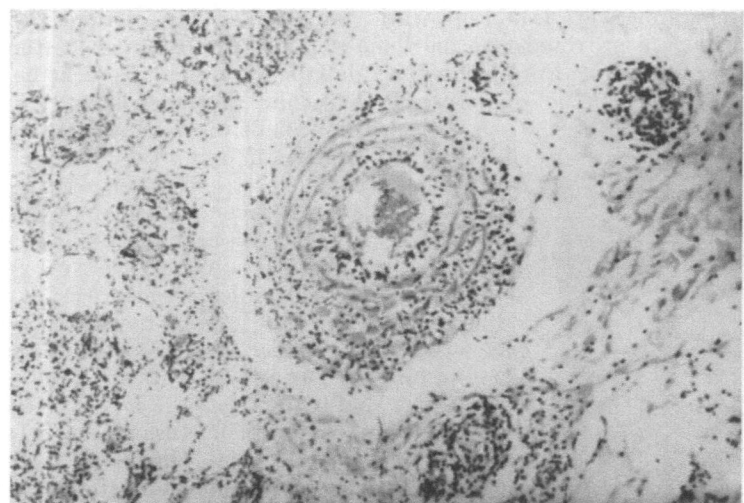

Abb. 18. Histiocytäre Aufräumgranulome

Klappe noch intakt ist (Abb. 13). Bei Insuffizienz folgen beträchtliche varicöse Erweiterungen (Abb. 14), das zugehörige phlebographische Bild sehen Sie hier (Abb. 15), ein weiteres in der Abb. 16.

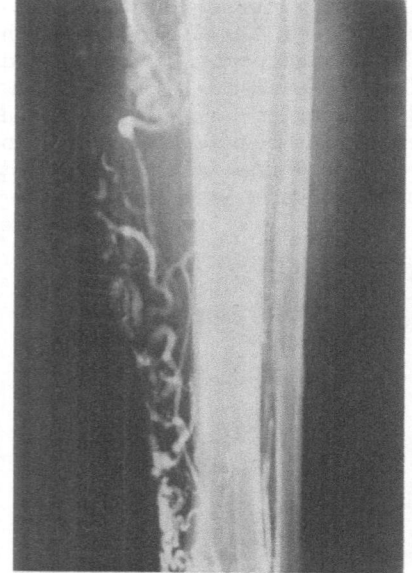

Abb. 19. Durchgängige, nicht obliterierte, subulceröse Varicenpolster

Unter diesen Prämissen wird es verständlich, daß trotz aller topischen Verschiedenheiten der Verschlüsse die Ulcera immer im selben knöchelnahen Bereich auftreten und nicht extrem acral, wie bei arteriellen Störungen. Es kommt hinzu, daß diese Region bei dem Mangel an Muskulatur auch noch eine arterielle Minderversorgung aufweist, wie mein Mitarbeiter FISCHER in Beatmungsversuchen gasanalytisch nachweisen konnte. Weiterhin wird aber auch klar, daß die tiefe intrafasciale Phlebothrombose immer, die oberflächliche extrafasciale Thrombophlebitis dagegen so gut wie nie ein Ödem zur Folge hat.

Im Ödemzusammenhang kommt auch dem zweiten ableitenden System, den Lymphgefäßen, besondere Bedeutung zu. Wir wissen, daß hochmolekulare Bestandteile des Interstitiums, die nicht in die Blutcapillaren rückdiffundieren können, genauso wie korpuskuläre Elemente, z. B. Ruß, vom Endothel der Lymphcapillaren aktiv aufgenommen werden und Flüssigkeit erst sekundär nachströmt. Diesbezügliche Resorptionsstörungen können unseres Erachtens z. B. bei NONNE-MILROY-MEIGE eine Rolle spielen. Für den Transport der Lymphe ist die Muskelpumpe jedoch noch entscheidender als beim Venensystem, kann doch Inaktivität alleine ohne pathologische Veränderungen schon zum Ödem führen, wie in den voll-

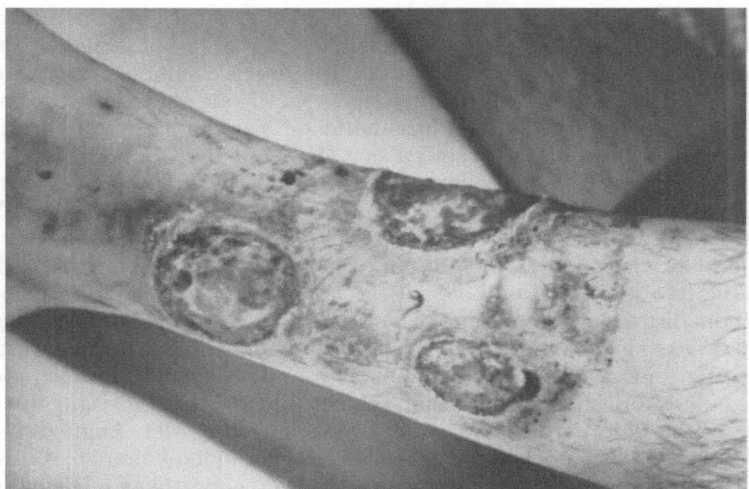

Abb. 20. Kombinationsulcera (arteriell, postthrombotisch, vasculitisch)

gepfropften Urlauberzügen des letzten
Krieges, bei den Bord- und Flugpassa-
gieren und den Fernsehern als „Fernseh-
bein".

Das Ödem hat auf die Dauer die Ver-
schwielung (Dermatosklerose) zur Folge
durch acelluläre Sklerose sowie durch
Fibrose infolge numerischer Faserver-
mehrung. Dieser Vorgang ist trotz tief-
greifender organischer Veränderungen reversibel, insbesondere auf die Kompres-
sions- und Verödungstherapie. hin. Weiterhin finden sich capilläre Thrombosen
(PROPPE) und Blutungen. Diese Mikro-
blutungen werden nicht wie Hämatome
(Makroblutungen) relativ schnell resorbiert, sondern lösen celluläre entzündliche Vorgänge mit Hämosiderinspeiche-
rung und nachfolgender zusätzlicher Me-
laninpigmentierung aus.

Superfizielle bzw. capillaritische Zustände führen zur Atrophie blanche, deren
netzförmig angeordnete Einzelelemente
histangischen Korrelationen im Sinne von
COMEL entsprechen, etwa dem Histion
LETTERERS.

Demgegenüber entspricht die tiefe
Vasculitis größeren tissulär-vasculären
Einheiten, die durch Endarterien im Sinne
von COHNHEIM repräsentiert werden und

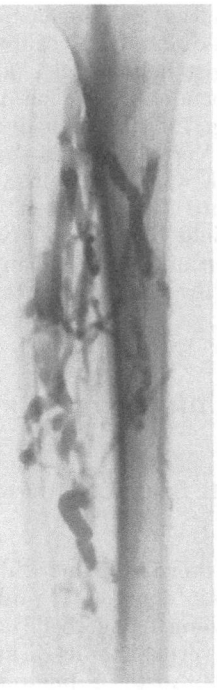

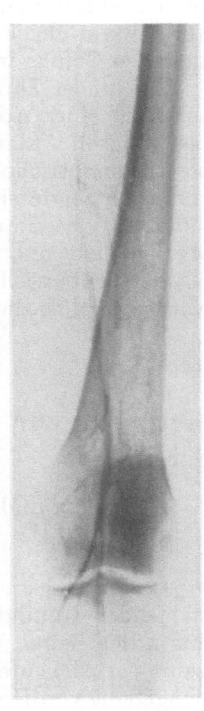

Abb. 21.
Phlebogramm zu
Abb. 20

Abb. 22. Arterio-
gramm zu Abb. 20.
Spasmus der Art.
tibial. (vgl. Art.
suralis!)

dadurch nur *einen* monomorphen Ablauf zulassen, der über die Fettgewebsnekrose
zu epitheloidzelligen (Abb. 17) und histiocytären (Abb. 18) Aufräumgranulomen

führt und nur ausnahmsweise zur Ulcusbildung. Umgekehrt findet man aber beim Ulcus cruris nur ganz selten tiefe Vasculitiden, dafür aber periphlebitische Prozesse, die wahrscheinlich bei der Pathogenese des Ulcus cruris ebenfalls mitwirken, selbst bei Durchgängigkeit der oberflächlichen Varicen. Große und tiefe Ulcera heilen überraschend schnell ab, wenn die durchlaufende Varice oberhalb und unterhalb verödet wird. Ich bin mit H. FISCHER der Meinung, daß die Abheilung erfolgt durch die Beseitigung adventitieller und periadventitieller Entzündungszustände im Bereich einer an sich durchgängigen Vene (Abb. 19). Unter diesen Voraussetzungen ist die Klinik der venösen Durchblutungsstörungen keineswegs so eindeutig und klar, wie es PAUL LINSER seinerzeit noch annehmen durfte. Es handelt sich keinesfalls um eine Krankheitsentität und schon gar nicht um eine anatomische Anomalie, vielmehr um ein Leiden mit ganz verschiedener Ätiologie und Pathogenese, das sich ständig zu verschiedenen Endzuständen fortentwickelt und weiterhin eine entscheidende Abhängigkeit von der Topik aufweist. So lehnt KOGOJ den Begriff des Ulcus varicosum schlechthin ab. Die Erfassung des Krankheitsbildes setzt den Vergleich des klinischen Aspektes der Angiographie und Histologie voraus, wozu noch eine Reihe von Meßmethoden kommen, die zum Teil erprobt, zum Teil in der Entwicklung begriffen, wertvolle Dienste leisten können.

Das abschließende Beispiel möge dies zeigen und darüber hinaus die Tatsache, daß die chron.-venöse Insuffizienz vor allem dann besonders schwere Bilder aufweist, wenn gleichzeitige Störungen im Bereich des arteriellen Systems und der kleineren Gefäße im Sinne der Vasculitis hinzukommen:

Ein junger Drogist bekam nach jahrelangem Phenacetin- und Nicotinabusus anläßlich einer Appendektomie eine Thrombose mit Lungenembolie. Es fanden sich klinisch Anfang 1965 beträchtliche therapieresistente Ulcera (Abb. 20) und postthrombotische Veränderungen bei der Phlebographie (Abb. 21). Arteriographisch zeigte sich wiederholt ein Spasmus der Art. tibial. ant. (Abb. 22). Die radioaktiv bestimmte Durchflußzeit war wiederholt verlängert. Hinzu kamen oberflächliche und tiefe Vasculitiden. Nach vorübergehender Rückbildung liegt der Kranke heute wieder mit dem gleichen Befund in der Klinik und von anderer Seite wurde ernstlich die Frage der Amputation erwogen.

Methoden zur Untersuchung zirkulatorischer Störungen der Beine

H. STORCK und E. STREHLER, Dermatologische Universitätsklinik Zürich (Schweiz)

Dermatologen, Internisten und Chirurgen interessieren sich zunehmend wegen steigender Häufigkeit der Gefäßkrankheiten für Prüfungsmethoden der Zirkulation der Beine. Wenn früher bei Dermatologen das venöse System überwertet wurde, wird heute vermehrt die Zirkulation als Ganzes betrachtet in ihrer Abhängigkeit von Herz, Aorta, Capillaren und Venen.

Wie überall in der modernen Medizin, ergänzen apparative Untersuchungsmethoden die auch in der Kreislaufpraxis immer noch fundamentalen unmittelbaren diagnostischen Maßnahmen des Beobachtens, Tastens, Fragens, Wissens und Denkens, die heute bereits in der Propaedeutik gelehrt werden. Die zur Verfügung stehenden apparativen zusätzlichen Methoden sind mehr oder weniger anspruchsvoll und ermöglichen zum Teil fortlaufende Registration. In der klinischen Dermatologie ist zweifellos den unblutigen Methoden der Vorzug zu geben.

1. Das arterielle Drucksystem

Ausgezeichnete Orientierung über Zustand und Funktion der großen und kleinen Arterien geben die durch Elektronenverstärker verbesserten und fortlaufend registrierenden physikalischen Methoden wie *Oscillographie, Plethysmographie,* und *Rheographie.* Messungen an den Zehen lassen als Suchmethode die Zirkulation des ganzen Beines beurteilen. Simultane Pulsregistrierungen an Zehen, Leisten und Carotis ermöglichen eine einwandfreie Form- und Zeitanalyse des zentralen und peripheren Pulses und damit Beurteilung individueller Besonderheiten des arteriellen Drucksystems. Die drei Methoden messen jedoch nicht genau dieselbe Funktion. Das Oszillogramm gibt Volumen- und Druckänderungen an und ist durch den äußeren Gegendruck verzögert und gedämpft. Das Photoplethysmogramm mißt Änderungen der Lichtdurchlässigkeit, die hauptsächlich durch Druck- und Volumenveränderungen und die Einstellung des Strömungswiderstandes bedingt sind. Das Rheogramm registriert Veränderungen der elektrischen Leitfähigkeit, die wahrscheinlich teils Volumenänderungen, teils aber auch Änderungen der Strömungsgeschwindigkeit widerspiegeln. Je nach der Kurvenform sagen sie aus, ob die pulsatorische Gefäßfunktion normal ist mit kurzer Anstiegszeit zum Gipfel und Vorhandensein der Dikrotie. Sklerose bringt kurze Anstiegszeit, fehlende Dikrotie, mit absteigendem Schenkel gegen oben konkav. Stenose erzeugt verlängerte Anstiegszeit, fehlende Dikrotie, gegen oben konvexen Abstieg. Völliger Verschluß mit Durchblutung via Kollateralen zeigt Kriechpuls oder vollständiges Fehlen der Ausschläge. Sämtliche Methoden geben nur qualitative, keine quantitativen Resultate, außer wenn sie mit Calorimetrie oder Verschlußplethysmographie kombiniert werden. Durch Erwärmung und Abkühlung läßt sich die Reagibilität der Gefäße beurteilen sowie auch unterscheiden, ob organische oder funktionelle Störungen vorliegen. Wir benützen an der Zürcher Klinik das Registriergerät nach VÖLKER-MATTHES, mit welchem die verschiedensten Kreislaufgrößen simultan registrierbar sind mit interessanten Aufschlüssen im Hinblick auf Praxis und Forschung. Für die Praxis genügen auch einfachere Geräte.

Die *Thermometrie* wurde technisch verbessert und erlaubt, Hauttemperaturen an mehreren Stellen gleichzeitig zu registrieren. Besonders aufschlußreich ist die Abtastung von oben nach unten zwecks Entdeckung von Temperaturstufen bei Verschlüssen oder Veränderungen nach medikamentöser Vasodilatation sowie nach kalten oder warmen Wasserbädern. Die Hauttemperatur reagiert aber träge auf die Umgebungstemperatur und innere Zirkulationsumstellungen. Bei umschriebenen Meßpunkten ist sie überdies von Zufälligkeiten abhängig, indem die Haut ein außerordentlich komplexes Temperaturmuster darbietet, wie die neuen Ergebnisse der Thermographie mittels flüssiger Kristalle zeigen. Die moderne Thermographie mittels besonderer Apparaturen vermittelt einen guten Überblick über Insuffizienz oder Vermehrung der Durchblutung. Die Thermographie mittels Cholesterinkristallen in flüssiger Phase mit temperaturabhängiger Farbreflexion verspricht eine wertvolle Methode zum Studium unterschiedlicher Durchblutungsmuster der peripheren Zirkulation zu werden.

Absolute Werte der Blutströmung pro Zeiteinheit und Gewebsmasse können indessen nur mit neueren, eichbaren, quantitativen, aber auch anspruchsvolleren Methoden gewonnen werden. Zu erwähnen sind hier die Verschluß- oder Segmentplethysmographie mit ihren zahlreichen Verbesserungen mittels elektronischer Verstärkung; ferner die Methoden, welche mit Verdünnung exogen zugeführter Faktoren arbeiten, z. B. Radioisotope, Farbstoffe, Kälte und Wärme wie Wärmeleitzahl, Calorimetrie. Oder schließlich Reflexion von eingestrahlter Energie, z. B. Ultraschallwellen zur unblutigen Messung der Blutströmungsgeschwindigkeit nach RUSHMER.

Den genauesten Überblick über die anatomischen Verhältnisse gibt die röntgenologische Angiographie. Es kommt die abdominale Aortographie in Frage zur Darstellung der Aorta, der A. iliaca und ihrer Seitenäste sowie die Arteriographie der Beine, mit Injektion des Kontrastmittels über dem Leistenband. Die rasch sich entwickelnde korrektive Gefäßchirurgie ist ohne diese, die anatomischen Defekte klar darstellenden Hilfsmittel nicht denkbar. Die Serienangiographie und die neueste Angiokinematographie gestatten heute zudem eine Beurteilung der Funktion. Solche Methoden wurden von WELLAUER u. Mitarb. entwickelt. Durch gleichzeitige Messungen von Kontrastmittelverdünnungen an zwei verschiedenen Stellen eines Gefäßes mittels der *Cinédensitometrie* oder der *Videodensitometrie* läßt sich der Durchfluß Q durch das betroffene Gefäß errechnen.

2. *Mikrozirkulation*

Die Methoden zur Beurteilung der qualitativen und quantitativen Verhältnisse der Mikrozirkulation in vivo an irgendeiner Stelle der Haut sind noch wenig entwickelt. Die direkteste Methode ist die Capillarmikroskopie, die aber nur an ausgewählten Stellen, wie Nagelfalz, Conjunctiven usw., größere Strecken der Capillaren verfolgen läßt.

Außer der bekannten histologischen Untersuchungsmethode bleiben für die Beurteilung der Capillarströmung, Brüchigkeit und Durchlässigkeit der Gefäße beim Menschen einige wenige Methoden, die teils auch die Verhältnisse der größeren Gefäße miterfassen. Es sind dies Temperaturmessung, Wärmeleitzahl, Farbverdünnung, Verteilung von fluorescierenden und radioaktiven Stoffen, Reflexplethysmographie, Stauungs- oder Saugglockenversuche.

3. *Das Venensystem*

Die Untersuchung der Venolen und Venen am Bein läßt sich durch die bekannten Teste nach TRENDELENBURG, PERTHES u. a. bezüglich Insuffizienz oberflächlicher, tiefer und kommunizierender Venen bewerkstelligen. Mit der einfachen Infrarotaufnahme stellen sich auch tiefere Venengeflechte als blaues Netz dar. Die Bilder erlauben eine Unterscheidung der arteriellen bräunlichen von den venösen bläulich gefärbten Gefäßen. Dieser Farbunterschied läßt sich in vitro am sauerstoff- oder kohlensäuregesättigten Blut, in vivo am Kaninchenohr oder an den beiden Herzhälften des Meerschweinchens beweisen.

Die exaktesten Aufschlüsse über Anatomie und Funktion der Venen ergibt zweifellos die Phlebographie, die am besten in zwei Phasen durchgeführt wird, nämlich erstens als retrograde Preßphlebographie, und zweitens als anterograde Phlebographie. Für besondere hämodynamische Fragestellungen lassen sich mit geeichten Wasserbehältern oder mit der modernen Segmentplethysmographie Volumen- und Druckmessungen an willkürlich gewählten Venenbezirken des Beines durchführen. Die moderne Elektronik erlaubt auch hier empfindliche, kontinuierliche Registrierungen. Speziell Venentonus und Venenmotorik finden neuerdings vermehrt Beachtung.

4. *Das Lymphsystem*

Die moderne Lymphographie ist ein zusätzliches wichtiges Hilfsmittel für die Beurteilung der Zirkulationsverhältnisse. Ohne diese sind primäre und sekundäre Störungen des Lymphsystems nicht sicher beurteilbar.

Auf Grund der Zürcher Erfahrungen möchten wir *zusammenfassend* folgendes sagen:

Die klinische Untersuchung mit einfachen Methoden läßt ein orientierendes Urteil zu über den Zustand von Herz, Arterien, Capillaren und Venen.

Mittels einfacher, unblutiger physikalischer Untersuchungen, wie Photo-plethysmographie, Oszillographie oder Rheographie, läßt sich der Zustand des arteriellen Systems bezüglich Sklerose, Stenose, Verschluß grob beurteilen. Besonders wertvolle Aufschlüsse geben auch Temperatur- und Druckabfall gegen die Peripherie.

Für genaue anatomische Beurteilung ist arterio- und Venographie, eventuell Lymphographie unumgänglich, wobei Serienangiographie oder die neu entwickelte Angiokinematographie in ausgewählten Fällen zusätzlich funktionelle Aussagen erlauben.

Absolute Durchblutungswerte werden mit Verschlußplethysmographie oder Segmentplethysmographie gewonnen. Absolute oder relative Blutströmungs-Meßdaten für wissenschaftliche Fragestellungen ergeben neuere Strömungsmesser auf Grund von Verteilung eingestrahlter Energie wie Wärme, Ultraschall oder Verdünnung von Farbstoffen sowie radioaktiver Isotopen. Thermographie erlaubt eine rasche Gesamtorientierung.

Arterial Reconstruction in Cutaneous Ischaemic Lesions

G. E. MAVOR and J. M. D. GALLOWAY, Aberdeen Royal Infirmary (Scotland)

Ischaemic lesions of the skin are of two types namely ischaemic ulceration and gangrene, the former often representing an earlier stage of the ischaemic process, with gangrene supervening later. In other cases gangrene of a greater or lesser extent develops without preceding ulceration.

Ischaemic ulceration results from deficient arterial circulation of the limb, continuity of the skin being broken spontaneously or as the result of trauma or infection. The underlying obliterative arterial disease is most frequently athero-sclerosis which is not uncommonly complicated by diabetes. In the younger age groups the cause is more frequently thromboangiitis obliterans. In contrast to venous ulcers the toes and heels and anterior surface of the tibia are the sites of predilection. Generally speaking the ulceration is peripheral and other manifestations of ischaemia, such as colour changes, coldness, intermittent claudication and absent arterial pulsation are in evidence. Rest pain is a frequent accompaniment and the two forewarn the onset of gangrene.

Gangrene

The classical pathological definition of gangrene is massive necrosis of tissue. LEARMONTH (1950) has stated that "the important feature of gangrenous tissue is that it is dead and therefore useless for there are no degrees of deadness". While both these statements are true they are none-the-less misleading. By the phrase 'massive necrosis' is meant macroscopic necrosis as opposed to microscopic necrosis, i.e. that an actual area of dead tissue is visible. However, this dead tissue may only involve the surface, namely the skin, and the deeper tissues have an adequate capillary bed, capable of allowing an adequate blood flow with sufficient gaseous and metabolic exchange for survival of the part, in the event of the causative lesion being corrected. This is obviously of fundamental importance and renders obsolete such statements as "once gangrene is established amputation in some form is inevitable". This accounts for the apparent reversibility of gangrene in some cases. The fact that gangrene does not inevitably mean amputation and the possibilities for limb salvage which are opened up in this way makes an accurate diagnosis of the cause of the gangrene essential. The causes of gangrene can be considered in three major groups (LEARMONTH):

1. Lesions of the efferent pathways — Arterial Disease.
2. Lesions of the afferent pathways — Venous Disease.
3. Lesions of the effective apparatus — Diseases of the Capillary Bed.

Table 1. *Causes of Gangrene of the Lower Limbs in 145 Patients*

Arterial		
Atherosclerosis with thrombosis		125
Main vessel occlusions	90	
Small vessel occlusions	11	
Main and small vessels occlusions	24	
Thromboangiitis obliterans		12
Embolism		6
Arterial Injury		4
Others		12
Venous		4

The relative frequence and the common forms of these diseases are shown in Tab. 1. It is apparent from this that narrowing or obliteration of the major arteries of the limb by atherosclerosis is the major cause of gangrene, accounting for about 70% of cases. Of these about 80% are suitable for some form of arterial reconstruction.

Clinical Patterns

The pattern of ulceration will serve to distinguish ischaemic lesions from other common causes of ulceration of the lower limb, notably venous ulceration. The type and distribution of gangrenous areas helps to distinguish the nature and site of the underlying pathology. Venous gangrene is usually extensive involving foot and leg and develops on a congested cyanosed limb, peripheral arterial pulses frequently being palpable. In gangrene due to arterial insufficiency the great toe is the most frequently and most severely affected in major arterial involvement in contrast to gangrene developing as a result of digital vessel thrombosis where the 4th and 5th toes are more often involved.

Arteriography

If the full potentialities for arterial reconstruction are to be realised it is essential that arteriography be employed routinely in the investigation of all cases of ischaemic ulceration and gangrene. No patient is too infirm to undergo this investigation. If a patient is fit enough to undergo major amputation, no matter how expeditiously it be performed, he is equally fit to undergo arteriography plus arterial reconstruction. The decision for or against arterial reconstruction remains a clinical one and can only be reached on the basis of a knowledge of the patient's condition as a whole, including his mental state. It cannot be decided, however, in the absence of the precise information which arteriography provides.

Segmental Involvement and Reconstruction

The segmental characteristics of atherosclerosis allow reconstructive surgery, and it is only with a knowledge of the natural history of the disease as it involves a given segment that the need for arterial reconstruction can be assessed.

Aorto-iliac Segment

Direct arterial surgery is reserved for the advanced case with severe narrowing. Although lesions at this level generally produce intermittent claudication without cutaneous ischaemia, ulceration and gangrene may result. Thrombo-endarterectomy is the operation of choice and in vessels of this size good results can be expected. Thus COCKETT (1956) reported that out of 37 aorto-iliac rebores only two showed late rethrombosis over a period from 9 months to 6 years.

Femoro-popliteal Segment

The nature and the extent of involvement of this segment as visualised by arteriography determines the type of arterial reconstruction which should be undertaken.

Vein Patch Graft

In the early stages of atherosclerotic involvement with either a stenosis, a short segment of narrowing, or a limited thrombosis, the whole involved segment being no more than 2.5 to 4 cm, autogenous vein patch grafting coupled with thrombo-intimectomy is a theoretically sound procedure. This procedure has proved successful in our hands, and thrombosis rate is low, only seven out of 51 cases. Theoretical risks of aneurysm formation are not confirmed, only occurring once in the 51 cases and this in a graft which was inserted under inadequate tension and where sepsis supervened in the early post-operative period. Less commonly vein patch grafts are employed in the treatment of more advanced disease. In such cases long patches up to 6 to 7 cm have been used and double patches have been used on three occasions. Here thrombosis is more common but it should be recognised that the aim of surgery in such cases is limited to improving an already poor outlook. Success in the use of vein patch grafting depends on accurate localisation of the lesion by operative arteriography, meticulous suture technique, with the vein being kept under adequate tension in both longitudinal and transverse directions.

Long Autogenous Vein Femoro-Popliteal Bypass

There is now general agreement that the long femoro-popliteal vein bypass is the surgical method of choice in the treatment of occlusion in the femoro-popliteal segment irrespective of the length of main vessel thrombosis. These grafts are from the common femoral to the popliteal arteries as far distally as possible. Such a procedure is feasible provided the popliteal artery is patent. An artery of small calibre or a poor run off are not contraindications to exploration. In such circumstances the popliteal artery is explored at the outset and if patent with even one small run of, a bypass graft is inserted. The improvement in the size of the popliteal artery and its branches at follow-up arteriography is often striking. Long term patency is to be expected with such grafts and the death rate is not so high as might be expected (Tab. 2). Malignant disease and coronary thrombosis are the common causes of death.

Table 2. *Autogenous vein Bypass 1959 to 1965* (For Advanced Femoro-Popliteal Disease)

Years	1959	1960	1961	1962	1963	1964	1965
Numbers	3	12	10	6	5	5	6
Deaths	0	2	0	2	1	0	0
Grafts thrombosed	0	2	3	3	0	0	0
Total	48 bypasses						
	5 deaths (3 grafts patent)						
	8 thrombosed (2 deaths)						

Arterial Homografts

Because of the success attending the use of autogenous vein bypass grafts arterial homografts have been reserved for the few cases where the saphenous vein is absent (as following surgery), grossly diseased, or where the patient's general condition would not permit a lengthy procedure.

Profunda Exploration

Where the profunda femoris is stenosed or where it is thrombosed in the presence of severe ischaemia, and where bypass grafting is not feasible, direct surgery to the profunda in the form of endarterectomy combined with vein patch grafting has been introduced, in an attempt to improve the collateral circulation. In a number of cases it has been possible to avoid major amputation by this means. This operation has been used where the popliteal artery has been so narrow or completely thrombosed, making a vein bypass graft impossible. Under such circumstances it must be appreciated that the outlook is limited.

Follow-up Arteriography

Follow-up arteriography is essential if the value of a reconstructive procedure is too determined, for clinical assessment is often inaccurate. Thus two patients whose long vein bypass grafts had functioned well for 1 and 3 years, reported with severe recurrence of symptoms. Clinical assessment would have classified this as graft thrombosis and a failure of reconstructive surgery. Arteriography revealed that severe stenosis of the common femoral artery proximal to the anastomosis was the causative lesion, the grafts being patent. Vein patch graft reconstruction was successful in both cases. Similarly we have seen arterial occlusion following a vein patch graft where arteriography has revealed that thrombosis resulted from progress of the disease in another area, the patched segment remaining patent.

Medical Treatment of Cutaneous Disorders of Vascular Origin

CL. HURIEZ and F. DESMONS, Clinique Universitaire de Lille (France)

Here we will describe the medical treatment of cutaneous disorders of vascular origin *(in which represent 18% of the 1800 patients in hospital in our department each year)*. It is based on the experience of more than 3000 ulcers, 1000 hypodermatitis, cutaneous lesions which remain of about 500 phlebitis and more than 200 elephantiasis.

In 25 years, we have shown the important role played by infection which is either secondary or primitive *(in the dermoepidermatitis or hypodermatitis even in superficial phlebitis)*.

1. The first common and indispensible period of the treatment will therefore be anti-infectious.

2. With ulcers, the second will be the stimulation of cicatrisation. With hypodermatitis, the struggle against the inflammatory element.

3. In any case, for all of them, *the correction of general metabolic disorders*.

4. And above all, so as to avoid a recurrence, the treatment of venous hypertension, post varicose, post phlebitic or of arterial insufficiency,

I. The Liquidation of the Infectious Factor

is assured by a local desinfection and by general antibiotics.

1. For the first we still use the *classical antiseptics:*

a) bactericidal solutions of potassium permanganate, methylene blue or eosine. Then, if there is no more eczema, an alcoholic solution of Milian violet or Dakin liquid. If there is excessive infection by the pyocyaneus bacillus, treatment with acetic acid or boracic acid at 2%;

b) amongst modern antiseptics, hexomedin is less sensitizing than mercurial solutions or quaternary ammoniums, of which we have shown the group sensitizing risks;

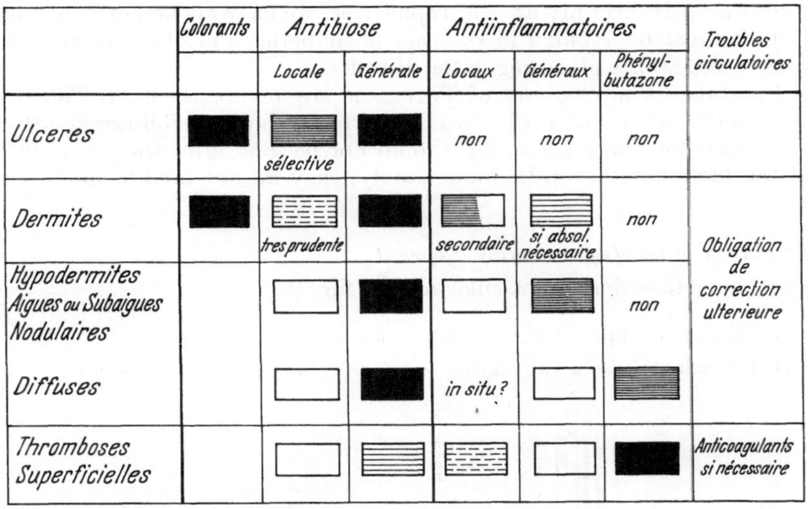

	Colorants	Antibiose		Antiinflammatoires			Troubles circulatoires
		Locale	Générale	Locaux	Généraux	Phényl-butazone	
Ulceres	■	▨ sélective	■	non	non	non	
Dermites	■	▨ tres prudente	■	◨ secondaire	▤ si absol. nécessaire	non	Obligation de correction ulterieure
Hypodermites Aigues ou Subaigues Nodulaires		□	■	□	▤	non	
Diffuses		□	■	in situ?	□	▤	
Thromboses Superficielles		□	▤	▤	□	■	Anticoagulants si nécessaire

Fig. 1

c) *local antibiotics* are effective but provide a risk of sensitization which makes us advise against those likely to be used in a general way (that is penicillin, tetracycline, chloramphenicol). Because of this we prefer to use framycetine and neomycine, polymyxine is expensive but must be used if there is the pyocyaneous bacillus;

2. *General antibiotics* are indispensable for us, in adequate doses, and must be given for 6 to 8 weeks in the case of long term ulcers. It can be shorter but just as useful in out-patients. The choice of antibiotics is at times guided by the antibiogram, above all after the sample taken by the peripheral puncture according to Thivolet technique.

Penicillin cannot be given without one first having assured that the patient has not already received nose or drops or penicillin ointment if some previous cure has not been tolerated, penicillin antibiotics will be search for derivatives of tetracycline are the most often used. In case of previous application of ointments containing these antibiotics, we prefer erythromycine or thiophenicol, which does not destroy the white globules as does chloramphenicol, when was without question the most active body.

II. Stimulation of Cicatrisation

only occurs after 10 to 15 days of treatment with antibiotics: the detersion of the superficial membrane is quickered by a mixture of alpha chymotrypsine and framycetine and then by a dry "tulle" with this antibiotic. A mixture of ester of malic, benzoic and salicylic acids was very stimulating, but this preparation (which is acerbine) offers a risk of sensitization of 8% to 10%, due to the propylene glycol which many of these preparations contain.

We have remained faithful to the application of compresses soaked by a solution of extract of digitalis. 200 units to the litre (DELMOTTE, HURIEZ, DESMONS), followed subsequently by applications of gelatine (Gelfloam spongel method), left in place for 4 to 5 days. This does not have the inconvenience of Burgraffs plasters which are too occlusive.

Placental implants (and not amniotic ones, injections being useless and ointments harmful) according to Filatof's technique, 5 to 8 times every fortnight with perfect asepsis certainly have a trophic role, we have spoken of biostimulines: in fact these must be avoided in the case of diabetics and obese people, as they determine or aggravate glyco regulator disorders.

The "postage stamp" *grafts* of THIERSCH are no longer used. The Brussels school uses them again. The antibiotic cover extends their possibilities greatly large, grafts, or pediculous ones (cross leg) should not be used after the age of 60 as, in spite of the fact that they take immediately, they do not hold in nine cases out of ten.

III. Treatment of the Inflammation Element

of cutaneous disorders of vascular origin (Fig. 2).

I. Hémodynamique = hypertension veineuse

II. Inflammatoire = la vascularite   *Progressive thrombosante*

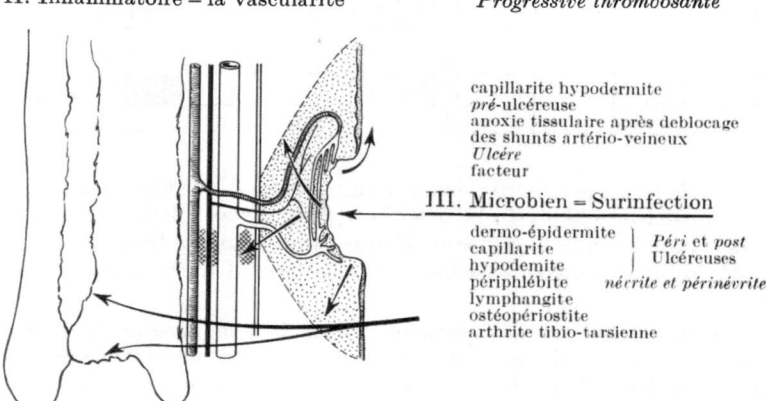

capillarite hypodermite
pré-ulcéreuse
anoxie tissulaire après deblocage
des shunts artério-veineux
Ulcére
facteur

III. Microbien = Surinfection

dermo-épidermite | *Péri* et *post*
capillarite | Ulcéreuses
hypodemite
périphlébite   *nécrite et périnévrite*
lymphangite
ostéopériostite
arthrite tibio-tarsienne

Fig. 2. Facteurs des douleurs dans les ulcéres d'origine veineuse

1. varicose eczemas are microbic ones. They obey the first phase of the treatment and at times necessitate corticoidal treatment, but only after liquidation of excessive infection;

2. peri-ulcerous eczemas benefit from the same treatment, but most often they succeed untimely sensitizing ointments — either —

antipruritic: antihistamine creams, notably with phenergan, the production of which has had to be suppressed for 20 years,

antialgetic-ointments containing derivatives of procaine *(containing just about the same risk of sensitization)*,

bacteriostatic-sulphonamides or antibiotics,

bactericidal-quaternary ammoniums, determining a group reaction, but also because of the benzoin contained in certain ointments,

stimulants which are too irritating,

corticoidal ointments used before liquidation of the infection, are likely to diffuse it gradually or in the form of secondary distant lesions.

Ulcerous eczema is the ideal trap into which practitioners can fall, and do what should not be done.

3. the subacute hypodermatitis benefits from rest and antibiotics. Big doses of vitamine C (injection of 10000 units daily for a month, if the maximum blood pressure is less than 17, then 2000 units daily for a month, then 1 g orally every day). If necessary suppositories of 250 mg of phenylbutazone can be used, twice a day for 2 to 3 weeks;

4. this same treatment can also be used for superficial thrombosis which generally does not need a treatment of anticoagulants as does deep phlebitis.

IV. Treatment of the Vascular Lesion

1. *venous hypertension* necessitates.

a) a long rest with the lower limbs raised for 1 to 2 weeks in the case of painful ulcers and hypodermatitis because they are very inflamed. As soon as the pain has be relieved, the ambulatory method is to be advised, but with means of contention: either the usual boots with Unna paste, the adhesive elastic plaster, or above all, the elastic bandage, which has an advantage over the elastic stocking (more aesthetic), that it can be readjusted to the size of the leg after a rest during the course of the day;

b) this contention is beneficial for all those with venous insufficiency. It is the only remedy for the "hopeless" cases (10%, very old patients with cardio-renal insufficiency). In the case of post-phlebitic patients with venous hypertension, it must be very slight. There is no treatment for superficial varicose veins, if it is not sure that the deep circulation is repermeabilized clinically or if necessary after phlebography. We have become very miserly about this, when the radiologist risks creating a supplementary ulcer. Associating an ascending phlebography with the flow of the current, and a retrograde phlebography, it is possible to see at times an obliteration of 10 to 25 cm. It is at times often to resect it, cause of rebel pains.

Venous hypertension of those with varicose veins, in normal deep circulation should be treated more actively. *The opposition of the sclerosis and stripping is the type of false problem which arises.*

c) *stripping after crossectomy* (of which surgeons speak) is suitable for large varicose veins at the failure of the valve of the arch of the internal saphenous vein and for varicose veins, whose course is rectilineal. The instrument for stripping should come out on heathly skin: if possible above the internal malleolus, otherwise higher up, below the knee;

d) on the other hand, if there is no incontinence of the ostial valve, if the varicose veins are of moderate size, or if they do not appear well systemized, then the *sclerosis* keeps all its indications. The quality of the results comes from a methodical progressive technique, whether from high to low, or from low to high, with daily injections. The French use more and more often sodium tetradecylsulfate, at 1% then 2% which is much less inconvenient than Urea Quinine. In any case, stripping only solves 60% to 75% of the cases of venous hypertension. Even if the patient is greatly relieved it is indispensable to harden scrupulously all distal or aberrant varicose veins. At the Congress of Phlebology at Aix la Chapelle we underlined that immediate results of all methods were good at the end of the first year, but were burdened with 20% to 30% less good results at the end of the

A   Traitement de fond des Arterites par Surcharge

I
Lutte contre l'athérome
Hygiène de vie — Pas de tabac
Régime hypolipidé
Lipotropes = Choline — Facteur lipocaic
Lipoconverseurs — Héparine
Hypocholestérolémiants
Coenzyme A   Stigmasterol

II
Traitement de l'insuffisance artérielle
Balneothérapie chaude
Vasodilatateurs = Ganglioplegiques — der methonium
Parasympathicomimétiques = Acetylcholine — Dilvasene
Sympatholytiques = Hydergine — Benzyl — Imidazoline
Musculotropes = Vasodil. actifs = Ronicol. Padutine-kalleone
Méthode electropneumatique = Syncardon
Cures hydrominérales = Royat — Bains carbogazeux

III
Lutte contre un diabète éventuel
Reduction hydrocarbonée
Insuline ou
Sulfamides hypoglycémiants

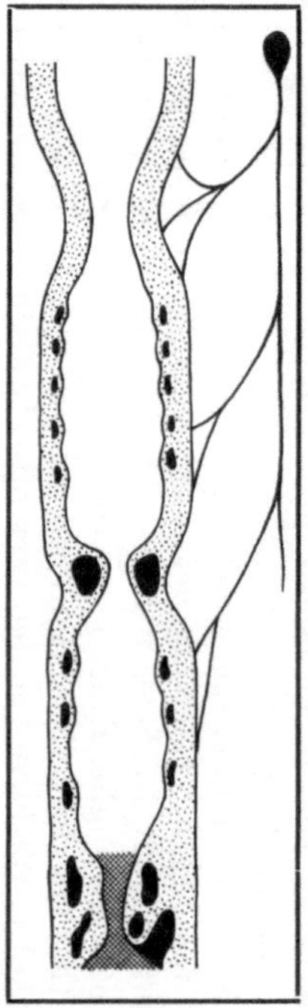

B   Traitement des Poussées Evolutives

I
Interventions hyperhemiantes
Contre le spasme

Cocaïne   *Sympathectomie*
Perifémorale   Perifémorale
Intrafémorale   ou
ou lombaire   lombaire
                           Surrenalectomie
Diathermie   Chaleur

Artériographies limitées aux cas chirurgicaux

II
Contre l'obstruction artérielle
Traitement anticoagulant (continu ?)
Heparine — Coumarine
Opérations restauratrices
Décortication bifurcation aortique
Artériectomie — Greffes limitées à des cas sélectionnes
By pass — Pontages fémoropoplites
avec opérations hyperhémiantes complémentaires

III
Contre la gangrène
Facteur Infectieux   = Antiseptiques de surface
                         Antibiose générale
Facteur Douleur   = Glace
                         Implant ultérieur
Amputation parfois encore nécessaire mais
le plus souvent retardée

Fig. 3. *Nécessité d'un Diagnostic Précoce et d'une Collaboration Medico. Radio. Chirurgicale*

second, 30% to 45% at the end of the third, if the patient does not receive, one month after the operation, all the complementary injections, which he needs at the reappearance of the slightest varicose vein;

e) thermal cures make those of our colleagues smile who come from countries where there are no springs with a great mineral content. French sufferers of venous hypertension know what a useful complement are the cures at Bagnoles de l'Orne, Aix en Provence, la Léchère or Barbotan.

2. *Diagram three* will suffice to class the justified action against *arterial insufficiency*; either this is incomplete with predominance of spasms or the obliteration has become complete, on a trunk, which is more or less important. Against the spasm, one has recourse moreso to lumbar infiltrations of Xylocaine without adrenalin, than to intra-arterial injections. One must not hesitate to consult the surgeon to realize direct action on the sympathetic nerve, when necessary. The taking of papaverin is always useful, and in my opinion is better than all the other medications, which above all have pretty names such as ,,sympathicolytiques, parasympathiconimétiques or vasculotropes". The thermal cures at Royat and also at Bains les Bains are not altogether without use. The *electropneumatic method* of the Syncardon has never been followed by disobstruction of the arteries, but it develops collateral circulation in a very beneficial way. Its association with lumbar infiltrations of the sympathetic nerve, with placental implants (which attenuate the pains of those suffering from arteritis) with the previous liquidation of infection by general antibiotherapy: here is a therapeutical method of which each isolated element is insufficient, but whose *methodical association has reduced by half the number of amputations for arterial ulcers during the last 10 years.*

3. Finally, the cutaneous consequences of *lymphatic involvement* can frequently be translated by dermatitis; sometimes current, sometimes verrucose, even in the type of vegetant pyodermatitis on the surface of elephantiasis. Be they of venous, lymphangitic or congenital origin, these lymphoedema are justiciable to a therapeutical method as follows.

a) A preparation by rest with raising of the lower limb, a dechlorinated diet and general antibiotics;

b) an elastic reduction by rolling a rubber tube from the tip of the toes to the thigh (van der Molen's method). This is only contra-indicated in elephantiasis after ganglionic blockage by radiotherapy or ganglionic curage after carcinoma of the external genital organs;

c) an elastic contention of the result is indispensable by elastic stockings, after many measurements at different levels.

V. Finally the treatment must include that *of general diseases which are associated* — correcting a diabetic, a strict diet for the overweight, hypolipidic diet for those with arteritis, which with only have prophylactic value when observed 20 years before the expiration of the atheroma, at times compensation of protidic defiency, following loss by the way of a long term ulcer. We shall not speak of *spleenectomy*, because of the rarity of spleenomegalic ulcers (less than 1 in 2000). These are the first truths; their justification is found, however, in the preliminary sentence of the report of ENJALBERT at the French Congress of Surgery in 1959. It is in the dermatological conception of the treatment of leg ulcers, that one must find the explanation for the absence of progress in the therapeutical methods of this disease.

I felt that this statement was an important offence to our speciality and it has been easy for me to show it, in an environment where I was at ease as former general teacher, and because for a quarter of a century, I have been a permanent advocate of the great cooperation between dermatologists and surgeons.

Leg ulcers, for a long time looked after by quacks, now interest phlebologists, radiologists and surgeons, to too great an extent. They have for a long time more or less interested dermatologists — and very often "less" than "more". The number of these in England is around 250 000 im a country of 50 million people.

Dermato-venerology had acquired a great consideration by the public powers, above all because of its efficacious struggle against venereal diseases, which had nothing verified nor entrancing about them. Our speciality does not lower, itself by not looking after a disease which is indeed commonplace, but which causes repercussions on the capacity of work of an individual, at times during decades and also on the national Budget, more than diseases, considered until now as social scourges. Exceptional diseases captivate us, and at times are even our diversion. To treat commonplace diseases, but above all, to treat them effectively, remains the duty of every doctor, even if he is a specialist.

Surgical Treatment of Venous Ulcers and Eczema of the Leg

K. Hæger, Malmö Allmänna Sjukhus (Sweden)

The terms venous ulcer and venous eczema have many synonyms, as for example stasis ulcer and eczema, hypostatic ulcer and eczema, simply leg ulcer and, unfortunately, also varicose ulcer and eczema. I would like to start with a short recapitulation of the anatomy and physiology of the veins in the leg: first in order to demonstrate the background to our method of treatment, and, secondly, to show that the term varicose ulcer or eczema is completely wrong and, in addition, also may lead to therapeutical errors.

The anatomy of the veins in the leg is demonstrated. You find that there are three different systems: the deep system represented by the three deep veins in the leg running together in the popliteal vein and the femoral vein; the superficial veins represented by the long and short saphenous veins, and the perforator system, which forms communications between the superficial and the deep venous systems.

Nobody knows if the mechanism for the development of an ulcer or an eczema is exactly the same. Probably there must be some reason why some people develop ulcers without any eczematous reaction, others get ulcer and eczema and still others get only eczema without ulcerations. As far as we know the difference cannot in all cases be attributed to allergy: there are allergic patients among all three categories.

The basic mechanism, however, is the same. The reason for both ulcers and eczema is an elevation of the tissue pressure in the skin and the subcutaneous layer. This high pressure is due to defectiveness in the valvular apparatus of the veins, particularly in the perforating veins. Normally the blood runs from the superficial system into the deep system via the perforators which all have valves. If this valvular mechanism is faulty the blood runs in the other direction and the high pressure from the deep veins is mediated to the skin, causing skin atrophy, edema and finally leg ulcers and/or eczema. Particularly severe high pressure is caused by those with defects also in the valves of the deep system, as is caused by, for instance, deep thrombosis of the leg.

In separate investigations from Sweden made by Arnoldi in Umeå and by myself we were able to prove with phlebography in all cases that there was a perforator incompetence in 100% of all cases with leg ulcers. Moreover, if this was eliminated by surgical operation, the rate of ulcer recurrences dramatically decreased. I shall come back to this later.

In cases of eczema also the perforators seem to play a decisive role. We were able to classify the eczema of the leg in four different types according to the localization. And when we compared these areas we found that they corresponded very well with the anatomical sites of perforator veins. We have found perforator incompetence in almost all cases of eczema too, but in this case there might be some doubt that plain superficial varices sometimes may be of pathogenetic interest. But I repeat that varicose veins, i. e. phlebectasies in the superficial veins, have nothing to do with the development of leg ulcers: hence the term varicose ulcer is wrong. At least in my country many patients have been operated upon, or subjected to sclerotherapy, for their varices on the indication that this should be of benefit for the ulcer. Follow-up investigations of these patients have shown, naturally, that there was no effect on the ulcers whatsoever.

To conclude: Leg ulcers and leg eczema are never, I repeat never, diseases sui generis — they are always symptoms of another disease. In 90% of the cases this disease is venous incompetence, and in 100% of these cases there is perforator insufficiency.

Then — what is the logical thing to do ? There is only one answer: eliminate the high venous pressure causing the ulcer or the eczema. And this is easily done by ligature of the perforators. Naturally many of these patients also have varicose veins and at the operation this disease should also be cured.

As you are well aware of the condition of the skin of these patients is very often not particularly tempting for a surgeon to deal with. Our rule is therefore to first heal the ulcer and the eczema by conservative means and then proceed with operation. There are many models of this preoperative treatments and I shall only present our standard method.

However, I would like to stress a few points. The most important in the preoperative treatment is an adequate compression, made by a very good elastic bandage and rubber foam. This compression must be just a little higher than the hypostatic pressure in the tissues, which causes the ulcer. It has been calculated that this pressure in most of the cases lies somewhere around 90 to 100 mm Hg — consequently the bandage should cause a pressure of at least that size. The pressure will be very different if the bandage is a good or bad one, or if it is applied by somebody who knows to deal with it or not. Another thing, which we in comparable series have found to be of distinct value is the administration of diuretics, which have been shown to decrease the healing time by combatting the edema. Edema should not be permitted in these cases: it compresses the small nutritive arteries which are so important for the course of healing.

Now, then —which are our results by this combined conservative and operative treatment ?

By the conservative treatment we have been able to heal 98% of all venous leg ulcers, and with 75% of the patients in their ordinary work. This figure may be thought to be fantastic and exaggerated. Some years ago I mentioned them in a meeting in Las Vegas, at which one dermatologist became so angry that he demonstratively left the audience. But, ladies and gentlemen, I can assure you that they are right. Furthermore: they are based on a material of several hundreds of leg ulcers, and they are corroborated by a material from Umeå in North Sweden, where ARNOLDI got the same results, using exactly the same principles.

Thus we can state, that we can heal almost all leg ulcers. But do they stay healed ? The recurrency rate after 3 to 6 years observation was about 16% in the postthrombotic legs and about 4% in the legs with only perforator incompetence.

We think that this is rather good for a disease which still by many is held to be incurable.

The operation for leg ulcer is rather simple and can be done ambulantly in most cases. Sick leave after operation usually will be about 3 or 4 weeks. Principally the same operation is done for cases with eczema: the difference is only which perforator should be ligated.

Results of operative eczema treatment: In this series we had 56 operated legs, 48 of which stayed free from eczema during an observation period from 1 to 6 years. The greater part of the series was observed more than 4 years.

These results seem rather good but, naturally, no far-reaching conclusions about the value of the operation can be reached from them alone. Let us, however, see what happens to another series. Due to unfortunate circumstances we have not always been able to operate upon these patients as soon as we would have liked to do it, namely as soon as we have got the skin in a favorable condition for surgery. 23 patients had to wait for their operation in 16 months or more. During this time three had one and four had two or more exacerbations of the eczema. During the 18 months following operation the same 23 patients showed only two recurrences! This I think may be taken as proof for the value of operative treatment in cases of eczema.

Crural ulcers and eczema has been called a crux medicorum. I hope to have been able to prove to you that dermatologists and surgeons together can achieve cure in most cases, and not only temporal but perennial healing of these common diseases.

Lymphedema of the Lower Extremities

J. BENINSON, Henry Ford Hospital, Detroit, Michigan (USA)

This report will deal primarily with genetic lymphedema (lymphatic dysplasia) of the lower extremities, some instances of secondary lymphatic obstructive disease of the lower extremities, and a new entity — recurrent acute toxic lymphangitis — at times associated with both of the above. The lymphedema due to leg ulcers will not be discussed here.

To date I have 107 cases of genetic lymphedema. 65 cases have been confirmed by radio-isotopic tracer, venographic and lymphangiographic studies and 42 were diagnosed clinically.

As dermatologists, we should be acquainted with these clinical pictures so that we can either treat or advise these patients.

A clinico-radiologic classification of the lymphedemas was initially suggested by me in 1962 [1] and revised slightly in 1966 [2] see table. Examples of some of these terms and the classification are illustrated by the following slides.

If the patient is willing to tolerate the temporary 2 to 4 months and rarely 6 months discoloration of the Evans blue dye one can readily demonstrate dermal backflow, dermal diffusion or chylous ascites. The subcutaneous injection of 0.25 ccm of the sterilized 0.5% Evans blue dye into the dorsum of the foot at the first and second web spaces between the first three toes using a tuberculin syringe and a 27 gauge needle 1/2 inch long is all that is necessary for this test. If your clinical judgment has been in error, the dye will probably dissipate within 3 to 6 weeks.

Patients who have pure genetic lymphedema of the aplastic type, regardless of their age, do not have lymphatic ectasias ("mossy foot") despite the severity of the condition. Since anatomically these patients lack a superficial lymphatic system, it is axiomatic that patients with superficial lymphatic aplasia never present with the clinical picture of "mossy foot".

Table. *Lymphedema*

Clinical	Radiological[a]
A. Genetic	Any admixture of the following features may be found in any one patient:
1. Lymphangial	1. Aplastic
(a) Milroy's—familial	2. Hypoplastic
(1) Congenital	3. Hyperplastic
(2) Tardive	4. Dermal backflow
(a) Pubertal	5. Chylous reflux
(b) Adult	6. Dermal diffusion
(b) Letessier's non-familial[b]	
(1) Congenital	
(2) Tardive	
(a) Pubertal	
(b) Adult	
2. Lymphangioma—primary	
(a) Simplex	
(b) Cavernous	
(c) Cystic (hygroma)	
3. A-V fistula	
4. Constricting bands	
5. Turner's and Bonnevie-Ullrich Syndromes	
6. Other	
B. Non-genetic	
1. Simple (clears when the artificial cause is relieved)	
2. Neoplastic	
3. Post-inflammatory organisms	
(a) Bacterial	
(b) Trichophytosis	
(c) Filariasis	
(d) Viral (?)	
4. Post-thrombophletibic	
5. Post-surgical	
6. Post-traumatic	
7. Post-paralytic	
8. Post-irradiative	
9. Lymphangioma—secondary	
(a) Simplex	
(b) Cavernous	
(c) Cystic	
10. Lymphangiosarcoma	
11. Neurofibromatosis	
12. Other	

Lymphedema

C. Combined—any admixture of A and B.

  [a] Most of these terms taken from Ref. 3.
  [b] Letessier's: This term for the non-familial type is suggested in honor of the man who recorded the first cases of genetic lymphedema. See Ref. 4.

Conversely, patient with hypoplastic, hyperplastic or normal superficial lymphatic systems can, following secondary factors (see table B — non-genetic), e.g. bacterial or mycotic infection, present with clinical pictures of lymphatic ectatic formations.

Suspecting genetic lymphedema one can check the afflicted extremity. About 15% have an unusually excessive sweating pattern. This usually affects the plantar aspect of the foot and may be present on portions of the dorsum of the foot, the inner leg, and/or inner thigh along the outflow tract of the superficial lymphatic system.

Less frequent features of lymphatic dysplasia are fullness of the right side of the face, below the zygoma; enlargement of the pudenda, particularly on the affected side; and lymphangiomas of the torso or upper extremities.

Congenital bands, in about 3% of the cases, are usually present above the ankle and almost never above the lower half of the leg. These are also seen in occasional instances of the Klippel-Trenaunay syndrome.

The dermatologist can be a very astute clinician if he sees a new-born who at birth or shortly thereafter has the top of one or both feet look like overstuffed pin-cushions. In one family that I am following, the mother's first question of the obstetrician is "Does my baby have 'fat feet'?" These children invariably have aplasia of the superficial lymphatics of the dorsa of their affected feet. Clinically, most of these babies have hypoplastic superficial lymphatics of the legs but a greater number of superficial lymphatics in their thighs. This clinical observation is in part corroborated by the Evans blue dye test. Lymphangiographic proof of these suggested anatomic features has not been pursued in the legs or thighs of these patients. In a Turner's or Bonnevie-Ullrich syndrome, the additional congenital aberrations make that differential unmistakable.

For definitive diagnosis, one must do the complete studies using venography, lymphangiography, and tracers to define the nature of the patient's lymphatic deficiency. Lacking these measures, however, does not mean that such patients cannot be treated. We have conducted these studies primarily to try to visualize the lymphatics, hoping that eventually a lymphatico-venous surgical by-pass could be accomplished. Reference to this work is cited in the bibliography [1, 2].

Obviously, the clinician is on firmer ground when he can substantiate his diagnosis prior to instituting therapy. Most of our patients have had correlated studies to corroborate the clinical diagnosis and then have undergone intermittent compression therapy [3] to decompress their affected limbs. Thereafter they were fitted with the appropriate pressure-gradient support [3] to control the degree of gravitational deficit present when they were up and about.

Over the past 14 years I have used pressure-gradient therapy [3, 4] in treating vascular problems of the lower extremities, torso and face. Because there is a practical limit to the amount of compression that can be built into the pressure-gradient supports made of bobbinet cloth, it is often necessary, at this time, to use one support over the other. In only one instance to date have I had to use three supports over each other and that was for the late stages of a pregnancy in a severe lymphatic dysplasia.

Under pressure-gradient therapy the "mossy foot" leafy excrescences tend to dry up, turn black and fall off. In one instance where many toes were involved I had to resort to strips of Ace bandages applied by the patient to his tolerance of local pressure to destroy these lesions as well. Complete obliteration of such excrescences at the most distal portions of the toes is almost impossible.

A heretofore unreported and not too unusual complication of lymphatic dysplasia or obstructive lymphedema is recurrent acute toxic lymphangitis [5]. All of us have seen cases of erysipelas and acute streptococcal lymphangitis.

A group of 15 patients that I have recently described do not fit these usual pictures, although elements of the above can occur. These patients usually present with sudden onset, within 1 to 2 h, of alternating chills and fever to 103 to 105.5, malaise, nausea, with or without vomiting, with occasional diarrhea, and about half of them go on to delirium and some to coma. Usually all of these symptoms precede tenderness and swelling of the extremity by as much as 6 to 36 h and rarely up to 72 h. After this lapse of time swelling of the extremity with or without any combination of rubor, localized cellulitis, bullae — either with our without hemorrhage, or specific tender areas occurs. One of these patients had what by history might have been red streaks but they were not present in the episode that I saw clinically.

Of this group, one had 2 and a second had 3 complete G.I. workups which were normal, and another had been treated for gout. All of them had been treated for acute thrombophlebitis because of their late presenting symptoms. One patient that had been treated repeatedly for acute thrombophlebitis, on phlebography showed completely normal veins.

About 20% reported a prodrome of stiffness, tenderness or pain in a small specific area of the extremity, e.g. the toe, the medial paramalleolar region or the groin. Patients in this group were adequately controlled by continuous oral penicillin therapy of either 200,000 or 400,000 units twice or three times a day and the use of pressure-gradient supports to minimize their edema. Intermittent compression pumping preceded the measuring for supports where necessary.

As for the pressures required in counterbalancing the lymphatic deficit, I have never seen an adult case of genetic lymphedema that could be controlled with less than 60 mm of mercury and many required double supports — 60 mm or 70 mm under 70 mm mercury supports. Children below 6 years of age usually get by with single supports of 30, 40 or 50 mm mercury compression because the gravitational pressure at their ankles is much lower.

Bibliography. 1. BENINSON, J., H. S. JACOBSON, W. R. EYLER, and L. A. DuSAULT: Preliminary report on genetic lymphedema as studied by venography, lymphangiography, and radio-isotopic tracers, NA_{22} and RISA. In: Progress in Angiology, Proceedings of the Internationalen Gespräches über Angiologie, 1962, pp. 114—122. Darmstadt: Dr. D. Steinkopff Verlag 1963. — 2. BENINSON, J., H. S. JACOBSON, W. R. EYLER, and L. A. DuSAULT: Vasc. Surg. 1, 43 (1967). — 3. BENINSON, J.: Angiology 12, 38 (1961). — 4. BENINSON, J.: Stasis Dermatitis and Stasis Ulcer. Current Therapy, pp. 483—485. CONN (ed.). Philadelphia: W. B. Saunders Co. 1958. — 5. BENINSON, J.: Superficial Lymphatics and Their Clinical Significance. Newer views of skin diseases, pp. 145—152. YAFFEE (ed.). Philadelphia: Little. Brown and Co. (Inc.) 1966.

Hipodermitis nodular subaguda migratiz

J. PIÑOL AGUADÉ, Cátedra y Escuela Profesional de Dermatologia y Venereología, Barcelona (España)

En 1956 dedicamos nuestra tesis doctoral a las afecciones inflamatorias de localización hipodérmica y entre 157 casos examinados escogimos 13 historias clínicas en las que se presentaba un proceso caracterizado por la aparición de nódulos que ofrecían un crecimiento excéntrico y llegaban a formar extensas placas. Las lesiones se distinguían claramente de otros procesos hipodérmicos por sus rasgos clínicos e histológicos. Este mismo año publicamos con VILANOVA en los Annales de Dermatologie et Syphiliographie una revisión de este síndrome al que dimos el nombre de "Hipodermitis nodular subaguda migratriz". Poco antes de salir a la luz nuestro trabajo apareció un artículo de BAFVERSTEDT en el que, con el nombre de "Erythema nodosum migrans", se describía un cuadro clínico similar o idéntico al estudiado por nosotros. Más tarde, esta misma afección ha sido estudiada entre otros por Ives Bureau y col. Rabbiosi, Fauvernier, Thiers, Perry y Winkel-mann, Pierini, Abulafia y Wainfield, Kerdel-Vegas, Poiares Baptista y Pierini.

En 1959 publicamos con Vilanova una nueva revisión de otras 19 observaciones y desde aquella fecha hemos podido observar 16 nuevos casos lo que hace un total de 49 observaciones personales. Se trata pues de un proceso relativamente frecuente en nuestros medios si se considera que durante este mismo periodo de 11 años se han observado en nuestro Servicio 247 vasculitis nodulares, 18 eritemas nudosos típicos y sólo 4 paniculitis de Pfeiffer-Weber-Christian.

La edad de aparición en nuestra serie oscilaba entre 9 y 65 años. Tan solo dos de los casos eran infantiles y la mayor parte correspondían a personas entre los 30 y 50 años. El predominio del sexo femenino foe evidente pues únicamente 4 de nuestras observaciones eran varones.

En 5 casos aparecieron las lesiones durante el embarazo y en 6 después de un pequeño traumatismo. En uno observamos este cuadro en una paciente afecta de enfermedad de Hodgkin. En 28 los nódulos se vieron precedidos por un episodio gripal, una faringitis o una discreta amigdalitis. El período precedente osciló entre 2 dias y varias semanas.

En su forma característica la erupción comienza por un nódulo hipodérmico del tamaño de un guisante a una cereza, inicialmente poco adherente a la piel que lo recubre, nódulo que puede acompañarse de notable edema perilesional. Después de unos dias de permanecer estacionario empieza a crecer formando una placa indurada de contornos redondeados o policíclicos que alcanza por regla general entre 10 y 15 cm de diámetro, pero que en ocasiones llega a ocupar la totalidad de la cara anterior, posterior o lateral de una pierna. Las placas crecen por extensión centrífuga y muchas veces serpiginosa, curando por uno de los bordes y progresando por el opuesto y otras veces por formación de nuevos nódulos en su periferia.

Una vez constituída la placa, adquiere induración esclerodermiforme y profunda en algún caso y en otros endurecimiento edematoso, superficial y papiráceo. El borde activo es más eritematoso que el centro que a veces es pálido o levemente rosado. La placa se resuelve después de un período de migración en un plazo que oscila entre unas semanas y unos meses dejando como reliquia discreta descamación o pigmentación. La enfermedad se prolonga por renovación de los elementos con intervalos libres de dias o semanas de forma que puede durar meses o incluso años. En nuestra serie, el promedio de duración es de 5 meses antes de ser tratados adecuadamente, pero en casos de evolución espontánea el promedio ha sido de un año y en un caso se prolongó durante 5 años. Pueden presentarse recidivas después de varios años libres de síntomas. Uno de nuestros casos las presentó después de 3 y de 9 años, otro recidivó a los 6 y finalmente una observación vista en 1954 presentó en 1967 un nuevo brote análogo al inicial.

En la inmensa mayoría de enfermos las lesiones se localizaron en una pierna situándose preferentemente en su cara anterior o bien en tobillos, dorso de pies o alrededor de la rodilla. En tres casos afectaron exclusivamente la cara posterior de la pierna donde forman grandes placas. Igualmente pueden observarse lesiones aisladas en muslos, regiones glúteas y antebrazos, estas últimas concomitantes con las de las piernas o bien presentándose después de estas.

Los diagnósticos establecidos durante nuestro examen fueron variables. La mayor parte de enfermos habian sido clasificados como vasculitis nodular, varicoflebitis, flebitis, erisipela o eritema nudoso. En 8 enfermos había sido sospechado un proceso inflamatorio óseo practicándoseles radiografía y 4 habían sido diagnosticados de reumatismo. En una enferma se había procedido a la extirpación e injerto de la zona indurada recidivando los nódulos en la vecindad del injerto poco después de ser intervenida. Excepcionalmente pueden las lesiones no tener tendencia extensiva con lo que la confusión con la vasculitis nodular es muy posible y el examen histológico es lo único que permite el diagnóstico. Esta eventualidad sucedió en dos enfermos. Si bien las lesiones no acostumbran ser dolorosas, en una de nuestras enfermas las molestias fueron tan acusadas y el edema y enrojecimiento tan aparatosos que fue ingresada en una clínica por sospecha de absceso permaneciendo hospitalizada varias semanas. Las lesiones localizadas en tobillo y dorso de pies ofrecen un acusado aspecto esclerodermiforme.

Por regla general los pacientes habían sido tratados previamente con antibióticos y esteroides que no mejoraron o mejoraron muy poco las lesiones y no evitaron las recidivas.

El estado general no acostumbra a estar afectado, y las pruebas de laboratorio son poco demostrativas. La V.S.G. sólo muy discretamente en un caso superaba los 50 mm la primera hora. El título de estreptolisinas era normal, salvo en 5 pacientes que presentaron cifras anormalmente elevadas. Esta determinación se realizó en 36 casos. No existían tampoco alteraciones del hemograma o proteínas que pudieran considerarse como características.

Las características primordiales del cuadro histológico consisten en la presencia de una capilaritis universal hipodérmica como lesión fundamental con infiltración inflamatoria histiocitaria, fibroblástica y monicitaria que se localiza exclusiva o predominantemente en los septos interlobulares del tejido adiposo. A esta lesión acompañan alteraciones más o menos acusadas de la colágena, tales como edema, fragmentación de las fibras, necrosis fibrinoide e incluso en algún caso esclerosis. Los endotelios vasculares están tumefactos y proliferados y son frecuentes las imágenes en *tourbillon* y la obstrucción de luces vasculares. Las grandes venas en cambio no muestran alteraciones aparentes. En un porcentaje elevado de casos se hallan también células gigantes que suponemos originadas a partir de la proliferación endotelial que llega a sobrepasar las dimensiones de los capilares dando lugar por tanto a una capilaritis giganto-celular. Nosotros no consideramos estas capilaritis y células gigantes absolutamente características de la hipodermitis nodular subaguda migratriz puesto que tantos unos como otros se hallan a veces en otros procesos hipodérmicos de las piernas pero en su conjunto el cuadro histológico es lo suficientemente característico para orientar el diagnóstico.

El diagnóstico diferencial debe establecerse con el eritema nudoso, la vasculitis nodular, la paniculitis de Pfeiffer-Weber-Christian y con otras hipodermitis. Algunos autores han indicado que este cuadro no es más que una variante del eritema nudoso, pero nosotros opinamos que posee una real personalidad y debe segregarse de este último, que en realidad no representa una entidad uniforme ni tiene etiología definida. Los puntos fundamentales de este diagnóstico diferencial serían los siguientes: 1. Al reves de lo que sucede en el eritema nudoso en la HNSM existe una fuerte predilección para la edad adulta y el sexo femenino; 2. Iniciación por una lesión aislada o muy escasas; 3. Falta de la simetría lesional característica de aquel; 4. Ausencia de afectación del estado general; 5. Tendencia extensiva de las lesiones; 6. Falta de aspecto contusiforme, incluso en casos de evolución aguda; 7. Evolución prolongada de las placas en contra de la relativa rapidez con que curan los nódulos del eritema nudoso; 8. Falta de respuestas a los medicamentos habitualmente activos en esta enfermedad y respuesta sistemática al yoduro potásico; 9. Falta de la multiplicidad etiológica observada en el eritema nudoso; 10. Estructura histológica con lesión fundamentalmente capilar y ausencia de interesamiento de grandes vasos y de nódulos de Miescher y 11. Mayor frecuencia en nuestros medios que el eritema nudoso típico.

Esta enfermedad cursa con rapidez con la administración de yoduro de potasio. Las dosis utilizadas por nosotros han oscilado entre 2 y 4 gr diarios. Por regla general a los 8 días ha desaparecido el edema y la infiltración y queda sólo un nódulo indurado residual que desaparece paulatinamente en unas 3 semanas. En algún caso la medicación ha tenido que prolongarse un mes y medio. Desconocemos el mecanismo de actuación de este medicamento.

Bibliografía. Bafverstedt, B.: Acta derm.-venereol. (Stockh.) **34,** 181 (1954). — Bureau, Y. J. Barriere, P. Litour et M. Veilhan: Bull. Soc. franç. Derm. Syph. **69,** 69 (1963). — Fauvernier, G.: Tesis Doctoral., Nantes 1963—1964. — Mazzini, M. A., y C. A. Castello: Rev. argent. Dermatosif. **48,** 125 (1964). — Kerdel-Vegas, F.: Hautarzt **17,** 116 (1966). — Pierini L. E.: Derm. ibero lat.-amer. **8,** 173 (1966). — Pierini, L. E., J. Abulafia y S. Mainfeld: Arch. argent. Dermatosif. **15,** 1, 105 (1965). — Poiares Baptista, A.: Hipodermite nodular subaguda migrans Congreso de Dermatólogos de Langua Portuguesa, Rio de Janeiro Octubre 1965. — Perry, H. O., and R. H. Winkelmann: Arch. Derm. Syph. (Chic.) **89,** 170 (1964). — Rabbiosi, C.: Minerva derm. **33,** 55 (1958). — Thiers, H., et J. Fayolle: Bull. Soc. franç. Derm. Syph. **69,** 501 (1963). — Vilanova, K., et J. Piñol Aguadé: Ann. Derm. Syph. (Paris) **83,** 369 (1956); — Brit. J. Derm. **71,** 45 (1959).

An Evaluation of Low Molecular Weight Dextran in Acrocyanosis and Acroscleroderma*

E. M. Farber, H. S. Zackheim and E. Aschheim, Department of Dermatology, Stanford University School of Medicine, Palo Alto, California (USA)

This report describes the use of low molecular weight dextran (LMWD) in two patients with acrocyanosis and in five patients with acroscleroderma.

Our knowledge of the pathophysiology of acrocyanosis is derived mainly from the work of Sir Thomas Lewis and Eugene Landis. They showed that the constriction or spasticity is found in the arterioles and that in this respect this condition differs from Raynaud's disease in which the spasticity extends to the digital arteries as well. However, acrocyanosis is also characterized by atonicity of the small venules, and presumably the cyanotic color of the skin is due to low rates of perfusion combined with a large vascular capacity. The arteriolar spasticity and low skin blood flow are readily abolished by total body heating of the subjects, and are associated with a corresponding change in skin color. However, since nerve blocks were ineffective in this regard, Lewis and Landis concluded that the disorder resides in the blood vessels themselves. Another argument in favor of this view is the circumstance that the blue coloration of the skin does not seem to correspond to any known distribution of nerves.

In our studies of four patients with acrocyanosis measurements were made of both digital blood flow and skin temperatures and were found to be much below normal (Fig. 1). Upon warming of the subjects by raising the ambient temperature the vaso-spasm was abolished. The skin temperatures reached body core temperature and the digital blood flow increased substantially (Fig. 2).

Considerable interest has developed in recent years as to the rheological effects and therapeutic possibilities of low molecular weight dextran (LMWD, mol. wt. 40,000). There is an increasing use of this polysaccharide in shock, vascular thromboses, vascular surgery, fat embolism and related conditions.

The reputed favorable effects of LMWD are attributed to the lessening of red blood cell and platelet aggregation and the lowering of blood viscosity. LMWD is

* This work was supported by USPHS Research Grant HE-03833-07-A2

said to increase red blood cell negativity causing mutual repulsion of the cells. GELIN [1] found no effect from LMWD on blood flow values in persons with normal erythrocyte sedimentation rates; however in persons with an ESR of over 80 mm/h LMWD produced an increase in blood flow.

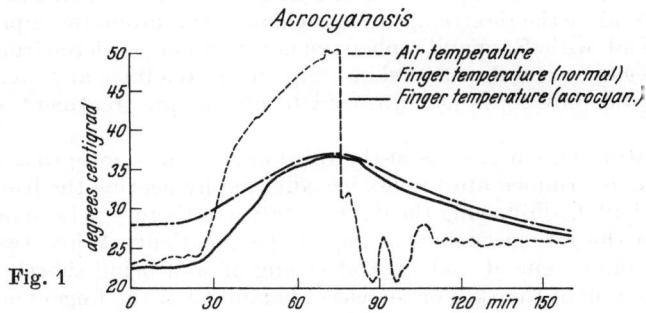

Fig. 1

Many of the claims for the effectiveness of LMWD have been disputed. FOLSE and COPE [2] believe that the volume expanding effect is more significant than its effect on blood fluidity. FLEMMA [3] found no preventive effect of LMWD on bioelectrically induced thromboses in dogs. PUTNAM [4] reported that both low molecular weight and regular dextran actually increase blood viscosity.

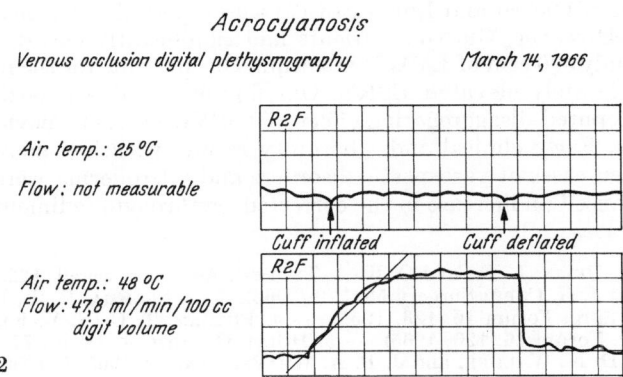

Fig. 2

Interest in the use of LMWD for vasospastic disorders and scleroderma was stimulated by the report of HOLTI [5] who claimed beneficial effects in ten of twelve patients with acrosclerosis receiving infusions of 2000 to 3000 ccm of LMWD. Increased skin temperatures, improved color and healing of finger-tip ulcers were noted. Similar benefits were claimed for "Raynaud's disease with obliterative changes". PRINGLE [6] found increased blood viscosity in Raynaud's disease. In early experiments LMWD lowered blood viscosity and improved the peripheral circulation.

We have administered low molecular weight dextran to two patients with primary acrocyanosis, two with Raynaud's phenomenon with early acroscleroderma, and three with moderate to marked acroscleroderma. All patients were hospitalized for 1 to 2 weeks and received 2000 to 3000 ccm of LMWD (10% Rheomacrodex in saline) in 48 to 72 h by continuous intravenous infusion. The patients have been followed for up to 9 weeks afterwards.

The two patients with acrocyanosis showed no improvement in their blood flow or skin temperature measurements after the dextran. There was likewise no change in their clinical condition.

One of the patients with Raynaud's phenomenon and early acrosclerosis, hospitalized for 2 weeks, showed improved blood flow and skin temperature readings for up to 5 weeks after the dextran. She also claimed symptomatic improvement. The second patient with Raynaud's phenomenon and early scleroderma showed moderately increased blood flow and skin temperature readings at 2 weeks, while still in the hospital, but these had dropped to almost pre-treatment values by 5 weeks.

Skin temperature measurements in the three cases of moderate to severe acrosleroderma were determined after reflex vasodilation by heating the feet or hands in warm water of 40 °C. Following the dextran infusion there was no significant or sustained rise in the measurements in any of these patients. While two claimed some subjective improvement and general feeling of well being shortly after the infusion, no softening of the skin or increased flexibility of the fingers or face was evident.

One interesting result of this study is that a majority of the patients showed an increase in the sedimentation rate following the LMWD infusion. This lasted for about a week and then gradually returned to pre-treatment levels. Six of seven patients had an increase in the uncorrected ESR, while one (initial ESR 47 mm/h) decreased. After correction of the ESR to a hematocrit of 45%, the ESR was still elevated in four, unchanged in two, and decreased in one. This contrasts with the report of GROTH and LOFSTROM [7] who reported a decrease in the ESR after LMWD. However, GROTH's patients had significantly elevated ESR's and they received only 500 ccm of LMWD in 30 min. Our patients for the most part had normal or moderately elevated ESR's. Our findings in this regard throw some doubt on the reputed disaggregating effect of LMWD on erythrocytes.

Conclusions. Early clinical and laboratory results with low molecular weight dextran in seven cases of vasospastic disorders and scleroderma were not impressive. LMWD caused an increase in the corrected erythrocyte sedimentation rate in four of seven cases.

References. 1. GELIN, L. E., and O. K. A. THOREN: Acta chir. scand. 122, 303 (1961). — 2. FOLSE, R., and J. G. COPE: Surgery 58, 779 (1965). — 3. FLEMMA, R. J., D. SILVER, and W. G. ANLYAN: Surg. Forum 16, 123 (1965). — 4. PUTNAM, T. C., S. V. KEVY, and R. L. REPLOGLE: Surg. Forum 16, 126 (1965). — 5. HOLTI, G.: Brit. J. Derm. 77, 560 (1965). — 6. PRINGLE, R., D. N. WALDER, and J. P. A. WEAVER: Lancet 1965, I, 1086. — 7. GROTH, C. G., and B. LOFSTROM: Acta chir. scand. 128, 1 (1964).

Free Communications

Oxygénothérapie locale dans les ulcères de jambe

W. RASIEWICZ et B. SZYMCZYK, Clinique Dermatologique de l'Académie Médicale Silésienne, Zabrze (Pologne)

La thérapie des ulcères de jambe est un problème complexe et difficile. Malgré l'abondance et diversité de méthodes de traitement les résultats sont décevants. Les recherches ultérieures sont alors bien indiquées.

Parmi les facteurs étio-pathogéniques, les troubles circulatoires locaux jouent — sans doute — le rôle prédominant, résultant parmi d'autres conséquences l'asphyxie locale. Cet état de choses indique thérapeutique améliorant la nutrition locale. Ainsi nous avons décidé d'essayer l'oxygène comme un agent curatif. La très intéressante publication de Chieregato et Pittoni (de la Clinique Dermatologique de Padoue) nous a fourni l'encouragement ultérieur.

Notre communication concerne le groupe de 20 femmes, agées de 30 jusqu'à 78, souffrant de vastes, torpides ulcères de jambe. Dans tous ces cas nous avons appliqué l'oxygénothérapie locale. Pour la réaliser on maintenait la jambe dans un sac de plastique dans lequel on securait un flux libre d'oxygène pur. Chaque procédure durait 3 h et le plein cours comportait 10 à 20 séances. Nous avons obtenu des suivants résultats de thérapie: a) une diminution de surface des ulcères de 70 à 80% dans onze cas. De ceux-ci on a constaté la guérison complète après l'intervalle de 1 à 2 semaines dans sept cas; b) une amélioration médiocre, c'est-à-dire la diminution des ulcères de 30 à 50%, fut constatée dans sept cas; c) enfin dans deux cas on n'a constaté un résultat quelconque. Seulement dans un unique cas nous avons observé la complication pendant la cure sous la forme d'allergisation secondaire.

Pour étudier le mécanisme d'action d'oxygène nous avons exécuté de suivants examens additionnels:

1. mesure de la température de la peau près des ulcères: seulement trois fois nous avons constaté une élévation marquée de la t°. Dans toutes autres occasions la fluctuation de la t° sous l'influence d'application d'oxygène était médiocre. 2. mesure de pH du fond des ulcères: nous n'avons constaté que des changements minimes de pH dans deux directions sous l'influence d'oxygène; 3. la composition de la flore bactérienne des ulcères était examinée avant et après la cure. Aucun changement significatif n'était constaté. 4. Dans huit cas de suivantes études histochimiques du tissu de granulation des ulcères étaient exécutées: a) la coloration PAS + alciane-bleu pour évaluer des mucopolysaccharides acides; b) la coloration avec carmine de Best pour évaluer le glycogène; c) la coloration selon Van Gieson pour examiner des fibres collagènes. Nous n'avons pas observé d'influence d'oxygénothérapie sur les résultats des études histochimiques sus-nommées.

Ainsi nos observations, qui correspondent à celles de Chieregato et Pittoni, encouragent à l'introduction d'oxygénothérapie locale dans le traitement des ulcères de jambe comme thérapeutique assez simple, exempte de danger et assurante de résultats favorables.

Bibliographie. 1. Cieregato, G., e. P. Pittoni: Minerva derm. **39,** 302 (1964).

Des aspects médico-sociaux et étio-pathogéniques de l'ulcère de jambe. L'importance de l'artério- et de la phlébographie dans l'ulcère dit variqueux

G. Nastase, Clinique Dermato-Vénérologique, et G. Chisleag, Clinique Radiologique, Iassy (Roumanie)

La fréquence de l'ulcère de jambe, la grande durée du traitement, la diminution de la capacité de résistance de l'organisme etc., font de ce syndrôme un problème médico-social. Ainsi, entre autres, en suivant 555 cas d'ulcère de jambe, on a constaté que la dépense de l'hospitalisation dépasse de 2,78 fois le barème des différentes dermatoses, tandis que 12,3% des cas ont nécessité des hospitalisations répétées. Cette situation est déterminée aussi par la complexité des facteurs étiopathogéniques qui s'imposent d'être recherchés et corrigés.

Par exemple, on doit tenir compte des lésions épidermiques, d'un éventuel eczéma périulcéreux (en réalité une dermite streptostaphylo-coccique) ou de la présence d'une capillarite, des éventuelles zones de sclérose environnant l'ulcère, l'existence d'une atrophie blanche, de l'œdème éléphantiasique, etc. D'ici, l'obligation d'un examen cardio-vasculaire, ainsi qu'une étude du réseau veineux. L'identification des segments avec périphlébite.

D'une grande importance apparaît alors l'examen radiographique des jambes. Ainsi une étude sur 124 cas, effectuée pendant l'époque de l'endémie de syphilis, a montré que 23,38% des malades ont présenté des lésions de périostite hyperplastique, tandis que 36,9% ont eu des analyses sérologiques positives pour la syphilis.

En continuant les recherches dans ce sens, dans le dernier temps sur 83 cas, dont 11,11% ont été positifs pour la syphilis, on a trouvé des modifications osseuses en 83,33% comme des appositions périostiques sous forme de manchons ou saillies mamelonnées et plus rarement sous forme de spicules, ainsi que le remaniement de la corticale.

L'examen des parties molles a relevé aussi des structures réticulaires à mailles transparentes, qui doivent être attribuées à la dégénérescence graisseuse du tissu conjonctif. De plus, des cordons variqueux, des calcifications artérielles et des nodules tissulaires calcifiés.

Dans l'ulcère dit variqueux s'impose l'étude des processus d'endothéillite (spécialement l'existence de ricketsioses dans les antécédents) ainsi que celui de l'altération du tissu conjonctif, recherche possible par des méthodes hystochimiques, regardant l'action des différentes enzymes, ainsi que les modifications des mucopolysaccharides dermiques. Aussi, ont été trouvées indispensables les recherches métaboliques en ce qui concerne le taux des protéines sanguines, qui sur 24 des cas ont été trouvées augmentées dans 13,3%, diminuées dans 8,7% et normales dans le reste. En même temps était présente l'inversion du rapport albumines/globulines, diminuées dans 62,5% et augmentées dans 37,5%.

A ne pas négliger les valeurs de la lipémie totale, qui dans nos cas a été augmentée en 18%, diminuée dans 11% et normale dans le reste; ainsi que le taux de la glycémie qui a été accrue dans 33% des cas tandis que la cholestérolémie a été augmentée dans 20%. Il est nécessaire de chercher les éventuels spasmes artériels et l'oscillométrie. Par exemple dans nos cas, nous avons constaté hyposphygmie dans 57,14%, normosphygmie dans 28,57% et hypersphygmie dans 14,28%. Tout à fait apparaît utile l'artério- et la phlébographie. Ainsi en exécutant des artériographies totales en série du membre inférieur pour poursuivre le régime circulatoire tant que du point morphologique que fonctionnel, des 14 malades examinés, nous avons constaté des modifications pathologiques à 11 des cas, provoqués dans 5 des cas par des obstructions artérielles (au niveau de la fémorale ou de la tibiale antérieure), tandis que 6 malades ont présenté des signes d'athéromathose.

De plus, on a constaté le retard de la progression de la substance de contraste dans huit cas et on a remarqué des anastomoses artérioveineuses au niveau de la hanche dans quatre cas.

Nous considérons la phlébographie nécessaire dans les varices hydrostatiques, qui peut mettre en évidence l'insuffisance valvulaire, le reflux veineux, le retard de la circulation veineuse, l'existence éventuelle de quelques communicantes, il faut aussi chercher les dilatations variqueuses autour des ulcérations, etc.

Dans les varices postphlébitiques on observe des obstructions par tromboses profondes, de la réperméabilisation du caillot, la perte de la fonction valvulaire des veines, qui permet le passage du sang de la circulation profonde dans la superficielle.

Nous avons démontré l'importance de la méthode de la phlébographie antérograde et rétrograde, cette dernière en position ortostatique ainsi que le cours et le reflux de la substance opaque dans des cas d'insuffisance des valvules. En même temps, s'il est nécessaire, il faut s'adresser à la lymphographie.

Dans leur ensemble, dans les cas d'ulcère de jambe, l'objectif principal est de mettre un diagnostic étiologique ainsi que de connaître les processus pathogéniques, pour diminuer les effets nocifs de ces manifestations.

Studies on the Healing Time of Leg Ulcers
A Clinical and Statistical Study Based on 200 In-Patients

A. Perdrup and J. Stene, Rudolph Bergh's Hospital, Copenhagen (Denmark)

An evaluation of the circulation in the lower extremities is necessary for diagnosis, choice of therapy and for the assessment of your therapy. A number of elaborate physiologic methods have been worked out which also could be used to assess the effect of some drug upon the peripheral circulation.

The dermatologists are, however, in the happy position of having among their clientele 1000 of patients with leg ulcers, a condition that before their naked eyes display the local circulatory condition, the effect and possibilities of treatment. The growth, the stagnation or the healing, in other words the variations of the area of the ulcer in relation to time must be a good indicator of the local circulation, if these variations are properly assessed. In the litearure you will find countless papers referring to the effect of this or that remedy on the healing of ulcers but conclusions are often drawn on loose premises.

At the Rudolph Bergh's hospital in Copenhagen we are trying to find the "healing curves of leg ulcers under a uniform standard treatment". The definition of "standard treatment" need some explanation: The Rudolph Bergh's hospital has for several decades been using about 50 of its beds for patients being dermatologically treated for leg ulcers of all kinds. These in-patients belong to the group with rather recalcitrant ulcers. The ulcers are topically treated with non-allergenic disinfective remedies, stasis is counteracted by elevation and by elastic bandages, some physical treatment is given for joints and muscles and manifest internal and other diseases are treated properly.

The main purpose of our efforts is now to consider to what extent the healing curves of leg ulcers thus treated are influenced by general conditions like sex, age, weight, a number of laboratory findings, a number of concomitant internal diseases and local conditions like the caracter of the ulcer, the induration of the surroundings, pulsations and rheography. We feel that we must necessarily have hold on these relations before it is possible to assess the effect of any treatment added to this simple "standard treatment" such as e.g. to evaluate the effect of hormones or other drugs postulated to affect favourably the peripheral circulation.

A series of 200 consecutive in-patients treated in our clinic during a year and a half are used for our calculations which, I must admit, are still in processing, so that I can only give some preliminary results. To illustrate examples of the many clinical circumstances which may influence the healing time I would like to show a few graphs and tables indicating the composition of the series with regard to:

Sex, age, weight, duration of the "ulcer-disease", anemia, findings of serum-electrophoresis, diseases hampering the gait, serious heart diseases, diabetes, hypertension, induration of the surroundings of the ulcers, survey of the findings of rheography.

The ulcers are measured by weekly planimetry of a pattern exactly drawn along the edge of the ulcer on transparent plastic foil.

The course of an ulcer must necessarily be an interaction between destructive and regenerative processes.

The destructive processes represent the sum of known and unknown influences of local and general disease, degeneration and age.

The regenerative processes are the sum of natural resistance and rebuilding capacities of the body and — I hope — of treatment. Here two main questions appear:

1. will it be possible to estimate the effect of some of these destructive processes ?,

2. will it be possible to assess the effect of treatment ?

This problem has been raised in collaboration with my statistical adviser Mr. JON STENE who has developed a mathematical model for healing curves of leg ulcers. Because time is short the explanation has been printed separately and distributed to the audience.

From the mathematical theory and the shown examples it appears that the constructed model fits the healing curves of many leg ulcers. The parameters are determined by the condition of the patients.

A Mathematical Model for Healing Curves of Leg Ulcers

J. STENE, Institute of Statistics, University of Copenhagen (Denmark)

The aim of this preliminary report is to construct and describe a mathematical model of the healing process of leg ulcers in each individual patient during his stay in hospital and to confront this model to real healings. It seems suitable to assume that the course of a leg ulcer is determined by two adverse processes, namely destructive processes tending to increase the area of the ulcer or to decelerate the healing and the regenerative processes tending against healing of the ulcer.

Denote the sum of the destructive processes at a certain moment by A_1 and their effect of a certain unit of the of these processes by λ_1.

Then the increase of the area of the ulcer which is caused by these processes in an infinitesimal period following the chosen moment is

$$\lambda_1 A_1 . \tag{1}$$

The regenerative processes operate in the opposite direction with an effect denoted by λ_2 per unit of ulcer-area. Denote the area of the ulcer at the same moment as before by A.

The reduction of this area caused by the healing processes in the same infinitesimal period is

$$\lambda_2 A \tag{2}$$

and the total change of the area of the ulcer within the period is then

$$\frac{dA}{dt} = \lambda_1 A_1 - \lambda_2 A \tag{3}$$

since the destructive processes increase the area and the regenerative processes decrease it. The hampering of the destructive processes is unobservable but may be considered hypothetically. This hampering is assumed to take place at a rate which is equal to its effect upon the area of the ulcer i.e. that the reduction in an infinitesimal period is proportional to their sum A_1 at a certain moment, i.e.

$$\frac{d A_1}{d t} = -\lambda_1 A_1 \tag{4}$$

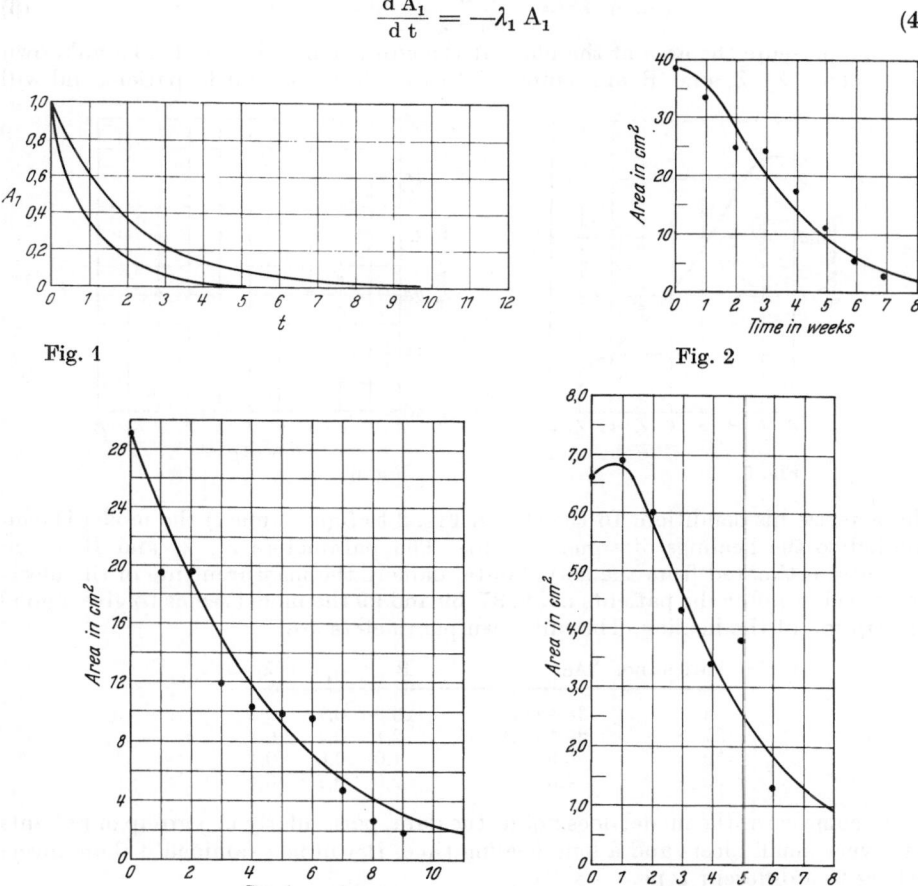

Fig. 1

Fig. 2

Fig. 3

Fig. 4

if this differential equation is solved, A_1, the sum of the destructive processes at a time t is

$$A_1 = -Be^{-\lambda_1 t} \tag{5}$$

where B, is the sum of the destructive processes at the time of the admittance to the hospital and e $= 2{,}718$ (the base number of the natural logarithms). A_1 as a function of the time t is represented in Fig. 1 where $B = 1$ and for the upper curve $\lambda_1 = 0{,}5$ and for the lower curve $\lambda_1 = 1{,}0$.

A large value of λ_1 implies that the hampering of the destructive processes is very efficient. A_1 given by (5) is the same as A_1 in (3) at the time t.

The idea of using the same parameter λ_1 to indicate the effect of a certain unit of the destructive process to increase the area of the ulcer and to indicate the rate of its hampering has no deeper meaning than to reduce the number of unknown parameters. By confronting the model to the actual material this hypothesis will be tested. If the destructive processes are supposed to be hampered at the given speed the area of the ulcer at the given time t will be given by the solution of the differential equation (3), namely

$$A = A_o \, e^{-\lambda_2 t} + \frac{B}{\lambda_1 - \lambda_2} \, (e^{-\lambda_2 t} - e^{-\lambda_1 t}) \, . \tag{6}$$

A_o represents the area of the ulcer at the admission to hospital. The unknown parameters, λ_1, λ_2 and B are supposed to vary from patient to patient and will

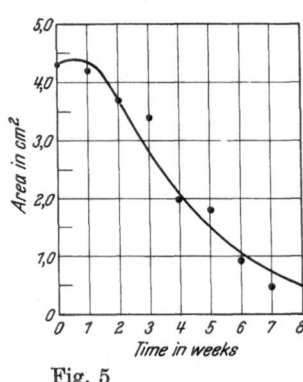

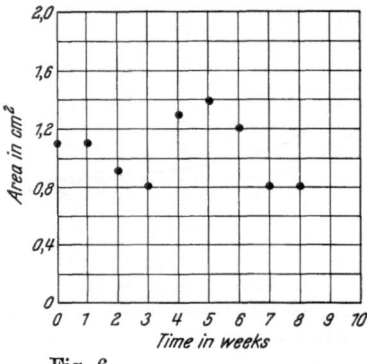

Fig. 5   Fig. 6

characterize his condition. In the shown Fig. 2 to 5 (see annex) the model is confronted to the healings of some patients. The parameters λ_1, λ_2 and B are in each case estimated from the actual data, namely the measurements of the ulcer-areas each we. For the patients no. 5, 37, 59 and 99 the model seems to give a good description of the healing. The unknown parameters are:

Patient no.	A_o	B	λ_1	λ_2
5	38,4 cm²	23,0	0,7	0,5
37	29,1 cm²	2,1	0,4	0,3
59	6,6 cm²	4,0	0,6	0,4
99	4,3 cm²	2,6	0,7	0,4

In some cases the model does not fit the data, particularly in a group of patients with very small ulcers and a long healing time. It will be examined if these ulcers belong to a different type.

Arterial Occlusion as a Cause of Gangrene and Ischemic Ulcerations of the Legs

R. G. Freeman and J. M. Knox, Department of Dermatology, Baylor University College of Medicine, Houston, Texas (USA)

Aortoiliac occlusion (Leriche syndrome), often the cause for gangrene and ischemic ulcerations of the legs and feet, was described in the 1920's. The original description included impotence and claudication and atropy of the hips and thighs, but today the term is used rather loosely to include femoral and popliteal occlusion. Although the disease was described four decades ago, restorative surgical treatment for it has been developed in the past decade by the pioneering work of Dr. Michael De Bakey of Baylor University College of Medicine.

Ischemia results from occlusion of the arteries by arteriosclerosis. Arterio-sclerosis begins with intimal proliferation and mural deposits of lipid-rich material, usually in the vicinity of bifurcations or near the origin of major branches. Thus the occlusion which usually develops insidiously, often involves only a segment of the artery. This segmental involvement makes restoration of adequate blood flow to the ischemic leg possible by vascular replacement, bypass reconstruction, or endarterectomy. The major areas of segmental localization are aortoiliac (Leriche syndrome), femoropopliteal, and popliteo-tibial. Occlusion in each of these areas can result in ischemic damage to the acral parts. The major cutaneous manifesta-tions of such vascular occlusion are gangrene of the digits and ulcers of the leg, ankle or foot which fail to heal. Often they are associated with pain, intermittent claudication and trophic changes of the skin including loss of appendages, atrophy, a glossy texture, hypertrophy of nails, and decreased skin temperature. The dorsalis pedis, posterior tibial, or both pulses will be diminished. The ischemic ulcers may occur on the foot in association with gangrene or may be more proximal on the lower leg.

Clinical Material

Over 2500 patients have undergone repair of segmental aortoiliac or femoral-popliteal occlusion by replacement or bypass reconstruction of vessels carried out by vascular surgeons in the Texas Medical Center. Of 2500 patients whose case histories were analyzed, 315 had major cutaneous manifestations with their arterial insufficiency. These included gangrene, ischemic ulcers, cold gray anesthetic foot, and cold edematous red foot. Many other patients had trophic skin changes of a minor nature. Of particular interest to the dermatologist was the finding of gangrene in 29%, and chronic ischemic ulcers resistant to conventional therapy in 18%. Gangrene was most often insidious in onset but occasionally developed rapidly and was more varied in onset than other skin changes. Ischemic ulcers always developed insidiously, often as the result of failure to heal after slight trauma. Characteristically ischemic ulcers will not respond well to any treatment before restoration of blood flow. Pain is a frequent and prominent symptom.

The majority of the 315 patients (62%) had either aortoiliac or femoral popliteal occlusion or both. The remaining 38% had distal popliteal-tibial occlusion, a location usually not amenable to correction by vascular surgery.

Results of Surgical Treatment

Restoration of blood flow carried out by vascular replacement or bypass reconstruction was successful in 73% of the femoral popliteal obstructions and 91% of aortoiliac obstructions. Gangrenous changes were halted with salvage of much of the extremity heretofore doomed to amputation. The ischemic ulcers which before had been resistant to any form of treatment now healed readily.

Discussion

Arteriosclerosis is one of the leading causes of death in the world today. One of its dermatologic manifestations is the production of ischemic changes as a result of segmental occlusion of the aortoiliac, femoral, popliteal, or popliteal-tibial arteries.

Gangrene and ischemic ulcers of the leg are common manifestations of this arterial occlusion and while gangrene is well known and widely recognized in association with arterial disease, the ischemic basis for ulcers of the leg and foot is often not recognized but attributed to stasis, trauma, or other reasons. Although the results of restorative vascular surgery in arterial occlusive disease has been widely publicized, many physicians still do not recognize the association between ischemic lesions of the leg and arterial occlusion in such a remote site as the aorta, iliac, or femoral arteries. This phenomenon is emphasized to dermatologists be-cause the majority of patients with gangrene and ischemic ulcers can be treated successfully by restoration of blood flow to the ischemic part.

Präventivmaßnahmen bei Rezidiven der Unterschenkelgeschwüre

B. Janoušek, H. Dlabalová und V. Rozsívalová, Karls Universität
Prag, Fakultät Hradec Králové, (Tschechoslowakei)

Bei zunehmendem Alter wächst ständig die Zahl der Kranken mit varicösen Unterschenkelgeschwüren und ihren Rezidiven an. Das Ulcus cruris und seine Rezidive werden zu einem ernsten gesundheitlich-ökonomischen Problem. Das führte uns im Jahre 1962 zu einer zielbewußten Prävenz der Rezidive und zu einer langfristigen Beobachtung, welche von den Präventivmaßnahmen die erfolgreichste wäre. Alle Kranken in observatione wurden in ein Dispensaire mit eigenen Vormerkblättern mit gründlicher Anamnese und Untersuchungsergebnissen (einschließlich angiologischem und Knochenbefund) übergeführt. Vor dem Rezidiv wurden die Kranken mit folgenden Präventivmaßnahmen geschützt:

1. Durch elastische Binden auf Gummischwamm über der Narbe gewickelt.
2. Durch elastische Binden ohne Schwamm.
3. Interne Verordnung von Dihydroergotoxin. Diese Methode wurde aber bald verlassen, weil sie sich nicht bewährt hatte.

Gleichzeitig beobachteten wir, wie sich bei Ausbruch des Rezidivs das Alter der Kranken, Obesität, schwere physische Arbeit, orthopädische Anomalien und Knochenveränderungen an den Unterschenkeln geltend machten.

Von 1962 bis Ende 1966 wurden auf diese Art 287 Kranke beobachtet, die in zwei Gruppen nach der Behandlungsmethode geteilt wurden (Tab. 1).

Tabelle 1. *Gesamtzahl der geheilten Kranken*

	Männer	Frauen	Insgesamt
Konservative Behandlung	64	138	202
Inselförmige Plastik	39	46	85
Insgesamt	103	184	287

Tabelle 2. *Durch Konservativbehandlung geheilte Kranke*

Präventive Maßnahmen	Anzahl der Kranken	Anzahl der Rezid.	%	Standard-fehler	Durchschnitts-zahl der Monate bis zum Rezidiv
Schwamm und Binde	50	9	18	5,4	16,5
Binde ohne Schwamm	83	35	42,16	5,4	9,5
Kontrollgruppe	69	41	59,42	5,9	7,5
Insgesamt	202	85	42,1		

Determinationskoeffizient für Schwamm und Binde — 10,1.

Tabelle 3. *Kranke geheilt mit inselförmiger Plastik*

Präventive Maßnahmen	Anzahl der Kranken	Anzahl der Rezid.	%	Standard-fehler	Durchschnitts-zahl der Monate bis zum Rezidiv
Schwamm und Binde	24	3	12,50	6,7	36
Binde ohne Schwamm	45	16	35,55	7,1	11
Kontrollgruppe	16	5	31,25	11,5	5
Insgesamt	85	24	28,23		

Determinationskoeffizient für Schwamm und Binde — 6,6.

Die Ergebnisse der Präventivmaßnahmen und die Einflüsse gewisser Faktoren bei der Entstehung von Rezidiven der Unterschenkelgeschwüre wurden statistisch mit der Methode der Monofaktordispersanalyse — modifiziert für Qualitativmerkmale — verarbeitet. Durch Berechnung erhielten wir den Determinationskoeffizienten[2], der den Einfluß des beobachteten Faktors auf das Resultat angibt. Eine Übersicht der Präventivergebnisse ist in den Tab. 2 und 3 angegeben.

Atrophie blanche

R. SANTLER, II. Universitäts-Hautklinik Wien (Österreich)

Wie wir schon in früheren Berichten, zum Teil in Übereinstimmung mit anderen Autoren (GONIN, GREITHER, HAUSER, NÖDL, TOURAINE), feststellen konnten, ist die Epidermis im Bereiche der Atrophie blanche meist verschmälert, der Papillarkörper abgeflacht bis völlig verstrichen. Die Hornschicht ist gut ausgebildet, Follikelöffnungen und Drüsenausführungsgänge sind, soweit noch vorhanden, mit Hornmassen ausgefüllt. Melanotisches Pigment ist vornehmlich in den Basalzellen nachzuweisen. Ein auffälliger Pigmentmangel konnte nicht festgestellt werden. Das in den oberflächlichen Cutisschichten gelegene Bindegewebe zeichnet sich einerseits durch eine ödematöse Auflockerung, andererseits durch Homogenisierung aus. Die tieferen Cutisschichten, die Subcutis und die Bindegewebssepten sind oftmals ausgeprägt fibrosiert. Die papillär und subpapillär gelegenen Gefäße vom Typ der Capillaren, Präcapillaren und Arteriolen lassen oftmals knäuelartig aneinandergelagerte Proliferationen erkennen. Innerhalb dieser Knäuelbildungen finden sich Capillaren, die durch zahlreiche, hellplasmatische Zellen vom Typ der Quellzellen auffallen. Eine perivasculäre entzündliche Infiltration fällt nicht auf, dagegen ist reichlich Blutpigment, besonders um diese Gefäßknäuelbildungen, aber auch entlang der Gefäße nach der Tiefe zu, ebenso um die Schweißdrüsen, zu beobachten. Die Arteriolen sind vielfach hyalinisiert. Die Arterien im Cutis und Subcutisbereich weisen ein eher enges Lumen auf. Hautanhangsgebilde fehlen oder sind zumindest rarefiziert, lediglich die Schweißdrüsen sind meist gut erhalten.

Durch entsprechende therapeutische Maßnahmen ist die Atrophie blanche zum Teil rückbildungsfähig. Die Weißfärbung, Ausdruck einer Mangeldurchblutung, weicht einer normalen Farbtönung.

Bioptisches Material ehemaliger Atrophie blanche Herde, histologisch untersucht, läßt einwandfrei faßbare Unterschiede fast nur an den Gefäßen erkennen. Die Gefäßknäuel sind jetzt verkleinert oder vollständig rückgebildet. Die Wand der Gefäße ist vielfach verdünnt, sog. Quellzellen sind nur mehr vereinzelt zu sehen. Die Capillaren zwischen den Knäuelbildungen, die vor der Behandlung nur spärlich anzutreffen waren, sind jetzt eher reichlich vorhanden.

Die beschriebenen Gefäßknäuelbildungen sind unseres Erachtens nicht als entzündliche oder eigengesetzlich wachsende Wucherungen aufzufassen, sondern vielmehr als Vorgänge, die übergeordneten Regulationen unterliegen. Solche können, z. B. auf die Atrophie blanche bezogen, hämodynamischer Natur sein, aber auch neurale und hormonelle Einflüsse sowie Stoffwechselstörungen sind in Betracht zu ziehen.

Da die mikroskopischen Veränderungen durch entsprechende therapeutische Maßnahmen rückbildbar sind, darf vorsichtig gefolgert werden, daß der Atrophie blanche eine Anpassungshyperplasie bestimmter Gefäßabschnitte bei einer Fehlsteuerung bzw. Dysfunktion bestimmter Organe oder Organsysteme zugrunde liegt, wobei nach Beseitigung einer oder mehrerer dieser ursächlichen Komponenten auch die Anpassungsvorgänge hinfällig werden.

Bei dem zur Debatte stehenden Krankheitsbild sind wir geneigt, der Gefäßknäuelbildung vorwiegend die Aufgabe zuzusprechen, das Blut bei hämodynamischen Störungen — in erster Linie bei Stauungszuständen — abzuleiten, und zwar durch Nebenschlüsse, die im Stande sind, den Capillarkreislauf gewisser Gefäßbezirke zu regulieren und vor Schaden zu schützen und die Zirkulation vor größeren Störungen zu bewahren.

Experimentell ist Clark und Clark die Neubildung von arterio-venösen Anastomosen unter bestimmten physiologischen und pathologischen Bedingungen gelungen. Sie nimmt nach Clark und Clark ihren Ausgang von einer Capillarschlinge, die in dem aussprossenden Gefäßnetz infolge einer unvermittelten Zunahme des Blutstromes in der zuführenden Arteriole sich erweitert, und leitet auf kürzestem und direktem Weg den größten Teil des Blutes von der erweiterten Arteriole in die nächste Vene ab, so daß die übrigen Capillarschlingen vorübergehend weniger durchströmt werden. Wir sind geneigt, der Atrophie blanche ähnliche Vorgänge zugrunde zu legen.

Stasis Dermatitis and Atrophie Blanche
A Clinicopathologic and Histochemical Study *

A. S. Marques, J. H. Graham, W. C. Johnson and H. R. Gray, The Skin and Cancer Hospital of Philadelphia and the Departments of Dermatology and Pathology, Temple University School of Medicine, Philadelphia (USA)

This study presents a comparative analysis of 50 patients with typical stasis dermatitis and 19 patients with atrophie blanche and is a continuation of previous studies of these diseases [1, 2]. Both diseases represent circulatory disorders of the legs with overlapping clinicopathologic features, but critical evaluation reveals significant distinguishing differences.

In stasis dermatitis, the primary lesions appeared as erythematous to bluish-purple, purpuric macules, and the subacute and chronic stages were edematous, eczematous, papular, scaly, and hyperpigmented. Varicose veins and relatively non-painful ulcerations were frequently present. Trauma and thrombophlebitis were often precipitating factors in producing ulcers which commonly occur in the region of the malleoli (Fig. 1).

Atrophie blanche is common in women and initially shows erythematous, telangiectatic, purpuric macules or papules with subsequent development of painful ulcerations located on the lower legs, ankles and dorsal surfaces of the feet (Fig. 2). The ulcers heal slowly and leave residual irregularly shaped white atrophic scars surrounded by a narrow telangiectatic, hyperpigmented border. Varicose veins and thrombophlebitis were not common associated diseases in patients with atrophie blanche. Exacerbations occurred during the summer months in patients with atrophie blanche, whereas, those with stasis dermatitis showed no seasonal variation.

Microscopically, stasis dermatitis is characterized by eczematous epidermal changes and pseudoepitheliomatous hyperplasia was observed in one-third of the

* This investigation was supported in part by Research Training Grant 2 A-5289 (C₅) from the National Institute of Arthritis and Metabolic Diseases, National Institutes of Health, Public Health Service, Bethesda, Maryland.

biopsies obtained from ulcer margins. In the corium, nodules of capillary-endo-thelial proliferation, vascular ectasia, fibrosis, inflammation, extravasated red blood cells, hemosiderin, and atrophy of pilosebaceous follicles were the usual features (Fig. 3). Intimal proliferation and thickening of arteries, arterioles,

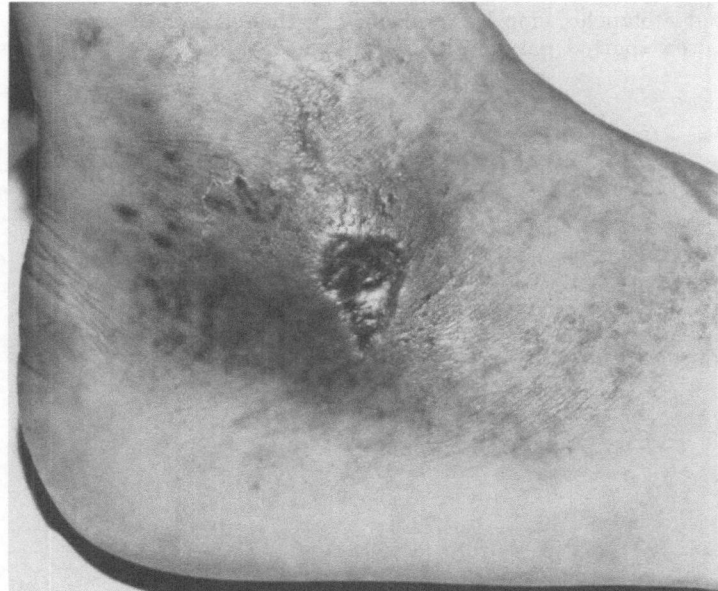

Fig. 1. Stasis dermatitis with ulceration

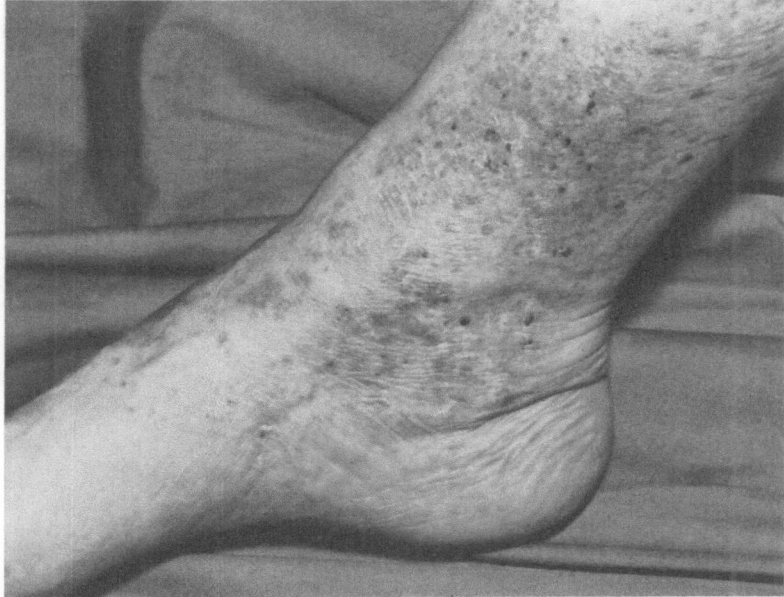

Fig. 2. Atrophie blanche showing new lesions of small purpuric macules and punched-out ulcers as well as old inactive white scars surrounded by hyperpigmentation

capillaries, venules and veins were observed. Fresh frozen thick sections stained
for alkaline-phosphatase showed the blood vessel changes consist of capillary-
endothelial proliferation, elongation, tortuosity, ectasia, and shunting (Fig. 4).
These changes give the spurious appearance of multiple vessels in a nodule when
seen in five to seven microns sections (Fig. 3).

In atrophie blanche, biopsies from early erythematous, telangiectatic, purpuric
lesions showed spotted parakeratosis, slight acanthosis, focal spongiosis, and V-

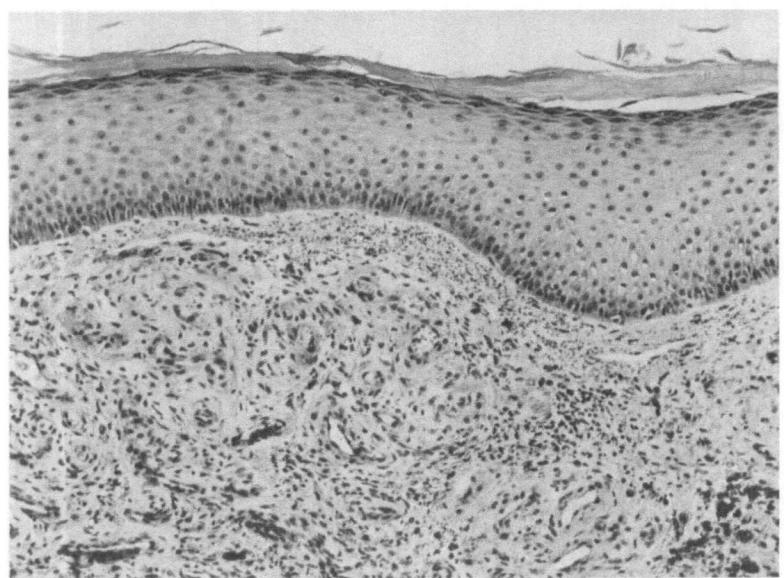

Fig. 3. Stasis dermatitis showing nodules of capillary-endothelial proliferation, inflammation,
fibrosis, and hemosiderin pigment. H and E, X 107

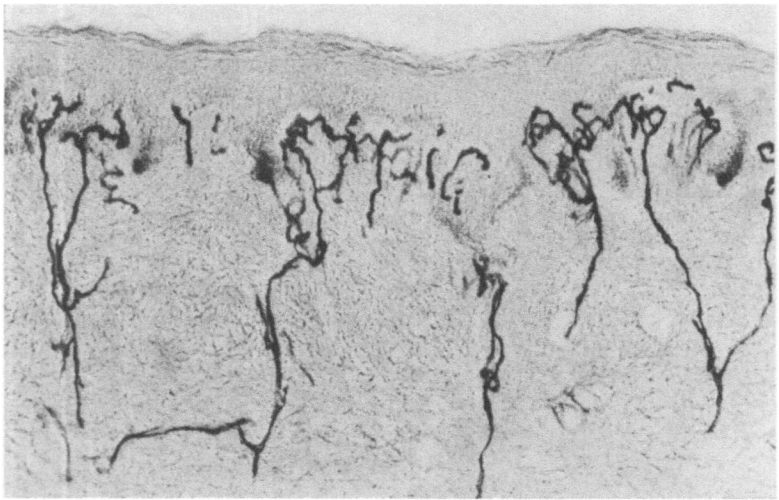

Fig. 4. Stasis dermatitis showing blood vessel changes of capillary-endothelial proliferation,
elongation, tortuosity, ectasia, and shunting. Alkaline-phosphatase, X 58

shaped areas of necrosis involving the epidermis and superficial corium (Fig. 5 A).
The necrotic epidermal cells stained acidophilically, and showed vacuolization,
spongiosis and loss of cohesion, but usually maintained their cell walls. Early
stages sometimes showed inflammation involving the perivascular stroma and
blood vessels walls (Fig. 5B). The blood vessels and sometimes adjacent stroma
showed eosinophilic-staining fibrinoid material (Figs. 5 A and 5 B) which was

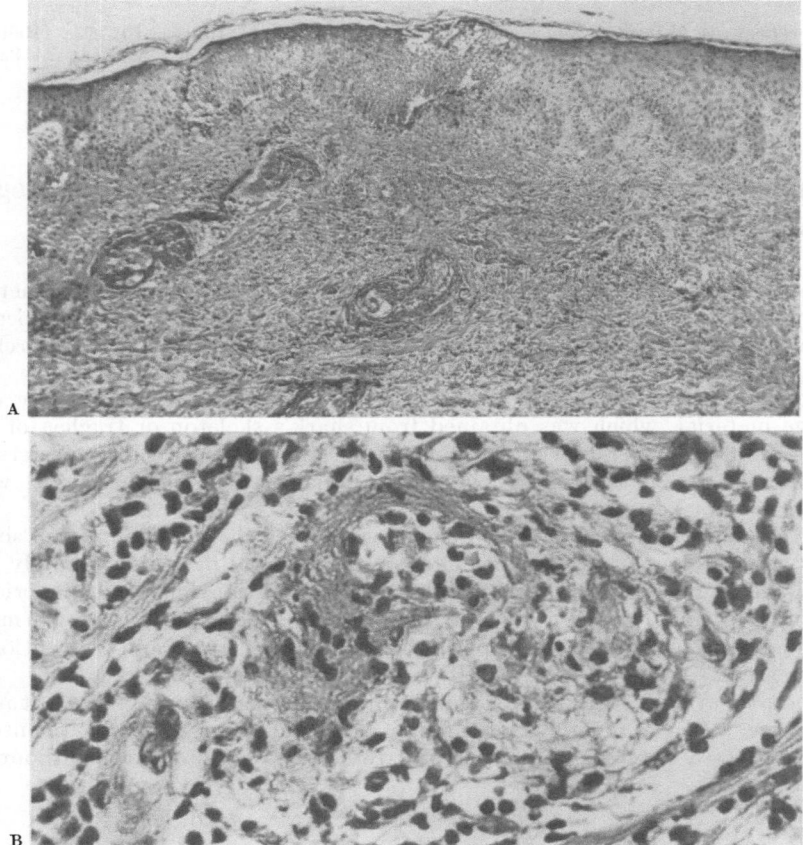

Fig. 5. Atrophie blanche. A, Fibrinoid material is present in blood vessel walls and lumina
in the corium immediately beneath a V-shaped area of necrosis involving the epidermis and
superficial corium. H and E, X 66. B, A higher power of Fig. 5 A showing fibrinoid change
of a vessel wall and cellular infiltration. H and E, X 445

red with Movat's pentachrome stain, blue with phosphotungstic acid hematoxylin,
and periodic acid-Schiff (PAS) positive and diastase resistant. Some of the superficial blood vessels showed fibrinoid thrombi in their lumina, and others were
dilated and engorged with red blood cells. The V-shaped areas of epidermal
necrosis and fibrinoid changes in the subjacent blood vessels and stroma indicate
that a segmental infarction had occurred.

Extravasated red blood cells, hemosiderin pigment, increased amounts of hyaluronic acid in the ground substance, and solid or reticulated PAS positive and
diastase resistant material in the superficial blood vessel walls, were present in both
diseases.

Stasis dermatitis represents a disease of arteries, arterioles, capillaries, venules and veins and there is a predilection for the disease to occur in men with pre-existing vascular diseases. The etiology of atrophie blanche is unknown, but there is a high association with other cutaneous and systemic diseases and the histopathologic features suggest a localized cutaneous hypersensitivity vasculitis. Although there are overlapping features in stasis dermatitis and atrophie blanche, observations indicate these diseases are distinct and separate entities.

References. 1. MARQUES, A. S., and J. H. GRAHAM: Lab. Invest. 15, 1138 (1966). — 2. GRAY, H. R., J. H. GRAHAM, W. C. JOHNSON, and C. F. BURGOON jr.: Arch. Derm. 93, 187 (1966).

Cutaneous Manifestations of Circulatory Disorders of the Legs

A. BOROTA, New York Medical College, New York (USA)

During the last 10 years we studied the effect of several therapeutic methods on decubitus and leg ulcers. Some of them are mentioned by previous speakers and non of them was so effective that we would have discontinued to search for better possibilities.

Recently — about 10 months ago — we started to use a powderized, dry, steril cartilage material, which was obtained from shark's skeleton or trachea of calfs or older animals. This material contains chondroitin mucoitin sulfuric esters and this supposed to be the repository of a granulation stimulating factor, which however has not been isolated.

The comparative study of more then 20 cases, with the same number of similar control cases gave more than satisfactory and in several patients strikingly good results. Although each case, being under our observation for a longer period of time, may serve as his own control, we performed comparative measurments, planometry and series of photographs in both cartilage treated and conventionally treated cases.

The application is simple and painless in almost every case. We did not notice side effects, allergic reactions or foreign body reactions. The treatment was interrupted in a few cases — for several reasons — and resumed without any untoward effect.

Neue Gesichtspunkte in der Behandlung venöser Durchblutungsstörungen

H. WEITGASSER, Ambulatorium für Dermatologie der Steiermärkischen Gebietskrankenkasse für Arbeiter und Angestellte in Graz (Österreich)

Funktionelle und organische Veränderungen am Venensystem der unteren Extremitäten führen zu den hartnäckigen Erkrankungen, deren schwierige therapeutische Beeinflußbarkeit allen denen, die sich mit diesen Leiden beschäftigen, nur zu bekannt ist.

Über die Ursachen dieser Veränderungen wurden jahrzehntelang verschiedenste, oft spekulative Theorien aufgestellt, angefangen von der Annahme einer Insuffizienz der Venenklappen, bis zu hormonellen Dysfunktionen einer oder mehrerer innersekretorischer Drüsen. Ferner wurden statische Momente, erbliche Faktoren, angeborene Bindegewebsschwäche, entzündliche oder degenerative Veränderungen der Venenwände und Störungen im Gleichgewicht innerhalb des vegetativen Nervensystems verantwortlich gemacht.

Immer jedoch waren es die Venen selbst, die man für das Auftreten der Erkrankungen beschuldigte, ohne jedoch die Frage beantworten zu können, wo am Gefäßsystem die auslösende Ursache zu suchen wäre. Diese Fragen klärten in eingehenden Untersuchungen GROTERJAHN u. SEYSS, RAPPERT, LUGER, O. MÜLLER u. a., wobei sie auch auf den arteriellen Schenkel der Endstrombahn hinwiesen und auf dessen Mitbeteiligung bei der Erkrankung der Venen aufmerksam machten. Bestätigung fand diese Annahme durch die vasographischen Beiträge VOGLERS, der die ursächliche Bedeutung arterieller Gefäßschäden für die Entstehung der Venenerweiterung nachweisen konnte.

Trotz dieser nun doch schon länger bekannten Tatsache beschränkte sich die medikamentöse Allgemeintherapie in der Hauptsache auf den Versuch, eine Tonisierung der Venen selbst durchzuführen, wobei der arterielle Teil in therapeutischer Hinsicht meist vernachlässigt wurde.

Ein unter der Versuchsbezeichnung DRA 363 von der Fa. Sandoz A.G. Basel herausgebrachtes Kombinationspräparat schien uns diesen Überlegungen zu entsprechen. Das Präparat enthält Dihydroergocristin sowie die bei der Behandlung von Venenleiden schon lange verwendeten Substanzen Rutin und Aesculin.

Das hier besonders interessierende *Dihydroergocristin* übt eine peripher-sympathico-adrenolytische Wirkung aus, wobei nach pharmakologischen Untersuchungen von FLÜCKIGER u. BALTHASAR an isolierten Venen und Aortenstreifen bei ersteren die tonisierende und bei letzteren die andrenolytische Wirkung überwiegt. Daraus kann ein synergistischer Effekt im Sinne einer besseren peripheren Gewebsdurchblutung abgeleitet werden. Dieser doppelte Angriffspunkt erscheint bei allen Zuständen, die durch eine Hypotonie gewisser Venenbezirke mit entsprechender Blutabsackung charakterisiert sind, wie varicöser Symptomenkomplex, venöses Ulcus crur. etc., therapeutisch wertvoll. In diesem Zusammenhang sei nochmals auf die Untersuchungen von VOGLER hingewiesen, der bei solchen Erkrankungen durch Serienangiographien das Vorhandensein von AV-Anastomosen nachweisen konnte, in deren Folge einerseits die distal gelegenen Capillargebiete eine Minderversorgung aufweisen, andererseits die Venen, welche durch die Anastomosen Blut unter arteriellem Druck aufzunehmen haben, dilatiert werden. Durch intraarterielle Verabfolgung einer Kombination von Dihydroergocornin, -cristin und -kryptin gelang es, den Kreislauf im untersuchten Abschnitt zu normalisieren und neben dem Schluß der arterio-venösen Anastomosen die periphere Strombahn zu eröffnen.

Rutin vermindert wie bekannt die Permeabilität der Capillaren. Für den in Frage stehenden Symptomenkomplex bedeutet dies, daß die gestaute Peripherie entlastet und das hypostatische Ödem beseitigt wird.

Aesculin, die dritte Komponente von DRA 363, unterstützt die Rutinwirkung, indem es ebenfalls die Permeabilität der Capillargefäße herabsetzt, wobei die Wirkung wahrscheinlich auf einer Hemmung der Hyaluronidase beruht, die durch Abbau der Hyaluronsäure in der interstitiellen Kittsubstanz die Permeabilität erhöht. Bei nur ambulant durchführbaren Untersuchungen ist schon die Beurteilung des Schweregrades einer Venenerkrankung an sich schwierig, zumal nicht selten dazu Diskrepanzen zwischen dem objektiven Befund und den subjektiven Angaben der Patienten bestehen. Wohl kann, wie oben erwähnt, in klassischen pharmakologischen Studien die Wirksamkeit des einen oder anderen Präparates auf das in Frage stehende Gefäßsystem nachgewiesen werden, wohl können im klinischen Rahmen bei statischen Patienten entsprechende Untersuchungen vor, während und nach der Behandlung durchgeführt werden, bei einer ambulanten Prüfung müssen diese Erfahrungen jedoch empirisch gefunden werden.

Diese Überlegungen waren vorauszuschicken, um aufzuzeigen, wie schwierig die Beurteilung der medikamentösen Behandlung venöser Durchblutungsstörungen auf breiter Basis ist.

Nun zu unseren eigenen Untersuchungen. Wir haben in einem Zeitraum von 2 Jahren das erwähnte Versuchspräparat DRA 363 vorwiegend bei Patienten mit folgenden Indikationen zur Anwendung gebracht: Prävaricöses Stadium, varicöser Symptomenkomplex mit und ohne Ulceration, postthrombotisches Syndrom.

Zunächst wurde in einer *Pilot-Study* an 39 Patienten das Präparat mit einer der Schwere des Falles angepaßten Dosierung von dreimal 1 bis dreimal 2 Dragées oder dreimal 20 bis dreimal 50 Tropfen täglich verabreicht. Im allgemeinen wurde zu Beginn höher dosiert, um dann im weiteren Verlauf auf die gerade notwendige Erhaltungsdosis herabzugehen. Die Behandlungsdauer erstreckte sich von 3 Wochen bis zu 8 bis 10 Wochen.

Die Verträglichkeit war gut, vereinzelt angegebene Magenbeschwerden konnten nach Rückgang der Dosis zum Abklingen gebracht werden. Bei drei Pat. war eine verlängerte Menstruation feststellbar, so daß wir bei Frauen, die in der Anamnese über Menstruationsbeschwerden klagten, in dieser Zeit das Präparat absetzten.

Bei 28 von den 39 Fällen war ein sehr guter bis guter Erfolg zu verzeichnen, bei sieben nur ein mäßiger und bei vier ein negativer bzw. waren diese Fälle nicht beurteilbar.

Um diese ermutigenden Ergebnisse zu erhärten, führten wir mangels anderer für die ambulante Praxis anwendbarer Untersuchungsmethoden eine *Doppelblindstudie* mit Placebo und *sequentialanalytischer Auswertung* durch. Es wurden hierzu Paare mit möglichst gleichem Alter, Geschlecht und vor allem gleicher Symptomatik gebildet, von denen kontemporär ein Pat. dreimal täglich 2 Dragées des Wirkstoffes und der andere dreimal täglich 2 Dragées des Placebos durch 3 Wochen einzunehmen hatte. Außer dieser Behandlung wurde nur die an der Ambulanz übliche Lokalbehandlung mit indifferenten Salben, Kompressionsverbänden usw. durchgeführt. Die Auswertung durch eine dritte Person, die nicht an den Untersuchungen beteiligt war, erfolgte an Hand des für die Sequentialanalyse bestehenden Schemas (2 α = 0,05), wobei jeweils beurteilt wurde, welcher Patient des Paares besser auf die bei ihm durchgeführte Behandlung angesprochen hatte.

Die Resultate wurden fortlaufend in ein Sequentialanalysennetz eingetragen. Die Studie wurde erst nach Überschreiten einer Grenze des Diagramms beendet. Paare mit gleicher Beurteilung der Wirkung wurden ausgeschlossen.

Nachdem dadurch der therapeutische Wert des Präparates mittels statistischer Methoden bewiesen werden konnte, kam das Präparat in einem *dritten Stadium* der Untersuchung in breiterem Umfang zur Anwendung.

Zusammenfassend läßt sich über das neue Kombinationspräparat DRA 363 sagen, daß aufbauend auf die neuen Erkenntnisse einer arterio-venösen Ursache der Venenerkrankungen, eine kausale Allgemeintherapie durchführbar ist. Die Untersuchungen von KOCH u. WIRTLER u. a. sowie unsere hier mitgeteilten bestätigen, daß eine konsequent durchgeführte Behandlung mit DRA 363 auch von Erfolg begleitet ist.

Angiolopathien und Unterschenkeldermatosen

N. KLÜKEN, Universitäts-Hautklinik Essen (Deutschland)

Das Verhalten der Durchblutung der Unterschenkel wird als lokalisationsdeterminierender Faktor für verschiedene Dermatosen angesehen. Dabei kann von dem so allgemein und unverbindlich gehaltenen Terminus Durchblutung in seinen möglichen Variationen die befriedigende Klärung solcher pathogenetischer Zusammenhänge nicht erwartet werden. Unter dem hier zur Diskussion stehenden

pathogenetischen Aspekt erfährt der Faktor Durchblutung, je nach Art der Zirkulationsstörung eine unterschiedliche, unter Umständen sogar gegensätzliche
Wertung.

So ist seit langem bekannt, daß venöse Leiden — wie der varicöse Symptomenkomplex oder das postthrombophlebitische Syndrom — zum lokalisations-deter-
minierenden Faktor werden. An sich an jeder beliebigen Lokalisation anzutreffende
Dermatosen können bei venösen Zirkulationsstörungen in deren Bereich bevorzugt
oder sogar ausschließlich auftreten. Als Beispiele seien der Lichen ruber planus und
die Psoriasis vulgaris ausschließlich im Verlauf von Varicen sowie der nur am
Unterschenkel beim Status varicosus lokalisierte Lupus vulgaris genannt. Der
pathogenetische Faktor unter dem Bilde des Lupus erythematosus-squamosus ist
in diesen Fällen nicht die Mangeldurchblutung, sondern eine durch gestörten venösen Rückfluß bedingte passive Hyperämie im Rahmen einer venösen Dekompensation, gerne auch als Stauung bezeichnet.

Mit solchen venösen Zirkulationsstörungen werden auch Hautveränderungen
aus dem Formenkreis des Ekzems in pathogenetischen Zusammenhang gebracht,
die sog. Stauungsdermatose. Dieser Terminus ist klinisch nicht klar zu umreißen,
und oft genug beobachtet man, daß irgendwelche Hautveränderungen bei der
venösen Dekompensation als Stauungsdermatose angesehen werden. Bei näherer
Differenzierung gelingt es meist, diese Hautveränderungen als eine Dermoepider-
mitis bzw. als ein mikrobielles Ekzem oder als ein allergisches Ekzem abzuklären.
Andererseits tritt längst nicht regelmäßig eine sog. Stauungsdermatose bei venöser
Dekompensation auf. Das chronisch-rezidivierende Erysipel ist ein weiteres Beispiel für eine Verknüpfung einer am Unterschenkel lokalisierten Dermatose mit der
venösen Rückflußstörung.

Bei Zuständen echter Mangeldurchblutung auf dem Boden vornehmlich arteriell lokalisierter Gefäßprozesse sind Dermatosen — abgesehen vielleicht von einer
Tinea pedis — nicht regelmäßig nachzuweisen. Aus dem bisher Gesagten ergibt
sich, daß venöse Leiden mit in der Epidermis bzw. im Corium lokalisierten Erkrankungen verknüpft sein können. Auf Grund eines solchen kombinierten Zusammentreffens gefäßbedingter Morbi mit den genannten Dermatosen wird der pathogenetische Zusammenhang als bewiesen angesehen und oft die sich hieraus er-
gebende Problematik übersehen. Denn wie häufig kommt doch eine venöse Dekompensation ohne diese erwähnten Dermatosen vor und warum? Diese Fragen
können zur Zeit noch nicht befriedigend beantwortet werden.

Eine analoge Problematik ergibt sich bei den Endstrombahnerkrankungen, den
Angiolopathien. Es gibt Krankheitsbilder, die wir den akrozyanotischen Zustands-
bildern zuordnen und die praktisch nie mit makromorphologischen Veränderungen
im Bereich der Cutis bzw. der Epidermis einhergehen, so bei der Acrocyanosis sui
generis oder der Erythrocyanosis crurum puellarum. Dies ist um so überraschender,
als bei diesen Krankheitszuständen eine ausgeprägte Hyperhidrosis vorliegt, die
doch als begünstigender Faktor bei der Entstehung gewisser Dermatosen, so der
Tinea, angesehen werden kann.

Im Gegensatz hierzu liegen bei der Dermatopathia cyanotica cruris (Rost), bei
der der Acrocyanosis analogem pathologisch-anatomischem Substrat des atonisch-
hypertonischen Symptomenkomplexes des obersten cutanen Gefäßgeflechtes regelmäßig Hautveränderungen vor, die sich in einer Verhornungsanomalie, nämlich in
einer grob-lamellösen Abhebung des Stratum corneum zeigt. Daneben besteht
flächenhaftes Nässen und Infiltration als Ausdruck exsudativer und proliferativer
Prozesse der Cutis.

Die pathogenetische Verknüpfung solcher cutanen Prozesse mit Zirkulationsstörungen in den Endstrombahnbereichen drängt sich auf Grund klinischer Fakten

zwar auf, ist aber in ihrer Beantwortung mehr als problematisch. Warum treten in einem Fall bei gleichem pathologisch-anatomischen Substrat der Endstrombahn-gefäße Hautveränderungen auf und warum im anderen Falle nicht? Zur Auslösung der epidermalen Erscheinungen bedarf es daher wohl noch anderer uns bislang noch unbekannter Gegebenheiten. Das pathologische Verhalten der Gefäße im Endstrombahnbereich kann daher nur als *ein* Realisationsfaktor angesehen werden, nicht aber als ausschließliches pathogenetisches Prinzip.

Noch schwieriger gestalten sich die pathogenetischen Zusammenhänge bei einer weiteren Angiolopathie, nämlich bei der Cyanosis circumscripta e lipoma. Das Krankheitsbild ist charakterisiert durch umschriebene Gefäßveränderungen, die denjenigen der akrozyanotischen Zustandsbilder entsprechen. Sie sind circumscript im zyanotisch veränderten Hautbereich über einer lipomartigen Wucherung des subcutanen Fettgewebes lokalisiert. Angiographisch findet man im Bereich dieser Veränderungen eine Vermehrung der Hautgefäße. Im Röntgenbild zeigt sich fast ein angiomartiger Charakter.

Auch bei dieser Angiolopathie drängt sich die Frage auf: Stehen die Gefäßveränderungen mit der umschriebenen Vergrößerung des subcutanen Fettgewebes in einem pathogenetischen Zusammenhang? Die Beantwortung dieser Frage ist auch deshalb so problematisch, weil unsere Kenntnisse um die Ätiopathogenese dieses Krankheitsbildes noch recht unzulänglich sind. Bei einer anderen Angiolopathie, nämlich der Erythrocyanosis crurum puellarum, ist konstitutionell die Tela subcutanea im Bereich der unteren Extremitäten gleichmäßig vermehrt und verdickt. Diesem konstitutionellen Faktor messen wir bei der Erythrocyanosis crurum puellarum eine pathogenetische Bedeutung bei. Bei der umschriebenen, lipomartigen Verdickung der Subcutis bei der Cyanosis circumscripta e lipoma möchten wir die Veränderungen der Endstrombahngefäße in Analogie zum vorhergenannten Krankheitsbild als in der Pathogenese sekundäres Geschehen ansehen.

The Pathogenesis of Nodular Panniculitis of Calves

P. BARTÁK, Dermatological Clinic, Faculty of Hygiene, Prague (Czechoslovakia)

The nodular Panniculitis of calves is considered an allergic vasculitis that is induced by traumatic or toxiallergic factors. Its pathogenesis has not been investigated more closely. We have gathered 50 cases and these facts have come out of their clinical and mainly pathohistological analysis:

1. the disease was manifested as violet, painful, indurated plaques localized mainly on side parts of the calves,

2. there were mainly affected women (45:5), most frequently in the forth decade,

3. 88% of patients were working standing in cold rooms or on a cold floor,

4. 78% of patients were suffering from frequent tonsillitis for their whole lives and in nine cases from rheumatism, too. The history of tuberculosis was with three patients,

5. just before the origin of the disease 74% of patients came through light feverish disease (cold, tonsillitis, flu),

6. the dominant pathohistological finding in all cases was vasculitis on little venules in the periphery parts of fat lobules. The changes were of various intensity from a simple oedema of endothelial cells and the erythrocytic extravasations to fibrinoid degeneration of the wall with granulomatosic formations of the neighbourhood and fibroplasia.

We consider the localisation of pathological vascular changes in the periphery of the fat lobules a very considerable one for the origin of the patho-histological picture. It is a known fact that the fat lobules is being supplied by means of the solitary adductive arteriole which is dipped into the fat lobule and is distributed very soon into the capillar network. It itself is connected into a rich venous network localised in the periphery of the fat lobule only.

This division has its functional consequenses that are manifested especially in the practice of plastic surgery.

This density of the venous network with the possibility of collaterals is the base of the difference between panniculitis and erythema induratum. We don't find any central necrosis typical for erythema induratum. But we do not mind that panniculitis and erythema induratum are two different diseases. On the contrary, we consider their substance to be identical. The difference between them lies in the fact only that the solitary adductive arteriole is affected by erythema induratum and its obliteration causes necessarily necrosis comprising variously large part in the middle of the fat lobule.

Our further laboratory and clinical findings confirm contemporary aspects that it is a matter of an allergic vasculitis. It originates on calves because of the fact that varicoses, permanent cold — especially with the women — and the width of poikilothermic cover of lower extremities form locus minoris resistentiae. It may be the seat of the allergic reaction just in the walls of little vessels in the periphery of the fat lobules. This is the way how the panniculitis on the calves originates.

This explanation seems to be in a considerably scale a mere simplification of the biological reality. Nevertheless it forms the fundamentals to which we can add further knowledge till the whole problem is cleared out.

We can take it for a starting point when looking for the substance and mutual relations of the other nodular calf-diseases.

Histopathological Studies on Inflammatory Nodular Diseases in Lower Leg, Especially Concerning on Vascular Change

T. MIYAZAWA, Department of Dermatology, Sendai Teishin Hospital, and Y. SASAI, Department of Dermatology, Tohoku University School of Medicine, Sendai (Japan)

The diseases of which the chief symptom is the inflammatory nodules in the lower leg were observed on the view-point of the vascular change in the dermal and subcutaneous layers, esp. in the subcutaneous layers, and the theory of circulatory disorder as the pathogenesis of these diseases was experimentally studied. In this report, the histopathological findings and the experimental results are presented.

The studies were made with 56 cases: the clinical diagnosis showed that 10 cases of erythema nodosum, 8 cases of erythema induratum, 36 cases of "intermediate type" and 2 cases of vasculitis allergica cutis. The cases with which Behcet's disease, Weber-Christian's disease and sarcoidosis had been proved were excluded.

1. Kind of affected Blood Vessel

The vascular involvement was found in all our cases. When the kind of affected vessels were classified, it was proved that the capillary tube was affected in

37 cases, the vein including the venule in 31 cases, the arteriole in 12 cases and the artery in 2 cases. The main histological differentiation between the artery and the vein depends upon the distribution of the elastic fibers in the tunica media. In the former the elastic fibers are not found while in the latter they are found to be annular.

2. Inflammation degree of Involvement of Vessel

The degree of involvement of vessels is not so great. In both the arteriole and vein the change of the intima is marked which develops the features of endothelial proliferation and intima thickening. The change of the tunica media and adventitia are not great, and the cellular infiltration is slight in most cases. The involvement of the vein is greater than that of the artery, and that is observed at the same time in one specimen. The capillary tube swells in most cases, and fibrinoid degeneration is found in seven cases among them. Fibrinoid degeneration is also found in a case of arteriolitis. Obliterative change is observed in ten cases; four cases show "granulomatous panphlebitis", while the other cases are full of blood cells.

3. Specific Histological Findings on Each Disease

It is difficult to differentiate between erythema nodosum and erythema induratum by a kind of the affected vessels and a greatness of the affected veins. The degree of vasculitis is greater in erythema induratum than that in erythema nodosum. As the remarkable findings of erythema induratum, a proliferation of capillary wall in the deep dermal and subcutaneous layers may be taken up. When this proliferation develops further, vascularization or degeneration may occur in the very part. If 36 cases of "intermediate type" are histologically examined on the basis of the degree of vasculitis, the presence of the proliferation of capillary wall and the nature of panniculitis, about half the number may be thought of as erythema induratum.

It may be possible that some of the cases in which obliterative phlebitis is found are diagnosed as erythema induratum, but it may be proper that most of them are diagnosed as vasculitis nodularis in due consideration of the clinical findings. From the above, the disease characterized by the presence of inflammatory nodules in lower leg may be classified into erythema nodosum, vasculitis nodularis and erythema induratum.

4. Exciting Factor of the Diseases

The above vascular change (the change in more often caused in the vein than in the artery and degree of vasculitis is not so great) and such the localization of the diseases as the lower leg being considered, the circulatory disorder may be thought of as the exciting factor of the diseases. When the blood vessel of pinna of the rabbit which was immunized by additional FREUND's complete adjuvant to BSA or guinea pig's serum is ligated, and the antigen is intravenously injected, the petechiae is observed in the peripheral area of the vessel which was ligated in 15 to 24 h. This phenomenon is almost controlled by giving vascular tonic, Etamsylate. The petechiae is not caused under the non-ligated condition. It is believed that this experimental result may suggest that the circulatory disorder must be a exciting factor of vascular involvement.

The Treatment of Tropical Ulcer with an Antibacterial Soap and Topically Applied Sugar

R. A. Osbourn, Department of Medicine (Division of Dermatology), Georgetown University Medical Center, Washington, D.C. (USA), B. Benjamin, University of the West Indies, Kingston (Jamaica), and B. E. Ellickson, Armour Research Laboratory, Chicago, Illinois (USA)

Tropical ulcer is a term that has been applied to a variety of ulcerative skin lesions occurring in the warmer climes. While these have included syphilis, yaws, cutaneous leishmaniasis, and cutaneous diphtheria, in the strict sense, it should apply to nonspecific pyogenic and phagedenic ulcerations occurring chiefly on the lower extremities in natives living in the tropics [1, 2].

A vivid description of such lesions has been given by Pillsbury et al. [3], "Their appearance is quite characteristic, having a remarkably circular outline, with a distinctly elevated and undermined bluish red border. The ulcer has been likened to a cup; a foul smelling mucopurulent slough, often blood-tinged, is generally present in the davity. Removal of the slough reveals granulation tissue".

The exciting cause is some type of trauma such as laceration, bruise abrasion, burn or insect bite. The predisposing causes are poor hygiene, malnutrition, vitamin deficiency, anemia, parasitic infestation and other chronic internal diseases. In the older age group stasis in the circulation of the lower extremities, often plays an important role in causation.

The bacterial flora of such ulcers exhibits a variety of organisms. *Staphylococcus aureus* and hemolytic streptococci are frequently found. Other organismus include *Escherichia coli*, *Pseudomonas pyocyaneus*, *Bacillus proteus* and the fusopirochetal organismus. However, not all of these latter have been shown to be pathogenic. Because of the infectious nature of tropical ulcer therapy has usually depended upon local or systemic use of antibiotics or both. When it was practical, therapy was also directed toward the underlying causes.

Since Barnes [4] in a dramatic exhibit showed remarkable healing of decubitus ulcers by the local use of sucrose (granulated sugar) even though in some cases the systemic disease of the patient had a hopeless prognosis, one of us felt such therapy might be of value in tropical ulcers. Because Barnes [4] found he got better results when he cleansed the ulcers with a detergent containing hexachlorophene, we decided to use a soap containing this agent as a part of our therapy.

The use of sugar in the therapy of ulcers did not originate with Barnes. There are occasional nonspecific references to its use in the older literature and Trimble [5] traced its use back to 1957, while Perelman [6] reported that it was used in 1941. More than 60 years ago Hostalrich [7] in French Indo China reported on the rapid healing of ulcers with 50% sugar solution. More recently Rostenberg et al. [8] have shown that sugar paste (containing about 30% sucrose) is beneficial in several types of skin ulcers including stasis and decubitus ulcers.

Method of Study

This study was undertaken in Kingston, Jamaica, because such ulcers are quite prevalent there. One factor which contributes to such a frequency is the use of reclaimed galvanized corrugated iron roofing for fencing. There are many sharp edges and nail holes in the metal, and children frequently traumatize their legs against same.

Since soap containing hexachlorophene was to be used, it was decided to do a double blind evaluation of such germicidal soap at the same time the sugar therapy was being evaluated. Accordingly, the soap manufacturer who cooperated in this study supplied number coded identical bars, one group containing 0.75% hexachlorophene and 0.75% 3,4,4, trichlorocarbanilide. The codes were not known to any of the investigators, nurses, nor obviously to the patients. The patients were divided into four groups for therapy and a fifth untreated control group. It was planned to study 100 patients but because of the difficulties in obtaining follow-up, only 72 patients completed the program. They were divided as follows:

Table 1

Group No.	No. of Cases	Type of Therapy
I	18	Control soap and sugar
II	14	Antibacterial soap and sugar
III	16	Control soap and dry dressing
IV	17	Antibacterial soap and dry dressing
V	5	Untreated controls
	2	Treated controls — acriflavin locally and penicillin I.M.

Technique

The use of sugar in ulcers is very simple. In very large ulcers some degree of debridement may be necessary but in most ulcers this is not really required. The lesions were cleansed with soap and water, gently dried with sterile gauze flats, then sugar in rather copious amount was applied and covered with sterile gauze. Ideally the dressing should be changed once a day, or if the lesion be very exudative, two or more times a day. However, in our case, it was only possible to change the dressings every other day.

Bacterial Culture

An attempt was made to culture every ulcer before and after therapy, but because of follow-up dufficulties, it was only possible to get such cultures in 42 cases. In most cases, the organism grown was coagulase positive Staphlococcus aureus. In several cases Echerichia coli was isolated, but we considered this to be nonpathogenic. The results of such cultures are given in Tab. 2.

Table 2

Group	No. of initial Cultures (Staph aureus)	No. of same which became negative on final culture	% Rendered Free of Pathogenic Bacteria
I (control soap)	12	6	50
II (antibacterial soap)	10	7	70
III (control soap)	8	3	37
IV (antibacterial soap)	12	8	75

Clinical Results

The patients were studied for a period of 8 weeks. Some of these patients healed in less than 8 weeks but those that did not heal in that period of time were considered treatment failures. The results are given in Tab. 3.

Table 3

Group	Therapy	No. of Cases	No. Healed	No. not Healed	% Healed
I	Control soap and sucrose	18	6	12	33.0
II	Antibacterial soap and sucrose	14	9	5	64.3
III	Control soap and dry dressing	16	6	10	37.5
IV	Antibacterial soap and dry dressing	17	9	8	53.0
V	Untreated controls	5	0	5	0
	Treated controls (Acriflavin locally Penicillin I.M.)	2	0	2	0

Discussion

There were several difficulties encountered in this study and therefore, this should be considered as a preliminary report. The cases were outpatients and were not under the controlled conditions such as the patients reported by BARNES [4]. The patients could not be seen every day; hence their dressings could not be changed as often as they should have been. Ideal therapy would have been to change dressing and put on fresh sugar every day or more often if necessary, expecially for the first 1 to 2 weeks. A great difficulty was experienced because of the coarseness of the sugar available for the study. The cases with which we were familiar had used the usual granulated sugar of the United States market and this was much finer than that which was obtained in Jamaica. Late in the study finer sugar was used and the clinical impression was that it promoted faster healing. In fact, in some cases the coarser sugar was found to be irritating.

However, in spite of these difficulties there was 64.3% healing in Group II. This was the group using the sugar and the antibacterial soap. The next best healing rate was in the group using the antibacterial soap and dry dressings (Group III). The groups using the soap without the antibacterial agents showed the poorest healing. These findings then indicate that sugar applied locally does promote healing of tropical ulcers, particularly when it is used in conjunction with cleansing of such ulcers by a containing hexachlorophene and trichlorocarbanilide. Since this was a double blind study, it is indicated that soap containing such antibacterial agents possess an advantage over the same soap without those agents in the type of therapy herein advocated.

References. 1. ANDREWS, G. A., and A. N. DOMONKOS: Diseases of the Skin, Ed. 5, pp. 229 to 230. Philadelphia: W. B. Saunders Co. 1963. — 2. ASH, J. E., and S. SPITZ: Pathology of Tropical Diseases, pp. 338—339. Philadelphia: W. B. Saunders Co. 1945. — 3. PILLSBURY, D. M., W. B. SHELLEY, and A. M. KLIGMAN: Dermatology, pp. 495—496. Philadelphia: W. B. Saunders Co. 1956. — 4. BARNES, J. W. (an Exhibit): Treatment of Skin and Soft Tissue Ulcers with Granulated Sugar, shown at Scientific Assembly of the Medical Society of the District of Columbia, Washington, D. C. Nov. 22—24, 1965. — 5. TRIMBLE, G. X.: J. Amer. med. Ass. **197**, 790 (1966). — 6. PERELMAN, H.: J. Amer. med. Ass. **198**, 489 (1966). — 7. HOSTALRICH, M.: Bull. Soc. Méd.-Chir. dl'Indo Chine (Hanoi et Haifong) **V**, 14 (1914). — 8. ROSTENBERG, A., E. R. WASSERMANN, and R. S. MEDANSKY: Arch. Derm. **78**, 94 (1958).

Main Theme VII   **Regeneration and Transplantation of the Skin**

Régénération et transplantation de la peau

Regeneración y transplantación de la piel

Regeneration und Transplantation der Haut

Organizer

FR. FLARER, Italy

Presidents

P. CERUTTI, Italy

H. EL HEFNAWI, U.A.R.

FR. KOGOJ, Yugoslavia

H. O. PERRY, USA

Delegate of the Organization Committee

A. LEINBROCK, Germany

Reports

Regeneration and Transplantation Experiments with Lower Vertebrate Skin as a Guide to Possible Endogenous Sources of Localised Pathogenesis in Man

I. W. WHIMSTER, Department of Pathology, St. Thomas's Hospital Medical School, London (England)

Introduction

Relatively seldom is the whole skin involved simultaneously and uniformly in any endogenous disease process. On the contrary it is usual for certain areas only to be involved, while other skin, apparently similar and immediately adjacent to the diseased areas, remains unaffected. Localised distributions of endogenous disease affecting internal organs have been studied by morbid anatomists since the beginning of pathology. Whenever the localisation has become explicable in terms of morbid anatomy and physiology the nature and pathogenesis of the disease has become better understood. For example, once the distribution of localised areas of necrosis are related anatomically to occlusive vascular lesions their pathogenesis is established as ischaemic. It can be stated as a broad generalisation that no endogenous disease which is characterised by a localised distribution of its lesions has yet had its pathogenesis satisfactorily explained until the cause of the localisation has first been determined. Skin provides the most numerous, varied and easily observed examples of localised distribution occurring in all types of endogenous disease. Almost nothing is known about the factors responsible for this localisation and there is no satisfactory understanding of the pathogenesis of any localised endogenous skin disease. These two fields of ignorance are directly related: the pathogenesis of localised skin disease will not be understood until its distribution can be explained. Understanding of all bodily mechanisms capable of causing localised variations in skin behaviour is an essential prelude to the search for sources of localised endogenous pathogenesis.

My research is based on this proposition. It is aimed at identifying whatever mechanisms exist within the vertebrate body whereby any area of its skin may be caused to behave differently from another, in any way, at any time, normally or abnormally.

Problems of Disease Distribution

1. Individual Small Focal Lesions. Most dermatoses consist basically of macules, papules or vesicles and variously grouped aggregates of them. Each individual lesion is an area of skin a few millimetres across, throughout which disease affects many thousands of cells. The disease may be of any type and the tissue predominantly affected may be dermal, epidermal or neuro-ectodermal, but yet the individual lesions are remarkably constant in size. Although skin tissues so commonly become diseased in circumscribed macular areas we recognise no such normal subdivisions of skin, intermediate between the single cell and the whole body.

Localised vascular occlusion may kill all the cells in a correspondingly focal area of skin, but this vascular form of pathogenic cutaneous subdivision is the only one we understand. The majority of dermatoses cannot be attributed to ischaemia, and therefore we require knowledge about some other forms of cutaneous subdivision which will explain the macular focality of non-ischaemic lesions.

2. Herpetiform Grouping. Multiple focal lesions are often not scattered evenly over the body but grouped. This grouping clearly reflects some aspect of pathogenesis which requires to be understood. If a lazy flea bites repeatedly without walking far between meals, the result is a herpetiform group of identical papules, separated by normal unbitten skin. What endogenous factor can be blamed for the herpetiform grouping of non-parasitic lesions ? In herpes zoster it can probably be attributed to the patterns of cutaneous innervation but very similar grouping occurs with other lesions whose neural associations are less obvious. To understand the pathogenesis of lesions which may show herpetiform grouping it is first necessary to establish the anatomical and physiological basis of the herpetiform areas themselves.

3. Linear and Segmental Grouping. More sophisticated than simple herpetiform grouping is the linear arrangement of focal lesions. Sometimes these lines appear segmental and sometimes not. At present there is no satisfactory explanation of what such linear patterns really represent and of how they come about. We therefore remain ignorant of the pathogenic mechanisms by which they can become exclusively involved in such a wide range of disease.

4. Regional Distribution. Certain endogenous lesions regularly affect characteristic regions and spare others. Acne vulgaris is a disease of pilo-sebaceous follicles but only of those on certain parts of the body. Many other endogenous diseases share with acne the habit of preferentially or exclusively affecting certain anatomical regions of skin. In no instance can we account precisely for this differential regional distribution. We cannot even explain the origin of the many normal and conspicuous regional differences in skin, such as those between the palm and the back of the hand. There are hair follicles on most parts of the body but we cannot say how those of the scalp always come to be different from those of the forehead and different again from the eyebrows. Until we can explain the origin of normal regional variations in skin we cannot hope to explain regional disease.

5. Symmetrical Distribution. The most challenging illustrations of our ignorance about disease distribution are those cases in which localised lesions appear with bilateral symmetry, which is too perfect to be fortuitous and yet cannot be attributed to exogenous factors. All the intrinsic skin tissues; epithelium, pigment cells and connective tissues; undergo their embryonic development separately on either side of the body. The cells of two symmetrical areas of skin, away from the midline, have had no direct contact with each other since the early cleavages of the ovum. We must seek an endogenous pathogenic mechanism which is capable of selectively afflicting two widely separated areas of skin, whose only common factor is that they occupy mirror image positions on the body.

Comparative Study

Since the same distribution patterns occur repeatedly, not only in different patients but in different diseases, it seems reasonable to suppose that their production is dependent on mechanisms which are universally present in man, though not apparent unless demonstrated by their selective involvment in disease.

Normal human skin shows no subdivision into macular units and no circumscribed herpetiform or linear areas. Intersegmental boundaries are imperceptible, and apart from regional differences there are few positive indications of bilateral symmetry.

Normal regional differences are established irreversibly in embryonic life and the other pathogenic types of distribution pattern appear only in the unpredictable circumstances of disease. The difficulty of investigating the origins of such patterns directly in man are therefore obvious; but the necessity of understanding them is paramount.

Lower vertebrates offer greater scope for the investigation of localised cutaneous differentials. No direct homology is claimed between the normal differentials of morphology and colour in animal skin and the diseases of man. It is suggested only that fundamentally similar mechanisms may be involved in bringing about the distribution of normal and abnormal localised cutaneous differentials.

Lower vertebrate skin is readily available for experiment. It shows normal subdivisions into small unit areas, each with some degree of structural and functional independence. It shows conspicuous and characteristic regional variations in colour and texture on different parts of the body, as well as more localised and circumscribed variations within these regions. It commonly shows linear patterns; and intersegmental boundaries are frequently visible, morphologically and as differences in colour. Furthermore, the skin of many animals shows a degree of bilateral symmetry in morphology and colour pattern which is almost perfect.

It is clear that in these animals there are bodily mechanisms capable of bringing about selective localised differences in the morphogenesis and function of intrinsic skin tissues. These differences are brought about with an immensely wide range of variations, but yet with such a precise degree of control that it is possible to identify almost any species of vertebrate by its patterns of cutaneous morphology and colour.

This combination of variation and control over the production of localised differentials in their skin makes these animals good subjects for investigating how such control is exercised.

Experimental Study

The greatest advantage of lower vertebrates over mammals and man for this kind of investigation is their ability to regenerate new skin, after full thickness excision, which is not only of almost normal texture and colour but which reproduces localised differentials which were present at the site before excision. The mechanism for producing these differentials is not something exclusive to a particular stage of embryonic development but present and potentially active throughout life. It can therefore be studied in adult animals.

The regeneration of localised differentials in new skin, formed after full thickness excision, suggests that the responsible mechanism does not originate within the skin itself, but projects its influence on the skin from deeper in the body. Transplantation experiments provide even more striking evidence of this unidentified deep source of site-specific cutaneous influence. In the toad *Bufo marinus* the dorsal skin is brown with glandular nodules and horny spines, while the ventral skin is almost white and relatively smooth. The epidermis, the dermis and the pigment cells are all formed and function differently in the two regions. Full thickness dorsal and ventral wounds regenerate new skin with the appropriate regional characteristics of colour and texture. When full thickness ventral skin is transplanted to the dorsum and a full thickness wound is made in the centre of this graft, the animal is left with a wound situated on the dorsum but marginated by ventral skin. The new skin which forms in this wound develops dorsal characteristics of colour and texture. Something emanating from the site of the wound dictates the way in which all the regenerating skin tissues will grow and differentiate, although this is opposite to the way of the marginal skin from which most of the regenerating tissues are derived.

These examples demonstrate the power and versatility of site-specific tissue-controlling mechanisms which can influence the skin. If similar mechanisms were present in the human body, and if parts of them functioned abnormally, they might account for some of the otherwise inexplicable distributions of apparently "spontaneous" endogenous localised lesions in skin. It is hoped that further investigation of these skin-controlling mechanisms, and attempts to determine their nature and source by experimental interference with their activity, will lead to their identification.

It will then become possible to look for their counterparts in the human body and to assess their possible role in the pathogenesis of localised endogenous disease.

The Cell Turnover of Human Epidermis

A. Tosti, Istituto di Dermatologia sperimentale dell'Università di Palermo (Italy)

According to the properties of its cells, the epidermis may be considered as a system composed by three compartments with distinct functional and topographic features: a stem compartment, formed of the basal layer whose mitotic activity represents the fundamental refurnishing of the whole system; an expanding compartment, corresponding to the deep spinous layer in which differentiation is still compatible with some mitotic activity; a terminal compartment, formed of the whole postmitotic cell population.

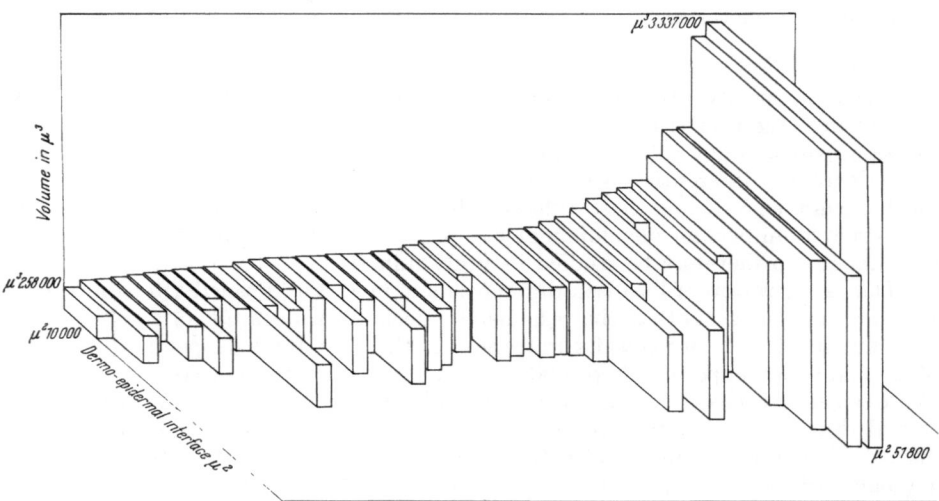

Fig. 1. Tissue volume and area of epidermal inner surface in 43 specimens of human epidermis ranged from hypoplasia to hyperacanthosis. Values referred to a 10.000 μ^2 area unit of keratinized surface

The term of steady balance has been used to mean the harmonic ratio between cell supply and cell elimination in the three compartments. This term, however, appears somewhat misleading because it may suggest the existence of a simple relation between regenerative activity and differentiation in the epidermis.

Several data are against the hypothesis of such a simple mechanism and in the present paper a theoretical model of the epidermal selfmaintenance is proposed on the basis of personal morphometric studies.

We will start by underlying the amplitude of the variations which can occur in some fundamental histometric properties as the volume of epidermis and the area of epidermal inner surface (dermoepithelial interface).

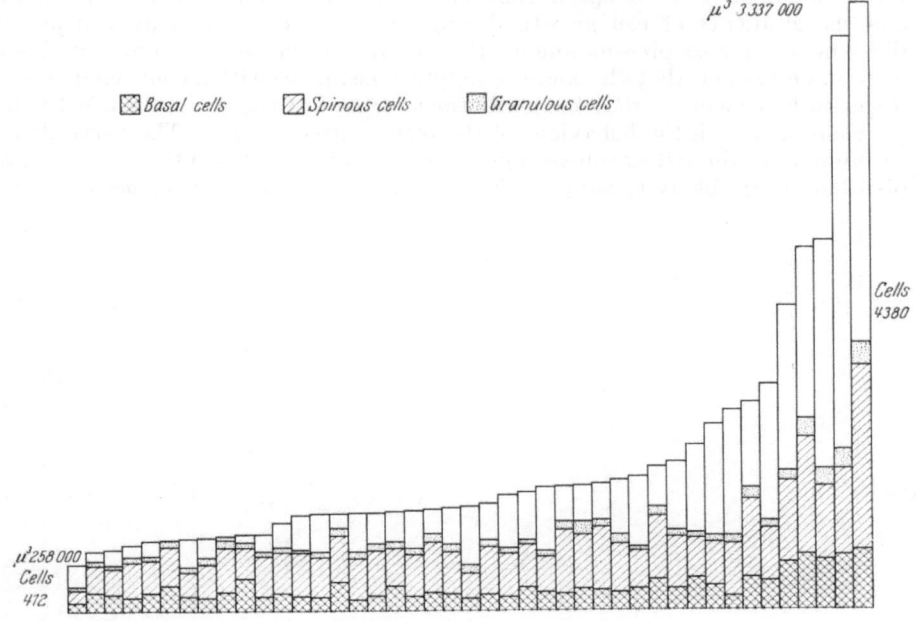

Fig. 2. Specimens as in diagramm 1

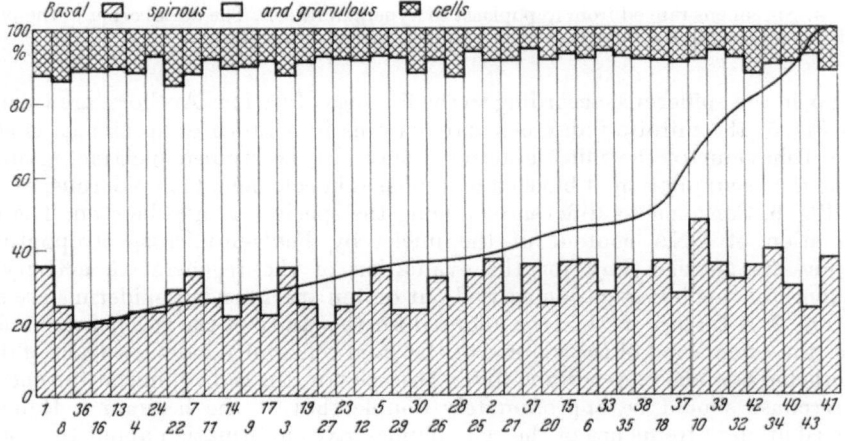

Fig. 3. Specimens as in diagramm 1

In Fig. 1, 43 specimens of interfollicular human epidermis, ranging from hypoplasia to hyperplasia are represented. Both the values of tissue volume (corneum is excluded) and dermoepithelial interface are referred to an area unit of keratinized surface. Obviously, the ample variations recorded (not ever related to each other) depend on differences in number and/or volume of the cell population. The number of the cells recorded in each specimen is shown in Fig. 2. The variations in the number of the cells affect sometimes the volume of the tissue, other times the area of dermoepithelial interface or both, according also to the quantitative repartition of the cells of the three compartments. This quantitative repartition in our series of specimens is shown in Fig. 3. As regards the cell volumes and the gradients of cell growth during the differentiative span, conspicuous differences are also present among the various specimens, as shown in Fig. 4. Now, if we assume that the keratin supply takes place with a continuous rating, it should be concluded that the oscillations of the histo- and cytometrical values are connected with the behaviour of the regenerative activity. The variability in the number of the mitoses in the epidermis, their frequent scantiness and uneven distribution are likely to support this conclusion. In the table, values of mitotic

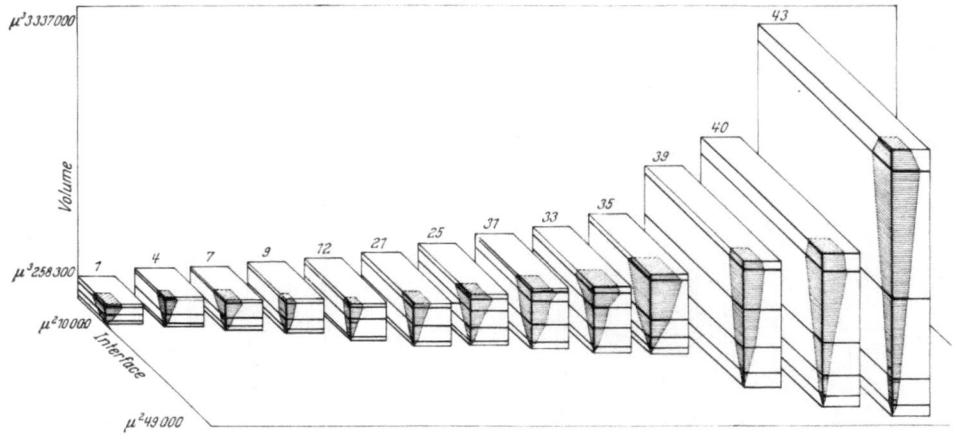

Fig. 4. Specimens ranged from hypoplasia to hyperakanthosis. The dark corner of the parallel-epipeds represents the increase of cell volumes during differentiation

index in the epidermis, according to the findings of various Authors, are tabulated. In Fig. 5, the mitotic index calculated by us in a range of specimens is shown. The behaviour of the mitotic activity may also be studied plotting against the time the accumulation of blocked metaphases in colchicinated epidermis, as shown in Fig. 6. Conspicuous differences among the specimens may be seen. The determination of DNA content of the nuclei by Feulgen-microspectrophotometry represents another way for the evaluation of the regenerative activity. The findings of this investigation carried out on ten specimens of epidermis are shown in Fig. 7. A further method we adopted for the study of the regenerative activity was the calculation of the volume of the stem cells ranged along a tract of dermo-epithelial boundary. According to the Driesch law, the cell volume at the end of the interphase should be approximately double that at the beginning. Hence, the distribution of frequence of the cell volumes gives information about the course of the mitotic activity. The diagram of Fig. 8 represents the distribution pattern of the stem cell volume in six specimens.

At last, the direction of the division axis of the mitoses in the basal layer helps in understanding the dynamics of the cell supply. The homotypic mitoses, with orizontal division axis, give two daughter cells to the basal layer. The hetero-typic mitoses, with vertical axis, give one cell to the basal layer and one to the spinous layer. The refurnishing of the stem and of the expansion compartment, therefore, is subjected to variations according to the two kinds of mitotic division, as reported in a previous work [1]. Moreover, the spinous layer can also be refurnished in a way other than by cell duplication, that is, by means of the direct transfer of basal cells as Flügelzellen.

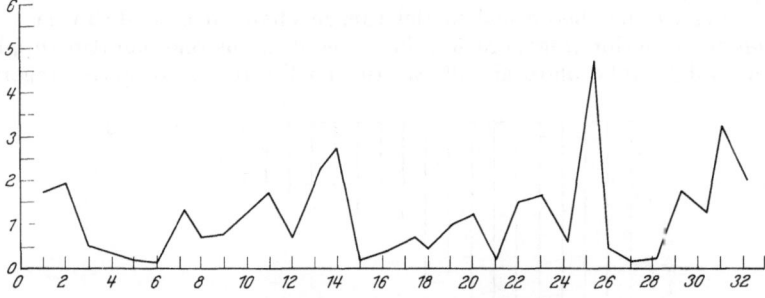

Fig. 5. ·Mitotic index in 35 specimens of human epidermis

Table. *Mitotic index in the epidermis according to the findings of various Authors*

THURINGER 1928	human	ear	0.0037	
	human	leg	0.0026	
	human	scalp	0.41	
ANDREW-ANDREW 1949	human	forearm	0.13	
KATZBERG 1952	human		0.20	
	human		0.45	aged subjects
· PINKUS 1952	human	forearm	1.59	
MEYER et al.	human	gingival mucosa	0.98	
	human		1.56	aged subjects
THURINGER 1928	human	prepuce	5.61	
COOPER-SCHIFF 1938	human	prepuce	5.48	night
	human	prepuce	3.02	day
COOPER 1939	human	prepuce	6.8	night
	human	prepuce	1.4	day
BRODERS-DUBLIN	human	prepuce	8.17	night
	human	prepuce	4.30	day
CARLETON 1933	mouse	abdomen	2.3	night
	mouse	abdomen	2	day
COOPER-FRANKLIN 1940	mouse	ear	1.45	
KNOWLTON-HAMPELMANN 1949	mouse	ear	1.69	
KNOWLTON-WIDNER 1950	mouse	ear	0.75	
COOPER-RELLER 1942	mouse	ear	0.8—1.5	
	mouse	ear	9.9	Methylcholanthrene treated
GLÜCKSMANN 1945	mouse	back	2	
	mouse	back	3.6	3—4 Benzpyrene treated
RUSCH et al. 1951	mouse	back	1.65	
	mouse	back	0.57	under starvation
RITCHIE et al. 1953	mouse	back	1.3	
	mouse	back	7.3—11.1	after croton oil
RELLER-COOPER 1944	mouse	ear	1.1	
	mouse	ear	0.9—2	after Methyl-chclanthrene
ANDREW-ANDREW 1949	rat	back, abdomen	0.58	
HENRY et al. 1952	rabbit	oral mucosa	5.1	
THURINGER 1939	cat	pad	2.37	

From what has been said above, we are lead to conclude that the mitotic activity in the epidermis is characterized by an irregular succession of mitotic waves. During the periods between a mitotic wave and another, however, the keratin supply cannot be lowered below a given level, otherwise the protective properties of the tissue should be affected. Hence, we must admit that in connection to the alternating rest and reviviscence of the reproductive activity, a complex economy takes place in the tissue and acts as regulating mechanism.

According to our theoretical model this mechanism consists in converting a discontinuous function (regeneration) into a continuous one (keratin supply). The conversion might take place as follows: during the phases of active regeneration

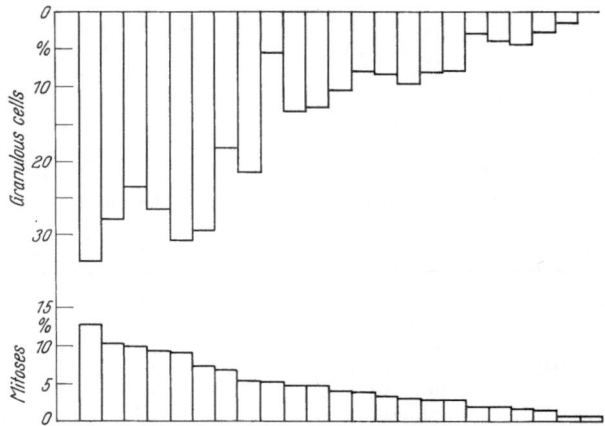

Fig. 6. The specimens are disposed according to the extent of accumulation of colchicinated mitoses (lower histogram). The corresponding percent increase of granulous cells is reported in the specular histogram

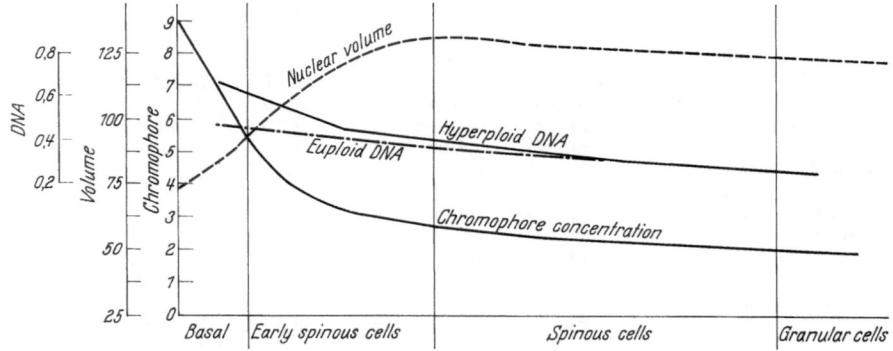

Fig. 7. Nuclear volumes, chromophore concentration, and DNA content in arbitrary units measured in human epidermis by Feulgen microspectrophotometry

the cells resulting from mitotic waves are stored in the deeper layers and, as consequence of the increase of the cell population, the extent of the dermoepithelial interface and the tissue volume are increased. When the mitotic activity is lacking, the requirements of the tissue surface are fulfilled by means of the stored cells at the expense of the papillarity and of the thickness of the tissue. As consequence of this, the epidermis undergoes alternating phases of expansion and contraction of its histometrical values. Admittedly, definite limits are imposed to such a mechanism. For instance, after a prolonged rest of the mitotic activity the ratio between keratinized surface and dermoepithelial interface can be lowered down to a value equal to one. Such a low ratio results from a severely decreased amount of the cell population of the stem compartment and in these conditions the selfmaintenance of the system depend on a closely restricted balance between cell supply and keratin refurnishing.

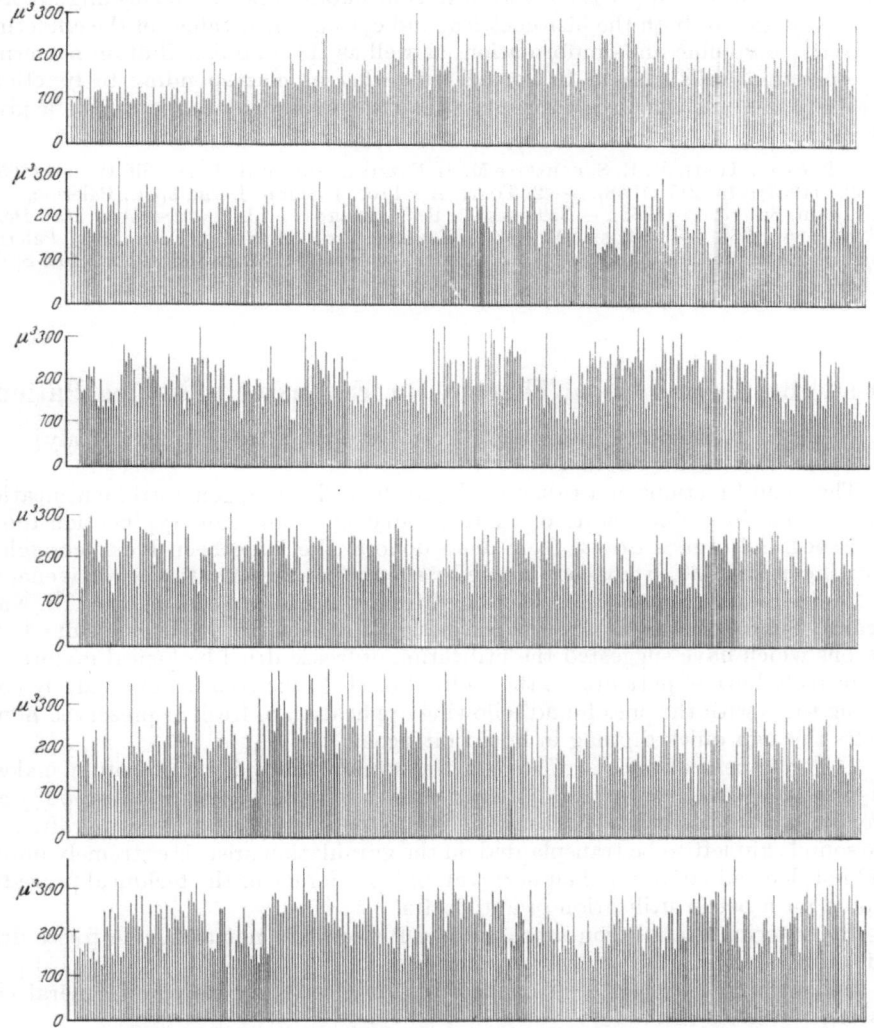

Fig. 8. Volumes of 300 basal cells ranged along a tract of dermoepithelial boundary in six specimens

The corresponding morphologic pattern is the one of the hypoplasic epidermis in which an elevated mitotic index may often be found. In spite of it, the cell supply is strongly lowered because of the reduced number of stem cells per area unit of epidermal surface. As the balance becomes defective the features of the senile icthyosis, i.e., are realised. Turning to the opposite condition, if a protracted mitotic activation occurs, the amount of intermitotic cells increases as well as the papillarity and the volume of the tissue. Over a given limit of hyperplasia (corresponding, according to our findings, to an interface/surface ratio around 4 to 5) the proximo-distal polarity of the epidermis may be lost as in pseudo-epitheliomatous hyperplasia.

Consequently, it can be suggested that the mechanism by which the discontinuous mitotic supply is converted in continuous keratin refurnishing involves the modulation of both the histometrical and cytometrical values of the epidermis. If so, tissue volume and conformation, as well as size and distribution pattern of the epidermal cells, should be considered rather as corresponding to functional phases of the epidermal cell turnover than as permanent properties of a given epidermis.

References. Tosti, A., R. Scerrato e M. L. Fazzini: Ann. ital. Derm. Sif 12, 233 (1957); 12, 327 (1957); 13, 217 (1958). — 2. Tosti, A.: Proc. I Symp. Derm. sper., Palermo, Ann. ital. Derm. Sif. 13, 47 (1958). — 3. Tosti, A., R. Scerrato e M. L. Fazzini: Ann. ital. Derm. Sif. 14, 185 (1959). — 4. Tosti, A., e M. L. Fazzini: Proc. II. Symp. Derm. sper., Palermo. Ann. ital. Derm. Sif. 15, 53 (1960). — 5. Tosti, A., e. M. L. Fazzini: Proc. II. Int. Symp. Dermat., Brno, 109, 1965.

Tissue Banks and Local Therapy for Extensively Burned Patients

G. Dogo, Istituto di Chirurgia Plastica, Ospedale Civile, Padova (Italy)

The main functions of a tissue bank are the collection, genetical identification, preservation in a viable state or by freeze-drying — and now typification too — of tissues and organs drawn from dead donors. We have been lucky enough to experiment with 30 extensively burned patients the therapeutical effectiveness of freeze-dried skin from cadavers obtained from the Tissue Bank of the U.S. Navy Medical School (Bethesda). My paper is aimed at reporting briefly about: 1. the reasons which have suggested the utilization of freeze-dried biological material on extensively burned patients; 2. the method used; 3. the results obtained, by comparing these with the ones found following application of fresh or preserved homografts through quick dipping in liquid nitrogen.

1. The beneficial effects of urgent transfusion therapies quite often make it possible to operate on burned patients with destruction areas equal to 50% and over of their body surface. In these patients, the possibility of obtain grafts from the sound skin left to be transplanted on the granulation areas is extremely limited and not determinative for their survival, independently of the technical procedure chosen for a better utilization of autografts.

By covering granulation areas with well-tolerated, not antigenic freeze-dried skin from cadavers, two objects are pursued, i.e.:

a) deferring heavy surgery on patients in a seriously impaired general condition;

b) avoiding losses of organic liquid, blood, proteins and salts, from granulation areas, controlling infections and limiting the pain due to contact with non-biological dressing material.

2. The method used is an extremely simple one. The freeze-dried skin, rehydrated immediately before using them, are applied on the granulation areas up to total covering and kept in place by a slightly compressing bandage. That requires no form of anesthesia. At the first dressing — carried out after 5 days — the tissues eventually destroyed by infectious causes or on account of enzymathic activities are replaced by other tissue. That is done also at the second, third, fourth, and fifth dressing, so as to secure a constant covering of granulation areas.

3. The results obtained went much farther than the objects we had proposed to ourselves. In fact, not only does the freeze-dried skin prove to be an excellent biological dressing, but it fulfils the function of a sliding bridge for the epithelium from the sound margins towards the center of the lesion. After each application of freeze-dried skin, it is possible to observe a gradual, progressive decrease in the size of granulation areas, until total, non-cicatricial healing of the injured area. This healing has been defined as guided or piloted.

The skin regeneration thus induced takes place by means of elementary skin provided with a thin epidermis, with a slight cohesion of the horny layer and dermo-epidermal connections without or scarcely provided with papillae and inter-posing dermal gems. It is a skin with the essential morphological characters of a normal fetus between the 6th and 9th month's life, with no signs of glands and hair and absolutely deprived of scar retraction facts.

Homologous skin from living or dead donors have been utilized for covering extensively burned patients by previously preserving them through direct immersion in liquid nitrogen. The material thus preserved has, however, the drawback of being quickly destroyed, which limits the protective and therapeutical effects to a much shorter time than the one offered by freeze-dried skin.

The adoption of fresh homografts in extensively burned patients emphasizes the importance of tissue banks in modern repairing surgery. The antigenic stresses caused by living homografts on multitransfused organisms are such as to induce dramatic immunity conditions sometimes incompatible with the patient's survival. It is only by previously checking the degree of tissue compatibility between the donor and the recipient that it is possible to utilize fresh homografts clinically. Today we can preserve large quantities of skin tissues in a viable state, for months or years, by gradually subtracting heat and subsequently immersing in liquid nitrogen.

This biological material — genetically identified, i.e. previously typified — is, in my opinion, the only one which can offer a therapeutical alternative to the adoption of freeze-dried skin. Once again, then, it is from tissue banks that we derive new prospects for treatment in this complex sphere of pathology, with the suggestion of the suitability of living or dead donors as contributors to saving extensively burned patients.

Transplantation of Normal Skin to Pathologic Skin

N. ORENTREICH, New York University School of Medicine, Dept. of Dermatology, New York (USA)

1. Introduction

Autografts of skin have been used in animals to study aging, hair growth, the hair growth cycle, pigment formation, wound healing, and immunity. Exchange autografts have been used in man to study vitiligo, amyloidosis, morphea, scleroderma, acrodermatitis chronica atrophicans, allergic eczematous contact dermatitis, fixed drug eruptions, hyperidrosis, psoriasis, androgenetic alopecia (male pattern alopecia and diffuse hair loss in women), alopecia areata, and alopecia cicatrisata. The effects of autografts have been observed following plastic repairs for lupus erythematosus.

2. Methods

The technique of multiple transposition of skin punch free grafts was devised to study some factors in the pathogenesis of dermatological disorders. After local anesthesia, and appropriate surgical preparation of the skin, which included washing, shaving and cleansing with alcohol, four full thickness circular excisions were made with specially designed Orentreich punches. These punches have a stainless steel cylinder cup, with a sharpened rim, attached at its base to a mandril type handle 3 mm in diameter and knurled for good gripping between the first and second fingers. One twirl between the fingers rotates the punch three to four revolutions and permits easy, clean, controlled round excisions in the skin. Two circular grafts were excised from a site of persistent disease, and two circular specimens were excised from a normal site.

The grafts were removed, making certain that the excision was carried well below the dermis into the subcutaneous fat and below the hair follicles when they were present. Each graft was trimmed of excess fat, and of the galea aponeurotica if present. The grafts were then transplanted in the following manner: 1. a normal graft was transplanted to a normal site; 2. a normal graft was transplanted to an affected site; 3. an affected graft was transplanted to a normal site, and 4. an affected graft was transplanted to an affected site.

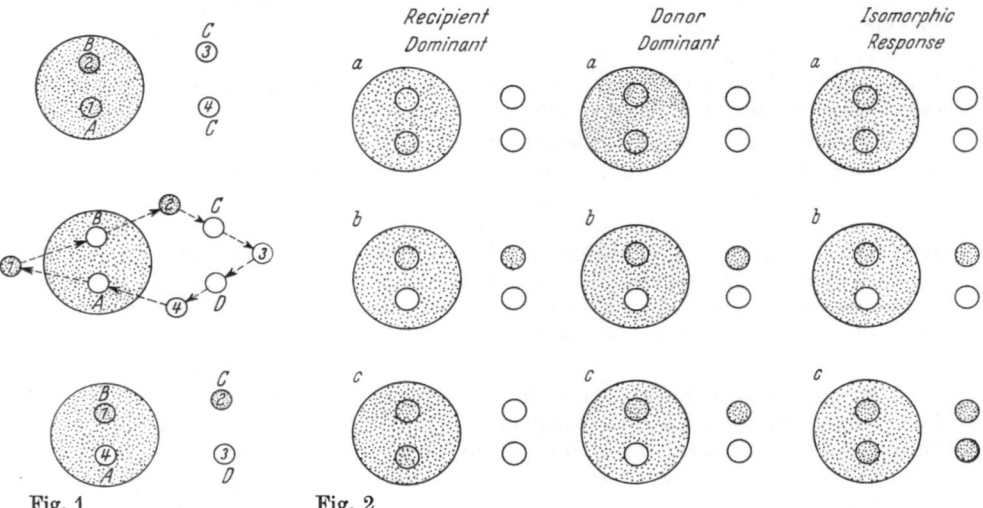

Fig. 1   Fig. 2

Fig. 1. The large stippled circle represents the dermatologic disorder. Punch grafts 1, 2, 3, and 4 are taken at site A, B, C, and D. The grafts are removed and transplanted in clockwise fashion: 1 to B (an affected graft to an affected site). 2 to C (an affected graft to a normal site), 3 to D (a normal graft to a normal site), and 4 to A (a normal graft to an affected site)

Fig. 2. The stippled areas represent the dermatologic disorder: a) depicts the time when the punch incisions were performed; b) shows the grafts immediately after they were transplanted in a clockwise fashion; and c) represents the fate of the grafts after a period of timer

Wherever feasible the grafts were transposed in clockwise fashion (Fig. 1).

Care was taken to set the grafts so that the possible growth of the hair would be in the desirable direction. Hemostasis was obtained by direct pressure for 20 to 30 min.

Fixation of the graft was accomplished by fibrin clot. Occasional fixation with perforated porous tape, collodion or sutures was used. Grafts up to 6 mm rarely required sutures. The 12 mm grafts were all sutured in place. The sutures were inserted into the surrounding skin near the graft and carried over the graft. No suturing was done into or under the graft. Sutures and other dressings were removed after the 6. to 9. day.

3. Results

1000 of these autografting procedures have been performed over the past 13 years. The grafts under 5 mm in diameter invariably took and showed little or no effects of transplantation. The larger grafts occasionally fibrosed. The larger the graft the greater and more certain the fibrosis and the poorer the take. For best results and to insure the integrity of the graft, they should be 4 mm in diameter and smaller. Though split thickness grafts have been studied the results reported in this paper refer only to full thickness skin grafts.

Immediately following transplantation the grafts were avascular and anesthetic. Within 24 h they showed some signs of revascularization and within 48 to 72 h active revascularization was evident. Superficial crusting occurred and separated in 10 to 14 days. Hair if present invariably fell out in 1 month. An occasional hair did not fall out. The hair shaft thinned, but its growing phase was only affected and not interrupted. The hair continued to grow and the hair shaft diameter returned to normal. This usually occurred at the rim of a graft where rapid revascularization could take place and was frequently seen in single hair follicle transplantation procedures.

The terms donor dominant, recipient dominant, and isomorphic response were used to describe the following conditions; when the transposed grafted skin maintained its integrity and characteristics independent of the recipient site it was donor dominant; when the transposed grafted skin took on the characteristics of the recipient site it was recipient dominant; when all the transposed sites took on the characteristics of the dermatologic disorder it was considered an isomorphic response (Fig. 2).

4. Discussion

The use of autografts as a research tool has helped our understanding of many physiologic and pathologic phenomena of the skin. Previous studies had occasionally failed or had produced contradictory result. Moreover, confusion had resulted from transplants that had failed to take or had been only partially successful. Therefore the multiple controls of the present technique were instituted. Donor dominance occurred in the following dermatologic disorders:

Androgenetic alopecia; male pattern alopecia; diffuse alopecia in women.
Alopecia areata.
Alopecia cicatrisata, end stages of pseudopelade; lichen plano-pilaris.
Hair growth cycle.
Amyloidosis, localized.
Recipient dominance occurred in the following dermatologic disorders:
Vitiligo.
Allergic eczematous contact dermatitis.
Fixed drug eruptions.
Lupus erythematosus.
Morphea.
Acrodermatitis atrophicans.
An isomorphic response occurred in psoriasis.

Skin grafts growing hair were implanted at the edge of a receding hairline. In 10 years of observation following the grafting the hairline continued to recede at its preordained pace. The grafts, however, continued to show hair growth, greater and greater distances being manifest between the hair of the graft and continued recession of the hairline. Moreover, the hair growth of the grafts appeared unimpaired.

32*

Cultivation and Regeneration of Normal and Psoriatic Cells

B. Lagerholm, Department of Dermatology, Korolinska sjukhuset, Stockholm (Sweden)

Throughout the psoriatic epidermis the cells are characterized by a paucity of tonofilaments, by few and poorly developed, desmosomes, by the abundance of mitochondria, Golgi apparatuses and membrane-bound and free particles which presumably are ribosomes.

In order to facilitate experimental investigations on the nature and differentiation of the tonofilamentous system in normal and psoriatic epidermis and on the other cellular changes observed in psoriatic epidermal cells tissue cultures of psoriatic skin and of unaffected epidermis were prepared. Successful growth in in Leighton tubes of both kinds of specimens was obtained by using a medium of 70% medium 199, 20% human serum and 10% chick embryo extract and a modification of the technique described by Frøland (1961) [3] and Hall (1964) [5].

Before incubation the dermis was removed from the specimens by microdissection under a stereomicroscope.

After equal periods of culture the newly formed areas of the psoriatic primary explants were larger than those of the explants of unaffected epidermis. The submicroscopic cytoplasmic structural organization of the cell aggregates, in the outgrowth of 5 and 9 weeks old primary tissue cultures from normal skin and unaffected skin of psoriatic patients, is characterized by the presence of a large amount dispersed tonofilaments which seems to surpass that of non-cultured epidermal cells, suggesting an excessive synthesis of tonofilament during the culturing periods. Whereas the masses of tonofilaments are mainly dispersed at random in the cytoplasm of the cells from the outgrowth of 5 weeks old primary cultures, a grouping of the tonofilaments into loosely aggregated bundles similar to that seen in non-cultured cells seems to be common in the outgrowth of explants cultured for 9 weeks.

The cells of the outgrowth areas from the two groups of primary cultures of normal skin are connected by numerous intercellular bridges. The structure of the desmosomes of the cells of the outgrowths is undistinguishable from that of not cultured normal epidermis.

The cytoplasm of the psoriatic cells cultured for 5 and 9 weeks respectively is relatively rich in tonofilaments, when compared with that of non-cultured, psoriatic epidermal cells. The cytoplasm of the psoriatic cells from the outgrowth of primary explants contained, however, considerably less tonofilamentous material than did the cytoplasm of the cells of normal epidermis cultured under identical conditions. Thus, after 9 weeks of culturing both the cells from the outgrowth of normal skin and those from the outgrowth of psoriatic explants were found actively engaged in tonofilament synthesis which facilitated the identification of these cells as epidermal cells.

Another study was undertaken to investigate whether the cells of long term subcultures of pure epidermis could maintain the capacity of tonofilament synthesis in the absence of the influence of connective tissue. The mutual influence of epithelial and mesenchymal tissues on differentiation — or on suppression on dedifferentiation has been described for many different systems of organ culture e.g. by Champy (1913) [1] and Grobstein (1959) [4].

The purpose of this study was furthermore to determine whether a permanent difference in the capacity to synthesize tonofilaments, between normal and psoriatic cells, is preserved in long term subcultures. The subcultures were prepared from the outgrowths of primary cultures, 5 weeks of age, of psoriatic and normal epidermis and thus consisted of small cell aggregates of newly formed cells. The newly formed areas of the psoriatic subculture explants were larger than those of the explants of the unaffected epidermis after equal periods of subculture indicating that the growth rate of the primary explants is maintained. The cytoplasm of the cells in the outgrowth of the 35 week old subcultures prepared from 5 week old primary cultures of normal epidermis, as it appears after glutaraldehyde-osmium tetroxide fixation, is rich in tonofilamentous material mainly grouped into loosely arranged bundles forming a network. Bundles oriented towards the desmosomes are seen and in certain places the tonofilaments can be followed into irregular masses with stronger electron scattering properties resembling keratohyalin. The individual tonofilaments are clearly distinguishable in the bundles.

The subcultured psoriatic cells are poor in tonofilamentous material and are connected by fewer desmosomes.

The experiments on long-term tissue subcultures revealed that the capacity of tonofilament synthesis and the difference in the capacity between cultured normal and psoriatic cells is preserved.

References. 1. CHAMPY, CHR.: Bibliogr. Anat. **23**, 184 (1913). — 2. CHAMPY, CHR.: C. R. Mém. Soc. Biol. **76**, 31 (1914). — 3. FRØLAND, A.: Acta path. microbiol. scand. **53**, 319 (1961). — 4. GROBSTEIN, C.: The Cell (BRACHET, J., and A. E. MIROKY, eds.) I, 441 (1959). — 5. HALL, B.: Acta paediat. (Uppsala) Suppl. **154**, (1964).

Reactions Between Skin Grafts and Hosts

A. CASTERMANS, G. DEGIOVANNI, A. M. HAENEN-SEVERYNS and G. LEJEUNE, Department of Surgery, University of Liège (Belgium)

One aspect only of the vast problem of the relationships between skin grafts and hosts will be discussed, namely that observed in case of histoimcompatibility between host and graft. That phenomenon has been most extensively studied with skin allografts, that means grafts exchanged between genetically different members of the same species, mainly in the mouse. In that particular situation skin allografts behave for 5 or 6 days just like autografts that survive indefinitely. But after 6 days allografts start becoming oedematous, cyanotic, haemorrhagic and finally ulcerate and die after about 10 days.

The cause of the death of the graft is a reaction of the host versus the graft and immunologic in nature. The most important effectors of the reaction are lymphocytes. The reaction of the host against the allogeneic graft differs from conventional immune reaction by certain features, particularly a longer delay between the antigenic stimulus (here the skin graft) and the host response. 100 h after the subcutaneous injection of allogeneic lymphoid cells, a peak of immunoblasts is observed among the cells leaving the lymph node draining the area of injection. After challenge by allogeneic skin grafts, a significant rise in the number of immunoblasts does not appear before 200 h (J. G. HALL, 1967). That latent period is probably necessary for the setting up of new lymphatic and vascular pathways to the graft, that would be required for the transport of the large molecular size graft antigens. Those antigens, called transplantation antigens, have focused our attention for several years.

Since the basic finding by BILLINGHAM, BRENT and MEDAWAR (1956) that subcellular fractions could immunize against grafts, many workers have tried to solve the problem of the chemical nature and the biological rôle of these antigens. Preliminary studies have described some properties of these antigens: their great lability for most chemical reagents and enzymes, their insolubility in saline, their gross chemical analysis: a complex of proteins, lipids and sugars, and their localization to membrane structures of the cell. Different ways for extracting and concentrating the antigens have been worked out. Most of them yielded the antigenic matter in a particulate or finely suspended stabilized form. But any important step in the identification of the transplantation antigens was soon proved to be impossible as long as those antigens were insoluble for the thorough chemical and physical investigation of a substance requires it to be at first made soluble. A second reason for solubilizing the antigens was that such a state of the antigenic matter seems essential for inducing a specific tolerance to allografts. This is still a working hypothesis but it has received some support from observations showing that a particulate preparation of antigens is more propitious than a stabilized suspension for eliciting sensitization to skin allografts and that the subcutaneous route of injection is more adequate than the peritoneal route and this one more than the intravenous one for the same purpose (MEDAWAR, 1963). That last observation emphasizes the rôle of the focal reaction in the onset of the sensitization to allografts.

Soluble antigens when introduced by the intravenous or even intraperitoneal route would not provoke any focal reaction but would be immediately and widely distributed in the organism. Actually the first attempts to induce tolerance by means of a finely suspended antigen did succeed in prolonging the survival of skin allografts. Yet similar studies using truly soluble antigens are urgently needed.

In our laboratory solubilization of transplantation antigens has been investigated from two different approaches. The first one consisted in the solubilization of an already concentrated particulate antigen, the second one in the systematic search of a right away soluble preparation.

In the first procedure cells were homogenized in NaCl 0,15 M and all deoxyribonucleoproteins and most of the ribonucleoproteins were discarded from the extract. The extract was then submitted to successive incubations with trypsin and RNase, allowing the removal of some additional RNA and an important amount of inactive proteins. The residue was extracted by 20 volumes of the mixture: tris buffer pH 7.54, 20% n-butanol (V/V). That treatment provided three fractions: a lower aqueous phase, an upper organic solvent phase and an intermediate phase. The antigenic matter present in the aqueous phase remained active and soluble after dialysis against water, but the level of the immunogenic activity recovered at the end of the procedure was much lower than that of the starting material. No doubt that loss of activity was due to a denaturation of the antigenic molecules. It was even suggested that certain antigenic determinants could be selectively destroyed. That method was therefore discarded as being inadequate for attempts of inducing tolerance. A total antigen was indeed required for such a purpose.

The second approach aims at getting a soluble preparation from the start and keeping at the same time most of the activity. The best results have been achieved by the extraction of the cells in a blender of the cylinder and piston type in high viscosity media, namely 0.25 M sucrose. The antigenic matter has been concentrated by centrifugation and solubilized by sonication. After discarding the insoluble by centrifugation, the preparation was fractionated by chromatography on a Sephadex G 200 column. The whole antigenic activity was recovered as a single peak representing roughly one third of the material absorbed on the column. That fraction was soluble and was constituted of proteins, lipids and small amounts of glucose and nucleotides. It is still a complex mixture but the method described here has the great advantage to provide a very active and soluble transplantation antigen in a very short time.

References. BILLINGHAM, R. E., L. BRENT, and P. B. MEDAWAR: Nature (Lond.) **178**, 514 (1956). — HALL, J. G.: Proceedings of the Symposium on Cell Bound Immunity, University of Liège 1967. — MEDAWAR, P. B.: Transplant. Bull. **1**, 21 (1963).

Indikationen und Ergebnisse von Transplantationen bei Dermatosen

H. C. FRIEDERICH, Univ.-Hautklinik Tübingen (Deutschland)

Die Dermatologie ist nicht nur aus historischer Sicht, sondern überdies auch rein sachlich aus ihrer Grundkonzeption gleichermaßen ein Kind der inneren Medizin und der Chirurgie. Für den Bereich des Hautorgans und seiner Grenzfunktionen zwischen drinnen und draußen muß sie beider Interessen nachkommen, wenn sie nicht ihren durch diese Doppelgesichtigkeit entscheidend mitbestimmten, eigenständigen und sie in besonderer Weise auszeichnenden Charakter einbüßen will (KLEINE-NATROP). Damit gehört die operative Therapie des Dermatologen zur allgemeinen dermatologischen Klinik und Ausbildung. Sie besitzt keine größere Selbständigkeit, aber die gleiche Bedeutung wie sie die dermatologische Röntgentherapie, Mykologie, Andrologie, Serologie oder die Allergieforschung genießen. Allerdings sind ihr gewisse anatomische Grenzen gesetzt, die über die Behandlung von Epithel, Bindegewebe und zugehörigem Fettpolster nicht hinausgehen. Bei einer solchen grundsätzlichen Einstellung weitet sich die Zahl der plastischen Eingriffe und auch der Indikationen im Lauf der Jahre automatisch aus. An der Tübinger Klinik wurden zwischen 1952 und 1967 insgesamt 9915 Eingriffe ausgeführt, davon 1095 im Jahre 1966.

Beim Überblicken der OP-Statistik zeichnen sich fünf Methoden ab, die aus dermatologischer Indikation Anwendung finden: erstens die Dehnungsplastik, zweitens die V-Y-Plastik, drittens die Flügellappenplastik, viertens die Rotationslappenplastik, fünftens das Freihauttransplantat. Die Indikation zur Anwendung leitet sich aus der Lokalisation des Eingriffes, der damit notwendig werdenden Schnittführung und dem erwünschten postoperativen Zustand ab. Die Radikalität des Eingriffes bestimmt entscheidender die Technik als ästhetische Gesichtspunkte. Jede plastische Technik kann daher je nach der Einstellung des Operateurs bei der Ausrottung nahezu jeder Hautveränderung angewendet werden.

An der Spitze der Indikationen zur Hauttransplantation steht das Basaliom und das Spinaliom. 593 Kranke mit 737 Basaliomen wurden zwischen 1958 bis 1966 operativ plastisch versorgt. 630 davon wurden 1967 gemeinsam mit STUMPP nachuntersucht. Von 74 der Verstorbenen waren 55 bis zum Tod nachuntersucht. Die Todesursache stand nie in Zusammenhang mit der Hautkrankheit. 73 Kranke — neun davon waren kurzfristig nachuntersucht — kamen nicht zur Nachuntersuchung. Bei einer Kontrolle von mindestens 5, höchstens 8 Jahren blieben von 202 Kranken 181 (89,6%) rezidivfrei; nach 3 Jahren waren es 359 (92,8%) von 387 Kranken, die erscheinungsfrei blieben. Bei 50 Kranken, die Rezidive aufwiesen, ging eine Vorbehandlung (Rö, kaltkaustische Zerstörung) voraus. 39,1% der Rezidive ließen bei der histologischen Untersuchung erkennen, daß die Excision nicht im Gesunden erfolgte, 32,6% der Rezidive heilten wahrscheinlich aus den gleichen Gründen per secundam ab. In 51,3% der Rezidive lag histologisch ein sklerodermiformes Basaliom vor. Die Rezidivquote aller operativ behandelten sklerodermiformen Basaliome (146) lag bei 13,6% (20 Kranke). Dies bedeutet, daß die bei allen Basaliomen verwendete Sicherheitszone von 0,5 cm beim sklerodermiformen Basaliom auf 1 bis 1,5 cm zu erhöhen ist. Zieht man von der Zahl der operierten Basaliome die Kranken, die als „Rezidive nach Vorbehandlung" zur Operation überwiesen wurden, ab, zeigt sich, daß von 176 Kranken (5 Jahre beobachtet) 166 (94,3%), von 346 Kranken (3 Jahre beobachtet) 333 (96,2%) rezidivfrei blieben. Die Behauptung, daß eine Vorbehandlung die Rezidivquote der Operation beeinträchtigt, erscheint daher berechtigt; Rezidive traten durchschnittlich nach 23,8 Monaten auf. Die Nachbeobachtung von 259 operativ und kombiniert operativ radiologisch behandelten Spinaliomen ergab: Von 95 Kranken (5 Jahre beobachtet) blieben 85 (88,2%) rezidivfrei. Von 135 Kranken (3 Jahre beobachtet) blieben 153 (90,8%) erscheinungsfrei. Die Nachbeobachtung ausschließlich operativ versorgter Spinaliome ergab bessere Werte: Von 80 Spinaliomen (5 Jahre beobachtet) blieben 71 (87,3%) rezidivfrei. Von 148 Kranken (3 Jahre beobachtet) verblieben 135 erscheinungsfrei. Gliedert man diese Zahl noch weiter auf, so zeigt sich, daß von 67 primär operativ versorgten Kranken 63 (93,6%) während einer 5jährigen, von 127 Kranken 121 (95,1%) während einer 3jährigen Beobachtungszeit erscheinungsfrei blieben.

Wenn man die Deutung der Präcancerosen als Vorläufer der Krebsentsteher an der Haut bejaht, bietet sich die Entfernung mittels plastischer Eingriffe an. Ihre histologische Auswertung erlaubt die Antwort zur Frage, ob noch eine Präcancerose oder schon ein Carcinom vorliegt. Hierher gehört die Amputation des Lippenrots mit Neubildung aus der Mundschleimhaut im Rahmen der Entfernung von Präcancerosen, die Excision von Leukoplakien, die Entfernung der Keratomata senilia, in erster Linie aber die radikale Excision und nachfolgende plastische Deckung erwünschter und unerwünschter Rö-Folgezustände. Von 48 zwischen 1958 bis 1965 so behandelten Kranken konnte bei 46 durch Verschiebe- oder Freihauttransplantate ein dauernder Verschluß erzielt werden und damit die Eliminierung einer „obligatorischen" Präcancerose (HALTER).

Die operativ plastische Versorgung des Lupus vulgaris — der Boden für ein solches Vorgehen wurde ja erst im Zeitalter der Tuberculostatica reif (GOTTRON) — ist bei Arzneimittelunverträglichkeit oder unter dem Schutz von Chemotherapeutika die Methode der Wahl. NEISSERS Grundsatz, nach dem die erste Frage in der Lupusbehandlung die nach der chirurgischen Behandlung sein soll, besitzt im Zeitalter der Tuberculostatica besonderen Wert und Bedeutung.

Auch die chemotherapeutische Behandlung des Lupus erythematodes wird durch operativ-plastische Behandlung sinnvoll ergänzt und abgekürzt. Arzneimittelunverträglichkeit oder Störungen des Auges unter der Behandlung können die plastische Versorgung zur Methode der Wahl werden lassen.

Die Melanosis circumscripta präblastomatosa stellt eine der wichtigsten Indikationen für den plastischen Eingriff dar. Die histologische Kontrolle in Serienschnitten empfiehlt sich allerdings. Fehlen Zeichen maligner Entwicklung, ist die Behandlung — allerdings bei strikter Kontrolle der Kranken in den nachfolgenden 10 Jahren — abgeschlossen. Von 31 so behandelten Kranken blieben 28 in der Beobachtungszeit (6 Kranke $1/_2$ Jahr, 3 Kranke 2 Jahre, 5 Kranke 3 Jahre, 6 Kranke 4 Jahre, 1 Kranker 5 Jahre, 7 Kranke $5^1/_2$ Jahre) erscheinungsfrei (FRIEDERICH-SCHNEIDER JR.).

Naevuszellnaevi soll nur der plastisch versorgen, der in der Morphologie dieser Gebilde Erfahrung hat. Wir führen Totalexcisionen und Serienexcisionen sowie Freihauttransplantationen im Rahmen dieser Therapie durch. Von 1621 Naevuszellnaevi, entnommen bei 1383 Kranken zwischen 1947 und 1965, ist eine maligne postoperative Entartung im Anschluß an den Eingriff nie beobachtet worden.

Die Deckung von Naevi flammei des Gesichtes erfolgt entweder durch Serienexcisionen oder Freihauttransplantate. Die Technik steht im Einzelfall in Abhängigkeit von Ausdehnung und Begrenzung.

Der prothetischen Deckung des irreversiblen Haarverlustes durch eine Prothese ist stets — falls technisch möglich — eine einzeitige oder mehrzeitige Deckung vorzuziehen. Ob man diese mittels Heranbringen, Hineinschwenken benachbarter Hautareale, durch Dehnung oder Rotation durchführt oder die Orentreichsche Transplantation durchführt, hängt von der Auffassung des Einzelnen ab. Wir konnten jedenfalls über dem unterminierten Corium eine Haarwuchssteigerung beobachten, wenn intakte Haartalgdrüsensysteme vorlagen.

Eine weitere interessante Indikation stellt die circumscripte Sklerodermie dar. Bei radikaler Entfernung traten bisher nach Dehnungs-, Verschiebe- und Freihauttransplantationen keine Rezidive in den Operationswunden, dagegen in der Umgebung auf.

Eine weitere Indikation ist die Chondrodermatitis nodularis, die wir ausschließlich durch breite Keilexcision oder halbmondförmige Exstirpation mit Knorpelkürzung behandeln. 56 Kranke wurden 10 Jahre nachbeobachtet (v. SAWITZKI), einmal trat ein Rezidiv ein.

Zwei praktisch bedeutsame Indikationen des plastischen Eingriffes sind alte oder frisch erworbene Tätowierungen und Fußsohlenwarzen. Die Totalentfernung einer Tätowierung ohne Nachahmung der Konturen durch die OP-Narbe erfordert hohes Einfühlungsvermögen des Operierenden. Serienexcisionen sind die Methode der Wahl. Die Totalexcision der Fußsohlenwarze mit anschließender Thierschung ist eine einfache und brauchbare Methode. Die Deckung des Ulcus cruris im Anschluß an eine Varicenverödung (SCHNEIDER) bedeutet eine Verkürzung der Behandlungszeit.

Der Vorteil der im Vortrag geäußerten Einstellung liegt darin, daß erstens die gesamte Therapie nahezu einzeitig ausgeführt wird, zweitens am Ort der Erkrankung nur zarte Narben verbleiben. Es liegt Material für die histologische Untersuchung vor, viertens die Operation stellt nie eine Kontraindikation gegen eine eventuell notwendig werdende Röntgenbestrahlung dar.

Free Communications

Electron Microscopic Studies of Epithelial Growth and Keratinization in Cultures of Split-Thickness Adult Human Skin

PH. H. PROSE and A. E. FRIEDMAN-KIEN, New York University School of Medicine, Department of Pathology and Department of Dermatology, New York (USA)

In a previous report [1], a simple and successful method for culturing splitthickness adult human skin was described. An outgrowth of epidermal, or epidermal and fibroblastic cells, surrounded the explants. The cultures survived for up to 10 weeks, when the fibroblastic elements crowded out the epidermal cells.

In the experiment herein described, a biopsy specimen of skin was obtained from each of five adult male surgical patients. The specimens were cultured in plastic Petri dishes. One biopsy specimen was sacrificed after 6 days; the others, after 4 to 8 weeks. The cultures were processed for electron microscopy while still in their plastic dishes. After fixation in cold 3% glutaraldehyde in phosphate buffer, they were post-osmicated, dehydrated in graded alcohols and embedded in Epon. Thin sections, stained with uranyl acetate and lead citrate, were examined in a Siemens Elmiskop I.

The 6 day-old specimen showed a three to four fold increase in the thickness

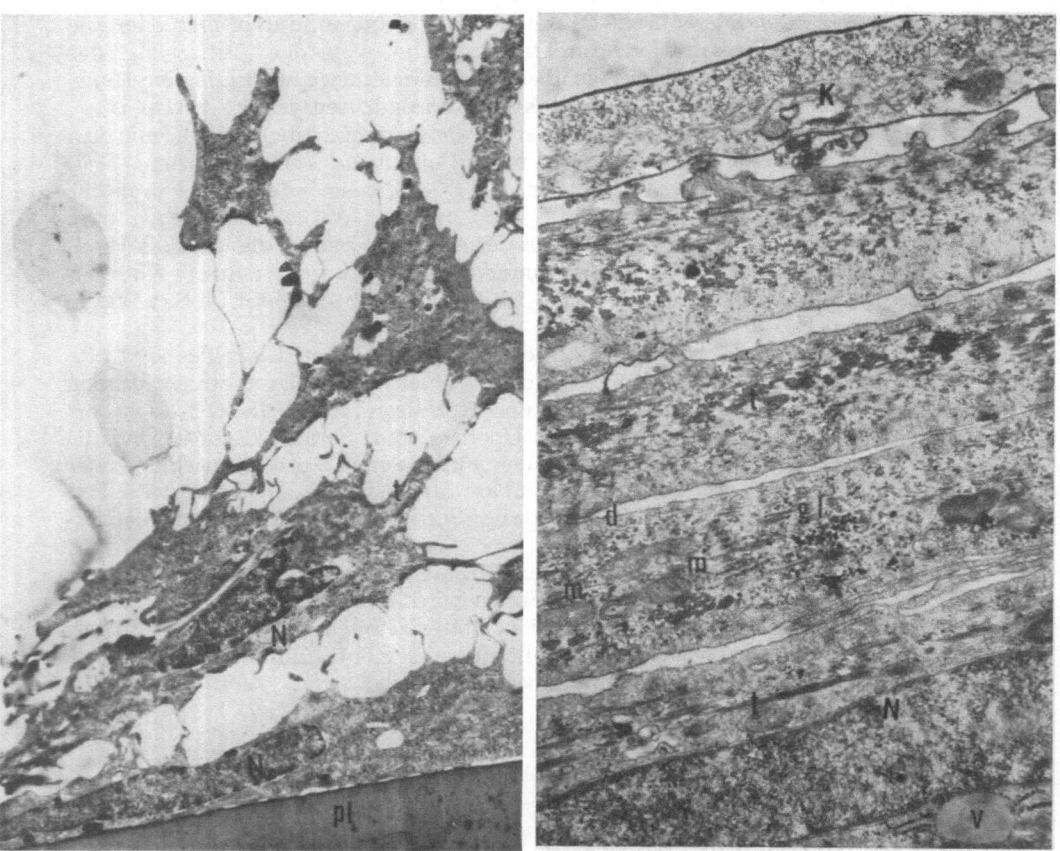

Fig. 1   Fig. 2

Fig. 1. Outgrowth in the 6 day-old culture, sectioned at right angles to the surface, showing a few layers of epidermal cells which grew from the explant (on the right, but not shown in the micrograph) onto the plastic dish (pl). The cells have a nucleus (N) and a moderately electron dense cytoplasm which contains ribonucleoprotein particles, tonofilaments (t), melanin granules and occasional mitochondria. The intercellular space is wide. x 4,800

Fig. 2. Outgrowth in a 7 week-old culture, sectioned at right angles to the surface of the culture, showing part of the stratified squamous epithelium which covered the surface of the plastic dish. The lower cells are not keratinized. The lowermost cell is tallest. It contains a nucleus (N), a lipid filled vacuole (v), tonofilaments (t), and rough surfaced endoplasmic reticulum on either side of the vacuole. Mitochondira (m), tonofilaments (t) (arranged in varied directions) and glycogen granules (gl) are shown in the remaining non-keratinized cells. No melanin granules were found in the outgrowth in the older cultures. A desmosome (d) is seen between two non-keratinized cells. The uppermost cell is keratinized (K). It is surrounded by a thick outer membrane and contains fibres. x 17,000

of the epidermis covering the explant. However, only a few layers of elongated and flattened epidermal cells appeared viable; these were located just above the corium. The epidermis covering the lateral edge of the explant was thin, four to six cells in depth. From this region, epidermal cells (containing tonofilaments ending on well structured desmosomes) grew and migrated in the following directions: a) upward, covering part of the keratin layer of the explant; b) downward, and then inward, encompassing the lateral resected margin and part of the undersurface of the explant, (epiboly); and c) downward and outward, investing a small area on the surface of the plastic dish (Fig. 1). In the region adjacent to the lateral resected margin of the explant, an epidermal cell in mitosis was found.

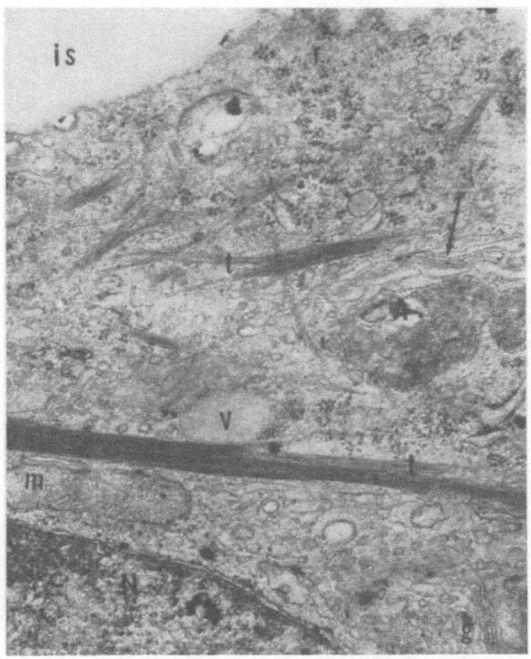

Fig. 3. Part of an epidermal cell in the mid-zone of a 7 week-old culture sectioned parallel to the surface of the culture. Part of the nucleus (N) is surrounded by a perinuclear "clear" zone which contains a mitochondrion (m), a Golgi apparatus (g), and vesicles. Agreggates of tonofilaments (t) are shown. A lipid filled (v) and an autophagic (A) vacuole, stacks of flattened vesicles surrounded by smooth surfaced endoplasmic reticulum (→), and ribonucleoprotein (r) particles are present in the cytoplasm. The intercellular space (is) is seen in the upper left part of the micrograph. x 21,000

In the 4 to 8 week-old cultures, the epidermis covering the explant was devitalized. The rete ridges were flat. The lateral resected margin of the explant was surrounded by cellular debris which contained lamellae of keratin fibers and a rare keratinized cell. The debris was covered by stratified squamous epithelium, up to 20 layers in depth. This epithelium was continuous with the epithelium (Fig. 2) that covered the surface of the plastic dish for a considerable distance.

The cells in the lower layers of the stratified epithelium were not keratinized. They were considerably elongated and flattened; their greatest diameters were found in sections that paralleled the surface of the culture. These cells resembled the epidermal cells in the lower stratum spinosum of grossly normal adult skin

(Fig. 3). They showed a perinuclear "clear" zone and a meshwork of electron dense tonofibers in the mid-zone of the cytoplasm. The tonofibers ended on desmosomes which are characteristic for squamous epithelium (Fig. 4). However, there were differences between the cultured cells and those in healthy skin. The cultured cells had a larger nucleus and perinuclear "clear" zone; their cytoplasm was denser and contained a greater number of ribonucleoprotein particles (often arranged in rosettes); and the cytoplasm of some of the cultured cells showed, either singly or in combination, clusters of glycogen granules, multivesicular bodies, autophagosomes, centrioles and microtubules.

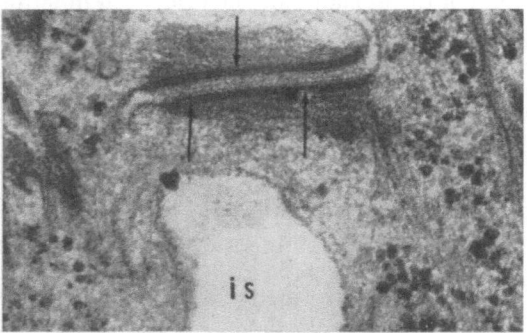

Fig. 4. A well structured desmosome (→) in the outgrowth in a 7 week-old culture sectioned at right angles to the surface. The cells lining the interspace (is) contain tonofilaments, ribonucleoprotein and glycogen particles. x 56,700

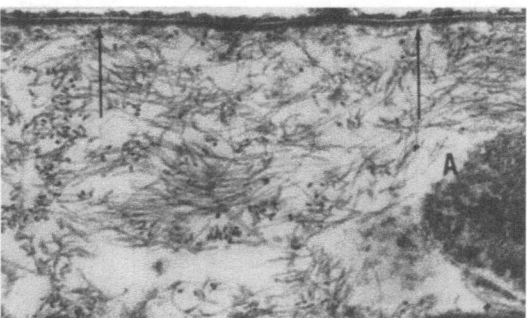

Fig. 5. Part of a keratinized cell in the outgrowth in a 7 week-old culture, sectioned at right angles to the surface of the culture. The outer cell membrane is trilaminar (→). The cytoplasm contains fibers arranged in varied directions and an autophagosome (A). x 41,800

The cells in the upper layers (one to ten cells in depth) were cornified (Fig.2). The transition between non-keratinized and cornified layers was abrupt. The cornified cells had a trilaminar outer cell membrane composed of a thin, outer and a thick, inner membrane with a thin, electron translucent space between (Fig. 5). The cytoplasm was "pale" and contained fibers, ($\sim$ 100 Å in diameter), arranged in varied directions. Some of these fibers were less electron dense than the tonofibers. Within the cytoplasm of some of the cornified cells, autophagosomes containing spiralled membranes, electron dense amorphous material, and remnants of cytoplasmic membranes were seen. No desmosomes were found between cornified cells.

At the outer edge of these cultures, the cells were not keratinized. The outer cytoplasmic membrane bordering the culture showed numerous long, branched villi. Multinucleated, giant epidermal cells were found in this region.

In summary, the explants in these cultures gave rise to outgrowths of stratified squamous epithelium. The progression from non-keratinized to keratinized cells resembled that seen in grossly normal adult skin. Elimination of cytoplasmic elements from keratinized cells was incomplete. It seems likely that this was, in part, accomplished by incorporation of these elements into autophagosomes, probably filled with digestive enzymes. Although nuclei were retained in some of the keratinized cells, these parakeratotic cells did not resemble those found in diseased skin, since they did not have an electron dense, amorphous cytoplasm.

Acknowledgements: This work was supported by a grant from the JOHN A. HARTFORD Foundation, Inc. and by a NIH training grant (TI-AM-5326).

Bibliography. 1. FRIEDMAN-KIEN, A. E., P. H. PROSE, H. LIEBHABER, and S. MORRILL: Nature (Lond.) **212**, 1583 (1966).

The Management of Extensive Full-thickness Burns by Skin Grafting

T. ANZAI, Kanto Labour Accident Hospital, Chofu, Tokyo (Japan)

In the local treatment of 3rd degree burn, we should perform débridement and autogenic skin grafting as early as possible; but when the burn is extensive the burn wound often forms a chronic ulcer because of the limited available donor area for skin graft and other associated difficulties.

Six cases of extensive full-thickness burns, which involved 15 to 28% of the body surface area, were treated successfully by wrapping the entire wounds with the skin graft.

In the case of extensive 3rd degree burn, protein is lost through the burn itself, and also the metabolism of the protein in the plasma is itself altered and, as a result, remarkable changes often occur within the level of the plasma protein. Concerning the protein fractions, albumin, which has smaller molecules, is lost more than globulin which has greater molecules. As long as the ulceration continues unhealed, protein will be continuously lost. Therefore, the hypoalbuminemia and hyperglobulinemia that usually develop with an extensive burn cannot be corrected completely until the ulceration heals completely.

In the early stage after burn, there occurs hemolytic anemia, and later always chronic anemia follows due to the blood loss at the burn wound, bleeding accompanying the débridement and disturbed hemopoietic ability. Therefore, to compensate for this situation, well planned blood transfusion is of course very important, but at the same time the coverage of the wound is indispensable.

Regarding the blood, plasma and albumin which is used in a copious amount against burn shock or in case of operation, the great problem is serum hepatitis which often reaches serious proportions. The problem is serious, because the treatment of burn cannot be accomplished without giving blood or plasma.

Concerning the skin autografting for the ulcer after burn, free grafting is done. The area with ulceration usually has infection, and under this circumstances, free graft which "takes" better than pedicle graft is preferable. After the free grafting for the general areas is completed, a pedicle graft may be tried for such a special region as the dorsal surface of a hand. Regarding the outlook and function of the free graft the thicker the graft is, the better is the result; but the rate of "take" decreases as the thickness increases. Therefore, we have chosen one ten-thousandth of an inch as the most appropriate thickness of the graft.

Now, concerning the process of grafting in our cases, we cautiously tried to cover the burn completely in each area. To close the entire areas of burn, two to four operations were usually sufficient.

Differently from ours, the postage stamp method has been conventionally popular, but we do not use this; not only because a scar or keloid might develop between the grafts giving an ugly look, but also because the cicatrical contracture disturbs the motor function.

To obtain split-thickness grafts, we used Padgett-Hood's dermatome and Brown's electric dermatome. We think the latter is more convenient as it works quickly and simply.

For fixing the graft, 3 M Steri-Strip Skin Closure was applied. By this means the fixation was excellent and the operation time could be greatly reduced.

In case of an extensive burn ulcer, the donor site is naturally limited making the autografting difficult. However, grafts can be taken repeatedly from the same site. We "took" a split-thickness graft two to three times from one spot. In such manner, we could cover the whole area of ulceration.

Les hétérogreffes animales:
Phénomènes de rejet des hétérogreffes répétées et des autogreffes secondaires

P. Laugier, M. Véron, J. C. Risold et V. Ellena, Clinique Dermatologique et Chaire de Microbiologie, Centre Hospitalier et Universitaire de Besançon (France)

Les résultats obtenus (Bromberg [1]) avec des greffes de peau animale (porc) chez des brûlés, nous ont incités à utiliser ce procédé pour hâter la cicatrisation d'ulcérations torpides [2,3]. La répétition successive des hétérogreffes aboutit à leur rejet de plus en plus rapide. Pour compléter la cicatrisation, nous avons remplacé les hétérogreffes par des autogreffes. Notre surprise fut grande de constater leur rejet immédiat comme s'il s'agissait encore d'une hétérogreffe. L'apparition de ce phénomène chez tous les malades nous laisse donc supposer qu'une sensibilisation acquise à la peau de porc entraîne pour le sujet une sensibilisation à sa propre peau. Pour vérifier ce fait, des tests sont faits en injectant dans le derme de la région deltoïdienne avant et après les greffes 0,1 à 0,2 ml de broyat antigénique; la réaction est lue 48 h après l'injection afin de ne tenir compte que des réactions de type retardé, et non pas des réactions allergiques précoces, d'ailleurs rares, pouvant être dûes au formol. Ces préparations antigéniques destinées à l'étude des réactions d'hypersensibilité cutanée sont réalisées soit à partir d'un mélange de peau de porc soit à partir de la peau d'un malade donné, en broyant pendant

Tableau 1. *Observations cliniques*

Malades	Nombre d'hétérogreffes	Autogreffes	Observations
21 malades hétérogreffes seules	de 1 à 7	0	avec bonne cicatrisation
3 malades témoins		1	bonne prise du greffon
7 malades hétérogreffes suivies autogreffes	de 1 à 5	1 rejetée	rejet de l'autogreffe

Tableau 2. *Expérimentation*

Malades	I.D. avant greffes avec antigène de		Nombre d'hétéro-greffes	Autogreffes	I.D. après greffes avec antigène de		Observations
	peau du malade	peau de porc			peau du malade	peau de porc	
1. M., Alice, 65 ans	0	++	4	rejetée	+	+++	
2. W., Clémence, 74 ans	+*	++	4	rejetée	++	+++	* Réaction positive avant toute greffe
3. J., Jeanne, 72 ans	0	+++	3	rejetée	+	+++	
4. A., Maria, 75 ans	++*	++	5	rejetée	++	++	* Avait reçu avant les 1ères intradermo. 3 hétéro-greffes lors d'une première hospitalisation
5. B., Marie, 74 ans	0	+++	3	rejetée	+	+++	
6. C., Jeanne, 73 ans	0	++	3	rejetée	++	+++	Rejet d'une autogreffe controlatérale après bonne prise et deux hétérogreffes sur la jambe de l'autre côté
7. B., Marguerite, 65 ans	+	++	3	rejetée	++	+++	Une deuxième autogreffe est éliminée beaucoup plus lentement
8. D., Marie, 80 ans	0	++	5	rejetée	++	++	
9. D., Jean, 56 ans	±*	+	3	bonne prise	0	++	* Avait reçu quatre hétérogreffes antérieures aux 1ères I.D.
10. V., Marcel, 37 ans			7	1è rejetée 2è rejetée plus lentement 3è bonne prise			

5 min avec un mixeur tournant à 5.000 tours/min environ 10 à 20 mm³ de tissu cutané dans 4 ml de tampon physiologique acide borique-borax, pH 8,6 (acide borique 0,2 M + borax 0,05 M). Le broyat est traité avec 1% de formol (formaldéhyde 30%) pendant 48 h à +4 °C.

Observations Cliniques (voir tableau détaillé)

Sur 38 sujets traités par hétérogreffes 17 ont eu ultérieurement des autogreffes. Dans 16 cas sur 17 les autogreffes ont été immédiatement rejetées; une a été parfaitement conservée. Dans un cas les autogreffes répétées sont de mieux en mieux puis parfaitement tolérées.

Discussion

Le phénomène de rejet des autogreffes pratiquées après une ou plusieurs hétérogreffes se retrouve dans 16 observations sur les 17 rapportées ici. Il semble donc s'agir d'un phénomène très fréquent, survenant chez la presque totalité de nos malades traités de cette façon.

Malgré un état trophique déficient et une vascularisation très mauvaise des téguments, l'autogreffe primitive donne de bons résultats chez l'ensemble des témoins n'ayant pas reçus d'hétérogreffes. On peut donc penser que le rejet de l'autogreffon placé secondairement sur un ulcère déjà traité par hétérogreffes est dû non pas à un état tissulaire local défavorable, mais à un processus immunitaire de portée générale. Cette hypothèse est corroborée par les faits suivants:

1. le rejet de l'autogreffon est d'autant plus rapide que le nombre d'hétérogreffes préalables est plus grand;

2. avant hétérogreffe, les malades ne présentent pas de réaction d'hypersensibilité cutanée à leur propre peau; après hétérogreffe (s) avec la peau de porc, ils réagissent par contre fortement aux antigènes de peau de porc et plus ou moins fortement aux antigènes de leur propre peau (observations n° 1, 3, 5, 6, 8);

3. le rejet d'un autogreffon placé sur un membre peut être déclenché à distance par des hétérogreffes faites sur un autre membre (observation n° 6).

Pour tenter d'expliquer le phénomène, nous proposons l'interprétation suivante. Au cours des greffes d'une part et au cours du traitement *in vitro* d'autre part (action possible du formol), la structure macromoléculaire de la peau humaine subirait une légère modification qui ferait apparaître un nouveau déterminant antigénique commun avec la peau de porc. Lors d'une hétérogreffe, les anticorps formés qui correspondent à ce déterminant antigénique commun, sont aptes à réagir fortement avec l'hétérogreffon et aussi, quoique plus faiblement, avec la peau humaine «modifiée», tant au niveau des intradermo-réactions que des autogreffons. En répétant les tentatives d'autogreffes post-hétérogreffes, nous avons d'ailleurs pu obtenir dans un cas (observation n° 10) un processus semblable à une désensibilisation spécifique, comme si les greffons autologues replacés plusieurs fois dans le lit des hétérogreffons finissaient par épuiser localement les anticorps anti-peau de porc; ce phénomène est bien en accord avec l'existence supposée d'une réaction croisée, au cours des greffes, entre les peaux de porc et d'homme. Une expérimentation sur le lapin est actuellement en cours; elle devrait nous permettre de vérifier la validité de nos hypothèses.

Bibliographie. 1. BROMBERG, B.: Presse méd. **73**, 227 (1965). — 2. LAUGIER, P., J. C. RISOLD, V. ELLENA, LALLEMAND et F. PEQUEGNOT: Strasbourg Méd. **10**, 855 (1965). — 3. LAUGIER, P., et J. C. RISOLD: 5e Congrès de dermatologie Yougoslave, p. 254—256. Zagreb, 26 juin 1965. — 4. MATHÉ, G., et J. L. AMIEL: La greffe. Aspects biologiques et cliniques. Paris: Masson 1962. — 5. FLARER, F., et G. C. CHIEREGATO: Dermatologica (Basel) **127**, 1 (1963). — 6. FLARER, F., e G. C. CHIEREGATO: Nota I, Minerva derm. Atti SIDES, **38**, 4, 472 (1963). — 7. FLARER, F., e G. C. CHIEREGATO: Nota II, Minerva derm. **39**, 95 (1964). — 8. FLARER, F., e G. C. CHIEREGATO: Minerva derm. **40**, 379 (1965). — 9. CAVALLO, G.: Folia allerg. (Roma) **12**, 5, 303 (1965). — 10. CAVALLO, C.: Riv. Ist. sieroter. ital. **39**, 1, 15 (1964).

Transplantation of Epithelial Cell Cultures and the Formation of an Epidermis

M. A. KARASEK, Department of Dermatology, Stanford University School of Medicine, Palo Alto, California (USA)

The application of epithelial cell cultures in the reconstruction of wounds has been an attractive possibility since the development of cell culture techniques and the growth of epithelial cells in cell culture. In 1952, BILLINGHAM and REYNOLDS demonstrated that sheets of epidermis and trypsinized suspensions of epithelial cells could be transplanted successfully [1]. After dissociation of 15-day mouse embryonic skin into individual cells, MASCONA reported that skin cells reaggregated, and that the aggregates differentiated into patches of skin with hair rudiments [2]. However, the behavior of postembryonic grafts of epithelial cells following a period of growth in cell culture has not been previously reported.

In 1964, our laboratory described some of the growth characteristics of the human skin epithelial cells in cell culture [3]. In contrast to a large number of cells that rapidly dedifferentiate to form a non-specific cell type, the epithelial cell retains many of the properties characteristic of the epithelial cell *in vivo*. The presence of tonofilaments and tonofibrils was demonstrated by electron microscopy, and a fibrous protein with the histochemical properties of keratin was isolated. Other cell characteristics, however, such as the formation of keratohyalin granules, were not observed. In order to determine if the absence of all histiospecific cell properties was a result of a permanent somatic variation in the epithelial cell after cell culture and therefore would preclude the possibility that cultured epithelial cells could be used for the reconstruction of an epidermis, we have studied the behavior of orthotopic grafts of epithelial cell suspensions after a limited period of cell culture.

Since wound contraction seriously interferes with the long-term study of transplanted cells, we have constructed a silicone rubber window that effectively prevents wound contraction and reepithelialization from a wound margin from taking place when this chamber is placed between the dermis and the muscle fascia (figure page 514). These chambers induce a minimal inflammatory response and are tolerated by rabbits.

Following transplantation of cells to the prepared graft site, sequential biopsies at weekly intervals show the following behavior of transplanted cells:

1. One week after transplantation, the epithelial cells proliferate to form a cell layer over the entire wound site that is three cells in thickness. There is a thin and irregular basement membrane, and no surface keratinization or a stratum granulosum.

2. Within 2 weeks, the cells have continued to grow, and the transplanted cells and their progeny form an epidermis that is five to ten cells in thickness. The epidermis continues to show a thin and irregular basement membrane. Suface keratinization occurs, and a stratum granulosum is present.

3. After 3 weeks, the epidermis becomes intensely hyperplastic and hyperkeratotic. The epidermis attains a thickness of 15 cells. The basement membrane continues to be thin and irregular.

4. In the remaining weeks of growth, a deterioration of the epidermis begins that eventually results in the presence of only occasional areas of a greatly altered epidermis.

The experiments described in this report have been carried out with rabbits. In other studies, silastic implants of correspondingly smaller dimensions have been constructed and successfully maintained in mice, rats, and guinea pigs. With the higher degree of genetic information available in mice, estimates of the genetic diversity of the epidermis appear possible. To the extent that morphologic and biochemical behavior of epithelial cells can be studied both *in vivo* and *in vitro* the stability of specific cell characteristics *in vitro* can be determined, and the development of methods to permit the eventual permanent reconstruction of an epidermis by epithelial cell cultures may be expected.

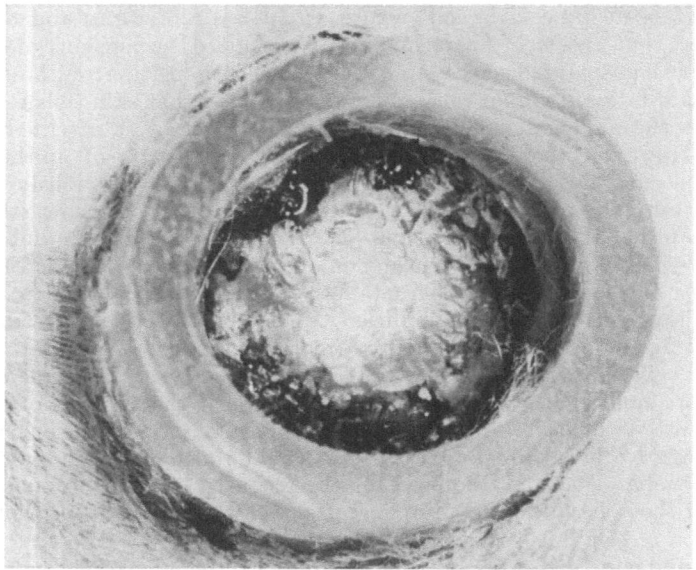

Fig. Silicone rubber window inserted between dermis and muscle fascia on back of New Zealand white rabbit. New growth of epidermis from transplanted epithelial cells is seen in center of window

References: 1. BILLINGHAM, R. E., and J. REYNOLDS: Brit. J. plast. Surg. 4, 25 (1952). — 2. MOSCONA, A. A.: Exp. Cell Res. 22, 455 (1961). — 3. KARASEK, M.: J. invest. Derm. 47, 533 (1966).

Influence of Genetic Relationship on Skin Homotransplantation Survival in Humans

R. CEPPELLINI, M. VISETTI and G. LEIGHEB, Institute of Medical Genetics and Department of Dermatology of the University of Turin (Italy)

It is now biologically accepted that histocompatibility factors are controlled by a genetic mechanism. With this in mind we set out to analyze the influence of genetic relationship on skin graft survival in humans. The study was carried out in healthy volunteers and 95 skin homografts were exchanged between unrelated donors, parents and children and siblings.

The grafts were round and of full skin thickness with diameter 12 mm. They were removed in sterile conditions and transplanted on the volar surface of the recipient's forearm.

Macroscopic and stereomicroscopic readings began on the 6. day. The onset of capillary thromboses, the visible expression of an irreversible bio-immunological reaction, was taken as the limit for graft survival time.

Mathematical analysis of the mean survival values of the three classes of grafts showed, in confirmation of theoretical hypotheses, that graft survival is shorter, the greater the genetic distance between donor and recipient. Between unrelated donors the mean was 11.9 ± 0.3 days, between parents and children 14.2 ± 0.7 and between siblings 15.1 ± 0.8.

These findings can be compared suggestively with the data in the Registry of Human Kidney Transplantation and confirm that kidney and skin transplants are controlled by the same immunogenetic law.

Extending our research we examined whether the ABO erythrocyte system affects the course of skin grafts since it is known that these erythrocyte antigens are present at skin level. Contrasting hypotheses have been advanced on this question (GRIFFITHS et al.; KUHNS et al.; RAPAPORT et al.; CEPPELLINI et al.).

DAUSSET et al. have recently reported that homografts from A subjects induced a white graft type of rejection in group O subjects who had been preimmunized against AB. We ourselves have studied the possible influence of some natural blood antigens on homografts of non-preimmunized individuals. Our research showed that histoincompatibility is greater in homografts carried out in group O recipients from donors with antigen A_1. The grafts may present early rejections or even white graft type of rejection (four observed cases). On the other hand we have observed no interaction between histocompatibility and the MN and Rh (D) erythrocyte systems.

The P 1—P 2 system proved to have an influence on homografts (10.8 days survival between P-incompatible unrelated donors and 12.4 days between P-compatible unrelated donors).

To conclude, we think that the results of our studies give further weight to the hypothesis that the test skin homograft is the most useful biological test for analyzing genetic distance and thereby the degree of histocompatibility between donor and recipient.

Über die klinische Anwendung homologer und heterologer Hauttransplantate

W. WITTELS, I. Universitäts-Hautklinik Wien (Österreich)

Die Kürze der zur Verfügung stehenden Zeit gestattet nur eine sehr knappe und gedrängte Darstellung des Themas. Homologe und heterologe Hauttransplantate können prinzipiell nur als eine vorübergehende Maßnahme in ihrer therapeutischen Anwendung angesehen werden. Während bei der homologen Transplantation von Mensch zu Mensch eine echte Einheilung für einen variablen Zeitraum stattfindet, ist vom heterologen Transplantat nur unter außergewöhnlich günstigen Umständen eine kurzzeitige, echte Einheilung zu erwarten. Als Kriterium der echten Einheilung ist das histo-morphologisch und histo-chemisch nachgewiesene Einsprossen von Capillaren in das Transplantat anzusehen, wie es unter anderem von K. WOLFF u. W. WITTELS aus der Klinik publiziert wurde (Dias). Unter den normalen Bedingungen der klinischen Anwendung erreicht man mit heterologen Transplantaten einen biologischen Wundverschluß für kurze Zeit, auf dessen Vorteile noch eingegangen wird.

33*

Auf Grund des Mitgeteilten sind somit die Indikationsgebiete homologer und heterologer Hautübertragungen abgegrenzt. Sie betreffen in erster Linie den Verschluß großflächiger, lebensbedrohender Wunden, wie er nach ausgedehnten, tiefen Verbrennungen auftritt, bei denen eine Erstversorgung mit Autotransplantaten infolge schlechten Allgemeinzustandes oder des Fehlens von Entnahmeflächen nicht möglich ist. Weiter hat sich das Homo- als auch das Heterotransplantat in der Therapie schlechtheilender Ulcerationen verschiedenster Genese an den unteren Extremitäten sehr bewährt. Das homologe Transplantat ist beim großflächigen Wundverschluß gegenüber dem heterologen unbedingt vorzuziehen, da seine Wirkung die des letztgenannten weitaus übertrifft. Die klinische Anwendung heterologer Hauttransplantate ist somit als letzte Notstandsmaßnahme beim Fehlen auto- und homologen Ersatzmaterials anzusehen.

Auf Grund eigener Erfahrungen an der von Prof. TAPPEINER geleiteten I. Universitäts-Hautklinik in Wien ist über den klinischen Wert dieser Transplantate wie folgt Stellung zu nehmen:

1. Die großflächige Homotransplantation von vital übertragenen Spalthautlappen, von Hautspendern 24 Std vor der Übertragung entnommen und bei +4°C refrigeriert, ergibt beim eigenen Krankengut von schwersten Verbrennungen eine echte Einheilung von 21 Tagen als Mittelwert. Die Einheilungsdauer kann durch die Gabe von Glucocorticosteroiden verlängert werden. Entschließt man sich zu dieser Maßnahme, ist ein kritisches Abwägen der Vor- und Nachteile der Steroidapplikation unbedingt nötig. Das Angehen der Homotransplantate ist in erster Linie von der Keimbesiedlung der Wundfläche abhängig. Gezielte lokale und allgemeine Antibioticavorbehandlung ist daher notwendig, wobei sich in letzter Zeit die lokale Gentamycintherapie mit Refobacin in Puder- und Salbenform sehr bewährt hat. Im Vergleich zum Heterotransplantat ist das Homotransplantat wesentlich anspruchsloser in seinen Anheilungsbedingungen. Für den genannten Zeitraum von etwa 3 Wochen ist das homologe vom autologen Transplantat klinisch nicht zu unterscheiden. Die schachbrettartige, wechselweise Auflage von Auto- und Homohautläppchen eignet sich zum endgültigen Wundverschluß ausgezeichnet und erlaubt es, mit einem Minimum von Autotransplantaten auszukommen.

2. Beim nicht behebbaren Mangel an homologem Hautmaterial sowie aus klinisch-experimentellem Interesse wurden Heterohauttransplantationen bei ausgedehnten Verbrennungen durchgeführt. Zwei Arten von Transplantaten kamen zur Anwendung. *Erstens* embryonale Kalbsvollhaut, entnommen von etwa 4 Monate alten Kalbsembryonen. Die Aufbewahrung erfolgte bei +4 °C in isotonen Breitbandantibioticalösungen. *Zweitens* Kollagenfolien der Fa. Braun, Melsungen, die uns zu Versuchszwecken zur Verfügung gestellt wurden. Diese werden aus Tierkollagen in bestimmten Verfahren hergestellt und sind steril abgepackt lange lagerfähig. Auf der Wunde aufgetragen, unterscheiden sie sich optisch kaum von Kalbshauttransplantationen. Mit beiden Transplantatarten ist lediglich eine Verklebung mit der Wundfläche im Sinne des biologischen Verbandes für etwa 5 bis 8 Tage zu erreichen. Das embryonale Kalbshauttransplantat fällt auf Grund der eigenen Erfahrungen der Proteolyse später anheim als die derzeitigen Chargen der Kollagenfolien. Der Effekt des biologischen Verbandes besteht in seiner Behinderung des Eiweißverlustes, Anregung der Epithelisierung bei gleichzeitiger Eindämmung der bakteriellen Wundbesiedlung und subjektiver Schmerzfreiheit.

Während der Haftdauer der Transplantate von durchschnittlich einer Woche ist eine merkbare Besserung im Allgemeinbefinden der Schwerstkranken festzustellen. Nach Auflösung der Transplantate oder deren Abstoßung in mumifiziertem Zustand ist das Wundgebiet gereinigt und gut durchblutet mit festen körnigen

Granulationen. Es befindet sich in einem idealen Zustand für eine nun nachfolgende Autotransplantation.

Die zweite Indikationsgruppe umfaßt schlechtheilende Ulcera, vorwiegend an den Unterschenkeln, deren Genese varicös, arteriovenös, trophisch und durch ionisierende Strahlen bedingt sein kann. Da an der Klinik von unserem Verbrennungskrankengut oft homologes als auch heterologes Transplantationsmaterial zur Verfügung stand, konnten wir die Wirkung dieser Transplantate an einem größeren Patientengut beobachten.

Homologe Transplantate wurden ein- bis höchstens zweimal übertragen, um keine Sensibilisierung zu provozieren. Heterologe Kalbshaut sowie Kollagenfolien konnten unbeschränkt oft übertragen werden, da embryonales Gewebe fast nie antigen wirkt, die Untersuchungen über mögliche Immunisierung mit Kollagenfolien sind noch im Gange.

Alle drei Transplantatarten zeigten einen ausgezeichneten Effekt hinsichtlich der Anregung der Epithelisierung und der Bildung eines gut durchbluteten, keimarmen Granulationsgewebes. Nachfolgende Autotransplantationen haben nach dieser Vorbehandlung eine viel höhere Anheilungsquote.

Zusammenfassend ist festzuhalten, daß die Hauthomotransplantation als lebensrettende Zwischenmaßnahme in der Therapie ausgedehnter Verbrennungen ihren festen Platz hat. Bisherige Versuche mit heterologen embryonalen Kalbshauttransplantaten verliefen ermutigend, die Anwendung industriell hergestellter Kollagenfolien wird kritisch weiterverfolgt und zeigt vielversprechende Anfangsergebnisse. Als Nebenindikationsgebiet hat sich die Anwendung homo- und heterologer Transplantate zur Verbesserung der Heilungstendenz schlecht heilender Ulcera verschiedener Genese ergeben.

Acid Mucopolysaccharide Synthesis in Scleredema

S. I. LAMBERG, Department of Dermatology, School of Medicine, University of Pennsylvania, Philadelphia (USA)

Recent histochemical and biochemical studies of scleredema have shown an accumulation of material in the corium which stains in the same way as an acid mucopolysaccharide (AMPS) and acts as either hyaluronic acid or chondroitin. The purpose of this study was to define the specific AMPS involved and to determine the dynamics of its accululation. Methods of organ culture, autoradiography and radio-chemical assay were utilized to compare incorporation of glucosamine (a component of hyaluronic acid) and incorporation of galactosamine (a component of chondroitin) into AMPS.

Two cases of scleredema and five controls were studied. Specimens of skin were obtained from both involved and more normal areas of the patients with scleredema and from the edge of wounds on the back and abdomen of controls undergoing elective surgery. 40 specimens from the two patients and 20 specimens from the controls were planted on organ culture dishes and incubated under standard conditions for 10 days.

Radiochromatographically-pure glucosamine-^{14}C and galactosamine-^{14}C were added in "pulses" of 2 days prior to the removal of each specimen. Part of the specimen was fixed, sectioned and dipped for autoradiography. The rest of the tissue and the culture media were separately weighed and digested, and the AMPS isolated by selective precipitation. Liquid scintillation counting, hyaluronidase digestion and electrophoresis were used to characterize the AMPS obtained. To minimize variables the only data compared were those within the same experimental "run" which included both scleredema and control skin. To eliminate laboratory prejudice all specimens were coded and all manipulations were performed at random. Only when the final date and counting were completed was the code broken and the specimens rearranged in sequence for evaluation.

Results. [14]C labeled AMPS derived from glucosamine-^{14}C was present in largest amounts in the tissue from involved areas of the two patients with scleredema; it was in a mid-range in the clinically normal areas of these patients and in smallest amounts in control skin from normal subjects. The galactosamine-^{14}C exposed specimens did not differ in their amount of uptake between involved, clinically normal and control skin. Since glucosamine is a component of hyaluronic acid and galactosamine of chondroitin, these findings suggest that the AMPS accumulated in scleredema is hyaluronic acid.

In order to learn whether differences in incorporation of the isotope were due to augmented production of AMPS or to stronger binding by the tissue, it was necessary to know the total production of labeled AMPS, including that which diffused into the media. A most striking difference was seen when concentrations of labeled AMPS in the tissue were compared to those in the media. There was a marked increase in amounts of incorporated glucosamine-^{14}C retained by tissue in scleredema as compared to controls; clinically uninvolved areas from the patient being intermediate. The media contained more counts than the tissue only in the control specimens.

Radioelectrophoresis showed that most of the glucosamine-^{14}C was incorporated into a material which traveled in the same location as hyaluronic acid. Hyaluronidase removed most of this labeling, further suggesting that the AMPS which accumulates in scleredema is mostly hyaluronic acid.

The studies presented here show that both scleredema skin and normal control skin synthesized large amounts of high molecular weight AMPS. However, the total production, including that which diffused into the media, was not much different. An important feature is that the AMPS diffuse into the growth media far more easily in control skin than in skin involved with scleredema. It is proposed, therefore, that the defect in scleredema is one of abnormal protein binding rather than overproduction of hyaluronic acid. The increased metachromasia in tissue sections may only be reflecting this binding.

La dynamique de la croissance des fibroblastes in vitro à partir des explants de peau humaine

M. GAVRILESCU, Centrul Dermato-Venerologic al M. S. P. S., Bucarest (Roumanie)

En vue d'obtenir des données sur la dynamique de la croissance des fibroblastes in vitro à partir des explants de peau, nous avons prélevé des fragments de peau normale à 21 sujets exempts de toute dermatose. La mise en culture des explants consiste soit à leur inclusion dans du plasma coagulé de coq, soit — selon le procédé de THERKELSEN — à leur maintien dans les tubes Leighton entre deux surfaces planes de verre (notamment des lamelles couvre-objet). Dans les deux cas le milieu nutritif se compose des éléments suivants: 70% d'un mélange en parties égales des solutions de HANKS et EARLE, 20% d'une solution de hydrolisé de

lactalbumine à 2,5%, 10% sérum frais de veau, 1% d'une solution M/5 de glutamine et des antibiotiques (pénicilline 400 U/ml et streptomycine 200 μg/ml). Les
préparés sont maintenus à l'étuve à 37 °C et par des contrôles journaliers on peut
suivre le développement des fibroblastes qui découle en plusieurs étapes.

Après une période de quiétude d'environ 2 jours, les premières manifestations
apparaissent sous l'aspect d'une *agitation plasmatique*. Tout près des explants, le
coagulum de plasma — qui jusqu'alors était d'une transparence homogène —
engendre de fines pseudo-striations, dûes probablement aux certaines modifications
subies par sa réfractilité. Les pseudo-striations, disposées isolément ou en faisceaux,
s'appendent au fragment de peau ou bien elles s'organisent en son voisinage;
elles s'éloignent par degrés, décrivant une trajectoire courbe, en arcade, concave
vers le fragment; à leurs extrémités elles s'éparpillent en éventail et disparaissent
imperceptiblement.

Un autre phénomène, secondaire à celui qui vient d'être décrit, est *l'agitation
cellulaire*. Elle s'exprime principalement par la migration des cellules qui se
séparent du fragment dont elles proviennent et duquel elles s'éloignent graduelle-
ment. Il s'agit de cellules isolées, rondes, de petite taille, ayant un contour
réfringent. La migration concerne à la fois une grande quantité de détritus
cellulaire et de fibriles conjonctives qui réalisent en ensemble des amas polymorphes, assez étendus, sur le pourtour des fragments.

L'agitation plasmatique et cellulaire, en tant que phénomènes prémonitoires,
n'indique pourtant pas l'imminence de la croissance in vitro, étant donné qu'ils
apparaissent même dans les cultures entièrement dépourvues d'activité proli-
férative.

Le premier signe indiquant la croissance des fibroblastes est l'apparition des
prolongements cytoplasmiques, en «touffe d'herbe», émergeant des fragments
inclus. Leur structure fusiforme, fibroblastique devient de plus en plus manifeste et
par leur accolement successif on assiste à la formation de faisceaux et d'arbori-
sations caractéristiques.

Une autre modalité indiquant le début de la croissance est la transformation
fibroblastique des cellules migrées, qui représentent à ce propos un potentiel
remarquable. Progressivement, toutes les cellules migrées se mettent en activité
comme par contamination de proche en proche. Au commencement, les cellules
fusiformes se disposent en directions variées, fortuites, mais dans les stades suivants, un certain courant dominant s'impose, faisant disparaître toute autre
direction à peine ébauchée. Assez souvent les pseudo-striations plasmatiques
dirigent l'évolution d'un faisceau dans leur propre sens.

En utilisant le procédé de THERKELSEN, nous avons obtenu une appréciation
sur la force de croissance des fibroblastes constitués en faisceau à direction déterminée. En examinant la marge de la lamelle couvre-objet on constate que les
faisceaux qui la cotoient parallèlement ne la dépassent pas, tandis que les faisceaux perpendiculaires sur cette marge aboutissent toujours à l'outre-passer, en
y créant de nouvelles colonies cellulaires à direction identique que le faisceau-
mère. Cela veut dire que la force qui imprime la direction à un faisceau de fibroblastes dans le sens de la longueur possède un pouvoir de progression supérieur
à la croissance en épaisseur de celui-ci.

Biologia de las heridas cutaneas

J. Sánchez-Muros y F. de Dulanto, Cátedra y Escuela Profesional de Dermatología Médico- Quirúrgica, Universidad de Granada (España)

I. Material y metodos

Estudiamos el proceso de reparación de las heridas cutáneas en los siguientes grupos de lesiones:

1. *Heridas incisas*, efectuadas en la región infraclavicular para obtener injertos de piel total destinados a la reparación de defectos faciales. Se suturaron con puntos en U de seda fina.

2. *Heridas excisas:* Zonas donadoras de injertos dermoepidermicos obtenidos con dermatomo o cuchilla.

3. *Zonas tratadas con abrasion rotatoria.* Las investigaciones se realizaron mediante numerosas pequeñas biopsias obtenidas a intervalos regulares a partir de la intervención hasta 25 dias después con cilindros cortantes especiales movidos electricamente. Las biopsias se incluyeron en parafina verificando series de cortes para lograr una visión tridimensional.

Además estudiamos numerosas cicatrices de heridas incisas y de zonas dadoras de injertos laminares de 1 a 3 años de antiguedad con el fin de precisar aspectos tardíos del proceso reparador.

II. Resultados

Las observaciones verificadas muestran diferencias considerables con las descripciones clásicas. En las heridas *incisas* la epidermis se invagina en profundidad sobre la superficie cruenta y forma densas proliferaciones acantósicas. También prolifera a lo largo de los hilos de sutura formando tubos o canales epiteliales que provocan intensas reacciones en la dermis. De estos fenómenos depende la cicatriz: estética o patológica y deben tenerse en cuenta en las técnicas quirúrgicas.

No hemos observado la formación de nuevos folículos pilosebáceos señalada en la bibliografía y a la que puede oponerse una observación clínica innegable: las cicatrices son lampiñas. No hay pruebas definitivas de la neoformación de folículos pilosebáceos en el ser humano después del nacimiento a diferencia de lo que sucede en los mamíferos inferiores.

En las heridas *excisas* y zonas tratadás con abrasión rotatoria la reparación se desarrolla a partir de: 1° la epidermis de los bordes de la herida y 2° la vaina epitelial externa de los folículos pilosebáceos y el conducto excretor de las glándulas sebáceas. Obtuvimos la impresión que la matriz del pelo, sus vainas epiteliales internas y las glandulas sudoríparas eccriñas no intervienen en la reparación de la epidermis de superficie y regeneran únicamente sus propias estructuras. El concepto de «Equipotencialidad de la célula epidermica» de Montagna tendría, por lo tanto, limitaciones al menos en el ser humano adulto. Son interesantes las relaciones entre *reparación y carcinogenesis*. En la epidermis en regeneración se observan aspectos morfológicamente similares a las etapas precoces de los carcinomas que desaparecen rápidamente. Estos datos pueden ser válidos para profundizar en el conocimiento de la carcinogénesis, como fracaso del control de la epidermis por la dermis. Esta situación entre otras sucede en los queratomas actínicos y es posible modificarla mediante la abrasión rotatoria.

Electron Microscopy of the Immunologically Competent Cells During Skin Homograft Rejection in the Rhesus Monkey (Macaca mulatta)

F. Allegra, M. Bell and L. Giacometti, Oregon Regional Primate Research Center, Beaverton, Oregon (USA)

Electron microscopists disagree on the definition and identification of the cells involved in rejection processes. Furthermore, to our knowledge, no one has investigated with the aid of electron microscopy, the immunologically competent cells acting in the skin during skin homografts rejection. The present study was undertaken in order to establish the type of cells occurring in the skin during homograft rejection in rhesus monkeys, using both light and electron microscopy. For light microscopy, biopsy specimens collected daily were fixed in Bouin's fluid, embedded in paraffin and stained with routine hematoxylin and eosin. For electron microscopy, specimens were obtained from first and second-set grafts, seven and five days respectively after grafting. They have been fixed in glutaraldehyde, postfixed in $O_s\ O_4$ and, after dehydration, embedded in Araldite.

Beginning with the 2nd to 3rd day after grafting, an increasing number of mononuclear cells was noticed. The pale-stained nuclei of these cells were large, oval or round and contained one or two nucleoli. They were surrounded by rims of basophilic cytoplasm and selectively located at the border zone between the graft and the host bed. From this zone they gradually invaded the deep and middle dermis of the grafted skin. This type of cell corresponds to the "reticulum cell" as defined by Fagraeus (1960) in "Mechanism of antibody formation", Ciba Foundation Symposium.

Four to five days after grafting, the above mentioned cells were joined by small lymphocytes. Few eosinophils, neutrophils, red blood cells and occasional plasma cells were seen among these cells. The above mentioned cells have been observed both during first and second-set graft rejection. The lymphocytes appeared earlier (three to four days) after the second-set graft.

The ultrastructure of the reticulum cell showed a rim of cytoplasm with ill-defined cytoplasmic organelles surrounding the large nucleus. Few elements of endoplasmic reticulum and free ribosomes were identified. Some of these cells had microtubules, which may indicate that they were capable of dividing. Lymphocytes, with large, round nuclei, some containing large nucleoli, were identified. Free ribosomes were abundant in the cytoplasm.

Seven days after first-set grafting, plasma cells were demonstrated, which had uniformly organized endoplasmic reticulum cisternae. Golgi elements had small dense granules associated with them. Mitochondria were numerous.

In the same preparation, seven days after first-set graft, the plasma cells showed both uniformly organized or dilated endoplasmic reticulum cisternae; moreover, the cytoplasm of the plasma cells having dilated endoplasmic reticulum cisternae was much more electron-opaque, thus giving further evidence of their secretory activity.

Five days after the second-set graft, plasma cells were encountered in which the endoplasmic reticulum cisternae were greatly distended.

A few days after first-and second-set grafting, many dermal cells are found in the grafted skin. Since these cells proliferate before the establishment of vascular connections with the host and are also found in autografts, it is likely that the reticulum cells originate and proliferate in the grafted tissue as a consequence of the inflammatory and reactive processes accompanying the rejection. In more advanced stages, both in first and second rejection, lymphocytes and plasma cells have been observed. These cells are probably of host origin and may enter the graft via the newly formed vessels, together with other circulating cells. They probably play a role in the formation, storage and secretion of cell-bound and humoral antibodies.

Zur Frage des Ausgangsmaterials der senilen Elastose
Licht- und elektronenmikroskopische Befunde

H. BERGER, Universitäts-Hautklinik Freiburg i. Br. (Deutschland)

Seit den grundlegenden Untersuchungen UNNAS (1894) wird darüber diskutiert, ob das für die senile Elastose typische Material aus kollagenen Fasern, aus elastischen Elementen oder aus beiden Bestandteilen und Retikulinfasern besteht. Bis in die jüngste Zeit existieren hierüber verschiedene Ansichten: So nehmen z. B. NIEBAUER und STOCKINGER auf Grund elektronenoptischer Untersuchungen an, daß bei der senilen Elastose „primär eine Schädigung des kollagenen Fasermaterials vorliegt, aus dem elektronendichtes Material zusammensintert, das dem Bild der senilen Elastose entspricht". Hingegen sind FEYRTER, FEYRTER u. NIEBAUER (1) bis (3), BRAUN-FALCO u. a. der Auffassung, daß die Strukturen elastischen Fasern von ungewöhnlicher Beschaffenheit entsprechen und daß die pathischen Veränderungen der elastischen Fasern zum Teil auf Veränderungen ihrer Hüll- und Kittmassen bzw. ihrer Mikrofibrillen beruhen [FEYRTER u. NIEBAUER, (2)]. STEIGLEDER vermutet, daß es sich um ein neugebildetes minderwertiges Bindegewebe handelt, das weder als Elastica noch als Kollagen anzusprechen ist.

Zur *elektronenmikroskopischen Untersuchung* gelangten insgesamt neun Gewebsstücke mit seniler Elastose und ein Kontrollpräparat aus klinisch bedeckt getragener Haut eines 21jährigen Mannes.

Im elektronenmikroskopischen Bild lassen sich verschiedene Degenerationsprodukte nachweisen, die auf Grund morphologischer Ähnlichkeit zum Teil auf das elastische Material zurückgeführt werden können (BERGER u. WALTER).

1. Fibrillen, die in ihrer Struktur den kollagenen Fibrillen ähneln, jedoch im Vergleich zu den unveränderten Kollagenfibrillen nicht so scharf begrenzt sind und keine so dichte Innenstruktur wie diese aufweisen. Die für die kollagenen Fibrillen typische periodische Querstreifung ist meist erkennbar, wenn auch manchmal verwaschen. Zwischen den Fibrillen liegt amorphes Material, dessen Herkunft nicht geklärt werden kann.

2. Faserförmige Strukturen, die wie elastische Fasern eine unregelmäßig verlaufende, elektronenoptisch dichte und scharfe Außenlinie aufweisen. Mit den elastischen Fasern hat diese Degenerationsform die homogene Matrix gemeinsam, in die stärker kontrastgebende punktförmige, fibrillenartige oder schollige Verdichtungen eingelagert sind. Die genannten Strukturen ähneln sehr den unveränderten elastischen Fasern, wie sie z. B. von SCHWARZ; SCHWARZ u. DETTMER; GIESE u. GIESEKING sowie von GIESEKING beschrieben sind. Allerdings erscheint die Struktur wesentlich vergröbert.

3. Ebenfalls faserförmige Strukturen, die mit den unter 2. beschriebenen große morphologische Ähnlichkeit haben (jedoch keine scharfe Außenlinie aufweisen). Wie diese besitzen sie fibrillenartige Einlagerungen verschiedener Dicke. Sie unter-

scheiden sich jedoch von den scharf begrenzten faserförmigen Strukturen durch den Besitz einer feingranulären „Matrix", in die unregelmäßig Hohlräume eingelagert sein können, die zur Umgebung hin scharf begrenzt sind. Die Bilder unter 2. und 3. haben eine erhebliche Ähnlichkeit mit denen, wie sie bei Schädigung der elastischen Fasern der Aorta beim experimentellen Lathyrismus (z. B. HARTMANN, SEIFERT u. BÖLSING; SEIFERT u. HARTMANN) beschrieben werden.

4. Eine Degenerationsform, die gekennzeichnet ist durch netzartige Strukturen, die aus elektronenoptisch leeren Räumen und aus einer dazwischenliegenden dichtgefügten, feingranulären Substanz bestehen. An manchen Stellen geht dieses netzartig angeordnete Material in wie Blasen aussehende Räume über, die mit einem homogenen Inhalt ausgefüllt und von einer elektronenoptisch dichten schmalen Außenzone umgeben sind.

Außer den als Degenerationsform beschriebenen degenerierenden kollagenen Fibrillen lassen sich die übrigen Degenerationsprodukte eindeutig weder auf elastisches Material noch auf Kollagen zurückführen. Auf Grund der morphologischen Ähnlichkeit der im elektronenoptischen Bild dichtbegrenzten faserförmigen Strukturen mit den elastischen Fasern ist es wahrscheinlich, daß sie aus diesen entstehen. Die nichtbegrenzten faserförmigen Strukturen (unter 3. aufgeführt) scheinen aus den dichtbegrenzten faserförmigen Strukturen hervorzugehen. Für diese Auffassung spricht, daß Zwischenformen gefunden wurden. Die als 4. Degenerationsform beschriebenen netzartig angeordneten Strukturen sind sowohl elastischen als auch kollagenen Fasern morphologisch zu unähnlich, als daß man einen unmittelbaren Übergang annehmen könnte. Möglicherweise sind hieran kollagene und elastische Fasern sowie die Mikrofibrillen der Grundsubstanz (HAUST) beteiligt bzw. Retikulinfibrillen.

Bei der Silberimprägnation der elektronenmikroskopischen Einzelschnitte nach MARX u. MÖLBERT hatte sich ergeben (BERGER u. HUNDEIKER), daß ein sehr differentes Kontrastierungsverhalten zwischen elastischen Fasern einerseits und kollagenen Fibrillen bzw. Retikulinfibrillen andererseits besteht. Innerhalb aktinisch-elastotischen Materials lassen sich mit dieser Methode nur zu einem sehr geringen Teil argyrophile Strukturen nachweisen, die nach Form und Größe kollagenem Material oder Retikulinfibrillen entsprechen. Der enge Kontakt bzw. das Einstrahlen versilberbarer Fasern von außen in elastische Fasern kann — entsprechend den Verhältnissen in unveränderter Haut (BERGER u. HUNDEIKER) — beobachtet werden.

Die Rutheniumrotkontrastierung (nach FASSKE u. STEINS) bzw. die Alcianblaumethode ergaben im Elektronenmikroskop zu wenig Kontrast.

Die durchgeführten lichtoptischen Untersuchungen, insbesondere mit Hilfe der Phosphorwolframräure-Hämatoxylinfärbung nach MALLORY, erlauben den Schluß, daß wahrscheinlich ein direkter Übergang von den elastischen zu den veränderten Fasern besteht. Mit der Mallory-Färbung hebt sich das veränderte Material vom elastischen ab, wohingegen es sich mit den üblicherweise für Elastica angewandten Färbeverfahren von diesen nicht unterscheiden läßt. Die Tatsache, daß durch äußere Einflüsse veränderte kollagene oder elastische Fasern stark von den normalen in ihrer morphologischen Struktur abweichen können, macht die Zuordnung der degenerierten Fasern bei der senilen Elastose zu dem kollagenen oder dem elastischen Fasersystem allerdings im Einzelfalle schwierig. Die Interpretation wird weiterhin dadurch erschwert, daß schon unter normalen Bedingungen die elastischen Fasern räumlich sehr eng mit den Kollagenfasern verknüpft sind.

Eng mit der Frage der senilen Elastose ist die nach der Entstehung der elastischen Fasern verbunden. Während wir über die Bildung der kollagenen Fasern recht gute Vorstellungen haben, ist über den Bildungsort elastischer Fasern

relativ wenig bekannt. Ebensowenig wissen wir Eindeutiges über den „Umsatz"
elastischen Materials und darüber, ob die Zellen, die die elastischen Fasern bilden,
zeitlebens diese Funktion in gleicher Weise erfüllen oder — mit zunehmendem
Alter — die Fähigkeit immer stärker eingeschränkt ist. Es gibt gewisse Indizien,
die hierfür sprechen könnten, wie z. B. die Angaben von HAYEK über den verminderten ¹⁴C-Einbau in das elastische Material der Lungen mit steigendem Alter
und das auffallend spärliche Vorkommen von elastischen Fasern in Granulations-
geweben. Wir selbst haben im subepidermalen Bindegewebsband über elastoti-
schen Herden (RITZENFELD) regelmäßig Fibroblasten gefunden, die elektronenmikroskopisch Zeichen intensiver Kollagenproduktion erkennen ließen. Vereinzelt
liegen Fibroblasten, insbesondere perivasculär, auch umschlossen von aktinisch-
elastotischem Material. Dieser Befund gewinnt an Bedeutung im Hinblick auf die
Ansichten STEIGLEDERS und SALFELDS über die Herkunft aktinisch-elastotischen
Materials. Die Ausreifung kollagener Fibrillen in dem neugebildeten Binde-
gewebsmaterial ist — wie Befunde an silberimprägnierten elektronenmikroskо-
pischen Schnitten zeigen — unvollständig. Das neugebildete Material lagert sich
an benachbartes elastotitisches an, das homogen erscheint und mit dem zuvor
unter 4. beschriebenen Material identisch ist. Phagocytose aktinisch-elastotischen
Materials wurde nicht gesehen, ebensowenig bisher Neubildung elastischer Fasern.

Literatur. BERGER, H., u. M. HUNDEIKER: Arch. klin. exp. Derm. **228**, 385 (1967). —
BERGER, H., u. M. WALTER: 11. Kongr. dtsch. Ges. Aesthet. Med. Münster, 21. Mai 1966;
Aesthet. Med. **16**, 121 (1967). — BRAUN-FALCO, O.: In: Hbd. d. Haut- und Geschl.-Kr.,
Ergänzungswerk I/2, p. 519—561. Berlin-Göttingen-Heidelberg: Springer 1964. — FASSKE,
H., u. I. STEINS: Z. wiss. Mikr. **67**, 47 (1965). — FEYRTER, F.: Frankfurt. Z. Path. **75**, 317 (1966).
— FEYRTER, F., u. G. NIEBAUER: (1) Z. Haut- u. Geschl.-Kr. **40**, 218 (1966); — (2) Derm.
Wschr. **152**, 1176 (1966); — (3) Med. Welt N. F. **17**, 2097 (1966). — GIESE, W., u. R. GIESE-
KING: Beitr. path. Anat. **117**, 17 (1957). — GIESEKING, R.: Veröffentl. aus der morpholo-
gischen Pathologie, Heft 72. Stuttgart: Fischer 1966. — HARTMANN, F., K. SEIFERT u. F.
BÖLSING: Z. Zellforsch. **59**, 358 (1963). — HAUST, M. D.: Amer. J. Path. **47**, 1113 (1965). —
HAYEK, H.: Münch. med. Wschr. **108**, 864 (1966). — MARX, R., u. E. MÖLBERT: J. Microscopie
4, 799 (1965). — NIEBAUER, G., u. L. STOCKINGER: Arch. klin. exp. Derm. **221**, 122 (1965). —
RITZENFELD, P.: Arch. klin. exp. Derm. **215**, 558 (1963). — SALFELD, K.: Disk.-Bem. zu
BERGER u. WALTER. — SEIFERT, K., u. F. HARTMANN: Z. Zellforsch. **59**, 878 (1963). —
STEIGLEDER, K. G.: Veränderungen der Haut im Alter. In: Alterskrankheiten, S. 356—380.
Hrsg. von G. SCHETTLER. Stuttgart: Thieme 1966. — SCHWARZ, W.: Arch. Biol. (Liège) **75**,
369 (1964). — SCHWARZ, W., u. N. DETTMER: Virchows Arch. path. Anat. **323**, 243 (1953). —
UNNA, P. G.: Mh. prakt. Derm. **19**, 397 (1894).

Epithelial and Fibroblast Tissue Culture Studies as a Trial to Understand the Action of Asiaticoside as a Healing and as a Fibrolytic Agent

H. EL-HEFNAWI, Cairo University (UAR)

The two actions of asiaticoside as a healing agent (reported by many authors)
and as a fibrolytic agent (EL-HEFNAWI 1962) seem contradictory. The present study
on epithelial and fibroblast tissue cultures is a trial to understand the action of
this drug on these two types of cells. The study of fibroblast tissue culture showed
that the activity of the fibroblast cells was markedly diminished in the presence of
asiaticoside and these cells finally shrivelled and died. The study on the epithelial
tissue culture slices of pig's skin (EL-HEFNAWI and MAY) showed a marked increase in the thickness of the prickle cell layer as a result of activity of the basal

cell layer. The fibroblasts in the dermis of the slices of pig's skin showed some changes too.

The work done on epithelial tissue culture: The powder of Madecassol (asiaticoside)* was added to the medium

1/3 m gm/ml	no action
2/3 m gm/ml	little action
1 m gm/ml	maximum effect

The effect of Madecassol was:

1. Increased vascularity of the dermis and a cellular reaction. 2. The fibrous tissue cells in the dermis show rounding of the fibroblasts. 3. Epidermal changes: parakeratosis, thickening of stratum corneum, vacuolization of the prickle cells and basophilic staining of the basal cell layer.

The work done on the fibroblast tissue culture: 1.25 mg/ml of asiaticoside emulsion was added to the fibroblast tissue culture solution. Only slight effect (a little rounding of some cells). Presumably higher than this would damage the cells. Less than 1.25 mg/ml had no apparent effect on the fibroblast cell. Tissue culture solution was used as control and showed no effect. Again, 0.01% (1 m gm/ml) of the soluble form of asiasticoside was added to the fibroblast tissue culture. Solution destroyed the sheet of the fibroblast cells. The same happened with higher concentrations. When 0.5 m gm/ml of the soluble asiaticoside was added, there was only slight effect. Less than 0.5 m gm/ml showed no effect at all.

The fibrolytic action of asiaticoside can explain many of the variable clinical results obtained by this drug:

1. *Cure of keloids and hypertrophic scars:* by stopping the activity of the fibroblasts.

2. *Healing of chronic ulcers:* by allowing better circulation of the ulcer area by dissolving the fibrous tissue bar around it.

3. *The beneficial action in the treatment of leprosy:* by dissolving the fibrous tissue in the nodules and around the affected nerves and hence allowing more intimate contact of the anti-leprotic agents and the Hansen's bacilli.

---

* Asiaticoside (Madecassol) was kindly supplied by Laboratoires La Roche Navarron-France.

Symposium 1   **Genodermatoses**

Génodermatoses

Genodermatosis

Genodermatosen

Organizer

S. Lapière, Belgium

Presidents

N. Danbolt, Norway

E. Hadida, France

J. Pierard, Belgium

H. W. Siemens, Netherlands

Delegate of the Organization Committee

U. W. Schnyder, Germany

Reports

Classification of Genodermatoses

D. Bloom, New York, N.Y. (USA)

Classification is a concept and working method of Medical Science which aims to change nosology from purely descriptive, morphological to that of biochemical etiological. While its ultimate task is to arrange diseases on the basis of etiologic factors its function consists essentially in acquisition of knowledge which leads to that basic information. Classification depends on all available knowledge which it utilizes to adjust and improve itself. It is thus dynamic and steadily changing.

In the field of genetically determined skin disorders science of genetics has been of great help in acquisition of knowledge and etiologic information. The revelation that gene action consists of different sequential biochemical steps, each of which is controlled by an enzyme, and that each disease is due, in the last instance, to a definite defect of chemical nature, has created a valuable investigative approach and has helped to clarify many obscure disorders.

However, etiologic classification of genodermatoses based on biochemical-enzymatic action of the gene is, at present impossible. For in most of these disorders this fundamental knowledge is incomplete or entirely lacking. Only in comparatively few disorders is this information available, namely, in the "inborn errors of metabolism", many of which involve also the skin. In others, only some of the underlying biochemical factors are known. Thus, in xanthoma tuberosum, it is hypercholesteremia, and in angiokeratoma corporis diffusum, lipid metabolic disturbance of the vascular wall is the known link in the gene action. The biochemical knowledge in these two dermatoses, although incomplete, is, nevertheless, of practical value. For it enables us to differentiate these disorders from others which they resemble clinically and histologically, namely, xanthoma tuberosum from other xanthomatous eruptions, and angiokeratoma corporis diffusum from angiokeratoma Mibelli.

In the inborn defects of structures of the dermis, still less biochemical information is available. Although we know that in pseudoxanthoma elasticum elastic tissue is defective, in Ehlers-Danlos syndrome there is collagen defect, and that Rendu-Osler-Weber disease is due to an inborn weakness of the vascular wall, the fundamental biochemical-enzymatic defect in these dermatoses is obscure. However, there is reason to expect that in these disorders also, additional basic biochemical knowledge will, some day, be obtained. Recent division of gargoylism into six types of mucopolysaccharidosis, on the basis of clinical, genetic and biochemical factors, is, I believe, a remarkable example of progress in etiologic elucidation of connective tissue disorders [1].

Until more fundamental biochemical knowledge is obtained, classification of genodermatoses has to be based on combination of clinical, morphologic and any available biochemical and genetic factors. The latter have proven particularly valuable. For knowledge of the mode of inheritance, whether autosomal or sex-linked, dominant or recessive, and information in regard to expressivity and penetrance of a disorder, yield important etiologic factors.

Thus in disorders of keratinization in which no basic biochemical knowledge is available, genetic factors in combination with clinical and morphologic features have proven useful criteria for classification. In the ichthyosis group, due a great deal to the genetic studies of Siemens [2], division in ichthyosis vulgaris and congenita, with erythroderma ichthyosiforme congenitale as a form of the latter, has proven satisfactory as a basis for classification. The bullous type of erythro-derma ichthyosiforme congenitale, which has been studied by LAPIERE [3], is, I believe, an entity, different from the non-bullous form, because of clinical, histologic and, particularly, genetic differences. In regard to this form of ichthyosis, recently termed "epidermolytic hyperkeratosis" [4], the opinion is expressed, that some systematized and even unilateral keratotic nevi are identical with this bullous disorder [5, 6]. This opinion is based on similarity of histopathologic features and on intrafamilial occurrence. It seems to me that this assumption may be erroneous. For identity of diseases cannot be assumed merely on the basis of histologic findings, particularly when there is a definite genetic difference. As to the intra-familial occurrence, one has to keep in mind that ichthyosis congenita as well as erythroderma ichthyosiforme congenitale, are known to change in appearance and assume a localized or linear configuration resembling keratotic nevi [7 to 9]. It is, therefore, necessary to have these patients observed from birth to adult life, in order to be certain that one is not dealing with a generalized form of ichthyosis which had assumed the appearance of a nevus.

In the other large and confusing group, namely, keratoderma palmare et plantare, an overall classification, based on clinical and genetic features with consideration of associated defects, was satisfactorily accomplished by FRANCE-SCHETTI and SCHNYDER [10].

The group of ectodermal dysplasias which involve mainly the epidermis and its appendages, has been studied by TOURAINE [11] and FRANCESCHETTI [12]. Here, a satisfactory overall classification is not feasible because of absolute lack of basic etiologic knowledge. Nevertheless, this group also yields some examples which illustrate the value of combined use of genetic and clinical criteria. For instance, hidrotic and anhidrotic ectodermal dysplasia have been established as two opposing entities, on the basis of clinical and genetic differences. Similarly, two different forms of "incontinentia pigmenti" were recognized: the "classic" Bloch-Sulzberger, and the "reticular" Naegeli type [12].

There is one disorder in this group which shows how new knowledge may bring an old entity into limelight and raise it to a position of medical importance. This disorder is the so-called "dyskeratosis congenita" [13], which has been linked to and even identified with Fanconi's syndrome, because of the high incidence of malignancy and blood dyscrasia [14 to 17]. It will be of interest to learn whether in this disorder also, chromosomal abnormality is present like in Fanconi's anemia.

In recent years new genodermatoses were recognized. Some of them are: "hereditary non-allergic angioneurotic edema" [18], "erythropoietic protopor-phyria" [19], and the syndrome of "congenital telangiectatic erythema and stunted growth" [20 to 22]. Their discovery and evaluation was possible because of the available biochemical and genetic knowledge. They illustrate also the close connec-tion of advances in basic science with progress in classification.

Conclusion. Although in most genodermatoses etiologic biochemical informa-tion is lacking, classification based on clinical and morphologic features combined with genetic factors, has proven very useful. Careful clinical and morphologic observation, and pedigree studies of affected families have not lost importance. On the contrary, advances in biochemical and genetic knowledge made them more valuable. One may expect that continued intensive study and progress in basic science will shed light on many obscure genodermatoses and thus make an etiologic classification possible.

References. 1. McKUSICK, V. A.: Heritable Disorders of Connective Tissue, 3rd. Ed. St. Louis 1966. — 2. SIEMENS, H. W.: Die Vererbung in der Ätiologie der Hautkrankheiten. In: Jadassohn's Handbuch der Haut- und Geschl.-Kr., Bd. 3. Berlin: Springer 1929. —

3. LAPIÈRE, S.: Ann. Derm. Syph. (Paris) 80, 597 (1953). — 4. FROST, P., and E. J. VAN SCOTT: Arch. Derm. 94, 113 (1966). — 5. BARKER, L. P., and W. SACHS: Arch. Derm. Syph. (Chic.) 67, 943 (1953). — 6. ZELIGMAN, I., and J. POMERANZ: Arch. Derm. 91, 120 (1965). — 7. SIEMENS, H. W.: Arch. Derm. Syph. (Berl.) 156, 624 (1928). — 8. DELACRÉTZ, J., and R.-M. LORÉTAN: Acta derm.-venereol. (Stockh.) 3, 659 (1957). — 9. LYELL, A., and C. H. WHITTLE: Acta derm.-venereol. (Stockh.) 667. — 10. FRANCESCHETTI, A., and U. W. SCHNYDER: Dermatologica (Basel) 120, 154 (1960). — 11. TOURAINE, A.: Presse méd. 62, 1289 (1957). — 12. FRANCESCHETTI, A.: Dermatologica (Basel) 106, 129 (1957). — 13. COSTELLO, M. J., and C. M. BUNCKE: Arch. Derm. 73, 123 (1956). — 14. BAZEX, A., et G. DUPRÉ: Ann. Derm. Syph. (Paris) 84, 497 (1957). — 15. EL NASI, and H. EL HAFNARI: Egypt. Med. Ass. 46/2, 1109 (1963). — 16. GORGOURAS, K.: Aust. J. Derm. 8, 31 (1965). — 17. SILVA, J. R. E.: Ann. Derm. Syph. (Paris) 93, 497 (1966). — 18. AUSTEN, K. F., and A. L. SHEFFER: New Engl. J. Med. 272, 649 (1965). — 19. MAGNUS, J. A.: Lancet 1961, 2, 448. — 20. BLOOM, D.: J. Pediat. 68, 103 (1966). — 21. SAWITSKY, A., D. BLOOM, and J. GERMAN: Ann. intern. Med. 65, 489 (1966). — 22. GERMAN, J., et L. P. CRIPPA: Ann. Génét. 9, 143 (1966).

Les génodermatoses bulleuses

S. LAPIÈRE, Clinique Dermatologique, Hôpital de Bavière, Université de Liège (Belgique)

Parmi les rapports qui vont suivre, les Dermatoses bulleuses génotypiques vont être envisagées successivement par U. W. SCHNYDER, par J. PIERARD et KINT et par J. R. SIMPSON.

Il nous a paru intéressant de les présenter d'abord dans leur ensemble comme BLOOM l'a fait pour les Génodermatoses en général, laissant à mes successeurs le soin de les reprendre en détail.

Ce travail, nous l'avions déjà publié il y a deux ans (1965); cependant, par la suite, beaucoup d'auteurs se sont intéressés au même sujet; j'ai souhaité présenter également leur point de vue.

Pas davantage que dans la plupart des autres Génodermatoses nous ne connaissons l'explication biochimique de ces déviations; nous nous en approchons semble-t-il dans le cas des Acrodermatites entéropathiques et de certaines Porphyries bulleuses.

En attendant, il nous faut donc les analyser soigneusement sur les autres plans c'est-à-dire clinique, morphologique et génétique et classer avec soin la valeur relative de ces caractères.

Compte tenu des toutes dernières acquisitions, nous continuons à les classer en quatre catégories:

Les Génodermatoses bulleuses par épidermolyse.

Les Génodermatoses bulleuses par dermolyse.

Les Génodermatoses bulleuses par dégénérescence granuleuse.

Les Génodermatoses bulleuses par acantholyse.

Les Génodermatoses bulleuses par épidermolyse

Nous y incorporons l'Epidermolyse bulleuse simple (KOEBNER), l'Epidermolyse létale (HERLITZ), ainsi que l'Acrodermatite entéropathique (DANBOLT et CLOSS). La symptômatologie clinique ainsi que l'évolution de ces trois affections sont nettement différentes ainsi que leur transmission héréditaire: mais ce qui les rapproche est leur image morphologique: celle-ci consiste en une altération primitive et essentielle du seul revêtement épidermique, tant que n'interviennent pas des complications infectieuses.

En ce qui concerne l'Epidermolyse congénitale simple de KOEBNER (E.B.S.K.) il semble régner un accord complet: ROBERTS et coll. (1960), LEVER (1961) et surtout PEARSON et SPARGO (1961) et PEARSON (1962) ont apporté des images convaincantes tant au microscope ordinaire qu'au microscope électronique. Seules les cellules épidermiques subissent le processus dégénératif; la membrane basale dans son entièreté reste adhérente à un derme normal. Cette affection se transmet en dominance.

L'Epidermolyse bulleuse létale de HERLITZ *(E.B.L.H.)*, au contraire, est sujette à de nombreuses controverses. Nous avons eu l'occasion d'en suivre deux cas jusqu'à l'évolution létale habituelle: deux soeurs, mortes la première à 6 mois et la seconde à 5 mois, malgré des soins très précis en collaboration avec notre Service Universitaire de Pédiatrie. Nos efforts conjugués n'ont pu les sauver d'une mort précoce; on n'observait pas d'état cicatriciel ni de kystes épidermiques.

La question en litige, discutée à perte de vue est celle-ci: l'E.B.L.H. doit-elle rester dans le cadre des Epidermolyses à côté de celle de KOEBNER, ou rentrer dans les Dermolyses (Epidermolyses bulleuses dystrophiques récessives).

Les arguments histopathologiques (LAPIÈRE et coll.), (PEARSON et coll.) montrent dans les cas de biopsies sur des bulles jeunes, des images superposables à celles de l'E.B.S.K., sans participation du derme. Il faut ajouter que dans les rares cas qui survivent plus longtemps, les images peuvent devenir moins nettes (SCHNYDER, KLUNKER, etc.). Faut-il s'en étonner si l'on tient compte du défaut non encore expliqué de guérison des ulcérations si superficielles dans les cas d'E.B.L.H. Cette affection se transmet en récessivité.

L'Acrodermatite entéropathique de DANBOLT *et* CLOSS, est intéressante à beaucoup de points de vue que nous ne saurions envisager ici. Selon sa morphologie, la situation des bulles, nous nous trouvons en présence, comme dans les deux Génodermatoses précédentes, d'une simple épidermolyse au-dessus de la membrane basale, avec intégrité du derme. C'est ce que nous avons conclu provisoirement de l'étude d'un cas observé par nous (1961). Nous attendons pour conclure, la relation d'autres examens histopathologiques que jusqu'à présent nous n'avons pas trouvés dans la littérature dermatologique.

Les Dermolyses bulleuses

Contrairement à ce qui se passe dans la catégorie précédente, le clivage bulleux se fait au niveau du derme, à la suite d'altérations localisées primitivement dans ce dernier, soit tout-à-fait en surface, soit plus profondément; le plancher de la bulle est constitué par du tissu collagène et élastique plus ou moins altéré; le toit est formé d'un épiderme primitivement intact doublé d'une membrane basale intacte ou non et même dans certains cas, d'une portion dermique (TRAPL, 1957; PEARSON, 1962). On comprend que dans ces conditions, contrairement au groupe précédent on doit s'attendre à des cicatrices soit hypertrophiques, soit atrophiques, d'intensité en rapport avec la profondeur et la durée du processus, mais aussi des kystes épidermiques ou grains de milium.

Diverses Génodermatoses bulleuses entrent dans cette catégorie de dermolyses:

1. Les Epidermolyses hyperplasiques ainsi que les types albopapuloïdes de PASINI (transmission en dominance). L'altération dermique est très superficielle. L'épiderme intact qui forme le toit de la bulle peut parfois montrer 1 sec bulle (SCHNYDER et coll., 1964; P. RITZENFELD, 1966) sous cornée; celle-ci est à mon avis une formation résiduelle à peu près éliminée d'une bulle plus ancienne (on rencontre des faits semblables dans les dermatoses polymorphes douloureuses de DUHRINGBROCQ, qui sont aussi des bulles par dermolyse).

2. Les Epidermolyses bulleuses polydysplasiques (transmission en récessivité). Les altérations du collagène et du tissu élastique sont très marquées et souvent profondes. Epiderme et membrane basale constituent le toit de la bulle et entraî-

nent parfois une portion du collagène (R. Pearson, 1962); même dans la peau non traumatisée on signale quelques altérations des fibres collagènes au microscope électronique.

3. Les porphyries cutanées bulleuses tardives semblent bien présenter un type semblable de dermolyse par formation de véritables bulles intrachoriales et bien entendu sclérosantes. Il nous semble évident que dans toutes ces dermolyses, l'intensité et la profondeur des altérations cicatricielles et mutilantes peuvent varier selon l'intensité de la sclérose.

Les Génodermatoses bulleuses par dégénérescence granuleuse

Celle-ci constitue une génodermatose dont l'autonomie par rapport aux ichtyoses congénitales et aux érythrodermies ichtyosiformes congénitales ne fait plus de doute.

En 1932 [Ann. Derm. Syph. Paris 3, 401 (1932)], nous avons proposé à l'occasion du premier cas de ce type que nous avons étudié, la dénomination d'Epidermolyse ichtyosiforme congénitale pour bien la séparer des autres érythrodermies ichtyosiformes congénitales. Cette proposition n'avait pas été suivie dans la littérature dermatologique. Nous n'avons pas insisté et continué de donner à ces cas le nom d'Erythrodermie ichtyosiforme bulleuse.

Revenant sur cette question (Ann. franç. Derm. Paris 1953 et 1957) nous avons pu montrer qu'il s'agissait d'une dégénérescence granuleuse des tonofibrilles avec préservation des ponts intercellulaires. Il y a donc bien épidermolyse d'un type spécial mais non acantholyse. Cette dernière affection se transmet en dominance alors que l'Erythrodermie ichtyosiforme non bulleuse se transmet en récessivité. Ce sont donc deux affections cliniquement, histologiquement et génétiquement bien séparées et non pas comme certains l'ont soutenu longtemps, une complication bulleuse infectieuse.

Tout récemment (1966 et 1967) E. R. Weibel et U. W. Schnyder ont confirmé, grâce au microscope électronique, l'Epidermolyse granuleuse avec persistance des desmosomes.

Cette dégénérescence granuleuse peut, lors de la transmission en dominance, présenter une expressivité très variable d'un cas à l'autre: tantôt généralisée incompatible avec la vie (forme létale), tantôt très étendue, tantôt atteignant surtout les grands plis, mais toujours on signale une atteinte palmoplantaire; ces dernières localisations peuvent être seules en cause (Gasser, 1964). Nicolau et Balus ont retrouvé cette dégénérescence granuleuse caractéristique (1959 et 1961) dans des naevi systématisés hyperkératosiques. Il n'est pas impossible que ces cas fassent partie d'une chaîne héréditaire du même type.

Tout récemment les auteurs américains P. Frost et E. V. van Scott (1966) sur le plan clinique ainsi que G. F. Wilgram et J. B. Caulfield (1966) au microscope électronique ont étudié des cas d'Erythrodermie Ichtyosiforme bulleuse et ont retrouvé la dénomination «d'Ichtyosiform Dermatolysis» et «d'Epidermolytic hyperkeratosis» que nous leur avions déjà donnée en 1932.

J. R. Simpson (1965) qui a confirmé notre séparation des Erythrodermies ichtyosiformes en deux formes tout-à-fait distinctes, les bulleuses et les non bulleuses, va reprendre cette question dans le rapport page 549.

Les Génodermatoses par acantholyse

Celles-ci ont trouvé leur expression dans le Pemphigus, bénin familial de Hailey-Hailey et dans la maladie de Darier.

L'idée du rapprochement entre ces deux dermatoses génotypiques et de leur séparation complète a autant de partisans que d'adversaires. Les citer tous ainsi que leurs arguments nous entraînerait trop loin. Des cas ont pu être considérés comme ayant présenté en même temps ou successivement les symptômes cliniques des deux affections et ont été cités notamment par DEGOS (1958) et par WINER et LOEB (1953). Une étude récente au microscope électronique par WILGRAM et coll. (1962) et ensuite par PIERARD et KINT (1964) ont montré que les lésions essentielles dans la maladie de H.H. est une rétraction des tonofibrilles et de leur accumulation autour des noyaux sans formation de kératohyaline avec comme suite la lyse des desmosomes qui s'y rapportent; cependant, PIERARD et KINT ont également démontré que si elle n'est pas aussi précoce ni aussi complète que dans la Maladie de DARIER, un début de kératinisation se voit quand même autour des noyaux.

KINT et PIERARD, ont insisté sur la kératinisation très complète et précoce observée dans les mêmes conditions dans la dyskératose folliculaire. Il n'y aurait entre les deux images qu'une différence de degré et de précocité; ce qui explique les analogies et les faits de passage ou les concomitances. La maladie de H.H. peut être regardée comme une génotypie semblable mais de moindre expressivité que la kératose folliculaire. Elles se transmettent d'ailleurs toutes deux en dominance. Nos collègues, PIERARD et KINT nous en donneront de plus amples détails dans leur rapport.

References. CAULFIELD, J. B., and J. F. WILGRAM: J. invest. Derm. 39, 307 (1962). — DANBOLT, N., and R. CLOSS: Acta derm.-venerol. (Stockh.) 23, 127 (1942). — DEGOS, R.: Dermatologie, p. 423, 446. Paris: Flammarion 1958. — DELACRETAZ, J., and R. M. LORETAN: Proceedings of the XIth International Congress on Dermatology, 1957. Acta derm.-venereol. (Stockh.) 3, 659 (1960). — FROST, P., and E. J. VAN SCOTT: Arch. Derm. 94, 113 (1966). — GASSER, U.: Thèse de la Clinique Dermatologique de Zurich (sous la direction de Storck, M., et U. W. SCHNYDER) 1964. — HAILEY, H., and H. HAILEY: Arch. Derm. Syph. (Chic.) 39, 679 (1939). — HERLITZ, C. W.: Acta paediat. (Uppsala) 17, 315 (1935). — KLUNKER, W.: Arch. klin. exp. Derm. 216, 74 (1963). — LAPIERE, S.: Ann. Derm. Syph. (Paris) 3, 401 (1932). 80, 597 (1953); 84, 5 (1957). — LAPIERE, S., et S. CASTERMANS-ELIAS: Arch. belges. Derm. 14, 101 (1958); 17, (1961). — LAPIERE, S., u. H. FIRKET: Hautarzt 15, 30 (1964). — LEVER, W. F.: Medicine (Baltimore) 32, 1 (1953). — NICOLAU, S. G., and L. BALUS: Derm.-Vener. (Buc.) 4, 307 (1959); — Derm. Wschr. 143, 462 (1961). — PEARSON, R. W.: J. invest. Derm. 39, 551 (1962). — PEARSON, R. W., and B. SPARGO: J. invest. Derm. 36, 213 (1964). — PIERARD, J., et A. KINT: Arch. belges Derm. 20, 40 (1964). — RITZENFELD, P.: Arch. klin. exp. Derm. 224, 128 (1966). — ROBERTS, M. H., R. S. HOWELL, J. L. BRAMHALL, and B. RAUBNER: Pediatrics 25, 283 (1960). — SCHNYDER, U. W., u. D. EICHHOFF: Arch. klin. exp. Derm. 218, 62 (1964). — SCHNYDER, U. W., E. C. JUNG, und T. SALAMON: Arch. klin. exp. Derm. 220, 38 (1964). — TOURAINE, A.: Ann. Derm. Syph. (Paris) 2, 309 (1942). — TRAPL, J.: Excerpta med. (Amst.), Sect. XIII, Vol. XI (XIth Internat. Congr. Dermat.) C 141, p. 80, 1957. — VOGEL, A., u. U. W. SCHNYDER: Dermatologica (Basel) 131, 81 (1965). — WEIBEL, E. R., u. U. W. SCHNYDER: Arch. klin. exp. Derm. 227, 341 (1967). — WILGRAM, J. F., and J. B. CAULFIELD: Arch. Derm. Syph. (Chic.) 94, 127 (1966). — WILGRAM, F., J. B. CAULFIELD, and W. F. LEVER: J. invest. Derm. 36, 373 (1962). — WINER, L. H., and A. J. LOEB: Arch. Derm. Syph. (Chic.) 67, 77 (1953).

Le test gémellaire dans les dermatoses héréditaires

L. GEDDA et R. CAVALIERI, Istituto di Genetica Medica, Università di Roma (Italie)

Dès que GALTON, en 1865, attira l'attention des rechercheurs sur la possibilité d'utiliser les jumeaux pour définir l'importance relative du milieu et de l'hérédité dans la détermination des caractères, les méthodologies gémellaires aussi bien que les études de génétique, ont subi une évolution qui nous permet, aujourd'hui, d'établir non seulement l'apport du génotype et des facteurs exogènes à des phénotypes déterminés, mais aussi la fréquence et la pénétrance des génotypes causaux.

Ces résultats sont obtenus généralement en comparant des séries de couples MZ et DZ, sur la base de coefficients statistiques différents, tels que le coefficient de corrélation, la mesure de la variance ou le pourcentage de concordance.

Bien que ces coefficients diffèrent, la valeur conceptuelle est toujours la même, c'est-à-dire que les différences dans un couple MZ peuvent être déterminées seulement par des agents péristatiques, tandis que les différences entre-couple des couples DZ représentent une différence d'origine génotypique et une différence d'origine péristatique.

La schématisation mathématique de ce principe, connue sous la formule d'HOLZINGER $H = \dfrac{V_{DZ} - V_{MZ}}{V_{DZ}}$ permet d'établir le quantum héréditaire H et, par différence, le quantum péristatique $E = 1 - H$ dans la détermination d'un caractère donné.

Avec de formules semblables, telles que celles d'HUITZINGA et de STERN, on peut obtenir les valeurs des fréquences p du génotype déterminant un caractère spécifique et la pénétrance y du caractère même.

En ce qui concerne l'application de la méthodologie gémellaire dans le domaine de l'hérédopathologie humaine, nous avons envisagé depuis longtemps une recherche spécifique dans le secteur de la pathologie dermatologique et, plus précisément, de la pathologie allergique.

Tableau 1

Asthme	MZ	DZ	Oculo-rhinite	MZ	DZ
Concordance par forme allergique	4	5	Concordance par forme allergique	26	27
Concordance par diathèse	0	10	Concordance par diathèse	0	17
Discordance	5	25	Discordance	16	50
Total	9	40	Total	42	94
H = 36%			H = 46%		

Urticaire	MZ	DZ	Eczéma	MZ	DZ
Concordance par forme allergique	31	40	Concordance par forme allergique	23	33
Concordance par diathèse	2	18	Concordance par diathèse	2	18
Discordance	21	64	Discordance	14	38
Total	60	122	Total	39	89
H = 43%			H = 35%		

Nous avons d'abord envisagé une recherche de masse dans un groupe de pathologie associée, c'est-à-dire la pathologie allergique.

A ce but nous avons analysé 2865 couples de jumeaux âgés de plus de 6 ans et classifiés dans la cartothèque de l'Institut Mendel. Les 1237 réponses qui ont été obtenues de ces 2865 couples sans appliquer aucun critérium séléctif constituent la base des élaborations successives.

La distribution du matériel par sexe et zygotisme peut être ainsi classifié:
133 couples MZ (59 ♂♂ et 74 ♀♀),
429 couples DZ (59 ♂♂, 95 ♀♀ et 275 ♂♀),
couples dont le zygotisme n'a pas été classifié (285 ♂♂ et 390 ♀♀).

Sur la base de ce matériel on a relevé et enregistré, pour chaque couple, les combinaisons présence/absence de formes allergiques précédemment classifiées, telles que Asthme, Oculo-rhinite, Eczéma, et Urticaire.

Les distributions des couples à zygotisme certifié selon la présence/absence des allergopathies considérées sont illustrées aux Tab. 1 à 4, où la voix « concordance par diathèse » indique la présence chez les jumeaux de deux différentes formes d'allergopathie. On a aussi indiqué les valeurs H des déterminations du quantum héréditaire calculées selon la formule d'HOLZINGER.

Les résultats de la recherche peuvent être classifiés dans la manière suivante:

1. La concordance d'incidence pour la même allergopathie est plus élevée chez les couples MZ et le nombre de jumeaux MZ concordants pour la même allergopathie est nettement supérieur aux MZ discordants.

2. Chez les couples MZ la concordance pour la même affection (concordance par forme allergique) n'augmente pas, même en tenant compte de la concordance pour les autres allergopathies (concordance par diathèse allergique), tandis que chez les couples DZ la concordance par diathèse a une incidence supérieure, bien que inférieure à la concordance par forme.

On peut donc affirmer que, en ce qui concerne les allergopathies, l'hérédité constitue le facteur responsable pour la prédisposition à la maladie, en tant que condition nécessaire, mais non suffisante.

On peut donc parler d'hérédité causale, différant de l'hérédité concausale, qui se manifeste à un certain moment sans qu'une concause péristatique spécifique intervienne. Nos observations nous permettent aussi de valoriser, au delà des termes d'une intuition vague, le concept de diathèse ou prédisposition héréditaire, ce qui permet la distribution, dans l'espace individuel et familial, d'une pathologie qui, bien que différenciée en clinique, est liée à un dénominateur pathogénétique commun. On doit donc parler de diathèse allergique.

Du point de vue pathogénétique nous pouvons avancer l'hypothèse que, étant donné la détermination génétique des anticorps, la prédisposition allergique héréditaire est, au moins partiellement, liée à ces facteurs génétiques.

La détermination génétique des allergopathies peut être démontrée par l'incidence familiale élevée des manifestations allergiques concernant le même organe et par la haute concordance pour la même affection allergique chez les jumeaux MZ.

Les difficultés de rilévation de séries de couples de jumeaux DZ, dont un au moins atteint par une affection dont les paramètres génétiques pouvaient être étudiés, ont souvent empêché l'application de la méthodologie interzygotique classique.

Avant d'arriver au domaine de la clinique gémellaire, nous avons étendu nos recherches à la pathologie dermatologique, à fin d'avoir une vision d'ensemble des formes de ces pathologies qui sont les plus fréquentes chez la population gémellaire et leur distribution chez les divers couples, en évaluant spécialement l'incidence chez les MZ vis-à-vis aux DZ et leur concordance ou discordance intra-couple.

Le Tab. 2 rapporte les différentes dermatoses trouvées chez un groupe de jumeaux qui se sont prêtés spontanément à notre observation.

Le Tab. 3 présente le rapport général des concordances et discordances chez les 84 conples observés.

Ces observations concordent avec les conclusions de plusieurs auteurs. En particulier, les concordances chez les MZ sont plus élevées que chez les DZ.

Tableau 2. *Distribution des cas par forme clinique (84 cas)*

Forme clinique	N.	Forme clinique	N.
Acné	26	Strophulus	1
Psoriasis	10	Xérodermie pigmentée	1
Séborrhée	10	Pityriasis rubra pilaire	1
Angiome	8	Pityriasis alba	1
Alopécie aréolaire	3	Perniosis	1
Vitiligo	4	Naevus pigmentaire hypertrophique	1
Kératose pilaire	2	Pseudoxanthome	1
Dermatite atopique	2	Ichtyose	1
Kératodermie	1	Pemphigous	1
Hypotrichose	1	Hypertrichose	1
Epidermolyse bulleuse	2	Hyperhidrose	1
Prurigo nodulaire	1	Urticaire pigmentaire	1
Erythrodermie de L.	1	Granulosis rubra nasi	1

Tableau 3. *Distribution des cas par concordance, sexe et zygotisme*

Sexe/Zygotisme	Couples concordants			Sexe/Zygotisme	Couples discordants		
	MZ	DZ	Total		MZ	DZ	Total
♂♂	13	3	16	♂♂	2	3	5
♀♀	13	11	24	♀♀	12	11	23
♂♀	—	3	3	♂♀	—	13	13
Total	26	17	43	Total	14	27	41

La concordance est plus élevée chez les MZ atteints par acné ou séborrhée. Au contraire, la discordance entre MZ et DZ atteints par psoriasis n'est pas significative. La même chose vaut pour les angiones, une discordance remarquable est présente chez les MZ.

Ces résultats concernent seulement les dermatoses à incidence plus élevée, car un jugement valide n'était pas possible lorsque la casistique était réduite.

L'introduction, en 1961, du test clinico-gémellaire de GEDDA a permis de prévenir les difficultés présentées par la valutation des données au moyen de la méthodologie interzygotique classique, en réduisant le rélèvement à un seul couple MZ et en comparant les deux jumeaux non comme des unités statistiques, mais comme deux univers.

Cette nouvelle disposition de l'expériment gémellaire est possible car une pathologie déterminée représente, généralement, un concept d'un ensemble variable de tableaux cliniques concordants pour les conditions de la maladie, mais discordants pour la présence, absence, intensité ou moment de la manifestation de nombreux symptômes non nécessaires.

Ce concept nous permet de donner une valeur de probabilité à tous les tableaux symptomatologiques et, par conséquent, de calculer la probabilité causale de concordance pour le même tableau de deux individus différents atteints par la maladie étudiée. On peut ainsi obtenir au moyen du compte de la probabilité causale de concordance, un terme de comparaison pour le rapport fréquent chez les couples de jumeaux, des tableaux symptomatologiques superposables.

L'exclusion de la casualité de la concordance peut être utilisée en deux directions diverses, selon que le zygotisme du couple étudié soit connu ou non. Si le zygotisme n'est pas connu, le test clinique-gémellaire en permet la détermination, la superposition des tableaux étant impossible dans les cas des couples DZ. Quand le zygotisme est connu et le couple est classifié MZ, le test clinique-gémellaire permet, au moyen du critérium sélectif de la concordance des symptômes, de déterminer les symptômes à causalité génotypique ou péristatique.

La conviction que le test clinique-gémellaire permet d'ultérieures recherches sur l'hérédité et la manifestation de la maladie nous a amenés à étudier un groupe de couples gémellaires MZ, afin d'évaluer non seulement les paramètres génétiques des maladies en question, mais aussi les modalités cliniques d'expression d'un génotype déterminé.

Notre nouvelle recherche présente donc des cas de jumeaux atteints par érythrocyanose, area celsi, acné et kératose pilaire, en tant que témoignage de nos téchniques de recherche.

Les cas étudiés avec le test clinique-gémellaire commencent avec un couple de jumelles atteintes par erythrocyanose, couple diagnostiqué MZ sur la base des données immunohématologiques aussi bien qu'anthropométriques.

Le tableau clinique de l'érythrocyanose chez ce couple a été analysé par rapport à des paramètres évolutifs auxquels nous avons attribué une probabilité déterminée par rapport à l'évolution clinique de la maladie dans sa manifestation la plus commune.

Dans le cas spécifique nous avons trouvé les paramètres suivants: évolution cyclique dans les périodes saisonniers, localisation différentielle, association avec d'autres expressions pathologiques, réactivité aux thérapies. Sur la base de la concordance de toutes ces observations, nous avons évalué une probabilité individuelle du tableau clinique en question (p = 0.032); une probabilité de concordance causale chez le couple dans le tableau clinique (p = 0.001).

Enfin, la probabilité pas élevée de concordance causale présente un conditionnement héréditaire particulier de l'érythrocyanose, non seulement pour la maladie en général, mais pour la période de manifestation, son écoulement et son évolution.

Le deuxième cas étudié par la méthodologie clinique-gémellaire concerne un couple de jumeaux atteints par areacelsi, couple diagnostiqué comme MZ selon les méthodes utilisées dans le cas précédent. Dans ce cas les paramètres ont été les suivants: période de manifestation, évolution et forme cliniques, neurodistonie associée. De ces paramètres résultaient discordantes la forme clinique, à plaques chez l'un des jumeaux et ophiasique chez l'autre, et l'évolution, chez l'un des jumeaux limitée à 2 ans, et prolongée chez l'autre pour plus de 10 ans.

Etant le compte de la probabilité du tableau clinique individuel limité seulement aux paramètres concordants, on a obtenu une valeur du 35%, donc une probabilité causale de concordance chez les jumeaux du 12.25%.

Enfin, la probabilité de concordance causale relativement élevée et les discordances de forme et d'évolution clinique soulignent l'existence d'un facteur héréditaire responsable de la pathologie ou d'un terrain prédisposant sur lequel est possible l'action de facteurs péristatiques capables de produire une variabilité de manifestation particulièrement vaste, ainsi que dans le cas décrit.

La troisième analyse clinique-gémellaire concernait un cas d'acné juvénile chez un couple de jumelles MZ.

Les paramètres du tableau clinique considérés dans ce cas ont été: période de manifestation, évolution clinique, incidence thérapeutique, complications et associations pathologiques. De ces paramètres on a trouvé concordance seulement pour la réactivité aux médicaments et pour la pathologie associée.

La probabilité de concordance causale pour ces deux paramètres, sur la base de la seule méthodologie décrite, conduisent à une valeur du 22%.

Enfin, l'analyse du tableau clinique du couple étudié, sur la base des données concernant les deux couples MZ déjà examinés, souligne l'existence de nombreux facteurs péristatiques concausaux dans la détermination des formes cliniques de l'acné juvénile, le facteur héréditaire de laquelle est réduit probablement à une forme de réactivité constitutionnelle aux agents péristatiques, ce qui est aussi confirmé par la réponse concordante à la thérapie.

Dans le quatrième cas le test clinique-gémellaire n'a pas été utilisé pour la définition des facteurs péristatiques et héréditaires de la maladie, dans le cas spécifique la kératose pilaire, mais pour la détermination du zygotisme chez un couple de jumeaux. Dans ce cas aussi, la méthodologie se base sur l'analyse du tableau clinique, ses aspects étant considérés en tant paramètres indépendantes.

Pour la kératose on a considéré les paramètres suivants: période de manifestation, pathologie associée, réponse aux thérapies.

Les deux tableaux cliniques, malgré la fréquence individuelle relativement non élevée de quelques aspects de la localisation, résultaient tout à fait superposables.

La concordance causale, évaluée par la méthodologie décrite, résultait de 2/100.000.

Enfin, la superposition pratique des tableaux cliniques chez les jumeaux peut être comparée à la concordance des données anthropométriques utilisées pour la diagnose de zygotisme.

La basse probabilité relevée nous permet donc d'affirmer que le couple examiné est MZ. Nous soulignons le fait que dans ce cas la réponse du test est double, parce que le diagnostic de monozygotisme comporte l'attribution à la kératose pilaire d'un conditionnement causé par le génotype seulement.

L'application du test gémellaire présenté nous permet quelques considérations d'ordre général sur l'utilité de cette méthodologie non seulement dans la recherche, mais aussi dans la clinique dermatologique. En effet, la méthodologie gémellaire, dans son actuation interzygotique classique, permet la résolution des problèmes concernant la détermination des paramètres génétiques principales d'une pathologie: ce qu'est souvent impossible dans la génétique humaine.

En outre, l'actuation clinique gémellaire permet de substituer au terme de comparaison moyen, un terme rigoureusement «ad hominem», comparaison qui présente normalement une sensibilité particulière pour la rilévation de la symptomatologie peu vérifiable.

Enfin, nous soulignons le fait que les comparaisons gémellaires, entre séries de couples à zygotisme différent ou entre jumeaux du même couple, permettent d'attribuer une valeur causale aux facteurs héréditaires et péristatiques des différentes pathologies, ce qui est d'importance fondamentale dans la dermatologie.

Epidermolysis bullosa hereditaria
Klinik, Histologie, Elektronenmikroskopie

U. W. SCHNYDER, Universitäts-Hautklinik Heidelberg (Deutschland)

Das Hauptsymptom der hereditären Epidermolysen ist die Blasenbildung. Klinisch kann man nicht-dystrophische und dystrophische Typen bzw. Formen unterscheiden. Klinisch-genetisch muß man heute mindestens acht Typen postulieren. Vier Typen werden autosomal-dominant und drei autosomal-recessiv vererbt, während die x-chromosomale Form bis jetzt nur in einer einzigen holländischen Familie beobachtet wurde. SCHNYDER, SALAMON u. JUNG [11] schlagen deshalb folgende klinisch-genetische Klassifizierung vor:

Tabelle. *Klinisch-genetische Klassifizierung der hereditären Epidermolysen*

Dermatologisches Leitkriterium	Bezeichnung der Krankheit	Erbgang
nicht vernarbend	Epidermolysis bullosa simplex Köbner Recurrent bullous eruption of the feet Weber-Cockayne	autosomal-dominant
vernarbend	Epidermolysis bullosa letalis Herlitz Epidermolysis bullosa dystrophica s. polydysplastica Hallopeau-Siemens Epidermolysis bullosa dystrophica ulcero- vegetans Nicolas, Moutot und Charlet	autosomal-recessiv
	Epidermolysis bullosa dystrophica s. hyperplastica Cockayne-Touraine Epidermolysis bullosa albo-papuloides Pasini	autosomal-dominant
	Dystrophia bullosa Typus maculatus Mendes da Costa-van der Valk	x-chromosomal-recessiv

Bei der *Epidermolysis bullosa simplex* entstehen die Blasen teils spontan, teils nach Reiben. Die Abheilung erfolgt immer ohne Narbenbildung. Prädilektionsstellen sind außer den Händen und Füßen der Stamm. Die „Recurrent bullous eruption of the feet Weber-Cockayne" ist wahrscheinlich nur eine klinische Variante der Epidermolysis bullosa simplex. Mit zunehmendem Alter nimmt die Intensität der Blasenbildung spontan ab. Der Allgemeinzustand solcher Patienten ist nicht beeinträchtigt; assoziierte Symptome fehlen, und die Lebenserwartung ist normal. Histologisch liegt eine intraepidermale Blase vor, die durch Desintegration der Basalzellen und der suprabasal gelegenen Malpighi-Zellen zustande kommt [8, 9, 11].

Die *dystrophischen Epidermolysen* gehen mit Nagelveränderungen, atrophischer und/oder hypertrophischer Narbenbildung sowie Milien einher. Die dominant-dystrophischen Epidermolysen sind sehr selten. Ob die dominant vererbte Epidermolysis bullosa hyperplastica und die Epidermolysis bullosa albopapuloïdea nosologisch verschiedene Entitäten darstellen, ist noch nicht geklärt [10]. Beide Typen haben eine normale Lebenserwartung und gehen ohne assoziierte Symptome einher, wenn man vom Fall LEINBROCK [7] absieht, der mit ulcero-vegetierenden Veränderungen und einer tardiven Hämangiomatose einherging. Nach den spärlichen Unterlagen zu schließen, ist die Blasenbildung teils intraepithelial, teils epidermolytisch [10].

Zu den recessiv-dystrophischen Epidermolysen gehören die letale Form (Herlitzsche Krankheit), ferner die sehr seltene ulcero-vegetierende Form und vor allem die relativ häufige polydysplastische Form.

Für die erbbiologischen Verhältnisse sei auf meine Darstellung im Jadassohnschen Handbuch Band VII [12] verwiesen. Die letale Form beginnt ohne dystrophische Veränderungen. Da in ein- und derselben Geschwisterschaft letale und polydysplastische Fälle auftreten können [5] und sich im 1. Lebensjahr die polydysplastische Epidermolyse klinisch nicht von der letalen Form zu unterscheiden braucht, ist die Eigenständigkeit der letalen Form bestritten worden. Sie stellt nach Ansicht des Autors die letale Variante der recessiven Epidermolysen dar. Charakteristisch für die Epidermolysis bullosa polydysplastica sind Nagelveränderungen, atrophische Narben, Klumphandbildung, Milien, Conjunctivalsynechien, Ektropien mit Hornhautdytrophien sowie Blasenbildung der Schleimhäute. In den letzten Jahren wurde vermehrt auf Oesophagusstenosen hingewiesen, die als Folge vernarbender bullöser Prozesse der Speiseröhrenmucosa aufgefaßt werden müssen [2, 16]. Die Schwere der Hauterscheinungen scheint kein Indicator für analoge Veränderungen im Bereich des Oesophagus zu sein, da nach unserer Erfahrung leichte Hauterscheinungen mit schwerer Stenose einhergehen können und umgekehrt. Im Kollektiv ist die Lebenserwartung der Epidermolysis polydysplastica nicht zuletzt wegen der Oesophagusstenose deutlich reduziert, worauf schon SIEMENS [13] hinwies. Häufig ist auch die Intelligenz vermindert, weshalb WATRIN, KISSEL u. BEUREY [15] diese Krankheit zu den neuroektodermalen Syndromen zählen.

Histologisch findet man eine Abhebung (Epidermolyse) der meist atrophischen Epidermis von der Cutis. Der Papillarkörper und die oberen Abschnitte der Cutis sind fibrös umgewandelt, oft entzündlich infiltriert und arm an elastischen Fasern [9, 11].

Elektronenmikroskopisch wurden in den letzten Jahren vor allem die letale und polydysplastische Epidermolyse untersucht. So fanden PEARSON [9], LAPIÈRE et al. [6], ferner BELLONE et al. [1] übereinstimmend bei der letalen Epidermolyse unregelmäßige Spaltbildungen zwischen den Basalzellen, Verschwinden der Halbdesmosomen und Tonofibrillen sowie eine Schädigung des Cytoplasmas der Basalzellen und der suprabasal gelegenen Malpighi-Zellen. Nicht einheitlicher Art sind hingegen die Beobachtungen bei polydysplastischen Epidermolysen. PEARSON [9] sah eine Desintegration des subepidermalen Kollagens, wobei die elektronenoptische Basalmembran vitalen Basalzellen anhaftete. Analoge Verhältnisse sahen auch VOGEL u. SCHNYDER [14]. Auch in unseren beiden Fällen dieser Art waren die Halbdesmosomen gut ausgebildet. In einem dritten Fall hingegen kam es im sog. „adepidermal space" zur Blasenbildung zwischen Basalzellen und Basalmembran. Die Blasenbildung ging mit degenerativen Veränderungen der Basalzellen sowie Schwund der Halbdesmosomen und Tonofilamente einher. Analoge Befunde publizierte kürzlich KOBAYASI [3].

Die elektronenmikroskopischen Befunde lassen daran denken, daß die Pathogenese der Blasenbildung bei den recessiven Epidermolysen nicht einheitlicher Natur ist. Bilder, wie sie bei letaler Epidermolyse erhoben wurden, kommen somit auch bei der polydysplastischen Epidermolyse vor [3, 14], während in der Mehrzahl dieser Fälle die Basalmembran den Basalzellen anliegt, ohne daß es zu einer wesentlichen Schädigung der Halbdesmosomen und Tonofibrillen in den Basalzellen kommt [9, 14]. Möglicherweise sind in solchen Fällen die Verankerungsfasern der Kollagenfibrillen anlagemäßig geschädigt. Sollten weitere ultrastrukturelle Untersuchungen die bisherigen Befunde bestätigen, so müßte die Frage gestellt werden, ob die klinisch-genetische Gruppe der recessiven Epidermolysen genetisch heterogener Art ist.

Literatur. 1. BELLONE, A. G., R. CAPUTO e F. CLEMENTI: G. ital. Derm. Sif. **106**, 135 (1965). — 2. BERGENHOLZ, A., O. OLSSON, T. ARWILL und N. R. LINDSTRÖM: Arch. klin. exp. Derm. **217**, 518 (1963). — 3. KOBAYASI, T.: Acta derm.-venereol. (Stockh.) **47**, 57 (1967). — 4. KOGOJ, FR.: In margine epidermolysis bullosae hereditariae. Jugosl. Akad. Znonosti i Umjetnosti, Zagreb 1966. — 5. KLUNKER, W.: Arch. klin. exp. Derm. **216**, 74 (1963). — 6. LAPIÈRE, S., S. CASTERMANS-ELIOAS und H. FIRKET: Hautarzt **15**, 30 (1964). — 7. LEINBROCK, A.: Hautarzt **7**, 395 (1956). — 8. LEVER, W. F.: Epidermolysis bullosa. In: J. JADASSOHN: Handbuch der Haut- und Geschlechtskrankheiten, Ergänzungswerk. Band II/2, 596. Berlin-Heidelberg-New York: Springer 1965. — 9. PEARSON, R. W.: J. invest. Derm. **39**, 551 (1962). — 10. SCHNYDER, U. W., u. D. EICHHOFF: Arch. klin. exp. Derm. (Im Druck). — 11. SCHNYDER, U. W., T. SALAMON und E. G. JUNG: Arch. klin. exp. Derm. **220**, 38 (1964). — 12. SCHNYDER, U. W.: Die hereditären Epidermolysen. In: J. JADASSOHN Handbuch für Haut- und Geschlechtskrankheiten, Ergänzungswerk, Band VII, 440, Berlin-Heidelberg-New York: Springer 1966. — 13. SIEMENS, H. W.: Arch. Derm. Syph. (Berl.) **143**, 390 (1923). — 14. VOGEL, A., u. U. W. SCNHYDER: Dermatologica (Basel) (Im Druck). — 15. WATRIN, J., P. KISSEL, BEUREY et J. BARBIER: Bull. Soc. franç. Derm. Syph. **60**, 66 (1953). — 16. WEY, W., u. U. W. SCNHYDER: Dermatologica (Basel) **128**, 173 (1964).

Le pemphigus familial bénin chronique et les formes bulleuses de la maladie de Darier

J. Piérard et A. Kint, Clinique Dermatologique, Université de Gand (Belgique)

Peu de maladies ont suscité dès leur apparition autant de controverses passionnées que le pemphigus familial bénin chronique. Pour les frères Hailey, il s'agissait d'une entité nosologique non encore décrite. Pour Pels et Goodman, ce n'était qu'une maladie de Darier à forme vésiculo-bulleuse. Ayres et Anderson reconnaissaient bientôt que leurs cas de «Recurrent herpetiform dermatitis repens» correspondaient à ceux des frères Hailey et l'opinion de Frank et Rein, Sachs et coll. etc., qui entrevoyaient des rapports entre la maladie de Hailey-Hailey et l'épidermolyse bulleuse, n'a pas été suivie. La discussion se limite donc aux thèses des Hailey et de Pels et Goodman.

Le problème n'est pas simple, en raison de la présence de vésicules et de bulles dans certains cas de dyskératose folliculaire. Ces formes sont connues depuis l'article de Boeck (1891) et de nombreuses publications sont venues confirmer les constatations de cet auteur. Mais, dans tous ces cas, la présence d'autres symptômes (papules kératosiques aux endroits classiques, au dos des mains etc.) vient étayer le diagnostic de maladie de Darier. D'autre part il n'est pas douteux — et ici nous partageons l'avis de Jablonska et Chorzelski — que des confusions ont été faites et que des malades atteints de pemphigus bénin familial ont été considérés comme présentant de la dyskératose folliculaire et, inversément, que des maladies de Darier avec bulles ont été étiquetées maladies de Hailey-Hailey.

Quoiqu'il en soit, la question demeure très discutée. Deux courants d'opinion s'affrontent.

La position des partisans de l'unité des deux affections se base principalement sur les données suivantes:

1. Le caractère familial et héréditaire commun aux deux affections. Dans les deux cas l'hérédité est dominante, généralement irrégulière, non liée au sexe. D'autre part, il y a également dans les deux maladies des cas isolés sans incidence familiale.

2. La ressemblance entre les deux maladies: la forme bulleuse de la dyskératose folliculaire affectionne le cou, les régions inguino-crurales et les aisselles, emplacements d'élection du pemphigus bénin familial.

3. La présence éventuelle de papules kératosiques autour des placards actifs de pemphigus familial bénin (Degos) ou après guérison de ceux-ci.

4. La coexistence chez le même sujet de lésions dont les unes ont l'aspect clinique et histologique de pemphigus bénin familial, les autres celui d'une maladie de Darier.

5. La constatation, faite per Degos, de la succession dans le temps d'une maladie de Darier et d'un pemphigus bénin familial.

6. Les caractères communs dans la structure histologique des deux maladies.

7. L'argument, invoqué par Pels et Goodman, que le diagnostic histologique de la maladie de Darier ne repose pas sur la présence de corps ronds et de grains, mais sur l'acanthose et la tendance aux fissures et aux espaces lacunaires.

8. Ce dernier argument serait assez paradoxal s'il n'existait pas, pour le compenser, des cas de maladie de Hailey-Hailey où le microscope révèle la présence de «grains» et même, exceptionnellement, de «corps ronds».

Toutefois tous ces arguments sont discutables. L'espace nous faisant défaut, nous nous efforcerons de résumer au maximum et sans citation de noms d'auteurs, les raisons qui nous incitent à admettre que le pemphigus bénin familial est une affection autonome.

1. Arguments cliniques

Si pour l'hérédité les données sont sensiblement les mêmes dans les deux affections, l'incidence familiale est différente. GRAHAM et HELWIG observent dans le pemphigus de Hailey-Hailey, un arrière plan familial trois fois plus élevé que dans la maladie de Darier. D'autre part, les enquêtes faites au Danemark (B. SVENDSEN et ALBRECTSEN; RAASCHOU-NIELSEN et REYMANN), et celle de BECKER et OBERMAYER, ont montré qu'il n'y a pas de mélange des deux affections dans une même famille.

L'âge du début: La maladie de Darier apparaît généralement au cours de l'enfance, même de la première enfance, ou de l'adolescence. Pour la maladie de Darier bulleuse, en particulier, on a décrit des cas existant à la naissance. — Pour le pemphigus bénin congénital, le début se place couramment chez l'adulte jeune, entre 16 et 35 ans, en moyenne vers la vingtième année.

L'évolution est différente. La maladie de Darier est chronique et progressivement extensive; il n'y a qu'une seule attaque et les rémissions éventuelles ne sont que partielles. — Le pemphigus familial bénin est une affection chronique à caractère intermittent; les poussées apparaissent brusquement, s'étendent rapidement et n'atteignent que des surfaces limitées. Il a un caractère saisonnier net et la rémission complète est possible.

Les *sensations subjectives* font défaut dans la maladie de Darier, sauf si les lésions sont végétantes et macérées. — Elles sont très prononcées dans la maladie de Hailey-Hailey, les malades se plaignant de prurit ou de sensations de brûlure et de cuisson.

L'aspect clinique. Dans la maladie de Darier classique, les lésions sont papuleuses, grisâtres, kératosiques; elles peuvent devenir végétantes, voire tumorales dans les plis. Dans le Darier bulleux, phlyctènes et croûtes séreuses ou purulentes se surajoutent aux papules présentes dans les régions séborrhéiques. Le signe de Nikolsky est négatif.

Les lésions du pemphigus familial bénin sont primitivement vésiculeuses ou bulleuses. Elles forment dans les grands plis et les endroits exposés aux frottements des nappes circonscrites par des contours arciformes et bordées par un fin ourlet d'épiderme macéré. Ces nappes sont parcourues de fissures sur lesquelles DEGOS a attiré l'attention. Le visage et le cuir chevelu sont épargnés. Parfois on découvre, au pourtour de certains placards, des papules ressemblant à celles de la maladie de Darier; nous reviendrons plus loin sur leur structure (voir cytologie). Le signe de Nikolsky est fréquemment présent au voisinage des placards.

Localisation des lésions. La dyskératose folliculaire envahit progressivement la plus grande partie du tégument, bien qu'il y ait des endroits d'élection: les régions dites «séborrhéiques». Les lésions bulleuses siègent de préférence dans les plis, comme les lésions de la maladie de Hailey-Hailey, mais il y a toujours des papules kératosiques typiques à d'autres endroits. — Quant au pemphigus bénin familial, qui occupe les faces latérales du cou, les aisselles, les aines et la région périnéale, et déborde rarement sur le tronc, il épargne le visage et le cuir chevelu.

Les papules kératosiques à aspect de verrues planes du dos des mains sont présentes dans les cas de dyskératose folliculaire de type bulleux que nous avons relevés dans la littérature; elles font, d'après nos lectures et notre propre expérience, constamment défaut dans le pemphigus familial bénin.

La kératodermie palmaire et plantaire est fréquente et variée dans ses aspects cliniques dans la maladie de Darier. Elle n'a pas été signalée dans la maladie de

Hailey-Hailey et nous n'en avons jamais observé. Il en est de même de *l'état des ongles* dont les anomalies décrites dans la dyskératose folliculaire font défaut dans le pemphigus bénin familial.

Relation avec les traumatismes. C'est surtout l'exposition au soleil et aux rayons U-V qui a été tenue pour responsable de l'éclosion de certains cas de maladie de Darier. Le traumatisme — en particulier les frottements — joue au contraire un rôle important dans la genèse des foyers de maladie de Hailey-Hailey; ce rôle s'objective d'ailleurs sous forme du signe de Nikolsky. Dans une intéressante étude expérimentale, T. CHORZELSKI a déclenché par des moyens multiples (mécaniques, physiques, toxiques, allergiques et bactériologiques) une acantholyse typique dans le pemphigus de Hailey-Hailey; dans la maladie de Darier, par contre, il n'a obtenu ni acantholyse, ni dyskératose.

Atteinte des muqueuses. Dans la dyskératose folliculaire, les altérations des muqueuses sont connues depuis longtemps. — Dans le pemphigus bénin familial, elles paraissent exceptionnelles.

Rapports avec des troubles psychiques et autres. De nombreux auteurs ont signalé l'existence d'anomalies psychiques dans la maladie de Darier: débilité mentale, idiotie, épilepsie, psychopathies, voire aliénation. — Jusqu'à présent, aucun de ces troubles psychiques ne paraît avoir été relevé dans la maladie de Hailey-Hailey. Il en est de même pour d'autres anomalies signalées par TOURAINE dans la maladie de Darier: hypoplasie génitale, amyotrophie, myopie, hypotrichose, ichtyose, etc.

2. *Arguments histologiques*

Il semble que les divergences d'opinion proviennent de la façon de concevoir la *dyskératose*. Nous pensons qu'en cette matière, il importe de s'en tenir à la conception de DARIER, dans laquelle interviennent la *ségrégation* des cellules, caractérisée par leur isolement des cellules voisines, la *desmolyse* ou perte de leur ponts d'union, et leur kératinisation prématurée et individuelle aboutissant à la formation de *corps ronds* et de *grains*. Or si on recense les cas de maladie de Darier comportant des bulles ou des vésicules et où un examen histologique a été pratiqué, on constate que les auteurs y relatent avec constance la présence de «corps ronds» et de «grains». La forme bulleuse est donc une dyskératose folliculaire authentique qui répond aux caractères microscopiques exigibles pour ce diagnostic; seule varie la dimension des lacunes suprabasales. Dès lors, le problème de la distinction histologique entre maladie de Darier bulleuse et maladie de Hailey-Hailey se réduit à celui du diagnostic différentiel entre maladie de Darier en général et maladie de Hailey-Hailey.

Dans la maladie de Darier, il s'agit d'une dyskératose typique avec ségrégation des cellules et desmolyse (acantholyse). On constate de l'acanthose, de la papillomatose, une hyperkératose déprimant l'épiderme en forme de cônes tronqués et la présence de fissures siégeant au-dessus de la germinative. Quelle que soit la dimension de celles-ci, simple fente ou vaste lacune, leur toit est un amas de cellules dyskératosiques surmonté d'une couche cornée contenant des «grains». Des «corps ronds» se voient dans les parois ou dans le toit de la lacune, surtout dans la granuleuse, parfois aussi dans le corps muqueux. Il n'y a pas de mitoses (Fig. 1).

Dans le pemphigus bénin familial, le caractère le plus saillant est la dislocation quasi complète du corps muqueux. Au-dessus de la basale qui prend parfois, comme dans la maladie de Darier, un aspect villeux, la fissure se ramifie dans toutes les directions, isolant des cellules acantholysées ou des blocs cellulaires dont la cohésion est précaire (Fig. 2). Dans la cavité ainsi formée, les cellules libérées s'arrondissent, augmentent légèrement de volume. Le toit de la bulle est généralement formé des rangées supérieures du corps muqueux surmontées d'une granuleuse et d'une couche cornée parakératosique. Il y a des mitoses dans les cellules flottant dans la cavité et en bordure de celle-ci.

Certains auteurs relèvent la présence de «corps ronds» dans le pemphigus des frères HAILEY. En réalité les «corps ronds» véritables sont exceptionnels. Mais on

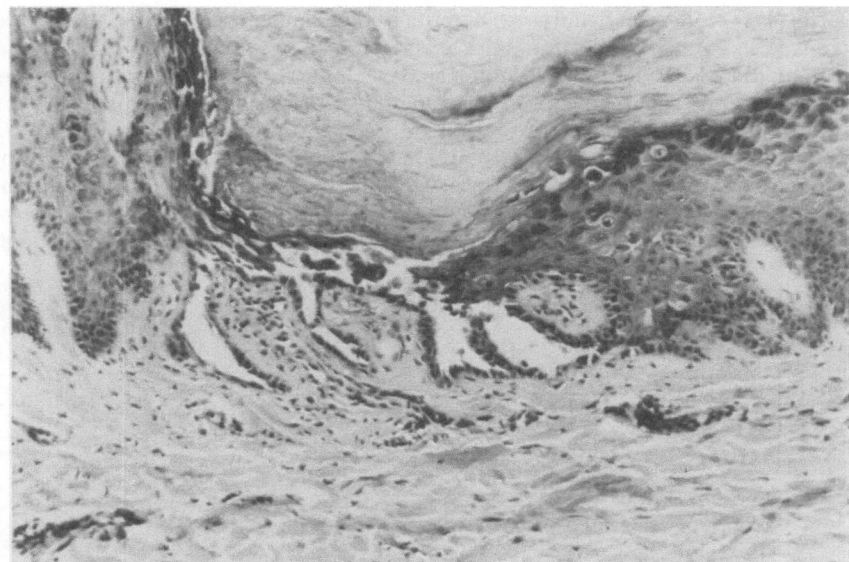

Fig. 1. Maladie de Darier. Hyperkératose en cône tronqué. Fissure supra-basale et allongement des papilles. Acanthose. Corps ronds et grains (HE, × 79)

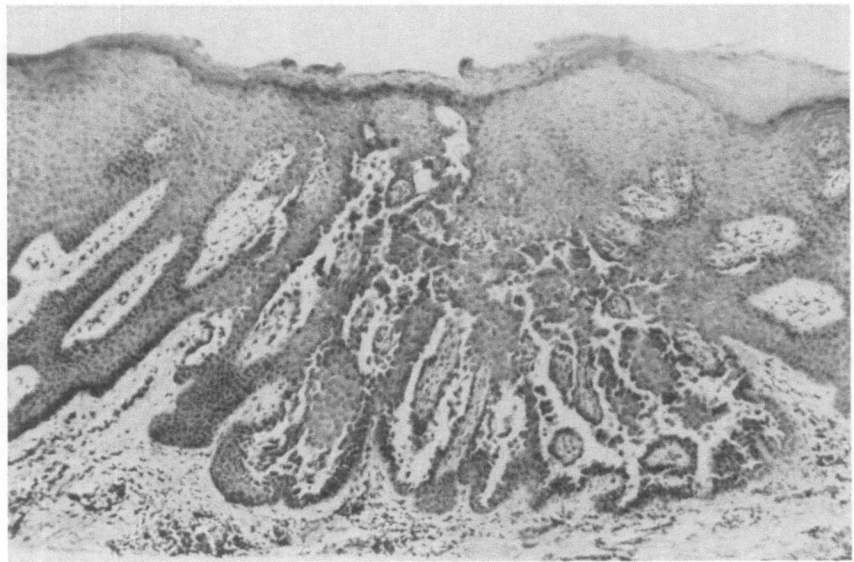

Fig. 2. Maladie de Hailey-Hailey. Acanthose avec papillomatose. Acantholyse avec dislocation complète du corps muqueux. Absence de corps ronds et de grains (HE, × 79)

trouve fréquemment, dans le corps muqueux, des cellules acantholysées dont le noyau est entouré d'une bande de cytoplasme éosinophile plus ou moins homogénéisé et fortement coloré. Le fort grossissement révèle toutefois que les limites cellulaires dépassent cette zone, qui se prolonge par une aire peu colorée aux contours assez flous, et la membrane réfringente à double contour fait constamment défaut.

Parfois les cellules acantholysées, troublées dans leur métabolisme, se nécrosent et le toit de la cavité est éliminé par l'exsudation.

La maladie de Darier, même bulleuse, est donc avant tout un trouble de la kératinisation, une sénescence précoce et atypique des cellules épineuses (DUPONT, JABLONSKA), aboutissant à la formation de «corps ronds» et de «grains». — Le pemphigus familial bénin par contre est conditionné par l'acantholyse. La plupart des cellules s'adaptent, paraissent conserver leur vitalité, ou tentent de compenser leur souffrance par une multiplication active. Toutefois la kératinisation est troublée; au minimum la couche cornée sera parakératosique, mais parfois le

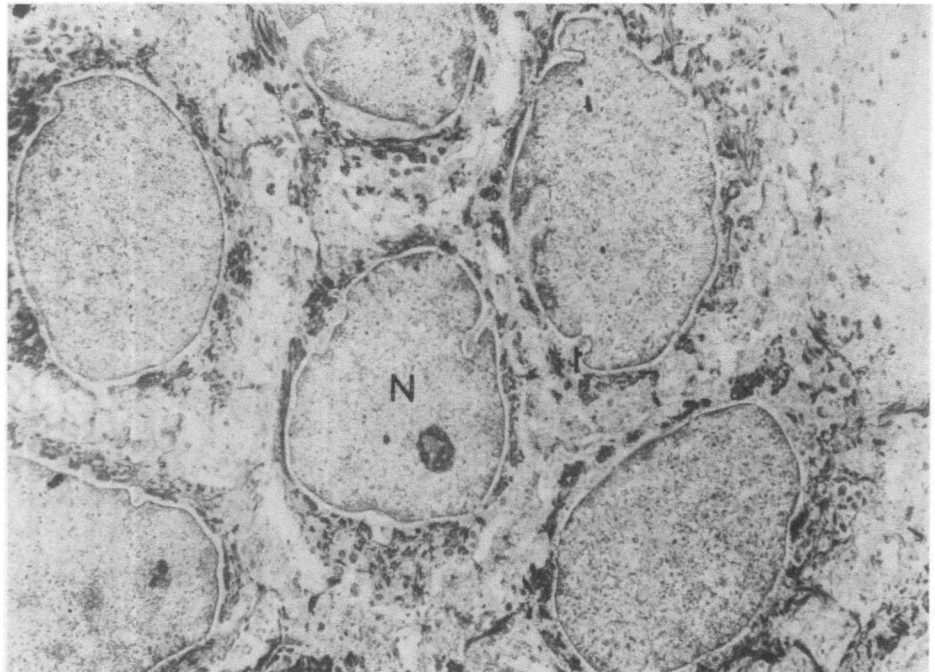

Fig. 3. Maladie de Darier. Corps muqueux en microscopie électronique. Disparition des desmosomes. Noyaux volumineux (N). Amas périnucléaires de faisceaux de tonofilaments (t) (× 6600)

processus conduit à la formation de quelques éléments ressemblant à des «grains». — Cependant ce dérèglement de la kératinisation est secondaire et nous verrons que le «grain» du pemphigus bénin familial n'a pas la même structure que celui de la dyskératose folliculaire.

3. Arguments tirés de la cytologie

Les frottis de dyskératose folliculaire montrent des cellules isolées ou en îlots. Au MAY-GRÜNWALD-GIEMSA elles ont un cytoplasme homogène légèrement bleuté et un noyau central assez gros, fortement teinté en violet.

Dans la maladie de Hailey-Hailey, les frottis contiennent de petits placards d'épiderme dont les éléments sont peu cohérents. Les cellules sont arrondies et possèdent un noyau généralement central, riche en chromatine et muni d'un nucléole dense. Autour du noyau se voit un anneau bleu pâle qui est à son tour entouré d'une bande périphérique bleu foncé ou violacé. Ces images sont donc différentes de celles qu'on trouve dans la maladie de Darier. Or, les frottis obtenus au départ des papules kératosiques qu'on observe parfois au pourtour des placards de pemphigus bénin familial, donnent une image cytologique de maladie de Hailey-Hailey et non de maladie de Darier.

4. Arguments histochimiques

Des diverses méthodes histochimiques utilisées*, seules la technique d'UNNA et BRACHET et la réaction de la leucine-aminopeptidase de BURSTONE nous ont fourni des données intéressantes.

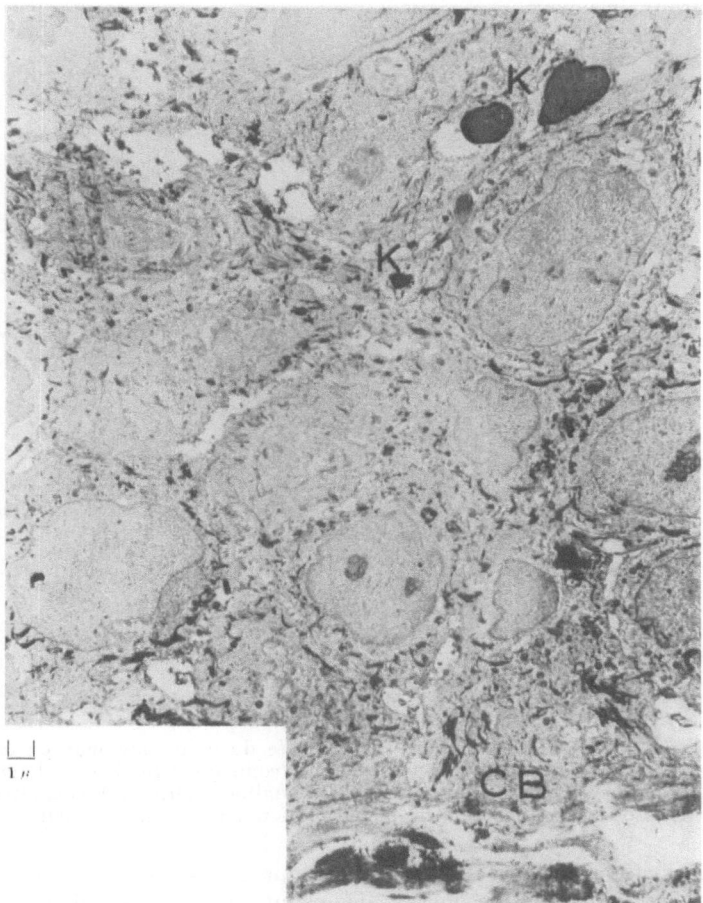

Fig. 4. Maladie de Darier (Microscopie électronique). Couche basale (CB) et partie inférieure du corps muqueux. Noter la présence de volumineux grains de kératohyaline (K) dans le corps muqueux inférieur (en haut et à droite) ($\times$ 3260)

L'acide ribonucléique est nettement augmenté dans les cellules acantholytiques de la maladie de Hailey-Hailey; la coloration la plus intense se situe au niveau de l'anneau périphérique du cytoplasme, tandis que la zone périnucléaire n'est que faiblement basophile. Dans la maladie de Darier les zones dyskératosiques de l'épiderme contiennent généralement moins d'ARN que le corps muqueux normal.

* P.A.S.; Hale-P.A.S.; bleu de toluïdine; méthode d'UNNA-BRACHET; FEULGEN; coloration de BARRNETT et SELIGMAN; lipides; enzymes.

La réaction de BURSTONE pour la mise en évidence de l'activité de la leucine aminopeptidase, n'offre aucune particularité dans les cas de maladie de Hailey-Hailey. — Dans la maladie
de Darier, le derme papillaire situé en dessous des zones dyskératosiques est fortement positif.

5. Arguments tirés de la microscopie électronique

L'examen au microscope électronique des cellules de la *maladie de* Darier
(sept cas) met en évidence les caractères suivants:

1. La rupture des attaches entre desmosomes et tonofibrilles. Ces dernières
abandonnent la périphérie des cellules pour se grouper en faisceaux et former une
couronne autour du noyau.

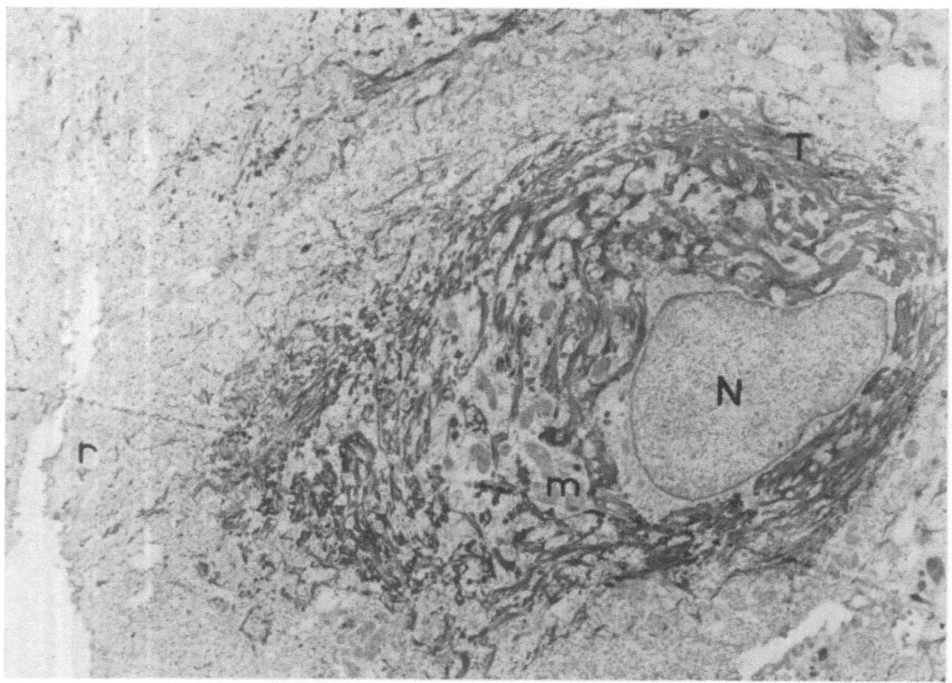

Fig. 5. Maladie de Hailey-Hailey. Cellule acantholysée du corps muqueux en microscopie
électronique. Noter le rapport nucléo-cytoplasmique (comparer avec Fig. 3), le groupement
péri-nucléaire des faisceaux de tonofilaments (T) et des mitochondries (m), l'exoplasme peuplé
de ribosomes (r) et presque complètement dépourvu de tonofilaments (× 6600)

2. La disparition — consécutive à cette rupture — d'un certain nombre de
desmosomes, d'où perte de la cohésion des cellules qui s'isolent et prennent une
forme arrondie. Cette desmolyse explique la formation de la lacune.

3. Une modification du rapport nucléo-cytoplasmique au profit du noyau, qui
occupe la plus grande partie de la cellule (Fig. 3).

4. La présence anormale de grains de kératohyaline, dans les couches inférieures
du corps muqueux de MALPIGHI, voire même dans la couche basale (Fig. 4).

5. La formation de «grains» par un processus d'homogénéisation cytoplasmique
et de dégénérescence nucléaire.

6. La formation de «corps ronds» réalisés par le groupement périnucléaire
d'épais faisceaux homogénéisés de tonofilaments, la présence de granules d'ODLAND
et de grains de kératohyaline (CAULFIELD et WILGRAM).

Dans *la maladie de* Hailey-Hailey (cinq cas), la première étape — séparation des tonofilaments et des desmosomes et groupement en couronne périnucléaire des faisceaux de tonofilaments — est apparemment la même, mais la suite est différente. L'acantholyse est plus accentuée, les desmosomes disparaissent, les cellules s'écartent les unes des autres; l'aire cellulaire s'agrandit et la modification du rapport nucléo-cytoplasmique se fait, cette fois au profit du cytoplasme dont la périphérie s'enrichit en ribosomes (Fig. 5). Une substance amorphe s'accumule dans certains espaces intercellulaires. Dans la suite, le cytoplasme périphérique se repeuplera de tonofibrilles néoformées qui vont alors remplir la cellule entière et qui procèdent probablement des ribosomes.

Cependant, l'évolution des cellules du corps muqueux supérieur ne paraît pas fondamentalement troublée. L'apparition de grains de kératohyaline au sommet de la couche épineuse crée une granuleuse; la couche cornée, formée de cellules de densités variées, s'écarte légèrement du type normal.

Notons la formation éventuelle de «grains», sous forme d'éléments où les tonofilaments acquièrent une densité extraordinaire. Ces grains-ci résultent par conséquent d'une kératinisation viciée du cytoplasme et leur morphologie est différente de celle des «grains» de DARIER.

En conclusion, nous pensons que la clinique, l'histologie, la cytologie et la microscopie électronique fournissent un faisceau d'arguments concordants qui permettent de considérer que la maladie de Hailey-Hailey est bien une affection autonome. Qu'il existe une certaine parenté entre elle et la dyskératose folliculaire, qu'il existe même quelques cas troublants, cela ne paraît pas douteux, mais nous pensons que la thèse de l'identité de la maladie de Hailey-Hailey et de la maladie de Darier bulleuse peut être rejetée.

Bibliographie. AYRES, S., and N. P. ANDERSON: Arch. Derm. Syph. (Chic.) **40**, 402 (1939). — BECKER, S. W.: Arch. Derm. Syph. (Chic.) **41**, 1170 (1940). — BOECK, C.: Arch. Derm. Syph. (Berl.) **23**, 857 (1891). — CAULFIELD, J. B., and G. F. WILGRAM: J. invest. Derm. **41**, 57 (1963). — CHORZELSKI, T.: Dermatologica (Basel) **124**, 21 (1962). — DARIER, J.: Ann. Derm. Syph. (Paris) 2ᵉ Série, X., 597 (1889); — Ann. Derm. Syph. (Paris) 3ᵉ Série **7**, 742 (1896). — DEGOS, R.: Dermatologie. Paris: Flammarion 1965. — DEGOS, R., et J. CIVATTE: Bull. Soc. franç. Derm. Syph. **67**, 854 (1960). — DUPONT, AD.: Ann. Derm. Syph. (Paris) **78**, 703 (1951); — Hautarzt **11**, 75 (1960). — FRANK, S. B., and CH. R. REIN: Arch. Derm. Syph. (Chic.) **45**, 1030 (1942). — GRAHAM, J. H., and E. B. HELWIG: Arch. Derm. **77**, 377 (1958). — HAILEY, H., and H. HAILEY: Arch. Derm. Syph. (Chic.) **39**, 679 (1939). — JABLONSKA, ST., u. T. CHORZELSKI: Dermatologica (Basel) **117**, 24 (1958). — PELS, I. R., and M. H. GOODMAN: Arch. Derm. Syph. (Chic.) **39**, 438 (1939). — RAASCHOU-NIELSEN, W., and F. REYMANN: Acta derm.-venereol. (Stockh.) **39**, 280 (1959). — SACHS, W., A. B. HYMAN, and M. B. GREY: Arch. Derm. Syph. (Chic.) **55**, 91 (1947). — SVENDSEN, I. B., and B. ALBRECTSEN: Acta derm.-venereol. (Stockh.) **39**, 256 (1959). — TOURAINE, L.: L'hérédité én médecine. Paris: Masson 1955.

The Different Forms of Ichthyosiform Erythrodermia

J. R. SIMPSON, Royal Devon and Exeter Hospital, Exeter (England)

Congenital Ichthyosiform Erythrodermia was first distinguished from Ichthyosis Vulgaris by BROCQ (1902) because the former is congenital and persistent, it usually features generalized erythema and always generalized hyperkeratosis, which is most marked on the greater flexures and often involves the palms and soles; abundant sebaceous secretion from the scalp and rapid growth of the nails and of the hair on scalp and limbs are also commonly seen. BROCQ noticed that some cases develop bullae which are flaccid, irregularly shaped, contain opalescent fluid, cause pain but no itching and leave no scars. They tend to occur less frequently as the subject grows older.

Although two of the cases Brocq discussed were studied histologically, one with and one without bullae, it was Lapière (1932) who first drew attention to the striking histological difference between the two forms of the disease, demonstrated that the changes peculiar to the bullous form are present even where there are no clinical bullae and affirmed that the two types are entirely distinct.

With regard to the hereditary characteristics Lapière (1957) noted that the bullous form was often dominant. This was supported by Heimendinger and Schnyder (1962) and by Greither (1964). Wells and Kerr (1965) have shown conclusively that the bullous form is inherited as an autosomal dominant, the non-bullous as an autosomal recessive, so that they can equally clearly be separated on a genetic basis.

The clinical difference between the two types may be summarized as follows. In the severe cases the bullous form shows extensive or total epidermal stripping from birth, as if the infant had been boiled, while the non-bullous form is covered with a thick carapace and has been termed Harlequin Foetus. In survivors and in the less severe cases the one form continues to develop bullae of varying size, with gradually diminishing frequency, about 25% continuing to do so until at least the age of 20 (Simpson, 1964); in the least severe cases the bullae may be so sparse and infrequent as scarcely to be noticed. The other form never produces bullae at all. The bullous cases generally begin to develop hyperkeratosis within the first year and even when bullae are not evident this form can usually be distinguished by the following points. The hyperkeratosis is less generalized and more friable, permitting easier observation of the underlying erythema. Small scales are shed abundantly and the skin is sometimes moist, particularly in the flexures. The face is less often involved and then only in the lower part. Moreover, in general, there is a tendency to improvement in adult life. In the non-bullous form the skin is uniformly dry, the hyperkeratosis is more widespread and often masks the erythema; the scales are large and dark and the upper part of the face is commonly involved, causing ectropion. There is little tendency to improvement.

The histological difference is even more striking. In the non-bullous form there is usually no more than a general increase in thickness in all layers of the epidermis. In the bullous form, however, there is extreme hyperkeratosis and moderate acanthosis. The basal layer is normal but the middle and upper parts of the malphighian layer show intra-cellular oedema, granular degeneration of the nuclei and cytoplasm and disappearance of many of the cell boundaries, forming large cavities of irregular size and shape, of which some are empty, some contain a much modified nucleus looking rather like a "corps rond" and some contain amorphous debris. These changes are continued into the granular layer and to a less extent into the horny layer. They are found in all areas but are much more obvious in sections taken from the sites of the bullae.

Difficulty has arisen because it has been known for many years that some solid verrucous epidermal naevi of the hystrix type show histological appearances identical with those just described, even though the patients have never had bullae. Barker and Sachs (1953) reported a girl with bullous congenital ichthyosiform erythrodermia whose father had such a neavus. For this reason some authors have suggested the term epidermolytic hyperkeratosis to include both these conditions.

Electron microscopic studies by Wilgram and Caulfield (1966) on these special epidermal naevi and by Weibel and Schnyder (1966) on bullous ichthyosiform erythrodermia have confirmed the histological similarity between these two conditions and their difference from other hyperkeratotic abnormalities. Briefly the main features are an excess of tonofilaments and keratohyalin granules which are aggregated into large masses and an increase in number of ribosomes and mitochondria. The desmosomes are normal. This suggests that the hyperkeratosis is due to a faster rate of production and migration of epidermal cells rather than to a slower rate of shedding of the horny cells.

References BARKER, L. P., and W. SACHS: Arch. Derm. Syph. (Chic.) **67**, 443 (1953). — BROCQ, L.: Ann. Derm. Syph. (Paris) **3**, 1 (1902). — GREITHER, A.: Dermatologica (Basel) **128**, 464 (1964). — HEIMENDINGER, J., u. U. W. SCHNYDER: Helv. paediat. Acta **17**, 47 (1962). — LAPIÈRE, S.: Ann. Derm. Syph. (Paris) **3**, 401 (1932); **84**, 5 (1957). — SIMPSON, J. R.: Trans. St. Johns Hosp. derm. Soc. (Lond.) **50**, 93 (1964). — WEIBEL, E. R., and U. W. SCHNYDER: Arch. klin. exp. Derm. **225**, 286 (1966). — WELLS, R. S., and C. B. KERR: Arch. Derm. Syph. (Chic.) **92**, 1 (1965). — WILGRAM, G. F., and J. B. CAULFIELD: Arch. Derm. Syph. (Chic.) **94**, 127 (1966).

Xeroderma pigmentosum

E. HADIDA, F. G. MARILL et J. SAYAG, Clinique Dermatologique Hôtel-Dieu, Faculté de Médecine de Marseille (France)

A la lumière de 50 observations personnelles, de 18 observations mises à notre disposition, de 14 autres publiées en Afrique du Nord et des documents recueillis dans la littérature, nous voudrions résumer les données essentielles relatives à l'étude clinique, histologique, étio-pathogénique et thérapeutique du xeroderma pigmentosum (X.P.).

Manifestations cutanées. — Le X.P. évolue en trois phases: érythémateuse et pigmentée, atrophique et télangiectasique, néoplasique. Chez nos malades l'affection s'est exprimée par des lésions très classiques. Nous voudrions cependant signaler une particularité. Chez une quinzaine de sujets, nous avons trouvé au niveau de la région lombaire, qui est à l'abri de la lumière, un semis de taches lenticulaires achromiques, avec peu ou pas d'atrophie.

La dégénérescence maligne se manifeste inéluctablement mais dans des délais très variables, en moyenne au bout de 2 ans d'évolution. Dans la généralité des cas il s'agit d'épithéliomas baso-cellulaires, spino-cellulaires ou métatypiques. Du point de vue clinique ces épithéliomas se traduisent par des productions verruqueuses, des tumeurs végétantes, ou par des ulcérations qui peuvent devenir térébrantes. Il se produit parfois des métastases ganglionnaires. Par contre, dans la règle, il n'y a pas de métastases viscérales. En dehors des épithéliomas on observe, mais beaucoup plus rarement, des mélanomes malins et des sarcomes. La gravité du X.P. est liée au développement des tumeurs malignes, dont l'évolution est du reste très variable. Il en est dont la marche est relativement lente, mais il en est qui revêtent parfois une allure galopante.

Chez nos malades, les formations dégénérées se sont constituées avec une fréquence considérable, aussi bien par le nombre de sujets atteints que par le nombre de tumeurs observés sur un même individu (jusqu'à 13 chez un malade).

Manifestations oculaires. — Sur 48 observations, nous avons relevé une atteinte oculaire dans 40 cas: des lésions palpébrales 36 fois; des lésions conjonctivales 21 fois; des lésions cornéennes 25 fois; des lésions du globe oculaire 5 fois; des tumeurs oculaires 20 fois (dont 7 au niveau du limbe). C'est souvent que ces lésions se trouvaient associées chez un même malade.

Manifestations neuro-psychiques. — Nous avons pu mettre en évidence une atteinte psychique dans une importante proportion de cas; arriération mentale, degrés variables d'imbécilité, idiotie, altérations des tracés électro-encéphalographiques.

Troubles endocriniens et somatiques. — Chez quelques sujets nous avons observé un retard de l'évolution sexuelle. Nous avons également noté dans certains cas un état d'infantilisme harmonieux.

Anatomie pathologique. — Il n'existe aucun signe histologique pathognomonique de X.P. C'est un ensemble d'altérations qui permet d'évoquer le diagnostic. Diverses variétés de tumeurs bénignes et toutes les formes de cancers cutanés peuvent être observées. Chez nos malades nous avons pratiqué des examens histologiques essentiellement sur les formations tumorales. Cependant nous disposons de 16 biopsies de peau «xérodermique» non dégénérée dont deux effectuées sur des zones non insolées. Voici le bilan de nos constatations. L'image est identique qu'il s'agisse de peau couverte ou de peau exposée au soleil: l'épiderme est tantôt hyperacanthosique, tantôt atrophique, réduit à une on deux assises cellulaires. La basale parfois détruite, souvent rectiligne, contient par endroits une grande quantité de mélanine qui déborde sur les assises profondes du corps muqueux. Un infiltrat lympho-histiocytaire occupe le derme superficiel, se disposant avec prédilection autour des vaisseaux ou volontiers «en bande» sous-épithéliale. De nombreux mélanophores parsèment le corps papillaire; mais la mélanine peut se disposer en dehors des histiocytes. Une sclérose plus ou moins importante selon l'âge des lésions, peut remanier la structure du derme. La trame élastique présente d'importantes altérations: fragmentation, raréfaction, parfois même disparition complète. Les annexes sébacées et sudoripares s'atrophient progressivement.

Répartition géographique et raciale. — Le X.P. se voit en tous lieux. Il se rencontre avec une fréquence certaine en Afrique du Nord. Il s'observerait fréquemment chez les juifs, encore que les chiffres soient très variables suivant les statistiques. Parmi 80 malades dont nous faisons état dans ce travail, 2 seulement sont européens, aucun n'est d'origine juive, 78 sont musulmans.

Age. — Chez nos malades, les premières atteintes se sont marquées précocement dans 34 cas sur 42 avant 8 ans; 26 fois sur 42 entre les premiers mois de la vie et 2 ans environ.

Sexe. — Sur 80 malades, 56 appartiennent au sexe masculin, 24 au sexe féminin.

Hérédité. — Le X.P. est une affection familiale héréditaire, une génodermatose qui dans la règle se transmet en récessivité simple. Nos observations donnent à penser que la transmission en récessivité sexuelle est peut-être moins rare qu'il n'est classique de l'admettre.

Actino-sensibilité et radio-sensibilité. — En dépit de données discordantes aussi bien du point de vue expérimental que clinique, la tendance générale est d'admettre que les malades atteints de X.P. présentent une hypersensibilité aux radiations. Ce sont les radiations de courte longueur d'onde, les U.V. et plus encore les rayons X qui se montrent nocifs. Aussi incrimine-t-on pour expliquer cette hypersensibilité, une fragilité cutanée congénitale. Enfin mentionnons l'hypothèse suivant laquelle le X.P. serait lié à une erreur congénitale du métabolisme soufré.

Mesures d'eugénisme. — La maladie se transmettant généralement en récessivité simple, il est classique de déconseiller les mariages consanguins.

Protection contre les rayons actiniques. — Utiliser des médications photoprotectrices. Certains auteurs ont souligné les avantages des sels de chloroquine; nous les avons utilisés chez de nombreux malades, en cures prolongées, sans bénéfice franchement appréciable.

Traitement anti-inflammatoire. — Nous avons eu recours à la corticothérapie chez de nombreux xerodermiques; nous avons noté l'action anti-inflammatoire du traitement mais n'avons pas obtenu en définitive de résultats dignes d'être retenus.

Traitement préventif et curatif des dégénérescences. — Des auteurs ont utilisé les psoralens dans de rares cas de X.P., mais il faut être circonspect en ce qui concerne l'emploi de ce traitement. On a récemment signalé l'action prophylactique du phosphore radio-actif sur la dégénérescence, mais le recul du temps est insuffisant pour autoriser une conclusion à cet égard. Actuellement la conduite à tenir la meilleure consiste à surveiller méticuleusement les malades atteints de X.P. pour saisir et détruire dès leur apparition les foyers de dégénérescence.

Free Communications

Importance génétique et clinique des altérations atypiques du fond de l'oeil dans le syndrome de Groenblad et Strandberg (pseudo-xanthome élastique et stries angioïdes)

A. FRANCESCHETTI, Genève (Suisse)

Les stries angioïdes du fond d'oeil, décrites pour la première fois par DOYNE (1889), ont toujours suscité un très grand intérêt et la littérature sur ce sujet est énorme (FRANCESCHETTI et coll., 1963). C'est le mérite de GROENBLAD et STRAND-BERG (1929) d'avoir attiré l'attention sur l'association de pseudo-xanthome élastique et de stries angioïdes. C'est pour cette raison que FRANCESCHETTI (1934) a proposé d'appeler cette association d'atteinte élective du tissu élastique cutané

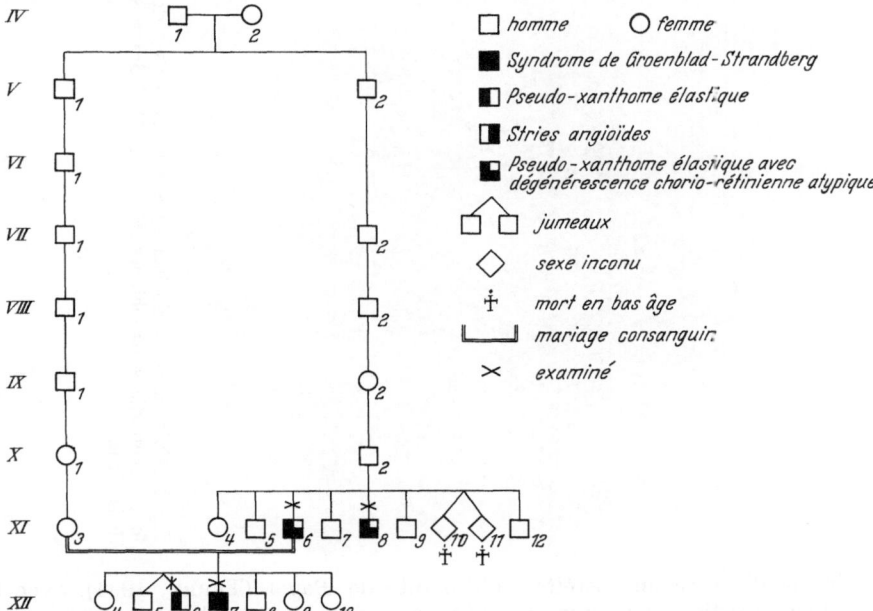

Fig. 1. Syndrome de Groenblad-Strandberg (Pseudo-xanthome élastique de la peau et stries angioïdes de la rétine) avec dégénérescence chorio-rétinienne atypique chez deux membres de la XIe génération. Manifestation typique dans la XIIe génération avec consanguinité des parents. [Extrait de l'arbre généalogique publié par F. AMMANN et F. MARTY, J. Génét. hum. **11**, 228 (1962)]

et oculaire, *Syndrome de* Groenblad et Strandberg, dénomination qui a l'avantage de pouvoir inclure les cas où il existe d'autres altérations oculaires que les stries angioïdes classiques. Ce n'est que plus tard que l'on a mentionné l'associa-

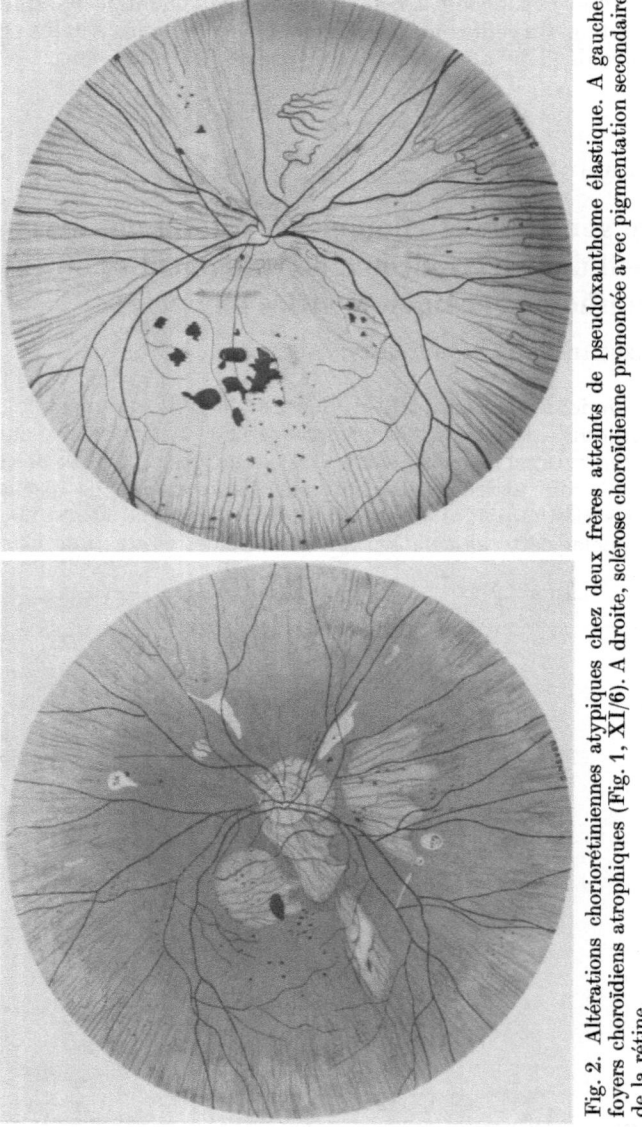

Fig. 2. Altérations choriorétiniennes atypiques chez deux frères atteints de pseudoxanthome élastique. A gauche, foyers choroïdiens atrophiques (Fig. 1, XI/6). A droite, sclérose choroïdienne prononcée avec pigmentation secondaire de la rétine.

tion fréquente avec une ostéite déformante de Paget (Terry, 1934), avec les altérations cardio-vasculaires et l'hypertension (élastorrhexie systématisée, Touraine, 1941) et finalement avec l'anémie à cellules falciformes (drépanocytose, Geeraets et Dupont Guerry III, 1960). Soulignons que les lésions qui sont à l'origine des stries angioïdes, sont localisées dans la membrane élastique de Bruch.

Si les stries angioïdes constituent l'élément type de l'affection, elles peuvent parfois être accompagnées, précédées ou remplacées par d'autres lésions du fond d'œil, comme CALHOUN (1927) l'a signalé le premier.

1. Les lésions maculaires: hémorragies, taches atrophiques et pigmentaires

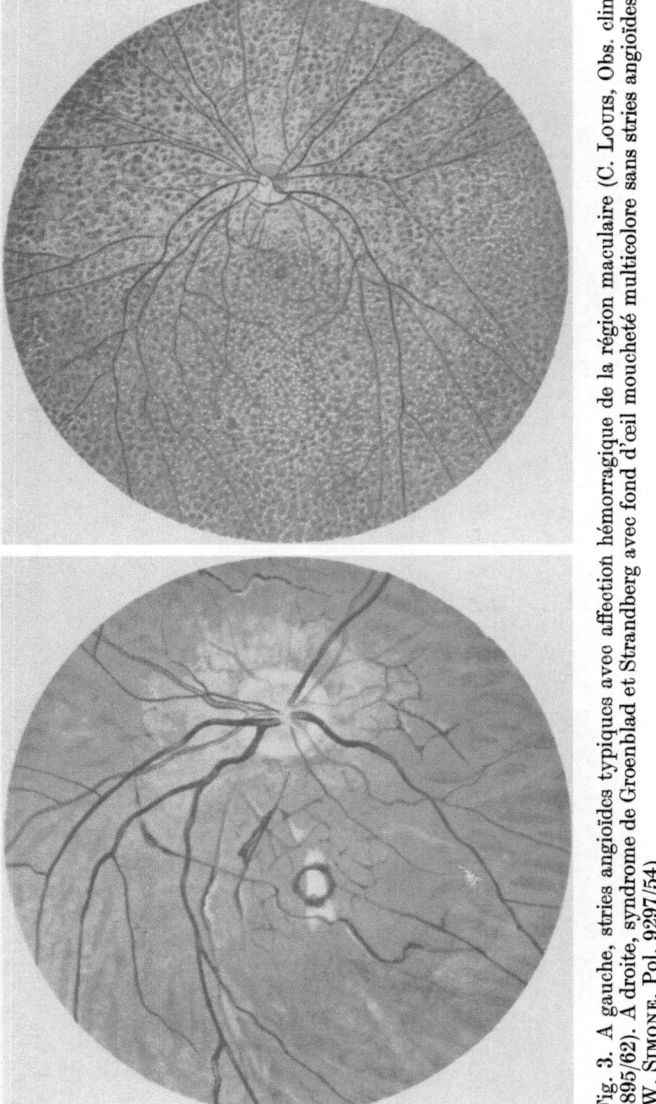

Fig. 3. A gauche, stries angioïdes typiques avec affection hémorragique de la région maculaire (C. LOUIS, Obs. clin. 4895/62). A droite, syndrome de Groenblad et Strandberg avec fond d'œil moucheté multicolore sans stries angioïdes. (W. SIMONE, Pol. 9297/54)

sont très fréquentes. Elles ressemblent souvent à la dégénérescence disciforme sénile.

2. *Foyers d'atrophie choroïdienne* rappelant des cicatrices de chorio-rétinite. Parfois il s'agit uniquement de foyers pigmentaires au pôle postérieur. Nous avons eu l'occasion d'observer chez deux frères âgés respectivement de 71 et 66 ans (arbre généalogique XI/6 et XI/8 Fig. 1), de grands placards atrophiques, jaunâtres

et pigmentés au pôle postérieur, ressemblant à la dystrophie pseudo-inflammatoire de Sorsby (Fig. 2). Le diagnostic exact n'a pu être posé que par la découverte chez le fils de l'un d'eux (XII/7) de stries angioïdes typiques et d'un pseudo-xanthome

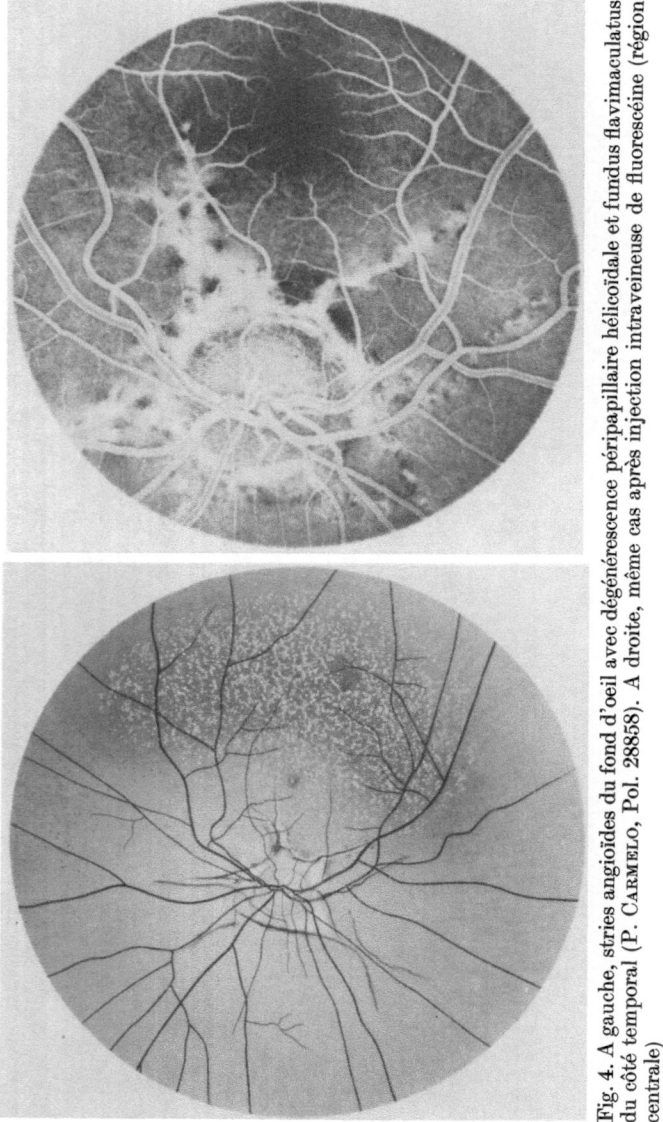

Fig. 4. A gauche, stries angioïdes du fond d'oeil avec dégénérescence péripapillaire hélicoïdale et fundus flavimaculatus du côté temporal (P. CARMELO, Pol. 28858). A droite, même cas après injection intraveineuse de fluorescéine (région centrale)

élastique chez les trois malades. Un frère du fils présente des stries angioïdes mais pas de pseudo-xanthome, ce qui montre que la pénétrance pour les différents symptômes du Syndrome de Groenblad et Strandberg est variable. Le fait que le père atteint a épousé une cousine éloignée, (XII/6) explique l'apparition du Syndrome de Groenblad et Strandberg chez le fils. On se trouve ainsi, en présence d'une pseudo-dominance.

3. L'élastose rétinienne évolue presque toujours vers la *sclérose choroïdienne* (Fig. 2) qui accompagne ou remplace la dégénérescence maculaire disciforme, complication presque habituelle des hémorragies maculaires (Fig. 3).

4. Une autre variété d'altérations rétiniennes est le *fond d'oeil moucheté multicolore* (BISCHLER, 1955). Toute la rétine est parsemée de mouchetures pigmentées associées à un pointillé blanchâtre (Fig. 3).

5. A côté des stries angioïdes ou à leur place, on peut trouver aussi des *verrucosités hyalines de la papille* ou des *drusen de la lame vitrée* qui peuvent prendre l'aspect d'une rétinopathie ponctuée albescente.

6. Il est probable que dans un certain nombre de cas, il ne s'agissait pas de drusen de la lame vitrée, mais d'altérations du type du *fundus flavimaculatus* (FRANCESCHETTI, 1962). En effet, ces derniers temps nous avons observé trois cas où il existait des altérations localisées typiques, du type *fundus flavimaculatus* (Fig. 4).

Tout récemment, l'ophtalmoscopie après injection intra-veineuse de fluorescéine et l'histologie ont révélé que dans le fundus flavimaculatus, il ne s'agit pas de drusen de la lame vitrée mais d'altérations au niveau de l'épithélium pigmentaire (Fig. 4).

Finalement, on peut trouver une dégénérescence péripapillaire hélicoïdale (FRANCESCHETTI, 1962), comme le montre la Fig. 4. D'autres cas semblables sont d'ailleurs cités dans la littérature (FRANCESCHETTI et coll., 1963, vol. I, p. 623). Il résulte de cet exposé que les manifestations oculaires du Syndrome de Groenblad et Strandberg sont souvent atypiques. Il faut donc, dans tous ces cas, faire un examen systématique de la peau et surtout des recherches génétiques, afin de ne pas risquer de méconnaître l'affection générale responsable.

Littérature. Pour la bibliographie, voir: FRANCESCHETTI, A., J. FRANÇOIS et J. BABEL: Les hérédodégénérescences chorio-rétiniennes, 2 vol.; Paris: Masson 1963. — Travaux récents mentionnés dans le texte: AMMANN, F., D. KLEIN, and A. FRANCESCHETTI: J. Neurol. Sci. **2**, 183 (1965). — AMMANN, F., u. F. MARTY: Arch. Klaus-Stift. Vererb.-Forsch. **37**, 50 (1962); — J. Génét. hum. **11**, 221 (1962). — FRANCESCHETTI, A.: Über tapetoretinale Degenerationen im Kindesalter. III. Fortbildungskurs dtsch. ophthal. Ges. 1962, p. 107—129. Stuttgart: F. Enke 1963. — FRANCESCHETTI, A., F. AMMANN, W. JADASSOHN et R. PAILLARD: Dermatologica (Basel) **127**, 148 (1963).

The Necessity of Distinguishing Four Types of Acanthosis Nigricans

H. OLLENDORFF CURTH, Department of Dermatology, College of Physicians & Surgeons, Columbia University, New York (USA)

Since the last International Congress of Dermatology, where I stressed the necessity of distinguishing three types of acanthosis nigricans, new information has led to the recognition of a fourth type. The new type belongs to that main form which is not associated with a malignant tumor and, therefore, is benign in a broad sense of the word.

I. Other benign types not associated with a malignant tumor are:

a) truly "benign" acanthosis nigricans, which is a rare dermatosis, greatly resembling ichthyosis hystrix. It follows irregular dominance. There are no accompanying endocrine disorders. Although benign, it may greatly disfigure the patient. Surgical treatment has proved highly successful in a generalized case. A movie describing the various surgical techniques employed is being shown here.

b) pseudo acanthosis nigricans, which is mostly seen in brunette or colored individuals. It is not uncommon, is acquired, and dependent on an underlying cause such as obesity, acromegaly, and gigantism. The obesity may or may not be due to an endocrine disorder. Some of the causes leading to obesity are reversible. In such cases loss of weight is accompanied by regression of the dermatosis. The term "pseudo" indicates that we are dealing with a phenocopy of benign acanthosis nigricans. If the term seems objectionable to some observers, they must realize that the terms "secondary" or "acquired" are not applicable, because malignant acanthosis nigricans is also acquired and may be secondary. In the tropics even non-obese individuals may develop pseudo acanthosis nigricans from constant maceration, perspiration, and friction.

c) In the new type, only recently recognized, acanthosis nigricans is part of a syndrome.

Table. *Acanthosis nigricans as part of a syndrome*

Syndrome	Inheritance
Bloom's syndrome	Recessive
Crouzon's syndrome	Sporadic cases or dominant
Seip's syndrome	Recessive
Insulin-resistant Diabetes	Sporadic cases
Rud's syndrome	Recessive or sporadic cases
Degenerative disorder of	Recessive or sporadic cases
Deafness	Sporadic cases

Among the various syndromes listed here (table) with their mode of inheritance are:

1. Bloom's syndrome (dwarfism with lupus erythematosus-like cutaneous changes). Acanthosis nigricans in the axillas appeared in childhood or at puberty.

2. Crouzon's syndrome (cranofacial dyostosis). One female patient had the dermatosis since puberty, the other since childhood.

3. Seip's syndrome (lipodystrophy, muscular hypertrophy, and accelerated osseous maturation). Consanguinity and multiple affected siblings have been reported.

4. Insulin-resistant diabetes. Acanthosis nigricans may develop at the onset of the diabetes or at puberty. Since insulin-resistant diabetes may also accompany lipodystrophy patients with insulin resistant diabetes may belong to the syndrome listed under 3.

5. Rud's syndrome (infantilism, tetany, epilepsy, anemia, and mental retardation). Acanthosis nigricans greatly resembles ichthyosis hystrix.

6. A degenerative disorder of the pyramidal tracts. Acanthosis nigricans has been present since childhood.

In chondrodystrophy and phenylketonuria the association with acanthosis nigricans may be coincidental.

II. In *malignant acanthosis nigricans* high malignancy of the associated tumor has been observed in almost all cases. However, one of my patients, an 86 year old Negro, is still well 3 years after the removal of an adenocarcinoma of the sigmoid colon. Before the cancer had caused any symptoms mild progression of the dermatosis prompted me to order a barium enema, which revealed the tumor.

ACKERMANN and LANTIS reported on the association of acanthosis nigricans with Hodgkin's disease. The authors believe that a causal relationship exists between the two, especially since the dermatosis regressed following radiation of the chest. The presence of an adenocarcinoma, however, cannot be completely ruled out without prolonged observation of the patient, operations, or an autopsy. Systemic steroid therapy may improve the dermatosis.

Angiokeratoma Corporis Diffusum Fabry

W. P. DE GROOT, Binnen Gasthuis, Amsterdam (The Netherlands)

Angiokeratoma corporis diffusum has been diagnosed in 29 Dutch patients, belonging to six families. In one family 15 cases are known, in another 7. Both pedigrees are in accordance with X-chromosomal heredity. The three brothers

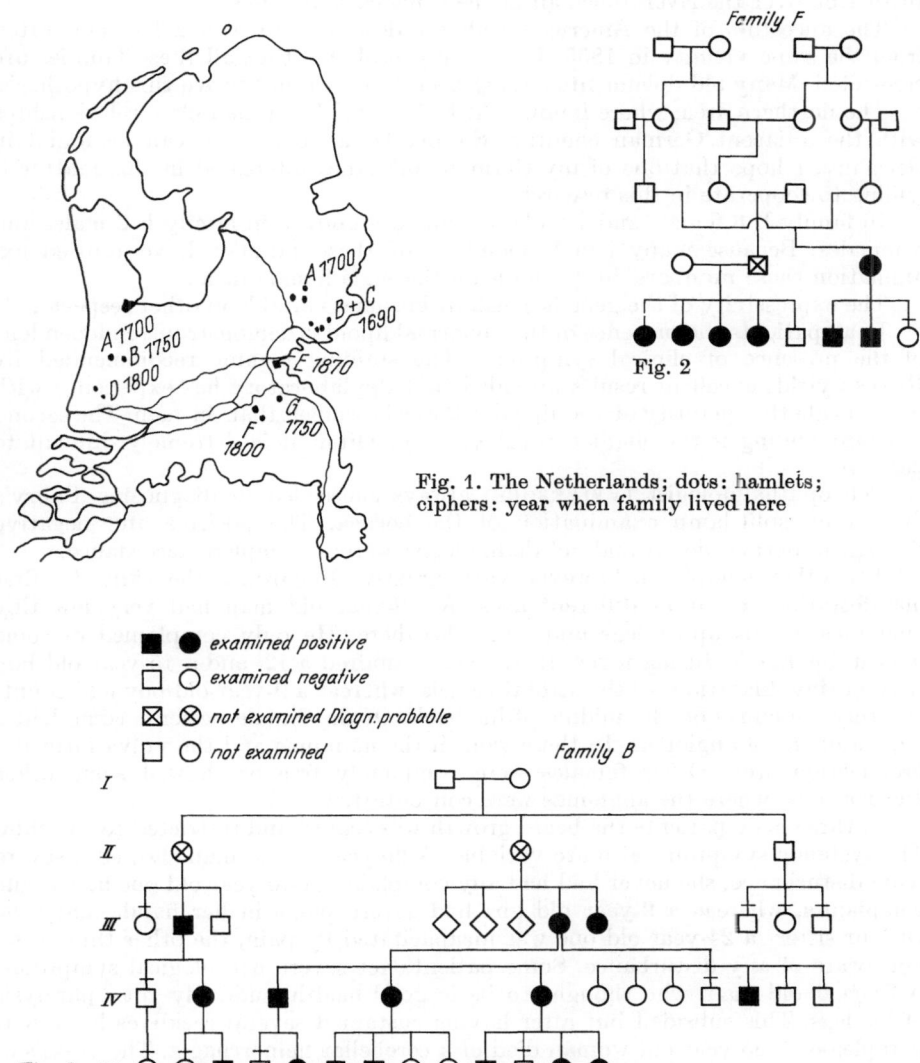

Fig. 1. The Netherlands; dots: hamlets; ciphers: year when family lived here

■ ● examined positive
☐̄ Ō examined negative
⊠ ⊗ not examined Diagn.probable
☐ ○ not examined

Fig. 2

Fig. 3

described by RUITER belong to a third family. In each of the other families one isolated case has been found as yet.

The ancestors of two of these families (B, C) lived in 1690 in the same hamlet in an isolated district, near the German border. A third family (A) lived in the same time in the same neighbourhood. This area was thinly inhabitated, so probably these three families are related. This part of Holland was Roman Catholic territory. The adjacent Dutch provinces were protestant except the region to the south. Marriage between protestants and catholics was then extremely rare. The different religions formed a major impediment for social contacts, whereas the rivers between the two catholic areas didn't raise an important obstacle. Now the fourth family (E) lived just over the Rhine, the fifth (F) a bit further on over the river Maas, all in the same catholic diocese.

The ancestors of the American pedigree described by OPITZ had emigrated from the same vicinity in 1856. It is highly probable that all these families are connected. Many old documents having been lost I cannot prove this hypothesis.

The northern area, where families A, B, C and E lived, had close relationships with the adjacent German country. So maybe a connection can be found in Germany. I hope that one of my German colleagues interested in this matter is willing to cooperate in this research.

In family B 8 female and 7 male patients are known, in family F 2 males and 5 females. Because many female members of these families have refused examination these numbers do not indicate the male-female ratio.

The expressivity of the gene is constant in some, variable in other respects.

In all patients the presence of the abnormal lipoid is demonstrable independent of the presence of clinical symptoms. The staining technic recommended by RUITER yields excellent results provided that the laboratory has experience with it. As a rule the quantity of the lipoid is lower in women than in men. The second constant finding is the slight corneal opacity. Often it is extremely difficult to perceive.

The ophthalmologist (VELZEBOER) always succeeded in diagnosing Fabry's disease by split-lamp examination of the cornea. The positive and negative findings of dermatologist and ophthalmologist were in complete accordance.

The other symptoms however vary greatly. Regarding the skin the first manifestations occur at different ages. A 19-year old man had very few tiny angiomas on his upper legs and none elsewhere. He only complained of some pain in his hands during fever. In the same kindred a 12- and a 15-year old boy showed tiny dilatations of the scrotal vessels, whereas a 9-year old boy had countless tiny angiomas on the middle of his back. Of the female patients some had a large amount of angiomas. In these women the mammae and the vulva formed a predilection area. Other females were completely free or showed some other localizations, where the angiomas were concentrated.

In three male patients the beard growth was scanty and restricted to the chin. The systemic symptoms also are variable. A 60-year old woman showed a severe renal disturbance, she never had had any complaint. A 40-year old one had vague complaints, whereas a 9-year old girl had severe pains in her hands and legs. Of four sisters a 24-year old one was incapacitated by pain, the other three were not aware of any disturbance. Some patients get severe neurological symptoms. A 31-year old man, who thought to be in good health, suddenly got a paralysis of his legs. This subsided but after having sustained several recidives he now is paraplegic. A 55-year old woman died of a cerebellar hemorrhagia. The vessels of the cerebellum were stuffed with the lipoid. The hemorrhagia probably was a result of this storage. A male patient developed an internal deafness on his 35th year. Other patients show little or no neurological symptoms.

Studies on Ichthyosis Vulgaris

Y. Igarashi, K. Ueda and K. Iwashita, Department of Dermatology, Kyoto
Prefectural University of Medicine, Kyoto (Japan)

The epidermis of ichthyosis vulgaris was studies in 18 cases microautoradiographically, histochemically and electron microscopically. Two techniques were carried out for microautoradiographic study, i.e. (1) Labeling in vitro: Specimens were incubated in 1 ml of Eagle's medium with 1 μC ^{3}H-thymidine for 3 h (DNA synthesis), with 2 μC ^{3}H-uridine for 40 min to 6 h (RNA synthesis) and 30 to 70 μC ^{3}H-amino acids (glycine, methionine, tyrosine, phenylalanine, valine and leucine) for 1 to 6 h (amino acid metabolism), (2) local labeling (estimation of life-span of epidermal cell): following intraepidermal giving 0.1 ml of 25 μC ^{3}H-thymidine per 0.1 ml of physiological saline solution at several sites of the area to be examined, the labeled cells were traced in serial biopsy specimens taken at intervals.

Results: ^{3}H-thymidine labeled exclusively the nuclei of basal cells as seen in normal epidermis, but its labeling index was a little greater than that of normal. The life-span of the epidermal cell was almost normal, i.e. ^{3}H-thymidine labeled cell migrated to the top of nucleated strata from basal layer for 14 days. Incorporation of ^{3}H-amino acids such as tyrosine, phenylalanine, valine and leucine seen over the lower layer in normal epidermis, was here observed also over the upper spinous layer, showing more compact density of the silver grain. Although it is difficult how to interpret such increase of labeling index and abnormal incorporation of amino acids, this may be attributed to the prolongation of DNA synthesizing duration provided genetically, and to the aberrant function of epidermal cell in the upper layer, if remotely thought.

RNA synthesis in the spinous cells was not so reduced by examination using either modified Bertalanffy's technique or ^{3}H-uridine autoradiography. There existed histochemically only traces of glycogen, a little amount of phospholipids studied by Okamoto's method and a fairly weak activity of nonspecific esterase as well as acid phosphatase in the epidermis.

The extremely flat horny cells which were confirmed most distinctly under the electron microscope, contained PAS-positive substances and were arranged compactly each other. This PAS-positive substance may play a role for one of possible factors for decreased shedding of horny material as a cementing substance.

In histochemical study using Barrnett-Seligman's method, -SH groups were distributed more concentrated, -SS- bonds were less concentrated in the horny layer than those of normal. It was noteworthy that such higher concentration of -SH groups in the horny layer was not actually due to the reaction of cytoplasm, but in the horny layer was not actually due to the reaction of cytoplasm, but of membrane of horny cell.

Furthermore it was noticeable that the activity of cysteine desulphurase which stain wine-red by Jarrett's technic, was found here moderately in the horny layer, while it was detectable neither in the normal horny layer nor in the hyperkeratotic layer of other diseases. Primarily, this cysteine desulphurase is one of the factors responsible for the marked reduction of cysteine-SH to the pyruvate. So it will be considered that the most amount of -SH groups in the membrane of horny cell is derived from cysteine.

The so-called keratogenous zone could be distinctly demonstrated as a bandlike structure just beneath the horny layer, showing the most pronounced activity of cysteine desulphurase, the fairly intensive labeling from ^{3}H-glycine, the especially rich presence of -SH groups and the peculiar electron microscopic findings of unique feature, i.e. a part of tonofibrils showed an intermediate density between tonofibril and keratohyalin granule, above which transitional cells scattered.

Further, under the electron microscope, tonofibrils were extremely disorganized as to their directions in the spinous layer, which was slightly richer in mitochondria and RNP than the normal. Thus it was indicated that the cellular metabolism was not so reduced, corresponding to the autoradiographic observation by ^{3}H-uridine and the histochemical finding by Bertalanffy's technic. The acid phosphatase activity confirmed electron microscopically using modified Gomori's method by HOLT, was localized particularly intensive in the transitional cells, and more strong in the horny layer with compact keratin pattern than that with loose keratin pattern.

The insensible water loss of the skin was measured for ten cases by cup method using Karl Fischer's apparatus, it was decreased beyond the normal limit in four cases and fairly decreased within the normal range in five cases, and only one case showed the perfectly normal value.

A Genetic Study of X-Linked Ichthyosis in Israel

L. ZIPROWSKI, A. FEINSTEIN and A. ADAM, Departments of Dermatology and Human Genetics, Tel-Aviv University Medical School, Government Hospital Tel Hashomer (Israel), and RUTH SANGER, R. R. RACE, M.R.C. Blood Group Research Unit, The Lister Institute, London (England)

A survey of the Jewish population of Israel has so far revealed 30 families, in which ichthyosis vulgaris segregates in a characteristic X-linked manner. In an additional 42 families, this mode of inheritance seems likely or possible, but not proved. All these families belong to the various communities with approximate proportionality to their percentages in the total population. In all, we have seen 125 ichthyotic males within the typical X-linked families. Therefore, our estimate for the prevalence of ichthyosis of the X-linked type in the Jewish communities is at least 1:9500 males.

There is as yet no estimate for the prevalence of X-linked ichthyosis among non-Jewish Israelis, nor for other forms of ichthyosis in Israel. Our impression, however, is that the X-linked form may account for about 50% of all cases of ichthyosis vulgaris. This is a considerably higher proportion than previously estimated for other populations.

In some of the typical pedigrees of the X-linked variety, certain mild manifestations were seen in the skin of heterozygous females. These manifestations were confined to the lower extensor surfaces of the legs, and were seen during the winter and spring months only. Fig. 1 shows a section through the affected area of the skin of one of these obligatory heterozygotes, where hyperkeratosis and absence of the granular layer in some regions can be seen. The manifestations of ichthyosis in heterozygous females may vary widely, from dry skin to temporary mild ichthyosis, and were recorded in 39 out of 88 heterozygotes examined during last winter and spring. Similar findings among a large group of normal women occurred much less frequently. As far as we know this finding in heterozygotes has not been previously recorded. It may be useful sometimes for the diagnosis of the genetic variety of ichthyosis and hence for genetic counselling. This partial and variable expressivity of the gene is similar to what has been described for other X-linked recessive genes in heterozygous females.

Another aspect of X-linked ichthyosis which is being investigated, is its linkage relations to other genetic traits, governed by loci of the X chromosome, in an attempt to construct a genetic map of the chromosome. This study is done by examining all available and potentially informative members of these families, for several "genetic markers" of the X chromosome. These markers are: the Xg blood groups, glucose-6-phosphate dehydrogenase (g6pd) deficiency of the erythrocytes and protan and deutan colorblindness. The combinations and recombinations of these traits with ichthyosis among the members of the families are then analyzed statistically; the calculated recombination frequencies provide an idea of the distances and sequence of the respective loci along the chromosome.

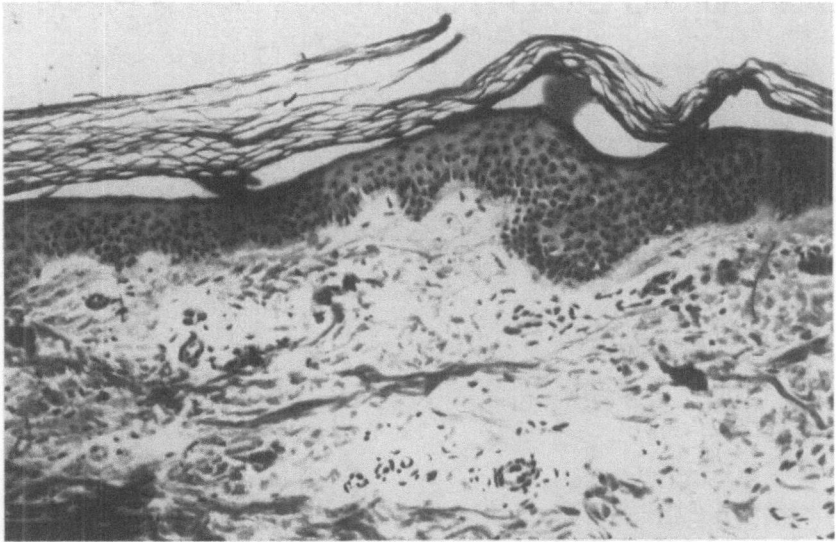

Fig. 1. A section through affected area of the skin of a heterozygous female

Among our 30 families with typical X-linked ichthyosis there were 16 informative ones, namely families which segregated for ichthyosis and for one or more of the other X-linked traits.

The data obtained so far confirm the conclusion of KERR, WELLS and SANGER (1964), that the loci of ichthyosis and of Xg are within measurable distance of each other. Our data improve the previous estimate; the most likely recombination fraction for the total Israeli data is 0.11, with narrow confidence limits. This corresponds to a map distance of 11 centimorgans. Fig. 2 illustrates this close linkage between ichthyosis and the Xg blood groups: in this family 5 ichthyotics are Xg-negative and 4 non-ichthyotics are Xg-positive. There is only one apparent recombinant, an Xg-positive ichthyotic (R).

In addition, our accumulating data suggest measurable linkage between ichthyosis and g6pd, but a loose and probably unmeasurable linkage between ichthyosis and the two loci of color-vision, protan and deutan. These findings are illustrated in Figs. 3, 4 and 5; Fig. 3 shows a family suggesting close linkage between ichthyosis and g6pd, where there are four non-recombinants and only one recombinant: the two ichthyotics with normal g6pd, and the two non-ichthyotics with

36 *

g6pd deficiency are either similar or dissimilar to their maternal grandfather, regarding the two traits, and are, therefore, non-recombinants. The single recombinant is the eldest grandson, who is similar to his grandfather in only one of the traits.

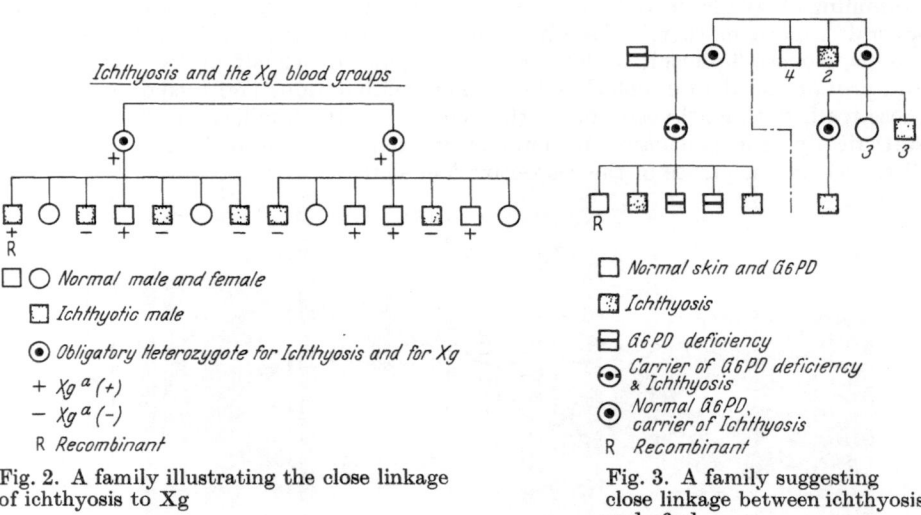

Ichthyosis and G6PD deficiency

☐ *Normal skin and G6PD*

▦ *Ichthyosis*

⊟ *G6PD deficiency*

⊙ *Carrier of G6PD deficiency & Ichthyosis*

⊙ *Normal G6PD, carrier of Ichthyosis*

R *Recombinant*

Fig. 3. A family suggesting close linkage between ichthyosis and g6pd

Ichthyosis and the Xg blood groups

☐○ *Normal male and female*

☐ *Ichthyotic male*

⊙ *Obligatory Heterozygote for Ichthyosis and for Xg*

+ *Xg ᵃ (+)*

− *Xg ᵃ (−)*

R *Recombinant*

Fig. 2. A family illustrating the close linkage of ichthyosis to Xg

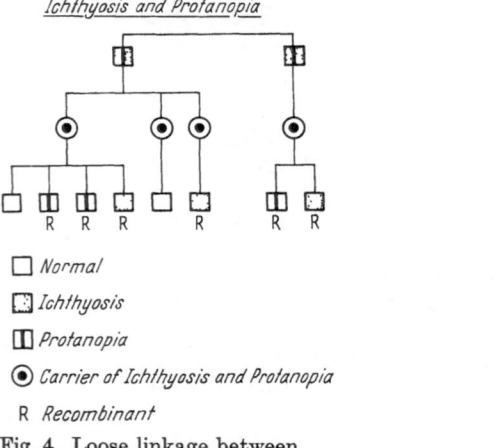

Ichthyosis and Protanopia

☐ *Normal*

▦ *Ichthyosis*

▥ *Protanopia*

⊙ *Carrier of Ichthyosis and Protanopia*

R *Recombinant*

Fig. 4. Loose linkage between ichthyosis and protanopia

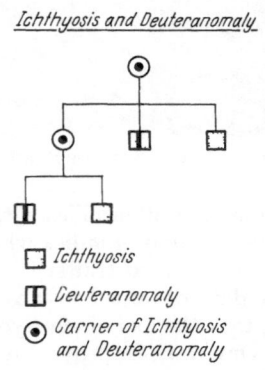

Ichthyosis and Deuteranomaly

☐ *Ichthyosis*

▥ *Deuteranomaly*

⊙ *Carrier of Ichthyosis and Deuteranomaly*

Fig. 5. Loose linkage between ichthyosis and deuteranomaly

Fig. 4 strongly suggests that the loci for ichthyosis and protanopia are too far away from each other in the X chromosome, for the distance to be measured: in this family there are two non-recombinants and six recombinants; the first two being different from the maternal grandfathers in both respects, the latter six being like the grandfathers in one trait but different in the other.

Fig. 5 shows a family with recombination between ichthyosis and deuteranomaly, again suggesting that the genes are far apart: colorblindness seems to segregate independently of ichthyosis.

The latter data, for ichthyosis and g6pd, and for ichthyosis and the two color-vision loci, are not yet sufficient to estimate the respective recombination fractions; but if this trend is confirmed by the study of further families, these three linkage relationships may adumbrate unrealized mechanisms, because the loci for g6pd, protan and deutan are known to be close to each other.

When combined with other linkage studies, our data suggest that the locus of ichthyosis lies between the locus of Xg on one side, and those of g6pd, protan and deutan on the other. According to previous studies, all these loci are probably located on the short arm of the X-chromosome.

Our study is still in progress and we hope that we shall eventually be able to define more accurately the positions of these genes in relation to each other.

References. ADAM, A., L. ZIPRKOWSKI, A. FEINSTEIN, R. SANGER, and R. R. RACE: Lancet **1966** I, 877. — KERR, C. B., R. S. WELLS, and R. SANGER: Lancet **1964** II, 1369. — LINDSTEN, J., M. FRACCARO, P. E. POLANI, J. L. HAMERTON, R SANGER, and R. R. RACE: Nature (Lond.) **197**, 648 (1963).

Atrophodermie folliculaire, proliférations baso-cellulaires et hypotrichose

B. CHRISTOL, A. DUPRÉ et A. BAZEX, Clinique Dermatologique, Hôpital la Grave, Toulouse (France)

L'atrophodermie folliculaire est un nouveau type de lésion élémentaire décrit pour la première fois par MIESCHER en 1944.

Cliniquement l'atrophodermie folliculaire réalise de petites dépressions cupuliformes centrées sur l'ostium folliculaire, véritable image en négatif du spinulosisme. Elle réalise un aspect en peau de pécari. On dirait que la peau a été piquée par une épingle. Ces dépressions sont très nettes sur le dos des mains, ainsi que sur le visage où elles réalisent un aspect cicatriciel particulier.

La signification nosologique de l'atrophodermie folliculaire est très spéciale. Elle traduit l'existence d'une tare génotypique complexe et grave en raison de ses multiples associations morbides. L'atrophodermie folliculaire n'est jamais un symptôme isolé: elle s'intègre toujours dans le tableau d'une génodermatose et d'une génodystrophie complexe et grave.

Le type de la génodystrophie varie selon les cas: aucune observation n'est superposable aux autres. Par ordre chronologique nous citerons les cinq travaux relevés dans la littérature:

G. MIESCHER. Atypische Chondrodystrophie, Typus Morguino, kombiniert mit follikulärer Atrophodermie. Dermatologica (Basel), **89**, 38 (1944). Enfant de 7 ans présente des plaques d'alopécie atrophique et de l'atrophodermie folliculaire sur le tronc et les extrémités. Les troubles associés étaient: une cyphoscoliose, une lordose, une luxation de la hanche, une raccourcissement des deux bras.

H. O. CURTH. Follicular atrophoderma and pseudo-pelade associated with chondrodystrophia calcifians congenita. J. invest. Derm. **13**, 233 (1949). L'auteur présente trois observations personnelles: *Obs. 1:* enfant de 8 ans de race jaune présentant dès sa naissance une éruption croûteuse sur le corps et le cuir chevelu. Au bout de quelques semaines les croûtes tombent et l'enfant gardera une atrophodermie folliculaire sur le corps et une alopécie cicatricielle. *Obs. 2:* une fillette de 9 ans présente une atrophodermie folliculaire, une pseudo-pelade, une incontinentia pigmenti, une cataracte, une cyphoscoliose, etc. Tous les frères de la mère ont une tête asymétrique, l'enfant d'un cousin est né sans bras et sans jambes. *Obs. 3:* il s'agit de la mère du cas précédent âgée de 37 ans. Elle a une atrophodermie folliculaire sur les bras et le dos, un raccourcissement du bras gauche. Une de ses filles âgée de 6 ans est de petite taille et présente une incontinentia pigmenti, une pseudo-pelade, a le côté droit plus court ainsi qu'une atrophodermie folliculaire.

A. BAZEX, A. DUPRÉ et B. CHRISTOL. Atrophodermie folliculaire, proliférations baso-cellulaires et hypotrichose. Bull. Soc. franç Derm. Syph. 71, 206 (1964). — Ann. Derm. Syph. (Paris) 93, 241 (1966). — Présentation de quatre frères ayant trois ordres d'anomalies constitutionnelles: 1. Une atrophodermie folliculaire prédominant au niveau des mains et du visage. 2. Une alopécie soit de type triangulaire, soit de type diffus, soit de type pseudo-pelade de Brocq. 3. Des proliférations basocellulaires certaines bénignes (naeviques) d'autre malignes (épithéliomas).

P. CAUBET. Génodermatose complexe. Bull. Soc. franç Derm. Syph. 71, 753 (1964) — P. LE COULANT, L. TEXIER, J. M. TAMISIER et P. CAUBET. Atrophodermie folliculaire, kystes épidermiques et hypotrichose (Réunion de Toulouse du 22 avril 1967). Le travail porte sur 12 cas familiaux (7 hommes et 5 femmes). Les sujets atteints présentent: une trichorrexie noueuse, des kystes sébacés et des grains de milium, une atrophodermie folliculaire du dos des mains.

O. BRAUN-FALCO et S. MARGHESCU. Über eine systematisierte follikuläre Atrophodermie mit Keratosis palmoplantaris dissipata und Keratosis follicularis. Hautarzt 18, 13 (1967). Un homme de 23 ans présente: 1. Une hyperidrose palmoplantaire. 2. Une atrophodermie folliculaire du dos, du côté droit du thorax, du cuir chevelu, du bras gauche et des genoux, disposée en bandes ramifiées ou en plaques. 3. Une kératose palmo-plantaire avec des dépressions cratériformes contenant le plus souvent un bouchon hyperkératosique. 4. Une kératose folliculaire des bras et des cuisses.

Ces observations peuvent être rapprochées mais non assimilées à d'autres observations: 1. Observation de naevi baso-cellulaires associés à des dyskératoses ponctuées palmo-plantaires (WARD; HOWEL, ANDERON et CLENDON; ABRAHAMS): 2. Observations publiées sous la dénomination d'«atrophia maculosa varioliformis cutis» (HEIDINGSFELS; SENEAR; CORRISON et ROYS).

En résumé: l'atrophodermie folliculaire, symptôme spécifique, apparemment sans importance pathologique, simple petite disgrâce inesthétique, est en réalité un symptôme très péjoratif par sa signification génotypique puisqu'il dénote l'existence d'une tare familiale grave et puisqu'il s'associe à des manifestations morbides redoutables, squelettiques ou épithéliomateuses.

Genetic Analysis of Erythropoietic Protoporphyria (EPP) the Erythrocyte Fluorescence Method

K. D. WUEPPER and J. H. EPSTEIN, Division of Dermatology, University of California School of Medicine, San Francisco, California (USA)

Erythropoietic protoporphyria is now recognized with increasing frequency, particularly in children with photosensitivity. Since 1961, when MAGNUS and his associates described this disease in the English literature, nearly 70 patients have been reported. In this disease, protoporphyrin is increased in red cells and feces but the urine is normal. Protoporphyrin III (Type 9) is apparently produced in excess in erythropoietic tissues.

In previous genetic studies, slightly increased red cell protoporphyrins have been described in some family members. However, in many families, red cell protoporphyrins have been normal. We describe here increased numbers of red-fluorescing erythrocytes in asymptomatic relatives of patients with protoporphyria; this abnormality is apparently transmitted as a Mendelian dominant. We chose to study red cell fluorescence because of the speed, simplicity, and general availability of this technique.

We studied 11 patients with protoporphyria and 51 relatives in five kindreds of eight of these patients. There were 93 controls; these included six patients with porphyria cutanea tarda and four patients with variegate porphyria. In addition, there were 13 patients with other sun-sensitive problems. The remainder of the controls represented disorders not related to sun sensitivity. The details of the fluorescent procedure have been described. Briefly, heparinized blood at 1:1 to

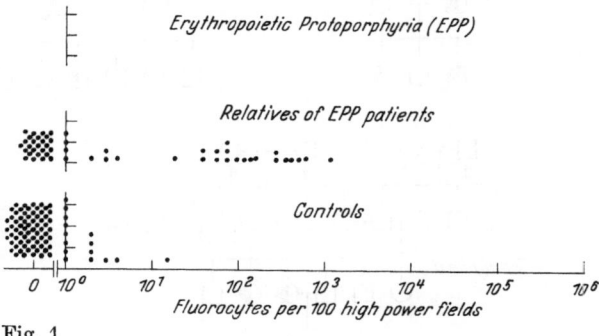

Fig. 1

1:1,000 dilutions is examined at 400 x magnification in 100 fields in an ultraviolet microscope with BG-12 primary and 500 nm secondary filters. Approximately one million erythrocytes are observed and the number of fluorocytes are determined. Red-cell protoporphyrins were assayed by the method of GRINSTEIN and WINTROBE.

The results of the tests (Fig. 1) were five or less in 92 control specimens; the result was 15 in one person. Identical patterns of red-cell fluorescence were observed in the eleven patients with protoporphyria. 17 to 24% of circulating erythrocytes fluoresced. All gradations of intensity of fluorescence were observed, that is from bright to soft red. Actual counts revealed from 230,000 to 350,000 fluorocytes per 100 high power fields. Red-cell protoporphyrins examined chemically ranged from 460 to 4,060 mcg per 100 ml packed cells.

19 relatives of the patients with erythropoietic protoporphyria showed increased numbers of fluorescing erythrocytes. The abnormal counts ranged from 20 to slightly over 4,000 with a mean of 581 fluorocytes per 100 high power fields. Red-cell protoporphyrins were within normal limits (less than 55 mcg per 100 ml) in all relatives.

In the pedigrees of the five families (Fig. 2), affected individuals are illustrated by completely darkened symbols; the propositus is indicated by an arrow. Relatives with increased fluorocytes were considered "carriers" and are shown by half-darkened symbols. The fluorocyte abnormality is present in a single parent in the first four families. This may be from mother or father to son or daughter. In family Gra., both parents have increased numbers of fluorocytes. Moreover, siblings of each parent were found to have increased fluorocytes. This apparently represents the union of two persons dominant for the abnormal trait. Both children born to these parents had protoporphyria; the 3 year old girl was completely asymptomatic

and did not have sun sensitivity despite hours of mid-day sun exposure. There were
no miscarriages in this family.

In these families, carriers ranged from 4 months to 77 years of age. Children of
parents with normal counts were normal; whereas of 23 children born to carriers,
5 had protoporphyria and 8 were carriers. Three of four offspring of affected
individuals were "carriers".

By the method reported here, a presumptive diagnosis of EPP and an estimate
of relatives who may transmit the disease can be made. Four of the eleven patients
with protoporphyria reported here were presumptively diagnosed by this method;

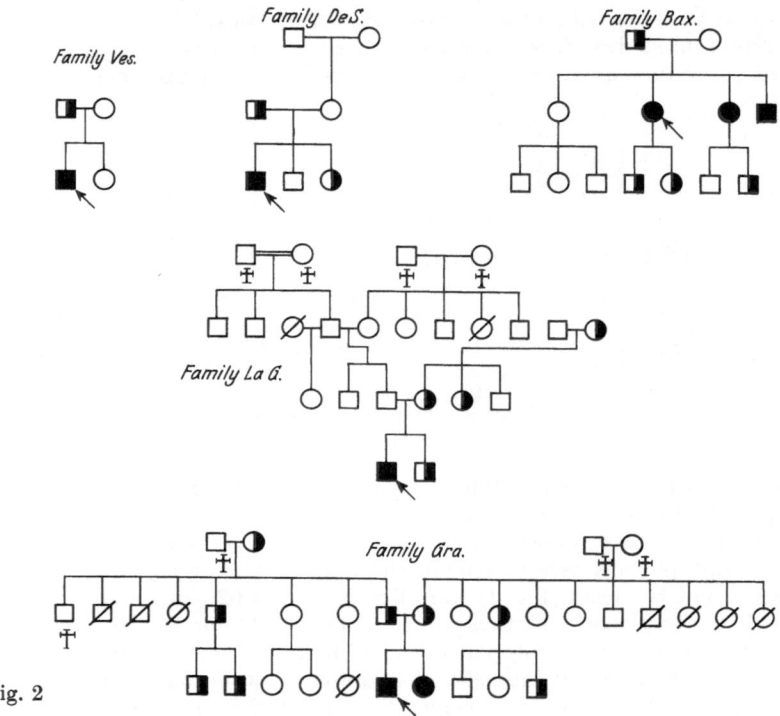

Fig. 2

nine others were excluded by the test. Chemical determination of red-cell protoporphyrins confirmed the presumptive diagnoses in all.

The gene frequency for EPP is unknown; however, from the studies of HAEGER-
ARONSON and her associates, it is at least 1 in 300,000. Linkage studies by LANGHOF
et al. have shown no association with ABO or Rh blood groups.

Since all circulating erythrocytes do not fluoresce, it is possible that protoporphyrin not incorporated into heme-protein is lost during red-cell aging. Alternatively, two populations of red-cell precursors may exist; in one, protoporphyrin
may be produced in excess.

A rapid, semi-quantitative fluorescent method was used to determine fluorocytes in patients with protoporphyria and their relatives. The fluorocyte abnormality is transmitted as a simple Mendelian dominant. In offspring who have markedly increased numbers of fluorescing cells and red-cell protoporphyrins, photosensitivity phenomena occur. The factors which affect the magnitude of this cell population and, ultimately, erythropoietic protoporphyria remain to be elucidated.

Erythropoietic Protoporphyria — a Family Study

E. M. DONALDSON, A. D. DONALDSON and C. RIMINGTON, Department of Dermatology, North Staffordshire Hospital Centre, Stoke-on-Trent (England)

"I am too much i' the sun" — Hamlet

Erythropoietic protoporphyria (E.P.P.) is an inborn error of porphyrin metabolism characterised by an excess of protoporphyrin in the red blood cells. The cardinal symptom is photosensitivity shown by an unpleasant burning sensation, usually beginning in childhood and associated with diverse physical signs on skin exposed to sunshine. Erythema and oedema are most common, but urticaria, purpura, and episodes of vesiculation and crusting are recorded. Chronic skin changes persisting and progressing between acute attacks are most often seen on the dorsa of hands, especially over the knuckles, but also on the nose, cheeks, and lips. Thickening of skin with inconspicuous papules, pitted or linear scars, and furrows resembling rhagades are the salient features. *Diagnosis* rests on the characteristic biochemical findings — excess protoporphyrin in erythrocytes; consistently normal urine; and raised faecal protoporphyrin and coproporphyrin in some but not in all patients. Conversely, the "biochemical markers" of raised blood and stool protoporphyrin may be present without clinical photosensitivity. *Family study:* The proband (case 15 in Family Tree) was seen in 1961 and a diagnosis of E.P.P. was confirmed.

The family comprising 90 members in five generations was studied, 58 being available for examination. Results are shown on Family Tree. The clinical and biochemical findings show that E.P.P. in this family may occur in several patterns:

Group 1: Photosensitive (7). Raised protoporphyrin in blood and stool 6. No biochemical abnormality at age 6 years 1.

Group 2: Non-photosensitive carriers

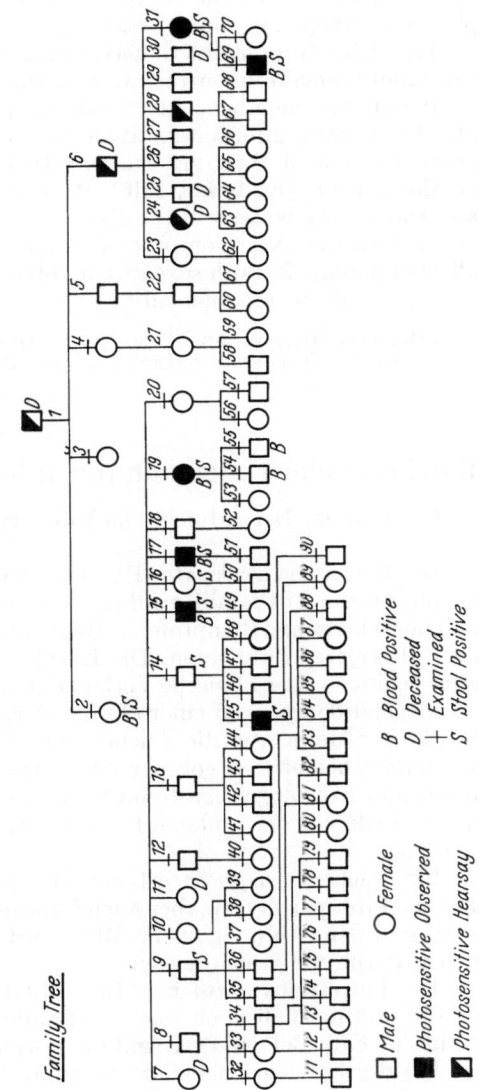

(6). Raised protoporphyrin levels in blood and stool 1. Raised protoporphyrin levels in blood only 2. Raised protoporphyrin levels in stool only 3.

Group 3: Photosensitive by hearsay (4). Clear historical evidence of classical photosensitivity.

Discussion: The affected members show a remarkably uniform clinical picture. A burning sensation and swelling following exposure to sun are the salient features; objective changes are as a rule minimal or absent in the intervals between attacks. The family shows gradations from overt and classical E.P.P. with photosensitivity and abnormal porphyrin levels in blood and faeces to symptomless biochemical "carriers". Between these extremes lie members showing minimal symptoms with gross to minimal changes in porphyrin metabolism. The oldest living member, aged 85 years, shows the complete biochemical stigmata of the disorder without photosensitivity, i.e. clinical latency.

Transition from latent to active disease has not been recorded; the children of this family remain under review with this possibility in mind.

In only two members may the degree of photosensitivity have declined in later life. The genetic information available to date, including the present study, supports the view of HAEGER-ARONSEN that transmission is by a simple autosomal dominant gene. Our family fulfils the criteria required for this type of inheritance and which may be seen in the Family Tree viz.

1. With the exception of case 1, all affected members are known to have an affected parent. 2. Both sexes are involved. 3. There is clear evidence that at least three generations are affected.

References. DONALDSON, E. M., A. D. DONALDSON, and C. RIMINGTON: Brit. med. J. 1967, I, 659. — HAEGER-ARONSEN, B.: Amer. J. Med. 35 450 (1963).

Biochemische Untersuchungen bei Porphyria variegata

G. ZIEGLER, Dermatologische Universitätsklinik Basel (Schweiz)

Die Porphyria variegata (PV) [1] ist eine selbständige Form der hepatischen Porphyrie. Sie tritt familiär auf und vereint Lichtempfindlichkeit mit abdominalen und neurologischen Symptomen. Haut- und interne Symptome können gleichzeitig oder alternierend auftreten. Die Krankheit kann schon im frühen Erwachsenenalter beginnen. Der klinische Verlauf entsprach bei fünf untersuchten Patientinnen vorwiegend demjenigen einer akuten Porphyrie (AIP) mit und ohne Lähmungen. Ein junger Mann wies die Zeichen einer Porphyria cutanea tarda (PCT) auf. Die PV unterscheidet sich von der AIP durch die viel bessere Prognose der abdominalen und neurologischen Symptome, aber auch biochemisch unterschieden sich unsere Fälle von den anderen Porphyrien. Darüber soll in diesem Beitrag berichtet werden.

Eine sichere Diagnose erlaubt die quantitative Porphyrinuntersuchung der Faeces. Protoporphyrin, aber auch Coproporphyrin werden immer stark vermehrt ausgeschieden. Abb. 1 gibt die Mittelwerte der Stuhlporphyrine bei den verschiedenen Porphyrieformen wieder.

Die Porphyrinvorstufen (ALA, PBG) im Urin sind im akuten Anfall stark erhöht und normalisieren sich vollständig in der Remission. Dies ist bei der AIP nicht der Fall. Bei der PCT sind die Porphyrinvorstufen im Urin kaum vermehrt.

Bei der konventionellen Extraktion der Urinporphyrine [2] fällt der relativ große Anteil an ätherlöslichen Porphyrinen auf, wie wir ihn bei der AIP und PCT nicht finden. Bei der hochspannungselektrophoretischen Auftrennung der Porphyrine [3] kommt dies noch besser zum Ausdruck. Abb. 2 zeigt, daß jeder einzelnen Form der hepatischen Porphyrie ein bestimmtes Porphyrinausscheidungsmuster zukommt, wobei bei der PV der hohe Anteil an Porphyrinen mit vier und acht Carboxylgruppen auffällt, während bei der AIP nur 8-COOH-Porphyrine und bei der PCT 7-COOH- und 8-COOH-Porphyrine im Vordergrund stehen.

In unserem Einzugsgebiet ist die PV fast so häufig wie die AIP. Eine genaue biochemische Abklärung lohnt sich deshalb in jedem Fall.

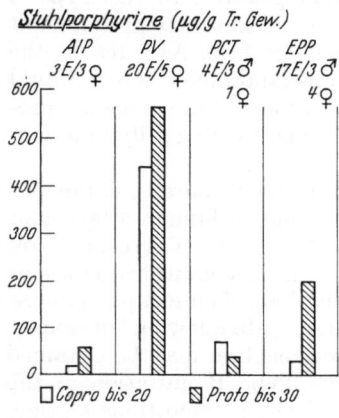 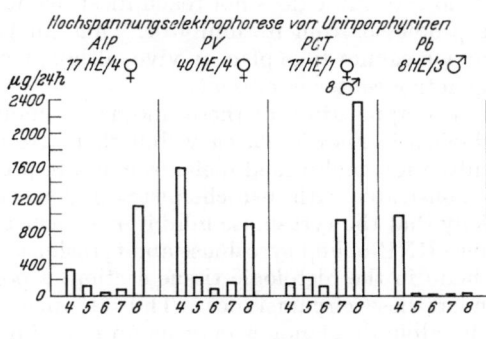

Abb. 1   Abb. 2

Abb. 1. Mittelwerte der quant. Stuhlextraktionen bei akuter Porphyrie (AIP), Porphyria variegata (PV), Porphyria cutanea tarda (PCT) und erythropoet. Protoporphyrie (EPP). Normalwerte für Copro- und Protoporphyrin unten

Abb. 2. Mittelwerte der quant. Hochspannungselektrophoresen bei akuter Porphyrie (AIP), Porphyria variegata (PV), Porphyria cutanea tarda (PCT) und Blei-Porphyrinurie. Normalwerte: 4-COOH-Porphyrine (Coproporphyrin) bis 120 μg/24 Std, 8-COOH-Porphyrine (Uroporphyrin) bis 30 μg/24 Std

Literatur. 1. GOLDBERG, A., and C. RIMINGTON: Diseases of Porphyrin Metabolism. Springfield (Ill.): Charles C. Thomas 1962. — 2. RIMINGTON, C.: Quantitative Determination of Porphobilinogen and Porphyrins in urine and faeces. Chemical Pathologists, broadsheet No. 36 (new series) 1961. — 3. CLOTTEN, R., u. A. CLOTTEN: Hochspannungselektrophorese. Stuttgart: Thieme 1962.

The Molecular Cause of Albinism

G. F. WILGRAM, Dermatologic Genetics Laboratory, New England Medical Center Hospitals, Boston, Massachusetts (USA)

In the Type A mutation of the S 91 mouse melanoma the enzyme tyrosinase seems to be completely deleted, because tyrosinase is not extractable and melanosomes cannot be detected with electron microscopy. A fully functioning inhibitor is present. In the Type B mutation of the S 91 mouse melanoma, an albino tyrosinase is extractable and a few melanosomes are detectable with electron microscopy. The ultrastructure of these few albino melanosomes is different from that of the abundant melanosomes in the wild pigmented strain. Tyrosinase activity can be demonstrated in vitro after the inhibitor is removed by cell fractionation. Both the RNP-bound and the freely soluble forms of this albino enzyme are susceptible in vitro to the normally present inhibitor. We also believe that through mutation a small change took place in the protein carrier of the albino enzyme, as detected by refined electrophoresis. The active center of the mutant enzyme does not seem to be altered since the Michaelis constant is almost identical to that of the wild enzyme. In the wild pigmented strain, tyrosinase apparently "aggregates" itself into melanosomes where the enzyme is protected from its inhibitor. Therefore, despite the presence of an inhibitor, tyrosinase activity can be shown in the whole tumor as well as in whole homogenates. In the Type B albino mutant the small change in the protein carrier of the enzyme does not allow the "aggregation" of albino tyrosinase into melanosomes. As a result, the albino tyrosinase does not reach its stable form in the melanosome where it would be protected from its inhibitor. Thus, melanosome formation and melanin production cannot take place in vivo, although albino tyrosinase with a fully functioning active center is present.

The application of these findings in mouse and hamster tumors to cutaneous albinism in man is not easy, but there are indications that in human albino hair bulbs a few malformed melanosomes are present and that traces of tyrosinase are demonstrable with histochemistry under favorable substrate conditions. It seems likely that the tyrosinase inhibitor is washed out during histochemical procedures. Since RNP-bound tyrosinase and tyrosinase "aggregated" into a few melanosomes, remain in the histologic tissue section, a positive dopa reaction may be obtained under these circumstances. Thus it appears that the Type B mutation in the S 91 albino melanoma may be an experimental model of the conditions as they prevail in albinism in man.

Zum Mechanismus der Aktivitätsminderung der Phosphoglucose-Isomerase in Erythrocyten von Kranken mit florider Psoriasis vulgaris

H. HOLZMANN und B. MORSCHES, Universitäts-Hautklinik Mainz (Deutschland)

Substrate des Kohlenhydratstoffwechsels in der Haut von Kranken mit Psoriasis vulgaris (Ps.v.) wurden schon 1933 durch MONACELLI und später durch MONACELLI u. RIBUFFO (1952) bestimmt. Dabei stellten die Autoren einen erhöhten Gehalt an reduzierenden Substanzen mit der Methode nach HAGEDORN-JENSEN fest. Im weiteren wurde erstmals von GRÜNEBERG und SZAKALL (1959) über ein vermehrtes Vorkommen von Pentosen innerhalb der wasserlöslichen Komponenten psoriatischer Schuppen berichtet, was im folgenden mehrfach bestätigt wurde. HASEGAWA [3] konnte außerdem einen erhöhten Glucose-6-Phosphatgehalt in psoriatischer Epidermis nachweisen.

Neuerdings wurden auch Aktivitätsmuster von Enzymen des Kohlenhydratstoffwechsels in der befallenen Epidermis von Kranken mit Ps.v. untersucht. So konnten RASSNER [9] sowie HALPRIN u. OHKAWARA [2] einen Aktivitätsanstieg dieser Enzyme feststellen. Nach RASSNER beträgt die Aktivitätssteigerung bei den glykolytischen Enzymen durchschnittlich 75%, bei den NADP-spezifischen Dehydrogenasen des Pentosephosphatcyclus jedoch 250%.

Diese Befunde weisen auf eine Steigerung des Substratdurchflusses im Pentosephosphatcyclus und einen mäßig erhöhten Substratdurchfluß in der Glykolyse hin. Somit liegt eine Verschiebung der Proportionen des Glucoseabbaues zugunsten des Pentosephosphatcyclus in der Psoriatikerhaut vor.

Die klinisch bekannte Manifestationsverstärkung und auch Erstmanifestation der Ps.v. durch Chloroquin und der bisher einzige reproduzierbare pathologische

Befund an Erythrocyten bei solchen Merkmalsträgern, nämlich der Nachweis eines gesteigert ablaufenden Pentosephosphatcyclus durch MALINA (1961) u. a. [1], war Ausgangspunkt unserer Untersuchungen. So hat einer von uns (H.) Aktivitätsmuster von Enzymen sowie Substrate und Kosubstrate des Kohlenhydratstoffwechsels und den Einfluß von Chloroquin auf den Kohlenhydratstoffwechsel in Erythrocyten von Kranken mit Ps.v. untersucht [4].

Es ergab sich als Hauptbefund ein nur während der floriden Phase nachweisbarer Enzymmangel der Phosphoglucose-Isomerase (PGI) mit Substratanstau von Glucose-6-Phosphat, der sich nach Glucoseinkubation unter Chlorquinbelastung bei Psoriatikern erheblich verstärkt, bei Kontrollpersonen jedoch deutlich vermindert. Als Folge liegt ein vermutlich kompensatorisch gesteigerter Kohlenhydratabbau über den Pentosephosphatcyclus bei funktionell erhaltener Glykolyse vor. Dabei ist unverkennbar, daß wesentliche Vorgänge des Kohlenhydratstoffwechsels in Erythrocyten und Epidermiszellen bei Psoriatikern gleichsinnig verlaufen. Es gelang somit, die nachgewiesene Sensitivität der Psoriatiker-Erythrocyten gegenüber Chloroquin*, die ihr klinisch-empirisches Korrelat bei entsprechenden Anlageträgern nach Chloroquinaufnahme hat, an der bezeichneten labilen Stoffwechselstelle zu lokalisieren. Diese Sensitivität wird von uns als pharmakogenetische Wirkung aufgefaßt.

Unsere weiteren Untersuchungen galten dem Mechanismus der Aktivitätsminderung der PGI in Erythrocyten von Kranken mit florider Ps.v. Sie ergaben, daß die Syntheserate des Enzymproteins nicht beeinflußt wird, da durch Inkubation der Psoriatikererythrocyten mit isotonen Lösungen die verminderte PGI-Aktivität auf Normwerte ansteigt. Weiterhin weist die Erythrocyten-PGI von Kontrollpersonen und Psoriatikern keine Unterschiede hinsichtlich Michaeliskonstante und pH-Optimum auf [5]. Auch agargelelektrophoretisch zeigte sich hinsichtlich der PGI aus Erythro-, Leuko- und Thrombocyten von Normalpersonen und floriden Psoriatikern sowie aus psoriatischem Schuppenhomogenat keinerlei Unterschied [6]. Daraus kann geschlossen werden, daß größere mit den hier angewandten Methoden erfaßbare strukturelle Unterschiede zwischen der PGI von Kontrollpersonen und Psoriatikern nicht vorliegen. Demgegenüber ergab sich in verschiedenen Hämolysatverdünnungen bei Kontrollpersonen eine der Verdünnung weitgehend entsprechende Abnahme der PGI-Aktivitäten, während bei floriden Psoriatikern dieser Aktivitätsabfall geringer ist, als es dem Verdünnungsgrad entspricht. Dies läßt auf einen „Hemmkörper" schließen, dessen Wirkung bei Verdünnung stärker zurückgeht als die PGI-Aktivität [5]. Einen weiteren Hinweis für einen „Hemmkörper" erbrachten Versuche, in denen festgestellt werden konnte, daß die PGI-Aktivitäten in Mischhämolysaten von Kontrollpersonen und Psoriatikern sich nicht additiv zusammensetzen. sondern unter den theoretischen Erwartungswerten liegen. Der im Psoriatiker-Hämolysat vorliegende „Hemmkörper" beeinflußt also die PGI-Aktivitäten im Hämolysat der Kontrollperson [7]. Während über die Natur dieses „Hemmkörpers" noch keine weiteren Aussagen gemacht werden können, machen jedoch Dialyseversuche eine niedermolekulare Verbindung, wie z. B. 6-Phosphogluconat, dessen Hemmwirkung auf die PGI bekannt ist, unwahrscheinlich [5].

Der Nachweis einer signifikanten Aktivitätsminderung der PGI gelang uns ebenfalls in Thrombocyten, nicht in Leukocyten von floriden Psoriatikern [8], was vermutlich präparationsbedingt sein dürfte.

Auf Grund dessen glauben wir, daß floride Psoriatiker eine generalisierte Störung des Kohlenhydratstoffwechsels aufweisen — Vergleiche zum Köbner-

---

* Übrigens wird Chloroquin bevorzugt in der Epidermis abgelagert [10].

phänomen drängen sich hierbei auf —, deren Umsetzung in ein morphisches Substrat nur an der Haut, möglicherweise auch an der Synovia erfolgt. Der Nachweis einer pharmakogenetischen Wirkung des Chloroquins auf den Kohlenhydratstoffwechsel des Psoriatiker-Erythrocyten stellt hierbei eine direkte Verbindung zur erblichen Verankerung dieser Krankheit dar. Wir nehmen daher an, daß das Primärereignis der psoriatischen Reaktion sich sowohl an den epidermalen wie cutanen Abschnitten zugleich bzw. koordiniert abspielt und von einer übergeordneten Stelle gesteuert wird.

Literatur. 1. BIELICKÝ, T., L. MALINA, and J. SONKA: Acta derm.-venereol. (Stockh.) 46, 72 (1966). — 2. HALPRIN, K. M., and A. OHKAWARA: J. invest. Derm. 46, 51 (1966). — 3. HASEGAWA, J.: The Root of Psoriasis. Read before the American Dermatological Association. Coca Raton, Florida, February 27, 1965. — 4. HOLZMANN, H.: Arch. klin. exp. Derm. 225, 231 (1966). — 5. HOLZMANN, H., u. B. MORSCHES: Arch. klin. exp. Derm. 228, 52 (1967). — 6. HOLZMANN, H., u. B. MORSCHES: Arch. klin. exp. Derm. 228, 171 (1967). — 7. HOLZMANN, H., u. B. MORSCHES: Hautarzt 18, 229 (1967). — 8. HOLZMANN, H., B. MORSCHES und W. OHLER: Klin. Wschr. 45, 319 (1967). — 9. RASSNER, G.: Arch. klin. exp. Derm. 226, 111 (1966). — 10. SHAFFER, B., M. M. CAHN, and E. J. LEVY: J. invest. Derm. 30, 341 (1958). Weitere Literatur s. [4].

Lichtdermatosen mit Hyperaminoacidurien

P. H. CLODI, I. Medizinische Universitätsklinik Wien (Österreich)

Die in den letzten Jahren mehrfach nachgewiesenen Hyperaminoacidurien bei verschiedenen Formen der Lichtdermatosen (Hartnup-Syndrom, Xeroderma pigmentosum und Hydroa vacciniforme) rechtfertigen es, diese Erkrankungen gemeinsam zu besprechen.

Bei den Fällen von Hartnup-Syndrom, von denen bis jetzt nur wenig über 20 Fälle bekannt sind, wird als konstantes Symptom eine Hyperaminoacidurie gefunden; weitere Symptome sind die Lichtdermatose, die bei vermehrter Sonnenbestrahlung auftritt, cerebellare Symptome und eine nicht ständig nachweisbare Indolaceturie. Es scheint sich dabei um eine Störung zu handeln, die sowohl die Tryptophanresorption im Dünndarm, die Rückresorption in den Nierentubuli und vielleicht auch den Intermediärstoffwechsel betrifft. In der Niere werden nur die Monoaminomonocarbonsäuren nicht rückresorbiert, im Dünndarm ist für Tryptophan und Tyrosin eine Resorptionsstörung nachgewiesen worden. Glutamylacrylglycin wurde bei einem Teil der Fälle gefunden. Nach Tryptophanbelastung findet man im Harn ein gegenüber dem Normalen stark verzögertes Ansteigen eines Tryptophanmetaboliten (3. Indol-Essigsäure), es kommt jedoch zu einer zeitlich verlängerten Ausscheidung, offenbar weil durch bakteriellen Abbau des nichtresorbierten, in den Dickdarm gelangenden Tryptophans große Mengen von Abbauprodukten aufgenommen werden. Antibiotica sollen diese Ausscheidung durch Hemmung des Bakterienwachstums und damit des Abbaues hemmen. Der von uns publizierte Fall zeigte alle biochemischen Symptome, war aber hinsichtlich der dermatologischen Symptomatik verschieden, insoferne als diese dem Poikiloderma congenitum Rothmund-Thomson glich. Eine Störung des Porphyrinstoffwechsels war nicht nachzuweisen.

Bei weiteren Untersuchungen aller zur Beobachtung gelangenden Lichtdermatosen wurde bei zwei Fällen von Hydroa vacciniformis deutliche Vermehrung der Harnaminosäureausscheidung gefunden, wobei eine auffällige Histidinvermehrung registriert wurde. Der Mechanismus dieser Hyperaminoacidurie konnte nicht weiter aufgeklärt werden.

Bei einem Fall von Xeroderma pigmentosum fanden wir, so wie auch schon bei einigen Fällen der Literatur berichtet, eine auffällige Vermehrung der Harnaminosäureausscheidung, die jedoch nicht konstant war, zusätzlich zu dieser Hyperaminoacidurie waren jedoch auch neurologische Symptome vorhanden, die sehr ähnlich jenen des de-Synctis-Cacchione-Syndromes waren; bei diesen Fällen wurde aber keine Hyperaminoacidurie festgestellt. Andererseits wurde bei jenen Fällen von Xeroderma pigmentosum, bei denen die Hyperaminoacidurie gefunden wurde, eine neurologische Symptomatik nicht beschrieben bzw. von HARRIS und KEET auf briefliche Anfrage ausdrücklich verneint. Es erscheint möglich, daß der von uns publizierte Fall hinsichtlich seiner Symptomatik mit Symptomen, die bisher nur getrennt bei dieser Erkrankung beschrieben wurden, eine Sonderstellung einnimmt, bzw. daß verschiedene ätiologische Ursachen Xeroderma pigmentosum hervorrufen können, wobei die Begleitsymptome verschieden sein können. Die Hyperaminoacidurie ist jedoch bei Xeroderma pigmentosum viel weniger typisch als beim Hartnup-Syndrom.

Da in letzter Zeit mehrfach Zusammenhänge zwischen intestinalen Erkrankungen und Hauterkrankungen beschrieben wurden, sollte auf Lichtdermatosen hingewiesen werden, die wenigstens zum Teil neben anderer interner Symptomatik eine intestinale Resorptionsstörung zeigen.

Literatur. CLODI, P. H., E. DEUTSCH und G. NIEBAUER: Arch. klin. exp. Derm. **218**, 165 (1964). — Wien. klin. Wschr. **76**, 623 (1964). — CLODI, P. H., F. WEWALKA und E. ZWEYMÜLLER: Z. Kinderheilk. **93**, 223 (1965). — HARRIS, L. C., and P. M. KEET: J. Pediat. **57**, 759 (1960). — MILNE, M. D.: Brit. med. J. **1964**, I, 327. — SHUSTER, S., and J. MARKS: Lancet **1965**, I, 1367). — WELSS, G. G.: Brit. med. J. **1962**, II, 937.

Zur Klinik und Chromosomenanalyse der V. Phakomatose

G. VELTMAN und S. ADARI, Universitäts-Hautklinik Bonn (Deutschland)

Die V. Phakomatose ist eine frühembryonale Entwicklungsstörung, die durch multiple, als Basalzellnaevi, Naevobasaliome oder Naevus epitheliomatosus multiplex bezeichnete Hautveränderungen charakterisiert ist und mit Entwicklungsstörungen anderer Organsysteme, vor allem mit naevoiden Erscheinungen am Zentralnervensystem und am Auge und mit Geschwulstbildungen auf naevoider Grundlage sowie weiteren assoziierten Entwicklungsstörungen wie z. B. Mandibularcysten, Knochenanomalien einhergeht.

Histologisch zeigt der Basalzellnaevus Zellwucherungen von basalzellähnlichen Elementen ohne Intercellularbrücken. Es gibt keine feingeweblichen Merkmale, die eine sichere Abgrenzung vom Basaliom erlauben.

Bericht über vier Patienten mit einer V. Phakomatose

Fall 1. G. B., 18 Jahre: Hasenscharte, Wolfsrachen, Gaumenspalte, je eine akzessorische Mamille. Mit 18 Monaten laufen, mit 6 Jahren undeutlich sprechen. Hilfsschule ohne Erfolg. Seit dem 3. Lebensjahr zunehmende Knotenbildungen im Bereich des gesamten Integuments: Basalzellartige, netz- und strangförmige Wucherungen mit zahlreichen, zum Teil ulcerierten Horncysten. Kraniofaciale Dysplasie, Strabismus divergens und chronische Blepharo-Conjunctivitis auf Grund einer Hyperopie. Imbezillität. Dysdiadochokinese. Knochensystem: Geringe Pneumatisation der Stirnhöhlen, stark ausgebildete Impressionen, wuchtiges dorsum sellae. 13 Rippenpaare mit Fehlbildungen einzelner Rippen (Brückenbildungen, Defektbildungen). Linkskonvexe Skoliose der oberen Brustwirbelsäule mit Subluxation einzelner Wirbel nach rechts, Verschmälerung der Zwischenwirbelräume. 4. Brustwirbelkörper keilförmig abgeflacht. Nach rechts gekrümmtes Os sacrum. 7 HWK, 13 BWK, 5 LWK, 5 KWK, 4 Steißbeinwirbel, Spaltbildung im Wirbelbogen 6. HWK.

Völlige Verschattung der rechten Kieferhöhle, rechter Augenbogen deutlich nach cranial eingedrückt, retinierter sowie hochgelagerter Eckzahn. Follikuläre Cyste im Bereich des rechten Oberkiefers.

Fall 2. K. P., 9 Jahre: Mit 2 Jahren laufen, mit 3 Jahren sprechen. 2 Jahre Hilfsschule, da nur unartikulierte Sprache, Sprachheilschule. Gesicht, Ohren, Rücken, Brust, typische Tumoren im Sinne von histologisch gesicherten Basalzellnaevi. Schlierige Glaskörperdestruktion links. Oberkiefercyste links.

Fall 3. C. L., 72 Jahre: Von drei Kindern leidet ein Sohn (Fall 4) an den gleichen Hautveränderungen. Gesicht, Hals, Stamm, erbsen- bis linsengroße Tumoren, zum Teil zentral ulceriert. Undifferenzierte, oberflächliche, teils solide, teils cystische Basaliome.

Fall 4. P. L., 49 Jahre: Im Bereich des gesamten Integumentes zahlreiche linsen- bis pfennigstückgroße Knoten: Teil cystische, teils adenoide, oberflächlich undifferenzierte, sog. pagetoide Basaliome.

Fall 3 und 4 müssen wohl als *abortive Formen der V. Phakomatose* aufgefaßt werden, bei denen das eine oder andere Symptom fehlt oder weniger ausgeprägt sein kann, während die Fälle 1 und 2 alle Anzeichen einer V. Phakomatose aufweisen.

Die *Chromosomenanalyse* (Lymphocyten, Haut, Wandung einer Kiefercyste und ein Hauttumor) ließ bei keinem der vier Fälle mit V. Phakomatose eine Chromosomenanomalie erkennen (Path. Inst. der Universität Bonn: Prof. Dr. GROPP).

Incidence of Anti-Nuclear Antibodies Among First-Degree Relatives of Patients with Chronic Discoid Lupus, Systemic Lupus and Normal Subjects

C. MARCH, N. ROTHFIELD and N. PACE, New York University Medical School, New York (USA)

The relationship of chronic discoid lupus erythematosus (CDLE) to systemic lupus erythematosus (SLE) is controversial. Some authorities think that these two entities are part of the same disease. Others (including ourselves) feel that there are enough dissimilarities in the type of abnormalities found among patients with these two entities as to warrant their being differentiated. A small number (no more than 3%) of patients with CDLE also have SLE, and approximately 15% of patients with SLE display lesions of CDLE; families in which several members have these two diseases or some related abnormality have been described. This tends to show that both SLE and CDLE probably occur on a genetic basis.

In an attempt to further delineate the genetic background of patients with CDLE and SLE, a study of the incidence of anti-nuclear antibodies and other serum globulin abnormalities was performed on first-degree relatives of patients with CDLE, with SLE and of normal subjects.

Materials and Methods. Patients and Relatives

The patients whose families were studied were attending the clinics of Bellevue Hospital and the Skin and Cancer Unit of New York University Medical Center. Considerable effort was devoted to include all of the living first-degree relatives of the patients in the study.

The group of relatives of CDLE patients (24 propositi) comprised 86 individuals. The group of relatives of SLE patients (35 propositi) included 62 individuals. In addition, in order to provide controls, the relatives of 15 normal subjects matched for sex, race and age with the CDLE propositi, were also investigated, thus providing a group of 35 control subjects.

Laboratory Methods

Laboratory determinations included the following:

Serum paper-electrophoresis for determination of gamma-globulins. Figure ober 20% gamma-globulins were considered abnormal.

Latex-fixation test for rheumatoid factor.

Serologic tests for syphilis (Mazzini, VDRL, Kline, Rein-Bossack) as well as Reiter protein complement-fixation test (RPCF) whenever any of the other tests were positive.

Indirect fluorescent anti-nuclear antibody (ANF) test using mouse-liver sections as source of nuclei. The pattern of fluorescence was noted in positive specimens.

Results (Table)

Examination of table reveals the following:

1. There was greater incidence of hyper-gamma-globulinemia among relatives of CDLE patients (17.5%) than among relatives of SLE patients (9.7%) and "normals" (5.7%). Examination of detailed data showed that of 15 hyper-gamma-globulinemic CDLE relatives, about one-half (7) occurred in three families while the rest were scattered occurences, as were the hyper-gamma-globulinemics found among SLE relatives and normals.

2. The "biologic false-positive tests" (BFP) for syphilis were equally frequent among the three groups. It must be noted, however, that in all three groups, there was "family clustering" of BFP reactors. The significance of this finding is unknown and warrants further study.

Table. *Serologic findings in first degree relatives of CDLE, SLE and normal subjects*

	Increased gamma-globulins		Latex fix over 1:80		"False-positive" Serology		Antinuclear factor over 1 +	
86 Relatives of CDLE (24 propositi)								
Females 44	11	25.0%	2	4.5%	4	9.0%	2	4.5%
Males 42	4	9.5%	1	2.4%	3	7.1%	0	0.0%
Total 86	15	17.5%	3	3.5%	7	8.1%	2	2.3%
62 Relatives of SLE (35 propositi)								
Females 33	6	18.0%	1	3.0%	2	6.0%	5	15.1%
Males 29	0	0.0%	0	0.0%	2	6.9%	2	6.9%
Total 62	6	9.7%	1	1.6%	4	6.4%	7	11.3%
35 Relatives of Normals (15 propositi)								
Females 19	2	10.5%	0	0.0%	0	0.0%	1	5.3%
Males 16	0	0.0%	0	0.0%	2	12.4%	0	0.0%
Total 35	2	5.7%	0	0.0%	2	5.7%	1	2.9%

3. The presence of ANF was markedly higher among SLE relatives (11.5%) than among CDLE relatives or normals (2.3% and 2.9% respectively). There was no clustering among family members. There were equal numbers of speckled and diffuse patterns of fluorescence among all groups.

4. Females among all three groups of relatives are regularly more often affected by hyper-gamma-globulinemia and presence of ANF. This ist not the case for BFP.

5. Examination of the detailed data failed to reveal any difference in age-related distribution in any of the categories.

Discussion

A number of studies have indicated varying incidence of abnormalities in the sera of relatives of patients with systemic lupus erythematosus. These abnormalities include the presence of the rheumatoid factor, of biologic false-positive serology, hyper-gamma-globulinemia, and the presence of antinuclear antibodies. The incidence of antinuclear factors reported by different investigators varies considerably. This is no doubt due in greater part to the differences in techniques used to elicit the presence of these globulins.

Until the present study, no systematic survey of relatives of patients with CDLE has been reported. Familial CDLE with asymptomatic familial hyper-gamma-globulinemia [1] and CDLE with presence of LE cell phenomena in an asymptomatic relative [2] have been described.

In order to compare several groups of subjects adequately, it is necessary that the tests be performed in the same laboratory, using the same methods with each group. Our results indicate that there is a real difference in the incidence of antinuclear factors among the relatives of patients with CDLE and the relatives of patients with SLE. The incidence of the antinuclear factors is four times higher in relatives of SLE patients than in relatives of CDLE patients. The incidence of these factors in relatives of CDLE patients is not different from that prevailing among "normal" controls. This may indicate a different genetic background between CDLE and SLE, as has been suggested previously [3, 4]. Our study again shows that the incidence of antinuclear factor is much higher in females than in males. This is also true for the incidence of hyper-gamma-globulinemia. The suggestion that some sex-linked abnormalities in the immune mechanisms were responsible for the high female/male ratio in SLE was made previously by us [4].

The clustering of hyper-gamma-globulinemia as well as of BFP test among certain families (unrelated to each other or to the presence of ANF) also indicates that genetic factors may account for these abnormalities.

We wish to express our thanks to Dr. R. MENDEZ BRYAN of the University of Puerto Rico School of Medicine for collecting the sera of a number of the relatives studied.

References. 1. GALLO, R. C., and D. L. FORDE: Arch. intern. Med. **117**, 629 (1966). — 2. BENCZE, G., L. LAKATOS, and K. SIPOS: Acta rheum. scand. **10**, 221 (1964). — 3. BECK, J. S., and N. R. ROWELL: Quart. J. Med. **35**, 119 (1966). — 4. ROTHFIELD, N., C. H. MARCH, P. MIESCHER, and C. McEWEN: New Engl. J. Med. **269**, 1155 (1963).

Electrocardiographic Abnormalities in a Family with Generalized Lentigo

R. J. WALTHER, B. POLANSKY and I. A. GROTS, Boston University School of Medicine, Boston, Massachusetts (USA)

This communication presents a family of four, three members of which have a widespread cutaneous pigmentary disorder and unexplained abnormalities of the electrocardiogram. None of the subjects have had cardiovascular symptoms at any time.

The family came to our attention when the propositus, a boy of 11 years, was referred to the Pediatric Heart Clinic of the Boston City Hospital for evaluation of a cardiac murmur detected by the school physician. Positive physical findings were limited to the skin and the cardiovascular system. The entire cutaneous surface showed myriads of dark brown, smooth macules of varying size, most numerous on the trunk, and of somewhat sparser distribution on the distal portions of the extremities. Some of these lesions had been present at birth but most had appeared during infancy. The hairy scalp, face, palms, soles, genitalia, and external ear canals were involved, but the accessible mucous membranes were spared.

Examination of the heart revealed a grade II harsh, short systolic murmur, heard best at the left lower sternal border. An electrocardiogram and vectorcardiogram, the latter according to the cube system, demonstrated a superiorly oriented QRS frontal axis and changes usually seen in inferior myocardial necrosis. There was also incomplete right bundle branch block and diffusely abnormal T-wave changes. The QRS loop of the vectorcardiogram initiated anteriorly, to the right, and the main body of the loop was displaced superiorly and to the right. Catheterization of the right side of the heart was normal. Dye injection into the ascending aorta revealed the origin of two main coronary arteries but contrast was inadequate for further detail.

The sister of the propositus, aged 13 years, was examined because of similar cutaneous lesions. Although there were noticeably fewer pigmented macules, their distribution was essentially the same as that seen in the propositus. Physical examination of the cardiovascular system revealed no abnormalities, but the electrocardiogram demonstrated left axis deviation of minus 50 degrees. The QRS loop of the vector cardiogram showed initiation anteriorly and slightly to the left, whereas the main portion of the loop was deviated posteriorly and superiorly.

The mother, a 37-year-old housewife, was also examined. Identical cutaneous findings of widespread, deeply pigmented macules which spared the accessible mucous membranes were noted. An additional feature were several areas of vitiligo of recent onset. Other positive findings were confined to the cardiovascular system. There was a grade III rough systolic murmur and click at the second and third intercostal spaces at the left sternal border. The second sound at the pulmonic area was decreased in intensity. The electrocardiogram suggested a degree of right bundle branch block with associated necrosis of the interventricular septum and inferior surface. The vectorcardiogram showed a loss of the initial septal forces in the horizontal plane suggesting incomplete right bundle branch block with septal necrosis. The main body of the QRS loop was displaced superiorly and to the right. Catheterization of the right side of the heart revealed mild pulmonary stenosis.

The family history was non-contributory. All living maternal relatives including the grandparents of the propositus were examined but failed to reveal cardiac or cutaneous findings similar to those described above. There was no known pigmentary anomaly on the paternal side of the family.

Several cutaneous biopsies were obtained from the pigmented lesions of the propositus and the mother, revealing the identical histologic picture of lentigo.

We believe that, at least from the dermatologic point of view, our patients fall into the category of generalized lentigo described by ZEISLER and BECKER (Ref.). Although the clinical and histologic findings of the skin lesions were similar in our patients and those reviewed by the above authors, the latter did not record any abnormal cardiac manifestations.

A familial conduction defect seems the most likely explanation for the cardiac abnormalities observed in our patients. Idiopathic hypertrophic subaortic stenosis might be considered in the differential diagnosis and cannot be positively excluded, but the arterial and aortic pulse contours and the physical and X-ray findings described in the majority of patients with muscular subaortic stenosis were lacking in our cases. The evidence presented relative to our patients would favor a primary conduction abnormality rather than a myocardiopathy.

In summary, three patients in two generations of a family having a syndrome

37*

consisting of generalized lentigo and unexplained electrocardiographic abnormalities are described. The appearance of this disorder in a mother and her two children suggests a genetic transmission by an autosomal dominant mode. A search through the literature for similar cases has yielded no results.

Supported in part by: Training Grant (5 TO1 AMO 5295-07) National Institute of Arthritis and Metabolic Diseases, United States Public Health Services.

Reference. Zeisler, C. P., and S. W. Becker: Arch. Derm. Syph. (Chic.) **33**, 109 (1936)

Pachyonychia Congenita

C. B. Viziam, R. Mathai, A. Mammen and Z. Isaac, Dept. of Dermatology and Venerology, Christian Medical College Hospital, Vellore (India)

Jadosshon and Lewandowsky first described Pachyonychia Congenita in 1907. Subsequently several authors have reported on this disease. From the review of literature it is gathered that Pachyonychia Congenita is a congenital dyskeratotic condition affecting the skin and mucous membranes. In addition some authors have reported associated congenital diseases like Ichthyosis, Ectodermal defects and Epidermolysis Bullosum Simplex. We have three cases of Pachyonychia Congenita:

Case No. 1. Male — 18 years. Showed at birth dystrophic nails, leucokeratosis of mouth, follicular keratosis and hyperkeratosis of palms and soles. No family history of similar disease.

Case No. 2. Male — 5 years. Born to consanguine parents. Showed at birth clinical manifestations similar to Case No. 1. In addition showed kinky hair and vesiculobullous eruptions. No family history of similar disease.

Case No. 3. Male — 6 years. Born to consanguine parents. showed at birth clinical manifestations similar to Case No. 2. One brother had similar disease from birth but died at the age of 5.

The purpose of this paper is to point out the basic pathological feature which is responsible for the various clinical manifestations of Pachyonychia Congenita.

The basic defect seems to be *abnormal keratinization*. This is manifested in three different structures:

1. *Normal keratinizing structures:* resulting in hyperkeratosis of skin particularly around joints, palms and soles, follicular hyperkeratosis and kinking of hair. Kinky hair is never seen in Indian Population and probably represents a genetic anomaly in this situation. Hyperkeratosis is the cause of eccrine poral plugging and sweat retension blisters. This is most prominent on hands and feet. In the past these blisters were reported as Epidermolysis bullosum simplex.

2. *Partially keratinizing nail bed:* resulting in complete keratinization and subungual keratosis. Nail bed epithelium shows prominent granular layers. Interestingly there are sweat ducts seen in the nail bed. The granular layers and sweat ducts are seen in the nail bed epithelium before and after avulsion of the dystrophic nails. The ectopic eccrine sweat gland and the vicarious keratinization of nail bed are probably developmental anomalies.

3. *Non-keratinizing oral mucosa:* showing leucokeratosis with the presence of granular layer. This is also probably a developmental anomaly having vicarious keratinization.

In summary, attempt is made to show that abnormal keratinization is the basic defect responsible for various clinical manifestations of Pachyonychia Congenita. The abnormality lies in hyperkeratinization and anomalous keratinization. Kinking of hair is generally a genetic anomaly. The ectopic eccrine sweat gland in the nail bed is a developmental anomaly. The vesiculo-bullous eruptions are sweat retention blisters and not epidermolysis bullosum.

Estudios citogeneticos en dermatologia

J. ESTELLER, J. PIÑOL AGUADÉ, A. ALIAGA y E. GIMFERRER, Universidades de Valencia y Barcelona (España)

Con objeto de ampliar los conocimientos sobre la real importancia de los estudios citogenéticos en Dermatología hemos realizado la investigación de los cariotipos de sangre periférica de una serie de 160 pacientes con procesos dermatológicos de diversa indole. En esta comunicación se exponen los resultados obtenidos y se efectúa en algun caso la comparación con datos proporcionados por otros autores y que han ido apareciendo en la literatura. Las afecciones cutáneas estudiadas por nosotros pueden clasificarse de la siguiente forma:

1. Facomatosis

a) *Enfermedad de v. Recklinghausen.* Fueron examinados los cariotipos de un total de 5 enfermos. En 4 de los casos se halló un número de cromosomas completamente normal. El quinto paciente, una mujer que padecía además de la sintomatología tipica de la neurofibromatosis una luxacion recidivante de codo, oligofrenia y comunicación interauricular de tipo ostium-secundum presentaba un cariograma anormal. De esta enferma fueron examinadas 100 células yugales por el método de PAPANICOLAU y de ellas 27 eran cromatin-positivas y 9 presentaban dos corpúsculos de BARR. En el cariotipo existía un cromosoma extra que tenía las características de los del grupo 6-X-12. Fue clasificado como gonosoma X, debido a la existencia de dos corpúsculos de BARR en el frotis bucal.

b) *Enfermedad de Pringle-Bourneville.* Se examinaron los cariotipos de 4 casos sin que ninguno de ellos ofreciese cariograma anormal.

c) *Síndrome de Stürge-Weber.* Se estudió un conjunto de 16 casos y en ninguno de ellos pudo comprobarse imágenes que recordasen la trisomia descrita por HAYWARD a BOWERS (1962) en un enfermo, o la trisomia parcial estudiada por PATAU y colab. (1962) en otro paciente. En todos nuestros casos el número y disposición de los cromosomas era normal.

2. Conectivopatias congenitas

Se practicó el cariotipo de 3 enfermos de síndrome de Ehlers Danlos y de los padres de uno de los pacientes no pudiendo comprobarse anomalías en ninguno de los examinados. En otro enfermo con sintomatología cutáneo-articular propia del síndrome de Ehlers Danlos pero con rasgos esquelèticos correspondientes a un síndrome de Marfan el cariograma era normal y no pudimos evidenciar las anomalías cromosómicas (satélites gigantes) descritas por TJIO, PUCK y ROBINSON (1959). Igualmente normal era el cariotipo de una enferma con *cutis laxa* congénita, así como el de una pacciente con artrochalasis circunscrita con lesiones cutáneas limitadas a la zona con laxitud articular.

3. Enfermedades del metabolismo

Dos casos de porfiria crónica del adulto y uno de porfiria variegata con sintomatología cutánea muy aparatosa y mutilaciones de las partes acras en la que (las alteraciones cutáneas aparecieron a los pocos meses después del nacimiento) con intensa eliminacion de porfobilinògeno, todos ofrecían cariotipos sin alteraciones.

4. Anomalias de la queratinizacion

Se han estudiado 7 casos de ictiosis vulgar, 2 de eritrodermia ictiosiforme congénita, uno de síndrome de Sjogren-Larson y 2 hermanos con síndrome de Refsum.

En todos ellos el recuento de cromosomas no presentaba anormalidades y tampoco existían alteraciones morfológicas de los mismos. Un nevus sistematizado generalizado, del tipo de ictiosis hystrix tambien presentaba cariograma normal.

Se examinaron igualmente 4 queratodermias palmo-plantares, 2 de ellas de tipo Unna-Thost, otra de tipo Brauer y otra con seudo-ainhum (keratodermia mutilans Vohwinkel), esta última de un enfermo que tenía antecedentes familiares de neoplasias viscerales y falleció de neoplasia pulmonar. En todos ellos el examen de cromosomas proporcionó cifras normales.

Tres casos de enfermedad de Darier, uno de ellos con marcada oligofrenia no presentaban tampoco alteraciones del cariotipo.

5. Hiperplasias, aplasias, atrofias y distrofias cutaneas

En la casuística se comprende un síndrome de François-Hallermann-Streiff, 3 casos de síndrome de Rothmund-Thomson y 6 pacientes de xeroderma pigmentosum. Todos estos casos ofrecieron igualmente cariotipos normales, excepto un enfermo de xeroderma pigmentosum que presentó un número anormal de cromosomas: 46/47 XX. El cromosoma en exceso pertenecía al grupo de los pequeños acrocéntricos del grupo G de la clasificación de Patau (grupos 21-22 de la de Denver). Era por tanto esta enferma un mosaico normal/trisomìa G.

6. Enfermedades ampollosas congenitas

Fueron estudiados un total de 6 epidermolisis, 2 de ellos con epidermolisis ampollosa distrófica y los restantes de epidermolisis ampollosa simple. No pudieron detectarse anomalías cromosómicas.

7. Alteraciones pigmentarias

En nuestra casuística consta un caso de vitiligo y otro de síndrome de Peutz-Jeghers. En este último fueron examinadas igualmente la madre y una tía materna. En todos los casos no se pudieron comprobar anomalìas.

8. Anomalias congenitas de anejos

Una hiperqueratosis congenita ungueal y 2 casos de monilethrix de nuestra serie tenían cariotipos normales.

9. Afecciones vasculares

Un caso de enfermedad de Rendu-Osler no ofrecìa anomalías en el número de cromosomas. Un angioma de la nuca aparecido en un oligofrènico con discretos rasgos mongoloides fue motivo de su consulta en nuestro Servicio. Este enfermo presentaba un mosaico 46/47 XY con cromosoma extra del grupo 21-22.

10. Nevus y tumores

En nuestra serie figuran 2 casos de nevus en slip con nevus pigmentarios profusos, un caso de hidradenomas eruptivos, uno de melanoma maligno, un paciente de nevus basocelular y un enfermo de nevus organoide de gran extension que abarcaba la mitad del cuero cabelludo y parte de la cara. En todos estos casos no pudieron comprobarse anomalías del recuento de los cromosomas.

11. Psoriasis

La estadística abarca un total de 40 casos de psoriasis, algunos de ellos familiares en los que el cariotipo era completamente normal.

12. Eczema

En esta serie se comprenden 6 casos de eczema atópico con claros antecedentes familiares en los que el cariograma era normal. Figura tan solo un caso de eczema seborreico en una niña de 11 años, con oligofrenia discreta y sin malformaciones evidentes. En esta paciente pudo constatarse un cariotipo anómalo correspondiente a una trisomìa del cromosoma X (superfemale XXX). No consideramos significativo este dato en relacion a su proceso cutáneo.

13. Otras afecciones estudiadas

Nuestra serie comprende además un caso de atresia auris, uno de fistula de conducto tireogloso, uno de mastocitosis nodular, 2 casos de reticulosis malignas, 2 de pitiriasis rubra pilaris, un caso de dermatomiositis, 2 de lupus eritematoso familiar y 4 de alopecia areata familiar. En todos ellos el cariograma resultó completamente normal. Una paciente que consultò por un impétigo y a la que en la exploracion pudimos constatar la existencia de pterygium de cuello, corta estatura y falta de desarrollo genital presentaba un número de cromosomas normal. Esta enferma no pudo sin embargo ser estudiada con detencion.

Über den Erbgang einiger Formen von palmo-plantarer Keratose in Zusammenhang mit ihrem erbbiologischen und nosologischen Konzept

E. I. Bologa, Krankenhaus für Haut- und Geschlechtskrankheiten, Brasov (Rumänien)

Die Variabilität der klinischen Formen, das Fehlen einer ätiologischen Einteilung und die Verschiedenartigkeit ihrer erblichen Übertragung führen bei den der Gruppe der Genodermatosen angehörenden palmo-plantaren Keratosen zu besonderen Schwierigkeiten.

Auf Grund einiger Beobachtungen, die durch genaue Familienuntersuchungen, die alle lebenden Individuen der Sippe erfaßten, erhalten wurden, möchten wir zu einer besseren Kenntnis dieses Kapitels der Genodermatologie beitragen und stellen fest, daß eine Orientierung und Klassifizierung mittels heredopathologischer Kriterien noch nicht möglich ist, sondern nur auf dem Wege von statistischen, die auf genauen genealogischen Studien, also auf Untersuchungen der Familienpathologie basieren, realisiert werden kann.

Beginnend mit den systematischen, auf H. Siemens und A. Touraine zurückgehenden Studien über die Vererbung der Hautkrankheiten, wurde eine Anzahl von Daten erzielt, die trotz ihres stellenweise diskutablen Charakters doch Ausgangspunkte für die genaue Kenntnis des Problems darstellen.

So wurde bezüglich des Vererbungsmodus festgestellt, daß die leichten Formen (ichtyosis vulgaris) im allgemeinen dominant, die schweren Formen (ichtyosis kongenitale letale) dagegen recessiv vererbt werden.

Die Verhältnisse komplizieren sich im Falle der palmo-plantaren Keratosen, die ursprünglich eine einheitliche nosologische Gruppe bildeten, wobei die verschiedenen klinischen Abarten als Formen der gleichen Grundkrankheit angesehen wurden.

Nach den klinisch-genetischen Untersuchungen von Franceschetti und Schnyder umfaßt diese Gruppe wenigstens fünf voneinander unabhängige klinische Formen, die autosomal-dominant vererbt werden:

1. Keratosis diffusa circumscripta Thost-Unna,
2. Keratosis palmo-plantaris striata-linearia,

3. Keratosis palmo-plantaris papulosa s.maculosa,
4. Keratosis extremitatum progrediens Greither,
5. Keratosis palmo-plantaris multilans.

Dazu fügen die Autoren noch drei verschiedene autosomal-recessive Formen hinzu:

1. Keratosis palmo-plantaris transgrediens (Meleda),
2. Keratosis palmo-plantaris diffusa Papillon-Lefévre,
3. Keratosis palmo-plantaris circumscripta (syndrom Hanhart).

Ebenso wie auch im Falle der bullösen Erkrankungen stellen die Verhornungsstörungen der Haut innerhalb ihrer recessiven Formen nur ein Symptom einer systematisierten Entwicklungsstörung dar.

Die Feststellung, nach der verschiedene genetische Defekte klinisch sehr ähnliche Veränderungen hervorrufen können, führte zu neuen Gruppenbildungen von analogen oder ähnlichen Krankheiten. Für die einen ist die Klassifikation, die auf dem Modus der Vererbung basiert, derjenigen, die sich nach dem klinischen Aspekt richtet, vorzuziehen.

Bezüglich der familiären Häufung werden immer mehr Beobachtungen von Einzelfällen mitgeteilt, die für die recessive Vererbung charakteristischer sein sollen. Ein solcher Tatbestand müßte zur Vorsicht bezüglich der Einreihung oder Nichteinreihung einer Krankheit in die familiären Erkrankungen führen.

Es darf nicht vergessen werden, daß bis heute spezifische Hautkrankheiten auf Grund von Chromosomenanomalien nicht bekannt geworden sind, so wie dies bei den Mißbildungen der Fall ist, die bekanntlich in ihrer Vererbung nicht den Mendelschen Regeln folgen.

Der moderne Hautarzt muß die erbliche Variabilität in Betracht ziehen und beobachten (und zwar sowohl als klinischen Aspekt, als auch als Vererbungsmodus), eingedenk der Möglichkeit der Existenz von auslösenden hereditären Defekten, die durch verschiedene auslösende Faktoren (z. B. latente hereditäre enzymatische Defekte, manifest geworden nach Verabreichung von besonderen Medikamenten) in Bewegung gesetzt werden können.

Das Mitwirken von exo- oder endogenen Faktoren bei der Entstehung einer palmo-plantaren Keratose erklärt und gibt dem Versuch· von GRACIANSKY, eine ätiologische Klassifikation zu schaffen, seine Berechtigung.

Innerhalb dieses Problems der hereditär beeinflußten, die Krankheit erzeugenden Faktoren, unterscheidet VOGEL neben den Erbkrankheiten durch Mutation eines einzigen Gens (papulöse palmo-plantare Keratose) auch diejenigen durch Chromosomenabwegigkeiten (Mongolismus) sowie eine dritte Kategorie durch Zusammenwirken einiger dispositioneller, hereditärer und Umweltsfaktoren (wie z. B. wahrscheinlich bei der Psoriasis).

Auch nach der Beobachtung von TOURAINE können die angeborenen Krankheiten bei der Geburt manifest sein oder latent bleiben, um in den ersten Lebensjahren oder später zu erscheinen.

Bezüglich der palmo-plantaren Keratosen, die er in die Gruppe mit sicherer regelmäßiger Dominanz einreiht, unterscheidet TOURAINE innerhalb der di- oder polyhybriden Formen:

a) eine sexuelle Dominanz, mit Vorwiegen des männlichen Geschlechtes,
b) eine sexuelle Dominanz, mit Vorwiegen des weiblichen Geschlechtes,
c) eine sichere einfache Recessivität (Meleda),
d) eine wahrscheinliche einfache Recessivität.

Nach diesem Autor stellen die palmo-plantaren Keratosen nur ein Element innerhalb der Polykeratosen dar und sind immer der Ausdruck von Anomalien, die durch zahlreiche Faktoren bedingt sind.

Hier muß an die Einteilung der Keratosen von SIEMENS erinnert werden, die drei Gruppen umfaßt: idiopathische, idiodispositionelle und paratypische Keratosen. Bei den atypischen Formen ist die Dominanz ungewiß, wobei hie und da eine Recessivität beobachtet werden kann.

Bei der Besprechung der nosologischen Einheit der palmo-plantaren Keratosen hebt MONCORPS hervor, daß die streifenförmigen Formen sich zu diffusen Formen entwickeln können oder daß sie in anderen Fällen das Endstadium derselben darstellen können. Nach dieser Auffassung ist die streifenförmige Form nur eine Variante der gleichen Grundkrankheit. MONCORPS stellte noch bei den streifen- und inselförmigen Keratosen eine deutliche Abhängigkeit von auslösenden mechanischen Faktoren fest.

Besprechung einiger Fälle

Im Sinne der obigen Daten ergaben die von uns studierten Fälle folgende Beobachtungen:

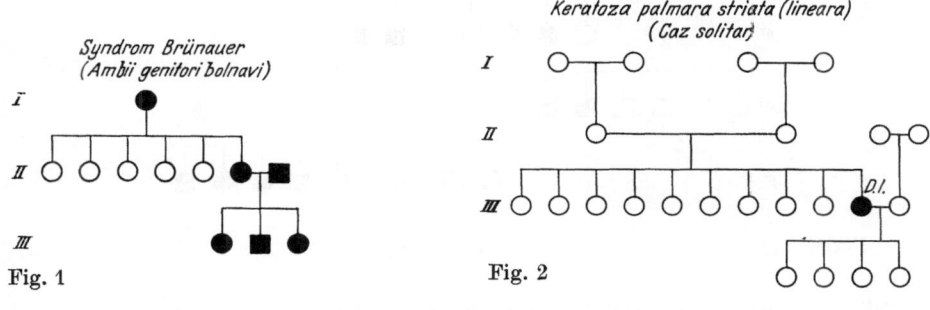

Fig. 1

Fig. 2

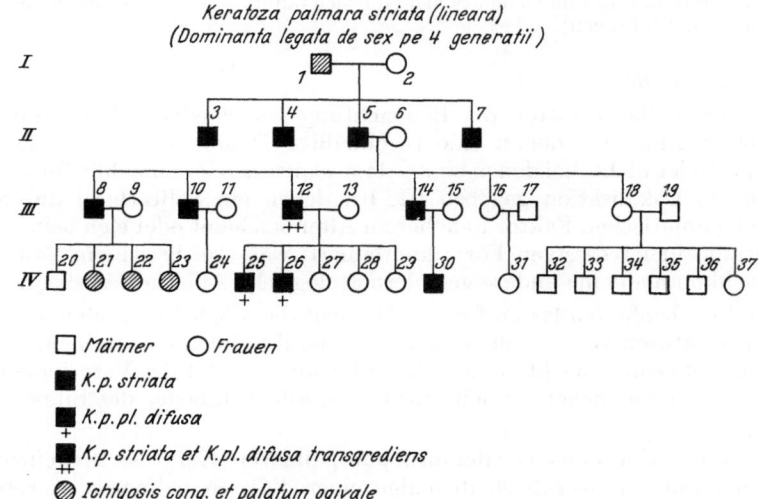

Fig. 3

Fall 1. Ein Brünauer Syndrom (keratosis palmo-plantaris mit hogyvalem Gaumen) beobachtet durch drei Generationen, dominant, nicht geschlechtsgebunden übertragen, bei dem beide Elternpaare in der zweiten Generation die Krankheit aufwiesen.

Fall 2. Eine ausschließlich palmare Keratose, Einzelfall innerhalb von vier Generationen, im Alter von 22 Jahren aufgetreten, und zwar nach Beginn der Tätigkeit als Faßbinder. Das ständige mechanische Trauma erscheint in diesem Fall als auslösender Faktor bei einer hereditären, bis dahin latenten Veranlagung und gebunden an die Gegenwart einer manifesten essentiellen palmaren Keratose.

Fall 3. Eine streifenförmige palmare Keratose mit dominanter Vererbung, gebunden an das männliche Geschlecht durch vier Generationen und bei 37 Familienmitgliedern. Dabei findet sich in einem Fall gleichzeitig eine transgrediente plantare Keratose, bei zwei Kindern eine diffuse palmare Keratose, sowie bei drei weiteren (weiblichen) Kindern, eine ichtyosis congenita mit hogyvalem Gaumen, während die Mutter keinerlei sichtbare Mitbeteiligung der Haut aufwies.

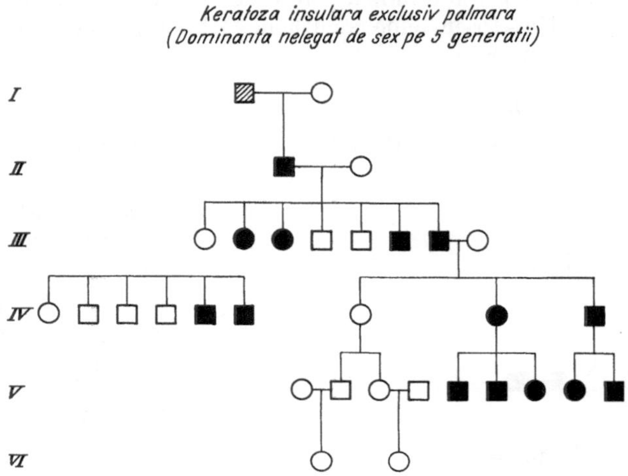

Keratoza insulara exclusiv palmara
(Dominanta nelegat de sex pe 5 generatii)

Fig. 4

Fall 4. Der letzte Fall zeigt eine inselförmige, ausschließlich plantare Keratose mit dominanter Vererbung. In fünf Generationen fand sich unter 32 Individuen die Krankheit bei 15 (10 Männer und 5 Frauen).

Diskussion der Fälle

Diese vier Fälle gestatten die Beobachtung verschiedener Modalitäten erblicher Übertragung, bei denen eine regelmäßige Dominanz an das Geschlecht gebunden ist oder nicht, bei denen eine palmo-plantare oder ausschließlich palmare oder plantare Lokalisation gegeben ist, bei denen ein Solitärherd durch einen exogenen traumatischen Faktor in höherem Alter erscheint oder sich beim gleichen Kranken mit einer recessiven Form kombiniert, während bei einem Fall bei den ersten Nachkommen eine andere genodermatologische Affektion vorliegt.

Solche Gegebenheiten lassen für den Moment die Möglichkeit offen, die palmo-plantaren Keratosen vom nosologischen Standpunkt global einzureihen, wobei die Einreihung auf Grund des klinischen Aspektes und der Art der Vererbung erfolgt, die mittels Familienanchete erzielt wurde, die alle Mitglieder der Sippe erfassen muß.

Die Kombination einer streifenförmigen palmaren Keratose mit einer transgredienten plantaren Keratose, diejenige einer diffusen palmaren Keratose bei zwei Kindern, deren Vater eine streifenförmige Form aufweist, oder das Auftreten bei drei weiblichen Kindern einer ichthyosis congenita, deren Mutter vom dermatologischen Standpunkt gesund ist, deren Vater jedoch eine streifenförmige palmare Keratose aufweist, stellen offene Probleme dar auf dem weiten und komplizierten Gebiet der Genodermatologie im allgemeinen und auf dem der palmoplantaren Keratosen im besonderen.

Disseminated Superficial Actinic Porokeratosis

M. E. Chernosky and R. G. Freeman, Department of Dermatology, Baylor University College of Medicine, Houston, Texas (USA),
D. E. Anderson, The University of Texas M. D. Anderson Hospital and Tumor Institute, Houston, Texas (USA)

Recent studies [1, 2] indicate that disseminated superficial actinic porokeratosis (DSAP) is probably a distinct entity and differs in many ways from classical porokeratosis (Mibelli). DSAP is characterized by multiple, small, superficial, annular or circinate, keratotic, anhidrotic lesions, which are surrounded by a slightly raised border. They have not been observed on mucous membranes or the palms and soles. Their bilateral distribution is limited to sun exposed areas of skin. Sun exposure frequently produces pruritus and exacerbation of the lesions. The condition is not rare particularly in geographic areas with large amounts of sun exposure, although apparently the condition is not widely recognized. Follicular keratotic papules with central depressions are present in some lesions. Although the centers of most lesions are atrophic, central thickening and erythema at times give an appearance similar to advanced actinic keratoses or squamous cell carcinoma.

The histologic feature essential for diagnosis of porokeratoris is the cornoid lamella, a column of lighter staining stratum corneum containing parakeratotic cells beginning in the malpighian layer and extending upward through the granular and keratin layers. This may be very faint and is found at the margin of the lesion, bordering a center which is usually atrophic.

A genetic investigation of DSAP has recently been initiated. The results to date indicate that the condition is equally frequent in examined males and females and is inherited as a classic autosomal dominant.

Interestingly, in the 31 index patients previously studied clinically [1, 2] 24 were females and seven were males, a ratio of 3.4 to 1. This predominance of females is probably because women are most likely to seek aid for the minor cosmetic defects produced. In addition, genetic findings show absence of a significant sex difference in the affection-rate of DSAP among examined individuals. These findings are distinctly different from those for classic porokeratosis (Mibelli), which is reported to occur three times as frequently in men as in women [3].

Our genetic investigation also indicates that age has a profound influence on the affection-rate of DSAP. The condition is observed in only 9% of examined individuals younger than age 20 years, compared to over 50% for individuals 20 year of age or older.

Clinical exacerbation following natural or experimental ultraviolet light irradiation [2], distribution of lesions limited to sun exposed areas of skin, appearance of lesions late in life after prolonged sun exposure, and frequent clinical and histologic similarities to true actinic keratoses indicate that actinic irradiation plays an important role in the pathogenesis of DSAP. Moreover, the absence of lesions on the mucous membranes, palms and soles, and their equal frequency in males and females further indicate that DSAP differs from classic porokeratosis (Mibelli) and probably constitutes a distinct hereditary entity.

Bibliography. 1. Chernosky, M. E.: Southern. Med. J. **59**, 289 (1966). — 2. Chernosky, M. E., and R. G. Freeman: Disseminated Superficial Actinic Porokeratosis (DSAP). Arch. Derm. **96**, 611 (1967). — 3. Butterworth, T., and L. P. Stream: Clinical Genodermatology, pp. 26—28. Baltimore: Williams and Wilkins 1962.

Werner's Syndrome
Report of a Case with Postmortem Findings

Y. Hamada, Namazu City Hospital, Shizuoka-Ken (Japan)

History. A 51 year-old carpenter was hospitalized for repeated epistaxis arhythmia and anemia. His father died at 40 years of age following a trauma of arm and his mother died at 80 years of age. Both had almost normal stature. He had six brothers and sisters and one of his elder brother who died at the age of 40 from pulmonary tuberculosis had small stature, cataract, premature gray hair and baldness. Patient had married with healthy woman at the age of 30 but had no children. He had first noticed emaciation and high-pitched voice at the age of 18. Loss and graying of hair increased at the age of 28. Cataract bothside were operated at the age of 30.

Physical Examinations. He was poorly developed, 150 cm tall, weighed 29 kg. He appeared about 20 years older than his age of 51 and responded in a husky, high-pitched voice. No microdontia. Kidneys were not palpable. Prostate, testis and epididymis were atrophic. On examination no edema, cyanosis and tele-angiectasia were seen. Pigmentation and depigmentation were found on ear lobules and back of nose. The face was characteristically altered by moderate micrognathia and by wrinkled skin on forehead and perioral region. His hair was gray and white on the scalp except for parietal region and was almost absent in *axillae* and pubic region. Seborrheic scales were seen on scalp. The skin of extensor surface of extremities especially of forearms, legs and feet was taut and stretched over the wasted underlying subcutaneous tissues. Hypertrophy and koilonychia were seen in all finger nails and onycholysis was seen in right third finger nail. Ulcers of varying in size were found on back of left foot and sole.

Laboratory Data. Complete blood count, liver and kidney function, serum cholesterol and serology were normal. Serum protein 6.0 g/dl and A/G was 0.7. Hypercalcinemia 7.3 — 6.8 m Eq/L, BMR + 21%. Eosinophilic response following intramuscular administration of ACTH was — 14%. The roentgenograms showed osteoporosis in ribs and bone of extremities. Decalcification was noticed in metatarsal and digital bones. Sclerosis was noticed in patella and sesamoidal bones. Calcium deposit was seen in elbow joints, forearm, patella, tibia, calcaneum, navicular and medial cuneiform bones. Sella turcica and skull were normal. Electromyogram normal. Biopsy was made from the back of right foot. The epidermis showed atrophy, edema, loss of epidermal processes and slight increase of pigment. In the corium hypertrophy of small blood vessel wall and the reduction of capillary lumen were seen. Slight perivascular round cell infiltration was seen. Degeneration of collagen bundles was not distinct. Atrophy of subcutaneous fat tissue and sweat gland was manifest.

Hospital Course. The patient treated at first for pulmonary tuberculosis about 8 months and then treated almost symptomatically for ophthalmological and dermatological complaints. About 1 year after admission his temperature rose 39.6 °C accompaning vomitting, dyspnea, arhythmia and incontinence of urine. He died on Oct. 19, 1965.

Autopsy. Autopsy was performed 2 h postmortem by the author.

1. The skin appeared atrophic, gray hair was distinct. Several ulcers were found on the bony processes of the right foot. Microscopically atrophy is seen in epidermis, cutis and cutaneous appendages.

2. The hypophysis. No abnormality in the proportion of the cells. Vacuole formation, atrophy or liquefaction of protoplasma. The adrenals. Cortex was

markedly atrophied. Blood vessels of capsule was sclerotic. The testis. Atrophy or
loss of the epithelium of tubules. Interstitial cell was increased.

3. The aorta. Loss of elasticity was noticed and easily ruptured. Hypertrophy
of intima, hydropic swelling of media.

4. The lungs. Diffuse fibrosis of right upper lobe including old pulmonary
tuberculosis. Bronchopneumonia in right lower lobe. Partial hypertrophy and
adhesion of right pleura seemed to be the result of poor development of bronchial
musculatures.

5. The heart. Hypertrophy of left ventricle. Myocardial edema.

6. The liver. Weighed 750 g.

7. The kidneys. Multiple cysts in right kidney.

8. The prostate. Reduced in size.

9. The Spleen. Slight fibrosis.

10. The brain and the digestive apparatus. Grossly unremarkable.

Unklassifizierte fleckenhafte Atrophie der Haut
bei zwei Schwestern
Capillaritis maculo — keratotica atrophicans familiaris

R. ILEA und M. PAVEL, Krankenhaus für Erwachsene, Arad (Rumänien)

Wir möchten zwei kranke Schwestern vorstellen, die an einem fleckenhaften
livid-atrophischen und keratotischen Ausschlag an den Beinen, Armen und im
Gesicht leiden. Die Krankheit begann vor 11 Jahren bei einem und vor 14 Jahren
bei dem anderen Fall, 2 Jahre nach der Menopause, mit Erscheinung von kleinen
Keratosen, unter denen mit der Zeit atrophische, rote Flecken erschienen, die bei
Orthostatismus, bei Kälte und bei Wärme sichtbarer werden und beim Druck ver-
blassen. Die Krankheit hat einen langsamen, jahrelangen progressiven Verlauf
(bemerkt von uns in den letzten 8 Jahren). Bei einem Fall Schwindelanfälle
labyrintischen Ursprungs. (Vorgeschichte: Masern, Scharlach, Bauchtyphus,
Malaria und Lungen-Tbc.)

Status praesens. In den distalen zwei Dritteln der Beine sind rote Flecken mit
atrophischer Oberfläche von 3 bis 5 mm Durchmesser sichtbar, manche von einer
leicht entfernbaren kollodiumähnlichen Keratose bedeckt. Durch die verdünnte
Epidermis in der Mitte der Flecken erkennt man eine rote angiomatöse Zone,
während der Umfang blaß und von einem filiformen scuamös-keratotischen Rand
begrenzt ist. Neben diesen sind andere kollodiumschichtähnliche keratotische
Elemente sichtbar, nach deren Entfernung man weiß-atrophische Flecken neben
anderen braun-roten papulösen erkennen kann. Auf den Streckseiten der Arme
und im Gesicht erkennt man geringere, nur keratotische Ausschläge.

Histologie: Hyperkeratotische Atrophie der Epidermis, Verschwinden der
Papillen, Ödem der Dermalschicht mit Homogenisierung und Zupfen der Kollagenfasern. Die Capillaren sind pseudoangiomatös erweitert, limphoide Infiltration
um die Gefäße. Die Wände der Muskulärarteriolen weisen einen lacunären Aspekt
in „Lichtungen" der Media und Endothelitis auf. Die Untersuchung der Phospho-
lipiden nach BACKER in den Lichtungen der Arteriolenwände blieb negativ. PAS,
Mucicarmin, Kongo-Rot, Sudan III, Silberimprägnationen gaben keine besonderen Ergebnisse. Mit Toluidin-blau nur in der fünften Excision eines papulösen
Elementes Mastzellenhäufung (25/Herd), und dieser Befund war negativ in den

vier vorigen Biopsien. Bei Orzein konnte man eine schwere Beteiligung des elastischen Gewebes feststellen.

Laborbefunde. Mikroagglutination nach GIROUD für Rickettsia prowazecki, R. mooseri, R. conori, R. burneti und pararickettsien negativ. Gesamte Lipämie 1165 und 1240; Cholesterolämie 278 und 288 mg-%. Bei drei von sechs Mitgliedern in zwei Generationen der Familie Hypo-Gamma-Globulinämie (3 bis 7,5%) und Steigerung der Alpha-1 (6 bis 8%) und der Alpha-2 (10 bis 12,5%). Capillarotoxischer Test stark positiv.

Wir möchten die Aufmerksamkeit auf folgendes lenken:

1. Das familiäre Auftreten der Krankheit.

2. Das Erscheinen nach der Menopause.

3. Jahrelanger progressiver Verlauf.

4. Polymorphismus der Eflorescenzen: kleine Keratosen, maculöse Atrophie, blaß an der Peripherie, zentral angiomatöse ohne arboreszente Telangiektasien, neben papulösen Ausschlägen. Es ist ein klinisches Bild, das ganz verschieden ist von dem monomorphischen Aspekt das Telangiectasie en plaques der Franzosen.

5. Histologisch: Hyperkeratotische Atrophie der Epidermis, pseudoangiomatöse Erweiterung der Capillaren in der Papillarschicht, vacuoläre Schädigung der Muskulärarteriolenwände.

6. Pathologische Befunde der Lipämie, Proteinogramm und des capillarotoxischen Testes.

7. Eine Rickettsiose wurde ausgeschlossen, ohne eine andere infektiöse, toxische oder allergische Ätiologie feststellen zu können.

8. Als Folgerung, auf Grund von oben erwähnten Kriterien, konnten wir das morpho-klinische Syndrom von anderen, wie Telangiectasie en plaques, Telangiectasia macularis eruptiva persistans Parkes-Weber, Angiokeratomen, primäre und sekundäre Atrophien, trennen und es als eine distrophische Capillaropathie mit atrophischem Ausgang betrachten, bei dem familiär bedingte endokrino-metaboische Faktoren mitwirken.

Pyodermatitis

Affections cutanées dues aux pyogènes

Afecciones cutáneas producidas por agentes piógenos

Pyodermien

Organizer

CL. LIVINGOOD, USA

Presidents

R. F. BETTLEY, Great Britain

FR. KERDEL VEGAS, Venezuela

A. MIDANA, Italy

L. POPOFF, Bulgaria

Delegate of the Organization Committee

H. RÖCKL, Germany

Reports

The Etiology of Pitted Keratolysis*

D. Taplin and N. Zaias, Department of Dermatology, University of Miami School of Medicine, Miami, Florida (USA)

Introduction

Pitted keratolysis is a common superficial infection of the plantar and occasionally palmar surfaces producing crateriform pits in the stratum corneum, which may be small and discrete or coalesce to form large irregular patches of superficial erosion [1]. Most cases are asymptomatic, but under tropical conditions among indigenous populations it has been reported to produce symptoms severe enough to require medical treatment.

Biopsies in every case reveal Gram positive filamentous and diphtheroid-like organisms in the stratum corneum and confined to the areas of keratolysis. Acton and McGuire [2] believed the causative organism to be a member of the Actinomycetales, and called it *Actinomyces keratolyticus*. Having examined the reference strain of their organism, we are convinced that it is in fact a member of the genus *Micromonospora*, a saprophyte of mud and soil.

We report here the results of studies which indicate that the common forms of this disease, at least in the United States are caused by a member of the genus *Corynebacterium*. The limitations of time permit only the most brief description of these studies, which will be reported in detail elsewhere.

Methods

In five cases of typical Pitted Keratolysis the surface of the soles were cleansed with 70% Ethyl alcohol, and scrapings were made from the pits and adjacent intact stratum corneum. All scrapings were homogenized in broth with a tissue grinder, and the homogenate plated on a battery of culture media, both anaerobically and aerobically. Similar methods were used to retrieve organisms from experimentally induced infections.

Results

In five cases of typical Pitted Keratolysis of the soles, an organism was isolated from the pits which was not recovered from the adjacent skin. Occasionally, only a few colonies were isolated, but in nine attempts to isolate the organism, it was the predominant growth on anaerobic cultures on five occasions.

Description of Causative Organism

Cultural characteristics. Within 3 to 5 days on Brain Heart Infusion Agar incubated at 37 °C in a mixture of pure nitrogen containing 5 to 10% CO_2, minute, irregular, colorless colonies were seen which under the microscope showed filamentous growth into the agar at the periphery and under the colonies. On further incubation in air, or on aerobic subculture, these minute filamentous micro colonies developed into creamy white to tan, circular, convex to pulvinate colonies with entire margins, composed of Gram positive diphtheroid organisms. In early stages of aerobic growth, these domed colonies could be scraped away to reveal the filamentous growth in the agar underneath the colony. The diphtheroids and filaments were Gram positive and non-motile. Subcultures of the aerobic diphtheroid

* This study was supported in part by the Office of the Surgeon General, Department of the Army, under the sponsorship of the Commission on Cutaneous Diseases of the Armed Forces Epidemiology Board, and by the Dermatology Foundation of Miami.

forms to nitrogen/CO_2 or CO_2/ air atmospheres again stimulated a tendency to filamentous growth in early stages of incubation.

Serological Studies. Antisera produced in rabbits by intravenous injections of formalised and washed cells from the first isolate we obtained, agglutinated by direct slide method all subsequent isolates. There were no cross reactions with other known skin diphtheroids, including *C. minutissimum* or *C. acnes.* Ouchterlony gel immunodiffusion studies revealed at least two soluble extracellular antigens which were not shared by *C. minutissimum, C. acnes,* or oleate-dependent skin diphtheroids. No precipitin bands were observed when antisera to *C. minutissimum* and C. acnes were tested against soluble antigens derived from our organisms.

Microscopic characteristics. Gram stained smears from cultures showed Gram positive bacteria with variable morphology, varying from small diphtheroid forms to filaments with a tendency to form branches, depending on the cultural environment and nutrition. Occasional club forms were seen. The microscopic dimensions were consistent with other known species of *Corynebacteria.*

Biochemical characteristics. The organisms were catalase positive, urease positive, methyl red and Voges Prauskauer negative, indol negative, Citrate negative, and did not reduce nitrates. Positive reactions for lysine decarboxylase were noted by the Pathotec paper strip method. Carbohydrates were not attacked either oxidatively or fermentatively in any of the standard carbohydrate media, but growth was poor and the possibility exists that carbohydrates might be utilized in a suitable medium. Carbohydrates were incorporated into a wide variety of chemically defined and non defined enriched media but growth was poor in all, and no carbohydrates were attacked.

DNA-Analysis. Analysis of the DNA from five typical isolates, kindly performed by Prof. MANLEY MANDEL of the University of Texas gave a mean value for percent Guanine/Cytosine of 59.4. This is consistent with a corynebacterium and sufficiently far removed to exclude *Nocardia, Mycobacteria,* and *Listeria.* It is also different from *C. acnes* (48% G. C.) and *C. minutissimum* (71% G. C.) *Actinomyces* is ruled out on the grounds of capacity for aerobic growth and positive catalase test.

Artificial Infections

Typical lesions of Pitted Keratolysis were reproduced in two male and two female subjects. The skin of the heels was cleansed with 70% alcohol and dried. Heavy inoculations of a pure, fresh culture were made by scraping the growth directly from an agar plate on to one heel. The other heel was similarly treated, but no culture was applied. Both heels were covered by a small occlusive patch of polyethylene sheeting, and strapped with adhesive tape. 6 days later all subjects had developed typical lesions of Pitted Keratolysis, which continued to spread, as long as the heel was occluded. No lesions developed under the control patch on the other heel. The organism was recovered in culture from all cases, and proved to be identical serologically and morphologically to the inoculated strains. No positive cultures were obtained from the control heels.

Discussion

The organism which we have isolated repeatedly from our cases of Pitted Keratolysis appears to be an aerobic *Corynebacterium* species. All isolates are similar in essential characteristics, and appear to be serologically distinct from the most commonly isolated diphtheroids from the skin. It is most easily recognised on primary isolation by examining Brain Heart Infusion Agar plates under the low power of a microscope. It also grows on routine sheep blood agar and Brain Heart Infusion Agar, but the larger colonies and diphtheroid morphology make it difficult to recognize from other skin diphtheroids.

KOCH's postulates were fulfilled and the microscopic characteristics of the artificial lesions were identical to the naturally occuring infections.

We have biopsied one case of severe pitting of the soles in which the organisms seen in histological sections were not compatible with a *Corynebacterium*, so that we would entertain the possibility that not all cases of Pitted Keratolysis are due to the organism described in this report. All other biopsies examined from 15 cases are compatible with a corynebacterium. Our experience with many strains of skin diphtheroids lead us to believe that filamentous growth and branching are not in themselves sufficient justification to remove an organism from the genus *Corynebacterium*. The apparently abundant urease produced by all strains of our organism is of interest, and this, together with the direct slide agglutination, proved of value in differentiating them from many other skin diphtheroids.

Acknowledgements: We wish to record with appreciation the outstanding technical assistance of Miß GLORIA JEAN SINGLER.

References. 1. ZAIAS, N., D. TAPLIN, and G. REBELL: Arch. Derm. **92**, 151 (1965). — 2. ACTON, H. W., and C. McGUIRE: Indian med. Gaz. **65**, 61 (1930).

Bacterial Flora — The Role of Local and Environmental Factors

J. M. KNOX, M. E. McBRIDE and W. C. DUNCAN, Department of Dermatology, Baylor University College of Medicine, Houston, Texas (USA)

It has been observed that the incidence of superficial skin infection is greater in hot humid climates. Most pathogenic microorganisms have an optimum temperature for growth which approximates body temperature. Certain cutaneous pathogens are found to have temperature optimums slightly lower than 37 °C, corresponding to the surface temperature, 31° to 32 °C, rather than core temperature.

Regardless of these slight differences in optima, it is well known that bacteria proliferate more rapidly in a warm, moist environment. It was of interest, therefore, to determine the extent that environmental changes in temperature affect the normal skin flora of man, and thus determine factors in the physiological dependence of the cutaneous flora. We have studied the problem by examining the changes in skin populations of individuals under experimental conditions in a climate-controlled chamber. Later the effect of varying the humidity will be studied.

The experimental procedure was as follows: Two groups of ten men were studied: One at 32 °C with 90% humidity and the second at 21 °C with 90% humidity. Bacterial cultures were taken from the back, groin, hands and feet in duplicate, using identical areas on the right and left sides of the body. The number of bacteria per square centimeter of skin was calculated for each culture. Each subject was cultured upon entering the climate chamber, after 15 h under the experimental conditions, and again before leaving the chamber at 63 h. After their return to a natural environment follow-up cultures were taken from every subject at 24 h and 96 h.

A comparison of the skin bacterial populations of the two groups of subjects during and after 63 h at 32 °C and 21 °C are shown in a series of scattergrams. The log of each bacterial count per square centimeter is represented by an open

dot for the 21 °C group and a solid dot for the 32° C group. Each calculation is
from the mean of the right and left sides, six counts having been performed on each
culture. Fig. 1 shows the changes that occur in the skin populations of the back at

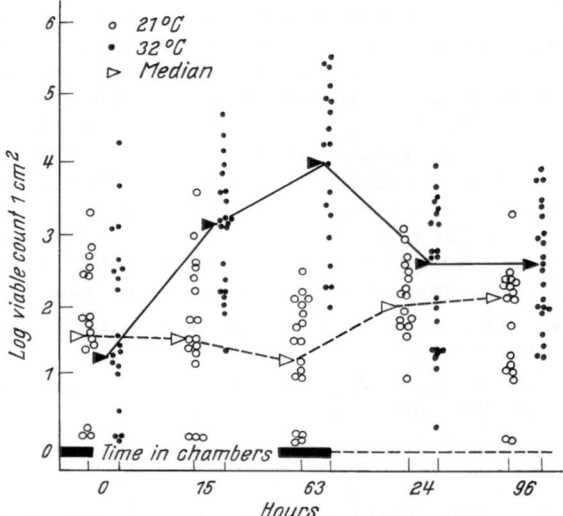

Fig. 1. Comparison of bacterial skin populations of the back during a 63 h period at 21 °C
and 32 °C

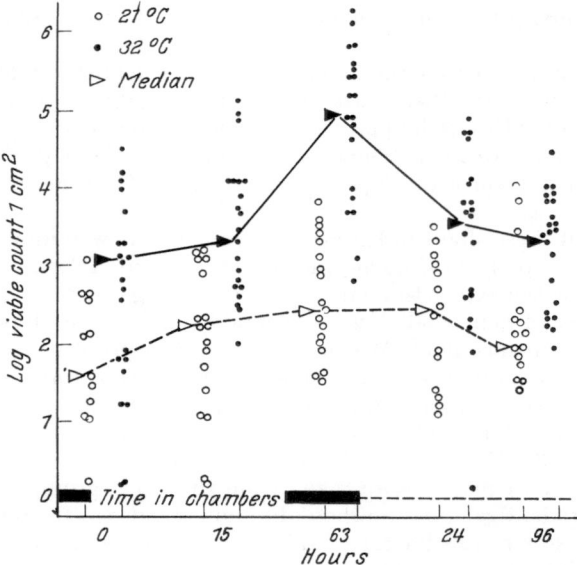

Fig. 2. Comparison of bacterial skin populations of the groin during a 63 h period at 21 °C
and 32 °C

32 °C and 90% humidity, as compared to individuals at 21 °C and 90% humidity.
The medians indicated by the arrow are within log 0.4 bacteria per square centimeter of skin at the initiation of the experiment though the counts from both
groups are distributed over a wide range throughout the experimental period. By

comparing the medians of the 21 °C group throughout the experimental period it can be seen that the medians vary only within log 1.0 bacteria per square centimeter of skin. At 32 °C however, the counts increase by a log 2.8 bacteria per

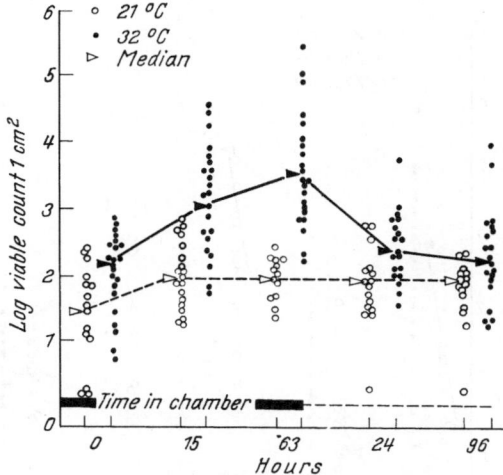

Fig. 3. Comparison of bacterial skin populations of the hands during a 63 h period at 21 °C and 32 °C

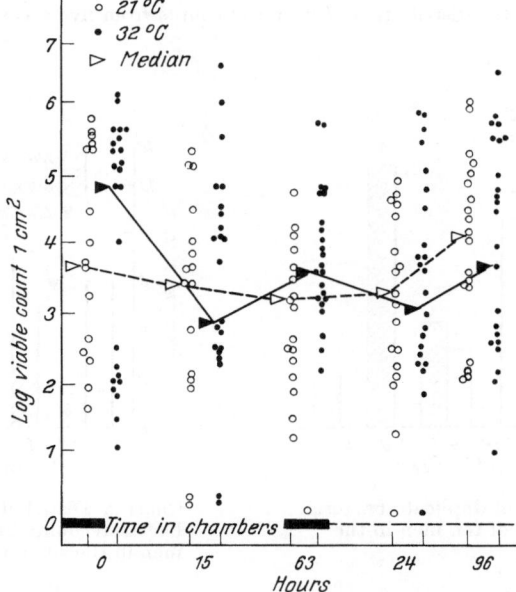

Fig. 4. Comparison of bacterial skin populations of the feet during a 63 h period at 21 °C and 32 °C

square centimeter after 63 h in the chamber with a decline following the subjects' return to a natural environment. Comparable results can be seen for the groin in Fig. 2 and the hands in Fig. 3 despite the fact that hand washing was permitted during the experiment. The feet, however, failed to show similar increases in bacterial populations at 32 °C as shown in Fig. 4. A wider distribution of count is noted for feet and with the exception of the initial high count obtained at 32 °C there are no significant differences between the medians of the two groups.

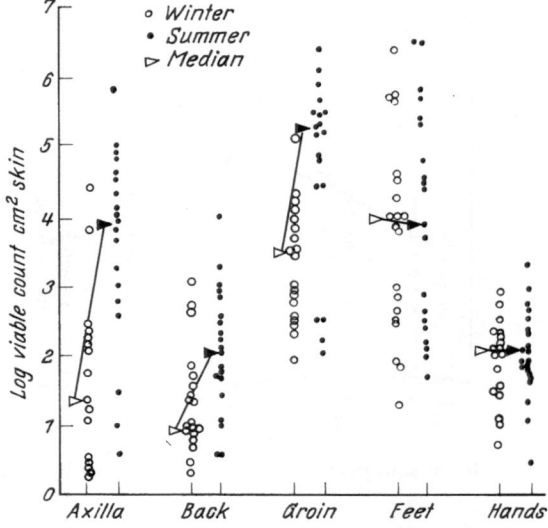

Fig. 5. Comparison of the distribution of bacterial counts from five areas of the body in the winter and in summer

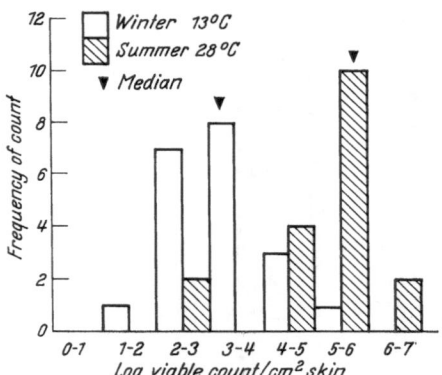

Chart 1. Distribution of duplicate bacterial counts from the groin of ten men in the summer and winter

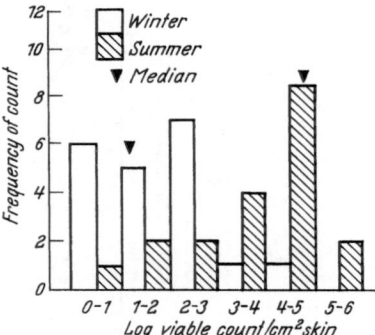

Chart 2. Distribution of duplicate bacterial counts from the axillae of ten men in the summer and winter

It was concluded from this study that bacterial skin populations in certain areas of the body, namely, the back, the groin, and the hands increase with increasing temperatures. Generally speaking, there was no qualitative change in the bacterial flora, just quantitative. Hydration of the skin was encouraged by the high percentage of humidity (90%); therefore, only temperature was varied under the conditions of this experiment.

To determine if the increases in bacterial skin populations noted under experimental conditions of temperature occurred in the natural environment, a group of ten sailors were studied in their natural environment at two extremes our of local temperature during the winter (average 12 °C) and summer (average 28 °C). Bacterial cultures were taken from the hands, feet, back and groin as described

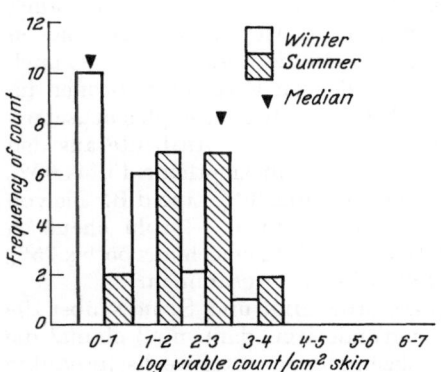

Chart 3. Distribution of duplicate bacterial counts from the backs of ten men in the summer and winter

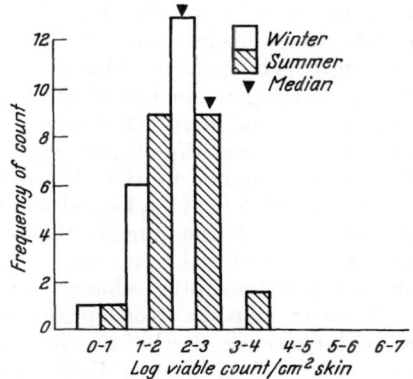

Chart 4. Distribution of duplicate bacterial counts from the hands of ten men in the summer and winter

above. The scattergram (Fig. 5) summarizes all the results with each count per square centimeter of skin being represented by a dot. The increased bacterial counts during the summer sampling period can be readily observed for the axilla, back, and groin, while the hands and feet are unaffected by the environmental temperature change.

These results can be expressed in another way as is shown in the subsequent figures. The comparison of the distribution of bacterial counts from each body area in summer and in winter have been tabulated. The bacterial populations from the groin are presented in Chart 1, the white representing counts taken during the winter months and the black indicating the results from the summer. It can be seen that the greatest number of bacterial counts from the winter range between the log values of two and four per square centimeter of skin while in the summer the greatest number of counts were within the range of log values between five and six per square centimeter of skin. The medians for each group is

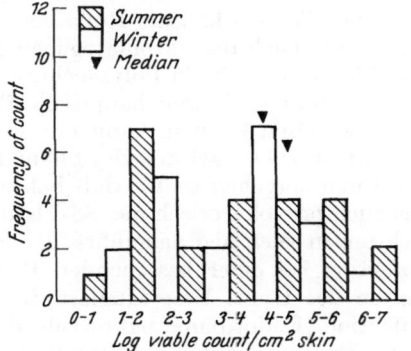

Chart 5. Distribution of duplicate bacterial counts from the feet of ten men in the summer and winter

indicated by an arrow and the differences between summer and winter can be clearly observed. Charts Nos. 2 and 3 showing the results of the axillae and back respectively also demonstrate increased bacterial populations in the summer. On the other hand, Charts Nos. 4 and 5 are the results of the hands and feet respectively and show no difference with increased summer temperatures.

Polysaccharidfraktionen von Bakterien in ihrer Bedeutung für die Haut

J. Meyer-Rohn, Universitäts-Hautklinik Hamburg (Deutschland)

Polysaccharidfraktionen werden aus Endotoxinen vornehmlich gramnegativer Keime (Salmonella, Brucella, Shigella, Escherichia, Serratia), aber auch grampositiver Keime und Tuberkelbakterien isoliert. Gegenüber der eigenen fermentartigen Natur der klassischen Toxine aktivieren die Endotoxine, also auch die aus ihnen gewonnenen Polysaccharide eine Fülle von Fermentreaktionen im Organismus, die den bekannten „Abwehrreaktionen" teilweise gleichzusetzen sind. Der genuine Endotoxinkomplex kann in 5 bis 10%iger Ausbeute aus den Bakterien gewonnen werden. Er enthält je nach Gewinnungsmethode 45 bis 60% Polysaccharid, 5 bis 15% Lipoid A, 15 bis 20% Protein und 10% Lipoid B. Die von Westphal nach der Phenol-Wasserextraktion gewonnenen — wohl chemisch am saubersten charakterisierten — Lipopolysaccharide setzen sich aus 55 bis 75% phosphorylierten Polysaccharid und 25 bis 45% Lipoid A zusammen.

I. Wenn man die Konzeption von Robert, Miescher und Storck über die Entstehungsweise des bakteriellen Ekzems zugrunde legt, dann muß einmal die Tatsache, daß es lebende Keime sind, die ekzematogene Stoffwechselprodukte bilden, zum anderen die Tatsache, daß das Ekzem nach Eliminierung der Keime zur Abheilung kommen kann, auf den Gedanken lenken, daß auch Stoffe der Bakterienleiber selbst an der Entstehung des mikrobiellen Ekzems beteiligt sein könnten. So hatte uns Westphal entgegenkommenderweise einen Staphylokokkenstamm chemisch so weit aufgearbeitet, daß wir eine Fraktion, die ein Polysaccharid und Nucleinsäure enthielt, bei Patienten mit mikrobiellem Ekzem im Epicutantest nach vorheriger Skarifikation testen konnten: Wenngleich die positiven Reaktionen überwogen, so waren die Ergebnisse bei einem Vergleich mit Nichtekzematikern nicht signifikant; Bakterienpolysacchariden kann auf keinen Fall die alleinige kausale Rolle beim mikrobiellen Ekzem zugesprochen werden. Die Frage nach der ekzematogenen Natur der aus Staphylokokken gewonnenen Teichinsäure, auch ein Polysaccharid, bedarf noch der Klärung.

II. Ob und wie weit bakterielle Polysaccharide Shwartzman-Sanarelli-Phänomene auslösen können, kann nur vermutet, aber nie bewiesen werden, weil ein experimenteller Nachweis des Phänomens am Menschen nicht möglich ist. Manche Faktoren sprechen dafür, daß bakterielle Polysaccharide sowohl präparatorisch als auch provokatorisch das SS-Phänomen auszulösen vermögen. Nur zwei Beobachtungen seien hier angeführt: Erstens nach einer sekundär aufgetretenen Coliinfektion bei einer bestehenden Hauttuberkulose kommt es zu Geschwürsprozessen der Haut. Hier fungiert die Tuberkulose als Präparation und die Coliinfektion (Endotoxine, bakterielle Polysaccharide) als Provokation. Zweitens bei einer Pyodermia chronica papillaris et exulcerans kommt es nach Penicillinbehandlung zu hämorrhagischen Nekrosen. Hier wirken die durch die Penicillintherapie freigesetzten Bakterientoxine oder auch Endotoxine (Polysaccharide) präparatorisch und eine hinzugetretene Proteusinfektion provokatorisch. Nach Storck, Proppe, Richter, Gougerot und anderen Autoren lassen sich verschiedene Krankheitsbilder als SS-Phänomene deuten: Unklare Geschwürsprozesse, Pemphigus acutus febrilis gravis, Purpura fulminans nach Scharlach, profuse Hautblutungen bei Meningo- und Pneumokokkensepsis und vielleicht auch die thrombotische Mikroangiopathie von Moschcowitz.

III. Bevor auf therapeutische Möglichkeiten durch bakterielle Polysaccharide eingegangen wird, müssen die Antwortreaktionen des Organismus auf intravenöse

Gaben von Lipopolysacchariden dargelegt werden. Diese Reaktionen sind zum
Teil richtungsweisend für die Indikationsstellung.

Fieber tritt 1 Std nach der Injektion ein mit einem Maximum nach 3 Std und
anschließendem lytischen Abfall.

Im Blutbild erscheint dabei eine initiale Leukopenie, der eine *Granulocytose*
mit Linksverschiebung folgt. Normalisierung des Blutbildes erfolgt binnen 24 Std.

Es kommt zu einer *Steigerung des Phagocytoseindex* und der *unspezifischen
Resistenz* des Organismus gegenüber pathogenen Keimen. Nach Untersuchungen
ROWLEYS mit P 32 markierten Lipopolysacchariden findet mit der Zunahme der
unspezifischen Immunität eine Steigerung der Phagocytosefähigkeit der Zellen des
RES statt.

Schließlich kommt es zu einer *Stimulierung des Properdinsystems* und zur
Aktivierung der fibrinolytischen Aktivität im Vollblut.

Alle Antwortreaktionen sind durch unzählige Untersuchungen fest unter-
mauert und jederzeit reproduzierbar.

Der Gedanke der Reizkörpertherapie reicht schon ins Altertum zurück. Aber
erst WAGNER-JAUREGG, HOFF und PFEIFFER schufen ihr durch ihre grundlegenden
Arbeiten einen festen Platz in der wissenschaftlichen Medizin. Absolut neu an den
Lipopolysacchariden WESTPHALS ist die Tatsache, daß diese chemisch wohldefi-
nierten Stoffe nach Gewichtseinheiten in Gamma-Größe dosiert werden können,
was dem Therapeuten wesentlich mehr Sicherheit gibt, im Gegensatz zu den
früher benutzten unkontrollierbaren und teilweise undefinierten Substanzen.

Im Rahmen dieser Ausführungen kann nur ein Überblick gegeben werden,
welche Krankheitsbilder aus dem Bereich der Dermato-Venerologie aussichtsreich
mit Lipopolysacchariden behandelt werden können. Dabei muß einschränkend
betont werden, daß eine Objektivierung von Heilerfolgen gerade hier außerordentlich problematisch ist.

Aus der Gruppe der Ekzeme sind das endogene und das mikrobielle Ekzem zu
nennen.

Die chronische Urticaria, bei der keine auslösenden Noxen zu eruieren sind,
spricht teilweise gut an. Die gute Beeinflussung chronischer Thrombophlebitiden
kann auf die Aktivierung der fibrinolytischen Aktivität im Vollblut durch Lipopolysaccharide zurückgeführt werden. Beim chronisch rezidivierenden Erysipel,
der Furunkulose und der Pyodermia chronica papillaris et exulcerans können mit
einer kombinierten gezielten Antibioticatherapie und Lipopolysacchariden gute
Erfolge erzielt werden. Hier kommt es bekanntlich auf eine Steigerung der unspezifischen Resistenz an. Auf dem Gebiet der Venerologie sind es die unspezifische
Urethritis, Epididymitis und Prostatitis, die — auch wieder in Kombination mit
Antibiotica oder anderen bewährten Therapieformen — gut auf Lipopolysaccharide ansprechen.

Insgesamt übersehen wir ein Krankengut von über 2500 Fällen, die in den
vergangenen 10 Jahren stationär mit Lipopolysacchariden behandelt worden sind.
Die Verträglichkeit ist im allgemeinen gut. Leichtes Frösteln, Unbehaglichkeit,
Kopf- und Gliederschmerzen sind als Begleiterscheinungen des Fiebers nicht zu
ernsthaften Nebenwirkungen zu zählen. Bei empfindlichen Patienten können die
durch das Fieber bedingten Nebenerscheinungen und das Fieber selbst durch
Antipyretika gedämpft werden, ohne die erwünschten Systemreaktionen zu beeinflussen. Allergien oder hyperergisch anaphylaktische Reaktionen wurden bisher
in keinem Fall beobachtet. Kontraindikationen sind schwere Organschäden,
Nebenniereninsuffizienz, exsudative Lungentuberkulose, Magenulcus und Schwangerschaft. Als Altersgrenze für die Therapie mit Lipopolysacchariden sollte das
60. Lebensjahr gelten.

Staphylococcal Strain 502-A in the Treatment of Recurrent Furunculosis

H. I. MAIBACH and W. G. STRAUSS, Division of Dermatology, University of California School of Medicine, San Francisco, California (USA)

Fortunately, chronic furunculosis is an uncommon disease; in those individuals or families so involved, it may however, persist for many years. Previous attempts to break the cycle with staphylococcal toxoids, nasal and systemic antibiotics, and topical germicides, have either failed or never been given a controlled assay. The natural history of the disease is such that long-term follow-up is required to ascertain if therapy has been successful, as relapses occur months to years later.

H. SHINEFIELD introduced the concept of bacterial interference for the prophylaxis of staphylococcal infection in the newborn. In a series of well-controlled and well-documented studies, he and his colleagues demonstrated that newborns could be artificially colonized with a less virulent strain of staphylococcus and thus prevent serious staphylococcal disease with the prevalent hospital staphylococci such as phage type 80/81.

We have applied similar methods in the treatment of chronic furunculosis and have reported previously on our first patient [STRAUSS, W. G., H. I. MAIBACH, and V. HURST: Purposeful change of staphylococcal phage types in a patient with furunculosis. J. Amer. med. Ass. 191, 759 (1965)]. The criteria for selection is a patient in otherwise good health with a minimal history of 1 year of recurrent boils. Cultures are made of representative body sites including the nose, throat, back, groin, buttocks, and rectum to determine the site of staphylococcal carriage. Generally the nose and throat are the most common sites with the buttocks the next most common. The patients are treated with full doses of a synthetic penicillin (such as oxacillin) for 5 days. The site of staphylococcal carriage (usually the nose, but sometimes the buttocks) is treated with a topical antibiotic. On the 6th through 10th days, the nares and any skin carriage site are inoculated daily with one drop of a fresh overnight broth culture of staphylococcus strain 502-A. This is a minimum of 10^6 organisms. SHINEFIELD originally chose this strain from a nurse carrier in their nursery whose strain had never produced disease in the newborn nursery.

In the 4 years of follow-up with over 15 patients having greater than 1 year follow-up, we have had success in all patients. Half of the people had to be recolonized two or more times before the 502-A strain took. When it did take, the cycle of boils stopped. Long term follow-up and the treatment of many cases will be required to further confirm its long-term efficacy and safety.

Some Observations on the Normal Cutaneous Flora of Different Age Groups

M. J. MARPLES, Department of Microbiology, University of Otago (New Zealand)

Although there have been many investigations into the normal flora of the skin, the majority has involved only the glabrous skin, and the subjects have been young adults. The study recorded below was carried out on 410 healthy individuals whose ages ranged from 4 days to 98 years. This report is based on work undertaken by the Mycology Unit of the Department of Microbiology, the results of which were presented by Dr. DOROTHY SOMERVILLE as a thesis for the degree of Ph.D.

Materials and Methods

Three areas representative of the general skin surface namely the forehead, the dorsum of the hand and the dorsum of the foot were sampled. In addition, the following special cutaneous areas were selected: external ear, nostrils, axilla, nail folds, and first and fourth interdigital spaces of the foot. Gum swabs were also collected from all subjects and in the infants rectal and umbilical swabs were added to the samples.

The age distribution of the subjects investigated is shown in the table. Females outnumbered males among the premature infants and the geriatric patients, but in other groups the numbers were approximately equal.

Sampling for the presence of bacteria and yeasts was carried out using broth moistened swabs. Primary isolations were made on blood agar plates, incubated at 37 °C for 48 h. Among the adults, scrapings from the interdigital spaces of the feet were examined by direct microscopy and by culture for the presence of fungal pathogens.

Results

Coagulase negative staphylococci and micrococci were recovered from virtually all cutaneous sites of all individuals, as were diphtheroids in all but the two infant groups. Other species varied in their distribution with age and in some cases with sex. The table shows the percentage of subjects carrying various marker species somewhere on the skin. Figures in parentheses indicate carriage on the general skin surface.

Considerable differences in incidence occurred in different age groups, and many of these are statistically significant. Cutaneous carriage of coagulase positive staphylococci did not entirely reflect nasal carriage of these organisms. *Staph. aureus* was isolated from the nostrils of 28% of infants, 40% of all adults and 65% of children, but in 43.4% of subjects the phage type of the nasal isolate did not correspond with that of the cutaneous strain. This result differed from findings reported elsewhere (RIDLEY, 1959; WILLIAMS, 1963). *Staph. aureus* was isolated significantly more frequently from the axilla of premature infants than from all other age groups (p < 0.001).

Sarcina appeared to be a true member of the cutaneous flora of children and was regularly isolated from all cutaneous areas. In adults this organism showed a sex difference in its distribution. It was isolated from some cutaneous site in 68.8% of males and from 40.7% females (p < 0.001). Non-haemolytic and alpha haemolytic streptococci were mainly isolated from the nostrils but were frequently found on the glabrous skin of the younger age groups. Beta haemolytic streptococci were scanty in all sites and only four isolates were assigned to Group A. Coliform organisms were rarely isolated except in the infant groups. *E. coli* was isolated from the umbilicus of 40% infants and from the axilla of 22% premature and 45% full term babies.

The distribution of members of the tribe Mimeae was of considerable interest. *Mima polymorpha* was isolated from some skin site, usually the toe webs, of 33.8% and *Herellea vaginicola* from 11.3% of children. Mimeae were also found significantly more frequently on the skin of male adults (19%) than of females (3.2% p < 0.001). TAPLIN and his colleagues (1963) have noted the importance of these organisms in the microbial communities inhabiting the axilla and the toe webs of males.

Candida albicans was isolated from the gums of 24.0% of premature and 3.9% of full-term infants, from 31.3% of children, 22.9% of young and 44.5% of elderly adults. The yeast was not isolated from the general skin surface of children

Table. % *Skin Carriage of Various Micro-organisms in Different Age Groups*

Age Groups	Staph. aureus	Sarcina spp.	Alpha haemolytic streptococci and pneumococci	Beta haemolytic streptococci	Gram positive bacilli	Neisseria spp.	Gram negative bacilli Lac +	Lac −	Mima and Herellea	Candida albicans
50 premature infants 4—9 days	60.0 (40.0)	4.0 (—)	58.0 (46.0)	22.0 (12.0)	18.0 (4.0)	4.0 (2.0)	54.0 (10.0)	— (—)	— (—)	18.0 (14.0)
51 full-term infants 4—7 days	47.1 (25.7)	5.9 (2.0)	82.3 (58.8)	9.8 (3.9)	25.5 (7.8)	13.7 (7.8)	56.9 (7.8)	9.8 (2.0)	— (—)	7.8 (3.9)
80 children 3—12 years	76.3 (38.8)	87.5 (68.8)	67.5 (43.8)	5.0 (2.5)	93.8 (60.0)	55.0 (31.3)	2.5 (2.5)	5.0 (1.3)	41.3 (20.0)	3.8 (—)
166 young adults 17—45 years	41.0 (16.4)	54.2 (34.8)	21.1 (13.4)	4.2 (1.8)	62.6 (37.2)	44.0 (19.4)	9.0 (1.2)	10.2 (1.8)	9.0 (3.0)	3.6 (—)
63 elderly adults 60—98 years	42.9 (22.2)	30.2 (20.0)	38.1 (15.9)	6.4 (4.8)	79.4 (27.0)	46.0 (25.4)	3.2 (1.6)	23.8 (1.6)	6.4 (3.2)	20.6 (7.9)

Figures in parentheses show % carriage on the glabrous skin.

or young adults but 3.8% children and 3.6% young adults carried it in one of the special areas. The organism was however recovered from the skin of 14.0% infants and 20.6% geriatric patients and in both groups was found not infrequently on the glabrous skin. The difference in incidence between infants and geriatrics and the other age groups is significant ($p < 0.001$). Dermatophytes are not included in the table. They were isolated from the feet of 16.3% young and 16.7% elderly males but from only 2.3% of all adult females. The difference is significant ($0.001 < p < 0.01$).

Discussion

There have been many studies of the anatomical and physiological characters of the human skin, and it has been shown that the cutaneous habitat varies not only in different areas of the body but also in different climates and with age and sex (ROTHMAN, 1954; MARPLES, 1965). It is therefore not surprising that the microbial community living on the skin should have a composition which varies with the age and sex of the host and with the bodily site which it inhabits. When a pathogenic organism alights on the skin it must compete with the resident flora for its essential requirements. Its success may well depend on the qualitative and quantitative attributes of the resident community which are affected by the age and sex of the host.

Acknowledgements. It is a pleasure to record my gratitude to Dr. DOROTHY SOMERVILLE for her work in the present study. My thanks are also due to the Medical Research Council of New Zealand and to E. R. Squibb & Son for financial assistance, and to the doctors who gave me permission to examine their patients.

References. MARPLES, M. J.: The Ecology of the Human Skin. Springfield (Ill.): Charles C. Thomas 1965. — RIDLEY, M.: Brit. med. J. **1959** I, 270. — ROTHMAN, S.: Physiology and Biochemistry of the Skin. Chicago: University Press 1954. — TAPLIN, D., G. REBELL, and N. ZAIAS: J. Amer. med. Ass. **186**, 952 (1963). — WILLIAMS, R. E. O.: Bact. Rev. **27**, 56 (1963).

Free Communications

Über die Dynamik der Zusammensetzung der Bakterienflora auf der Haut

A. TODOROV und P. POPCHRISTOV, Universitäts-Hautklinik Sofia (Bulgarien)

Am XI. Internationalen Kongreß in Stockholm 1957* haben wir über die Rolle der normalen Bakterienflora auf der Haut, im Mund und in der Urethra und von ihrer antibakteriellen Schutzrolle berichtet. Damals haben wir mitgeteilt, daß die normale Bakterienflora auf den oben genannten Körperregionen auf einem breiten Spektrum von pathogenen und apathogenen Mikroorganismen antagonistisch wirkt. Für diese gesetzmäßig festgestellte Tatsache muß man dem theoretischen und praktischem Standpunkt Rechnung tragen.

Bei unseren weiteren Untersuchungen über die Zusammensetzung und die biologische Rolle der Bakterienflora auf der Haut, im Mund und in der Urethra haben wir neue Fakten festgestellt, die Gegenstand dieser Mitteilung sind.

Vor allem haben wir uns eigenes Kriterium von der Zusammensetzung der sog. normalen Bakterienflora auf der Haut ausgearbeitet. Grundfehler bei den

---

* P. POPCHRISTOV and IV. BOGDANOV. Proceedings, volume III. Symposia 1 bis 16. Stockholm 1958.

bisherigen Untersuchungen ist, daß man die Resultate von einmaligen Untersuchungen bei vielen Personen summiert, anstatt dynamisch die Zusammensetzung der Bakterienflora auf längere Zeit bei ein und denselben Personen zu untersuchen.

Bei der dynamischen Untersuchung der Bakterienflora auf der Haut der Finger bei 342 gesunden Personen während einem Jahr haben wir folgende Mikroorganismen festgestellt:

I. Gruppe: Medizinisches Personal (Krankenschwester, Laborantinnen, Krankenpflegerinnen) 20. Staphylococcus albus non haemolyticus in 100% der Fälle, Sarzinen 58.2%, Gram-positive Bakterien 50,3%, Staphylococcus albus haemolyticus 47,3%, Streptococcus 29,7%, Staph. aureua n. haemolyt. 14,5%, Staph. aureus haemolyt. 10,3%, Gram-negative Bakterien in einzelnen Fällen.

II. Gruppe: 252 Personen mit nicht exsudativen juckenden Dermatosen. Staph. albus n. haemolyticus 100%, Gram-positive Bakterien 95%, Sarzinen 92%, Staph. albus haemolyticus 31,3%, Streptococcus 16,1%, Staph. aureus haemolyt. 12,4%, Staph. aureus n. haemolyt. 10,3%, Gram-negative Bakterien in einzelnen Fällen.

III. Gruppe: 47 Kursteilnehmerinnen. Staph. albus n. haemolyticus 100%, Sarzinen 85%, Gram-positive Bakterien 78%, Gram-negative Bakterien, Streptokokken u. a. in einzelnen Fällen.

IV. Gruppe: 23 Kinder aus einem Kindergarten. Staph. albus n. haemolyt. 100%, Sarzinen 95%, Gram-positive Bakterien 78%, Gram-negative Bakterien, Streptokokken u. a. in einzelnen Fällen.

Wie aus den Untersuchungen ersichtlich ist, werden in allen Fällen weiße nicht hämolytische Staphylokokken isoliert, gefolgt von Sarzinen und Gram-positiven Bakterien. Das stellt, unserer Auffassung nach, die normale Bakterienflora der Haut dar. Andere Bakterienarten werden seltener, in einzelnen Fällen und unbeständig isoliert.

Ähnliche Resultate von der Bakterienflora der Urethra haben wir am Ersten Symposium über die nicht gonorrhoischen Urethritiden in Montreal* 1959 mitgeteilt. Auch im Mund haben wir als ständige Bewohner apathogene Staphylokokken und Gram-positive Bakterien gefunden.

Parallel durchgeführte Untersuchungen über den Antagonismus der normalen Bakterienflora auf der Haut, im Mund und in der Urethra zeigen, daß der Hauptträger dieser antagonistischen, antibiotischen Eigenschaften der Staphylococcus albus non haemolyticus ist.

Auf Grund der ausgeführten Untersuchungen sind wir der Meinung, daß die ständige Zusammensetzung der Bakterienarten auf der Haut, im Mund und in der Urethra sehr beschränkt ist. Die auf diese Organe gelangenden pathogenen und apathogenen Mikroorganismen sind vorübergehende, zufällige Bewohner, die von der Haut durch die verschiedenen Schutzmechanismen und besonders durch die antibiotischen Eigenschaften der ständigen Bewohner der Haut, d. h. die weißen nicht hämolytischen Staphylokokken (Staph. epidermidis), beseitigt und vernichtet werden. Gleichzeitig wollen wir darauf hinweisen, daß beim Händewaschen fast alle Bakterienarten von der Haut beseitigt werden, nicht aber die weißen Staphylokokken.

Die oben angeführten Angaben über die Zusammensetzung und die antibiotische Rolle der normalen Mikroflora können Anlaß geben für eine neue Deutung mit praktischen Schlußfolgerungen über die Pathogenese mancher Pyodermien, Urethritiden und Stomatitiden. Vielleicht könnten sie als Dysbakterie aufgefaßt

---

* POPCHRISTOV, P., and S. NEYTCHEV, I. Canad. sympos. Montreal 1959.

werden. Wir haben z. B. festgestellt, daß die stark verstaubte Haut der Arbeiter in den Steinkohlengruben zu einer stark ausgedrückten Dysbakterie, bzw. zur Inhibierung der antagonistischen Eigenschaften der normalen Bakterienflora führt, was oft Pyodermien zur Folge hat.

Bei der Höhenklimatherapie bessern sich die antibakteriellen Schutzmecha nismen der Haut nicht nur durch die Besserung des Säuremantels der Haut, sondern auch durch die Änderung der Bakterienflora vom Zustand der Dysbakterie zum Zustand der Eubakterie.

Keloidal Folliculitis of the Neck in Mongolism

E. Kocsard, J. E. Moulton and F. Ofner, Department of Public Health, Lidcombe Hospital, Sydney (Australia)

More than a dozen inmates suffering from Scabies Norvegica were discovered in a mental hospital for male patients (Kocsard et al., 1960, 1967). All of them were mongols. As could be expected we found in the same environment numerous

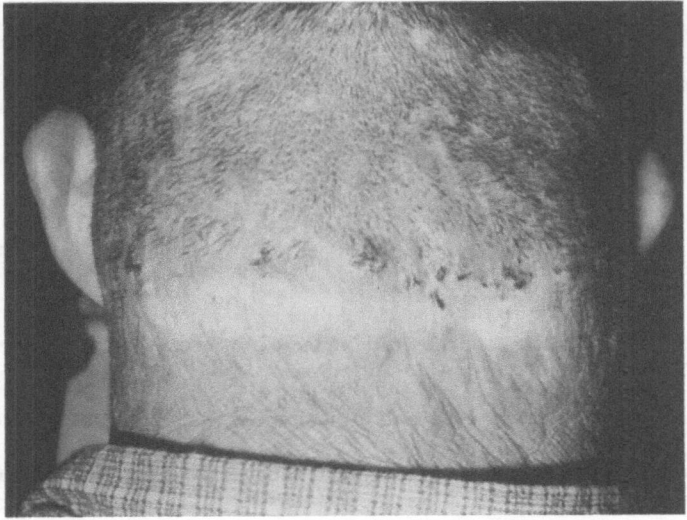

Fig. 1. Folliculitis keloidalis in a mongol patient showing numerous compound hairs and considerable scar formation

other patients showing characteristic lesions of ordinary scabies and of pyoderma. About 50% of the mongols of the hospital — were suffering from Folliculitis keloidalis (F. K.) of the neck. Some of these had scabies and other types of pyogenic lesions at the same time. There was also a high incidence of scars due to follicular pyodermas, over the trunk and the chest. These scars were usually hypertrophic but in some patients had an anetodermic appearance.

All mongoloid patients with F. K. had thick necks and many compound follicles were seen over the scalp of the neck. Bacteriological studies of the lesions demonstrated the presence of Staphylococcus aureus and beta haemolytic Strepto-coccus of Lancefield group A. The staphylococci were coagulase positive and of the phage type 80, 81 and 53. In several cases the staphylococci were not typable.

Two of the most severely affected patients underwent surgical excision of the skin of the affected region, followed by plastic repair (MOULTON). On histological examination of the removed skin area the classical changes of the chronic stage of F. K. were observed. There was follicular destruction. A heavy infiltrate of plasma cells, lymphocytes and histiocytes was present with plasma cells predominating. There were many foreign body giant cells very often arranged in vertical columns corresponding to the destroyed hair follicles.

Following the discovery of the Norvegian scabies cases and the energetic measures undertaken to eradicate scabies and pyoderma, there was a decline of the incidence of the above dermatoses and the F. K. cases became much less

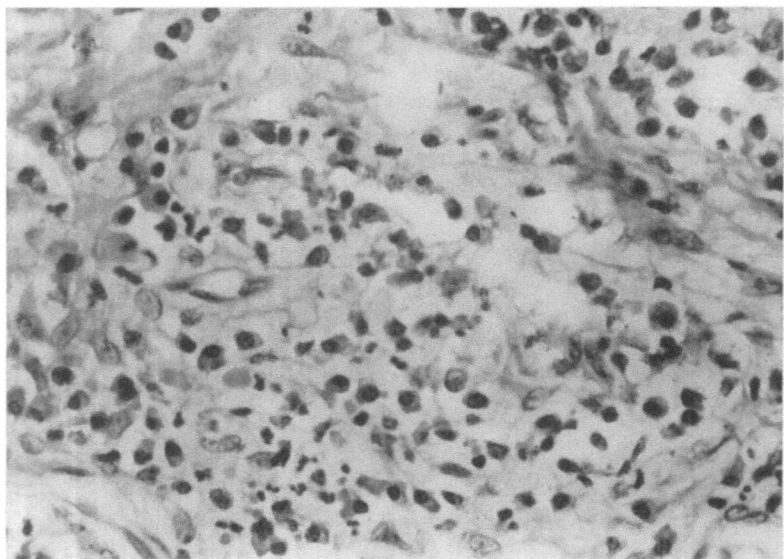

Fig. 2. Chronic inflammatory infiltrate with numerous plasma cells, characteristic of the chronic stage of the condition

florid losing the signs of the acute inflammation and showing only the scars of the progressed condition.

One of us (OFNER) had occasion to visit another Institution for mental defectives, having 55 mongols. In this second Institution there were no cases of scabies nor of pyoderma and not one of the mongols had F. K. of the neck. Another sporadic case of F. K. has been reported to us by Dr. J. B. CAHILL of Sydney affecting a mongol who was not hospitalized.

Discussion

According to the literature F. K. does not seem to be a frequent finding in mongols and is usually not mentioned when the skin manifestations and complications of mongolism are considered. KRINER and DAITSCH (1958) reported a 39 years old mongol patient with the condition and mentioned that the same patient had also lesions of anetoderma of SCHWEININGER and BUZZI over the neck and the shoulders.

As mentioned above we have observed similar atrophic or hypertrophic scars in our patients. These were probably the end results of follicular pyodermic lesions.

According to PILLSBURY et al. (1956) negroes are the usual victims of F. K. A thick neck and compound hairs (polytrichia) are the usual predisposing factors. It has been repeatedly stressed by many that compound follicles, many hairs emerging from the same follicular orifice, are predisposing to follicular infections (LOEWENTHAL L. J. A., 1947; H. PINKUS, 1951; OBERSTE-LEHN, 1957). PILLSBURY et al. (1956) say "Infection is a sequel to the crowding of several hairs in a common follicular orifice".

A thick neck is a characteristic of patients affected by F. K. It was reported by HALL (1966) that "an excess skin of the back of the neck is seen in about 80% of newborn mongoloid infants". Our patients with F. K. had also this thick neck characteristic of mongolism.

As generally in chronic pyodermas in F. K. one has to stress the terrain on which the infection develops. Mongols seem to be predisposed to the development of F. K. The association of a high incidence of scabies and pyodermas in the mental institution where we discovered the high incidence of F. K. shows the importance of the pyogenic factor in triggering off the condition.

Acknowledgements. This investigation was conducted under the auspices of the Unit of Clinical Investigation, Lidcombe Hospital. It is a pleasant duty to acknowledge the cooperation of the Medical Superintendent and the Staff of Peat and Milson Island Hospital and of Dr. GWEN SAX.

References. HALL, B.: Clin. pediat. (Bologna) **5**, 4 (1966). — KOCSARD, E.: Cutis **3**, 41 (1967). — KOCSARD, E., J. L. COLES, and F. OFNER: Aust. J. Derm. **5**, 235 (1960). — KRINER, J., and J. DAITSCH: Arch. argent. Derm. **8**, 323 (1958). — LOEWENTHAL, L. J. A.: J. invest. Derm. **8**, 263 (1947). — OBERSTE-LEHN, H.: Arch. klin. exp. Derm. **206**, 506 (1957). — PILLSBURY, SHELLEY, and KLIGMAN: J. invest. Derm. **17**, 291 (1951).

Die Auswertung der Einwirkung des Staphylokokken-Anatoxins bei der Therapie und Diagnostik der Staphylokokken-Hautkrankheiten

J. LAŃCUCKI, J. SAMOS, Z. JÓZEFCZYK und E. STANOWSKA, JKP-WAM, Warschau (Polen)

Das Staphylokokken-Anatoxin aus den Stämmen des Staphylococcus albus 0-15 Moskwa und des Staphylococcus aureus Wood 46 London wurde in der Therapie chronischer und resistenter Staphylokokken-Hautkrankheiten angewandt: in 117 Fällen von Furunculosis, in 15 von Hidradenitis axillaris, Sycosis, 41 von Folliculitis und 52 von Acne phlegmonosa und pustulosa mit gleichzeitiger Staphylokokkeninfektion, insgesamt bei 225 Männern in ähnlichen Existenzbedingungen, die keine andere Behandlung bekommen haben; die behandelten Männer waren im Alter von 21 bis 22 Jahren.

Bei den Behandelten, sowie bei gesunder Kontrollgruppe, wurden Hautteste mit Staphylokokken-Anatoxin, Streptolysin, Histamin, Adrenalin und Trafuril durchgeführt. Außerdem wurden bestimmt Antistaphylolysin und Antistreptolysin sowie die Blutmorphologie, die Senkungsreaktion, Zahl der Thrombocyten sowie der Fibrinogenspiegel, Fibrynolysin und Proteinogramm.

In den Kulturen wurden meist antibioticaresistente Stämme von Staphylococcus aureus (Coagulase +), seltener von Staphylococcus albus, erhalten. Das Anatoxin wurde subcutan in Dosen von 0,2 bis 0,3 ml, einmal monatlich, verabreicht.

Die Verträglichkeit der Behandlung war gut. Bei 40% der Kranken traten nach 24 Std subfebrile Reaktion und bei 70% eine Aussaat abortiver Folliculitiden, bzw. eine Verschlechterung der Krankheitsherde ein. Die Entzündung nach der Impfung war am stärksten nach 48 Std ausgeprägt. Die größte Lokalentzündung nach der Impfung wurde bei Kranken mit Furunculosis und Hidradenitis festgestellt, bei 15% dieser Personen wurden sogar sterile Abscesse beobachtet.

Während 1¹/₂jähriger Kontrolle wurden bei 30% der Kranken mitFurunkulose und Hidradenitis sowie bei 17% der Kranken mit Sycosis staphylococcica keine Rezidive festgestellt. Bei Acne phlegmonosa und pustulosa wurde kein therapeutischer Erfolg erzielt.

Intracutane Teste mit dem Staphylokokken-Anatoxin waren am stärksten nach 24 Std und dauerten bis 48 Std. Die stärkste Reaktion war bei den Kranken mit Furunkulose. Teste, durchgeführt 14 Tage nach der Impfung, waren stärker bei allen Kranken sowie auch bei Gesunden. Intracutane Staphylolysin-, Adrenalin- und Histaminteste, sowie der epidermale Trafuriltest, bleiben unverändert. 3 Tage nach der Impfung wurde meist eine Leukocytose mit Lymphopenie und 14 Tage nach der Impfung eine geringe Lymphocytose festgestellt. Die Zahl der Thrombocyten war unverändert. Die Senkungsreaktion war am 3. Tag erhöht.

Die Untersuchung des Spiegels von Asta und ASO ist vor der Impfung, 14 Tage nach der Impfung und dann in Abständen von einem Monat durchgeführt worden. Der Ausgangsspiegel (bei Gesunden 0,5 bis 2) bei den Kranken vor Staphylokokkeninjektionen war zwischen 1,5 bis 2, betrug dagegen bei 43% der Furunkulosefälle und bei 25% Hidradenitis axillaris 3 bis 5. Nach dem 12. und 20. Tag nach der Impfung steigt der Spiegel von Asta bis 5 bis 8 (maximal 20) — bei 50% Furunkulosefälle, Hidradenitis axillaris und Sycosis staphylogenes, bei 42% Acne phlegmonosa und pustulosa und bei 70% der Gesunden. Nach weiteren Impfungen ist die Steigerung des Astaspiegels nicht so intensiv wie nach der ersten Impfung. Nach der ersten Impfung blieb der erhöhte Astaspiegel 3 bis 4 Monate und nach der zweiten Impfung 6 bis 8 Monate. Bei 40% der Kranken mit hohem Astaspiegel wurde eine stärkere Lokalreaktion festgestellt und bei 30% der Kranken ein positiver Anatoxintest. Bei Furunkulose und Hidradenitis wurde die Steigerung der Astawerte von einer klinischen Besserung begleitet. Die Impfungen haben keinen Einfluß auf den ASO-Spiegel verübt.

Nach der Impfung tritt eine Erhöhung des Globulin- (besonders Alpha und Beta) und eine Senkung des Albuminspiegels ein. Bei einer großen Zahl der Kranken mit hohem Astaausgangsspiegel ist eine Vermehrung von IgM- bei normalen oder öfters gesenkten IgG-Werten festgestellt worden. Nach einem längeren Zeitabstand nach der Impfung — unabhängig von dem Ausgangsspiegel — kam es zu einer Erhöhung der IgG-Werte. Der Fibrinogenspiegel ist niedriger, und die Zeit der Fibrinolyse verkürzt.

Schlußfolgerungen

1. Das Anatoxin hat einen guten therapeutischen Effekt bei Furunkulose und Hidradenitis, besonders in den Fällen, bei welchen parallel die Asta- und die IgG-Werte größer sind.

2. Die Hautreaktion auf Staphylokokken-Anatoxin ist bei chronischen Staphylokokken-Hautkrankheiten stärker. Die Einführung des Staphylokokken-Anatoxins intensiviert diese Hautreaktionen, wobei sie auch keinen Einfluß auf Streptolysintest aufweist.

3. Klinische Besserung, bei gleichzeitiger Erhöhung des Asta-Spiegels, Senkung der Fibrinogenwerte, Verkürzung der Zeit der Fibrinolyse, Intensivierung der Staphylokokken-Anatoxinhautreaktion und Fehlen der Wirkung auf die Streptolysin-Histamin-Adrenalin- und Trafurilreaktion sowie auf den ASO-Spiegel beweisen, daß eine spezifische und immune Wirkung des Staphylokokken-Anatoxins besteht.

Die Erysipelfrage. I. Allergologische und immunologische Untersuchungen an Erysipelkranken

E. Rajka, S. Korossy, J. Böszörményi, J. Szita und M. Gózony, II. Hautabteilung, Krankenhaus Kun-Gasse, Hautabteilung István-Spital, Impfstoffproduktions- und Forschungsinstitut Human, Budapest (Ungarn)

Zur Klärung des Pathomechanismus des streptogenen Erysipels (E) wurden bei 81 E- und 253 Kontrollpatienten (mit nicht streptogenen Erkrankungen) *intracutane* Proben und *serologische* Reaktionen durchgeführt. Zur intracutanen Probe dienten verschiedene Antigene, und zwar eine *polyvalente Streptococcus-(Str)-Vaccine*, hergestellt aus am häufigsten vorkommenden Typen der Str-Gruppe A, ferner Streptolysin O, Streptokinase und ein thermostabiler Faktor. Die Zahl der mit der Str-Vaccine erzielten *positiven Spättypreaktionen* übersteigt zwar bei den *Erstinfizierten* die der Kontrollen (51 gegen 30%), die Zahl der positiven Reaktionen erreicht jedoch bei den *Rezidivfällen* kaum die der Kontrollfälle (27 gegen 30%). Dies läßt die Folgerung zu, daß die bei der E-Gruppe gefundenen positiven Werte nicht so sehr dem erysipelatösen Prozeß, sondern den früheren Str-Infektionen zuzuschreiben sind. Die Zahl der mit den *Enzymantigenen* erzielten Spättypreaktionen schwankte im Durchschnitt zwischen 29 und 48%.

Die Zahl der positiven *serologischen* Reaktionen (Titer über 250 Einheiten) übertrifft bei E die der Kontrollen beträchtlich: bei Antistreptolysin-O 65 gegen 42% und bei Antistreptokinase 45 gegen 18%. Bemerkt sei, daß in 24% der E-Fälle weder Hautreaktionen vorhanden waren, noch der Titer der humoralen Antikörper die normale obere Grenze übertrat.

Aus 115 E-Fällen konnten *21-β-hämolysierende Str-Stämme* isoliert werden, die — beinahe zu gleichen Verhältnissen — den *A-, C-* und *G-Gruppen* zugehörten. In der A-Gruppe wurden *sechs Typen* festgestellt (3, 8, 12, 13, 24, 25). Im Laufe der *Virulenzbestimmung* stellte sich heraus, daß diese Str-Stämme zumeist *avirulent*, bzw. zum Teil nur *mäßig virulent* waren und M-Protein nicht enthielten.

Mit Rücksicht darauf, daß 1. die Zahl der positiven Spättypreaktionen bei den Rezidivfällen unter der der Kontrollen blieb, 2. eine *echte Immunität* nicht auftritt (häufige Rezidiven), 3. trotz der *avirulenten* Stämme die schweren Symptome des E auftreten, stellten wir die Hypothese auf, daß es sich bei Erysipelas um einen *Immundefekt*, vor allem der zellenvermittelten Spättypsensibilisierung, handelt.

Die Erysipelfrage. II. Resultate der Streptococcus-Vaccinetherapie bei rezidivierenden Erysipelkranken

S. Korossy, E. Rajka, J. Böszörményi und M. Gózony, II. Hautabteilung, Krankenhaus Kun-Gasse, Hautabteilung István-Spital, Impfstoffproduktions- und Forschungsinstitut Human, Budapest (Ungarn)

69 wiederholt (2- bis 72mal) rezidivierende Erysipel-(E)-Kranke wurden mit einer polyvalenten Streptococcus-(Str)-Vaccine, die aus in Ungarn am häufigsten vorkommenden, M-Protein enthaltenden und gegen weiße Mäuse virulenten 14 Typen der Gruppe A hergestellt war, immunisiert. Die meisten erhielten sechs *immunisierende* und sechs „*erinnernde*" Injektionen. Es handelte sich nicht um Erzielung einer *Grundimmunität*, sondern um *sekundäre Stimulierung* einer durch mehrfache frühere Str-Infektionen induzierten Immunität. Zieht man den *zeitlichen*

Rhythmus der Rezidive in Betracht, so blieben, nach einer Beobachtungszeit von 8 bis 27 Monaten, bei 29 Patienten (42%) im Durchschnitt 4,5 Rezidive aus, während bei 22 (32%) trotz der Behandlung *Rückfälle* auftraten. Bei 18 (26%) waren die Rezidive noch nicht fällig, und sie traten auch im Laufe der Beobachtungszeit nicht auf.

Die *Immunlage* wurde während der Vaccinetherapie durch Hautproben mit der Str-Vaccine und mit einem thermostabilen Antigen, außerdem durch Bestimmungen des Antistreptolysin- und Antistreptokinasetiters verfolgt. Erstere gingen nach mäßigem Anstieg zurück, letztere stiegen deutlich an.

Die häufigen Rezidiven weisen auf einen *Immundefekt* hin, und zwar sind die auf die angewendete, M-Proteinantigene enthaltende Str-Vaccine gelieferten mangelhaften Immunantworten, indem trotz der Behandlung fast die Hälfte der derzeit bewertbaren Fälle (43%) rezidivierte, möglicherweise auf einen (vielleicht genetisch determinierten) relativen Defekt des Lymphsystems zurückzuführen. Bei der anderen, größeren Hälfte (57%) blieben jedoch die Rückfälle aus; wir sind der Ansicht, daß in diesen Fällen nicht so sehr eine Stimulierung der geschwächten Immunreaktivität der E-Kranken, als eher die Wiedererweckung einer durch frühere virulente Str-Infektion hervorgerufene Immunität mitgespielt hat.

Bacterial Etiology of Superficial Pyoderma in the Middle East*

A. S. DAJANI, F. S. FARAH and A. K. KURBAN, Department of Pediatrics and Division of Dermatology (Department of Medicine) of the American University of Beirut and the American University Hospital, Beirut (Lebanon)

The bacterial etiology of 90 consecutive cases of acute superficial pyoderma was investigated between April and November, 1966. The subjects were patients at the American University Hospital in Beirut, Lebanon, and included 56 children and 34 adults.

Material for culture was obtained from the skin lesions by means of a sterile swab after cleansing of the surrounding area with 70% alcohol and removal of any dry scabs. The swabs were inoculated onto rabbit blood agar plates and into Pike's selective medium. After 18 to 24 h incubation of the latter medium, subcultures were made onto blood agar plates. Throat swabs were also obtained from all the patients and were processed in a similar manner. All plates were read after 24 h incubation at 37 °C. Bacterial isolates were identified and then stored at —65 °C for further testing.

Identification of group A beta-hemolytic streptococci was performed using the bacitracin disc method of MAXTED and grouping was confirmed serologically according to Landefield's technique. Group A streptococci were classified by the agglutination technique for T-protein as well as by M-protein typing. The tube test was performed for assessing coagulase production by staphylococci. Phage typing was performed by standard techniques. Antibiotic sensitivities were determined by using a single low-potency disc.

The various organisms isolated from the skin lesions and their relative frequency are shown in the table. Staphylococci were the most commonly isolated organisms, and were recovered from 80% of the cases. In 11%, coagulase negative staphylococci were recovered and these were sensitive to all antibiotics tested.

* Supported by a grant from the Research Committee of the Faculties of Medical Sciences of the American University of Beirut.

All *S. aureus* isolates were coagulase positive. 49 (80%) of the staphylococci could be phage-typed. The most frequent reaction (40%) was with multiple phages of group II, among which phage type 71 was the most prevalent. Phage patterns belonging to groups I, III or other phage patterns occured in equal frequency (approximately 20% each). Only 15% of the *S. aureus* strains were sensitive to 2 units penicillin discs, whereas all were sensitive to 2 units Gentamicin and 97% were sensitive to 2 units Neomycin.

Table. *Organisms isolated from 90 cases of superficial pyoderma*

Organism	Number	Percentage
beta-hemolytic streptococcus	16	18%
Staphylococcus aureus	36	40%
beta-hemolytic streptococcus and S. aureus	26	29%
Staphylococcus albus	10	11%
Gram-negative rods	2	2%

B-hemolytic streptococci were recovered from 47% of the skin lesion cultures, either singly (18%) or in association with staphylococci (29%). The frequency of isolation of streptococci from mixed cultures was similar in Pike's medium and on blood agar plates. All but one of the streptococcal isolates belonged to Lancefield's group A, the one exception being a group C. Agglutination with T-antisera was performed on 37 strains, and a typable reaction was observed in 36 of these. The most common T-reaction was with Impetigo 19 antiserum (45%), with a relatively equal distribution observed among the other types (viz. 1, 4, 6, 11, 12, 14, 28 and 3/13/B 3264). M-protein typing was performed on 36 of the strains. Identification of types by this technique was obtained in 19 strains (52%) with most of the Impetigo 19 strains (T-reaction) failing to type by this technique. Of the M-protein typable strains, 5 reacted with type 25 antiserum, 4 with type 12 antiserum, 2 each with types 11 and 33 antisera, and one each with types 2, 5, 6, 8 and 29.

Analysis of throat cultures revealed that only three cases had positive cultures for group A-B-hemolytic streptococci. None of the patients had clinical evidence of pharyngitis, and all were children. There was no clinical evidence of nephritis in any of the cases. Treatment of all lesions was achieved by the use of topical Gentamicin or Neomycin with favorable results. Details of the comparative use of these agents has been published previously.

The results of this study indicate that *S. aureus* and group A-B-hemolytic streptococci are the major etiologic agents encountered in superficial pyodermas in the Middle East. A preponderance of specific staphylococcal phage types as well as certain streptococcal T-types in skin lesions has been observed in this series. This correlates with the experience of other investigators on cases seen in the United States and England. The surprisingly low recovery of streptococci from throat cultures of patients reported in this study may suggest that streptococcal skin infection may not necessarily be accompanied by streptococcal pharyngitis.

L'Influence de l'infection sur la marche du psoriasis

M. ZAJFEN et B. EJMONT-SKRZYPCZYK, Service Dermatologique du 2ᵉ Hôpital Central Clinique à Varsovie (Pologne)

Tenant compte des données bien contradictoires des auteurs scandinaves (NORRLIND, NØRHOLM-PEDERSEN, SONCK et WIDHOLM; HÄRÖ et coll.), allemands (GRÜNEBERG et CONRADI; ZAUN et HEITE), français (HURIEZ et coll.), italiens

(ZINA et BONU) en ce qui concerne le rôle de l'infection comme agent provoquant ou exacerbant le psoriasis, nous avons examiné le même problème dans nos conditions et dans un milieu homogène, c'est à dire chez les sujets du même sexe, du même âge et vivant dans la même région géographique de la Pologne centrale. Nous avons soumis à notre examen trois groupes de sujets à 50 personnes chacun, dont: un groupe de personnes complètement saines, hommes de 19 à 21 ans; un autre groupe de malades psoriatiques, eux aussi hommes du même âge; enfin un troisième groupe hétérogène composé de personnes des deux sexes et de divers âge, atteintes du psoriasis. Ainsi le premier et le troisième groupe ont été des groupes de contrôle, tandis que le deuxième groupe a été le groupe examiné. Chez les sujets de tous les groupes ont été examinés: le taux des antistreptolysines O (ASO) dans le sérum sanguin, l'état général de santé, les amygdales, parfois les sinus. L'évaluation du taux des ASO sériques a été effectuée selon deux méthodes: l'une de TODD, l'autre d'après BADIN et CABAU afin d'éliminer les phénomènes de la non-spécificité des taux trop élevés. Dans le premier groupe (hommes sains) nous avons évalué les limites du taux normal des ASO à niveau de 170 unités de TODD. Dans ce groupe 14% des examinés ont surpassé ces valeurs. Dans le deuxième groupe (hommes psoriatiques) 28% des examinés ont surpassé la limite de 170 unités de TODD. Dans le même groupe nous avons établi que chez dix sujets (20%) le psoriasis avait été précédé par une amygdalite aiguë. Dans le troisième groupe neuf sujets (18%) ont surpassé la valeur de 170 unités des ASO et le pourcentage de cas précédés d'une amygdalite aiguë a été le même: 18%.

Groupes et leur composition	Taux des antistreptolysines 0 sériques						Valeur moyenne du taux des ASO	Nombre de cas	
	0 à 24 un.	25 à 49 un.	50 à 99 un.	100 à 149 un.	150 à 199 un.	200 à 299 un.		après une angine	surpassant 170 u.
I. Hommes sains, 19—21 ans.	1	7	17	14	8	3	109 ± 8	0	7
II. Malades, du même âge et sexe	1	6	13	10	12	8	131 ± 10	10	14
III. Divers malades psor.	2	7	14	14	8	5	115 ± 9	9	9

Les différences de la valeur moyenne du taux des ASO entre les trois groupes ne sont qu'apparentes. Une analyse statistique de ces données nous a convaincus que contrairement à ce qu'affirmaient quelques auteurs, les taux élevés des ASO ne sont aucunement attachés au psoriasis comme tel et qu'ils ne sont qu'une expression plus ou moins exacte d'une infection streptococcique subie.

Quant au rôle de l'infection comme agent provocateur responsable de l'exacerbation du psoriasis, notre travail l'affirme d'une façon très nette. Il en résulte que la prophylaxie des maladies infectieuses dans des ensembles comme écoles, pensions, casernes etc. pourrait contribuer à la prophylaxie des récidives du psoriasis. D'autre part l'exacerbation du psoriasis n'est due que dans 20% de cas à l'infection, ce qui nous interdit de maximaliser le rôle des infections. D'autres facteurs (climatique, psychique, alimentaire, toxique etc.) doivent être pris en considération et examinés et leur rôle respectif expliqué.

Antiovulatorios en el tratamiento del acné juvenil

M. Ahumada, L. Neumann y E. Ortega, Centro Médico "La Raza",
Mexico D. F. (Mexico)

Parece hoy totalmente admitido que los factores patogénicos fundamentales del acné vulgar juvenil son la hiperplasia de las glándulas sebáceas y la excesiva queratinización del ostium folicular [1, 2, 8 a 11], a los que pueden añadirse otros factores (siempre secundarios), tales como la infección y la inflamación [9, 10].

El predominio de uno u otro factor patogénico fundamental da origen a los diferentes tipos clínicos de acné (papuloso, pustuloso, quístico, etc.) [1].

La hipersecreción sebácea que se observa en el acné juvenil, se debe a que bajo el estímulo hormonal se activa la división mitótica de las células basales de la glándula. La presencia de esta hipersecresión en la pubertad, es prueba de la existencia de una estrecha relación entre la hormonas sexuales, principalmente los andrógenos y las glándulas sebáceas [2, 5 a 7].

Los estudios realizados por Strauss y col. han demostrado con claridad que los estrógenos pueden de hecho, atrofiar las glándulas sebáceas. Sin embargo, las cantidades requeridas para lograr este objeto son seguidas invariablemente de efectos no deseables: ginecomastia y disminución de la líbido en el hombre, hemorragia e irregularidad en el ciclo menstrual en la mujer [12, 13]. Los trastornos menstruales son extremadamente raros cuando se utilizan asociaciones de estrógenos y derivados progestacionales a las dosis habitualmente señaladas como anovulatorios [1, 2, 4, 14].

Así se ha generalizado el tratamiento del acné con productos hormonales en pacientes del sexo femenino y puede decirse que con su empleo se logran buenos resultados sin el inconveniente de las alteraciones menstruales [1, 2, 3, 6].

Material y Metodo

Se eligieron 74 mujeres entre 14 y 30 años de edad que presentaban acné juvenil. La mayoría (62) fueron sometidas previamente, durante períodos que varían de 3 meses a 1 año, a otros tratamientos *No Hormonales*, principalmente dietéticos e higiénicos.

El tratamiento hormonal consistió en administrar 80 microgramos de 3 metil eter de etinil estradiol* del 5 al 25° día del ciclo menstrual, agregando 1.0 miligramos de 6-cloro — 6-dehidro 17 acetoxi progesterona 21 acetato** del 16 al 25° día del mismo ciclo bajo el método secuencial llamado 11 + 10, durante un período de 8 a 12 ciclos consecutivos.

El tratamiento hormonal se instituyó como único tratamiento del acné y se mantuvo ciclo tras ciclo consecutivamente, hasta lograr la mejoría objetiva y subjetiva. Después se prolongó durante un ciclo más y se suspendió, recomendando a nuestras pacientes solamente aseo local con jabón neutro, una vez al día. Nunca combinamos ningún otro tratamiento ni dieta durante la administración del tratamiento hormonal secuencial.

Todas las pacientes fueron revisadas clínicamente durante los períodos de sangrado-menstrual (o del sangrado por deprivación).

Durante la revisión clínica, se registró el efecto de los tratamientos sobre la sintomatología del padecimiento y sobre el ciclo menstrual, así como los efectos colaterales.

Resultados

En el cuadro 1 se observaron las características clínicas de nuestras 74 pacientes de 14 a 30 años de edad; el tiempo de evolución del acné juvenil fue de 53.6 meses (con extremos de 3 a 120 meses); 15 de ellas presentaban acné grado I, 33 en grado II, 10 en grado III y 16 en grado IV.

---

* Mestranol-Syntex.
** Acetato de Clormadinona-Syntex.

Cuadro 1. *Caracteristicas clinicas*

Numero de casos	Edad (Años)	Tiempo de evolucion del padecimiento	Acné juvenil		Area corporal afectado (%)	Padecimientos concomitantes	(Casos)
			Grado	No. de pacientes			
74	14 a 30	3 a 120 meses	I	15	10—30	Obesidad	11
			II	33		Pre-diabetes (Tolerancia a la glucosa)	6
			III	10		Alopecia difusa	5
			IV	16		Psoriasis en placas	1
Promedios: 23 años		53.6 meses			16%		

Como promedio el 16 por ciento (10 a 30%) del área corporal estaba afectada por el padecimiento que se asentaba en las zonas corporales habituales: cara, pecho y espalda.

La obesidad (más del 30% sobre el peso ideal de acuerdo con la edad y la estatura) fué el padecimiento concomitante mas frecuente en nuestro grupo (11 casos), seguida por Pre-diabetes (6 casos) diagnosticada con pruebas de tolerancia a la glucosa y Alopecia difusa (5 casos), un caso presentaba Psoriasis en placas.

Cuadro 2. *Tratamiento anterior (no hormonal)*

Tratamiento (S) Empleado (S)	No. de casos	Duracion del tratamiento	Mejoria obtenida	Promedio %
1. Dieta 1500 calorias baja en CHO y Lípidos. Higiene local con jabón neutro	32	3—12 meses	15—50	26
2. Antibióticos Sistémicos	15	8—30 días	30—50	40
3. Lociones astringentes y queratolíticas	8	3—12 meses	30—60	40
4. Vitamina A.	5	30—60 días	7—20	15
5. Sedantes Nerviosos	2	15—60 días	5—15	10

Antes de iniciar el tratamiento hormonal secuencial (11 + 10) con Acetato de Clormadinona y Mestranol, 62 pacientes habían sido sometidas a diferentes tratamientos No Hormonales, durante períodos de 15 días a 12 meses. De estas, 32 pacientes habían recibido dieta hipocalórica (1500 calorías), pobre en grasas y carbohidratos durante 3 a 12 meses, y habían obtenido mejorías del 15 al 50% que en promedio fue de 26%; otras 15 enfermas fueron sometidas a tratamiento con antibióticos sistémicos a dosis bajas (Tetraciclina 500 mg/día) obteniendo una mejoría de 30 a 50% con promedio de 40%. Este mismo índice de mejoría (40%) se obtuvo en 8 pacientes que habían recibido lociones astringentes y queratolíticas. En 5 pacientes a las que administramos Vitamina A durante 4 a 8 semanas, la mejoría fue de solo 15% y en 2 pacientes que recibieron solamente sedantes nerviosos, la mejoría fue del 10%.

En el cuadro 3 hemos hecho un resumen de los resultados que se obtuvieron en estas mismas pacientes de acné cuando recibieron tratamiento hormonal secuencial (11 + 10) como única terapéutica, en comparación con la mejoría obtenida con los diferentes tratamientos previos No Hormonales. Como se puede observar, se aumentó el grupo con 12 pacientes de nuevo ingreso que nunca habían recibido ningún tratamiento para su padecimiento.

Para calificar la mejoría, se delimitó una área de 2 cm cuadrados en la zona más afectada por el padecimiento y se contó el número de elementos dermatológicos presentes, anotando la observación en hojas especiales de evolución individual que fueron tabuladas al final del experimento.

Durante las consultas períodicas, ignoramos cualquier mejoría sobre el estado del padecimiento al iniciar el tratamiento que significara menos del 50%. A partir de este momento, registramos cualquier mejoría por pequeña que fuera.

Para facilitar la apreciación, hemos calculado el promedio de mejoría por grupo integrado el promedio al número entero más inmediato, superior o inferior (ejemplo: 8.7 = 90 ó 8.3 = 80).

El grupo que presentaba acné grado I, logró un 50% de mejoría, promedio en el tercer ciclo de tratamiento hormonal secuencial 11 + 10 y a partir de ese momento, el progreso fue notable y rápido. En el VII ciclo de tratamiento, todas las pacientes habían mejorado 100%. El tratamiento se suspendió en todas las pacientes al terminar el ciclo VIII.

El grupo que presentaba acné grado II, alcanzó un 50% de mejoría en el IV ciclo. Sin embargo, todas las pacientes, al igual que en el grupo anterior, alcanzaron 100% de mejoría en el ciclo VII y para el ciclo VIII todas suspendieron el tratamiento.

Algunas de nuestras pacientes, con acné grados III y IV, alcanzaron 100% de mejoría. Sin embargo, los grupos solo alcanzaron un promedio de 90% en XII ciclos de tratamiento, mejoría que ya se había logrado en algunos casos en el ciclo IX y X respectivamente.

En el cuadro 4, hemos resumido la evolución de los principales síntomas, objetivo que presentaban nuestras pacientes, anotando en cada casilla el número de casos que presentaban el síntoma, en orden descendiente.

La seborrea desapareció en la mayoría de las pacientes mas rápidamente que los comedones y éstos, con más rapidez que las pápulas y las pústulas. Los abscesos,

Cuadro 3. *Tratamiento hormonal secuencial*

Grado de Acné	N° de Casos	Promedio de Mejoría (%) Obtenida con Tratamientos No Hormonales	Ciclos de Tratamiento (Promedio de Mejoria en %)											
			I	II	III	IV	V	VI	VII	VIII	IX	X	XI	XII
I	15	30 (5—60)			50	70	80	90	100	100				
II	33	20 (5—40)				50	60	80	100	100				
III	10	10 (0—20)							70	80	90	90	90	90
IV	16	5 (0—10)							50	70	80	90	90	90

La mejoria fué calificada contando el N° de lesiones existentes que desaparecieron, y la aparición de nuevas lesiones en una area de 2 cm² en la zona mas afectada al iniciar la observación.

aunque solo lo presentaron 23 casos al iniciar el tratamiento, fue uno de los síntomas más rebeldes y esta observación es quizá la indicación para agregar antibióticos sistémicos en los pacientes que presentan estos elementos. Como es natural,
aumentó el número de pacientes con cicatrices residuales.

Cuadro 4. *Evolución de la sintomatología*

	Antes de iniciar el Tratamiento Hormonal Secuencial	Numero de Casos que presentan el Sintoma Ciclos De Tratamiento:											
		I	II	III	IV	V	VI	VII	VIII	IX	X	XI	XII
Seborrea	74	74	74	60	44	15	7	7	7	7	7	7	7
Come-dones	74	74	74	74	69	61	54	26	26	19	7	7	7
Papulas	74	74	74	67	60	45	33	21	18	5	2	0	
Pustulas	62	62	62	62	62	60	53	34	22	18	7	7	2
Eritema	39	39	30	25	20	15	8	8	6	4	0		
Absesos	23	23	23	23	23	20	20	19	16	13	8	3	3
Quistes	21	21	21	21	21	21	21	18	14	10	8	8	8
Costras	10	9	6	5	3	0							
Cicatrices	40	40	40	42	47	49	52	58	58	59	61	61	61

Cuadro 5. *Ritmo menstrual*

Duración del Ciclo	Antes	Durante el tratamiento Hormonal Secuencial			
		En el Ciclo III	En el Ciclo VI	En el Ciclo IX	En el Ciclo XII
menos de (<) 25 dias	11	4	4	1	
25—35 dias	18	40	38	19	21
mas de (>) 35 dias	32	22	26	4	3
Irregular	13	8	6	2	2
Dismenorrea	54	16	6	0	3

Las observaciones sobre el ritmo menstrual y la dismenorrea que registramos
en el cuadro 5, indica la frecuencia con que las pacientes de acné presentan
alteraciones de la función del aparato reproductor.

Más de la mitad de nuestras pacientes, 45 casos, presentaban ciclos de más de
35 días o eran irregulares, 11 pacientes tenían ciclos de 24 días o menos y solamente
18 de ellas tenían ciclos que se pueden considerar normales (25 a 35 días).

Al examinar este parámetro en el ciclo III, encontramos que el número de
pacientes con ciclos normales se había duplicado (40 casos) y esta situación se
mantuvo en los ciclos VI, IX y XII, aunque en estos dos últimus, el número total
de pacientes es menor, ya que todos los casos con acné grados I y II habían
suspendido el tratamiento.

Casi dos terceras partes del grupo de enfermas (54 casos) presentaban dismenorrea al iniciar la terapia hormonal secuencial 11 + 10. En el ciclo III el
número se había reducido a una quinta parte de las pacientes del grupo y para el
ciclo VI solamente 6 pacientes presentaban al síndrome, lo que indica que el 90%
de las pacientes de dismenorrea se benefician con este tipo de terapia. Ninguno de
nuestros casos presentó dismenorrea en el ciclo IX, pero si se presentó en 3 pacientes en el ciclo XII.

Conclusiones

El tratamiento hormonal secuencial 11 + 10 con 80 microgramos de Mestranol del 5° al 25° día del ciclo, más un miligramo de Acetato de Clormadinona del día 16° al 25° del mismo ciclo, es más efectivo por si solo para el tratamiento del acné juvenil que los tratamientos 1 y 3 *No Hormonales*, utilizados por nosotros en 40 mujeres jóvenes con acné juvenil.

No consideramos de valor comparativo en este estudio, la experiencia previa con los tratamientos 2, 4, 5 en 22 pacientes, ya que el tiempo de tratamiento *No Hormonal* fue muy corto.

La efectividad de la terapia hormonal secuencial 11 + 10 no se ve influenciada por la más o menos cronicidad del acné juvenil, pero si está en relación directa con el grado del padecimiento.

Se confirma en la clínica la hipótesis experimental de otros autores que la administración de estrógenos es de primordial importancia en el tratamiento del acné para suprimir la hiperplasia glandular y la consiguiente hipersecreción sebácea y que el agregar compuestos progestacionales impide los efectos indeseables en las pacientes del sexo femenino con acné [1, 2, 4, 14].

En nuestras manos, el tratamiento estrogénico del acné es el de elección en las mujeres que presentan el padecimiento. Sin embargo, en los casos con infección agregada, es quizás aconsejable la administración de antibióticos sistémicos para acelerar la mejoría.

En nuestro grupo, la mayoría de las pacientes presentaban alteraciones del ritmo menstrual y dismenorrea. La terapia hormonal secuencial corrigió estas alteraciones en la mayoría de los casos.

Bibliographic References. 1. AHUMADA, P. M.: Rev. Fac. Med. **6 (11)**, 715 (1964). — 2. ANDREWS, W. C.: Fertil. and Steril. **15**, 75 (1964). — 3. BERGER, R. A.: Arch. Derm. **89**, 898 (1964). — 4. BORGLIN, N. E.: Int. J. Fertil. **9**, 17 (1964). — 5. GARCIA, C. R.: Int. J. Fertil. **9**. 95 (1964). — 6. MALKINSON, F. D.: Illinois med. J. **124**, 420 (1963). — 7. SULZBERGER, M. B., and V. H. WITTEN: Med. Clin. N. Amer. **35**, 373 (1951). — 8. STRAUSS, J. S., and P. E. POCHI: Arch. Derm. **86**, 757 (1962). — 9. STRAUSS, J. S., and P. E. POCHI: J. Amer. med. Ass. **190**, 815 (1964). — 10. STRAUSS, J. S., and A. M. KLIGNAN: Arch. Derm. **82**, 779 (1960). — 11. STRAUSS, J. S.: J. clin. Endocr. **21**, 215 (1961). — 12. TORRE, C.: J. Amer. med. Ass. **164**, 1447 (1957). — 13. WALKER, R.: J. Obstet. Gynec. **4**, 83 (1964). — 14. WONSKER, B. A.: Sth. med. J. (Bgham. Ala.) **57**, 917 (1964).

Dermatoses, Nervous System and Psychotic Origin

Dermatoses, système nerveux et psychisme

Dermatosis, sistema nervioso y psiquismo

Die Bedeutung nervöser und psychischer Faktoren für die Entstehung von Hautkrankheiten

Organizer

J. GAY PRIETO, Spain

Presidents

M. M. BOLGERT, France

AD. DUPONT, Belgium

A. KAMINSKY, Argentina

M. E. OBERMAYER, USA

Delegate of the Organization Committee

C. CARRIÉ, Germany

Reports

Haut und Nervensystem in klinischer Sicht

G. W. KORTING, Universitäts-Hautklinik Mainz (Deutschland)

Der bisher lichtoptisch angenommene syncytiale Zusammenhang des peripheren Nervensystems ist zum Teil durch elektronenoptische Untersuchungen in Frage gestellt. Andererseits ist nunmehr elektronenmikroskopisch die Innervation der Talgdrüsen gesichert, was klinisch z. B. für die Annahme einer kontinuierlich-nervalen Genese des „Salbengesichtes" bedeutsam ist. Grundsätzlich ist aber das vegetative Gesamtsystem nerval, hormonal und cellulär regulierbar. Weniger direkt effektorisch erfaßt wird dergestalt hingegen das Bindegewebssystem, wenn wir auch andererseits in der Sklerodermie eine neurovasculär induzierte Verschiebung der Kollagenfraktionen erblicken möchten. Sodann ist klinisch bedeutsam der funktionelle Antagonismus zwischen neurohormonellem und vegetativem System in der Haut: Das erstere dient einerseits der Freisetzung von Aminen, das letztere der Aktivierung katecholaminartiger Anteile (WIEDMANN). Die Hauptbedeutung des vegetativen Nervensystems wurde lange Zeit als wesentlich für die Durchströmungsregulation angesehen. Jedoch hat die Hypothese eines aktiven Vasomotorenspiels der Capillaren der Nachuntersuchung nicht standgehalten (ILLIG). Die Hautgefäße unterstehen vermutlich nur dem Sympathicus: Die Vasoconstriction ist ein direkt gesteuerter Vorgang und die Vasodilatation das Resultat einer Lockerung des vasoconstrictorischen Tonus. Das Sinneserlebnis des Schmerzes als sinnvoller Warner, z. B. von Tumoren, wie etwa dem Glomustumor, dem Leiomyom, manchem Neurinom oder dem ekkrinen Spiradenom, tritt dem Dermatologen nur selten entgegen. Wenig bekannt ist in diesem Zusammenhang das Ortnersche Zeichen, das Kältegefühl am Thorax bei Aortenlues. Zusammenhänge zwischen vegetativem Nervensystem und Immunität werden heute nur insofern für möglich gehalten als eben die Antikörperproduktion von vegetativ-nervösen Einflüssen abhängen könnte, so beispielsweise das Arthussche und Shwartzmansche Phänomen vom sympathischen Nervenstrang (LUKASIAK u. Mitarb.), während umgekehrt eine periphere anaphylaktoide Reaktion Hirngefäße und -parenchym beteiligen kann (ERIKSSON u. SÖDERBERG). Was klinische Sonderbilder angeht, so ist die Feersche Neurose des Kleinkindes als neuroallergische Quecksilberspätreaktion enträtselt und damit weitgehend als morbus sui generis aufgegeben. Bei der sog. familiären Dysautonomie, dem Syndrom von RILEY u. DAY, liegen offenbar hauptsächlich Destruktionen der Substantia reticularis, weniger auch von Hypothalamus und Kleinhirn, sowie funktionelle Störungen im Katecholaminstoffwechsel vor. Als klinische Beispiele für eine periphere neurocutane Symptomatik ist neben der „glossy skin" auf die sklerodermiformen Hautzustände nach peripherer Nervenverletzung oder bei Arbeitern mit Preßluftwerkzeugen hinzuweisen. Ähnliches sieht man aber auch bei der amyotrophischen Lateralsklerose. Im übrigen lassen sich aber bei der circumscripten Sklerodermie die einzelnen Sklerodermiefelder kaum jemals bestimmten spinalen Veränderungen oder röntgenologisch faßbaren Abweichungen zuordnen. Bei der Reflexdystrophie des Schulter-Hand-Syndroms begegnen wir neben vasomotorisch-trophischen Störungen ebenfalls wiederum glatter Atrophie oder subcutaner Sklerose. Angiotrophoneurosen sind als Dekubitalulcerationen, z. B. infolge Bandscheibenläsion, im Nasenflügelbereich als Folge einer Alkoholinjektion in das Ganglion Gasseri, im Fersen- oder Gaumenbereich vor allem bei Tabes dorsalis, Diabetes mellitus, Lepra, weniger auch bei multipler Sklerose und Syringomyelie, geläufig. Die charakteristischen Hautsymptome der

Syringomyelie — succulente Ödeme, warzenförmige Efflorescenzen und torpide Ulcerationen — erwartet man bekanntlich vorzugsweise im Bereich der oberen, die tabetischen Atrophien eher im Bereich der unteren Extremitäten. Vor allem trifft man aber bei dieser Krankheit des Mucius Scaevola auf das sog. „panaris analgésique", also auf eine torpide „dermatologische" Paronychie, vergleichbar etwa dem „panaris mélanique", der Paronychie bei Lues congenita oder Lues I, bei progressiver Sklerodermie oder durch Soor. Wichtig als Pseudo-Syringomyelie ist vor allem die familiäre Akropathia ulceromutilans, das Thévenard-Syndrom. Hinzuweisen wäre sodann noch auf die sog. Hypoglossuszunge und das Karpaltunnelsyndrom. Hemilaterale Hauterscheinungsbilder, wie sie z. B. als bullöse Eruption nach Ictus apoplecticus auftreten können, finden sich z. B. als Hyperhidrose nach Sympathektomie oder als Hemitrichose nach Durchschneidung der Hinterwurzel. Halbseitige chronisch-intermittierende Gesichtsschwellungen können auf eine parasympathische Funktionsstörung im Ganglion pterygopalatinum hindeuten (FEGELER) und einem Melkersson-Rosenthal-Syndrom ähneln. Posttraumatischvegetativ kann auch ein Naevus flammeus im Trigeminusgebiet auftreten (FEGELER), während die hemifaciale lokale Panatrophie ja schon seit 1846 als v. Rombergsche Krankheit bekannt ist. Offenbar abhängig von zentralen Faktoren und nicht seitenbeschränkt im Gesichtsbereich sind alsdann das sog. periorale Syndrom nach FISCHER-BRÜGGE und SUNDER-PLASSMANN, als Ausdruck gesicherter bulbopontiner oder mesencephaler Beeinträchtigung (z. B. nach cerebraler Myelographie). Blickdiagnostisch wichtig sind sodann der postencephalitische braune Stirnring und das Herthogesche Augenbrauenzeichen als endokrin-vegetativ gesteuertes Syndrom (Myxödem, Thallium, Lues II, endogenes Ekzem). Damit kommen wir zu den sog. Lähr-Sölderschen Linien, die den lateralen Brauenbezirk dem 3. Segmentbereich zuordnen, bzw. zu der Schmetterlingslokalisation mancher Dermatosen (Scharlachgesicht, Typus rusticanus, Lupus erythematodes, Rosacea, aber auch endogenes Ekzem). Jedoch lassen sich ansonsten Ekzemfiguren nur selten einzelnen Dermatosen zuordnen (auffällige Lokalisationsbesonderheiten im Bereich schlaffer Paresen nach Polio, bei Syringomyelie, wiederum bei Schulter-Hand-Syndrom, in einem Ischiasterrain). Besonders sinnfällig und nicht allzu selten sind Ekzemreaktionen bei Schädigung des Nervus cutaneus lateralis, also bei der sog. Meralgia paraesthetica oder in Gestalt der „Dermatitis suboccipitalis", in der sich die besondere neurale Reaktionsfähigkeit der Nackenhaut abzeichnet, bei welcher bei Durchschneidung der 2. Cervicalwurzel die Hautsensibilität völlig ausfällt (WIEHL). Im übrigen sind segmentär ausgebreitete Dermatosen keineswegs selten zu beobachten. Erwähnt seien aus der eigenen Kasuistik der letzten Zeit ein Naevus flammeus oder eine Vitiligo in der Verteilung des Schulter-Hand-Syndroms, M. Recklinghausen und Herpes zoster im selben Segment, Ekzemreaktionen im Bereich eines Tabesgürtels oder auch Arzneiexantheme im Verlauf einer Headschen Zone. Den Paradefall für die Bedeutung segmentaler Reflexvorgänge für die Ausbreitung von Hautkrankheitszuständen stellt jedoch die segmentäre Dermatose schlechthin, der Herpes zoster, wobei die Häufigkeit einer Gürtelrose im Trigeminusbezirk sowie der Segmente C^3 und C^4, der Dermatome des N. phrenicus, insonderheit auf die viscero-cutane Relation hinweisen (HAUSER). Gelegentlich kann auch eine Urticaria spinal-segmentär, z. B. bei Wirbelfrakturen, wenn auch nur kurzfristig, in Erscheinung treten. Hinsichtlich neurocutaner Syntropien sei zunächst auf die dermatologische Randsymptomatik bei der mongoloiden Abartung (einschließlich Alopecia areata, Cheilitis und Lingua scrotalis usw.), auf das Leitsymptom der ichthyosiformen Hautbeschaffenheit bei Oligophrenien verschiedener Genese und nicht zuletzt auf die xerodermische Idiotie von DE SANCTIS und CACCHIONI hingewiesen. Nur kursorischer Erwähnung bedarf in diesem Kreise der

Formenkreis der neurocutanen Systemkrankheiten, wie er von VAN DER HOEVE als Phakomatosen zusammengefaßt wurde. Hervorgekehrt bei der Neurofibromatose Recklinghausen seien hier lediglich die peristatische Beeinflußbarkeit des Phaenotypus, z. B. durch Pubertät oder Schwangerschaft, das Vorkommen reiner Pigmentfälle (Typus Leschke, ,,axillary freckling", CROWE) sowie die Frage der vasculären Neurofibromatose, bei der es sich nach FEYRTER um eine Neurofibromatose der Gefäße selbst, nach REUBI um eine eigentümliche Gefäßkrankheit bei der Neurofibromatose handelt. Wenig bekannt ist auch, daß den Recklinghausen-Kranken — analog der Facies dermatomyositica — ein träumerischer, müder, schläfriger Gesichtsausdruck eignet, wie ihn RILLE eingehend charakterisiert hat. Bei der 2. Phakomatose, dem M. Pringle-Bourneville, ist im Hirnbereich hauptsächlich die Gegend der Basalganglien betroffen, wie aus dem Autopsiebericht über 31 solcher Beobachtungen von REED, NICKEL und CAMPTON hervorgeht. Das Sturge-Weber-Syndrom kennzeichnen cerebrale Jackson-Anfälle, Hemiplegien, Migräne, auch Oligophrenie. Bei der v. Hippel-Lindauschen Krankheit finden sich intrakranielle Gefäßwucherungen. Bei dem Ataxie-Teleangiektasie-Syndrom der belgischen Neurologin LOUIS-BAR beobachtet man darüber hinaus Café-au-lait-Flecke oder andere Pigmentveränderungen. Als 5. Phakomatose führt man neuerdings die multiplen familiär auftretenden Basalzellnaevi mit blastomatösen Erscheinungen am Zentralnervensystem. Als weitere neurocutane Syndrome wären schließlich auch der Ota-Naevus, die Tourainesche centrofaciale Lentiginose (Epilepsie, Oligophrenie, Hemiparese) sowie die Pigmentflecken-Polypose vom Typus Peutz-Jeghers-Klostermann aufzuführen. Aber auch bei der Incontinentia pigmenti finden sich selbst, wenn man das Schrifttum durchgeht, bei ein Drittel der Fälle Little-Symptome, Schwachsinn oder Krämpfe. Als Melanophakomatose finden wir bei der neurocutanen Melanoblastose Touraine neben multiplen Hautpigmentmälern als neurologische Akzente Hydrocephalus, Meningismus, eventuell auch die Kombination mit Neurofibromatose oder Syringomyelie. Schließlich liegen aber bei einer ganzen Reihe klassischer Hautkrankheitszustände bekanntlich bedeutsame Nervenveränderungen vor, wofür exemplarisch nur auf die kennzeichnende Proliferation des vegetativen Endnetzes bei der Prurigo nodularis Hyde, auf die Hautnervenveränderungen bei Pellagra (ROSENTOUL, KORTING) zu erinnern wäre. Aber auch bei der progressiven Sklerodermie liegt bekanntlich eine Reihe sicherlich beachtlicher, und zwar nicht nur zentraler (EEG!), sondern auch periphernervöser Befunde vor (JOHN, ORMEA). Und selbst bei der Akrodermatitis chronica atrophicans ist es — bei aller Würdigung der Transplantationsergebnisse der letzten Zeit — um die Erfassung nervöser Substrate keineswegs ruhig geworden (HOPF: bei 37 von 92 Fällen neurologische Komplikationen). Fernerhin könnte auch in solchem Zusammenhang beim endogenen Ekzem bzw. der Neurodermitis disseminata auf deren vegetativ-dysregulative Struktur eingegangen werden, die das Erscheinungsbildliche bei diesem Leiden als gestaltlichen Ausdruck eines zentral wie peripher vorbereiteten funktionellen Naevus, z. B. in Gestalt einer Oligobradyhidrosis, zentraler hyporegulativer Starre und vor allem einer exquisiten peripheren Tendenz zur Vasoconstriction, interpretieren läßt (Einzelheiten s. bei KORTING). Tierexperimentelle Untersuchungen von HENSEL u. Mitarb. haben bei Kühlungsversuchen des Hypothalamus der Katze eine lineare Funktion zwischen zentraler Reizung und Konstriktion der Hautgefäße ergeben. Angesichts solcher klinisch-nosologischen Eindrücke müssen das äußere Integument und das Nervensystem geradezu als eine funktionell zusammengehörige Gewebsformation erscheinen. So gesehen gehört mithin die Erfassung individualer neurocutaner Wechselwirkungen mit zur vordringlichen Aufgabe ärztlich-diagnostischer Bemühungen.

Structure des fibres amyéliniques du système nerveux cutané *

AD. DUPONT et A. BOURLOND, Clinique Dermatologique de l'Université de Louvain, Hôpital St. Pierre, Louvain (Belgique)

Au cours de nos recherches sur l'innervation cutanée, nous nous sommes attachés à l'analyse des voies amyéliniques. Nous avons pu à l'aide de techniques argentiques ou histochimiques en reconnaitre l'architecture générale mais c'est leur étude au microscope électronique qui nous a permis de comprendre leur structure intime.

Les techniques d'imprégnation au carbonate d'argent ammoniacal font apparaitre à côté des gros troncs nerveux et des terminaisons sensitives des filaments rubanés qui se ramifient et s'anastomosent par endroits en un réseau complexe. Ces filaments sont constitués par une lame protoplasmique renfermant une délicate résille de fines fibrilles argyrophiles et des vacuoles. Dans certains d'entre eux seulement un neurite bien individualisé est reconnaissable. L'absence apparente de celui-ci pourrait être due à l'imperfection des techniques incapables de rendre visibles des éléments trop minces. Ainsi que nous le dirons plus loin, nos recherches en microscopie électronique confirment cette interprétation. La théorie du neurone de Cajal trouve ainsi sa confirmation. Le réseau amyélinique enveloppe étroitement les glandes sudoripares, les muscles lisses, les artérioles et les poils. Quelques éléments semblables s'observent également dans le derme superficiel.

La simplicité et la spécificité des réactions de Gomori en font un procédé de choix pour la mise en évidence des voies amyéliniques dans la mesure où celles-ci sont chargées de cholinestérases. D'autre part, le contraste des images est excellent; il permet même de contrecolorer les coupes. Malheureusement, cette technique n'apporte guère de renseignements quant à la composition intime des fibres car le précipité de sulfure de cuivre s'étale presque uniformément sur toute l'épaisseur des éléments nerveux. L'innervation des glandes sudoripares et des vaisseaux entre autre apparait d'une richesse exceptionnelle. Soulignons l'existence sous l'épiderme de fibres dont l'épaisseur et la distribution sont celles des fibres argyrophiles.

Les méthodes histochimiques proposées pour l'étude des voies adrénergiques se sont entre nos mains avérées décevantes. Leur spécificité et leur sensibilité sont en effet insuffisantes. Le technique de fluorescence de FALCK leur est de loin supérieure bien que sa complexité technique limite son utilisation à des laboratoires bien équipés. Les neurites chargés de catécholamines prennent l'aspect de filaments moniliformes très minces, isolés ou réunis en faisceaux; ils suivent les vaisseaux et les muscles lisses. La fluorescence primaire ou secondaire de divers constituants dermiques est génante; elle ne compromet pas cependant la valeur de la technique.

La microscopie électronique fait apparaitre avec une parfaite netteté la structure intime des fibres amyéliniques. Celles-ci se composent d'un nombre variable de neurites et de cellules schwanniennes. Les neurites, dont le nombre va de deux ou trois à 15 ou 20, sont des cylindres réguliers, disposés en faisceaux parallèles. Ils sont logés dans des replis des cellules schwanniennes de la manière dont le tube digestif est enfermé dans les expansions du péritoine. Ils apparaissent comme suspendus dans un sac dont les parois en s'accolant forment un mésaxone. Ils ne sont donc point inclus dans le protoplasme lemnoblastique comme le laissent supposer les colorations ordinaires. Une membrane basale recouvre le tout; elle ne pénètre pas dans les mésaxones.

Plusieurs unités semblables sont rassemblées dans les petits nerfs dermiques; elles sont séparées par des fibres de réticuline. L'enveloppe périneurale est formée

---

* Chargé de Recherches du Fonds National de la Recherche Scientifique de Belgique.

de plusieurs lamelles cytoplasmiques recouvertes d'une membrane basale et isolées les unes des autres par une trame discrète de réticuline. Il n'existe pas ou il n'existe que de rares fibres myéliniques dans ces troncs nerveux dermiques. Le microscope électronique permet ainsi de comprendre les échecs de la microscopie optique: un nombre relativement élevé d'axones sont rassemblés dans un faible espace et ils ont souvent un diamètre égal ou inférieur au pouvoir de résolution des microscopes ordinaires. De plus, ils sont accompagnés de fibres de réticuline et de membranes

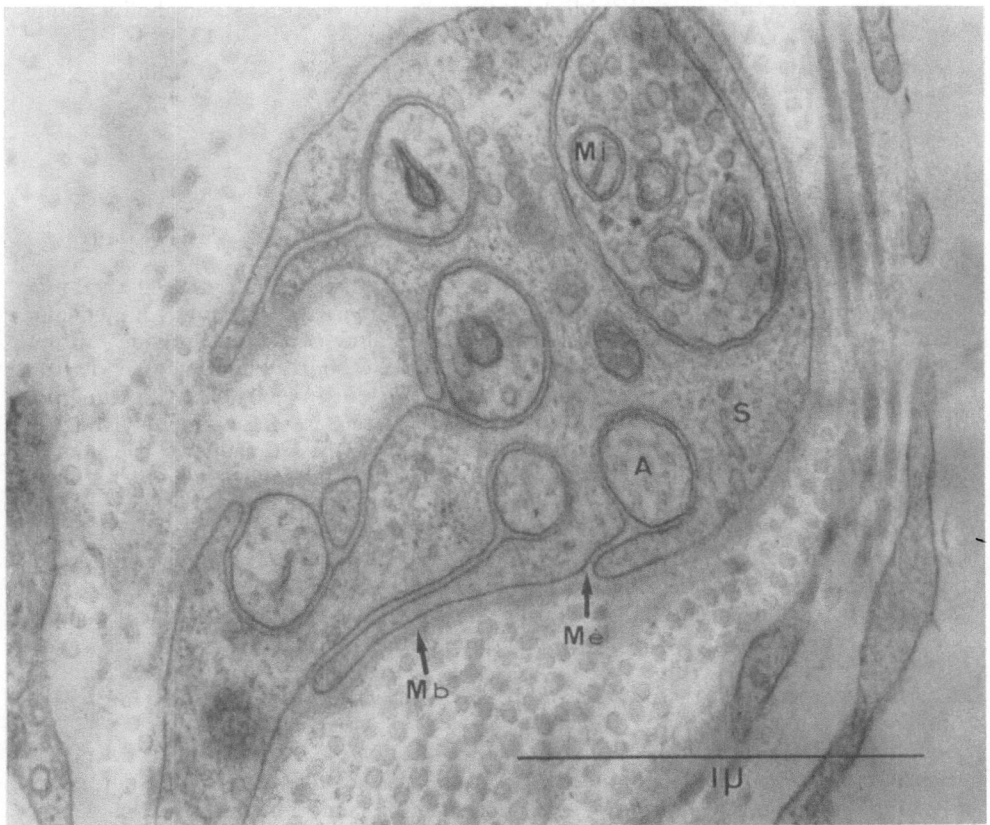

Fig. Fibre amyélinique du derme papillaire comportant six axones (A) de diamètre variable, parfois chargés de mitochondries (Mi); les mésaxones (Mé) sont de longueur inégale. La membrane basale (Mb) apparait nettement tout autour de la cellule schwannienne (S). Il n'existe pas ici de gaine périneurale. ($\times$ 80000; réduit de %)

basales en proportion plus grande qu'on ne l'imaginait autrefois. Les fibres amyéliniques, au voisinage des glandes, des muscles lisses et des vaisseaux perdent leur gaine périneurale et s'appliquent étroitement sur les organes effecteurs. L'analyse détaillée des modalités neuro-effectrices sortirait du cadre de cet exposé. Sous l'épiderme, il existe des unités très grêles, dépourvues souvent d'enveloppe périneurale, ne comptant que deux ou trois axones mais toujours recouvertes d'une membrane basale. Leur disposition permet de les identifier aux fibres argyrophiles et cholinestérase-positives observées au même niveau. Ces fibres, à notre expérience, ne contractent pas de rapports particuliers avec les cellules basales ou avec les mélanocytes; elles ne pénètrent pas dans l'épiderme. Il est intéressant de noter que les fibres dites de TIMOFEEV, voisines des corpuscules tactiles de WAGNER-MEISSNER, présentent le même aspect. On avait admis autrefois que ces fibres amyéliniques sousépithéliales représentaient des voies végétatives; nous croyons plutôt que la majorité est de nature sensitive.

Ainsi donc la microscopie électronique, grâce à son pouvoir de résolution, permet une étude précise des voies amyéliniques. Nul doute que, combinée à des techniques histochimiques, elle permettra d'analyser les modalités des articulations synaptiques végétatives et d'établir la nature sensitive ou végétative, cholinergique ou adrénergique de chaque neurite considéré isolément.

Bibliographie DUPONT, AD.: Arch. belges Derm. 1967 (Sous presse). — BOURLOND, A.: Arch. belges Derm. 1967 (Sous presse).

Dermatologie psychosomatique

P. DE GRACIANSKY et O. DE POLIGNY, Hôpital Saint-Louis, Paris (France)

Un fait frappe d'emblée dans l'approche psychosomatique des sujets atteints de dermatoses: leur réticence à se situer par rapport à la lésion, face au médecin. Par le jeu de mécanismes divers ils ont tendance à éluder tout dialogue mettant en cause la signification de la dermatose. Cette véritable «barrière cutanée» constitue souvent un obstacle infranchissable à la poursuite d'une investigation approfondie. Une première raison de cette résistance est le caractère immédiatement visible de la lésion. Si le malade se tait, c'est que par sa lésion, il a déjà parlé. De plus la dermatose est exposée aux regards donc aux jugements éventuellement malveillants d'autrui: le dialogue risquerait de réveiller les angoisses sociales. D'autre part, la lésion qui constamment se voit, se touche, se sent, se rappelle en permanence à l'attention du sujet et entraîne, de ce fait, une atteinte narcissique particulière qui bloque le sujet sur lui-même, rappelant certains mécanismes des psychoses. Cette double frustration narcissique et sociale surinvestit le pouvoir du médecin dont la guérison est attendue sur un mode quasi magique.

Il a été attribué à la peau de multiples significations qui demandent à être interprétées.

1. La peau participerait à l'*expression des émotions*. En fait, la peau n'exprime rien par elle-même: les phénomènes secrétoires et vasomoteurs qui s'y déroulent ne sont qu'une des composantes périphériques de l'émotion qui envahit la personnalité.

2. La peau représenterait *une frontière avec le milieu extérieur*. En réalité, il n'y a pas un en-dedans et un en-dehors du corps séparés par la peau: seul existe un «corps phénoménal» (MERLEAU PONTY) insérant à chaque instant le corps dans le monde et conférant un sens à l'un et à l'autre.

3. Le peau aurait *un rôle protecteur*. En fait il n'est nullement démontré qu'une manifestation pathologique cutanée puisse être en elle-même un moyen de protection et permette une sorte d'évacuation, dite «décharge d'urgence». Par contre, la peau joue le rôle d'un symbolisme protecteur, car l'enfant, ayant reçu de la Mère des gratifications multiples par l'intermédiaire de la peau, celle-ci s'intègre secondairement à une fonction protectrice, liée à la notion de sécurité conférée par la Mère. Ce symbolisme protecteur peut entrer en conflit avec différentes fonctions érogènes de la peau et avec les différents symbolismes que la personnalité peut ultérieurement conférer aux vêtements.

4. *Le rôle érogène* de la peau est bien connu. Un certain nombre de pulsions: scoptophilie, exhibitionisme, sadisme, masochisme, activités de type masturbatoire, se manifestent au niveau de la peau ou d'une lésion cutanée. Plus importante est la relation de la peau avec les activités auto-érotiques. Celles-ci peuvent impliquer la peau dans le jeu musculaire et la mettre ainsi en liaison avec des structures archaïques (morcellement, pithiatisme, hystérie) ayant ou non un sens pour la personnalité. Le contenu psychologique de ces structures peut avoir ou non, selon les cas, un rapport de sens avec la réalité.

Les classifications des maladies cutanées, vues sous l'angle psychosomatique, qu'elles soient à point de départ dermatologique ou psychologique paraissent artificielles. On peut en effet à propos de chaque dermatose soulever toute la problématique génitale ou prégénitale des sujets. Inversement, à chaque perturbation psychique peuvent correspondre d'innombrables manifestations cutanées. Ni l'une ni l'autre de ces classifications ne tient compte de deux éléments essentiels: la signification que la manifestation cutanée revêt pour la personnalité et d'autre part les bouleversements qui en résultent. En fonction de ces données on peut proposer la classification suivante.

1. *Les dermatoses provoquées* (dermatoses par artéfact, trichotillomanie, onychophagie, etc.) posent le problème du choix de l'organe. La signification de la lésion varie suivant son siège, sa forme et le degré d'atteinte de la personnalité. Dans certains cas la signification est évidente: il s'agit de simulations diverses. Ailleurs, la lésion sert d'exutoire permettant à la personnalité d'exprimer une pulsion partielle, tel l'exhibitionisme ou sa répression érotisée comme parfois dans l'acné excoriée. Dans certaines mutilations la lésion peut avoir une valeur de symbole demandant à être explicitée. Elle peut enfin traduire une tentative destinée à exprimer soit une agressivité (essai d'effraction à l'intérieur du corps pour le supprimer), soit, au contraire, être un mode de défense pour faire exister le corps, notamment dans les cas où un prurit intense lui est associé.

2. *Les «psycho-endodermatoses»* sont caractérisées par le déplacement sur une zone cutanée normale ou à peine atteinte, de tensions intrapsychiques importantes. La peau ou les muqueuses sont l'objet de préoccupations obsédantes sans proportion avec la lésion objective. Elles sont le siège de sensations (gêne, paresthésies, prurit, etc.). Ainsi sont constituées les diverses phobies cutanées somatisant la peur de la mort. L'examen psychologique des sujets retrouve en effet une peur pathologique de la mort plus ou moins camouflée. Les phobies cutanées sont à distinguer des phobies proprement névrotiques classiques, telle la phobie du toucher, la peur de contaminer, la peur des choses sales, etc. où la peau ne s'intègre dans la phobie que d'une manière indirecte par l'acte du toucher, objet de préoccupations obsédantes des sujets. Ces deux types de phobies peuvent s'intriquer chez un même malade. Il importera de préciser pour les principales phobies: phobies des microbes, de la syphilis, du cancer, etc. la part que prend chacun des deux types.

3. *Le prurit*, survenant en peau apparemment saine, ou accompagnant dans certains cas une lésion dermatologique, est, dans son essence un mode de défense pathologique. Il vise à colmater l'angoisse primordiale de morcellement, qui se manifeste à la périphérie, et dont on prouve l'existence par l'étude des phantasmes des malades. Ultérieurement il revêt des significations multiples, dépendant des pulsions diverses et des réactions de la personnalité à l'égard de ces pulsions. Ces significations varient selon le siège du prurit.

4. *Les «psycho-exodermatoses»* comportent par définition la présence d'une lésion dermatologique. Il conviendrait d'abord de préciser si et comment des tensions intra-psychiques, des irruptions pulsionnelles contre lesquelles l'organisme

lutte par des contre-investissements puissants, des émotions supprimées, contenues ou refoulées, peuvent intervenir dans la genèse d'une maladie cutanée. D'autre part, l'apparition de la lésion peut bouleverser la personnalité qui lui confère un sens. La frustration liée à la lésion entraîne un type particulier de régression conduisant le sujet à intérioriser les conflits. La dermatose est impliquée dans ce remaniement structural de la personnalité. Ces bouleversements rendent difficile l'appréciation exacte du traumatisme ayant provoqué la dermatose et l'état antérieur de la personnalité. Le caractère localisé ou généralisé de la dermatose quel qu'en soit le type est un élément important pour la classification.

A. *Dans les psycho-exodermatoses localisées* la lésion permet souvent de saturer les pulsions interdites (exhibitionisme, agressivité, etc.) un certain équilibre se crée ainsi entre la personnalité et la lésion qui peut de ce fait se trouver pérennisée. L'existence de cet équilibre explique l'importance en pareil cas de la résistance cutanée étudiée au début. Ailleurs, comme dans certaines alopécies, apparaissent d'autres causes de difficultés. L'intensité de la frustration et la valeur symbolique de la lésion entraînent de tels bouleversements qu'il devient particulièrement diffic ile d'affirmer la valeur étiologique des éléments psychologiques révélés par l'examen.

B. *Les psycho-exodermatoses généralisées* ont en commun des limitations sociales parfois massives qui grèvent lourdement l'existence des sujets. Lorsque la dermatose apparait dans les premiers mois de l'existence (comme l'eczéma constitutionnel dit atopique) et quelle que soit l'attitude de la mère ou de ses substituts, elle entraine une fixation pathologique à ces derniers. La peau participe directement à la vie affective. Un cercle vicieux peut se créer entre les lésions cutanées et les perturbations psychologiques. Lorsque la dermatose apparait chez l'adulte (comme dans le psoriasis généralisé) son étendue, sa laideur, sa chronicité, provoquent une régression massive de la personnalité qui réinvestit les objets antérieurs, et peut y rester fixée. Dans les deux cas cette fixation rend la personnalité dépendante à l'égard de ces objets ou de leurs substituts dont des gratifications sont attendues d'où la recherche de bénéfices secondaires (hospitalisme, recherche de pension, etc.).

Alteraciones cutáneas con interacción mental

A. KAMINSKY, Profesor Adjunto de Dermatología, Universidad de Buenos Aires (Argentina)

Los correlatores que nos preceden y siguen, han estudiado las relaciones entre sistema nervioso, piel y nervios periféricos, o agotado el estudio de la dermatología psicosomática. Como ya lo establecieron MACLEOD, WITTKÖWER y MARGOLIN, dentro de la metodología psicosomática "se requiere que el investigador establezca fronteras artificiales dentro del campo total de su experiencia observable". Hemos delimitado nuestra frontera a la inter-relación o inter-acción entre enfermedades mentales y cutáneas, y a una clasificación que nos permita ubicar el tema entre agrupaciones conexas. Concretando nuestra investigación, hemos seleccionado algunos de los textos fundamentales dentro de la literatura habitual y vemos que no es excesivo el interés por la proyección cutánea de la psicosis o por los estados mentales relacionados con las dermatosis reactivas.

En su libro "Medicina Psicosomática" WITTKOWER y col., en 1954, dedicaron un capítulo — a cargo de SEITZ — a los aspectos psicológicos de las enfermedades de la piel, y en su clásico tratado de 1953 sobre "Factores Emocionales de las Enfermedades Cutáneas", sobre 203 páginas de texto sólo hay 14 para el capítulo

"Piel y Psicosis". Estas no están incluídas en el libro de Flanders Dunbar sobre "Diagnóstico Psicosomático".

En su tratado "Emociones y Alteraciones Somáticas" el mismo autor incluye ya unas 20 páginas sobre 750 de texto. OBERMAYER, en "Medicina Psicocutánea" — cuya edición española yo he prolongado — reproduce, entre otras, las clasificaciones de LEWIS y CORMIA, la clasificación anatómica de TOURAINE, la de BRANDT, y esencialmente la de SULZBERGER y BAER. OBERMAYER, por su parte, crea tres capítulos: "Dermato-neurosis verdaderas", "Dermatosis en las cuales los factores emocionales constituyen habitualmente un elemento importante" y "Distintas dermatosis con elementos psíquicos". LÓPEZ IBOR, especializado en medicina psicosomática, enfatiza sus dificultades diciendo que "el problema de la causalidad psíquica es demasiado limitado y confuso". Son clásicos los trabajos de BOLGERT y otros autores franceses y de distintas escuelas Europeas. El excelente libro de Psiquiatría de VALLEJO NÁGERA, sobre 1000 páginas es probable que sume dos de ellas como total de manifestaciones cutáneas. Un aporte muy interesante es el de QUIROGA que, en el tomo dedicado al maestro CROSTI, sintetiza la acción de los factores psicógenos en dermatología.

Para nuestro relato hemos reajustado las nomenclaturas de SULZBERGER y BAER, la de QUIROGA y la de OBERMAYER, integrándolas con las dermatosis reactivas con efecto psíquico y las enfermedades mentales con proyección cutánea. Creo que los dermatólogos necesitamos, para mejor comprensión de estos problemas, recordar definiciones ampliatorias: Estamos hablando de dermatosis reactivas, de interacción y de interreacción, de psíquico, de mental, de somático, de vivencia, de psico-emocional, etc.

Reacción. Desde el punto de vista médico es toda acción orgánica que tiende a combatir o detener la influencia de un agente patógeno. La *reacción* en psiquiatría:

a) *Reacción biológica:* es la del cerebro ante los distintos estímulos orgánicos exógenos o endógenos.

Reacción exógena: es la constante presentación de ciertos síndromes psíquicos agudos consecutivamente a la actuación de determinados agentes patógenos externos, en especial toxi-infecciosos. Por toxinas metabólicas que actúan como eslabones intermedios se establece la psicosis: amencia, estupor, delirio, confusión, estado crepuscular, etc. (psicosis traumáticas, tóxicas, sintomáticas, orgánicas).

Reacción endógena: es la que moviliza una psicosis bio-hereditaria genotípica constitucional por la actuación de agentes patógenos externos (esquizofrenia, paranoia, psicosis maníaco-depresiva, epilepsia, oligofrenia).

b) Además de la reacción biológica existe la *reacción psicogenética:* es la desviación de un proceso psicológico de su desarrollo normal, por la intervención de una vivencia que actúa etiológicamente o variando las manifestaciones clínicas del síndrome.

Vivencia — "Hecho de experiencia que con participación consciente o inconsciente del individuo se incorpora a su personalidad".

Psiquiatría — de "psyche" (alma) e "iatreia" (curación), o sea la ciencia que tiene por objeto el estudio de las enfermedades mentales.

Psicosis — Nombre general de las enfermedades mentales.

Enfermedad psíquica — Enfermedad somática con preferente participación cerebral.

Somático — Aplícase a lo que es material o corpóreo en un ser vivo.

Emoción finalmente, es un "estado de ánimo que se caracteriza por una conmoción orgánica consiguiente a sensaciones, ideas o recuerdos, que trae consigo fenómenos viscerales que el sujeto percibe y que se traduce a veces por gestos, actitudes, risa, llanto, etc" (VALLEJO NÁGERA).

Resumiendo, creemos que la inter-acción psíquica, psicosomática, neurológica, emocional y cutánea puede ser esquematizada en las siguientes agrupaciones: 1. Dermatosis psicógenas determinables por factores psicoemocionales; 2. Dermatosis modificables por factores psicoemocionales; 3. Dermatosis por inter-reacción cutáneo-neuro-mental.

En el primer capítulo general tenemos así dermatosis reactivas como respuesta a estímulos que pudiendo ser específicas son en general, inespecíficas, sintomáticas o sindromáticas, pero que tienen como denominador común la posibilidad de una neta relación entre la causa y el efecto. En el segundo grupo se reúnen dermatosis en las que los factores psicoemocionales pueden tener una expresión somática pero que, en general, es cuestionable la inter-relación y reacción entre ambos elementos. Finalmente, la tercera agrupación comprende dermatosis que provocan una respuesta psiconeurológica reactiva, procesos mentales y psico-neurosis que se integran con cuadros cutáneos en algún momento de su evolución y formas de enfermedad psico-neurológica y cutánea que se alternan, coexisten o se integran formando en ocasiones verdaderos círculos patológicos donde la inter-reacción es subcontinua o continua.

Esta revisión de nomenclaturas dermatológicas y psico-neurológicas puede ser, entonces, esquematizada de cierta manera. Enfáticamente establecemos que la única tarea original es de compilación y reajuste. La información corresponde a los autores citados al comienzo con sus clasificaciones respectivas y la mayor parte de lo que corresponde a "Psiquiatría" está parcial o textualmente reproducido del libro de VALLEJO NÁGERA y adaptado a nuestra necesidad didáctica dermatológica.

1. *Dermatosis psicógenas determinables por factores psicoemocionales*

a) *Con respuesta vascular:* 1. Rubor; 2. Palidez; 3. Cianosis; 4. Livedos; 5. Hemorragias.

b) *Con respuesta edematosa predominante:* 1. Urticaria; 2. Edema angioneurótico; 3. Dermografismo.

c) *Con respuesta pigmentaria predominante:* 1. Melanodermias; 2. Leucodermias.

d) *Con respuesta exudativa predominante:* Dermatitis eczematoidea, atópica o por contacto en las que los mediadores químicos desempeñan un papel importante (histamina, acetilcolina, serotonina, etc.).

e) *Con respuesta secretoria o excretoria predominante sudoral: ecrina o apocrina, sebácea, etc.*

f) *Con respuesta pruriginosa predominante:* 1. Prurito y prúrigos; 2. Liquenificación; 3. Neurodermatitis diseminada (influencia de dermatitis atópica).

g) *Con respuesta epidermopoyética predominante (influencia genética:)* 1. Psoriasis; 2. Eczematides o dermatitis seborreicas (influencia del substrato).

h) *Con respuesta pilosa predominante:* 1. Hipertricosis e hirsutismo; 2. Alopecia areata.

2. *Dermatosis modificables por factores psicoemocionales*

a) Acné; b) Liquen ruber plano; c) Herpes simple; d) Herpes zoster; e) Vitiligo; f) Rosácea; g) "oid" dermatitis; h) Con menor intensidad, otras numerosas dermatosis.

3. *Dermatosis por inter-reacción cutáneo-neuro-mental*

a) *Interacción reactiva psico-cutánea con expresión subjetiva:*
1. Alteración de la sensibilidad (anestesia, hiperestesia, disestesia, causalgia).
2. Dermatofobias (cancerofobia, sifilofobia, ácarofobia).

b) *Interacción reactiva psico-cutánea con expresión objetiva:*

1. Dermatomanías (onicofagia, tricotilomanía, titilomanía).
2. Patomimias (excoriaciones neuróticas, dermatosis facticias).
c) *Interacción reactiva psico-cutánea con expresión dermatológica:*
1. Oligofrenia (nevos, vitíligo, gerodermia, flaccidez cutánea, alteraciones de la sensibilidad, mixedema hipotiroideo).
2. Epilepsia (mordeduras, heridas y cicatrices traumáticas, modificaciones del espesor topográfico de la piel, hipoestesias).
3. Psicosis maníaco-depresiva (secuelas cutáneas de traumatismos y autoagresiones, prurito, lesiones de rascado, fenómenos vasomotores, cianosis, acroparestesias; depresión reactiva endógena y exógena, histérica, etc. en manía y melancolía).
4. Síndromes paranoicos (patomimias, tatuajes, etc.).
5. Psicosis esquizofrénicas (pliegues faciales anormales por gesticulación paramímica y paratímica, ecoprexia del "autismo" (lesiones por repetición de movimientos), hiperqueratosis, erosiones, ulceraciones, esfacelos, autolesiones del negativismo: intertrigos, micosis, pliegues del estupor catatónico y de las estereotipias de actitud; alucinaciones cenestésicas con pirodermia, reptación, farmacodermias locales, etc.; trastornos vasomotores: edemas, eritemas y cianosis de los catatónicos y dementes precoces, seborrea fluente facial, hiperhidrosis, bromhidrosis, trastornos tróficos cutáneos, mutilaciones y amputaciones en los obsesivos-impulsivos).
6. Psicosis sintomáticas:
A) Psicosis de las erisipelas cefálicas.
B) Psicosis en la evolución de las enfermedades exantemáticas (tifus).
C) Psicosis de las colagenopatías cutáneo-articulares (lupus eritematoso).
D) Neurosis de ansiedad de los pruritos genitales.
E) Psicosis pelagrosas (según GREGORY hay 7 tipos: neurastenia, demencia estupurosa, amencia, delirium tremens, catatonía, psicosis de angustia y locura maníaco-represiva. MAYER da tres grupos: demencia aguda, amencia y delirio. agudo. Para BABCOCK: mutismo y estupor, tendencia al suicidio y depresión)
F) Psicosis de las porfirias (según BINGEL: angustia, intranquilidad, depresión, tendencia al suicidio, estados confusionales, delirios, psicosis de Korsahov).
G. Psicosis sifilítica (incipientes: hipocondria, sifilofobia, neurastenia; sífilis cerebro-espinal, basilar, vascular cerebral, alucinosis, psicosis tabética, parálisis general, etc.).
7. Psicosis involutivas:
A) Psicosis senil: gerodermia, hiperqueratosis, prurito, prúrigo, lesiones de rascado, patomimias.
B) Demencia arteriosclerótica: parestesias, prurito, excoriaciones, erosiones, ulceraciones, esfacelos.
8. Reacciones psicogenéticas: reacción patomímica patológica, sinistrosis, excoriaciones, erosiones, ulceraciones, esfacelos.
9. Expresiones reactivas más características: encefalitis y herpes simple, psicosis y urticaria, ulceraciones neurotróficas por enfermedades del sistema nervioso central o de los nervios periféricos (siringomielia, polineuritis, traumatismos, tumores, nevos, etc.), manifestaciones mucosas y semimucosas de las enfermedades neuropsíquicas (glosodinia, glosopirosis, lesiones traumáticas, etc.).
10. Psicosis por dermatosis crónicas deformantes (lepra, tuberculosis, esclerosis sistémicas progresivas, psoriasis, lupus eritematoso fijo, micosis profundas, etc.).
11. Enfermedades genéticas o congénitas con proyección psíquica, neurológica y/o cutánea (síndrome de hipoplasia dérmica focal con microcefalia y retardo mental), síndrome de Sturge-Weber (epilepsia, retardo mental, hemiplejía contralateral y angiomatosis encéfalo-facial), síndrome del ganglio geniculado, síndrome de sudor gustatorio, hipertrofia hemifacial o unilateral (retardo mental), etc.,

telangiectasia hemorrágica hereditaria con participación cerebro-espinal, hialinosis de la piel y mucosas con calcificaciones cerebrales y epilepsia, hipertrofia de los edentados, incontinentia pigmenti (40% incluye retardo mental, micro e hidro-cefalia, parálisis y convulsiones), síndrome de Melkersson-Rosenthal, con sintomas neurológicos, neurofibromatosis de Recklinghausen (retardo mental, epilepsia, tu-mores), síndrome de Gorlin (con nevos basocelulares, meduloblastomas, etc.), síndrome de Romberg (con hemiatrofia facial, epilepsia, etc.).

12. Neurosis histéricas, de ansiedad, obsesivas, etc. (signos neurotróficos, ede-mas, eritemas, flictenas hemorrágicas, estigmas), urticarias, hiperhidrosis, quera-tosis pilar, impulsiones, compulsiones y manías con lesiones auto-determinadas.

13. Dermatosis por terapéuticas psiconeurológicas (hidantoína, etc.) y psicosis por terapéuticas dermatológicas (corticoides, etc.).

De este catálogo fragmentario se deduce lo que hemos querido enfatizar en nuestro relato. Las interacciones e inter-reacciones neuro-psíquicas y cutáneas son hechos en plena investigación pero constituyendo una realidad innegable. En lo que respecta a las inter-reacciones cutáneo-mentales afirmamos que su conocimiento y difusión debe motivar trabajos experimentales y de investigación. Siguiendo la comparación de GUY DE CHAULIAC, ese capítulo es como un niño sobre los hombros del gigante psico-cutáneo. Ve lo mismo, pero más allá y con proyecciones de futuro.

Rehabilitation in Dermatologic Therapy

H. M. ROBINSON, Division of Dermatology, University of Maryland, School of Medicine, Baltimore (USA)

Prolonged and disabling illness may be productive of inertia. At times the loss of motivation may be so great that some patients lose the desire to perform any type of gainful occupation, even after restoration to good health. The physician responsible for an individual's medical care, should also be concerned with his eventual retiurn to an employable state. It is frequently necessary to utilize organized rehabilitation procedures to accomplish this objective.

The rehabilitation program has as its objective the assistance of handicapped or injured individuals to achieve physical, social, emotional, and economic inde-pendence. To achieve this goal, there must be collaboration by the members of the rehabilitation unit composed of a physician, clinical psychologist, social worker, and vocational counselor. Through the team approach, the patient will be provided with expert medical care, psychological evaluation, physical restoration and voca-tional counseling. The success of this procedure for a specific individual will depend on the extent to which the handicap can be removed by medical care, the intellec-tual capacity of the patient, his motivation and emotional adjustment to the situation.

The problem of rehabilitation has been neglected by dermatologists but not by other medical specialties. Rehabilitation agencies are doing excellent work in the care of patients with arthritis, cardiac disorders, speech defects, orthopedic dis-orders, neurologic lesions and amputees, but facilities have not been developed for the care of patients with chronic skin eruptions of occupational or non-occupational origin.

An eruption which develops as a result of contact with sensitizing substances or primary irritants may incapacitate the patient for a much longer period of time than the time loss produced by a fractured femur. A cosmetic defect may also be an economic hazard. Dermatologists and other physicians must awaken to the realization that well motivated patients with chronic skin eruptions are better candidates for rehabilitation procedures than many of those afflicted with cerebral palsy, chronic arthritis and other disabling conditions.

Early diagnosis and prompt referral for the institution of rehabilitation procedures lessen the chance of failure. Not all patients are suitable candidates for rehabilitation but prolonged delay in evaluation and institution of proper care frequently mean loss of motivation. Medical care, social service evaluation, psychological studies and vocational guidance can be performed simultaneously. Most patients with cutaneous lesions accepted for rehabilitation procedures can be treated on an out-patient status.

Training in the highly specialized field of rehabilitation should be part of every medical school curriculum. Medical school affiliated hospitals and other medical centers which have good training programs should be encouraged to establish comprehensive rehabilitation centers as part of the training program. A well trained competent dermatologist must be included in such a program and serve as an important part of the medical team. He will not only give expert medical care to patients under his supervision but will be able to dispel the feat and ignorance uniformed persons have regarding cuteanous lesions.

Rehabilitation should be started on the day the diagnosis is made and the nature of the condition carefully explained to the patient. It is especially important to institute the procedures as early as possible in patients who have congenital defects.

The dermatologist who participates in the team approach must have knowledge of the basic principles of rehabilitation and function as part of the unit rather than as an individual. A properly oriented social service worker will determine the patient's socio-economic status. The clinical psychologist will report on the motivation and mental capacity of the patient as well as his peronality traits, academic achievements and aptitude. The vocational counselor will test the patient's aptitude for work and determine his ability to perform skilled, semi-skilled, clerical or service work. The dermatologist will study the condition from all aspects and prescribe the necessary therapy. These studies may require the ancillary services of trained laboratory personnel, a psychiatrist, an internist, or plastic surgeon. The process of rehabilitation must not be deferred until the eruption has been cleared or the lesion removed, but active and intelligent therapy should be continually administered while the patient is being trained to insure his economic independence. The processes of medical care and rehabilitation must integrate to provide the necessary comprehensive service.

The medical criteriae for employability vary to a large extent with the type, location and the extent of the eruption. Extensive lesions may limit the patient's physical ability to function and in such instances it will be necessary to restrict activity until involution of the condition permits the return to work. In many instances, particularly in the case of some recalcitrant eruptions, it will be essential to have the patient perform some type of gainful occupation to avoid the development of inertia. Decisions relative to employability from the medical standpoint will depend on the considered judgement of a competent dermatologist.

At the completion of initial studies on each patient, it is essential that the members of the rehabilitation team hold a conference to compare information. The results of psychological testing, vocational testing, social service studies and the response to medical care, are of value in the determination of future steps to be taken. The information is pooled, digested, and a decision made relative to the course necessary in the rehabilitation of each specific patient. During the follow-up period, this type of staff conference should be repeated periodically to determine the success of the prescribed procedures and to alter methods when necessary.

To initiate a program such as this, it is essential to provide for education in rehabilitation for general practitioners, industrial physicians, industrial clinics, insurance claim agencies, social service departments and other agencies concerned with health and welfare. The purpose of the seminar is to demonstrate that the primary purpose of the rehabilitation effort is to return the patient to a normal way of life and wage earning potential.

Rehabilitation embodies the democratic ideals which assume that each individual is unique, entitled to the right to participate in all aspects of life, and should contribute to society to the fullest extent of his capacity. In the future, the dermatologist must play a greater role in this type of operation.

Witchdoctors and their Ways

C. M. Ross, 303 Medical Centre, Pretoria (South Africa)

I speak as a breaker of idols and as a destroyer of images.

Of all the legends of Africa, there are none more often told, yet further from the truth, than those about witchdoctors. It is my purpose to correct these misconceptions and to present a true picture of the witchdoctor's role, training, methods, remedies and dress. It is a grave mistake to think of him as a power for evil, casting spells on all who cross his path. The word "witch" has unfortunate associations. He is, in fact, a combination of priest, wise man and healer, who opposes and exercises evil spirits and who, by primitive psychotherapy, bolstered up by placebos, attempts to right wrongs and heal the sick brought to him.

To understand his role, you must grasp the African conception that all deaths, except from old age or in battle, are unnatural, and are brought about by disturbed or discontented spirits. The same applies to disease and to such catastrophies as fire, theft, the straying of cattle or the destruction of huts by lightning. The African worships his ancestors, particularly his dead grandparents, and his religion obliges him to offer many sacrifices and tokens of respect to those who have passed away. If he forgets, then the spirits will torment him until the oversight has been corrected. In time of need, traditionally reared Africans turn to their dead as those of other religions turn to God, believing that happy, contented spirits will protect, and unhappy spirits punish them. When disaster befalls them, they take their problem to the witchdoctor, who listens to their story, decides where they have gone wrong, and offers a solution or a cure. In so doing he may choose to present his opinion while in a trance, or confirm it by throwing his set of divining bones. It is perhaps because these techniques are so different from our own that he is thought a charlatan; but is he, when both he and his subjects believe implicitly in what he does, when he has undergone a long and complicated course of instruction to fit him to do it, and when his results suggest that he successfully practises an aspect of psychotherapy we do not utilise or fully understand ?

The Training of a Witchdoctor. Though female witchdoctors are known, most of them are men; the sons, grandsons, and great-grandsons of those who have practised the calling from time immemorial. A diviner-to-be first passes through a stage of mental change, in which he becomes possessed by a spirit. His symptoms during this period closely resemble those of schizophrenia. From being apparently robust and healthy, he becomes delicate, fastidious about food, and given to complaining of pains in various parts of his body. He may have convulsions or enter trancelike states. He will certainly be tormented by vivid dreams. At this stage, he will be taken as a patient to an established witchdoctor. The witchdoctor usually recognises that his patient is suffering from Ukuthwasa, the "witchdoctor's disease", the illness from which all who are to enter the calling must suffer. Having made the diagnosis, the witchdoctor accepts him as both patient and initiate, and treats him without fee. His treatment and training are synonymous and simultaneous, the relationship resembling that of a westernised patient undergoing psychoanalysis. But there the resemblance ends, as in African culture the "cured" patient emerges not only with insight into his own con-

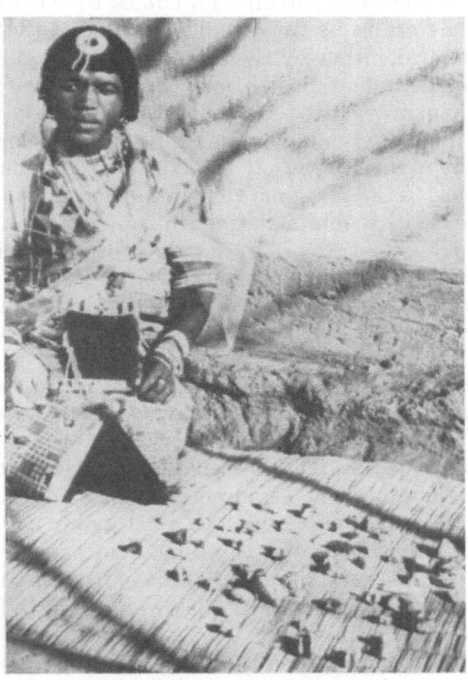

dition, but with the training and knowledge to deal with the problems of others. On his return from treatment, the patient is said to have developed anew, and the words used to describe his return — Uthwasile Ukuthwasa — are also those used for the re-appearance of the new moon. Before he assumes his new role and position, he gives evidence of the knowledge and powers which he has acquired by performing some appropriately impressive supernatural feat. When divining, it is usual for him to enter into a trance. In such a trance he is possessed and guided by his own particular spirit, just as western spiritualist mediums claim to be.

The Technique of Divination. A consultation consists of questions put by the witchdoctor and answers given by the patient or his family. The nature and tone of the answer indicates whether the diviner is "hot" or "cold" on the trail of the solution. When he is "hot", the response is excited, affirmative and spontaneous. When "cold" it is automatic and unenthu-

Fig. A witchdoctor in his exotic costume. He is seated behind a reed mat, on which he has thrown his divining bones

siastic. Gradually, by this method of elimination and deduction, the diviner will learn from his client the reason for his visit, and the suspected cause. Though many clients are fully conscious that it is they themselves who supply the information and diagnosis by the vehemence of their replies, this type of divination is extremely popular, and Africans find strong emotional satisfaction in participating in the consultation; a close resemblance to abreaction.

Not all diviners require assistance from their clients. Some look into bowls of water or crystal balls; others are ventriloquists who possess "talking calabashes"; and some use divining instruments known as Mankgonyane. These, reminiscent of Aaron's rod in the Bible, are manipulated by slight and invisible pressure of the fingers, and made to point to suspects. Such techniques were and are used in trials by ordeal, to put blame on likely culprits; and guilty or not, what chance had they once they had been "found out" by such supernatural and therefore "infallible" methods ?

Once the diagnosis has been made, it is confirmed by the throwing of bones, which also assist in the choice of a remedy. These divining sets, which are shown in this slide, consist of numerous paired bones and other objects. Pairs are used to represent both sexes. Formerly, the two most important pairs of bones were made of ivory. With ivory scarce nowadays, other tusks, bones or hardwood may be used. One side of these bones is plain, and the other is marked with dots or rings. They usually taper toward one end, and the "females" are notched. The other pairs of bones represent the Methopo or totem animals of tribes or clans, and are the astraguli of various small animals. They are kept in a skin bag. When they are used for divining, the person who comes to ask for this service sweeps the ground where they are to be thrown. The ground is then covered with a mat and the bones are thrown, either by the diviner, or, more rarely, by the client. They are held in both hands, elbows down, and thrown forward. The diviner then carefully examines them in order to see the position they have taken. The bones do not always "speak", i.e. give a readable combination. They may have to be thrown repeatedly. When the diviner sees that the bones have fallen into a satisfactory position, he praises that "fall" for some time, and then explains to his client that the bones have confirmed his findings and will now guide his treatment, just as we lean on X-ray plates for support in our diagnoses. He then gives a charm or a medicine to the client, or suggests a sacrifice, and receives a fee from him in exchange. The fee varies according to the service, from a few shillings to a goat or a cow. It is interesting to note that the patients do not go in fear of being punished if they fail to pay; but that they try to pay, for fear that if they don't, the doctor would withdraw the virtue from what he has given them, thus leaving it useless; or that when they next needed him, he would refuse them help.

The Remedies. A great variety of plants, insects and parts of animals are used as remedies. They are usually carried loose in the witchdoctor's bags, although materials such as insects, which would suffer from being knocked about, are wrapped in paper or cloth, or stored in a container such as a small glass bottle, a tin or a matchbox. Prepared medicines in the form of powder or ointment are carried in similar receptacles, or in calabashes. Many of the strongest medicines are used by the witchdoctor on his own person, to fortify and protect him and to ensure his success in practice.

Many doctors possess an undoubted knowledge not only of psychology, but of the medicinal and poisonous effects of plants. Most of their medicines, however, undergo prolonged burning by fire before use, and are so charred that they must presumably work only as placebos, though verification of this generalisation by clinical trial is clearly desirable, and is work on which I am presently engaged.

Ritual Murder. The provision of ingredients for the most powerful remedies had much to do with ritual murders. These ingredients were made from human parts. Due to the hanging of all those tried and found guilty of any connection with such crimes, they are now largely a thing of the past. Such remedies had magical as well as pharmaceutical properties, and their chief function was to create and maintain confidence and relieve anxiety. A man would no longer worry about his health, nor a warrior about his victory in battle, if felt that he had a medicine powerful enough to attain it for him.

Such medicines were kept in the horns or Lenaka of small animals and on being rubbed into incisions made in the skin, conferred their powers on the user. The two chief types were known as Ditlo and Diretlo. Ditlo was made from flesh obtained from enemies killed in warfare, and was used to make warriors fearless. Diretlo was made from the bodies of persons thought to possess specific attributes considered essential for the particular medicine. These persons were killed so that the murderers, by use of the medicine, would themselves acquire these attributes. These were particularly gruesome murders, as the flesh, usually the skin and muscles of the whole face, the penis and breasts, was cut from the victims while they were still alive.

The Witchdoctor's Dress. The witchdoctor's dress is impressive and exotic, and serves an important psychological function in establishing his power and prestige. In many instances, it conforms to a pattern set down to comply with the requirements of the particular spirit which possesses him. The garments are usually buried with the witchdoctor when he dies, so that each initiate has to collect his own set. Where variations occur, some doctors have told me that they were guided in their choice by information given to them by ancestors who appeared to them in dreams, or by their bones. When they are not acting in their professional capacity, witchdoctors are ordinary members of the tribe, ploughing and planting. They do not live a life apart, nor dress differently, but are members of the community, fulfilling when the need arises, a special function dependent upon their special knowledge and training. Like ourselves, they fill this role with a varying measure of success; but unlike us, their art still retains its secrets and its glamour. The Readers' Digest has not yet brought their clients to a position where they may be more up to date than the doctor himself.

Witchdoctors, like medicine itself, require a lifetime of study. Ladies and gentlemen, in the few minutes allotted to me here, I have tried to lift one corner of the veil that surrounds these enigmatic, legendary and fascinating figures.

Free Communications

Some Experimental Observations of Psychosomatic Aspects of Allergic Skin Disorders

K. Higuchi, Department of Dermatology, Kyushu University School of Medicine, Fukuoka (Japan)

Our first experiment dealt with male high school students who were said to develop contagious dermatitis by touching the lacquer tree or the wax tree. A subject was blindholded and a harmless chestnut tree was applied to the right arm and the suggestion was given that this was a wax tree. The left arm was touched with a wax tree with the suggestion that this was a chestnut. Then, 30 min later, no reaction was observed in the arm where a wax tree was applied, while dermatitis appeared on the other arm where a chestnut tree was applied with the suggestion that it was a wax tree. 3 h later, papules on the right arm increased markedly.

In another subject, the extract of the wax tree was applied to the flexor surface of both forearms, telling the subject that the right spot was the extract of the wax tree and the left spot was harmless fluid. 71 h later, flushing and papules appeared only on the right side. On the 6th day the inflammation spread all over the right forearm, and nothing appeared on the left side.

As the final step, we performed the experiment of inducing dermatitis by the conditioning procedure. The raw extract of lacquer tree colored by methylene blue was applied to different spots on the left and right forearms of the subject once daily without explanation as to the nature of the fluid.

The blue color being the conditioning stimulus, the auto-suggestive conditioning was strengthened by repeating this procedure. When such a conditioning was thought to have been built up, the blue-colored control solution was applied on the right forearm. 1 day later, red macules and papules could be seen right under the blue color of the fifth spot (this is control). 4 days later, there appeared small vesicles in this spot. The following day, a crust was formed.

A biopsy specimen was taken from this pathological tissue induced by conditioning. As a control, a biopsy specimen was taken from one spot of the left forearm where dermatitis of almost identical severity was induced by the application of the extract. The comparison between the pathological changes induced by the extract and those induced by the control fluid revealed no essential differences.

According to the comprehensive results of 51 subjects who completed the series of such experiments, in 18 subjects dermatitis was thought to have developed predominantly due to allergic reaction, and that is 35.5% of the total. But as many as 26 subjects, that is 51%, showed no reactions when they did not know that they were touching the noxious trees, and they brought out their reactions only when they were aware of touching those trees, or suggestions were given. The subjects who showed no reactions not only to suggestion but also to the actual contact with the noxious trees of which they were fully aware, numbered 5, that is 13.7%.

These data have led us to envisage the possibility of inhibiting allergic symptoms by eliminating auto-suggestive fear to noxious trees. 13 subjects, who are hypersensitive to these trees and highly suggestible, were chosen for such a therapeutic experiment. They were trained to overcome their fear by being exposed to the threat of noxious trees of gradually increasing degree under completely relaxed condition. After the completion of such a "psychophysiological desensitization", all subjects became non-reactive to the actual contact with those trees.

Basing it upon the same idea, psychosomatic aspects of solar dermatitis have been experimentally studied in several cases. Two typical cases will be demonstrated. The skin pathology of a patient with solar dermatitis was examined after his arm was exposed to sunbeams. This was compared with the pathological finding of his skin, which was induced by waking suggestion that his arm was exposed to sunbeams. There could not be found no essential differences between the two specimens. In the histology of a case of cholinergic urticaria examined after he was given the hypnotic suggestion of being placed in very warm room, definite urticarial changes could be observed.

The above-mentioned "psychophysiological desensitization" is being applied to such allergic skin disorders with considerable success. Results of these experiments suggest that the significance of autosuggestive factors in the course of allergic skin disorders should be re-evaluated.

Psychothérapies et traitements classiques dans les dermatoses psychosomatiques

P. PICHOT et S. LAMBERGEON, Paris (France)

Les dermatoses psychosomatiques, de par leur nature même, posent le problème de la nécessité d'utiliser soit une méthode médicale classique, soit une méthode psychothérapique, soit les deux associées.

Du fait de l'origine psychogène de ces maladies, il serait logique de penser à leur curabilité par des méthodes psychothérapiques. En réalité, ces modes réactionnels de défense que constituent les affections psychosomatiques demandent à être maniés avec extrêmement.de prudence, en dermatologie comme dans les autres domaines de la pathologie, étant donnés les risques de décompensation que peut entraîner une psychothérapie intempestive.

Cette prudence ne doit pas conduire à nier la nécessité d'une approche psychologique de ces dermatoses. Ce serait oublier qu'outre l'action topique des traitements locaux par exemple, et dont l'indication précise est le travail propre du dermatologiste, l'attitude thérapeutique, le «geste thérapeutique» sont déjà un acte psychothérapique qui contient une teinte de réassurance et contribue à gratifier le malade sur le plan psychologique affectif, aussi bien que sur le plan somatique. La «relation malade-médecin» est une relation de dépendance momentanée où le malade s'en remet — provisoirement — à celui qui sait. Cela explique le succès de certaines thérapeutiques classiques quand elles sont appliquées pour la première fois, et leur échec quand elles sont à nouveau utilisées lors d'une poussée ultérieure de la maladie. C'est essentiellement un «effet placebo». Mais nous n'insisterons pas sur l'aspect psychothérapique de l'acte médical classique, qui a déjà fait l'objet de nombreuses études.

Un certain nombre de dermatoses psycho-somatiques ne pourront cependant avoir d'autre traitement efficace que psychothérapique. La *psychothérapie* seule a des indications précises. Elle pourra être proposée dans deux cas:

1. Une dermatose fonctionnelle accompagnant une névrose d'angoisse plus ou moins apparente, et dont elle est le signe principal. Ainsi, *l'Hyperidrose*, fréquente et souvent passagère à l'adolescence (et même dans l'enfance), peut devenir un symptôme primordial, envahissant, inhibant. C'est son caractère de symptôme inhibant qui pourra faire accepter au patient, et même lui faire désirer une psychothérapie. *L'érythème pudique*, lui aussi, et qui s'accompagne toujours d'une névrose d'angoisse, peut envahir le champ de conscience au point de devenir un véritable symptôme phobique, qui doit donc être traité comme tel.

2. *Une névrose phobique* à thème cutané ou capillaire, telle que la peur de la chute des cheveux. Ce sont ces malades, hommes ou femmes, dont la peur d'un symptôme minime, voire d'un état simplement physiologique devient une préoccupation constante, et qui vont de dermatologiste en dermatologiste sans trouver que très passagèrement une accalmie à leur angoisse.

3. Nous ne parlerons pas des *symptômes hallucinatoires*, souvent d'ailleurs non évidents: les parasitophobies sont parfois des phobies simples, mais le plus souvent des délires hallucinatoires qu'au début les malades camouflent plus ou moins consciemment. Ils sont du domaine de la psychiatrie et relèvent d'une thérapeutique psychiatrique; encore faut-il les reconnaître.

4. Les indications de psychothérapie dans les dermatoses psychosomatiques vraies telles le psoriasis sont beaucoup plus délicates. Du fait de la fragilité des mécanismes de défense dans ses maladies, une psychothérapie de type analytique est en général contre-indiquée car elle risque d'entraîner des phénomènes de décompensation. La psychothérapie se sera conseillée que dans les cas où la dermatose accompagne une névrose caractérisée (agoraphobie par exemple). En dehors de ces cas, il sera prudent de s'en tenir aux traitement classiques, associés ou non aux traitements nervins.

Nous en arrivons donc aux cas, où, au traitement local classique devra être associé un psychotrope. Le choix de l'agent chimiothérapique est important, et fait en fonction de la teinte dominante de la structure psychologique; tendance obsessionnelle, dépressive, phobique ou hypocondriaque. Des nombreux psychotropes dont nous disposons, seuls les psycholeptiques et les psychoanaleptiques pourront être utilisés, les psychodysleptiques n'ayant d'indication qu'en psychiatrie pure.

Ce sont essentiellement les neuroleptiques qui sont employés dans les dermatoses psychosomatiques et tout spécialement leur action sur le symptôme prurit qui accompagne nombre de ces dermatoses. Les composés de la chlorpromazine sont maintenant d'utilisation courante en dermatologie, tant pour leur action sur les lésions prurigineuses que pour leur action spécifique dans les maladies telles que la pelade. De nouveaux neuroleptiques peuvent être utilisés, tels que le Levomepromazine (Nozinan), aussi sympatholitique et anti-adrénergique que la chlorpromazine, mais qui présentent certains phénomènes d'intolérance comme la sensibilisation à la lumière au même titre que la chlorpromazine. Les tranquillisants proprement dits sont maintenant d'utilisation courante, trop courante même. Nous ferons une place à part à l'alimémazine ou Théralène dont l'action anti-prurigineuse est bien connue maintenant.

Les psychoanaleptiques sont d'un emploi plus restreint en dermatologie. Nous pouvons assimiler aux anti-dépresseurs l'isoniazide ou Rimifon dont on a pu constater les effet d'excitation euphorique et c'est dans ce sens qu'il a pu être utilisé dans une affection le plus souvent d'étiologie psychosomatique : le lichen plan. Enfin l'imipramine (Tofranil) est souvent utile, à petites doses, chez les petits déprimés et chez les vieillards.

Nous ferons une place à part à l'utilisation de la narco-analyse, que nous considérons comme le traitement spécifique d'un certain nombre de dermatoses psychosomatiques vraies quand la psychothérapie est contre-indiquée et que les traitements classiques et nervins sont insuffisants ou inefficaces. Elles constituent à la fois une chimiothérapie par l'action spécifique de la substance utilisée — (Penthiobarbital sodique par exemple) et une psychothérapie. Grâce à cette double action, il est possible de venir à bout de pelades décalvantes anciennes et rebelles, de lichen plans généralisés ayant résisté aux traitements classiques tant dermatologiques que nervins, de psoriasis ayant épuisé les thérapeutiques courantes, d'eczéma atopiques aggravés par des circonstances émotionnelles traumatisantes, enfin de prurits névropathiques accompagnant les névroses traumatiques en particulier. Bien que de maniement délicat, la narco-analyse reste la thérapeutique de choix en dermatologie psychosomatique.

Lichen ruber planus und Psyche

R. WEITZ und G. VELTMAN, Universitäts-Hautklinik Bonn (Deutschland)

Die Frage nach einer Beziehung zwischen Lichen ruber planus und Psyche ist im Gefolge der Entwicklung der psychosomatischen Medizin wieder mehr in den Vordergrund gerückt. Im folgenden wird versucht, aus einem Vergleich der Lichen ruber planus-Frequenz während der Kriegsjahre mit der Anzahl der Erkrankungsfälle in der Nachkriegs- und Friedenszeit und mit Hilfe einer gezielten Patientenbefragung Rückschlüsse auf die Bedeutung psychischer Einflüsse beim Entstehen des Lichen ruber planus zu ziehen.

Die Ansicht, daß affektive Reize für das Auftreten des Lichen ruber planus allein oder doch wenigstens *hauptverantwortlich* sind, es sich hierbei also um eine „funktionelle Krankheit", eine „Hautneurose" handelt, basiert einmal auf der Anschauung, daß nicht die Hautveränderung juckt, sondern der Juckreiz der Eruption immer vorausgeht und setzt zudem voraus, daß der Übergang von sog.

funktionellen Syndromen in organische Krankheiten möglich ist. Beide Voraussetzungen dürften indessen bis heute nicht mit Sicherheit bewiesen sein, so daß es keinen zuverlässigen Anhaltspunkt dafür gibt, daß der Lichen ruber planus als eine ihrem Wesen nach spezifisch physische Erkrankung eingeordnet werden müßte.

Die psychosomatische Medizin geht demgegenüber von einer multifaktoriellen Aetiologie der entsprechenden Hautleiden aus, d. h. die psychosomatische Erkrankung ist als das Ergebnis des Zusammentreffens mehrerer, unter Umständen auf verschiedener Ebene liegender Faktoren anzusehen. So könnten z. B. psychische Einflüsse für den Ausbruch oder die Abheilung einer Krankheit von Bedeutung sein, der zwar eine somatische Ursache zugrunde liege, deren Aktivierung jedoch durch emotionelle Impulse erleichtert werde.

Für den Lichen ruber planus z. B. wird die Ansicht vertreten, daß an Lichen ruber planus Erkrankte leicht überaus nervöse Menschen mit einer Fehleinstellung zur Umwelt auf Grund von inneren Konflikten, Schwierigkeiten und Hemmungen seien. Statistische Untersuchungen einer Umfrage der Univ.-Hautklinik Bonn bestätigen die Erhebungen der Mayo-Klinik (ALTMANN u. PERRY) und ergeben keinen Anhalt dafür, daß eine nervöse = vegetativ labile Grundstimmung besonders stark ausgeprägt ist. Zudem muß bei derartigen Überlegungen beachtet werden, daß langdauernde und entstellende, ihrem Wesen nach unbekannte Hautveränderungen mit subjektiven Störungen eine psychische Belastung darstellen, die ihren Ausdruck in einer seelischen Fehlhaltung des Patienten finden können.

Schließlich könnte ein Lichen ruber planus im Anschluß an seelische Erregungen (länger dauernde Belastungen des Nervensystems, ungewöhnlich starke und anspannende geistige Anstrengungen, familiäre oder berufliche Sorgen, Ärger, unvorhersehbare, die ganze Persönlichkeit zutiefst erschütternde, schockartige Ereignisse) auftreten, wobei den psychischen Insulten die Funktion eines auslösenden Momentes, etwa im Sinne eines psychogenen Köbner-Effektes bei vorhandenem somatischem Faktor-Lichendisposition, zukäme. Die Zahl dieser zum Teil sehr eindrucksvollen Beobachtungen bildet jedoch — so bestechend sie auch im Einzelfall sein mögen — eine verschwindende Minderheit und ist somit ohne tatsächliche Bedeutung, da sie kaum über das Maß eines zufälligen Zusammentreffens beider Ereignisse hinausgehen dürfte. Auch eine Umfrage bei 76 Lichen ruber planus-Patienten der Univ.-Hautklinik Bonn ergab keine diesbezüglichen Befunde. $63 = 83\%$ der Patienten lebten zur Zeit des Krankheitsbeginnes nach ihren eigenen Angaben in normalen und nur $8 = 10,5\%$ in gespannten und $5 = 6,5\%$ in sehr schwierigen häuslichen und beruflichen Verhältnissen. In den Krankengeschichten der 539 Lichen ruber planus-Kranken von 1939 bis 1963 fand sich lediglich in einem einzigen Fall eine in bezug auf einen psychischen Affekt spontan vorgebrachte positive Anamnese.

Auch während der Kriegsjahre 1914 bis 1918 und der Kriegs- und Notzeit der Jahre 1939 bis 1946 war der Lichen ruber planus mit Sicherheit nicht häufiger als in den Nachkriegsjahren, so daß psychische Faktoren für die Entstehung des Lichen ruber planus kaum angenommen, ja nicht einmal wahrscheinlich gemacht werden können.

41*

A Controlled Experiment in the Psycho-Therapy of Psoriasis

G. H. V. CLARKE and P. J. ASHURST, Manchester and Salford Hospital, Manchester (England)

That psychological factors can bring on psoriasis seems well attested. We are all familiar with patients who develop psoriasis, or become much worse following car accidents, surgical operations, or psychic trauma, such as the surgeon who develops psoriasis when his wife runs away with a butcher!

Can these factors work the other way? Can good fortune bring a cure? Claims have been made for hypnosis and for suggestion. We have heard of cases recovering after an operation and a recurrence being successfully treated by a mock operation with a shallow skin incision. We have had a schizophrenic patient with obstinate psoriasis who was cured by electro-convulsive therapy.

It is necessary to distinguish between those cases where the suggestion of cure is mediated through an operator — either by hypnosis or by the "healing touch", and those brought about by pure suggestion without the intervention of an operator.

In the first experiment an impressive diathermy spark was demonstrated against a metal object and with the electric current then reduced to zero, a patch of psoriasis was outlined by the diathermy probe. This was repeated on the same patch after 2 weeks and once more after a further 2 weeks. The following results were obtained:

14 *cases*
- 2 cases ... All lesions no change
- 3 cases ... All lesions worse
- 4 cases ... All lesions better
- 1 case ... No change at first then all worse
- 1 case ... Worse at first then better
- 2 cases ... Better at first then worse
- 1 case ... No change at first then better.

There was no case in which the treated lesions got better while the untreated remained stationary or got worse.

The second investigation involves pure suggestion without the intervention of an operator. If the patient has had in the past a reliable method of treatment for his psoriasis and one which, from his past experience, he believes will cure his disease, he can be given a similar seeming but placebo treatment. We have such a treatment in Methotrexate. This drug can produce a dramatic result through not infrequently the disease relapses. It was these relapsed cases which were selected for placebo treatment. What happened:

24 *cases*
- 4 cases ... Responded dramatically
- 2 cases ... Responded partially
- 11 cases ... Showed no change
- 5 cases ... Showed a good initial response but relapsed and became worse while still on placebo
- 2 cases ... Became worse

Of ten cases that showed no response to the placebo, eight responded rapidly to a second course of Methotrexate and two more slowly. The four that responded dramatically to the placebo had been of long standing and would seem to prove that "suggestion" is effective.

There is, however, another possible explanation. If psoriasis is a cyclic disease exhibiting a circadian rhythm, waxing and waning, the results of suggestion would depend on which phase of the cycle it is applied. If the disease is waning cure occurs and vice versa. The process may be represented graphically by an harmonic sine wave curve as shown:

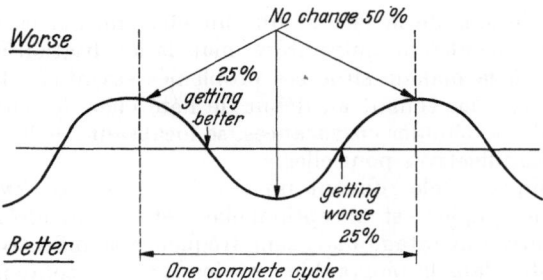

In such a rhythmic disease we would expect the numbers getting better to be balanced by those getting worse and, roughly, double the number to remain stationary — with a cure rate of 25%.

The present series are rather few for statistical validity but the numbers getting better and worse balance in both investigations while in the second the numbers showing no change are roughly double those getting better or worse. The cure rate is 25% which is the usual placebo level. We have to show a greater rate of cure than the placebo effect to prove "suggestion" is operating.

We should then, consider psoriasis a rhythmic disease affected by unknown factors but in which suggestion is not an effective curative agent.

Etude psychologique clinique et paraclinique des psoriasiques

M. SOULE, J. M. PIRET, J. NOEL, G. HUREL et M. BOLGERT, Hôpital St. Louis Paris (France)

Nous nous proposons d'exposer les raisons qui, au cours d'une étude de plus de quinze ans, nous ont convaincus que le psoriasis doit être inclus dans le groupe des affections maintenant classiquement reconnues comme très souvent psychosomatiques, telles que l'asthme ou l'ulcère gastrique.

Les anciens auteurs avaient décrit depuis longtemps l'apparition de poussées psoriasiques à la suite de *vives émotions*, mais ces cas étaient exceptionnels. Vers 1950, l'étude de 108 malades nous montrait que des faits analogues se retrouvaient souvent, pour peu qu'on ne se contentait pas de noter les plus spectaculaires. En 1955, était publié le bilan de l'examen psychologique de 200 psoriasiques, et l'étude de plusieurs centaines d'autres cas s'est poursuivie depuis.

L'examen clinique impose certaines exigences: ambiance adaptée, de préférence en tête à tête, et surtout disponibilité du médecin à prolonger et au besoin répéter l'entretien. Il est pourtant fondamental, permettant seul de découvrir les *coïncidences chronologiques*, évocatrices du caractère psychologique des facteurs déterminant les lésions, qui peuvent se répéter à chaque poussée de la dermatose; de préciser les dynamismes mis en cause par des évènements apparemment anodins, souvent simples changements de situation professionnelle ou familiale. Parfois ceux-ci semblent au premier abord favorables au malade et il faut les replacer dans le contexte biographique pour comprendre leur caractère pathogène. Selon notre expérience, de tels mécanismes psychosomatiques interviennent dans plus de la moitié des cas.

Une fois sur cinq environ, la *localisation* des lésions semble en rapport avec le type de difficultés auxquelles le malade se trouve affronté: *professionnelles* lors des lésions des membres, *sexuelles* lors des lésions génitales, *affectives* au sens large du terme lors des lésions de la face et du cuir chevelu. Certes les conflits sous-jacents sont généralement d'un autre ordre, mais la localisation indique fréquemment le domaine où le malade situe ses problèmes essentiels. De même avons-nous vu plusieurs cas, survenant au début de l'été chez de jeunes femmes préoccupées à l'idée de se dénuder en vacances, se localisant sur les parties du corps particulièrement significatives pour elles.

L'examen clinique révèle souvent un *terrain mental particulier*. L'existence de troubles psychologiques est exceptionnelle, celle de syndrômes névrotiques typiques se rencontre davantage mais sans fréquence significative. Par contre, il est habituel de noter dans la biographie certains types de comportement particuliers quoique non franchement pathologiques. Le plus courant combine la restriction des ambitions et une adaptation sereine à des situations médiocres, avec absence de toute expression d'agressivité. Parfois s'y ajoute une attirance spéciale vers la nature, et certains de ces malades guérissent spontanément au cours des vacances. Ces *structures caractérielles obsessionnelles* sans névrose proprement dite nous paraissent de beaucoup les plus fréquentes. D'autres tableaux peuvent se présenter, l'*anxiété* s'exprimer plus directememt par exemple.

Dès 1955, le RORSCHACH et le *TAT* étaient appliqués à 79 psoriasiques comparativement à 78 atteints d'autres dermatoses et 51 sujets sains. Au RORSCHACH on notait un mode d'aperception dominé par les détails, le fréquent refus d'une planche au moins; des réponses estompages, des réponses anatomiques et des réponses de symétrie beaucoup plus nombreuses que la normale. Le TAT était généralement abordé avec une attitude de critique et de défense contre les planches évitant au sujet de se laisser entrainer aux interprétations et aux fantasmes qu'elles induisent normalement.

Nous avons enfin appliqué récemment à 50 psoriasiques choisis au hasard le *test du MMPI*, choisi pour son objectivité et l'absence d'intervention de l'examinateur. Il est apparu que le groupe différait de la population normale de façon significative à moins de .01 après calcul des t de Student sur divers points: l'élévation des trois notes Pa, Pt et Sc avec maximum en Pt, l'élévation moindre de Dl moindre encore de Pd et accessoirement de Si chez les hommes.

Nous ne pouvons nous étendre ici sur l'interprétation de ces résultats évoquant ceux des psychiasthéniques sans leur être pourtant superposables. Il nous paraît en tout cas remarquable qu'un groupe constitué sur le seul critère de la présence du psoriasis se révèle significativement différencié par ce test.

Bibliographie. BOLGERT, M., et M. SOULÉ: Sem. Hôp. Paris 51, 1251 (1955); — Théories psychogènes du psoriasis; hypothèses; arguments cliniques. Sem. Hôp. Paris 31, 1261 (1955). — NOEL, J., M. SOULE et M. BOLGERT: Sem. Hôp. Paris 31, 1267 (1955). — PIRET, J. M., G. HUREL et M. BOLGERT: Bull. Soc. franç. Derm. Syph. 1967 (Sous presse).

Genetic Neurological Disorders of Choreoathetosis and Cerebellar Ataxia with Important Dermatological Findings

W. B. REED, University of California, Medical School, Los Angeles, California (USA)

A dermatologic consultation is necessary for many genetic neurologic disorders, particularly those that demonstrate cerebellar ataxia and choreoathetosis. Most of these disorders are comparatively rare, with an autosomal recessive inheritance pattern, and they are often not cited in the standard dermatologic texts.

Choreoathetosis results from a dysfunction of the basal ganglia, while ataxia is sometimes cerebellar in origin. However, these two neurologic signs are usually closely associated (table).

Disorder	Cerebellar Ataxia	Choreo-athetosis	Inheritance
1. Ataxia-telangiectasia	Yes.	Yes	Autosomal recessive
2. Xerodermic Idiocy of de Sanctis and Cacchione	No	Yes	Autosomal recessive
3. Cockayne's syndrome	Yes	Yes	Autosomal recessive
4. Juvenile gout with choreoathetosis	No	Yes	Sex-linked
5. Refsum's disease	Yes	No	Autosomal recessive
6. Myoclonic Epilepsy of Unverricht and Lundborg	Yes	Yes	Autosomal recessive
7. Hartnup disease	Yes	No	Autosomal recessive
8. Phenylketonuria	No	Yes	Autosomal recessive
9. Wilson's disease (hepatolenticular degeneration)	No	Yes	Autosomal recessive
10. Hallervorden-Spatz syndrome	No	Yes	Autosomal recessive
11. Albinism (CROSS-McKUSICK)	No	Yes	Autosomal recessive

Ataxia-Telangiectasia

The cardial features of ataxia-telangiectasia are progressive cerebellar ataxia beginning in infancy, progressive telangiectasia beginning on the exposed bulbar conjunctiva, tendency to sino-pulmonary infections leading to bronchiectasis, apraxia of eye movements simulating ophthalmoplegia, and high familial incidence [1, 2].

Other less striking features are unusual facial and postural attitudes, variable choreo-athetoid or tic-like movements, occasional myoclonic jerks, cerebellar speech, drooling, internal strabismus, and growth retardation. Although mental deficiency is not a feature of the early stages of the disease, the I.Q. scores invariably drop below normal levels as the disease progresses.

Autopsy findings indicate that more than half of the patients with this disorder die from chronic pulmonary disease, while most of the remainder die from lympho-reticular malignancies [1, 3].

The cutaneous telangiectasia is first noted in the ears, across the butterfly area of the face and bridge of the nose and peri-orbitally. With increasing age the face becomes more involved with extension to the neck, dorsa of the hands and feet, and in the antecubital and popliteal areas. The pattern of the telangiectasia suggests that the areas of greatest sun exposure are the most affected. The ears become inelastic and the skin of the face becomes hidebound, similar to scleroderma.

In a study of 22 patients, cafe-au-lait spots were seen in four and areas of depigmentation (partial albinism) were noted in eight [4]. In some of the older patients sclerodermatous changes were present. Cutaneous malignancies were found in patients over 21 years of age. Patients with ataxia-telangiectasia have poor resistance to skin infections, whether it is of bacterial, viral or fungal origin. Typical atopic dermatitis was noted in two patients and nummular eczema in another.

Several authors [5, 6, 7, 8, 9] have demonstrated a deficiency of immune globulin-A in patients with ataxia-telangiectasia, suggesting that these patients may lack the ability to cope with infections. At autopsy, an absence or hypoplasia of the thymus has been noted, but other lymphatic structures including the spleen may be reduced. Contact sensititazion is reduced in these patients, indicating a further immunological defect.

Recent autopsies [10] have revealed severe degeneration of the cerebellar cortex and loss of myelinated nerve fibers in the posterior columns of the spinal cord. However, examination of the peripheral nervous system also revealed degenerative changes in the posterior root and autonomic ganglia. In addition, degenerative changes were noted in the liver, lungs, pancreas and the pituitary; these changes were similar to those seen with vitamin E deficiency in animals and with congenital biliary atresia in man.

Xerodermic Idiocy of de Sanctis and Cacchione

De Sanctis and Cacchione [11] described three brothers with idiocy, xeroderma pigmentosum, testicular hypoplasia, and retarded skeletal development. The postmortem examination of one revealed grossly a small brain and microscopically gliosis and loss of neurons in the frontal and temporal cortex. None had epilepsy. Elsasser and associates [12] noted that 41 of the 286 patients reported with xeroderma pigmentosum up to 1949 had evidence of mental and growth deficiencies. Among their 20 patients, Larmande and Timsit [13] found a 60 to 80% definite incidence of mental deficiency, stunted growth, and electroencephalographic irregularities. Nearly all the reported patients have demonstrated the clinical picture first observed by De Sanctis and Cacchione [14].

1. Xeroderma pigmentosum, sun sensitivity, and early development of cutaneous malignancies (before the age of three, in two of my patients).

2. Microcephaly with progressive mental deterioration (usually mental deficiency and spastic paralysis).

3. Gonadal underdevelopment.

4. Dwarfism, delay in bone maturation and congenital deformities.

5. Recessive inheritance.

6. Increased incidence of abortions in mothers.

Cockayne's Syndrome

Cockayne's syndrome has so far been described only in English patients. Mac Donald and assoc. [15] summarized the features as a clinical onset in the second year of life after a normal infancy, dwarfism with kyphosis and ankylosis, disproportionately long extremities, long hands and feet, lipodystrophy of the face, mental deficiency, light sensitivity, retinitis pigmentosa, partial deafness, cerebellar ataxia, cyanotic extremities and carious teeth. This is a relentleessly progressive neurological disorder, and terminally the patients are blind, deaf and paralyzed. Neuropathologically there is cerebral and cerebellar atrophy with secondary enlargement of the ventricles. Microscopically there is a loss of neurons through the brain [16]. There is a dermatitis on the sun-exposed parts of the body. "butterfly area" of the face is the most severely involved, suggesting a picture of lupus erythematosus.

Familial Gout with Choreoathetosis

The juvenile gout syndrome occurs in young males who have a persistent hyperuricemia without other signs of clinical gout. They have an athetoid cerebral palsy, usually appearing in the first month of life [17, 18, 19]. Self-mutilation of the face, particularly the lower lip, and of the hands is a prominent feature, and these patients often must be restrained. There is increased urinary uric acid excretion, and increased uric acid pool and an increased incorporation of labeled glycine into uric acid when given intravenously. Two uricosuric drugs, probenecid and allopurinol, easily reduce the serum uric acid levels, and this is often reflected clinically by less irritability and self-destruction. However, I have observed mentally disturbed patients with similar destructive tendencies who had normal uric acid levels. The disorder appears to have a sex-linked inheritance.

Heredopathia Atactica Polyneuritiformis (Refsum's Disease)

In 1949 REFSUM and assoc. [20] described a disorder in Norway in which ichthyosis may be an important part. These patients, not mentally deficient, have a progressive disease characterized by a hypertrophic polyneuritis involving the motor and sensory nerves, retinitis pigmentosa, cerebellar ataxia, nonspecific EKG changes, and nerve deafness. There are also skeletal abnormalities [20, 21, 22]. The protein content of the cerebrospinal fluid is increased, with an albumino-cytologic dissociation. An abnormal fatty acid, linked perhaps to the metabolism of cholesterol, has been found in the serum and body tissues of these patients [22], and may be the cause of the ichthyosis. The ichthyosis develops in mid-childhood at the same time as the peripheral neuropathy. The inheritance is autosomal recessive.

Myoclonic Epilepsy of UNVERRICHT *and* LUNDBORG

The onset of this disorder occurs between 6 and 13 years of age, and is charac-terized by progressively severe convulsions. Later mental deficiency, dementia and cerebellar ataxia develop. Abnormal deposits of acid muco-polysaccharides have been demonstrated in the central nervous system, retina, cardiac muscle and liver [23]. A patient with this disorder was found to have papules and nodules behind both ears, as well as indurated thickened skin on both forearms. A biopsy revealed large amounts of acid mucopolysaccharides [24].

Hartnup Disease

This autoxomal recessive disorder is named after a family in which four of eight children had a hereditary pellagra-like skin rash aggravated by sunlight, a temporary cerebellar ataxia, slight to moderate mental deficiency and a charac-teristic aminoaciduria [25]. These children were the result of a first cousin marriage. One of the patients reported by the HALVORSENS [26] had premature graying of the hair. The metabolic defect apparently lies in the transport of tryptophan in the proximal renal tubules, and possibly across the cells of the jejunum [27].

Phenylketonuria (PKU)

This is probably the most common metabolic disorder found among patients in mental institutions. Phenylketonuria is characterized by mental deficiency, epilepsy and skin changes, primarily decreased pigmentation. This is particuarly striking amont Japanese patients, who have brown hair instead of black. Part-ington noted that six of 36 patients had generalized infantile eczema between the first and fourth months of life. Five other children in his study had dry skin with repeated nonspecific rashes. Sunlight sensitivity is often a problem, and some patients become highly sensitized to the phenothiazine compounds. Early detec-tion of PKU is being widely stressed, since the early institution of diets low in phenylalanine may decrease the brain damage. These patients cannot convert phenylalanine to tyrosine, resulting in abnormally high serum levels of this compound, which progressively results in destruction of cerebral cells. There is no abnormality in the metabolism of tyrosine [28]. One can promote pigmentation in patients with PKU. If these individuals are given increased amounts of tryosine in the diet or if phenylalanine is decreased, more tyrosine is converged to melanin and their hair and skin become darker [29].

Pigmentation Disorders

Increased skin pigmentation has been noted with various intracranial disorders (encephalitis, schizophrenia, Fanconi syndrome, Schilder's disease). It has also been noted in WILSON's hepatolenticular degeneration, a disorder of copper metabolism, and in Hallervorden-Spatz syndrome, a disorder of iron metabolism in the brain. The pigmentation has perhaps resulted from an increase in the melanocyte-stimulating hormone, but in WILSON's disease and Hallervorden-Spatz syndromes, perhaps also from the faulty control of the involved cations [30]. CROSS, McKUSICK and BREEN [31] recently described three living siblings with mental deficiency, spastic diplegia, cutaneous hyperpigmentation and multiple ocular anomalies. They had slow writhing movements of the hands and fingers. Conspicuously, cerebellar signs were absent. The children were members of an inbred Amish family, and the inheritance is autosomal recessive.

References. 1. BODERÍ E.í and R. P. SEDGWICK: Univ. Southern Calif. Med. Bull. **9,** 15 (1957). — 2. BODER, E., and R. P. SEDGWICK: Pediatrics **21,** 526 (1958). — 3. BODER, E., and R. P. SEDGWICK: Little Club Clin. Develop. Med. 8, 110 (1963). — 4. REED, W. B., W. L. EPSTEIN, E. BODER, and R. P. SEDGWICK: J. Amer. med. Ass. **1955,** 746 (1966). — 5. PETERSON, R. D. A., W. D. KELLY, and R. A. GOOD: Lancet **1964 I,** 1189. — 6. FIREMAN, P., BOESMAN, and D. GITLIN: Lancet **1964 I,** 1193. — 7. YOUNG, R. R., K. F. AUSTEN, and W. H. MOSER: Medicine (Baltimore) **43,** 423 (1964). — 8. EISEN, A. H.: New Engl. J. Med. **272,** 18 (1965). — 9. ROSENTHAL, I. R., A. S. MARKOWITZ, and R. MEDENIS: Amer. J. Dis. Child. **110,** 69 (1965). — 10. SOLITAIRE, G. B., and V. F. LOPEZ: Neurology (Minneap.) **17,** 23 (1967). — 11. DE SANCTIS, C., and A. CACCHIONE: Riv. sper. Freniat **56,** 269 (1932). — 12. ELSASSER, G., O. FREUSBERG, and F. THEML: Arch. Derm. Syph. (Chic.) **188,** 651 (1955). — 13. LARMANDE, A., and E. TIMSIT: Acta. XVII Concil Ophthal. (1954), **3,** 1643 (1955). — 14. REED, W. B., S. B. MAY, and W. R. NICKEL: Arch. Derm. **91,** 224 (1965). — 15. MAC DONALD, W. B., K. D. FITCH, and T. C. LEWIS: Pediatrics **25,** 997 (1960). — 16. PADDISON, R. M.: Derm. Tropica **2,** 195 (1964). — 17. LESCH, M., and W. L. NYHAN: Amer. J. Med. **36,** 561 (1964). — 18. HOEFNAGEL, D.: J. ment. Defic. Res. **9,** 69 (1965). — 19. MICHENER, W. M.: Amer. J. Dis. Child. **113,** 195 (1967). — 20. REFSUM, S., L. SALOMONSEN, and M. SKATVEDT: J. Pediat. **35,** 335 (1949). — 21. ARDOUIN, M.: Bull. Soc. franç. Ophtal. **76,** 137 (1963). — 22. DEREUX, J.: Rev. neurol. **109,** 599 (1963). — 23. HARRIMAN, D. G., and J. H. MILLAR: Brain **78,** 325 (1955). — 24. MEDVED, A., W. C. PETERSON, and R. U. JOHNSON: Arch. Derm. **95,** 206 (1967). — 25. BARON, D. N.: Lancet **1956, II,** 421. — 26. HALVORSEN, K., and S. HALVORSEN: Pediatrics **31,** 29 (1963). — 27. SCRIVNER, R. C.: New Engl. J. Med. **273,** 530 (1965). — 28. JERVIS, G. A.: Proc. Soc. exp. Biol. (N.Y.) **82,** 514 (1953). — 29. HASSEN, C. W., and L. A. BRUNSTING: Arch. Derm. **79,** 458 (1959). — 30. DERBES, V. J., G. FLEMING, and S. W. BECKER jr.: Arch. Derm. **72,** 13 (1955). — 31. CROSS, H. E., V. A. McKUSICK, and W. BREEN: J. Pediat. **70,** 398 (1967).

Segmentale Innervation und Hautkrankheiten

W. HAUSER, Universitäts-Hautklinik Bonn (Deutschland)

Für die Lokalisation und Pathogenese zahlreicher Dermatosen sind segmental-reflektorische Vorgänge von entscheidender Bedeutung. Es handelt sich dabei vornehmlich um viscero-cutane Reflexe, die von chronisch alterierten oder erkrankten Visceralorganen verursacht werden und zu vasomotorischen Irritationen in den segmental zugeordneten Dermatomen führen. So zeigen Headsche Zonen Abblassung oder Cyanose (HANSEN), Verstärkung des Dermographismus, der Histaminquaddel und der Kantharidenblase sowie Herabsetzung der Capillarresistenz. Es ist naheliegend, daß solche segmental-reflektorischen vasomotorischen Alterationen für die Pathogenese von Dermatosen von Bedeutung sind. GOTTRON hat gezeigt, daß ein peristatischer Zustand der terminalen Strombahn mit Strömungsverlangsamung Voraussetzung für die Manifestation verschiedenster Hautkrankheiten ist. In Headschen Zonen finden sich solche Alterationen der Endstrombahn. Es ist daher zu erwarten, daß sich viele Prozesse an der Haut in Headschen Zonen und damit segmental gebunden manifestieren. Dies kann in eigenen Untersuchungen bestätigt werden.

Für die folgenden Ausführungen ist wesentlich, daß man die Topographie der Segmente und die segmentale Zuordnung der Visceralorgane kennt. Dabei sind besonders die Dermatome C 3, 4 im Hals-Schultergürtelbereich zu beachten. Sie können als Hautprojektionsfelder des N. phrenicus reflektorische Impulse nicht nur von Thorakalorganen, sondern auch von Bauch-, vornehmlich Oberbauchorganen erhalten. Daraus erklärt sich bei vielen Dermatosen der häufige Befall des Halses und Schultergürtelbereiches. Dies ist um so eindrucksvoller, als zwischen C 4 und Th 2 eine Hiatuslinie besteht. Die dazwischenliegenden Segmente C 5 bis Th 2 finden sich nicht am Stamm, sondern an den Armen. *Hiatuslinien* sind von besonderem Interesse: Sie können Begrenzung von Krankheitsprozessen darstellen, oder in ihnen können sich Dermatosen in striärer Form manifestieren (z. B. Lichen striatus). Da sich in die phrenicuszugehörigen Dermatome von den verschiedensten Visceralorganen Reflexe projizieren können, wird die Hals-Schultergürtelregion besonders häufig reflektorisch irritiert und damit auch von Dermatosen besonders häufig betroffen. Ähnliches gilt für das Ausbreitungsgebiet der ersten Äste des N. trigeminus. Auch dieses kann erfahrungsgemäß von den verschiedensten Visceralorganen reflektorisch irritiert werden.

Im folgenden sei auf eigene Beobachtungen von Dermatosen mit segmentalreflektorischer Bindung hingewiesen. Aus Zeitgründen kann auf Herpes zoster und Typhus abdominalis nicht eingegangen werden. Ich verweise auf meine diesbezüglichen Publikationen.

Von weiteren Krankheitsbildern soll nun ein Teil erörtert werden:

Urticaria: In C 3,4, also an Hals und Schultergürtelgegend lokalisiert, z. B. bei *Asthma bronchiale.* Manifestation in den dem Uterus zugeordneten Dermatomen an Unterbauch und Oberschenkelinnenseiten bei *gynäkologischen Prozessen* einschließlich *Gravidität.*

Schwangerschaftsdermatosen: Impetigo herpetiformis oder *Herpes gestationis* sind bevorzugt in Hautarealen lokalisiert, die auch den Lumbalsegmenten zugeordnet sind. Die Lokalisation an Unterbauch und Oberschenkeln ist zwar bekannt, jedoch ist diese bislang nicht unter segmental-reflektorischer Sicht gedeutet worden.

Basaliome: Beobachtung mit Manifestation in C 4 rechts bei vorhergegangener rechtsseitiger Lungentuberkulose ($2^1/_2$ Jahre Pneumothorax rechts). Ausbreitung von medial nach lateral unter Respektierung der Hiatuslinie C 4/Th 2. Basaliome in oberen Lumbalsegmenten bei gynäkologischer Anamnese wurden von mir wiederholt beobachtet. *Häufigste Manifestation von Basaliomen sind im Gesicht die oberen zwei Drittel. Es handelt sich dabei weitgehend um die Ausbreitungsgebiete der ersten Äste des N. trigeminus oder um Projektionsfelder vom Trigeminuskerngebiet aus.* Für die Manifestation des Basalioms hat übrigens NÖDL auf die Bedeutung neurovaculärer Störungen in der Endstrombahn hingewiesen. Seine Auffassung wird durch die eigenen Untersuchungen bestätigt.

Pityriasis versicolor: Maßgeblich sind auch hier segmental-reflektorische Vorgänge mit bevorzugter Lokalisation im Bereich von C 3,4 (Hals-Schultergürtelbereich). Nach chronischen Krankheitsprozessen oder deren Folgezuständen an Thorax- und Bauchorganen ist zu fahnden.

Soormykose: Eigene Beobachtung mit exquisit segmentaler Zuordnung bei einem Mediastinaltumor und einem Soorbefall des Darmes sei als Beispiel für die segmental-reflektorische Bindung von Dermatosen angeführt.

Sog. Reticulosarkomatose Gottron: Auch hier konnte bei eigenen Beobachtungen eine auffällige Bindung an die ersten Äste des N. trigeminus sowie an C 3,4 oder anderweitige dermatomgebundene Zuordnung zu Visceralorganprozessen beobachtet werden.

Dermatomyositis: Haut- und Muskelveränderungen zeigen eine bemerkenswerte segmentale Bindung. Hierzu einige Beispiele: Die *pelerinenartige Anordnung* der Hautveränderungen im Hals-Schultergürtelbereich entspricht den Dermatomen C 3,4, also den Hautprojektionsfeldern des N.phrenicus. Von hier aus deszendieren die Hauterscheinungen auf die Außenseiten der Arme. Dies entspricht den benachbarten Dermatomen C 5, 6, 7, 8.

Für die Muskulatur gilt Analoges: Zunächst ist der Schultergürtel betroffen, später der Arm. Diese sind alle cervical versorgt, ebenso wie Zwerchfell und Herz, so daß deren Mitbeteiligung aus segmental-reflektorischer Sicht durchaus verständlich ist. Wenn im Gesicht primär Stirn, *Ober*lider, Nase und vorderer Anteil des behaarten Kopfes betroffen werden, so entspricht dies wiederum dem Ausbreitungsgebiet der ersten Trigeminusäste. Auch schmetterlingsförmige zentrofaciale Anordnung der Erytheme kommt vor. Diese ist reflektorisch über das Trigeminuskerngebiet erklärbar. Die Dermatomyositis ist auf Grund der segmentalen Bindungen nur als Zweitkrankheit bei einem Grundleiden verständlich. Dieses bedingt reflektorisch segmental gebundene peristatische Kreislaufstörungen und damit hypoxämische degenerative Schäden der anliegenden Gewebe. *Dabei liegt also ein viscero-cutanes und in gleichen Segmenten sich abspielendes visceromuskuläres Reflexgeschehen zugrunde, das durch unterschiedliche viscerale Prozesse (Tumor, entzündliche Prozesse) bedingt wird.*

Die dargestellten Beispiele zeigen durch Erkennung segmentalreflektorischer Vorgänge bei der Manifestation von Dermatosen ein bislang nicht beachtetes Prinzip der Pathogenese von Hautkrankheiten.

Literatur. HAUSER, W.: Fortschr. Med. 85, 571 (1967). — Z. Haut- u. Geschl. Kr. 1968 (Im Druck). Dort Abbildungen zu dem Referat und weitere Literaturangaben.

Untersuchungen über den Zustand des vegetativen Nervensystems bei Urticaria-Kranken

St. CHLEBAROV, Kinderkrankenhaus Seehospiz „Kaiserin-Friedrich", Norderney (Deutschland)

Ausgehend von der Tatsache, daß bei der Urticaria oft Funktionsstörungen des vegetativen Nervensystems vorliegen, haben wir bei 155 an Urticaria leidenden Männern mittels der titrierenden Mediaphorese mit steigenden Verdünnungen von Adrenalin- und Acetylcholinlösung die Reagibilität der Hautvasomotorenfunktion und damit den Zustand des Sympathicus (S-R) und Parasympathicus (P-R) festgestellt. Hierbei ergaben sich vier Gruppen — mit Hypersympathose (S-Gruppe = 105), Hyperparasympathose (P-Gruppe = 21), mit normaler Reagibilität (N-Gruppe = 26) und Hyperreagibilität beider Teile des VNS (SP-Gruppe = 3).

Am stärksten war das mittlere Alter (21 bis 50) von der Krankheit betroffen.

Auch das Aussehen der Quaddeln ist je nach der Gruppe verschieden. Bei den extremen Fällen der S-Gruppe sind sie blaß, bei Patienten mit deutlicher Hyperparasympathose erythematös, wo mittlere Titer vorliegen, zeigen sie meist eine livide Farbnuance.

In der S- und N-Gruppe finden wir bei über 70% der Kranken einen chronischen, bei 62% der P-Gruppe einen akuten Verlauf (Krankheitsdauer bis zu 3 Monaten) vor. Diese Ergebnisse veranlassen uns zu wiederholen, daß die chronische und typisch neurogen verlaufende Urticaria einen sympathicomimetischen Mechanismus hat, während die antigenbedingte in der Mehrzahl der Fälle akut verläuft und eine parasympathicomimetische Organisation besitzt.

Die meisten Kranken leiden an der unbestimmten Form der Urticaria. Die Kombination mit Oedema Quincke fanden wir am häufigsten in der S-Gruppe (35 Fälle = 22,5%) oder bei insgesamt 48 Fällen (31%, verteilt auf alle Gruppen). Die durch physikalische Faktoren hervorgerufene Urticaria ist ebenfalls nur in der S-Gruppe vorzufinden. Bei etwa 45% war der erste provozierende Faktor nicht feststellbar, bei den übrigen 55% wurden verschiedene Ursachen eruiert. Am häufigsten waren hierbei die Nahrungsmittelallergene, die jedoch nach der Chronifizierung als Reizfaktoren zu betrachten sind, auf die der Kranke mit einer urticariellen Reaktion antwortet. Epicutan-, Intracutan- und Pricktestungen haben uns nur selten zum tatsächlichen ätiologischen Agens geführt.

Das Suchen nach bakteriellen oder parasitären Foci ist dagegen von großer Bedeutung. In der S-Gruppe fanden wir bei 49 von 74 untersuchten Patienten einen oder mehrere Fokalherde, in der P-Gruppe bei 12 von 16 und in der N-Gruppe bei 11 von 18 Probanden. Alle drei Patienten der SP-Gruppe zeigten das Vorliegen eines Focus. Der Antistreptolysintiter war bei 12 von 62 Fällen positiv. Von den insgesamt 85 untersuchten Patienten waren bei 15 (17,5%) Wurmeier vorhanden. Es muß auf die geringe Anzahl der positiven Ergebnisse in der S-Gruppe hingewiesen werden.

Mit Hilfe der titrierenden Histaminophorese haben wir bei 127 Patienten die Histaminreagibilität (H-R) der Haut festgestellt und sie mit der neurovegetativen Reagibilität derselben verglichen. In der S-Gruppe sind die Titer der H-R verhältnismäßig niedrig im Gegensatz zur P-Gruppe, wo sie in Richtung der höheren Werte verschoben sind und parallel zur P-R verlaufen. Dieser parallele Verlauf der H-R zur P-R findet sich auch in der N- und SP-Gruppe.

Den Übergang von der antigenbedingten (akuten) in die neurogenbedingte (chronische) Form der Urticaria erklären wir uns durch das Bestehen des Mechanismus der somatovegetativen Engraphie, bei der das vegetative Nervensystem Spuren von früher provozierten Reaktionen beibehält. Gleichzeitig beginnt die engraphierte Reaktion sich unter vollkommen unspezifischen Reizen zu entwickeln. Der Kranke beginnt auf Reize, die keinerlei antigenen Charakter mehr besitzen, mit dem klinischen Bild einer Urticaria zu reagieren. Die entscheidende Rolle der somatovegetativen Engraphie bei der Polyallergisierung und Chronifizierung der Urticaria ist als Verlust der spezifischen Signalwirkung der Antigene zu betrachten.

Die Behandlung bestand in dem Versuch, durch Beeinflussung der neurovegetativen Reaktionslage in einer oder der anderen Richtung mit der Veränderung der Ausgangswerte auch eine Besserung der Erkrankung zu erzielen.

Bei den Kranken mit erhöhter S-R wandten wir hauptsächlich eine sympathicolytische Therapie mit Ergotamin und Rimifon, 1 bis 3 Monate lang, neben der Herdsanierung an. Die Behandlung der P-Gruppe bezweckte eine parasympathicolytische bzw. antiallergische Wirkung durch Calcium gluconicum je eine Ampulle à 10 cm³ i.v. und i.m. (gleichzeitig) morgens und abends (vier Ampullen in 24 Std) + Vitamin C oder manchmal durch Antihistaminica oder Sandosten-Calcium in Kombination mit Extr. belladonnae 0,01 + Ephedrin 0,02 und Pepton 0,5, dreimal täglich. Die Kranken der N-Gruppe behandelten wir mit Sympathicolytica bzw. Parasympathicolytica. Von den drei Kranken der SP-Gruppe führten wir bei einem eine sympathicolytische, bei einem anderen eine antiparasitäre Behandlung erfolgreich durch.

Durch diese vorwiegend sympathicolytische oder parasympathicolytische Behandlung wurde die neurovegetative Reagibilität der Haut in Richtung Norm verschoben, was wir bei 54 Kranken objektiv nachweisen konnten.

Abschließend erlauben wir uns, eine Ergänzung und Präzisierung der Nomenklatur der Urticaria vorzuschlagen. Wir würden diejenige Form der Erkrankung, die in die S-Gruppe eingeordnet wurde, einen mehr oder weniger chronischen Verlauf und eine Art von unspezifischer Überempfindlichkeit aufweist sowie einen adrenergischen Mechanismus besitzt, als *Urticaria atopica* oder *adrenergische Urticaria* und jene, die der extremen P-Gruppe angehört, einen überwiegend akuten Verlauf aufweist, spezifisch monoallergisch ist und einen cholinergischen Mechanismus besitzt, als *Urticaria allergica* oder *cholinergische Urticaria* bezeichnen.

Neuropsychiatric Manifestations in Xeroderma Pigmentosum

M. S. ABDEL GAWAD, Dept. of Psychiatry, and
H. EL-HEFNAWI, Dept. of Dermatology, Cairo University (UAR)

The correlation between the skin lesion in Xeroderma Pigmentosum and the neuropsychiatric manifestations present in some cases has been studied in 33 patients.

The following abnormalities were detected on clinical neurological examination. Familial choreiform tremors, defective speech and stuttering were present in two siblings. Familial deaf-mutism in one patient. Residual facial palsy with fine tremors of facial muscles in another patient. Eight patients had eye complications interfering with visual perception, the eye is embryologically a bud of nervous tissue.

Electroencephalography (E.E.G.) was done for 30 patients. Definite abnormalities were detected in four cases and mild changes were present in further six cases.

Psychometric studies using the Progressive Matrices, the Porteus Maze and the Seguin Form Board as well as the clinical assessment of intellectual capacity was carried out. The results showed that 33% of cases studied were mentally subnormal and 18% were mentally dull and backward. In the general population, the incidence rate is 1% and 3% respectively. It appears that mental subnormality is almost an integral part of the Xeroderma Pigmentosum Syndrome (X.D.P.) since it was manifested in one degree or the other in approximately 50% of the x.d.p. patients in contrast to 4% of the general population. None of the 33 cases studied, however, suffered from mental deficiency amounting to idiocy. Thus, our results do not substantiate the postulation of DE SANCTIS and CACCHIONE of "Xerodermic Idiocy".

The correlation between severity of the skin lesion and the neuropsychiatric abnormalities in x.d.p. has not yet been thoroughly investigated. In syphilis, it appears, however, that individuals and races who develop a sharp primary and secondary reaction to the infection are less likely to develop neurosyphilis than those who react less severely. Thus, in syphilis a negative correlation exists between the severity of skin lesion and that of the nervous system. In the present investigation we tried to find whether the same observation holds true in x.d.p. by studying the correlation between the degree of skin atrophy and the severity of neuropsychiatric manifestations. Analysis of the results showed that a positive correlation seems to exist between the degree of skin atrophy and the severity of mental subnormality. Thus, 65% of patients who are intellectualy below average (Grades IV & V) suffer from a moderate or severe degree of skin atrophy, while 40% only of those who are above average in intellectual capacity (Grade II) and 54% of patients with average intellectual capacity (Grade III) are similarly affected.

Equally well, a positive correlation seems also to exist between the degree of skin atrophy and the severity of E.E.G. abnormality. Thus, 75% of the patients with definite E.E.G. abnormality suffer from a moderate or severe degree of skin atrophy, while 52% only of those with normal E.E.G. and 65% of patients whose E.E.G. show mild abnormality are similarly affected.

We are of the same opinion as DE SANCTIS and CACCIONE that in the Xeroderma Pigmentosum Syndrome, changes in both skin and brain might be due to a congenital defect of the ectodermal tissue. We believe that the variation in the clinical picture could, however, be attributed to variation in the degree of gene penetration or manifestation.

The discrepancy in response of the skin and nervous system which are of the same embryological origin may be attributed to the nature of the etiological factor whether it is an exogenous infection as in syphilis or a genetically determined abnormality as in x.d.p.

Andrology (Masculine Impotence and Sterility)

Andrologie (impuissance et stérilité masculines)

Andrología (impotencia y esterilidad masculinas)

Andrologie (Impotenz und Sterilität des Mannes)

Organizer*

C. G. SCHIRREN, Germany

Presidents

R. CERNEA, Italy

R. ELIASSON, Sweden

K. LEJMAN, Poland

O. STEENO, Belgium

Delegate of the Organization Committee

J. HARTUNG, Germany

---

* Chairmann during the session: C. SCHIRREN, Hamburg

Experimental Andrology

Reports

Biochemische Untersuchungen an Spermaplasma unter Berücksichtigung des Prostaglandins und seiner klinischen Bedeutung

R. ELIASSON, Physiologisches Institut, Karolinska Institutet, Stockholm (Schweden)

Biochemische Analysen der *Samenflüssigkeit* können wertvolle Auskünfte über die funktionelle Kapazität der männlichen akzessorischen Geschlechtsdrüsen geben. Da die Sekretion dieser Drüsen direkt von der Produktion männlicher Geschlechtshormone in den Testikeln abhängig ist, gibt die Zusammensetzung der Samenflüssigkeit ein gutes Bild von der Androgeneinsonderung. Wertvolle Beiträge zum Verständnis dieser Zusammenhänge sind von deutschen Forschern wie NOWAKOWSKI, DOEPFMER und SCHIRREN (s. KIMMIG et al., 1967; MANN, 1967) geliefert worden.

In unserem Fertilitätslaboratorium im Karolinska Institutet, Stockholm, haben wir uns besonders für die Funktion der männlichen Geschlechtsdrüsen unter normalen und pathologischen Bedingungen interessiert. Ich werde mich auf zwei Fragestellungen beschränken, nämlich:

1. biochemische Veränderungen im Zusammenhang mit Erkrankungen in Prostata und Samenbläschen;

2. den Zusammenhang zwischen der Produktion von Fructose und Prostaglandin in den Samenbläschen.

Die Patienten, um die es hier geht, sind alle von einem erfahrenen Urologen, Dr. GÖSTA LEANDER, Stockholm, untersucht worden, und in den meisten Fällen liegen bakteriologische und cytologische Analysen von ausgepreßtem Prostatasekret der Patienten vor. Die Diagnose „bakterieller Prostatit" hat stets eine positive Bakterienzüchtung und spezifische cytologische Veränderungen erfordert. Die cytologischen Untersuchungen sind von Dr. E. JOHANNISSON durchgeführt worden. Die biochemischen Analysen umfassen saure Phosphatase, Cholesterol, Zink und Milchsäurendehydrogenase (aus der Prostata) und Fructose (aus den Samenbläschen).

Eine Biochemie gilt als normal, wenn die Fructose mehr als oder gleich 150 mg/100 ml, die saure Phosphatase mehr als oder gleich 20000 IE/ml und Cholesterol mehr als oder gleich 30 mg/100 ml beträgt.

17 Patienten mit akuter oder chronischer bakterieller Prostatitis zeigten, mit zwei Ausnahmen, ein stark pathologisches biochemisches Muster sowie in 85% auch ein stark pathologisches Spermiogram. Die zwei Patienten mit der normalen Biochemie waren die einzigen mit Gonokokken im Prostatasekret.

Von den 32 Patienten, deren Prostatitis als klinisch ausgeheilt angesehen wurde, zeigten etwa die Hälfte eine Biochemie mit pathologischen Werten, wenn die Beobachtungszeit kürzer als 1 Jahr war, während keiner der neun Patienten mit einer längeren Beobachtungszeit als 2 Jahre eine pathologische Spermabiochemie aufwies.

Besonders interessant ist, daß unter den 54 Patienten, die den Arzt aufsuchten, auf Grund ähnlicher Symptome wie bei einer Prostatitis, bei denen man aber mit klinischen, bakteriologischen und cytologischen Untersuchungen keine objektiven

42*

Kriteria für Erkrankungen von Prostata oder Samenbläschen finden konnte, etwa die Hälfte pathologische Werte in Spermamorphologie und Spermabiochemie aufwiesen.

Die Zink- und Cholesterolanalysen zeigten eine sehr gute Korrelation mit den Analysen von saurer Phosphatase, während eine ähnliche Korrelation zwischen saurer Phosphatase und Milchsäurendehydrogenase nicht vorkam.

Wie bekannt, ist Prostaglandin der Sammelname für eine Gruppe pharmakodynamisch sehr aktiver Fettsäuren. In der menschlichen Samenflüssigkeit hat man bisher 13 verschiedene Prostaglandine isolieren können. Im Hinblick darauf, daß die Prostaglandinaktivität in der Samenflüssigkeit normaliter sehr hoch ist sowie daß diese Substanzen einen starken Einfluß auf die Motorik der nicht schwangeren Gebärmutter ausüben, ist es wahrscheinlich, daß die Prostaglandine im Samen für die Fortpflanzung des Menschen von Bedeutung sind (s. ELIASSON u. EULER, 1967).

Der Prostaglandingehalt ist durchschnittlich niedriger in Ejaculaten von Männern mit herabgesetzter Fertilität als in Ejaculaten von fertilen Männern. Die Bedeutung dieser Beobachtung ist noch nicht klar, aber es ist denkbar, daß ein niedriger Prostaglandingehalt immer mit anderen biochemischen Veränderungen im Seminalplasma verbunden ist. Gegen diesen Hintergrund ist es von Interesse, daß Dr. MARC BYGDEMAN und ich kürzlich Patienten hatten, die einen niedrigen Fructosegehalt aber normalen Prostaglandinspiegel bzw. niedrigen Prostaglandinspiegel aber normale Werte für Fructose aufwiesen.

Die Tatsache, daß der Prostaglandingehalt im Samen nicht mit der Konzentration anderer routinemäßig bestimmter Stoffe parallel läuft, läßt es wünschenswert erscheinen, Prostaglandinanalysen in die Untersuchungen eingehen zu lassen, welche den Zusammenhang zwischen der Fertilität und den biologischen Eigenschaften des Seminalplasma beleuchten sollen. Leider sind jedoch diese Analysen noch allzu kompliziert, um routinemäßig ausgenützt werden zu können.

Die Ergebnisse unserer Studien deuten darauf hin, daß biochemische Analysen des Spermaplasma wertvolle Informationen liefern, nicht nur im Zusammenhang mit Untersuchungen über die männliche Fertilität, sondern auch für Untersuchungen verschiedener Formen von Funktionsstörungen in den männlichen Geschlechtsdrüsen.

Literatur. VON EULER, U. S., and R. ELIASSON: Prostaglandins. Academic Press 1967 (In press). — KIMMIG, J., O. STEENO und C. SCHIRREN: Internist 8, 25 (1967). — MANN, T.: Ciba Foundation Colloquia on Endocrinology 16, 233 (1967).

On the Adrenal Origin of Dehydroepiandrosterone in Human Seminal Plasma

O. STEENO, C. SCHIRREN, W. HEYNS and P. DE MOOR, Rega Instituut, Laboratorium voor Experimentele Geneeskunde, Leuven (Belgium), and Andrologische Abteilung der Hautklinik, Universitäts-Krankenhaus Hamburg-Eppendorf (Deutschland)

The first reports on the presence of androgens in human ejaculate are very controversial. In the *same* pool of semen, HUIS IN'T VELD [1] found only atypical Zimmermann chromogens, while DIRSCHERL and BREUER [2] supposed that the substance they obtained in the neutral cetonic fraction was specific. They did, however, not confirm this finding in a later publication [3]. In 1963, RABOCH and coll. [4] failed to identify androgens by means of paper chromatography. Recently then, DIRSCHERL and BREUER [5] isolated dehydroepiandrosterone (3-beta-hydroxy-Δ^5-androsten-17-one) in the concentration of 6.9 μg per 100 ml semen.

We have been able to confirm the presence of solvolysable dehydroepiandrosterone (DHEA) in semen by means of gas chromatography [6]. The levels of dehydroepiandrosterone we found were about five times higher than those found by DIRSCHERL and BREUER [5] and were similar in normal men and in men in various states of sub- and infertility. This made us think that the DHEA in seminal plasma was of adrenocortical and not of testicular origin as postulated by DIRSCHERL and BREUER [5]. In order to settle this question, dynamic exploration tests were performed.

Table 1. *Dehydroepiandrosterone (µg per 100 ml) in human seminal plasma before and after dexamethasone administration*

No	before	after	% change
1	19.8	8.8	— 55.4
2	52.9	19.6	— 63.0
3	52.6	27.9	— 47.0
4	39.5	20.7	— 47.6
5	16.2	6.9	— 57.5
6	60.2	19.8	— 67.2
7	43.4	16.1	— 63.0
mean ± S.D.	40.7 ± 16.9	17.1 ± 7.2	

In a first step, dexamethasone (0.75 mg twice a day for 6 days) was given to seven patients with normospermia and DHEA was measured in semen collected by masturbation before and during this adrenocortical suppression. The values obtained were corrected for losses throughout the procedure by adding tracer amounts of tritiated DHEA-sulfate to the samples. As can be seen in Tab. 1, the DHEA-levels in semen significantly decreased from 40.7 ± 16.9 (S.D.) to 17.1 ± 7.2 μg per 100 ml (P < 0.005), i.e. a decrease of 58%.

In a second step, DHEA-determinations were done on semen samples of patients with hypo- or slight oligozoospermia, treated with serum gonadotropins (2.000 I.U. twice a week for 3 weeks). Semen was collected before and 1 or 2 days after the last injection. The values obtained are given in Tab. 2. No change in DHEA-concentration could be observed under these circumstances.

Table 2. *Dehydroepiandrosterone (µg per 100 ml) in human seminal plasma before and after serum gonadotropin therapy*

No	before	after
1	42.5	42.1
2	11.6	12.7
3	56.1	50.7
4	33.6	33.3
5	29.1	26.9
mean ± S. D.	34.6 ± 16.4	33.1 ± 14.5

The presented data fully support our hypothesis that dehydroepiandrosterone in human seminal plasma is of adrenal origin. It seems likely that this DHEA is extracted from the blood stream by the glandular structures of the seminal vesicles. Further studies with chorionic gonadotropins are in progress.

This work has been supported by a Grant from the Lalor Foundation, Wilmington, Delaware, USA.

References. 1. HUIS in't VELD, L. G.: Acta endocr. (Kbh.) **16**, 257 (1954). — 2. DIRSCHERL, W., and H. BREUER: Acta endocr. (Kbh.)**16**, 248 (1954). — 3. DIRSCHERL, W., and H. BREUER: Acta endocr. (Kbh.) **19**, 30 (1955). — 4. RABOCH, J., I. GREGOROVÁ, and K. ŘEŽÁBEK: J. clin. Endocr. **23**, 521 (1963). — 5. DIRSCHERL, W., and H. BREUER: Acta endocr. **44**, 403 (1963). — 6. STEENO, O., C. SCHIRREN, W. HEYNS, and P. DEMOOR: J. clin. Endocr. **26**, 353 (1966).

Oestrogene im menschlichen Sperma

C. SCHIRREN, Universitäts-Hautklinik Hamburg (Deutschland)

Im Rahmen der andrologischen Grundlagenforschung auf dem Gebiete der Biochemie des Spermaplasmas wurden die Gesamtoestrogene nach der Methode von ITTEICH bestimmt (zum Teil gemeinsam mit HASCHKE). Uns interessierte dabei besonders die Frage eines Zusammenhanges zwischen Gesamtoestrogengehalt und Spermatozoenzahl; dieses Problem war für eine Klärung der Ätiologie der postpuberalen Leydig-Zellinsuffizienz von Bedeutung.

Es wurde sowohl Frischspermaplasma als auch Tiefkühlspermaplasma untersucht. Pro Ejaculat kam jeweils 1,0 ml Spermaplasma zur Verwendung. Es ließ sich keinerlei Unterschied zwischen den Oestrogenwerten von Frischsperma und Tiefkühlsperma nachweisen.

Tabelle 1. *Übersicht der Oestrogenwerte im Frischsperma und und im Tiefkühlsperma (in μg/ml)*

Diagnose	Frischsperma	Tiefkühlsperma
Normospermie	0,048	0,048
Hypozoospermie	0,049	0,043
Oligospermie	0,034	0,035
Aspermie	0,033	0,035

Auch bei einer differenzierten Aufarbeitung des Spermas und Bestimmung der Oestrogene im scharf zentrifugierten Spermaplasmaüberstand wie im spermatozoenhaltigen Sediment war eine Oestrogenaktivität nachzuweisen. Der höhere Prozentsatz im Sediment kann u. a. darauf beruhen, daß durch den Zentrifugierungsvorgang selbst eine Zerstörung von Spermatozoen und damit eine weitere Freisetzung von intracellulär vorhandenen Oestrogenen erfolgte.

Tabelle 2. *Oestrogenaktivität verschiedener Spermaanteile (in μg/ml)*

Gesamtsperma	Sediment	Überstand
1. 0,056	0,047	0,041
2. 0,039	0,033	0,027
3. 0,061	0,041	0,045

Aus diesen Befunden geht hervor, daß die Oestrogene nicht nur an die Spermatozoen gekoppelt sein können, wie es von MCCULLAGH u. SCHAFFENBURG (1951) auf Grund ihrer Tierversuche mit gewaschenen Spermatozoen angenommen wurde, sondern daß sich auch im Spermaplasma selbst Oestrogene befinden. Das geht z. B. auch daraus hervor, daß bei Patienten mit einer Aspermie auf Grund eines Verschlusses der ableitenden Samenwege ebenfalls eine Oestrogenaktivität nachweisbar war; hier dürften die Oestrogene also über den Blutweg aus dem Hoden via Bläschendrüsen und Prostata in das Sperma gelangen. Wenn sich eine deutliche Differenz in der Oestrogenaktivität bei spermatozoenhaltigem und spermatozoenfreiem Spermaplasma ergeben hat, so beweist das ein Vorhandensein von Oestrogenen an bzw. in den Spermatozoen.

Diskussion. Über die Bildungsstätte der Oestrogene kann auf Grund unserer Versuche keine Aussage gemacht werden. Nach DICZFALUSY u. LAURITZEN (1961) nimmt man an, daß sie in den Leydigschen Zwischenzellen entstehen; hier wird offensichtlich ein Teil synthetisiert, während der andere Teil durch Umwandlung aus den ebenfalls dort gebildeten Androgenen entstehen soll. Nach den Perfusions-untersuchungen am Hengsthoden mit markiertem Acetat ist anzunehmen, daß der Hoden zunächst Oestron synthetisiert (NYMAN, GEIGER u. GOLDZIEHER, 1959).

Wenn wir festgestellt haben, daß mit Abnahme der Spermatozoenzahl auch ein Absinken der Oestrogenaktivität resultiert, so ergibt sich dennoch, daß auch bei völligem Fehlen von Spermatozoen immer noch eine relativ hohe Oestrogenaktivität vorhanden ist. Unter Berücksichtigung der „Transport-Funktion" der Spermatozoen für die Oestrogene muß man demnach den Schluß ziehen, daß auch andere Eiweißkörper des Spermaplasmas für den Transport der Oestrogene verantwortlich sein dürften.

Literatur. DICZFALUSY. E., u. CH. LAURITZEN: Oestrogene beim Menschen. Berlin-Göttingen-Heidelberg: Springer 1961. — ITTRICH, G.: Zbl. Gynäk. **80**, 429 (1960). — McCULLAGH, E. P., and C. A. SCHAFFENBURG: J. clin. Endocr. **11**, 403 (1951). — NYMAN, M., J. GEIGER, and J. W. GOLDZIEHER: J. biol. Chem. **234**, 16 (1954). — SCHIRREN, C.: Fertilitätsstörungen beim Manne. Diagnostik, Biochemie des Spermaplasmas, Hormontherapie. Stuttgart: F. Enke 1961.

Neue Ergebnisse der Immunologie des Spermaplasma

W. P. HERRMANN, Univ.-Hautklinik Hamburg-Eppendorf und Univ.-Hautklinik Köln (Deutschland)

Die Samenflüssigkeit des Mannes enthält etwa 4 bis 6% Eiweiß [4, 5, 8], das zum größten Teil aus den Samenbläschen stammt und sich elektrophoretisch in mehrere Fraktionen auftrennen läßt. Etwa 60% dieser Proteine sind dialysierbar, so daß Zweifel aufgetaucht sind, ob es sich durchweg um echte Proteine handelt [1].

Von den nicht dialysierbaren Fraktionen weiß man seit langem, daß sie Albumin enthalten [7]. Nach Einengung der Samenflüssigkeit mittels Druckfiltration fanden LEITHOFF u. LEITHOFF vier weitere Bluteiweißkörper, von denen einer als Transferrin, ein zweiter als Gamma-G-Globulin identifiziert werden konnte; die beiden anderen wurden als $\beta_2 A$ (IgA) und $\beta_2 M$ (IgM) angesprochen, doch konnte nicht zweifelsfrei entschieden werden, ob es sich tatsächlich um diese Immunglobuline gehandelt hat.

Eigene Untersuchungen mit der zweidimensionalen Immunodiffusion nach OUCHTHERLONY haben ergeben, daß noch weitere Bluteiweißkörper im Seminalplasma enthalten sind, und zwar α_1-Seromucoid, α_1-Glykoprotein und $\alpha_1 A$-Globulin (Antitrypsin). IgM konnte nicht nachgewiesen werden, während IgA sich mit einem spezifischen Antiserum eindeutig darstellen ließ.

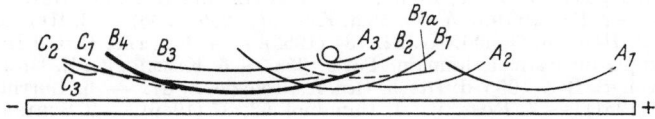

Mit Antiseren gegen menschliche Bluteiweißkörper erhält man in der Immunelektrophorese gewöhnlich nur zwei, bestenfalls drei Präcipitate im Bereich von Albumin, Transferrin und Gamma-Globulin. Verwendet man aber spezifisch gegen Spermaplasma gerichtete Antiseren von Kaninchen, dann lassen sich wenigstens acht bis neun, mit einigen Immunseren bis zu elf Fraktionen unterscheiden. Diese Fraktionen sind nicht dialysierbar; man kann daher annehmen, daß es sich um Proteine handelt. Ihre elektrophoretische Beweglichkeit erstreckt sich — gemessen an der der Serumproteine — vom Albumin- bis in den Gamma-Globulinbereich.

Da die Mehrzahl von ihnen substratspezifisch ist, haben wir sie mit den Symbolen A_1—$_3$, B_1—$_4$ und C_1—$_3$ bezeichnet, um eine Verwechslung mit Bluteiweißkörpern zu vermeiden [2, 3].

Vergleicht man Immunopherogramme vom Sekret der Samenbläschen, dem Ejaculat von Patienten mit Verschlußaspermie und normalem Seminalplasma miteinander, dann zeigen sich Unterschiede, aus denen auf die Herkunft der einzelnen Fraktionen geschlossen werden kann. Danach dürften die Fraktionen A_1, A_3, B_{1a}, B_2 und C_1 aus den Samenbläschen, B_1, B_4 und C_2 aus der Prostata und vielleicht aus den Cowperschen Drüsen, und die Fraktionen A_2 und C_3 möglicherweise sogar aus den Hoden bzw. Nebenhoden stammen.

Bisher konnte nur bei drei dieser Fraktionen eine Antigengemeinschaft mit Bluteiweißkörpern nachgewiesen werden, obgleich manche der gegen Spermaplasma gerichteten Kaninchenseren auch noch andere Serumproteine zu präcipitieren vermögen. Eine solche Antigengemeinschaft ist bis jetzt nur zwischen den Fraktionen C_2 und Gamma-Globulin, A_1 und Albumin sowie zwischen B_2 und einem α_2-Globulin nachgewiesen worden, das wir bis vor kurzem für Cöruloplasmin gehalten haben.

Die Fraktion B_2 ließ sich nämlich mit einem spezifisch gegen Cöruloplasmin gerichteten Kaninchenserum der Fa. Hyland gut darstellen. Es gelang allerdings nicht, in dieser Fraktion Kupfer nachzuweisen, obwohl das Seminalplasma nach Befunden von NETH ganz erhebliche Mengen an Kupfer enthält, und auch eine Phenoloxydasereaktion war mit der Fraktion B_2 nicht zu erzielen. Weitere Untersuchungen haben nun gezeigt, daß das seiner Zeit von der Fa. Hyland bezogene Antiserum nicht monospezifisch war. Es enthielt einen zweiten Antikörper gegen ein Begleitprotein aus dem Bereich der α_2-Globuline, das bislang noch nicht identifiziert werden konnte. Die ursprünglich angenommene immunologische Verwandtschaft zwischen der Fraktion B_2 und dem Cöruloplasmin beruhte in Wirklichkeit auf einer Antigengemeinschaft mit diesem Begleitprotein.

Dieser Irrtum, so betrüblich er zunächst war, hat uns jedoch zu einer außerordentlich interessanten Beobachtung verholfen, nämlich zu der Erkenntnis, daß die Fraktion B_2 in zwei Varianten auftritt, die wir als Typ I und Typ II bezeichnet haben: der Typ I stellt sich als sichelförmiges Präcipitat direkt neben der Auftragsstelle dar, Typ II ist langgestreckt und reicht sehr viel weiter zur Anode hin.

Eine Korrelation dieser Typen zu irgendwelchen Fertilitätsstörungen ließ sich nicht feststellen. An einer Serie von insgesamt 119 Ejaculaten, die zusammen mit Herrn SCHIRREN untersucht wurden, hat sich vielmehr gezeigt, daß diese beiden Typen in einem Verhältnis von ziemlich genau 2:1 vorkommen, und das deutet darauf hin, daß es sich möglicherweise um ein genabhängiges System handelt.

Literatur. 1. HERMANN, G., W. LICHT, H. J. KEUTEL und E. KRUG: Naturwissenschaften **45**, 268 (1958). — 2. HERRMANN, W. P.: Med. Klin. **61**, 1286 (1966). — 3. HERRMANN, W. P., u. C. SCHIRREN: Z. Haut- u. Geschl.-Kr. **34**, 134 (1963). — 4. KEUTEL, H. G.: In: La fonction spermatogénétique du testicule humain. Paris 1958. — 5. KIMMIG, J.: Z. Urol., Sonderband Hamburger Kongr. Ber. 1955 d. Dtsch. Ges. f. Urologie, S. 87. — 6. LEITHOFF, H.: Med. Welt **21**, 1137 (1961). — 7. ROSS. V.: J. Immunol. **52**, 87 (1946). — 8. SCHIRREN, C.: Derm. Wschr. **141**, 228 (1960).

Neuere morphologische Untersuchungen an Hodenzellen

H.-J. Bandmann, Dermatologische Klinik der Universität München (Deutschland)

Der Histologe, welcher ein Hodenbild andrologisch auswerten will, kann und soll sich an zwei Sätze halten:

1. Isomorphie ist nicht gleich Isogenie.

2. Je ausdifferenzierter eine Zelle der spermiogenetischen Reihe ist, desto früher erliegt sie einer Schädigung.

Der Begriff Isomorphie soll hier bewußt pragmatisch angewendet werden. Sicher zeigen die Kerne der verschiedenen Präspermatidengruppen (G. Hertwig) und der Spermatocytenarten (Bandmann, 1965) verschiedene, jedoch nur statistisch nach genauen Messungen zu erfassende Größenunterschiede. Auf diese Beobachtungen kann der diagnostizierende Histologe keine Rücksicht nehmen. Für ihn haben die unentwickelte Hodenzelle, die Spermatogonie und der Spermatocyt I ebenso ein gleiches Aussehen wie der Präspermatid I und der Präspermatid II.

Für unsere These und für die gesamte Spermatogenese des Hodens besonders interessant ist aber die Tatsache, daß sich im unentwickelten kindlichen Hoden und der Cryptorche morphologisch nur eine Zellrasse feststellen läßt, d. h., daß sich auch Sertolizellen und die Präspermatogonien isomorph verhalten. Sie haben beide die Gestalt der Zelle, welche im Hoden des Erwachsenen als Sertolizelle angesprochen wird. Könnte man bei der Cryptorche diese Beobachtung noch so deuten, als ob nur die sehr resistente Sertolizelle dem Wärmeschaden widersteht, so ist uns diese Deutung des Hodenbildes beim Kind verschlossen. Es ist bis heute eine offene Frage, ob die Sertolizelle und die Spermatogonie sich gemeinsam aus einer Zelle entwickeln (Stieve) oder ob hier zwei völlig verschiedene Zellrassen, recht unterschiedlicher Herkunft (Stark), nur die gleiche Gestalt besitzen. Denken wir doch daran, daß das Sertolizellsyndrom nur dann ein Recht auf Eigenständigkeit hätte, wenn man den zweiten Gedanken unter Beweis stellen könnte (Bandmann, 1966).

Im Erwachsenenhoden bilden sich aus Sertolizellen jedenfalls nach unserer jetzigen Kenntnis keine Zellen der Spermatogenese aus.

Zum zweiten Satz zunächst eine genaue Erläuterung: Die Spermatohistogenese, d. h. die Reifung der Zellen aus der Präspermatide II über die Spermatide zum Spermatozoon, ist allen Schädigungen gegenüber sehr viel empfindlicher als die Spermatocytogenese: Die Reifeteilung und die Differenzierung durch Teilung von der Spermatogonie zum Spermatocyten und zur Präspermatide I ist weniger empfindlich.

Für den Histopathologen ist es ein gewohntes Bild, wenn er in einem geschädigten Hoden nur noch die Spermatocytogenese, nicht aber mehr die Spermatohistogenese beobachtet. Er spricht dann von einem Stop der Spermatogenese auf Höhe der Spermatocyten oder von einer Hodenatrophie II°. Den stärksten Widerstand allen Schädigungen gegenüber leisten die Sertolizellen und die Leydigschen Zwischenzellen. Die letzteren überstehen sogar eine Homotransplantation über viele Jahre (Romeis).

Wir erinnern uns daran, daß es außerdem noch Hodenschäden gibt, bei welchen von den Tubuli nur noch die bindegewebigen Wände übrigbleiben, also auch die Sertolizellen verschwunden, die Leydigschen Zellen aber immer noch, oft sogar „relativ" hyperplastisch anzutreffen sind. Wir wollen in diesem andrologischen Vortrag nicht auf die bekannten Hodenbilder beim M. Klinefelter und bei den endokrinologischen Affektionen eingehen.

Zum Schluß dieses kleinen Referates sollte ein Vorschlag zur Vereinfachung der verschiedenen Grade der Hodenparenchymschädigung stehen, der uns biologisch verständlich und morphologisch einfacher dünkt, als die bisherige Einteilung in die verschiedenen Grade der Hodenatrophie:

1. Hodenparenchymschädigung mit Aufhebung der Spermatohistogenese,
2. Hodenparenchymschädigung mit Aufhebung der Spermatocytogenese,
3. Hodenparenchymschädigung mit völliger Tubulusatrophie.

Diese einfachen histologischen Diagnosen erfordern dann natürlich die Korrelation mit den übrigen andrologischen Befunden. Wir sind uns klar darüber, daß Hodenbiopsien nur dann repräsentative histologische Bilder liefern, wenn das Gewebe diffus geschädigt ist. Herdförmige Schäden können wir mit der Hodenbiopsie nicht verbindlich erfassen (s. LANZ und NEUHÄUSER).

Literatur. BANDMANN, H. J.: Kernmessungen an Zellen der Spermatogenese. Neue Ergebnisse der Andrologie. Berlin-Heidelberg-New York: Springer 1965; — Arch. klin. exp. Derm. **227**, 688 (1966). — HERTWIG, G.: Z. mikr.-anat. Forsch. **33**, 373 (1933). — LANZ, T., u. G. NEUHÄUSER: Z. Anat. Entwickl.-Gesch. **123**, 462 (1963). — ROMEIS, B.: Klin. Wschr. **12**, 42 (1933); — Anat. Anz. **84**, 24 (1943). — STARK, D.: Embryologie, 2. Aufl. Stuttgart: Thieme 1965. — STIEVE, H.: Männliche Genitalorgane. Bd. VII/2 des Hdb. Mikroskopische Anatomie des Menschen. Hrsg. von W. v. MÖLLENDORF. Berlin: Springer 1930.

Free Communications

Basische Proteine in Spermienköpfen fertiler und infertiler Männer

W. MEYHÖFER, Universitäts-Hautklinik Gießen (Deutschland)

Basische Kernproteine sind mit der Desoxyribonucleinsäure (DNS) im Kern derart verbunden, daß die phosphorischen Gruppen der DNS-Doppelhelix durch basische Aminogruppen neutralisiert werden. Es wird angenommen, daß die Anzahl basischer Proteingruppen der Anzahl saurer Phosphatgruppen der DNS entspricht. Basische Proteine sind durch Säuren aus dem Zellkern extrahierbar und werden als Histone bzw. Protamine bezeichnet. Der Hauptanteil der basischen Nucleoproteine sind arginin- und lysinreiches Histon bzw. Protamin. Das Verhältnis von Histon zu DNS wird als konstant angesehen. Man nimmt an, daß die Histone Genregulatoren, sind bzw. daß die Histone durch Hemmung der DNS-abhängigen RNS-Synthese „Gen-Verdränger" (MURRAY) darstellen. ALFERT u. GESCHWIND haben eine Methode für die selektive Färbung von basischen Proteinen vorgeschlagen, die einfach anzuwenden und angemessen spezifisch ist.

Zur Frage des Gehaltes von basischen Proteinen in Spermatozoenköpfen aus Ejaculaten von fertilen und klinisch sub- oder infertilen Männern wurden mittels der Fastgreen-pH-8,2-Cytophotometrie halbquantitative Bestimmungen von basischen Proteinen in unserer Klinik vorgenommen. Aus den gleichen Ejaculaten erfolgten DNS-Bestimmungen mittels der Feulgen-Cytophotometrie. Aus diesen Untersuchungen berichten wir über Ergebnisse, die aus Ejaculaten von 20 Männern gewonnen wurden. Insgesamt wurden 2000 Zellmessungen nach der Fastgreen-pH-8,2-Färbung und 2000 nach der klassischen Feulgen-Schiff-Reaktion ausgeführt. Zehn dieser untersuchten Ejaculate waren von Männern, deren Ehefrauen Aborte zwischen mens II und IV erlitten hatten. Die Messungen erfolgten am Barr & Stroud-Photometer für Fastgreen-pH-8,2 bei der Wellenlänge 635 nm, für Feulgen

bei 570 nm. Für die statistische Auswertung der Meßergebnisse mit Signifikanz-
berechnung wurde der „t"-Test angewandt.

Die Ergebnisse lassen sich in mehrere Gruppen unterteilen:

1. Eine Vermehrung der basischen Proteine und der DNS jeweils gegenüber der
Norm wurde bei fünf Patienten gefunden. In dieser Gruppe haben Ehefrauen von
drei Patienten Fehlgeburten durchgemacht. Die klinischen Untersuchungen zeigten in vier Fällen Teratospermien, kombiniert mit Zahl- oder Bewegungsvermin-
derungen der Spermatozoen. In einem Falle bestand eine sog. Normospermie.

2. Vermehrung der Histonproteine, keine Veränderung der DNS gegenüber der
Norm bei einem Patienten. Im Ejaculat Oligospermie mit Fehlgeburten bei der
Ehefrau mens III.

3. Bei einem Patienten sahen wir eine Vermehrung der basischen Proteine
gegenüber der Norm und eine Verminderung der DNS. Im Ejaculat bestand eine
Teratospermie.

4. Die nächste Gruppe umfaßt drei Patienten, bei denen eine Vermehrung der
DNS und eine Verminderung der basischen Proteine abzulesen war. Die Ehefrauen
von zwei Patienten haben Fehlgeburten erlitten.

5. Im weiteren eine Gruppe mit vier Patienten, bei denen die DNS unverändert
gegenüber der Norm war, die basischen Proteine vermindert gefunden wurden.
Auch hier bei drei Patienten Fehlgeburten bei der Ehefrau.

In den zwei letztgenannten Gruppen sind vier Polyspermien, zwei sog. Normospermien und eine Hypo-Asthenospermie enthalten.

6. In der letzten Gruppe sind drei Patienten aufgeführt, die Verminderungen
von DNS und basischen Proteinen zeigten. Im ersten Falle bei kleinen Rund-
spermatozoen, im zweiten Fall bei einer Nekrospermie mit fast ausschließlich
amorphen Zellen und im dritten Fall bei einer Hypospermie mit Fehlgeburten bei
der Ehefrau.

7. Ejaculate von 3 Männern mit Normospermien, in deren Ehen Kinder geboren waren, wurden zu Kontrollen bei den jeweiligen Untersuchungen herangezogen.

Zusammenfassend möchten wir sagen, daß wir bei fertilen Männern bei den
basischen Proteinen nach Fastgreen-Färbung im Mittelwert 19% niedrigere Ab-
sorptionsarbeitseinheiten als nach Feulgen-Färbung fanden (s. Bahr: 20% bei
Bullenspermatozoen). Bei klinisch infertilen bzw. subfertilen Männern war bei
insgesamt acht Patienten ein konstantes Verhältnis von Histon zu DNS zu finden,
d. h. eine Vermehrung von DNS entsprach einer Vermehrung von Histon bzw.
umgekehrt, während bei den übrigen Patienten keine entsprechende Relation zu
finden war. Wie wir bereits 1962 bei ultraviolett-mikrospektrophotometrischen
Untersuchungen feststellen konnten, zeigte der Gehalt an Proteinen in den Spermatozoenköpfen aus Ejaculaten subfertiler Männer starke Schwankungen. Hierauf
wurden die stärkeren Streuungen im DNS-Gehalt bei der Ultraviolett- gegenüber
der Feulgen-Cytophotometrie angenommen. Die jetzigen Untersuchungen bestätigen diese Annahme.

Atomabsorptions-spektrometrische Untersuchungen des Magnesium- und Zinkgehaltes im Hoden und Prostatagewebe sowie im Ejaculat des Menschen

R. HERRMANN, W. KNOTH und W. MEYHÖFER, Universitäts-Hautklinik Gießen (Deutschland)

Bei orientierenden Untersuchungen fanden wir einen erhöhten Zinkgehalt im Ejaculat. Unsere Ergebnisse waren nur zum Teil mit den Befunden anderer Autoren vergleichbar. Die Durchsicht der einschlägigen Literatur ergab, daß man bisher vorwiegend mit chemischen Bestimmungsmethoden arbeitete.

Wir stellten uns die Aufgabe, mit dem relativ neuen, sehr genauen, spezifischen und zugleich zeitsparenden Verfahren, der Atom-Absorptionsspektrometrie, die vorliegenden Befunde zu überprüfen. Gleichzeitig sollte das Verhältnis von Magnesium zu Zink im Ejaculat sowie im Prostata- und Hodengewebe bestimmt werden.

Untersuchungsmethode und Material

1. *Meßanordnung*. Die Abbildung zeigt das Prinzip des Atomabsorptionsverfahrens.

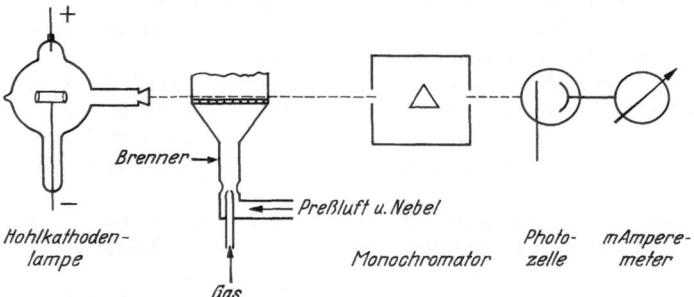

Abb. Schemazeichnung des Atomabsorptionsverfahrens

Die verdünnte Probe wird in einer Flamme zerstäubt, wobei das Material verdampft und dissoziiert. Die freigewordenen gasförmigen Atome werden mit der Atomabsorption nachgewiesen. Die Eichung erfolgt mit Lösungen entsprechender, aber bekannter Zusammensetzung. Beim Vorliegen von geraden Eichkurven sind die gemessenen Analysenextinktionen E_a und die Eichextinktionen E_e den zugehörigen Konzentrationen c_a bzw. c_e direkt proportional:

$$\frac{Ea}{Ee} = \frac{ca}{ce} \quad \text{oder: } ca = ce\,\frac{Ea}{Ee}.$$

2. *Untersuchungsmaterial*. Für die Gewebsmessungen wurde von 0,5 bis 1 g Feuchtgewebe ausgegangen. Es standen, abgesehen von je zwölf Gewebsproben für Vorversuche, jeweils 19 Gewebsproben für die endgültigen Versuche zur Verfügung, die 19- bis 68jährigen Sektionsfällen entnommen waren. Abgesehen von Hoden- und Prostatageweben werden zum Vergleich auch Leber und Pankreas untersucht. Das Durchschnittsalter der Fälle lag bei 50,5 Jahren. Die 100 untersuchten Ejaculate wurden durch Masturbation nach 5- bis 8tägiger Karenz gewonnen.

3. *Aufbereitung des Materials*. Die Gewebsproben wurden getrocknet, verascht und mit verdünnter Salzsäure wieder aufgenommen und direkt dem Flammenphotometer zugeführt. Die Ejaculate konnten nach entsprechender Verdünnung direkt flammenphotometrisch gemessen werden.

Ergebnisse

Die in mg/100 g Feuchtgewicht bei Gewebeuntersuchungen bzw. in mg/100 ml Ejaculat angegebenen Magnesium- und Zinkkonzentrationen ersieht man aus der folgenden Tabelle:

Organ bzw. Körperflüssigkeit	Zahl der Fälle	Mittlere Elementkonzentration und die Standardabweichung in mg/100 g Frischgewicht bzw. in mg/100 ml Ejaculat	
		Mg	Zn
Hoden	19 (+ 12)	6,7 ± 0,7	1,6 ± 0,4
Prostata	19 (+ 12)	8,3 ± 0,8	9,4 ± 1,6
Ejaculat (alle Fälle)	100	8,1 ± 4,1	17,2 ± 6,8
Untergruppen:			
Normospermie	26	8,1 ± 3,0	17,1 ± 6,1
Polyspermie	2	11,4 ± 0,8	21,2 ± 0,6
Oligospermie	8	8,2 ± 4,9	16,6 ± 6,6
Aspermie	8	7,4 ± 1,2	15,4 ± 4,3

Weitere Untergruppen sind hier nicht aufgeführt. Siehe dazu die Arbeit von LIEBIG

Zum Vergleich:			
Leber	19 (+ 12)	10,4 ± 1,6	7,7 ± 2,3
Pankreas	19 (+ 12)	8,0 ± 1,0	2,6 ± 0,5

Diskussion

Ein Teil unserer Ergebnisse bestätigt qualitativ die bisherigen Befunde von Voruntersuchungen. Die gefundenen Zinkkonzentrationen liegen deutlich niedriger als die bisher in der Literatur angegebenen. Bei einigen unserer Magnesiumergebnisse sind vergleichbare Literaturangaben noch nicht bekannt. Eine Beziehung zwischen den Samenqualitäten einerseits und den Magnesium- und Zinkkonzentrationen andererseits können wir nicht immer feststellen. Für Zink war das schon früher von VASTERLING, VOLKMANN, SCHIRREN und BELTERMANN gefunden worden. — Bei acht Fällen mit Aspermie liegt bei uns der Zinkgehalt 10,5% höher als das Mittel der Normwerte. SCHIRREN u. Mitarb. fanden in 23 Fällen von Aspermie einen um 18,1% höheren Zinkgehalt als es dem normalen Mittelwert entspricht. Der Vergleich der Zn- und Mg-Konzentrationen im Ejaculat vom eigenen Material ergibt, daß bei einem hohen Zn-Gehalt auch der Mg-Gehalt hoch ist. Der dazu errechnete Korrelationskoeffizient liegt bei 0,7, was einer mittelstarken Korrelation entspricht. Unsere Fälle mit Oligoastheno-, Astheno- und Teratospermie sind in der Arbeit von LIEBIG berücksichtigt. Aus Zeitgründen können wir auf diese Befunde hier nicht eingehen.

Bei den Gewebsuntersuchungen ergeben sich erhebliche Unterschiede zwischen dem Zinkgehalt des Hodens und der Prostata (KNOTH, VASTERLING). Wenn man die gefundenen Werte mit denjenigen der anderen Organe vergleicht, so besitzt das Hodengewebe sowohl den geringsten Zink- als auch den niedrigsten Magnesiumgehalt.

Hervorzuheben ist, daß die höchsten Zinkwerte, auch im Vergleich zu den Untersuchungsbefunden der Leber und des Pankreas, im Prostatagewebe vorliegen. Es kann angenommen werden, daß die gemessenen Zinkkonzentrationen im Ejaculat wahrscheinlich nicht aus dem testiculären Gewebe, sondern aus den Anhangdrüsen der Samenwege und zumindest im großen Teil aus der Prostata stammen. Die atomabsorptions-spektrometrische Untersuchung des Prostatasekrets steht noch aus.

Literatur. BELTERMANN, R.: Experimentelle Untersuchungen zur Bestimmung des Zn-Gehaltes im menschlichen Sperma. Inaugural-Dissertation, Hamburg 1961. — HERRMANN, R.: Z. klin. Chem. **3,** 178 (1965). — KNOTH, W.: Diskussionsbemerkung zum Vortrag H. W.

VASTERLING. Arch. klin. exp. Derm. **213**, 764 (1961). — LIEBIG, D.: Flammenphotometrische Bestimmung des Zink- und Magnesiumgehaltes im Spermaplasma des Menschen. Inaugural-Dissertation, Gießen 1967 (In Vorbereitung). — PORTEN, R.: Absorptionsflammenphotometrische Messungen der Konzentration von Magnesium und Zink in Leber, Pankreas, Prostata und Hoden des Menschen. Dissertation, Gießen 1966. — SCHIRREN, C.: Klinische und experimentelle Untersuchungen zur Diagnostik der Fertilitätsstörungen des Mannes und ihrer Therapie mit Hormonen. Habilitationsschrift, Hamburg 1960. — VASTERLING, H. W.: Arch. klin. exp. Derm. **213**, 759 (1961). — VOLKMANN, H.-D.: Das Zink im Sperma des Menschen. Dissertation, Göttingen 1961.

Zur Bedeutung der Prostaglandine im humanen Seminalplasma

H.-C. STURDE, Klinik und Poliklinik für Hautkrankheiten am Klinikum Essen der Universität Münster (Deutschland)

Die Prostaglandine wurden erstmals durch v. EULER [1934 (1, 2)] und unabhängig von ihm durch GOLDBLATT (1933, 1935) aus dem menschlichen Sperma isoliert. Weitere analytische Untersuchungen führten schließlich zur Trennung mehrerer Verbindungen, bei denen es sich um ungesättigte Fettsäuren handelt [ELIASSON, 1959; SAMUELSSON, 1963; BERGSTRÖM, 1949; BERGSTRÖM u. SJÖVALL, 1957, 1960 (1, 2); BERGSTRÖM, RYHAGE, SAMUELSSON u. SJÖVALL, 1962; BERGSTRÖM, KRABISCH, SAMUELSSON u. SJÖVALL, 1962 sowie HAMBERG u. SAMUELSSON, 1966). Die hervorstechendste Eigenschaft dieser körpereigenen Wirkstoffe ist ihre Fähigkeit, den Blutdruck zu senken und glatte Muskulatur zu kontrahieren. Die große Menge an Prostaglandinen in der Samenflüssigkeit des Mannes läßt vermuten, daß ihnen innerhalb der Fertilitätsmechanismen eine Bedeutung zukommt. Beziehungen zwischen dem Prostaglandingehalt des Spermas und der männlichen Fertilität sind daher durchaus denkbar. Der erste Hinweis dieser Art findet sich bei v. EULER (1949). Er berichtete, daß in Fällen von Sterilität der Prostaglandinspiegel des menschlichen Samens erniedrigt gefunden wurde. Weiterhin haben ELIASSON (1959), HAWKINS u. LABRUM (1961) sowie HORTON u. THOMPSON (1964) die Aktivität von Samen an der glatten Muskulatur verschiedener Tierorgane gemessen. Ganz allgemein stellten sie dabei fest, daß das Sperma von Männern mit normaler Fertilität mehr Prostaglandine enthält als das einiger Proben von infertilen Männern. Der Versuch, Beziehungen zwischen der Größenordnung der glattmuskelstimulierenden Wirkung des Seminalplasmas und anderen Eigenschaften des zugehörigen Spermas herzustellen, führte aber bislang zu keinen eindeutigen Ergebnissen (ASPLUND, 1947, 1949).

Für die Bestimmung der glattmuskelkontrahierenden Prostaglandine im Seminalplasma erwies sich uns der isolierte überlebende Meerschweinchendarm als am besten geeignet. Die pharmakodynamische Wirkung dieser Verbindungen bewegt sich dabei in der gleichen beachtlichen Größenordnung wie diejenige von Histamin, Acetylcholin und Oxytocin. Mit dieser biologischen Arbeitsmethode haben wir den Gehalt von Samenproben an Prostaglandinen vergleichsweise gemessen. Als Äquivalent diente Beta-Imidazoläthylamin (Histamin). Die hier angegebenen Zahlenwerte beziehen sich auf einen Histaminquotienten (Histaminäquivalent : Spermavolumen). Dieser Quotient gibt Aufschluß über die Größenordnung der glattmuskelstimulierenden Aktivität der überprüften Samenprobe und ist bei der von uns gewählten Versuchsanordnung mit dem Prostaglandingehalt (Prostaglandinspiegel) gleichzusetzen.

Das im Sperma enthaltene, ebenfalls muskelaktive Cholin wurde durch einen Atropinzusatz zur Tyrodelösung (Nährmedium für den isolierten überlebenden

Meerschweinchendarm) blockiert. Das außerdem in der Samenflüssigkeit vorkommende Histamin reicht nach unseren experimentellen Erfahrungen im allgemeinen nicht aus, um nachweisbare (störende) Kontraktionen der Darmmuskulatur auszulösen. Die Herstellung eines mehr oder minder gereinigten Prostaglandinpräparates aus jeder Samenprobe erwies sich auf Grund von Vorversuchen als nicht notwendig. Wir verwendeten daher zentrifugiertes, weitgehend zellfreies, mit Aqua destillata 1:5 verdünntes Seminalplasma. Außerdem ließen sich die Proben bis zur Prostaglandinbestimmung ohne Verlust ihrer pharmakodynamischen Aktivität bei — 20 °C einfrieren.

Aus unserem Arbeitsprogramm stellen wir die Ejaculatuntersuchungen von 80 Männern vor. 50 davon hatten unsere Klinik zur Fertilitätsuntersuchung wegen einer sterilen Ehe aufgesucht (Dauer der sterilen Ehe im Durchschnitt 4,1 Jahre). Im angefertigten Spermatogramm wiesen alle eine Normospermie auf (= Gruppe I, Probanden ohne Kinder). Zum Vergleich diente uns eine Gruppe von 30 nachweislich fertilen Männern, deren Sperma neben den sonstigen Eigenschaften auch auf seinen Gehalt an Prostaglandinen untersucht wurde (= Gruppe II, Probanden mit Kindern).

Die Ergebnisse der Prostaglandinbestimmung im Seminalplasma ergaben folgende Befunde: Bei der Gruppe I (Probanden ohne Kinder) fand sich ein durchschnittlicher Prostaglandinwert von 1,23 (Histaminquotient), bei der Gruppe II (Probanden mit Kindern) hingegen ein Histaminquotient von 3,65. Der Prostaglandinspiegel betrug demnach bei den offenbar zeugungsfähigen Männern gegenüber den Probanden ohne Kinder fast das Dreifache.

Während wir bei den Männern aus sterilen Ehen (Gruppe I) bewußt nur diejenigen mit einer Normospermie für diese Gegenüberstellung ausgesucht haben, fanden sich unter den nachweislich fertilen Männern drei Oligospermien (Spermienzahl zwischen 8 und 20 Mill/ml) und sechs Hypospermien (Spermienzahl von 27 bis 39 Mill/ml). Diese Fälle wiesen jedoch alle einen besonders hohen Prostaglandinspiegel auf (durchschnittlicher Histaminquotient 4,4!). Einer der Probanden mit einer Oligospermie (Spremienzahl um 10 Mill/ml, Spermavolumen zwischen 3 und 4 ml) wurde vor kurzem wieder Vater. Damit stimmen die Beobachtungen von HAWKINS u. LABRUM (1961) überein, die über zwei Männer mit einer Oligospermie bei gleichzeitig relativ hohem Prostaglandingehalt des Samens berichteten und deren Ehefrauen gravid wurden. Diese Befunde weisen auf recht enge Beziehungen der Prostaglandine zur männlichen Fertilität hin, auch wenn ihre physiologische Bedeutung zur Zeit noch nicht klar erkennbar ist. Der Gehalt der Samenflüssigkeit an Prostaglandinen bildet unseres Erachtens einen beachtenswerten Faktor für die Beurteilung der Fertilität eines Spermas. Ist der Prostaglandinspiegel niedrig, so kann das anscheinend bereits die Fruchtbarkeit des Mannes beeinträchtigen.

Literatur. ASPLUND, J.: Acta physiol. scand. **13**, 109 (1947). — BERGSTRÖM, S.: Nord. Med. **42**, 1465 (1949). — BERGSTRÖM, S., and J. SJÖVALL: Acta chem. scand. **11**, 1086 (1957); — (1) Acta chem. scand. **14**, 1693 (1960); — (2) Acta chem. scand. **14**, 1701 (1960). — BERGSTRÖM, S., R. RYHAGE, D. SAMUELSSON, and J. SJÖVALL: Acta chem. scand. **16**, 501 (1962). — BERGSTRÖM, S., L. KRABISCH, D. SAMUELSSON, and J. SJÖVALL: Acta chem. scand. **16**, 969 (1962). — ELIASSON, R.: Acta physiol. scand. **158**, 1 (1959). — EULER, U. S. v.: (1) J. Physiol. (Lond.) **89**, 102 (1934); — (2) Naunyn-Schmiedeberg's Arch. exp. Path. Pharmak. **175**, 78 (1934). — GOLDBLATT, M. W.: Chem. Indust. **52**, 1056 (1933); — J. Physiol. (Lond.) **84**, 208 (1935). — HAMBERG, M.. and B. SAMUELSSON: J. biol. Chem. **241**, 257 (1966). — HAWKINS, D. F., and A. H. LABRUM: J. Reprod. Fertil. **2**, 1 (1961). — HORTON, E. W., and G. J. THOMPSON: Brit. J. Pharmacol. **22**, 183 (1964). — SAMUELSSON, B.: J. biol. Chem. **238**, 3229 (1963).

Vergleichende licht- und elektronenmikroskopische Untersuchungen an Hodenbiopsien von infertilen Männern

H. Schmalbruch, Institut für Biophysik und Elektronenmikroskopie der Universität Düsseldorf, und O. P. Hornstein, Universitäts-Hautklinik Erlangen (Deutschland)

Elektronenmikroskopische Untersuchungen des normalen menschlichen Hodens sind im Vergleich zu anderen Organen noch ziemlich selten [7, 12, 2, 16, 22, 20]. Unseres Wissens fehlen sie von pathologisch veränderten Hoden. Dieses hat seinen Grund in der Empfindlichkeit des Materials, besonders der Leydigschen Zwischenzellen, deren Struktur sich bei der Fixierung im Stück stets verändert.

Material und Methode: Wir verarbeiteten Biopsiematerial von 16 Patienten, die teils wegen Infertilität, teils wegen Potenzstörungen zur Untersuchung kamen. Unter verschiedenen prä- und postpuberalen Formen des Hypogonadismus waren auch ein schlecht eingestellter Diabetiker und mehrere Fälle von Klinefelter-Syndrom. Als Vergleich dienten normale Hoden von Patienten mit Verschluß-aspermie. Die Biopsien wurden unter Lokalanästhesie des Periorchiums entnommen.

Die lichtmikroskopische Untersuchung erfolgte an 5 µ dicken Paraffinschnitten der in Bouinscher Lösung fixierten, verschieden gefärbten Gewebspartikel. Für die Elektronenmikroskopie wurde das Material unmittelbar nach Entnahme in gepuffertem 1% OsO_4 fixiert, nach Entwässerung mit Aceton in Vestopal W eingebettet, mit Glasmessern geschnitten und im Siemens-Übermikroskop bei 60 kV ohne Nachkontrastierung der Schnitte untersucht.

Unsere elektronenmikroskopischen Untersuchungen beziehen sich auf folgende Konstituenten des Hodengewebes:
1. Die interstitiellen Leydig-Zellen (und Capillaren);
2. Die bindegewebige Tubuluswandung;
3. Die Sertolischen Stützzellen.

Die *Leydig-Zellen* enthalten reichliches agranuläres Reticulum, das bei unseren Biopsien in 0,05 bis 0,5 µ großen Bläschen vorliegt. Neben Fettpartikeln und Pigment finden sich zahlreiche große Mitochondrien. Weiter enthalten die Leydig-Zellen wechselnd viele Reinkesche Kristalloide, die je nach Schnittrichtung entweder einen gitterförmigen oder linearen Aufbau mit elektronendichten Punkten oder Linien im Abstand von etwa 20 nm zeigen. Es handelt sich um Eiweiß-kristalle, die offenbar in einem bisher unbekannten Zusammenhang mit der Androgensynthese stehen. Wie wir früher gezeigt haben [10], sind sie bei mangelhafter Hormonbildung statistisch signifikant verringert.

Tubuluswandung: Sie besteht aus zwei Fibrocytenschichten, die locker miteinander verbunden sind. Sertoli-Zellen und Spermatogonien werden gegen die Tubuluswand von einer Basalmembran begrenzt. Diese macht im Lauf der Hodenreifung eine Verdickung auf etwa 0,5 µ durch. Es entwickeln sich pilzförmige, oft mehrere µ in die anliegende Sertoli-Zelle vordringende, knopfförmige, lamelläre Einstülpungen.

Beim präpuberalen sekundären Hypogonadismus bleibt die Basalmembran mehr oder minder in ihrem unreifen, infantilen Status. Bei postpuberalen Tubulusschäden ist mehr der bindegewebige Anteil der Wandung verändert. Bei der Fibrosklerose bestehen vermehrte, durch seitliche Fortsätze verzahnte Fibrocyten, zwischen denen feingranuläres Material liegt. Innere und äußere Zellschicht können weit auseinanderrücken mit einem elektronenmikroskopisch fast leeren Zwischenraum. Im Hoden eines Diabetikers nimmt das erwähnte feingranuläre Material die ganze Tubulusbreite ein. Wahrscheinlich handelt es sich bei dieser granulären Substanz um sog. Hyalin.

Die *Sertoli-Zellen* enthalten neben zahlreichen kleinen Mitochondrien wenig granuläres und viel agranuläres Reticulum [2, 20]. Im Grundplasma lassen sich, neben Glykogen, die lichtmikroskopisch als Spangaro-Kristalle bekannten Filamente nachweisen. Die Sertoli-Zellen bilden kein Syncytium. Von den Spermatogonien sind sie leicht durch ihren Fettgehalt zu unterscheiden (kleine, stark osmiophile Triglyceridtropfen und große, von einer Membran begrenzte „Liposomen" [9]). Im unreifen Hoden sind Liposomen und Neutralfetttropfen vermindert. Beim Diabetiker sind die ersteren enorm vermehrt und vergrößert.

Nach heutiger Auffassung dient das granuläre Reticulum der Eiweißsynthese der Zelle, während das agranuläre in manchen Zellen mit Steroidstoffwechsel vorkommt (z. B. in den Leydig-Zellen und in den Zellen der NNR). Das Überwiegen des agranulären Reticulums sowie die Veränderungen der Liposomen bei Diabetes (mit klinischem Androgenmangel) lassen eine Bedeutung der Sertoli-Zellen im Steroidstoffwechsel vermuten (vgl. auch frühere Versuche von TEILUM [24] und McCULLAGH et al. [17]). Wir möchten jedoch betonen, daß die Frage einer eigenen Hormonproduktion der Sertoli-Zellen rein morphologisch wohl nicht zu entscheiden ist.

Literatur. 1. AAGENAES, O., and H. MOE: Diabetes **10**, 253 (1961). — 2. BAWA, S. R.: J. Ultrastruct. Res. **9**, 459 (1963). — 3. BIAWA, C. G., G. DYRDA, G. GENEST, and S. A. BENCOSME: Amer. J. Path. **44**, 349 (1964). — 4. BRÖCKELMANN, J.: Z. Zellforsch. **64**, 429 (1964). — 5. CHRISTENSEN, A. K.: J. cell. Biol. **26**, 911 (1965). — 6. CRABO, B.: Z. Zellforsch. **61**, 587 (1963). — 7. FAWCETT, D. W., and M. H. BURGOS: Ciba Foundation Colloquia in Ageing **2**, 86 (1956). — 8. FUCHS, U.: Frankfurt. Z. Path. **73**, 318 (1964). — 9. GUSEK, W., u. H. BUSS: Frankfurt. Z. Path. **75**, 172 (1966). — 10. HORNSTEIN, O., H. EIFEL und O. MITTMANN: Arch. klin. exp. Derm. **225**, 1 (1966). — 11. HORNSTEIN, O., u. H. EIFEL: Arch. klin. exp. Derm. **225**, 440 (1966). — 12. HORSTMANN, E.: Z. Zellforsch. **54**, 68 (1961). — 13. IRVINE, E., J. F. RINEHART, J. E. MORTIMORE, and J. HOPPER jr.: Amer. J. Path. **32**, 647 (1956). — 14. JONES, A. L., and D. W. FAWCETT: J. Histochem. Cytochem. **14**, 215 (1966). — 15. KIMMELSTIEL, P., G. OSAWA, and J. BERES: Amer. J. clin. Path. **45**, 21 (1966). — 16. MANCINI, R. E., O. VILAR, M. PERES DES CERRO y J. C. LAVIERI: Acta physiol. lat.-amer. **14**, 382 (1964). — 17. McCULLAGH, E. P., and F. J. HRUBY: J. clin. Endocr. **9**, 113 (1949). — 18. McMILLAN, D. E., D. L. BREITHAUPT, W. ROSENAU, J. C. LEE, and P. H. FORSHAM: Diabetes **15**, 251 (1966). — 19. MURAKAMI, M.: Zellforsch. **72**, 139 (1966). — 20. NAGANO, T.: Z. Zellforsch. **73**, 89 (1960). — 21. PALADF, G. E.: J. exp. Med. **95**, 285 (1952). — 22. SCHMIDT, F. C.: Z. Zellforsch. **63**, 707 (1964). — 23. SCHWARZ, W., H. J. MERKER und G. SUCHOWSKY: Virchows Arch. path. Anat. **335**, 165 (1962). — 24. TEILUM, G.: Acta endocr. (Kbh.) **4**, 43 (1950). — 25. TONUTTI, E.: KAUFMANN-STAEMMLER: Lehrbuch spez. patho. Anat. Bd. I/2, pp. 1306—1323. Berlin: de Gruyter & Co. 1956. — 26. VILAR, O., A. STEINBERGER und E. STEINBERGER: Z. Zellforsch. **74**, 529 (1966).

Clinical and Therapeutical Andrology

Reports

Ursachen der Impotentia coeundi

R. CERNEA, Mailand (Italien)

Unter Impotentia coeundi verstehen wir die Schwierigkeit, eine befriedigende Erektion, Ejaculation und Libido zu erreichen. Aus praktischen Gründen zieht man im allgemeinen vor, die verschiedenen Formen der Impotentia in zwei große Hauptgruppen, die „organischen" und die „funktionellen" oder „psychischen" einzuteilen. Diese Einteilung ist heute nicht mehr haltbar, denn die Bezeichnung „funktionell" richtet den Blick allzu stark auf körperliche Vorgänge und läßt zu wenig Raum für die begleitenden psychischen Prozesse. Der Begriff „psychogen"

legt allzu sehr den Gedanken an ein vom Körper unabhängiges Seelenleben nahe,
ein Postulat, das im Rahmen dieser Betrachtungen unnötig ist. Auch in Fällen, in
denen das Organische anscheinend eine überwältigend große Rolle spielt (z. B. Ka-
stration), hat das psychische Moment eine gewisse Bedeutung. Nur wenn man Fälle,
bei denen gar keine organischen Veränderungen vorzuliegen scheinen, als psycho-
gene Impotenz bezeichnet, so ist das ein Fehler unserer heutigen Untersuchungsmethoden, denn es läßt sich ja denken, daß eine wirkliche Impotenz niemals ohne
organische Unterlage auftreten kann. Denn tatsächlich sind Körper und Seele
nichts anderes als zwei verschiedene Betrachtungsweisen unseres Organismus.
Wir können uns einen seelischen Prozeß nicht ohne entsprechende körperliche
Veränderungen denken. Von den organischen Ursachen der Impotentia coeundi
wären zu nennen: Mißbildungen (Hermaphroditismus, Kriptorchismus, Phimose),
krankhafte Veränderungen und Verletzungen des Penis, des Musculus bulbo oder
ischio-cavernosus, neurologische Ursachen als Begleitsymptome von Nerven-
leiden (Tabes, multiple Sklerose, Syringomyelie); ebenfalls erworbene Entzün-
dungen der Harnröhre und Prostata, Über- und Unterfunktion von innersekretorischen Drüsen (Hoden, Hypophyse, Thyreoidea, Pancreas und Nebenniere).
Soviel man weiß, reagieren die verschiedenen innersekretorischen Drüsen sehr
empfindsam auf rein psychische Einwirkungen. Durch langwährenden psychischen
Druck kann also eine Vermehrung oder Verminderung bestimmter Hormone zustande kommen, wodurch wiederum auf die Psyche eingewirkt wird. Die Regulation funktioneller Abläufe geschieht nicht nur neural, sondern auch hormonal.
Das übergeordnete Zentrum ist das Nervensystem. Von seinem Einfluß hängt es
vorwiegend ab, in welcher Menge Hormon gebildet wird und ob und wann es
ausgeschieden wird. Das gilt für das autonome und für das vegetative Nervensystem. Im einzelnen Fall ist es nicht beweisbar, wer die Führung übernimmt. Es
wird zu wenig berücksichtigt, daß die Sexualfunktion der Hypophyse einer weitgehenden psychischen Beeinflussung unterworfen ist. Sexuelle Triebregungen
gehen von Impulsen des Zwischenhirns aus und sind weitgehend vom Großhirn
gesteuert. Aber auch die rein somatischen Vorgänge in den Geschlechtsorganen
unterliegen Einwirkungen der vegetativen Steuerung des Gehirns. Die Koppelung
des vegetativen Nervensystems mit dem endokrinen System ist sehr eng, allgemein schon dadurch, daß Vagus und Sympathicus über die hormonähnlichen
intermediären Wirkstoffe ihren Einfluß ausüben — auf der einen Seite Acetylcholin und Histamin, auf der anderen Seite Adrenalin. Das vegetative Nervensystem reguliert mit Hilfe dieser beiden Stoffe alle dem Willen unterworfenen
Funktionen. Die Leistungsfähigkeit des Menschen ist erst dann in Frage gestellt,
wenn die Leistung betont verlangt wird. Nun beginnt auch schon der Mechanismus
der sog. ,,Erwartungsangst'' eine Rolle zu spielen. Sobald die Situation eine
Sexualleistung erwartet, muß sich ja die ähnliche Erwartung eines Mißerfolges
geltend machen.

Heute sind wir durch exakte Analyse in der Lage, fast alles diagnostizieren zu
können. Das Hormon, das im Hoden gebildet wird, ist Testosteron. Es wirkt auf
die im Hoden selbst stattfindende Spermiogenese ein, kommt in die Blutbahn,
wirkt auf die sexuellen Anhangsdrüsen (Prostata, Samenblase) und entfaltet seine
Wirkung im ganzen Organismus. Schließlich wird es in abgebauter Form im Harn
ausgeschieden. Im Harn läßt es sich durch eine Gruppenreaktion als Steroid mit
einer Ketongruppe an der C-17-Stellung erfassen. Für diese Keto-C-17 Steroide
gibt es auch die Nebenniere als Quelle.

Hält man sich an die Symptome: Überempfindlichkeit, Schwindelerscheinun-
gen bis zum plötzlichen Übergang von der horizontalen zur vertikalen Lage, allgemeine Ermüdbarkeit, lokalisierte Kopfschmerzen, besonders im Hinterkopf,

Schlappheit selbst morgens, nachdem man ausgeschlafen hat, so wird man bei einem Mann zwischen 40—55 Jahren auch bei einem Blutdruck von 120/80 mit der Diagnose Hypotonie nicht fehlgehen. Diese geschilderten Symptome stellen einen typischen Fall von Vagusneurose eines hormonal insuffizienten Mannes dar: die Kreislaufhypotonie oder auch Dysharmonie bei einem hypophysär erschöpften Manne, der bisher über einen reichlichen Hormonvorrat und ein klares Übergewicht seines sympathischen Systems bedenkenlos verfügt. Speziell auf unserem Gebiet wird man aus der Angabe, daß niemals morgens, sondern immer erst nach dem Mittagessen und dem Kaffee das Bedürfnis zum Geschlechtsverkehr bestanden habe, Hypotonie vermuten. Tatsächlich findet man so Hypotonie und Erektionsschwäche häufig vereint.

Man würde den Sinn der Potenzstörungen mißverstehen, wenn man die Sexualität von der Gesamtpersönlichkeit loslösen wollte. Bei einer genauen Untersuchung zeigt sich fast jede Form von Potenzstörung als Ausdruck eines neurotischen Lebensstils. Eine irgendwann einmal auftretende Potenzstörung braucht an sich noch kein neurotisches Symptom zu sein, auch wenn eine organische Grundlage nicht nachweisbar ist. Aber eine einmal aufgetretene Potenzstörung kann unter bestimmten Bedingungen leicht neurotisch fixiert werden. Jede Zeit hat ihre charakteristische Thematik und stellt den Menschen vor spezifische Fragen. Aber nicht alle Menschen einer Epoche leben in der selben Zeit. Sie leben vielmehr gleichzeitig in verschiedenen Zeitaltern. Es gibt Gruppen, die sich die Problematik bereits überholter und von der geistigen Spitzengruppe schon gelöster Lebensfragen erhalten haben. So ist es zu erklären, warum wir Neurosen begegnen, deren Thematik im Grunde schon überholt ist. Solche Menschen machen jetzt die Krisen durch, die etwa die Väter überwunden haben. Deshalb äußert sich das Bild der Neurose einer Epoche bunt und in keiner Weise uniform. Treten temporär in einer Praxis die gleichen Neuroseformen auf, so ist das ein Zeichen dafür, daß eine große Zahl von Menschen mit einer spezifischen Thematik des Lebens nicht fertig wird. Für die Hemmungen der Psyche — d. h. der Neurosen — sind zwei Dinge charakteristisch: einmal die Störung des Menschen in seinem Verhältnis zu sich selbst und zweitens sein Verhältnis zu den Mitmenschen.

Störungen der erektiven Potenz können auch darauf beruhen, daß einer der Partner Spielformen des Vollzuges wünscht, oder von ihnen abhängig ist, die dem anderen unbekannt oder ungewöhnlich sind, weil er sie für abnorm hält, während es sich in Wahrheit nur um Differenzierungen und Varianten der Ars amandi handelt. Hier hilft nur eine Ausräumung von Vorurteilen, denn beim Kulturmenschen sind sexuelle Abweichungen beinahe ein normaler Bestandteil des Trieblebens.

Viele Männer kastrieren sich selbst, indem sie sich mit einer vorzeitigen Impotenz abfinden. Die Schuld trägt hier die eigene Ehefrau.

Gewisse Gifte, wie z. B. Arsen, Blei, Genußmittel, haben auch eine schädliche Wirkung auf die sexuellen Funktionen. Alkohol, viel Nicotin, Opium, Cocain, Morphin sowie Schlafmittel stumpfen ebenfalls den Sexualdrang ab, Abusus von Neuroleptica, Tranquilizern desgleichen. Die amerikanischen Statistiken wie auch die europäischen erwähnen einen immer mehr steigenden Gebrauch von seiten der männlichen Jugend von Tranquilizern, aufpeitschenden Mitteln der Benzedringruppe, sowie von Appetitzüglern. Alle diese Präparate bringen eine Abstumpfung der Libido und eine regelrechte Impotentia coeundi mit sich.

Die Impotentia coeundi ist also als ein Zivilisationsschaden zu betrachten.

Successful Treatment of Azoospermia with Human Gonadotropins

CH. A. JOËL, The Institute for Research and Treatment of Infertility at the State and Municipal Hospitals, the Medical Centre and the University of Tel Aviv (Israel)

The treatment of male fertility disorders, especially those where only isolated spermiocytogenetic cells are found in the ejaculate — i.e. Azoospermias — has only rarely been successful. MAC LEOD et al. (1964) report on the restoration of spermiogenesis after treatment with human menopausal gonadotropin (HMG — trade name Pergonal 500) in a man who had undergone partial hypophysectomy. They were guided by the example of GEMZELL and KJESSLER who in a similar case were able to remove infertility by using a gonadotropic extract from the pituitary glands. Then, in 1965 MOR and his associates reported three successfully treated cases of Azoospermia, using H.M.G. and H.C.G. (human chorionic gonadotropin, trade name Chorigon), while LUNENFELD et al. reported another two cases. In 1967 POLISHUK et al. reported on a total of 23 cases, 6 with Azoospermia, 14 with Oligospermia and 3 with Hypokinesis. In one of the six cases of Azoospermia spermiogenesis was induced to the extent of 5 million sperms per cc and a mobility of 40%.

Unfortunately the spermiocytogram was not taken into account. In four of the 14 Oligospermias the condition of the sperms could be improved and one case resulted in pregnancy.

In all cases FSH values and the genitalia were normal. The authors rightly do not consider the results obtained very encouraging.

Material and Methods

In this report we shall deal only with fertility disorders connected with Azoospermia and Aspermia, whereas a further group of patients with light to severe Oligozoospermia will be treated in a separate report.

In 15 patients aged 21 to 34, two to three and sometimes more sperm examinations were performed before treatment as well as hormone determinations, such as 17 KS, FSH, and the usual blood tests. In addition testicle biopsies were carried out. In the three successful cases two further biopsies were performed after treatment. The patients were given 60 to 70 injections of HMG (Human Menopausal Gonadotropin-Pergonal 500) and the same number of injections of HCG (Human Chorionic Gonadotropin-Chorigon, 2500 J.U.) within a period of 13 to 14 weeks. Of the three patients two are still unmarried. Since the symptoms and findings in all these three cases were practically the same, as was the treatment, and as they have been described in detail elsewhere (2) we shall here discuss only the one case where successful fertilization occurred after treatment and a normal child was born.

Results

This was the case of a 31 year old man of asthenic constitution who had been treated by us since 1961. He first consulted us because he was suffering greatly from a distinct absence of secondary sex characteristics and impotentia coeundi. The anamnesis showed that he had never been seriously ill. Genital examination showed hypoplastic testicles with a longitudinal diameter of 3.5 cm on the right and 3.0 cm on the left inside the scrotum. The epididymis was small, the penis 8 cm long with a circumference of 12 cm and without abnormalities. The seminal vesicles and the prostate were likewise normal. The state of the testicles was indicative of hypogonadism. In several repeated semen examinations isolated spermatogonia were occasionally found after strong centrifugation — i.e. Azoospermia. The blood tests showed normal values. Hormone determination showed that the FSH contained less than 33 R.U. per liter and the 17 KS — 8.5 mg/24 h. Testicle biopsy showed seminiferous tubules of small diameter, basal membrane partly thickened and isolated spermatogonia between the Sertoli cells and in the lumen. The interstitial tissue was edematous or dense with few Leydig cells and occasionally thickened vessel membranes (Fig. 1). Because of the low 17-KS values the patient was given twice weekly injections of 50 mg testosterone isobutyrate crystals over 10 weeks. For the first time in his life normal intercourse became possible. From then until March 1965 he received, as required, 100 to 200 mg testosterone-isobutyrate crystals every 2,3 or 5 months. After this treatment his beard started growing slightly (the patient shaved 2 to 3 times a week) accompanied by an ample growth of public hair.

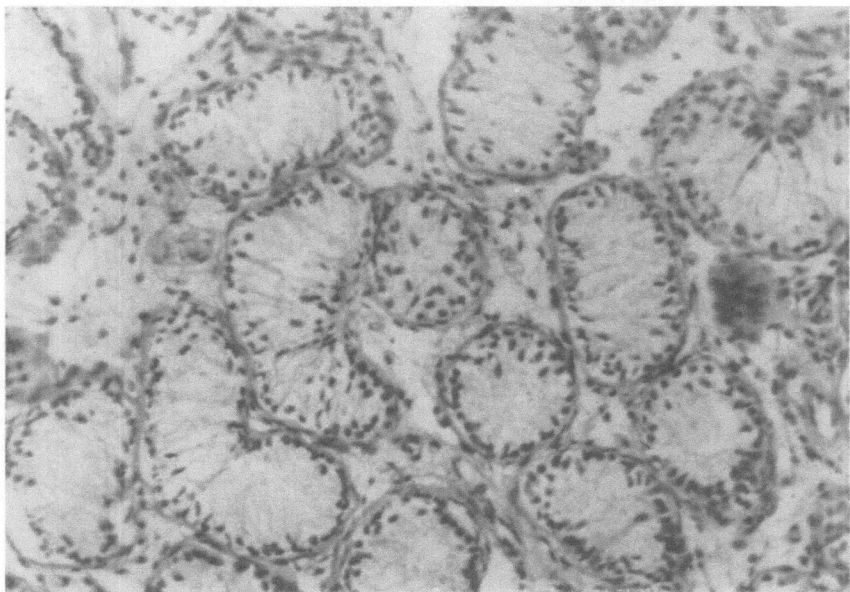

Fig. 1. Testicle biopsy before treatment: Small seminiferous tubules. Basal membrane partly thickened. Isolated spermatogonia between Sertoli-cells. Interstitial tissue edematous or dense with few Leydig-cells. Atrophy grade three. Magnification 560

The patient married in 1963. Two sperm examinations and a testicle biopsy performed on 13th May, 1965 showed the same results as described before. The hormone investigation of 18th March, 1965 carried out by the highly accurate kaolin method showed only traces of FSH and 17 KS — 9.2 mg/24 h.

The patient was accordingly given 65 injections of HMG, Pergonal 500, and a similar number of injections of HCG-Chorigon, 2500 I.U., within 13 weeks. The results were as follows: the sperm examination of 20th June, 1965 showed a quantity of 3 cc with 60% mobility 1 h after ejaculation by the Nativetest and 65% by the Eosine test; after 4 h 30 and 40%, respectively, and after 24 h, 0 and 5%, respectively. The number of sperms was 22 million per cc, a total of 66 million. The spermiocytogram showed 63% normal and 27% pathological sperms, and 10% spermiocytogenetic cells. Fructose content at 2,500 γ/ml was normal.

Accordingly the picture was one of slight Oligozoospermia with low secretion of pathological sperms, and increased number of spermiocytogenetic cells and slightly reduced motility in the native test, with normokinesis in the eosine test.

The hormone values were FSH — 10 M.U./24 h, 17 KS — 12 mg/24 h. The results of the testicle biopsy showed that the seminiferous tubules had a medium

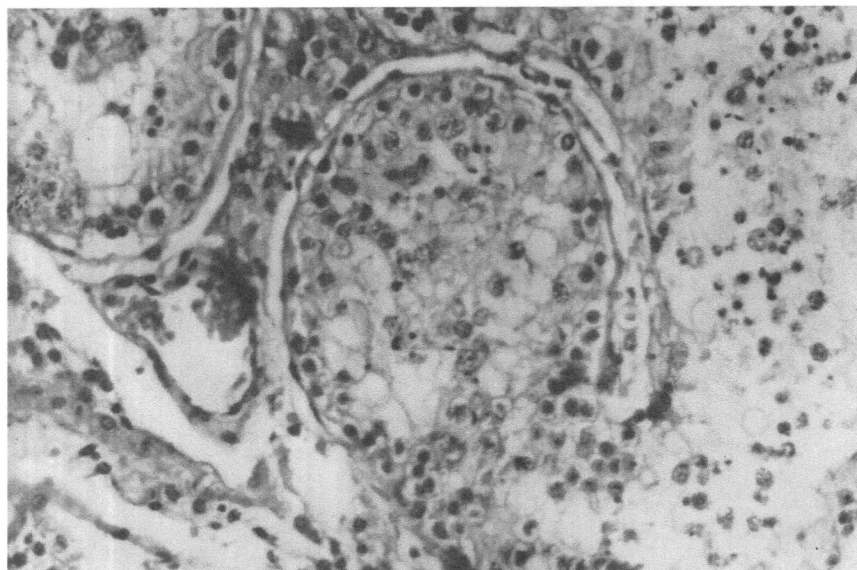

Fig. 2. Testicle biopsy after the first treatment with HMG and HCG: Seminiferous tubules with a medium diameter. Basal membrane thin. Spermiogenetic tissue, mainly spermatogonia between Sertoli-cells and spermatocytes rather few spermatids and sperms. Interstitial tissue normal. Hypospermatogenesis grade one till two. Magnification 560 ×

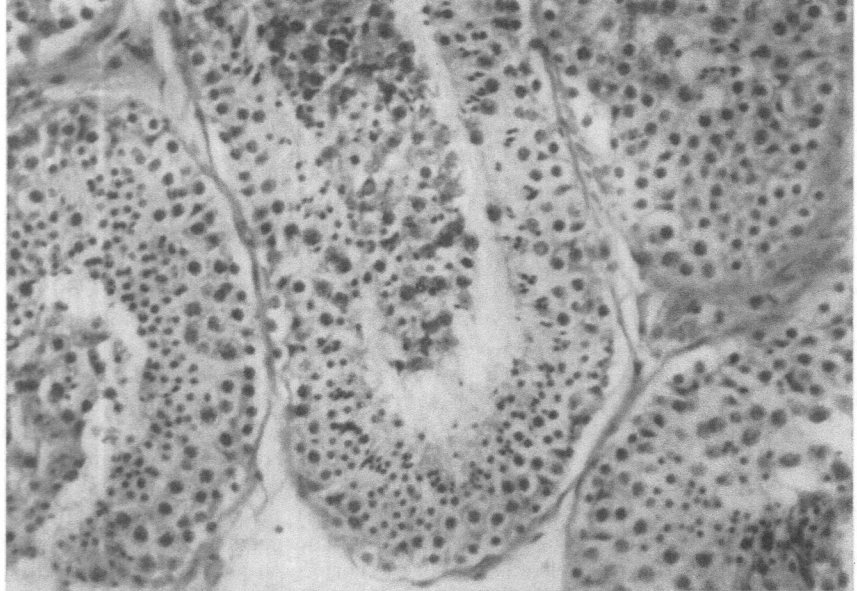

Fig. 3. Testicle biopsy after the second treatment with HMG and HCG: Seminiferous tubules with a large diameter. Spermiogenetic tissue with all stages of spermiogenesis, including many sperms. Interstitial tissue normal. Magnification 560 ×

diameter, the basal membrane was thin, the spermiogenetic tissue, between the Sertoli cells, contained mainly spermatogonia and spermatocytes with rather few spermatids and sperms. The interstitial tissue was normal. According to our nomenclature this corresponds to hypospermogenesis grade 1 to 2 (Fig. 2).

In the light of these results additional similar treatment with 65 injections of Pergonal 500 and Chorigon 2500 I.U. was administered for 13 weeks.

Results: Sperm examination of 25th September 1965 — quantity 3.5 cc; motility — after 1 h 75% by the native test and 80% by the eosine test; after 4 h — 45 and 50%, respectively; after 24 h — 0 and 10%, respectively. The sperm number was 78 millions per cc, — a total of 273 million. The spermiocytogram showed 78% normal, 18% pathological sperms and 4% spermiocytogenetic cells. Fructose contents was 3200 γ/ml, i.e. normal. This means that the semen was perfectly normal. Hormone values: FSH 20 MU/24 h, 17 KS —13.2 mg/24 h. Testicle Biopsy: The seminiferous tubules usually had a large diameter while the basal membrane was thin. The spermiogenetic tissue showed all stages of spermiogenesis, including numerous sperms. Thus the testicular tissue was normal (Fig. 3).

3 months after termination of the second course of treatment the patient's wife became pregnant. The last menstruation was on 5th February, 1966. On 13th November 1966 a healthy boy weighing 3,800 g was born.

Conclusions. Only a few years ago there still were only isolated reports of a successful treatment of Azoospermia.

Thanks to the fact that nowadays by the kaolin method even slight traces of FSH may be determined, and thanks to the production of HMG on an industrial scale, new methods of treatment have become possible, especially of female fertility disturbances where ovulation can be successfully induced.

In seven cases of Azoospermia we were in three cases able to induce spermiogenesis and bring it up to the normal. In one of these patients who was married this eventually resulted in the birth of a boy. In four further patients with Azoospermia without hypogonadism and almost normal FSH values the treatment failed. Similarly unsuccessful were our efforts in eight cases of Aspermia. Present experience — of my own and others — with the use of human gonadotropins in men is still too limited to arrive at a final conclusion. Nevertheless it seems justified, especially in Azoospermias, where former therapeutic measures proved of no avail, to try out treatment with human gonadotropins. These patients have nothing to lose and can only profit because sometimes their infertility can indeed be removed.

Literature. GEMZELL, C. A., and B. KJESSLER: Lancet **1964**, I, 644. — JOEL, C. A.: Harefuah **71**, 281 (1966). — LUNENFELD, B., A. MOR, M. MANI, and N. ZIMBERG: Clinica Europea **4**, 169 (1965). — MAC LEOD, J., A. PASIANOS, and B. S. RAY: Lancet **1964**, I, 1196 .— MOR, A., M. MANI, B. LUNENFELD, and E. RABAU: Harefuah **69**, 43 (1965). — POLISHUK, W. Z., Z. PALTI, and A. LAUFER: Fertil. and Steril. **18**, 127 (1967).

Uses and Abuses of Gonadotrophins in the Male

G. HELLINGA, Amsterdam (The Netherlands)

Although we don't know for certain how many gonadotropic hormones are in existance, in the male we distinguish two different gonadotropic actions. The so-called FSH-gonadotrophin (comparable to the follicle stimulating hormone in the female) acts on the spermatogenetic tissue. LH-gonadotrophin (comparable to the luteinizing hormone in the female) stimulates the cells of Leydig to the production of testosterone. Commercial gonadotrophins have both these activities in different proportions. Rich in FSH-activity are H.M.G., from the urine of post-menopausal nomen, and P.M.S. from the serum of pregnant mares. Chorion gonadotrophin from the urine of pregnant women has mainly LH-activity. The extracts from human pituitary glands have both FSH- and LH-activity.

There are several possibilities for the application of gonadotrophins in the male, to prevent or to cure disturbances in fertility.

1. Testicular Maldescent

Signs of degeneration appear already in the undescended testicles of boys from the age of 6 years and lasting damage thereof begins at the age of 10. So we now aim to correct cases of maldescent at about 10 years of age. Before referring to surgery, treatment with chorion gonadotrophin should always be tried, if there is a possibility of succes.

2. Retarded Puberty

When there are not as yet signs of secundary sexual development in boys of about 14 years of age, one should try to obtain a "priming effect" by a short-term treatment either with androgens or with chorion gonadotrophins.

3. Hypogonadotropic Hypogonadism

In this group, a careful selection of the patients is necessary to prevent deceptions.

a) Sometimes, in patients with the infantile type of hypogonadism the testicular biopsy reveals tubules with undeveloped spermatogenetic tissue. Stimulation with FSH- and LH-gonadotrophins may result in the developement of a normal androgenetic function with normal fertility. It is even possible that in this type of patient a priming effect is obtained and that the treatment may be discontinued after one or two courses. I have seen this happen in a patient when the treatment was started when he was already 32 years old.

b) Quite a few successes are reported in the literature, concerning patients who have lost their gonadotropic activity during or after the age of puberty. This may be because of an encephalitis, destruction of the pituitary gland by a tumor or because of hypophysectomy. Both FSH- and LH-gonadotrophins have to be used.

c) Less frequent are the so-called "fertile eunuchs", who are most often "eunuchoids" however. These patients lack spontaneous LH-activity, whereas the FSH-activity of the pituitary gland is normal. The testicular biopsy shows hypospermatogenesis in an otherwise healthy spermatogenetic tissue. Treatment with LH-gonadotrophins or with testosterone results in normal sex urge and potency and the patients then have fertile semen. As soon as the treatment is discontinued, they have a complete relapse (if not, then they belong to group a) (infantile type of hypogonadism).

Most patients with complete hypogonadism, even those with a very low output of gonadotrophins, have testes smaller than beansize, which are not able to react to gonadotropic stimulation. Treatment with androgens will restore sex urge and the developement of secundary sexual characteristics. There is no use in giving gonadotrophins.

4. Hypogonadotropic Oligo-asthenozoospermia

Many patients with seminal deficiencies of all kinds are treated with gonadotrophins, without a sound and logical base. In our experience there is no sense in treating a man with LH-gonadotrophins as long as his androgenic function is normal. Treatment with FSH-gonadotrophins should be restricted to the following group of patients:

a) the testes should be of fairly normal size;

b) in the semen, a low density and low motility should not be accompanied by an increase in the number of abnormal head forms;

c) the output of gonadotrophins in the urine should be low;

d) local anomalies (for instance a varicocele) or general disabilities of any kind should be ruled out.

If so desired, I will give you particulars about the dosages and the results of our follow-up study.

5. Teratozoospermia

Patients with teratozoospermia (semen with low density, low motility and a high number of abnormal headforms) rarely have a gonadotropic deficiency. Most often, the output of gonadotrophins is rather high (probably as a result of "non-consumption" by the seminiferous tissue), so there is no sense in treating these patients with gonadotrophins. A well known manner of treatment (if there is no demonstrable local or general cause for the subfertility) is to try for a rebound effect after the inhibition of the spermatogenesis with high doses of testosterone. This has the disadvantage however, that some of the patients, after having reached the stage of azoospermia, do never recover completely, and a number of patients will end up worse than they were, instead of having a rebound phenomenon. Apparently, during the stage of inhibition of the endogenous gonadotrophins, damage occurs to the spermatogenetic tissue, as has been shown in testicular biopsies by several authors. Dr. EVERTSE from Organon suggested many years ago that the addition of FSH-gonadotrophin (Gestyl) might be able to prevent the local damage. This proved to be true. We could prove in twelve patients who submitted to a testicular biopsy before and after the injections (after 6 weeks) that the signs of degeneration in the testicular tubules were absolutely absent (Everse-effect). There was no thickening of the basal membranes, no kariorexis or kariolysis. Since we add Gestyl injections to the testosterone, we never see a lasting damage from our trials to get a rebound effect.

I regret to say that the percentage of patients who show a "two-point-improvement" and also the percentage of pregnancies are not increased by the addition of Gestyl. About half of the patients show a significant improvement. In the follow-up study of 1960 we found in 225 patients 31 % pregnancies in the patients who were improved, against 18 % in those who did not show a two-point improvoment.

6. The Overproduction Effect

Lastly, there is a treatment known as the Overproduction effect, which, as far as I know, has been introduced by HOHLWEG. He gave testosterone together with LH-gonadotrophin. This should maintain the function of the cells of Leydig during the inhibition of the endogenous LH-production by the testosterone. After cessation of the therapy this should lead to an increased hormone production and so to an improvement of the spermatogenesis. I have to admit that the theoretical background seems to me rather dubious; I have no personal experience with this treatment.

All in all we can say that there are a number of good indications for the treatment of males with infertility or subfertility with certain kinds of gonadotrophins. However, results can only be expected, when the patients are carefully screened and selected.

Nicht-hormonale Substanzen in der Behandlung der männlichen Infertilität

W. NIKOLOWSKI, Hautklinik der Stadt Augsburg (Deutschland)

Ausgehend von den Resultaten andrologischer Sprechstunden (negative Auslese!) kann man gegenwärtig allenfalls in 10 bis 15% aller Fälle von infertilitas et subfertilitas virilis mit befriedigenden Erfolgen rechnen [44]. Obwohl therapeutisch der Verabfolgung von Hormonen (Testosteron, Gonadotropine) der erste Platz gebührt, sollten die nicht-hormonalen Behandlungsmöglichkeiten nicht vernachlässigt werden.

Unter den nichthormonalen Substanzen rangieren die *Vitamine* an der Spitze — unter diesen das Vitamin E (= Tokopherol).

Der sich auf die Fertilität bzw. Sterilität erstreckende, für den Menschen nicht unbestrittene Effekt des Vitamins E ist ein Teil seines komplexen Wirkungsmechanismus [28, 29] und dürfte mit der Gonadotropinbildung zusammenhängen [63]. Als gesichert kann u. a. gelten, daß beim männlichen Vitamin-E-Mangeltier eine Reduzierung des Keimepithels bis auf die Sertoli-Zellen stattfindet, daß unter Vitamin-E-Zufuhr die Produktion der corticotropen [58], thyreotropen [53] und gonadotropen [34] Vorderlappenhormone gesteigert wird, daß nach Wärmeschädigung der Testes im Tierversuch der Repopulationsgrad unter Tokopherol größer ist als nach Choriongonadotropin oder Serumgonadotropin und Testosteron [23] und daß ein im Säugetierejaculat nachweisbares Antiagglutinin in einer abspaltbaren Gruppe neben Schwefelsäureester und Zucker auch Alpha-Tokopherol enthält [26].

Neben einer Reihe negativer Beurteilungen des Vitamin-E-Effektes bei männlichen Fertilitätsstörungen (z. B. [8, 18, 30, 31, 62]) liegen zahlreiche Empfehlungen vor, z. B. (chronologische Reihenfolge) Anwendung bei nicht neuropathisch bedingter Sterilität [11, 12]; Stimulierung der exkretorischen Hodenfunktion durch Vitamin E in Kombination mit Hypophysenvorderlappen-Gesamtextrakt [32]; Heilung von Impotentia coeundi und generandi durch Behandlung mit Vorderlappenextrakt, einem Testes-Yohimbin-Kombinationspräparat und nachfolgender Vitaminverabfolgung [51]; Einleitung jeder Subfertilitätstherapie mit Vitamin E [55]; Zunahme der spontan beweglichen Spermien [9]; regelmäßige Anhebung der Spermiogenese bei 30 mg Vitamin E für 3 Monate [4]; vielfach günstiger Einfluß [6]; Tages- und Gesamtdosen entscheiden über Erfolg oder Mißerfolg [21]; hormonsparender Effekt des Tokopherols, daher Anwendung im Beginn und im Intervall bei jeder Fertilitätsbehandlung [35]; Warnung vor relativer Überdosierung [35, 36, 38]; häufiger Nachweis erniedrigter Serum-Tokopherolspiegel bei Störungen der Sexualfunktionen [13]; Vitamin E als Differential-Prognosticum [37]; Zunahme der Spermienmotilität bzw. -vitalität [57]; Vitamin E wichtiges, vielleicht wesentliches Adjuvans bei Fertilitätskuren [7]; vielfach erniedrigte Serum-Tokopherolwerte bei den tubulären, v. a. bei der inkretorisch-exkretorischen Insuffizienz [1]; Vitamin E wertvoll bei Oligozoospermie täglich 50 bis 100 mg [10]; Zunahme der Spermienquantität unter Vitamin E zuverlässiger erreichbar als nach Testosteron oder Gonadotropin [2].

Zusammenfassend kann empfohlen werden, jede Behandlung bei In- oder Subfertilität mit Vitamin E zu beginnen und die Dosis (anfänglich) dem Grade der tubulären Insuffizienz anzupassen, z. B. 10 bis 20 mg Tokopherol bei Ausgangswerten von weniger als 20000000 Spermien/ml, 60 bis 100 mg bei 20- bis 40000000 Sp./ml, 100 mg (und mehr) bei 40- bis 60000000 Sp./ml, insgesamt pro Kur (durchschnittlich 2 Monate) 600 bis 1800 — 3600 — 6000 mg [39, 40, 41, 42, 43, 44, 45, 46, 47, 48].

Die Anwendung von *Vitamin A* bei der exkretorischen Hodeninsuffizienz läßt sich tierexperimentell gut begründen; denn bei Vitamin-A-frei ernährten Ratten tritt nach etwa 1 Monat völlige Atrophie des Keimepithels unter Erhaltenbleiben der für Ernährung und Regeneration bedeutsamen Sertoli-Zellen auf [25]. Negativen Bewertungen des Vitamin-A-Effektes bei männlichen Fertilitätsstörungen (z. B. [3, 19, 20]) stehen eine Reihe positiver Berichte gegenüber, z. B. Zunahme von Spermienzahl und -motilität bei Tagesdosen zwischen 30 und 50000 IE, Abnahme bei Dosen von 100 bis 200000 IE [33]; günstig bei Spermiogenesehemmungen geringen Grades [50]; 1 bis 6 Monate täglich 50 bis 200000 IE, zum Teil kein Einfluß, zum überwiegenden Teil jedoch Besserung und Empfängnis [52]; 3 Monate täglich 50 bis 100000 IE, zusätzlich Hormontherapie, überwiegend Anhebung bzw. Konzeption [57]; zum Teil erfolgreich [64]; Zunahme des Ejaculatvolumens, qualitative Normalisierung der Spermiogenese [22]; abgesehen von Zuständen nach Dystrophie keine Beziehung zwischen Vitamin-A-Gehalt im Serum und Grad der tubulären Störung, gelegentlich allerdings Spiegelanstieg nach Testosteron [1].

Zusammenfassend kann die (zusätzliche) Vitamin-A-Medikation versucht werden nach Abheilung entzündlicher (Rest)-Zustände, nach Anastomosenoperation und bei vorhandener, jedoch verlangsamter Spontanregeneration, z. B. nach hormonaler Bremstherapie [49].

Die Verabfolgung von *Vitamin B* — entweder sämtlicher oder einzelner Faktoren — wird verschiedentlich empfohlen (z. B. [54]). Die angegebene Stimulierung der Motilität (20% aller Fälle) konnte in eigenen Beobachtungsreihen nicht bestätigt werden.

Dem *Vitamin C* wird bei mehrmonatiger hochdosierter Zuführung (täglich 1,0 bis 2,0) ein positiver Einfluß auf Quantität und Qualität der Spermiogenese zugesprochen [3], was nicht in Abrede gestellt werden kann.

Über andere Vitamine liegen keine verwertbaren Resultate vor. Die Aufsehen erregenden Erfolge nach Verabfolgung von Vitamin T Goetsch [61] sind offenbar nicht nachgeprüft worden.

Da ein (latenter) Hyperoestrogenismus gelegentlich in ursächlichen Zusammenhang mit einer Subfertilität gebracht wird und da *lipotrope Substanzen* in der Leber den Abbau des endogen gebildeten (weiblichen) Hormons beschleunigen, ist ein entsprechender Therapieversuch vertretbar [15, 16, 14, 60].

Gelegentliche Mitteilungen über Stimulierung der Spermiogenese durch *Antibiotica* [59] sind vermutlich auf Ausheilung von — den Spermienstoffwechsel beeinträchtigenden — akut- und vor allem chronisch-entzündlichen Krankheits-(Rest-)Zuständen in den abführenden Samenwegen und namentlich in den akzessorischen Geschlechtsdrüsen zu beziehen. Obwohl derartige Adnexitiden usw. bei weniger als 10% der wegen Kinderwunsches den Andrologen aufsuchenden Männern die (wesentliche) Ursache der Subfertilität darstellen [44], sollte stets danach gefahndet werden [27, 24]; denn die nach Erregertestung einzuleitende antibiotische Therapie hat — in Verbindung mit einer schulmäßigen Prostatitis-usw. -Behandlung — eine relativ hohe Erfolgsquote, und zwar nicht nur bei derartig bedingter Oligo- oder Asthenozoospermie, sondern auch bei Teratozoospermie [43].

Die Verabfolgung von *Spasmolytica* (dreimal täglich 15 mg Belladonna bzw. dreimal 40 mg Papaverin durchgehend für 6 Wochen oder lediglich vom 4. bis 14. Tage des Cyclus der Ehefrau) wurde unter Hinweis auf die mögliche Bedeutung spastischer Zustände im Bereiche der glatten Muskulatur der männlichen Genitalorgane für eine unvollständige Entleerung der Samenwege bei der Ejaculation und eine so bedingte Herabsetzung von Zahl und Motilität der Spermien empfohlen [17]. Indikationen können also darstellen Oligozoo-, Astheno- und Oligo-Asthenozoo-Spermieformen — nicht jedoch eine Teratozoospermie. Die zahlenmäßig noch wenig umfassenden eigenen Beobachtungen (lediglich cyclusgerechte Behandlung mit Papaverin) bestätigen, daß bei mittleren Oligozoospermieformen eine Erhöhung der Spermiendichte möglich ist.

Abschließend kann gesagt werden, daß trotz der — statistisch gesehen — wenig günstigen Prognose der Mehrzahl männlicher Fertilitätsstörungen eine Behandlung bzw. ein Behandlungsversuch (nach entsprechender Belehrung über Aussichten und zeitliche Begrenzung) bei jedem Manne gerechtfertigt ist, bei welchem sich im Ejaculat oder im Hodenparenchym überhaupt noch eine spermiogenetische Aktivität nachweisen läßt [46].

Nach Unterrichtung über allgemeine Verhaltungsmaßnahmen [43] sollten nichthormonale Substanzen im Rahmen des Behandlungsplanes sinnvoll eingesetzt werden, d. h. namentlich im Beginn und im Intervall. Das gilt um so mehr, als einmal in einer andrologischen Sprechstunde überwiegend Männer ohne inkretorische, vielmehr mit rein exkretorischer Hodeninsuffizienz zur Untersuchung kommen und zum anderen unerwünschte Nebenwirkungen weitgehend fehlen. Für die Verordnung von Vitamin E sprechen darüber hinaus sein hormonsparender Effekt und sein hoher differentialprognostischer Wert.

Literatur. 1. ADAM, W., u. W. NIKOLOWSKI: Proc. II. World Congr. Fert. Ster., Bd. I, S. 219. Neapel 1956. — 2. AWENDER, R. L.: Behandlung männlicher Fertilitätsstörungen. Inaug.-Diss., Tübingen 1961. — 3. BALLERIO, C., u. A. GIAROLO: Gynéc. prat. 4, 95 (1953). — 4. BLAHAK: Zit. n. SWYER. — 5. BOEMINGHAUS, H., u. H. KLOSTERHALFEN: Z. Urol. 51, 249 (1958). — 6. BOHNSTEDT, R. M., u. J. WAGNER: Ärztl. Wschr. 1949, 460. — 7. CLOTTEN, R.: Ärztl. Forsch. 1954, I, 109. — 8. DOEPFMER, R.: Derm. Wschr. 145, 185 (1962). — 9. FARRIS, E. J.: Ann. N.Y. Acad. Sci. 52, 409 (1949). — 10. GERTLER, W.: Dtsch. Gesundh.-Wes. 1960, 1871. — 11. GIERHAKE. E.: Klin. Wschr. 1936, 220. — 12. GIERHAKE, E.: Münch. med. Wschr. 1936, 1720. — 13. GIESE, H., u. R. BECKMANN: Med. Welt 1951, 1172. — 14. GLASS: Disk. z. Heckel u. McDonald. Fertil. and Steril. 3, 49 (1952). — 15. GOLDMAN, J.: Fertil. and Steril. 1, 259 (1950). — 16. HARTMANN, I., R. HERTEL, G. SCHULZE und H. WELLMER: Naunyn-Schmiedeberg's Arch. exp. Path. Pharmak. 214, 152 (1951). — 17. HELLINGA, G.: Spasmolytica in der Therapie von Fertilitätsstörungen. In: Neue Ergebnisse der Andrologie, hrsg. von C. SCHIRREN, Berlin-Heidelberg-New York: Springer 1965. — 18. HERBRAND u. LAEMMER: Zit. n. GIESE u. BECKMANN. — 19. HORNE, H. W., and CH. L. MADDOCK: Fertil. and Steril. 1, 123 (1956). — 20. JANSON, PH.: Hippokrates (Stuttg.) 1956, 470. — 21. KAISER, B.: Medizinische 1950, 1516. — 22. KAR, J. K., and R. M. KAPADIA: Indian. J. Med. Sci. 8, 625 (1954). — 23. KIESSLING, W.: Hautarzt 13, 11 (1962). — 24. KIESSLING, W.: Z. Haut- u. Geschl.-Kr. 38, 198 (1965). — 25. KÜTTNER, H.: Frankfurt. Z. Path. 54, 113 (1940). — 26. LINDAHL, P. E., and J. E. KIHLSTRÖM: Nature (Lond.) 174, 600 (1954). — 27. LUDVIK, W.: Wien. med. Wschr. 1964, 825. — 28. MARKEES, S.: Int. Z. Vitamin-forsch. 22, 335 (1950). — 29. MARKEES, S.: Dtsch. med. Wschr. 1956, 976. — 30. MEYHÖFER, W.: Derm. Wschr. 145, 187 (1962). — 31. MILLER, W. H., and A. M. DESSERT: Ann. N.Y. Accad. Sci. 52, 167 (1959). — 32. MÖNCH, G. L.: Mschr. Geburtsh. Gynäk. 105, 154 (1937). — 33. NARPOZZI: Riv. Ostet. Ginec. 36, 254 (1949). — 34. NEGRO, u. SCOPINARO: Zit. n. CLOTTEN. — 35. NIKOLOWSKI, W.: Therap. d. Gegenw. 1950, 329. — 36. NIKOLOWSKI, W.: Z. Urol. 43, 94 (1950). — 37. NIKOLOWSKI, W.: Therapiewoche 1951/52, 10/11. — 38. NIKOLOWSKI, W.: Strahlentherapie 87, 113 (1952). — 39. NIKOLOWSKI, W.: Therapiewoche 1955/56, 23/24. — 40. NIKOLOWSKI, W.: Dtsch. med. Wschr. 1958, 984. — 41. NIKOLOWSKI, W.: Med. Klin. 1960, 415. — 42. NIKOLOWSKI, W.: Med. Welt 1961, 1130. — 43. NIKOLOWSKI, W.: Die Zeugungsfähigkeit des Mannes und ihre Störungen. In: Dermatologie u. Venerologie, hrsg. v. GOTTRON, u. SCHÖNFELD, Bd. I/2. Stuttgart: Thieme 1962. — 44. NIKOLOWSKI, W.: Hautarzt 13, 377 (1962). — 45. NIKOLOWSKI, W.: Derm. Wschr. 145, 189 (1962). — 46. NIKOLOWSKI, W.: Derm. Wschr. 152, 722 (1966). — 47. NIKOLOWSKI, W.: Münch. med. Wschr. 1967, 913. — 48. NIKOLOWSKI, W., and W. ADAM: Proc. II. World Congr. Fertil. Steril., Bd. II, 729, Neapel 1956. — 49. NIKOLOWSKI, W., and W. ADAM: Proc. II. World Congr. Fertil. Steril. Bd. II, 770. Neapel 1956. — 50. PILLAY, A. P.: J. Sexology 1953, 51. — 51. RITTER, H.: Med. Welt 1937, 504. — 52. RÜTTE, U. v.: Gynaecologia (Basel) 135, 83 (1953). — 53. SCHNEIDER, E.: Med. Klin. 1939, 499. — 54. SINGHER, H. O., and E. T. TYLER: Proc. II. World Congr. Fertil. Steril. Neapel 1956. — 55. STEMMER,

W.: Med. Welt **1940**, 375. — 56. Swyer: Brit. J. Nutr. **3**, 100 (1949). — 57. Tschumi, R.: Gynaecologia (Basel) **135**, 87 (1953). — 58. Tonutti, E.: Int. Z. Vitamin-forsch. **13**, 1 (1943). — 59. Tremblay, E. C., P. Destouches et N. Karatchenzeff: Presse méd. **1953**, 292. — 60. Tyler, E. T., and H. O. Singher: J. Amer. med. Ass. **1956**, 91. — 61. Urgell, M.: Proc. II. World Congr. Fertil. Steril., II. Bd., 778. Neapel 1956. — 62. Valle, u. Segere: Zit. n. Giese, u. Beckmann. — 63. Verzar, F.: Exper. Befunde f. eine Theorie d. Angriffspunktes von Vit. E. In: Vitamina E Atti de terzo Congresso Intern., Venezia 1955 (Verona 1956). — 64 Wenner, R.: Ther. Umsch. **1954**, 88.

Free Communications

Klinische, histologische und endokrinologische Untersuchungen beim „idiopathischen" Hyperoestrogenismus

M. F. Hofmann, G. Pozzo und M. Cristofolini, Clinica Dermatologica dell' Università, Mailand, und Ospedale Civile, Trient (Italien)

Bei 100 Fällen von männlicher Hypofertilität bzw. Sterilität wurden folgende Untersuchungen angestellt:

Krankengeschichte und genaue klinische Untersuchung unter Zugrundelegung eines Fragebogens.

Spermiogramm (Ejaculatvolumen, Spermienzahl/ml, quali- und quantitative Motilität, Morphologie).

Hormone im 24-Std-Harn: 17 Ketosteroide, 17 Hydroxycorticosteroide, Phenolsteroide, Gonadotropine.

Bei gewissen Fällen dynamische Hormonuntersuchungen: Wiederholung der Dosierung der 17 Ketosteroide und Phenolsteroide nach Stimulierung mit 5000 Chorion-Gonadotropineinheiten/Tag während 3 Tagen.

Dosierung des basalen Plasmakortisols, nach ACTH-Reiz und nach Dexamethasoninhibition.

Routinelaborprüfungen: Blutsenkung, Elektrolyte, Protidogramm, Blutzucker, Glucosebelastungskurve.

Radiographie des Schädels, speziell des Türkensattels (sella turcica).

Radiographie gewisser Skeletabschnitte zur Untersuchung der Knochenentwicklung und Suche nach Osteoporose.

Psychiatrische Untersuchung (beim Klinefelter-Syndrom und besonderen Fällen).

Bei diesen Untersuchungen fielen 15 Patienten mit folgenden Charasteristiken auf:

Junge kräftige Männer; kein chronischer Äthylismus; kein eunuchoider Habitus; bedeutungslose Anamnese, insbesondere keine klinisch ersichtlichen Leberschäden; Serumlabilität und Protidogramm normal.

Hypofertilität: Spermienzahl/ml 2 bis 10 Millionen; Motilität 10 bis 30%; normale Spermien 50 bis 70%; Hodenbiopsie: Verarmung der spermiogenetischen Linie, zum Teil mit Spermiogenesestop; Basalmembran mehr oder weniger verdickt.

Hormone im Harn: Zunahme der Phenolsteroide, insbesondere nach Chorion-Gonadotropinstimulierung; übrige Hormone im Normalbereich.

Glucosebelastungskurve: eindeutige Erhöhung des hyperglykämischen Dreiecks von Labbe und Thepenier; Blutzucker an sich normal.

Zusammenfassend handelte es sich um kräftige junge Männer mit einer Alteration der Spermiogenese auf Grund einer Verarmung der spermiogenetischen Linie, mit verdickter Basalmembran, pathologischer Blutzuckerbelastungskurve, erhöhter Phenolsteroidausscheidung wahrscheinlich primärer Art, da keine so beachtlichen Leberschäden bestanden, daß ein fehlender Abbau der Oestrogene angenommen werden könnte.

Diese Befunde sind noch schwer zu interpretieren. Eine Bestätigung und eine Klärung für diese Fälle kann wahrscheinlich nach Dosierung der Plasmahormone mittels Gaschromatographie erfolgen, eine Methode, von der wir hoffen, sie baldigst in unsere Prüfungen einschließen zu können.

Spermaqualität und Konzeptionsrate

R. KADEN, Hautklinik der Freien Universität im Rudolf Virchow-Krankenhaus Berlin (Deutschland)

Über die Bewertung spermatologischer Befunde hinsichtlich Beurteilung des Zeugungsvermögens ist man sich bekanntlich nicht einig. MacLEOD u. GOLD (1951) haben zwar nach größeren Reihenuntersuchungen recht überzeugende Richtlinien für die Bewertung spermatologischer Befunde aufgestellt, jedoch gibt es nur wenig Beobachtungen über jenes Krankengut, das wegen jahrelanger ungewollter Kinderlosigkeit in der andrologischen Sprechstunde anzutreffen ist (SCHIRREN u. BUNGE, 1964). Bei der Behandlung erstrebt man erfahrungsgemäß als Nahziel eine Verbesserung der Samenqualität, die in diesen Fällen nur dann einen Wert hat, wenn sich eine entsprechende Verbesserung der Konzeptionschance nachweisen läßt [SCHIRREN, 1965; KADEN, 1966, (1, 2)].

Deshalb sind am eigenen Krankengut sowohl die Therapiewirkung auf das Spermiogramm in Kontrolluntersuchungen festgestellt als auch die Ehen auf Eintritt von Schwangerschaften in katamnestischen Explorationen überprüft worden.

Eigene Untersuchungen

Bei allen Vorhaben sind grundsätzlich nur spermatologisch fertile oder subfertile Männer berücksichtigt worden, da der Nachweis einer totalen Infertilität praktisch ein unabänderlicher Status ist (MOLNAR, 1963). Für die spermatologischen Kontrollen nach Hormontherapie sind 45 subfertile Männer eliminiert worden. Die Therapie bestand aus 3monatigen Kuren überwiegend mit insgesamt 18000 IE Gonadotropin und 800 mg Methyltestosteron bzw. 1600 mg Methylandrostanolon. Vor und nach der Therapie ist jeweils Ejaculat nach 5tägiger Karenzzeit per masturbationem für die spermatologische Untersuchung gewonnen worden.

Die Behandlungsergebnisse lassen sich durch Vergleich der Kontrollspermiogramme mit den Anfangsspermiogrammen nachweisen. Für diese Arbeit ist das Interesse lediglich auf Dichte, Motilität und Normalmorphologie der Spermien beschränkt worden. In einer graphischen Darstellung (Abb. 1) ist die wertmäßige Verbesserung der Einzelfaktoren auf der Plusseite und die Verschlechterung auf der Minusseite ablesbar. Bei Ordnung in Gruppen mit zunehmender Spermiendichte finden sich bei den Faktoren der *Dichte* und *Motilität* die eindrucksvollsten Veränderungen durch deutliche Verbesserungen in den mittleren Bereichen. Dagegen sind extrem schlechte Qualitäten der Hormontherapie offensichtlich kaum zugänglich.

Bei den katamnestischen Explorationen über Konzeptionen in den folgenden 4 Jahren nach der andrologischen Erstuntersuchung des Ehemannes haben sich die Befunde von 152 Ehen, die folgende Vorbedingungen erfüllten, verwerten lassen: Mehrjährige Ehe mit durchschnittlich 3jähriger ungewollter Kinderlosigkeit, spermatologische Beurteilung mit fertil oder subfertil (ausgeschlossen Infertilität), Ehefrau gynäkologisch angeblich empfängnisfähig, mehrjährige (mindestens 1 Jahr, höchstens 4 Jahre) Nachbeobachtungszeit und unveränderter Kinderwunsch.

Bei durchschnittlich 3jähriger ungewollter Kinderlosigkeit ist es in 41 Ehen trotz spermatologischer Fertilität des Ehemannes nur zu 13 = 32% Konzeptionen gekommen. In 111 Ehen mit subfertil beurteilten Ehemännern ist die Konzeptionsrate mit 29 = 26% Konzeptionen lediglich um 6% geringer. Die Resultate bei hormonbehandelten bzw. unbehandelten Ehemännern lassen mit 27% bzw.

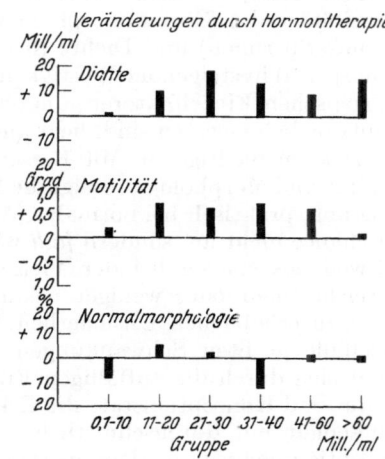

Abb. 1. Veränderungen spermatologischer Einzelfaktoren innerhalb Gruppen zunehmender Spermiendichte nach eins bis zwei kombinierten Gonadotropin-Testosteronkuren. Mittelwerte von 45 Patienten

Tabelle. *Konzeptionen bei 3jähriger Kinderlosigkeit, geordnet nach spermatologischer Fertilität und Subfertilität*

Fertilität (41 Ehen)		Subfertilität (111 Ehen)
	behandelt	21/78 = 27%
	unbehandelt	8/33 = 24%
13 = 32%	insgesamt	29 = 26%

24% eine unwesentliche Verbesserung durch die Behandlung erkennen (Tab.). Bei Zugrundelegung des üblichen Bewertungsmaßstabes erscheint die Konzeptionsrate von lediglich 32% bei spermatologisch fertil bewerteten Ehemännern unerklärlich

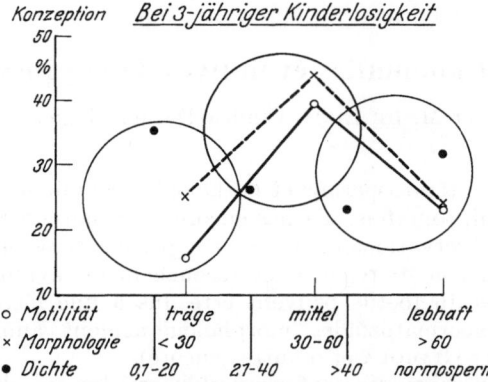

Abb. 2. Konzeptionsraten bei 3jähriger Kinderlosigkeit nach spermatologischen Einzelfaktoren in steigender Wertigkeit. Mußmaßliche Konzeptionschance nach gruppaler Zusammenfassung

gering, zumal bei gesunden Ehepartnern innerhalb eines Jahres mindestens etwa 75 bis 90% Konzeptionen zu erwarten sind (HEINKE u. DOEPFMER, 1960). Man darf jedoch nicht übersehen, daß vorliegendes Krankengut eine spezielle, wenn nicht *negative Auswahl* darstellt, da die andrologische Vorgeschichte dieser Männer durch eine mehrjährige ungewollt sterile Ehe belastet ist.

Es fragt sich nun, welche der spermatologischen Einzelfaktoren im Zusammenhang mit der gesamtspermatologischen Situation den größten Einfluß auf die Konzeptionsrate haben. Bei graphischer Darstellung dieser Verhältnisse (Abb. 2) sind Angaben verwendet worden, denen die katamnestisch ermittelten Konzeptionen innerhalb Gruppen gleicher spermatologischer Einzelfaktoren, wie Motilität (drei Intensitätsgrade), Normalmorphologie (unter 30, 30 bis 60 und über 60% normal geformte Spermien) und Dichte (0,1 bis 20, 21 bis 40, über 40 Millionen/ml und normosperm) in steigender Wertigkeit zugrunde liegen. Bei den schlechtesten spermatologischen Einzelfaktoren, die offenbar für die bisherige Kinderlosigkeit mitverantwortlich gewesen sind, liegt auch die Konzeptionsrate in der Nachbeobachtungszeit am niedrigsten. Mit Besserung der Spermaqualität, im besonderen der Motilität und Morphologie, steigt die Konzeptionsrate konkordant an. Bei weiterer Besserung, praktisch bei normalen Wertigkeiten, hält die Steigerung der Konzeptionschance nicht an, sondern *fällt* wider Erwarten ab.

Zweifellos spielen bei der Vielschichtigkeit des konzeptionellen Geschehens zahlreiche mehr oder weniger bekannte Imponderabilien eine große Rolle und führen zu erheblichen Unsicherheitsfaktoren, so daß die Konzeptionschance im Einzelfalle größten Schwankungen unterworfen ist (KADEN, 1967). Immerhin drängt sich durch die auffälligen Ergebnisse der Beziehungen zwischen Spermaqualität und Konzeptionsrate die Erklärung auf, daß im speziellen andrologischen Krankengut mit durchschnittlich mehrjähriger ungewollter Kinderlosigkeit die Konzeptionschance aus dem spermatologischen Befund nach *anderen Maßstäben* zu beurteilen ist als bei anamnestisch unbelasteten Männern.

Literatur. HEINKE, E., u. R. DOEPFMER: In: MARCHIONINI, A.: Erg.-Werk. Hdb. Haut-u. Geschl.-Kr. Bd. VI, Teil 3. Berlin-Göttingen-Heidelberg: Springer 1960. — KADEN, R.: (1) Vortrag 5. Tagg. dtsch. Ges. Fertilität. Regensburg 1966; — (2) Forsch. Prax. Fortb. (Med) 17, 219 (1966); — Vortrag 1. Europ. Kongreß Fertilität u. Sterilität, Venedig 1967. — MACLEOD, J., and R. GOLD: J. Urol. (Baltimore) 66, 436 (1951). — MOLNAR, J.: Allgemeine Spermatologie. Budapest: Verlag Ungar. Akademie d. Wissenschaften 1963. — SCHIRREN, C.: In: C. SCHIRREN: Neue Ergebnisse der Andrologie, S. 64. Berlin-Heidelberg-New York: Springer 1965. — SCHIRREN, C., u. U. BUNGE: Med. Welt 1964, 2343.

Tératospermie et anomalies évolutives de la grossesse

A. MONTAGNANI, et M. DE LUCA, Clinica Dermatologicà dell'Universita di Napoli (Italie)

Les rapports entre tératospermie et pathologie gravidique constituent un problème important, qui, toutefois, n'a pas encore été éclairci dans tous ses aspects.

De nombreuses observations cliniques et expérimentales ont confirmé que, en certains cas, les avortements répétés, les accouchements avant terme, les malformations congénitales du foetus peuvent être dus à une fécondation de l'ovule effectuée par des spermatozoïdes morphologiquement anormaux (HINGLAIS, LEGROS, BALLERIO et GIAROLA et d'autres encore).

Après un examen soigneusement conduit parmi les cas observés au sujet du sperme au Centre de Sexologie de la Clinique Dermatologiques de Naples, une donnée est apparue, en accord avec ce qui a été désormais accepté par presque tous les Aa., c'est-à-dire: un sujet du sexe masculin peut être fertile quand le nombre de spermatozoïdes par cc n'est pas inférieur à 20 millions, pourvu que le plasma séminal et les némaspermes mêmes répondent aux paramètres de la physiologie (pH, viscosité, activités enzymatiques, fructose, morphologie, activité cinétique, etc.).

De plus, en soumettant à l'examen des sujets sûrement fertiles nous avons remarqué que le plus fort pourcentage de formes némaspermiques anormales encore compatibles avec la fertilité, est résulté être le 35%, plus élevé que celui qui est admis par d'autres Aa. (LANE-ROBERTS, WEISSMANN, etc.).

Nous basant sur ces données et sur les signalations des Aa. précédemment cités, nous avons examiné 130 sujets dont les épouses déclaraient une histoire d'avortements répétés, d'accouchements avant terme avec foetus morts, accouchements à terme avec foetus prémorts ou foetus vivants mais non viables ou présentant de graves malformations; nous avons fait cet examen avec le but de vérifier la possibilité d'un rapport causal entre anomalies morphologiques des némaspermes et anomalies gravidiques que nous venons de rapporter, naturellement en l'absence de conditions pathologiques de la mère qui auraient pu justifier à elles seules ces mêmes anomalies.

Nous avons donc réparti de la façon suivante les 130 cas examinés:

1. Oligozoospermie ($<$ de 20 000 000 de spermatozoïdes/cc) .... 5 cas
2. Normospermie (20/100 000 000 de spermatozoïdes/cc) .... 80 cas
3. Hyperspermie ($>$ de 100 000 000 de spermatozoïdes/cc) .... 45 cas

$n°$ 130 cas

Pour ce qui concerne le type des mouvements, nous avons distingués deux groupes:

1. $n°$ 120 cas avec spermatozoïdes doués de mouvements en prévalence progressifs;
2. $n°$ 10 cas avec spermatozoïdes doués de mouvements en prévalence sussultoires et rotatoires

Sur la base de l'examen morphologique exécuté sur des frottis colorés à la carbolfuxine à environ 3000 grossissements et ensuite sur la base des formules relatives (spermiocitogramme), nous avons déduit les données suivantes, qui concernent de plus près le but de notre étude:

1. Spermiocitogramme normal (formes anormales $<$ de 35% .... $n°$ 15 cas
2. Spermiocitogramme anormal (formes anormales $>$ 39—81% .... $n°$ 115 cas

Environ 89% de nos patients, donc, présentaient un tableau plu ou moins grave de tératospermie: cette donnée nous semble avoir un intérêt particulier si l'on tient compte que, chez ces mêmes patients, la concentration et l'activité cinétique des némaspermes apparaissait normales ou, de toute façon, dans les limites de la normalité.

De l'examen des relatives fiches cliniques il n'a pas été possible d'identifier un rapport précis entre degré et type de tératospermie d'un côté et nombre ou type d'anomalies du décours gravidique de l'autre. C'est pourquoi la seule conclusion que, pour le moment, il nous semble possible de tirer de notre étude est qu'il existe certainement un lien, probablement causal, entre altérations morphostructurelles des spermatozoïdes et anomalies de la grossesse ou du produit de la conception. Nous voudrions donc souligner le concept que l'examen séminal du mari doit être pratiqué non seulement quand un couple apparaît stérile, mais aussi quand la femme, tout en concevant, ne réussit pas, systématiquement, à porter à terme physiologiquement ses grossesses.

Les troubles de l'éjaculation — Observations cliniques

G. Santori, Centro Italiano di Sessuologia, Roma (Italie)

Les troubles de l'éjaculation, bien que fréquemment observés, sont encore très mal connus, soit au point de vue de leur pathogenèse qu'au point de vue de leur thérapie. Le plus connu entre eux est sans doute la «eiaculatio praecox». Lorsque l'éjaculation a lieu «ante portas» l'e.p. rend le coït impossible mais, dans la plupart des cas, ce n'est pas le problème de la «impotentia coeundi» qui se pose, mais celui de la desharmonie sexuelle. L'homme trouve maintes fois sa satisfaction sexuelle, tout en regrettant la rapidité de l'éjaculation, mais c'est surtout la femme qui en ressent les conséquences, parce que le coït est trop rapide pour qu'elle puisse atteindre l'orgasme. On pense très souvent que l'é.p. soit un trouble d'origine seulement psychique et c'est pour cela que l'on conseille la psychothérapie.

Personellement, je ne suis pas d'accord avec cette interprétation exclusiviste, bien que je reconnaisse la très grande importance des facteurs psychiques dans tout phénomène sexuel — y compris celui de l'éjaculation. Je crois toutefois que d'autres élements interviennent dans la génèse de l'e.p.: y aurait-il peut-être dans certains sujets un plus grand nombre de corpuscules sensitifs? ou bien pourrait-on penser à un accroissement de leur sensibilité ou de la sensibilité des centres nerveux? Quoi qu'il en soit, la psychothérapie est souvent inefficace et d'autre part c'est bien difficile qu'elle puisse être pratiquée par la plupart des sujets, en tenant compte du temps et de l'argent nécessaires pour son accomplissement.

Pourvu qu'il s'agisse d'une e.p. sans aucun trouble de l'érection, les traitements médicaux seront souvent très utiles. On obtient de bons résultats avec les inhibiteurs de la monoaminoxydase (I.M.A.O.): le Marplan, par exemple est, dans ce group de médicaments, l'un des plus fréquemment employé, mais il ne faut pas oublier qu'il s'agit là de substances qui ne sont pas dépourvues de toxicité.

Bien plus simple et inoffensif est le traitement externe avec des pommades anesthésiantes, pourvu que leur composition soit bien choisie. Selon mon expérience, la pommade à la xylocaine 5% est peut-être la plus efficace.

Si l'e.p. est importante presque seulement au point de vue de l'harmonie sexuelle, la «impotentia eiaculandi» doit être envisagée dand le même temps au point de vue de la stérilité conjugale. Le chapitre de l'i.e. est très mal connu et beaucoup de médecins n'en connaissent pas même l'existence. Le cadre clinique qui s'observe avec une relative fréquence est celui de la «eiaculatio seiuncta». Dans cette condition le sujet n'est pas capable d'éjaculer ni dans le coït, ni dans la masturbation; dans quelques cas, toutefois, une masturbation très énergique et très prolongée peut aboutir à l'éjaculation. Mais ce qui caractérise l'e.s. c'est le fait que l'éjaculation spontanée se produit sans aucune difficulté pendant le sommeil: il s'agit donc évidemment d'un trouble fonctionnel. La e.s. guérit parfois après une psychothérapie ou même sans aucun traitement; mais dans beaucoup de sujets toute thérapie reste inefficace.

Personellement, j'en ai observé une vingtaine de cas: l'un d'eux est très curieux parce que le patient, bien que très intelligent et instruit dans d'autres domaines, était d'une ignorance sexuelle absolue, et il s'était adressé au médecin uniquement parce qu'il n'avait pas encore d'enfants après deux années de vie conjugale! Je me permets de rappeler ici un autre de mes cas, dans lequel on pourrait parler d'une «eiaculatio seiuncta» relative: cet homme ne pouvait jamais éjaculer dans le coït avec son épouse, tandis que l'éjaculation était possible avec une autre femme.

Mais la «impotentia eiaculandi» peut avoir elle aussi une cause organique: l'i.e.

est alors absolue, c'est-à-dire que dans ces cas là l'éjaculation ne survient jamais, ni dans la vie consciente ni pendant le sommeil. C'est une condition beaucoup plus rare à observer que l'e-seiuncta, et elle peut être la conséquence d'un fait traumatique ou bien d'une maladie.

J'en ai observé un cas après une méningomyélite; mais il faut aussi rappeler la possibilité d'une origine yatrogène, à la suite, par exemple, d'une intervention chirurgicale sur le sympathique abdominal.

Un troisième aspect de l'i.e. est celui dans lequel l'orgasme est conservé, mais sans qu'il soit accompagné d'éjaculation. Cette condition s'observe parfois dans les sujets traités avec la thyoridazine (MELLERIL) et cesse alors après l'interruption du traitement; on l'observe aussi dans les prostatectomisés, dans lesquels toutefois il s'agit plutôt d'une éjaculation rétrograde (dans la vessie) que d'un manque de l'éjaculation. Mais il faut savoir que ce trouble très particulier de l'éjaculation peut s'observer aussi sans aucune intervention médico-chirurgicale ou maladie préalable, et son origine est alors très obscure.

J'en connais un cas que je suis désormais de beaucoup d'années et qui me fut adressé avec la diagnose de azoospermie. Le sujet ne soupçonnait pas même d'avoir un trouble de l'éjaculation, dès que ses rapports conjugaux étaient tout à fait satisfaisants, bien que stériles. Il fit analyser ce qu'il croyait être son sperme (en fait c'était seulement la sécrétion des glandes de COWPER!) et il reçut par l'analyste une réponse négative. Mais lorsque j'examinai au microscope le sédiment de l'urine émise après un massage prostato-vésiculaire, j'eu la surprise de voir un très grand nombre de spermatozoïdes. Au contraire, l'urine émise après le coït ne contenait pas de spermatozoïdes, ce qui démontre qu'il ne s'agissait pas d'éjaculation rétrograde. Peut-être ce dernier type d'i.e. est exceptionnel seulement en apparence; la présence d'orgasme peut en effet masquer l'absence d'une vraie éjaculation.

Impuissance organique par dystrophies spinales congénitales (Spina bifida occulta et spondylolisthésis)

J. SIAGE, Département de Dermato-Vénérologie à la Faculté de Médecine Damas (Syrie)

L'impuissance d'origine organique, par malformations spinales congénitales, n'occupe pas dans la littérature médicale la place qu'elle mérite. Cette négligence si regrettable, d'un problème aussi angoissant, ne peut que livrer au charlatanisme, un champ libre pour des manoeuvres et ordonnances dont le moins qu'on puisse dire qu'elles sont répréhensibles.

L'impuissance, même vue sous l'angle scientifique continue à être considérée du domaine de la médecine psychosomatique, et hormis les cas flagrants de traumatismes ou d'inflamations, la tendance des esprits universitaires, imbus de finalisme naturel, est de reléguer au second plan une étiologie organique dans la genèse de ce syndrome. Et pourtant, malgré le zèle de la nature à sauvegarder une fonction dont dépendent ces nobles desseins, dans la perpétuité de l'espèce, il doit y avoir des états d'impuissances organiques par dystrophies congénitales.

L'étude que nous vous soumettons repose sur quarante cas d'impuissance, que nous avons recueillis au courant des deux dernières années. Ces cas comprennent, sans aucun triage, tous les patients qui nous ont consulté pour un état d'impuissance. Tous étaient bien constitués, et ne présentaient aucune tare organique

apparente, et n'avaient jamais été atteints de maladies infectieuses à répercussions
génitales. Aussi, tous présentaient-ils les caractères sexuels secondaires au complet.

Les examens de laboratoire qui leur furent effectués concernaient surtout la
syphilis et le diabète. Tous en étaient indemnes. La radiographie de la colonne
dorso-lombo-sacrée, à laquelle nous les avons tous soumis, nous a donné les constatations suivantes:

Spina bifida occulta	18 cas, soit 45%
Spondylolisthésis	6 cas, soit 15%
Malformations diverses	6 cas, soit 15%

Ces malformations se répartissent ainsi:

Turgescence des disques	3 cas
Pincement de l'espace lombosacré	2 cas
Sacralisation du 5ème lombaire	1 cas
Normaux	10 cas, soit 25%

L'âge de ceux des deux premières catégories, que nous retenons pour notre
étude, et qui forment les 60% des cas, se répartissait entre 20 et 30 ans. Sept
d'entre eux s'étaient mariés et venaient consulter pour une consommation manquée. Dans les commémoratives des 24 cas à lésions spinales, nous avons relevé les
symptômes suivants:

1. Libido normale;
2. Absence ou rareté de pollutions nocturnes;
3. Absence ou faiblesse d'érection au réveil;
4. L'érection provoquée par les vaso-dilatateurs, totalement déficiente, ou faiblement esquissée.

Quant à la troisième catégorie, dont les lésions spinales peuvent être considérées
acquises, et qui formeraient avec les deux premières catégories un pourcentage de
75% des cas, le syndrome d'impuissance avait un cycle épisodique, irrégulier, en
concordance probablement avec les répercussions douloureuses de leurs lésions.

Mais ceux de la quatrième catégorie, à la colonne vertébrale normale, étaient
tous des inquiets, irritables, phobiques, à coefficient neuro-psychique prononcé,
ce qui nous permet d'attribuer leur invalidité instable, à un reflexe conditionné
quelconque. Leur fonction génésique n'était perturbée qu'au stade de l'intro-
mission.

De l'exposé de ces faits, nous pouvons présumer, que l'impuissance dans les
première et deuxième catégories, provenait d'un défaut dans le système neuro-
vasculaire, qui préside à la vaso-dilatation des artères, et par suite à la tumescence
des tissus érectiles.

L'innervation organo-végétative des organes génitaux érectiles, est fournie par
les nerfs caverneux, qui viennent du plexus hypogastrique. Parmi les branches
afférentes de ce plexus, se trouvent des rameaux qui se détachent des racines du
plexus honteux, et qui proviennent des 2ème, 3ème et 4ème branches antérieures
des nerfs sacrés. Ces derniers rameaux constituent les nerfs érecteurs de ECKHARD,
qui se constituent par les émergences du S1, S2, S3, et dont l'excitation provoque
la vaso-dilatation de l'artère dorsale, de la verge et des artères caverneuses.

Le reflexe neuro-vasculaire dilatateur, qui est sous la dépendance directe des
nerfs érecteurs issus des ganglions sacrés, peut se trouver perturbé par une lésion
nerveuse congénitale, parallèle à la lésion osseuse dans les cas de spina bifida et de
spondylolisthésis, et cette malformation nerveuse, qui atteint ce relais parasympathique, rend toute médication vaso-dilatatrice aléatoire.

Le traitement que nous avons préconisé, sont les points de feu (ignipuncture)
sur les émergences nerveuses lombosacrées en dix séances répétées une fois tous
les deux jours. Les résultats de cette médication empirique ne sont pas spectacu-

laires, et nous ne savons pas si des interventions locales par injections épidurales, ou par décompression, peuvent avoir de meilleurs résultats.

De l'aperçu précédent, nous avons tiré les conclusions suivantes:

1. En ne retenant que nos cas d'impuissance à Spina bifida et Spondylolisthésis, nous atteignons le pourcentage de 60%. Ces deux anomalies ne sont que pour 20% chez les individus pris au hasard [1]. Ce haut pourcentage n'est donc pas fortuit dans nos cas d'impuissance.

2. Les dystrophies spinales congénitales, agiraient par altération du relais parasympathique sacré, qui forme le ganglion de Eckhard, et préside à la tumescence des organes érectiles, par altération, agénésie, ou compression concomitantes.

3. Les critères symptomatique, de cette impuissance organique. sont: l'absence (ou faiblesse) de l'érection matinale, de la pollution nocturne, et de l'érection provoquée par les parasympaticomimétiques.

4. La constatation d'une lésion dystrophique spinale, confirme le diagnostic d'impuissance organique, de pronostic fonctionnel très réservé.

5. Le traitement par ignipunture sur les émergences des racines lombo-sacrées ne semble pouvoir avoir qu'un effet palliatif.

Références. 1. Roentgen Diagnostics James T. Case (1952). — Bors, E. C.: Urol. Surv. **10**, 191 (1960). — 2. Gill, G. G., and H. L. White: Clin. Orthop. **5**, 66 (1955). — 3. Roen, P. R.: Impotence **1965**, 2576.

Endocrine Function of the Testes, Gonadotropic Activity and Genetic Sex in Male Infertility

L. Andreassi, Clinica Dermatologica dell'Università di Siena (Italy)

Our knowledge on male infertility is remarkably enlarged in these last years. The introduction of testicular biopsy has contributed in a decisive way. However this investigation has not been accepted at least in our country, in usual practice, especially for the opposition of patients who only exceptionally accept to submit themselves to the collection of the gonadal parenchyma. For this reason in the diagnosis of male infertility some simple investigations become more acceptable, which may constitute a useful and important complement of the examination of the sperm. We are referring to the study of the genetic sex and to the exploration of the androgenic and gonadotropic function, investigations carried out as a routine in our Clinic.

Our case report includes 41 subjects varying in age from 21 to 41 years all suffering from an insufficient tubular function revealed by the examination of the sperm and which may be classified in one of the following forms: oligospermia, azoospermia, astenospermia, necrospermia and teratospermia.

In 28 of these patients it was possible to find out the cause of the tubular damage, ascribable to cryptorchidism, varicocele, funicular torsion, previous parotitic orchitis, traumatic orchitis etc. In the other cases an etiological explanation was not possible.

In all these subjects the dosage of the urinary 17-ketosteroids (17-KS) was carried out, after a warm acid hydrolysis by a previous addition of hexamine in order to inhibit the formation of pigments and by extraction of metabolites with ethyl ether. On the total extract, by means of Zimmermann's reaction, the dosage of 17-KS was carried out, before and after treatment with digitonine in order to evaluate also the precipitable fraction with this substance. In some cases we have carried out the stimulation test with gonadotropin, in others that of the suprarenal block with dexamethasone.

For the dosage of urinary gonadotropin we have employed a variation of the immunological method of WIDE, concentrating beforehand 100 times gonadotropin by means of kaolin adsorption and subsequently by reacting proper scalar dilutions of the concentrated extract with an anti-HCG immune serum and with a sensitizing latex with HCG, which, as is known, immunologically behaves like LH.

The sexual chromatin was systematically searched on the desquamation cells of the oral mucous membrane and in granulocytes of the peripheral blood. The study of the genetic sex was moreover carried out by means of the examination of the karyogram on cultures of peripheral blood lymphocytes stimulated with phytohemoagglutinin and operating a block of mitoses with colchicine.

These last investigations gave us the possibility of finding out two typical cases of Klinefelter's syndrome with positive sexual chromatin and with a karyogram of the XXY type. In all other patients the percentage of Barr's bodies and of drumsticks was in any case lower respectively than 3% and 1% and the karyogram perfectly normal.

The urinary 17-KS were found in the majority of cases within normal limits with a similar behaviour of the separable fraction with digitonin. Only in one case of Klinefelter's syndrome, in one of eunuchoidism and in other five of oligo- and azoospermia due to unknown cause, we found the 17-KS clearly lower than normal. In some subjects with low values of these metabolites, the administration of 10.000 U. of LH gonadotropin was followed by an increase of the 17-KS elimination of more than 5 mg in 24 h. The data regarding the dosage of gonadotropin have revealed an increased urinary output of this hormone in one case of Klinefelter's syndrome and in one of eunuchoidism and moreover in other six patients suffering from oligo- and azoospermia due to unknown cause.

No agreement of values between the urinary output of gonadotropin and that of 17-KS was found, exception made of a case of Klinefelter's syndrome and of one of eunuchoidism, in whom a low elimination of 17-KS was associated with a similar low value of urinary gonadotropin.

On the basis of the data obtained from the hormonal dosage we have systematically instituted in our patients a hormonal treatment aiming to correct the deficit found, with the hexogenous intake of the missing factor. The results were extremely gratifying as in a significant percentage of cases an improvement of the tubular function was obtained, revealed by the fertility index.

In conclusion on the basis of our results we think, that apart from testicular biopsy, in each case of male infertility the dosage of gonadotropins and of 17-KS, the research of sexual chromatin and the analysis of the karyogram should be carried out. These investigations in fact may give useful data not only for diagnostic scope but also for a rational therapy.

Essais de traitement endocrinien de l'infertilité due à des altérations testiculaires

L. SEMMOLA, Clinique Dermatologique de l'Université de Florence (Italie)

Le traitement gonadotropinique de la stérilité masculine due à une altération de la gamétogénèse n'a pas été uniformément évalué dans ses effets, tant par les AA. qui ont recouru à des gonadotropines d'origine animale (PMS) que par ceux qui ont recouru aux gonadotropines humaines (HCG et UMG). Abstraction faite des critères d'évaluation, l'inégalité des résultats s'explique: 1. par l'importance variable de l'altération séminale; 2. par la nature des différentes causes morbigènes; 3. par les différents types de gonadotropines utilisées. Le traitement gonadotropinique qui trouve tout naturellement sa première indication dans les hypogonadismes hypogonadotropiques, a été également employé dans les déficiences séminales dues à des lésions directes du testicule. Même dans la plus récente expérimentation avec des gonadotropines humaines, on a relevé tantôt des résultats négatifs ou faibles [1 à 6], tantôt des résultats positifs quoique inconstants ou rares, confirmés parfois par une grossesse [7 à 16].

Sur 302 individus, appartenant à des couples stériles depuis 2 à 12 ans, on a soumis à un traitement gonadotropinique 14 azoospermiques et 24 oligozoospermiques de gravité variable et d'âge compris entre 25 et 45 ans. La fonction gamétogène était supprimée ou compromise par suite d'altérations testiculaires primitives ou d'altérations consécutives à une activité gonadotropinique déficiente. En l'absence de déficiences androgènes, on n'a administré que PMS ou HMG. Chez cinq eunucoïdes (signes cliniques et de laboratoire évidents, éjaculat de faible volume) on a associé HCG. Examens séminaux répétés 2 à 6 fois.

Traitement avec PMS. Chez 10 azoospermiques (2 eunucoïdismes, 3 hypogonadismes normoandrogènes, 1 reliquat d'orchite parotidique, 3 cryptorchidismes, 1 dû aux rayons X): deux cycles de 20 injections en 20 jours de 1000 U.I. de PMS, à six mois de distance; chez les eunucoïdes, association de six injections par cycle de HCG de 2500 U.I. Résultat: dans aucun examen séminal on n'a relevé de spermatozoïdes. Chez 17 oligozoospermiques (1 eunucoïdisme, 13 hypogonadismes normoandrogènes, 1 monocryptorchidisme, 1 reliquat d'orchite parotidique, 1 reliquat d'orchite traumatique), le même traitement a été appliqué, en deux cycles de PMS, avec association de HCG uniquement dans le cas d'eunucoïdisme. A l'oligozoospermie (dans cinq cas au-dessous de 1 M/cc et dans 12 de 11 à 18 M/cc) étaient associées de l'asthénozoospermie et de la dyszoospermie à divers degrés. Résultat: augmentation de la population spermatozoïque de 10 à 20%, avec de faibles améliorations de la cinèse et de la morphologie, dans 8 cas sur 17; pas de changement dans 7 cas; aggravation dans 2 cas; pour 3 des 8 cas améliorés, aggravation en un second temps par rapport aux données de départ.

Traitement avec HMG. Chez onze sujets, on a injecté en 70 jours 30 flacons de Pergonal 500 (à action, comme l'on sait, surtout folliculostimulante). On n'a associé HCG que dans deux cas d'eunucoïdisme (un flacon de 2500 U-I. tous les 5 jours). Sur quatre azoospermiques (2 par eunucoïdisme, 1 par cryptorchidisme, 1 dû aux rayons X), seul ce dernier a présenté 90 jours après le début du traitement l'apparition de spermatozoïdes dans le sperme (1 M/cc, motilité basale 15%, atypie morphologique 60%). Cet azoospermique avait quatre ans auparavant répondu négativement au PMS. Chez sept oligozoospermiques: deux cryptorchides avec une concentration spermatozoïque d'environ 1 M/cc n'ont présenté aucune variation séminale; cinq hypogonadiques normoandrogènes, avec des concentrations spermatozoïques de 7 à 18 M/cc ont bien réagi au traitement avec des accroissements de la population spermatozoïque allant de 50 à 150%, avec une amélioration de la cinèse et de la morphologie (90 et 120 jours après le début du traitement).

Ainsi, dans nos recherches, conformément à ce qui avait été observé par d'autres AA., l'action stimulante du HMG sur la gamétogénèse est apparue supérieure à celle du PMS. La différence a été expliquée par l'absence de l'apparition, après HMG, d'antigonadotropines lesquelles font suite à l'introduction dans l'organisme humain de gonadotropines hétérologues quoique pour peu de temps. Avec l'HMG, il est au contraire possible de prolonger pendant longtemps la

stimulation des structures séminifères; et cela d'après les observations [17] selon
lesquelles la durée du cycle de la gamétogénèse chez l'homme est d'environ 74 jours.
   Cette action du HMG, qu'elle s'applique aux spermatogones [18] ou qu'elle se
limite à favoriser la maturation des spermatides primaires à spermatozoïdes [19],
présente un intérêt biologique certain. Sur le plan clinique, l'on n'a pas obtenu la
preuve de la fertilité par le moyen d'une grossesse, même dans les cas où le sperme
était devenu normal ou presque. Les conditions de suppression ou de réduction de
la gamétogénèse dans la multiforme pathologie spontanée du testicule sont trop
différentes par rapport à la situation quasi expérimentale du testicule chez l'homme
hypophysectomisé, chez qui l'on a obtenu [18, 19] la restauration de la fonction
gamétogène en corrigeant avec des gonadotropines humaines la déficience hor-
monique spécifique qui a fait suite à l'opération.

   Bibliographie. 1. Schoysman, R.: Bull. Soc. roy. belge Gynéc. Obstét. (1964). — 2. Delle
Piane, G., e S. Gaffuri: Simp. Int. Roma. Clinica Europea 1965. — 3. Paulsen, C. A.:
Proc. of Med. VI Pan-Amer. Congress of Endocr., Mexico City 1965. — 4. Forbes, A.:
Obstet. Gynec. Digest (1966). — 5. Mroueh, A., B. Lytton, and N. Kase: J. clin. Endocr.
(1967). — 6. Mauleon: In: Docum. Geigy, 1° semestre (1967). — 7. Debiasi, E.: Simp. Int.
Roma, Clinica Europea 1965. — 8. Lunenfeld, B.: Simp. Int. Roma, Clinica Europea 1965. —
9. Pasetto, N.: Simp. Int. Roma. Clinica Europea 1965. — 10. Abelli, G., e M. Falagario:
Attual. Ostet. Ginec. (1966). — 11. Marchesi, F.: Congr. Urologia. Taormina 1966. —
12. Lunenfeld, B.: Simp. Hôp. Necker, Paris (1966). — 13. Polishuk, W. Z.: Fertil. and
Steril. (1967). — 14. Herres: In Docum. Geigy, 1° sem. (1967). — 15. Schirren: In: Docum.
Geigy, 1° sem. (1967). — 16. Comminos: In: Docum. Geigy, 1° sem. (1967). — 17. Heller,
C. G., and Y. Clermont: Recent Progr. Hormone Res. (1964). — 18. Mac Leod, J.: Simp.
Int. Roma, Clinica Europea 1965. — 19. Gemzell, C. A., e B. Kjessler: Lancet **1964**.

Die Therapie des Klinefelter-Syndroms

H. Niermann, Hautklinik der Universität Münster (Deutschland)

   Man weiß heute, daß das Klinefelter-Syndrom eine häufige Krankheit ist.
Nach Untersuchungen von Moore u. Mitarb. (1959), MacLean u. Mitarb. (1961)
sowie Bergemann (1961) bei insgesamt 6801 männlichen Neugeborenen wurden
18 chromatinpositive Fälle (0,26%) gefunden. Auf annähernd 400 männliche Ge-
burten kommt somit ein Klinefelter-Fall. Bei dem eigenen Krankengut von 3800
seit 1954 auf Zeugungsfähigkeit untersuchten Männern wurden 100 Patienten mit
einem Klinefelter-Syndrom beobachtet, d. h. 2,6%. Unter 665 Patienten mit
Azoo- oder Aspermie waren 100 Klinefelter-Patienten, d. h. 15%. Die klinischen
Symptome wie eunuchoider Habitus, Gynäkomastie, Behaarungsanomalien oder
Schwachsinn sind variabel. Nach Beobachtungen bei den eigenen 100 Klinefelter-
Patienten sind nach der Pubertät als konstante Symptome anzusehen die atrophischen Hoden, Azoo- bzw. Aspermie, Hypergonadotropinurie, histologische,
hochgradige Tubulusatrophie mit Leydig-Zellhyperplasie, chromatinpositives
Kerngeschlecht und die XXY-Chromosomenanomalie.
   Seit der ersten Beschreibung dieses Syndroms 1942 von Klinefelter, Reifen-
stein u. Albright über den 1956 von mehreren Autoren gleichzeitig festgestellten
chromatinpositiven Kerngeschlechtsbefund und die 1959 durch Ford u. Mitarb.
sowie Stewart nachgewiesene Geschlechtschromosomenanomalie in einer XXY-
Anordnung hat man sich bei dem Klinefelter-Syndrom zunächst mehr mit der
Ätiologie, Pathogenese und Symptomatik beschäftigt. Die Häufigkeit dieser
Krankheit bedingt, daß man jetzt auch der Therapie besondere Beachtung
schenken muß.

In die andrologische Sprechstunde kommt der Klinefelter-Patient meist wegen *Kinderlosigkeit* in der Ehe. Wegen der Azoo- bzw. Aspermie bei hochgradiger Tubulusatrophie ist eine Behandlung der Impotentia generandi erfolglos. Dies sollte man möglichst bald dem Patienten mitteilen und ihm die Adoption eines Kindes empfehlen. Oftmals tritt bei den Klinefelter-Patienten zusätzlich zur Impotentia generandi vorzeitig eine mehr oder weniger starke Impotentia coeundi auf. Diese läßt sich meist günstig durch eine Substitutionstherapie mit männlichem Keimdrüsenhormon beeinflussen.

Von größerer praktischer, häufig aber nicht beachteter Bedeutung ist die durch das Androgendefizit der Klinefelter-Patienten bedingte, meist bereits im 4. Lebensjahrzehnt auftretende *Osteoporose*. Diese ist bevorzugt lokalisiert im Bereich der Lendenwirbel- und unteren Brustwirbelkörper. Sie wird oft als rheumatische Arthritis, Lumbago, Ischias und dergleichen mehr fehlgedeutet und fehlbehandelt. Von 16 eigenen röntgenologisch untersuchten Patienten, die über 25 Jahre alt waren, hatten acht Männer eine Osteoporose. Das Durchschnittsalter dieser Patienten betrug 31 Jahre.

Bei dem ältesten, 39jährigen Patienten mußte wegen Osteoporose mit Wirbelkörpereinbrüchen eine stationäre Behandlung erfolgen. Kyphosen und Knochenschmerzen können sogar zu einer frühzeitigen Erwerbsunfähigkeit führen. Man muß vom 30. Lebensjahr an bei Klinefelter-Patienten stets röntgenologische Untersuchungen vor allem der Wirbelsäule auf Vorliegen einer Osteoporose durchführen. Eine weitere Folge des Androgendefizits ist eine allgemeine, durch Störung des Eiweißstoffwechsels bedingte Schwäche der Muskulatur.

Die *Gynäkomastie* ist nicht immer vorhanden, sie kann, stärker ausgeprägt, für den Patienten sehr störend sein. Hormonal ist sie nicht beeinflußbar. Vor allem bei Hochgradigkeit und Schmerzhaftigkeit muß operative Behandlung empfohlen werden. Der spärliche oder fehlende Bartwuchs kann durch Testosteroneinreibungen gebessert werden.

Wichtig ist die möglichst *frühzeitige Erkennung* des Klinefelter-Syndroms. Primär läßt sich bei Knaben bis zur Pubertät das Klinefelter-Syndrom noch nicht eindeutig nachweisen. Man weiß beispielsweise, daß Klinefelter-Patienten wie auch sonst Knaben vor der Pubertät altersentsprechend niedrige Gonadotropinwerte haben. Der histologische Befund von Hodengewebsproben eines eigenen 13jährigen Klinefelter-Patienten stimmte mit dem eines gleichaltrigen Gesunden weitgehend überein. Auch die klinischen Symptome wie Gynäkomastie oder Eunuchoidismus treten, wenn überhaupt, erst nach der Pubertät auf. 5 von 17 eigenen jugendlichen Klinefelter-Patienten bis zum 20. Lebensjahr zeigten röntgenologisch eine Retardierung der Knochenreifung. Bei einem Teil der Klinefelter-Patienten kann das Lebensalter der Mütter während ihrer Geburt als Ursache für die non-disjunction der X-Chromosomen angesehen werden. Nach Angaben von FERGUSON-SMITH (1959), WALTER u. Mitarb. (1958), LENZ (1959) und NIERMANN (1963) waren bei 27 von 131 Klinefelter-Fällen (20,6%) die Mütter bei der Geburt über 40 Jahre alt.

Lediglich positives Kerngeschlecht und Chromosomenanomalie sind bereits seit Geburt vorhanden. Nun wird man nicht bei jedem Knaben sofort nach der Geburt Kerngeschlechts- und Chromosomenuntersuchungen durchführen wollen. Bei Knaben vielleicht vom 6. Lebensjahr an, die an Schwachsinn, Wuchsanomalien oder auch Kryptorchismus leiden, sollte man aber doch die leicht durchzuführende Kerngeschlechtsbestimmung aus Mundepithelien oder Leukocyten vornehmen. Die Leydig-Zellinsuffizienz und somit das Androgendefizit macht sich erst von der Pubertät ab bemerkbar. Ab dann muß die Substitutionstherapie mit männlichem Keimdrüsenhormon je 250 mg in 3monatigen Abständen erfolgen. Bei noch späterer Erkennung und eventueller Impotentia coeundi und vor allem Osteoporose

muß 250 mg Testosteron in 4wöchigen Abständen unter Zusatz von Calcium und
Vitamin D gegeben werden.

Zusammenfassend muß betont werden, daß man sich keineswegs auf die
Diagnose des Klinefelter-Syndroms beschränken darf. Durch das Androgendefizit
bedingte Störungen der Potentia coeundi, Gynäkomastie, fehlender oder spärlicher
Bartwuchs, Stoffwechselstörungen mit Muskelschwäche und Osteoporose machen
eine frühzeitige Substitutionstherapie mit männlichem Keimdrüsenhormon erforderlich. Die Impotentia generandi läßt sich nicht beeinflussen.

Die Gonadotropine menschlicher Herkunft in der Behandlung der männlichen Unfruchtbarkeit

P. CERUTTI und M. DE LUCA, Clinica Dermatologica dell'Università, Neapel
(Italien)

Für die Behandlung der männlichen Unfruchtbarkeit sowie der ungenügenden
Fruchtbarkeit, bedingt durch sekundäre Alterationen der Gonaden, ist, wie bekannt, die Verabreichung von Gonadotropin, insbesondere des FSH-Types, von
ganz besonderer Bedeutung. Die Ergebnisse, die mit dieser Therapie erzielt werden
können, sind oft enttäuschend, vor allem weil die uns zur Verfügung stehenden
Gonadotropine bis vor einigen Jahren tierischen Ursprungs waren, was zur Folge
hatte, daß eine verlängerte Gonadotropinverabreichung das Auftreten von Antikörpern verursacht und somit die therapeutische Aktivität neutralisiert.

Um diesem Übelstand abzuhelfen, ist man zur Isolierung von aus dem Harn
von Frauen in der Menopause (HMG) extrahierten gonadotropischen Hormonen
(MMG), FSH-Typ, übergegangen.

Die von zahlreichen Autoren berichteten guten Ergebnisse, welche mit diesen
Gonadotropinen in der männlichen Samenpathologie erzielt wurden, haben uns
veranlaßt, eine Versuchsreihe bei den Patienten des Sexuologischen Zentrums der
Dermatologischen Klinik zu Neapel durchzuführen. Unsere bisherige Kasuistik
bezieht sich, wie aus der Tabelle ersichtlich, auf 24 Patienten, die folgendermaßen
unterteilt werden können:

1. Azoospermie	2 Fälle	
2. Schwere Oligozoospermie	8 Fälle	
3. Oligozoospermie mittleren und schweren	9 Fälle	
4. Asthen-Diszoospermie	5 Fälle	

Alle Patienten sind gemäß des nachfolgenden therapeutischen Schemas behandelt worden: 500 Einheiten MMG: 70 Phiolen pro tägliche Einspritzung.
2500 Einheiten MCG: 1 Phiole jeden 10. Tag (7 Phiolen). Die Kontrollsamenunter-
suchung ist 30 Tage nach Beendigung der Behandlung durchgeführt worden. Man
kann die Ergebnisse folgendermaßen schematisieren:

1. *Negativ* bei drei Fällen, in denen das Samenbild praktisch unverändert geblieben ist.

2. *Gering* bei sechs Fällen, in denen die Besserung nur einige Parameter interessiert hat.

3. *Gut* bei elf Fällen, in denen eine deutlichere Neigung zur Normalisierung des
Samenbildes aufgetreten ist.

4. *Sehr gut* bei vier Fällen, in denen auf eine deutliche Besserung aller oder fast
aller Parameter kurze Zeit später eine Schwangerschaft folgte.

Unsere nur wenig Fälle umfassende bisherige Kasuistik erlaubt uns keine genaue Bewertung der threapeutischen Wirksamkeit des MMG, vor allem was die zeitliche Stabilität der erzielten Ergebnisse anbetrifft. Auf jeden Fall scheint es

Fall N°	Spermie Vol./ml.		Spermatozoiden /mm³		Abnormale formen %		Bewegungen		Anfangs- beweglich- keit		Fruktose		Ergebnis
	vor	nach	vor	nach	vor	nach	vor	nach	vor	nach	vor	nach	
1	8	8	Abwesend	Abwesend	"	"	" "	" "	"	"	540	450	O
2	5	6	Abwesend	Abwesend	"	"	" "	" "	"	"	430	550	O
3	4	5	300	46.000	78	44	KREISFÖRMIG	GRADLINIG	20%	90%	180	460	+++
4	4.5	4	400	5.700	57	37	KREISFÖRMIG	GRADLINIG	20%	30%	180	460	++
5	6	6	500	42.000	66	50	KREIS.-ZUCK.	GRADLINIG	30%	60%	580	840	++
6	2.5	4	525	13.000	50	48	KREISE-ZUCK.	IDEM	70%	70%	330	400	+
7	3.5	4	600	10.000	48	40	ZUCKEND	IDEM	30%	40%	500	620	+
8	3.5	3.8	6.500	18.000	43	35	GRADLINIG	IDEM	40%	80%	280	520	++
9	6	6	7.000	10.000	63	48	GRADL.-KREISF	GRADLINIG	30%	50%	360	990	++
10	5	5	10.000	11.500	56	50	GRADLINIG	IDEM	50%	50%	300	580	O
11	5	5	14.000	28.000	75	72	KREISF.-ZUCK.	IDEM	60%	70%	650	600	+
12	4	5	15.200	34.000	54	33	KREISF.-ZUCK.	GRADLINIG	40%	60%	190	380	+++
13	2	2.8	15.600	26.000	39	28	GRADL.-ZUCK.	IDEM	40%	60%	270	530	++
14	3	3	16.000	17.000	44	43	ZUCKEND	GRADLINIG	20%	40%	580	400	+
15	3.6	4	16.600	28.000	48	40	KREISF-ZUCK.	GRADLINIG	35%	45%	680	650	++
16	3	4	17.000	46.000	77	50	KREISF.-ZUCK.	IDEM	70%	80%	630	730	++
17	2.5	3.8	17.200	28.000	41	34	GRADLINIG	IDEM	50%	50%	520	550	++
18	3	4	17.800	56.000	51	51	GRADLINIG	IDEM	45%	70%	190	450	+++
19	3.2	4.4	18.300	29.000	53	43	GRADL.-KREISF.	IDEM	20%	70%	420	580	++
20	3	4	30.000	20.000	33	26	GRADL.-KREISF.	IDEM	60%	60%	670	930	+
21	2.2	3	45.000	68.000	61	41	ZUCK.-KREISF.	IDEM	60%	60%	680	860	+++
22	2.5	3	50.000	55.000	78	46	GRADL.-ZUCK.	IDEM	30%	65%	320	600	++
23	3	2	66.000	72.000	52	33	GRADL.-KREISF.	IDEM	60%	90%	465	730	++
24	2	4	84.000	100.000	40	35	ZUCK.-KREISF.	IDEM	70%	70%	590	460	+

uns, daß wir, an Hand einer akuraten Analyse der Ergebnisse selber, die folgenden Schlußfolgerungen ziehen können:

1. Die am meisten und am beständigsten von dem MMG-Gonadotropin beeinflußten Parameter sind hier in abnehmender Serie: a) Anzahl der Nemaspermen; b) Morphologie der Nemaspermen; c) plasmatische Fluctosekonzentration; d) Beweglichkeitsgrad der Nemaspermen; e) Art der Bewegung der Nemaspermen; f) Ausmaß des Ejaculates.

2. Nur bei den Azoospermiefällen erzielte die durchgeführte Therapie keinerlei Wirkung; auf der anderen Seite erhielten wir überraschende Besserungen bei den Fällen, in denen die anfänglichen Samenverhältnisse wenig Hoffnung auf Erfolg versprachen.

3. Es besteht ohne Zweifel eine wesentliche Ungleichheit in der Art und Weise, wie jedes einzelne Individuum auf die Therapie reagiert, Ungleichheit, welche es nicht erlaubt, einen proportionellen Zusammenhang zwischen dem anfänglichen Samenbild und den Ergebnissen, die man mit dieser Therapie erzielen kann, ausfindig zu machen.

Enzymatic Activities on Nucleic Acids and their Derivatives in Human Seminal Plasma

P. Santoianni and G. Argenziano, Dermatology Clinic, University of Naples (Italy)

The studies carried out up to date on a peculiar group of enzymes occurring in the seminal plasma enable to outline a scheme of the so-called seminal nucleolytic system (Fig.).

Together with nucleases (Zamenhof), is present a high ATPase activity (Mann, 1945) and a nucleotide pyrophosphatase, which hydrolyzes some dinucleotides into mononucleotides. The acid phosphatase, beside acting as a phosphomono-esterase on 2'- and 3'-nucleotides, has another point of attack in the system, on ribose-5'-phosphate. A key-position we believe is holded by the abundant

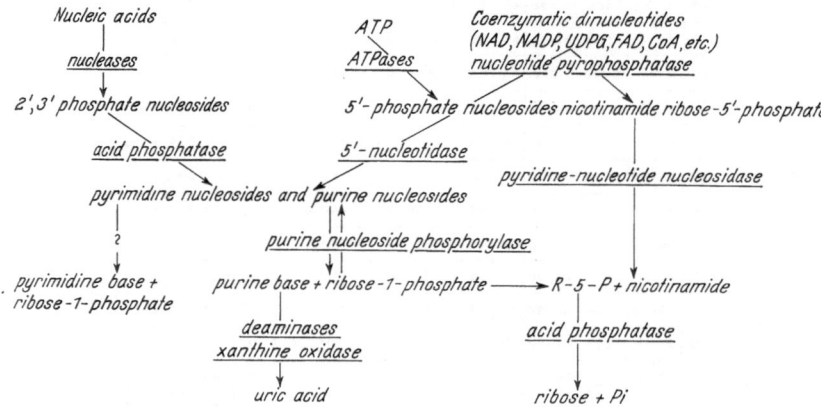

Fig. *A tentative scheme of the nucleolytic system of seminal plasma*

5'-nucleotidase (Reis, Santoianni and Farina), enzyme which specifically de-phosphorylates mononucleotides phosphorylated in position 5'.

Remarkably interesting are the enzyme acting on coenzymatic pyridine-dinucleotides (NAD or "DPN" and NADP or "TPN") or on the nicotinamide mononucleotide (Santoianni e Leone, Santoianni e d'Alessio). This pyridine-nucleotide nucleosidase liberates nicotinamide from NAD ("NADase") or from NADP ("NADPase"); while from nicotinamide mononucleotide is yielded ribose-5'-phosphate, furtherly split by acid phosphatase, as mentioned.

The liberation from nucleosides of ribose-1'-phosphate and of the purine base takes place by nucleoside phosphorylase [Santoianni, 1959, (1); Cerutti e Santoianni, 1959] enzyme most likely acting after a deaminase, which we found in other mammals [Leone and Santoianni, (1)], but not in man (Cerutti and Santoianni, 1959). The deamination and eventual oxidation of the purine bases yield uric acid through hypoxanthine and xanthine [Leone and Santoianni, (2)].

Beside the disposal of catabolites of nucleic acids, this group of enzymes, there-fore, makes ATP and coenzyme dinucleotides (NAD, NADP, FAD, etc.) undergo a true coenzyme-destroying action of seminal plasma.

Though the patrimony of nucleolytic enzymes of the seminal plasma can be expression of the high general metabolic and secretory activity of the accessory glands, a specific function should be recognized to the equilibrium of the various reactions catalized by the system.

The occurrence of alterations of some of these enzymes in pathological seminal conditions was by us investigated. In regard to purine-nucleoside phosphorylase was found a decrease of activity in asteno-and oligozoospermic ejaculates (CERUTTI and SANTOIANNI, 1960). Nevertheless it was not possible, also in the present investigation, to estabilish a more precise relation between clinical and enzymatic impairement. A more extensive knowledge of the physiological role of the nucleolytic system is apparently needed.

The elimination and inactivation of breakdown products of nucleic acids of the spermatozoa functionally damaged or of coenzymes is the most obvious function, but an anabolic and biosynthetic one seems also likely. There are some data supporting this view: 1. nucleosidephosphorylase normally operates synthesis of nucleosides; 2. acid phosphatase shows a transferase activity and can form nucleotides from nucleosides and organic phosphate (SCHNEIDER and LORING); 3. the sperm contains a polynucleotide-phosphorylase, capable of the synthesis of polynucleotides from smaller compounds, like nucleotide diphosphates (HAKIM).

Discussing the role of these enzymes we think should be taken into consideration that biometabolic exchanges occur between sperm cells and seminal plasma, made possible by the high permeability and filiform structure of the sperm cell. Exchanges can also take place at coenzymatic and enzymatic level. It is in this connection intriguing to note that some enzymes like pyridine nucleosidase, which generally occur in a form tightly bonded to the cellular structures, are present viceversa in a soluble form in the seminal plasma.

Furthermore, a toxic pharmacologic action may be brought about by several substances on some enzymes (e.g. the inhibitory action on acid phosphatase of the polymeric phosphate of hesperidin) (BELING) or on some coenzymes (e.g. the formation of an inactive compound from pyridine coenzymes (NAD, NADP) with isonicotylhydrazide (INI) (SANTOIANNI, 1959, 2) or histamine (ABDEL-LATIF and ALIVISATOS) by the action of pyridine-nucleotide nucleosidase).

Alterations of the physiological medium of the spermatozoa might well explain some pathologic conditions, like asteno- and necro-zoospermia.

The study of the two main enzymatic systems of the seminal plasma (the "fibrinolytic" and the "nucleolytic" ones) holds, in our opinion. a primary importance for the clarification of sperm and fertility alterations, detectable or not morphologically.

References. ABDEL-LATIF, A. A., and S. G. A. ALIVISATOS: J. biol. Chem. 237, 500 (1962). — BELING, C. G., and E. DICZFALYSY: Biochem. J. 71, 229 (1959). — CERUTTI, P.. u. P. SANTOI-ANNI: Arch. klin. exp. Derm. 211, 127 (1960); — Dermatologia (Napoli) 10, 136 (1959). — HAKIM, A. A.: Nature (Lond.) 183, 334 (1959). — LEONE, E., e P. SANTOIANNI: (1) G. Biochim. 6, 226 (1957); — (2) Boll. Soc. ital. Biol. sper. 33, 670 (1957). — MANN, T.: Biochem. J. 39. 451 (1945). — SANTOIANNI, P.: (1) Boll. Soc. ital. Biol. sper. 35, 905 (1959); — (2) Dermatologia (Napoli) 10, 182 (1959). —SANTOIANNI, P., e G. D'ALESSIO: Boll. Soc. ital. Biol. sper. 35, 1908 (1959). — SANTOIANNI, P., e E. FARINA: Boll. Soc. ital. Biol. sper. 35, 911 (1959). — SANTOIANNI, P., e E. LEONE: Boll. Soc. ital. Biol. sper. 34, 1943 (1958). — SCHNEIDER, A. J., and H. S. LORING: J. biol. Chem. 220, 129 (1956). — REIS, J.: Enzymologia 2, 183 (1937). — ZAMENHOF, S.: Nature (Lond.) 165, 756 (1950).

Ein neuer Gesichtspunkt endokriner-normospermatischer Infertilität

St. Ilca, C. Dodica und Z. Ioanovici, Klinisch-chemisches Laboratorium, Lugoj (Rumänien)

Im allgemeinen wird die männliche Infertilität auf spermatologische, hoden-bioptische und gonadal-endokrinopatische Änderungen zurückgeführt.

In der letzten Gruppe findet auch die normospermatische Infertilität ihren Platz. Für diese Subjekte wurden verschiedene Versuche unternommen, um eine wissenschaftlich begründete Erklärung zu sichern. Die Komplexität der hierbei angetroffenen Phänomene, ihre Verkettung, konnte aber bisher nicht restlos erfaßt werden.

Wir möchten hier auf einen neuen Aspekt endokrin-normospermatischer Infertilität hinweisen, ohne dabei den Anspruch einer richtigen Erklärung zu erheben. Vielmehr sollen diese Beobachtungen dazu dienen, in dieser Richtung weitere Untersuchungen anzuspornen.

Von den 109 von uns untersuchten männlichen infertilen Subjekten boten fünf das Bild einer normospermatischen Infertilität. Die Ehepartner wiesen keinerlei anatomische oder endokrine Störungen auf. Eine der Frauen hatte aus der ersten Ehe zwei Kinder. Einer der Untersuchten männlichen Subjekte befand sich bereits in der vierten Ehe, er löste drei Ehen wegen einer angeblichen Sterilität der Frauen auf. Alle fünf Subjekte wiesen ein normales Spermatogramm auf. Wir versuchten daher bei diesen, das Verhältnis Harnoestrogene-Harn 17-Hydroxycorticoide zu bestimmen, um festzustellen, ob nicht eine deutliche Verschiebung vorliegt.

Wie aus unserer Arbeit zu ersehen ist, entsprechen zwischen 18 bis 40 Jahren für 1 γ Harnoestrogene 400 γ Harn-17-Hydroxycorticoide (als Mittelwert für Männer). Als normale Grenzen fanden wir 370 bis 460 γ 17-Hydroxycorticoide.

Drei von den fünf untersuchten Subjekten wiesen ein normales Verhältnis auf. Bei zwei fanden wir aber eine auffallende Verschiebung des Verhältnisses, und zwar entsprach bei diesen für 1 γ Harnoestrogen 260 bzw. 310 γ Harn-17-Hydroxycorticoide. Die 24-Std-Entleerung von Harnoestrogenen sowie der Harn-17-Hydroxycorticoide lagen zwar bei diesen zwei Subjekten zwischen den üblichen — leider zu weitgesteckten — Normalgrenzen, ihr Verhältnis entsprach aber durchaus nicht den von uns beobachteten Normalgrenzen. Beide Subjekte wiesen eine zwischen den Normalgrenzen schwankende 17-Ketosteroidausscheidung auf. Auch die Fraktionierung der 17-Ketosteroide gab keinen weiteren Aufschluß, das Verhältnis Androsteron/Etiocholanon lag ebenfalls zwischen den normalen Grenzen. Demgegenüber lag aber der Fructosegehalt des Spermaplasmas — trotz der normospermatischen Lage — unter der normalen Grenze. Eine Testosteronbehandlung blieb erfolglos, denn der Fructosegehalt als auch das Verhältnis Harnoestrogene/Harn-17-Hydroxycorticoide blieben unverändert. Danach wurden beide Subjekte gleichzeitig mit Testosteron und Cortison behandelt. Bereits nach 3 Behandlungswochen erreichten so die Fructosewerte wie auch das Verhältnis Oestrogene/17-Hydroxycorticoide die normalen Grenzen. Nach dem Absetzen der Behandlung sanken die Werte wieder ab. Bei einem dieser Subjekte blieb der konkrete Erfolg nicht aus, nach mehreren Behandlungsperioden blieb die Frau schwanger. Beim zweiten Subjekt blieb der Erfolg aus. Ob hier noch andere Faktoren am Mißerfolg mitgewirkt haben, blieb uns verborgen.

In dieser Situation liegt es nahe, im Mißverhältnis Oestrogene/Corticoide eine Erklärung zu suchen, denn eine gegenseitige Beeinflussung dieser Hormone ist nicht abzuleugnen. Bei einer erniedrigten Corticoidsekretion und bei einem gleichbleibenden Oestrogenspiegel wirken sich die Oestrogene negativ auf den Fructosegehalt des Spermaplasmas aus und verhindern dadurch den normalen Ablauf der zur normalen Fertilität notwendigen Entwicklung.

Natürlich ist es nicht möglich, auf einen einzigen erfolgreichen Fall eine Therapie aufzubauen. Auch ist bei diesem Subjekt die Mitwirkung eines ,,Zufalles'' vorläufig nicht auszuschließen. Nur weitere ausgedehnte Forschungen, weitere therapeutische Erfolge in ähnlichen Fällen, würden die Hypothese der Mitwirkung eines bloßen Zufalles weitgehend entkräften.

XIII. Congressus Internationalis Dermatologiae

XIII. Congressus Internationalis

Dermatologiae

31.7. – 5. 8. 1967 / München

Editors: W. Jadassohn and C. G. Schirren

Volume 3

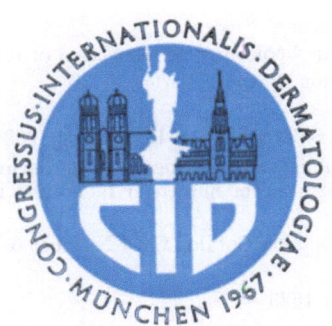

Springer-Verlag Berlin Heidelberg GmbH 1968

Additional material to this book can be downloaded from http://extras.springer.com

ISBN 978-3-642-49455-0   ISBN 978-3-642-49735-3 (eBook)
DOI 10.1007/978-3-642-49735-3

All rights reserved
No part of this book may be translated or reproduced in any form without written
permission from Springer-Verlag

© by Springer-Verlag Berlin Heidelberg 1968
Originally published by Springer-Verlag Berlin-Heidelberg New York in 1968
Softcover reprint of the hardcover 1st edition 1968

Library of Congress Catalog Card Number 68-8552

Title Number 1523

The reproduction of general descriptive names, trade names, trade marks, etc. in this
publication, even when there is no special identification mark, is not to be taken as a sign
that such names, as understood by the Trade Marks and Merchandise Marks Law,
may accordingly be freely used by anyone

Photos: pages *1—128:* L. Heigl, H. Giessner, R. Pröhl and W. Gerstenbrey

Volume 1   page

Preface . . . .   VII—X
Congressus Internationales Dermatologiae   XII
Contents . . . .   XIII—XXXIX
Organization, Addresses and Course of the Congress . . . .   *1—128*
Main-Theme I—VII . . . .   1—525
Symposium 1—4 . . . .   527—703

Volume 2

Symposium 5—15 . . . .   705—1375
Case Presentations and Fundamentals on Film . . . .   1377—1382
Scientific Exhibition . . . .   1385—1591
Authors Index . . . .   1592—1598

Contents   Volume 2

Symposium 5: Malignant Reticuloses and Lymphomas

Reports

Histopathologic and Hematologic Changes in Malignant Lymphomas and Reticuloses.
H. MONTGOMERY and R. K. WINKELMANN   707

Zur Nosologie und Einteilung der Reticulosen, Reticulosarkomatosen und verwandter
Krankheitsbilder unter Berücksichtigung cytophotometrischer Untersuchungen.
W. KNOTH   712

Patología y clínica de los reticulolinfomas óculopalpebrales. P. H. MAGNIN, M. C.
MORGENFELD and R. L. CABRINI   714

The Identity and Treatment of the Lymphoma Mycosis fungoides. M. A. LUTZNER .   720

Free Communications

Klinik und Histopathologie der malignen Reticulosen. K. W. MACH   721

Cytological Studies on Lymphoma with Electronmicroscopy. H. FUJITA   724

Cutaneous Lymphoblastoma, Spontaneous Involution of Tumours. D. MAJCAN, D.
STEVANOVIĆ and B. LALEVIĆ   725

Blood Vessel Morphology in the Reticuloses. T. J. RYAN   727

Generalized Giant-Cell Reticulohistiocytosis (Lipoid Dermatoarthritis) — Clinical and
Histopathological Study of two Cases. P. NAZZARO, U. GRANELLI and A. BIGNAMI .   728

Malignant Development in Mastocytosis. F. SAGHER and Z. EVEN-PAZ   729

Sézary Syndrome. G. L. ROCHA, F. SANTOS, R. AZULAY and A. PETRARCA DE MESQUITA   731

Mycosis Fungoides. — Mode of Presentation of 55 Cases. P. D. SAMMAN   733

Cytological Diagnosis in Mycosis Fungoides. E. BREHMER-ANDERSSON and U. BRUNK   735

Triacetyl 6-Azauridine in Mycosis Fungoides. CH. J. MCDONALD, P. CALABRESI and
R. C. DE CONTI   739

Ultrastructure de l'angio-réticulo-sarcomatose cutanée: Maladie de Kaposi. E. CALAS,
H. BONNEAU and J. P. CESARINI   741

Zur Entität des sog. Morbus Kaposi. G. OEHLSCHLAEGEL   745

Les localisations cutanées spécifiques de la maladie de Waldenstroem. H. BARRIERE, P.
LITOUX and B. BUREAU   747

Esquisse de la physionomie de l'angio-sarcomatose de Kaposi en Algérie (A propos de
25 observations personelles). F. G. MARILL, E. HADIDA and J. SAYAG   748

Intérêt de la lymphographie dans les hématodermies. M. DANA, R. BOURDON, V. BISMUTH
and J. P. DESPREZ-CURELY   750

Radiothérapie des hémoréticulopathies malignes. R. BOURDON and M. DANA   752

page

Symposium 6: Cosmetology; Biology and Pathology of the Hair

Cosmetology

Reports

Recherches sur le mécanisme d'action des antiperspirants. R. Brun, N. Hunziker and
P. Evdos 755
Hair Dyes. A. Rostenberg and G. Kass 758

Free Communications

International Dermatology and the World of Cosmetics. E. W. Brauer 761
Hormonal and Microbial Influences on the Sebaceous Follicles in Acne. P. E. Pochi . . 762

Biology and Pathology of the Human Hair

Reports

Development of the Human Hair Follicle. — Biology and Pathology of the Human
Hair. F. Serri 763
Alopecia areata, Basic Notions. G. Moretti, A. Rebora, E. Rampini, F. Crovato and
C. Cipriani 765
Klinik und Therapie der Alopecia areata. R. Schuppli 769
Causes actuelles des alopécies féminines diffuses. E. Sidi †, J. Bourgeois-Spinasse
and J. Arouète 771

Free Communications

Propiedades depilatoria y citotóxica de la seleno-cistationina. F. Kerdel-Vegas. . . 775
Control of Mammalian Hair Growth: Studies with a Cell-Free Protein Synthesizing
System. I. M. Freedberg 776
The Effects of Various Pathologic Conditions of the Scalp upon Hair Melanogenesis and
Hair Growth. W. Kostanecki 780
The Histological Changes in Idiopathic Premature Vertex Baldness in Women.
I. Martin-Scott 781
The Normal Trichogram of People Beyond 50 Years but Apparently not Bald.
J. M. Barman, I. Astore and V. Pecoraro 783
Microscopic Studies of Pili Annulati. V. H. Price, R. S. Thomas and F. T. Jones . . 786
Rate of Hair Growth. M. Saitoh, M. Uzuka, M. Sakamoto and T. Kobori 788
Chronical Female Alopecia. M. Binazzi 791
Le problème des états pseudopeladiques ou pseudopeladoïdes dans le cadre des alopécies
cicatricielles. M. Juon 793
La pelade, maladie psychosomatique. S. Lambergeon 795
Biological Depth Dose Studies in Electron Beam Therapy: Effects on Anagen Mouse
Hairs. L. H. Lanzl and F. D. Malkinson 796
Elektronenmikroskopische Befunde an den peritrichialen Nervenfasern des mensch-
lichen Haarfollikels. C. Orfanos 798
Die Behandlung der Alopecia areata im Kindesalter. J. Tomášková 801
Untersuchungen über die Veränderungen des Haares der Augenbrauen bei endogenem
Ekzem. H. Langhof† and M. Munteanu 803

Symposium 7: Mycoses (Superficial and Deep)

Reports

Untersuchungen über die Zuverlässigkeit eines „in vitro"-Lymphocytentests zwecks
Nachweises einer Dermatophyteninfektion. H. Götz 807
Effects of Human Body Fluids on Candida albicans. V. D. Newcomer, J. W. Landau,
N. Dabrowa and M. L. Fenster 813

page

Histoplasmose Africaine. R. VANBREUSEGHEM 817

Micetomas y actinomicosis. A. GONZÁLEZ OCHOA 819

Pathogenesis of South American Blastomycosis (Lutz's Mycosis). A. PADILHA-GON-
ÇALVES 824

Nouvelles acquisitions sur le mécanisme d'action de la Griséofulvine. P. PINETTI . . 826

Free Communications

Les onychomycoses. G. ACHTEN 828

Aspects particuliers de l'épidermomycose causée par epidermophyton floccosum.
I. ALTERAS and I. COJOCARU 830

Ultraestructura y citoquímica de la Candida albicans. L. F. MONTES and V. S. CON-
STANTINE 831

Keloidal Blastomycosis (Jorge Lobo's Disease). S. FRAGA and J. LISBÔA MIRANDA . . 831

A Look at Mycetoma in India. B. B. GOKHALE, A. A. PADHYE and M. J. THIRUMALACHAR 833

Esporotricosis, estudio clínico epidemiológico. V. C. JARAMILLO, G. C. VÉLEZ, A. R.
MORENO, I. R. PIZANO and A. C. CORTÉS 835

Favus Infection in Iraq. G. F. RAHIM 837

La macrocheilite de la blastomycose Sud-Américaine. J. RAMOS-SILVA and A. PADILHA-
GONÇALVES 839

Experiencias en cuatro casos de cromoblastomicosis y su tratamiento. F. A. OCAMPO,
R. T. PEREZ and R. V. VICTORIA 841

Quelques aspects de la mycose de Lane-Pedroso (chromoblastomycose ou chromomycose) dans la région Amazonique (Brésil). D. SILVA 842

Survey of the Mycoses in U.A.R. K. EL ZAWAHRY and M. EL ZAWAHRY 847

Main Transmission Routes of Spread of Trichophyton Mentagrophytes var. gran.-
Infection from a Natural Focus to Man in a Foothill Region. L. CHMEL, J. BUCHVALD
and M. VALENTOVÁ 851

Beitrag zum Problem tiefer anorectaler Mykosen. O. MALE 852

Flore dermatomycosique actuelle dans la région d'Athènes et sensibilité des souches isolées à la griséofulvine. C. KANITAKIS, U. MARCELOU-KINTI and CHR. GEORGIADIS . . 854

Biological, Sanitarian and Environmental Factors in Dermatomycoses. D. TRICHO-
POULOS, O. MARSELOU-KINTI and A. POLYCHRONOPOULOU 856

New Experiments on Culture, Immunology and Inoculation. J. DE AZEVEDO CARNEIRO,
R. D. AZULAY and L. M. C. DE ANDRADE 858

Sensibilisations de la peau par les dermatophytes. I. COJOCARU, I. ALTERAS and L.
DULAMITĂ 859

La valeur du milieu Gluzman modifié par Condrea dans la préparation de la trichophytine. V. COSTEA, M. CARNIOL, M. LAŽAR and M. ILIES 861

Onychomycose due à alternaria tenuis. J. DELACRÉTAZ and D. GRIGORIOU 863

Fungus-Allergy and its Skin Manifestations. E. FEJÉR 864

The Mycologic Laboratory Specimen. The Collection, Inoculation, and Culture Methods.
H. C. GOLDBERG 866

Tinea Versicolor: The Electron Microscopic Morphology of the Genera Malassezia and
Pityrosporum. F. M. KEDDIE 867

Effect of the Immunosuppressive Agent, Cyclophosphamide, on Experimental Systemic
Coccidioidomycosis. J. W. LANDAU, L. INDIANER and V. D. NEWCOMER 872

Enzyme des Kohlenhydratstoffwechsels bei Dermatophyten. W. MEINHOF and G.
RASSNER 876

Microsporum Nanum as a Cause of Human Infections. J. F. MULLINS and C. J. WILLIS 877

Les dermatophytes du sol en Bulgarie. P. POPCHRISTOV, V. BALABANOFF, T. FILKOV and
P. USUNOV 879

L'ultrastructure des grains dans les maduromycoses provoquée par Monosporium apiospermum. M. STOIAN and A. AVRAM 881

page

On the Mycomimetic Pictures Found in Mycologic Examinations. P. SBERNA   883

Zur fermentativen Leistung von Fadenpilzen. W. ADAM   884

Parenté antigénique et localisation des antigènes dans le genre Candida: Etude par immunofluorescence. P. RIMBAUD, J.-M. BASTIDE, M. BASTIDE and J. ALLEGRINI .   886

Essais de marquage de Candida albicans par radioisotopes. Etude de leur distribution dans l'organisme du lapin. S. ANTONESCU   892

Observations of the Treatment of Superficial Mycosis in South-East Europe with CO_2 Snow (Method Haxthausen). M. BRNIČEVIĆ   893

La contamination staphylococcique des trichophyties suppurées. Résultats d'une thérapie combinée: Griséofulvine, antibiotiques antimicrobiennes et traitement local. I. CAPUSAN, P. BALOSU and N. MAIER   895

Tratamiento de las tiñas on Griseofulvina. M. P. MIGUENS   896

Sporotrichosis Recurrens Cicatrisans (Repeating Self-Healing Sporotrichosis). R. N. MIRANDA   898

Traitement expérimental des mycoses cutanées superficielles par l'Amphotéricine B. D. PERYASSÚ and G. LÖWY   900

Experimentelle Grundlagen der externen antimykotischen Therapie. W. RAAB . . .   901

Über den Einfluß von Moronal (-Nystatin) auf den Zellstoffwechsel von Candida albicans (Autoradiographische Untersuchungen). M. RAHMANN-ESSER and F. FEGELER . .   903

Mechanism of Antifungal Action of Potassium Iodide on Sporotrichosis. H. URABE, T. NAGASHIMA and K. NAKASHIMA   907

Fissured Nipples of Lactating Females and its Relation to Candida Infection. A. M. EL MOFTY, R. MEHAREB, H. M. EL KOMY and C. D. JEFFRIES   908

Symposium 8: Malignant Melanomas

Reports

Melanin Biosynthesis in Melanomas. T. B. FITZPATRICK   913

Mélanoses neurocutanées of Touraine. T. KAWAMURA, S. IKEDA, S. NODA, S. ISHIZU and T. NAKAJIMA   915

La mélanose circonscrite précancereuse de Hutchinson-Dubreuilh (M.H.D.). B. DUPERRAT and J. M. MASCARO   917

Spontaneous Regression of Malignant Melanoma. L. BOWDEN   918

Elektrometrie zur Früherkennung von malignanten Melanomen. N. MELCZER   925

The Surgical Treatment of Malignant Melanoma. R. W. RAVEN   926

Die Behandlung des malignen Melanoms mit schnellen Elektronen eines 15 MeV-Betatrons. G. F. KLOSTERMANN   928

Histologische Diagnostik der Melanome. J. J. HERZBERG   933

Free Communications

Benign Juvenile Melanoma. — Several Selected Aspects from a Study of 51 Lesions. R. ANDRADE   936

Über das Verhalten der Melanomzellen in vitro. B. ROHDE   938

Production of Melanomas in Hairless Mice with Ultraviolet Light. J. H. EPSTEIN, W. L. EPSTEIN and T. NAKAI   939

Effects of Depigmenting Agents on Melanocytes and Melanogenesis. M. A. PATHAK, G. SZABÓ, E. FRENK, S. S. BLEEHEN, Y. HORI and T. B. FITZPATRICK   941

Dopa in Melanoma. H. RORSMAN   942

Multiple Forms of Tyrosinase from Mammalian Melanoma. J. B. BURNETT and H. SEILER   943

370 Mélanomes malins. — Statistiques et pronostic. J. M. SIMONART   944

A propos de 400 mélanomes malins cutanés. C. DUFOURMENTEL, R. MOULY and J. GLICENSTEIN   946

page

Zur Häufigkeit des malignen Melanoms. Ergebnis einer Umfrage. H. KÄSTNER, P.
JORDAN and G. FORCK 948

Lentigo Maligna and Malignant Melanoma. R. JACKSON 949

Un diagnostic différentiel important des mélanomes. L'Angiokératome noir.
G. E. GOETSCHEL 951

Les noevocarcinomes de l'enfant. R. MOULY, CL. DUFOURMENTEL and J. GLICENSTEIN 954

Nevus y melanomas malignos. L. A. RUEDA 955

Early Diagnosis of Melanoblastoma with the Aid of Electrometric, Thermo-Differential
and ^{32}P Uptake Test. A. GULBERT 957

Histologische Befunde beim transplantierten Melanom des Menschen. H. GARTMANN 958

Veränderungen bei inoculierten Melanocyten. KH. WOEBER and O. GRÜTZ † 960

Macromolecular Differentiation of Melanocytic and Nevocytic Malignant Melanomas.
Y. MISHIMA 961

Investigación de células tumorales en sangre periférica en enfermos con melanoma
maligno. A. ALIAGA and J. CALAP 968

Some Mechanisms of Pox Virus Oncolysis in Malignant Melanoma. A Review of 50 Cases.
G. W. MILTON and M. LANE BROWN 970

Richtlinien und unsere Erfahrungen in der Behandlung des malignen Melanoms.
GY. KÁRPÁTI, T. VENKEI, Ö. BIHARI, GY. NÉMETH and A. GULBERT 973

Observations concernant la prophylaxie et le traitement du mélanome malin.
E. UJVÁRY and I. KREPSZ 974

Données relatives au problème de la possibilité de dissémination après l'irradiation aux
rayons X dans les cas du mélanome malin. T. VENKEI and Ö. BIHARI 975

The Uptake of Radioactively Labelled Compounds by Malignant Melanoma. M. S. BLOIS 976

Sensitization to X-Irradiation of Melanoma Cells Using Alpha-MSH. M. LANE BROWN
·and G. W. MILTON 978

Symposium 9: Physiology of the Skin

Reports

Enzyme und Physiologie der Haut. G. K. STEIGLEDER 983

Collagen Metabolism in Skin. CH. M. LAPIÈRE 986

Physiological Response of Human Skin to Ultraviolet Light. M. A. EVERETT and R. L.
OLSON 988

The Clinical Significance of a Comparative Approach to the Physiology of Hair Growth.
A. J. ROOK 993

Physiologie der Hautoberfläche. Die relative Bedeutung verschiedener Befunde.
F. HERRMANN 995

Some Remarks on the Barrier Function of the Epidermis. J. HORÁČEK 999

Le pouvoir tampon de la peau. H. THIERS 1002

Free Communications

Studies of Some Glycolytic Pathways in the Skin of Rats Under Experimental Conditions. G. RABBIOSI and A. GIANNETTI 1003

Plasma Kinin Formation and Human Inflammation. H. ZACHARIAE, J. MALMQUIST,
J. A. OATES and W. PETTINGER 1006

Synthesis of Unique Proteins in Epidermal Keratinization. I. A. BERNSTEIN 1008

Mechanism of Water Binding in Stratum Corneum. J. D. MIDDLETON 1010

Studies on the Epidermal Keratinization of the Human Fetus in vitro with Special
References to the Electron Microscopic and Autoradiographic Observation.
K. OKAMURA, K. IWASHITA and K. UEDA 1012

page

The Envelope of Epidermal Horny Cells. A. G. MATOLTSY 1014

Follicular Hyperkeratinization Induced in the Rabbit Ear by Human Skin Surface Lipids. A. L. LORINCZ, H. KRIZEK and S. BROWN 1016

The Influence of Dimethyl Sulphoxide, Dimethyl Acetamide and Dimethyl Formamide on the Epidermal Barrier to Water. H. BAKER 1017

Die hygrometrische Aufzeichnung der Hydromeiose und das Abtrocknen der Hornschicht als Maß ihrer physiologischen Qualität. J. ROVENSKÝ and J. ZÁHEJSKÝ . . 1020

Physiologische Antiperspirants. H. P. FIEDLER 1022

Sodium Secretion and Reabsorption by the Eccrine Sweat Gland. R. L. DOBSON . . 1024

The Insensible Water Loss and Skin Temperature. F. A. J. THIELE and K. G. VAN SENDEN 1025

The Fine Structure of the Sebaceous Gland of the Adult Female Rat After Receiving Sexual Hormones. Y. SATO and M. MOROHASHI 1028

The in vivo Study of Cutaneous Lipogenesis. G. LIPKIN and V. R. WHEATLEY 1029

Physiology of Human Sebaceous Glands-Hormonal Control Mechanisms. J. S. STRAUSS 1031

Le contrôle hormonal de la glande sébacée chez l'homme. M. BONELLI, E. ALESSI, C. TOMASINI and S. PICCININI 1033

Der Einfluß des Hautoberflächenmilieus auf Staphylococcus aureus. E. MÜLLER . . . 1036

The pH and the Bacterial Flora of Normal Skin Under Fluocinolone-Plastic Occlusion Treatment. E. A. KNUDSEN 1038

The Alkali Neutralization Capacity of Human Skin in vivo. K. SCHUTTER 1041

Über ultraviolett-absorbierende Verbindungen im Wasserlöslichen epidermaler Verhornungsprodukte. E. SCHWARZ 1043

Ultraviolettes Licht als Stimulus für Kininbildung in menschlicher Haut. R. K. WINKELMANN, J. EPSTEIN and K. WOLFF 1045

Sur la réponse vasculaire biphasique au siège de l'érythème dû aux radiations ultraviolettes. Existe-t-il une réponse plus élémentaire que l'érythème? G. ZINA and A. BENEDETTO 1047

A Cutaneous Role in the Regulation of the Body's Carbohydrate Milieu. R. M. FUSARO and J. A. JOHNSON 1048

Research on Sialic Acid in the Human Skin. A. GIANNETTI and G. RABBIOSI 1050

Mepyramine and Adrenergic Neurone. B. S. VERMA and O. D. GULATI 1053

Lysosomes and the Skin. R. L. OLSON, R. NORDQUIST, J. NORDQUIST and M. A. EVERETT 1056

Modificaciones clínicas e histológicas de la reacción tuberculínica bajo la acción local del valerato de betametasona en cura oclusiva. A. CASALÁ, C. BIANCHI, O. BIANCHI, S. STRINGA and O. ROQUÉ 1060

The Significance of Low Serum Iron Levels in the Causation of Itching. I. B. SNEDDON and M. GARRETTS 1061

Comparatively Study on the Effects of Corticosteroids, Resochine and Synopene on the Arthus's Phenomenon in Rabbits. B. BAJDEKOV, K. BERTCHEV, B. BOJKOV and I. ISMIROV 1063

Die Adenosintriphosphatase der normalen menschlichen Haut. C. ENE-POPESCU . . 1064

Symposium 10: Effects of Radiation on the Skin

Reports

Radiobiologie cutanée. P. VAN CANEGHEM 1069

Strahlenwirkung im Hautbereich in Abhängigkeit von der verwendeten Strahlenqualität. A. PROPPE 1070

Strahlenwirkung im Hautbereich in Abhängigkeit von der verwendeten Strahlenqualität. F. WACHSMANN 1074

page

Indications dermatologiques du traitement ionisant. Traitement ionisant des épithéliomas et des mélanomes malins à l'aide de techniques de radio-sensibilisation nouvelles.
E. G. Scolari 1078

Indications thérapeutiques des substances radioactives en dermatologie. B. Pierquin 1081

Algunos rasgos ultraestructurales de las radiolesiones. J. Cabré 1083

Preliminary Investigative Studies of the Laser Treatment of Angiomas. L. Goldman,
R. J. Rockwell jr. and R. Meyer 1084

Free Communications

The Treatment of Skin Tumours with Radium and Hyperbaric Oxygen. C. Vallecchi
and G. Mantellassi 1087

Nouvelle technique de Radiumthérapie en oxygène hyperbaryque. M. Nannelli and
G. Mantellassi 1088

Acute Effects of Irradiation on the Skin. — A Histochemical and Chemical Study.
A. K. Kurban and F. S. Farah. 1090

Biochemische Untersuchungen an Serum und Hauteiweißen von Ratten nach Röntgenbestrahlung. O.-E. Rodermund 1091

Radiations et tissu élastique cutané. M. Ledoux-Corbusier 1093

Problemas del uso de los rayos grenz en los negros y en los mulatos. M. A. Contreras 1094

Tierexperimentelles zur Röntgenfernbestrahlung der Haut. M. Betetto 1096

Dermatological Observations in the A-Bomb Survivors of Hiroshima and Nagasaki,
Japan. M.-L. T. Johnson, T. Taura and P. B. Gregory 1097

Studies on Induction, Persistence and Recovery of Radiation Damage in Proliferative
(Anagen) and Non-proliferative (Telogen) Rodent Hair Cell Populations. F. D. Malkinson and M. L. Griem 1099

Autoradiographische Untersuchungen zur epidermalen Proliferation unter physiologischen, pathologischen und experimentellen Bedingungen mit Tritium-markierten
Nucleosiden. W. Born 1101

Histochimie des enzymes des follicules irradiés du cobaye. A. Kint and J. de Bersaques 1103

Untersuchungen zur experimentellen Photosensibilisierung mit Sulfanilamid und
Phenothiazinen. K. Schwarz, J. Rothenstein and M. Schwarz-Speck 1106

Light is an Aetiological Factor for Certain Dermatoses in U.A.R. M. el Zawahry. . 1107

Heliotherapie und ihr Einfluß auf die Aktivität mancher Enzyme bei Psoriasiskranken.
N. Balevska, J. Petkov, G. Mustakov, S. Jowev, N. Zlatkov and G. Tomov . . 1110

The Action Spectrum of Erythema Induced by Ultraviolet Radiation. Preliminary
Report. D. Berger, F. Urbach and R. E. Davies 1112

The Absorption Spectrum of the Stratum Corneum as the Natural Sunscreen of Human
Skin. A. R. H. B. Verhagen 1118

Prurigo actínico. F. Londoño 1122

Psoralen Therapy of Vitiligo in the Tropics. T. L. Fleisher 1124

Zur Kombinationsbehandlung der Mycosis fungoides mit Röntgenstrahlen und Spindelgiften. A. Wiskemann 1125

Photochemical Movement of Cholesterol in Skin. E. W. Rauschkolb and J. M. Knox 1126

Symposium 11: Immunology in Dermatology

Reports

Aetiology of Some Autoimmune Diseases. N. R. Rowell 1131

Aspects immunologiques du lupus érythémateux aigu dissémine. J. Thivolet . . . 1134

Autoimmunity in Pemphigus. T. Chorzelski 1135

Immunology of Acne Vulgaris. Dermal Hypersensitivity and Circulating Antibody
Levels to Corynbacterium Acnes. S. M. Puhvel, T. H. Sternberg and R. M.
Reisner 1136

page

Zur Immunologie in der Dermatologie. J. Kimmig 1139

The Role of the Basophil in the Immune Response. W. B. Shelley 1143

Free Communications

Classes of Immunoglobulins Associated with Skin Sensitizing Properties. M. J. Fellner
and R. L. Baer 1144

Patterns of Skin Fluorescence in Lupus Erythematosus. R. H. Cormane 1146

Delayed Hypersensitivity Responses in Immunologic Deficiency States. W. L. Epstein 1148

Antikörpermangelsyndrome und Hautveränderungen. G. Brehm 1149

Zur Frage der Antigenspezifität von 2,4-Dinitrochlorbenzol-Epidermis-Conjugaten im
Meerschweinchenversuch. F. Klaschka 1151

Antinuclear Factors in Clinical Dermatology. J. S. Beck, N. R. Rowell and T. E.
Anderson 1153

Vasoactive Substances at Sites of Cutaneous Allergies. Th. M. Inderbitzin and P. J.
Grob 1154

Application de la technique d'immunofluorescence en dermatologie. Y. Montet, J.
Duheille and J. Beurey 1156

Experimental Studies on the Pathogenesis of Acantholysis in Pemphigus. P. J. Grob
and Th. M. Inderbitzin 1158

Autoantibodies in Pemphigus Foliaceus. T. A. Furtado, A. O. Lima, G. O. Andrade
and O. Seabra 1159

L'apport de l'immuno-fluorescence dans la mise en évidence du rôle de l'allergie à
Candida albicans dans certaines dermatoses communes. P. Temime, M. Benne,
M. Lebeuf, J. P. Marchand and Ph. Latourelle 1162

Recherches électrophorétiques et immunophorétiques en moyens gélifiés sur protéines
de muscle strié dans différentes collagénoses d'intérêt dermatologique. G. Martina
and A. Midana 1168

Immunoelektrophorese der Serumproteine bei akuten und chronischen Formen des
Erythematodes. T. Bielický, L. Malina and J. Opplt 1170

Immunologic Defect of the Skin in Lymphadenopathy. Y. Noguchi, K. Ishiwara,
M. Higuchi and S. Yoshida 1171

Immunologische Untersuchungen von Lymphocytenkulturen. Eine diagnostische
Methode in der Dermatologie. H. J. Heitmann 1174

Mechanisms of Anaphylaxis. M. W. Greaves 1176

The Immunochemical Basis of the Urticarial Reaction. F. S. Farah and A. K. Kurban 1176

The Release of Serotonin in Hypersensitivity States. J. S. Comaish 1179

Réactions sérologiques et terrain d'allergie humorale en dermatologie. Cl. Mikol and
M. Renoux 1180

Experimentelle Untersuchungen zur Desensibilisierung und Immunotoleranz gegen
niedermolekulare Allergene. K. H. Schulz 1181

Experimentelle Sensibilisierung mit drei- und sechswertigem Chrom. M. Schwarz-
Speck 1183

Zur Frage autoallergischer Reaktionen bei der Neurodermitis. B. Kopecká, E. Sorkin,
S. Borelli and Å. Fjelde 1185

Delayed Reactivity to Bacterial, Mold and Viral Allergens in Atopic Dermatitis.
G. Rajka 1187

Das Shwartzman-Phänomen, eine dem Arthus-Phänomen ähnliche, pseudo-immuno-
logische Reaktion der Haut auf Endotoxin. I. Kunick and L. Illig 1187

Immunological Aspects of the Aldrich's Syndrome. G. Iacovacci, S. Ungari and F.
Aiuti 1189

Mise en évidence d'anticorps circulants dans les manifestations cutanées de l'allergie à
la pénicilline. J. Paupe and Cl. Mikol 1190

Heutige Diagnostik der Penicillinallergie. P. Michailov and N. Berowa 1191

page

Symposium 12: The Skin and Internal Disease

Reports

Erythropoietic Protoporphyria. I. A. MAGNUS 1195

Xanthomatoses et maladies systémiques. A. BAZEX, A. DUPRÉ and B. CHRISTOL . . 1197

Skin Disorders in Relation to Malabsorption. G. C. WELLS 1200

Further Studies on Acrodermatitis Enteropathica. N. DANBOLT 1202

A New Classification for Lupus Erythematosus. J. R. HASERICK 1204

Angiokeratoma Corporis Diffusum. H. J. WALLACE 1207

Consideration of the Etiology of Pyoderma Gangrenosum. H. O. PERRY and P. DIDIS-HEIM 1208

Free Communications

A Cutaneous Affection from Malabsorption. A. BACCAREDDA-BOY and F. CROVATO . . 1212

Hauterscheinungen bei Colitis ulcerosa. H. REICH 1214

Crohn's Disease Associated with Cutaneous Lesions. G. A. GRANT PETERKIN 1214

Lung Function in Patients with Cutaneous Vasculitis. M. CATTERALL 1215

Atteinte du rein au cours des allergides nodulaires dermiques de Gougerot. ST. BOULLE and J. GUILAINE 1217

Therapie der Porphyria cutanea tarda (Ergebnisse in 9 Jahren). H. IPPEN 1218

Hautreaktionen bei rheumatischen Erkrankungen. E. WOHLSTEIN 1219

Studies on Iron Metabolism in the Porphyria Cutanea Tarda (P.C.T.). L. LEVI, C. L. MENEGHINI, F. SPINELLI-RESSI and C. A. BETTINELLI 1222

Krankhafte Zusammenhänge zwischen Leber und Haut in "Porphyria cutanea tarda". P. TÎRLEA and I. CĂPUSAN 1222

Schistosomiasis (Bilharziasis) der Haut. C. M. HASSELMANN 1224

Schistosomal Infestation of the Skin. A. M. EL MOFTY 1224

The Hepatitis Associated with Infantile Papular Acrodermatitis. V. A. PUCCINELLI . . 1228

Zum Krankheitsbild des Myxoedema circumscriptum praetibiale. CHR. EBERHARTINGER 1229

Natural Course of Various Types of Scleroderma. A. Follow-up-Study over a Period of 20 Years. Z. STAVA 1230

Preparation and Application of Lesional Casts in the Study of Cutaneous Disease. D. A. ROE 1231

Perorale Kreatinbelastung bei Haut- und Muskelerkrankungen. H. W. KREYSEL and M. JÄNNER 1232

Liquen rojo plano de la mucosa bucal. Su asociación con diabetes. Nuevas observaciones. D. GRINSPAN, J. DÍAZ, L. O. VILLAPOL, J. SCHNEIDERMAN, R. BERDICHESKY, D. PALESE and J. FAERMAN 1234

Sarcoidosis with Cicatricial Alopecia Resembling Generalized Discoid Lupus Erythematosus. L. S. SAUTER 1235

Dermatological Aspects of Crohn's Disease. D. I. MCCALLUM and P. D. C. KINMONT 1237

A propos du syndrôme de Winterbauer (Syndrôme C.R.S.T.). A. PUISSANT, E. LECLERCQ and F. VANBREMEERSCH 1238

Acanthosis Nigricans. — A Clinical Manifestation of Internal Disorders. T. YASUDA, SH. NISHIYAMA and SH. TSUYUKI 1240

Glucorrhoea. Is this Pre-diabetes? J. R. G. AGIUS 1241

Hormonelle Untersuchungen und Behandlungsmethoden bei Acne vulgaris. F. TÓTH and L. NÉKÁM 1243

Vorkommen von Paraproteinämie bei Pyoderma gangraenosum. H. RÖCKL 1244

Zur Problematik der Arthropathia psoriatica. F. VLČEK, M. ZBOJANOVA, G. NIEPEL and Z. SITAY 1246

page

Quelques observations sur l'élimination urinaire des cétostéroïdes dans l'acnée féminine. R. DUMITRIU, M. HAISUC, L. REITER, M. HONTARU and A. COSER 1248

The Seborrhoic Symptom Complex.— The Expression of a Disturbed Intestinal Malutilization of Vitamin B 12 as Proven by Measuring the Radioactivity after Administration of Co 60 Vitamin B 12. W. A. CASPER 1249

Diabetes and Impetigo Contagiosa (Passage from one Diabetic Family to Another Diabetic Family Via a Related Cousin Carrier). B. R. HEARST 1251

Dermatitis uraemica Rössle. H. FISCHER 1252

Symposium 13: Bullous Dermatoses

Reports

Zur Klinik bullöser Eruptionen (Exklusive bullöse Genodermatosen). J. TAPPEINER 1257

Herpes Zoster and Nonmalignant Disease. L. H. WINER and E. T. WRIGHT 1259

Producción experimental de ampollas; su correlacción con los cambios estructurales en las dermatosis ampollosas. D. J. GÓMEZ ORBANEJA 1262

La maladie de Duhring-Brocq à grosses bulles dite «pemphigoïde de Brocq», après la cinquantaine. P. LE COULANT, L. TEXIER and P. BORAUD 1264

Subcorneal Pustular Dermatosis. A review after 10 years. D. S. WILKINSON 1266

Bullous Lesions in Patients with Internal Disorders. E. SKOG 1267

Corticosteroid Treatment of Pemphigus. C. T. NELSON 1270

Friction Blisters Produced under Controlled Conditions. TH. A. CORTESE jr., T. B. GRIFFIN and M. B. SULZBERGER 1273

Free Communications

Experimental Investigations on the Acantholysis Induced by Staphylococcus pyogens. Comparative Study with the Acantholysis on Pemphigus. B. ZILBERBERG . . . 1275

An Electron Microscopic Study of Cutaneous and Oral Pemphigus Vulgaris. K. HASHIMOTO 1278

Localización de gamma globulina IgG y complemento (C'3) en la epidermis de enfermos de Pénfigo vulgar. S. STRINGA, C. BIANCHI, A. CASALA, C. INGLESINI and O. BIANCHI 1283

Dermatite Bulleuse Mucosynéchante et Atrophiante. A. G. BELLONE, M. F. HOFMANN and G. CAPUTO 1285

Experimental Friction Blisters: Histological Investigation. K. FUKUYAMA and TH. A. CORTESE jr. 1288

Etude de la composition protéique du liquide des bulles dans les dermatoses bulleuses. G. MOULIN and Y. MANUEL 1289

Nouvelles observations sur le phénomène citochémiotatique dans la bulle du pemphigus. P. SERTOLI 1291

Hepatische Porphyrien: Veränderungen der Serumenzymaktivitäten und hämatologischen Befunde beim Menschen und bei der Ratte. H. PIETSCHMANN and W. RAAB . 1293

Interessante, bei den an bullösen Dermatosen leidenden Kranken erhobene hämatologische und gastroenterologische Befunde. V. ROZSÍVALOVÁ, F. MATĚJA, B. FIXA and O. KOMÁRKOVÁ 1294

The Treatment of Porphyria Cutanea Tarda by Chelation. G. A. HUNTER and G. F. DONALD 1296

Toxic Epidermal Necrolysis. M. B. LEWIS 1297

Acute Epidermal Necrolysis (Ritter-Lyell). — The Scalded Skin Syndrome. P. J. KOBLENZER 1298

The Ultrastructure of Acantholysis in Lichen Planus. L. FRY and F. R. JOHNSON . . 1301

page

Symposium 14: Mycobacterial Infections of the Skin

Reports

Etude biologique récente dans la lèpre: Analogies antigéniques et séro-diagnostic de la lèpre par immunofluorescence sur bacille de Stefansky. F.-P. MERKLEN and F. COTTENOT 1305

Las formas submicroscópicas del m. leprae. J. GAY PRIETO and G. GABINO 1306

Die gegenwärtige Epidemologie und Bakteriologie der Hauttuberkulose in der Bundesrepublik Deutschland. F. EHRING 1308

Mykobakterienbefunde bei den sog. Tuberkuliden. N. SIMON 1312

Thalidomide in Lepra Reaction and in Hansen's Disease. J. SHESKIN, F. SAGHER, M. DORFMAN and J. CONVIT 1314

Free Communications

Geographical Distribution of Skin Tuberkulosis, Leprosy and Sarcoidosis in Japan. K. KITAMURA 1316

A propos des tuberculoses cutanées — leur classification — leur diagnostic biologique — leur traitement. M. BOLGERT and P. L. DELAIRE 1317

Lupus Vulgaris Gigantea Caused by Mycobacterium Avium. J. V. CHRISTIANSEN . . 1319

Atypical Acid fast Micro-Organisms in Scleroderma. A. R. CANTWELL, E. CRAGGS, J. W. WILSON and F. SWATEK 1320

Nature of the Antigen Responsible for the Kveim Reaction in Sarcoidosis. R. KOOIJ and J. W. VAN WAVEREN HOGERVORST 1322

Present Position of BCG Vaccination against Leprosy. L. M. BECHELLI 1323

Über die pigmentierten Naevi bei lepromatösen Leprakranken. Y. ISHIBASHI and T. KAWAMURA 1325

Mise en évidence du bacille de Hansen dans les lèpres apparemment abacillaires. F. COTTENOT, F.-P. MERKLEN and TRINH THI KIM MONG DON 1326

The Frequency of Intracellular Lipid in the Several Structureal Types of Leprosy. R. D. AZULAY and L. C. DE ANDRADE 1328

Cutaneous Response of Leprosy Patients to Living and Heated Mycobacterium Leprae Cultures on the Olitzki-Gershon Medium. M. DORFMAN, F. SAGHER, J. SHESKIN and A. L. OLITZKI 1329

Serum Immunoglobulin Changes in Leprosy and Tuberculosis. SOO DUK LIM and R. M. FUSARO 1332

Nuevos avances terapéuticos en lepra. J. C. GATTI, J. E. CARDAMA and L. M. BALINA 1334

Double Reversal of the Tuberculin Reaction in Sarcoidosis. S. H. SILVERS and F. S. GLICKMAN 1335

Clinical Applications of Shepard's Mouse Foot Pad Technique. P. FASAL and L. LEVY 1337

Impétigo herpétiforme Hébra Kaposi ou Psoriasis pustuleux généralisé (chez une femme âgée de 22 ans, apparu au cours de 5e mois de sa 2e grossesse). R. SAMII 1339

Symposium 15: Iatrogenic Diseases in Dermatology

Reports

Dermatosis iatrogénicas. Definición, patogénia, clasificación. M. I. QUIROGA 1343

The Aetiology of Toxic Epidermal Necrolysis. A. LYELL 1346

Iatrogenic Disease Due to Physical Treatment. A. N. DOMONKOS 1347

Eruptions du type L. E. et syndromes lupiques provoqués par des médicaments. CH. GRUPPER and G. A. C. MARCEL 1349

Dermatoses des traitements antidiabétiques. J. BEUREY, P. JEANDIDIER and A. BERMONT 1352

Iatrogenic Dyschromies. H. MÖLLER 1355

page

Free Communications

Photosensitive Dermatitis as an Iatrogenic Disease. T. Kobori and H. Araki 1357

Les accidents cutanés de l'allergie humorale médicamenteuse. Intérêt du test de Shelley. J. Maleville, H. Bergoend and A. Basset 1359

La thésaurismose cutanée par polyvinylpyrrolidone (PVP). J. M. Lachapelle . . . 1362

Mascaras pigmentarias como expresión iatrogénica a dosis altas y prolongadas de feniotiacina y derivados en el control de afecciones psiquiatricas. E. B. Molina Leguizamón, A. A. Cordero and E. Follmann 1363

Necrolisis Epidermica Toxica. — Observaciones sobre 12 Casos. A. Cortés Cortés and V. Cárdenas Jaramillo 1371

Dermatosis por anovulatorios. Y. Ortiz 1373

Case Presentations and Fundamentals on Film

Second International Film Presentation of the Institute for Dermatologic Communication and Education

Keratosis Follicularis (Darier's Disease). N. Karltorp and St. Floderus 1379

Congenital Ichthyosiform Erythroderma. K. Rehtijärvi, K. Kuokkanen and P. Karma 1379

Xeroderma Pigmentosum. H. el Hefnawi 1379

Metastasizing Basal Cell Carcinoma. C. Ch. Thomas 1380

The Nevoid Basal Cell Carcinoma Syndrome. J. B. Howell and D. E. Anderson . . 1380

Gold Leaf Treatment of Cutaneous Ulcers. N. M. Kanof 1380

Diagnosis of Latent Psoriasis. G. Holti 1380

Surgical Treatment of Benign Acanthosis Nigricans. H. Ollendorff Curth 1380

Pellagra and other Avitaminoses in the Bantu. M. Rose 1381

Lupus Erythematosus. D. L. Tuffanelli and W. B. Reed 1381

Lipoid Proteinosis. R. M. Caplan 1381

Acrodermatitis Chronica Atrophicans (Herxheimer). F. Herrmann and O. Schultka . 1381

Granulomatous Dermo-Hypodermitis with Progressive Atrophy. J. Convit, Fr. Kerdel-Vegas and M. F. Allende 1381

Report of the Institute for Dermatologic Communication and Education to the International Committee of Dermatology 1382

Scientific Exhibition

Clinical Dermatology

Die spontane Heilungsquote der Blutschwämme und die daraus zu ziehenden Schlüsse für die Prognose und Therapie. G. F. Klostermann 1387

Spontanverlauf der Säuglingshämangiome. A. Proppe and H. Hauss 1387

Laser Surgery of Angiomas with Special Reference to Port-Wine Angiomas. L. Goldman, E. J. Ritter, R. J. Rockwell jr., R. Meyer, B. Henderson and K. Wm. Kitzmiller 1388

Therapie hypercholesterinämischer Xanthomatosen. N. Zöllner, M. Gudenzi and G. Wolfram 1390

Proteolytic Enzyme Treatment of Skin Ulcers. M. C. Spencer 1393

Chemosurgery for the Microscopically Controlled Excision of Skin Cancer. Fr. E. Mohs 1393

Multiple Punch Autografts for the Alopecias. D. B. Stough 1394

Evaluation of Parental Methotrexate for Intractable Psoriasis. Ch. P. Defeo, A. Allyn and S. Eisenberg 1394

Zur Wirkung des hochalpinen Klimas in der atopischen konstitutionellen Neurodermitis. S. Borelli, H. Brenn, St. Chlebarov, C. Ene-Popescu, H. Gehrken, B. Kopecka, P. Michailov and H. Vossieck. 1395

Klimatherapie von Hautkrankheiten an der Nordsee. W. Pürschel 1397

page

Die Verbrennung — ein dermatologisches Problem. Komplikationen, Therapie und Prophylaxe. G. WEBER and H. JURSCH 1400

A New Principle in Topical Corticosteroid Treatment. G. HAGERMAN 1406

Casus rari muco-cutanei. A. GREITHER and O. HORNSTEIN 1408

Visualization in Dermatology. K. K. MUSTAKALLIO 1409

Examen radiographique des tissus cutanés et sous-cutanés normaux et pathologiques. CH. GROS, A. BASSET, S. SCHRAUB, J. MALEVILLE, E. GROSSHANS and E. HEID . . 1409

Klassifizierung der Ichthyosen. U. W. SCHNYDER and B. KONRÁD 1411

Andrologie in Klinik und Praxis. C. SCHIRREN and H. GRELL 1413

Papulonecrotic and Acneiform Tuberculids. C. E. SONCK 1413

Exhibit on Genodermatoses. L. ZIPRKOWSKI 1418

A Case of Congenital Erythropoietic Porphyria. K. YAMAMOTO 1420

Contact Allergy in Scandinavia. B. MAGNUSSON, S.-G. BLOHM, S. FREGERT, N. HJORTH, G. HØVDING, V. PIRILÄ and E. SKOG 1421

Klinische Pharmakologie des neuen Histaminblockers Tavegil. L. KERP and H. KASEMIR 1425

Hautveränderungen und Antikörper-Mangelsyndrome. G. BREHM 1426

L'allergie de contact. J. FOUSSEREAU 1429

Chamber Test Method. V. PIRILÄ and L. FÖRSTRÖM 1430

Erythropoietic Protoporphyria. R. M. FUSARO, W. J. RUNGE, E. S. PETERKA. M. O. JAFFE, E. W. GOLTZ and C. J. WATSON 1432

Gegenüberstellung von Angiomatosis Kaposi (Sarcoma idiopathicum haemorrhagicum multiplex) und Stewart-Treves-Syndrom (Sarcoma angioplasticum in elephantiasi). H. TELLER and H. KRÜGER 1435

Une affection liée au sexe: la gérodermie ostéodysplasique. D. KLEIN, F. BAMATTER, A. FRANCESCHETTI, G. BOREUX, J. E. W. BROCHER and P. HOLENSTEIN 1443

Elektronenmikroskopische, histochemische und polarisationsoptische Untersuchungen bei Pemphigus familiaris benignus (Hailey u. Hailey). F. NÜRNBERGER and G. MÜLLER 1444

Pemphigus Benignus Chronicus and Keratosis Palmo-plantaris in a Finnish Family. C. E. SONCK 1444

Shibi-Gatchaki-Syndrome. Y. KATABIRA 1447

Cas Cliniques. A. BASSET 1448

Gnathostomiasis Cutis. Yangtze Edema in China and Similar Migrating Intermittent Swellings of the Skin in Japan, Both Due to Gnathostoma Spinigerum Owen, 1836. K. KITAMURA 1449

Plusieures dermatoses. G. SAKELLARIOU 1450

Seltene Hautkrankheiten. G. HARGITA 1451

Angiokeratoma corporis diffusum Fabry. R. DENK 1459

Die primäre Hautreaktion nach infektiösem Tsetsefliegenstich bei der afrikanischen Schlafkrankheit. H. E. KRAMPITZ 1459

Amoebiasis Skin Manifestations. TH. DOXIADES and J. CAPETANAKIS 1462

Skin Diseases in Arabian Countries: Certain Notes and Comments. M. EL ZAWAHRY . 1464

Die Tumormetastasierung von der Haut und in die Haut. H. DREPPER and F. EHRING 1465

Zur Pathologie cutaner Lymphgefäße. J. TAPPEINER and L. PFLEGER 1467

Neuere Aspekte zur Histopathologie der Alopecia areata. W. THIES and CH. FISCHER 1469

Befund Langerhans-ähnlicher Zellen in den Hauterscheinungen der Reticuloendotheliose von Letterer-Siwe. V. PUCCINELLI, F. GIANOTTI and R. CAPUTO 1472

Tetracycline Fluorescence in Squamous Cell Carcinoma. H. J. DONSKY and G. R. MIKHAIL 1474

Concept of the Molecular Cause of Albinism. G. F. WILGRAM 1475

Xeroderma pigmentosum. H. EL HEFNAWI 1476

Skin Tuberculosis, Leprosy, Cutaneous Leishmanosis, Favus. M. A. MALEKI 1476

page

Experimental Dermatology

A Cutaneous Rôle in the Regulation of the Body's Carbohydrate Milieu. R. M. FUSARO and J. A. JOHNSON 1477

The Interplay of Opposites. Immunological Reactions in the Skin. TH. M. INDERBITZIN and P. J. GROB 1480

Autoradiographic Studies on Psoriatic Epidermis. S. SOTOMATSU, Y. IGARASHI and Y. OOSHIMA 1481

Die Mastzelle. A. SCHAUER 1483

Electronmicroscopy of Merkel's Tastzelle. K. K. MUSTAKALLIO and U. KIISTALA . . . 1493

Bilddemonstration zur mikroskopischen Anatomie des Haarfollikels im Verlauf des Haarcyclus. H.-J. BANDMANN and K. BOSSE 1493

Zur Ultrastruktur des menschlichen Haarfollikels. V. PUCCINELLI and R. CAPUTO . . . 1494

Zur licht- und elektronenoptischen Struktur der Nerven am Haar. E. HAGEN and G. NIEBAUER. 1495

Neuere Entwicklung der dermatologischen Virusforschung. TH. NASEMANN 1499

Recent Observations on Langerhans Cells. K. WOLFF, R. K. WINKELMANN and K. HOLUBAR 1502

Malignant Melanomas: Subcellular Differentiation of Nevocytic and Melanocytic Ontogeny. Y. MISHIMA 1505

Epidermal Melanin Unit. M. A. PATHAK, G. SZABÓ, T. B. FITZPATRICK, Y. HORI, S. S. BLEEHEN, E. FRENK, M. MIYAMOTO, M. SEIJI and A. BREATHNACH 1506

Dermo-Epidermal Separation by Suction. N. KIISTALA and K. K. MUSTAKALLIO . . 1513

Comparative Study with the Acantholysis in Pemphigus. Experimental Investigations on the Acantholysis Induced by the Staphylococcus pyogenes. B. ZILBERBERG . . 1513

Pathophysiologie allergischer Dermatosen. G. STÜTTGEN, I. GIGLI and F. HERRMANN 1514

Das mikrobielle Ekzem. H. RÖCKL, F. SCHRÖPL, E. MÜLLER and G. PETER 1516

Experimental Eczema of the Guinea Pig. N. HUNZIKER 1518

Terpentinöl-Intoxikation bei Arbeitern einer Schuhcreme-Fabrik verursacht durch d-Alpha-Pinen. F. NÜRNBERGER 1522

Enzymaktivitätsmuster im Serum und in Erythrozyten bei verschiedenen Hautkrankheiten. H. HOLZMANN, B. MORSCHES, G. W. KORTING and R. DENK 1524

Immunofluorescence Studies of the Skin. R. H. CORMANE, E. H. BAART DE LA FAILLE, J. B. VAN DER MEER, A. A. W. TEN HAVE-OPBROEK and W. W. MUIJS VAN DE MOER 1524

Herkunft der mononucleären Entzündungszellen (Makrophagen) bei der unspezifischen Entzündung (Untersuchungen am Rebuck'schen Hautfenster bei der Ratte). M. BEGEMANN 1531

Unspezifische und spezifische Wirkstoffe bei allergischen Reaktionen der Cutis. G. STÜTTGEN, J. GIGLI and F. HERRMANN 1531

Allergens of Quinone Structure. K. H. SCHULZ, P. SCHMIDT and H. GRELL 1531

Methode zur Hornschichtdickenmessung in vivo. F. KLASCHKA and R. A. KRAUSE . . 1533

Dermatological and Immunological Aspects of Cryoglobulinaemia. K. K. MUSTAKALLIO and O. WAGNER 1534

R.U.V., X-Ray and Alpha-particles Micrography of the Skin. A. TOSTI 1535

L'Exploration thermographique en dermatologie. CH. GROS, C. VROUSOS, J. ALT and A. BASSET 1539

The History of the Dermatological Section of the Royal Society of Medicine. T. J. RYAN, Y. M. CLAYTON, E. J. MOYNAHAN, J. F. KENNEDY, P. POLANI and I. A. MAGNUS . . 1541

Zellphysiologische Aspekte der Psoriasis vulgaris. O. BRAUN-FALCO, E. CHRISTOPHERS, S. MARGHESCU, D. PETZOLDT, G. RASSNER and M. RUPEC 1546

Mycology

Mikroskopische Demonstration von Fadenpilzen und Hefen. H. BRAUN and C. SCHÖNBORN 1550

page

Faserzerstörung durch Dermatophyten und keratinophile Pilze. L. KREMPL-LAMPRECHT 1550

Dermatophyten und ihre Hauptfruchtformen. G. A. DEVRIES and L. KREMPL-LAMPRECHT 1555

Serological Relationship of the Dermatophytes of Emmons-Conant-System. H. PALDROK and K. R. SUNDSTRÖM 1556

Adaptationsphasen der Dermatophyten in Zusammenhang mit ihrer Klassifikation. V. A. BALABANOFF 1556

Epidemiologische Analyse des Vorkommens von Dermatophyten in der Slowakei. L. CHMEL. 1560

Einige biochemische Eigenschaften der Isothiocyanate. A. BOJANOVSKÁ 1560

Trichofytocid Spofa® (5% p-bromphenylisothiocyanat) bei der Behandlung von Trichophytosis. L. CHMEL, M. VALENTOVÁ and J. BUCHVALD 1561

Histopathomorphologische Befunde der Haut nach der Applikation von Trichophytocid. L. CHMEL and A. BOJANOVSKÁ 1561

Chromomycosis Caused by a New Species Chmelia slovaca. L. CHMEL, I. KOCHOVÁ and A. BOJANOVSKÁ 1562

The Third Case of Chromomycosis in the Territory of Czechoslovakia. L. CHMEL, I. KOCHOVÁ, A. BOJANOVSKÁ and B. KONRÁD 1563

Pilzerkrankungen innerer Organe. T. WEGMANN 1563

Survey of Mycoses in U.A.R. M. EL ZAWAHRY 1564

Clinical Diagnosis of Onychotrichophytosis. J. ALKIEWICZ and W. SOWINSKI 1564

Favic Infections in the Surroundings of Göttingen. M. KIRSCH-NIETZKI 1566

Pilzinfektionen im Bereich des Auges. D. H. HOFFMANN 1566

Parasitic Forms of the Causative Fungi in the Cutaneous and Visceral Lesions of Chromoblastomycosis. R. FUKUSHIRO and S. KAGAWA 1568

Chromomycosis (in the World and in Finland). T. PUTKONEN 1570

Relations entre formes cliniques et espèces mycologiques. A. BASSET et M. BASSET . 1570

Dermatomykosen bei Säugetieren. H. KRAFT 1570

Mykosen bei Tieren (Befall durch Aspergillus, verschiedene Dermatophyten und Alternaria). H. KRAFT 1572

Maduromykose beim Pferd. B. SCHIEFER and B. GEDEK 1573

Beitrag zur Mykologie der Systemmykosen: Histoplasmose und Kryptokokkose. H. KARUGA. 1574

Vorkommen von Dermatophyten im Boden und bei Tieren als mögliche Infektionsquellen. D. JANKE 1577

Trichophytie und Blastomykose. Zs. HERPAY 1580

Ultrastructure of Dermatophytes. W. MEINHOF and W. VOGELL 1581

Infektionen durch Candida albicans. J. THURNER 1584

Quantitative Methoden der Antimykotikaprüfung. W. DITTMAR 1586

Enzymhistochemische Untersuchungen an Dermatophyten. K. HOLUBAR and O. MALE 1590

Dermatophyten und Schimmelpilze. B. BRAUN, H. RIETH and C. FINGER 1590

Additional Demonstrations

Kollegheft der Vorlesung von F. VON HEBRA, geschrieben von F. CURTI, zur Verfügung gestellt von O. GRUMBACH unter Vermittlung von O. GANS 1590

Histopathology of Leprosy. M. L. BRUBAKER and P. FASAL 1590

Antibiotics and the Placebo Reaction in Acne. R. C. SAVIN and M. CHANCO-TURNER . 1590

Authors Index 1592

Malignant Reticuloses and Lymphomas

**Hémoréticulopathies malignes
(réticuloses malignes, lymphomes malins)**

**Hemoretículopatias malignas
(Reticulosis y linfamas malignos)**

Maligne Retikulosen der Haut

Organizer

F. SAGHER, Israel

Presidents

P. DE GRACIANSKY, France

I. KATZENELLENBOGEN, Israel

H. MONTGOMERY, USA

A. MUSGER, Austria

Delegate of the Organization Committee

H. W. SPIER, Germany

Reports

Histopathologic and Hematologic Changes in Malignant Lymphomas and Reticuloses

H. MONTGOMERY and R. K. WINKELMANN, Mayo Clinic and Mayo Foundation: Section of Dermatology, Rochester, Minnesota (USA)

We are pleased and honored to participate in this symposium on malignant lymphomas and reticuloses, a subject in which one of us has been interested for almost 50 years. The background has been reviewed in a recently published book [1] and in some more recent reports [2 to 7].

Opinions differ in different countries regarding classification, terminology, etc. of the whole group of conditions being considered in this symposium. Even in a single institution, on final analysis of the results of clinical, histopathological, bone marrow, touch smear, and other laboratory examinations, a case may be interpreted differently among senior consultants in various specialties such as pathology, hematology, and dermatology and require further observation over a longer period. As long as the unknown factor in regard to cancer, precancerous dermatoses, histiocytosis X, Kaposi's sarcoma, etc. remains to be determined and the prognosis of these conditions varies greatly, relating at times more to extent of involvement than to histopathology, it would seem best to classify according to clinical syndromes and to simplify the many synonymous terms for the same condition.

It is our concept, which may be a minority opinion, that persistent and repeated irritation or trauma can eventually induce a malignant neoplasm. By this, we would include certain of the lymphoma-reticulosis group and all the so-called precancerous group as defined in the dermatopathology text [1]. This corresponds to the transformation of hyperplastic reticulosis to malignant reticulosis as described by DEGOS. Up to a certain point there is a reversible reaction, depending on the carcinogenic agent involved — for example, whether experimental carcinogenesis in mice or rats or arsenic in humans. DEGOS has emphasized and described cases of mycosis fungoides in which there was an antecedent history of eczema or psoriasis. Our experience agrees with this and, although these cases are rare, it emphasizes the relationship between repeated inflammation and trauma and eventual malignancy.

We believe that, in a significant number of cases, mycosis fungoides (excluding the fulminating d'emblee type which from the beginning is reticulum sarcoma) eventuates in one or another of the malignant lymphomas or reticuloses with typical biopsy findings. WINKELMANN regarded cases of exfoliative dermatitis or erythroderma in the later decades of life, associated with reticular lymphocytes with a benign folded nucleus, as Sezary's syndrome rather than true Alibert type of mycosis fungoides. MONTGOMERY still believes, contrary to Bluefarb and others, that mycosis fungoides may start out as an exfoliative erythroderma. On the other hand, the Sezary cell and syndrome have been so clearly defined in recent years that they belong as part of the whole symposium that we are discussing. Our definition at present is "reticular lymphocytic premalignant dermal reticulosis producing erythroderma and often reticulemia." Recent electron microscopic studies also distinguish between the two conditions.

There is not time to go into borderline conditions such as histiocytosis X (eosinophilic granulomas of skin and bone) and possibly some cases of Hand-Schüller-Christian and Letterer-Siwe disease (benign granulomatous histiocytic

45*

processes); however, the latter can act like a malignant lymphoma. The same applies to Hodgkin's disease, including the paragranulomatous, granulomatous, and malignant forms as defined in the recent literature.

It therefore becomes important to correlate various clinical, histopathologic, histochemical, and other laboratory findings to arrive at a diagnosis in a given

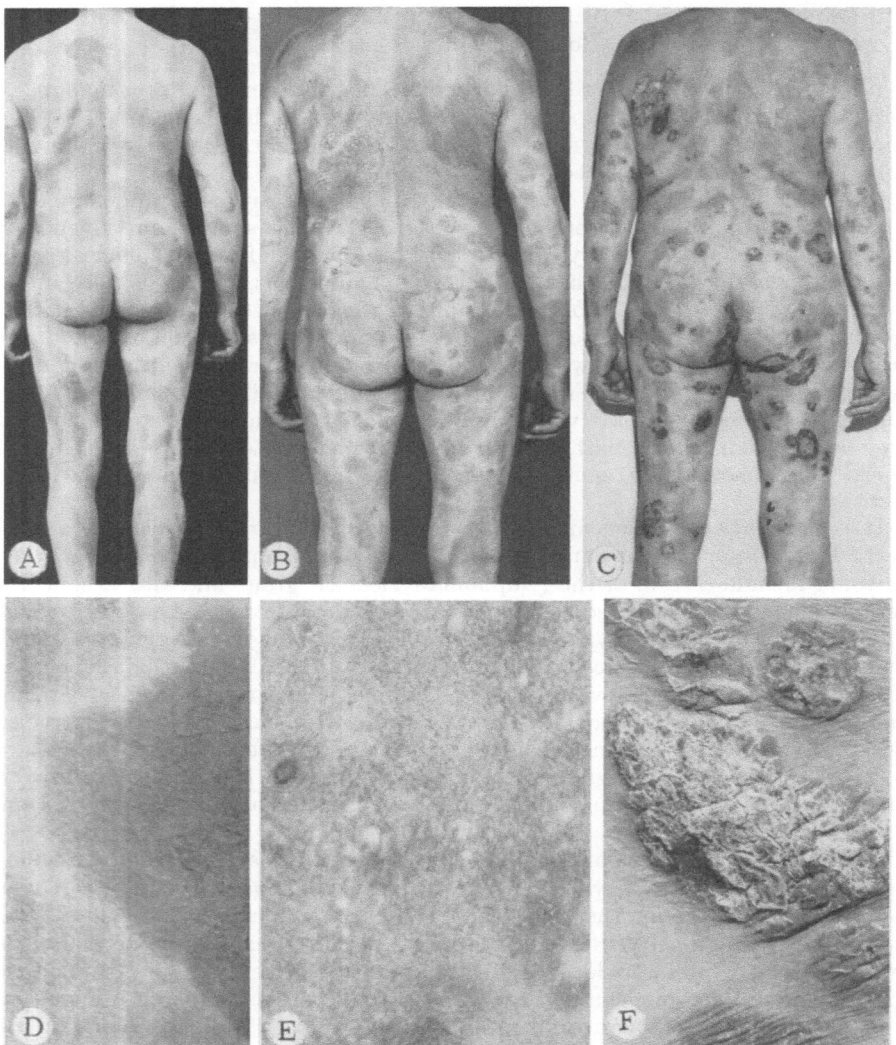

Fig. 1. (Case 1.) *A*, Premycotic and indurated plaques when first seen in 1937. *B* and *C*, Appearance on return for further treatment in 1946 and 1963. *D*, Premycotic plaques, leg, 1937. *E*, Poikilodermatous changes in 1946 below axilla. *F*, Indurated psoriasiform plaques in 1953

case. This provides not only cytohistologic classification but also some prognostic classification.

The concept of Kaposi's sarcoma in relation to lymphomas and reticuloendothelial system diseases has been discussed [6] and it was suggested that Kaposi's sarcoma is closely related to the lymphomas or reticuloses.

Mycosis Fungoides

We believe that the first changes in mycosis fungoides may frequently occur in the cutis and that epidermal changes including Pautrier microabscesses are not essential for diagnosis. We define mycosis fungoides as related to the large-plaque type of parapsoriasis, not the parapsoriasis of the small-plaque type described by

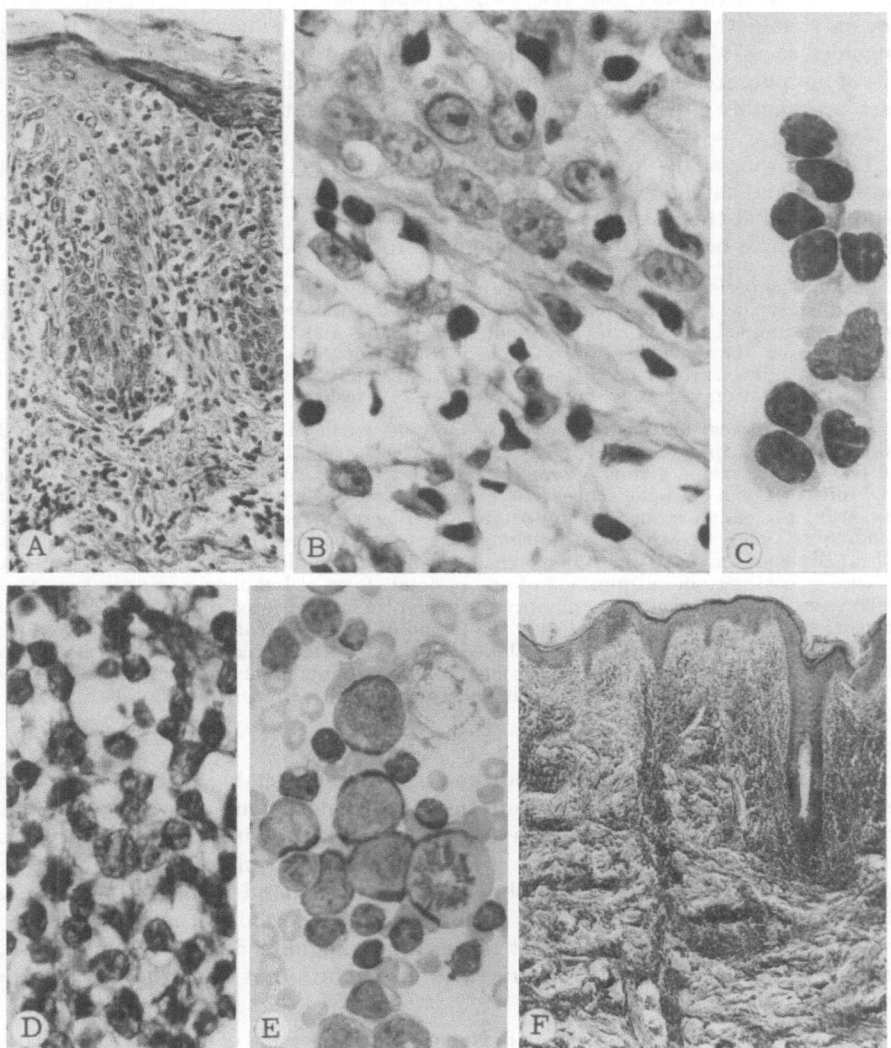

Fig. 2. *A*, *B* and *C*, Mycosis fungoides (case 1). *A*, Typical histologic picture in lesion from middle of back in 1937. (Hematoxylin and eosin; × 220.) *B*, Biopsy in 1957. Note migration of pyknotic cells through epidermis. (Hematoxylin and eosin; × 800.) *C*, Touch smear in 1957, showing immature cells with grooving. (Wright's stain; × 850.) *D*, Lymphosarcoma in a 46-year-old man who had bilateral cervical adenopathy for 6 years with erythema of scalp for 1 year. Biopsy of lymph node revealed lymphosarcoma 1 year later. Nodule from scalp showed lymphomatous, nonspecific infiltrate. (Hematoxylin and eosin; × 600.) *E*, Touch smear from same case as *D* shows immature leukocytes and mitotic figure. (Wright's stain; 600.) *F*, Lymphatic leukemia (exfoliative stage). Biopsy reveals lack of involvement of epidermis and dense infiltrate in cutis, also in narrow strands. (Hematoxylin and eosin; × 45)

Brocq. The large-plaque type, described by Degos and assoc. and with many of his colleagues in Belgium and elsewhere, with poikilodermoid features is what Lane of New Haven and later Oliver and others in Chicago called "premycotic mycosis fungoides."

Although many pathologists do not recognize the term "mycosis fungoides" and confuse it with other reticuloses and lymphomas, their view is limited because they only make their observations at the autopsy table. The percentage of mycosis fungoides cases which eventually become reticulum cell sarcoma or some other type of lymphosarcoma is very difficult to determine. All cases of mycosis fungoides must presumably have the same premalignant potential yet many cases never express it.

The following slides demonstrate the approach from the benign to the malignant lymphoma and reticuloses. I do this purposely to emphasize what my co-author demonstrated at the last International Congress in an exhibit — that cytology and histology define benign as well as malignant forms of reticular disease.

Case 1. The patient, a man, was 49 years old when he first was seen at the Mayo Clinic in 1937; he had typical mycosis fungoides. He had noted the first plaque when he was 17 years old. He was reexamined at this clinic through 1963 (Fig. 1 and 2). At no time was there any hematologic or other evidence of systemic involvement. The condition was controlled for 27 years by judicious roentgen therapy. The patient finally died at age 76 at home. No postmortem examination was done, but the mycosis fungoides was still under control.

Case 2. A 25-year-old medical student was seen at the Mayo Clinic in November 1926 and was shown at the Minnesota Dermatological Society meeting where Drs. P. A. O'Leary and Henry Michelson, among others, thought that the patient had parapsoriasis en plaque but Professor Gans read the biopsies as early mycosis fungoides. The onset was $6^1/_2$ years previously, as a circumscribed scaling patch. A full-blown mycosis fungoides then developed, including at times an exfoliative erythroderma with poikilodermatous changes and large infiltrated plaques and, at times, hemorrhagic elements. He died 20 years later without any evidence at postmortem examination of any systemic form of lymphoma or reticulosis. Over the 20 years, he had continued to practice medicine. He had repeated roentgen therapy. Some lesions received more than 4,000 R over the period of 20 years. Numerous biopsies were performed, and toward the end, some of the sections looked more like reticulum cell sarcoma but without evidence at postmortem examination of systemic involvement. I might add that in both cases of mycosis fungoides, touch smears were positive for immature cells.

Sezary's Syndrome

In many respects, Sezary's syndrome is indistinguishable from mycosis fungoides. Sezary described many syndromes of reticulosis, but we wish to limit the use of his name to the form of lymphocytic reticulosis (with or without erythroderma). Histologic and hemocytologic studies of the peripheral blood and touch smears reveal more reticular lymphocytes than are found in other lymphomas. There is usually a fatal outcome within a 5-year period without evidence of systemic reticulosis. We believe that this is a premalignant dermal reticulosis with a special cell type and are not surprised at the evolution of this syndrome toward typical lymphoma.

Case 3. A 74-year-old man was seen in November 1959 because of eczema and exfoliative dermatitis of 1 year's duration, diagnosed at first as possible mycosis fungoides or leukemia cutis. The diagnosis later was changed to Sezary's syndrome (Fig. 3 A, B, and C). The patient responded to treatment with chlorambucil (Leukeran) and steroids and he died of a cerebrovascular accident in July 1963; there was no postmortem examination.

Hodgkin's Disease

Hodgkin's disease rarely shows specific cutaneous changes. It usually recurs as a simple toxic pruritus with excoriation, but it may be of primary cutaneous origin, either as an exfoliative dermatitis or in the form of ulcers or nodules.

Case 4. The patient, a 45-year-old woman, had exfoliative Hodgkin's disease with many nodules on the face and scalp (Fig. 3 D) resembling those of monocytic reticulosis; she died of Hodgkin's disease 4 years later (Fig. 3 E).

Space does not permit giving case histories but we wish to emphasize that occasionally both mycosis fungoides and Hodgkin's disease may eventuate in

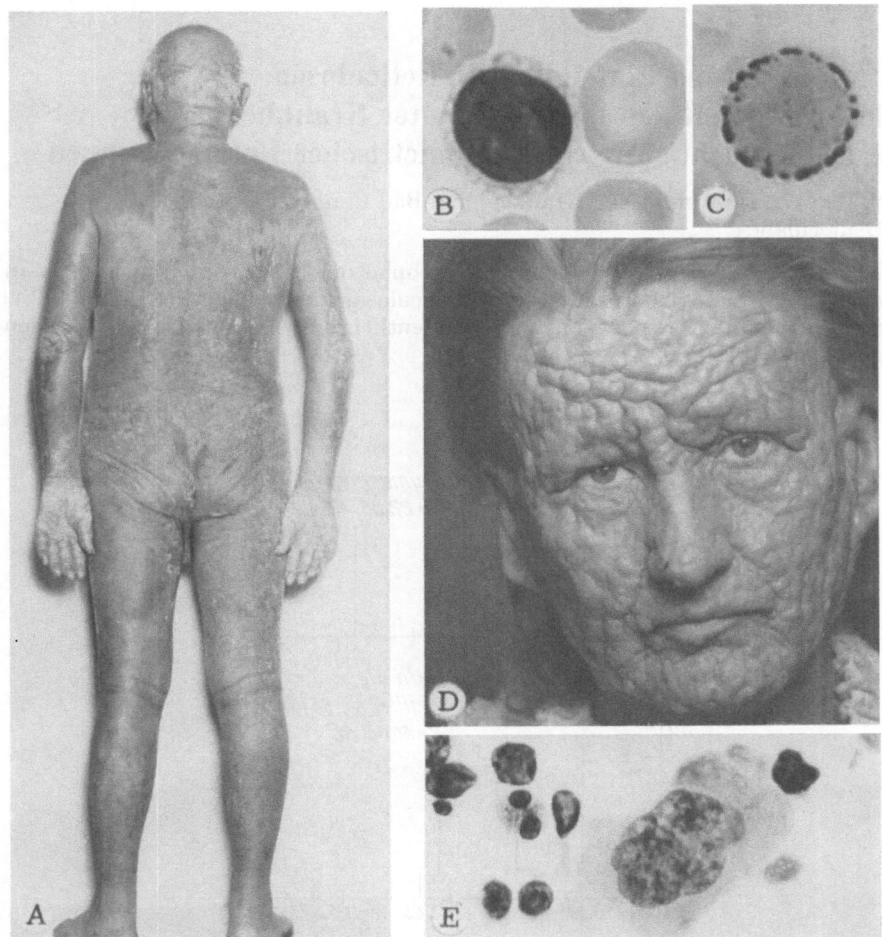

Fig. 3. *A*, *B* and *C*, Malignant erythroderma in Sezary's syndrome (case 3). *B* and *C*, Typical Sezary cells in peripheral blood. *B*, Wright's stain. ($\times$ 1,800.) *C*, PAS-positive cytoplasmic granules. ($\times$ 1,800.) *D* (case 4), Patient (45 years old) had exfoliative Hodgkin's disease with many nodules of face and scalp. *E*, Touch smear of cutaneous biopsy, same case as *D*, showing typical Sternberg-Reed cell. ($\times$ 850)

reticulum cell sarcoma and also that acute fulminating reticuloses may simulate the clinical appearance of mycosis fungoides. The acute forms of reticuloses and lymphomas with undifferentiated stem or blast cells, whether of primary cutaneous or, more frequently, of systemic origin, usually have a fulminating and fatal course.

References. 1. MONTGOMERY, H.: Cutaneous Lymphoma and Malignant Reticuloses. In: Dermatopathology, vol. 2, p. 1203. New York: Hoeber 1967. — 2. ALLEN, A. C.: The Skin: A Clinicopathological Treatise. Ed. 2, p. 1182. New York: Grune & Stratton 1967. — 3. GELLER,

W., and M. J. LACHER: Med. Clin. N. Amer. **50**, 819 (1966). — 4. O'BRIAN, P. H., and R. D. BRASFIELD: Cancer (Philad.) **19**, 1497 (1966). — 5. RAPPAPORT, H.: Tumors of the Hematopoietic System. In: Atlas of Tumor Pathology, Section III, Fascicle 8. Washington, D.C.: Armed Forces Institute of Pathology 1966. — 6. REYNOLDS, W. A., R. K. WINKELMANN, and E. H. SOULE: Medicine (Baltimore) **44**, 419 (1965). — 7. Symposium on Reticuloses. Neoplasma (Bratisl.) **13**, 453 (1966)

Zur Nosologie und Einteilung der Reticulosen, Reticulosarkomatosen und verwandter Krankheitsbilder unter Berücksichtigung cytophotometrischer Untersuchungen*

W. KNOTH, Hautklinik im Krankenhaus Bad Cannstatt, Stuttgart (Deutschland)

Im folgenden berichten wir über neue cytophotometrische Untersuchungen an Reticulose-, Reticulosarkomatose- und Reticulosarkomkranken. Die Ergebnisse erweitern die mit W. SANDRITTER 1965 veröffentlichten DNS-Messungen an Zellen einschlägiger Fälle.

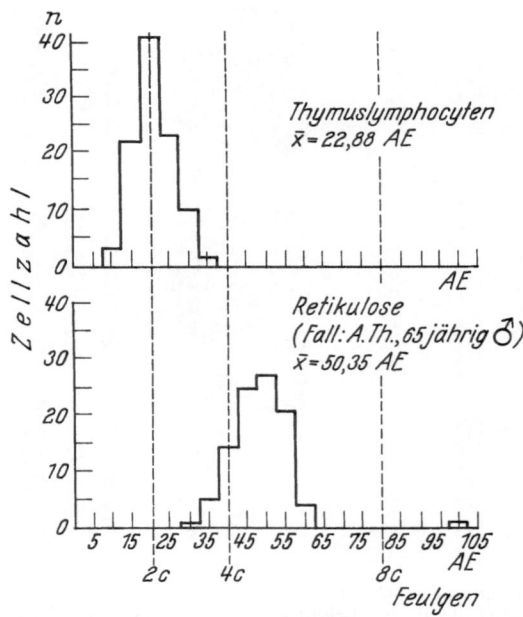

Abb. 1.   Cytophotometrisches DNS-Verteilungsdiagramm (Feulgen-Reaktion). Normale menschliche Thymuslymphocyten (oben), Reticulosezellen eines 65jährigen Mannes (unten). 2 c, 4 c und 8 c = diploider, tetraploider und oktoploider Meßwert. Ordinate: n Zellzahl; Abszisse: AE Arbeitseinheiten

Bei fünf Kranken mit entsprechenden Hauterscheinungen nahmen wir an Feulgen- und Fastgreen (pH 8,2)-gefärbten Zellausstrichen die Desoxyribonucleinsäure(DNS)- bzw. Histonproteinmessungen mit einem integrierenden Mikrodensitometer vor. Zur Kontrolle standen menschliche Thymuslymphocyten und zum

---

* Mit Unterstützung der Deutschen Forschungsgemeinschaft. Die Untersuchungen wurden in der Universitäts-Hautklinik Gießen durchgeführt.

Vergleich Ausstriche von zwei polymorphzelligen Hautsarkomen zur Verfügung. Insgesamt wurden über 1500 Zellen gemessen. Zur statistischen Sicherung der Meßergebnisse wandten wir nach Festlegung der mittleren Streuung und der Mittelwerte die Student-Signifikanzberechnung (P-Test) an.

Ergebnisse

Alle fünf Krankheitsfälle ergaben in den nach FEULGEN gefärbten Zellausstrichen ein ähnliches DNS-Verteilungsmuster mit Mittelwerten der Meßergebnisse von $\bar{x} = 50{,}35$ bis $56{,}14$ Arbeitseinheiten (AE). Die mituntersuchten Thymuslymphocyten lagen demgegenüber zwischen $\bar{x} = 22{,}88$ bis $25{,}43$ AE (s. Abb. 1 und 2).

Bedeutend höhere Mittelwerte der AE konnten wir bei den polymorphzelligen Sarkomen feststellen. Außerdem war das DNS-Muster hier abartiger und bis zu irregulären Polyploidiestufen verteilt.

Die cytophotometrische Untersuchung der Fastgreen-Präparate von vier Fällen ergab in bezug auf die Thymuslymphocyten und die Zellen der Reticulose-, Reticulosarkomatose- und Reticulosarkomkranken ein differenzierteres Bild. Die Mittelwerte der Meßergebnisse lagen bei $\bar{x} = 14{,}91$ (Reticulose), $17{,}21$ (Reticulosarkomatose), $17{,}85$ und $18{,}31$ AE (Reticulosarkome) (s. Abb. 3).

Den dazugehörigen Kontrollwert der Thymuslymphocyten ermittelten wir mit $\bar{x} = 10{,}53$ AE.

Über das Ergebnis der statistischen Prüfung aller Untersuchungszahlen wird an anderer Stelle berichtet.

Diskussion

Die nach Feulgen-Färbung durchgeführten cytophotometrischen DNS-Messungen fielen bei fünf Kranken mit Hauterscheinungen der Reticulose, der Reticulosarkomatose und des Reticulosarkoms entgegen unseren Erwartungen nicht stark unterschiedlich aus. Vorwiegend zeigte sich ein gering hypertetraploides Verteilungsmuster ohne erhebliche Irregularität.

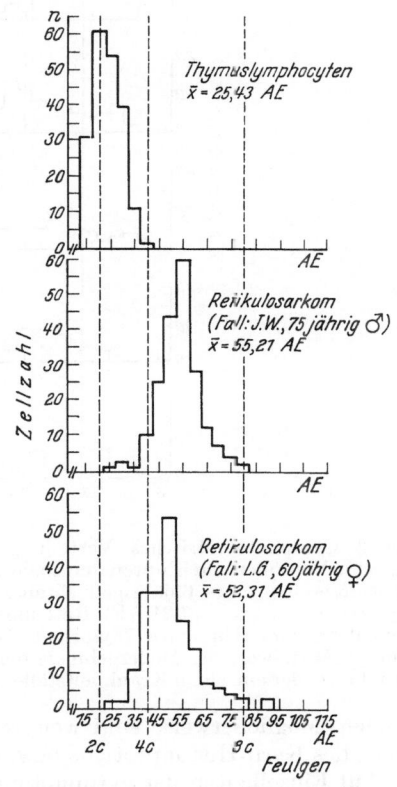

Abb. 2. Cytophotometrisches DNS-Verteilungsdiagramm (Feulgen-Reaktion). Von oben nach unten: normale menschliche Thymuslymphocyten, Reticulosarkomzellen eines 75jährigen Mannes, Reticulosarkomzellen einer 60jährigen Frau. Zeichenerklärung: siehe Abb. 1

Dagegen konnten bei den Histonproteinbestimmungen in den Zellkernen der entsprechenden Patienten auffälligere Abartigkeiten gefunden werden. Die Meßergebnisse der Fastgreen-Präparate waren besonders gegenüber den AE-Werten der Thymuslymphocyten abnorm.

Der Vergleich zwischen den zeitlich koordinierten DNS-Bestimmungen an Reticulose-, Reticulosarkomatose- und Reticulosarkomzellen sowie solchen polymorphzelliger Hautsarkome erbrachte ein grundsätzlich verschiedenes Verhalten beider Gruppen. Die polymorphzelligen Sarkome zeichneten sich durch ein sehr unregelmäßiges, breitstreuendes DNS-Verteilungsmuster aus.

Auf Grund der vorgelegten cytophotometrischen DNS-Untersuchungen gelingt es bis jetzt noch nicht, mit einer gewissen Regelmäßigkeit zwischen den einzelnen Formen reticulo-histiocytärer Geschwulsterkrankungen deutliche Zäsuren zu er-

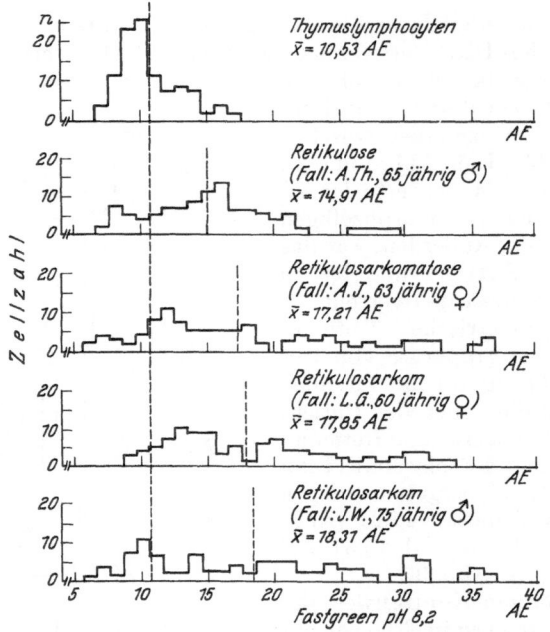

Abb. 3. Cytophotometrisches Verteilungsdiagramm des Histonproteingehaltes (Fastgreen pH 8,2). Von oben nach unten: normale menschliche Thymuslymphocyten ($\bar{x}$ = 10,53 AE), Reticulosezellen eines 65jährigen Mannes ($\bar{x}$ = 14,91 AE), Reticulosarkomatosezellen einer 63jährigen Frau ($\bar{x}$ = 17,21 AE), Reticulosarkomzellen einer 60jährigen Frau ($\bar{x}$ = 17,85 AE), Reticulosarkomzellen eines 75jährigen Mannes ($\bar{x}$ = 18,31 AE). Durchgehend gestrichelte Linie = Mittelwert der Meßergebnisse der Thymuslymphocyten; kurz gestrichelte Linien = Mittelwerte der einzelnen Krankheitsfälle. Ordinate: n Zellzahl; Abszisse: AE Arbeitseinheiten

kennen. Möglicherweise sind weitere Messungen, namentlich der basischen Proteine, des Kern-Histonproteins usw. ergiebiger.

Auf Einzelheiten der cytophotometrischen, histologischen und klinischen Befunde der angesprochenen Krankheitsfälle unter Berücksichtigung der Nosologie und Einteilung mußte aus Zeitgründen verzichtet werden.

Literatur. KNOTH, W., u. W. SANDRITTER: Arch. klin. exp. Derm. **223**, 217 (1965).

Patología y clínica de los reticulolinfomas óculopalpebrales

P. H. MAGNIN, M. C. MORGENFELD y R. L. CABRINI, Cátedra de Dermatologia, Hospital Ramos Metia, Buenos Aires (Argentina)

En el transcurso de doce años se estudiaron trece casos de reticulolinfomas óculopalpebrales. La bibliografía es escasa y salvo excepciones se refiere al relato de observaciones únicas o de recopilación [1]. Nuestros casos con sus características más importantes están resumidos en el cuadro No. 1. Del análisis del mismo surge:

Tabla de linfomas palpebrales oculopalpebrales

N°	Edad	Sexo	Tiempo de evolucion	Muerte	Tipo de linfoma	Tratamiento	Iniciacion localizado	sistémico	leucemia	Antecedentes	Localizacion DER. C.	IZQ. C.	Observaciones
1	24	F	33 m	NO	Linfoblástico	Rayos X	SI	NO	NO	conjuntivitis catarral recidivante	X	X	Curada
2	71	M	8 m	SI	Linfoblástico-linfocítico	Rayos X y citoestáticos	SI	SI	SI	conjuntivitis catarral recidivante	X	X	
3	4	F	10 m	SI	Linfoblástico	Rayos X y citoestáticos	SI	SI	NO	conjuntivitis catarral recidivante	X	X	Evolución muy agresiva
4	63	M	15 m	NO	Linfoblástico reticular	Co⁶⁰	SI	SI	NO	Edema Facial		X	
5	29	M	8 m	SI	Linfoblástico	citoestat. y corticoesteroides	NO	SI	NO	—	X	X	Hijo muerto de leucemia
6	75	F	48 m	NO	Linfoblástico	Rayos X	NO	SI	NO	—	X	X	Curada
7	43	M	96 m	NO	Folicular	citoestat. y Rayos X	NO	SI	NO	—	X	X	Curada
8	45	F	108 m	NO	Linfoblástico	Rayos X y citostáticos	NO	SI	NO	—	X	X	Curada
9	57	M	72 m	SI	Linfoblástico	Rayos X y citostáticos	NO	SI	NO	—	X	X	Muerte. insuficiencia cardiaca
10	37	M	144 m	SI	Linfocítico	citostáticos y Rayos X corticoesteroides	NO	SI	NO	—	X	X	
11	61	M	24 m	NO	Linfocítico		SI	NO	NO	conjuntivitis catarral recidivante		X	
12	38	F	20 m	NO	Linfocítico	Rayos X	SI	NO	NO	conjuntivitis catarral recidivante			
13	30	M	30 m	NO	Linfoblástico	Telecoblatot.	NO	SI	NO	conjuntivitis catarral recidivante	X		

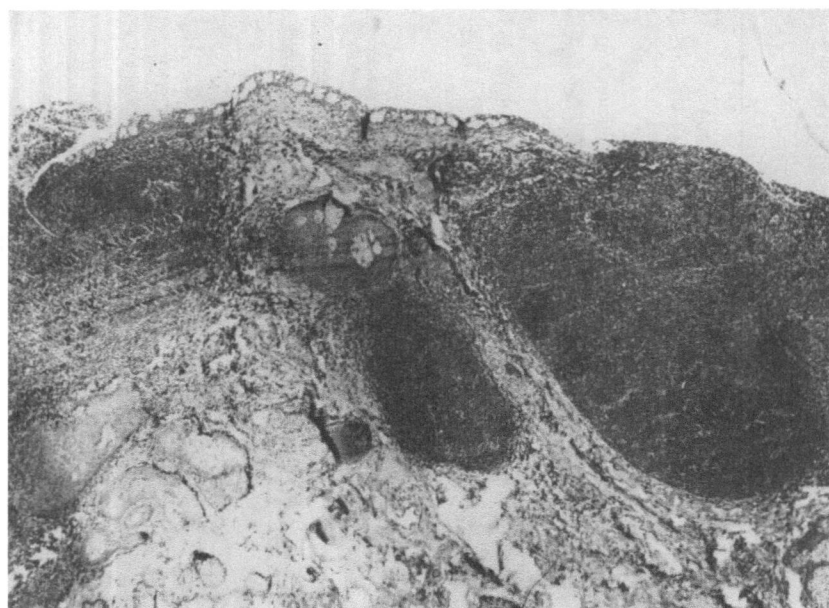

Fig. 2. En este caso se observa como el linfoma ha constituido nódulos que crecen prolapsando la conjuntiva (H. E. × 15)

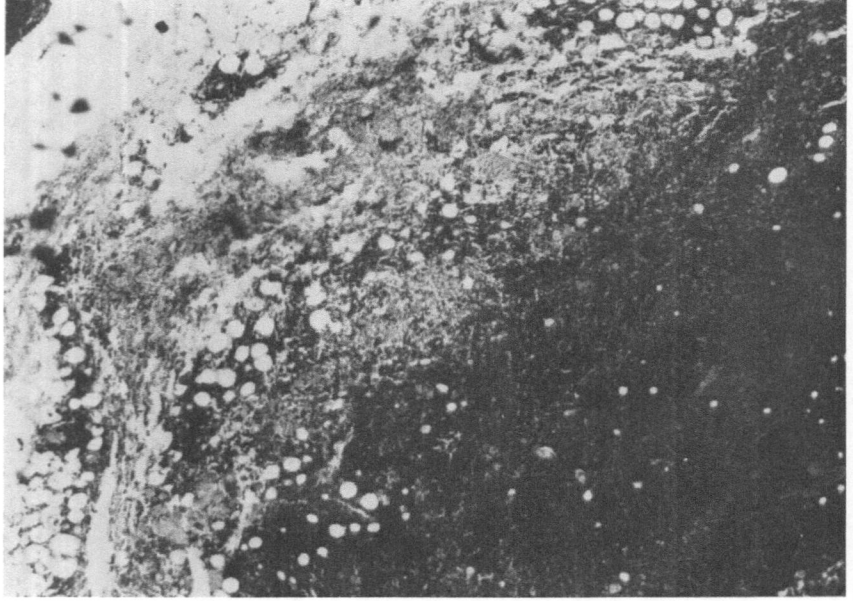

Fig. 1. Infiltración linfomatosa de tipo difusa que se traduce por una tumoración local (H. E. × 15)

1. Edad: oscila entre 4 y 75 años (x̄: 44).

2. Sexo: ocho hombres y cinco mujeres.

3. Tiempo de evolución: entre 8 y 144 meses (x̄: 50 meses) de los cuales los cinco que murieron alcanzaron un promedio de 48 meses de sobrevida.

4. Tipos de linfomas: 8 linfoblásticos puros, 1 linfoblástico-reticular, 3 linfocíticos y 1 macrofolicular.

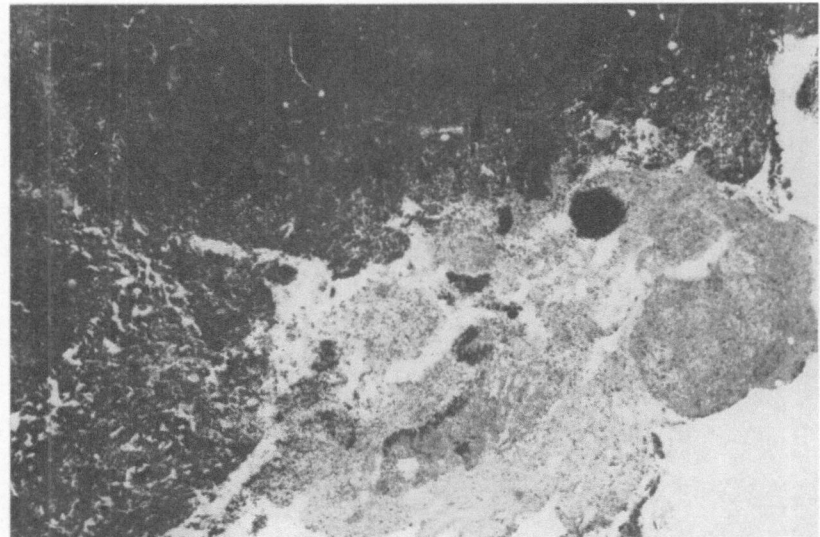

Fig. 4. Area de una proliferación subconjuntival densa que posee un extenso sector necrótico (H. E. × 15)

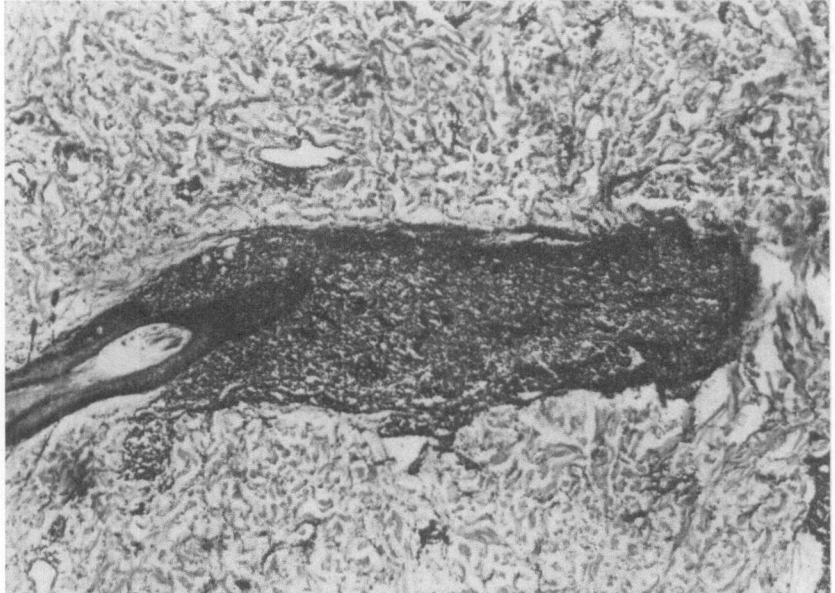

Fig. 3. A veces el estudio histológico solo permite el linfoma en estructuras anexiales vecinas (H. E. × 15)

5. Forma de iniciación: en 6 el comienzo fue localizado en la región óculopalpebral; en los 7 restantes apareció como una de las manifestaciones sistémicas.

6. La terminación leucémica se observó en dos casos.

7. En 3 reticulolinfomas óculopalpebrales de la serie linfoblástica (casos 1, 2 y 3) y en 2 linfocíticos (casos 11 y 12) se observaron manifestaciones de conjuntivitis catarral recidivante en los dos años que precedieron al desarrollo tumoral.

8. Tratamiento: 5 casos con roentgenterapia exclusivamente, 6 casos con roentgenterapia y citoestáticos y 2 con citoestáticos y corticoesteroides.

9. En cuatro casos existen elementos que permiten considerar la aparente curación del proceso.

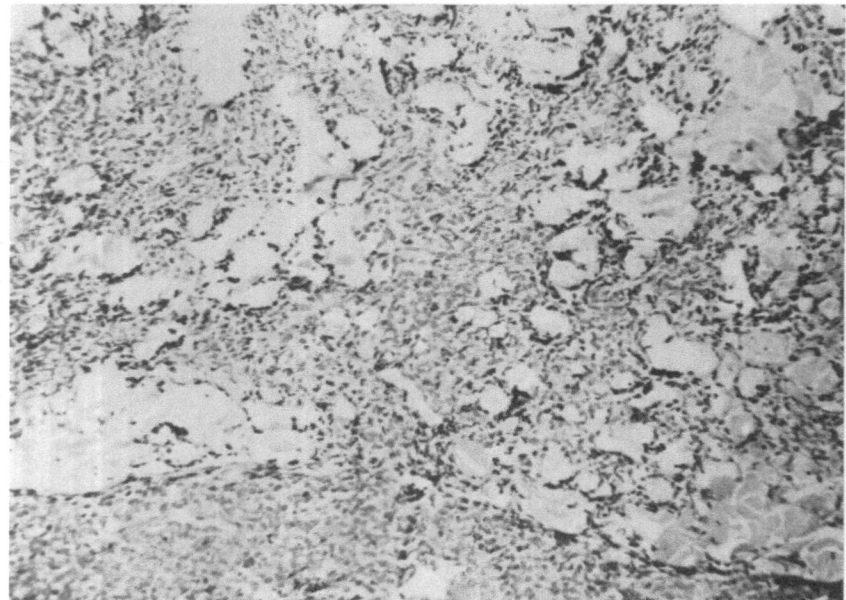

Fig. 5. El linfoma infiltra activamente el conectivo y ha provocado un proceso de hialinosis (H. E. × 15)

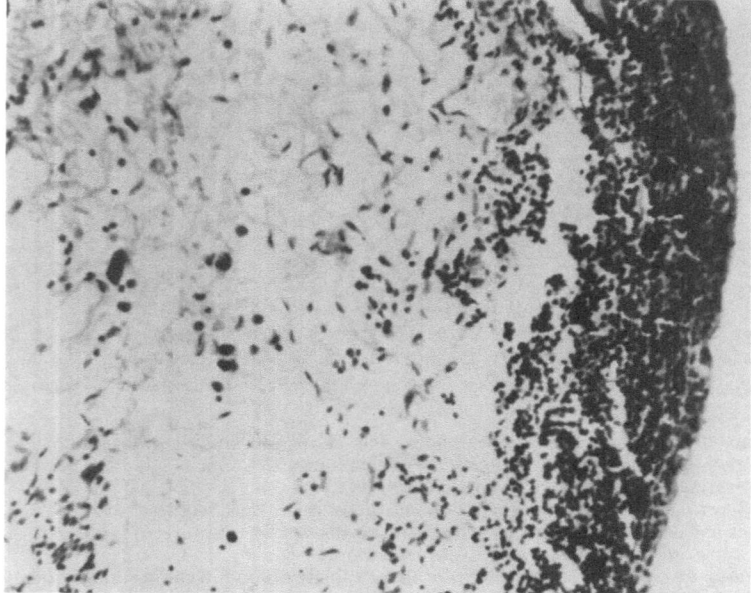

Fig. 6. En la microfotografía se observa la infiltración linfoidea por debajo del epitelio conjuntival (H. E.)

Discusión

Por su forma de comienzo en seis enfermos el linfoma se había iniciado en la conjuntiva palpebral mientras en los siete restantes dicha localización apareció en el transcurso evolutivo de formas generalizadas de preferencia ganglionares. Del primer grupo fallecieron dos enfermos, uno con transformación leucémica (caso 2) y otro con generalización sistémica (caso 3). Se infiere que la forma localizada óculopalpebral no implica deducción pronóstica.

En un trabajo anterior [1] llamamos la atención sobre el antecedente de conjuntivitis catarral recidivante precediendo a los reticulolinfomas óculopalpebrales. En esta serie cinco enfermos presentaron la misma manifestación entre los 18 y 24 meses previos a la aparición del tumor.

La histopatología de la serie de 13 linfomas nos mostró en algunos un índice mitótico elevado y en otros bajo. Los focos de necrobiosis y necrosis se asociaron por lo general a las formas de crecimiento difuso y compactante (Fig. 4).

Se analizó con particular cuidado la actividad macrofágica por el especial significado que parece tener en la evolución de los linfomas [2]. En nuestras observaciones el índice de macrofagia fue bajo, lo que indicaría tendencia evolutiva poco agresiva.

El predominio linfoblástico fue evidente, aunque en algunos casos se observaron células reticulares y/o linfocitos. La disposición del infiltrado en la mucosa conjuntival y piel fue la siguiente:

1. masa compacta de proliferación linfoide que desplazando la estructura vecina, se tradujo clínicamente como una tumoración (Fig. 1).

2. con crecimiento menos denso los infiltrados linfoides constituyeron estructuras seudofoliculares llegando a prolapsar la mucosa conjuntival (Fig. 2).

3. crecimiento linfomatoso perivascular o/y perianexial (Fig. 3).

El comportamiento local del linfoma mostró que el crecimiento difuso se acompañaba de focos de necrosis y que al crecer en el tejido conectivo vecino provocaba un proceso activo de fibrosis e hialinización (Fig. 5).

La terapéutica en once de los casos fue la roentgenterapia sola o asociada mientras que dos enfermos recibieron quimioterapia como único tratamiento en una etapa de la enfermedad.

Los resultados en cuanto a la lesión ocular se refiere, fueron satisfactorios salvo en uno de gran agresividad tratado con Leukeran, Natulan, Endoxan y Corticoesteroides (caso 5). El otro caso, con diagnóstico previo de linfoma macrofolicular, medicado con Clorambucil logró una regresión satisfactoria de la lesión ocular lo que se explica porque la enfermedad de BRILL-SYMMERS es muy sensible a ese derivado de las mostazas nitrogenadas.

Creemos que la escasez de información sobre la incidencia de la localización en párpados respecto a otros sitios es debida a que los estudios estadísticos efectuados en ese sentido son en gran parte producto de protocolos de necropsias. Por otro lado a excepción del trabajo de MCGAVIC los datos obtenidos son la suma de observaciones de distintos autores. SCHULZ y HEATH encuentran un 0,9% de linfomas de conjuntivas en 1676 casos y ASH 1,02% de 1173. RICHMOND y col. estudian 690 autopsias de linfomas malignos y no relatan manifestaciones oculares.

Referencias. 1. MAGNIN, P. H., y M. MORGENFELD: Rev. argent. Dermatosif. 50, 1 (1966). — 2. MORGENFELD, M. C., F. SCHAJOWICZ y R. L. CABRINI: 2° Congr. Argent. Hematol., 22 noviembre 1966, Córdoba, Argentina. La bibliografía completa consultada figura en los trabajos mencionados.

The Identity and Treatment of the Lymphoma Mycosis fungoides

M. A. Lutzner, Dermatology Branch, National Cancer Institute, National Institutes of Health, Bethesda, Maryland (USA)

Since the earliest description of mycosis fungoides by Alibert in the 1800's students of this disease have posed many questions. Is mycosis fungoides a neoplastic disease of the lympho-reticular system ? From what cell does the neoplasm arise ? In its early phases, when it manifests non-specifically as a pruritic eczematous or psoriasoform dermatitis, is it already established as a neoplasm, or instead do these skin changes predispose in some way to the development of the not yet established neoplasm ? Do the lesions of parapsoriasis en plaque and parapsoriasis variegata develop into mycosis fungoides or are they mycosis fungoides at their onset ? Can mycosis fungoides convert to leukemia, Hodgkin's disease, reticulum cell sarcoma, or lymphosarcoma ?

A prime reason for the plethora of questions and for the enigma cloaking mycosis fungoides is the lack of clear-cut cytologic criteria for the identification of the neoplastic cell or cells in mycosis fungoides. Instead, histologic diagnosis in this disease, at present, depends upon the recognition of architectural changes in the epidermis; that is, Darier-Pautrier's microabscesses. And diagnosis depends upon changes in the composition of the dermal cell population — a pleomorphic cellular infiltrate containing atypical cells known as the mycosis fungoides (MF) cell. The MF cell can often not be clearly identified with existing histologic methods. Perhaps the situation could be compared to the problems that would be faced in diagnosing Hodgkin's disease in the absence of the pathognomonic Reed-Sternberg cell.

Recently, we have used the electron microscope to study tissue from 28 patients clinically suspected to have mycosis fungoides. Skin biopsies from all 28 were compatible with the diagnosis of mycosis fungoides. From this study a cell has emerged with characteristic cytologic ultrastructural features. This cell is 15 to 30 micra in diameter and posesses a bizarre nucleus which is lobulated, indented and drawn into ribbons and threads. This cell has been found in the skin, lymph nodes, and occasionally in blood of these patients. It has not been found in a variety of other skin lesions studied, and at the moment it appears specific for mycosis fungoides.

Using these ultrastructural criteria we attempted to answer some of the questions which have been posed. Skin from one patient with persistant pityriasis rosea-like lesions, from one with parapsoriasis variegata, and from one with parapsoriasis en plaque was studied. Standard histologic sections showed only non-specific dermatitis, but characteristic MF cells were found in all these patients using the electron microscope.

Eleven lymph nodes were studied from these patients. Six nodes had been diagnosed by standard histologic methods as dermatopathic lymphadenopathy, two as lymphosarcoma, two as reticulum cell sarcoma, and one as a malignant lymphoma. Using the electron microscope we found MF cells in ten of eleven nodes. The five patients with nodes diagnosed as various types of malignant lymphoma might have been considered, without this new information, to have converted from mycosis fungoides to other types of malignant lymphoma.

Chemical and radiation therapy is available which can reverse the progressive course of mycosis fungoides, but no treatment at present can be considered predictably curative. Chemotherapeutic agents such as cytoxan and methotrexate have proven to be effective to some extent. But what is needed is a drug which can effectively irradicate the neoplastic cells of mycosis fungoides.

Free Communications

Klinik und Histopathologie der malignen Reticulosen

K. W. MACH, I. Universitäts-Hautklinik Wien (Österreich)

Die Bezeichnung Reticulose wird heute vielfach als übergeordneter Begriff verwendet, der verschiedene bekannte Krankheitsgruppen zusammenfaßt. Wir verstehen darunter jedoch ein streng umrissenes Krankheitsbild, welches durch eine Vermehrung der Bestandteile des reticulo-histiocytären Systems zustande kommt. Durch die besondere Wachstumsart sowie ihre systemgebundene Ausbreitung unterscheiden sie sich deutlich von den malignen Tumoren. Ebenso sind sie gegen jene Infiltrate abzugrenzen, die auf reaktiver Grundlage entstehen und reversibel sind.

In den letzten 20 Jahren konnten wir an der I. Universitäts-Hautklinik in Wien 21 Fälle von Reticulosen beobachten. Davon wurden 13 Fälle ursprünglich anderen Diagnosen, wie Retothelsarkom bzw. Lymphosarkom, zugeordnet. Auf Grund klinischer Beobachtung sowie zahlreicher aufeinanderfolgender Biopsien in zeitlichen Intervallen mußten die Diagnosen berichtigt werden.

Klinisch bieten diese Fälle je nach Verlaufsart ein verschiedenes Erscheinungsbild und gleichen in ihrem Aussehen weitgehend den Hautveränderungen bei den Leukosen. Die akuten und subakuten Formen erscheinen als Erythrodermien. Diese Form ist auch unter der Bezeichnung Sézary-Syndrom bekannt. Die chronischen zeigen hingegen flache Infiltrate oder zahlreiche kleine Tumoren, die meist eine bestimmte Größe nicht überschreiten. Innerhalb einer längeren Beobachtungszeit zeigen sie vorübergehende Remissionen, die jedoch stets von neuen Schüben abgelöst werden. Die Krankheitsdauer erstreckt sich oft über Jahrzehnte.

Histologisch zeigen sie eine weitgehende Monomorphie. Das Gewebe ist überwiegend aus Reticulumzellen aufgebaut, die entweder als kleine lymphoide Reticulumzellen in netzartigen Verbänden oder als große Reticulumzellen in Erscheinung treten. Oft findet man auch Mischformen mit großen und kleinen Reticulumzellen. Manche Fälle enthalten auch Plasmazellen, Mastzellen oder eosinophile Leukocyten, wobei das Mischungsverhältnis sehr unterschiedlich ist. Ebenso ist die Verteilung der Zellen unregelmäßig, so daß man oft Herde mit Plasmazellen oder stellenweise vermehrt eosinophile Leukocyten beobachten kann, die in seltenen Fällen das histologische Bild beherrschen.

Bei alleiniger Beurteilung des Infiltrates bereitet die Abgrenzung gegenüber dem Lymphosarkom und Retothelsarkom außerordentliche Schwierigkeiten. Wenn man jedoch das Hauptaugenmerk auf das umgebende kollagene Bindegewebe legt, so zeigt dies bei den Reticulosen ein auffallend konstantes Verhalten, welches die Diagnose erheblich erleichtert. Selbst jene Fälle, bei denen innerhalb einer längeren Beobachtungsperiode eine Veränderung in der Histomorphologie der Infiltrate beobachtet werden konnte, zeigte das angrenzende Bindegewebe stets dieselben Veränderungen. Diese bestehen aus einem Umbau des normalen benachbarten fibrillären Bindegewebes, der in zwei verschiedenen Arten in Erscheinung treten kann.

Die eine Form ist durch eine enorme Proliferationstendenz der Bindegewebszellen gekennzeichnet (Abb. 1). Es kommt zur fibroblastenartigen Anschwellung der Fibrocyten. Die Bindegewebszellen zeigen ovale, blasse chromatinarme Kerne mit ein bis zwei Kernkörperchen. Das Cytoplasma ist im histologischen Präparat nur schwer erkennbar. Lediglich in den Bindegewebslücken oder in cytologischen Präparaten (Abb. 2) wird ein blasses, feingranuliertes Cytoplasma sichtbar, das oft

wie ein Segel zipfelförmig begrenzt und an benachbarten kollagenen Fasern be-
festigt ist. Die Fibroblasten sind in ihrer Anzahl stark vermehrt und bilden
in den infiltratnahen Zonen des Bindegewebes zum Teil Ansammlungen, die an
Epitheloidzellknötchen erinnern. Die kollagenen Fasern lassen häufig die Anord-

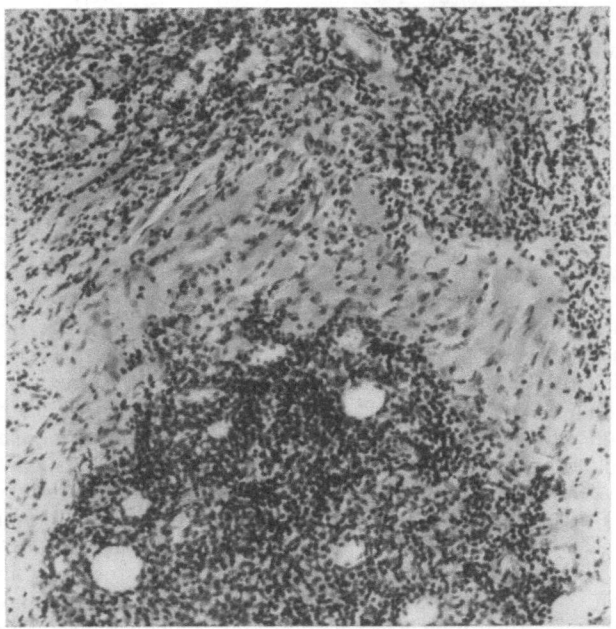

Abb. 1. Reticulose; 65jährige Frau. Zwischen den Herden zeigt sich ein fibroblastenreiches
Bindegewebe mit parallel angeordneten Fasern, die vorwiegend senkrecht zu den Infiltratgrenzen ausgerichtet sind (40×)

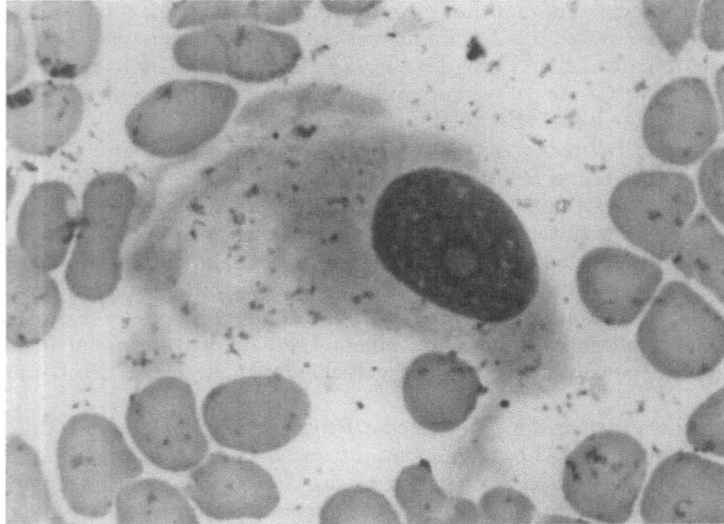

Abb. 2. Reticulose; 69jähriger Mann. Fibroblast mit deutlichen Kernkörperchen und reichlich
entwickeltem Cytoplasma (Tupfpräparat 400×)

nung zu einzelnen Bündeln vermissen und sind in parallelen, oft welligen Zügen eher unregelmäßig angeordnet. Mitunter hat man den Eindruck einer ödematösen Durchtränkung, ebenso lassen sich vereinzelt basophil tingierte Areale erkennen, wie man dies in jungem neugebildetem Bindegewebe findet.

Die zweite Art des Umbaues im umgebenden Bindegewebe kann bei den Reticulosen dann beobachtet werden, wenn die Proliferationstendenz des fibrillären Bindegewebes nicht so stark ausgeprägt ist und die kollagenen Fibrillen zu Bündeln

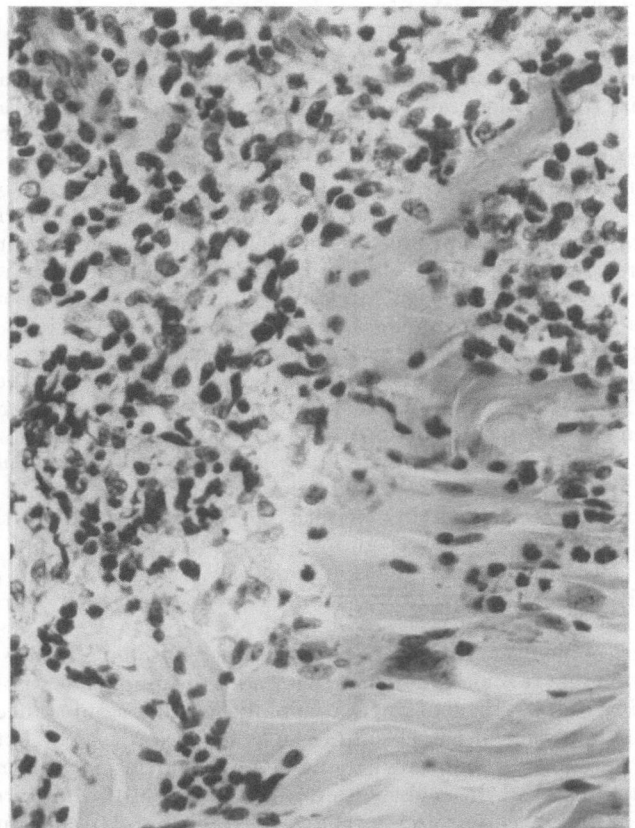

Abb. 3. Reticulose; 53jähriger Mann. Die kollagenen Bündel verlaufen senkrecht zur Infiltratgrenze. In der Grenzzone lösen sich die kollagenen Bündel in ein spinnwebenähnliches Netzwerk auf. Die infiltratnahen Bindegewebszellen sind fibroblastenartig vergrößert (100×)

angeordnet sind. Hier ziehen die Bündel zum Großteil senkrecht gegen die Infiltratgrenzen. Eine zirkuläre bzw. tangentiale Anordnung der einzelnen Bündel findet man nur selten. Knapp bevor die kollagenen Bündel die Infiltratgrenze erreichen, splittern sie sich meist in unregelmäßig angeordnete feinste Fasern auf, die wie ein Spinnwebennetz zwischen den Enden der kollagenen Bündel und den Infiltratzellen ausgebreitet sind (Abb. 3).

Die Bindegewebszellen sind mit ihrer Längsachse ebenso wie die kollagenen Bündel vorwiegend senkrecht zu den Infiltratgrenzen ausgerichtet. Falls die Fibrocyten in normaler oder nur leicht vermehrter Anzahl vorhanden sind und nicht die vorher aufgezeigten Proliferationsmerkmale aufweisen, so sind zumindest die dem

Infiltrat unmittelbar benachbarten Bindegewebszellen fibroblastenähnlich ange-
schwollen (Abb. 3).

Diese Zellart ist auch stets in cytologischen Tupfpräparaten (Abb. 2) nachweisbar und bildet ein wichtiges differentialdiagnostisches Merkmal.

Cytological Studies on Lymphoma with Electronmicroscopy

H. Fujita, Dept. of Dermatology, Yamaguchi University, Ube (Japan)

We have made this study with special reference to two problems. The first
problem is this: from what kind of cell do the tumor cells in the cutaneous lesion
of lymphoma originate ? Namely, do the tumor cells originate from lymphatic cell,
from reticulum cell or from histiocyte ? And the second problem is this: what kind of
nature and what kind of genesis do argyrophilic fibers around the tumor cells have ?
The present report concerns the electronmicroscopic investigation of the tumor cells
in the lesion of lymphoma, in order to make clear these unsettled problems.

As the correlative study to the electronmicroscopic investigation, we performed
the light microscopic investigation, dividing the biopsied tumor tissues into two
parts. One part was used to make stamped specimen for the light microscopic
investigation; namely, Giemsa stain, supravital stain with neutralred-Janusgreen,
and phagocytosis test of India ink were made. Another part of biopsied tissue was
fixed in 4 to 6.25% Glutaraldehyde, then refixed in 1% osmic acid, and embedded
in Epoxy resin 812. Ultrathin sections were stained with 2% uranyl acetate, and
4% lead citric acid. Then, we investigated electronmicroscopically, comparing with
the results of the above-mentioned light microscopic observations.

By this study, we clarified that majority of the tumor cells in the lesions of
reticulum-cell lymphoma were reticulum-cell-typed tumor cells and lymphocyte-
typed tumor cells. Besides these predominant cells, we found light- and electron
microscopically histiocyte-typed cells, monocyte-typed cells and fibroblast-typed
cells exist.

Light microscopic observation of Giemsa stained specimen from a case of reticulum cell lymphoma revealed that there were a lot of tumor cells whose cytoplasm
showed ovoid areas which contained basophilic granular substances. Electron-
microscopic examination of the lesion of the same case revealed that these areas
were electron less dense vacuoles with one-layered limiting membrane, about 0.4
to 2.6 μ in diameter. And these vacuoles were considered to be cysternally dilated
smooth surfaced endoplasmic reticula. They were often found to contain many virus-
like particles. These particles were ovoid in shape and about 130 mμ in diameter.
And they were found to possess electron dense nucleoid structure in their center.

Light microscopic examination of the Giemsa stained specimens of another case
of reticulum-cell lymphoma revealed that there were numerous tumor cells whose
nuclei showed ovoid areas. And these ovoid areas were slightly less basophilic than
the surrounding chromatin. Electronicmicroscopic examination of the lesion of the
same case revealed that these tumor cells were of reticulum-cell type with well
developed rough surfaced endoplasmic reticula, and their nuclei possessed small
ovoid bodies about 100 mμ in diameter. These small ovoid bodies were revealed to
contain electron dense granular substances. Their electron density was higher than
that of the surrounding chromatin.

Then, we investigated electronmicroscopically the nature and genesis of argyrophilic fibers around the tumor cells. Argyrophilic fibers were considered to be
composed of at least following elements.

1. Fine filaments adjacent to the cytoplasmic membrane of reticulum cells.
2. Fine filaments around perithelial cells of blood vessels.
3. Electron dense, dendrite-like process of reticulum-cell-typed cells.
4. Very narrow and long cytoplasmic process of fibroblast-typed cells whose cytoplasm were packed with numerous fine filaments.
5. Electron dense, fibrous substance possibly originated from degenerated tumor cells.

Cutaneous Lymphoblastoma, Spontaneous Involution of Tumours

D. MAJCAN, D. STEVANOVIĆ and B. LALEVIĆ, Departement of Dermatology, University of Beograd (Yugoslavia)

The spontaneous disappearance of malignancy in a human represents a rarity. It is estimated that only in 1 in 80,000 or 100,000 patients does such a possibility occur. Among these skin malignancies are exeptional.

During the last 5 years we have observed four patients with lymphoblastoma. Because of the shortage of time we shall give here only the indispensable data of patients illustrating by slides and commenting clinical and histological pictures of active lesions as well as sites of spontaneous involution.

In the first patient, a woman aged 26, with reticulum cell sarcoma currettage of tumours which were "exophytic" brought about complete healing of these sites. Another dermal tumour spontaneously dissappeared leaving a histiocytoma like tumour. During the last 2 years no new tumours developed.

In the second patient, a man aged 36 with lymphoblastic lymphoma, spontaneous involution occurred only in some tumours. The patient succumbed after 2 years of follow up. Spontaneous involution was evidenced by the increased growth of fibroblasts and the greater amount of collagen bundles among which lymphoid cells and histiocytes were seen.

The third patient aged 32 was developing new tumours within a period of approximately 15 months. The duration of each tumour was 7 to 9 months. Histologically lymphoblastics cells in larger plages and round blood vessels were seen. In involuted tumours plages were replaced by collagen while less infiltrate was present round blood vessels.

Tumours so far 30 in number in the fourth patient, a boy aged 10, were slowly appearing within the last 3 years. More than half of them have already disappeared — usual duration of single tumours being 8 to 15 months.

Tumours were characterized by an infiltrate of immature lymphocytes. At the sites of spontaneous involution hardly any pathologic cells were present; replacement by collagen was evident.

Discussion. In a series of 168 malignancies (of which 67 were observed during 1950 or later) in which cure, spontaneous involution or only regression were observed, clear cell carcinoma of the kidney, bladder tumours and sympathoblastoma were most often encountered; one multiple skin sarcoma of the face (in 1866) and three sarcoma of the back (1902, 1927 and 1936 resp.), the later two stated as being "fibrosarcoma" were included among them.

Apart from the unusual course, tumours in our first patient were also unusual in their appearance. The tendency of tumour growth was clearly exophytic, except in the last one, where it was intradermal and infiltrating.

The later tumour during its involutory phase was very reminiscent of histiocytoma; at another examination 6 months later this infiltration had completely dissappeared, leaving only a thin scar.

While histologic differentiation between neoplasia and inflammatory hyperplasia in the reticular tissue is difficult and the response of the reticulo-lymphoid system to a specific agent in many cutaneous diseases known, it is hardly possible that this case represents only an inflammatory condition with local reticulum cell hyperplasia. Neither could it be included in the group "benign disseminated reticulosis". The more infiltrating tumour, last to appear, also suggests the real nature of the condition. It looked as if, until the appearance of the last tumour, only the upper dermis took part in the reticular proliferation, which part, together with the tumour was scraped off by the curettage.

While in the first patient after a follow-up of almost 1 year no new tumours appeared, in the second, besides some tumours which have spontaneously involuted, new tumours, some of which were more destructive, were continiosly appearing necessitating X-ray treatment. The histopathologic evidence of spontaneous regression of the examined tumour was manifested by considerable augmentation of fibroblasts and collagen.

Regression of neoplasms during radiation, antimitotic and hormonal therapy, beside cytolitic and antimitotic action, is also partly acsribed to connective tissue alteration. Fibrosis was also the probable factor of the spontaneous involution of the mentioned small tumour in the first patient; on the site of a previous tumour only a hard dermo-hipodermal mass, size of a pea, on clinical examination easily passing for "nodular subepidermal fibrosis", was present. An inflammatory process often precedes the later condition; spontaneous involution occasionally occurs in it, leaving a somewhat atrophic scar.

In the third and fourth patient dissappearance of pathologic cells and their replacement by collagen was the histologic finding of the spontaneously involuted tumours.

It is to be supposed that the spontaneous dissappearance of the tumour besides many unknown immunologic factors, was also the result of the progressive fibrosis with possible obliteration of the tumour cells — a similar mechanism being involved in the healing phase of another, but benign, "reticulosis" — sarcoidosis. Thus in our case, beside an abnormal proliferation of the lymphoid group of the stem cell responsible for the tumour, a hyperplasia of the reticulo-histiocytic cell group with the increased formation of fibroblasts and collagen occured. That malignant proliferation of more groups in the same patient also occurs, resulting in e.g. monocytic lymphoid and myelocytic leukemia, is well known.

Mention should be made here, though not suggesting a direct relationship, of the so-called fibre forming reticulosarcomata formed of cells with intermingled fibers or in a matrix of plentiful reticulin or collagen fibers. The course and follow-up of such cases might contribute to more knowledge of the possible role played by these fibres in the spontaneous involution of some tumours in lymphoma.

Our first case is very similar to that reported by BLUEFARB. It also corresponds to Gottron's "Retothelsarcomatose", i.e. "Retothelsarcom" with autochthonous successive multicentric growth. GRACIANSKY also cites cases with spontaneous involution of "Reticulosarcomatoses".

It is better to regard our cases as examples of only spontaneous regression of some tumours and not involution of the malignancy. Their prognosis depends on the time of the involvement of the life important internal organs.

Investigation into the mechanism and reasons for spontaneous regression of some tumours of the skin, were it only for a limited period of the evolution of lymphosarcoma, the problem of the "indolent-benign" type of Hodgkin's disease differing histologically from the classical form mainly in the percentage of reticular cells and lymphocytes, with the presence of Sternberg-Reed cells in both are without doubt justified.

Blood Vessel Morphology in the Reticuloses

T. J. RYAN, St. John's Hospital for Diseases of the Skin, London (England)

Redness is one of the most characteristic features of the skin in the reticuloses. A complete understanding of the reticuloses requires that the redness should be explained. Using a stereoscopic microscope a study has been made of the surface patterns of the microcirculation of the skin in patients with the following diseases:

Generalised erythroderma associated with chronic lymphatic leukaemia (1), Hodgkin's disease (2), Sezary syndrome (1). Localised erythroderma in mycosis fungoides (7), parakeratosis variegata (2), parapsoriasis-en-plaques (4), pityriasis lichenoides chronica (2), lymphocytoma (2), suspected pre-reticulotic erythro- derma (6), and these were compared with the appearances in normal skin, psoriasis, lichen planus and a variety of other skin disorders.

The cause of the redness is usually immediately apparent. In areas of hypertrophy there is proliferation of the blood vessels. They elongate, coil and like all actively growing capillaries they become more fragile and may bleed or allow a few red cells to escape into the tissues when compressed. The normal orientation of the capillaries towards the epidermis is frequently disturbed.

In areas of atrophy the redness is due to exposure of the horizontal sub-papillary plexus. In normal skin this plexus is obscured by the tissue fluid formed from the papillary vessels. In atrophy the papillary vessels are absorbed (RYAN, 1966). The vessels of the exposed horizontal plexus are less permeable and fragile than the papillary vessels in hypertrophic skin.

The epidermis is usually hypertrophic in areas where there is proliferation of the blood vessels. In areas of vascular atrophy the epidermis appears thin and poorly nourished.

The knowledge that infiltrates do not occur without prior endothelial change is essential to the understanding of the reticuloses. The factors which cause stickiness of the endothelium to leucocytes are often the same as those factors which cause endothelial hypertrophy (CLARK and CLARK, 1935).

One of the functions of white cell infiltrates is to control those factors which are responsible for inflammatory states. White cells remove bacteria and necrotic tissues and in so doing reduce the activity of capillary endothelium i.e. the response of the endothelium to the damaged tissue which is responsible for the arrival of white cells in the vicinity.

Normally, no more white cells arrive in an inflamed area than is necessary to control the inflammation and prevent the extravascular stimulus from causing further stickiness of the endothelium to leucocytes.

Normal tissues show on histology a mild degree of infiltration by leucocytes. There is evidence that white cells are continually passing through the tissues from endothelium to lymphatic channels (HALL and MORRIS, 1966). It is likely that the normal growth and aging processes of the epidermis release a continuous mild stimulus to its vasculature. This stimulus is controlled by the inhibitory phagocytic properties of the white cells which move into the tissues and surround the blood vessels when the stimulus is excessive (RYAN, 1967).

It is necessary to ask, how can a disordered white cell, in a disease such as chronic lymphatic leukaemia, cause widespread proliferation of the epidermis and vascular endothelium?

Studies of white cell function in the reticuloses suggest that they are under active and not over active. Thus in some of these diseases the following are reported (BLUEFARB, 1959; DAMESHEK, 1967): 1. Increased susceptibility to infection.

2. Decreased delayed hypersensitivity reactions. 3. Depressed in vitro response to phytohaemagglutinin.

If these cells are functionless then they may be unable to control the endothelial response to tissue stimuli. Excessive infiltration is then inevitable.

The patterns that result from the imbalance of tissue relationships will depend on the proportion of white cells that are functionless. Random distribution of white cells, 50% of which are non-reactive, will cause hypertrophy in some areas and atrophy in others.

The cause of the non-reactivity may be an intrinsic gene defect or it may be a disordered response of the cell to its surroundings. This latter is known to occur when a lymphocyte develops tolerance in the presence of antigen excess. Many of the dermatoses believed to encourage the development of reticuloses are possibly providers of excess antigen.

The chronicity of the disorder partly depends on the strength of the factor stimulating endothelium. If it causes only slight changes in endothelium the infiltration will be only slight. The evidence of SANDERSON and DAVIES (1963) that lytic activity is proportional to histocompatible antigenicity may be relevant. A more chronic disorder may be due to the failure of a white cell to respond to a weak antigen which has only a weak effect on endothelium.

References. BLUEFARB, S. M.: Cutaneous manifestations of the Malignant Lymphomas, p. 515. Springfield (Ill): Charles C. Thomas 1959. — CLARK, E. R., and E. L. CLARK: Amer. J. Anat. 57, 385 (1935). — DAMESHEK, W.: Blood 29, 566 (1967). — HALL, J. G., and B. MORRIS: Quart. J. exp. Physiol. 48, 235 (1963). — RYAN, T. J.: Geront. clin. (Basel) 8, 327 (1966); — In a "Teach in" on factors controlling the blood supply of the epidermis 79, 1 (1967). — SANDERSON, A. R., and D. A. L. DAVIES: Nature (Lond.) 200, 32 (1963).

Generalized Giant-Cell Reticulohistiocytosis (Lipoid Dermatoarthritis) Clinical and Histopathological Study of two Cases

P. NAZZARO, U. GRANELLI and A. BIGNAMI, Institute of Dermatology "S. Gallicano Hospital", Rome (Italy)

Generalized giant-cell reticulohistiocytosis (G.G.R.), a disease of unknown etiology, is characterized by mucocutaneous nodules and severe progressive polyarthritis; histopathological findings in the skin and the joints are diagnostic, showing a proliferation of mono and multinucleated histiocytic giant cells with intensely PAS positive cytoplasm.

Only 28 well documented examples of this condition have been so far described in the literature, not including cases with solitary nodules showing the same histological picture of G.G.R. It is not known whether these cases are a forme fruste of the disease under discussion or not related at a 11. We have recently observed two cases, the second one we were able to follow for 10 years [G. ital. Derm. Sif. 4, 285, (1963)]. In the first case the disease occurred in a woman with cancer of the breast and multiple cutaneous metastasis; in the same biopsy of the skin solid nests of cancer cells and the typical histiocytic cells of giant-cell reticulohistiocytosis were found. It is interesting to note that in two other cases of the literature cancer has been found associated with G.G.R.: adenocarcinoma of the colon in the case first described by CARO and SENEAR and successively illustrated in its further course by GOLTZ and LAYMON; neoplastic carcinoma probably originating in the lung in the thirdt case observed by WARING and EVANS.

In the second case skin lesions were very extensive and there was a nodular eruption in the oral mucosa as well. In both cases joint changes had a progressive course with the clinical picture of osteoarthritis mutilans.

Histological examination of the skin, joints and oral mucosa showed large mono and multi-nucleated histiocytic cells which gave a strongly positive PAS reaction and stained grayish with Sudan black; the staining disappeared after lipid extraction with hot pyridine. Reactions for glycogen and metachromasia with toluidine blue were negative.

In conclusion the histochemical data appeared to indicate that the material contained in the giant-cells was a glycolipid. In the second case trypanblue was injected into one of the skin nodules: phagocytosis of this vital stain was not observed up to 2 h after the injection.

In both cases there was a regression of skin changes following corticosteroid therapy. The first patient died in a state of cachexy with generalized cancer of the breast 2 years after the onset of multicentric reticulohistiocytosis: the cutaneous nodules of this condition were no more present at the time of her death.

The second patient was seen 6 years after the beginning of the disease and she was found completely cured. She had no more fever and she had gained weight. The mucocutaneous nodules which were particularly numerous in this condition had disappeared. In the radiographs there was an increased density around the punched-out lesions of the phalanges and carpal bones. Pain and swelling in the joints of the hands and feet were no more present.

Malignant Development in Mastocytosis

F. SAGHER and Z. EVEN-PAZ, Department of Dermatology and Venereology, Hadassah University Hospital, Jerusalem (Israel)

Until about 15 years ago urticaria pigmentosa was generally considered to be a rare and benign disease which was limited to the skin. This was so in spite of the fact that a few of the earlier reports, mainly by authors of the French school, had suggested that the condition might be related to a disorder of the blood or of some other system. The search for systemic involvement in this disease was greatly stimulated by the finding of widespread mast cell infiltrations in the internal organs, on the post-mortem examination of a child by ELLIS in 1949; and received further impetus following the detection of roentgenographic bone changes in an adult patient.

Up to the year 1952 a total of only six or seven cases had been reported in which the possibility of systemic involvement was suggested. Since that date, to our knowledge, about 150 cases with this possibility have been recorded. These comprise cases reported in the literature, cases reported to the central registry for mastocytosis set up at the Department of Dermatology of the Hadassah Hebrew University Hospital in Jerusalem, Israel, and patients observed in that department. This talk presents some of the findings, as well as some speculations, arising out of a review of these cases.

Systemic mastocytosis may involve many different organs and tissues, but the most commonly affected are the liver, spleen, lymph nodes, hemopoietic tissue and bones. The mast cells may also appear in the peripheral blood. Mast cell infiltration of the gastrointestinal tract has also been detected, and may be more common than is yet appreciated.

The finding of increased numbers of mast cells in the bone marrow is the most frequent basis for proving the diagnosis of systemic mast cell disease. It occurred in nearly 90% of the "proved" cases. The increase may be slight (from 2 to 5%), or mast cells may almost completely replace the normal bone marrow. Fibrosis of the bone marrow may occur, and then it may be difficult or impossible to obtain a satisfactory smear or to detect mast cells in the material aspirated. A study of a section of bone is usually more reliable for diagnostic purpose. The finding of a slight to moderate increase in the number of mast cells in the bone marrow is not, in itself, so gloomy a prognostic sign as is enlargement of the liver and spleen. A fatal outcome occurred in 35% of the cases.

Over 90 cases of mastocytosis with roentgenographic abnormalities of bone structure have so far been reported. It is possible that about 10% of all patients with mastocytosis have bone lesions, and this figure rises to approximately 70% of those who have the systemic form of the disease. The roentgenographic changes in the bones are not specific, and represent both osteoporotic and osteosclerotic processes. There are two main types of roentgenographic appearances: "diffuse-type" changes and "circumscribed-type" changes.

The data may be summarized as follows:

1. Roentgenographic bone changes are present in at least two-thirds of all cases of systemic mastocytosis.

2. The incidence of diffuse-type bone changes exceeds that of the circumscribed type.

3. When diffuse-type bone lesions are present, other evidence suggesting the presence of systemic involvement is frequent, but it is rare in cases with circumscribed-type bone lesions.

4. Diffuse-type bone lesions occur predominantly in adults. About half of the patients with this type of bone involvement were over 50 years of age.

5. Diffuse-type bone lesions were present in 50% of the fatal cases. 18% of all cases in which there were diffuse-type bone lesions terminated fatally.

A disturbance in the peripheral blood is common in systemic mastocytosis, and occurred in 62% of the cases. However, no characteristic pattern of blood change can be associated with the disease.

Tissue mast cells were present in the peripheral blood of eleven patients, or 16% of those with the systemic form of the disease. In five cases there was an associated eosinophilia. In nine out of these eleven patients, the disease terminated fatally.

The development of leukemia or of a related malignant condition affecting the tissues of the reticuloendothelial system is the main hazard faced by patients suffering from mastocytosis. Such disturbances were present in at least 20 out of the 26 fatal cases reviewed and were found in nearly one quarter of all the cases of 'proved' systemic mastocytosis. It is therefore not possible to claim that coincidence is responsible for the association, even though no regular pattern has emerged with regard to the type of leukemia or other malignant disturbance which may develop. These have so far included: tissue mast cell leukemia; monocytic leukemia; myeloid leukemia and chloroma; lymphatic leukemia; acute hemocytoblastic leukemia; myelofibrosis; polycythemia rubra vera; reticulum cell sarcoma; and Hodgkin's disease.

These developments and associations may reflect the close interrelationship which exists between the different cells of the reticuloendothelial system.

It is possible that the mast cell disturbance itself may be the factor which 'triggers off' a further chain of events leading to the malignant condition. This might depend on the biochemical content of the mast cells, or be connected with physical invasion and replacement of tissue, either by mast cells or by fibrous or bony material laid down under their influence. Replacement of the blood-forming bone marrow by this process, visible roentgenographically as osteosclerotic and osteoporotic changes, might lead to anemia, leukopenia and thrombocytopenia. Concomitant damage to the liver and spleen may reinforce these effects. The remaining hemopoietic tissue may then undergo hyperplasia, and extramedullary blood forming sites may develop; these changes could lead to leukocytosis and a leukemoid reaction, or to polycythemia. In the struggle to maintain an adequate supply of blood cells for the body, immature cell forms may be thrown out into the peripheral blood stream to produce an erythroleukoblastic reaction. Finally, the hyperplastic response may result in the development of a true leukemia.

When systemic involvement has been proved, the disease may nevertheless be, and remain, benign, but it possibly may take a malignant course in perhaps as many as one-third of these patients.

The duration of the disease in those cases in which it finally proved fatal was studied. Death occurred within 2 years of the onset of the disease in 50% of the cases, and within 10 years in another 30%.

It is worth noting that four (16%) out of the 25 fatal cases of systemic masto-cytosis were reported from hospitals in Israel. This may have been fortuitous, but, if not, it would suggest that many cases of malignant mastocytosis remain undiagnosed. There is no reason to except a disproportionately high percentage of fatal cases of mastocytosis in this small country with a population of approxi-mately two and half million. On the same basis, one might have expected several thousand cases to have occurred in the world as a whole.

To conclude, our conception of urticaria pigmentosa or mastocytosis, has therefore changed radically during the past 15 years, and our knowledge of this disease is still being added to. There is a need for a greater awareness among internists, hematologists and pathologists, as well as among dermatologists, of the many forms the disease may take, and of the necessity for very full investigation of these patients, including their periodic re-examination.

Sézary Syndrome

G. L. Rocha, F. Santos, R. Azulay and A. Petrarca de Mesquita, University of Guanabara, Rio de Janeiro (Brazil)

Since 1938 when Sézary and Bouvain [1] have presented the first case of an erythroderma with monstruous cells in the dermis and peripheral blood, some other cases have been enlisted in the literature [2, 3, 4, 5, 6].

Although the Sézary syndrome should be classified according to definitive symptoms and findings, that number is larger than should be, because the concept has been erroneouly enlarged.

The diagnosis of Sézary syndrome, has to be made, on the following require-ments: erythrodermic exfoliative process, mostly pruritic, associated with cutane-ous infiltrate composed of large atypical mononuclear cell, together with other cells, but very prominent in the dermis; presence of a large mononuclear cell, in the peripheral blood in association with high elevated leukocyte count. This atypical mononuclear cell presents a diastase-resistant P.A.S. material in the cytoplasm

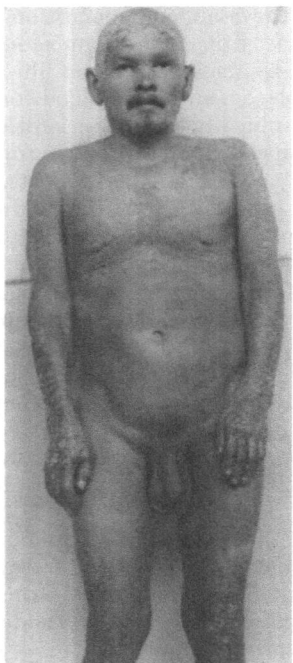

Fig. 1. Generalised
erythrodermic process

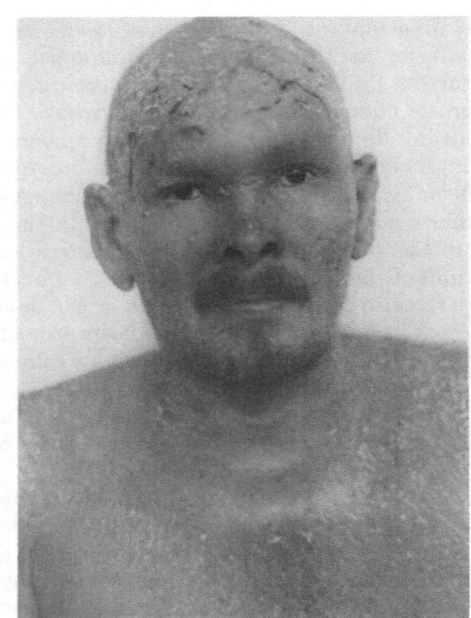

Fig. 2. Scaling, alopecia, edema
(moustache not touched)

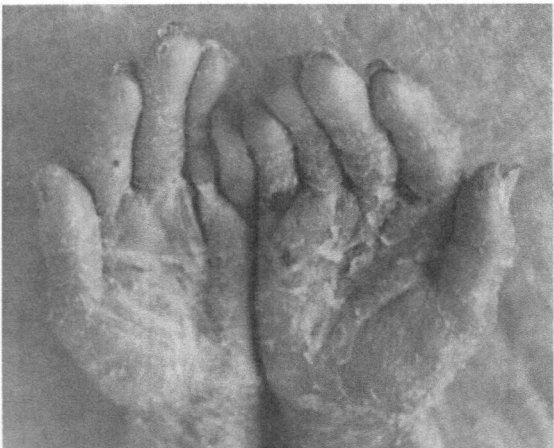

Fig. 3. Keratoderma of palms and soles

of the cells, as we could demonstrate; general good health; bone marrow smears
without anormalities; benign superficial lymphadenopathy; diffuse alopecia
(moustache not touched in our patient) keratoderma of palm and soles; ungueal
distrophies; edema is another feature, sometimes prominent; there is no involve-

ment of other organs; long course of the process; treatment with steroids and cytotoxic agents have yielded temporary relief in our patient.

These patients seems to have a fairly good course, during 5 years (our patient has 3 years of follow-up). Our patient had not pigmentary changes. Trying to fullfill more requirements for this diagnosis, one of us (G.L.R.) has performed with Dr. E. Dudova, a cariotype of our patient, that result normal. Under fluorescent microscopy (stain of Orange Acridine), we have observed a great number of immature cells, with very small cytoplasm and voluminous nucleus; this thin layer of cytoplasm showed an intense red fluorescence (Dr. P. de Mello). The overflow of the Sezary syndrome cases to other pathological status of the lympho-reticular system, if pertinent, gives to them the important and perhaps transient label of a syndrome, in its essence.

Case report. J.F.A., 40 years old male, white, married, farmer, living in Rio de Janeiro State, Brasil. First consultation in the Dermatological Clinic (Prof. Portugal), in May, 27, 1966, because of intense erythrodermic process with edeme and scaling (Fig. 1, 2 und 3) all over the body; pruritus not proeminent. By 1964, 2 years ago, starts the disease with maculo-erythematous lesions in the left forearm; from then many scattered lesions have became an erythrderma, 2 months later.

Physical examination revealed enlarged lymph nodes, with normal spleen and liver. In association with the erythroderma, there was alopecia (not of the moustache and slight in the pubis), hyperkeratosis of palms and soles, as well nail distrophies. The leukocyte count was 25.000 mm² of blood, with many atypical mononuclear cells (31%). Bone marrow reported as normal. Smears made a that time showed the PAS material in the large mononuclear cells, as we showed in the Ecktachrome.

Biopsies taken from different areas. One has to pay attention when examining the smears, for this special cellular type. The pathological specimens showed an intense cellular infiltration, uniforme and monomorphous composed chiefly of reticular cells and large mononuclear cells. There was no epidermal lesion. Biopsy taken from the superciliar area, when stained by PAS Alcian Blue, showed a mucinous appearance covering the whole follicle. Touch smears showed the presence of large cells, comparable with those of the peripheral blood.

References. 1. Sézary, A., et Y. Bouvrain: Bull. Soc. franç. Derm. Syph. **45**, 254 (1938). — 2. Pierini, L. E., J. Abulafia y A. Carvalho: III. Congresso Ibero-Latino Americano de Dermatologia, Memorias, p. 96. Mexico 1959. — 3. Mazzini, M. A., A. Scaletzky, E. L. Jonquieres, R. Psenne y O. Salti: V. Congresso Ibero-Latino Americano de Dermatologia, Memorias, p. 991. Buenos-Aires 1963. — 4. Taswell, H. F., and R. K. Winkelmann: J. Amer. med. Ass. **177**, 465 (1962). — 5. Baccaredda, A.: Arch. Derm. Syph. (Chic.) **179**, 209 (1939). — 6. Fleishmajer, R., and S. Eisenberg: Arch. Derm. **89**, 9 (1964).

Mycosis Fungoides — Mode of Presentation of 55 Cases

P. D. Samman, Westminster Hospital and St. John's Hospital for Diseases of the Skin, London (England)

A register of reticuloses and premycotic eruptions was started at St. John's Hospital for Diseases of the Skin in 1960, and all patients whose names have been included in the register are followed either by correspondence or personal interview once a year or more frequently to assess the progress of their disease. A preliminary report was made in 1964 when the number of patients on the register was 126. There are now more than 300 names on the list. Although the majority of patients come from the London area, many are resident in other parts of the country. All patients are seen by the clinician in charge of the survey who makes a diagnosis and registers the name. If a reticulosis develops later, on a premycotic eruption, the register is amended accordingly.

The present report deals with 55 patients who can be categorized as mycosis fungoides, and it will be seen from the table that the mode of onset varies widely, although the majority present in one of two ways either as the classical Alibert type or via poikiloderma atrophicans vasculare, or a form of parapsoriasis closely resembling it.

	Male	Female	Total
Classical (Alibert type)	14	10	24
i.e. Eczematous patches of irregular shape and colour, some patches becoming infiltrated			
Via poikiloderma atrophicans vasculare	3	7	10
Via poikiloderma — like eruptions			
(Parapsoriasis en plaques malignant type. Some lesions show reticulation)	6	1	7
Via parapsoriasis en plaques no lesions showing reticulation	2	0	2
Via erythroderma	1	1	2
With following mucinosis	2	0	2
Ulcerating nodules (no eczematous patches)	1	0	1
Infiltrated plaques (no eczematous patches)	3	1	4
Purpuric lesions predominating	2	0	2
Classical but very rapid	0	1	1
	34	21	55

Although the classical variety usually begins in middle life, we have seen a number of cases where it has started before the age of 20, and is well developed by this age, with infiltrations and incipient tumour formation. Progress in the majority of cases is very slow, 20 years or more, but in one case was very rapid. The same is true of poikiloderma atrophicans vasculare, most starting in middle life, but a number before the age of 20. The youngest had his first skin lesions at the age of 2 years and showed good evidence of mycosis fungoides by the age of 14. Even when the disease begins in childhood the progress is still very slow. The alternative name for poikilderma atrophicans vasculare is parapsoriasis lichenoides and this is perhaps a better name as it can include those cases of parapsoriasis en plaques with some reticulate patches which behave similarly. The reticulation in these patients can usually be detected within 2 or 3 years of onset of symptoms and more than half of them eventually progress to a reticulosis usually mycosis fungoides. It is very unusual for parapsoriasis en plaques to progress to a reticulosis without passing through a stage where some lesions are reticulate.

Cases presenting with erythroderma are very uncommon but there is no doubt that they are genuine.

We have seen no undoubted case of tumours developing without some evidence of pre-existing skin disease but the cases which present as infiltrated plaques or small ulcerating nodules, could perhaps be regarded as the tumour d'emblée variant. We have of course, seen a number of patients presenting with tumours which histologically were sarcomatous and are therefore, not included with mycosis fungoides.

Purpura is uncommon in mycosis fungoides but was presenting feature in two cases, and in one of these it closely resembled a carbromal eruption.

Patches of follicular mucinosis are quite common during the course of the disease but generally only form a minor part of the eruption; in two patients however, it was the presenting feature and it was some months before there was other evidence of mycosis fungoides.

Cytological Diagnosis in Mycosis Fungoides

E. Brehmer-Andersson and U. Brunk, Departments of Pathology and Cytology, University of Lund (Sweden)

A new method for the cytological diagnosis of mycosis fungoides, after tape stripping has been described by Brehmer-Andersson and Brunk in 1967. Ordinary commercial adhesive tape is used. New pieces of tape are repeatedly

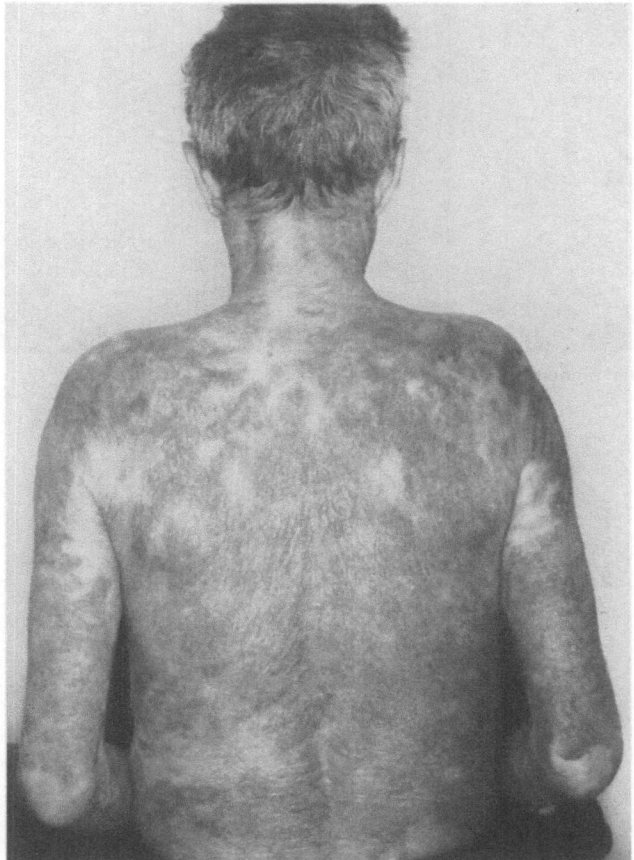

Fig. 1. Widespread, eczematous skin changes

applied to and stripped off from the skin lesions until oozing appears. Smears are then obtained by firmly pressing a microscope slide against the oozing surface. The slide is immediately placed in 96% ethyl alcohol. The smears are fixed for at least 1 h and then stained with Mayer's haematoxylin and eosin. This procedure is applicable to both plaques and tumours as well as eczematous lesions.

However, if patients are treated with local cortico-steroids under plastic occlusion or receive oral cortico-steroids it can be impossible to obtain smears. This is probably because the oedema in the epidermis, on which the method depends, disappears as a result of the cortico-steroid treatment.

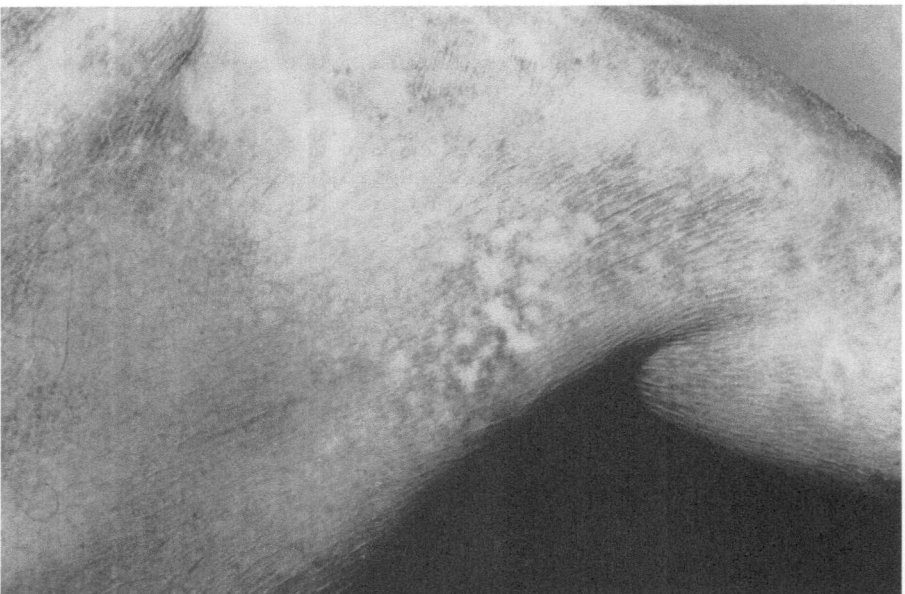

Fig. 2. Reticular pigmentation in the axilla

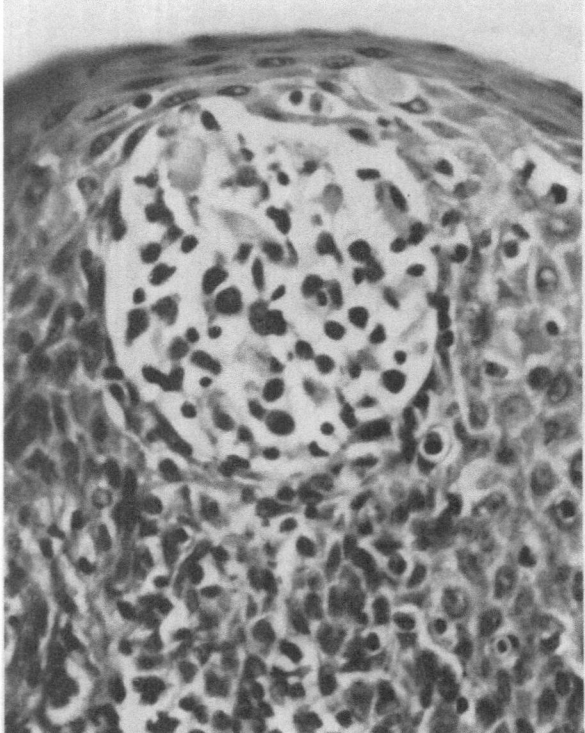

Fig. 3. Pautrier abscess in the epidermis, v. Gieson × 400

So far eight untreated cases with a clinical diagnosis of mycosis fungoides have been examined by the tape-stripping method. In five of the cases the diagnosis had been verified with skin biopsies. In the remaining three the biopsy could only give a suspicion of malignancy. In seven cases, smears showed numerous well preserved cells, and enabled a definite diagnosis of malignancy even in two of the histologically only suspected cases. In the third histologically uncertain case, scanty but well preserved swollen histiocytes and inflammatory cells were obtained. No atypical reticulum cells were found. The findings indicated a benign lesion.

One of the cases will be discussed in detail. The patient is a 65 year old lumberjack with at least a 15 year history of progressive eczematous skin changes. Periodically he had had severe itching. The epidermis is thin and easily broken. On account of the skin disease he was pensioned 3 years ago. His general condition, however, is good. He has been under the observation of a dermatologist since 1960, who already then suspected a diagnosis of mycosis fungoides. In February 1966 he was examined at the dermatology department. At that time the skin changes involved the trunk and extremities except for small irregular areas of normal skin. The lesions consisted mainly of a thin slightly scaley infiltrate, grey-brown-blue in colour due to the marked pigmentation. Between the strongly pigmented parts there were small scattered areas with reddish papules, giving a more active appearance (Fig. 1). In both axillae, the otherwise normal skin showed reticular pigmentation (Fig. 2). Some thicker, lichenified lesions were found on the thighs, extremities and waist area. The palms and soles showed hyperkeratosis.

In both inguinal areas there were some firm, slightly enlarged lymph glands. The liver and spleen were not palpable. The blood picture as well as X-ray examinations of chest and gastrointestinal tract were normal. Cytological puncture biopsy of the right inguinal glands showed reactive adenopathy. Previous lymph gland biopsies performed in 1964 and 1965, gave the diagnosis of dermatopathic lymphadenitis.

Between 1960 and 1966 nine skin biopsies were performed. All biopsies histologically showed a dense cell infiltrate made up of large, swollen, often pigment-laden histiocytes, round cells and leucocytes, but no atypical cells. The infiltrate was situated in the upper part of the corium and invaded the epidermis. In some biopsies the epidermis contained vesicles as in subacute dermatitis. Retrospectively some small Pautrier abscesses with suspected atypical cells were found in a biopsy from 1964 (Fig. 3). The exact nature of these cells, however, was difficult to recognize. In this case the diagnosis of a malignant lymphoma-mycosis fungoides could not be made from the histological picture alone.

In autumn 1966 imprint smears were made after tape stripping from two thick, lichenified lesions, one thin pigmented and one thin reddish infiltrate. No cell material was obtained from the lichenified lesions. The other two gave abundant and well preserved cells.

The imprint smears showed a definite malignant picture with many uniform atypical reticulum cells with irregular nuclei and an irregular patchy chromatin pattern. Occasionally some extreme cell types including tumour giant cells of Reed-Sternberg type as well as more normal histiocyte-like cells with delicate chromatin and abundant cytoplasm were found (Figs. 4 and 5).

Later investigation has included a preliminary cytochemical analysis of the cell material for some hydrolytic and oxidative enzyme systems: alkaline phosphatase, acid phosphatase, unspecific esterase, lactic acid dehydrogenase, succinic acid dehydrogenase, TPNH-diaphorase and DPNH-diaphorase.

As shown in this investigation the cytological method can confirm the diagnosis of mycosis fungoides in a number of cases, where the histological examination has only aroused a suspicion of malignancy. It may also be possible to rule out a clinical suspicion of malignant disease.

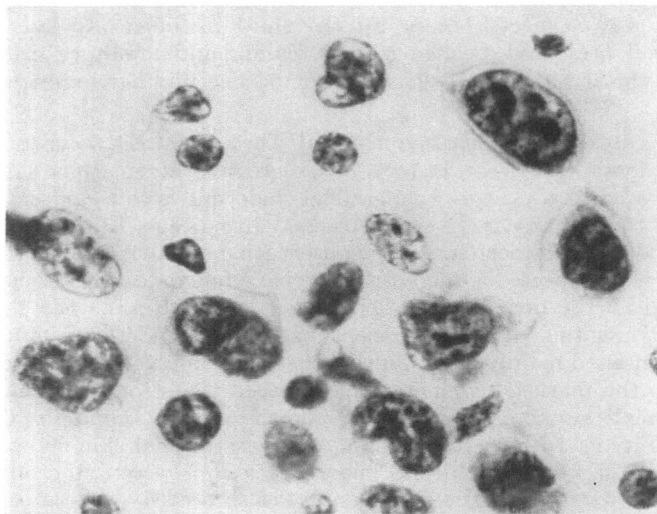

Fig. 4. Many atypical reticular cells together with scattered histiocytes. Haematoxylin-eosin × 1000

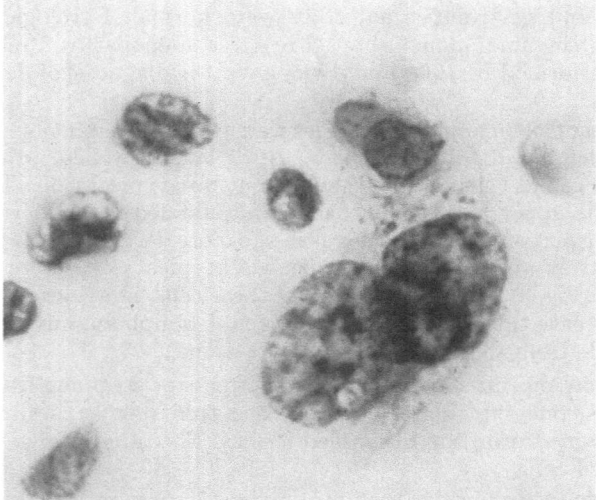

Fig. 5. Tumour giant cell of Reed-Sternberg type. Haematoxylin-eosin × 1000

In addition, systematic cytological examination including cytochemical studies of smears from patients with mycosis fungoides in different stages may show whether the invading cells in this disease have any characteristic morphology and enzymatic pattern.

Reference. BREHMER-ANDERSSON, E., and U. BRUNK: Acta derm. venereol. (Stockh.) 47, 177 (1967).

Triacetyl 6-Azauridine in Mycosis Fungoides*

Ch. J. McDonald, P. Calabresi and R. C. DeConti, Departments of Medicine and Pharmacology, Yale University School of Medicine, New Haven, Connecticut (USA)

Mycosis fungoides is a neoplastic disease of the lymphoreticular system primarily affecting the skin. In a large proportion of cases visceral organs are also involved. Three clinical and histological stages of the disease are recognized. They occur both singly and in various combinations. These stages have significant prognostic and therapeutic implications. Stage I, the eczematous or erythematous "premycotic" stage is the least malignant and is compatable with considerable longevity. The response of this type of disease to most forms of therapy is good. The infiltrative plaque form (Stage II), and the tumorous and ulcerative form (Stage III) are usually quite resistant to therapy.

The current treatment of mycosis fungoides like that of most generalized lymphomas is palliative. Electron beam therapy has been quite successful in alleviating the skin manifestations of this disease. However, this form of therapy has limitations. Instruments capable of emitting the necessary quality of electrons are extremely rare. We are aware of only four or five such machines operational in the entire United States. As is true with all forms of radiation therapy, there is a maximum tolerable skin dose of electrons beyond which there is irreparable skin damage. Topical and systemic corticosteroids, alkylating agents, and the vinca alkaloids have been used with varying results. To date, the most successful chemotherapeutic agent used in large numbers of patients has been antimetabolite methotrexate [1].

Zaruba et al., described objective evidence of disease remission in three patients treated with intravenous 6-azauridine (AZUR) [2]. Later, Calabresi and Turner described improvement in the clinical status of two patients with mycosis fungoides who received oral triacetyl-6-azauridine (TAZUR) [3]. We are now reporting our experience with seven patients. These patients constitute part of a continuing study, at the Yale University School of Medicine, of the effects of TAZUR in psoriasis and mycosis fungoides.

TAZUR is the triacetylated form of the nucleoside AZUR. The principal action of AZUR in mammalian systems is the intracellular inhibition of pyrimidine nucleotide synthesis. The metabolically formed 5' phosphate of 6-azauridine, i.e., azauridylic acid, competitively limits the access of the enzyme orotidylate decarboxylase to the normal substrate orotidylic acid. As a result, the *de novo* synthesis of uridylic acid does not occur, and in turn, the synthesis of nucleic acids is inhibited. Thus, malignant cells will not grow or reproduce.

Results. Six of the seven patients experienced clinical improvement for variable periods of time. Three of the six had complete clearing of disease; two of these have remained in clinical remission while on drug therapy for 5 and 18 months. The third patient in this group has continued to take TAZUR, but has required retreatment with electrons. In this individual, TAZUR apparently has prolonged the interval of time between courses of electron therapy. Of the three other patients who achieved partial remission, TAZUR was discontinued in one because of CNS symptoms. This patient is currently being treated with intralesional steroids and a combination of superficial x-ray and electrons. Another patient in this group has been readmitted to the hospital for more intensive TAZUR

* Supported by Grants (T 4 CA 5138-05, 5 MOI-FR-00038, CA 8341-02, CA 50944-06 of the U. S. Public Health Service, The Olsen Memorial Fund and Calbiochem Company.

47*

therapy in an attempt to better control her disease. In the third patient who was treated in the early phase of this study, lack of adequate supplies of drug necessitated termination of therapy after two courses of treatment. Both this patient and the one nonresponsive individual have succumbed to the disease.

TAZUR has significantly fewer toxic manifestations than other antineoplastic drugs. Leukopenia, thrombocytopenia, hair loss, gastrointestinal symptoms, aphthous ulcerations, and lower gastrointestinal lesions are not observed with TAZUR. In a total of 46 patients treated with this drug, abnormalities of liver and kidney function have not been detected.

The most common toxic manifestation to date is a mild to moderate reduction in hematocrit and red cell count. Both are alleviated by reduction in drug dosage or cessation of therapy. Five of 46 patients have developed symptoms of CNS toxicity. Specifically, these are drowsiness, myoclonic movements of the extremities and hyperreflexia. Cessation of oral therapy for 5 to 7 days eliminates these signs and symptoms. Generally, they do not reappear when oral therapy is reinstituted. Intravenous administration of 6-AZUR in the neurotoxic patient, after termination of oral TAZUR, is not accompanied by similar clinical manifestations.

Table. *Triacetyl 6-Azauridine (Tazur) in Mycosis Fungoides*

Case Number Age, Sex	Stage	Previous Therapy	Clinical Response to TAZUR	Subsequent Course
1. (70, M)	I	Systemic Corticosteroids	Complete remission after 6 weeks	Remission maintained for 18 months without other therapy
2. (50, F)	II	None	Complete remission after 6 weeks	Remission maintained for 5 months without other therapy
3. (37, F)	II	Methotrexate Corticosteroids Electron beam therapy × 3	Complete remission after 2 weeks	Relapse after 12 weeks on TAZUR. Required additional electron beam therapy. Interval between courses of electrons prolonged by TAZUR
4. (67, F)	II	Cytoxan, HN 2 Corticosteroids Methotrexate Electron beam therapy × 2	Partial remission after 3 weeks	Relapse after 6 weeks on TAZUR
5. (77, F)	II	Corticosteroids, Electron beam therapy Grenz ray Vinblastine, Methotrexate Superficial x-ray	Partial remission after 4 weeks	Relapse shortly after termination of drug. Subsequent control with repeated course of TAZUR
6. (48, M)	II	Electron beam therapy Chlorambucil Corticosteroids	Partial response after 4 weeks	Partial response lasting 4 months without maintenance therapy
7. (67, M)	III	Superficial x-ray Methotrexate	None	Deceased

In summary, it has been shown that TAZUR is a relatively safe and effective antineoplastic agent which may be of value in the treatment of patients with mycosis fungoides, either alone or in combination with electron beam therapy.

References. 1. WRIGHT, J. C.: Cancer (Philad.) 17, 1045 (1964). — 2. ZARUBA, F., A. KUTA, and J. ELLIS: Lancet 1963 I, 275. — 3. CALABRESI, P., and R. W. TURNER: Ann. intern. Med. 64, 352 (1966).

Ultrastructure de l'angio-réticulo-sarcomatose cutanée: Maladie de Kaposi*

E. Calas, H. Bonneau et J. P. Cesarini**, Groupe de Recherches Scientifiques sur les Tumeurs Humaines, Laboratoire de Microscopie Electronique du Centre Régional de Lutte contre le Cancer de Marseille (France)

De nombreux travaux ont mis en évidence la très grande fréquence de la maladie de Kaposi autour du Bassin Méditerranéen et en Afrique [1, 2, 3, 4]. Degos [5] a fait ressortir qu'il s'agissait plus d'un facteur géographique que d'un facteur ethnique. Bacconnier [6] dans une thèse remarquable a colligé 24 observations: 16 de ces malades atteints de cette affection ont voyagé, 11 ayant passé l'équateur. Notre matériel d'étude provient de ces mêmes malades. Depuis quelques années, la maladie de Kaposi a fait l'objet de nombreuses études ultra-structurales: Yodaiken (1962) [7], Pepler (1962) [8], Hashimoto et Lever (1964) [9], Mikko-Niemi et Mustakallio (1965) [10], Mottaz et Zellickson (1966) [11]. Ces travaux ont apporté des précisions importantes concernant la morphologie, la structure cellulaire et la morphogénèse de ces lésions. Nous avons donc axé notre travail sur la recherche au microscope électronique de signes révélateurs d'un contact viral, et sur l'histogénèse de la prolifération tumorale.

Matériel et méthode

Nous avons résumé par un tableau les cas étudiés

6 Cas	N° Thèse Bacconnier	Age	Origine	17 Biopsies	
1	MAG...		65 ans	Marseille	2 AL — 2 NL	J. Bonnet, E. Calas Marseille
2	SAD...	Obs. 7	60 ans	Algérie	AL — NL AL — NL	P. Temime Marseille
3	GAL...	Obs. 5	68 ans	Malte	AL avant Cs.th.NL NL après Cs.th.	J. Bonnet, E. Calas Marseille
4	TAS...	Obs. 22	44 ans	Corse	NL	J. Bonnet, E. Calas Marseille
5	PIE...	Obs. 11	73 ans	Corse	AL — NL NL	J. Bonnet, E. Calas Marseille
6	GUA...		60 ans	Naples	NL AL	E. Calas, A. Florens Marseille

AL = Ancienne lésion; NL = Nouvelle lésion; Cs th. = Cesium thérapie

Tous les prélèvements pour le microscope électronique ont fait l'objet d'un contrôle soigneux par examen au microscope photonique de coupes semi-fines et des coupes après inclusions à la parafine.

Les prélèvements pour la microscopie électronique ont subi immédiatement une double fixation: glutaraldéhyde [12] suivi du tétra-oxyde d'osmium. Après deshydratation par alcool ou acétone, ils sont inclus en Araldite [13] ou Araldite-Epon. Effectuées à l'ultrotome Leitz, les coupes fines sont examinées après contraste à l'acétate d'uranyl et au citrate de plomb [14], au microscope électronique Hitachi HS 7 S.

---

* Travail réalisé grâce à une subvention du Fond d'action sanitaire et social de la Caisse Régionale de Sécurité Sociale du Sud-Est, et du Groupement des Entreprises Françaises pour la lutte contre le cancer.
** Avec la collaboration technique de J. Ingrand, J. P. Duhal.

Résultat — Discussion

Aucun virus n'a pu être mis en évidence dans le matériel étudié que ce soit dans les lésions récentes, anciennes ou en pleines récidives après traitement. Nous avons recherché dans les noyaux, les cytoplasmes, les lumières vasculaires et les espaces intercellulaires des signes indirects traduisant le passage de virus à un moment de l'existence de la cellule. Aucun aspect de ségrégation nucléolaire [15], aucun gigantisme mitochondrial [16] n'a été décelable. Par contre, nous avons remarqué la présence dans tous les prélèvements d'un matériel intra-nucléaire dont la structure a déjà fait l'objet de publications dans d'autres espèces vivantes [17, 18] (Fig. 1). Ce sont des inclusions parfois finement fibrillaires contenant quelques granulations denses de la taille d'un ribosome, ces inclusions ont 0,5 à 1 micron de diamètre. Le plus souvent unique dans une coupe de noyau, nous les avons retrouvées au nombre de quatre et même cinq dans les lésions jeunes ou en récidive. Selon certains auteurs ces inclusions seraient en rapport avec une activité nucléaire encore indéterminée. Nous ne pouvons que signaler ici ce fait. Pour préciser l'histogénèse des cellules présentes dans les proliférations tumorales, nous nous sommes livrés à une étude systématique des hématies que nous avons trouvées dans tous les prélèvements en quantité variable. Certaines de ces hématies sont dans la lumière de vaisseaux capillaires, de structure très classique [19] dont les noyaux bombent fortement dans la lumière et qui sont entourés d'une membrane basale bien distincte et de cellules de type péricytaire caractéristiques (Fig. 2). D'autres hématies sont au contraire noyées dans un collagène dense sans structure cellulaire visible à proximité. Enfin, et c'est le plus intéressant, nous avons trouvé des hématies au milieu de structure cellulaire formée de plusieurs cellules non jointives entre-elles, à la membrane basale inexistante ou à peine ébauchées, ce qui permet de classer ces figures soit dans les capillaires de type embryonnaire, soit d'envisager une véritable attirance des cellules de type réticulo-endothélial pour les globules rouges extravasés (Fig. 5). Dans ce cas, les cytoplasmes sont très développés et le réticulum endoplasmique particulièrement abondant: sa dilatation implique une idée de fonctionnement intense. Nos clichés montrent sans discussion que du collagène à tous les stades de sa formation s'insinue entre les globules rouges et la ceinture cellulaire: (Fig. 3). Les contacts étroits entre hématies et cellules de type fibroblastique sont très particuliers et évoquent le phénomène d'immuno-cytoadhérence [20]: (Fig. 4). Ce phénomène, compte tenu des propriétés tinctoriales des cellules du système réticulo-endothélial [21] permet d'évoquer une origine réticulaire des cellules présentes dans la tumeur. Il n'est donc pas interdit de penser qu'en marge d'une population de vaisseaux bien structurés, il se produise une élaboration de structure para-vasculaire formée par les cellules de type réticulo-hystiocitaire plus ou moins différenciées entourant les hématies extravasées. L'aboutissement général de ce processus est la phagocytose d'éléments rouges que l'on retrouve dans les cellules sous forme de figure de type «myélinique» dans les lésions anciennes cicatricielles.

En conclusion: Si aucun élément viral, ni aucune trace virale n'est directement visible au microscope électronique, comme cela d'ailleurs était prévisible par analogie avec certains modèles d'oncogénèse virale chez l'animal [18]; certaines structures permettent de penser que les hématies pourraient presenter en surface des protéines douées d'un tactisme pour les cellules réticulaires libres. Ces cellules produiraient la néo-angiogénèse. Par ailleurs, leur différenciation réaliserait les images de réticulose de la maladie de Kaposi (Fig. 6). L'évolution finale, en effet, de cette maladie se fait très fréquemment vers le lympho-sarcome ou le réticulo-sarcome. La maladie de Kaposi serait donc une réticulose angiogène [22]

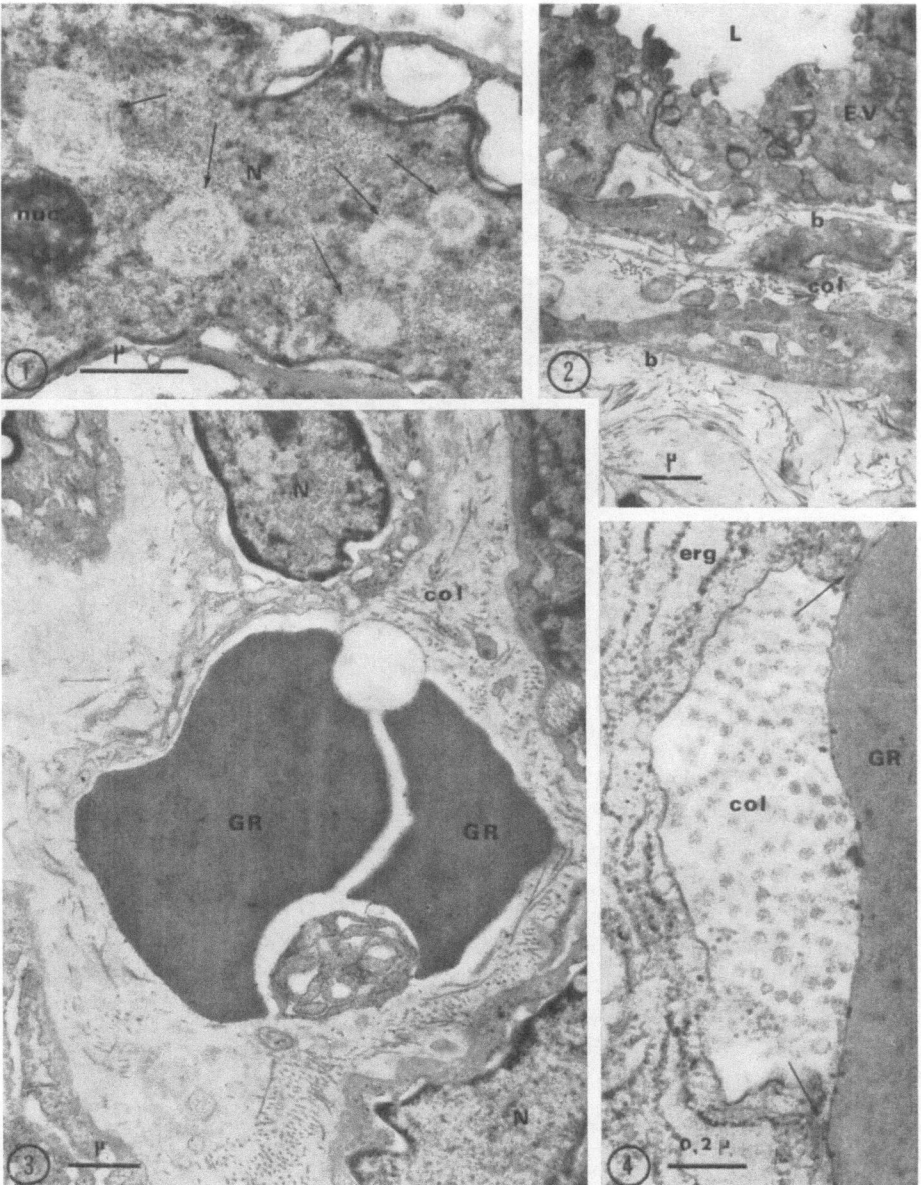

Fig. 1. Maladie de Kaposi, cas n° 3 après césium thérapie. Noyau (N) de cellule réticulaire.
On notera un nucléole (nuc) de structure normale et la présence de 5 inclusions fibrillaires (→)

Fig. 2. Maladie de Kaposi, cas n° 3. Paroi vasculaire de structure normale. L'endothélium
vasculaire (EV) repose sur une basale (b) bien individualisée. Du collagène (col) s'insinue entre
l'endothélium et les péricytes. Lumière vasculaire (L)

Fig. 3. Maladie de Kaposi, cas n° 3 après césium thérapie. Les hématies (GR) sont entourées
par des cellules. Le collagène (col) s'insinue entre celles-ci et les globules rouges. Noyau (N)

Fig. 4. Maladie de Kaposi, cas n° 5. Contact entre cellule de type réticulaire à l'ergastoplasme
(erg) bien développé et une hématie (GR). Les (→) montrent que l'espace entre les cellules
(100 A°) est comblé par un matériel finement dense aux électrons. Entre les cellules est inclu
du collagène (col)

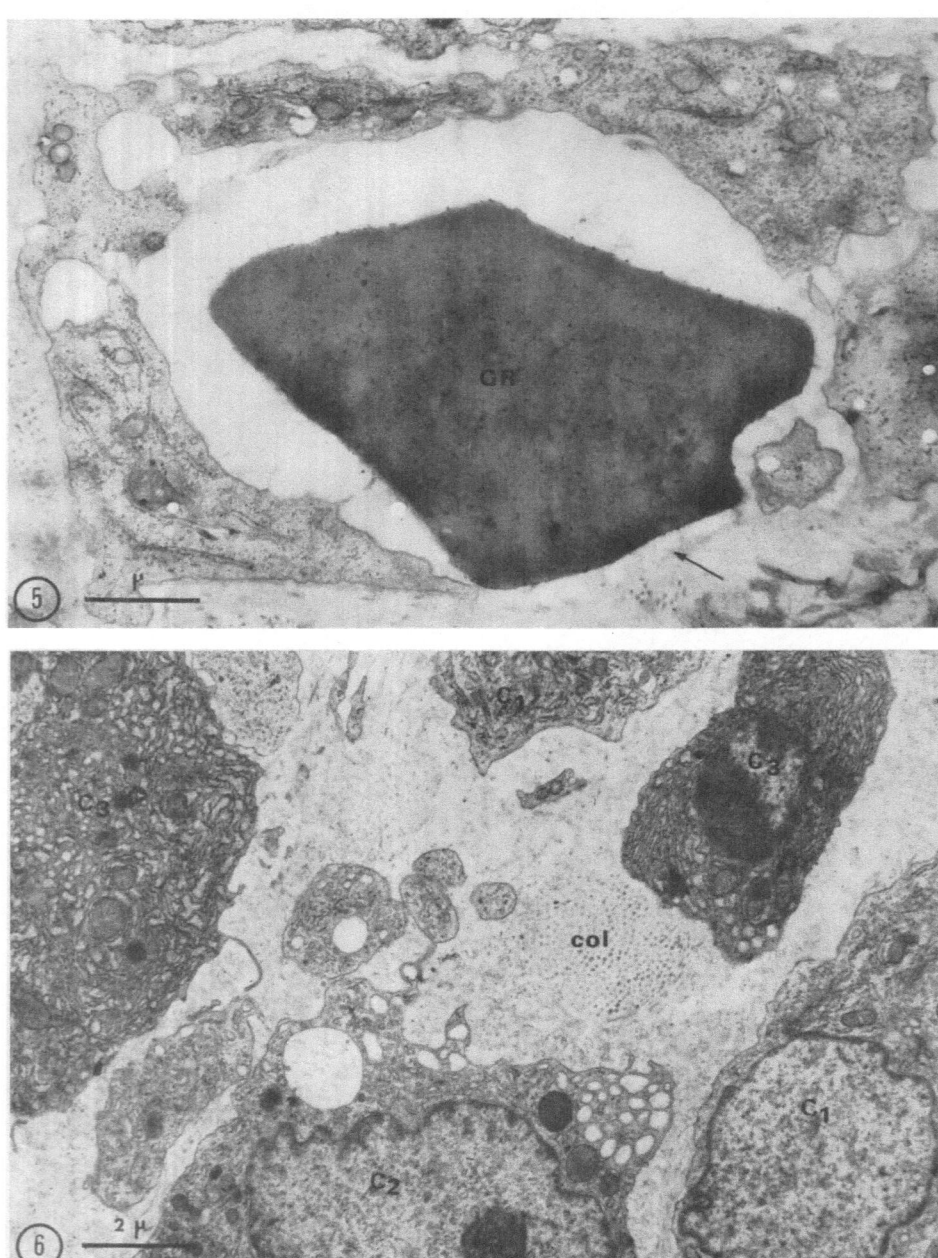

Fig. 5. Maladie de Kaposi, cas n° 6. Une hématie est entourée emcomplètent par les proliférations cellulaires réalisant un aspect de pseudo-vaisseau. On notera l'absence de basale. L'hématie est en contact direct (→) avec les milieux interstitiels

Fig. 6. Maladie de Kaposi, cas n° 1. Aspect général de la prolifération cellulaire montrant des cellules réticulaires à des stades progressifs de leur différenciation: C 1, C 2, C 3. Collagène (col.)

et le terme d'angio-réticulo-sarcomatose cutané rend bien compte de sa malignité terminale.

Bibliographie. 1. Temime, P.: Encyclopédie médico-chirurgicale-dermatologie 1962. — 2. Calas, E., et M. Pierron: Bull. Soc. franç. Derm. Syph. 1962. — 3. Bonnet, J., et E. Calas: Bull. Soc. franç. Derm. Syph. 1966. — 4. Paoli, J., H. Payan, H. Bonneau, R. Lieutaud et G. de The: Sem. Hôp. (Paris) 18, 183 (1960). — 5. Degos, R., R. Touraine, J. Civatte, S. Belaich et D. Fracek: Ann. Derm. Syph. (Paris) 91, 113 (1964). — 6. Bacconnier, J.: Contribution à l'étude de la maladie de Kaposi. In thèse, Marseille 1966. — 7. Yodaiken, R. E.: S. Afr. med. J. 36, 989 (1962). — 8. Pepler, M. J., and J. J. Theron: J. Path. Bact. 83, 521 (1962). — 9. Hashimoto, K., and W. F. Lever: J. invest. Derm. 43, 539 (1964). — 10. Mikko Niemi, K. K., and Mustakallio: Acta path. microbiol. scand. 63, 567 (1965). — 11. Mottaz, J. H., and A. S. Zellickson: Acta derm.-venereol. (Stockh.) 146, 195 (1966). — 12. Sabatini, D. D., K. Bensch, and R. J. Barnett: J. cell. Biol. 17, 19 (1963). — 13. Glauert, A. M., and R. H. Glauert: J. biophys. biochem. Cytol. 4, 191 (1958). — 14. Reynolds, E. S.: J. cell. Biol. 18, 208 (1963). — 15. Jezequel, A. M., M. M. Shreeve, and J. W. Steiner: Lab. Invest. 16, 287 (1967). — 16. Bernhard, W., and P. Tournier: Int. J. Cancer 1, 61 (1966). — 17. Buttner, D. W.: Z. mikro.-anat. Zellforsch. 77, 589 (1967). — 18. Bonneau, H., J. P. Cesarini, A. M. Lherisson, M. Berebbi et I. Varette: Soc. Biol. 28, 2 (1967) In press. — 19. Poirier, J., et H. Anh. Nguyen: Presse méd. 75, 469 (1967). — 20. Pavlovsky, S., G. Biozzi et J. L. Binet: J. Microscopie 6, 74 (1967). — 21. Dayan, A. D., and P. D. Lewis: Nature (Lond.) 123, 889 (1967). — 22. Margarot, J., P. Rimbaud et P. Cazal: Sem. Hôp. (Paris) 24, 6 (1948).

Zur Entität des sog. Morbus Kaposi

G. Oehlschlaegel, Dermatologische Klinik und Poliklinik der Universität Würzburg (Deutschland)

Die klinische und morphologische Vielgestaltigkeit der vor 100 Jahren von Kaposi als „Idiopathisches multiples Pigmentsarkom der Haut" beschriebenen Krankheit führte wohl zu einer entsprechenden Vielzahl von Auffassungen, doch zu keiner befriedigenden Kenntnis der nosologischen Stellung der Krankheit. Hierfür spricht eine Unzahl von Synonyma.

Es ist somit naheliegend, daß bei den Interpretationen, die von den extremen Polen der Sarkomnatur bis zur gutartigen Angiomatose reichen, eine Vielzahl von Beobachtungen erfolgte, die nicht dem beschriebenen Krankheitsbild entsprachen. Die Krankheit wurde also zu weit gefaßt oder überhaupt fehldiagnostiziert. Im Gegensatz hierzu mußte eine kritische Haltung zu der Frage führen, ob es denn den sog. Morbus Kaposi (M.K.) als Entität überhaupt gäbe. Diese Frage muß bejaht werden und soll nach Substraktion der Krankheitsbilder, die mit dem M.K. sicher nichts gemein haben, später begründet werden.

Scharf zu trennen vom M.K. ist die zirkulationsbedingte sog. reaktive Angiomatose der Unterschenkel, die zum Teil unter dem Bild der atrophie blanche verläuft. Wenn schon in klinischer Hinsicht möglicherweise einem M.K. ähnlich, so zeigt doch die histologische Untersuchung wesentliche Unterschiede beider Krankheitsbilder, als die Gefäßneubildung in kleineren umschriebenen Arealen vorliegt, die entfernt in ihrer Anordnung an Formen capillärer Angiome erinnern und wie diese als Gefäßregulationen im Sinne pathologischer Anpassung aufgefaßt werden müßten. Auch könnte eine sicher reaktive Angiomatose, die wir bei Obturation kleinerer Hautgefäße nach Eiweißpräcipitation bei Kryofibrinogenämie beobachten konnten, Anlaß zur Fehldiagnose geben. Auch ein Fall eines Rhabdomyosarkoms mit multiplen Knotenbildungen bot zunächst Anlaß zur Verwechslung. Selbst auf einer Tagung wurden an diesem Fall neben dem M.K. die verschiedensten Diagnosen gestellt. Diese Beispiele mögen genügen, auf

Fehldeutungen aufmerksam zu machen, ohne daß damit Anspruch auf Vollständigkeit der Differentialdiagnose gestellt würde.

Wodurch ist nun aber der M.K. charakterisiert, und wie ist die Krankheit definierbar? Das Verhaltensprinzip der primär multipel, jedoch auch gelegentlich der Metastasierung fähigen Krankheit ist als semimaligne zu bezeichnen. Das feingewebliche Bild spricht für die Auffassung einer „exquisit angioplastischen Neubildung" — ich zitiere VON ALBERTINI — „wobei die undifferenzierten Geschwulstabschnitte das Bild eines zellreichen Spindelzellsarkomes vortäuschen, in der Tat aber einen mesenchymalen Schwamm bilden, aus dem durch differenzierende Umformung ein feinporöses Capillarnetzwerk hervorgeht. In diesem kommt anscheinend keine Zirkulation zustande, die roten Blutkörperchen bleiben in den Maschen liegen und hämolysieren. Das freiwerdende Blut wird von den Geschwulstzellen phagocytiert". Soweit VON ALBERTINI.

Mit dieser treffenden Beschreibung ist bereits indirekt herausgestellt, worin prinzipiell eine Abgrenzung zu gutartigen Gefäßgeschwülsten und der sog. reaktiven Angiomatose liegt. Der grundsätzliche Unterschied liegt darin, daß den genannten Gefäßneubildungen komplexe organoide Teileinheiten zugrunde liegen. Diese entsprechen somit einem höheren Grad der Reife. Hingegen finden wir beim M.K. diese gestaltliche Gliederung nicht verwirklicht, als ein vorherrschender Aufbau aus komplexen Teileinheiten nicht vorliegt.

Wenn man die von BOLCK herausgearbeitete definierende Interpretation des Endotheliombegriffes zugrunde legt, muß zweifelsohne der M.K. als Endotheliom aufgefaßt werden. Die Begründung hierfür liegt im Nachweis des abstrahierten Prinzips der inneren Hohlraumbildung, wobei aber — was charakteristisch für Endotheliome ist — lediglich eine einfache örtliche Gliederung verwirklicht wird. In dieser Gliederung ist das Hauptmerkmal der Endotheliome zu erblicken. Allerdings gilt die Einschränkung, daß diese Gestaltsstufe nicht nur nachgewiesen sein muß, sondern vorherrscht und somit das Wesentliche darstellt.

Die sog. proteusartige Vielgestaltigkeit der Endotheliome ist im gegebenen Fall nichts anderes, als daß einerseits Tendenzen zur höheren Gliederung, andererseits zu tieferen Gestaltsstufen wirksam werden. Das heißt, daß die erstgenannte Potenz zu komplexen gestaltlichen Einheiten als nicht dominierender Teilerscheinung führen kann, wobei als Sonderfall Gefäßstrukturen entwickelt werden. Die zweitgenannte Möglichkeit bildet als ebenso nichtdominierende Teilerscheinung gleichmäßig aufgegliederte Zellmassen aus. Somit ist eine Abgrenzung nach „oben" zu gutartigen Gefäßtumoren gegeben und nach „unten" zu den angioplastischen Sarkomen.

Erlauben Sie mir zum Schluß noch ein kurzes Wort zur Histogenese, worin letztlich die Begründung für die Aufnahme dieser Ausführungen im Rahmen dieses Symposions liegt. Die Überlegungen zur Histogenese können nur gedanklicher Art sein und weniger vom Optischen abgeleitet werden, zumal Gleichartigkeit oder Ähnlichkeit nicht unbedingt histogenetische Identität bedeutet.

Man sollte davon ausgehen, daß das gemeinsame Keimlager für Bindegewebe und Blutgefäße, von HUECK als primitives Gefäßmesenchym bezeichnet, im reticulären Bindegewebe liegt. Es ist meines Erachtens völlig müßig, sich darüber zu streiten, ob somit den inneren Deckzellen — also Endothel — oder reticulär gelagerten Adventitialzellen — Retothel — die alleinige oder vorherrschende Rolle zukommt. Mit gebotener Zurückhaltung könnten dann auch Rundzellinfiltrate mit den verschiedenen Differenzierungsmöglichkeiten des Mesenchyms ihre Aufklärung finden.

Ich fasse somit zusammen: Der sog. M.K., der sowohl klinisch als auch histologisch wahrscheinlich zu häufig diagnostiziert wird, ist ein Endotheliom und somit semimaligne. Innerhalb der Endotheliomgruppe ist die Krankheit im wesentlichen charakterisiert durch ein schwammartiges mesenchymales Netzwerk, das einerseits wirbelartig angeordnete, an Fibrosarkom oder Spindelzellsarkom erinnernde Struktur ausbildet und durch besondere Umbildung zu mehr oder weniger ausgebildeten Gefäßräumen führt. Die Betonung der ersten genannten Eigenart bringt eine Näherung zum angioplastischen Sarkom, die gefäßbildende Tendenz eine Näherung zu gutartigen gefäßbildenden Tumoren oder mit Gefäßneubildung einhergehenden Anpassungshyperplasien.

Literatur. v. ALBERTINI, A.: Histologische Geschwulstdiagnostik. Stuttgart: Thieme 1955. — BOLCK, F.: Die Endotheliome. Leipzig: Thieme 1952. — HUECK, W.: Morphologische Pathologie. Leipzig: Thieme 1937.

Les localisations cutanées spécifiques de la maladie de Waldenstroem

H. BARRIERE, P. LITOUX et B. BUREAU, Clinique Dermatologique, Faculté de Médecine de Nantes (France)

On décrit diverses formes viscérales de la maladie de Waldenström. C'est ainsi que les lésions peuvent prédominer au niveau du revêtement cutané où existent des lésions constituées par des infiltrats spécifiques de la maladie, créant en quelque sorte une forme cutanée de cette affection. Nous avons retrouvé de telles lésions dans deux cas personnels:

Dans le premier de ceux-ci, il s'agissait d'un homme chez lequel s'était établie progressivement une infiltration massive et diffuse de coloration rouge violacée, de consistance ferme, déformant et boursoufflant tout le visage, envahissant également les oreilles. A ces lésions cutanées s'associent des lésions muqueuses sous la forme d'une infiltration importante au niveau de la voûte palatine ainsi que des infiltrats plus limités de la base de la langue et enfin, une infiltration de la muqueuse nasale au niveau des cornets moyens et inférieurs. Ces lésions ont évolué lentement vers la régression spontanée, tandis que l'état général restait floride.

Chez le second malade, l'aspect clinique était différent. Il s'agissait d'une femme présentant deux tuméfactions assez volumineuses l'une siégeant au niveau du poignet droit formant une sorte de véritable tumeur arrondie, rouge violacée, très dure et apparue dès le début des troubles de la malade. Secondairement était apparue une tuméfaction également dure, importante, au niveau de l'angle de la machoire formant à ce niveau un placard irrégulier, sans participation épidermique. Une radiothérapie locale a amené la fonte de ces lésions, mais l'état général de la malade a été en s'aggravant et celle-ci a succombé à son affection.

La biopsie de ces lésions cutanées montre un infiltrat dermique massif, respectant une bande dans le derme papillaire, constituée à la fois de lymphocytes et de cellules de taille un peu plus grande, de forme arrondie, à noyau excentré, à chromatine moyennement dense.

Chez ces deux malades les examens biologiques en particulier, immuno-électrophorèse et ultra-centrifugation confirment de façon indiscutable la macro-globulinémie primitive de Waldenström.

Nous pouvons rapprocher de ces deux observations personnelles cinq autres comparables: celles de GOTTRON (2), REVOL, BOTHIER, MICHON. L'ensemble de ces observations permet de décrire les localisations cutanées de la maladie de

Waldenström. Celles-ci se caractérisent soit par des tumeurs localisées, soit par des infiltrations diffuses, dures ou tout au moins fermes, d'une coloration rouge violacée dont l'aspect évoque assez les lésions observées au cours de réticulose cutanée. Par contre, l'existence des mêmes infiltrations au niveau de la muqueuse comme en présentait notre premier malade reste plus exceptionnelle.

L'histologie apporte un argument important pour authentifier ces lésions, en montrant d'une part un infiltrat cellulaire important ménageant le derme superficiel, mais s'étendant jusqu'à l'hypoderme et entraînant une destruction plus ou moins complète à son niveau du tissu conjonctif.

Les cellules de l'infiltrat semblent ainsi siéger dans un réseau délimité par de larges mailles. GOTTRON a signalé une réaction P.A.S. positive du conjonctif. Au niveau de ces infiltrats l'aspect des cellules est également très évocateur puisqu'à côté de lymphocytes caractéristiques on rencontre des cellules de taille un peu plus grande, à noyau clair et à situation excentrée. Des ilots de plasmocytes authentiques peuvent se rencontrer (REVOL).

Il nous semble que l'existence d'une telle infiltration cutanée où l'on retrouve les cellules lympho-plasmocytaires caractéristiques de l'affection, soit un argument supplémentaire pour considérer que le phénomène cellulaire est primitif et que ce sont précisément ces cellules particulières qui sécrètent une globuline anormale. Cette pathogènie rapprochant la maladie de Waldenström de la maladie de Kahler où l'on considère également que le rôle essentiel est celui d'un plasmocyte anormal sécrétant. On tend d'ailleurs à rapprocher dans une origine commune, plasmocytes, cellules lympho-plasmocytaires et lymphocytes proprement dit.

Enfin, l'existence de ces lésions cutanées ne paraît pas être un argument de pronostic quant à l'évolution de la maladie de Waldenström puisqu'elle a été très différente chez nos deux malades, apparemment résolutive chez l'un, sévère chez l'autre.

Esquisse de la physionomie de l'angio-sarcomatose de Kaposi en Algérie
(A propos de 25 observations personelles)

F. G. MARILL, E. HADIDA et J. SAYAG, Clinique Dermatologique, Marseille (France)

Depuis une vingtaine d'années, l'attention des milieux médicaux est attirée sur les caractères que l'angio-sarcomatose de Kaposi revêt en Afrique noire, assez particuliers pour avoir provoqué la tenue à Kampala, en 1961, d'un *Symposium* consacré à l'étude de cette question. A partir des travaux présentés à ces assises, il s'est établi que la maladie de Kaposi comporte effectivement, lorsqu'elle affecte les Noirs résidant en Afrique infra-saharienne, des modalités qui ne sont pas habituellement les siennes en d'autres contrées. Nous avons donc pensé qu'il serait intéressant, en nous fondant sur 25 observations personnelles, d'esquisser l'image de l'angio-sarcomatose en Algérie, c'est à dire dans un pays d'Afrique septentrionale et de population en presque totalité blanche et méditerranéenne.

Sur les 25 malades en question, à savoir 24 hommes et 1 femme, 17 étaient âgés de 50 à 73 ans, dont 10 de 67 à 73 ans; 2 seulement étaient des hommes jeunes: 20 et 28 ans; un seul adolescent de 15 ans; aucun enfant. Pour 24 de ces patients, la première localisation s'était établie sur les membres et plus spécialement, pour

20 d'entre eux, sur les extrémités, avec une nette prédilection pour les pieds. Ces premières manifestations n'offraient le plus généralement aucune particularité méritant d'être citée.

Passé quelques mois, les altérations cutanées se présentaient sous les deux aspects bien connus d'éléments angiomateux et de verrucosités plus ou moins volumineuses, s'associant selon des combinaisons variables, siégeant électivement sur les membres, et sur leurs extrémités. Ces lésions n'étaient ulcérées que chez cinq malades: ulcérations peu étendues et peu profondes. Seuls deux patients portaient des tumeurs. L'œdème constituait un symptôme d'accompagnement très fréquent, présent chez 17 sujets. Retenons l'atteinte de la muqueuse buccale dans deux cas.

Certaines manifestations laissaient admettre la notion d'une extension profonde du processus angio-sarcomateux: chez un malade, tumeur du larynx histologiquement vérifié et aire d'hypervascularisation du trigone vésical; chez cinq autres, images radiologiques d'altérations osseuses allant de l'aspect d'ostéolyse en mailles à celui d'érosion; chez trois autres encore, adénopathies inguinales, solitaires ou associées à des adénopathies médiastinales, l'évolution, chez l'un de ces sujets, s'étant orientée dans la voie du sarcome vrai.

Du contexte clinique peu de faits intéressants sont à citer: association au diabète sucré; tuberculose pulmonaire évolutive chez un adolescent; insuffisance cardiaque rapidement progressive, peut-être favorisée par la compression de l'artère pulmonaire par une adénopathie médiastinale; enfin, sur le plan dermatologique, association à un vitiligo.

Les examens biologiques de routine n'ont fait apparaître aucune donnée particulière.

Pour ces 25 observations nous avons pratiqué 36 biopsies cutanées et une biopsie ganglionnaire. L'aspect histologique est tout à fait classique sur 28 préparations. Les lésions suivantes s'associent à des degrés divers: prolifération angiomateuse capillaire et lymphatique, prolifération fibroblastique, infiltrat inflammatoire polymorphe, hémorragies récentes ou anciennes sous forme d'hématies ou d'hémosidérine (PERLS ou TURNBULL). L'image est également typique au niveau du ganglion kaposien. Dans huit cas, le microscope montre des lésions angio-granulomateuses qui ne permettraient pas d'affirmer l'angiosarcomatose de Kaposi, si l'aspect clinique ne s'accordait avec cette hypothèse ou si des biopsies itératives ne venaient confirmer ultérieurement le diagnostic. Par conséquent, pas de physionomie histologique qui soit particulière à la maladie de Kaposi rencontrée en Algérie.

De ces 25 sujets, 19 ont été soumis à une antibiothérapie, 17 par pénicilline, à des doses totales comprises pour 10 entre 40 et 120 millions d'unités, et avec, pour 8, association à divers autres antibiotiques: aucune action n'a été constatée sur les lésions cutanées, sauf dans un cas où le seul effet se serait marqué par l'affaissement d'une grosse tubérosité. Les seuls résultats favorables, encore que temporaires, ont été obtenus de la radiothérapie.

Sauf dans un cas où l'angio-sarcomatose s'est transformée cliniquement et histologiquement au point d'évoquer la sarcomatose vraie, elle a évolué chez tous les autres malades sous une forme lente. Deux malades seulement ont été vus dans les 3 mois qui ont suivi l'apparition des premières lésions cutanées; 14 ont été examinés de 2 à plusieurs années après le début de leur maladie; 5 ont été revus dans les délais allant de 1 à 6 ans après le premier examen: dans aucun cas la progression des accidents n'a adopté une allure alarmante.

Pour en terminer, deux séries d'indications chiffrées s'agencent pour donner une notion de la fréquence de l'angio-sarcomatose en Algérie. De 1950 à 1961, soit en 12 années, nous avons reçu dans deux services hospitaliers très spécialisés, à Alger et à Constantine, sur un total de 18637 patients présentant des affections cutanées diverses, 18 sujets atteints de maladie de Kaposi, et 396 malades porteurs d'épithélioma de la peau. De 1950 à 1960, soit en 11 années, J. BRÉHANT et Mme J. MUSSINI-MONTPELLIER font état de quatre cas d'angio-sarcomatose sur les 7849 tumeurs malignes détectées par l'ensemble du Réseau algérien de lutte contre le cancer, parmi lesquelles 6597 épithéliomas et 511 sarcomes au total, et 2210 tumeurs malignes de la peau.

En définitive donc, il semble bien que l'angio-sarcomatose de Kaposi revêt en Algérie, par l'ensemble de ses manifestations, la forme qu'il est classique de lui reconnaitre en Europe.

Intérêt de la lymphographie dans les hématodermies

M. DANA, R. BOURDON, V. BISMUTH et J. P. DESPREZ-CURELY, Service Central de Radiologie, Hôpital St. Louis, Paris (France)

La participation du système lymphatique au cours des hématodermies est une notion bien connue. C'est le cas en particulier au cours de la Maladie de Hodgkin, des réticulo et lymphosarcomes, des leucémides, du mycosis fongoïde et de la Maladie de Kaposi. Ces atteintes ganglionnaires posent plusieurs problèmes que la lymphographie permet dans une certaine mesure de résoudre.

1. Celui de leur dépistage: si des adénopathies superficielles sont faciles à déceler, il n'en est pas de même des localisations profondes, en dehors des cas où elles entraînent des signes indirects (compressions vasculaires, douleurs, déviation ou compression d'un organe).

2. Celui de leur nature: en effet, la découverte de ganglions ne signifie pas forcément le caractère spécifique, car il peut s'agir de ganglions inflammatoires, en particulier liés au grattage. Les aspects lymphographiques actuellement bien connus permettent souvent de différencier la nature tumorale, hémoréticulopathique ou simplement inflammatoire d'un ganglion [4]. C'est ainsi que la lymphographie permet avec moins de 10% d'erreur de distinguer: ganglion normal, ganglion inflammatoire, sarcomatose ganglionnaire, leucose chronique, lymphogranulomatose maligne. Ceci est d'autant plus intéressant que quelquefois il n'y a pas de lésion superficielle accessible à l'histologie, ou il n'y a à la biopsie que des lésions douteuses ou non spécifiques. L'histologie des ganglions elle-même est sujette à une erreur de 10% comme l'a montré la lecture à l'aveugle faite au Symposium International sur la Maladie de Hodgkin en 1965 à Paris [11].

3. Celui de l'extension de la Maladie: il semble exister une relation entre l'extension anatomique de la maladie lors de la première poussée et son pronostic. On a ainsi démontré que les formes loco-régionales de Maladie de Hodgkin sans atteinte de l'autre côté du diaphragme ont un bien meilleur pronostic que les formes étendues [9 à 11]. La même notion semble valable pour les lympho et réticulosarcomes [5].

4. Celui de leur traitement. La lymphographie est un document précieux pour le radiothérapeute qui peut ainsi dessiner avec exactitude des champs prenant l'ensemble des ganglions pathologiques et épargnant au maximum les organes sains [3].

5. Celui de leur surveillance après traitement. La surveillance des ganglions opacifiés par lymphographie permet de dépister précocément une récidive [3, 4].

Résultats de la lymphographie au cours des Hématodermies à l'Hôpital Saint-Louis

Nous ne nous étendrons pas sur la technique d'opacification des lymphatiques [7], ni sur les incidents minimes et rarissimes (sur 2000 lymphographies) moyennant quelques précautions [6]. La critique concernant le risque théorique d'une dissémination ne paraît pas devoir être prise en considération: l'injection se fait non dans la tumeur, mais dans un lymphatique sain indépendant d'elle; même s'il existe une atteinte ganglionnaire, l'injection poussée avec douceur n'entraîne pas plus de risque de dissémination qu'il n'en existe spontanément, la légère pression de la seringue n'étant pas transmise aux ganglions grâce à l'élasticité des lymphatiques; la rupture des lymphatiques est un accident rare dû à une injection trop rapide. Du reste, sur les dizaines de milliers de lymphographies pratiquées dans le monde, aucune n'apporte une observation indiscutable de dissémination par la lymphographie, telle que métastases du parenchyme pulmonaire succédant à une miliaire lipiodolée.

1. Dans six cas de Leucose Lymphoïde Chronique avec manifestations cutanées, nous avons observé dans tous les cas une atteinte massive et globale des chaînes ganglionnaires profondes lombaires et iliaques. La persistance de l'opacification pendant plusieurs mois ou années permet de suivre l'évolution et en particulier la régression sous chimiothérapie.

2. Dans la Maladie de Hodgkin. Dans six cas, il s'agit de L.G.M. certaine — la lymphographie montre cinq fois sur six une atteinte ganglionnaire profonde. Sur l'ensemble des cas de Maladie de Hodgkin ayant subi cet examen (156 cas) on note la fréquence suivante d'atteinte profonde décelée à la lymphographie [1, 2].

	Nombre	Lymphographies pathologiques
Formes sus diaphragmatiques		
Stade I	29	7 (20%)
Stade II	36	20 (38%)
Formes sous diaphragmatiques		
Stade I	2	2
Stade II	1	2
F. sus et sous diaphragmatiques		
Stade III	57	34

Ceci montre la très grande fréquence des atteintes ganglionnaires profondes dans les formes sous diaphragmatiques. Il montre aussi qu'une très forte proportion de formes apparemment locales ou loco-régionales sus diaphragmatiques sont en réalité des formes diffuses (20 à 38%). La méconnaissance de ces atteintes à distance conduisant à des échecs thérapeutiques.

3. Nous avons également pratiqué des lymphographies au cours d'autres Hématodermies. 1 cas de mycosis fongoïde: aspect normal; 1 cas de Réticulose Histiocytaire Maligne: aspect normal; 1 cas de réticulosarcome: aspect normal; 1 cas de Maladie de Kaposi: l'aspect est pathologique, mais très particulier, intermédiaire entre celui de la Maladie de Hodgkin et les aspects inflammatoires: ganglions augmentés de volume, à contours polycycliques, d'opacification piquetée, mais de façon grossière et irrégulière avec des micro-lacunes; 1 cas de sarcoïdose de Besnier-Boeck-Schaumann montrant également un aspect atypique.

Bibliographie. 1. BISMUTH, V., J. BERNAGEAU, J. P. DESPREZ-CURELY et R. BOURDON: Sem. Hôp. Paris 40, 2311 (1964). — 2. BOURDON, R., J. P. DESPREZ-CURELY, V. BISMUTH. M. DANA et P. MARKOVITS: N.R.F.H. 6, 32 (1966). — 3. DANA, M., J. P. DESPREZ-CURELY. V. BISMUTH et R. BOURDON: J. Radiol. Électrol. 47, 804 (1966). — 4. DANA, M., J. P. DESPREZ-CURELY, V. BISMUTH et R. BOURDON: Ann. Radiol. 7, 555 (1964). — 5. DANCOT, H.: Influence de la radiothérapie sur l'évolution des lympho et des réticulosarcomes. J. Radiol. A paraître. — 6. DESPREZ-CURELY, J. P., V. BISMUTH, A. LAUGIER et J. DESCAMPS: Ann. Radiol. 5, 577 (1962). — 7. DESRPEZ-CURELY, J. P., et V. BISMUTH: Coeur et Médecine intern. 3, 369 (1964). — 8. DUPERRAT, B., R. BOURDON, J. P. DESPREZ-CURELY, J. D. PICARD et M. DANA: Bull. Soc.

franç. Derm. Syph. **70**, 932 (1960). — 9. KAPLAN. H. S.: Radiology **78**, 553 (1962). — 10. PETERS, V., and K. C. H. MEDDLEMISS: Amer. J. Roentgenol. **79**, 114 (1958). — 11. Symposium International sur la radiothérapie de la Maladie de Hodgkin (Paris, le 15. 2. 65). J. Radiol. **47**, 1 (1966).

Radiothérapie des hémoréticulopathies malignes

R. BOURDON et M. DANA, Service Central de Radiologie, Hôpital St. Louis, Paris (France)

Au cours des Hématodermies, le traitement fait souvent appel à l'irradiation des localisations cutanées, celle-ci est faite selon des modalités classiques (Mycosis fongoïde, leucémides, Maladie de Kaposi, réticulose maligne, Maladie de Hodgkin) avec un rayonnement dont la pénétration est adaptée à l'épaisseur des lésions [1, 2].

Mais la pratique systématique des lymphographies a montré la fréquence des atteintes ganglionnaires profondes [10]. Il semble dès lors logique d'en faire l'irradiation chaque fois qu'elles sont mises en évidence. Une autre notion semble se dégager: certaines de ces affections comme la maladie de Hodgkin semblant se propager de proche en proche, il semble préférable d'irradier non seulement le territoire ganglionnaire atteint, mais les territoires voisins. Ces irradiations sont réalisées au mieux par télécobalthérapie par grands champs, qui permet malgré se difficulté une grande rigueur et évite les risques de sur et sous dosage à la jonction de petits champs jointifs [3, 4].

Des gamma-radiographies de contrôle (figures) sont faites avec le rayonnement même du Cobalt 60 pour vérifier que les limites de l'irradiation sont satisfaisantes.

Si l'atteinte cutanée est limitée et localisée, l'irradiation vigoureuse de l'ensemble des territoires ganglionnaires tributaires fait espérer la guérison dans certains cas de cette maladie. En effet, ces traitements semblent apporter près de 50% de guérison à 10 ans dans les formes loco-régionales de la Maladie de Hodgkin [5, 6, 7, 9, 10, 11].

Bibliographie. 1. BOURDON, R., M. DANA, F. BEIX et D. FLORI: Clinique (Paris) **LXI**, 619 (1966). — 2. DANA, M.: Presse méd. **23**, 1143; **24**, 1207. — 3. DANA, M., R. BIGOT et R. BOURDON: Rev. méd. **11**, 585 (1966). — 4. DANA, H., J. P. DESPREZ-CURELY, V. BISMUTH et R. BOURDON: J. Radiol. Electrol. **47**, 804 (1966). — 5. EASSON, E. C., and M. H. RUSSEL: Brit. med. J. **1**, 704; **2**, 114, 115 (1963). — 6. JELLIFFE, A. M.: Clin. Radiol. **16**, 274 (1965). — 7. KAPLAN, H. S.: Radiology **78**, 553 (1962). — 8. LAUGIER, A., H. J. SCHLIENGER, G. JULLIARD et R. LE FUR: Rev. Prat. (Paris) **XVI**, 895 (1966). — 9. PETERS, V., and K. C. H. MEDDLEMISS: Amer. J. Roentgenol. **79**, 114 (1958). — 10. Symposium International sur la radiothérapie de la Maladie de Hodgkin (Paris 10 15. 2. 65). Radiol. **47**, 1 (1966). — 11. TUBIANA, M., A. J. LAUGIER, M. J. SCHLIENGER et G. JUILLARD: Rev. Prat. (Paris) **16**, 911 (1966).

Cosmetology; Biology and Pathology of the Hair

Cosmétologie; biologie et pathologie du cheveu

Cosmética; biología y patología del cabello

Kosmetik; Biologie und Pathologie des Haarwachstums

Organizer

M. B. Sulzberger, USA

Presidents

A. A. Cordero, Argentina

I. T. Ingram, Great Britain

A. Rostenberg, USA

S. Shuster, Great Britain

Delegate of the Organization Committee

Fr. Herrmann, Germany

Cosmetology

Reports

Recherches sur le mécanisme d'action des antiperspirants* **

R. Brun, N. Hunziker et P. Evdos, Clinique Universitaire de Dermatologie, Genève (Suisse)

Quoique les antiperspirants à action locale (parasympatholytiques exclus) soient utilisés très couramment par le grand public, le mécanisme par lequel ils suppriment ou diminuent la sécrétion sudorale est encore problématique. D'une manière générale on admet que cet effet est dû à l'action astringente des antiperspirants. On constate effectivement que tous les produits qui sont connus pour leur efficacité dans ce domaine sont des astringents, c'est-à-dire des substances qui dénaturent les protéines par un processus physico-chimique. Partant de là, on peut se demander si tous les astringents ont une action anhidrotique sur la peau. Nos expériences résumées dans le tableau montrent que ce n'est pas le cas et que même des produits reconnus pour leur très forte action dénaturante sur le protéines n'ont pas d'activité antisudorale (par ex. acide sulfosalicylique, acide phosphotungstique). Donc il semble bien que si la propriété de dénaturer les protéines est nécessaire, elle n'est pas la seule en cause dans ce phénomène.

Tableau. *Effet anhidrotique de certains produits appliqués localement sur le bras*

	Conc.	Nombre de cas	Transpiration par rapport au contrôle		
			égale	diminuée	annulée
Chlorure d'aluminium	Mol.	33	1	17	15
Sulfate d'aluminium	Mol.	6	6	—	—
Nitrate d'aluminium	Mol.	5	—	3	2
Acéto-tartrate d'Al	10%	5	4	1	—
Chlorure de magnésium	Mol.	8	4	2	2
Acide phosphotungstique	Sat.	5	5	—	—
Acide sulfosalicylique	10%	4	4	—	—
Acide tannique	10%	3	3	—	—
Acide trichloracétique	5%	12	—	3	9

En 1949, Sulzberger, Zak et Herrmann montraient qu'après traitement des aisselles par une crème au sulfate d'aluminium et démonstration de la réduction nette de la transpiration axillaire, on décèle histologiquement des altérations au niveau des acini: inflammation, désintégration de l'épithélium, résidus cellulaires dans les canaux. Il est cependant curieux de constater que ce phénomène est limité aux acini des glandes sudoripares apocrines. En effet, les acini des glandes eccrines sont tout à fait normaux selon ces auteurs et ce n'est que la partie supérieure du canal excréteur des glandes eccrines qui présente quelques altérations.

En ce qui nous concerne, nous n'avons pas constaté d'altérations des glandes eccrines dans des biopsies prélevées sur des emplacements de la peau glabre traités au chlorure d'aluminium et où l'anhidrose totale ou presque avait été démontrée auparavant par des tests.

* Recherches sur la transpiration. 17ème comm.
** Ce travail a bénéficié d'un subside du Fonds National Suisse de la Recherche Scientifique.

A la suite des travaux de O'BRIEN sur les divers types de miliaria, l'hypothèse de l'occlusion des pores (poral closure) pour expliquer l'état d'anhidrose due aux antiperspirants fut invoquée par de nombreux auteurs. Commentant les travaux de SHELLEY en particulier, lequel démontra que de nombreux facteurs physiques ou chimiques pouvaient provoquer l'anhidrose, ROTHMAN pense que l'hyperkératose est une réaction générale de réponse à bien des agressions modérées au cours desquelles la peau est irritée.

L'irritation, c'est-à-dire l'inflammation, serait donc à la base du phénomène de l'hyperkératose qui provoque l'occlusion des pores.

La question du mécanisme d'action de ces antiperspirants n'est pas encore résolue et il nous a semblé que d'autres types d'expériences pourraient faire avancer la solution de ce problème.

Nous avons par exemple appliqué du chlorure d'aluminium sur le flanc du cobaye et, effectivement, ce traitement provoque la formation d'une forte hyperkératose accompagnée d'acanthose (Fig. 1a). Cette expérience parle en faveur de la capacité de ce produit de modifier la kératinisation et éventuellement de provoquer chez l'homme, par extension, l'occlusion des pores.

Ceci est d'autant plus remarquable que le sulfate d'aluminium, contrairement au chlorure, s'est montré inefficace dans nos expérience sur l'inhibition de la sudation sur le bras de l'homme. Or, parallèlement, ce sulfate n'a provoqué ni hyperkératose, ni acanthose, chez le cobaye (Fig. 1b). Avec ces deux sels d'aluminium, on constate une corrélation frappante entre l'effet anhidrotique chez l'homme et l'action kératogène chez le cobaye.

Enfin, nous aimerions insister sur une curieuse constatation faite chez l'homme:

En 1957, nous avons remarqué que si l'effet anhidrotique du chlorure d'aluminium était constaté régulièrement sur les personnes âgées de moins de 60 ans, par contre cet effet était quasiment nul si l'âge des sujets de l'expérience dépassait 60 ans.

Ce phénomène pourrait également parler en faveur de l'hypothèse de l'occlusion des pores à condition d'admettre qu'à partir d'un certain âge la peau de l'homme perd sa capacité de réagir en produisant cette kératose particulière qui mène à l'occlusion des canaux excréteurs.

Enfin, reprenant partiellement les expériences de PAPA et KLIGMAN, nous avons effectué sur des emplacements rendus anhidrotiques par le chlorure d'aluminium un stripping de la couche cornée jusqu'à la couche luisante. Si quelques cas montrèrent bien après ce stripping un rétablissement de la sécrétion sudorale, ceci en accord avec l'hypothèse de bouchons cornés superficiels, nous fûmes surpris de constater que dans la majorité de nos sujets d'expérience, le stripping ne modifie pas l'anhidrose provoquée par le chlorure d'aluminium. Ceci semble démontrer que si l'anhidrose est provoquée par l'occlusion du canal de la glande, il ne s'agit pas obligatoirement d'un bouchon corné superficiel.

D'un autre côté, il nous a paru intéressant d'étudier parallèlement à nos travaux avec le chlorure d'aluminium un autre produit qui selon PAPA et KLIGMAN a également une action anhidrotique: l'acide trichloracétique. Utilisant non pas la méthode des compresses sous pansement plastique imperméable, mais l'application biquotidienne pendant 2 jours de la solution d'acide trichloracétique à 5% dans l'eau au moyen d'un tampon, comme nous l'avions fait pour le chlorure d'aluminium, nous avons effectivement constaté sur le bras une très bonne action anhidrotique de ce produit (Fig. 2a). Contrairement à ce que l'on pourrait penser, ce traitement ne provoque aucune irritation, ce qui n'est pas le cas avec le chlorure d'aluminium. Par contre, tandis que ce dernier avait provoqué sur le cobaye une forte acanthose, accompagnée d'hyperkératose, il n'en est rien de l'acide trichloracétique qui visiblement ne modifie pas la peau du cobaye ni macroscopiquement, ni histologiquement (Fig. 1c).

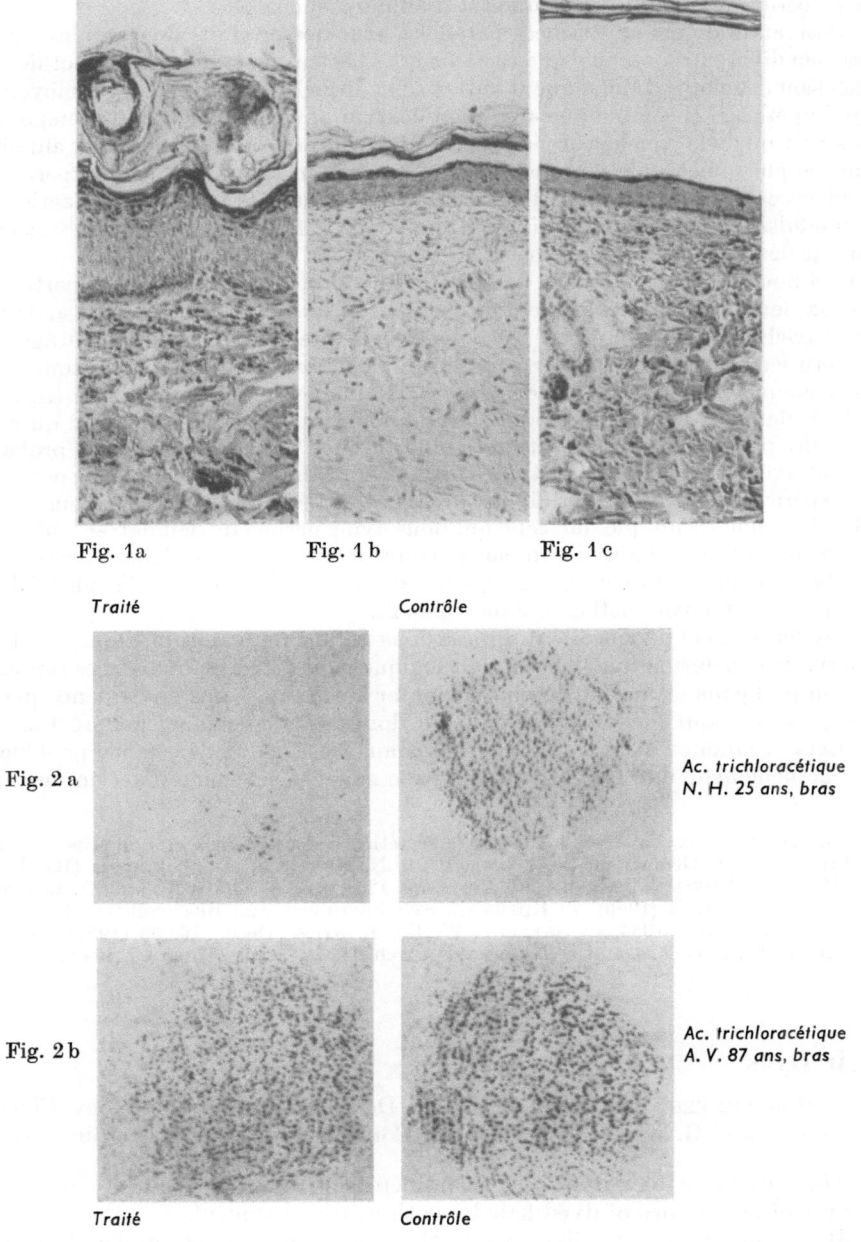

Fig. 1a   Fig. 1b   Fig. 1c

Traité   *Contrôle*

Fig. 2a

Ac. trichloracétique
N. H. 25 ans, bras

Fig. 2b

Ac. trichloracétique
A. V. 87 ans, bras

Traité   *Contrôle*

Malgré son manque d'effet hyperkératosique chez le cobaye, l'acide trichloracétique produit le même phénomène d'absence d'activité anhidrotique sur les personnes de plus de 60 ans (Fig. 2b), phénomène déjà constaté avec le chlorure d'aluminium. Enfin reprenant avec l'acide trichloracétique les expériences de stripping de la peau du bras traité, on constate que si sur la moitié des sujets on rétablit bien la fonction sudorale, sur l'autre moitié par contre, l'enlèvement de la couche cornée ne modifie en rien l'état d'anhidrose locale.

Ainsi, au fil de ces expériences parallèles avec des produits de formules chimiques bien différentes, on voit que certains faits parlent en faveur de l'hypothèse de l'occlusion des pores, tandis que d'autres sont difficiles à interpréter au moyen de cette hypothèse. Il semble que si la modification apportée par les antiperspirants à la structure de la couche cornée superficielle peut être la cause de l'effet anhidrotique, ce phénomène n'est probablement pas seul en cause. D'autres expériences seront nécessaires pour tenter d'élucider complètement le mécanisme d'action de ces produits antiperspirants qui, est-il besoin de le rappeler, sont utilisés chaque jour par des millions de personnes.

Ceci nous montre qu'à côté de l'intérêt théorique que peuvent comporter ces travaux, leur aspect pratique ne doit pas pour autant être négligé. C'est ainsi que l'acide trichloracétique présente du point de vue pratique plusieurs avantages sur le chlorure d'aluminium. En particulier celui de n'être pas irritant et surtout de ne pas provoquer une destruction des étoffes, comme le démontre le scorch-test.

Mais dans ce domaine pratique, c'est surtout au niveau de l'aisselle qu'il est nécessaire de démontrer une activité anhidrotique. Vu les résultats très probants obtenus avec l'acide trichloracétique sur la peau glabre, nous avons donc entrepris des expériences avec ce produit au niveau des aisselles. Pour cela nous avons utilisé la même technique que celle qui nous avait permis de démontrer l'effet très efficace du chlorure d'aluminium sur la transpiration axillaire. Mais, contre toute attente et malgré l'adjonction d'un agent tensio-actif à la solution*, l'acide trichloracétique s'est montré inefficace dans l'aisselle.

Ces dernières expériences entreprises dans un but purement pratique n'ont pas abouti à la conclusion que l'on pouvait logiquement attendre. Mais elles représentent un problème et un fait de plus à ajouter à ceux déjà mis en évidence par les divers auteurs qui ont travaillé dans ce domaine. Cependant, malgré tous ces résultats accumulés depuis de nombreuses années, il ne nous est pas possible de tirer actuellement une conclusion définitive sur le mécanisme d'action des antiperspirants.

Littérature. BRUN, R.: Recherches sur la sécrétion sudorale et la sécrétion sébacée. Thèse No 1219, Univ. de Genève 1954. — BRUN, R., u. N. HUNZIKER: Dermatologica (Basel) **114**. 177 (1957). — O'BRIEN, J. P.: Brit. J. Derm. **59**, 125 (1947). — PAPA, C., and A. KLIGMAN: J. invest. Derm. **47**, 1 (1966). — ROTHMAN, ST.: Physiology and Biochemistry of the Skin. Chicago: Univ. Press 1954. — SHELLEY, W. B.: J. invest. Derm. **16**, 53 (1951). — SULZBERGER, M. B., F. G. ZAK and F. HERRMANN: Arch. Derm. Syph. (Chic.) **60**, 404 (1949).

Hair Dyes

A. ROSTENBERG, University of Illinois, Department of Dermatology, Chicago, Illinois, and G. KASS, Alberto-Culver Company, Melrose Park, Illinois (USA)

The variety of hair dyes and their increasing usage continue to proliferate because of acceptance of dyed hair by both men and women.

Hair colorants can be divided into three categories: 1. vegetable, 2. mineral, 3. organic (synthetic).

---

* Nous remercions vivement le Dr. W. WEISS, Koblenz, de nous avoir conseillé et procuré du Sulfetal C 90, mouillant compatible avec l'acide trichloracétique.

The first two of these are, to a large measure, obsolete. The only vegetable dye that is still occasionally used is henna, a derivative from a shrub which grows in the mid-east (Lawsonia spp.). Henna is probably the safest of hair dyes; but, unfortunately, produces an artificial, unappealing shade of red. It is to be emphasized that henna produces only a red color. If a hair colorant produces a color other than red it is either not henna or it is henna plus something else.

Practically the only mineral dye still in use is lead. This is marketed as a solution of lead acetate. The product is to be brushed on the hair, producing a film of lead sulfide, which gradually darkens it; consequently, these dyes are known as progressive dyes. The advantages of these dyes is that they can be used in the home, they are easy to apply, they are quite safe; but they yield only drab, unnatural shades of brown.

This then brings us to the organic, or synthetic, dyes, which completely dominate the market. These can be divided into three sub-groups, namely: permanent, semi-permanent, and temporary.

Tab. 1 illustrates in a synoptic form the salient features of the color materials in each category.

Table 1

Permanent	Semi-Permanent	Temporary
Dye intermediate	Complete dye — many textile dyes	Complete dye — many acid rinses
Oxidation	No oxidation	No oxidation
Deep penetration	Modest penetration	Surface coating
All shades	Deficient in black or browns	Deficient in blacks or browns
Can bleach and dye simultaneously	Must pre-bleach	Must pre-bleach
Same color on virgin and non-virgin hair	Requires special formulation for non-virgin hair	Same color on virgin and non-virgin hair
Lasts until hair grows out	Lasts 4 to 5 shampoos	Lasts 1 shampoo
1 reaction in 50,000 or more applications	1 reaction in 100,000 or more applications Safety of solvents ?	Safe as use certified dyes

The permanent dyes, which are also known as oxidation type dyes, are the oldest category of organic hair dyes and, consequently, the one with which the greatest experience has been had. Their advantages are that any shade of hair color can be produced, including all natural shades. Further, the hair can be lightened in color at the same time that the dye is applied. These dyes are applied as dye intermediates and require oxidation to produce the color. The usual oxidant is peroxide, often in an ammoniacal solution. By virtue of the small size of the molecules of the dye intermediates, they are able to penetrate between the scales that comprise the outer cuticle of the hair shaft and also enter into the intermicellar spaces, so that they completely permeate the shaft. After oxidation, the molecules are converted into large dye molecules which are trapped within the shaft. This achieves the permanent effect, which is both an advantage and a disadvantage. It is an advantage in that the color will persist throughout an indefinite number of shampoos; but as the hair grows out the newly emerging portion of the hair is of the color that the person was genetically endowed with; and hence a "touch-up job" is required in order to make this portion of the hair blend in. It is a disadvantage in that if the woman wishes to change her hair color she either has to wait until the hair grows out or she has to have the old color bleached. The latter treatment is often quite damaging to the hair, making it quite brittle and also often capricious with respect to further dye applications.

In general, these products are paraphenylenediamine or paratoluylenediamine derivatives; but modern formulations are complicated mixtures with many ingredients.

At one time there was a considerable hazard attached to the use of these dyes; but in our opinion this is no longer the case. Tab. 2 gives the principal reasons for the increased safety of these products.

Table 2. *Increased safety of oxidation hair dyes*

1. Increased purity of dye intermediates
2. Increased efficiency of oxidation
3. Improved technics of application

A conservative estimate is that there is not more than one reaction in 50,000 applications. It is wise — and in the United States mandatory — to do a patch test prior to *each* application of the dye.

For a variety of reasons the cosmetic manufacturer has been endeavoring to develop dyes which will not stay fixed to the hair for as long a period. As Tab. 1 indicates, such dyes can be divided into semi-permanent and temporary; however, the distinction between these two types is less clear-cut than between them and the oxidation type.

The cosmetic chemist has often attempted to use textile dyes for dyeing human hair; but, unfortunately, most textile dyes would not penetrate the hair shaft, except under conditions that are not possible to use on a living person. Recent developments both of the dyes themselves and, more particularly, of solvent mixtures have succeeded in producing products which penetrate at room temperature; and a considerable range of colors in the semi-permanent category has been developed.

The advantage of these dyes is that they will persist through only four or five shampoos, so that the woman can rapidly change her hair color if she so desires. Their disadvantages are that if the woman wishes a lighter shade the hair must be pre-bleached and usually special formulations of the dye are required to produce the desired shade. The absorption and substantivity of a dye is apparently different in bleached hair and in virgin hair. Further, it is not possible to produce natural blacks or browns with these dyes. While there has not been the experience with these dyes that there has been with oxidation type dyes, nevertheless they have had a considerable usage and appear to be quite safe. A conservative estimate is that there is not more than one reaction in 100,000 applications. It is, however, to be realized that this is a developing field and new dyes and new solvent systems will be introduced; and experience alone will determine how safe these products are.

The final category of temporary dyes refers, in general, to dyes that are applied in acid solution; hence, they are often referred to as acid rinses; however, this is not true of all of the dyes in the temporary category. The dyes in this group apparently barely penetrate the shaft, so that they are capable of being removed by one or at most two shampoos. Their advantages and disadvantages are the same as in the semi-permanent dyes. Practically all the dyes in this category are quite safe in that they are dyes that have been certified by the U.S. Food and Drug Administration for use in cosmetics, meaning that extensive toxicologic and dermatologic experience has been had with them.

Free Communications

International Dermatology and the World of Cosmetics

E. W. BRAUER, Clinical Dermatology, New York University Schools of Medicine, New York (USA)

The use of cosmetics and toiletries is as old as recorded time; the magnitude of consumption is directly proportional to the standard of living and the cultural development of a particular society. Beginning modestly with the infant who is introduced to soaps, lubricating and cleansing oils and dusting powders, individual experience soon blooms in both sexes to the employment of sundry preparations for improved hygiene and personal adornment. With the possible exception of clothing, the products of the cosmetic and toiletries industry account for the greatest dermal exposure to the consumer population — by incidence as well as surface area.

Viewed in this light, the record of public safety for this branch of trade is commendable. The credit for this achievement is shared by many.

1. The cosmetic chemist who recognizes the biologic requirements and limitations of the skin and succeeds in formulating products within these dimensions.

2. The pharmacologist who develops practical parameters for measuring and extrapolating biologic response.

3. The dermatologist who understands best the intricate behavior of the skin in health and disease; who offers guidance to others in how to preserve the former by avoiding agents that may lead to the latter; who explains why it is that some agents may cause the skin to react in an unusual manner.

4. Government through its powers of regulation and enforcement achieves compliance from all interested parties for the greater public good.

The extent and degree of governmental control varies widely among nations of the world. Non-uniform, sometimes arbitrary, often archaic, — these regulations may be destructive and self-defeating. As an example, one need only cite the attitude toward hair dyes. In some nations paratoluylene diamine (PTD) is permitted but paraphenylene diamine (PPD) is not. In others, both are allowed. Such contradiction can not be the result of sound, mature, balanced scientific reasoning. The basic structure of these compounds is identical. As one would expect, in sensitized individuals they cross react on skin patch test. Purified materials coupled with refined manufacturing and marketing procedures are responsible for the present low incidence of skin reactions with hair dyes. The same low incidence exists in the PPD countries as in the PTD countries, — except that PTD gives poorer color quality.

While, in the foreseeable future, boundaries between nations will remain, from an economic and scientific viewpoint they have been under erosion for years. For illustration one need only to mention the European Common Market, air-travel between continents at the speed of sound, and the immediate sharing of world-wide events via audio-visual satellite communication.

The modernization of regulatory codes pertaining to cosmetics is inevitable. Revision presently is underway or partially achieved in several countries. Harmonization of such legislation by the Common Market Nations is actually a provision of the Treaty of Rome.

If good regulations are to be written in the future, all interested parties must be consulted and represented at the conference table.

Industry is indirectly represented through the International Federation of Societies of Cosmetic Chemists. The pharmacologists in Europe have organized an advisory Committee on Chronic Toxicity Hazards, also known as Eurotox. Both groups work with governmental agencies. But where are the dermatologists? Advisory medical opinion of only a passive nature is available to governments through the structure of the World Health Organization or the World Medical Association.

In establishing codes to assure the safety of cosmetics and toiletries, questions and problems of particular dermatologic significance do occur. The responsibility for their solution must rest with dermatologists — representatives of International Dermatology. It must not be abdicated to others by default.

As an international body, our reason for existence must go beyond that of exchanging ideas with each other every 5 years. Consideration should be given to the establishment of a permanent working committee. It must be an active unit that functions between Congresses and represents International Dermatology wherever the voice of our special medical discipline is required.

Hormonal and Microbial Influences on the Sebaceous Follicles in Acne

P. E. Pochi, Dept. of Dermatology, Boston University School of Medicine, Boston, Mass. (USA)

The hormonal influence on the sebaceous follicle is principally an androgenic one. The sebaceous gland is stimulated directly and sensitively by endogenous or exogenous androgen. Progesterone, in physiologic amounts, has no detectable effect on the human sebaceous gland. In acne vulgaris, sebaceous gland secretion is found to be greater than normal in most instances. In addition, the more severe cases show greater glandular activity than the less severe cases. Hormonal imbalance has often been mentioned as a possible cause for the increased sebaceous gland activity in acne vulgaris. However, it has been determined that the plasma concentration of testosterone and the 24-h-urinary excretion of testosterone, the body's most potent androgenic steroid, are not increased in patients with acne vulgaris when compared to age-matched normal control subjects. Therefore, the explanation for the increased secretion of sebum in acne is still unknown. In addition, there is no convincing evidence that acne vulgaris is either accompanied by estrogen deficiency or is associated with estrogen deficient states. In fact it has been shown that in males with acne the plasma concentration of estradiol-17-beta and of estrone is significantly higher than in subjects of comparable age without acne. The reason for this abnormal finding is not clear. However, it may possibly be the result of increased adrenal estrogen production in view of the fact that it had been previously demonstrated that acne patients show abnormally high urinary excretion of 17-hydroxycorticosteroids following corticotropin stimulation. Despite the fact that androgen production does not appear to be abnormal in acne, estrogen may be utilized in the therapy of this disease through its suppression of endogenous androgen secretion. In males, such treatment is usually contraindicated because of undesirable feminizing effects which invariably ensue. A convenient method of estrogen treatment is the cyclic use of combined estrogen-progestin ovulation-inhibiting drugs. Sebaceous gland suppression from the estrogen in these agents occurs slowly, and clinical improvement is not usually apparent until at least two or three cycles of drug therapy are completed.

The influence of skin bacteria upon the sebaceous follicle is not entirely clear in relation to the pathogenesis of acne vulgaris. The generally satisfactory response of this disease to the systemic administration of antibacterial agents suggests that a definitive relationship might exist. However, since acne vulgaris is not an infection and since the disorder is often helped by treatment with relatively small doses of antibiotic, the explanation for the antibiotic's beneficial effect in acne is probably a different one from that of an anti-infective action. It has been demonstrated that tetracycline treatment does not decrease the amount of sebum produced by the sebaceous gland. However, it has also been shown that the free fatty acid concentration of the surface sebum is significantly reduced by the oral administration of tetracycline, even in doses as low as 250 mg daily. The same result can be observed with other tetracycline compounds and with erythromycin. However, penicillin and sulfonamides fail to produce this effect. As the free fatty acids are highly irritating to the skin and are likely responsible for the formation of many inflammatory papules and pustules in acne vulgaris, a decrease in their concentration from broad-spectrum antibiotic treatment probably explains why these drugs are effective. The mechanism by which this effect is produced is unknown, but it is possible that the antibiotic acts by inhibiting the intrafollicular resident bacterial population, particularly the anaerobic diphtheroid, *Corynebacterium acnes*. These bacteria, which are sensitive *in vitro* to the action of broad-spectrum antibiotics, possess the capability of releasing free fatty acids from sebum. However, it is also possible that the reduction of the free fatty acid concentration within the sebaceous follicle is not related at all to bacterial suppression but instead is due to other mechanisms such as suppression of esterase activity of the follicular epithelium.

Biology and Pathology of the Human Hair

Reports

Development of the Human Hair Follicle
Biology and Pathology of the Human Hair*

F. SERRI, Department of Dermatology, University of Pavia (Italy)

The earliest development of hair follicles occurs as early as 9 weeks and is manifested as a palisade of cells at various points in the basal layer. These cell aggregates are always accompained by the alignment and concentration of the subjacent mesenchymal cells, which are very rich in alkaline phosphatase. Later, an accumulation of deeply basophilic nuclei in the basal layer forms a slight projection of the epidermis into the dermis. This swelling is free of glycogen and is separated from the dermis by a distinct basal membrane which is PAS positive and diastase resistant. The number of mesenchymal cells and fibroblasts beneath the hair germ increases, forming the anlage of the hair papilla; this will subsequently increase in size and in its content of alkaline phosphatase. Meanwhile, the hair germ becomes larger by a proliferation of its own cells and no longer at the expense of the basal cells of the epidermis. The elongation of the presumptive follicle into the mesenchyme takes an oblique direction, its movement apparently directed by the cluster of mesenchymal cells which accumulate beneath it and around it. The

* This study was partially supported by a grant from C.N.¹R. — Contract N. 115.0633.0.1346.⁴

outermost cells of this peg are columnar and compact with a radial arrangement, the inner cells tend to be arranged longitudinally and are less regularly aligned. As the hair peg develops further, its advancing extremity becomes bulbous and gradually grows around and envelops the mass of mesodermal cells at its base establishing a true papilla. When the hair follicle has attained the bulbous "hair peg" stage, two epithelial swellings of columnar cells appear on the posterior wall. The lower hemispherical, larger one, rich in glycogen, is the bulge to which the arrector pilorum muscle will later become attached. During fetal life the bulge becomes even larger; at the end of fetal life, however, the bulge is very small. The upper swelling, usually smaller than the bulge, but at times more evident in the early stages of development, is the anlage of the sebaceous gland. A third bud above the sebaceous gland, the rudiment of an apocrine gland, later appears on the posterior surface of the follicular infundibulum in many follicles. The anlagen of apocrine glands develop anywhere on the body and not only on the axilla, mons pubis, external auditory meatus, eyelids, circumanal area, areola and nipple of the breast, labia minora, prepuce and scrotum. They are particularly common on the scalp, nape, face, chest, adbomen, back, and legs, both in the Negro and in the Caucasian (SERRI, 1962). As the bulbous hair peg grows downward, the inner cells of the solid cord proliferate upward within the epidermis establishing the anlage of the hair canal above the sebaceous gland and the infundibulum. Meanwhile, the mesodermal cells adjacent to the posterior surface of the hair follicle, where the three knobs are formed, align themselves parallel to that surface at some distance from the bulge. These cells, surrounded by richly metachromatic ground substance, are the anlagen of the arrector pilorum muscle. Later the muscle cells change their direction and make contact with the bulge. At this stage ground substance of the dermis and presumptive hypodermis, and the fatty layer, all contain large amounts of glycogen.

When the anlagen of sebaceous glands appear on the posterior surface of the hair pegs, they are solid hemispherical protuberances composed of columnar or round cells at the periphery, and ovoid or flattened at the center, all containing a moderate amount of glycogen. The size of the anlage is variable according to the region in which the hair follicle is located. At times it is even smaller than the bud of the apocrine gland. Soon the cells in the center of the knob lose glycogen, become larger and acquire a foamy appearance as they accumulate droplets of lipids, and the cytoplasm becomes retiform. This process proceds rapidly from the center to the periphery of the round or flask-shaped gland, with the result that the largest and clearest cells in the center break down and those at the periphery remain unchanged and rich in glycogen. Not all cells undergo sebaceous differentiation.

When the gland is longer, it can be divided into a bulbous part, the head, and a narrower part, the neck, connecting it with the infundibulum of the follicle; the neck is not always clearly visible in the sections. Sebaceous differentiation and decay proceed from the cells of the bulbous part to those in the center of the neck, and finally to the cells of the infundibulum and pilary canal, forming a narrow pathway of lipidized cells, strongly colored with Sudan Black, going up from the sebaceous gland to the epidermis.

In the beginning, however, the gland has no duct. The latter appears first as a ridge-like septum which separates the hair canal from the newly formed keratinizing sebaceous duct. The early appearance of keratohyalin granules and keratin in the cells of the solid cord that grow upward into the epidermis from the infundibulum plays an important role in the formation of the hair canal. The hair canal is often long and pursues a prolonged course through the epidermis. Sometimes, and particularly in the Negro, it is nearly tangential to it. It appears to be an independent formation within the epidermis and present only in fetal skin, at least in its upper part. The lower part will participate in the formation of the "intra-epidermal infundibular unit" of the adult skin.

From their earliest differentiation at 13 to 15 weeks of fetal life, the sebaceous glands are large and functional; the sebum forms a part of the vernix caseosa. Growth of sebaceous buds takes place from the peripheral layer of cells of all portions of the gland. Evidence of this is manifested by the relative frequency of mitoses in these cells. The buds undergo sebaceous differentiation and become new sebaceous units. The gland becomes multiacinar with great variability in size and shape according to the area in which the follicle is located.

At the end of fetal life the sebaceous glands are well developed and large over the entire surface of the skin, but particularly in those areas in which later in adult life there will be the most glandular activity. After birth the size of the sebaceous glands is rapidly reduced and they enlarge and become actively functional again only at puberty.

Several enzymes have been demonstrated in the hair follicles and particularly in the sebaceous glands from early fetal life: amylophosphorylase, acid phosphotase, esterases, succinic dehydrogenase, monoamine oxidase, cytochrome oxidase, aminopeptidase, betaglucoronidase. The presence of so many enzymatic activities is a clear demonstration that the differetiating cell is capable of elaborating a multitude of chemical substances which are involved in the formation of hair and sebum.

(The paper has been illustrated by a large number of color slides.)

Alopecia areata, Basic Notions

G. MORETTI, A. REBORA, E. RAMPINI, F. CROVATO and C. CIPRIANI, Department of Dermatology, University of Genoa (Italy)

In our studies in Hair Biopathology [18, 21, 23, 24] we have also examined some morphofunctional aspects of alopecia areata, both in its "initial", "state", "healing" patches* and in apparently normal contralateral skin [2].

Material and Methods

For each set of investigations the normal or pathologic skin specimens used were obtained from similar sites in subjects of comparable sex and age: a) The total volume of all sebaceous glands annexed to the same two most centrally located follicular groups within each serial section was calculated by means of a histologic-reconstructive technique [22]. b) Fresh frozen sections were stained with an alkaline phosphatase technique to reveal arterioles and capillaries [17, 26]. c) The oxygen uptake $\mu l/h$ in 50 mm^2 of skin surface was gauged with a standard manometric technique [27]. d) Histamine was evaluated with the Feldberg-Loeser chemical-biological [12] and the Johnson microchemical techniques [15]. e) All data were statistically analyzed for SEM and t-test [13].

Results

a) The sebaceous glands' volume (table) in normal and contralateral skin was practically the same; in "state" alopecic skin, however, it was 47% lower. A division by volume into five arbitrary equal groups furthermore revealed a general

---

* Clinically classified according to SABOURAUD [28].

increase of the intermediate sizes in contralateral skin and a definite tendency to disappear in the higher groups in alopecic skin [22].

b) As to the blood vessels, in contralateral skin (Fig. 2) they occasionally revealed some enzymatic diffusion and a loss of sharp contours; these events were

Fig. 1   Fig. 2   Fig. 3

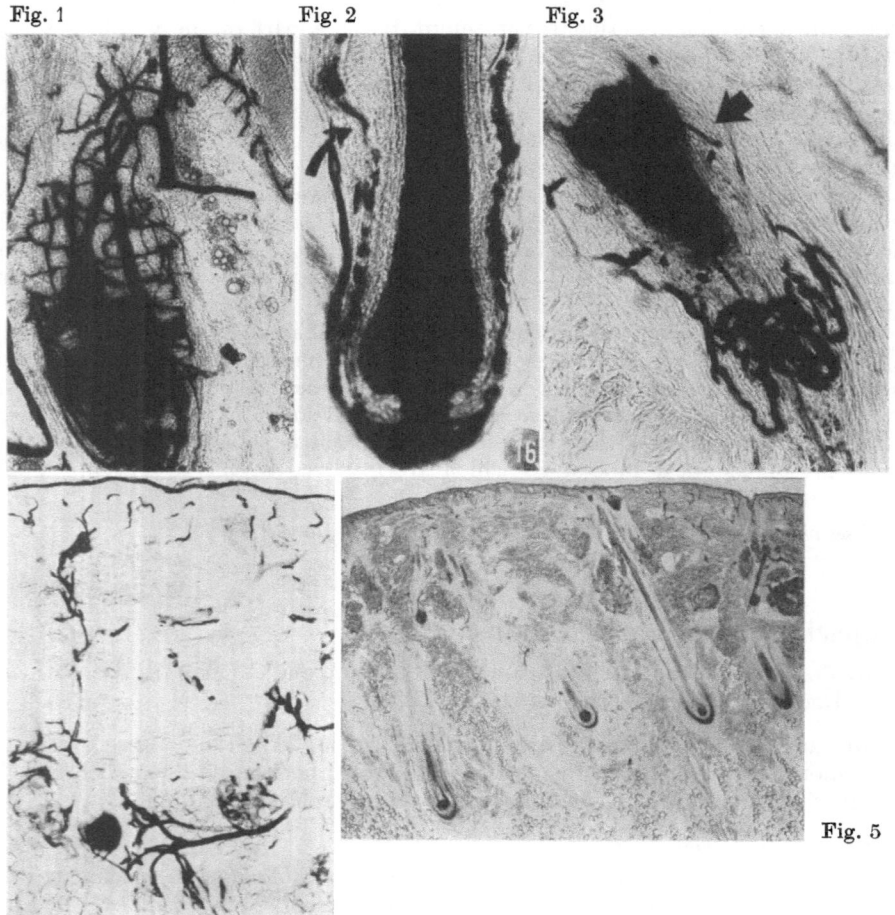

Fig. 5

Fig. 4

chiefly limited to the "transient" perifollicular* and papillary networks surrounding some diversely altered hairs [26]. In the "initial" (Fig. 3) patches the "external vascular belt"** maintains most of its anastomoses with the perifollicular networks, while beneath the hair papillae the so-called "ferment topf" and characteristic "strumpf wendung" aspects [16 to 26] are to be seen.

In "state" (Fig. 4) patches the "transient" perifollicular network disappears either partially or completely; the "external vascular belt"** looses most of the anastomoses with the "permanent" network* of hair whose relatively intact

---

* i.e. the vessels either permanently surrounding the upper third of the follicle or embracing the lower two thirds of growing hairs which disappear in Catagen and Telogen (Fig. 1) [20].
** i.e. all plexuses contained between the dermoepidermal line and the lower papillary dermis [20 to 26].

Table

Stage of Patch (SABOURAUD [28])	Oxygen Uptake		Histamine content				Sebaceous Glands' Volume		
			Feldberg-Loeser (12) technique		Johnson (15) technique				
	Nr. of subjects	μl/h/50 mm²	Nr. of subjects	γ/g d.w.	Nr. of subjects	γ/g f.w.	Nr. of subjects	conventional ml.	Division in Volume Groups (in conventional ml)
Initial	7 (7)	31.2 (48.9)	3 ♀ (4)	24.1 (38.1)	6 (7)	12.5 (22.0)	—	—	
State	7 (7)	30.8 (40.8)	2 ♀ (3)	20.7 (42.6)	2 ♀+ 3 (5)	9.6 (21.3)	8 (10)	107.3 (204.4)	
Healing	5 (5)	42.8 (37.2)	—	—	5 (5)	19.2 (22.1)	—	—	
Contralateral to Initial & State	6 (6)	33.7 (44.5)	2 (7)	24.6 (40.1)	7 (12)	14.2 (21.7)	6 (10)	201.5 (204.4)	
Contralateral to Healing	3 (3)	51.8 (38.4)	—	—	2 (5)	20.0 (22.1)	—	—	

(♀) = pools

conv. ml
0-40
40-80
80-120
120-160
160 and further
0 10 20 30 40 50 60 70 %

withe:
% of glands in normal subjects
grey:
% of glands in contralateral areas
black:
% of glands in "state" patches

Values from normal subjects are given in brackets. For statistical analysis and other informations see: BACCAREDDA-BOY A., et al.: L'alopecia areata. Minerva Derm. vol. 38 (suppl. to Nr. 1), p. 193—405 (1963).

meshes, however, still embrace the miniature follicles [26]. Finally, beneath the highly dystrophic follicles only a ball-shaped intensely reactive papilla is present; this is apparently nourished by a few capillaries originating from the nearest follicular vessels [26]. In "healing" (Fig. 5) patches, the reorganization of the meshes, which is initially restricted to a few fine capillaries and anastomoses with the "external vascular belt", follows the regrowth of corresponding hairs [26].

c) The oxygen uptake (table) in skin contralateral to both "initial" and "state" patches was 24% lower than normal; on the contrary in skin contralateral to "healing" patches it was 35% higher [27].

The "initial" and "state" patches showed respectively a 24% and 36% decrease of oxygen consumption; in "healing" patches the uptake was practically the same as in the control group [27].

d) The histamine content (table) with both methods decreased slightly in skin contralateral to the patches, and revealed a consistently progressive fall in "initial" and "state" patches [19]. With the Johnson method, for instance, histamine levels went from 21 to 22 γ/g f.w. in the control groups to 14.2 in skin contralateral to the "initial" patches and 9.6 in the "state" patches. The amine level tended to return to normality, however, both in the healing patches and in the surrounding hairy skin [19]. The loss of histamine apparently extended beyond the scalp: in four patients with alopecic scalps, the histamine content diminished even in the glabrous and apparently intact skin of the clavicular region; further, within the alopecic areas of three patients with patches on the whole of their skin, the amine level was lower than normal [19].

Discussion

It is to be concluded that in alopecia areata the whole scalp is affected, and perhaps the entire skin participates in the disease.

This is clearly proved by the changed volume of the sebaceous glands, the perifollicular blood vessels' scattered alterations, and the impaired carbohydrate and histamine metabolisms in the apparently healthy skin contralateral to the patches and, outside the scalp area, by the lower skin histamine content. Alopecia "areata" therefore is not at all "areata".

Further, in Area Celsi whenever the predisposing and conditioning local and general factors are present the hair loss or hair growth may be mediated (as perhaps in animals with collective hair growth), either alternatively or simultaneously, by some inhibiting or stimulating metabolites carried through the blood [1, 6, 8, 9, 10, 21].

This seems to be suggested by:

1. The generalized involvement of skin whose morphofunctional alterations are clearly evident even outside the scalp area.

2. The ascertained coexistence of psychic, neurovegetative, hormonal, etc. alterations [3, 7, 11, 25].

3. The gross analogy between hairs' modifications in Alopecia areata and in drug provoked hair loss [4, 29].

Lastly as regards the pathodynamic of the disease, the alterations of perifollicular vessels, and the notable oxygen-uptake decrease as well as the histamine loss, temporarily establish a particular morphofunctional situation within the patch. This is similar to that observed in the skin of some animals when their coat goes simultaneously from anagen to telogen [5]. In fact for some time at least all hairs may be found in telogen even in alopecic patches. Alopecia areata, in other words, becomes, as JACQUET says, a "hair wave in a limited space" [14].

Literature. 1. ARGYRIS, T. S., and B. F. ARGYRIS: Anat. Rec. **142**, 139 (1962). -- 2. BACCAREDDA-BOY, A.: Minerva derm. **38**, 193 (1963). — 3. BERTAMINO, R., E. RAMPINI e G. RUFFINI: Minerva derm. **38**, 342 (1963). — 4. BRAUN-FALCO, O.: Arch. klin. exp. Derm. **212**, 194 (1961). — 5. BRAUN-FALCO, O., e R. RASSNER: Minerva derm. **38**, 235 (1963). — 6. BULLOUGH, W. S., and E. B. LAURENCE: Exp. Cell. Res. **33**, 176 (1964). — 7. CAPPELLI, E.: Minerva derm. **38**, 209 (1963). — 8. CHASE, H. B., and G. J. EATON: Ann. N. Y. Acad. Sci. **83**, 365 (1959). — 9. DAVIS, B. K.: Nature (Lond.) **193**, 1304 (1962). — 10. EBLING, F. J., and G. R. HERVEY: J. Embryol. exp. Morph. **12**, 425 (1964). — 11. FARRIS, G., G. MORETTI e R. BERTAMINO: Minerva derm. **38**, 350 (1963). — 12. FELDBERG, W., and A. A. LOESER: J. Physiol. (Lond.) **126**, 296 (1954). — 13. FISHER, R. A.: Statistical methods for research workers (ital. translt.), Turin: UTET 1948. — 14. JACQUET, L., quoted by A. BACCAREDDA-BOY: Minerva derm. **38**, 404 (1963). — 15. JOHNSON, H. A.: Arch. Derm. Syph. (Chic.) **72**, 307 (1955). — 16. KLINGMÜLLER, G.: Hautarzt **9**, 176 (1958). — 17. MONTAGNA, W., and R. A. ELLIS: J. nat. Cancer Inst. **19**, 451 (1957). — 18. MORETTI, G.: Das Haar In: Die normale und pathologische Physiologie der Haut, by STÜTTGEN, G., S. 506. Stuttgart: Fischer 1965. — 19. MORETTI, G.: Minerva derm. **38**, 322 (1963). — 20. MORETTI, G.: Histology and histochemistry of skin blood vessels In: J. JADASSOHN: Handbuch der Haut u. Geschlechts-Krankh., Erg.-Werk. Berlin-Heidelberg-New York: Springer 1968. — 21. MORETTI, G., C. GIACOMETTI, V. BOIDO, and A. REBORA: J. invest. Derm. **40**, 205 (1963). — 22. MORETTI, G., A. REBORA e E. RAMPINI: Minerva derm. **38**, 246 (1963). — 23. MORETTI, G., A. REBORA, C. GIACOMETTI, V. BOIDO, E. RAMPINI, and C. CIPRIANI: J. invest. Derm. **46**, 231 (1966). — 24. MORETTI, G., C. CIPRIANI, A. REBORA, E. RAMPINI, and F. CROVATO: J. invest. Derm. In press. — 25. MÜLLER, S. A., and R. K. WINKELMANN: Arch. Derm. Syph. (Chic.) **88**, 290 (1963). — 26. RAMPINI, E., G. MORETTI e A. REBORA: Minerva derm. **38**, 290 (1963). — 27. REBORA, A., G. MORETTI e E. RAMPINI: Minerva derm. **38**, 312 (1963). — 28. SABOURAUD, R.: Les pelades et alopécies en aires. Paris: Masson 1929. — 29. VAN SCOTT, E. J.: In: MONTAGNA, W., and R. A. ELLIS: The biology of hair growth. New York: Academic Press 1963.

Klinik und Therapie der Alopecia areata

R. SCHUPPLI, Dermatologische Universitätsklinik Basel (Schweiz)

Obwohl in den letzten Jahren verschiedene zusammenfassende Arbeiten über die Alopecia areata erschienen sind und diese Krankheit auch das Thema verschiedener Kongresse gewesen ist, ist der Fortschritt in der Erkennung der Ursache dieser Krankheit äußerst geringfügig. Abgesehen von der besseren therapeutischen Beeinflußbarkeit einzelner Fälle durch die modernen Arzneimittel, entspricht der Stand unserer Kenntnisse auf diesem Gebiet demjenigen vor Jahrzehnten. Es ist deshalb ein Referat über das Thema der Klinik und Therapie der Alopecia areata unbefriedigend, und es kann sich hier nur darum handeln, neuere Arbeiten kritisch zu sichten und im übrigen schon Bekanntes zu referieren.

Statistische Feststellungen zeigen, daß etwa 2 bis 4% aller Patienten, die zum Dermatologen gehen, ihn wegen einer Alopecia areata aufsuchen. Ein Geschlechtsunterschied läßt sich nicht feststellen. Familiäres Vorkommen wird mit 10% angegeben. Die Alopecia areata ist eine Krankheit der Jugendlichen, 30% aller Fälle treten vor dem 10. Lebensjahr auf. Die totale Alopecia ist bei Kindern häufiger als bei Erwachsenen. Nach dem 60. Lebensjahr ist die Krankheit äußerst selten. Auch bei Haustieren und Wildtieren scheint die Alopecia areata vorzukommen. Diese Beobachtungen dürften für die Beurteilung der Genese von Interesse sein. In gewissen Kollektiven ist die Alopecia areata häufiger. So wurde sie bei 1000 Mongoloiden in 13⁰/₀₀, in Anstalten, in denen psychisch abnorme Kinder, speziell Epileptiker, untergebracht waren, in 2% aller Kinder gefunden.

Das klinische Bild der Alopecia areata ist so bekannt, daß es nicht erörtert zu werden braucht. Daß rein klinisch die Areata in drei Typen — die maligne Form, die Ophiasis oder bandförmige Form und die Areata vulgaris — eingeteilt wird, ist ebenfalls bekannt. Neuartig sind hingegen Versuche, eine Differenzierung der klinischen Formen auf Grund des Verlaufs und der Gesamtsituation vorzunehmen. So unterscheidet IKEDA vier Typen der Alopecia areata: 1. den schnell heilenden, gewöhnlichen Typus, 2. den prähypertonischen Typus, 3. den atopischen Typus und 4. den endokrinen Typus. Diese vier Formen unterscheiden sich durch den Verlauf, indem z. B. der gewöhnliche Typus meist nicht länger als 6 Monate dauert, während die anderen Formen, die mit Störungen interner Organe verbunden sind, länger zu dauern pflegen. Weiter unterscheiden sie sich durch die familiäre Disposition zu Hypertonie, durch die allergische Anamnese, durch Störungen innerer Organe wie Magenulcus und Diabetes. Als Ursache des weitaus häufigsten gewöhnlichen Typus werden psychische Stress-Situationen gefunden, die allerdings sehr vage begründet sind.

Besonderes Augenmerk wird Begleitkrankheiten gewidmet. Dabei ist es sehr schwer, eine statistische Korrelation herauszufinden und festzustellen, ob ein bestimmtes Zusammentreffen der Alopecia areata mit inneren Krankheiten zufällig oder durch eine ätiologische Zusammengehörigkeit bedingt ist. Dies dürfte für die in 7% der Fälle vorhandenen Nagelveränderungen zutreffen. Das Auftreten von Katarakten bei Alopecia areata wird auf eine generalisierte Störung des Ektoderms zurückgeführt. Caries und Foci anderer Art sollen ebenfalls eine Rolle spielen. Bemerkenswert ist der relativ hohe Anteil allergischer Krankheiten bei Kindern mit Alopecia areata totalis. Daraus allerdings abzuleiten, daß es sich bei der Alopecia areata um eine Autoimmunkrankheit handle, ist kaum angängig. Besondere Aufmerksamkeit ist den endokrinen Verhältnissen bei der Alopecia areata geschenkt worden. Die Untersuchungen der Schilddrüsen- und der Ovarialfunktion zeigen meist normale Verhältnisse. Auch die Verwertung der Nebennierenrindenhormone scheint nicht abnorm zu sein. Besonders schwierig sind die Zusammenhänge zwischen vegetativem Nervensystem und Alopecia areata zu objektivieren. Während Untersuchungen des Elektroencephalogramms bei solchen Patienten keine verwertbaren Anomalien ergeben haben, lassen sich histologisch in der Haut degenerative Veränderungen des Vegetativums feststellen. Die Prüfung der Zirkulation zeigt einen veränderten Tonus der peripheren Gefäße und kapillarmikroskopisch einen Spasmus der Capillaren. Schwierig ist die Feststellung des Zusammenhangs psychischer Änderungen und emotioneller Faktoren mit Alopecia areata. Sichere Beobachtungen sind selten, und der Spekulation dafür ein weites Feld offen.

Die Theorie der infektiösen Genese der Alopecia areata erhält durch die Beobachtung von MARSHALL, der eine Alopecia areata nach Zeckenbiß auftreten sah, neuen Auftrieb. Der Nachweis von Staphylokokken im Randgebiet von Areataherden gelang IKEDA in 37 von 80 Fällen. Dies läßt ebenfalls an eine infektiöse Genese denken, obgleich hier zu sagen ist, daß weder externe antibakterielle Therapie noch Antibiotica bei Alopecia areata wirksam sind.

Die Therapie der Alopecia areata hat durch die Applikation von Corticosteroiden eine Bereicherung erfahren, wobei allerdings ihr Effekt kurzdauernd ist und durch eine auf längere Sicht wirksamere Therapie ergänzt werden sollte. Im Prinzip sind sowohl ACTH wie alle Corticoide gleich wirksam, Voraussetzung ist eine genügend hohe Dosis. Deshalb hat sich Dexamethason, das am schnellsten Nebenwirkungen zeigt, am wirksamsten erwiesen. Immerhin ist zu sagen, daß 30% der Patienten auch auf diese Therapie nicht reagieren, während etwa 50% nur zeitweise, solange das Mittel gegeben wird, ansprechen, und nur bei etwa 10 bis 20% aller Fälle ein Dauererfolg erzielt werden kann. Die lokale Behandlung der Alopecia areata mit Fluocinolon unter Okklusivverband hat sich als eine praktisch durchführbare Methode erwiesen. Sie ist wohl den lokalen Cortisoninjektionen vorzuziehen. WEBER hat gesehen, daß die Kombination von Vitamin D intern und

extern von Nicotinsäureestern wesentlich bessere Erfolgschancen hat als langdauernde Corticosteroidtherapie. Die Anwendung von Thyreoideahormon und
anderen Organhormonen hat versagt. Die von italienischen Autoren empfohlene
Therapie mit Bucky-Strahlen dürfte wohl nicht allgemein angewendet werden.

Zusammenfassend muß der Stand unserer Kenntnisse über die Ursache der
Alopecia areata als höchst unbefriedigend bezeichnet werden. Sowohl Grundlagenforschung auf diesem Gebiet als auch eine genaue klinische Beobachtung solcher
Patienten sind notwendig, damit mehr Licht in das Dunkel unserer Kenntnisse
gebracht werden kann.

Literatur. IKEDA, T.: Dermatologica (Basel) **131**, 421 (1965); — Acta derm. (Kyoto) **60**,
118 mit englischer Zusammenfassung (1965). — MARSHALL, J.: Dermatologica (Basel) **135**,
60 (1967). — WEBER, G., u. C. KARNOP: Derm. Wschr. **149**, 457 (1964).

Causes actuelles des alopécies féminines diffuses

E. SIDI †, J. BOURGEOIS-SPINASSE et J. AROUETE, Service de Dermato-Allergie
du Docteur Edwin Sidi Fondation A. de Rothschild, Paris (France)

Mesdames, Messieurs, je vous prie tout d'abord de ne voir en moi que le porte-
parole, ému et reconnaissant, du Docteur EDWIN SIDI, notre Chef de Service si
brusquement disparu il y a quelques mois et qui devait lui-même vous présenter
ce rapport sur les étiologies possibles des alopécies féminines diffuses.

Au cours de ces dernières années, la plupart des dermatologistes, constatant la
fréquence accrue et la chronicité de ces alopécies, se sont attachés à la recherche de
leurs causes. De nombreuses enquêtes ont été conduites notamment par les Doc-
teurs SULZBERGER et WITTEN, et par nous-mêmes depuis 1958. Vous en connaissez
les résultats. Ce rapport n'a donc d'autre objet que de vous rendre compte très
simplement d'une expérience qui se fonde aujourd'hui sur l'observation de plus
de 2.000 malades.

Certes, toutes les statistiques ne sont pas d'égale valeur, mais lorsqu'elles
portent sur de grands nombres, nous pouvons en attendre la confirmation ou le
démenti de nos impressions cliniques.

Ainsi avons-nous pu mettre en évidence la rareté relative des alopécies diffuses
aiguës, puisque 232, soit 11% seulement de nos malades ont présenté des affections datant de moins d'un an. Nous ne parlerons pas d'ailleurs de ces formes
aiguës, profuses certes, parfois même impressionnantes, mais de courte durée et
d'étiologie bien connue, qui surviennent couramment deux mois après une infection aiguë, un accouchement et peuvent être aussi d'origine toxique, syphilitique
ou encore consécutive à une intervention chirurgicale. Elles ont toujours existé et
ne présentent aucune gravité puisqu'elles guérissent spontanément en quelques
mois.

Notre propos est seulement de traiter devant vous de l'étiologie des alopécies
féminines diffuses chroniques, qui durent depuis plusieurs années et représentent
89% des malades venus à notre consultation.

Ces alopécies surviennent le plus souvent chez des jeunes femmes. Voici le
pourcentage établi suivant l'âge d'apparition: 52% entre 20 et 40 ans, avec un
maximum de fréquence de 30 à 35 ans.

Elles s'installent progressivement si lentement même qu'au début la malade ne
s'en inquiète pas, quelquefois sur un cuir chevelu sec, mais le plus souvent après
une séborrhée intense, ainsi 69% de nos malades se sont plaintes d'avoir les

49*

cheveux huileux, agglutinés avant le 5ème jour qui suit le shampooing. On vérifie plus rarement la présence de pityriasis et d'eczéma séborrhéique.

La chute est alors diffuse sur tout le cuir chevelu avec souvent, un éclaircissement plus marqué au niveau des tempes et du vertex où les cheveux repoussent plus grêles. Cet éclaircissement peut même devenir impressionnant et le cuir chevelu apparaît par transparence uniquement recouvert de quelques mèches provenant d'une lisière de cheveux en bordure du front.

Toutefois, dans un petit nombre de cas, 21%, l'alopécie reste uniquement localisée à la région frontopariétale et la séborrhée est alors beaucoup plus rare. Cette photo montre clairement la fréquence de la séborrhée suivant la topographie de l'alopécie.

Quelles sont les causes le plus fréquemment incriminées? Suivant notre statistique, elles se répartissent en gros de la façon suivante:

Causes externes	5%
Etat général	
Amaigrissement	} 9%
Affections chroniques	
Causes endocriniennes	28%
Dystonies neuro-végétatives	46%
Causes indéterminées	12%

Ecartons d'emblée les causes externes, d'ailleurs exceptionnelles puisque nous n'avons pu leur imputer que 5% des cas. On a trop souvent, en effet, attribué aux traumatismes subis par la chevelure des alopécies qui ne sont en réalité que des ruptures du cheveu plus ou moins près de sa racine. Le crêpage, les applications de laque, les permanentes trop frisées, les décolorations successives, les shampooings secs, le tiraillement par des rouleaux ou autre objet destinés à modifier la direction naturelle du cheveu; ne sont responsables que de cassures passagères sans gravité puisqu'il suffit pour y remédier d'éviter le traumatisme originel.

La seule cause externe que l'on puisse incriminer est à notre avis, l'abus des shampooings. Il y a 20 ans les femmes se lavaient les cheveux toutes les 3 ou 4 semaines avec du savon de Marseille ou du savon liquide. Aujourd'hui, en raison sans doute des coiffures modernes, leurs visites chez le coiffeur sont hebdomadaires et surtout les shampooings utilisés sont à base d'alcool gras sulfoné dont l'action détergente bien connue provoque un afflux de séborrhée. Dans l'espoir d'y remédier, elles font des shampooings de plus en plus fréquents. 375 sur 1741 malades, soit 21%, nous ont avoué se laver les cheveux tous les 4 ou 5 jours, certaines même tous les jours. Or, chaque shampooing, chaque dégraissage du cuir chevelu, incite la glande sébacée à secréter à nouveau et celle-ci à la longue s'hypertrophie.

Cette action hypertrophiante de certains shampooings sur les glandes sébacées a d'ailleurs été constatée histologiquement sur l'animal. Après avoir soumis quelques lapins à des shampooings renouvelés tous les deux jours, on s'est aperçu au bout de 3 semaines, soit après dix shampooings environ, que leurs glandes sébacées avaient décuplé de volume.

Mais ces shampooings trop détergents et trop fréquemment répétés, ne font, selon nous, qu'aggraver les alopécies séborrhéiques. Les véritables causes sont internes: parfois un mauvais état général ou un déséquilibre hormonal, bien plus souvent, des troubles neuro-végétatifs.

Certaines affections responsables d'alopécies aiguës passagères peuvent en effet provoquer parfois, des alopécies plus durables et souvent même chroniques, je veux parler de certaines cures d'amaigrissement prolongées obtenues par l'absorption d'amphétamine et de diurétiques, de grossesses trop rapprochées, de certaines affections chroniques, ou de traitements de longue durée par certains médicaments comme les anti-mitotiques.

Diffuses et parfois associées à des troubles des phanères, ces alopécies évoluent souvent sans interruption pendant des mois et ne s'améliorent que lentement avec la reprise d'un meilleur état général. Toutefois, ces diverses causes demeurent très rares et ne sont à considérer, nous l'avons vu que dans 9% des cas.

Les causes endocriniennes paraissent beaucoup plus fréquentes. Elles seraient, d'après nos observations, responsables de 28% des cas.

Personne ne conteste d'ailleurs l'importance des sécrétions hormonales dans la physio-pathologie du système pileux: il est bien connu que certains syndromes endocriniens tels que les déséquilibres thyroïdiens, hypophysaires ou surrénaux s'accompagnent d'alopécie, parfois même d'une raréfaction de tout le système pileux ou d'hypertrichose. En particulier le rôle de la sécrétion d'androgènes a toujours été considérée comme essentielle dans l'alopécie séborrhéique de l'homme jeune. Chez la femme, bien que nous ayons très rarement pu mettre en évidence une augmentation des stéroïdes urinaires — 6 cas sur 41 — nous pensons que cette dysendocrinie peut également être responsable de certaines alopécies. Le Docteur REINBERG qui s'est occupé de ces dosages de notre Service considère que la quantité de testostérone produite par un ovaire pathologique peut être suffisante pour déterminer une hypertrichose ou une alopécie sans pour autant augmenter l'excrétion des 17 céto-stéroïdes.

En tous cas, il est certain que nous avons vu se développer chez 20% de nos malades des alopécies de «type masculin» à la suite d'administration d'androgènes ou même simplement de stéroïdes anabolisants soit disant non virilisants.

Ces alopécies toujours localisées au niveau des tempes et du vertex peuvent s'accompagner de séborrhée, mais il arrive souvent notamment chez des femmes ayant dépassé la quarantaine, traitées pour des fibromes ou des troubles méno-pausiques, que la séborrhée soit totalement absente et que l'alopécie androgénique se forme par un processus atrophique, sur un cuir chevelu absolument sec.

Le traitement d'hormones mâles n'a d'ailleurs pas besoin d'être intensif ou prolongé, ses effets dépendent essentiellement d'une sensibilité individuelle. Il suffit parfois d'une seule injection pour déterminer l'apparition d'alopécies qui peuvent évoluer ensuite inexorablement pendant des années. SMITH et WELLS n'ont-ils pas soutenu que chez les sujets prédisposés la présence d'androgènes joue un rôle déterminant dans l'apparition de l'alopécie, non dans sa persistance ?

Certes, l'administration d'hormones mâles n'est pas seule en cause et bien d'autres facteurs doivent intervenir. Nous pensons notamment à une prédisposition constitutionnelle héréditaire qui peut être responsable de l'extension et de la durée de l'alopécie, à la nature plus ou moins résistante du système pileux qui réagira à l'incitation hormonale par une alopécie comme par une hypertrichose, et sans doute aussi à une certaine réceptivité cutanée qui semble dépendre d'une action enzymatique locale.

D'autre part, nous avons remarqué que l'administration de stéroïdes progestatifs ou de gonadotrophines peut aussi provoquer ce même type d'alopécie masculine. Le rôle de premier plan que joue la progestérone dans la biosynthèse des hormones stéroïdes est d'ailleurs bien connu: chacun sait qu'elle donne naissance à la desoxycorticostérone et à la 17 deshydroxyprogestérone dont la dégradation oxydative est probablement le processus principal de la formation des androgènes et aussi, que sa sécrétion est elle-même réglée par les gonadotrophines.

Par contre — et bien que sur ce point notre expérience soit encore trop récente — il ne nous semble pas que les lutéomymétiques de synthèse utilisés pour la contraception en association avec un oestrogène soient responsables de telles alopécies.

Enfin, contrairement à ce que pensent de nombreux auteurs nous n'avons jamais constaté une inhibition très marquée de la séborrhée par administration d'oestrogènes. L'amélioration tant de la séborrhée que de l'alopécie que l'on peut noter dès les premières semaines de la grossesse, nous avait en effet incités à traiter

certaines alopécies séborrhéiques d'origine endocrinienne, par des applications locales ou l'administration per os d'oestrogènes. Or, nous n'avons jamais pu déterminer
une freination notable de la séborrhée. Les doses utilisées par nous étaient elles trop
faibles et l'imprégnation oestrogénique insuffisante ? C'est possible, mais dans certains cas, nous avons, au contraire, observé une recrudescence. Peut-on attribuer
celle-ci à une métabolisation de certaine oestrogènes en stéroïdes androgéniques ?

Si les troubles endocriniens sont assurément un facteur important d'alopécie,
les déséquilibres neurotoniques, liés d'ailleurs souvent à des troubles hormonaux,
demeurent à nos yeux la cause majeure des séborrhées. En ne tenant compte que
des déséquilibres nerveux évidents, nous les avons incriminés dans 46% des cas.

Nous avons en effet remarqué que les chocs émotifs, les contrariétés répétées,
la sensation d'insécurité, les dystonies neuro-végétatives avec insomnie, mélancolie,
anorexie, les états dépressifs par surmenage professionnel, sont autant de causes
possibles d'alopécies, généralement diffuses et toujours séborrhéiques. Ces séborrhées s'accompagnent le plus souvent d'une hypersécrétion sudorale qui confirme
encore leur origine diencéphalique. Désespérément chroniques, elles augmentent
par leurs effets psychiques l'instabilité neurotonique du sujet, déterminant parfois
de véritables névroses. De la séborrhée ou de la dépression, quelle est celle qui
donne naissance à l'autre ? Il est souvent difficile de le préciser. Ce qui est sûr c'est
qu'elles exercent l'une sur l'autre une action aggravante. En outre, les thérapeutiques qui paraissent indiquées, n'ont bien souvent, ici encore, d'autre résultat
qu'une aggravation des symptômes. Chez nos malades présentant des dépressions
nerveuses — qui sont assez nombreuses puisqu'elles constituent 32% de ces in-
stables neurotoniques, soit 14% de nos consultantes — nous avons souvent constaté des poussées aiguës d'acné et de séborrhée à la suite de médications psychotropes. Car si certaines de ces médications semblent inopérantes sur la séborrhée,
d'autres en revanche provoquent non seulement une hypersécrétion sudorale mais
aussi une exagération très marquée de la sécrétion sébacée.

Il faut bien reconnaître d'ailleurs, que quelle que soit l'étiologie de l'alopécie,
aucun traitement local ou interne ne nous a donné jusqu'à présent entière satisfaction. Les traitements généraux sont aussi nombreux qu'inefficaces: nous avons
renoncé aux traitements hormonaux car les doses faibles d'oestrogènes nous paraissent inactives ou aggravantes et nous n'avons jamais pu obtenir par des doses
plus élevées une imprégnation oestrogénique suffisante sans entraîner en même
temps des effets au niveau des récepteurs génitaux. Mais l'état nerveux de ces malades doit être soigné, ne serait-ce que pour éviter les effets psychiques de l'alopécie
et pour cela, les sédatifs légers nous semblent préférables aux neuroleptiques.

Nous prescrivons surtout des traitements symptomatiques, telle la cystéine à
forte dose associée suivant les cas à la vitamine A, au Calcium, à la vitamine D 2,
ou à certaines médications lipotropes.

Mais nos conseils sont aussi d'action locale et plus encore d'abstention: éviter
les brossages, les massages trop violents, les traitements locaux à base de lotion
capillaire dégraissante, surtout espacer les shampooings et les choisir aussi peu
détergents que possible. On remplacera même avantageusement les shampooings
par des savons ou des pseudo-savons en poudre à base de cystéine.

Pour conclure, je dirai que la fréquence accrue de ces alopécies féminines
diffuses ne nous paraît pas contestable. On ne saurait en effet l'expliquer seulement
par certaines facilités ou certains impératifs de la vie moderne. C'est bien leur
étiopathogénie qu'il nous faut rechercher. Et celle-ci demeure très complexe,
dépendant à la fois d'une prédisposition constitutionnelle héréditaire, de troubles
endocriniens et surtout de troubles neurotoniques qui, liés au mode de vie moderne,
constituent, à notre avis, la cause de loin la plus fréquente.

Free Communications

Propiedades depilatoria y citotóxica de la seleno-cistationina

F. Kerdel-Vegas, Dept. de Dermatología, Hospital Vargas y Universidad Central de Venezuela, Caracas (Venezuela)

Durante muchos años se ha reconocido el efecto depilatorio en humanos, ocasionado por la ingestión de las semillas del árbol denominado en Venezuela "Coco de Mono" *(Lecythis ollaria)*. La intoxicación observada consta de una fase aguda, con náuseas, vómitos y diarrea, y de síntomas ulteriores entre los cuales, los más marcados y constantes son los calambres musculares y la caída difusa del cabello. El *defluvium capillorum*, se observa principalmente en el cuero cabelludo, aun cuando en los casos severos se extiende a la barba y al vello corporal. Ocurre entre una y tres semanas después de la ingestión de las almendras. Hemos podido reunir siete casos bien documentados, en la literatura médica venezolana. Aparentemente no se han observado casos semejantes en otros países tropicales del hemisferio occidental, a pesar de la amplia distribución de la especie *Lecythis*, desde Costa Rica (en Centro América) hasta un paralelo que pasa al Norte de Rio de Janeiro, en Brasil. También en Venezuela, la ingestión de estas semillas no siempre producía caída del pelo, y esta irregularidad del comportamiento se prestaba a diferentes interpretaciones. Por ello fue necesario procurarnos semillas provenientes de un árbol, comprobadamente responsable del fenómeno descrito.

La hipótesis de trabajo con la cual iniciamos nuestras investigaciones se basaba en la probabilidad de que la sustancia activa capaz de ocasionar la caída del cabello, fuese simultáneamente un agente citotóxico, ya que algunos de estos productos producen un *defluvium capillorum* como efecto secundario indeseable. Para verificar esta hipótesis de trabajo utilizamos (en colaboración con el Dr. Lewis Aronow) un simple método de bioensayo, mediante cultivo de tejidos (fibroblastos de ratón). El material purificado, cristalino, obtenido a partir del extracto acuoso de las semillas de "Coco de Mono" se identificó como seleno-cistationina (cistaselenonina), o sea, el ácido L-2-amino-4- (L-2-amino-2-carboxietil) selenobutírico. La actividad biológica de esta sustancia fue exactamente equivalente a la del extracto acuoso previamente utilizado, produciendo una inhibición de un 50% en el crecimiento de los fibroblastos, con una concentración de 3—5 $\mu g_{/}$ml de medio de cultivo. Los efectos tóxicos *in vitro*, tanto de extractos crudos de las semillas, como de la seleno-cistationina purificada, se pueden revertir mediante la adición de l-cistina al medio de cultivo. Aparentemente, toda la actividad biológica de los extractos acuosos crudos de las semillas, se puede atribuir — en bases cuantitativas — al aminoácido seleno-cistationina.

En relación al mecanismo de acción de la seleno-cistationina parece lógico, al nivel de nuestros actuales conocimientos, que siendo un análogo (conteniendo selenio) del aminoacido azufrado cistationina, interfiera en la utilización del aminoácido (también azufrado) l-cisteína, indispensable en la síntesis proteica. En los cultivos de tejidos, la restricción de cisteína utilizable, lleva a una detención del crecimiento celular. Sin embargo la caída del pelo observada después de la ingestión de semillas de "coco de mono" puede ser debida al efecto citotóxico de la seleno-cistationina en las células del folículo piloso, pero con más probabilidad a la interferencia en la utilización de la cisteína por dichas células en la formación de la queratina dura del pelo, que como es bien sabido, se encuentra allí en cantidades apreciables y es de vital importancia en el proceso de la queratinización.

La administración por vía bucal y parenteral de los extractos acuosos activos de las semillas de "coco de mono", en ratones albinos, demuestra su acción depilatoria, impidiendo la repoblación pilosa de áreas especialmente depiladas con pinzas, e histopatológicamente se observan las siguientes alteraciones: atrofia y desaparición de las glándulas sebáceas, atrofia marcada de la epidermis, edema y hemorragia intraalveolar de los pulmones, focos necróticos en el hígado y bazo, congestión sinusoidal importante de las glándulas suprarrenales.

El problema de la acumulación del selenio y su síntesis en seleno-cistationina por parte de diversas plantas, entre ellas algunas muy importantes por su utilización como alimentos, tal es el caso del maíz y del ajonjolí, puede llegar a constituir un verdadero problema de salud pública, ya que de esta manera sería eventualmente ingerido por sectores importantes de la población.

Control of Mammalian Hair Growth: Studies with a Cell-Free Protein Synthesizing System

I. M. FREEDBERG, Department of Dermatology, Beth Israel Hospital, Boston, Massachusetts (USA)

During the past several years our laboratory has been studying protein synthesis in keratinizing tissues. Today, I shall discuss the biochemical mechanism and controls of protein synthesis in isolated mammalian hair root cells. Previously shaven, anaesthetized animals are painted with commercial latex paint. Within 30 min the paint dries and after 2 to 12 h attains the consistency and tensile strength of an elastic band. The latex sheet is then cut into strips and removed from the animal. The hair shafts are caught in and removed with the latex so that the animals are essentially totally epilated. The hair roots may be harvested from the latex sheets with a scalpel and subjected to further preparative procedures. Although the specimen contains much fully keratinized hair, the root cells are readily apparent. These cells are packed with ribosomes, many of which are closely aligned around filaments.

Table 1. *Hair Root Cell-Free Protein Synthesis*

Requirements	High Speed Supernatant Fraction
Particle Fraction	150,000 g supernatant fraction of hair root homo-
High Speed Supernatant Fraction	genate concentrated and run over Sephadex G-25.
ATP	
GTP	
Mg^{++}	

Particle Fraction
1. Homogenized hair roots centrifuged at 15,000 g to remove unbroken cells, debris, filaments, nuclei and mitochondria. Supernatant centrifuged at 150,000 g (60 min) yields pellet: *Microsomes*.
2. Homogenized hair roots centrifuged at 600 μg. Pellet of unbroken cells, debris, filament and nuclei washed and centrifuged at 600 g. Pellet extracted twice with 0.5% desoxycholate and recentrifuged at 600 g (10 min). Supernatant centrifuged at 150,000 g (60 min) yields pellet: *Nuclear pellet ribosomes*.
3. Hair roots washed in buffer. Extracted with 0.5% desoxycholate and centrifuged at 15,000 g. Supernatant centrifuged over sucrose at 150,000 g (60 min) yields pellet: *Extracted ribosomes*.

Tab. 1 summarizes the preparative techniques and incubation conditions required for cell-free protein synthesis in this tissue. Synthesis occurs when one of several different types of particle fraction obtained from the hair root cells is incubated in the presence of labeled amino acids, with a soluble fraction derived from the cell sap of the same tissue. ATP and GTP are required for full activity as is a magnesium concentration of 5 millimolar. Neither an ATP generating system nor a source of exogenous amino acids are necessary. We have used three different types of particle fraction for the studies. Microsomes obtained from the post-mitochondrial fraction of homogenized hair root cells may be separated from the cell sap by high speed centrifugation and used in incorporation experiments. This is the method used most commonly for similiar studies in other organ systems and is the system we have utilized most frequently. Our recent studies with epidermal protein synthesis, however, have indicated that in the epidermis the majority of protein synthesis occurs on ribosomes which sediment with the nuclear pellet at low forces and can be freed from the pellet by desoxycholate extraction. This technique yields what we have called nuclear pellet ribosomes. Finally, we have obtained from both hair roots and

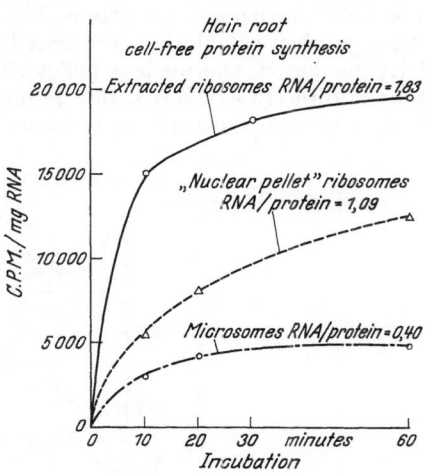

Fig. 1. Hair root cell-free protein synthesis. Particle fractions prepared as indicated were incubated with hair root high speed supernatant fraction

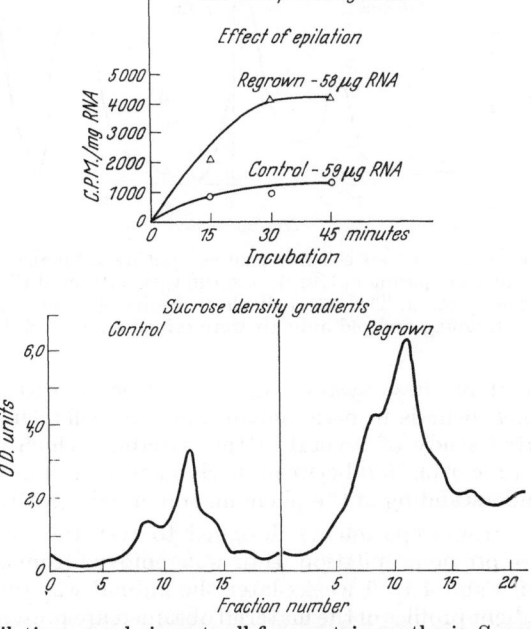

Fig. 2. Effects of epilation upon hair root cell-free protein synthesis. Sucrose density gradients were linear from 30% sucrose toward the left to 10% sucrose toward the right. The prominent peak in tubes 11 and 12 corresponds to 80s monomeric ribosomes. The incorporation experiment (top) was run with microsomes and hair root high speed supernatant fraction

epidermis an active particle fraction by direct extraction of the non-homogenized tissue with desoxycholate. We have referred to these as extracted ribosomes.

Fig. 1 displays the relative activities of the three types of particles in a cell-free amino acid incorporating system. The microsomes, in the bottom line, are active although when calculations are based upon counts incorporated per milligram of RNA incubated, the nuclear pellet ribosomes are approximately twice as active and the directly extracted, non homogenized particles five times as active. The RNA to protein ratios of the particles rise in parallel with their activity.

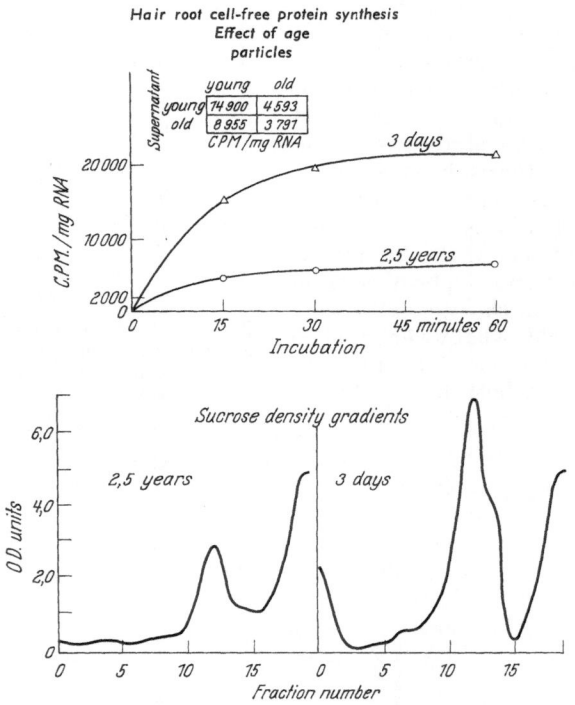

Fig. 3. Effects of age upon hair root cell-free protein synthesis. Sucrose density gradients as in Fig. 2. The incorporation experiments (top) were run with extracted ribosomes and hair root high speed supernatant fraction. The insert displays results of incorporation experiments in which components from young and old animals were mixed as indicated

The development of these systems has permitted investigation of the early steps of protein biosynthesis in mammalian hair root cells. Of equal importance, they have permitted study of several of the variables which affect hair growth in vivo. We sought a correlation between in vivo effects and in vitro results in the hope that some understanding of the phenomenon of hair growth would follow.

Fig. 2 is drawn from experiments designed to test the effect upon cell-free protein synthesis of previous epilation. Hair was removed from one-half of the skin of adult guinea pigs and 4 to 5 weeks later the animal was totally epilated with latex. Density gradient profiles of the material obtained are presented on the bottom of the slide. Production of synchronous growth in these follicles which are natively dyssynchronous results in a larger amount of ribosomal material being obtained from each follicle. The graph at the top indicates an additional change. The incorporation per unit amount of ribosomes incubated is significantly increased. There are more particles and each shows enhanced incorporating activity.

On the following figure are similiar data obtained from guinea pig hair when age variables are studied. The amount of ribosomes obtained from the follicles of 3 day old guinea pigs is much higher than that obtained from 2.5 year old animals. The gradient profiles reflecting the type of ribosomes in each case are essentially similiar. As noted at the top of the figure, the ribosomes from young animals are more active on the basis of counts incorporated per milligram RNA than are those from the older specimens. The insert in the upper left corner portrays results of experiments in which the components from young and old specimens were mixed prior to incubation. Both particle and supernatant fractions contributed to the enhanced activity present in young tissue.

Tab. 2 is drawn from experiments in which rat hair root cells were studied. These data are displayed in relative terms only since actual incorporation varies widely in experiments which are done at different times. Both the total synthetic capacity and the specific activity of components isolated from adult animals are high. During pregnancy, perhaps corresponding to the clinically evident change in hair growth which occurs, *in vitro* incorporation decreases and eventually totally stops post-partum at which time ribosomes are not extractable from the follicles. Following birth, few ribosomes are extractable and no incorporation occurs. At six weeks, however, the number of ribosomes increases and the synthetic capacity of the particles is above normal.

Table 2. *Rat Hair Root Cell-Free Amino Acid Incorporation*

	Synthetic Capacity (counts/animal)	Specific Activity (counts/mg RNA)	RNA/Protein Ratio	Gradient Pattern
Adult Male	+++	+++	1.96 (Ext. Ribo.)	Normal
Adult Female	+++	+++	0.88 (Micro.)	Normal
Pregnant Female				
Early	+	++	0.36 (Micro.)	Normal
Term	+	+	—	—
Post Partum	0	0	—	No ribosomes
Newborn				
2 weeks	0	0	0.74 (Micro.)	Normal
				Few Ribosomes
3 weeks	0	0	—	—
4 weeks	0	0	1.06 (Micro.)	—
6 weeks	++++	++++	1.19 (Micro.)	Normal
11 weeks	—	—	--	Normal
				Many Ribosomes

In summary, a cell free system derived from mammalian hair root cells has been used to measure protein synthesis under various conditions. Regrowing cells and young cells show enhanced synthetic capacity due to both quantitative and qualitative phenomena. Incorporation in hair roots derived from pregnant and post partum rats is inhibited. Follicles from newborn rats are also inactive although at 6 weeks of age, root cells demonstrate enhanced incorporation associated with a marked increase in the number of extractable ribosomes. The content of ribosomes in hair root cells may be one of the mechanisms which control mammalian hair growth.

The Effects of Various Pathologic Conditions of the Scalp upon Hair Melanogenesis and Hair Growth

W. KOSTANECKI, Department of Dermatology, Warsaw Medical School (Poland)

In the cases of thallium poisoning one observes hyperpigmentations in the anagen hair roots and catagen clubs. The latter are still detectable in telogen clubs after the stage of follicular involution. Analogous hyperpigmentations were also found in the generally scarce roots of growing hairs, clubs and/or adjacent parts of catagen and telogen hairs respectively, in some patients with the following pathologic conditions:

in the patients receiving cyclophosphamide,

in alopecia areata,

in tinea capitis caused by trichophyton (deep type), furuncles and some other pyodermas — in the hairs derived from the vicinity of the lesions.

Table. *State of the hair roots in the vicinity of skin lesions in various diseases*

Diagnosis	No. of cases	Duration of the disease	No. of cases showing anagen synchronisation of hair cycle	Catagen counts	No. of cases with melanin deposits in the roots of growing hairs	non growing hairs
Tinea capitis due to trichophyton (deep type)	10	1—3 mth.	2	5, 6, 8, 9, 11, 15, 16, 18, 21, 25	2	4
Mycosis fungoides Tumors	3	1—3 mth.	0	15, 18, 37	3	3
Furuncle	2	10—12 days	0	15, 30	—	—
Pyoderma vegetans	3	3—4 mth.	0	15, 20, 45	1	2
Tinea capitis due to trichophyton (superficial type)	5	1—2 mth.	1	3, 4, 5, 7, 25	—	1
Erythroderma	3	1—3 mth.	0	10, 15, 21	—	—
Pemphigus vulgaris	1	2 mth.	0	31	—	1

In several pathologic conditions such hyperpigmentations were observed only in the clubs and /or proximal parts of catagen and subsequently telogen hair roots. These include:

secondary recidivant syphilis,

tinea capitis caused by trichophyton (superficial type),

single cases of diffuse hair-loss in women and male pattern baldness (catagen and telogen count in these patients was remarkably high also in the border region of the scalp),

after application of 5% ammoniated mercury ointment,

following parenteral bismuth therapy,

after topical application of barium sulfide.

Hyperpigmentations of the catagen hair roots occurred after x-ray irradiations. The above mentioned hyperpigmentations which appear as dark deposits, also in the polarized light, loose their colour when treated with 25% solution of hydrogen peroxide. Sections of the hyperpigmented parts of hairs are darker then sections of distal non-pigmented parts which proves that we are dealing with melanin.

Deep inflammatory conditions of the scalp often cause precocious onset of the catagen phase in numerous hair follicles close to skin lesions, which is not so frequent in the superficial inflammations. This phenomenon might play a significant role in the tendency of the deep type of tinea capitis to self-healing. Inflammation may cause the anagen synchronisation of hair cycle around skin lesions. The hyperpigmentations always arise during anagen phase. Their appearance usually coincides with hair growth disturbances such as dystrophy or sometimes dysplasia or precocious onset of follicular involution. In certain conditions only the last possibility is involved. If the hair continues to grow after melanin deposits have appeared it will become depigmented. The factor which initially enhances melanogenesis, afterwards acts as it's inhibitcr. The presence of melanin deposits in the roots of growing hairs is always accompanied by hair growth disturbance of the type of effluvium anagenicum, telogenicum or mixtum.

The above data suggest among others that:

1. the differential diagnosis of thallium poisoning must include several diverse conditions,

2. a number of factors influencing epidermal melanogenesis do affect production of the hair pigment as well.

Our findings are yet another proof of the hair being an excellent model for the study of melanogenesis.

The Histological Changes in Idiopathic Premature Vertex Baldness in Women

I. Martin-Scott, Hospitals in Hertfordshire and Bedfordshire (England)

Hypothesis

It is suggested that this type of hair thinning in young women is caused by the excessive use of, or an abnormal reaction to, soapless detergent shampoos, which have been used almost universally during the last 20 years. The site of hair loss co-incides with the area of maximum shampoo friction. In supporting this theory it would seem essential to demonstrate that the histo-pathological changes are in keeping with a very low-grade inflammatory reaction on the scalp surface, which will finally lead to fibrosis and irreversible hair loss.

Selection of Cases

From the original number of cases I decided to exclude cases who had previously suffered from any type of hair loss and cases with anaemia, possible sex-hormone imbalance or hypothyroidism. I also excluded cases where physical causes could be blamed for their hair-loss. In other words their vertex hair thinning was entirely idiopathic. My series of cases by these stringent criteria was thus reduced to a total of 25. All these cases had used soapless shampoos since adolescence, and most washed their hair several times weekly. Since this condition only affects a relatively small proportion of women using soapless shampoos I wondered if this could be due to an acquired epidermal sensitivity to any of the four most commonly used chemicals contained in soapless shampoos in Great Britain. Occlusive 48 h patch-tests were therefore done in most cases, and one third of those so tested gave a positive mild reaction to either sodium lauryl sulphate or tri-ethanolamine lauryl sulphate both used in a 1% aqueous solution.

Histological Changes

The histology of most common skin diseases can be diagnosed with some certainty, but this is impossible in sections from female vertex alopecia, where the microscopic changes are most variable. The examination of a single section could easily be inconclusive, as the pathological changes may even vary in different parts of one single section. It is only after the study of many serial sections and the use of differential staining that one obtains some idea of the pathological picture, which in general terms resembles the changes in mice after frequent applications of a detergent to their pelts over a prolonged period. The histological changes do not seem to be directly influenced by the age of the patient nor the duration of the disease. Thus a woman who has had the trouble for 10 years may reveal the same histological picture as another case of recent origin.

The commonest changes seen were as follows:

1. Paucity of hair follicles.

2. Moderate general scalp surface hyperkeratosis, with a normal epidermis showing no evidence of atrophy.

3. This hyperkeratosis was increased at the mouths of the hair follicles, either forming a "goblet" plugging, or uniform hyperkeratosis extending down the follicles to the sebaceous glands.

4. Hyperkeratosis was also a feature of the sweat pores sometimes associated with either dilatation or complete absence of the sweat ducts.

5. The sebaceous glands were usually normal, but sometimes showed hypertrophy. Where general scarring occurred they later became involved, as did the hair muscles.

6. The elastic fibres in most cases showed a marked increase in the sub-papillary layer and especially around the necks of the hair follicles, as though strangling them. The hair papillae of these same follicles remained normally healthy, indicating the main onslaught was from the scalp surface. This intrusion of elastic tissue seemed to progress down the follicle to surround its appendages at a later stage.

7. There was no evidence of any acute inflammatory response nor surface organisms. Para-keratosis, eczema and peri-vascular infiltration were exceptional findings.

Conclusion

The histological changes are in accord with the frequent applications of a mildly noxious substance to the scalp surface, which devoids it of its protective sebum, and hence these glands hypertrophy. The main portals of entry of the detergent are the hair follicles and sweat ducts which react by producing more keratin. The general picture indicates a mechanism of defence to a lowgrade surface irritant to which a few women react abnormally and develop this familiar clinical picture of vertex cicatricial alopecia.

The Normal Trichogram of People Beyond 50 Years but Apparently not Bald

J. M. Barman, Dept. of Biophisic. Facultad de Medicina; I. Astore, Facultad de Odontología, and V. Pecoraro, Dept. of Dermatology. Facultad de Medicina. Universidad Nacional del Litoral. Rosario, Santa Fe (Argentina)

Introduction

In previous works we have dealt with the normal trichogram of newborn [1], prepuberal children [2], and adults [3] and with the normal evolution of the hair since its development in the fetus until 40 weeks of extrauterine life [4]. We will now try to establish the conditions of normality of the trichogram after 50 years of age, in persons apparently not bald.

The hairs of human scalp deteriorate variably along with ageing. Senile alopecia [5] and the histologic modifications that undergoes the hair of the scalp, at least in males [5], with the advance of age, so demonstrate it.

In individuals older than 50 years hairs deterioration is variable and generally marked; however a certain number of persons in this age group apparently do not deteriorate the hair scalp.

Materials and Method

The esencial characteristics of the trichogram (density: n° cms^{-2} — thickness of the hair — speed of growth, hair cycle) were studied in the central and peripherical regions of the scalp, coronal and frontal and parietals and occipital regions of a group of 36 apparently normal caucasian individuals. — There were nine women ranging from 54 to 76 years of age — medium 63.4, S.D. 7 and 27 men ranging from 50 to 83 years of age — medium 60.5, S.D. 5.2. — The men were subdivided in two groups: a) from 50 to 59.9 years of age — M: 54, S.D. 3.1 and b) from 60 to 83 years of age — M: 67, S.D. 6.8. — The mean age of the whole group was 61.5 with a standard deviation of 5.5. — The parietal regions were analized together since their reciprocal differences did not justify a separation; their values are thus expressed by the mean of both. — Since after 50 years of age the majority of the individuals, specially males, present a pronounced deterioration of the scalp hair, the present group has been selected among those persons whose scalp hair made them comparable to a normal average adult. — The results obtained in this investigation were compared with those previously known of a group constituted by younger adults, from 16 to 46 years of age [3]. — The method and technic of the trichogram have been previously described [6].

Results

The results obtained and their correlations are expressed in the graphs and tables.

Density. If we consider the scalp as a whole in either sex and in any age or group of the population studied, there is a striking dispersion in density — from 87 to 330 hairs per square centimeter — with a medium of 162.8 and a standard error (S.D.) of 12.7.

In the female group the range was of 87 to 215 — M: 147, S.A. 10.4. In the first male subgroup — 50 to 59.9 years — the range was of 104 to 330 — M: 178, S.E. 13.4 and in the second — 60 to 83 years — it was of 90 to 270, M: 161, S.E. 13.6. In the whole male group density was 168.5, S.E. 13.4.

Comparing the density of the whole scalp of this group with that of a group of adults from 16 to 46 years of age a significative reduction of density is apparent in the older group. Women's hair density is slightly less than that of males and in this last group density decreases with age.

In each one of the regions studied the persons beyond 50 years of age present a significative decrease in density if compared with the group of younger adults of both sexes. This reduction is more marked in the parietals and occipital regions.

The comparison between women and men over 50 years shows that women present a lesser hair density than men. This is so in all the scalp regions, the least density in both groups being present in the parietal regions.

Speed of Growth

The speed of growth of the scalp hair as a whole and of each scalp region in particular is less than that of younger adults, being significantly less in the central regions, particularly in the coronal region. The population studied presents no differences either between age or sex groups. The speed of growth varies slightly and irregularly in males as age advances.

Thickness

The relative proportion of thick hairs in the scalp as a whole is greater in adults over 50 years than in younger adults, while medium and thin hairs are less.

Comparing the relative proportions of thickness, by regions, between young and over 50 years adults a relative predominance of thick hairs is seen in all regions in the later. There are similarities between the two groups in frontal and coronal regions and significative differences in parietal and occipital regions.

Comparing the relative proportions of thick, medium and thin hairs in the entire scalp and among particular regions in the group beyond 50 years, slight, insignificant differences exist except for the coronal regions. In this region a relative dominance of thick hair over medium and thin hairs is seen in the sub-group between 50 to 59.9 years.

In the group of males beyond 50 years there are no differences of thickness in the entire scalp or within single regions but central and peripheral regions are very similar among themselves respectively.

Except for the coronal region there are no differences in the distribution of the percentages of thicknesses either in the entire scalp or among particular regions between males and females over 50 years.

Hair Cycle

The percentage of hairs in quiescence was computed together for catagens and telogens and expressed as telogens. Considering the scalp as a whole, the number of telogens showed a range between 3 and 51% in females and between 0 and 87% in males. The ranges for the respective subgroup of males were 0 to 87% for the subgroup of 50 to 59.9 years and from 0 to 58% for the subgroup of 60 to 83 years. In the group of adults below 46 years the range was 13 to 23 %.

To make the comparison between the total group of adults over 50 years and the group below 46 years and among the subgroups easier a graph is shown. The total group of adults over 50 years has a greater percentage of hairs in telogen in the entire scalp than the group of adults below 46 years. On analyzing the number of telogens between males and females over 50 years it is shown than the former have a greater number of telogens.

Within the subgroup of males, that from 60 to 83 years has a significatively lesser percentage of telogens than the subgroup from 50 to 59.9 years.

Upon analyzing the number of telogens by regions we see once more the different behaviour of the central and peripherical regions. On both groups of persons over 50 years and below 46 years, the number of telogens is lesser in the peripherical regions. The comparative study between adults over 50 years and below 46 years, by regions, shows that in people over 50 years the percentage of telogens in the frontal and coronal regions is significatively greater that in adults below 46 years while the proportion is less in the parietals and occipital regions. The comparative analysis by regions of the proportions of telogens between males and females over 50 years shows a significatively greater percentage in males in the frontal and coronal regions and similarities in the parietals and occipital regions.

Discussion

The formation of the forehead [7] before birth and its progressive extension with the advance of age together with the gradual involution of hairs demonstrated by the constant increase of intermediate and residual hairs since prepuberty [8] — makes the arrival to an advanced age of a group, certainly not minimal, of individuals with an apparently complete scalp hair, illogical.

This fact is also of occasional observation in other biological systems and must have an explanation in the infinite variety of the genetic mosaic that the species harbours in the chromosomes. Other factors — humoral, etc. have to be considered eventually co-participants.

The shift of the percentages in the dispersion of thickness in favour of the thick hairs is only apparently contradictory. One has to bear in mind that in these individuals the hairs that did not receive the genetic information necessary to persist, in its regression, have reduced their magnitude below the limit of efficiency of the method. This hypothesis could explain the reduction in density with the progress of age and also the shift in the proportions of the thickness. What has been said only differs in magnitude (number of unaffected hairs) from what happens in a relatively advanced bald person in whom, side by side with sparse, thick, apparently normal hairs, a great many of other are reduced to a practically invisible fuzz.

Along the path of suppositions and according with findings of daily practice: baldness, diffuse feminine alopecia, it is to be assumed that for circumstances of fortuite genetic combinations or for the multiplicity of genetic factors that bear over the trophic status of the hairs, an appreciable number of hairs harbour a genetic information related to a particular constitution that determines its persistence.

This assumption does not contradicts with the increase in the proportion of telogens with ageing since it has been demonstrated that the total duration of the cycles is reduced with age [3] and that not in every person and circumstances the repetition of the cycles bring an involution of equal magnitude.

Another apparently contradictory fact is seen in the subgroup of person 60 to 83 years old. Their number of telogens is lesser than in the other groups. This can be interpreted assuming that at this age the thin hairs — of which practically 90% are in telogen [9] — have suffered a regression of such magnitude that they no longer can be detected by direct observation of the scalp.

The important fact of the different biological behavior between central and peripherical regions that is very marked since the early formation of hairs — fetal and post-natal —, despite decreassing with the progress of age in a more or less neat way, persist even in persons older than 50 years in the majority of variables studied such as growth, distribution of thicknesses and phases of the cycle.

This phenomenon together with the various facts previously mentioned brings in the final conclusion that the principal role in the evolution of the hair in general and of the scalp hair in particular, in every moment of the life, is played by the genetic constitution.

The similarity of the characteristics of the scalp hair of women and men with the advance of age appears logical if it is born in mind that at this age of life, hormonal, humoral and other conditions tend to level off.

References. 1. PECORARO, V., I. ASTORE, and J. M. BARMAN: J. invest. Derm. **43**, 145 (1964). — 2. PECORARO, V., I. ASTORE, J. M. BARMAN, and C. I. ARAUJO: J. invest. Derm. **42**, 427 (1964). — 3. BARMAN, J. M., I. ASTORE, and V. PECORARO: J. invest. Derm. **44**, 233 (1965). — 4. BARMAN, J. M., V. PECORARO, and I. ASTORE: J. invest. Derm. (In press). — 5. ELLIS, R.: Ageing of the human male scalp. The Biology of Hair Growth, pp. 469—485. New York: Academic Press 1958. — 6. BARMAN, J. M., V. PECORARO, and I. ASTORE: J. invest. Derm. **42**, 421 (1964). — 7. HAMILTON, J. B.: Ann. N.Y. Acad. Sci. **53**, 708 (1951). — 8. To be published. — 9. To be published.

Microscopic Studies of Pili Annulati

V. H. PRICE, R. S. THOMAS and F. T. JONES, Division of Dermatology, University of California Medical Center, San Francisco (USA), and Wool and Mohair Laboratory, U.S. Department of Agriculture, Albany, California (USA)

Pili annulati, or ringed hair, is a rare anomaly of uncertain etiology in which the hair shafts characteristically show light and dark bands when viewed with reflected light. As described previously, the banding is caused by light scattered from periodically occurring clusters of abnormal, air-filled cavities within the hair [1]. This report presents our light- and electron-microscopic results obtained preliminary to more extensive ultrastructural studies, and confirms the ascribed basis of the anomaly. In addition, we describe a new type of ringed hair, here called pseudo-pili annulati, which has an entirely different basis.

Fig. 1 shows hair with classical pili annulati under reflected light, and demonstrates the typical banding. The bright regions correspond to the clusters of air-filled cavities. These bright regions appear dark when viewed with transmitted light (Fig. 3, upper). Between the abnormal dark areas, or in lengths of the hair not afflicted by obvious banding, the gross appearance resembles that of normal hair (Fig. 3, lower). The cavities can be readily filled by soaking the hair in water, and this greatly diminishes the banded appearance. Evidently the banding is due to scattering and total internal reflection of light from the microscopically irregular interfaces between the keratin (refractive index about 1.55) and the air of the cavities (refractive index 1.00). Light microscopy of cross sections through cavity regions shows the fiber riddled with many small spaces of one micron or less, and an occasional larger space of several microns (Fig. 4). Normal hair, excluding the medulla, is relatively free of such spaces (Fig. 5). Electron micrographs of cross sections show that the spaces occur between intact macrofibrils and apparently also between cortical cells (Fig. 6). In normal hair, the cortex is much more compact (Fig. 7).

Fig. 2 shows hair with pseudo-pili annulati under reflected light. The strikingly banded appearance here is not due to any internal anomaly; inner structure of this hair is apparently quite normal. Rather, banding results from a periodic flattening of the hair shaft, with the flattened external surfaces acting as little mirrors to preferentially reflect the light at certain angles and not others. The flattening and

---

Fig. 1. Pili annulati by reflected light

Fig. 2. Pseudo-pili annulati by reflected light

Fig. 3. Hair shafts by transmitted light. Upper: pili annulati (blonde hair). Lower: normal blond hair.

Fig. 4. Cross sections of hair with pili annulati

Fig. 5. Cross sections of normal medullated hair

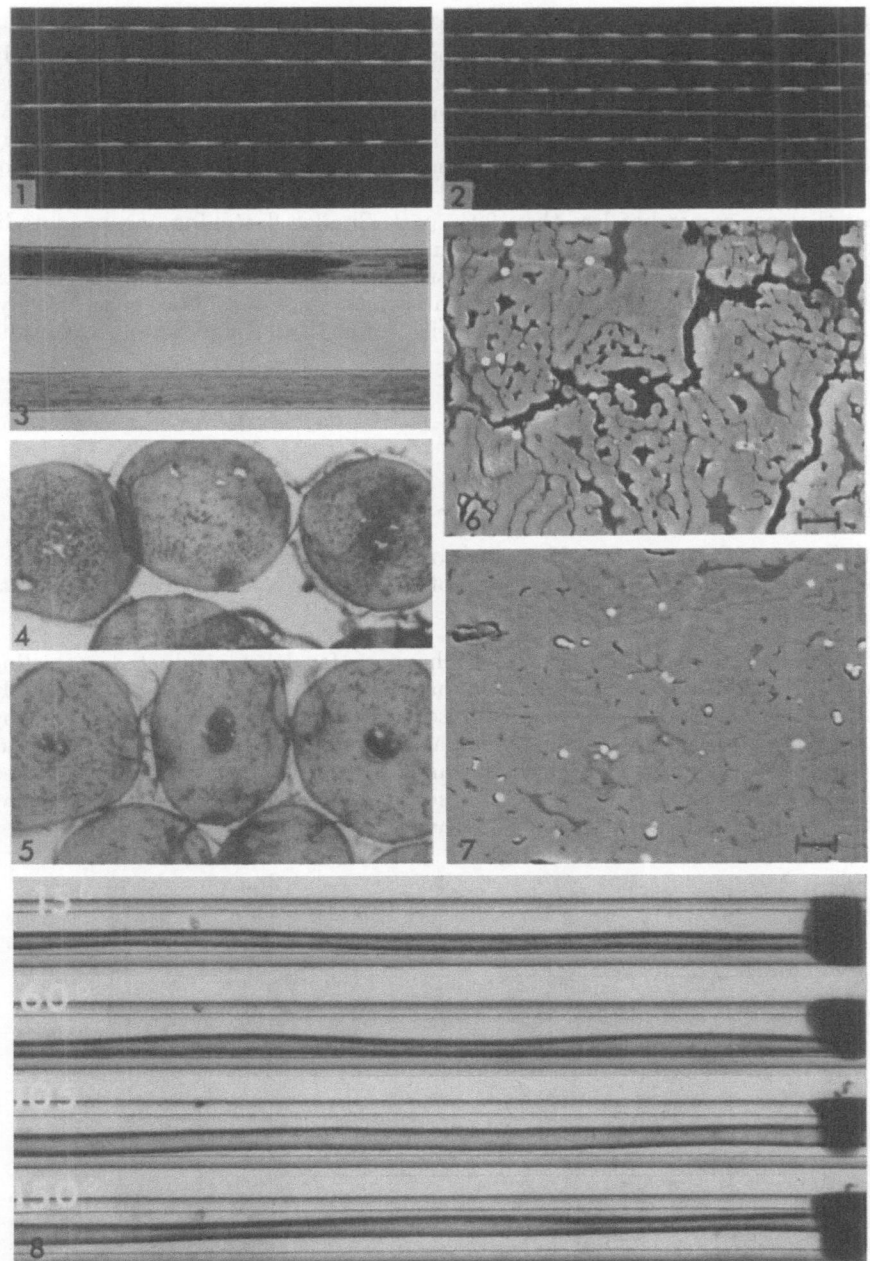

Fig. 1 to 5 (for legends see page 786)

Fig. 6. Electron micrograph of pili annulati cross section showing hair cortex (with added polystyrene latex calibration particles, and shadowing). Reverse contrast print. Magnification scale represents 1 micron

Fig. 7. Electron micrograph of normal hair cortex cross section. (Shadowed. No polystyrene; white particles are melanin.) Reverse contrast print. Magnification scale represents 1 micron

Fig. 8. Pseudo-pili annulati hair shaft in capillary tube rotated to various angles

its variations are easily seen by rotating the hair through 180 degrees. A typical specimen is seen in Fig. 8. At 15° rotation, the hair shaft diameter is relatively uniform and narrow. At 60° rotation, periodic widening and narrowing are obvious. At 105° rotation, the diameter again appears relatively uniform but wide. At 150° rotation, obvious widening and narrowing are again present but are exactly out of phase with the periodicity seen in the 60° position. Evidently the fiber is not simply twisted; instead its form is produced by periodic flattening in two alternating planes that are somewhat less than 90° apart. Similar flattening occurs sporadically in normal hair but not with the extensive periodicity seen here.

In addition to microscopic examination, both types of ringed hair have been subjected to amino-acid analyses, electron paramagnetic resonance spectroscopy, and stress-strain tests with an Instron tensile tester. In all these procedures, results are similar to those of normal hair.

Reference. 1. CADY, L. D., and M. TROTTER: Arch. Derm. Syph. (Chic.) **6**, 301 (1922).

Rate of Hair Growth

M. SAITOH, M. UZUKA and M. SAKAMOTO, Shiseido Chemical Research Laboratory, T. KOBORI, Department of Dermatology, Tokyo Teishin Hospital (Japan)

Studies on the rate of hair growth have so far been conducted regarding animals, especially sheep. Those on human hairs are few in number, probably because of various inconveniences for observation and, for want of a method by which to measure the rate of hair growth accurately and in a short period to time. We have recently developed a method using a capillary and successfully measured the rate of human hair growth and studied its governing factors. The following are the results obtained by this new method.

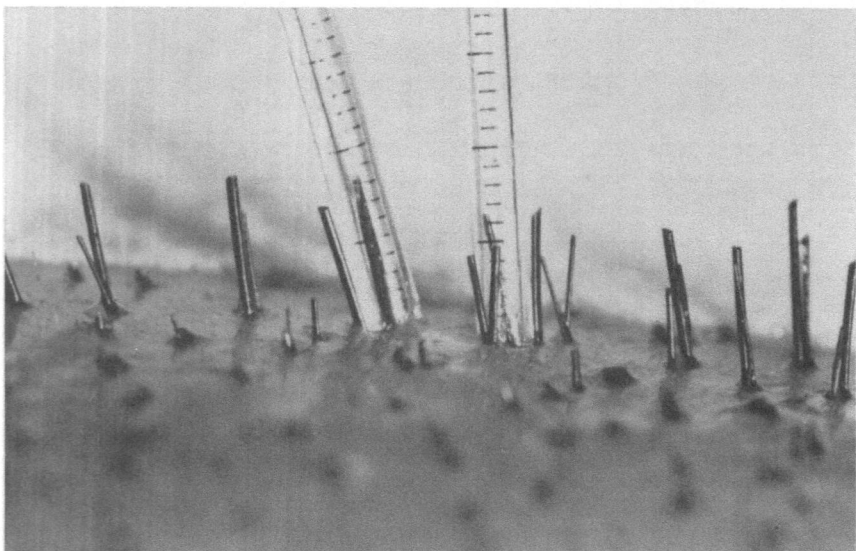

Fig. 1. Hairs and capillary tubes applied

1. Method of Measurement — Capillary Method —. Our new measuring method consists in fitting a capillary tube of glass around a growing hair, whose end is properly cut. The capillary is graduated at every 0.2 mm (Fig. 1). Hair is inserted into the capillary and the capillary tube gently pressed into the skin deep enough to reach the root of the hair. The hair in the capillary is magnified 25 times and measured by means of Zeiss Dermascope.

Features of the Capillary Method: a) Daily measurement is possible, b) Measurement can be done very precisely $\bar{R}/d^2 = 0.017$ mm, c) Measurement of the rate of hair growth in a short period of time is possible, d) The maximum error in measurement is within $\pm 0.82\%$ between 0 and 40 °C in temperature, and 0 and 100% in humidity.

2. Regional Differences in the Rate of Hair Growth. By means of the method just described, the rate of hair growth was measured in the following regions: vertex, temple, chin and chest. The comparison of the data obtained in this way from the four different regions will show that the vertex hairs (0.45 mm/day in female, 0.44 mm/day in male) are the

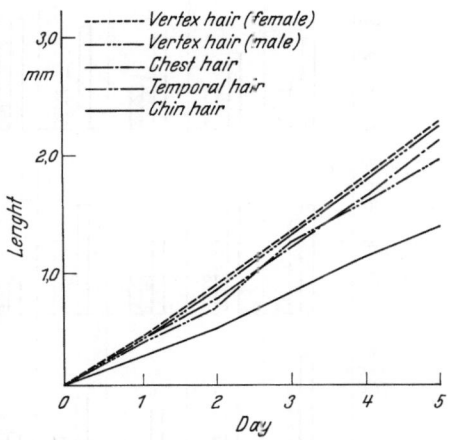

Fig. 2. Regional differences in hair growth

fastest to grow, followed by chest hairs, (0.40 mm/day) and temporal hairs (0.39 mm/day) and that the beards (0.27 mm/day) are much slower in growth than the others (Fig. 2).

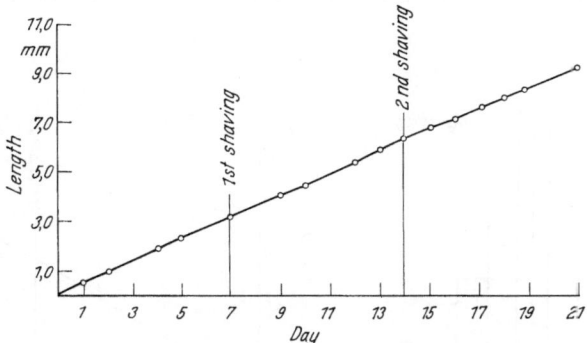

Fig. 3. Effect of shaving. Overall result with 66 hairs of eleven individuals

3. Effect of Shaving on Hair Growth. It is generally believed that shaving makes the hair thicker. Opinions, however, are divided in this regard. While BERTHOLD, REMESOW, SEYMOUR, FUCHS, TANINO, ARAKAWA and others state that shaving more or less expedite the growth of hair, BISCHOFF, TROTTER, CHASE, PINCUS, MONTAGNA and others deny any relation between shaving and thickening. A total of 66 chest hairs of eleven male individuals were first examined, and their rate of growth was measured. They were then shaved twice, with a 7 day's interval. Examinations of their growth before and after each shaving have proved that the rate of hair growth was unaffected (Fig. 3).

4. *Difference of the Rates of Diurnal and Nocturnal Hair Growth.* To this question there has been no established theory. LUBOW claims that hairs grow faster during the night. On the contrary, FUCHS, ROTHMAN and others support a "daytime

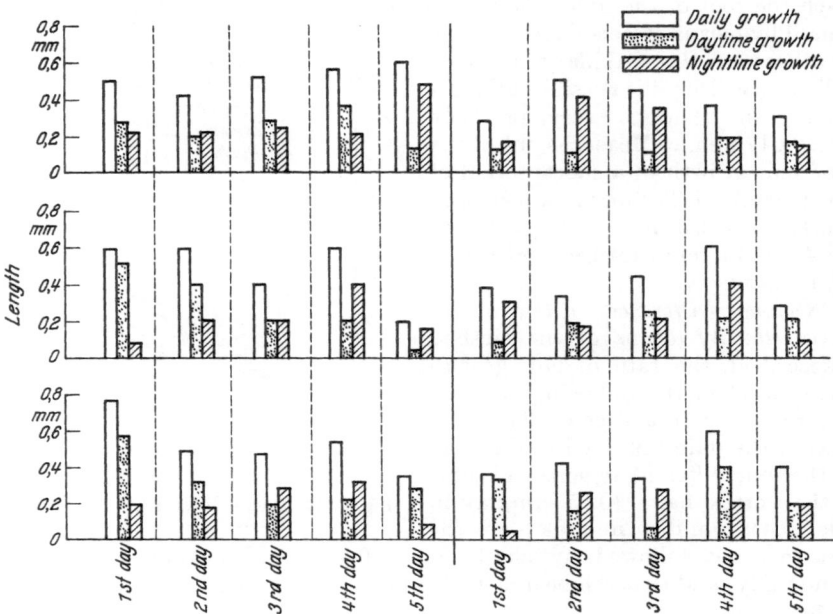

Fig. 4. Hair growth during daytime and nighttime. 19-years-old male, vertex hairs

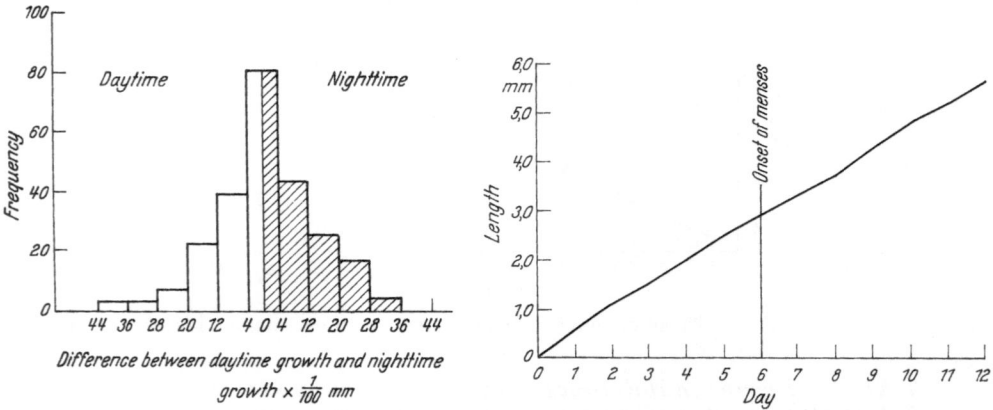

Fig. 5. Distribution of the variations in the mode of hair growth. Overall results of measurement by day and by night n = 25 b

Fig. 6. Influence of the menses on hairgrowth. Overall result with 30 hairs of six individuals

theory", and BULLOUGH and CHASE say that no such difference exists. In our study, a total of 70 hairs on the heads of six individuals of both sexes were measured over several days. We defined the period from 9 a.m. to 9 p.m. as "daytime", and that from 9 p.m. to 9 a.m. as "nighttime" for the sake of comparison. Fig. 4 is the result of daytime and nighttime measurements conducted over 5 days on six hairs of a 19-year-old male. It is readily seen that the growth rate is very variable, according to the day and the individual hair, and also we can say that neither "daytime" nor "nighttime" is the contributing factor in the rate of hair growth. Other word there is no significant difference in the rates of diurnal and nocturnal hair growth. All other hairs likewise examined showed similar tendencies. This histogram (Fig. 5) shows the variations in the mode of hair growth in a total of 256 examples, and represents the differences in the rate of growth during the day and night. The shaded portion indicates where the growth was greater during the night and the unshaded where the growth was greater during the day. As can be seen from the histogram, a normal distribution pattern is obtained with the peak at the center from which it can be deducted that there is no significant difference.

5. *Influence of the Menses on Hair Growth.* Hormones are considered to be a major governing factor of hair growth. From this point, we examined the rate of hair growth during menstruation. The rate of growth of 30 hairs of six females were studied before and after the menstruation. The individual as well as the overall result is not suggestive of any influence of the menses on hair growth (Fig. 6).

6. *Cinematographic Observation of the Actual Growth of Hairs.* The actual growth of hairs was recorded by time-lapse photography in three regions: temple, chin, and vertex. A fixed part of head was photographed over 48 h, with one exposure in every 15 min. The 192-frame series of ultra closeups has been cinematographically processed by means of animation technique. In this sequence on temporal hair growth, it will be recognized that each hair grows at a fairly constant speed. Similarly, the hair growth on the chin is also at near constant rate. On the vertex, secretion of sebum and perspiration can be observable.

Chronical Female Alopecia

M. BINAZZI, Clinica Dermosifilopatica, Università degli Studi, Perugia (Italy)

Over the last few years I have observed about 400 cases of chronical female alopecia generically of a genetic-dysendocrinal type. These are women between 16 and 54 years, often nulliparous or pauciparous, and the disease is familial in about 60% of them. Most are fair-complexioned and under 30, with a picture of "alopécie seborrhéique féminine"; then, there are older women with a picture of "alopécie féminine du vertex", that is with male characteristics (some of these had previously had "alopécie seborrhéique"). — Finally there are women with thinning and dystrophy of the hair, mainly without seborrhea. On examination, the hair shows about 40% of telogen, with little difference among the various forms. A metabolic-hormone study was performed on 200 patients, and I found, especially among the younger women, numerous subjects with emotional tensions, neuro-vegetative dystonia, a lively reaction of the hypotalamic centres and decrease of sexual appetite; they also had reduced oestrogenuria (without modifications in the relationship between the components), an increase of the pregnandiol complex (higher in the proliferation phase in patients with "alopécie seborrhéique", higher in the secretion phase in patients with "alopécie du vertex"), an increase of 17-ketosteroids (especially in the secretion phase and with a prevailing suprarenal rate), and, finally, a regular fluctuation of the corticoids.

I have interpreted these cases as hypoestrogenic female alopecia, thinking that a reduced or deviated ovary function may favour the appearance of some alterations of the biosynthesis of the suprarenal hormones (and therefore, in part, also of the pregnandiol complex), and also that a defect of the cortisol hormone in regulating the hypophysarian corticotropin may make the situation worse in the suprarenal and in the ovarian glands. In smaller groups, the elimination of hormones was normal, or there was a strong increase of 17-ketosteroids with prevailing suprarenal rate. Clinically these cases had male-type alopecia, hypertrichosis and acne.

In 8 cases the hormones were altogether reduced, especially the 11-oxy-steroids and the 17-ketosteroids. Finally, some carriers of serious, diffuse alopecia, little or non seborrheic, had clinical and biological signs of hyperthyroidism.

We are now studying the blood and urine levels of testosterone and epi-testosterone of our patients. In the secretion phase, we have found some hypo-estrogenic alopecia with normal testosterone excretion and some diffuse alopecia with normal excretion of the previously mentioned hormones and of testosterone.

A more or less marked reduction of the iron level in the blood, without anemia and nearly always with an increase of the copper level, resulted sometimes, almost exclusively in carriers of hypoestrogenic alopeciae with a picture of "alopécie seborrhéique".

In the structural examination there were no evident differences between the cases of genetic-dysendocrinal type and cases where such characteristics were lacking. Besides the known lesions, I found regressive injuries, such as a reduction and/or dystrophy of the elastic tissue and of the anagen figures. I also found acid mucopolysaccharides within the perifollicular connective tissue, as well as moderate angio-inflammatory lesions. In the alopeciae caused by hyperthyroidism, I found hyperkeratosis, hypotrophy of the sweat glands and limited alterations of the mucopolysaccharides.

In the treatment of hypoestrogenic alopecia, in its early phase and as far as the nature and size of the above-mentioned injuries allow, placental extracts and ovarian lysates have sometimes been useful, and I have had good results from repeated cycles of prednisone or dexamethasone for 15 to 20 days, followed by injections of diencephalic extracts.

The aim of this treatment was to reduce the hypophysarian corticotropin, to reactivate the gonadotropin function and to normalize the activity of the hypo-thalamic centres. I have had better results with 6 to 12 cycles of the less virilizing oral contraceptives, or of sequential treatment, preceded by dexa-methasone, accompanied by an antidystonic drug acting on the hypothalamus, and then followed by diencephalic extracts.

Oral contraceptives and the sequential treatment are used for their actions of contribution and substitution, as well as for their "rebound effect", and now, in order to create an oestrogenic climate, 0.1 or 0.2 mg a day of ethynilestradiol are added. 15 patients, some of whom had not responded to previous treatments, are now treated in this way and the results are encouraging.

Oral contraceptives have also been useful for the alopeciae caused by primitive androgenous hyperincretion. However, they have been unsuccessful in various cases in which the genetic basis and hormonal factors were not evident. The specific therapy is moderately active upon the alopecia caused by hyperthyroidism.

Le problème des états pseudopeladiques ou pseudopeladoïdes dans le cadre des alopécies cicatricielles

M. Juon, Lausanne (la Suisse)

Une récente publication Dermatologica (Basel) **133**, 60—75 (1966) a bouti aux conclusions suivantes:

1. Que des affections fort diverses peuvent réaliser le tableau clinique d'un état pseudopeladique (E.P.P.).

2. Que chaque cas peut, au cours de son évolution, présenter des aspects fort différents et changeants, qu'il existe par conséquent un *polymorphisme extrême*.

3. Qu'assez souvent, ni l'aspect clinique, ni l'examen histologique, ni le trichogramme, en l'absence de symptômes pathologiques sur le cuir chevelu ou sur la peau, ne permettent un diagnostic étiologique exact. (Ce sont précisément ces cas qui figurent dans beaucoup de travaux comme des pseudopelades authentiques).

4. *Conclusion:* La pseudopelade de Brocq, dans la conception de son auteur n'existe pas en tant que maladie autonome.

La communication d'aujourd'hui est destinée à exposer devant un auditoire international cette conception originale et pertinente dûe à l'école française (Degos et coll.), à la justifier et à discuter les points et problèmes qui demandent encore des recherches complémentaires.

ad. 1. *Cette polyétiologie* des états pseudopeladiques est aujourd'hui, grâce au travail de Degos et coll., aux nombreuses publications suscitées par lui dont notre récent travail, devenu un fait acquis et adopté par un grand nombre de dermatologues. *Les états pseudopeladiques* sont réalisés par les *folliculites décalvantes*, type Quinquaud, certaines formes d'infections streptococciques chez l'enfant, le groupe des folliculites ou folliculoses kératosiques comprenant le Lichen plan, Lichen spinulosus, le syndrome de Graham-Little-Lassueur, le Psoriasis (?), la sclérodermie, l'alopezia mucinosa et plus rarement la tuberculose, la lèpre, des traumatismes etc., ceci avec une grande diversité dans leur évolution. Ainsi, la *folliculite décalvante de Quinquaud* et certains cas d'impetigo streptococcique peuvent réaliser, au cours de leur évolution, un E.P.P. typique. Preuve à l'appui notre cas No. 2 à évolution extrêmement rapide. Un deuxième groupe comprend trois affections, liées par une parenté étiologique probable: le Lichen plan, Lichen spinulosis, le syndrome de Graham-Little. Le premier trop classique pour mériter une mention spéciale, son D.D. avec le lupus erythémateux est souvent difficile, mais peut être facilité par la coexistence de lésions cutanées. *Certains cas atypiques* comme notre cas No. 3 montrent une coexistance d'un Lichen plan avec lésions kératosiques de la peau, erythème et squames périfoliculaires au cuir chevelu évoluant vers un E.P.P. très particulier. Un autre, réalisant le tableau d'un Graham-Little, montre un E.P.P. associé à un état spinulosique du dos et un Lichen plan des muqueuses. Certains cas, atteints exclusivement de lésions spinulosiques ou kératosiques, non inflammatoires du follicule pileux évoluent vers un E.P.P. Trois cas de *Psoriasis*, vérifiés cliniquement et par l'examen histologique évoluent vers un E.P.P. observations dont nous attendons confirmation ou infirmation. Différentes observations (Degos, Grupper) signalent des E.P.P. consécutifs à une sclerodermie ou acrosclérose, Pinkus. Grupper, Meneghini à une alopezia mucinosa localisée au cuir chevelu, d'autres à une tuberculose, lèpre, traumatisme etc. du cuir chevelu (Degos). Dans tous ces cas, un diagnostic étiologique a pu être établi.

ad. 2. *Le Polymorphisme évolutif* existe au même titre dans les E.P.P. comme dans les P.P.B. sensu stricto et complique singulièrement le diagnostic étiologique.

Il est d'observation courante que certains aspects cliniques — la configuration particulière des plaques glabres, l'aspect et les lésions de leur surface (erythème, kératose et squames perifolliculaires) — s'effacent et laissent la place à un état cicatriciel banal. Tout au plus trouve-t-on encore certaines lésions évolutives à la périphérie des plaques cicatricielles. Pour un grand nombre de ces cas, un diagnostic étiologique devient impossible.

ad. 3. *Concerne la pseudopelade de Brocq sensu stricto ou alopézia atrophicans,* elle comporte le 30% des cas dans la statistique de DEGOS et un même pourcentage pour un nombre resteint de nos observations. BROCQ, sous un nom «criticable» en fait une maladie autonome. Sa description initiale fait mention de caractères cliniques caractéristiques comme l'apparition insidieuse de taches alopéciques d'un blanc ivoire, atrophique ou cicatricielles, dépourvues de tout duvet et d'orifices folliculaires. Ces taches se constituent d'emblée sans lésion préalable, avec absence de folliculites à la périphérie. Il existe parfois une légère teinte rose ou un point rouge autour de chaque poil atteint. BROCQ et SABOURAUD signalent également l'aspect particulier des racines des poils atteints, frappant par leur pigmentation excessive. Son apparition est insidieuse, son évolution chronique ou rapide, presque toujours progressive. Les plaques s'agrandissent, se fusionnent et forment de larges aires cicatricielles avec persistance de quelques touffes de poils sains. Dans la suite, ce même auteur admet l'existence d'une couleur variant du blanc-rose — rouge-vif à la périphérie des plaques et d'une sorte de gaine cornée périfolliculaire. Photinos signale comme non-exceptionnel la présence d'une fine desquamation et BROCQ lui-même admet plus tard la coexistence de folliculites suppurées à la périphérie. Tous ces symptômes s'observent également dans les E.P.P. Plusieurs de nos cas, dont l'étiologie a pu être confirmée, montrent également ces «symptômes pseudopeladiques» (DEGOS-JUON). Ce ne sont donc, en définitive, pas de critères valables pour affirmer l'authenticité de cette affection.

L'histologie, malgré les description classiques de LENGLET, MIESCHER et LENGGENHAGER, DUPERRAT, ne permet elle non plus d'affirmer cette autonomie. Des aspects en tout point semblables peuvent être réalisés dans les E.P.P. consécutifs à un Lichen plan, un lupus erythémateux etc. La P.P.B. perd ainsi, progressivement, son authenticité étiologique et clinique.

Que représentent finalement, du point de vue étiologique et nosologique ces 30% de cas «cryptogénétiques», appelés provisoirement «pseudopeladiques»? Il est difficile de répondre à cette question à l'heure actuelle, les critères cliniques et histologiques étant sujets à caution et non valables pour leur accorder une authenticité nosologique. Pour résoudre ce problème, chaque cas doit être soumis dès le début de son évolution à un examen local et général approfondi. Les prélèvements (biopsie et poils) sont à examiner selon les méthodes histologiques, histochimiques et bactériologiques modernes. Le comportement biologique des racines atteintes, à l'égard des Antibiotiques et Corticostéroïdes seront également susceptibles de donner des indications intéressantes. Une synthèse d'un grand nombre de cas ainsi examinés permettra un jour de connaître la véritable étiologie de cette affection et de réduire sensiblement le pourcentage des P.P.B. «cryptogénétiques» au profit des états pseudopeladiques étiologiquement classés.

En conclusion: La notion des E.P.P. à étiologie définie est acquise et remplace aujourd'hui celle de la pseudopelade en tant que maladie autonome. La qualification comme E.P.P. consécutif à une des affections à évolution cicatricielle repose sur leur configuration morphologique et les distingue d'une alopécie cicatricielle banale consécutive aux mêmes affections. 30% des cas posent encore aujourd'hui un problème non résolu. Enfin, états pseudopeladiques et cryptogéniques représentent un problème clinique, étiologique et thérapeutique d'une grande importance. Le dépistage et l'identification précoce permettront dans l'avenir un traitement spécifique valable pour les affections à étiologie définie (E.P.P.), un traitement à tenter par Antibiotiques et Corticostéroïdes pour les P.P.B. Ainsi conçu, le prognostic aujourd'hui si sévère de ces affections, sera moins redoutable dans un avenir prochain.

La pelade, maladie psychosomatique

S. Lambergeon, Hôpital Sainte-Anne, Paris (France)

Une étude psychosomatique des peladiques portant maintenant sur 15 ans d'expérience nous permet avec une conviction accrue de considérer la pelade comme le type même de la maladie psychosomatique. Il ne nous est pas possible en quelques minutes d'analyser en détail les nouveaux cas que nous avons eu l'occasion d'étudier. Nous résumerons simplement les points communs rencontrés dans ces différents cas, pour en arriver avec plus de détails aux conséquences thérapeutiques de nos constatations. Précisons, en outre, que les cas étudiés sont des cas de pelade décalvante totale avec ou sans généralisation à tout le système pileux, et où les traitements classiques avaient échoués. L'étude de chaque cas a porté sur l'histoire vécue du malade èt de sa maladie, sur le matériel psychologique (fantasmes, rêves, dessins d'enfants, etc.) apporté au cours des entretiens, sur les tests psycho-métriques.

La nature psychogène de la maladie est marquée par les circonstances d'apparition:

Le traumatisme psychique est constant, parfois apparemment minime, souvent grave. Sa teinte affective est importante à noter car il s'agit d'une situation entraînant une sentiment d'abandon, de rupture, de coupure par perte, physique ou morale, d'un être plus ou moins cher (mort, abandon, séparation définitive ou non), que cela survienne dans la vie sentimentale, familiale ou professionnelle.

Le retentissement de la circonstance occasionnelle sur les mécanismes psychologiques profonds est important: la rupture de la relation objectale, de la relation à autrui réactive des sentiments de frustration et par voie de conséquence une agressivité violente et jusqu'alors refoulée et non investie que le sujet retourne contre lui-même sur un mode masochiste.

Nous noterons, chez la femme, une situation très particulière au moment d'apparition d'une pelade décalvante: la grossesse. Les pelades gravidiques ou post-gravidiques sont en effet fréquentes, et pourraient plaider en faveur d'une origine endocrinienne de la maladie. En fait, on retrouve dans les implications psychologiques sous-jacentes le même sentiment de rupture, de coupure.

Le contexte psychologique ne permet que rarement la constatation d'une perturbation quelconque. L'angoisse, par exemple, est souvent peu importante apparemment, souvent niée même vis-à-vis de la pelade. Ces malades présentent en effet des mécanismes de défense rigides contre leurs affects, et à la mesure de leurs pulsions agressives mal investies dans des activités autorisées par un Surmoi sévère. Mais, et cela commande une très grande prudence dans l'approche psychologique de ces malades, les risques de décompensation sont grands, qui feront basculer le malade dans une psychose grave.

Les tests psycho-métriques montrent en effet, chez des sujets ayant presque tous d'ailleurs un niveau intellectuel élevé, une rigidité affective importante accompagnant des difficultés sur le plan de la relation à autrui par immaturité affective et des mécanismes d'inhibition.

La rigidité et la fragilité affective de ces malades conduisent à des considérations thérapeutiques importantes.

Le facteur «réassurance», dans la conduite du traitement quelqu'il soit, est
extrêmement important. Il est donc essentiel, et tous les dermatologistes, même
les plus hostiles à la théorie psychosomatique, le savent, qu'une bonne relation
médecin-malade s'établisse. C'est une relation «à distance», le malade mettant
entre lui et le médecin une barrière très subtile de bonne volonté souvent teintée
d'opposition discrète. Cette relation «à distance» respectée permet le plus souvent,
au début d'une pelade, un arrêt rapide de l'évolution et la guérison par les moyens
classiques habituels.

La nature psychogène de la maladie explique l'action certaine de certains
neuroleptiques tels que la Chlorpromazine, ou des Centrophenoxines (Lucidril);
mais aussi, dans les cas graves de grande pelade décalvante, de la narcothérapie
que nous considérons comme le traitement de choix en particulier après échec des
traitements classiques.

Au rythme d'une séance par semaine, parfois deux au début du traitement,
l'injection intra-veineuse de 10 cc de Penthiobarbital sodique entraîne un sommeil
d'une demi-heure à une heure, permettant de lever dans un premier stade la tension
nerveuse ainsi que l'insomnie qui accompagne très souvent la maladie. Le duvet
apparaît en général après huit ou dix narcoses, et la repousse des cheveux normaux
se fera peu à peu. Peu à peu aussi il sera possible d'établir un contact psychothérapique vrai, souvent impossible au départ, malgré l'apparence de bonne
volonté du patient. Au décours de la narcose, celui-ci pourra parler plus volontiers
de ses difficultés.

Nous en venons donc à l'approche psychothérapique de ces malades. Il nous
paraît, d'une façon générale, tout à fait contre-indiqué de faire une psychothérapie
de type psychanalytique chez ces sujets dont le Moi est fragile, tiraillé entre des
pulsions agressives intenses et un Surmoi tyrannique. Ce ne peut être qu'une
psychothérapie de soutien et menée avec la plus grande prudence.

Il peut arriver que le ou la malade accepte mal les narcoses. Dans ces cas, nous
avons conseillé des méthodes de relaxation, avec de bons résultats mais infiniment
plus longs à obtenir. Une technique de relaxation pourra d'ailleurs être indiquée
pour prolonger l'action d'une narcothérapie. De passive, la levée de la tension
nerveuse devient active, provoquée par la malade elle-même sous la conduite du
psychothérapeute.

Nous considérons que toutes les pelades décalvantes doivent guérir, seules
resteront un échec les pelades de psychotiques: la guérison du symptôme pelade
chez ces malades est exceptionnelle, même après amélioration de l'état psychotique.

Biological Depth Dose Studies in Electron Beam Therapy: Effects on Anagen Mouse Hairs*

L. H. LANZL and F. D. MALKINSON, Department of Radiology, Department of
Medicine (Section of Dermatology), and the Argonne Cancer Research Hospital**, Chicago, Illinois (USA)

The experiments reported here were undertaken to help elucidate the "skin-
sparing" effects that have been observed when high-energy electrons are used for

* This work was supported in part by United States Public Health Service Grant RH
00280-04, Division of Radiological Health.
** Operated by The University of Chicago for the United States Atomic Energy Commision.

cancer therapy. "Skin-sparing" refers to the observation that a higher dose of electrons is required to produce the same degree of erythema caused by exposure to 200 kv X-rays.

TAPLEY and FLETCHER have stated: "It is apparent that the skin-sparing effect with the electron beam is greater than can be explained by the demonstrated RBE of 0.8 to 0.9 for electrons compared with kilovoltage radiation, and may be attributed in part to the build-up factor." The experiments described in this paper are limited to a study of the build-up factor, utilizing physical and biological systems of dosimetry.

Physical Methods and Results

The electron source was the linear accelerator at the Argonne Cancer Research Hospital, The University of Chicago. This is a traveling-wave type of accelerator which was operated at an electron beam energy of 20 MeV.

The physical methods used to study dose build-up require systems of spatial resolution of about 0.5 mm since the electron beam is of the scanning type. To determine the average dose at depths near the surface, detailed measurements need to be made at the peaks and troughs of the dose distributions. Thermoluminescent dosimetry using lithium-fluoride crystals of mesh size between 100 and 200 satisfied this requirement.

Covered Teflon discs containing the lithium fluoride crystals were used as the absorbing media. The Teflon discs, centered in a 10×10 cm field, were scanned at a delivered dose of approximately 200 rads. The crystals were then processed and measured. The surface dose was observed to be 88% of the plateau dose which, for these measurements with a 20 MeV electron beam, starts at approximately 1.7 cm below the surface and appears to extend to a depth of at least 2.5 cm.

Biological Method and Results

The requirements for a satisfactory biological method of assessing buildup-include quantitation, small spatial resolution, and use of the same system on the surface as in the tissue depth. Growing hairs in the mouse provide a system compatible with all of these requirements, since hair damage can be measured on one flank at the surface and on the opposite flank — about 2.5 cm distant — in the depth or at the plateau of the build-up curve.

All studies were carried out in 3 month old female Carworth Farms No 1 mice according to the following technique. In this mouse strain anagen lasts 17 to 20 days. Initially, all animals were plucked widely over both flanks, and 24 days later, when hairs were in telogen, the mice were replucked. 12 days later (12th day of anagen) groups of 8 to 26 animals received a single dose of radiation under sodium pentobarbital anesthesia. For this procedure each animal was placed in the left lateral position with the right flank exposed to the radiation source. Through-radiation was given so that the average body thickness of 2.5 cm separated entry (right flank) and exit (left flank) treatment portals. 48 h after irradiation (14th day of anagen), all animals were given 3 to 5 μC of ^{3}H-DL-serine intravenously. On the 24th day hairs from both flanks of each mouse were plucked for study.

Hair samples were weighed and placed in a combustion apparatus in the presence of oxygen. Volatile materials were removed in a high vacuum system and radioactivity in the remaining material was assayed as tritiated water in a liquid scintillation spectrometer. Throughout the study hair samples from control and irradiated sites were studied individually for each animal in all experimental groups.

The radiation source was the same as that described in the section on physical methods.

Low-dose exposure (300 rads) depressed serine uptake in hair almost equally at entry and exit portals (table). At moderate doses of 500 to 600 rads, reduced incorporation of serine at the beam entry site was further lowered by 15% on average at the exit portal (table).

Reduced Levels of ^{3}H-DL-Serine in Mouse Hair Following Electron Beam Irradiation in Anagen. Percentages are Expressed as an Average Ratio of DPM/mg of the Beam Entry Side (R) to the Beam Exit Side (L) for Each Individual Animal

Dose (Rads)	Animals	DPM/mgL (Beam Exit Side)	DPM/mgR (Beam Entry Side)	R/L%	Standard Error of the Mean
300	8	2340	2044	95	13
500	9	2619	2978	118	12
600	26	322	365	113	4
No radiation (control group)	7	3131	3097	100	4

Discussion

Serine is incorporated into keratin and into cytoplasmic and nuclear proteins in hair matrix cells. Since protein synthesis is a radiosensitive process, impaired uptake of serine is a useful indicator of radiation injury to hair.

Experimental findings for the groups of mice receiving 500 or 600 rads (table) reveal that impairment of ^{3}H-DL-serine incorporation and protein synthesis on the exit side is about 15% greater than at the beam entrance site. The difference correlates well with the 12% higher plateau dose measured by physical means. The higher plateau dose is due to the well-established build-up phenomenon. It is quite possible, however, that hair damage does not exhibit the same quantitative response to radiation reflected by the degree of cutaneous inflammation and erythema produced. Clinical impressions of skin-sparing effects greater than 12 to 15% would most likely reflect a skin-specific RBE, perhaps primarily related to vascular reactivity, and not a substantially different build-up factor from that described above. These studies do indicate, however, that, with the instantaneous dose rates in use for pencil beam scanning, and at the dose levels studied, the physically and biologically measured build-up are in substantial agreement. Moreover, even though the linear energy transfer (LET) cannot be expected to be identical at the surface as compared with the depth, this difference has not produced a significantly different RBE at the two positions for the biological indicator used.

Elektronenmikroskopische Befunde an den peritrichialen Nervenfasern des menschlichen Haarfollikels

C. ORFANOS, Univ.-Hautklinik Köln (Deutschland)

Das menschliche Haar hat nicht nur kosmetische Bedeutung, sondern auch eine Sinnesfunktion. Im Elektronenmikroskop finden sich Hinweise dafür, daß das Haar bzw. der Haarfollikel für die Aufnahme von mechanischen Stimuli, die die behaarte Haut treffen, eine wesentliche Rolle spielen.

Auf Grund eines umfangreichen Schrifttums wissen wir, daß der Haarfollikel mit Nerven reichlich versorgt wird. Besonders in der Höhe der Talgdrüse lassen sich, nach den Untersuchungen von KADAHOFF, WEDDELL, WINKELMANN, MONTAGNA und vielen anderen, mehrere Nervenfasern nachweisen, die im Verhältnis zur Achse des Follikels zum Teil *longitudinal*, zum Teil *transversal* verlaufen. Die transversalen sollen auf dem Follikelepithel, die longitudinalen zwischen den Epithelzellen liegen.

Diese Gegend haben wir im Elektronenmikroskop untersucht. Untersuchungsmaterial war die normale behaarte Haut vier gesunder Probanden, im besonderen die Kopfhaut. Wir fanden im Corium zwischen den Haarfollikeln größere polyaxonale Nerven, die von Endo-, Peri- und Epineurium umgeben werden. Diese Nerven enthalten dünne und dicke Axone.

Dicke Axone innervieren den glatten Haarmuskel, den *M. arrector pili*. Es sind cholinergische und wahrscheinlich auch adrenergische Nervenfasern, die in „en-passant"-Synapsen mehrere Muskelzellen gleichzeitig versorgen.

Ähnliche Axone kommen auch in unmittelbarer Nähe der *Talgdrüse* vor. Sie treten nicht in das Drüsenepithel ein, sondern reichen nur bis an die Basalmembran heran, ohne sie zu durchbrechen. In diesen Regionen finden sich oft helle mitochondrienreiche Zellen, die sich von den Zellen des sezernierenden Drüsenepithels unterscheiden lassen. Welche Rolle sie im Talgdrüsenepithel spielen, ist noch Gegenstand weiterer Untersuchungen.

Dünnere Axone finden sich in der Nähe des *Follikelepithels*, zwischen langgezogenen Bindegewebszellen und dem peritrichialen Kollagen. Es scheint, daß hiervon Zweige ausgehen, die lanzettenförmig bis an die Basalmembran des Follikelepithels herantreten und Kontakt mit den Basalzellen der äußeren Wurzelscheide aufnehmen.

Sie sind dort mit kleinen Mitochondrien prall gefüllt und von modifizierten Schwann-Zellen umgeben. Modifiziert deshalb, weil ihre Membran eine pinocytotische Aktivität zeigt, die sonst nicht üblich ist. Diese Kontaktstellen zwischen Follikelepithelzellen und Nerven des Coriums haben wir als *epithelio-neurale Verbindungen* bezeichnet.

Was läßt sich nun aus der Morphologie über die Funktion der epithelio-neuralen Verbindungen sagen?

Manche Ähnlichkeiten zu den Befunden von PEASE u. QUILLIAM, CAUNA u. ROSS, ANDRES, YAMAMOTO u. a. lassen uns vermuten, daß es sich um *Receptoren* handelt, die mechanische Reize registrieren. Der Reichtum an Mitochondrien weist auf die Möglichkeit hin, mechanische Stimuli in *Generatorpotentiale* zu transduzieren. Solche Ansammlungen von Mitochondrien finden sich auch in anderen Receptoren der Haut, z. B. in den Meißnerschen Korpuskeln und in den Vater-Pacinischen Körperchen. In allen diesen Organen werden in mitochondrienreichen *Dendriten* und in direkter Abhängigkeit von der Reizgröße Generatorpotentiale gebildet; überschreiten die Generatorpotentiale einen bestimmten Schwellenwert, so lösen sie *Neuritenpotentiale* konstanter Amplitude aus, die von größeren myelinhaltigen Nerven übernommen und saltatorisch zentralwärts fortgeleitet werden.

Berücksichtigt man mit BODIAN und RUSKA bei der Bezeichnung solcher Strukturen die jeweilige Richtung der Erregungsleitung, so dürfte man nicht von *End-Organen*, wie bei den neuromuskulären Verbindungen, sondern von *Start- Organen* sprechen (s. Abbildung). End-Organe sind durch synaptische Vesikel als Merkmal der *Erregungsübertragung* gekennzeichnet, Start-Organe hingegen durch Mitochondrien als Merkmal der *Erregungsbildung*. Die epithelio-neuralen Verbindungen sind offenbar ein solches Start-Organ. Sie registrieren Bewegungen des Haares, die sich auf das Follikelepithel übertragen. Das Haar selbst wirkt dabei als Hebelarm.

Zum Schluß noch ein Wort zur Frage, ob im menschlichen Haarfollikel auch *intra*-epitheliale Nerven vorkommen:

Zwischen den Zellen der äußeren Wurzelscheide fanden wir oft, öfter als in der Epidermis, rundliche Profile, die Axonen entsprechen könnten.

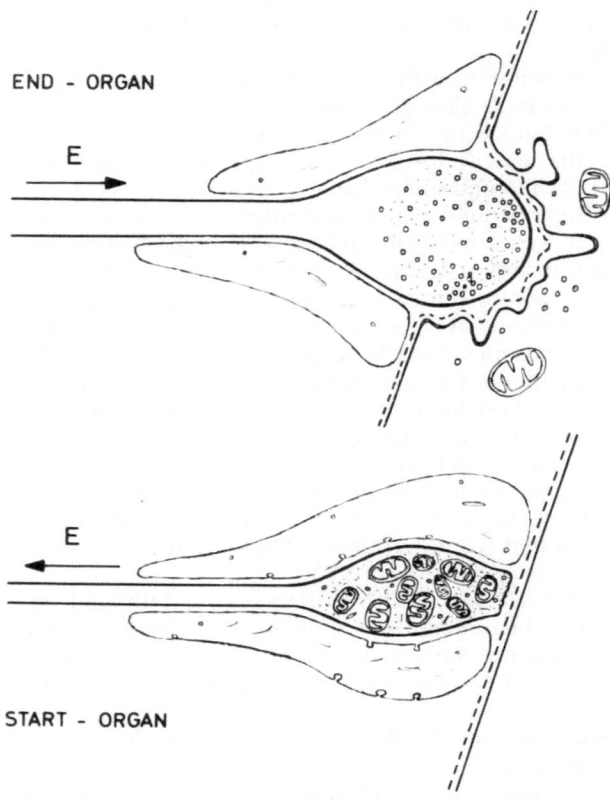

Es ist jedoch im Elektronenmikroskop schwer zu entscheiden, ob es tatsächlich Axone sind oder Ausläufer dendritischer Zellelemente des Epithels. Zumindest ein Teil davon sind solche Ausläufer, denn sie enthalten die charakteristischen „stäbchenförmigen" Profile des endoplasmatischen Reticulums, die in Axonen nicht vorkommen.

Sinneszellen schließlich, wie sie in den Sinushaaren verschiedener Tiere (ANDRES) vorkommen, haben wir in den Follikeln menschlicher Kopfhaare nicht gefunden.

Literatur. KADANOFF, D.: Z. Zellforsch. **6**, 631 (1928). — ORFANOS, C.: Arch. klin. exp. Derm. **228**, 421 (1967). — RUSKA, H.: Pers. Mitteilung 1966. — WINKELMANN, R. K.: Ann. N.Y. Acad. Sci. **83**, 400 (1957). — Weitere Lit. s. ORFANOS (1967).

Die Behandlung der Alopecia areata im Kindesalter

J. Tomášková, Univ.-Hautklinik Prag (Tschechoslowakei)

Es geht um eine relativ häufige Erkrankung. Das Vorkommen wird von verschiedenen Autoren in der Grenze von 1,2 bis 2,9% sämtlicher Dermatosen angegeben (Rothmann, Walker u. a.), in den letzten Jahren um etwas mehr. Saubouraud u. Crocker geben das Frequenzmaximum im Schulalter und zwischen dem 20. und 30. Lebensjahr an. Dem entspricht auch unsere Statistik. In den Jahren 1964 bis 1965 sind durch die Kinderambulanz der I. Hautklinik des Prof. Konopík in Prag 3200 neue Patienten gegangen; hiervon wurde die Alopecia areata bei 63 Kindern, das sind 3,9%, festgestellt. Diese verhältnismäßig hohe Anzahl ist höchstwahrscheinlich durch die fachmännische Selektion in den Gesundheitszentren gegeben, sie stimmt jedoch auffallend mit der zunehmenden Anzahl von Psychoneurosen im Kindesalter (Anderson) überein. Diese schließt Kranke im Alter von 4½ bis zu 15 Jahren ein. Das Verhältnis der beiden Geschlechter ist fast 1:1, nämlich 32 Knaben und 31 Mädchen. Darin sind wir mit den Angaben von Wais und Kepler einig, die eine Überlegenheit von Mädchen erst in der postpubertalen Zeit verzeichneten.

46 Fälle hatten einen quoad sanationem benignen Verlauf. Dreimal ist im Prepubertalalter Ophiasis vorgekommen, und bei zwei Kindern ging es um isolierte Alopecia areata in den Augenbrauen und zehn hatten totale, insgesamt maligne Alopecien. Mit den ersten Erscheinungen kamen 52 Kinder, bei der ersten Rezidive vier und bei der zweiten Rezidive zwei. Die Erkrankung vor der Untersuchung bei uns dauerte weniger als ein halbes Jahr bei 28 Kindern, ½ bis 5 Jahre bei 17 Kindern; bei den anderen konnte man die Dauer nicht genau feststellen. Alle Kinder wurden sowohl in somatischer als auch in psychischer Hinsicht untersucht; der Neurologe, der Psychiater, eventuell der Psychologe und der Endokrinologe wurden konsultiert.

Einige Kinder wurden hospitalisiert, die meisten jedoch ambulant behandelt. Wir haben den Blutdruck, Cholesterol, K, Na, alkalische Phosphatasen, 17-Ketosteroide, eventuell auch 17-Hydroxycorticosteroide und Steroidspektrum untersucht, ferner haben wir eine Röntgenaufnahme der Sella und des Handgelenks vorgenommen.

Die endokrinologische Untersuchung war insgesamt negativ. Psychische Probleme waren häufig vorhanden. 14 Kinder, d. h. 21% sämtlicher Fälle, zeigten verschiedene Störungen im Verhalten, ein Kind hatte Tick und Cephalalgie, bei 3 Kindern wurde Spasmofilie festgestellt, 3 waren ausgesprochen psychoneurotisch, 2 hatten Epilepsie mit einem typischen Befund auf das Elektronencephalogramm. Zwei Kinder waren pathologisch klein gewachsen, zweimal handelte es sich gleichzeitig um die Dawnov-Krankheit. Bei vier Kranken haben wir Vitiligo gefunden, zwei Kinder hatten atopisches Ekzem. Fast bei einer Hälfte der Fälle waren die Nägel verändert: Grübchen, Querfurchen und Zersplitterung. Die Katarakte wurde bei drei Kranken mit totaler Alopecia gefunden. Bei einem Kind handelte es sich um die unvollständige ectodermale Dystrophie.

Juon und eine Reihe anderer Autoren halten die Alopecia areata für eine das ganze Integument betreffende metabolische Störung (namentlich die Dysenzymatose). Uns ist es jedoch nicht gelungen, durch laufende Methoden eine metabolische Störung nachzuweisen, bloß zweimal hatten wir bereits vor Beginn der Behandlung höheren Cholesterol, ohne daß eine Hypothyreose nachgewiesen wurde.

Nach Stüttgen und Goertz haben endokrine Faktoren nur modifizierenden Einfluß auf den Verlauf der Krankheit. In unserem Kollektiv ging es nur zweimal um eine klare Hypothyreose. Eine viel größere Betonung wird auf die Konstitution und die psychischen Einflüsse über Corticodiencephalon und vagosympatische Wege zu den Gewebeeffektoren gelegt. Wir sind zweimal der familiären Form von Alopecia areata begegnet (Vater und Sohn, Mutter und Tochter). Ein Knabe hatte gleichzeitig Epilepsie, war jedoch geistig nicht verlangsamt, und bei seinem alopetischen Vater bewegte sich das Elektroencephalogramm in den Grenzen der Normen, so daß wir diesen Fall nicht als typisches Moyhan's-Syndrom einreihen können.

Zwölfmal ging dem Entstehen von Alopecia eine fieberhafte Infektionskrankheit voraus, was den neuen Ansichten über die Aufgabe des Hypotalamus als zentralem Faktor (ABDERHALDEN, HUME) entspricht. Eine Kopfverletzung ging in einem Fall vorher, zweimal entstand die Alopecia nach einem schweren geistigen Trauma. Einer fokalen Infektion sind wir in zwei Fällen begegnet. Bei einem kam es zur Heilung nach einer Tonsilektomie, der zweite hatte den Befund eines hemolytischen Streptococcus im Hals und wurde nach einer massiven PNC-Behandlung ausgeheilt.

Die Beschwerlichkeit der ätiologischen Analyse bei der Alopecia areata und deren spontane Tendenz zum Rücktritt sind die Ursachen, warum es eine ganze Reihe von Behandlungsmethoden gibt und die meisten derselben von deren Autoren als erfolgreich bewertet werden.

Lediglich längere Beobachtungen und Verfolgen des Trichogramms werden uns zeigen, ob durch die Behandlung die reversible Gegebenheit oder eine schwere Dystrophie der Haarwurzeln getroffen werden. Bei einer areaten Alopecia zeigt nämlich das Trichogramm insgesamt telogenes Haar und dystrophisches, anagenes Haar, und der steigende Glykogeninhalt ist das Zeichen der Heilung. Die Situation verschlechtert der Umstand, daß der kosmetische Nachteil zu einem Minderwertigkeitskomplex bei den Kindern führt und somit der Grund zu einer weiteren Rezidive oder Verschlechterung sein kann.

Deshalb bemühen wir uns, die Therapie durch ein beruhigendes, optimistisch gestimmtes Gespräch zu beginnen. Eine Milieuänderung ist passend. Die Besserung des Gesamtzustandes kann durch Hydrotherapie, ausreichenden Schlaf, eine an Eiweißstoff und Vitamin reiche Nahrung erzielt werden. Eine Beruhigung kann man im Anfang durch Zentralsedative (Vallium, Librium) unterstützen. Als Vitaminbehandlung haben wir B 12 in der Dosierung von 300 γ zweimal wöchentlich, oftmals mit Thyreoidin kombiniert, gewählt, bei gleichzeitiger Seborrhoe haben wir B 6, d. h. Pyridoxin, verabreicht, bei fettsüchtigen Kindern, in der Prepubertät und bei nachgewiesener Hypothyreose Thyreoidin mit Bepanthen kombiniert.

Bei totalen Alopecien hat sich am besten die Kombination Triamcinolon mit Stenolon bewährt. Wir haben 1 bis 2 mg auf 1 kg Gewicht pro Tag, Stenolon 1 bis 3 mg jeden 2. Tag verabreicht. Nach Haarerscheinung haben wir die Dosis herabgesetzt und die Behandlung höchstens ein halbes Jahr lang durchgeführt. Bei länger dauernder Verabreichung der Kombination von anabolischen und katabolischen Corticoiden erfolgte eine Steigerung von Leukocyten, einmal eine Blutdruckerhöhung, zweimal eine mäßige Cholesterolsteigerung, und zweimal äußerte sich eine prediabetische Kurve nach der Glucose. Einmal entstand die Facies lunata. Gleichzeitig wurden 60% Kinder ausgeheilt (viermal kam es im Laufe von 2 Jahren zu Rezidiven). Die nachwachsenden Haare zeigten sich normal. Sieben totale Alopecien blieben refraktär gegen die Therapie, bei drei hatten wir Erfolg bei der Kombination von Triamcinolon mit Grisovin. Lokal haben wir uns auf Bestrahlung mit der Bucky-Lampe zweimal à 400 r beschränkt.

Die Prognose bei totalen Alopecien erscheint nicht günstig; laufende Typen des Haarausfalles heilten innerhalb von 1 bis 2 Jahren, und zwar um so rascher, je jünger das befallene Kind war.

Literatur. Barman, J., V. Pecoraro, and I. Astore: J. invest. Derm. **6**, 421 (1964). — Barman, J. M., L. Astore, and V. Pecoraro: J. invest. Derm. **4**, 233 (1965). — Belezos, N. K.: Dermatologica (Basel) **4**, 176 (1965). — Fleck, F., u. M. Fleck: Die Haarkrankheiten des Menschen. Berlin: Verlag Volk und Gesundheit 1962. — Juon, M.: Zbl. Haut- u. Geschl.-Kr. **119**, 1 (1965). — Leider, N.: Practical pediatric dermatology. St. Louis: C. V. Mosby Comp. 1961. — Müller, S. A., and R. K. Wickelmann: Arch. Derm. **88**, 290 (1963). — Olivetti, L., e D. Bubola: G. ital. Derm. Sif. **105**, 689 (1964). — Perlmann, H. H.: Pediatric dermatology Chicago: The Year Book Publishers 1961. — Pecoraro, V., I. Astore, J. Barman, and C. I. Araujo: J. invest. Derm. **42**, 427 (1964). — Pozzo, G.: G. ital. Derm. Sif. **105**, 431 (1964).

Untersuchungen über die Veränderungen des Haares der Augenbrauen bei endogenem Ekzem

H. Langhof †, Universitätshautklinik Jena (Deutschland), und M. Munteanu, Universitätshautklinik Jassy (Rumänien)

Die Verdünnung des seitlichen Teils der Augenbrauen wird als ein häufiges und dadurch wichtiges Zeichen betrachtet hinsichtlich des endogenen Ekzems (G. W. Korting). Einige Verfasser (Brandt, E. Hoffmann, Urbach, Schönfeld, von Korting angeführt) legen eine mechanische Ursache diesem Symptom bei, indem sie es als eine Folge des Kratzens auslegen. Andere (Rost u. Marchionini; Polemann u. Peltzer) schreiben, daß infolge der verschiedenen anatomo-physiologischen Bedingungen, nämlich der inneren und äußeren Teile der Augenbrauen, manche endokrino-vegetativen Ursachen im Laufe des endogenen Ekzems besonders über die Haareswurzeln, die auf dem seitlichen Teil der Augenbraue sich befinden, wirkten. Aus diesen Gründen haben wir uns vorgenommen zu untersuchen, ob nicht einige morpho-dimensionale Besonderheiten des Haares dieser Gegend bei den Ekzematikern vorhanden seien; dadurch könnte man vielleicht irgendeine Aufklärung dieses Problems bringen.

Stoff und Methode

Unsere Untersuchungen beziehen sich auf 27 Kranke, die mit verschiedenen Dermatosen behaftet waren und die zugleich an den äußeren Teilen der Augenbrauen oder an anderen behaarten Körperstellen eine auffällige Verdünnung des Haarwuches zeigten. Von diesen Fällen hatten acht die Diagnose: endogenes Ekzem. Wir führten morphologische und mikrometrische Untersuchungen (Ocularmesser Zeiss) durch. Anschließend erfolgte die Auswertung der Untersuchungsergebnisse durch Vergleich der Haare der verschiedenen Körperregionen mit den Haaren aus den äußeren Teilen der Augenbrauen, unter gleichzeitiger Berücksichtigung anderer dermatologischer Veränderungen.

Ergebnisse

Die morphologischen Gegebenheiten der untersuchten Haare wie auch die Veränderungen in den verschiedenen Phasen der Haarentwicklung werden als bekannt vorausgesetzt und nicht als morpho-dimensionale Veränderungen der Haare von Ekzematikern betrachtet.

Wir sind aber überrascht, Änderungen des Durchmessers des Haarschaftes zu finden, die auf eine kleine spindelförmige Zone begrenzt sind und an das Aussehen von Trichoclasia Nodosa oder Monylethrix erinnern.

Diese Verdickungen werden vor allem am Gipfel des jungen Augenbrauenhaares bemerkt, das eben erst aus dem Follikel hervorgegangen ist. Manchmal befinden sich mehrere Knoten (zwei bis drei) auf ein und demselben Haar.

51*

Um eine etwaige traumatische Ursache àuszuschließen, wurden diese Veränderungen mit denen des Haares aus der Trichoptilomania und aus der Alopecia mecanica verglichen, welche bei den Kindern durch Reibung des Kopfes am Kissen stattfindet, wobei der mechanische Faktor sicher eintritt.

In diesen Fällen aber, obwohl sie auch begrenzt vorkommen, sind die dimensionalen Veränderungen doch nicht spindelförmig, sondern unregelmäßig, winkelig, und an dieser Stelle bemerkt man immer die Bruchlinie (Abb. 3).

Das mit solchen Knoten versehene Augenbrauenhaar erscheint mit einem sehr verweiteten und pigmentierten Haarmark, während die Corticale sehr begrenzt ist.

Obwohl an dieser Stelle der Haarhalm vergrößert erscheint, sind doch diese Knoten — weil sie nicht durch eine größere Keratinbeifügung entstehen —, anstatt eine größere Widerständigkeit zu haben, leicht zerbrechlich, und folglich wird ein kleiner Traumatism das Haar brechen.

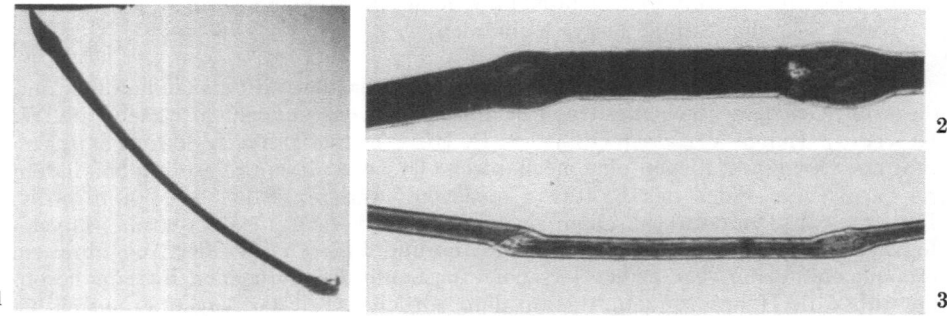

Abb. 1. Die spindelförmige Vergrößerung an dem Gipfel des jungen Haares

Abb. 2. Zwei spindelförmige Knötchen auf demselben Haar

Abb. 3. Zwei traumatische unregelmäßige und winkelige Vergrößerungen. Man sieht die Bruchlinie

Die Häufigkeit dieser Veränderungen geht aus den folgenden Daten hervor: a) Bei den 17 Fällen mit verschiedenen Dermatosen, waren nur bei zwei Kranken die spindelförmigen Vergrößerungen gefunden worden; b) bei den acht Fällen von endogenem Ekzem waren sechsmal die Veränderungen an der äußeren und zweimal auch an der inneren Seite der Augenbrauen bemerkt worden.

Zusammenfassend kann man eine Reihe von Eigenarten festhalten, die das laterale Augenbrauenhaar bei den Ekzematikern aufweist:

1. Die spindelförmigen Knoten sind am Gipfel des jungen Haares lokalisiert (Abb. 1). 2. Manchmal werden zwei bis drei Veränderungen auf einem Haar bemerkt (Abb. 2). 3. Diese Veränderungen fehlen bei den Haaren von anderen Körperstellen des Kranken. 4. Die äußeren Teile der Augenbrauen weisen ausgeprägte Zonen von Alopecia auf; dies kann jedenfalls nicht allein durch traumatisches Brechen des Haares erklärt werden. Diese Beweisgründe veranlassen uns zu der Annahme, daß die dimensionalen Veränderungen der seitlichen Augenbrauen bei den Ekzematikern ursprünglich und struktural sein werden.

Abschließend kann man sagen, daß die beiden folgenden Mechanismen anscheinend die Verdünnung des lateralen Augenbrauenhaares bei den Ekzematikern hervorrufen: Die traumatische Ursache wirkt auf ein gebrechlich gewordenes Haar, das bereits durch den ekzematösen Boden verändert worden war.

Mycoses (Superficial and Deep)

Mycoses (superficielles et profondes)

Micosis (superficiales y profundas)

Oberflächliche und tiefe Mykosen

Organizer

J. RAMOS E SILVA, Brazil

Presidents

L. P. EREAUX, Canada

K. ITO, Japan

P. RIMBAUD, France

W. J. WILSON, USA

Delegate of the Organization Committee

H. GÖTZ, Germany

Reports

Untersuchungen über die Zuverlässigkeit eines „in vitro"-Lymphocytentests zwecks Nachweises einer Dermatophyteninfektion

H. Götz, Klinik und Poliklinik für Hautkrankheiten am Klinikum Essen der Ruhr-Universität Bochum (Deutschland)

In der medizinischen Mykologie ist allgemein bekannt, daß nach einer Infektion des Organismus durch pathogene Pilze Sensibilisierungen eintreten, die durch bestimmte Untersuchungsmethoden (Agglutinationstest, Präcipitation im Agar-Gel, Komplementbindungsvermögen, Intracutanreaktionen u. a.) nachgewiesen werden können. Ihnen allen haftet der Nachteil an, daß sie in manchen Fällen auch zu falsch positiven Reaktionen führen können.

Seit geraumer Zeit beschäftigen wir uns an unserer Klinik mit immunbiologischen Studien, bei denen die Methode der Kultivierung von Lymphocyten des peripheren Blutes angewendet wird. Besondere Verdienste haben sich hierbei als erste Hirschhorn u. Mitarb. erworben. Bringt man unter bestimmten Bedingungen das Antigen eines kompetent sensibilisierten Menschen mit dessen in vitro gezüchteten Lymphocyten in Kontakt, so beobachtet man im gefärbten Lymphocytenausstrich merkwürdige Veränderungen. In den ohne Zusatz des Antigens gezüchteten Kontrollymphocyten fehlen sie. Dabei handelt es sich um die Bildung großer lymphoblastenähnlicher oder monocytenartiger Zellen, in deren Kernen nucleoliartige Chromatinverdichtungen auftreten. Insbesondere aber werden Mitosen in verschiedenen Stadien (Prophase, Metaphase, Anaphase, Telophase) angetroffen. Zudem pflegen in solchen „positiven" Kulturen die meisten Granulocyten zugrunde zu gehen. Alle diese Veränderungen fehlen, wenn zwar eine Sensibilisierung vorliegt, ein zugegebenes Antigen zu den „in vitro"-Lymphocyten aber nicht kompetent ist.

Aus diesen Ausführungen folgt, daß man im Prinzip durch die Zugabe suspekter Antigene zu den gezüchteten Lymphocyten eines sensibilisierten Menschen eine gestellte Verdachtsdiagnose klären oder erhärten kann. Voraussetzung ist natürlich, daß bei verwandten Krankheitsbildern Kreuzsensibilisierungen den Wert des Testes nicht verringern. In einer früheren Untersuchung (Götz u. Heitmann) konnten wir zunächst nachweisen, daß die geschilderte „in vitro"-Reaktion der Lymphocyten eines durch Dermatophyten sensibilisierten Patienten (Tinea oder Trichophytie) positiv ausfällt, wenn Trichophytin als Allergen hinzugefügt wird.

Darüber hinaus interessierte nun die Frage, ob dieser positive Ausfall streng spezifisch ist, oder ob wir auch dann die charakteristischen Lymphocytenveränderungen finden, wenn wir Antigene andersartiger Pilze zu den Zellkulturen hinzugeben. Da sich die Forschung auf diesem Gebiet noch in voller Entwicklung befindet, kam es uns jetzt nicht darauf an, unsere Untersuchungen sofort quantitativ zu untermauern, sondern zunächst qualitativ abzuklären. Dermatophyteninfektionen spielen in unseren geographischen Breiten die wichtigste Rolle. Ziel der vorliegenden Studie war es daher zu prüfen, ob der „in vitro"-Lymphocytentest tatsächlich zum Nachweis einer Sensibilisierung der Haut durch Dermatophyten herangezogen werden kann, ohne daß andererseits verwandte Pilzantigene (Candidin, Aspergillin) oder Pilzprodukte (Penicillin) gleichfalls zu positiven Reaktionen führen.

Auf die Technik will ich aus Zeitersparnisgründen nicht näher eingehen und verweise diesbezüglich auf die Arbeit meines Mitarbeiters Heitmann „Zur Methodik der Lymphocytenkultur als Allergietest". Nur soviel sei zum Verständnis der folgenden Ausführungen gesagt, daß wir als positiven Kontrolltest immer das Verhalten der „in vitro"-Lymphocyten des zu untersuchenden Patienten nach Kontakt mit Phytohämagglutinin (1:10) heranzogen. Bei normalem Ablauf des Testes muß dieser immer positiv ausfallen.

In der Abb. 1 sehen wir das Ergebnis bebrüteter Lymphocyten bei negativem Ausfall. Die Granulocyten sind zum großen Teil erhalten, die Lymphocyten zeigen sich im wesentlichen unverändert. Mitosen sind nirgends zu erkennen. In der Abb. 2 haben wir ein positives Ergebnis vor Augen. Die geschilderten Mitosen, teils in Pro-, teils in Metaphase, sind unübersehbar. Große lymphoblastenähnliche Zellen treten gleichfalls hervor. Besonders schöne Mitosebilder in der Metaphase sind in der Abb. 3 wiedergegeben. Schließlich sind in der Abb. 4 die schon mehrfach zitierten, für den positiven Ausfall des Testes gleichfalls so wichtigen mononucleären oder lymphoblastenartigen Zellen mit disseminierten Chromatinpartikeln im Kern dargestellt.

Hat man häufig die unter dem Einfluß eines Antigens entstandenen Veränderungen an kompetenten Lymphocyten zu beurteilen, dann empfiehlt sich eine gewisse Normierung, um möglichst vergleichbare Resultate zu erhalten. Zu diesem Zwecke haben wir an unserer Klinik in der nächsten Abb. 5 die Zellformen zusammengestellt und sie von a bis f bezeichnet, denen wir immer wieder im mikroskopischen Ausstrichpräparat begegnen. Den Beurteilungen zugrunde liegt der Durchmesser der Zellen in μ. Wie schon in den Abb. 3 und 4 gezeigt, besitzen die Mitosen (a) und die auffallenden lymphoblastenartigen Transformierungen (b) den größten Durchmesser. Die Morphologie der Zellen c bis f ist in der Abb. 5 beschrieben. Bis auf die starke Verminderung der Granulocyten bei positivem Ausfall des Tests kommt ihrer Anzahl keine entscheidende Bedeutung zu.

Aus jeder „in vitro"-Lymphocytenkultur zählten wir 1000 Zellen nach dem Schema der Abb. 5 aus. Insgesamt wurden 9 Personen untersucht, davon 3 Kontrollpersonen (2mal Psoriasis vulgaris, 1mal Spinaliom der Unterlippe) und 7 pilzkranke Patienten (1mal Trichophytia capitis, 1mal Tinea pedum et unguium, 3mal Candidiasis, 1mal Aspergillom). Bei diesen Untersuchungen ist ein erheblicher Arbeitsaufwand erforderlich. Insgesamt legten wir 51 Kulturen an (Dauer jeder Kultur 4 Tage), beurteilten 102 Präparate und gewannen die Ergebnisse nach Beurteilung und Differenzierung von 49500 Zellen.

In den folgenden Tabellen ersehen Sie die Ergebnisse, die wir an jeweils einem charakteristischen Befund demonstrieren.

Nach der Tab. 1 verliefen mit Ausnahme der Kontrollkultur sämtliche Kulturen negativ.

Nach der Tab. 2 fiel nur diejenige Lymphocytenkultur positiv aus, der das Antigen Trichophytin zugesetzt worden war.

Nach der Tab. 3 fiel nur diejenige Lymphocytenkultur positiv aus, der das Antigen Candidin zugegeben worden war.

Nach der Tab. 4 fielen nur diejenigen Lymphocytenkulturen positiv aus, denen die Antigene Trichophytin und Candidin zugesetzt worden waren.

Nach der Tab. 5 fielen nur diejenigen Lymphocytenkulturen positiv aus, denen die Antigene Aspergillin und Candidin zugegeben worden waren.

Beurteilung: Die erhaltenen Ergebnisse sprechen in dem Sinne, daß der Ausfall der Lymphocytenkulturen spezifisch ist. Kreuzreaktionen konnten nicht beobachtet werden. Eine Sensibilisierung durch ein Dermatophyton läßt sich sicher bestätigen. Differentialdiagnostisch müßte die Anwendung der „in vitro"-Lymphocytenkulturmethoden besonders in den Ländern erfolgversprechend sein, in denen häufiger Systemmykosen wie Histoplasmose, Blastomykose, Coccidioidomykose, Kryptokokkose usw. beobachtet werden.

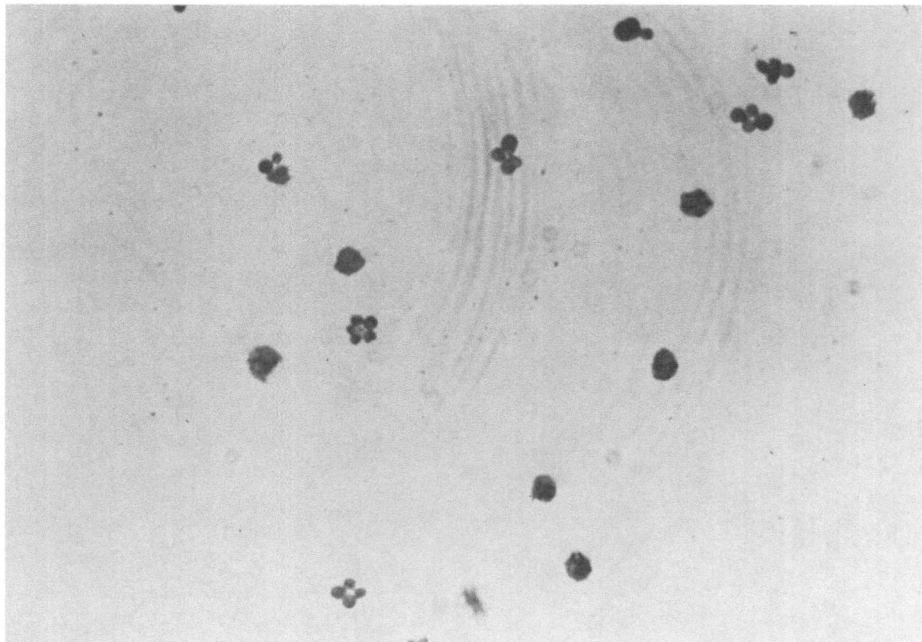

Abb. 1. Lymphocytenkultur bei negativem Ausfall. Granulocyten zum großen Teil erhalten, Lymphocyten im wesentlichen unverändert

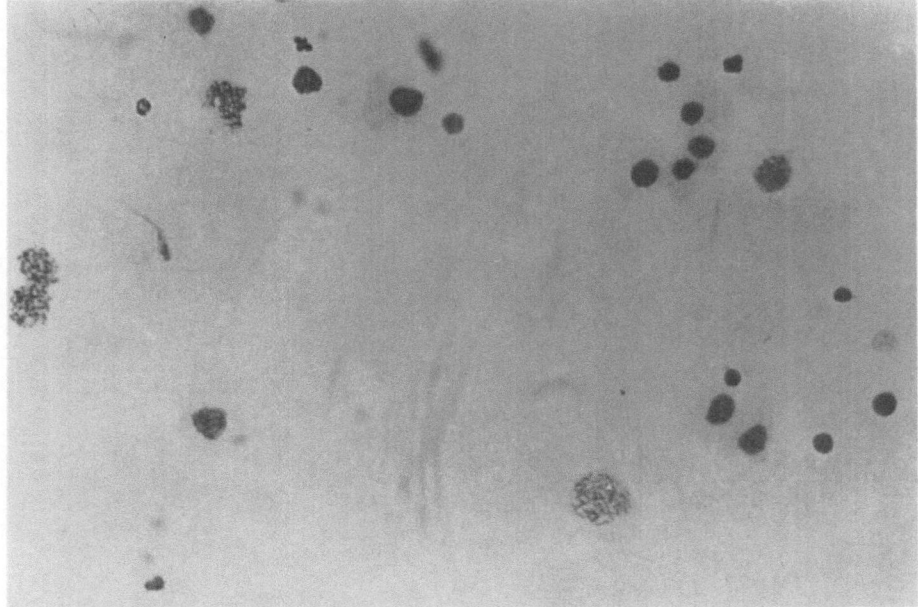

Abb. 2. Lymphocytenkultur bei positivem Ausfall. Neben charakteristischen Mitosen große lymphoblastenartige Zellen

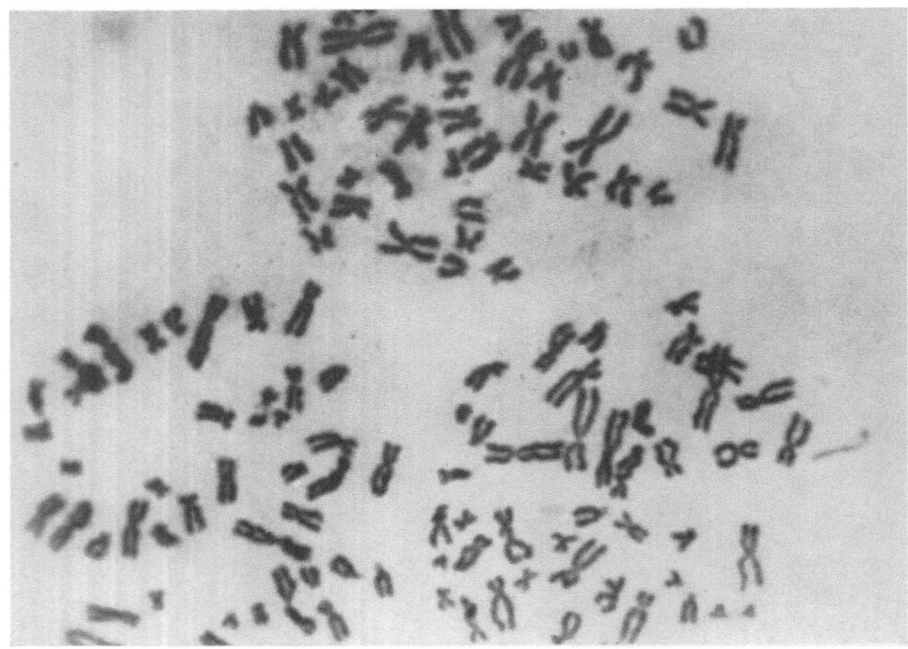

Abb. 3. Mehrere Mitosen in der Metaphase

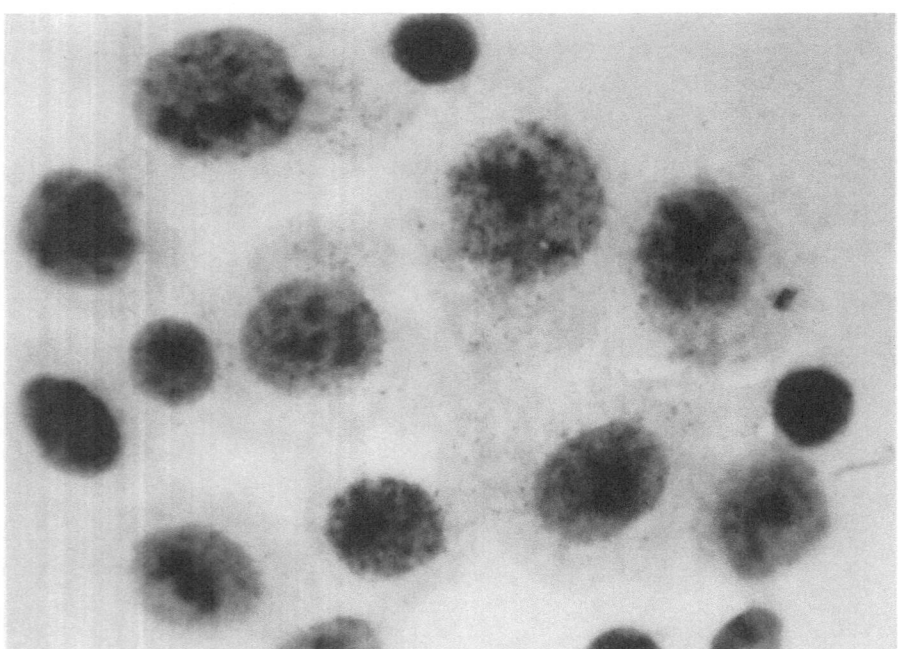

Abb. 4. Für den positiven Ausfall charakteristische, große lymphoblastenartige Zellen (∅ der Kerne 14 μ)

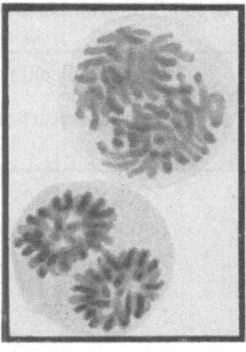 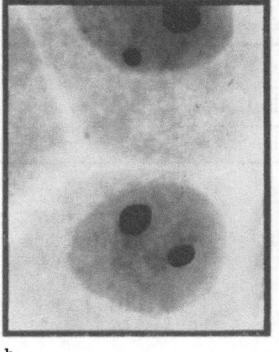 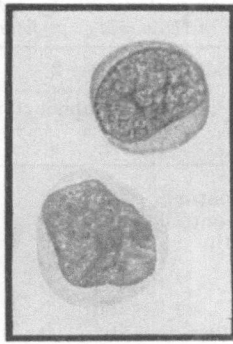

a   b   c

a *Mitosen.* Teilweise gut ausgebreitete Chromosomen, teilweise dicht und innerhalb von Zellen gelagerte Chromosomen, ∅ 16 μ
b *Lymphoblasten.* Besonders große mononucleäre Elemente mit nucleoliartigem Chromatinverdichtungen in den Kernen, ∅ 14 μ
c *Lymphoblasten.* Mittelgroße mononucleäre Elemente, bei denen nucleoliartige Chromatinverdichtungen in den Kernen kaum auffallen, ∅ 10 μ

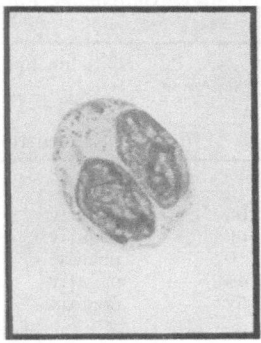 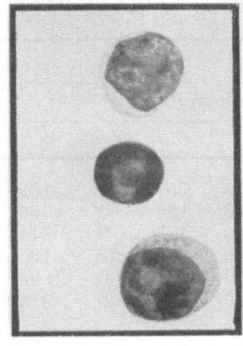 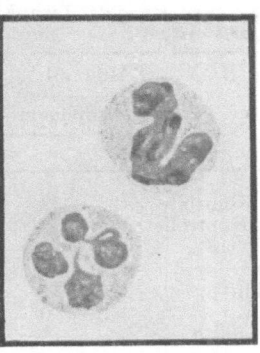

d   e   f

d *zwei- und mehrkernige* Zellen. Große Elemente, die teilweise den Eindruck einer lymphoblastenähnlichen Transformation erwecken, ∅ 6 μ
e *Lymphocyten.* Kleine mononucleäre Elemente mit intensiv gefärbten Kernen
f *Segment-Stabkernige.* Neutrophile Granulocyten (ganz vereinzelt eosinophile Zeller.)

Abb. 5. Zellformen, denen wir bei positivem Ausfall der Lymphocytenkultur im gefärbten Ausstrich begegnen

Tabelle 1. *Auswertung der Lymphocytenkulturen eines nicht sensibilisierten Patienten (Psoriasis vulgaris)*

Name: A. B.	Alter: 39							Geschlecht: ♂
	Lymphocytenkulturen							
	Nr.	a	b	c	d	e	f	(g)	Gesamturteil
positive Kontrolle	442	17	44	447	16	441	35	—	positiv
negative Kontrolle	441	0	0	87	0	604	309	—	negativ
Trichophytin	444	0	0	128	0	639	233	—	negativ
Candidin	443	0	0	154	0	840	6	—	negativ
Aspergillin	446	0	0	204	0	367	429	—	negativ
Penicillin	447	0	0	161	0	297	542	—	negativ
(Tuberkulin)	448	0	0	163	0	389	448	—	negativ

Hauttestungen: Trichophytin (intracut.): 1:300 ∅
Candidin (intracut.):   1:100 ∅

Tabelle 2. *Auswertung von Lymphocytenkulturen eines gegen Trichophytin sensibilisierten Patienten (Trichophytia superficialis capitis)*

Name: E. Sch.	Alter: 2							Geschlecht: ♂
	Lymphocytenkulturen							Gesamturteil
	Nr.	a	b	c	d	e	f	(g)	
positive Kontrolle	461	3	21	502	18	402	54	—	positiv
negative Kontrolle	462	0	3	152	0	620	225	—	negativ
Trichophytin	463	6	15	595	5	330	49	—	positiv
Candidin	464	(0	0	114	0	864	22)	—	negativ
Aspergillin	466	0	0	53	0	904	43	—	negativ
Penicillin	465	0	0	117	0	725	158	—	negativ
(Tuberkulin)	467	0	0	313	0	523	164	—	negativ

Hauttestungen: Trichophytin (intracut.): 1:300+++
Mykol. Unters.: Trichophyton verrucosum

Tabelle 3. *Auswertung der Lymphocytenkulturen eines gegen Candidin sensibilisierten Patienten (Candidiasis oris)*

Name: A. S.	Alter: 61							Geschlecht: ♂
	Lymphocytenkulturen							
	Nr.	a	b	c	d	e	f	(g)	Gesamturteil
positive Kontrolle	422	32	45	707	14	199	3	—	positiv
negative Kontrolle	421	0	0	124	0	766	108	—	negativ
Trichophytin	423	0	0	127	0	814	59	—	negativ
Candidin	424	25	132	619	29	195	0	—	positiv
Aspergillin	426	1	0	59	0	894	46	—	negativ
Penicillin	425	0	0	105	0	843	52	—	negativ
(Tuberkulin)									

Hauttestungen: Trichophytin (intracut.): 1:300 negativ
Candidin (intracut.): 1:300 Rötung und Knötchenbildung
Mykol. Unters.: Candida albicans

Tabelle 4. *Auswertung der Lymphocytenkulturen eines gegen Trichophytin (Tinea pedum et unguium) und Candidin (Candidiasis manuum et unguium) sensibilisierten Patienten*

Name: B. T.	Alter: 40							Geschlecht: ♂
	Lymphocytenkulturen							
	Nr.	a	b	c	d	e	f	(g)	Gesamturteil
positive Kontrollen	571	23	61	466	14	341	95	—	positiv
negative Kontrollen	572	0	0	127	0	674	199	—	negativ
Trichophytin	573	21	161	444	2	284	88	—	positiv
Candidin	574	11	50	493	5	362	79	—	positiv
Aspergillin	575	0	0	119	0	563	318	—	negativ
Penicillin									
(Tuberkulin)									

Hauttestungen: Trichophytin (intracut.): 1:300 ++ (Rötung und Knötchen)
Candidin (intracut.): 1:200 ∅ — 1:50 (+)
Aspergillin (intracut.): 1:200 ∅
Mykol. Unters.: Füße: Trichophyton rubrum et mentagrophytes; Hände: Candida parapsilosis

Tabelle 5. *Auswertung der Lymphocytenkulturen eines gegen Aspergillin (Aspergillom der Lunge) und gegen Candidin (Candidiasis pulmonum) sensibilisierten Patienten*

Name: H. M.	Alter: 62								Geschlecht: ♀
	Lymphocytenkulturen								
	Nr.	a	b	c	d	e	f	(g)	Gesamturteil
positive Kontrolle	481	3	39	373	2	519	64	—	positiv
negative Kontrolle	482	0	0	143	0	410	447	—	negativ
Trichophytin	483	0	0	173	0	375	452	—	negativ
Candidin	484	2	56	166	2	777	0	—	positiv
Aspergillin	485	4	66	335	4	584	7	—	positiv
Penicillin (Tuberkulin)	486	0	0	102	0	778	120	—	negativ

Hauttestungen: Candidin (intracut.):   1:300 ++
              Aspergillin (intracut.):   1:200 ∅ — 1:50 +
Mykolog. Unt.: Sputum: Aspergillus fumigatus, Aspergillus niger, Candida mycoderma

Bei der technischen Anfertigung der Zellkulturen sei besonders meinem Mitarbeiter H. J. HEITMANN, darüber hinaus der Deutschen Forschungsgemeinschaft für ihre finanzielle Unterstützung gedankt.

Literatur. FALK, C. A.: Acta derm.-venereol. (Stockh.) **28**, 342 (1948). — GÖTZ, H., u. H. J. HEITMANN: Hautarzt **18**, 23 (1967). — GÖTZ, H., u. W. THIES: Arch. Derm. Syph. (Berl.) **194**, 91 (1952). — HEITMANN. H. J.: Hautarzt **18**, 152 (1967). — HIRSCHHORN, K., F. BACH, R. L. KOLODNY, I. FIRSCHEIN, and N. HASHEM: Science **142**, 1185 (1963).

Effects of Human Body Fluids on Candida albicans*

V. D. NEWCOMER, J. W. LANDAU, N. DABROWA and M. L. FENSTER, Department of Medicine, Division of Dermatology, University of California, School of Medicine, Los Angeles, California (USA), and Medical Service, Veterans Administration Center, General Medical and Surgical Hospital, Los Angeles, California (USA)

Candida albicans is frequently found as a saprophyte in the oral cavity, gastrointestinal tract, and vaginal area of healthy individuals. This fungus, however, is capable of producing a spectrum of diseases ranging from commonly encountered local superficial cutaneous infections to fatal fulminating systemic infections. The presence of active anti-fungal components in normal human serum has been proposed as an explanation for the usual limitation of *C. albicans*, as either a saprophyte or a pathogen, to the surfaces of the skin and mucous membranes.

Inhibitory effects of normal human serum on the growth of *C. albicans* have been demonstrated with *in vitro* systems utilizing turbidimetric [1] and quantitative plating technics [2]. The evidence includes a decreased turbidity after incubation of a suspension of *C. albicans* in media containing serum compared with that of a similar suspension in media without serum, and a reduction in the number of colonies of *C. albicans* after incubation in serum compared with the number at the onset.

Another property of human serum is the induction of blastospores of *C. albicans* to form filaments or "germ tubes" when incubated in it for 3 h a 37 C [3]. This

* This study was supported in part by USPHS Grants TI AI 52-08, TI AM 5265-07, Al-06048-03, and by the Dermatologic Research Foundation of California, Inc.

phenomenon has been utilized as the basis of a laboratory test to distinguish *C. albicans* from other members of the genus Candida. The rapid formation of filaments also occurs when *C. albicans* is injected into mice [4]. *C. albicans* unlike most dimorphic fungi is commonly found as pseudomycelia, true mycelia, and blastospores in tissues of patients with clinical candidiasis and animals with experimental candidiasis. The significance of this rapid formation of germ tubes in serum has not been clarified and the question is incompletely resolved whether this represents inhibition or enhancement of subsequent growth.

Investigations in this laboratory have been directed at defining the factors in body fluids that influence the formation of germ tubes and the development of colonies of *C. albicans* [5 to 8]. This report will review salient previous observations with human serum and summarize results of recent experiments with saliva, urine, and cerebrospinal fluid.

Materials and Methods

Body fluids were centrifuged after collection, separated from the sediment, stored at 4 C, and used within one week. Sera were obtained from fasting donors. Saliva was collected without artificial stimulation at least 3 h post prandial in the morning. Urines were routine morning specimens. Their specific gravity ranged from 1.012 to 1.029 and the pH from five to seven. None contained protein or glucose detectable with routine methods. Cerebrospinal fluid was obtained by lumbar puncture performed for a variety of clinical indications. The protein in the fluid ranged from 19 to 163 mg per 100 ml. At least ten different specimens of each body fluid were examined in each experiment.

The procedure for determination of percentage of germ tubes consisted of dispensing 0.5 ml of a test medium into a sterile tube and inoculating with 0.05 ml of a fresh suspension of *C. albicans* containing approximately 10^7 cells per ml. After incubation for 3 h at 37 C, permanent slides were made, 200 cells counted, and the percentage of germ tubes and budding cells recorded.

The quantitative plating technic was performed by pipetting 0.9 ml of test medium into a sterile tube and inoculating with 0.1 ml of a fresh suspension of *C. albicans* to produce a final concentration of 2×10^2 cells per ml. After 72 h of incubation at 37 C, samples were withdrawn, suitably diluted, and cultured on Sabouraud dextrose agar. These plates were incubated for 48 h at 37 C and the number of colonies (viable particles) per ml of serum recorded.

Standard statistical tests were employed and a probability of $p < 0.05$ was considered statistically significant.

Experimental Results

The property of serum responsible for the rapid formation of germ tubes was characterized as heat-stable, independent of complement, not removed by dialysis, and unrelated to Candida agglutinins and precipitins. It was, however, absorbed by viable and non-viable cells of *C. albicans*. It was found to be present to approximately the same extent in sera from normal donors, maternity patients, newborn infants, and various medical patients. It occurred to a lesser extent in plasma Fraction II (gamma globulin) than in normal control sera. The cumulative evidence indicates that the factor (or factors) in serum is not related to classical antibody.

The serum protein transferrin functions principally in the transport of iron but also adversely influences the formation of germ tubes. Iron is bound to a portion of the transferrin and the remainder of the transferrin is termed unsaturated. Sera were examined before and after the addition of sufficient iron as ferrous ammonium sulfate to produce 100% and 200% saturation of transferrin. In all instances significantly, more germ tubes developed in the sera with 100% saturation than in the sera with unsaturated transferrin. No additional increase occurred with further saturation of transferrin to 200%. The achievement of 100% saturation of transferrin after oral ingestion of 2 g of ferrous sulfate resulted in maximum germ tube formation in the postingestion serum with no further increase following the direct addition of iron to the serum. The addition of the iron-chelating agent, desferrioxamine B, to sera with 100% saturated transferrin produced a significant reduction in the percentage of germ tubes. Presumably unsaturated transferrin binds iron ordinarily utilized in the metabolism of *C. albicans*. The mechanism responsible for the increase in germ tube formation following the addition of iron to serum is the removal of the inhibitory activity of unsaturated transferrin by saturation of this protein with iron.

Physiologic saline as a diluent adversely influences the formation of germ tubes. Sera were progressively diluted to 75, 50, 25, and 5% with physiologic saline and with distilled water. A significant progressive decrease in percentage of germ tubes followed dilution of each serum with increasing proportions of physiologic saline. This finding can not be attributed to a reduction in available nutrients since comparable decreases did not occur in serum similarly diluted with distilled water. A significant decrease in the percentage of germ tubes in sera diluted with distilled water compared with that in undiluted sera was not attained until the serum concentration was reduced to 5%. When sera were diluted with saline containing 0.2% dextrose, the percentage of germ tubes was significantly higher than that in sera diluted with saline alone but not significantly different from that in sera diluted with distilled water. Sera were also examined after dilution to 50% and 5% with various solutions containing the same concentration of sodium or potassium ion (0.15 M) as in physiologic saline. The percentage of germ tubes was less in sera diluted with $NaCl$, NaH_2PO_4, Na_2SO_4, and $NaNO_3$ than in sera diluted with the potassium salt of each compound at both dilutions.

Several comparative studies of the number of colonies developing in sera were performed. The findings of these studies paralleled those of germ tube studies in some but not all instances. An increase in the number of colonies was also observed after saturation of transferrin with iron and a decrease also followed the subsequent addition of desferrioxamine B. The inhibitory effect of physiologic saline on development of colonies was relative rather than absolute. It was demonstrated by comparing the number of colonies from sera diluted to 5% with physiologic saline with the increased number of colonies from sera similarly diluted with distilled water. An increase in the number of colonies also followed the addition of dextrose to sera diluted to 5% with physiologic saline. In other instances, however, the number of colonies increased following a modification of serum that produced a decrease in the percentage of germ tubes. This occurred in sera diluted to 5% with distilled water or with the solutions of NaH_2PO_4 or KH_2PO_4 compared with the findings in undiluted sera. The increased number of colonies developing in sera diluted to 5% with distilled water compared with that in undiluted sera illustrates that the activity of the antifungal factor in human sera, in respect to development of colonies, can be removed by dilution.

The property of human serum which promotes the formation of germ tubes by *C. albicans* is not identical to that which limits the development of colonies. Procedures which either increase or decrease the percentage of germ tubes may produce an increase in the number of colonies.

The absence of any definite relationship between the percentage of germ tubes and the number of colonies in human serum also extends to *C. albicans* incubated in other media. Using the same procedures, approximately 10^6 colonies developed in both Sabouraud broth and tissue culture Medium 199. In the former medium, a low percentage of germ tubes and a high percentage of budding cells developed whereas in the latter a high percentage of germ tubes and a low percentage of budding cells developed.

A summary of the effects on *C. albicans* of saliva, urine, cerebrospinal fluid, and control fluids is presented in the table. None of these body fluids was identical in its activity to serum. Both saliva and urine in contrast to cerebrospinal fluid and serum supported the luxurious development of colonies. The formation of germ tubes progressed very well in serum and saliva, somewhat less in urine, and least in cerebrospinal fluid. The formation of germ tubes and development of colonies in tissue culture Medium 199 resembled most closely that in saliva whereas the pattern in Sabouraud broth was unique.

Table. *Effects of various body fluids and control media on the formation of germ tubes and development of colonies*

Media	Percentage of Germ Tubes[a]	Number of Colonies per ml after 72 h[b]
Saliva	57	10^6
Urine	30	10^6
Cerebrospinal fluid	< 5	10^2
Serum	61	10^3
Tissue culture Medium 199	60	10^6
Sabouraud broth	< 5	10^6

[a] representative simultaneously performed studies
[b] mean of at least ten determinations.

Extensive studies of serum and saliva from a patient with *Candida* granuloma have not disclosed any apparent defect in the activity of these body fluids on *C. albicans*. The single exception was that a very low percentage of germ tubes occurred in one serum obtained while the patient was receiving amphotericin B. In this same patient, quantitative immunoglobulin values, isohemagglutinin titers, and response to typhoid and diphtheria immunizations were all within normal limits. Antibodies with precipitating, agglutinating, and phagocytosis-promoting activities were present in the serum. A possible deficit in delayed hypersensitivity response was the only suggestive clue to the unusual susceptibility of this patient to *C. albicans*.

Conclusions

The existence in normal human serum of *in vitro* inhibitory activity against *C. albicans* as demonstrable by quantitative colony counting or turbidimetric technics is well established by studies from this laboratory [6, 7] and others [1, 2]. Unsaturated transferrin and sodium chloride are probably only two of several factors in serum which are capable of limiting growth as measured by number of colonies. An unidentified small protein or polypeptide may be another [2]. Induction of formation of germ tubes appears to be a distinct activity of serum and can not be directly correlated with development of colonies.

The actual value in identifying patients with increased susceptibility to candidiasis has not been established for any of the procedures studied in this laboratory. Experience with the tests in patients, however, has not been exhaustive. Decreased inhibitory activity of serum against *C. albicans* as indicated by various procedures of others has been observed in isolated instances [1, 2, 9, 10]. Comparison of these various procedures is complicated by differences in the number of yeast cells in the initial inoculum, the time and temperature of incubation, and the criterion of inhibition.

Saliva, urine, and cerebrospinal fluid differ from serum either in their effects on the formation of germ tubes or development of colonies. Other studies are not available for direct comparison. Agglutinins [11] against *C. albicans* using immunofluorescent technics and an inhibitor [12] against *Cryptococcus neoformans* have been identified in human saliva. Continuing studies are currently in progress in this laboratory to define the mechanisms and significance of the effects of human body fluids on *C. albicans*.

Bibliography. 1. Roth, F. J., and M. I. Goldstein: J. invest. Derm. **36**, 383 (1961). — 2. Louria, D. B., and R. G. Brayton: Nature (Lond.) **201**, 309 (1964). — 3. Reynolds, R., and A. Braude: Clin. Res. Proc. **4**, 40 (1956). — 4. Hill, D. W., and P. L. Gebhardt: Proc. Soc. exp. Biol. (N.Y.) **92**, 640 (1956). — 5. Landau, J. W., N. Dabrowa, and V. D. Newcomer: J. invest. Derm. **44**, 171 (1965). — 6. Landau, J. W., N. Dabrowa, V. D. Newcomer, and J. R. Rowe: J. invest. Derm. **43**, 473 (1964). — 7. Dabrowa, N., J. W. Landau, and V. D. Newcomer: J. invest. Derm. **45**, 368 (1965). — 8. Newcomer, V. D., J. W. Landau, R. Lehman, N. Dabrowa, and A. Fujiwara: Arch. Derm. **93**, 149 (1966). — 9. Janke, D.: Ärztl Wschr. **10**, 349 (1955). — 10. Heite, H. J., A. Buck, and C. Lehmann: Dermatologica (Basel) **128**, 350 (1964). — 11. Lehner, T.: Arch. oral Biol. **10**, 975 (1965). — 12. Igel, H. J., and R. P. Bolande: J. infect. Dis. **116**, 75 (1966).

Histoplasmose Africaine

E. Vanbreuseghem, Prince Leopold Institute for Tropical Medicine, Anvers (Belgique)

L'histoplasmose africaine est une mycose décrite pour la première fois en 1952 par A. Dubois et R. Vanbreuseghem. Le premier cas avait été décrit la même année par A. Dubois, P. G. Janssens et P. Brutsaert. Elle est causée par un champignon appartenant à la classe des adélomycètes: *Histoplasma duboisii* Vanbreuseghem 1952.

A l'opposé de l'histoplasmose causée par *Histoplasma capsulatum* Darling 1906 qui est cosmopolite l'histoplasmose africaine est non seulement africaine mais encore localisée géographiquement au centre ouest africain.

L'histoplasmose africaine atteint les ganglions, les os, les articulations, la peau, les muqueuses et parfois se généralise. A l'encontre de l'histoplasmose américaine elle semble respecter étrangement les poumons. Par contre alors que la peau est rarement atteinte dans l'histoplasmose américaine, elle l'est presque toujours dans l'histoplasmose africaine. Nous signalions récemment (Vanbreuseghem, 1964) que sur 43 cas publiés, 33 présentaient des lésions cutanées mais nous insistions sur le fait qu'il n'était pas certain que les autres n'en avaient pas ou n'auraient pas pu en avoir.

Dans un travail sous presse R. Renoirte, J. L. Michaux, F. Gatti et R. Vanbreuseghem (1967) décrivent 13 nouveaux cas de l'affection. Malgré une symptomatologie très variée dans aucun cas les lésions cutanées ne font défaut.

Les lésions cutanées dans l'histoplasmose africaine ont deux localisations majeures: le tronc et la face. C'est d'ailleurs à ces deux régions que correspondent les lésions profondes le plus communément observées. Pour être plus précis, signalons cependant que sur 33 cas les lésions cutanées sont situées vingt cinq fois au tronc, dix huit fois à la tête, huit fois aux bras, six fois à la cuisse, six fois à la jambe, quatre fois aux avant-bras, une fois à la main et jamais aux pieds. Des localisations uniques sur le tronc ont été observées onze fois, sur la tête cinq fois, sur les avant bras trois fois, sur les jambes deux fois et une seule fois sur la main.

Nous avons réparti les lésions observées dans l'histoplasmose africaine en cinq groupes (Vanbreuseghem, 1964). Peut-être vaut-il mieux les envisager sous sept aspects différents:

a) des papules,	e) des fistules,
b) des ulcères,	f) des cicatrices,
c) des nodules,	g) des modifications pigmentaires.
d) des abcès,	

a) Les *papules* sont observées le plus souvent sur le tronc et le visage. Quand elles sont fraîches elles ont la couleur de la peau. Elles sont rondes ou ovales, décrites comme hémisphériques ou lenticulaires. Elles sont petites — quelques millimètres — ou grandes — 10 à 20 mm. Il est rare qu'elles disparaissent sans plus. Généralement elles vont s'ulcérer plus ou moins, se vésiculiser, proliférer en chou-fleur, prendre l'«apparence de chair crue» (G. H. V. CLARKE, J. WALKER et R. WINSTON, 1953). Beaucoup d'auteurs ont retrouvé des lésions qui simulent le *molluscum contagiosum* comme A. BASSET semble avoir été le premier à le décrire avec ses collaborateurs X. SERAFINO, M. LARIVIERE, P. HOCQUET, R. CAMAIN, M. BASSET et E. GOUDOTE (1962). En réalité ce sont de petites papules qui s'ulcèrent en leur centre assez superficiellement et qui prennent ainsi un aspect ombiliqué. Les papules pourront également être le point de départ d'une ulcération beaucoup plus vaste.

b) Les *ulcères*, nous venons de le voir peuvent résulter d'une ulcération des papules. Ils peuvent être petits ou grands, souvent de formes irrégulières, fongueux, plus exubérants que profonds, formant parfois des végétations massives qui suscitent presqu'immanquablement le diagnostic de néoplasie. L'origine des ulcères est variée: traumatisme accidentel ou chirurgical, ouverture à la peau de lésions profondes ganglionnaires ou osseuses. On aurait tort croyons-nous de les considérer comme le résultat d'une inoculation d'origine externe encore que celle-ci ne soit pas exclue. En fait la peau des malades peut être à ce point infiltrée par le parasite que le moindre traumatisme peut être à l'origine d'une ulcération.

c) Les *nodules* sont rarement décrits dans l'histoplasmose africaine et cela tient sans doute au fait que les lésions ont toujours tendance à perdre leurs limites, à s'étendre. BASSET et al. (1962) ont vu des «éléments dermo-épidermiques noueux» et des «éléments hypodermiques gommeux»; ils ont vu encore des «tuméfactions ... de la taille d'un pois à une noix, ... fermes, élastiques, indolores, irrégulières, légèrement lobulées». R. VAN LAETHEM, A. THIJS et R. VANBREUSEGHEM (1959) ont décrit des «nodules sous-cutanés, aplatis, de la grosseur d'un grain de café ...». Ils peuvent être très nombreux: une cinquantaine dans le cas de BASSET et al. (1962), 236 dans l'observation de R. VAN LAETHEM et al. (1959). MICHAUX et al. (1967) ont dû pour les distinguer des nodules onchocercosiques avoir recours à l'examen histologique. Ils coexistent généralement avec des papules, des ulcères ou encore avec des abcès.

d) Les *abcès* sont parmi les plus fréquentes des lésions que l'on peut percevoir sous la peau. Ils sont remplis d'un pus jaunâtre assez bien lié et toujours très riche en formes duboisii*. Ils peuvent se fistuliser à la peau. Nous concluions notre article de 1964 en écrivant qu'ils «nous apparaissent le plus souvent comme un exutoire de lésions osseuses» et nous insistions «sur la nécessité de pratiquer toujours un examen radiologique qui souvent décelera une lésion osseuse à leur voisinage». Le travail que nous publions actuellement avec MICHAUX et al. (1967) ne fait que confirmer cette opinion.

e) Les *fistules* résultent de l'ouverture à la peau d'abcès ou de ganglions, soit spontanément soit sous l'action du bistouri. Elles peuvent être la source d'une vaste ulcération ou guérir en laissant une cicatrice dépigmentée.

f) Les *cicatrices* sont consécutives à la guérison de fistules ou d'ulcères. Elles sont généralement déprimées ou hypertrophiques et souvent légèrement chéloïdiennes chez les malades de peau noire qui constituent la majorité des cas.

g) Des *troubles de la pigmentation* ne semblent pas avoir beaucoup attiré l'atten-

---

* Nous avons nommé forme duboisii la forme mûre de *l'Histoplasma duboisii* et forme capsulatum la forme jeune de ce champignon. Beaucoup d'auteurs parlent de «grandes formes» pour la première et parlent de «petites formes» pour désigner *Histoplasma capsulatum*.

tion des auteurs jusqu'ici et nous ne pourrions affirmer qu'ils soient fréquents. MICHAUX et al. (1967) en ont observé soit au cours de la cicatrisation — dépigmentation ivoire — soit au cours de la guérison de papules. D'autre part A. O. LUCAS (1967) a attiré notre attention sur un liseré noirâtre qui entoure fréquemment les ulcérations histoplasmosiques. Il lui attribuait une grande valeur diagnostique.

Nous avons la conviction que les lésions cutanées de l'histoplasmose sont encore très mal connues. Nous connaissons essentiellement celles qui se développent chez des malades dont l'histoplasmose est suffisamment développée pour qu'ils soient amenés à consulter ce qui entraine souvent une hospitalisation. Nous pensons que beaucoup de lésions banales d'histoplasmose simulent d'autres conditions dermatologiques. Comme le rappelait récemment encore A. BASSET, M. BASSET et P. HOCQUET (1963) les lésions de l'histoplasmose africaine sont extrêmement polymorphes.

Le diagnostic mycologique est extrêmement aisé car on trouve toujours dans les lésions une grande quantité de cellules ovalaires isolées, parfois disposées en courtes chaînettes dans les vieilles lésions. Ces formes duboisii mesurent 10 à 13 microns de longueur sur 7 à 8 microns de large. La culture est aisée et réussit parfaitement sur milieu de Sabouraud à 25°, voire à la température du laboratoire. L'examen histologique montre d'abondantes cellules géantes renfermant *H. duboisii*. Cette particularité, par rapport à l'histoplasmose à *H. capsulatum* où l'on ne trouve guère que des histiocytes a été constatée dès 1953 par A. DUBOIS et R. VANBREUSEGHEM et confirmée ultérieurement par tous ceux qui se sont occupés de la question.

Références. BASSET, A., X. SERAFINO, M. LARIVIERE, P. HOCQUET, R. CAMAIN, M. BASSET et E. GOUDOTE: Bull. Soc. méd. Afr. noire Langue franç. **7**, 71 (1962). — BASSET, A., M. BASSET et P. HOCQUET: Bull. Soc. franç. Derm. Syph. **70**, 61 (1963). — CLARKE, G. H. V., J. WALKER, and R. M. WINSTON. J. trop. Med. Hyg. **56**, 277 (1953). — DUBOIS, A., P. G. JANSSENS et P. BRUTSAERT: Ann. Soc. belge Méd. trop. **32**, 569 (1952). — DUBOIS, A., et R. VANBREUSEGHEM: Bull. Acad. roy. Méd. Belg. VIe série, **17**, II, 551 (1952). — DUBOIS, A., et R. VANBREUSEGHEM: Ann. Soc. belge Méd. trop. **33**, 383 (1953). — LUCAS, A. O.: Communication personnelle. — RENOIRTE, R., J. L. MICHAUX, F. GATTI et R. VANBREUSEGHEM: Bull. Acad. roy. Méd. Belg. VII. série 7, 5—6: 465, (1967). — VAN LAETHEM, R., A. THYS et R. VANBREUSEGHEM: Ann. Soc. belge Méd. trop. **39**, 319 (1959). — VANBREUSEGHEM, R.: Ann. Soc. belge Méd. trop. **44**, 1037 (1964); — Bull. Acad. roy. Méd. Belg. VIIe série. 4, 545 (1964); — Maroc Médical 1967. Sous presse; — In: DUBOIS, A., P. G. JANSSENS et P. BRUTSAERT: N.B.: On trouvera une liste de références très abondante sinon exhaustive dans les travaux de R. VANBREUSEGHEM de 1964 et 1967.

Micetomas y actinomicosis

A. GONZÁLEZ OCHOA, Departamento de Dermatología Tropical, Instituto de Salubridad y Enfermedades Tropicales, México (Mexico)

Las tumoraciones fistulosas crónicas en las que el hongo causante forma cúmulos de micelio o microcolonias, denominados granos reciben el nombre de Micetoma. Estas lesiones pueden ser causadas por especies del grupo de los Actinomycetes, excepto *Nocardia asteroides* que origina Nocardiasis*, o por mohos pertenecientes a diferentes géneros.

---

* La nocardiasis comprende las infecciones de meningo-encéfalo, pulmón y tejido subcutáneo en las que el agente etiológico, *N. asteroides*, se presenta como cortos trechos de micelio y elementos bacilares ácido resistentes.

52*

No obstante que el término micetoma, creado por VANDYKE-CARTER [1] desde 1874 tiene prioridad, y que la clasificación propuesta por CHALMERS y ARCHIBALD [2] en una serie de estudios publicados de 1916 a 1918 comprenden con precisión y claridad a los micetomas, el afán tan común en dermatología y micología médica, de introducir sin justificación sinonimias y cambios ha originado confusión en este capítulo tan simple.

Dicha clasificación puesta al día en lo que se refiere a los agentes etiológicos encontrados posteriormente, y a la actual nomenclatura de esos microorganismos, se presenta en el Cuadro. Los dos tipos de micetoma: el *actinomicético* y el *maduromicósico* están condicionados por dos tipos diferentes de granos, debidos a un Actinomycete en el primero, y a un moho en el segundo; los Actinomycetes causantes de micetoma corresponden a especies anaerobias: género *Actinomyces*, o a especies aerobias: géneros *Nocardia* y *Streptomyces*. Los mohos corresponden a multitud de géneros de lo más diversos.

Cuadro. *Clasificación de los micetomas de* CHALMERS y ARCHIBALD

Actinomicetico .... (Causado por Actinomycetes)	Anaerobios	*Actinomyces*	A. israeli (Actinomicosis) A. bovis
	Aerobios	*Nocardia*	N. brasiliensis N. caviae
		Streptomyces	S. madurae S. Pelletieri S. somaliensis
Maduromicosico .... (Causado por Mohos)		*Madurella*	M. mycetomi M. grisea
		Cephalosporium	C. recifei C. hgranulomatis C. falciforme
		Leptosphaeria senegalensis *Curvularia lunata* *Pyrenochaeta romeroi* *Allescheria boydii* *Neotestudina rosatti* *Phialophora jeanselmei*	
		Aspergillus sp. *Penicillium sp.*	} dudosa autenticidad

Pasaremos por alto los conceptos clásicos obviando repetir lo sobradamente conocido para referirnos a los criterios y aportaciones recientes por lo que se refiere a repartición geográfica y frecuencia, agentes etiológicos, aspectos clínicos en relación con la patogenia y reproducción experimental del micetoma, valoración de los procedimientos diagnósticos y tratamiento.

La clásica actinomicosis lógicamente debe quedar comprendida dentro del micetoma por tratarse de tumoraciones fistulosas con granos, criterio del que participan numerosos autores. Las razones para considerarla en capítulo separado del micetoma estriban en su repartición geográfica cosmopolita y en su patogenia, condicionadas ambas por la fuente endógena de su agente etiológico, así como por tener tratamiento especial.

I. Repartición geográfica y frecuencia de los micetomas

El micetoma actinomicético por anaerobios o actinomicosis es cosmopolita y de aparición esporádica dada la fuente endógena de *A. israeli*.

La disminución cada vez mayor de casos de actinomicosis ha sido observada en diversos países, lo que parece estar en relación con el uso cada día mayor de sulfonamidas y de antibióticos, así como por la mayor higiene bucal en lo que se refiere a la localización maxilo-facial.

El micetoma actinomicético por especies de Actinomycetes aerobios y el maduromicósico, ambos de fuente exógena, han sido encontrados en todos los continentes, pero evidentemente son padecimientos condicionados a las situaciones ecológicas de las regiones tropicales y subtropicales; sin embargo su frecuencia es muy desigual en países climatológicamente similares de un mismo Continente, aún sin considerar el mayor o menor interés que exista en su descubrimiento.

En el Continente Europeo, descontando la actinomicosis, solamente han sido observados unos cuantos casos esporádicos.

En América constituye una de las micosis de mayor importancia desde México hasta Argentina, siendo más o menos frecuente según los diversos países; así en México, Centroamérica, Venezuela, Colombia, y Brasil es un padecimiento de todos los días, por el contrario en Chile es muy raro.

En Africa la sensacional comunicación de ABBOT [3], la información recabada por EMMONS [4], la reciente exploración de MURRAY [5], así como otras numerosas comunicaciones, ponen de manifiesto que Africa es el Continente del micetoma, aunque con la misma disparidad de incidencia según los diferentes países. Mientras que en el Sudán fueron observados 3265 nuevos casos tan solo en el período 1961/1962 [4]; en el Congo sería raro según VANBREUSEGHEM [6].

En Asia y Oceanía de acuerdo con la información que le fue proporcionada a MARIAT [7] no constituiría problema, puesto que en el período de 1940 a 1960 se habrían registrado treinta casos en Asia y seis en Oceanía. Esto es poco probable ya que la India clásicamente es el país del micetoma, y según S. C. DESEAI (comunicación personal, 1967) en Bombay es sumamente común.

II. Micetomas Actinomicéticos

a) *Por Actinomycetes anaerobios* (Actinomicosis). — El *consensus* de los autores acepta que el micetoma actinomicético por anaerobios es debido a la especie *israeli* en el hombre, y en el animal a la especie *bovis*. Ambas pueden distinguirse por procedimientos bioquímicos e inmunológicos. Es más frecuente en el sexo masculino entre las décadas 3a y 4a de la vida; raro en el niño; no tiene predominancia por raza o actividad, pero se han señalado muchos casos en toxicómanos. En la localización máxilo-facial el padecimiento es de fácil identificación generalmente; pero cuando asienta en tórax o abdomen el cuadro clínico es muy similar al micetoma actinomicético por aerobios, particularmente al debido a *N. brasiliensis* una vez que ha penetrado a pulmón y, lo que es raro, a cavidad abdominal; sin embargo la anamnesis precisando el inicio del proceso, interno o visceral en la infección por *A. israeli*, y externo o de paredes en la de *N. brasiliensis* y desde luego, la determinativa del actinomycete establecen la diferenciación. La evolución es crónica, como en el resto de los micetomas, pero se han descrito casos de apendicitis aguda por *A. israeli*. No son raros los supuestos aislamientos de *A. israeli* que corresponden a contaminantes bacterianos (Corynebacterium), reconociéndose las bacterias por la blandura de las colonias y la falta de filamentización ramificada. En casos muy graves en los que hay una diseminación aguda los granos son escasos, observándose por el contrario filamentos ramificados aislados en forma abundante. El fenómeno íntimo del porqué *A. israeli*, saprofítico de la cavidad bucal, y probablemente de pulmón y región ceco-apendicular, adquiera virulencia es desconocido; tal vez el desequilibrio de las poblaciones microbianas tenga significación como se infiere de que la localización máxilo-facial se inicia a partir de un absceso dentario, y además

por la importancia que tienen las bacterias de asociación en su evolución y tratamiento. En algunos casos el padecimiento persiste, empeora o no responde a los
medicamentos específicos, debido a la asociación bacteriana.

b) *Por Actinomycetes aerobios.* — En el Continente Americano predomina
marcadamente el micetoma actinomicético sobre el maduromicósico. Participamos
del criterio de Emmons et al. [8] al excluir *N. asteroides* como agente del micetoma.
Recientemente observamos que cuatro cepas que habíamos aislado de micetoma y
catalogado como *asteroides* corresponden a *N. caviae*; este mismo hecho sobre
supuestas cepas de *N. asteriodes* que correspondieron a *N. caviae* fue reportado
anteriormente por Gordon y Mihm [9]. *N. brasiliensis* es el agente de la inmensa
mayoría de los casos americanos de micetoma. En México y en los países Centro-
americanos se aisla entre el 90 y 95% de los micetomas. De los *Streptomyces*,
madurae representa alguna importancia, en cuanto a *Pelletieri* y *somaliensis* son
excepcionales. Contrariamente a lo que acontece en América, en Africa predomina
el micetoma maduromicósico en general; sin embargo, en algunos países los actinomycetes aerobios son también importantes pero su repartición es inversa a la
americana; en Africa *N. brasiliensis* es la excepción mientras que *S. somaliensis* y
S. Pelletieri prácticamente cubren la patología del micetoma actinomicético.

III. Micetomas maduromicósicos

Como se mencionó, estos micetomas son raros en América y es interesante que
exceptuando *Alescheria* y *Cephalosporium* que son cosmopolitas, los mohos frecuentes en América se encuentran raramente en Africa; como es el caso de *M.
grisea.* Salvo *L. senegalensis, C. lunata* y *N. rosatti* el resto de los hongos descritos
como agentes de micetoma maduromicósico han sido aislados una que otra vez y
en uno o varios países americanos. En el Continente Africano *M. mycetomi* es
responsable de la mayoría de los casos, viniendo en segundo lugar *L. senegalensis*,
que es propio de Africa, lo mismo que *C. lunata* y *N. rosatti*. Los demás mohos
descritos se encuentran con menor frecuencia.

IV. Sintomatología en relación con la Patogenia y reproducción experimental

Una vez que el agente etiológico del micetoma actinomicético por aerobios o del
maduromicósico penetra a los tejidos, al través de una solución de continuidad de
la piel o vehiculado por algún cuerpo extraño ocasiona una lesión mínima que
perdura en forma quiescente por un tiempo más o menos prolongado. Los filamentos del hongo, alojados en este medio hostil que son los tejidos, lentamente se
multiplican y desarrollan, emitiendo más y más ramificaciones. El micelio se ve
costreñido por las células tisulares obligándole a apelotonarse formando los granos,
en un principio sin masas o clamidosporas; posteriormente alrededor de los filamentos de la periferia se depositan substancias proteínicas constituyendo las masas.
A medida que el micelio continúa multiplicándose sensibiliza los tejidos y esta
sensibilización hace que pierdan poder defensivo contra el hongo, y por consecuencia permitan su multiplicación y extensión; este fenómeno parece realizarse
en forma geométrica de manera que a mayor número de lesiones mayor sensibilización, y mientras más se sensibiliza el tejido, mayor es la facilidad para el desarrollo
de nuevos focos.

Los infiltrados granulomatosos alrededor de los granos terminan en microabscesos, y los cortos trechos de micelio que no pudieron ser destruidos dan origen
a nuevos granos. Los microabscesos forman túneles que comunican entre sí
extendiéndose radialmente; cuando estos túneles llegan a la superficie forman los
nódulos que se abren por múltiples orificios los que al fusionarse forman el orificio
de la fístula y las ulceraciones. Los trayectos fistulosos se rodean de tejido con-

juntivo que al esclerosarse produce un acortamiento, lo que trae por consecuencia que los elementos del micetoma, el nódulo, el orificio fistuloso, la ulceración o la costra o cicatriz, aparezcan en el centro de una depresión. La misma formación de conjuntivo que rodea microabscesos y fístulas va constituyendo la tumoración, condicionándole su dureza característica. Esa fibrosis ocasiona un marcado compromiso circulatorio, más bien que endarteritis como menciona COCKSHOTT [10], lo que dificulta el aporte de los fármacos en el tratamiento.

En el hueso se origina una periostitis que produce caries con osteolisis y osteoformación, y al penetrar forma cavidades rodeadas de hiperostosis, de mayor o menor tamaño, dando una imagen en panal.

Esta situación patogénica conforma el cuadro clínico del micetoma, existiendo como en cualquier otro padecimiento modalidades hasta cierto punto en función de la especie causante, pero manteniendo prácticamente un cuadro tan monomorfo como no se observa en otra micosis.

Hemos podido seguir paso a paso la patogenia expuesta al obtener la reproducción del micetoma al través de la inoculación de *N. brasiliensis* en la almohadilla plantar del ratón [11]. Esta inoculación produce una tumoración crónica fistulosa con granos, sin tendencia espontánea a la curación, que se extiende por contiguidad invadiendo hueso fundamentalmente es decir, un micetoma igual al humano. La significación de este estudio implica la posibilidad, de investigar fármacos activos para su tratamiento; y más aún, dado el parentezco inmunológico y terapéutico de *N. brasiliensis* con *Mycobacterium leprae* este micetoma experimental podría utilizarse para la investigación de leprostáticos.

V. Diagnóstico

El cuadro clínico tan definido permite establecer fácilmente la hipótesis de micetoma, y más fácil aún es su comprobación al observar los granos en la supuración. La histología, radiología e inmunología no aumentan las posibilidades de identificar el micetoma, y menos aún en los casos tempranos. El diagnóstico histopatológico depende del hallazgo de los granos, siendo más aleatorio que el examen microscópico directo de la supuración. La radiología muestra lesiones orientadoras pero no características, en los casos avanzados. La inmunología a la fecha, depende de la abundancia de los diversos anticuerpos, la que está correlacionada con la cantidad de tejido enfermo.

VI. Tratamiento

El micetoma actinomicético por anaerobios o actinomicosis, como es sabido tiene tratamiento específico en las sulfamidas, los antibióticos, bacterianos y la diamino-difenil-sulfona (DDS). Los casos resistentes deben ser tratados con varios fármacos a la vez, seleccionándoles en función de su actividad contra las bacterias de asociación previo antibiograma.

Para el micetoma actinomicético por aerobios, particularmente el de *N. brasiliensis*, se emplean la DDS y las sulfamidas, prefiriéndose las de eliminación lenta, pero los resultados son aleatorios. Al revisar la literatura se encuentran numerosas comunicaciones de autores que se apresuran a comunicar los éxitos de tratamiento, pero no reportan los fracasos. En sesenta casos de micetoma actinomicético por *N. brasiliensis* que tratamos con la sulfamida Ro 4 4-4393/2 (Fanasil "Roche") [12], con diferentes esquemas, pero todos a dosis mayores que las aconsejadas en los padecimientos bacterianos, y sostenido durante dos a cuatro años, los resultados acusaron curación clínica en el 30% de los casos, mejoría evidente en 60%, y fracasos en el 30%, observándose hasta cierto punto una relación entre la extensión de las lesiones, el ataque óseo, y la magnitud de las dosis.

Tomando en cuenta la fibrosis que compromete la vascularización en la zona enferma, ensayamos el suministro intraarterial de la misma sulfanilamida en la extremidad afectada, en dosis muy altas, continuando con el suministro oral una vez que descendían los niveles sanguíneos del fármaco obtenidos con la perfusión [13]. Para este tratamiento seleccionamos doce enfermos candidatos a la amputación en vista de la intensidad de las lesiones en tejidos blandos y óseos, a los que se les perfundieron cantidades que variaron de 4 a 8 Gms obteniéndose sulfidemias, al terminar la perfusión, de 24 a 40 mg-%, y haciendo de uno a tres tratamientos. Aunque no es posible obtener conclusiones los resultados son muy favorables ya que en algunos casos obtuvimos la curación a corto plazo. El caso que se muestra en las fotografías, con un micetoma de veinte años de evolución y marcado ataque óseo, curó en cinco meses.

En los casos avanzados de micetoma actinomicético por *N. brasiliensis*, en los debidos a *Streptomyces*, y sobre todo en los de micetoma maduromicósico, por ahora no existe tratamiento seguro y deben someterse a la amputación. La resección tendrá que practicarse a gran distancia de la lesión aparente, ya que no es raro observar la reaparición del micetoma en el muñón.

El problema del micetoma por actinomycetes aerobios y por mohos continúa en pie, y su posible solución dependerá del hallazgo de fármacos realmente activos, y lo que es más, de la educación del campesino en el que se observa el padecimiento con mayor frecuencia, y del médico para que sea capaz de hacer un diagnóstico temprano.

Pathogenesis of South American Blastomycosis (Lutz's Mycosis)

A. Padilha-Gonçalves, Escola de Medicina e Cirurgia do Rio de Janeiro and Department of Dermatology of the Policlinica Geral do Rio de Janeiro (Brasil)

South American blastomycosis is a systemic disease, usually, with chronic evolution and severe prognosis. It ends by death, unless adequately treated. There are no records of spontaneous cure. Nevertheless, the higher incidence of positive paracoccidioidin intradermic tests in persons living in endemic areas of the disease make us believe that some cases could have had an overlooked Lutz's mycosis that had healed spontaneously.

It is prevalent in the Americas, chiefly in South America, but as it also occurs in Central and North America and as a few cases were reported from Europe and Africa, some authors, including myself, would rather call it Lutz's mycosis, at the same time, dealing with the geographic distribution and enhancing the pioneer work of Lutz's, the Brazilian scientist who first described the disease. The contagion of this mycosis is unknown.

There are no reports of cases of the disease due to direct contact from man to man. The few reports of it's occurrence in members of a family may be due to the existence, in them, of a congenital immunological defect responsible for a higher receptivity to the Paracoccidioides brasiliensis present in the life ambient of the family. Until now Paracoccidioides brasiliensis was not found in parasitic activity in animals, and only recently it was isolated from samples of soil. The mycosis is prevalent in males, from 20 to 50 years of age, and in persons who are in close contact with nature. The principal portal or portals of entry are still hypothetical.

The most frequent lesions are tegumentary (oropharyngeal or cutaneous), ganglionary and pulmonary. Nevertheless, lesions of Lutz's mycosis may be found in any site of the body either before or specially when, after following its natural history, the disease reaches its final stages of generalization.

Particular attention should be given to the frequent and almost pathognomonic oropharyngeal exulcerative lardaceous lesions with small granulations and small hemorragic spots on its surface. This type of lesion is a very helpful due to the diagnosis of the disease. Since the fungus is easily found in the lesions, the diagnosis of Lutz's mycosis is comparatively easy to be confirmed, whenever one has in mind the possibility of it. On the other hand, the cultures of the Paracoccidioides are difficult to be obtained. Avoiding to discuss the arguments pro or against the prevalence of the tegumentary, pulmonary or intestinal portal of entry, the invasive route of Paracoccidioides brasiliensis is suggested to be as follows. Once entering in the body whatever the portal of entry may be, the Paracoccidioides, developing or not a local lesion, will reach the regional lymph nodes. The germinal center of these lymph nodes will answer with hyperplasia and proliferation followed, at first, by a tuberculoid nodular granuloma. Then necrosis appears and/or a polymorphous infiltration with a great number of plasmocytes. The granuloma and the other lesions may spread throughout the lymph node. The macroscopic expression is of a small almost imperceptible sub-clinical adenopathy or of a clinical adenopathy of medium or severe intensity with sinus draining through the skin. Still, via lymphatic vessels the parasite reaches the cava vein and the right heart who pumps it to the lungs. Via pulmonary vein it goes from the lungs to the left heart being then hematogenically disseminated through all the body tissues and organs. This schedule explains the high incidence of pulmonary lesions which occur in around 80% of the cases. It emphazises, also, the important role played by the lymphatic tissue and system, in the pathogenesis of Lutz's mycosis, either in the dissemination of the disease or in the defensive mechanism against it by means of phagocytic macrophages and of antibodies producers plasmocytes both, usually, present in great number in the affected lymph nodes. Lymph nodes lesions may be also originated hematogenically. Clinically normal or doubtfully affected lymph nodes as well as those severely enlarged may be found with Lutz's mycosis lesions in sites far from the tegumentary or visceral lesions.

There are also strange cases of generalized ganglionary Lutz's mycosis without any other detectable localization than those of the lymph nodes. The pathogenesis of these cases is difficult to explain. It is also very strange that, usually, in such clinical forms, the lungs are not affected. In the final stages of Lutz's mycosis, when intensive dissemination produces lesions in several organs and tissues, generalized ganglionary lesions are the rule. Actually, the pathogenesis and consequently the progressive character of the mycosis of Lutz's make apparent the failure of the attempts to classify it into clinical forms.

Nouvelles acquisitions sur le mécanisme d'action de la Griséofulvine

P. PINETTI, Clinica Dermosifilopatica, Centro di studi Micologici, Cagliari (Italie)

C'est une opinion encore très répandue que l'activité thérapeutique de la Griséofulvine dans le traitement des dermophytoses soit essentiellement due à l'accumulation de l'antibiotique dans les structures pilaires cornéifiées qui par cela même deviendraient inhabitables aux dermatophytes. Cette façon de voir le mécanisme d'action de la Griséofulvine, evidemment trop simpliste, ne fait compte que des aspects plus superficiels et marginaux du problème; elle doit être — à notre avis — considerée absolument erronée.

Aux argumentations et aux faits expérimentaux que, depuis 1960, nous avons à plusieures reprises portés à soutien de notre thèse, nous pouvons aujourd'hui en ajouter d'autres.

C'est incontestable qu'une partie de la Griséofulvine introduite par la voie orale se retrouve après quelque temps dans la peau et particulièrement dans les structures pilaires. GENTLES a prouvé que les poils des sujets traités par la Griséofulvine contient en effet une certaine quantité d'antibiotique et nous mêmes, avec LOSTIA, nous avons réussi à démontrer que ces poils restent longtemps réfractaires à l'infection dermatophytique in vitro. Ces faits sont incontestables, mais ils ne sont pas du tout suffisants à expliquer le mécanisme à travers lequel la Griséofulvine réalise son effet thérapeutique. Beaucoup de constatations cliniques et expérimentales nous conduisent à douter serieusement de l'existence réelle et de la valeur substantielle de la dite imprégnation griséofulvinique du poil. En effet la quantité de Griséofulvine que l'on peut isoler du poil est très petite: elle n'atteint qu'avec difficulté la dose minima qui «in vitro» est suffisante pour inhiber la croissance de certains dermatophytes plus sensibles, et ne représente que la 15°—20° partie de la dose nécessaire pour arrêter le développement des dermatophytes responsables habituels d'un grand nombre de dermophytoses humaines. Une grande partie de la Griséofulvine que l'on peut démontrer chimiquement dans le poil est en effet facilement extractible au moyen d'un simple traitement acqueux, ce qui veut dire qu'elle n'est pas fixée d'une façon stable aux éléments cornéifiés pilaires, mais peut être simplement déposée à leur surface. En plus, nous savons bien que la plus part de la Griséofulvine présente dans le poil est localisée dans la zone keratogène du bulbe pilaire dans un endroit, c'est à dire, où elle peut garder une concentration valide grâce à l'apport continu ématique.

Plusieur faits nous ont convaincu que l'activité antimycotique de la Griséofulvine n'est pas suffisante, toute seule, à réaliser son effet thérapeutique dans certaines dermatophytoses et que cette activité est un des nombreux facteurs, et peut être même pas le plus important, du processus de guérison dans lequel, au contraire, jouent un role fondamental les facteurs naturels de défense cutanée et tout un ensemble très complexe d'activités extra-antimycotiques qui intervient directement ou bien en activant ces derniers.

Suivant une interprétation personnelle de la pathogénèse des dermatophytoses que nous avons proposée il y a longtemps, le parasitage permanent qui est à la base de toutes infections dermatophytiques de l'épiderme et des poils, se réalise et se maintient grace au fait que, au niveau des zones kératogènes il se détermine une sorte d'équilibre dynamique entre la force expulsive naturelle des structures pilaires qui poussent, d'un côté, et la force invasive du mycelium qui prolifère, de l'autre. En conséquence la desquamation continue des couches épidermiques et l'allongement continu du poil représentent — a notre avis — des facteurs d'importance capitale dans le processus de guérison des dermophytoses. C'est évident que la rupture de l'équilibre dont nous avons parlé peut se déterminer sous l'action de deux types de facteurs: les uns qui font obstacle à la multiplication mycéliale — et c'est ici qu'entre en jeu l'action antifongique spécifique de la Griséofulvine bien qu'elle ne soit pas suffisante à réaliser un effet fungicide définitif — les autres qui activent les capacités naturelles de défense des structures cutanées.

Cette position théorique qui présuppose naturellement dans la Griséofulvine l'existence d'activités pharmacologiques tout à fait différentes de l'activité anti-mycotique, nous a poussés depuis longtemps à étudier avec une particulière attention certaines propriétés biologiques de cet antibiotique qui, tout en étant de quelque manière en relation avec l'activité antimycotique, en différent clairement et d'autres encore qui à l'activité antimycotique sont au contraire absolument étrangères. Nous ne pouvons naturellement n'en donner ici qu'une très courte notice.

Au sujet de l'interprétation que nous tachons de donner du mécanisme d'action thérapeutique de la Griséofulvine, un intérêt particulier présente à nos yeux l'influence que d'après nos recherches, l'antibiotique possède d'activer le rythme de croissance du poil humain. Les mesures systématiques que nous avons conduites avec une méthode rigoureusement standardisée sur des tronçons de poil obtenus par des rasages successifs périodiques effectués sur une même zone de cuir chevelu avant et pendant l'administration, ont mis en évidence une augmentation considérable du rythme de croissance d'environ du 10 à 20%. Ce fait a été confirmé récemment par les observations d'Haran qui prouvent dans des conditions analogues une augmentation évidente du rythme de renouvellement des cellules épidermiques. Il ne nous semble donc pas du tout hazardeux d'admettre comme hypothèse possible, que cette activation de la pilogenèse et de la régénération cellulaire épidermique, constitue un facteur capable d'intervenir validement dans la rupture de l'équilibre dynamique mycéte-hôte dont nous avons parlé tout à l'heure.

Des recherches récentes ont permis à moi et à mes collaborateurs de mettre en évidence encore d'autres importantes influences pharmacologiques que la Griséofulvine exerce sur certains phénomènes biologiques cutanés. Sous l'action de l'antibiotique, l'extension des réponses réactives à la tuberculine est, par exemple, réduite d'une manière sensible et constante. Agissant localement dans le derme la Griséofulvine influence dans un sens nettement négatif l'extension du pomphus hystaminique, réduit l'ampleur de l'halo érythémateux qui l'accompagne et encore exerce une activité inhibente sur la diffusion dermique de solutions colorées. Nous n'avons pas encore réussi à donner une explication satisfaisante de la nature réelle de ces phénomènes et la seule hypothèse que nous pouvons proposer au moment actuel c'est qu'ils soient de quelque manière en rapport avec l'activité du type anti-hystaminique que la Griséofulvine semble exercer dans certaines conditions expérimentales. En effet moi et mes collaborateurs nous avons réussi à prouver que l'antibiotique s'oppose à l'action contracturante de l'hystamine sur l'ileon isolé du cobaye.

Il ne faut pas oublier d'autre part que la Griséofulvine peut exercer une évidente action anti-inflammatoire. Les expériences de D'Arcy et collab. ont prouvé que dans les animaux d'expérience, l'administration de l'antibiotique inhibe la formation de tissu de granulation autour des corps étrangers introduits dans le derme et que ça se détermine avec un mécanisme qui, bien qu'encore inconnu, ne semble pas être du type cortisonique ni rapportable à une stimulation de l'axe surréno-hypophysaire.

Une importance particulière doit être enfin accordée à tout un ensemble très suggestif d'activités vasculaires qui, signalées au début par Fegeler et Fork, ont

été ensuite sujet de nombreuses expérimentations. Nous mêmes avec nos collaborateurs nous avons reussi à prouver que l'administration par la voie intrapéritonéale
de 100 mg/kg de Griséofulvine, s'oppose à l'action de l'ergotamine en empêchant
l'apparition de la nécrose ischémique avec amputation successive que cette substance provoque habituellement dans la queue du rat. Des recherches systématiques nous ont permis de prouver que l'administration de quantités adéquates de
Griséofulvine donne lieu dans les sujets normaux à une importante vasodilatation
dans le territoire artériolaire périférique, sans influer de manière appréciable sur la
pression artérielle systémique. Cette action vasculaire est d'autre part bien prouvée
par les résultats très satisfaisants que nous avons obtenus dans la cure de certaines
artériopaties oblitérantes des membres inférieurs.

La Griséofulvine est donc capable d'exercer, outre son activité spécifique anti-
fungique qui s'applique de manière quasi sélective aux dermatophytes, une série
d'activités pharmacologiques collatérales qui nous amènent à proposer une interprétation nouvelle du mécanisme d'action de la Griséofulvine dans le processus de
guérison des dermofitoses. Les propriétés pharmacologiques anti-inflammatoires,
anti-diachitiques, pilogénétiques et vasculaires dont nous avons parlés nous amènent
à avancer l'hypothèse que l'antibiotique intervient dans le mécanisme thérapeutique pas seulement dans un sens spécifiquement antimycotique, mais aussi d'une
façon aspécifique, en activant, c'est à dire, touts les facteurs naturels qui touchent
la formation, le renouvellement et l'accroissement physiologique des structures
cornéifiées qui, selon notre conception, jouent un rôle fondamental dans le processus de guérison des dermophytoses épidermiques et pilaires.

Free Communications

Les onychomycoses

G. ACHTEN, Clinique Dermatologique de l'Université de Bruxelles (Belgique)

Les observations effectuées sur 1.000 affections des ongles permettent les constatations suivantes en ce qui concerne les onychomycoses.

1. Les onychomycoses comprenant les affections à dermatophytes et à candida
représentent 25% des onychopathies observées.

2. Le diagnostic des onychomycoses est basé sur l'examen direct, la culture et
l'examen histologique.

3. La technique histologique qui a été exposée par ailleurs [1, 2] s'effectue sur
un prélèvement de l'extrémité unguéale qui est inclus directement dans la paraffine
et coupé au microtome en lamelles de 20 microns. Celles-ci après coloration au Mac
Manus et au bleu de toluidine sont montées comme une préparation histologique
normale. Cette technique permet de mettre en évidence les filaments mycéliens des
dermatophytes qui sont le plus souvent localisés au niveau de l'ongle ventral mais
peuvent s'observer dans l'ongle tout entier. Les levures sont également bien mises
en évidence à l'examen histologique soit au niveau de l'ongle ventral soit dans
l'épaisseur même de l'ongle sous la forme levurique ou sous la forme pseudo-
filamenteuse.

4. L'examen histologique est un moyen de diagnostic plus fidèle que la culture
et l'examen direct. Ces derniers ne sont positifs que dans 50% des cas alors que
l'histologie donne 90% de résultats favorables.

5. Deux tiers des onychomycoses sont causés par le candida, un tiers par les dermatophytes.

6. La levure la plus fréquemment en cause est le c. albicans. Le c. parapsilosis et tropicalis ont été également observés.

7. 20% des onychomycoses à candida sont cliniquement constitués par une onychose primitive avec onycholyse sans périonyxis, lésions en tous points comparables à l'onychose dermatophytique.

8. Les dermatophytes les plus fréquemment observés sont le trichophyton rubrum et le ctenomyces mentagrophytes.

9. On sait que l'ongle normal est composé de trois zones [1, 3, 4, 5]:

— l'ongle dorsal qui correspond à la lèvre supérieure de la matrice unguéale.

— l'ongle intermédiaire qui correspond à la lèvre inférieure de la matrice unguéale.

— l'ongle ventral qui correspond à la kératine du lit de l'ongle.

C'est l'ongle ventral qui, étant constitué de kératine molle, est le plus souvent envahi par le dermatophyte ou la levure.

10. Les trois zones unguéales ont par suite de leur structure même, des affinités différentes pour les colorants [1, 4].

Des modifications de ces affinités tinctorielles normales peuvent s'observer dans les onychomycoses à dermatophytes. Ces altérations peuvent être primitives ou secondaires. Primitives elles sont constituées par une modification de la kératine qui préexiste à son envahissement; secondaires elles sont le témoin d'une modification due à l'action du parasite lui-même; cette dernière est vraisemblablement d'origine enzymatique.

11. Des études effectuées in vitro par la mise en contact d'ongles normaux avec divers dermatophytes montrent [2]:

a) qu'il existe une relation entre la structure physico-chimique de la kératine et son envahissement par le dermatophyte. La kératine molle de l'ongle ventral se laisse plus facilement envahir que la kératine dure de l'ongle intermédiaire ou de l'ongle dorsal.

b) que la modification de la structure de la kératine par l'action de la chaleur, des alcalis, etc. permet une pénétration plus facile des dermatophytes.

c) que l'attaque de la kératine dure de l'ongle intermédiaire s'effectue différemment selon les dermatophytes en cause (organes perforateurs, filaments perforateurs). Ces organites particuliers apparaissent uniquement in vitro.

12. L'association des techniques histologiques et mycologiques permet d'envisager sous un aspect particulier:

a) le diagnostic des mycoses unguéales au laboratoire;

b) le rapport qui s'établit entre la structure de la kératine et la pénétration du parasite fungique;

c) la fréquence relativement grande des lésions à c. albicans et l'existence d'onychose levurique sans périonyxis;

d) la biologie particulière du parasite fungique en contact in vitro avec la kératine.

Bibliographie. 1. ACHTEN, G.: Dermatologica (Basel) **126**, 229 (1963); — Bull. Soc. franç. Derm. Syph. **71**, 579 (1964); Minerva derm. **40**, 431 (1965); — Dermat. (Paris) 12890 A. **10**, 1 (1967); — Histologie und Histochemie des Nagels. In: JADASSOHNS: Handbuch der Haut- und Geschlechtskrankheiten, Erg.-Werk, Bd. I/1. Berlin-Heidelberg-New York: Springer 1968. — 2. ACHTEN, G., et J. SIMONART: Ann. Derm. Syph. (Paris) **90**, 569 (1963); — Ann. Soc. belge Méd. trop. **44**, 755 (1964); — Mycopathologia (Den Haag) **27**, 193 (1965). — 3. HASHIMOTO, K., B. GROSS, R. NELSON, and W. LEVER: J. invest. Derm. **47**, 205 (1966). — 4. LEWIS, B.: Arch. Derm. **70**, 732 (1954). — 5. ZAIAS, N.: Arch. Derm. **87**, 37 (1963).

Aspects particuliers de l'épidermomycose causée par epidermophyton floccosum

I. Alteras et I. Cojocaru, Centre Dermato-vénéréologique, Bucarest (Roumanie)

C'était en 1913 quand le professeur Nicolau signalait, pour la première fois en Roumanie, la présence de l'Epidermophyton floccosum, pour lequel il proposait la dénomination d'«Epidermophyton plicarum», étant donné son siège de prédilection dans les plis. Dès lors, ce dermatophyte fut mentionné plusieurs fois dans les statistiques concernant l'évolution de la flore mycotique, en ne dépassant que très rarement 2% des infections à dermatophytes. Nos observations ont été faites sur 175 malades.

La plupart de nos cas, dont les mâles représentaient la majorité, provenaient du milieu urbain, où il y avait les conditions propices qui peuvent favoriser la transmission (bains public, piscines, salles de sport etc.). Quant à l'âge de nos malades, Epidermophyton floccosum affectait aussi bien l'enfant de 4 ans que le vieillard de 80 ans. Quoique la morphologie des colonies appartenant à cette espèce ne puissent pas nous offrir une variété d'interprétation, on ne pourrait dire la même chose sur le siège et le polymorphisme des lésions. En dehors des plis, dont les aines et les espaces interdigitaux des pieds figuraient, à proportion égale, pour deux tiers des cas environ, la présence d'Epidermophyton floccosum a été trouvé sur n'importe quelle région de la peau glabre. Citons par exemple la *région plantaire*, d'où cette espèce a été isolée chez 40 malades. Ça veut dire que ce territoire cutané n'est pas réservé exclusivement aux T. mentagrophytes ou T. rubrum, les principaux responsables de l'épidermophytie des pieds. Rappelons que Lloyd et Greer ont trouvé l'Epidermophyton floccosum beaucoup plus fréquemment aux pieds que dans la région inguinale).

A côté de la plante, la *face dorsale du pied* a été elle aussi atteinte par ce dermatophyte chez 7 de nos sujets. Chez 25% des malades, les lésions siégeaient tout le reste du tronc, à partir de la jambe jusqu'à la peau du crâne. L'atteinte des ongles a été observée chez 11 sujets dont deux seulement avec onychomycose des doigts. Pour une game si variée concernant la diversité des localisations choisies par l'Epidermophyton floccosum il lui fallait aussi une variété des manifestations cliniques, sinon comparables, mais au moins digne d'être signalée. L'aspect des lésions rencontrées chez nos malades était loin d'être monotone. En dehors du type commun de l'*eczéma marginé de Hebra*, considéré, au début de la mycologie médicale, comme une manifestation quasi-spécifique de l'Epidermophyton floccosum, tous les espects de l'*intertrigo*, dont l'expression clinique ne pouvait point suggérer l'appartenance étiologique, y ont été observés. Les localisations dans les espaces interdigitaux des doigts ou des orteils surtout, évoquaient par leur aspect, l'impression clinique d'une infection à Candida.

Un autre aspect clinique des lésions causées par Epidermophyton floccosum appartenait au type de la bien connue *épidermophytie des pieds* (tinea pedis), dont la plupart des cas à la forme sèche, habituellement rencontrée dans les infections à T. rubrum. Mais, la soit-disant «rubrophytie», dont certains auteurs font une entité à part n'est, en réalité, qu'une modalité d'expression clinique, réalisée par l'agression de plusieurs dermatophytes sur un terrain spécial, où l'évolution chronique de l'affection a son mot à dire.

L'aspect dyshidrosiforme de l'épidermophytie, à lésions vésiculo-bulleuses où l'Epidermophyton floccosum siégeait les paumes et les plantes a été observée, lui aussi, chez sept malades. En Roumanie, ce type de manifestations est plutôt réservé pour l'invasion de T. mentagrophytes. Il est encore à retenir la participation de l'Epidermophyton floccosum dans quatre cas de l'épidermophytie palmoplantaire, à l'aspect de «dysidrosis lamellaris sicca».

Chez douze malades les manifestations cliniques simulaient parfaitement le syndrôme de l'*eczéma numulaire*. Même l'aspect de la *neurodermite* était représenté, dans six cas (où seulement l'examen mycologique a permis d'établir la vraie éthiologie).

Un autre aspect particulier de l'infection à l'Epidermophyton floccosum a été observé chez deux sujets, qui présentaient des lésions semblables au *l'erythème polymorphe* en cocarde (la forme connue sous la dénomination d'*herpès iris*). Il vient encore un autre cas, dont l'éruption, assez curieuse, localisée dans la région médiosternale, offrait l'aspect des *eczématides figurées de Brocq*. Le type de *herpès circiné* (sous ses variables aspects qu'il puisse se manifester) a été provoqué par Epidermophyton floccosum chez 20% de nos malades. Il y avait, enfin, deux cas à lésions généralisées, dont l'un à l'aspect *verruqueux* et *végétant* et l'autre à l'aspect d'une *xérodermie*. Un cas à lésions verruqueuses, mais sans l'atteinte de la peau du crâne a été aussi rapporté par FISCHER et coll. en 1961.

L'avenir nous apportera, peut-être, d'autres surprises encore, en ce qui concerne les possibilités sans limites (croyons-nous) dont les dermatophytes sont capables de provoquer une game si variée des manifestations cliniques.

Ultraestructura y citoquimica de la Candida albicans

L. F. MONTES y V. S. CONSTANTINE, Department de Dermatologia, University of Alabama Medical Center, Birmingham, Alabama (USA)

Células de *C. albicans* cultivadas a temperatura ambiente, fueron estudiadas en cortes ultrafinos bajo el microscopio electrónico, y en extendidos después de incubarlas para localizar diferentes actividades enzimáticas. Para microscopia electrónica se fijaron en permanganato de litio (L. F. MONTES, J. invest. Derm. 45, 227 1965), se incluyeron en Araldite y se cortaron en un micrótomo Porter-Blum automático. Las observaciones se efectuaron en un microscopio RCA EMU3F y en un microscopio Philips 200. Las células de *C. albicans* poseen una gruesa pared celular (1000 hasta 1300 Å), una membrana plasmática con numerosas invaginaciones intracitoplásmicas, mitocondrias, vacuolas, reticulo endoplásmico bien desarrollado, nucleo y densos gránulos limitados por una membrana. Se describen las caracteristicas de cada una de estas organelas. Se presentan las observaciones efectuadas sobre la localización de varias actividades enzimáticas en células de *C. albicans* (Succino dehidrogenasa, tetrazolio reductasas, fosfatasa ácida, aminopeptidasa) con el microscopio óptico.

Keloidal Blastomycosis (Jorge Lobo's Disease)

S. FRAGA and J. LISBÔA MIRANDA, Rio de Janeiro (Brazil)

In 1931, JORGE LOBO [1] reported in Brazil the first case of this infection that can be defined as a chronic mycosis limited to the skin where the lesions present keloid-like aspect. The disease is caused by a fungus of still not clear systematic position and its name is also on dispute.

FONSECA and LEÃO [2], in 1940 were the first to name it as a new species — *Glenosporella Loboi*. ALMEIDA and LACAZ [3], in 1949 proposed *Paracoccidioides Loboi* and CIFERRI [4], in 1956 created *Loboa Loboi* for designating the parasite.

Possibly the fungus does not grow on any of the presently known culture media and the few claimed isolations were probably contamnants. Corroborating this supposition, MIRANDA [5] studying Carneiro's cultures [6], was able to verify that they produced abundant aspergillus fruiting heads on a media containing 40% saccharose. Otherwise same investigators [6, 7] suspect that the culture kept now as being the first isolation — *Glenosporella Loboi* is not anymore a transfer of the original, but a culture of *P. brasiliensis* mislabeled by inadvertence. Experimental infection in animals using material from human lesions was never obtained.

Geographic Distribution and Epidemiology. The disease is limited to the equatorial zone of the New World, mainly the Amazon area. The infection has been seen in adult white, mulattoes and indians, exceptionally in females.

Some patients correlate the original lesions to various injuries.

Clinical Picture. The disease is limited to the skin, without visceral dissemination. Seldom a residual lymphatic involvment has been described. The cutaneous lesions are isolated or confluent, firm nodules displaying the aspect of brownish or violaceous keloid-like tumors with smooth, glistening surfaces. By confluence they assume the aspect of lobulated tumors and may cover extensive areas. The surrounding skin does not show inflammatory reaction. Slight pruritus and local anesthesia are the only complaints. Localized or wide-spread skin lesions may occur. The disease has a very chronic course without affecting the patient's general health.

Morphology of the Parasite on the Lesions. It can be studied in fresh preparations or stained tissue sections. The microorganisms are round cells with thick, double contoured membranes, reproducing commonly by single bud and occasionally originating 2,3 or more buds. The parasites do not show great variation in size and their average diameter is 10 micra. The buds remain connected to the mother cell until their size are equalled. Some cells are deformed, others empty and still others show vacuoles in its interior. In stained sections, small short tubes connecting the buds to the mother cell are demonstrated. Cryptosporulation does not occur. Encircling some of the parasites one observes short radiating spines, constituted of granular PAS positive material, also stained by Gomori's reticuline and Gridley stain [8 to 11].

Histopathology. The histopathological changes are characteristic. There is atrophy of the epidermis and flattening of the rete pegs due to the pressure of dermal

	Keloidal blastomycosis	S. A. blastomycosis
Geographic distribution	Equatorial zone of the New World	South and Central America, Mexico
Clinical picture Evolution	Keloid-like lesions — chronic	Systemic involvement — progressive (membranes are mainly affected)
Treatment	No effective drug	Controled by sulpha and Amphotericin B
Histopathology	Predominantly histiocytic reaction. Abundant parasites	Proliferative and exsudative reaction. Less parasites
Morphology of parasite on tissue	Small variation in size. No cryptosporulation	Great variation in size. Cryptosporulation
Culture	Not obtained	Easily obtained
Animal inoculation from humans	Not obtained	Obtainable

infiltration. The dermis is occupied by a massive infiltration made up of great number of histiocytes with foamy appearance and giant cells. In frozen sections stained by Sudan III droplets of bi-refringent lipids are observed [8]. Collagenous and reticular fibers divided the affected area into lobules. The parasites are extremely abundant throughout the infiltrated areas.

Treatment. No drug has been effective in this infection. Stilbamidine, Amphotericin B or Sulphas compounds have been used without success. This disease is clearly distinct from S.A. Blastomycosis. In the following chart the chief differences between the two diseases are presented.

Case Report. A 70 year old male having the disease for the last 36 years contracted when living in the Amazon region. In 1963 the process had invaded the right arm up to the shoulder. X-ray treatment to the right wrist resulted in radiodermatitis that was then removed by surgery followed by skin grafting. Four years later the new skin showed innumerous islands of diseased tissue that eventually invaded the entire grafted area.

Clinically uninvolved areas already presented many organisms around the vessels and within connective tissue. Sections showed parasites apparently inside the blood vessels suggesting hematogenous route.

Bibliography. 1. Lobo, J.: Rev. méd. Pernambuco 1, 763 (1931). — 2. Fonseca Filho, O. Leão y A. E. Area: O agente etiológica da doença de Jorge Lobo 48, (3), 147 (1940). — 3. Almeida, F., y C. S. Lacaz: An. Fac. Med. Univ. S. Paulo 24, 5 (1948—49). — 4. Ciferri, R.: Trop. Med. Hyg. Sept. 1956. — 5. Miranda, J. L., and R. D. Azulay: Unpublished data (1954). — 6. Carneiro, L. S.: Contribuição ao estudo microbiológico do agente etiológico da Doença de Jorge Lobo. Tese. Imprensa Industrial. Recife-Pernambuco 1952. — 7. Fonseca Filho, O.: Therapy of fungus disease. An International Symposium, p. 56 (1955). Ed. by Thomas H. Sternberg. — 8. Fialho, A.: Hospital (Rio de J.) 14, 903 (1938). — 9. Guimarães, F. N., y D. G. Macedo: Contribuição ao estudo das blastomicoses na Amazonia 38, 223 (1950). — 10. Teixeira. G. A.: Hospital (Rio de J.) 62, 813 (1962). — 11. Emmons: Medical Mycology, p. 275. Philadelphia: Lea and Febiger 1963.

A Look at Mycetoma in India

B. B. Gokhale, Department of Dermatology, Sassoon General Hospitals, Poona-1 (India), and A. A. Padhye and M. J. Thirumalachar, Hindustan Antibiotics Research Laboratories, Pimpri, near Poona (India)

The term mycetoma implies a tumorous enlargement caused by a fungus infection. The characteristic clinical picture is produced by a variety of filamentous fungi belonging to different species and genera. Fungi causing mycetoma fall into two categories — Eumycetes and Schizomycetes. To avoid confusion it is better to qualify the term by signifying the type e.g. Actimomycotic mycetoma, Maduromycotic mycetoma etc.

The disease is endemic in certain parts of tropical zones and sporadic in subtropical climates. It is endemic in south and central India. Some cases have been reported from Bengal and Punjab. The first report was published from the department of dermatology, Sassoon Hospitals Poona in 1959 (Gokhale et al.) and second report in 1963 (Padhye et al.). The following cases have been reported from various places at various times:

Punja, G. (Calcutta, 1948) — Actinomycosis, cheek.
Ranawre, M. (Poona, 1951) — Actinomycosis lung.
Ranawre, M. (Poona, 1959) — Actinomycotic - pericarditis.
Kakoti, L., and N. Dey (Dibrugad-Assam, 1956) — Mycetoma.
Andleigh, H. (Jaipur, 1957) — Maduromycosis.
Banerji, B. (Calcutta, 1958) — Actinomycosis skin.
Banerji, A., et. al. (Calcutta, 1961) — Mycetoma.
Gaind, M. et al. (Poona, 1962) — Mycetoma.
Sanyal, M., and N. Basou (Calcutta, 1964) — Mycetoma.

This report presents 19 cases studied in Poona, India. Poona is situated in Western India on the Deccan plateau 18°—30' latitude and 73°—53' longitude. It is 101 km from Bombay (as the crow flies) and 564 m high above sea-level. The climate is dry during most parts of the year, and by reason of its elevation and dryness, Poona is cool during nights almost all round the year. The cold season is from November to February and the monsoon is from June to October. Maximum average temperature is 29—40 °C and the minimum average is 20 °C. The average rain fall is 76 cm.

The report includes cases described in 1959 and 1963. A detailed history was taken. Records of clinical examinations, laboratory and other investigations were maintained. Only those cases in which the causative organisms have been identified, are described.

An outline of the procedure of collecting granules will not be out of place. In very active or advanced cases collection of granules is a simple procedure. Very often the granules are collected from the dressings. However, in chronic cases with organisation of granulation tissue and localisation of inflammatory process, it is not always easy to recover the granules. To overcome this difficulty the following procedure may be adopted. The patent external os of the sinus is flushed with saline or an anesthetic. With this procedure the injected fluid is forced out from other intercommunicating sinuses pouring forth the granules. Some times a healthy area round about which multiple sinuses exist, is injected by using a thick bored needle. A local anesthetic is preferred because the procedure could be painful. On certain occasions when even this method fails and a therapeutic injection is adviced, uhyalase has been sed for the local injection as above. This loosens the dense organized tissue and releases the granules. The indicated therapeutic material is then injected locally. It is felt that local therapeutic injections yield better results than the same drug administered parenterally.

In 17 cases only foot was affected. In one instance a knee joint and in the remaining case a leg and foot was involved. 15 patients were male and four females. Amongst the males, all but two, were farm-workers. Out of the two one was a blacksmith and the other a labourer. Two of the females were farmworkers and two were housewives. All the patients were adults aged between 25 and 60 years.

Causative organisms were:	cases
Madurella mycetomi	7
Phialophora jeanselmi	2
Cephalosporium madurae	1
Nocardia asteroides	6
Actinomyces israeli	2
Madurella grisea	1

From the survey of the work done in this country and from our study, it is surmised that Madurella mycetomi, Nocardia species and Cephalosporium species are the predominant causative organisms.

It is obvious that most of our patients were farm-workers and foot was common site of lesion. The habit of going to work without foot-wear is an important factor in traumatic exposures. To India with an agrarian economy this is of great importance because amputation is an invariable rule in advanced cases of mycetoma. Thus there is an indication for a country wide survey of the disease and the etiologic agents. This will help the search for therapeutic agents.

May I take the liberty to add one interesting case of black granules caused by Cladosporium species, investigated after submission of the above report.

References. ANDLEIGH, H. S.: Mycopathologia (Den Haag) 8, 138 (1957). — BANERJEE, B. N.: Indian J. Derm. 3, 8 (1958). — BANERJEE, A. K., and S. P. BASU: Bull. Calcutta Sch. trop. Med. 9, 113 (1961). — GAIND, M. L., A. A. PADHYE, and M. J. THIRUMALACHER: Sabouraudia 1, 230 (1962). — Gokhale, B. B., A. A. Padhye, and M. J. Thirumalachar: Bull. Calcutta Sch. trop. Med. 7, 41 (1959). — Kakoti, L. M., and N. C. Dey: Indian J. med. Sci. 10, 889 (1956). — Padhye, A. A., B. B. Gokhale, and M. J. Thirumalachar: H. A. Bull. 5, 74 (1963). — Punja, G.: Indian med. Gaz. 83, 416 (1948). — Ranawre, M. M.: Indian J. med. Sci. 5, 63 (1951). — Ranawre, M. M., S. S. Kelkar, and J. Mordicai: Indian J. med. Sc. 13, 696 (1959). — Sanyal, M., and N. Basu: Bull. Calcutta Sch. trop. Med. 12, 115 (1964).

Esporotricosis, estudio clinico epidemiologico

V. C. Jaramillo, G. C. Vélez, A. R. Moreno, I. R. Pizano y A. C. Cortés, Universidad de Antioquia, Departmento de Medicina Interna, Dermatología, Medellin (Columbia)

Introduccion

En el presente trabajo los autores revisan 93 casos de esporotricosis que fueron observados durante un período de 8 años en la Facultad de Medicina de la Universidad de Antioquia en Medellín — Colombia — Suramérica.

Datos Epidemiologicos e Incidencia. El factor de más importancia en la incidencia fue el ocupacional como puede apreciarse en el cuadro 1. No parece tampoco

Cuadro 1

Ocupación	No. de Casos	%
Agricultores	38	41.0
Estudiantes	12	12.9
Oficios Domésticos	12	12.9
Obrero	9	
Albañil	6	
Zapatero	2	
Sacristán	2	
Comerciante	2	
Carnicero	2	
Vaquero	2	
Sin dato	6	
Total	93	

Quadro 2. *Distribucion por edades*

De 1 a 10 años	21
De 11 a 20 años	18
De 21 a 30 años	15
De 31 a 40 años	6
De 41 a 50 años	6
De 51 a 60 años	11
Mayores de 60 años	16
Total	93

Cuadro 3

Sexo	No. de Casos	%
Masculino	77	82.7
Femenino	16	17.3
Total	93	

Cuadro 4

Variedades Clínicas	No. de Casos	%
Epidérmica Superficial fija	66	71
Linfangítica	27	29
	93	100

Cuadro 5
Variedad Epidérmica — Formas Clinicas

Ulcerativa	27
Verrucosa	22
Eritemato-escamosa	15
Acneiforme	2
Total	66

Cuadro 6
Diagnóstico Diferencial

Esporotricosis
Cromoblastomicosis
T. B. C. Cutis
Leishmaniasis
Ca. Epidermoide
Piodermitis Vegetante
Granuloma inespecífico

Cuadro 7
Tratamiento

Yoduro de K. Oral
Yoduro de Na. I. V.
Griseofulvina

53*

existir predilección por la edad (cuadro 2) como lo demuestran los casos que
encontramos tanto en la primera infancia como en la edad senil. En cuanto al sexo
podemos notar (cuadro 3) una mayor incidencia en el sexo masculino, 77 casos
(82.2%). Sin embargo creemos que este hecho se debe más al tipo de trabajo que
ejecuta el hombre ya que es de anotar que en las mujeres campesinas sometidas
a oficios del campo, la enfermedad se presenta también con frecuencia. Así de los
16 casos nuestros presentados en mujeres, 12 eran campesinas. Generalmente se
encuentra el antecedente de abrasiones, pinchazos con vegetales etc., pero es de
anotar hay ocasiones en que no es posible por el interrogatorio encontrar antecedentes traumático alguno. En cuanto a las variedades clínicas mayores encontramos (cuadro 4) que 66 de nuestros casos, el 71%, correspondieron a la forma
epidérmica, superficial o fija y que sólo 27 casos, el 29%, presentaban la variedad
linfangítica que es la más común en la mayoría de los países. Fuera de esas dos
formas clínicas mayores queremos hacer mención de dos casos especiales que por
su atipicidad merecen consideración aparte. El primer paciente de estos presentaba compromiso de la extremidad superior izquierda de 20 años de duración.
Las lesiones eran escamo-costrosas sobre un fondo eritemato-ulcerativo. El otro
caso era el de un paciente con extensas lesiones vegetantes, papilomatosas, verrucosas, escamosas, de color rojo violáceo diseminadas en los miembros inferiores, las regiones glúteas y aún había lesiones en el dorso de la nariz y en el pabellón
auricular derecho. En el cuadro 5 se pueden apreciar las formas clínicas de la
variedad epidérmica:

	Casos
Ulcerativa	27
Verrucosa	22
Eritemato-escamosa	15
Acneiforme	2

Diagnostico

En todos nuestros casos el diagnóstico clínico de esporotricosis fue comprobado
por el cultivo del Sporotrichum schenkii.

Diagnostico Diferencial. La Esporotricosis entre nosotros simula muy de cerca
otras entidades. De ellas merecen especial mención la Cromoblastomicosis — con
ésta es frecuentemente casi imposible hacer el diagnóstico clínico especialmente
con las formas fijas, verrucosas de esporotricosis —; la T.B.C. verrucosa cutis; la
Leishmaniasis y más remotamente los carcinomas epidermoides, la piodermitis
vegetante y otros granulomas.

Debemos hacer hincapié sobre la forma linfangítica de la Leishmaniasis que
remeda casi en un todo y por todo la correspondiente forma linfangítica de la
esporotricosis. Sin embargo, desde el punto de vista clínico podemos decir que la
forma linfangítica de la leishmaniasis presenta nódulos pequeños, alineados, formando cordones de consistencia firme y que sólo excepcionalmente se ulceran.

Tratamiento. En todos nuestros casos los Yoduros produjeron la curación.
Generalmente los utilizamos por vía oral y sólo cuando hay gastralgia demasiado
marcada recurrimos a la forma intravenosa. La griseofulvina en nuestras manos
no dió nunca los resultados benéficos que han informado otros autores.

Resumen y Conclusiones. 1. Se presentan 93 casos de esporotricosis, el 71% de
los cuales pertenecía a la forma superficial, epidérmica o fija. 2. Se lama la atención sobre algunas formas atípicas de la esporotricosis las cuales se presentan en
diapositivas. 3. Se hace hincapié sobre la importancia del diagnóstico micológico
— el cultivo — ya que desde el punto de vista clínico muchos casos son indiferen-
ciables, especialmente, de la cromoblastomicosis y de la leishmaniasis linfangítica.

Favus Infection in Iraq

G. F. RAHIM, Skin Department, College of Medicine, University of Baghdad (Iraq)

Favus is a chronic dermatophytic infection of the scalp widely endemic among the urban and rural population of Iraq. It presents as two common clinical forms; the deeply invasive macro-scutulae type and the superficial milliary scutulae type.

The first, being the commonest type, commences with various sized scutulae over the vertex and spreads peripherally while the old lesions are drying in a cicatrix. The invasion of the scalp is relatively fast and the lesions which may vary in size between 3 to 20 mm involve the scalp quite deeply with severe local reaction which may spread eventually to the whole surface of the scalp.

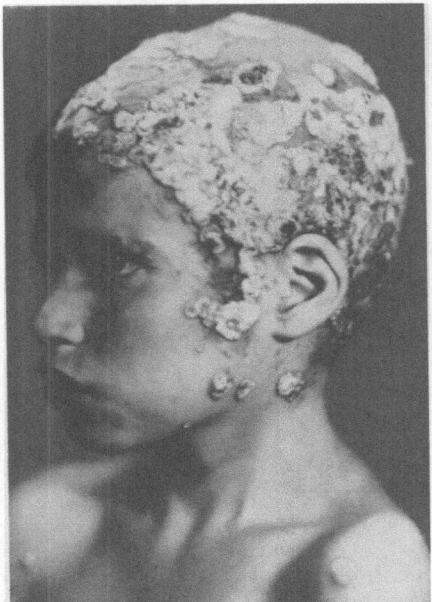 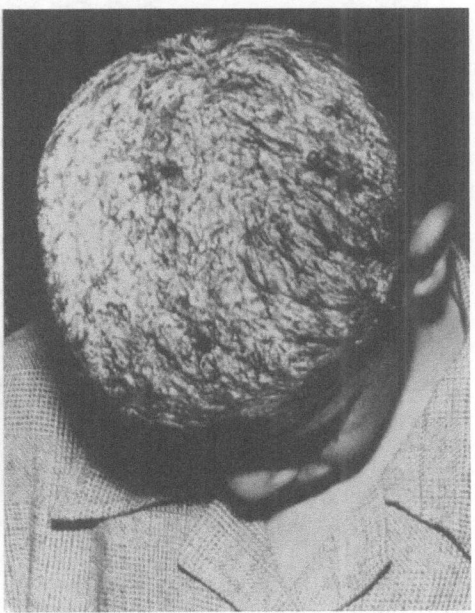

Fig. 1. Deeply invasive macro-scutulae type of Favus

Fig. 2. Superficial milliary scutulae type of Favus

The second type may pass unnoticed for long time and presents as various sized milliary scutulae surrounding the hair follicles. It progresses fairly slowly with less destruction than the first type. Affected hairs may grow normally and the longest fluorescing hair is about 10 μ.

Greenish hair flourescence is encountered in both types but every infected hair does not necessarily show fluorescence. Brilliant phosphorus-like fluorescence has also been observed mainly in the first type. Inflammatory reaction may occur in certain cases but no pyogenic or kerion like lesions have been observed. Favus of the glabrous skin is observed in 0.2 to 0.3% of infected cases, while Favus of the nails is encountered in 0.5 to 0.8% of cases of favus of the scalp.

It is possible to recognise a variable degree of characteristic facies in about 30 to 40% of favus patients. These facies are sufficiently marked to distinguish a favus patient in the street or in OPD attendance room.

Favus patients uniformly attend with their heads wrapped up. Males use a yashmagh (a native hair cover) while females use a black cloth cover. These usually cover the forehead down to the eyebrows and the pre-auricular hairy area.

On close examination these patient have a narrow oedematous forehead, protruded in front and flattened on the sides. The eyes are depressed and the mouth and chin seem elongated and protruding. The complexion is sallow. The face is pale clay in color with occasional patchy butterfly pigmentation. The patient appears intimidated worried and shy, trying to hide all his spots.

These characteristics occur mainly in children of 5 to 12 years of the rural districts with an extremely low standard of hygiene. Most of them exhibit extensive favus infection of the first type with a minimum duration of 2 to 4 years.

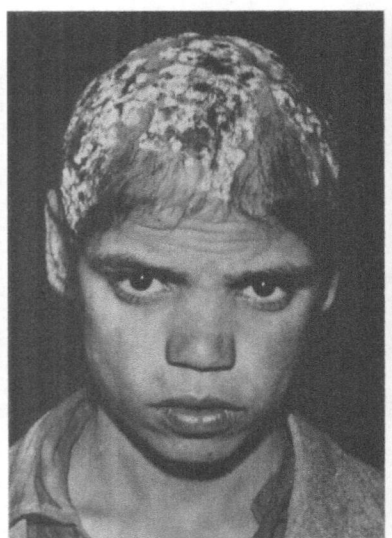 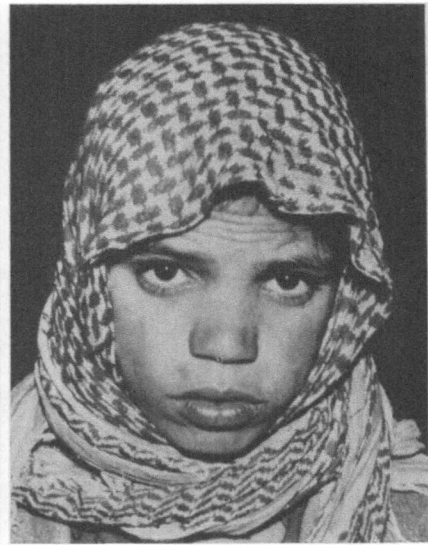

Fig. 3. Favus showing typical facies   Fig. 4. Same patient with a yashmagh

A comparative study has been made of one group of patients with the characteristic facies, another group without this facies and a third group of patients with tinea capitis due to other dermatophytes. The result of the investigation indicate that there is some degree of anaemia and leucocytosis in all cases of favus patients, most marked in those of the first group and in those cases with kerion celsi. The WBC differential count showed marked eosinophilia ranging from 3 to 30%. ESR varied between 10 to 90 mm. Serum proteins showed an appreciable hyperglobulinaemia with an accentuation of the A2-globulins. All these findings indicate that favus patients exhibit a toxaemic reaction due to tissue destruction which accounts as well to their bahavioral changes.

Ringworm of the scalp makes about 2% of the total attendence at the Skin OPD of the Republic Hospital, and favus constitutes about 76% of these cases or about 700 cases per year. The disease is invariably acquired in childhood, very often familial and frequently persists through adult life. The source of infection is often traced to a member in the family, to the neighbours or to the school.

Study of the flora of soil from the houses of infected patients did not reveal the presence of *T. schoenlini*. Viability of *T. schoenlini* in hairs stored at room temperature (7 to 45 °C) was shown to persist for a period of over $2^1/_2$ years. Infected hairs incorporated in various samples of soil showed total unrecovery by culture after 2 to 4 weeks. In further studies it was found that boiling or heating to 80°C for 5 min is lethal to the fungus, while the fungus could survive 70°C for 1 min, 0°C for 1 month and lypholisation. Soaps, detergents and antiseptics in common dilutions are not sufficiently fungicidal. Paint of tinct iodi mitis is sufficient to sterilise the skin, but a sprinkling of alcohol is of no use as a disinfectant.

La macrocheilite de la blastomycose Sud-Américaine

J. Ramos-Silva et A. Padilha-Gonçalves. Département de Dermatologie, Policlinique Générale, Rio de Janeiro (Brasil)

Les localisations buccales de la blastomycose sud-américaine (B.S.A.) sont très fréquentes et bien connues. Il n'avait pas échappé aux auteurs qui au Brésil ont commencé, il y a une soixantaine d'années, l'étude de cette grave maladie, la tuméfaction des lèvres (aspect lippu) parmi les manifestations cliniques de l'infection par Paracoccidioides brasiliensis.

Dans ce travail nous voulons, en reprenant l'étude de cette localisation de la maladie dans cinq cas de notre Service à la Policlinique Générale de Rio de Janeiro, sous le point de vue des idées actuelles, étudier non seulement la macrocheilite qui très souvent accompagne le processus inflammatoire actif avec des lésions ulcéro-végétantes siègeant tant à la face cutanée comme — et plus fréquemment, du coté muqueux des lèvres, mais aussi attirer l'attention sur les formes résiduelles de macrocheilite qui restent comme un reliquat plus ou moins durable après la guérison chimiothérapique de la B.S.A.

Comme l'on sait, Miescher a crée en 1945 sa macrocheilite granulomateuse essentielle, processus inflammatoire chronique de cause inconnue compromettant la lèvre inférieure (parfois aussi la lèvre supérieure), laquelle augmente de volume en raison d'un fort oedème inflammatoire et présente, à la surface, des rhagades de disposition radiaire. La biopsie montre un infiltrat cellulaire composé de lymphocytes et plásmocytes, avec des nodules épithélioïdes qui donnent l'impression d'une structure sarcoïdique.

Tableau 1. *Les macrocheilites*

1. Macrocheilite élephantiasique stréptococcique
2. Macrocheilite granulomateuse essentielle de Miescher
3. Macrocheilite du syndrome de Melkersson-Rosenthal
4. Macrocheilite du syndrome D'Ascher
5. Macrocheilites parasitaires
   - a) de la Leishmaniose
   - b) de la filariose
   - c) de la moniliase
   - d) de la blastomycose sud-americaine

Cette macrocheilite idiopathique peut se présenter isolée ou, en s'accompagnent d'une langue plicaturée et d'une paralysie faciale, constituer le syndrome de Melkersson-Rosenthal. D'un autre côté on a déjà signalé que certaines maladies parasitaires peuvent occasionner des aspects similaires à la macrocheilite de Miescher : la leishmaniose (Koch et Vilanova), la filariose (Gahlen et Gillman), la moniliase (Gerauer et Wiskemann). L'un de nous (A.P.G.), avait mentionné dès 1946, l'occurence dans certains cas de B.S.A., d'une cheilite glandulaire simple.

La forme hyperplasique de la cheilite glandulaire, a son tour, quand est accompagnée d'une grosse lèvre oedèmateuse, d'hypertrophie de la muqueuse nasale, d'épaississement des joues et de blépharochalase, constitue le syndrome d'Ascher.

Description sommaire de la macrocheilite de la B.S.A.

A. Clinique

Les lésions s'imposent à notre attention à la première vue, étant constituées par l'augmentation d'épaisseur, souvent énorme, de la lèvre inferieure et, parfois aussi, de la lèvre supérieure. Cet état est dû, d'un coté, à un gros oedème qui se répand au voisinage, aux joues et un peu aux ailes du nez, et de l'autre, à une infiltration cellulaire d'origine inflammatoire, dont la nature sera esquissée ensuite. Quand le processus est en pleine activité il y a quelques sillons radiaires et surtout des ulcérations dont le fond est discrètement végétant et en partie couvert d'un exsudat purulent adhérent, plus ou moins abondant, avec des points hémorragiques. Dans les formes résiduelles, plus importantes de notre point de vue, on trouve de l'oedème du type éléphantiasique, des cicatrices parfois dyschromiques, des lésions guéries de la peau ou de la muqueuse, parfois un peu de desquamation et dans les coupes, les altérations qu'on va detailler.

B. Histopathologie

Deux aspects principaux peuvent être rencontrés, séparément ou ensemble. Dans les cas en activité on peut rencontrer, à côté d'un infiltrat inflammatoire granulomateux, dense, polymorphe, contenant de nombreux plasmocytes, lymphocytes, histiocytes, polynucléaires, tant neutro comme éosinophiles — des véritables follicules tuberculoïdes composés de cellules épithélioïdes et de cellules géantes. Celles-ci abritent très souvent le Para coccidioides brasiliensis avec ses éléments

Tableau 2. *Macrocheilite de la blastomycose sud-américaine:* Oedème avec fibrose et infiltration cellulaire diffuse des lèvres:

Deux formes principales:
    a) Dans les cas en activité il y a des ulcérations et on trouve souvent au microscope le granulome typique de la B.S.A. contenant le parasite (Para coccidioides brasiliensis) dans des cellules géantes.
    b) Dans les cas résiduels (après chimiotherapie spécifique) on trouve des cicatrices parfois dyschromiques et atrophiques. Microscopiquement c'est une cheilite lympho-fibro-oedémateuse avec un infiltrat cellulaire d'inflammation diffuse chronique.

Tableau 3. *Tableau synoptique des observations*

N°[a]	durée de la maladie	type de la macro-cheilite	cheilite glandu-laire	autres localisations	recherche du parasite:	
					dans les coupes de la lèvre	examen extemporané à l'entrée
66.868	12 ans	résiduel	oui	nez, intérieur bouche	—	+
67.441	2 ans	résiduel	non	poumons; lésions disséminées peau	—	+
68.440	9 ans	actif	non	amygdales, glotte, ganglions cervicaux poumons	+	+
69.001	2 ans	actif	non	ganglions cervicaux, poumons	+	+
71.473	7 ans	actif	non	peau de la face	+	+

[a] Du Département de Dermatologie de la Policlinique Générale de Rio de Janeiro et Chaire de Clinique Dermatologique de l'Ecole de Médecine et Chirurgie (Prof. J. RAMOS-SILVA).

caractéristiques: cellules avec double contour, montrant parfois de la gemmulation périphérique. Dans les cas résiduels, guéris ou en train de guérir, les formations tuberculoïdes ne sont plus rencontrées, si bien que les lésions de cette macrocheilite soient les suivantes. L'épithélium est irrégulièrement épaissi avec des zones d'atrophie modérée, d'origine cicatricielle. Le derme se montre très oedémateux avec nombreux capillaires sanguins et lymphatiques très dilatés. Dans toute son extension on voit un infiltrat diffus, présentant parfois des agglomérations discrètes, de situation surtout péri-vasculaire. Cette infiltration est constituée de lymphocytes, plasmocytes, histiocytes, quelques éosinophiles et, exclusivement dans la zone papillaire, quelque mélanophores. Il y a augmentation nette de fibrocytes avec des zones plus ou moins étendues de fibrose; l'aspect est, en résumé, celui d'une cheilite lympho-fibro-oedèmateuse, avec, un infiltrat cellulaire d'inflammation diffuse chronique. Chez un de nos cas fut constatée la présence de petites glandes muqueuses hétérotopiques, montrant de l'hyperémie et entourées d'un infiltrat lymphocytaire notable.

Experiencias en cuatro casos de cromoblastomicosis y su tratamiento

F. A. OCAMPO, Hospital Regional del Instituto Mexicano del Seguro Social de Puebla, México, R. T. PEREZ, Patólogo del IMSS en Puebla, R. V. VICTORIA, Bacteriólogo del IMSS en Puebla y de la Facultad de Medicina (Mexico)

Se relatan las experiencias adquiridas, en cuatro casos de Cromoblastomicosis, localizados en una misma población del estado de Oaxaxa, México. De clima tropical, lamentable situación económica, nulas condiciones higiénicas y deficiente alimentación. De los pacientes estudiados, dos eran menores y dos adultos; tres del sexo masculino y uno del femenino. El tiempo de evolución del padecimiento oscilaba, entre uno y catorce años; la ocupación era la de cañero o conectada con el campo. En los dos primeros casos de un año de evolución, la micosis estaba localizada, a nuca en el primero y a antebrazo derecho en el segundo; las lesiones eran únicas, circulares, de 3 a 5 cm de díametro, verrucosas y color rojovioláceo. En los dos últimos casos de evolución crónica, la micosis se había diseminado. En el caso tres, abarcando rodilla, muslo y gluteo izquierdos; en el caso cuatro mano y tercio inferior de antebrazo derechos. Las lesiones extensas, formadas por coalescencia, eran verrucosas, color ocre o grisáceo. Existía hiperqueratosis, aumento de volumen de la extremidad infectada e impotencia funcional. El diagnóstico presuncional fué corroborado por los estudios micológicos e histopatológicos apropiados. El examen directo de las escamas, permitió observar células redondeadas, de color castaño, aisladas o en grupos y algunas tabicadas. En los cultivos se apreciaron colonias pardo-obscuras, aterciopeladas. En el estudio de las biopsias se observó en epidermis, hiperqueratosis, acantosis y papilomatosis; en la dermis dos tipos de reacción inflamatoria: la formación de granulomas y el infiltrado de linfocitos y de leucocitos polimorfo nucleares con formación de microabscesos. Las células multinucledas gigantes, tipo Langhans y las células fumagoides fueron identificadas. El microcultivo, permitió identificar la especie del hongo causal de los cuatro casos: Cladosporium carrionii. Para su tratamiento se empléo la hidrazina del ácido isonicotínico, en dosis de 10 mgrs. por kilogramo de peso, obteniendo los siguientes resultados: Caso uno, de un año de evolución: curación, en 7 meses;

Caso dos, de un año de evolución: Mejoría franca en 7 meses; Caso tres, de trece
años de evolución: mejoría en 5 meses de tratamiento; Caso cuatro, de catorce
años de evolución, mejoría en 6 meses de tratamiento.

Conclusión: 1.° Se identifica como agente causal de cuatro casos de Cromoblastomicosis a Cladosporium carrionii. 2.° Se emplea para su tratamiento a la
isoniazida, con resultados alentadores, que nuevas experiencias deberán robustecer
o desechar.

Quelques aspects de la mycose de Lane-Pedroso
(chromoblastomycose ou chromomycose)
dans la région Amazonique (Brésil)

D. SILVA, Clinique Dermatologique de la Faculté de Médicine, Université du
Pará (Brésil)

Dans un travail précédent [1], en 1954, on avait remarqué que la Mycose de
Lane-Pedroso était très fréquente dans la région amazonique, surtout dans l'Etat
du Pará et tout ça faisait prévoir que, d'ici à quelque temps nous aurions eu le plus
grand foyer mondial de cette maladie. Les études faites entre 1943/1954 on a
permis d'identifier 29 cas, malgré nous ne disposions pas jusqu'à cette époque là,
pratiquement, aucune condition de recherche. Après cette époque, avec l'installation du laboratoire de mycologie de la Clinique Dermatologique de la Faculté de
Médicine de l'Université du Pará, il a été possible d'étudier plus de 52 cas, pour un
total de 81, seulement dans l'Etat du Pará, que accrus aux 13 cas signalés dans les
autres Etats de la région amazonique, ça fait un total de 94 cas. Dans cette statistique nous ne prenons pas en considération les cas, que malgré les examens cliniques
et histologiques présentaient symptomatologie semblable à la mycose, mais ils ne
pouvaient pas être classés dans la même, par faute du parasite. Dans cette manière,
nous pouvons bien dire que nos prévisions étaient justes, quand on a signalé dans
un autre travail, que l'Etat du Pará était le plus grand foyer mondial de la maladie.
Comme il est connu, le Brésil présente presque le 40% de tous les cas classés dans
les statistiques mondiales, et l'Etat du Pará à sa fois, présente 39,6% de tous les
cas classés dans le Brésil même. Si nous faisons relation au cas/habitant, nous
aurions 1/22.802 pour l'Etat du Pará, mais si nous faisons relation avec toute la
région amazonique, la relation cas/habitants sera de 1/33.606. Avec des recherches
faites par des brésiliens, basées sur notre enquête, on a pu vérifier que la situation
nosologique de la chromoblastomycose dans l'Etat d'Amazonas, malgré la mycose
été rencontrée, ne constitue pas un foyer important. Tout ça constitue le résultat
des travaux de MORAIS, SOUZA FERREIRA et PINTO [2]. Donc il est bien prouvé
que le foyer de toute la région amazonique est l'Etat du Pará même, comme la
statistique peut démontrer. Dans l'Examen de 11.102 cas enregistrés dans la
Clinique Dermatologique de Faculté de Médicine du Pará, on est arrivé à la conclusion que le nombre de cas de mycose de Lane-Pedroso sont presque le même
de la sporotrichose, qui est la mycose rencontrée plus fréquemment.

Dans ordre d'importance, les mycoses plus fréquentes sont: 1. Sporotrichose,
2. Mycose de Lane-Pedroso, 3. Mycose de Lutz, 4. Mycose de Lobo.

La région amazonique qui pour ses caractéristiques physiques et géographiques
présente un climat chaud humide. La chromoblastomycose est peu fréquente dans
la région occidentale, où seulement quelque cas ont été signalés, et très fréquentés

Tableau. *Cas de la mycose de Lane-Pedroso, Pará — Brésil 1942 à 1966*

Rég. N°	Nom	Age	Sexe	Profession	Provenance	Localisation des lésions	Type des lésions	Temps de maladie	Diagnostic Mycologie	Diagnostic Histo-patho	Année
1	—	—	—	paysan	—	Pied-jambe G	verruqueuse	—	§§	+	1942
2	—	—	—	paysan	—	Pied-jambe D	verruqueuse	—	§§	+	1942
3	I.P.B.	52	♀	paysan	Bragança	Jambe D	verruqueuse	29 a	+	+	1952
4	M.C.R.	48	♀	blanchisseuse	Belém	Pied-jambe G	verruqueuse	15 a	D	+	1952
5	F.A.O.	—	♂	paysan	Pará	Pied-jambe G	verruqueuse	—	§§	+	1952
6	S.P.	—	♂	paysan	Pará	—	—	—	§§	+	1952
7	A.F.S.	—	♂	paysan	Ananindeua	Jambe G	verruqueuse	7 a	§§	+	1952
8	J.A.F.	42	♂	paysan	Pará	Pied-jambe G	verruqueuse	10 a	§§	+	1952
9	M.R.D.	56	♂	paysan	Belém	Pied G	verruqueuse	4 a	§§	+	1952
10	J.M.L.	57	♂	chaudronnier	N. Timboteua	Pied D	verruqueuse	10 a	§§	+	1952
11	M.J.S.	48	♂	paysan	Belém	Pied-jambe G	verruqueuse	6 a	+D	+	1952
12	P.V.C.	58	♂	maçon	Belém	Pied-jambe G	verruqueuse	25 a	§§	+	1952
13	R.C.B.	64	♂	vendeur	Bragança	Pied, jambe, genou D	verruqueuse	4 a	+D	+	1954
14	S.A.D.	52	♂	paysan	Vigia	Fesse	verruqueuse	10 a	+D	+	1954
15	F.P.O.	52	♂	paysan	Curralinho	Jambe, cuisse G	verruqueuse	4 a	§§	+	1954
16	A.P.F.	13	♂	paysan	Bragança	Pied D	ulc. verruqueuse	2 a	+D	+	1954
17	R.C.B.	63	♂	paysan	St. Luzia	Pied-jambe D	ulc. verruqueuse	30 a	§§	+	1954
18	M.R.P.	54	♂	paysan	Curuçá	Jambe D	ulc. verruqueuse	4 a	+D	+	1954
19	B.P.	36	♂	paysan	Barcarena	Jambe G	eczémateuse	3 a	§§	+	1954
20	B.S.G.	63	♂	paysan	Ourém	Pied D	ulc. verruqueuse	10 a	§§	+	1954
21	S.F.	56	♂	paysan	Acará	Jambe D	papillomateuse	30 a	+D	+	1954
22	R.F.A.	52	♂	paysan	Portel	Pied, jambe et cuisse D	verruqueuse	4 a	§§	+	1954
23	M.M.S.	74	♂	paysan	Pará	Jambe D	verruqueuse	1 a	§§	+	1954
24	H.C.	52	♂	paysan	Pará	Pied D	ulc. verruqueuse	5 a	§§	+	1954
25	R.V.O.	—	♂	paysan	Pará	Pied-jambe G	papillomateuse	—	§§	+	1954
26	J.A.F.	—	♂	paysan	Pará	Jambe G	—	—	§§	+	1954
27	J.N.C.	—	♂	paysan	—	—	—	—	§§	+	1954
28	J.T.P.	—	♂	paysan	—	—	—	—	§§	+	1954
29	O.P.J.	31	♂	paysan	Ig. Açú	Fesse D	verruqueuse	9 a	§§	+	1954
30	S.S.P.	59	♂	paysan	São Miguel	Pied D	papillomateuse	13 a	+D	§	1957
31	A.B.R.	50	♂	paysan	Vigia	Pied D	verruqueuse	3 a	+D	+	1957
32	C.V.A.	44	♂	paysan	Gastanhal	Pied D	ver. papillomateuse	15 a	§§	+	1957
33	A.A.A.	31	♂	paysan	Jari	Pied-jambe D	verruqueuse	8 m	+D	§	1957

Tableau (continuation)

Rég. N°	Nom	Age	Sexe	Profession	Provenance	Localisation des lésions	Type des lésions	Temps de maladie	Diagnostic Mycologie	Diagnostic Histo-patho	Année
34	M. J. S.	60	♂	paysan	Timboteua	Pied-jambe D	papillomateuse	10 a	+D	+	1957
35	R. S. C.	32	♂	paysan	Ourém	Pied D	verruqueuse	9 m	§	+	1957
36	J. B. S.	65	♂	paysan	Barcarena	Pied D	verruqueuse	10 a	§	+	1957
37	P. S. S.	40	♂	paysan	Ig. Açú	Pied G	verruqueuse	3 a	§	+	1957
38	O. S.	29	♀	femme de ménage	Belém	Pied G	verruqueuse	6 a	§	+	1957
39	M. M. R.	57	♂	paysan	Belém	Pied-jambe G	ver. papillomateuse	3 a	§	+	1957
40	F. B. A.	44	♂	paysan	Marabá	Pied-jambe G	ulc. verruqueuse	3 a	+D	§	1957
41	G. R. S.	58	♂	paysan	Ourém	Pied G	papillomateuse	2 a	+D	+	1957
42	L. A. 0.199	62	♀	femme de ménage	Belém	Pied D	ver. papillomateuse	4 a	+D	§	1957
43	L. F. A. 2.280	47	♂	paysan	Coqueiro	Hemitoraxe D	lupoïde	15 a	+D Culture:P. Pedrosoi	+	1958
44	M. M. R. 1.104	57	♂	paysan	Belém	Pied G	ver. papillomateuse	3 a	+D	§	1959
45	A. B. S. 3.495	50	♂	paysan	S. Miguel	Pied-jambe G	verruqueuse	14 a	+D	+	1959
46	R. N. P. 2.738	55	♂	paysan	Barcarena	Jambe D	verruqueuse	10 a	+D Culture: P. Pedrosoi	+	1959
47	J. M. S. 3.569	77	♂	paysan	Capanema	Pied-jambe D	papillomateuse	4 a	+D	§	1960
48	F. C. G. 3.716	50	♂	paysan	Belém	Jambe D	ulc. verruqueuse	16 a	+D Culture: P. Pedrosoi	§	1960
49	P. B. A. 3.786	60	♂	paysan	Anhanga	Pied, jambe, cuisse D	ver. papillomateuse	10 a	+D	§	1960
50	J. B. S. 3.850	35	♂	paysan	Imperatris-MA.	Pied, jambe, cuisse D	verruqueuse	1 a 4 m	+D	§	1960
51	R. F. S. 4.781	48	♂	paysan	Capanema	Pied D	ver. papillomateuse	2 a	§	+	1961
52	E. S. B. 5.394	55	♂	paysan	Primavera	Pied, jambe D	verruqueuse	15 a	§	+	1962

Tableau (continuation)

Rég. N°	Nom	Age	Sexe	Profession	Provenance	Localisation des lésions	Type des lésions	Temps de maladie	Diagnostic Mycologie	Histo-patho	Année
53	R. C.	40	♂	paysan	Barcarena	Pied, jambe, cuisse G	verruqueuse	5 a	+ D Culture: P. Pedrosol	§§	1962
54	A. M. C. 5.551	38	♂	paysan	Ananindeua	Jambe G	ulc. verruqueuse	8 a	+ D	§§	1962
55	A. F. R. 5.385	30	♀	femme de menage	Primavera	Pied G	verruqueuse	6 m	+ D	§§	1962
56	A. F. R. 5.668	53	♂	paysan	S. Caetano	Pied-jambe D	verruqueuse	29 a	§	+	1962
57	R. P. S. 6.849	37	♂	paysan	Ourém	Pied D	verruqueuse	10 a	+ D Culture: P. Pedrosoi	§§	1963
58	J. N. M.093	59	♂	paysan	Castanhal	Jambe G	verruqueuse	12 a	+ D Culture: P. Pedrosoi	§§	1964
59	P. P. D. 7.062	16	♀	étudiante	Belém	Coude D	verruqueuse	1 a	+ D	§§	1964
60	C. S. R. 7.639	57	♂	paysan	Vigia	Pied G	ulc. verruqueuse	12 a	+ D	§§	1964
61	J. B. S. 8.052	28	♂	paysan	Monção-MA.	Jambe G	ulc. verruqueuse	4 a	+ D	§§	1964
62	D. R. P.	50	♂	paysan	Abaetetuba	Jambe G	ulc. verruqueuse	4 a	+ D	+	1964
63	C. L. A. 8.166	42	♀	paysan	Breves	Genou D	verruqueuse	4 m	+ D	§§	1964
64	M. M. S. 8.779	45	♂	paysan	Gastanhal	Pied D	ulc. verruqueuse	6 a	+ D Culture: P. Pedrosoi	§§	1965
65	R. S. R. 8.755	30	♂	paysan	Bragança	Jambe G	verruqueuse	3 a	+ D Culture: P. Pedrosoi	§§	1965
66	J. M. C. 9.013	40	♂	paysan	Marajó	Pied, jambe, cuisse G	verruqueuse	20 a	+ D Culture: P. Pedrosoi	+	1965
67	J. B. S. 9.035	57	♂	paysan	Belém	Pied D	verruqueuse	18 a	+ D	§§	1965

Tableau (continuation)

Rég. N°	Nom	Age	Sexe	Profession	Provenance	Localisation des lésions	Type des lésions	Temps de maladie	Diagnostic Mycologie	Histo-patho	Année
68	B. F. 9.113	54	♂	paysan	Cândico Mendes-MA.	Pied-jambe D	verruqueuse	9 a	+ D	§	1965
69	B. S. L 9.116	37	♂	paysan	Bujaru	Pied-jambe G	ulc. verruqueuse	2 a	§	+	1965
70	A. G. S. 9.329	47	♂	marchand	Castanhal	Jambe D et G	verruqueuse	6 a	+ D	+	1965
71	N. F. 9.525	32	♂	paysan	Cametá	Coude G	verruqueuse	10 a	+ D	§	1965
72	M. S. Q. 10.028	48	♀	paysan	Breves	Jambe D	verruqueuse	20 a	+ D Culture: P. Pedrosoi	+	1966
73	M. A. C. 10.894	69	♂	paysan	Altamira	Pied-jambe D	verruqueuse	18 a	+ D Culture: P. Pedrosoi	+	1966
74	J. C. O. 10.766	86	♂	paysan	Salinópolis	Pied D	verruqueuse	2 a	+ D	+	1966
75	D. C. 10.157	63	♂	paysan	Cururupu	Pied D	verruqueuse	2 a	+ D Culture: P. Pedrosoi	+	1966
76	C. R. S. 10.191	60	♂	paysan	Belém	Pied D	ulc. verruqueuse	13 a	+ D	§	1966
77	M. M. P. 10.622	53	♂	charpentier	Parintins-AM	Pied-jambe D	verruqueuse	17 a	+ D Culture: P. Pedrosoi	§	1966
78	J. R. S. 10.074	36	♂	chauffeur	Cap. Poço	Genou, cuisse D	verruqueuse	10 a	+ D Culture: P. Pedrosoi	+	1966
79	F. W. S. 11.362	44	♂	paysan	Sta. Maria	Main D	ver. papillomateuse	25 a	+ D Culture: P. Pedrosoi	§	1966
80	J. L. S. 11.219	60	♀	femme de ménage	Belém	Bras D	ver. eczémateuse	5 m	+ D	+	1966
81	M. J. F.	33	♂	paysan	Belém	Pied G	verruqueuse	5 a	+ D	§	1966

§ = Non faite + = Positif D = Examen direct

dans la région orientale fait inexplicable du moment, que toute la région présente le même caractère écologique.

Selon le type clinique, les 81 cas sont aussi classés:

1. Végétantes .... 73 cas,
   a) verruqueuse .... 59 cas,
   b) papillomateuse .... 14 cas.

Des 73 cas,. 12 peuvent être classés aussi dans le sous-type éléphantiasique-cicatriciel.

Des cas pourraient être considérés mixtes, pour la présence des lésions verruqueuses et papillomateuses en même temps.

Beaucoup des malades présentaient aussi des lésions ulcéreuses.

2. Tuberculeuse (lupoïde) ..... 1 cas,
3. Eczémateuse .... 1 cas,
4. Sans référence .... 4 cas.

Nous n'avons pas enregistré les types syphiloïde, sarcoïde, psoriasiforme et maduromycosiforme. Des 81 cas, seulement en 16 il a été possible déterminer l'agent responsable: 15 identifiés comme Phialophora pedrosoi et un comme Phialophora verrucosa. Pour les études faites, nous pouvons arriver à la conclusion que le Phialophora pedrosoi est le plus répandue dans la région. Les autres cas ont été diagnostiqués par les examens directs ou par les examens histopatologiques.

Bibliographie. 1. SILVA, D. B.: Aspecto atual do Tema. Tese, Ed. Rev. Veter., Belém/Pará 1954. — 2. MORAIS, M. P., J. L. SOUZA FERREIRA y M. N. PINTO: Rev. méd. farm. cir. **306**, 1 (1963).

Survey of the Mycoses in U.A.R.

K. EL ZAWAHRY and M. EL ZAWAHRY, Kasr-el-Aini Faculty of Medicine, Cairo University (U.A.R.)

Fungi are prevalent in our country (U.A.R.) and in the Arabian countries which have more or less the same climatic state. The superficial fungus infections, i.e., the dermatomycoses are most common while the deep mycoses although present in our patients yet on a limited scale.

Dermatomycoses

Examination of 2000 patients revealed that superficial fungus infection is present in 395 cases with an incidence of 19.75% among the whole of our dermatoses. The commonest of the superficial group is ringworm of the scalp (tinea capitis) and 111 were found out of the 2000 cases with an incidence of 5.55% of the whole of our skin ailments. Out of the 111 patient 52 were males and 59 were females, i.e., it is equal in both sexes. Most of the cases are due to trichophyton violaceum and to less extent other species. Kerion and the inflammatory forms of ringworm are not so commonly seen as in the past and only four cases of kerion (Fig. 1) were met with. Favus is more prevalent in the village where it is the most common fungus infection of the scalp, even cases of favus of the body (Fig. 2) may be met with. On the body the achorion schoenleini attaches itself to a lanugo hair with the formation of sulphur cups or it may be seen in another clinical variety which is favus herpeticus in which minute vesicles rupture to display the sulphus cups. A rare third clinical variety of favus of the body is a patch of tinea-like appearance

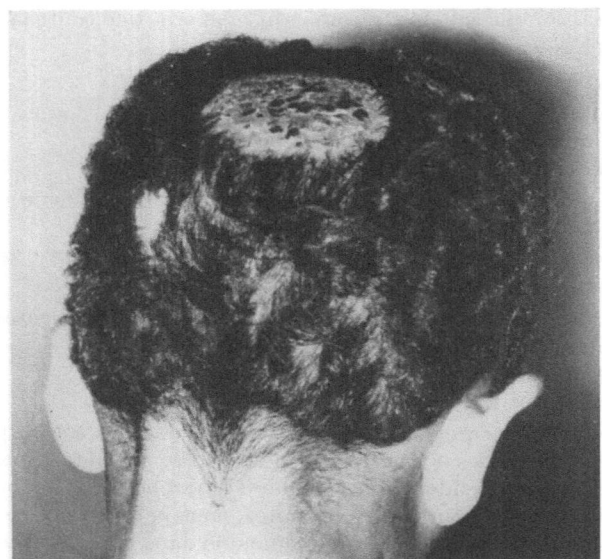

Fig. 1. Kerion

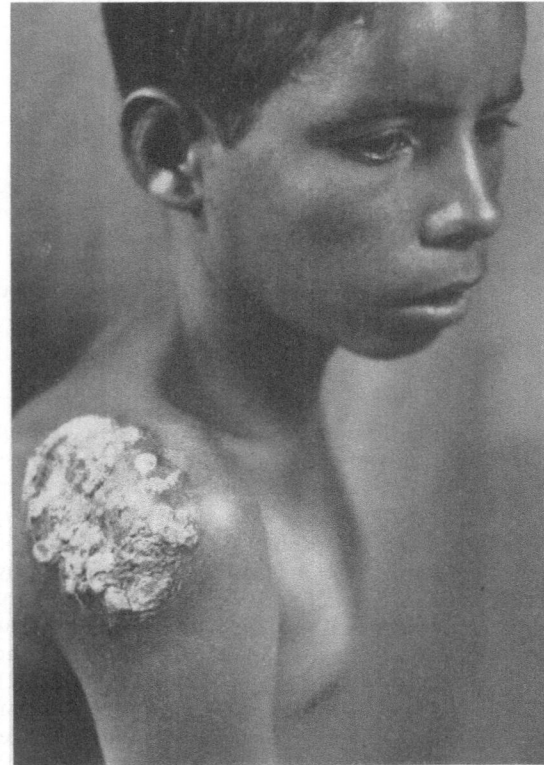

Fig. 2. Favus of the body

but on microscopical and cultural examination an achorion is present and not other fungi. Tinea versicolour comes next in frequency and 70 cases were found, this means an incidence of 3.5%, 38 were males and 32 females.

Erosio interdigitalis and erosio interdigitalis blastomycetica cases were 62, i.e., 3.1% of whom 45 were males and 17 were females. Some of the cases are severe and accompanied with foot infection and acute lymphadenitis. Tinea cruris was present in 46 patient, 36 males and only 10 of the females. The incidence in female patients may be higher than that, but the fall is due to the fact that they may not admit themselves to clinical examination. The incidence of tinea cruris is 2.3%. Eczematoid ringworm of hands and feet was noticed in 35 patient, 8 males and 27 females with an incidence of 1.75%. The clinical varieties, other than erosio interdigitalis, were the acute vesico-bullous form, the scaly and chronic hyperkeratotic variety. Onychomycosis was seen in 16 patient, 2 males and 14 females with an incidence of 0.8%. If we consider the fungus infection of the hands and feet as a whole we find it more common in females simply because of washing and house-holding and this reminds us with the term "washer-woman's hands". On the whole my practice with Griseofulvin in hand and feet fungus infection is not very encouraging.

Only one case of each of tinea barbae and erythrasma were met with in the series and I noticed that erythrasma does not respond to the recently suggested antibiotics.

Deep Mycoses

These are not so frequently seen in our patients nowadays and the most commonly encountered are blastomycosis, actinomycosis and maduromycosis.

Blastomycosis: This is the most prevalent deep mycotic infection in our patients. It is a group of clinico-pathological reactions characterised by the production of granulomatous lesions in the skin, and a special type of deep abscesses in deep structures, and in other cases by wide systemic spread. The condition although was first described by GILCHRIST in America in 1894 and North American, South American and European types have been described, yet cases are reported from all over the world and in our country blastomycosis is not very rare. The cases reported in our clinics are mostly cutaneous and not systemic blastomycosis. Also the cases reported are of the primary cutaneous infection. i.e., infection lies in the epidermis and upper layer of dermis and they are not of the secondary cutaneous form where infection starts in subcutaneous tissue and in deep cutis. Five cases of primary cutaneous blastomycosis were met with in the series studied and they were of the papulo-ulcerative and the papillomatous subvarieties (Fig. 3).

Actinomycosis: Used to be common in the past, but nowadays the condition is exremely rare. Only two cases were found among the 2000 patients examined, one belongs to the cervico-facial while the other belongs to the thoracic variety. Prior to that report we reported primary cutaneous actinomycosis affecting the leg of an adult male and caused by actinomyces bovis. Such primary cutaneous infection with actinomycosis is very rare and most of the reported cases are secondary to an underlying focus of infection and include cervico-facial, thoracic and abdominal clinical varieties.

Maduromycosis: Madura foot was prevailing in our villages and many of our farmers used to get it as they used to work bare-footed. At the present the incidence is infrequent and the causative agents are quite variable. Among the many causative agents are actinomycetes, i.e., nocardia madurae (the bacteria-like fungi) with a more hopeful prognosis and treatment is more liable to succeed. Other causative pathogens are aspergillus or some other true fungi. With the filamentous or weed-mould fungi, the condition is more serious and they do not respond to chemotherapeutic or antibiotic agents. Two cases of maduromycosis that belong to the last group were included in the survey (Fig. 4).

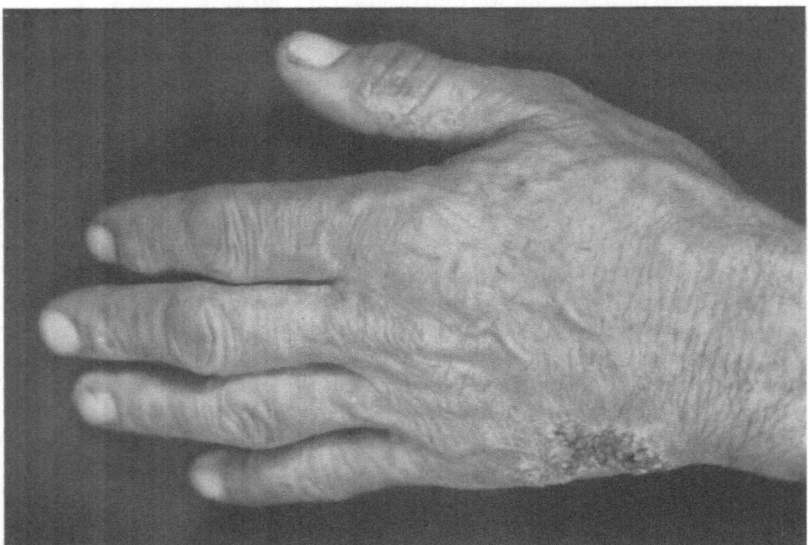

Fig. 3. Blastomycosis

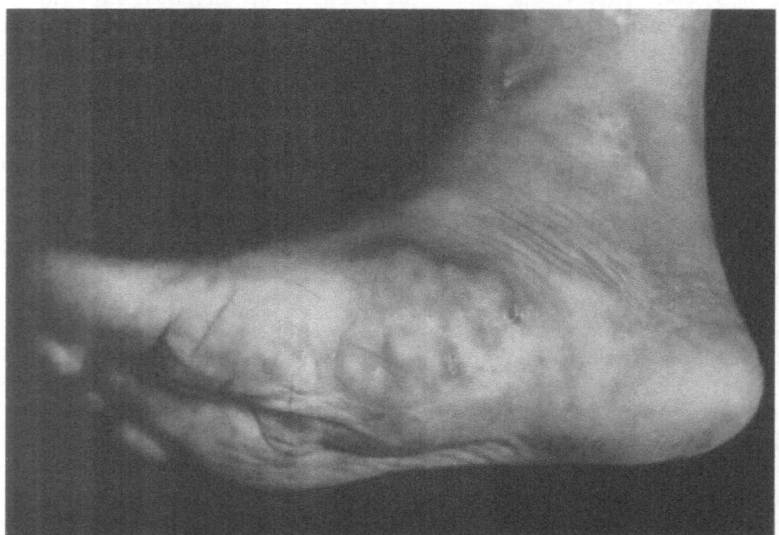

Fig. 4. Maduromycosis

References. SEIF EL NASR, H., and M. EL. ZAWAHRY: Indian J. Derm. **2**, 73 (1957). — ZAWAHRY, M. EL.: J. Egypt. med. Ass. **46**, 78 (1963); — J. Egypt. med. Ass. **47**, 1051 (1963); — Skin Diseases in Arabian Countries, 1, 2 and 3, 1963, 1964 and 1967, Cairo.

Main Transmission Routes of Spread of Trichophyton Mentagrophytes var. gran.-Infection from a Natural Focus to Man in a Foothill Region

L. Chmel, J. Buchvald and M. Valentová, Department of Dermatology, School of Medicine, Comenius University, Bratislava (Czechoslovakia)

The way of life of small rodents — the main reservoir of T. mentagrophytes var. gran.-infections — is regulated by natural factors. Man's indirect contact with these animals depends both on the degree to which he, by his own way of life and work, intrudes into their biotopes, and on the measure to which they penetrate farm buildings and even man's dwellings.

In the survey area we caught altogether 1210 rodents of 12 different species. The most frequent was Mus musculus 262, Apodemus flavicollis 228, Apodemus sylvaticus 153, Microtus arvalis 223, Clethrionomys glareolus 212 and Sorex araneus 78 times. The last two were the most frequent hosts to T. mentagrophytes, i.e. in 6.1 and 6.4% respectively.

Migration of rodents from their natural habitat into farm buildings at the onset of winter is conditioned by their indispensable search for food and shelter and results in an intense concentration of various species in restricted areas which at the same time become in winter the main work-places of agricultural workers.

A catch of rodents in farmer-workers' dwellings, granaries and barns showed considerable differences both as regards their numbers and composition. In the agricultural workers' habitations practically only M. musculus was found. In the other localities under survey, i.e. granaries and barns, where in each case 2000 traps had been set by stages, the representation differed widely. Out of a total of 325 rodents, 43% were caught in granaries and 57% in barns. Besides a quantitative difference there was a qualitative one, too. Only three species of rodents were found in granaries: M. musculus (114), hemisynanthropes Ap. sylvaticus (22) and Ap. flavicollis (4), whereas in barns there were six species: M. musculus (103), Ap. sylvaticus (35), Ap. flavicollis (3) and three exoanthropic species: Cl. glareolus (17), M. arvalis (16) and S. araneus (11).

While, the presence of rodents in granaries may be considered as accidental, in their search for food, their concentration in barns shows a more stable pattern related probably to nidification, shelter, a greater protection against domestic animals, a favourable microclimate and finally, food. As regards their composition we found here, in contrast to barns, also the exoanthropic species from nearby forests; these, because of timidity, keep away from dwellings and granaries.

Under these circumstances then, we may consider barns-farmers' most important work-place in winter — not only as a site of the greatest concentration of the most diverse rodents, but also their more stable haunts, a place of exchange of ektoparasites and at the same time a place where stored fodder and litter-straw become most contaminated by dermatophytes. In winter (December to March) we found 30.6% of caught rodents in farm buildings infested with dermatophytes which explicitly exceeds their 22.8% infestation in the months of May to July. Epidemiologically, barns may be counted as the principal foci of T. mentagrophytes infection. Here, natural and social factors are involved, those helping in infection transfer from foci in nature to man's environment, the others deriving from man's type of work and mode of dress, etc.

The relationship between the spread of infection and type of work may be judged from the fact that out of 445 workers in charge of animals, 72% were infected with T. verrucosum and only 28% with T. mentagrophytes var. gran.,

while out of 137 of those employed in plant production, T. mentagrophytes was
involved in 77% and T. verrucosum in 23% of cases. The relation between clothing
and localisation of T. mentagrophytes infection on the human skin is proved also
by analysis of 619 cases. Unprotected or inadequately protected parts of the
human body offer readiest access to dermatophytes from contaminated fodder and
litter in barns. An analysis showed the forearms to be affected most frequently
(23.4%), hands with wrists (19.1%). While in men the hands and wrists were
infected about equally (19.8 and 19.5% respectively), in women infection of the
forearms predominates (28.0%). However, the most striking disproportion was
seen in face infection (21.7% in men, 5.6% in women), while the shanks were
affected as much as 26.2% in women and only 3.9% in men.

Beitrag zum Problem tiefer anorectaler Mykosen

O. MALE, I. Univ. Hautklinik Wien (Österreich)

Im folgenden wird über eine Reihe tiefer Mykosen des Anorectalbereiches berichtet, die ätiologisch zwar überaus heterogen sind, in pathogenetischer, sympto-
matischer, diagnostischer und therapeutischer Hinsicht jedoch zahlreiche so weitgehend parallele Züge aufweisen, daß ihre gemeinsame Besprechung gerechtfertigt
scheint. Zunächst sollen an Hand einiger besonders charakteristischer Fälle unseres Krankengutes die klinischen Belange dargelegt, anschließend die pathogenetischen Aspekte der Mykosegruppe erörtert werden.

Fall 1 betrifft einen 1945 geborenen Studenten, bei dem 1964 chirurgischerseits
ein fistulierendes Sacraldermoid festgestellt und umgehend excidiert wurde. Die
histologische Befundung ergab in der Tiefe des Dermoides Drusen, die bei stärkerer
Vergrößerung deutlich die typischen Merkmale eines Strahlenpilzes erkennen
ließen. Trotz entsprechender Therapie kam es 4 Wochen postoperativ zum Wieder-
aufbrechen der Excisionswunde und unter zunehmenden Entzündungserscheinun-
gen zur raschen Entwicklung infiltrativer, vegetierender und fistulierender Veränderungen, weshalb der Patient im Herbst 1964 an unserer Klinik stationiert
wurde. Die Untersuchung des Fistelsekretes ergab zwar keine Drusen, jedoch ließ
sich unter geeigneten Bedingungen unschwer Actinomyces israelii kultivieren.
(Auf die Therapie wird später summarisch eingegangen.)

Bei Fall 2 handelt es sich um einen 1925 geborenen Büroangestellten, der seit
seinem 15. Lebensjahr an einer schweren Acne conglobata des Rückens litt, die
sich allmählich caudalwärts ausbreitete. Als die Veränderungen die Gesäßfurche
erreicht hatten, kam es perianal zur Ausbildung zunehmend heftiger Entzündungs-
und Infiltrationserscheinungen, die nach 4jährigem, völlig therapieresistentem
Verlauf zur Inkontinenz und schließlich zur Arbeitsunfähigkeit führten. Die interne Durchuntersuchung ergab außer einer BSR um 120 sowie einer Leukocytose
von rund 9000 keine abnormen Befunde. Histologisch fanden sich die Zeichen einer
chronischen, unspezifischen Entzündung mit multiplen Einschmelzungsherden,
die vereinzelt Pilzelemente enthielten. Die letzteren erwiesen sich bei Züchtung als
Torulopsis famata, die im Gewebe in Reinkultur vorlag, im Fistelsekret von
Protus vulgaris und Staph. aureus begleitet war.

Ebenfalls auf Basis einer Acne conglobata entstanden und nosologisch weitgehend gleichartig sind die beiden folgenden Fälle, die nur gestreift werden sollen.
Als Erreger wurde neben diversen banalen Keimen im ersten Fall Candida albicans und C. parapsilosis, im zweiten Fall Torulopsis sphaerica nachgewiesen.

Als Besonderheiten verdienen noch drei weitere Fälle Erwähnung. Eine sekundäre Aspergillose, eine Cryptococcose mit letalem Ausgang und die seltene Form einer Sporotrichose, die sich nach Kontakt mit Gras und Blättern in paraanalen Fistelgängen entwickelte.

Bei vergleichender Gegenüberstellung der einzelnen Krankheitsbilder zeigt sich, daß diese trotz ihrer weitgehenden ätiologischen Differentheit zahlreiche nosologische Parallelen aufweisen, die auf gemeinsame oder wenigstens verwandte pathogenetische Grundlagen hinweisen.

In erster Linie ist hervorzuheben, daß es sich bei den geschilderten Krankheitsbildern mit Ausnahme einer Aktinomykose durchwegs um sekundäre Geschehen handelte. Wie ausgeführt, lagen den mykotischen Prozessen regelmäßig disponierende, bzw. resistenzmindernde lokale oder allgemeine Störungen, wie paraanale Fistelgänge, Acne conglobata-Herde, eine Sebocystomatosis, ein Status seborrhoicus u. ä., zugrunde.

Die Anorectalregion stellt offenbar eine Prädilektionslokalisation dar. Dies geht einerseits aus den Angaben des Schrifttums, andererseits aus dem Krankengut unserer Klinik hervor. Neben den genannten elf Fällen wurden im gleichen Zeitraum nur drei vergleichbare Mykosen in anderer Lokalisation beobachtet.

Als weiteres gemeinsames Merkmal ist das Geschlecht hervorzuheben. Im gegenständlichen Kollektiv handelt es sich ausnahmslos um männliche Patienten. In analogen Zusammenstellungen der Literatur wird zwar auch über weibliche Fälle berichtet, jedoch sind diese mit Abstand in der Minderzahl.

Der Verlauf ist fast regelmäßig überaus chronisch und erstreckt sich bei unbehandelten Fällen über Jahre und Jahrzehnte. Spontanheilungen kamen in unserem Kollektiv nicht vor und werden bei vergleichbaren Fällen auch im Schrifttum nicht angegeben.

Die Folgezustände sind relativ gleichartig. Im allgemeinen kommt es nach unterschiedlicher Dauer des Prozesses zur zunehmenden Infiltration, vorwiegend der fossa ischiorectalis, und schließlich zur Zerstörung des M. sphincter ani, dadurch zur Inkontinenz und (weiteren) Superinfektion mit Darmkeimen. Es ist bemerkenswert, daß es auch bei außergewöhnlicher In- und Extensität der Erscheinungen sowie nach jahrelangem Verlauf nie zur Ausbildung einer Amyloidose oder einer Sepsis kam.

Der in praktischer Hinsicht wichtigste gemeinsame Wesenszug der besprochenen Mykoseformen ist ihre durchwegs weitgehende Therapieresistenz. Trotz der ätiologischen und graduellen Unterschiedlichkeit unserer Fälle erwiesen sich sämtliche medikamentösen bzw. konservativen Maßnahmen — wie etwa Amphotericin B, Antibiotica, u. a. bis zu 60 Mio E Penicillin pro die, Gamma-Globuline, Vaccine, Röntgenbestrahlungen und ähnliches — ausnahmslos als unzulänglich. Ebenso wie dies bei analogen Mykoseformen im Schrifttum hervorgehoben wird, wurde damit lediglich eine passagere Besserung, aber nie eine Heilung erzielt. Hingegen konnten mit Ausnahme der Cryptococcose alle übrigen Fälle durch Excision der Veränderungen und plastische Versorgung des Defektes (funktionell) wiederhergestellt werden.

Zweck der Ausführungen war es, die Kenntnisse über die anorectalen Mykosen durch einige besonders gelagerte Formen zu erweitern und insbesondere auf die ausgezeichneten Erfolge der chirurgischen Behandlung hinzuweisen, die um so problemloser und aussichtsreicher ist, je früher sie angewandt wird.

Flore dermatomycosique actuelle dans la région d'Athènes et sensibilité des souches isolées à la griséofulvine

C. KANITAKIS, U. MARCELOU-KINTI et CHR. GEORGIADIS, Clinique Universitaire des Maladies Cutanées et Vénériennes de la Faculté-Hôpital « Andreas Syggros » Athènes (Grèce)

Dans le présent travail nous avons voulu étudier:

1. La fréquence des Dermatophytes chez les malades de la Clinique Universitaire des Maladies Cutanées et Vénériennes de la Faculté d'Athènes depuis Janvier 1966, en comparaison des résultats obtenus par d'autres auteurs (LOUIZIDOU, 1938; SAKELLARIOU, 1959; MARCELOU-KINTI, KANELLIS, 1964) et des anciennes statistiques de la Clinique, pour constater s'il existe une diminution de leur fréquence, après l'avénement de la griséofulvine.

2. La localisation et l'aspect clinique des dermatomycoses observées.

3. L'identification des champignons isolés, pour constater s'il existe un changement de l'espèce, phénomène observé dans d'autres pays (RIVALIER, 1956; POPCHRISTOV et col., 1964; GÖTZ, 1952).

4. Les résultats thérapeutiques obtenus par l'administration de la griséofulvine, ainsi que l'action de cet antibiotique in vitro sur les souches isolées.

Matériel et Technique. Chez tous les malades suspects d'une Dermatomycose nous avons pratiqué un examen microscopique direct d'une part et une culture du matériel recueilli d'autre part. Pour l'examen direct des poils et des ongles nous avons appliqué la méthode de TOH à 40% et du Lactophénol et pour les squames de la peau, la coloration au bleu de Methylène. Les cultures du matériel pathologique ont été pratiqués sur gelose de SABOURAUD glucosé additionée de Pénicilline, Streptomycine et Actidione. L'identification des souches isolées s'est basée sur les caractères morphologiques macroscopiques et microscopiques. Pour l'étude des caractères microscopiques on a fait des cultures sur lame selon la méthode de RIVALIER et SEYDEL.

Pour le traitement de nos malades 10 à 12 mg par kg de poids et par jour de griséofulvine microcrystalisée ont été administrés. Pour l'étude de la sensibilité à la griséofulvine in vitro des souches isolées, nous avons appliqué une méthode simple, en incorporant l'antibiotique dans la gelose de SABOURAUD en raison de 1,25; 2,5; 5; 7,5; 10; 15; 20; 30 et 40 γ par cm³ du milieu.

Résultats. 1. Parmi les 20.061 nouveaux consultants de la Clinique pendant les 17 derniers mois, 1370 ont été retenus comme suspects d'une Dermatomycose. De ceux-là 550 étaient négatifs à l'examen direct et à la culture, tandis que 820 étaient positifs (4% du total des consultants).

2. Parmi les 820 malades présentant une dermatomycose, 578 souffraient de Teignes du cuir chevelu, 5 de la barbe, 65 d'eczéma marginé de Hebra, 50 de dermatomycose des pieds, 67 d'Hérpes circiné, 43 de dysidrose des pieds, 7 de lésions étendues du corps et 5 d'onychomycose, localisations qui toutes prenaient les aspects cliniques déjà connus (Tab. 1).

L'identification des champignons isolés a montré 340 souches de M. canis (41,47%), 17 M. gypseum (2,07%), 54 T. rubrum (6,58%), 273 T. violaceum (33,29%), 7 T. sulfureum (0,85%), 17 T. tonsurans (2,07%), 16 T. mentagrophytes (1,95%), 3 T. rosaceum (0,36%), 15 T. schoenleini (1,85%), 78 Epidermophyton floccosum (9,51%) (Tab. 1).

La plus grande partie des 816 malades a été traitée à la griséofulvine. Parmi ceux que nous avons pu suivre, quatre ont résisté au traitement et ont donné un examen direct et une culture positifs après un traitement de 2 mois.

En ce qui concerne la sensibilité in vitro des souches isolées, nous avons pu constater que 339 souches du M. canis, toutes les souches du M. gypseum, du T. sulfureum, du T. mentagrophytes, du T. rosaceum, ont été sensibles in vitro à la griseofulvine à une concentration de 2,5 γ tandis qu'à 1,25 ont donné un léger développement. Les souches du T. rubrum, du T. tonsurans, E. floccosum ont donné un développement très léger aux concentrations de 1,25 et 2,5 γ. Les souches appartenant au T. schoenleini ont été sensibles à 5 γ, tandis que aux 2,5 et 1,25 ont donné un léger développement (Tab. 3).

Tableau 1. *Cas des Dermatomycoses observées à la Clinique des Maladies Cutanées et Vénériennes de la Faculté d'Athènes de 1. 1. 1966 à 31. 5. 1967 et leur localisation*

Espèce de Dermatophytes	Cuir chevelu	Lésions de la Barbe	Eczéma marginé de Hebra	Dermatomycoses des pieds	Herpés circiné	Dysidrose des pieds	Lésions étendues du corps	Onychomycoses	Total	Pourcentage
M. canis	283	—	8	2	39	3	2	3	340	41,47
M. gypseum	13	—	1	—	2	1	—	—	177	2,07
T. rubrum	—	1	12	20	1	18	2	—	54	6,58
T. violaceum	251	—	2	—	19	—	1	—	273	33,29
T. sulfureum	2	—	4	—	1	—	—	—	7	0,85
T. tonsurans	7	1	6	—	3	—	—	—	17	2,07
T. mentagrop.	10	3	—	—	2	—	1	—	16	1,95
T. rosaceum	—	—	3	—	—	—	—	—	3	0,36
T. schoenleini	12	—	—	—	—	—	1	2	15	1,85
E. floccosum	—	—	29	28	—	21	—	—	78	9,51
Nombre de cas	578	5	65	50	67	43	7	5	820	%

Tableau 2. *Fréquence des Dermatomycoses de 1961 à 1967*

Année	Nombre Total des Consultants Cas	Cas Positifs		Cas d'Achorion		Autres Dermatomycoses	
		Nombre	%	Nombre	%	Nombre	%
1961	16.855	1035	6,14	23	0,14	1012	6,09
1962	17.816	856	4,80	35	0,19	821	4,61
1963	17.723	1041	5,89	29	0,16	1012	5,65
1964	16.413	864	5,27	30	0,18	834	5,08
1965	16.252	617	3,92	21	0,12	596	3,67
1966	11.562	592	5,12	6	0,05	586	5,07
1967	8.499	228	2,67	9	0,11	219	2,58

1. 1. à 31. 5.

Tableau 3. *Sensibilité à la griseofulvine des Dermatophytes isolés*

Espèce de Dermatophyte	Nombre de souches	0	0,62	1,25	2,5	5	7,5	10	15 γ
M. canis	329	++++ ++	+	0	0	0	0	0	
M. gypseum	17	++++ ++	+	0	0	0	0	0	
T. rubrum	54	++++ ++	+	+	0	0	0	0	
T. violaceum	273	++++ +++	++	+	0	0	0	0	
T. sulfureum	7	++++ ++	+	0	0	0	0	0	
T. tonsurans	17	++++ ++	+	+	0	0	H		
T. mentagrophytes	16	++++ ++	+	0	0	0	0	0	
T. rosaceum	3	++++ ++	+	0	0	0	0	0	
T. schoenleini	15	++++ +++	++	+	0	0	0	0	
E. floccosum	78	++++ +++	+	+	0	0	0	0	
M. canis	1	++++ +++	+++	+++	++	+	0	0	

Une souche de M. canis isolée du cuir chevelu d'un des quatre malades qui ont résisté au traitement a résisté in vitro à une concentration de 7,5 γ de griséofulvine.

Discussion — Conclusions. Des résultats obtenus dans ce travail nous pouvons tirer les conclusions suivantes:

1. La fréquence des Dermatomycoses chez nos consultants commence à diminuer, depuis les deux dernières années (Tab. 2).

2. La localisation et l'aspect clinique des Dermatomycoses n'a pas sensiblement changé.

3. Ainsi que dans d'autres pays il y a à Athènes un changement de l'espèce, notamment une diminution de la fréquence du T. schoenleini et du T. violaceum.

4. Le traitement à la griséofulvine est très efficace, fait, qui marche de pair avec la sensibilité des dermatophytes in vitro. Néanmoins nous avons constaté quatre cas d'échec thérapeutique in vivo et une résistance élevée in vitro, constations qui doivent nous rendre attentifs pour l'avenir.

Biological, Sanitarian and Environmental Factors in Dermatomycoses

D. TRICHOPOULOS, O. MARSELOU-KINTI and A. POLYCHRONOPOULOU,
Department of Hygiene and Epidemiology of the University of Athens (Greece)

The laboratory of Hygiene of the University of Athens under the direction of Professor V. G. VALAORAS organized and accomplished between the years 1963 to 1966 an extensive survey concerning the general health status of school children in Greece. The Survey covered a representative sample of 6155 school-children from all the regions of this Country. In a previous analysis, based on a smaller number of children, particular characteristics of the frequency of dermatomycoses for the whole Greece and its different departments were given. In the present study an effort was made to evaluate the effects of some biological, sanitarian and environmental factors on the frequency of dermatomycoses of the scalp.

I. Biological factors

a) *Sex.* The frequency of dermatomycoses is much higher among the males than among the females. This is a constant finding for all the ages (Tab. 1).

b) *Age.* The frequency shows a marked decrease when the age increases, this holds true for both sexes (Tab. 1).

Table 1. *Prevalence of dermatomycoses of the scalp according to age and sex. Absolute numbers and proportions*

Age in years	Males			Females		
	Total	Positive	⁰/₀₀	Total	Positive	⁰/₀₀
—8	797	37	46,4	711	10	14,1
8—9	969	28	28,9	909	4	4,4
10+	1.442	20	13,9	1.327	5	3,8
Total	3.208	85	26,5	2.947	19	6,5

c) *Hair color.* It has been suggested that the dermatomycoses of the scalp are more frequent among the brown than among the fair-haired. The hair colour, adjusted with the more constant eye-colour was known for 103 children for which the diagnosis of dermatomycoses of the scalp was made. Among them they were 84 brown and 19 fair-haired, that is a proportion of 81.6%. This percentage is higher than the one found in a sub-sample of 2.808 healthy children (2.115 were brown-haired or 75.3%). The difference is not highly significant (0.05 < p < 0.10) but the finding seems to be worth of a further investigation.

II. Environmental factors

a) *Climate*. A slightly higher frequency was found in the southern departments of Greece (Peloponnesos and Crete 27.7$^0/_{00}$) as compared with the northern ones (Thessaly, Epirus, Macedonia, Thrace 21.2$^0/_{00}$). The climate of the first mentioned areas is known to be warmer and more humid. However, the existing difference is not able to support by itself any reasonable supposition as far as the effects of climat on the frequency of dermatomycoses is concerned.

b) *Seasons of the year*. Seasonal variation in the prevalence of dermatomycoses was not proven to exist.

c) *Type of Dermatomycoses*. 40 successful cultivations were accomplished. According to them 26 of the cases were due to Trichophyton Violaceum (65%), 10 to Microsporon canis (25%), 2 to Trichophyton mentagrophytes (5%) and 2 to Achorion shoenleini (5%).

d) *Special soil contamination*. Soil cultivations were attempted in a case of epidemic outbreak, caused by Trichophyton Violaceum. The soil cultivation revealed the existence of Microsporon gypseum (44%), Microsporon cookei (20%), Chr. keratinofilum (24%) etc. Consequently, no relation existed between soil contamination and the scalp dermatomycoses. This should be expected for all our cases, because none of them was due to geophillic fungus.

III. Sanitarian factors

a) *Health Status*. The effect that the health status has upon the frequency of dermatomycoses is well known. In our survey the region with the higher standard of living (Attica) has a 5 to 10 times lower frequency than the other regions of the country.

Table 2. *Frequency of dermatomycoses of the scalp $^0/_{00}$, according to the age in years and the individual cleanness in arbitrary scoring (0 = fairly clean, 1 = dirty, 2 = very dirty)*

| Indiv. Cleanness | Age in Years | | | | | | | | | | | |
| | −8 | | | 8—9 | | | 10+ | | | Total | | |
	Exam. Chil.	Posi- tive	$^0/_{00}$	Exam. Chil.	Posi- tive	$^0/_{00}$	Exam. Chil.	Posi- tive	$^0/_{00}$	Exam. Chil.	Posi- tive	$^0/_{00}$
0	466	7	15,0	488	1	2,1	859	1	1,2	1813	9	5,0
1	564	21	37,2	659	9	13,7	800	10	12,5	2023	40	19,8
2	223	14	62,8	344	14	40,7	483	12	24,8	1050	40	38,1
Total	1253	42	33,5	1491	24	16,1	2142	23	10,7	4886	89	18,2

b) *Individual cleanness*. In order to evaluate the effect of the individual cleanness on the frequency of dermatomycoses, Tab. 2 was constructed. In this table the examined and the suffering children were cross-classified according to their age and individual cleanness. The last one was determined for 4886 children and it was arbitrary scored with 0, 1 or 2; zero meaning child fairly clean and two child very dirty. It becomes obvious that the individual cleanness has a very marked effect upon the frequency of dermatomycoses and that this holds true for all the ages under consideration. It is however interesting to note that in the younger ages the frequency in the "very dirty" group is 4 times higher than that in the "fairly clean" group; while in the older ages the corresponding ratio is 20. This fact indicates that the individual cleanness is a much more important factor for the older than for the younger ages.

New Experiments on Culture, Immunology and Inoculation

J. DE AZEVEDO CARNEIRO, Hospital de Clínicas Pedro Ernesto, Faculdade de Ciências Médicas, Universidade do Estado da Guanabara (Brasil), R. D. AZULAY, Faculdade de Medicina, Universidade Federal Fluminense (Brasil), and L. M. C. DE ANDRADE, Department of Pathology of the Instituto de Leprologia, Rio de Janeiro (Brasil)

In 1931, JORGE LOBO [1] described a new disease: Keloid-like Blastomycosis. He isolated from that first case a fungus which was studied by FONSECA FILHO and AREA LEÃO [2] who classified it as Glenosporella Loboi. Up to now no more than a few dozen of cases have been described by several authors. Cultures and experimental inoculations have been tried, by different authors, without any success. Recently we have studied a new case [3] which was presented to the XXII Annual Meeting of Brazilian Dermatologist held in Rio de Janeiro, 1965. Material from the skin lesion of this case permitted us to make the following experiments:

1. Culture: Hundreds of very small pieces of skin lesion were inoculated in Sabouraud medium. A few drops of peanut oil were mixed to the medium. In two media having that oil a fungus was isolated having the same features observed in the unique culture obtained from that first case. Subcultures have been obtained — for more than 21 months. The cultures are yellowish and coremioid in Sabouraud and whitish in Czapeck-Dox. The fungus grows better at room temperature. Microscopic examination of the culture shows:

1. Round, thick-walled, double contour refractile cells measuring 6 to 12 micra in diameter.

2. Hyphae with aleuriospore; the hyphae are 5 to 100 micra long and the aleuriospore have thick and refractile walls.

3. Arthrospores of several sizes and shapes either isolated or catenulate.

4. Dissociated hyphae, some thin and other thick-walled, with double contour, 5 to 300 micra long. The shortest hyphae resemble Fusarium spores, which are frequent in subcultures of Czapeck medium; most of these Fusarium-like elements present buddings.

In the subsequent subcultures in Sabouraud and Czapeck-Dox media predominate the Fusarium-like hyphae and in potato-agar medium predominate aleuriospores and the round forms.

2. Immunology: As one knows the lesions of Lobo's Blastomycosis has tremendous amount of parasites. An antigen — Lobine — was prepared *ad modum* lepromin. A piece of lesion was triturated with saline water, heated at $100°$ during 30 min and phenicated at $0,5\%$. Three types of lobine were prepared:

Lobine I: the proportion of fresh tissue to saline water was $1:5$.

Lobine II: that proportion was $1:20$.

Lobine III: Supernatant liquid after centrifugation.

Intradermic tests were made with these three lobines in one patient of Lobo's Blastomycosis, one of Lutz's Blastomycosis and four with other dermatosis. Readings were made in 48 h, 7, 15 and 21 days. The results were not conclusive; a larger number of cases must be tested.

3. Experimental inoculations: There were made in man and animals.

Inoculation in man: It was done in the forearm of the patient himself by scarification and multipuncture with fresh tissue of the patient lesion. Plastic dressing covered the inoculations for 48 h. No lesion developped during a follow-up of 1 year.

Animal inoculation: A triturated material of skin lesion in saline water was inoculated in white rats, mice, rabbits and guinea-pigs by the following vias: testicle, foot-pads, peritoneum and ear. Two rats presented microscopic lesions of the testicle showing a granuloma with round forms of parasites just like one sees in human lesions.

A group of animals was inoculated with our culture. One rat presented — granuloma of the testicle with some scarce round forms of parasites. Another rat presented in the foot-pads filamentous hyphae stained by methylene blue.

Conclusions. The A. A. succeeded in isolating from a case of Lobo's Blastomycosis a fungus having the same features as described by FONSECA and LEÃO for the first case. Antigens (Lobine) prepared with human material were tested in one patient of Lobo's Blastomycosis and five cases of other dermatosis; the results were not conclusive. Inoculations in the testicle, foot-pads, peritoneum and ear of white rats, rabbits, guinea-pigs and mice suggest a positive reproduction of the disease. Inoculations made in the patient himself were negative.

Bibliography: 1. LOBO, J.: Rev. méd. Pernambuco 1, 763 (1931). — 2. FONSECA FILHO, O., and A. LEÃO: Med. Cir. Brasil. 48, 143 (1940). — 3. AZULAY, R. D.: Micose de Jorge Lobo. Documentário dos casos clínicos e clínico-patológicos da XXII Reunião dos Dermato-sifilógrafos Brasileiros.

Sensibilisations de la peau par les dermatophytes

I. COJOCARU, I. ALTERAS et L. DULAMITĂ, Centre Dermato-Vénérologique, Bucarest (Roumanie)

Le nombre des cas à sensibilisations cutanées dues aux agents mycosiques vient retenir de plus en plus notre attention. Au Centre Dermato-Vénérologique on pense toujours à cette possibilité, surtout quand il s'agit d'une dermatose allergique. Les sujets apparement sains peuvent être aussi sensibilisés, l'allergie étant alors décélée seulement par les intradermoréactions. Il y en a encore les sensibilisations créées par une infection mycosique antérieure, maintenant guérie [25].

L'éruption allergique peut siéger soit l'ancienne lésion [15], où les parasites font maintenant défaut, soit n'importe quelle endroit, en voisinage ou même plus loin [14] (LONGHIN), l'allergène s'étant deplacé du foyer primitif, par voie hématogène ou lymphatique [6].

Chez 24% de nos 315 malades aux dermatoses allergiques, on a trouvé une épidermophytie des pieds, dont ils ignoraient l'existence et qui pouvait être incriminée à l'origine des éruptions allergiques.

Afin d'étudier plus minutieusement la liaison possible entre l'infection mycosique et la présence d'une éruption allergique, nous avons poursuivi de nouvelles investigations mycologiques et immunoallergologiques sur un lot de 122 malades.

La présence de Trichophyton mentagrophytes var. interdigitale a été trouvée pour la plupart des cas, correspondant d'ailleurs aux résultats positifs des intradermoréactions (60% des cas) à l'antigène respectif. Le potentiel sensibilisateur de Tr. rubrum a été plus réduit.

En ce qui concerne les formes cliniques des sensibilisations cutanées, l'eczéma occupe la première place, pour 60% des cas à dermatoses allergiques examinées. Pour le reste, nous avons observé des névrodermites, des eczématides like purpura, des urticaires. Voici les résultats de nos observations:

1. Sur un lot de 70 malades aux manifestations cutanées d'origine allergique et porteurs d'une épidermophytie, décélée par la présence du parasite à l'examen directe et cultures, les épreuves immunoallergologiques ont été positives dans un pourcentage important des cas. Ainsi, les intradermoréactions à la trichophytine standard ont été positives dans 41% des cas. De même, les hémaglutinations passives à l'épidermophytine ont mis en évidence la présence des anticorps sériques pour 20,3% des cas. Des résultats pareils ont été enregistrés pour les tests de fixation du complément. Le transphère passif des anticorps (chez les cobayes) confirmaient à son tour les données mentionées plus haut.

2. Sur le deuxième lot, de 27 malades à l'épidermophytie des pieds, mais dépourvus de manifestations de sensibilisation cutanée, le pourcentage des tests immunoallergologiques positives a été beaucoup plus réduit. Ainsi, on a trouvé une hémaglutination positive en deux cas seulement, tandis que le nombre des réactions sérologiques négatives a été de 18. De même, la fixation du complément à la trichophytine a donné deux réactions positives du total de 20. Le transphère passif des anticorps a revélé seulement un cas positif, à l'antigène utilisé.

3. Sur le lot témoin, de 25 sujets, indemnes d'infections mycosiques ou d'une éruption allergique, les épreuves immunoallergologiques venaient de confirmer les résultats négatifs des examens mycologiques.

Il y a donc une différence notable entre les données obtenues par suite des investigations sur les malades appartenant au premier groupe (épidermophytie et sensibilisation cutanée) et les deux autres groupes étudiés. Les tests immuno-allergologiques ont été négatifs sur le lot témoin. Un pourcentage réduit des cas positifs a été noté pour les malades à épidermophytie, mais sans phénomènes de sensibilisation. Le pourcentage des intradermiréactions et des réactions sérologiques positives a été assez élevé chez les malades présentant aussi une épidermophytie et une dermatose allergique.

Le traitement désensibilisant à l'aide des antigènes mycosiques a donné des importantes améliorations et même des guérisons durables, à condition que le traitement soit prolongé jusqu'à la complète disparition du foyer mycosique dépisté. Sur 16 malades ainsi traités et contrôlés après, on a constaté une amélioration importante dans sept cas, l'effacement des lésions à la sortie de l'hôpital dans deux cas et guérison définitive dans cinq cas. La persistance, quoique discrète, des lésions a été notée chez deux malades.

Un aspect plus particulier de la sensibilisation cutanée causée par les agents mycosiques concernait le prurit allergique d'origine mycosique, où les intradermoréactions ont été positives. Le traitement désensibilisant par la trichophytine, ainsi que le traitement local des lésions mycosiques ont rendu possible la disparition définitive du prurit.

Quant aux manifestations à type d'allergides mycosiques, nous avons obtenu des résultats semblables aux données récemment rapportées dans la littérature [16, 20, 22]. Le traitement par la trichophytine, ainsi que le traitement antimycosique local a conduit à la disparition du certains lésions de l'hypodermite nodulaire des jambes. Le résultat obtenu a été durable.

Un autre aspect étudié a envisagé l'action de la sensibilisation dermatophytique préparant le terrain pour le développement d'une dermatose professionnelle expliqué par le phénomène des polysensibilisations successives (NICOLAU et BĂDĂNOIU [18]). Nous avons poursuivi le cas d'un maçon, présentant une dermite des mains causée par le ciment et, chez qui on a trouvé aussi une épidermophytie des pieds. L'intradermoréaction à la trichophytine a été positive. Le traitement spécifique par trichophytine, associé au traitement local des lésions cutanées mycosiques a donné de bons résultats.

En conclusion, les faits présentés ci-haut montrent la nécessité d'une recherche systématique de l'existence possible d'une infection mycosique chez les malades atteints de certaines éruptions de type allergique, de même que l'utilité, en pareil cas, des traitements destinés à stériliser le foyer mycosique, associée à des désensibilisations spécifique.

Bibliographie. 1. CAP, J., and J. JANULA: Čs. Derm. **1**, 317 (1958). — 2. COJOCARU, I., et M. HONTARU: Le rôle de l'épidermophytie des pieds dans l'étio-pathogénie de certaines dermatoses allergiques. Du vol. „Omagui lui Stefan Gh. Nicolau" ed. de l'Académie, Bucarest, 1963, p. 333—338. — 3. COJOCARU, I., I. ALTERAS et AL. BĂDĂNOIU: Quelques données immunoallergologiques sur les sensibilisations cutanées causées par les dermatophytes. Travail présenté au Symposium international de dermatologie, Bratislava 1966. — 4. DEGOS, R., P. CHONBRAC et J. DUCHE: Ann. Derm. Syph. (Paris) **2**, 147 (1946). — 5. EVOLCEANU, R., A. AVRAM, I. ALTERAS et T. ROXIN: Dermatomicozele (Les dermatomycoses). Vol. Ed. med. Bucarest 1955. — 6. FEJER, A.: Acta allerg. (Kbh.) **13/5**, 424 (1959). — 7. GÖTZ, H.: Die Bedeutung der Dermatophyten als Erreger von Berufskrankheiten. Travail présenté au Symposium de dermatoses professionelles. Prague 1960. — 8. GAILYAVICHYUS, P., G. BORISEVICHENE et E. VALENTENE: Vestn. Derm. Vener. **9**, 28 (1965). — 9. GREKOVA, V.: Immunological studies of antigens from trichophytons. Travail présenté au Symposium international de dermatologie. Bratislava 1966. — 10. HEWITT, H., J. MEYER-SCHMID, P. DESRIQUES et J. SCLAFER: Bull. Soc. franç. Derm. Syph. **4**, 458 (1959). — 11. KISHI, S.: Jap. J. Derm. **7**, 161 (1957). — 12. KOJEVNIKOV, P. V.: Derm. Vener. (Buc.) **1**, 1 (1962). — 13. LEBEDEV, G. V.: Vestn. Derm. Vener. **2**, 46 (1961). — 14. LONGHIN, SC., AL. DIMITRESCU, and C. ENE-POPESCU: Derm. -Vener. (Buc.) **3**, 209 (1964). — 15. LONGHIN, SC.: Viața med. **13**, 723 (1962). — 16. LĂZĂRESCU, I.: Derm.-Vener. (Buc.) **6**, 539 (1962). — 17. GH. NICOLAU, ST.: Viața med. **6**, 363 (1963). — 18. NICOLAU, ST. GH., et AL. BĂDĂNOIU: L'importance des réactions d'ordre immun et allergique dans la pathologie cutanée. Le mécanisme du développement de ces phénomènes. Rapport présenté à la Conférence Nationale de Dermatologie. Bucarest 1963. — 19. NICOLAU, ST. GH., and AL. BĂDĂNOIU: Derm.-Vener. (Buc.) **1**, 1 (1960). — 20. RUTOWITSCH, M.: Bol. Centro de Estudio do Hospital dos servidores de Estado, **6**, 290 (1954); ref. Ann. Derm. Syph. (Paris) **6**, 707 (1957). — 21. SHOSTAK, L. I.: Vestn. Derm. Vener. **9**, 47 (1961). — 22. SZODORAY, L.: Further investigations concerning the mycotic pathogenesis of nodulare vasculitis of the leg. Travail présenté au Symposium international de dermatologie. Bratislava 1966. — 23. TÉMIME, P., P. CASTELAIN, J. PEIRAT, J. BESSON et M. BENNE: Bull. Soc. franç. Derm. Syph. **67**, 747 (1960). — 24. VANBREUSEGHEM, R.: Arch. belges Derm. **8**, 343 (1952). — 25. VILANOVA, X., et M. CASANOVAS: Ann. Derm. Syph. (Paris) **88**, 601 (1961). — 26. WOOD, S., and C. CRUICKSHANK: Brit. J. Derm. **8—9**, 329 (1962). — 27. JOSHIZUMI, M.: Jap. J. med. myck. **2/4**, 239 (1961).

La valeur du milieu Gluzman modifié par Condrea dans la préparation de la trichophytine

V. COSTEA, M. CARNIOL, M. LAZĂR et M. ILIES, Institut de Médecine et de Pharmacie, Clinique Dermato-Vénérologique, Jassy (Roumanie)

On sait que dans le traitement biologique des mycoses, l'extrait du matériel pathologique est plus efficace que celui d'une culture. Ceci nous a incités à nous demander si la fonction antigénique ne serait pas influencée, dans le sens de sa croissance, par l'utilisation d'un milieu de bouillon de viande pour la culture du trichophyton. Nous avons pensé aussi que ce milieu liquide pourrait se comporter lui-meme — après que la culture aura été mise de côté — comme un extrait trichophytique, puisque le parasite y a agi par des ferments afin de le rendre assimilable. Pour la stérilisation, nous avons choisi le filtrage (filtre d'asbeste EKS II) comme le meilleur moyen, remplaçant ainsi les antiseptiques qui pourraient avoir une influence défavorable sur la fonction antigénique.

Préparation de la trichphytine sur milieu Gluzman modifié par CONDREA

Nous avons utilisé le milieu Gluzman [4] modifié par P. CONDREA et collab. [1] (ce milieu administré comme tel par voie intradermique chez des sujets normaux s'est avéré moins réactogène que d'autres, tels que le bouillon maltosé ou à la peptone WITTE) dans lequel nous avons cultivé *Trichophyton gypseum asteroides* [2, 3]. Le milieu Gluzman* modifié par P. CONDREA est un mélange en parties égales de bouillon de viande de boeuf (une partie viande + deux parties eau) avec un hydrolysat acide (ClH 1,77 g-$^o/_{oo}$) à chaud, préparé avec la viande qui a servi à la preparation du bouillon (une partie viande pour six parties eau). On neutralise l'hydrolysat à chaud avec une solution de carbonate de sodium anhydre (170 g-$^o/_{oo}$). Ensuite on stérilise 30 min à la vapeur et 30 min à 110°. Pour l'utiliser on filtre, après refroidissement, sur de l'ouate. Le mélange en parts égales de bouillon et d'hydrolysat est corrigé pour le pH 7—7,2 qui précipite par chauffage 30 min à 120°. Le milieu ainsi obtenu est clarifié par filtrage sur du papier-filtre. On le répartit par 200 ml dans des flacons Erlenmayer de 1000 ml, en réalisant ainsi une surface d'aération à diamètre de 17 à 18 cm et une hauteur de la colonne de milieu de 20 mm. La stérilisation se fait à l'autoclave, 30 min à 110°. Les indices chimiques du milieu sont l'azote aminique 22 à 28 mg-%, azote total 230 à 260 mg-%, peptone 0,9 à 1,2 g-% et substances protéiques 1300 à 1600 mg-%. Le flacon ensemencé avec le *Trichophyton gypseum astéroïdes* est mis à incuber à 24 à 26°. Le 15-e jour on prend la culture et on filtre tout le contenu à travers du papier filtre, puis à travers un filtre stérilisant en asbeste (EKS II).

L'étude de la fonction antigénique de la trichophytine obtenue sur le milieu Gluzman modifié par CONDREA, en administration intradermique chez des sujets mycotiques et non mycotiques

Nous avons étudié la fonction antigénique de cette trichophytine en administration intradermique, par 0,2 ml d'une solution de $^1/_5$ serum physiologique, dans 78 cas de pilomycoses et 37 de dermatoses non mycotiques en la comparant avec la trichophytine obtenue de la masse mycélienne (culture deshydratée par l'acétone, triturée avec du sable de quartz et centrifugée à 13000 tours). Les réactions obtenues ont été notées: positive +++(plaque érythémato-oedémateuse avec un diamètre de 3 cm, qui s'est maintenue pendant 3 à 4 jours); positive ++ (plaque érythémato-oedémateuse de 2 cm); positive + (plaque faiblement congestive de maximum 1,5 cm, sans oedème) et douteuse± (congestion discrète de 0,5 cm qui disparaissait après 24 h). Dans 78 pilomycoses on a obtenu les réactions suivantes:

a) Trichophytie pyogène (Kerion Celse ou Sycosis parasitaire). Dans 26 cas les réactions pour les deux trichophytines ont été intensément positives.

b) Microsporie. Dans 36 cas on a obtenu avec la trichophytine préparée par nous trois réactions positives (+) et avec la trichophytine témoin 25 (14 + et 11 ++).

---

* Le milieu Gluzman est un mélange de bouillon de viande de cheval ou de boeuf (une partie viande + une partie eau) avec un hydrolysat acide (ClH 3,54 à 10,50 g-$^o/_{oo}$) à chaud, préparé avec la viande qui a servi à la préparation du bouillon (une part viande pour trois parts eau). L'hydrolysat est filtré chaud sur ouate. Il résulte un liquide trouble qu'on mélange en quantité égale au bouillon de viande. Le mélange est dilué avec une solution de ClNa 0,5% et mis à bouillir 15 min, après quoi on ajuste le pH à 6,8.

c) Favus. Dans 11 cas on a enregistré une réaction positive (+) et avec la trichophytine témoin 8 (5 + et 3 ++).

d) Trichophytie sèche. Dans cinq cas on a eu deux réactions positives (+), et avec la trichophytine témoin 3 (2 ++ et 1 +++).

Dans 37 dermatoses non mycotiques on a obtenu 6 réactions positives (2 + et 4 ++) et à la trichophytine témoin 23 (12 +, 9 ++ et 2 +++).

Conclusions. La trichophytine, représentée par le milieu Gluzman même, modifié par CONDREA, dans lequel on a cultivé *Trichophyton gypseum asteroides*, de même que celle préparée avec la masse mycélienne qui nous a servi de témoin, administrées par voie intradermique, produisent des réactions intensément positives dans tous les cas de trichophytie pyogène (Kerion Celse ou Sycosis parasitaire). Dans les cas de microsporie, de favus et de trichophytie sèche on a enregistré pour la trichophytine préparée sur le milieu Gluzman modifié par CONDREA des réactions positives dans un plus petit nombre de cas (environ six fois moins) que pour la trichophytine témoin, ce qui démontre une réduction de la sphère des réactions de groupe. Dans les dermatoses non mycotiques on a obtenu, comme avec d'autres trichophytines, des réactions positives mais en plus petite proportion (environ quatre fois moins) qu'avec la trichophytine témoin).

Bibliographie. 1. CONDREA, P., D. KAHAN, M. LAZĂR et N. LASCU: Arch. roum. Path. exp. **XVI**, 24 (1957). — 2. COSTEA, V., M. LAZĂR, M. CARNIOL et M. ILIES: Rev. Med.-chirurg. Iasi, Românìa, **2**, 429 (1961). — 3. COSTEA, V., M. CARNIOL, M. LAZĂR et M. ILIES: Rev. Med.-chirurg. Iasi, Românìa 4, 915 (1961). — 4. GLUZMAN, M. P., M. P. CERVIAKOV et G. M. STAROBINET: Ann. Inst. Mecinikov 2, 379 (1965).

Onychomycose due à alternaria tenuis

J. DELACRÉTAZ et D. GRIGORIOU, Clinique universitaire de dermato-vénérologie, Lausanne (Suisse)

C. R., homme de 35 ans, présente depuis quelques mois une affection des ongles des mains pour laquelle il a appliqué sans succès de nombreux traitements. Ce patient, botaniste de son état, entre professionnellement en contact avec différentes espèces de champignons parmi lesquels Alternaria tenuis, thielaviopsis basicola, cladosporium cladosporioides, etc.

L'examen clinique montre une atteinte des ongles du pouce, du médius, de l'index et de l'auriculaire gauches, ainsi que du pouce, de l'annulaire et du médius droits; leur bord libre est décollé, la lame unguéale est épaissie, la table externe est soulevée par le reste de la substance unguéale, devenue friable et poussiéreuse; elle présente des ponctuations et des stries. Les zones atteintes présentent une légère coloration jaunâtre, plus marquée dans le dépôt sous-unguéal. L'examen clinique général et les examens de sang ne montrent rien de particulier. A l'examen direct des ongles prélevés, on note de très rares spores, rondes à ovalaires et des filaments mycéliens segmentés, fragmentés, de couleur brun foncé.

Les cultures se sont développées sur les milieux de riz-gélosé et Sinlac mieux que sur le milieu de Sabouraud, additionné ou non de cyclohexemide. La température optima s'est révélée située entre 20 et 25 °C. La culture atteint sa maturité au bout de 4 à 5 jours. On voit alors des colonies rondes, légèrement surélevées, présentant parfois un bouton central ou une ombilication, poussiéreuse ou couverte d'un duvet brun grisâtre, entouré d'un hâlo gris jaunâtre de filaments radiés. Leur couleur est olivâtre, virant au brun foncé en vieillissant. Le pigment ne diffuse pas ou que très peu dans le milieu. Nous n'avons pas observé de pléomorphisme.

A l'examen microscopique des cultures, les filaments mycéliens, cylindriques, d'aspect hyalin ou bruns, sont plus fins et plus fortement ramifiés en profondeur qu'en surface; des conidiophores, courts, ramifiés et septés, insérés perpendiculairement à l'hyphe, portent une sorte de fuseaux brun foncé, qui, par bourgeonnement, forment des chaînes plus ou moins longues ou des grappes. Ces fuseaux, pluriseptés longitudinalement et transversalement, ont, à leur partie distale, un appendice clair; parvenus à maturité, ils se dissocient facilement.

Parmi les sucres, le champignon assimile bien le fructose, qui se révèle être sa meilleure alimentation hydrocarbonée. Comme source d'azote, il utilise bien l'urée et le nitrate de sodium, moins bien le sulfate d'ammonium, qui inhibe considérablement sa croissance; il utilise peu la L-leucine, la L-cystine et la méthionine, alors que les amides des acides monoaminodicarboxyliques (glutamine, asparagine) sont pour lui les meilleures sources d'azote polyvalentes.

Ces caractéristiques morphologiques et physiologiques nous permettent d'identifier la souche isolée comme étant Alternaria tenuis, HEES 1817. Les réactions sérologiques que nous avons effectuées (déviation du complément, sporoagglutination, immunofluorescence) sont demeurées négatives.

Le nombre de cas d'infections humaines provoquées par Alternaria que nous avons trouvées dans la littérature est très peu important: PÄTIÄLÄ et HÄRÖ rapportent un cas d'éruption dysidrotique des pieds; VILAS-BOAS et MARTINS, SCHNAPKA et GÖTZ rapportent des cas d'onychomycose. Toutefois dans le cas de SCHNAPKA et deux des cas de GÖTZ, il s'agissait d'une affection mixte dans laquelle le rôle de Alternaria, associée à un Trichophyton rubrum, est incertain; aussi pouvons-nous considérer notre cas d'onychomycose à Alternaria comme le troisième de la littérature, après celui de VILLAS-BOAS et MARTINS et l'un de ceux rapportés par GÖTZ.

Parasites habituels des végétaux, les champignons du genre Alternaria peuvent être pathogènes pour l'homme, probablement de façon moins exceptionnelle que la rareté des cas publiés ne pourrait le faire croire; une recherche systématique à ce sujet mériterait d'être entreprise.

Bibliographie. GÖTZ, H.: Zur Problematik der Schimmelpilze als pathogene Organismen. In: GRIMMER, H., u. H. RIETH: Krankheiten durch Schimmelpilze bei Mensch und Tier. Berlin-Heidelberg-New York: Springer 1965. — PÄTIÄLÄ, R., and S. HÄRÖ: Karstenia 1, 48 (1950). — SCHNAPKA, O.: Arch. klin. exp. Derm. **202**, 45 (1955). — VILAS-BOAS, N., et C. MARTINS: Ann. Derm. Syph. (Paris) **4**, 526 (1933).

Fungus-Allergy and its Skin Manifestations

E. FEJÉR, Skin Department of the Stephen Hospital, Budapest (Hungary)

The author exposes the question by reason of clinic, mycologic and allergologic analysis of many hundreds of cases. It is well known that the number of fungus-infections of the skin increased considerably all over the world. It accounts for the great frequency and clinical importance of the fungus-allergic diseases. The principal pathogenetic factors of these diseases are: 1. sensitizing *primary mycotic foci*, 2. *specific allergy* caused by these, 3. *specific and non-specific eliciting factors*, 4. *fungus-allergic clinical symptoms*.

1. Among the sensitizing primary foci the most important are

a) various forms of the *Tinea pedis*, but

b) the author by reason of his examinations does attach special importance to the *sensitizing effect of the onychomycosis* carrying for a long time through the matrix (nail-bed), which is rich in blood- and lymphatic vessels, its antigens into the organism,

c) the author does attach special importance *beside de flexural mycoses* to *the female genital mycosis* (mykosis vulvovaginalis), making up one of the most frequent primary foci of the fungus-allergic diseases occurring very often by women (ekzema et pruritus mykogenes). The sensitizing and eczematogenic action of the vaginal mycosis was proved with experimental examinations, clinical observations and therapeutical results obtained after the liquidation of the mycosis.

2. From the point of view of the aetiology all fungi having a sensitizing power may exert eczematogenic effect. In cases of Tinea pedis the sensitizing effect is exerted overwhelmingly by dermatophytes, while in female genital mycosis mainly by Blastomyces resp. various sorts of Candida, yet beside these fungi the sensitizing action of various mould fungi may have an important role, which independently or as co-infection are present in the primary focus. Thus for the diagnostics dermatophyton-, candida- and various mould fungi antigens must be used for the cutaneous test, giving importance both to the early and late reactions.

3. *The clinical symptoms* — on fungus-allergic terrain — are caused partly by fungus-antigens absorbed from the primary foci, yet non-specific stimuli may also be eliciting factors of these diseases, for the fungus-allergic terrain shows increased sensitivity to non-specific (physical, chemical and microbial) stimuli too. This group contains the fungus-allergic diseases produced by sunshine and ultraviolet rays.

4. Among the clinical manifestations of the fungus-allergy most important and frequent are:

a) *dyshidrosiform and eczematiform* manifestations (dyshidrosis and eczema mykogenes). It accounts for the great significance of fungus-allergy in the pathogeny of the eczematiform affections of fungus origin, which are wide-spread. Therefore in the aetiological diagnostics of the eczematiform affections it is necessary to try to find always the sensitizing fungus-foci, resp. fungus-allergy. The fungus-allergic dyshidrosis and eczema — as in general the "id"-reactions are mainly sterile eruptions, yet very often are taking place secondarily microbial superinfections.

b) *Pruritus allergicus mykogenes.* The author's widespread examinations are proving that fungus-allergy caused by mycotic foci (often multiple foci) may manifest itself in *general* or *regional* (perifocal) itching, that is *pruritus* may be very often the single symptom of fungus-allergy, moreover the author's investigations are proving, that behind of an important part of the cases of pruritus there are fungus-foci, resp. mycotic allergy. Therefore, in order to clear up the aetiology of the worrying itchings, which are very important in practice, it is necessary always to search for the possible mycotic foci and fungus-allergy too. This domain is, particularly, a fruitful subject both to the aetiological diagnostics and therapy.

c) *Neurodermatitis mykogenes.* According to the author's examinations as a manifestation of the fungus-allergy disseminated and circumscribed neurodermatitis can emerge too, furtheremore

d) *fungus-allergic* blepharoconjunctivitis and worryingly itchy *palpebral eczema*. After adequate examination of these stubborn affections their fungusallergic origin turns out often and the worrying processes frequently lasting for many years can be cured by liquidation of the above-mentioned primary foci.

Therapy. The knowledge of aetiology and pathogeny allows efficacious causal therapy of these affections. Its most important factors are: a) *liquidations of the mycotic foci,* b) *desensitizing treatment with specific antigens,* c) *antiseptic treatment of the possible secondary infections.*

Literature. FEJÉR, E.: Allergia mykogenes. In: FEJÉR, E., D. OLÁH, and S. SZATHMÁRY: Medical Mycology, 562—671. Budapest: Akadémiai Kiadó 1957 (hung.); — Pilzallergie. In: E. RAJKA: Allergie und allergische Erkrankungen, 2, 551—601. Budapest: Akademie Verlag 1959 (in germ.); — Pilzallergie und pilzallergische Krankheitsbilder. In: FEJER, E., D. OLÁH und S. SZATHMÁRY: Medizinische Mykologie und Pilzkrankheiten, 539—674. Budapest: Akademie Verlag 1966. (in germ. und russian) there detailed literature.

The Mycologic Laboratory Specimen. The Collection, Inoculation, and Culture Methods

H. C. GOLDBERG, Plainfield, N. J. (USA)

1. The location, of the area from which the specimen is taken: Fungal elements may be found in many areas of the involved skin surface. Nail clippings and scrapings taking as proximally as possible are most suitable for diseases of the nail. Debris under the nail should not be used. In scalp involvement fluorescent hairs should be plucked for examination. Since many fungus diseases of the hair do not fluoresce, the hairs of areas showing clinical involvement should be cut short, and the hair stubs and the involved skin areas scraped and collected for examination.

2. The manner in which the skin scrapings are collected: It is important to use a sharp scalpel with a small blade which can conveniently scrape skin scales from areas between the toes, the finger webs, as well as more accessible places. The area selected for taking the skin sample must be wiped free of debris which often covers and conceals fungal elements.

3. The amount of material taken and how it is planted and/or inoculated: The percentage of positive fungus examinations found in the laboratory specimens depends on the amount of the skin scrapings, hair, and/or nail clippings obtained for these tests. An easy method is to scrape large amounts of material on a slip of paper. As much of this is planted as our culture tube or plate will hold. In 100 positive culture examinations found when large amounts of material were planted, only 86 were positive when 1/3 of this amount of specimen material was simultaneously planted on another culture tube. It is helpful to directly scrape and plant material for culture on media in a petri dish. This provides a wide opening which is most useful in collecting specimen material from areas which usually provide only minimal amounts of tissue, such as the fingers, scalp, scrotum, and also from wet areas.

4. The direct microscopic examination: The addition of a few drops of Parker's superchrome ink to 30 ml of 15% potassium hydroxide solution makes it easier to find fungal elements when they are present. Other preparations are available, but this one has proven most useful for us. A green Wratten B filter No. 58 has also been helpful in giving better contrast for viewing.

5. The medium: We use Mycosel agar as our standard inoculation medium. This is made up of Sabouraud's medium, to which is added cyclohexamide, and chloramphenicol. The chloramphenicol is a broad spectrum antimicrobial agent. It effectively hinders the growth of bacteria on this medium and thus removes one group of organisms which has interferred with the growth and identification

of pathogenic fungi. The cyclohexamide is efficient in retarding the growth of the non-pathogenic organisms. Thus we are able to view the relatively uncomplicated growth of the pathogens of interest to us. Since it may take 2 to 4 weeks for some of the pathogens to grow on the various types of media which may be used, the gradual drying out of this material has affected the potential growth of many of these slow growing organisms. Various capped tubes or bottles have been used to keep the medium in ideal condition for laboratory use. In general the cap of these containers has been loosely replaced. To determine whether the growth of the organism is helped or retarded by the tightness of the cap replaced after the inoculation, cultures were tested as follows: Various fungi were inoculated on Mycosel agar and plain Sabouraud's agar. One set was tightly capped and one set was closed only with a cotton plug. Both sets grew about the same for the first 2 weeks. After that, the cultures in the tightly capped containers grew better since the medium did not dry out.

6. The temperature: Whereas the mycologist has been accustomed to keeping his cultures at room temperature [1, 2] which is excellent for the growth of the superficial dermatophytes, the bacteriologist has tended to grow these at 37 °C (99 °F). Placing cultures in an incubator at a constant 25 °C (77 °F), gives better results than haphazard fluctuating room temperatures.

7. Animal specimens for the laboratory: Since it is usually impractical to go to the animal or have it brought to the laboratory, an easy way to obtain such specimens is to have the animal combed with a "brush" [3]. The brush is sent to the laboratory and is pressed on culture media for growth. If the animal has a fungus involvement, a positive culture will usually develop.

Bibliography: 1. GEORG, L. K.: Amer. Acad. Derm. Syllabus Course in Mycology, p. 21, Part I, 3rd Ed., Univ. of S.C. School of Medicine 1955. — 2. PALDROK, H.: Acta derm.-venereol. (Stockh.) **35**, 1 (1955). — 3. GOLDBERG, H. C.: Arch. Derm. **92**, 103 (1965).

Tinea Versicolor: The Electron Microscopic Morphology of the Genera Malassezia and Pityrosporum*

F. M. KEDDIE, Department of Medicine, Division of Dermatology, University of California, Center for the Health Sciences, Los Angeles, California (USA)

The electron microscopic morphology of *Malassezia furfur* (ROBIN) BAILLON 1889, in the scales of tinea versicolor was reported in 1966 (KEDDIE). The morphology of this fungus *in vitro* has now been compared to that of the fungus in the human epidermis and found to be the same. Furthermore, electron microscopic examination of *Pitrosporum ovale* (BIZZOZERO) CAST. et CHALMERS, 1913, *Pityrosporum orbiculare* GORDON, 1951, *Pityrosporum canis* GUSTAFSON, 1954, and the cultures isolated by PANJA, in 1927, from the scales of tinea versicolor and from scales of the human scalp show them to have the same definitive type of cell wall construction and vegetative reproduction by budding and fission that characterize *Malassezia furfur*. PANJA stated that he had proved the two genera i.e. *Malassezia* and *Pityrosporum*, to be one class of organisms of the same genus. The genus *Malassezia* having been created first should have preference, hence *P. ovale* becomes *M. ovalis* (Bizz.) PANJA, 1928.

* These studies were supported by United States Public Health Service Special Fellowship Grant Nr. 1-F 3-AM-Z 4, 359-01 and Program Project Grant Nr. A 1-06048-03.

55*

The distinctive characteristics of the genus *Malassezia* (syn. *Pityrosporum*) are clearly shown in thin sections at magnifications of 5,000 to 40,000 times. The cell wall appears to be made up of delicate fibrils, sometimes compressed in layers, and sometimes separated from one another in regular sequences which correspond to protrusions into the cytoplasm. These protrusions, as seen in profile in sections examined in serial order, form ridges and furrows on the inner surface of the cell wall. Furthermore the ridges and furrows are slightly oblique to the long axis of the cell. Less frequent are finger-like protrusions of the cytoplasm which form small pits in the substance of the cell wall.

A second distinctive characteristic is the septal wall which serves to separate the bud from the parent cell. In serial sections this wall appears to grow inward from the peripheral wall at the level of the base of the bud. As the wall grows it begins to separate into two layers which mark out the future line of fission. Once the crosswalls are completed, the two cells are forced apart by the continued growth of these crosswalls which now form the walls of the new buds. The outer wall splits more or less completely apart, leaving edges that form a rim around the periphery of the crosswall.

Apart from the cell wall and the septum, these fungi have the usual cytoplasmic structures of other yeasts. The matrix, which is dense, is filled with ribosomes, mitochondria, a nucleus, vesicles of various sizes and complexity, and a well developed reticulum. The folds of the reticulum, which parallel the ridged contours of the cell wall, appear to arise as off-shoots from the nuclear envelope. The mitochondria contain inner membranes which sometimes appear to be lamellae and sometimes tubules.

Old and new isolates were examined. The old ones were those of PANJA isolated from the scales of the scalp (MRL 3073) and from tinea versicolor (MRL 3074) which had been maintained in the Mycological Reference Laboratory of the London School of Hygiene and Tropical Medicine since 1930; a strain of tinea flava (MRL 3075) isolated by Dr. E. C. SMITH in Lagos in 1928; and the type culture of *P. ovale* (CBS 1878) isolated by RHODA BENHAM in 1939. The recent isolates were strains of *P. canis* (CBS 1879 RDSVS 2079, 63a), four strains from patients with tinea versicolor (UCLA 6, 7, 14, 186 CBS 5634) and one from a patient with blepharitis (UCLA 26).

All the cultures examined were grown under the same conditions and prepared for electron microscopic examination at the same time, except for one culture which was allowed to grow until hyphae developed. Aside from the rather consistent differences in shape between the isolates from the human skin and from the ear wax of dogs, there is an added difference in the fact that the animal species does not require lipids for growth in culture. It is more difficult to separate the so-called *P. ovale* from the so-called *P. orbiculare* by morphology alone. It seems likely they will prove to be distinct species when they have been studied biochemically. The electron microscopic techniques of preparing thin sections which were examined in serial sequences have shown that the two genera *Malassezia* and *Pityrosporum* are alike in their structure and their vegetative reproduction, thus confirming Panja's reports of 1927, 1946, and 1962. Inasmuch as his cultures, though now 40 years old, present the same morphology as he described, we believe his work to be confirmed and concur with his statement that there should be one genus, namely *Malassezia*, for which *Pityrosporum* becomes a synonym.

The cultures were maintained in a fast phase of growth by transferring them every 5 days to fresh medium overlaid with olive oil. Before harvesting for electron microscopic preparation they were grown for 3 days without the oil. The cells were suspended in glutaraldehyde in cacodylate buffer solution, post-fixed in potassium permanganate solution followed by uranyl

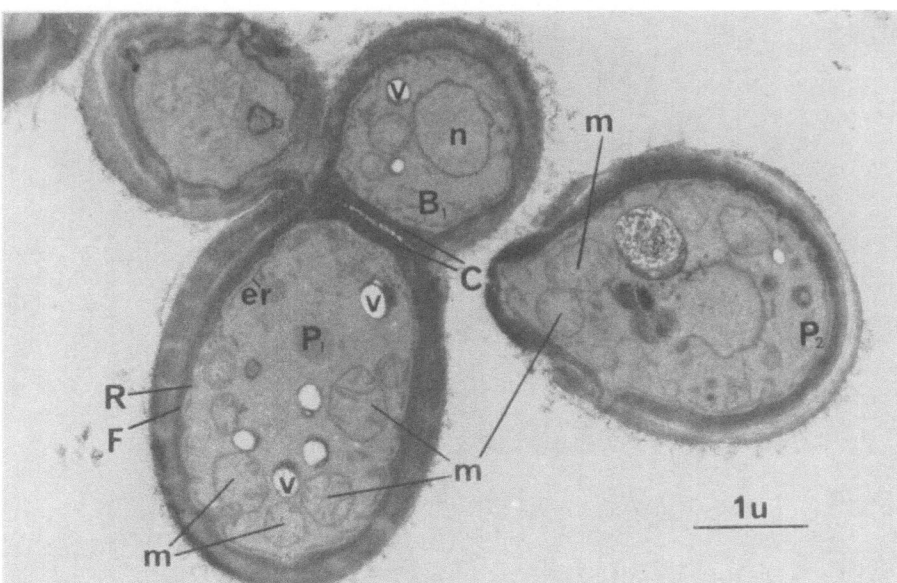

Fig. 1. P. orbiculare (CBS-5634) isolated from tinea versicolor. A parent cell (P-I) is separated from its bud (B-1) by two crosswalls (C) which join the outer wall at the junction (J) of the two cells. The cell walls are thick, their interior surfaces raised in a ridge (R) and furrow (F) pattern. The cell (P-2) is beginning to form a bud by extension of the cross wall (C). The cytoplasm of the cells contains a nucleus (n), mitochondria (m), vesicles (v), folds of endoplasmic reticulum (er), and is bounded by a cytoplasmic membrane

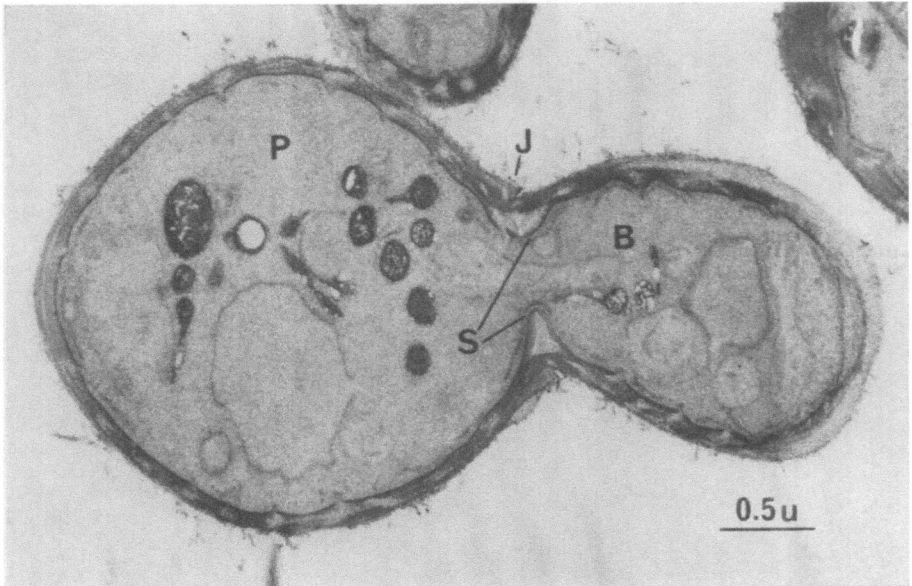

Fig. 2. P. orbiculare (UCLA-14) isolated from tinea versicolor. Here the septum (S) between the parent cell (P) and the bud (B) is beginning to grow in the form of a ring by extension of the inner lamellae of the cell wall at the junction of the two cells, which is marked by the rim (J) of the outer wall of the parent cell (P)

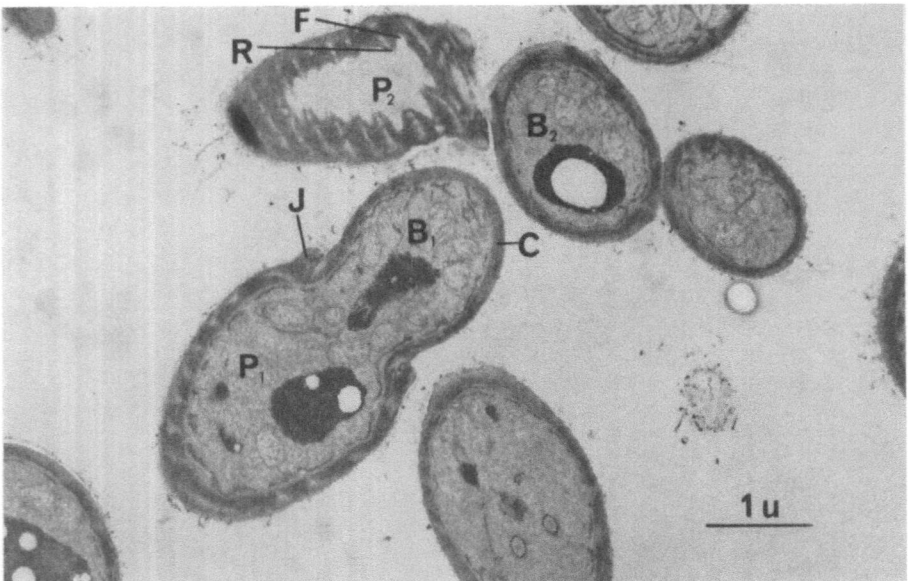

Fig. 3. P. ovale (CBS-1878), the type strain from scales of the human scalp. The parent cell (P-1) has formed a bud (B-1) by extension of the former cross wall (C). The broken ends of the parent cell form a rim at the junction (J) of the two cells. The septum has not yet begun to form. The bud (B-2) has already separated from its parent cell (P-2). The ridges (R) and furrows (F) of the cell wall lie oblique to the long axis of the cell. The cell wall is compressed in the furrows and loosely textured in the ridges

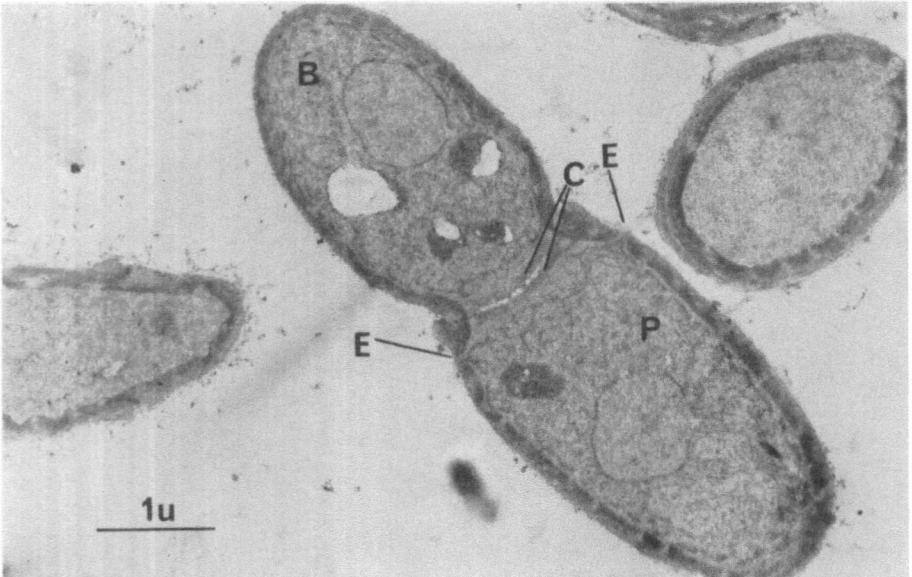

Fig. 4. P. ovale (CBS-1878). The parent cell (P) is separated from its bud (B) by a septum which has split into two crosswalls (C). The two finger-like protrusions of the cytoplasm (E), one on each side of the cell, extend almost to the outer surface of the cell wall

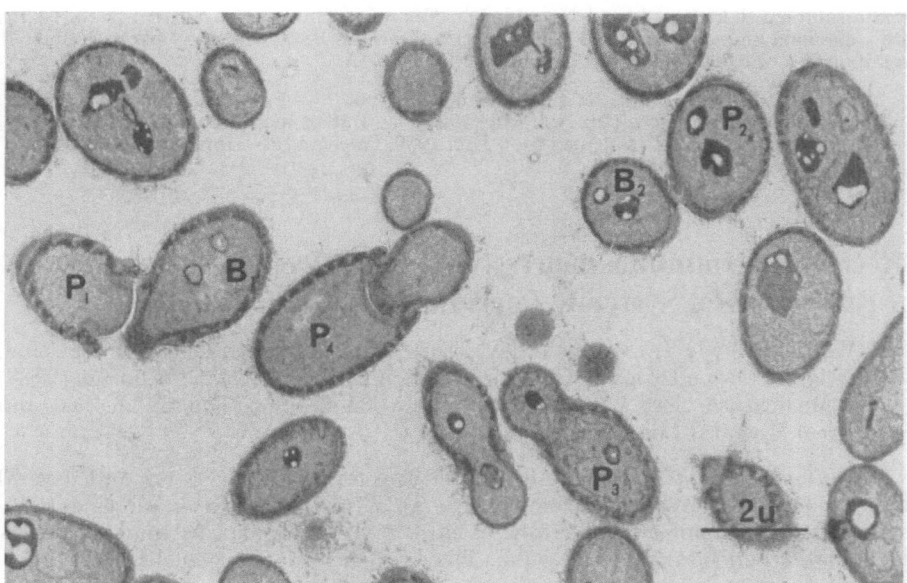

Fig. 5. P. canis (CBS-1879). A low power view of a number of cells in various stages of vegetative reproduction. Cells P-1 and P-2 have separated from their buds B-1 and B-2, except for
attachment of a portion of the outer wall. Cell P-3 is forming a bud and cell P-4 has a septum.
Other cells are seen in cross and oblique section

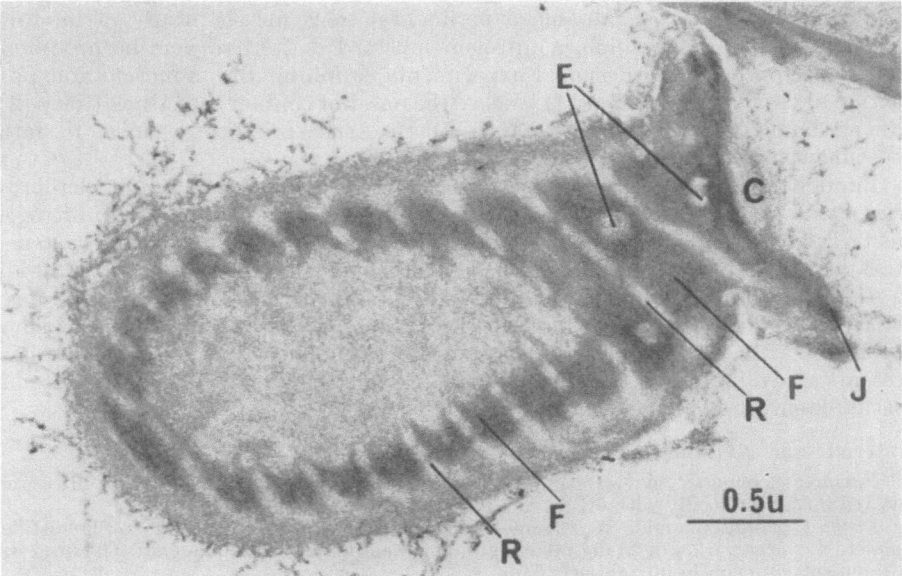

Fig. 6. P. canis (CBS-1879). A cell cut parallel to its long axis and through the substance of
the wall near the neck of the cell. The rim (J) is flared out and a bit of the crosswall (C) lies
in the cup of the rim. The ridges (R) and furrows (F) form a pattern of bands oblique to the
long axis of the cell. The finger-like extensions (E) of the cytoplasm show as holes in the dense
furrows (F)

acetate solution, dehydrated, and imbedded in Vestopal. Thin sections, cut in serial strips with a diamond knife, were stained with uranyl acetate and lead citrate and photographed at magnifications of 5,000 to 40,000 times in an Elmiskop IA.

References. KEDDIE, F. M.: Sabouraudia 5, 134 (1966). — PANJA, G.: Trans. 7th Cong. Far Eastern Assn. trop. Med. (1927) 2, 442 (1928); — Indian med. Gaz. 81, 305 (1946); — Proc. Symp. Sch. trop. Med., Calcutta 5—6 Feb. 1959. Calcutta Sch. trop. Med. 1962, 199.

Effect of the Immunosuppressive Agent, Cyclophosphamide, on Experimental Systemic Coccidioidomycosis*

J. W. LANDAU, L. INDIANER and V. D. NEWCOMER, Department of Medicine, Division of Dermatology, UCLA Medical School, Los Angeles, California (USA) and Medical Service, Veterans Administration Center, General Medical and Surgical Hospital Los Angeles, California (USA)

Coccidioides immitis is endemic to southwestern United States and several other areas of the Western Hemisphere. This fungus produces an essentially asymptomatic pulmonary infection in most individuals but in some instances disseminated and fatal disease results. The exact host defense mechanisms determining resistance to coccidioidomycosis are not established but such factors ae non-white race, male sex, and pregnancy are known to increase the severity of the disease.

Drugs with immunosuppressive activity are now used extensively in the treatment of neoplastic and "auto-immune" diseases and the prevention of homograft rejection following organ transplantation. Immunosuppressive agents have also proved to be valuable experimental tools for the study of immune responses. Cyclophosphamide, a nitrogen mustard derivative, has been demonstrated in appropriately designed experiments to inhibit the induction and production of circulating antibody [1], delay the onset of contact hypersensitivity [2], prolong homograft survival [3], and enhance susceptibility of mice to fatal experimental pulmonary aspergillosis [4].

Limited information is available concerning the influence of immunosuppressive agents on experimental coccidioidomycosis. Administration of nitrogen mustard to rabbits infected 7 weeks earlier with *C. immitis* slightly hastened their deaths and did not influence their complement-fixation titers [5]. Administration of cyclophosphamide, actinomycin-D, and methotrexate to mice 2 days before their subcutaneous inoculation with *C. immitis* did not affect the incidence of dissemination to internal organs or the local cellular response [6]. This report presents an evaluation of the effect of cyclophosphamide on the course of systemic coccidioidomycosis in the mouse.

Materials and Methods

Fungus: C. immitis, Silveira strain, was cultured as described previously [6]. Mice were injected intraperitoneally with 0.1 ml of a 0.5% suspension in saline.

Drug: Cyclophosphamide (Cytoxan^R-Mead Johnson) was dissolved in sterile distilled water to a concentration of 20 mg/ml and administered in a dose of 200 mg/kg. The drug was injected subcutaneously into the left flank.

Animals: Female albino mice weighing 18 to 20 g were divided into six groups each containing 40 mice with approximately the same distribution of weights. The mice were allowed commercial laboratory chow and water *ad libitum*. Four groups were infected with

* This study was supported in part by USPHS Grants Al-06048-03 and T1 AM 5265-07 and by the Dermatologic Research Foundation of California, Inc.

C. immitis. Cyclophosphamide was also administered to three of these groups. One group received the drug 4 days before infection, another 2 h before infection. and another 4 days after infection. The fourth infected group was given a subcutaneous saline injection and retained as a *C. immitis* Control group. A Drug Control group received a cyclophosphamide injection and an intraperitoneal saline injection. A Saline Control group received an intraperitoneal and a subcutaneous saline injection.

Hematologic Studies: Blood was obtained from the tail of twelve mice in the infected and saline control groups immediately before and 7 days after the time of infection. Blood was obtained from twelve mice in the drug control group on the third, 7., and 11. day after cyclophosphamide administration in order to have appropriate 7. day control values. The micro-hematocrit, white blood cell count, and differential cell count were determined for each mouse.

Autopsy: Mice in the four infected groups dying during the study were autopsied. Gross observations were recorded and samples of the liver, spleen, kidneys and lungs were cultured on Sabouraud dextrose agar. Sections of tissue for histologic study were obtained from several mice in each group dying between the 12. and 14. day of the experiment. The tissues were fixed in 10% formalin, sectioned, and stained with hematoxylin and eosin.

Statistics: The t test was used to compare means and the chi square test was used to compare numbers of surviving mice on a particular day. A probability of occurrence of $p < 0.05$ was considered statistically significant.

Results

The figure presents the percentages of surviving mice during the course of the study which was terminated 35 days after infection. All mice in the saline control group and all but two mice in the drug control group survived during this period. From the 11. day, onward the numbers of surviving mice in the groups given cyclophosphamide 2 h before and 4 days after infection were both significantly

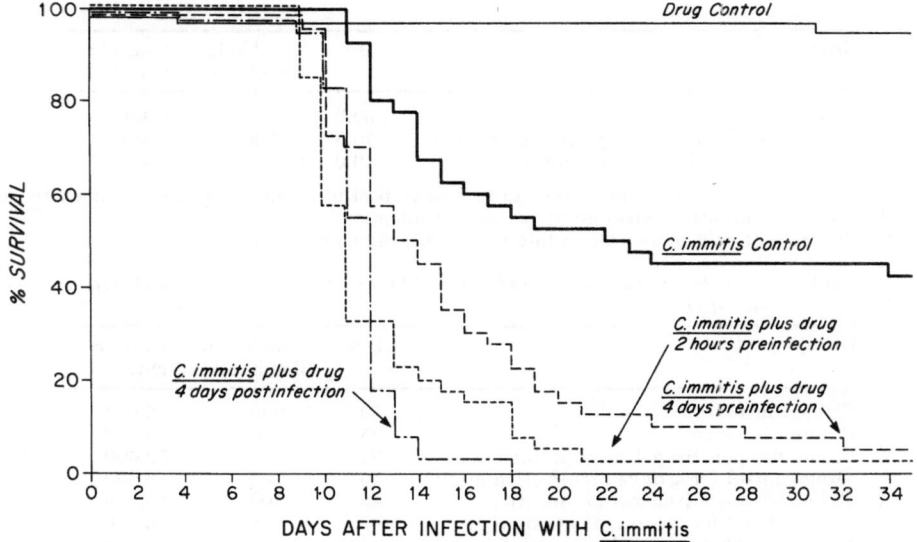

Fig. Effect of time of administration of cyclophosphamide on survival of mice infected with C. immitis

less than those in the *C. immitis* control group. The numbers of surviving mice in the group given cyclophosphamide 4 days before infection were significantly less than those in the *C. immitis* control group after the 15. day. Between the 12. to 20. day, significantly less mice survived in the group given cyclophosphamide 4 days after infection than in the group given cyclophosphamide 4 days before infection. The mean number of days of survival and the standard error

of the means of the *C. immitis* control group and the groups given cyclophosphamide 4 days before, 2 h before and 4 days after infections were 24.0 ± 1.3,
15.6 ± 1.0, 12.4 ± 0.7, and 11.6 ± 0.3 respectively. The differences between the
mean survival time of the *C. immitis* control group and that of each of the other
groups are significant. The difference between the mean survival times of the
group receiving cyclophosphamide 4 days before and 4 days after infection is also
significant.

Blood counts at the time of infection are presented in Tab. 1. The mean total,
leukocytes, granulocytes, and mononuclear cell counts at the time of infection
were significantly lower in the group given cyclophosphamide 4 days before
infection than in the other groups.

Blood counts performed 7 days later are presented in Tab. 2. The hematocrit
of the *C. immitis* control group was significantly lower than that of the saline
control group and the hematocrits of the infected groups given cyclophosphamide
4 days before or after infection were significantly lower than that of the *C. immitis*
control group. The granulocyte but not the total leukocyte count of the *C. immitis*
control group was significantly higher than that of the saline control group. The
total leukocyte and granulocyte counts of the two pretreated infected groups
were significantly higher than those of the *C. immitis* control group and their
respective drug control groups. The total leukocyte, granulocyte, and mononuclear cell counts of the *C. immitis* group treated after infection were significantly
lower than those of the *C. immitis* control group.

Table 1. *Hematocrits (mean %) and White Blood Cell Counts (mean cells/mm³)
at Time of Infection*

Group	Hct	Total White Blood Cells	Granulo-cytes[b]
C. immitis control[a]	50.0	13,800	2700
C. immitis plus drug 4 days preinfection	40.8	3,600	200
C. immitis plus drug 2 h preinfection	49.0	11,000	3000

[a] Saline control and C. immitis plus drug 4 days postinfection groups are assumed to be
similar to the C. immitis control group at time of infection.
[b] Mononuclear cells equal total white blood cells minus granulocytes.

Table 2. *Hematocrits (mean %) and White Blood Cells Counts (mean cells/mm³)
7 Days Postinfection*

Group	Hct	Total White Blood Cells	Granulo-cytes
Saline control	50	15,000	2,600
C. immitis control	45	15,400	5,500
C. immitis plus drug 4 days preinfection	39	41,500	30,000
Drug control for 4 days preinfection group[a]	50	15,200	6,800
C. immitis plus drug 2 h preinfection	45	21,700	15,200
Drug control for 2 h preinfection group[b]	49	13.000	6,400
C. immitis plus drug 4 days postinfection	41	1,500	50
Drug control for 4 days postinfection group[c]	48	3,200	200

[a, b, c] Blood obtained 11,7, and 3 days, respectively after cyclophosphamide administration
to provide appropriate control values.

The autopsies did not reveal any striking differences between the *C. immitis*
control and the three other infected groups. Granulomas were observed on gross
examination of each organ and cultures yielded *C. immitis* in almost every
instance. Microscopic examination of the few mice sampled revealed numerous
spherules in all sections with the exceptions that relatively fewer spherules were

observed in the liver and kidney from the *C. immitis* control group and the infected group given cyclophosphamide 2 h before infection. Infiltrates composed of granulocytes, lymphocytes, and histiocytes surrounded the spherules in all organs. The intensity of the infiltrate in the lung, liver, and kidney was relatively greater in the two *C. immitis* groups given cyclophosphamide 4 days before and after infection compared with the other two infected groups.

Discussion

These findings indicate that the administration of cyclophosphamide has a significantly adverse effect on the course of experimental coccidioidomycosis. This effect is not merely a result of non-specific inanition since almost all of the mice in the drug control group remained in good condition throughout the experiment.

Leukopenia associated with immunosuppressive therapy has been postulated to be a factor predisposing the host to certain fungous infections such as aspergillosis, candidiasis, cryptococcosis, and phycomycosis [7]. Significant leukopenia at the time or during the course of infection was demonstrated in two groups in this experiment. The third infected-drug treated group probably also was leukopenic at a time not sampled. Other studies in this laboratory have demonstrated that cyclophosphamide, as given in this experiment, regularly produces a leukopenia 1 to 5 days after its administration which is followed by a leukocytosis, principally a granulocytosis, persisting for several days.

The reason for the significantly more rapid deaths of the mice given cyclophosphamide after infection compared with those treated 4 days before infection is not readily apparent. A possible explanation is that the period of leukopenia in the former group corresponded with the onset of endospore formation [8]. The importance of timing of cyclophosphamide administration has also been demonstrated in suppression of homograft rejection [3] and antibody synthesis [1] in the mouse.

The leukopenia produced by cyclophosphamide can not be accepted without reservation as the sole reason for the adverse effect of this drug on experimental coccidioidomycosis since cyclophosphamide also inhibits a variety of humoral and cellular immune responses. Furthermore, mice with leukopenia induced by x-irradiation experienced milder *C. immitis* infections with less tissue damage than control infected mice [9]. The possibility that antileukemic drugs might suppress spherulation in humans has been hypothesized but preliminary use of nitrogen mustard as therapy for disseminated coccidioidomycosis in man produced equivocal results [10]. The histological findings in the current study, however, indicate that a slight increase rather than any decrease in spherulation was present in tissue from two of the infected-drug treated groups.

This study suggests that the use of immunosuppressive therapy in man may adversely affect active coccidioidomycosis and also implies that it may exacerbate quiescent infections. Statistical proof in man is not available but several such examples have been observed [11]. Most of these patients had also been treated with corticosteroids which have also been demonstrated to adversely affect experimental coccidioidomycosis [12]. Finally additional studies of the experimental model of animals treated with immunosuppressive agents before and after infection may prove useful in elucidating the various immune responses determining susceptibility and resistance to *C. immitis* and other fungous infections.

Bibliography. 1. FRISCH, A. W., and G. H. DAVIES: Cancer Res. **25**, 745 (1965). — 2. MAGUIRE, jr., H. C., and H. I. MAIBACH: J. invest. Derm. **37**, 427 (1961). — 3. FOX, M.: Transplant. Bull. **2**, 475 (1964). — 4. SIDRANSKY, H., E. VERNEY, and H. BEEDE: Arch. Path. **79**, 299 (1965). — 5. BROSBE, E. A., J. N. KIETZMAN, and N. B. KURNICK: J. Bact. **88**, 233 (1964). — 6. FENSTER, M., J. W. LANDAU, and V. D. NEWCOMER: Proc. 2nd Coccidioidomycosis

Symp., Univ. Arizona Press 1967, p. 381. — 7. BAKER, R. D.: Amer. J. clin. Path. **37**, 358 (1962). — 8. TARBET, J. E., E. T. WRIGHT, and V. D. NEWCOMER: Amer. J. Path. **28**, 901 (1952). — 9. BAKER, O., and A. I. BRAUDE: J. Lab. clin. Med. **47**, 169 (1956). — 10. KURNICK, N. B.: Trans. 3rd Ann. Meeting, Veterans Administration — Armed Forces Coccidioidomycosis Cooperative Study, p. 11, 1958. — 11. WILL, D. W., J. F. MURRAY, S. M. FINEGOLD, V. L. SUTTER, and B. F. FISHKIN: Amer. Rev. resp. Dis. **84**, 114 (1961). — 12. NEWCOMER, V. D., E. T. WRIGHT, J. E. TARBET, L. H. WINER, and T. H. STERNBERG: J. invest. Derm. **20**, 315 (1953).

Enzyme des Kohlenhydratstoffwechsels bei Dermatophyten

W. MEINHOF und G. RASSNER, Dermatologische Klinik und Poliklinik der Universität München (Deutschland)

Die Glucose nimmt bei den Dermatophyten ebenso wie bei den Hefen und bei tierischen Zellen eine zentrale Stellung im energieliefernden Stoffwechsel ein. JENSEN u. Mitarb. (1957), CHIN u. KNIGHT (1962) sowie CHATTAWAY u. Mitarb. (1960) haben gezeigt, daß Trichophyton mentagrophytes und Microsporum canis über Enzyme der Glykolyse, des Pentosephosphatcyclus und des Citronensäure-cyclus verfügen.

In unseren eigenen Untersuchungen konnten wir mit Hilfe biochemischer und histochemischer Methoden bei 29 verschiedenen Dermatophytenarten die folgenden Enzyme des energieliefernden Stoffwechsels bestimmen.

Hefen sind zur Energiegewinnung aus Glucose einerseits über den Weg der oxydativen Phosphorylierung und andererseits über die alkoholische Gärung befähigt. Bei tierischen Organismen wird unter anaeroben Bedingungen aus der Brenztraubensäure nicht Alkohol sondern Milchsäure gebildet. Die Endprodukte der alkoholischen bzw. der Milchsäuregärung entstehen unter Einwirkung der Enzyme Alkoholdehydrogenase und Lactatdehydrogenase. Da bei den Dermatophyten nach unseren Befunden Alkoholdehydrogenase und Lactatdehydrogenase nur in sehr geringer Aktivität vorliegen oder ganz fehlen, muß die Frage nach dem Endprodukt des anaeroben Glucoseabbaus hier noch offen bleiben.

Die Regulation der verschiedenen energieliefernden Stoffwechselwege ist bei der Hefe Saccharomyces cerevisiae einerseits von dem Sauerstoffangebot und zum andern auch von der Menge und der Art der zur Verfügung stehenden Kohlenhydrate abhängig (POLAKIS u. BARTLEY, 1955; POLAKIS u. Mitarb., 1965). Um einen näheren Einblick in die regulatorischen Vorgänge des Glucosemetabolismus der Dermatophyten zu erhalten, haben wir die Pilze mit verschieden hohen Glucosekonzentrationen und mit anderen Zuckern in einem synthetischen Nährmedium angezüchtet. Unter Verwendung biochemischer Methoden wurden die Aktivitäten einiger Enzyme des Glucosestoffwechsels bestimmt. In einer weiteren Versuchsreihe wurde das Sauerstoffangebot von 150 mg Hg auf einen Partialdruck von 120 mg Hg gesenkt. Bei Microsporum gypseum, das einmal in einem Medium mit 3% Glucose und zum andern mit 0,1% Glucose gezüchtet wurde, wird deutlich, daß bei höherem Glucoseangebot auch höhere Enzymaktivitäten zu finden sind. Nach Verwendung verschiedener Zucker im Nährmedium zeigt sich, daß die Glucose höhere Enzymaktivitäten bewirkt als Fructose oder Galaktose. Auch nach Anzucht mit Ribose oder Pyruvat als Kohlenstoffquelle fanden wir wesentlich geringere Enzymaktivitäten als mit dem glucosehaltigen Medium. Beim Verhalten der Enzymaktivitäten bei verringerter Sauerstoffspannung wird erkennbar, daß nicht nur die Enzyme des sauerstoffabhängigen Citronensäurecyclus sondern auch die Enzyme der Glykolyse durch Verringerung der normalen Sauerstoffspannung um ein Fünftel in ihrer Aktivität herabgesetzt werden.

Bei dem Versuch, die Enzyme des energieliefernden Stoffwechsels auch histochemisch unter verschiedenen Anzuchtbedingungen darzustellen, erhielten wir Befunde, die unseren biochemischen Untersuchungsergebnissen zunächst zu widersprechen scheinen. Ein reicher Gehalt des Nährmediums an Glucose (3%) ergab nur geringe enzymaktivitätanzeigende Formazanpräcipitate. Die niedrige Glucosekonzentration von 0,1% im Nährmedium führte bereits zu stärkeren Farbstoffniederschlägen. Der gleiche Effekt wurde auch durch Herabsetzung der Sauerstoffspannung bewirkt. Am deutlichsten zeigte sich eine Steigerung der histochemisch nachweisbaren Enzymaktivitäten bei Verwendung von Fructose, Galaktose oder Pyruvat anstelle der Glucose.

Eine gesicherte Erklärung für den Unterschied zwischen unseren biochemischen und unseren histochemischen Befunden können wir bisher nicht abgeben. Man muß jedoch bei der Gegenüberstellung histochemischer und biochemischer Befunde berücksichtigen, daß in dem ersteren Falle der Grad der Enzymaktivität aus der Dichte der Formazanpräcipitate geschätzt wird, daß jedoch die Aktivität nicht auf das Gesamtgewicht des Mycels oder dessen Proteingehalt bezogen wird. Das bedeutet aber, daß bei histochemischen Untersuchungen auch dann von einer starken Aktivität gesprochen wird, wenn diese nur topisch begrenzt auftritt, während bei biochemischen Untersuchungen stets die Gesamtaktivität bezogen auf die gesamte Pilzmenge berücksichtigt wird. Auf diese Weise können histochemisch intensiv dargestellte Enzymaktivitäten biochemisch als nur schwache Enzymaktivitäten erscheinen, wenn die Enzymaktivitäten unterschiedlich im Mycel verteilt vorliegen. Anhaltspunkte für ein derartiges Verhalten fanden sich vor allem bei Verwendung von Galaktose als Zucker anstelle von Glucose. Die histochemisch faßbaren Enzymaktivitäten liegen hier nur in einzelnen Kammern der Makrokonidien und in einzelnen Mycelabschnitten vor. Die Konzentrierung der Enzymaktivitäten in einzelnen Konidienkammern und Mycelabschnitten stellt möglicherweise einen Vorgang dar, der mit der vermehrten Bildung von Dauerformen (Konidien, Mycelsporen) in einer Mangelsituation in Zusammenhang steht.

Zusammenfassend läßt sich sagen, daß die kombinierte Anwendung biochemischer und histochemischer Untersuchungsmethoden zu Ergebnissen geführt hat, die auf Eigenheiten des Stoffwechsels der Glucose bei Dermatophyten hinweisen. Es bleibt zu überprüfen, ob Phänomene der adaptativen Enzymbildung hierbei von Bedeutung sind.

Unterstützt durch die Deutsche Forschungsgemeinschaft.

Microsporum Nanum as a Cause of Human Infections

J. F. MULLINS and C. J. WILLIS, University of Texas, Medical Branch, Galveston, Texas (USA)

The purpose of this presentation is to review the world literature regarding cases of tinea corporis caused by *Microsporum nanum*. As will be noted, *M. nanum* has been a fairly common pathogen of swine, producing lesions which are fairly consistent in morphology, evolution, and gross appearance. The tinea infection is of no specific importance to the health of the swine. In both of our cases [1], the tinea infections were of a rather nondescript morphology, and only a tentative diagnosis of a tinea corporis infection could be made initially. The lesions were inflamed and pruritic and of considerable concern to the patients.

A *Microsporum* with peculiar dwarf macroconidia was described by FUENTES et al. in 1954 [2]. It was the causative agent of an inflammatory tinea capitis on an 8-year-old Cuban boy. The hairs were Wood's light fluorescent, and the potassium hydroxide (KOH) preparation revealed air bubbles of a "favic type" of endothrix infection. The organism grew well on Sabouraud's dextrose agar and at 4 days was cottony white with the reverse side orange. In 11 days, the colony was a granular buff with the reverse side a deep brownish red. It required no special nutrition and was proved pathogenic to man and animals.

The organism pierced hair and elaborated abundant pearshaped echinulate macroconidia with one to three cells. There were few microconidia. Because of the physical and cultural characteristics, the organism was thought to be a variant of *M. gypseum* and was called *M. gypseum var nanum*.

A similar organism was isolated from a glabrous ringworm on an adult man 7 months later. Neither fungus changed physical characteristics over a period of years, and, in 1956, FUENTES [3] separated the organisms, assigning the species name *M. nanum*.

The third reported case appeared in the Mexican literature as a case of tinea corporis [4]. The first report of a case in the United states occurred in Mississippi in 1961. BROCK [5] reported the latter case of tinea capitis occurring on an 8-year-old boy. The organism isolated was identical with that described by FUENTES. BROCK reported no fluorescence or air bubbles in the hairs of his case. The lesions were treated topically and resolved within a few weeks.

Nannizzia obtusa, or the perfect state of *M. nanum*, was demonstrated by DAWSON and GENTLES [6]. These authors also noted cultures from Cuba and swine ringworm in Kenya, Africa.

In 1962, CARMICHAEL and REID [7] from Alberta, Canada, reported a case of tinea manum caused by *M. nqnum* occurring on a 7-year-old schoolgirl. Contact with farm animals, dogs, and cats was recorded, but no direct transmission was demonstrated. That same year, EVOLCEANU et al. [8] felt they had isolated *M. nanum* from Rumanian soil. This was subsequently identified as *Chrysosporium keratinophilum* [9]. AJELLO et al. [9] discussed two cases of tinea capitis and tinea corporis in the United States and a third case of tinea corporis in Australia which were previously unreported. In this fine review, the authors concluded that the clinical lesions were inflammatory, may or may not fluoresce, but were endothrixic without the usual well-formed mosaic of spores outside the hair shaft. They felt that the organism must have a swine habitat in which to propagate and that it is an active growing saprophyte when in the soil. The lesions produced on pigs are very chronic, slowly enlarging patches of scaling dermatitis which do not manifest much inflammation or alopecia and are mildly pruritic.

An outbreak of swine ringworm in Centre County, Pa, in 1864, caused by *M. nanum* was reported by BUBASH et al. [10]. GINTHER et al. [11, 12] also reported swine infections in Kansas, Kentucky, New Jersey, and Pennsylvania. Early in 1964, GINTHER and AJELLO [13] discussed the prevalence of this organism in the United States and recorded its isolation from soil and swine in twelce states, including Texas. GINTHER and AJELLO [13] felt that this was a relatively new infection in swine and not simply an increasing awareness of an already existing reservoir. One of their isolates from Texas originated in the area of Bellville, the geographic location of our cases.

Comment

It is of interest that the lesions produced by *M. nanum* in swine may go undetected until specifically pointed out to the owner by a veterinarian or investigator working in the field of swine mycology. In contrast, our two patients became symptomatic within 3 to 4 days after the initial onset of a clinically apparent lesion. The factors directly contributing to man's susceptibility to infection with *M. nanum*, a rather common pathogen of swine, cannot be stated at this time. *M. nanum* has a high degree of infectivity for swine. 1000 of people daily are in contact with infected swine, and it is our concluding opinion that *M. nanum* may represent a definite public health problem. It should be suspected as a causative agent whenever patients from a swine-raising region present with a diagnosis of tinea corporis.

References. 1. MULLINS, J. F:: Arch. Derm. **94**, 300 (1966). — 2. FUENTES, C. A., R. ABOULAFIA, and R. J. VIDAL: J. invest. Derm. **23**, 51 (1954). — 3. FUENTES. C. A.: Mycologia **48**, 613 (1956). — 4. BEIRANA, L., y M. MAGANNA- Bol. Derm. **4**, 11 (1960). — 5. BROCK, J. M.: Arch. Derm. **84**, 504 (1961). — 6. DAWSON, C. O., and J. C. GENTLES: Sabouraudia **1**, 49 (1961). — 7. CARMICHAEL, J. W., and J. F. REID: Mycopathologia (Den Haag) **17**, 49 (1961). — 8. EVOLCEANU, R., I. ALTERAS, and M. STOIAN: Mycopathologia (Den Haag) **19**, 24 (1963). — 9. AJELLO, L.: Mycologia **56**, 873 (1964). — 10. BUBASH, G. R., O. J. GINTHER, and L. AJELLO: Science **143**, 336 (1964). — 11. GINTHER, O. J., G. R. BUBASH, and L. AJELLO: Vet. Med. **59**, 79 (1964). — 12. GINTHER, O. J.: Vet. Med. **59**, 490 (1964). — 13. GINTHER, O. J., and L. AJELLO: J. Amer. vet. med. Ass. **146**, 363 (1964).

Les dermatophytes du sol en Bulgarie

P. POPCHRISTOV, V. BALABANOFF, T. FILKOV et P. USUNOV, Clinique Dermatologique de Sofia (Bulgarie)

Les dimensions de notre pays et notre organisation des services dermatologiques nous ont permis dès 1952 d'effectuer en Bulgarie une série d'études des dermatomycoses et des dermatophytes sur tout le territoire du pays.

Une circonstance particulièrement favorable pour nous, c'est que l'Institut des maladies cutanées et à présent la Clinique dermatologique de Sofia, dirigent scientifiquement tous les services dermatologiques du pays et tous les dermatologistes bulgares sont nos élèves.

Durant les années 1952 à 1958 nous avons effectué une étude détaillée sur la flore dermatophytique, de même que le dépistage et le traitement des pilomycoses dans tout le pays. Il y a 2 ans, nous travaillions en collaboration avec les autorités vétérinaires sur les dermatomycoses d'origine animale chez l'homme.

Au cours de ces études furent isolé en 1954, des lésions cutanées d'enfants jouant avec de la terre de parcs, le *Microsporum gypseum* et en 1962 du sol de grottes les formes parfaites et imparfaites de *Trichophyton terrestre* et de *Keratinomyces Ajelloi*, puis de cours d'étables *Microsporum gypseum* et sa forme parfaite *Nannizzia incurvata, Microsporum cookei* etc.

En 1964 furent entreprises des recherches systématiques des dermatophytes telluriques dans tous les districts du pays. Les résultas de ces investigations sont l'objet de notre communication.

De 3336 prélèvements de terres, réparties dans chaque distzict séparément (Tableau) c'est le *M. gypseum*, qui est isolé en premier lieu 1719 fois, suivi par *K. Ajelloi* 695, *T. terrestre* 269, *M. cookei* 78, *T. mentagrophytes* 26 et *T. vanbreuseghemii* 1 fois.

Les formes sexuées, rangées par l'ordre de leur fréquence sont: *A. quadrifidum, N. incurvata, A. uncinatum, N. cajetana* et *A. gertleri*. Les moissisures keratinophiles du genre *Chrysosporium, Ctenomyces* n'entrent pas en ce nombre.

C'est pour la première fois que furent isolés chez nous et la seconde fois en Europe après BÖHME, *T. vanbreuseghemii* et sa forme parfaite *A. gertleri. T. mentagrophytes* est rare dans le sol et fut isolé seulement 26 fois de biotopes visités par

Tableau

District	Nombre des prélèvements	Positifs	K. ajelloi	M. gypseum	M. cookei	T. terrestre	T. mentagrophytes	T. vanbreuseghemii
Varna	204	164	63	96	1	4		
Vratza	350	291	48	222	5	16		
Michailovgrad	166	146	28	102	4	12		
Plovdiv	417	399	52	216	5	126		
Sofia	411	304	107	156	9	32		
Vidin	150	105	14	57	2	32		1
Haskovo	303	267	100	139	9	12	7	
Pleven	328	283	111	118	39	10	5	
Blagoevgrad	41	27	14	5	1	2	5	
Tirnovo	416	336	126	232	1	1	6	
Chumen	450	371	25	339		4	3	
St. Zagora	100	64	7	37	2	18		
Total	3336	2787	695	1719	78	269	26	1

l'homme et les rongeurs. Il est présenté surtout par sa forme parfaite du type Arthroderma anascosporée ou abortive. Dans le peridium de quatre souches on observe des macroconidies munies de spirales.

Le nombre des isolements positifs est plus fréquent en automne et au printemps, dans les régions montagneuses, que dans les plaines. Le pourcentage plus élevé de *M. gypseum* peut être attribué aux conditions spécifiques d'élevage intensif.

Pareillement à nos investigations anterieures, *M. gypseum* prédomine dans les régions riches en matières organiques et phanères, visitées par l'homme et les animaux. Par contre, *T. terrestre*, en sa qualité de dermatophyte saprophyte moins exigeant, se trouve dans les sols arides et sableneux. *T. mentagrophytes*, en sa qualité de dermatophyte zooantropophile et non tellurique, est peu fréquent dans le sol. D'une manière générale, c'est les dermatophytes primitifs à morphologie complète, à un niveau d'adaptation parasitaire initiale, et non les dermatophytes pathogènes, qui font partie naturelle de la flore mycotique du sol.

Une comparaison faite entre le pourcentage des dermatophytes pathogènes-antropophiles et zoophiles dans les divers districts du pays (5000 cultures) et celui des dermatophytes telluriques dans les mêmes districts (3336 cultures), montre, qu'il n'existe pas un parallélisme ou une dépendance directe entre les agents de dermatomycoses et leurs prédécesseurs dans le sol.

Il faut noter cependant, que la forme de passage vers le parasitisme — *M. gypseum*, est la cause d'infections rares (45 cas dans nos investigations) et bien plus rarement encore *M. cookei* (5 cas du Dr. SCHICK). Ces infections surviennent surtout dans les professions de contact direct avec le sol — jardiniers, laboureurs, agronomes etc. Les céréales, les fourrages et autres matières de contact avec les rongeurs, sujets d'épizooties dermatophytiques, plutôt que le sol, ont été la cause d'infections par *T. mentagrophytes* et *T. quinckeanum*. Il s'agit d'agents mycotiques à un niveau de différenciation biologique plus élévé, dont l'habitat ordinaire sont les rongeurs ou leurs matières de contact et non le sol.

Conclusion. Cette étude présente un essai d'investigation des dermatophytes telluriques dans les districts d'un pays tout entier. Un parallélisme avec la flore de dermatophytes pathogènes, cause des dermatomycoses dans les mêmes districts n'existe pas. Une différence avec la flore dermatophytique des autres pays ne peut pas être constatée, si on ne compte pas certaines particularités spécifiques régionales.

L'ultrastructure des grains dans les maduromycoses provoquée par Monosporium apiospermum

M. Stoian et A. Avram, Centre Dermato-vénéréologique de Bucarest (Roumanie)

La microscopie électronique a été assez peu utilisée jusqu'à présent dans l'étude des ultrastructures de cellules fongiques et pas du tout dans celle de grains maduromycosiques. Pendant les dernières 5 années, en adaptant les techniques habituelles

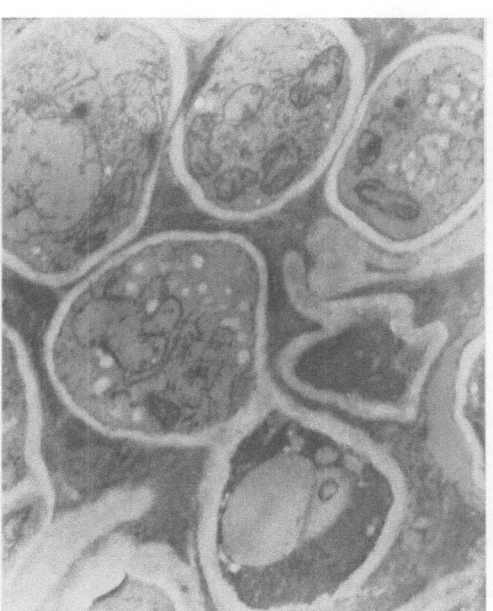
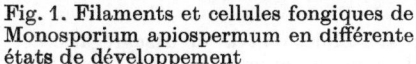

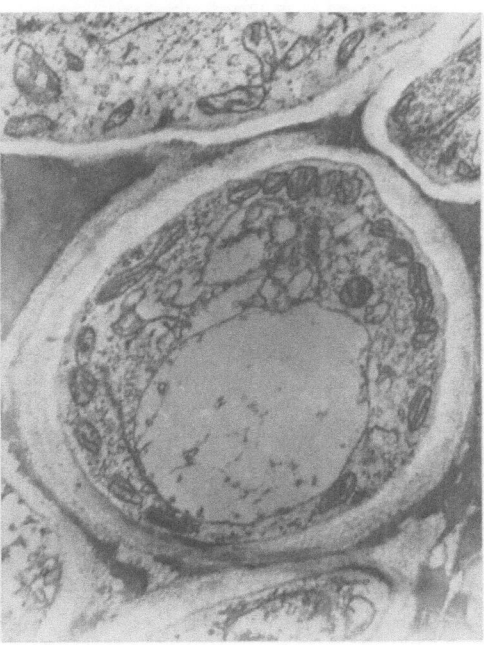

Fig. 1. Filaments et cellules fongiques de Monosporium apiospermum en différente états de développement

Fig. 2. Cellule de Monosporium a. vers le fin de la phase stationnaire tardive

de fixation, nous avons étudié au microscope électronique des grains provenant de trois cas de mycétome provoqués par le Monosporium apiospermum.

Dans les micrographies électroniques, ces grains apparaissent comme des agglomerations de filaments et de cellules fongiques (Fig. 1). Les cellules de Monosporium ont été surprises dans différentes états de développement, allant jusqu'à la désagrégation cellulaire.

On voit un très grand nombre de ces cellules munies de parois très grosses et fortement osmiophobes, contrastant avec un cytoplasme osmiophile contenant, à part le noyau, les éléments ultrastructuraux communs à toutes sortes de cellules, à savoir: un réticulum endoplasmique (très réduit d'habitude ici), de nombreuses mitochondries, des vacuoles et de granules lipidiques (Fig. 2). Le noyau, grand, arrondi ou ovale a une densité réduite par rapport au cytoplasma. La membrane nucléaire est très nette, mais quelques fois très sinueuse. Les mitochondries, ovales ou bien allongées ont des dimensions variables et se distinguent par leur orientation dans l'axe longitudinal de leurs membranes internes (les « cristae mitochondriae »), orientation caractéristique pour les champignons. Parfois les mitochondries sont disposées en couronne autour du noyau, ou bien près de la paroi cellulaire, dans leur phase stationnaire tardive. Dans les cellules en pleine évolution vers la phase stationnaire, par contre, les mitochondries sont plus grandes. Quelquefois on peut observer dans les cellules vieilles des formes très différentes dans lesquelles les crètes sont effacées, en même temps qu'une désagrégation mitochondriale (Fig. 1). Tous ces données attestent qu'une bonne partie des cellules constituant ces grains ne sont pas des formes de résistance, ainsi qu'elles étaient considéres par la mycologie

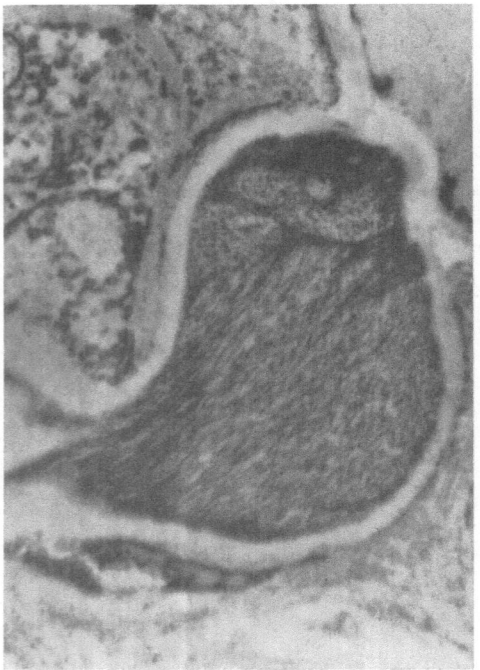

Fig. 3. Transformation fibrillaire du cyto-plasma d'une cellule de Monosporium a.

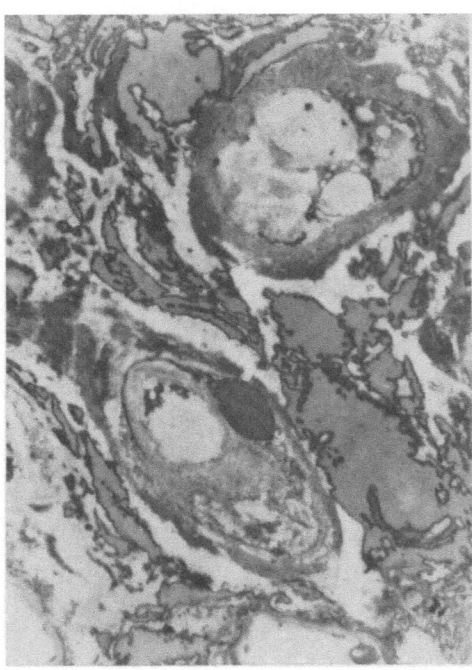

Fig. 4. Cellules en état de désagrégation et les bandelettes et les îlots d'une substance intercellulaire

classique, mais par contre des cellules en pleine développement et dotées d'un inépuisable potentiel régénératif. On observe toujours cette sorte de cellules sur-tout vers la surface des grains, tandis que leur centre est occupé seulement par de vieilles cellules en voie de dégénérescence. Alors (Fig. 4), leur cytoplasma est très raréfiée et parfois absente, l'intérieur de la cellule étant occupé par des débris in-formes et de grandes granules lipidiques. Quelquefois cet état est précédé par une transformation fibrillaire de leur cytoplasma (Fig. 3).

Quoique la paroi de ces cellules soit fort osmiophobe, on voit souvent qu'elle est constituée par de minces couches concentriques d'aspect fibrillaire très fines.

Parmi les cellules ou les debris cellulaires ci-dessus décrits, le microscope électronique nous permet d'observer la présence d'une substance, un peu plus dense que le cytoplasma, parsemée en bandelettes de forme et longueur très différentes (Fig. 4). Nous supposons que cette substance est une sorte de ciment que la microscopie conventionelle n'a pas eu la possibilité de le remarquer, quoique sa présence soit logiquement nécessaire.

À la périphérie des grains nous n'avons pas observé aucune membrane limitante, mais parfois des macrophages. Aucune section examinée ne nous a montré la présence de conidies caractéristiques pour cette espèce.

Par rapport aux les grains de Cephalosporium falciforme, un autre agent des maduromycoses à grains blancs, nous avons constaté certaines différences, qui feront l'objet d'un travail différent.

On the Mycomimetic Pictures Found in Mycologic Examinations

P. Sberna, Clinica Dermatologica dell' Università degli Studi Florence (Italiy)

The capacity of some biological and physiochemical phenomena of simulating images having the protean fungus structure is universally well known by the medical mycologist who must solve the problem of the real fungus structure of the microscopically observed images of specimens collected from suspected lesions. The interest on this subject was furnished by the observation of large number of images found in a case of a granuloma with abscess of the buttock which occurred in a syphilitic patient following the injection of fat-soluble bismuth preparation; these images were reproducing in a baffling way the morphological characteristics of the parasite Coccidioides immitis, but only after numerous and repeated observations and after the consideration of the clinical, biological, cultural data, a negative conclusion was reached from the mycological point of view. The above mentioned formations were a simple falsification simulating in a suggestive way fungus elements.

More frequently than expected, nature offers occasions to note the tendency of some substrata to assume fungus like structures. T. Benedek has called attention on some images simulating in a suggestive way the macroconidia of Microsporum and even images close to the peritecial formations which could wrongly be interpreted as perfect forms of multiplication with evident disrepute of the authority of the mycologist.

The diagnostic hesitation is easily solved by the missing internal structure of these formations. Their production occurs after precipitation in microcrystals of phenol and chloral hydrate contained in Aman's chlorallactophenol. This is a particular case of the so-called "crystal mimicry" frequently noticed in the mineral kingdom.

Another phenomenon should be briefly mentioned in the pathological material collected from the palmar and plantar regions that is the so called "mosaic fungi", pseudomycelial mosaic formations respecting the boundaries of the epitelial cells and caused, according to Stumpf, by the saponification of free fatty acids during maceration with potassium hydroxide. The transformation of these formations in rhombic cholesterol crystals owing to the action of cold 20% KOH has induced Davidson and Gregory to call them "cholesterol mosaic". The question of the possible fungus origin is not yet solved, as these crystals may occur, according to Vanbreuseghem, even in altered mycelial filaments. It is also known that they are not formed if the clarification is made in lactophenol.

The mycomimetic images observed in our case belong to another group of biological phenomena, like those due to foreign bodies; the clinical case regards a 30 year old woman, with latent syphilis in whom, after a course of intramuscular

injections of an oil suspended bismuth preparation, a deep abscess of the left
buttock occurred, followed by a successive hard infiltration of dermoipodermic
nodular elements, which reaching maturation, were discharging abundant semi-
solid, granular, thick yellowish material. Owing to the nodular component in the
dermo-hypodermic site suggesting actinomycosis, several mycologic examinations
of the discharged material and of the not yet sloughing nodular elements were
carried out.

The microscopic examination of the material in saline solution, in 20% KOH
and in chlorallactophenol-Coton blue, showed formations resembling in their particular morphological characteristics the cists or sporiferous sacs of Coccidioides
immitis; the sacs of various dimensions always show a well evident capsule, not
doubled, containing a great number of rounded elements of 2 to 5 micron in size,
never budding, thichly crowded suggesting typical Coccidioides spores. These
sporular elements do not regularly stain with blue coton and are PAS negative.
Some sporular elements had a long appendix simulating a germinative tube and
in some images showed a true twining of filaments but without well evident septa.
During manipulations some cysts became ruptured with elimination of sporular
elements and after drying these formations were altered and then they disappeared; some small formations resisted for few months in chlorallactophenol. The
histological examination showed amorphous and fatty material with numerous
polymorphonuclear neutrophils and large often polynucleated hysticocyte cells in
the peripherial zone and good lymphocyte infiltration. Repeated cultural examinations in Sabouraud's agar with antibiotics (penicillin, streptomycin and Actidione)
were always negative in contrast with the easy growth of Coccidioides immitis
(CIFERRI). Inoculation into guinea-pig, the skin test with coccidioidine were
negative. The clinical course in the first 4 months was varied but after another
2 months a complete cicatricial recovery was obtained, only with local treatment.

Numerous trials of artificially induced mycomimetic images using guinea-pig
brain and egg lecithin in KOH at 20% were done, obtaining various images which
are generally easily distinguished for their queer form and variable dimensions.
Infrequently images similar to those seen in our case are observed. The images
observed in our clinical case are probably due to the particular biological conditions only obtainable in vivo by the contact of a foreign body (lipoid) with living
tissues.

Zur fermentativen Leistung von Fadenpilzen

W. ADAM, Universitäts-Hautklinik Tübingen (Deutschland)

Die vorliegenden Untersuchungen wurden mit dem Ziel begonnen, zu quantitativen Aussagen über die Aktivität von Endoenzymen einiger Dermatophyten zu
gelangen. Es sollte ferner geprüft werden, ob und inwieweit Veränderungen des
Nährsubstrates zu einer Änderung auch der Aktivität von Endoenzymen führen,
wie das verschiedentlich an Ektoenzymen festgestellt wurde. Es sollte damit
gleichzeitig ein grob modellartiger Beitrag zu der von HANS RIETH angeschnittenen
Frage geliefert werden, wie weit in dem Wechselspiel zwischen Erreger und Wirt
Veränderungen des Wirtmilieus Änderungen des Dermatophyten nach sich ziehen
können.

Zu den Untersuchungen wurden aus Krankheitsherden frisch isolierte Stämme
von Trichophyton rubrum sowie der gipsigen und der flaumigen Variante von

Trichophyton mentagrophytes verwendet. Die Reinkulturen wurden je 6 bis 8 Tage auf Maltose- und dann auf 2%igen Pepton-Würzeagar gebracht, um optimale Wachstumsbedingungen zu erhalten. Die Kultivierung für die Fermentbestimmung erfolgte in einer 2%igen Peptonlösung mit unterschiedlichem Glucosegehalt in kleinen Portionen (40 ml) in einem kontinuierlich dreidimensional umschüttelnden Gerät, jeweils 6˙bis 8 Tage lang. Nach Abnutschen des Nährsubstrates wurde die Ernte zweimal gewaschen und dann zerkleinert.

Dabei zeigte sich, daß die *Technik des Aufschlusses* wesentlich die *Höhe der Fermentaktivität* bestimmte. Von den geprüften Verfahren (Homogenisatoren verschiedener Arbeitsweisen, Ultraschall, Rühren in hypertonischen Lösungen, Schütteln mit Glassplittern, Verwendung von Zelltrockenpulver) erwies sich uns das alte Zerreiben mit Quarzsand unter Kühlung als das schonenste und gleichzeitig das ergiebigste. Wie sehr der Modus des Aufschlusses die Resultate bestimmt, zeigt ein Vergleich: Zerreiben der Mycelien mit Quarzsand ergab gegenüber dem Schütteln einer Suspension mit ·Glassplittern etwa 30fach höhere Werte.

Qualitativ wurden in den zerkleinerten und wäßrig extrahierten Mycelien GOT, GPT, Aldolase und G-6-PDH nachgewiesen, LDH wurde nicht gefunden. Von den genannten Enzymen wurden zunächst GOT und GPT quantitativ bestimmt; hierzu mußten vorab die *optimalen Reaktionsbedingungen* ermittelt, d. h. Substrate und pH variiert werden. Hierbei wurde unter Variation von Asparagin die höchste GOT-Aktivität mit 112,039 mg Na-Asparagenat* in 3 ml 0,1 m Phosphatpuffers erhalten. Für die GPT-Bestimmung wurde unter Variation von Alanin die höchste Aktivität bei 65,92 mg in 3 ml 0,1 m Phosphatpuffers erzielt. Variation der Ketoglutarsäure unter Verwendung der angegebenen Substratoptima erbrachte für beide Fermentbestimmungen die günstigsten Resultate mit 0,1 ml 0,25 m Ketoglutarates. Als pH-Optimum wurde für die GOT-Bestimmung 7,7, für GPT 7,4 erhalten, wobei sich die letztgenannte Bestimmung als weniger pH-abhängig erwies.

Parallelansätze zur Kontrolle des *methodischen Fehlers* ergaben für die GOT-Bestimmung bei einem Mittelwert von 321,7 mU einen Variationskoeffizienten von 6,5%, für GPT bei einem Mittelwert von 412,1 mU eine Standardabweichung (V in %) von 4,5.

Nach diesen Voruntersuchungen wurden die *Endkulturen* der Dermatophyten zuckerfrei sowie mit unterschiedlichen Glucosemengen zum Basismedium einer 2%igen Peptonlösung angesetzt, der Zuckergehalt wurde von 0 bis 10% in Stufen von je 2% gesteigert. Dabei ergaben sich sowohl für GOT als für GPT kontinuierliche Aktivitätszunahmen bis zu einem Glucosegehalt von 6% mit einem deutlichen Abfall der Enzymaktivität bei Zuckerzusätzen von 8% und 10%. Der pH-Wert der Nährlösungen bewegte sich aus dem Alkalischen gegen den Neutralpunkt zu, er lag aber noch bei einem Glucosegehalt von 8% zwischen 7,0 und 7,6.

Bei einem Vergleich verschiedener, zu unterschiedlichen Zeiten und von verschiedenen Mykosen isolierter Dermatophytenstämme hinsichtlich ihrer *aktuellen Enzymaktivität* ergaben sich trotz der unmittelbar vorher erfolgten Stoffwechselanregung durch Vorzüchtung stark unterschiedliche Werte, die außerhalb jeder methodisch bedingten Schwankung liegen. Die primäre Stoffwechselintensität der Dermatophyten scheint demnach *schon von Stamm zu Stamm sehr unterschiedlich* zu sein. Dieser Sachverhalt macht es vorläufig unmöglich, verschiedene Dermatophytenarten hinsichtlich ihrer Transaminase (TA)-Aktivität miteinander zu vergleichen.

---

* Verwendet wurde das Natriumsalz der Asparaginsäure. Der Umrechnungsfaktor beträgt 1,17.

Die bisher skizzierten Untersuchungen haben gezeigt — und bestätigt —, daß Dermatophyten auf ein dosiert vermehrtes Nährstoffangebot mit einer Stoffwechselsteigerung reagieren, die sich u. a. mit der Bestimmung der TA-Aktivität schon frühzeitig erfassen läßt.

In den bisher beschriebenen Versuchen waren die Dermatophyten durch Vorzüchtung auf Maltose- und Pepton-Würzeagar auf das vermehrte Nährstoffangebot vorbereitet, d. h. *konditioniert* worden. Für spätere klinische Fragestellungen könnte unter Umständen bedeutungsvoller sein zu wissen, wie rasch und in welchem Umfang ein Dermatophyt mit seinem Stoffwechsel auf ein gesteigertes Nahrungsangebot reagieren kann, wenn er diesem nicht mit bereits entsprechend angeregtem Stoffwechsel, sondern aus dem gegenteiligen Milieu eines einseitigen — hier glucosefreien — Nährmediums heraus ausgesetzt wird. Es wurden deshalb Stämme der drei geprüften Dermatophyten je 6 Tage lang sowohl auf zuckerfreiem Peptonagar als auch auf einem 2% Glucose enthaltenden Würzeagar vorgezüchtet und dann in 2%ige Peptonlösungen mit einem Zusatz von 2% und 6% Glucose gebracht. Die TA-Bestimmungen erfolgten wie oben beschrieben.

Als *Ergebnis* dieser Versuchsserie läßt sich zunächst feststellen, daß die Dermatophytenernte bei allen Stämmen, die auf Würze-Dextrose-Agar vorgezüchtet waren, wesentlich *ergiebiger* war als bei den auf zuckerfreiem Medium kultivierten: Die Frischgewichte waren am Ende der 6tägigen Wachstumszeit in den bewegten Kölbchen 2,5 bis 4mal so hoch. Eine *Beziehung* zwischen Gewicht und Enzymaktivität ergab sich jedoch *nicht*. Vergleicht man dagegen die TA-Aktivitäten der Trichophyton mentagr.-Stämme in den 2% und 6% Glucose enthaltenden Endkulturen miteinander, so zeigt sich, daß nach Vorzüchtung auf Glucose-Würze das vermehrte (6%) Zuckerangebot zu einer erheblich höheren Enzymaktivität führt als nach Vorzüchtung auf zuckerfreiem Medium, daß sich also bei den auf Pepton vorgezüchteten Stämmen das hohe Glucoseangebot (noch) *nicht* in einer entsprechend gesteigerten TA-Aktivität äußert.

Der in diesem Versuch verwendete T. rubrum-Stamm verhielt sich jedoch anders: Er reagierte offenbar weniger empfindlich auf das Fehlen von Glucose im Nährboden; das höhere Zuckerangebot in der Endkultur führte nach beiden Vorzüchtungen zu *gleichsinnigen Erhöhungen* der TA-Aktivitäten. Daraus allerdings eine (dem Kliniker naheliegende) bessere Anpassungsfähigkeit von T. rubrum an veränderte Umweltbedingungen ableiten zu wollen, erscheint zumindest noch verfrüht.

Parenté antigénique et localisation des antigènes dans le genre Candida: Etude par immunofluorescence

P. RIMBAUD, J.-M. BASTIDE, M. BASTIDE et J. ALLEGRINI, Montpellier (France)

L'étude de la structure antigénique des Candida a été déjà réalisée par de nombreux chercheurs. Deux méthodes d'investigation ont surtout été utilisées dans ce but: l'agglutination par l'école japonaise (II) et l'immuno-électrophorèse par BIGUET et ses collaborateurs [5]. TSUCHIYA et coll. ont pu ainsi établir une classification de certaines levures et mettre en évidence sept groupes d'espèces en tenant compte de leur structure antigénique et de leur pouvoir de fermentation et d'assimilation des sucres. Avec l'application de la technique des anticorps fluorescents au domaine de la Mycologie médicale [7] une nouvelle voie de recherches fructueuses s'est révélée. A la suite des premiers travaux de GORDON [6], nous avons essayé de faire l'analyse antigénique de diverses espèces de *Candida* [2, 3, 4 et 9]. Dans ce premier travail, nous donnons les résultats obtenus dans la révélation et la localisation par immunofluorescence des antigènes de *Candida albicans* éventuellement communs à 28 espèces de *Candida*.

I. Matériel et méthodes

C. albicans (*LM 68*), *C. stellatoïdes* (*LM 121*) et *C. tropicalis* (*LM 123*) sont utilisés pour préparer des antigènes destinés à l'immunisation des animaux. Les autres souches de Candida proviennent de notre collection ou de mycothèques spécialisées. Leurs caractères morphologiques et biochimiques ont été rigoureusement contrôlés.

1. Préparation des antigènes

Trois types d'antigènes sont utilisés: cellulaire, pariétal et cytoplasmique.

a) *Antigène cellulaire:* C'est une suspension en eau salée à neuf de *Candida albicans* (LM 68) provenant d'une culture de 48 h sur milieu M.M. (I). Elle est numérée à la cellule compte-microbes.

b) *Antigènes pariétal et cytoplasmiques:* On prépare une masse microbienne par culture sur milieu M.M. en boite de Roux pendant 48 h. Cette masse microbienne est lavée deux fois à l'eau distillée stérile. Après centrifugation, le culot microbien est remis en suspension dans l'eau distillée stérile et il est broyé pendant 40 min au broyeur à billes de verres de type Braun. La destruction cellulaire obtenue est supérieure à 90%. Le broyat est centrifugé à 6.000 t/m pendant 15 min à +4°C. Le culot et le surnageant sont recueillis séparément. Le surnageant constitue l'antigène cytoplasmique, il est standardisé de telle sorte que 10 g de cet antigène correspondent à 1 g de cellules entières. Le culot constitué par les parois cellulaires de levures est lavé deux fois à l'eau distillée stérile. Il est remis en suspension dans l'eau distillée et constitue l'antigène patiétal. Il est standardisé de façon à ce que 10 g de cet antigène correspondent à 1 g de cellules entières.

2. Préparation des antisérums

Ces antigènes sont respectivement utilisés pour l'immunisation de trois lots de lapins.

a) *Sérum anti-levure entière:* Il est préparé par injection intraveineuse de la suspension de Candida albicans. On injecte 100×10^6 blastospores en douze injections réparties sur 5 semaines.

b) *Sérum anti-paroi et sérum anti-contenu cellulaire:* Ils sont préparés par injection intraveineuse respectivement de 5 ml d'antigène pariétal et de 6 ml d'antigène cytoplasmique en douze injections réparties sur 5 semaines. Après la période d'immunisation, le sang des animaux est recueillie par ponction cardiaque. Les sérums sont inactivés, répartis en flacons et congelés à −30 °C.

c) *Antisérums absorbés:* Divers antisérums spécifiques d'une seule fraction ou de plusieurs fractions antigéniques, selon la structure établie par TSUCHIYA, sont préparés d'après le tableau suivant:

Antisérums	Souche absorbante	Antisérum spécifique
Anti-Candida tropicalis	C. stellatoïdea	6
Anti-Candida albicans	C. stellatoïdea	6, 7
Anti-Candida stellatoïdea	C. guillermondi	5, 10, 32
Anti-Candida albicans	C. zeylanoïdes	5, 6, 7
Anti-Candida albicans	C. kruseï	3, 4, 6, 7

Les absorptions se font sur les antisérums inactivés dans lesquels on met en suspension la souche absorbante provenant d'une culture de 48 h sur milieu M.M. Les suspensions sont portées au bain-marie à agitation pendant 2 h à 37 °C, puis 12 h à +4 °C et enfin 2 h à 37 °C. Après ce traitement on centrifuge et on recueille le sérum surnageant dont on contrôle par agglutination sur lame l'absence d'anticorps correspondant à la souche absorbante. On poursuit les absorptions avec une nouvelle culture de 48 h si nécessaire.

3. *Réaction d'immunofluorescence*

La technique d'immunofluorescence utilisée dérive de celle de WELLER et COONS à l'isothiocyanate de fluorescéine. Afin d'assurer le contact parfait entre les antigènes et les anticorps mis en jeu et pour ne pas dénaturer les antigènes nous avons réalisé cette technique en tube, sans fixation préalable, selon la technique décrite dans une publication précédente [10]. Le schéma général est le suivant:

— mettre en suspension dans un tube à hémolyse d'une öse de platine de l'antigène à étudier provenant d'une culture de 48 h dans 0,1 ml du sérum anti-*Candida* à fixer. Laisser en contact pendant 45 min au bain-marie à 37 °C;

— faire deux lavages successifs au tampon phosphaté à pH 7,2 en s'aidant d'une centrifugation à 5.000 t/m;

— mettre en suspension le culot précédent dans deux gouttes de sérum antiglobuline de lapin marqué à l'isothiocyanate de fluorescéine. Laisser fixer pendant 30 min au bain-marie à 37 °C;

— laver deux fois au tampon à pH 7,2 avec centrifugation comme précédemment;

— faire un frottis à partir du culot ainsi obtenu, laisser sécher et observer au microscope à fluorescence.

Les différentes espèces de Candida examinés en immunofluorescence proviennent d'une culture de 48 h sur milieu M.M. Pour chaque espèce, la réaction est répétée quatre fois afin de s'assurer d'une bonne reproductibilité des résultats. Chaque essai comporte un témoin souche traité uniquement par le sérum anti-*Candida* ou par le sérum anti-globuline marquée pour éliminer les réactions dues à l'autofluorescence où à la fluorescence non spécifique. L'intensité de la fluorescence observée est appréciée selon l'échelle de valeur suivante:

0 ou ±	Fluorescence négative
+	Fluorescence médiocre
++	Fluorescence faiblement positive
+++ ou ++++	Fluorescence positive
+++++	Fluorescence fortement positive

II. Résultat et discussion

Parenté antigénique. L'étude comparative des réactions d'immunofluorescence entre divers sérums anti-*Candida albicans* et les 28 espèces de Candida utilisées est résumée dans le Tab. 1. La lecture de ces tableaux nous permet d'établir des degrés différents de parenté antigéniques entre *C. albicans* et les diverses espèces. Le groupe *C. tropicalis, C. claussenii, C. stellatoïdea* parait très proche de *C. albicans*. Ensuite vient le groupe *C. krusei, C. zeylanoïdes, C. guillermondii, C. macedoniensis, C. catenulata*, etc. Enfin le groupe *C. scottii, C. utilis, C. curvata, C. humicola* ne présente aucune parenté avec *C. albicans*.

En général, le sérum anti-paroi donne des réactions d'immunofluorescence légèrement plus fortes que celles obtenues avec le sérum anti-levure entière. Par contre, le sérum anti-contenu cellulaire est relativement peu antigénique vis à vis de C. albicans et de la plupart des espèces étudiées sauf *C. kruseï*, *C. zeylanoïdes*, *C. lipolytica*, *C. intermedia*, *C. pulcherrima*, *C. pelliculosa*, *C. utilis*.

Tableau 1. *Réactions d'immunofluorescence entre des sérums anti-Candida albicans et divers antigènes*

Antisérums Antigènes	C. albicans Levures vivantes	C. albicans Parois	C. albicans Contenus cellulaires
C. albicans (4 souches)	++++	++++	+
C. claussenii	++++	+++	++
C. tropicalis (4 souches)	+++	++++	+
C. stellatoïdea (3 souches)	+++	++++	+
C. kruseï (4 souches)	+++	+++	++
C. zeylanoïdes (2 souches)	+++	++	++
C. guilliermondii (3 souches)	+++	++	+
C. macedoniensis	++	+++	+
C. catenulata	++	+++	+
C. brumptii (2 souches)	++	++	+
C. mesenterica	++	++	
C. reukaufii	++	++	+
C. solani	++	+	+
C. parakrusei (2 souches)	++	++	+
C. parapsilosis (2 souches)	++	+	+
C. pseudotropicalis	+	++	±
C. lipolytica (2 souches)	+	+	++
C. intermedia	+	±	++
C. pulcherrima (2 souches)	±	±	++
C. robusta (2 souches)	+	+	+
C. mycoderma (2 souches)	+	+	+
C. rugosa (3 souches)	±	+	+
C. tenuis	+	+	±
C. pelliculosa (2 souches)	±	+	±
C. melinii	±	±	±
C. curvata	±	±	0
C. scottii	0	±	
C. utilis	0	0	±
C. humicola	0	0	0

Il est donc possible de penser que certaines fractions antigéniques communes avec C. albicans se retrouvent suivant les espèces soit dans la paroi, soit dans le cytoplasme de la cellule. Dans le but de vérifier cette hypothèse nous avons essayé d'utiliser des sérums anti-*Candida albicans* absorbés par C. kruseï, C. zeylanoïdes et C. stellatoïdea et qui par conséquent ne révèlent plus respectivement que les fractions 3, 4, 6 et 7 ou 5, 6 et 7 ou 6 et 7. Nous donnons dans le Tab. 2 les résultats obtenus par Immunofluorescence comparativement au sérum anti-*Candida albicans* non absorbé. On retrouve ainsi la présence des fractions 3, 4, 5, 6 et 7 ou seulement certaines d'entre elles dans la plupart des espèces conformément au schéma établi par Tsuchiya. En particulier, *C. zeylanoïdes* dont la structure antigénique est 1, 2, 3, 4, 13, 17 selon Tsuchiya donne une réaction positive avec l'anti-sérum 3, 4, 6, 7 et une réaction négative ou médiocre avec les anti-sérums 5, 6, 7 et 6, 7.

Toutefois certains de nos résultats ne confirment pas totalement la structure établie par l'école japonaise: *C. macedonensis* et C. pseudotropicalis, dont la structure est voisine (1, 8, 10, 28, 31) présentent des réactions d'immunofluorescence positives avec l'antisérum 5, 6, 7.

La fluorescence que nous avons observée dans toutes les réactions précédentes parait localisée à la surface des levures. Toutefois pour *C. albicans*, *C. claussenii* et

Tableau 2. *Réactions d'immunofluorescence entre un sérum anti-Candida albicans non adsorbé et adsorbé et divers antigènes*

Antisérums Antigènes	C. albicans non adsorbé	C. albicans adsorbé par C. stella-toïdea	C. albicans adsorbé par C. kriuseï	C. albicans adsorbé par C. zeyla-noïdes
C. albicans (4 souches)	++++	++	+++	+++
C. claussenii	++++	++	+++	++
C. tropicalis (3 souches)	+++	++	++	++
C. stellatoïdea (3 souches)	+++	±	++++	++
C. kruseï (4 souches)	+++	++	0	+++
C. zeylanoìdes (2 souches)	+++	+	+++	0
C. guilliermondii (3 souches)	+++	+	++	±
C. macedoniensis	++	++	+	++
C. catenulata	++	++	+	++
C. brumptii (2 souches)	++	+	±	+
C. mesenterica	++	+	++	+
C. reukaufii	++	+	++	+
C. solani	++	++	+	+
C. parakrusei (2 souches)	+	++	+	++
C. parapsilosis (2 souches)	++	++	++	+
C. pseudotropicalis	+	++	+	++
C. lipolytica (2 souches)	+	+	+	++
C. intermedia	+	±	±	+
C. pulcherrima (2 souches)	±	±	±	+
C. robusta (2 souches)	+	+	+	+
C. mycoderma (2 souches)	+	+	+	+
C. rugosa (3 souches)	±	±	+	+
C. tenuis	+	±	++	+
C. pelliculosa (2 souches)	±	+	±	0
C. melinii	±	±	±	0
C. curvata	±	±	±	0
C. scottii	0	0	0	±
C. utilis	0	±	0	+
C. humicola	0	0	0	0

C. tropicalis nous avons obtenu des images différentes. En effet ces trois espéces traitées par le sérum anti-5, 6, 7 ou anti 6, 7 montrent une fluorescence de surface et une fluorescence interne très localisée de même intensité. On peut penser, compte-tenu de la structure antigénique de ces espèces, que la fraction 6, et peut être la fraction 5, se trouve également réparties dans leur paroi et dans leur cytoplasme. Il est curieux de noter que le sérum anti-3, 4, 6, 7 ne donne pas cette fluorescence interne. Tout se passe comme si la réaction antigénique sur les sites 3 et 4, qui sont vraisemblablement pariétaux comme ont pu l'établir KEMP et SOLOTOROVSKY [8], empéchait l'accés aux sites 5 ou 6. Pour préciser la position de ces deux fractions nous avons préparé les sérums anti-5, 10, 32 et anti-6. Nous avons pu ainsi étudier par immunofluorescence leur localisation dans la paroi ou dans le cytoplasme de diverses espèces. Le Tab. 3 rendent compte des résultats obtenus. Pour chaque espèce examinée nous avons mis en rappel la structure antigénique établie par TSUCHIYA.

C. albicans, C. claussenii, C. tropicalis et C. parapsilosis possédent la fraction 5 à la fois dans leur paroi et dans leur cytoplasme. C. stellatoïdea, C. kruseï, C. catenulata, C. mycoderma et C. melinii présentent une localisation presque uniquement pariétale de la fraction 5. Notons que cette fraction est surtout intra-cytoplasmique chez C. pulcherrima.

La fraction 6 est répartie également en surface et dans le corps cellulaire de C. tropicalis et C. albicans. Elle parait de nature surtout pariétale chez C. claussenii.

Signalons enfin le comportement très particulier de *C. pulcherrima* et de *C. pelliculosa* qui montrent une fluorescence intra-cytoplasmique respectivement avec les sérums anti-6 et anti-5 alors que leur formule antigénique ne présente pas les fractions 6 ou 5.

Tableau 3. *Localisation cytologique de diverses fractions antigéniques*

Espèces	Structure Antigénique (selon TSUCHIYA)	Sérum Anti-Fraction 5, (10, 32)		Sérum Anti-Fraktion 6	
		Paroi	Cytoplasme	Paroi	Cytoplasme
C. albicans	1, 2, 3, 4, 5, 6, 7	++++	++	+++	++
C. claussenii	1, 2, 3, 4, 5, 6, 7	+++++	++	++++	+
C. tropicalis	1, 2, 3, 4, 5, 6	++++	++	++	++
C. stellatoïdea	1, 2, 3, 4, 5, 10, 32	+++	±	0	0
C. kruseï	1, 2, 5, (11), b	+++	±	±	±
C. guilliermondii	1, 2, 3, 4, 9	+	±	0	±
C. macedoniensis	1, 8, 10, 28, 31,(a)	±	±	±	±
C. catenulata	1, 2, 5, 11, b	+++	±	0	±
C. brumptii	1, 2, 19	±	0	±	0
C. mesenterica		++	0	±	0
C. reukaufii	1,2,(5),(11),(12),b,f	+	±	±	±
C. solani	1, 2, 5, 11, 12, 20, 21, 37	+	±	±	±
C. parakrusei	1, 2, 3, 5, 13, (14), (15), c	++	+	0	±
C. parapsilosis	1, 2, 3, 5, 13, (14), (15), c	+++	++	0	±
C. pseudotropicalis	1, 8, (10), 28, 31, a	±	±	±	±
C. lipolytica	1, 2,	±	±	±	±
C. pulcherrima	1, 2, 3, 5, 13, (14), (15), d	+	++	0	++
C. mycoderma	1, 2, 5, 11, 12	++++	±	0	0
C. rugosa	1,2,3,4,11 19,g	±	0	±	0
C. tenuis		++	+	0	0
C. pelliculosa	1,2,14,15,16,20	0	++	±	±
C. melinii	1,2,3,5,10,17,25	+++	+	±	0
C. utilis	1, (2), (14), (16), 17, c	0	±	±	±

La technique des anticorps fluorescents nous a permis de constituer des groupes d'espèces présentant une parenté plus ou moins proche de *C. albicans*. C'est ainsi que nous avons pu montrer l'étroite parenté de *C. albicans*, *C. tropicalis*, *C. claussenii* et C. stellaoïdea et au contraire le peu d'affinité qu'il existe entre *C. albicans*, *C. curvata*, *C. scottii*, *C. utilis* ou *C. humicola*. L'utilisation de sérum anti-paroi ou anti-contenu cellulaire met en évidence la très forte antigénicité de la paroi comparativement au cytoplasme lui-même sauf pour quelques espèces dont *C. pulcherrima*. A l'aide de sérums spécifiques d'une ou plusieurs fractions antigéniques, nous avons pu retrouver dans la plupart des cas la structure antigénique établie par TSUCHIYA.

De plus ces sérums spécifiques nous ont révélé la présence pariétale ou intracytoplasmique des antigènes 5 et 6. Mais la position de ces antigènes ne parait pas identique pour toutes les espèces qui les possédent: l'antigène 5 est pariétal et cytoplasmique chez *C. albicans*; il est pariétal chez *C. catenulata*, *C. mycoderma* ou *C. melinii* il est intra-cytoplasmique chez *C. pulcherrima* ou *C. pelliculosa*. De même la proportion relative d'une fraction antigénique donnée est variable d'une espèce à l'autre. C'est ainsi que le sérum anti-5 donne une réaction d'immunofluorescence très forte avec *C. claussenii* et *C. mycoderma* par exemple, et très faible avec *C.*

pulcherrima ou *C. solani*. Les deux premières espèces sont riches en fraction 5, les deux dernières en sont pauvres.

Enfin nous avons pu noter dans quelques cas certaines discordances entre nos résultats et ceux de Tsuchiya. Ces discordances ne sont pas profondes; elles sont certainement dues aux techniques différentes utilisées. En effet, même si les anti-corps fluorescents et les anticorps agglutinants concernent des sites antigéniques identiques de *Candida*, ce qui reste encore à démontrer, il est bien certain que leur «avidité» pour un site antigénique donné peut être totalement différente. Nos recherches se poursuivent dans ce sens et nous essayerons d'en élargir le cadre.

Bibliographie: 1. Bastide, M.: These Doct. Etat Pharm. Montpellier **49**, 85 (1965). — 2. Bastide J.-M., C. Bessiere, M. Bastide et J. Allegrini: Soc. franç. Mycologie médicale. Journées Montpelliéraines 1966. — 3. Bastide, J. M., J. Allegrini et M. Bastide: Soc. franç. Mycologie Médicale. Séance du 27 Janvier 1967. — 4. Bessiere, C., F.-M. Bastide, M. Bastide et J. Nakam: Trav. Soc. Pharm. Montpellier **25**, 256 (1965). — 5. Biguet, J., P. Tarn van Ky, and S. Andrieu: Mycopathol. et Mycol. **17**, 239 (1962). — 6. Gordon, M.-A.: Proc. Soc. exp. Biol. (N.Y.) **97**, 694 (1958). — 7. Kaplan, W., and L. Kaufman: Sabouraudia **1**, 137 (1961). — 8. Kemp, G., and M. Solotorovsky: J. Immunol. **93**, 305 (1964). — 9. Rimbaud, P., et J.-M. Bastide: Soc. franç. Derm. Syph. 1966, (Sous presse). — 10. Rimbaud, P., J.-M. Bastide, M. Bastide et J. Allegrini: XIIIéme Congrés des Sociétés de Pharmacie du Sud de la Loire, Marseille, Mai 1967 (Sous presse). — 11. Tsuchiya, T., Y. Fukazawa, and S. Kawakita: Mycopathol. et Mycol.

Essais de marquage de Candida albicans par radioisotopes. Etude de leur distribution dans l'organisme du lapin

S. Antonescu, IIe Clinique Dermatologique Bucarest (Roumanie)

Les recherches effectuées ont eu les buts suivants:

1. trouver des substances marquées avec des radioisotopes qui soient fixées par les cellules levuriques en quantités suffisantes pour permettre de poursuivre la distribution des cellules devenues radioactives dans l'organisme du lapin infecté expérimentalement;

2. l'étude par la méthode radioisotopique quantitative de certaines nécessités métaboliques de *Candida albicans*;

3. l'investigation en dynamique de la radioactivité sanguine et urinaire chez les lapins inoculés avec *C. albicans* marquée par des radioisotopes.

C. albicans cultivée sur des milieux contenant des principes nutritifs et des facteurs de croissance marqués par ^{32}P, ^{35}S, ^{14}C et ^{59}Fe fixe ces isotopes, devenant radioactive (après avoir été débarrassée de l'excès de radioisotopes du milieu de culture par des lavages et des centrifugationes successives, les cellules levuriques — à la différence du liquide de lavage — restent radioactives.

La quantité de radioisotopes fixés par les cultures de *C. albicans* varie en rapport avec les *nécessités métaboliques de la cellule mycélienne*, la concentration des radioisotopes dans le milieu et, probablement, avec la souche cultivée. Ainsi, le fer, la cystéine et la glycine sont fixés en quantités infimes (0.001 à 0.002 g-%), tandis que la métionine, la thiamine et le phosphate disodique sont fixés en quantités bien plus élevées (0,43 à 1,45 g-%) et suffisantes pour permettre la mise en évidence des cellules mycéliennes par la méthode autoradiographique.

Nous avons également réussi le double marquage des *C. albicans* et *C. krusei*, en les cultivant dans des milieux qui contenaient aussi bien du phosphate disodique ^{32}P, que de la méthionine ^{35}S.

Les inoculations par voie intraveineuse chez le lapin des cultures de *C. albicans* et de *C. krusei*, doublement marquées par du ^{32}P et ^{35}S et l'étude de la radio-activité des homogénats d'organe, ainsi que les histoautoradiographies des animaux qui ont succombés en 72 à 120 h (inoculés avec *C. albicans*), ou qui ont été sacrifiés après le même intervalle de temps (injectés avec *C. krusei*), ont permis les observations qui suivent:

1. les lapins inoculés avec *C. albicans* présentent une radioactivité sanguine (preuve de la septicémie candidienne), qu'on ne retrouve pas chez les lapins inoculés avec *C. krusei*;

2. la distribution des cellules levuriques dans l'organisme des lapins n'est pas homogène, l'indice topique variant d'organe à organe.

Les déterminations effectuées ont montré les valeurs suivantes: pour *C. albicans* — reins = 14,65; foie = 14,25; cerveau = 5,85; rate = 2,54; poumon = 1,5; sang = 1,36; myocarde = 0,54 et pour *C. krusei* — foie = 2,35; rate = 1,91; reins = 1,81; cerveau = 1,06; poumon = 1,02; myocarde = 0,31. Ces variations s'expliquent par l'affinité d'organe du microorganisme, reliée à la pathogénicité différente des souches, fait également attesté par les histoautoradiographies. Tandis que la souche pathogène *(C. albicans)* prolifère, réalisant des granulomes nodulaires, dans lesquels les cellules mycéliennes restent intègres, la souche non-pathogène *(C. krusei)* présente une dissémination relativement uniforme, subissant en même temps un procès de lyse des cellules mycéliennes, avec libération des substances marquées par radioisotopes et leur éventuelle élimination.

Les recherches comparatives sur la dynamique de la radioactivité sanguine et urinaire, dans les premières 48 h après l'inoculation des lapins à infection expérimentale avec *C. albicans* marquée avec ^{32}P et ^{35}S ont montré que la radioactivité sanguine est sensiblement plus élevée que celle urinaire; de même, tandis que la seconde se maintient à un niveau constant, la première subit des fluctuations marquées; sur le fond d'une radioactivité quasi-constante, apparaissent des crochets qui correspondent probablement aux décharges d'éléments fongiques des foyers viscéraux, dont le dernier exprime la décharge préagonique.

Ces faits indiquent la nécessité — lorsqu'il s'agit du diagnostic clinique de septicopyohémie candidienne — d'exécuter des hémocultures répétées à brefs intervalles. La présence des cellules levuriques dans l'urine apparaît comme un épiphénomène, explicable par l'existence de microabcès rénaux, accompagnés de rupture de la barrière glomérulaire et de l'élimination des éléments levuriques métastasés dans les reins. Cette levururie constante fait de l'uroculture un test utile pour le diagnostic de la septicémie candidienne, en cas de symptômes de glomérulonéphrite en foyer.

Observations of the Treatment of Superficial Mycosis in South-East Europe with CO_2Snow (Method-Haxthausen)

M. BRNIčEVIć, Department of Dermatology, General Hospital, Osijek (Yugoslavia)

In the year 1950 a well-known Danish dermatologist, Prof. HAXTHAUSEN from the University of Copenhagen, published his observations and results of the transformation of superficial trichophytosis into deep mycosis with local application of CO_2 snow (attempt at artificial immunization).

His essential idea was: "that Kerion formation is attended by processes of immunization which result in local healing. This immunity effects the disappearance of superficial patches of trichophytosis also without local treatment of these lesions."

So far it has been known, that with treatment of superficial mycosis by means of different ointment one can unintentionally cause inflammation and deep mycosis. This inflammation has plausibly indicated an animal origin of infection (zoophilic species) because of occurring in agricultural regions.

In the post-war circumstances this proposition inspired the hope, that this method would give one the opportunity of transforming deliberately and in controlled manner, not only superficial trichophytosis, but all the superficial mycosis into deep mycosis attended by processes of immunization. Especialy because he had previously treated 24 patients all successfully.

Our region (Osijek, Yugoslavia, South-East Europe) situated in the walley of the Danube is similar to Denmark as an agricultural land with many cattle-breeding farms.

However, this area has, in addition, a particular characteristic which is a consequence of historic development. Here through centuries was the border between Europe and the Turkish Empire. There were repeated migrations of people from subtropic regions of Nord Afrika and all the countries of Near-East to the South-East Europe. These migrations of people brought with them several infectious subtropic diseases such as the fungus disease Favus (it is a subtropic form of trichophytosis).

In this area the following cases of mycosis were treated with CO_2 snow:

a) All superficial mycosis of the hair on children: Trichophytosis and Favus (in our region there is no Microsporia).

b) All superficial mycosis on adults: Trichophytosis in the beard and Favus in the hair.

c) All cases of the trichophytosis on the smooth skin.

During this work it was noticed, that not one case of Favus in the hair reacted with inflammation after treatment with CO_2 snow. The cases of superficial trichophytosis reacted differently. Some cases reacted on the first freezing with CO_2 snow with inflammation, and some other cases did not react on repeated and prolonged freezing.

We could not find satisfactory explanation for this striking difference.

Last year nature itself provided a new experiment, which brought more light to clear up the problem of this different reaction.

A boy, 8 year old, was admitted in hospital ill with one focus of deep trichophytosis in the hair and many other focuses of superficial trichophytosis (the infection was from animal origin). In the meantime trichophytosis spread as an epidemic on many other boys in the neighbourhood.

On the freezing with CO_2 snow, the first cases of ill boys reacted with inflammation and superficial trichophytosis in the hair was transformed into deep mycosis with all its consequences. The last cases of this chain reaction, after several passages of infection from human being to human being, did not react any more with inflammation on this treatment.

As the results of the treatment of superficial mycosis of different ethiology with local application of CO_2 snow, we have come to these fairly plausible conclusions:

1. The cases of superficial mycosis of the hair and beard, whose infection originated from an animal, all reacted with inflammation as a true zoophilic species.

2. The cases of superficial mycosis from human origin, including Favus in the hair, did not react with inflammation as a true anthropophilic species.

3. Zoophilic species, after a number of passages on human beings, reacted no more as a zoophilic species, but like an anthropophilic species. It was evident, that they had undergone certain changes.

The difference in obtained results, between Denmark and South-East Europe, is a consequence of different pathogenic agents: in Denmark there are mostly zoophilic species, and in South-East Europe there are more anthropophilic species or zoophilic species with changed characteristics.

La contamination staphylococcique des trichophyties suppurées. Résultats d'une thérapie combinée: Griséofulvine, antibiotiques antimicrobiennes et traitement local

I. Capusan, P. Balosu et N. Maier, Clinique Dermatologique de Cluj (Roumanie)

La présence des staphylocoques dans les follicules pilo-sébacés a été rapportée par différents auteurs dans une proportion variable entre 25 et 90%. Nous avons donc considéré comme nécessaire d'entreprendre des recherches afin d'identifier la flore staphylococcique des trichophyties suppurées. Cette étude nous a paru d'autant plus importante, que les recherches microbiologiques jusqu'à présent ont été orientées presqu'exclusivement vers les agents mycotiques. Sans vouloir diminuer leur rôle étiologique primordial, nous avons considéré notre investigation d'actualité, par le fait que la griséofulvine se montre inactive contre les bactéries y compris les staphylocoques [1], ceux-ci pouvant maintenir le procès suppuratif de la trichophytie profonde [2 à 4].

Matériel et méthode: notre casuistique est formée par un nombre de 62 malades de trichophytie suppurée (kérions, sycosis...), internés dans notre clinique au cours de deux ans (1963 et 1964). Chaque cas a été diagnostiqué par l'aspect clinique et l'examen mycologique.

L'identification de la flore microbienne a été faite par des cultures sur gélose-sang, ensemencées dans le premier jour d'hospitalisation, avec le pus recolté des lésions non-ouvertes (pustules, abscès). Les souches ainsi isolées ont été identifiées par l'aspect macroscopique des colonies, ainsi que par l'examen microscopique. La pathogénité des staphylocoques a été appréciée à l'aide de la capacité de production du pigment, de l'hémolyse, ainsi que par les tests suivants: agglutination par le plasma humain, coagulation du plasma oxalaté, et pouvoir fibrinolytique. Ultérieurement nous avons effectué l'antibiogramme, par la méthode des rondelles.

Les résultats de nos recherches ont été condensés dans les tableaux suivants. Le premier donne les résultats de l'ensemencement, le second le comportement dans les tests de pathogénité:

Tableau 1

Ensemencements	Résultats	
	En chiffres absol.	%
Nombre total des malades	62	100
Cultures positives pour staph.	40	64
Tétragènes et cocci non-pathog.	5	8
Cultures demeurant stériles (ensemencements répétés)	17	27

Tableau 2

Caractéristiques des souches isolées	Résultats positifs	
	En chiffres absol.	%
Cultures positives pour staph.	40	64
Dont: souches hémolytiques	31	50
souches chromogènes (dorées)	21	34
souches agglut. par le plasma	15	24
souches coagulant le plasma	12	19
souches lysant la fibrine	5	8

Pour compléter le Tab. 2, nous relatons qu'un nombre de 18 souches (presqu'un tiers des cas), ont présenté une positivité à trois tests de pathogénité, simultanément.

La contamination staphylococcique est donc présente dans environ deux tiers des cas de trichophytie suppurée, dans un tiers des cas avec des germes d'une pathogénité marquée. Cette constatation nous a orientés vers la nécessité d'une thérapie antibiotique complexe, en ajoutant à la griséofulvine des antibiotiques antimicrobiennes.

Tableau 3

Antibiotique	Sensibilité
Pénicilline	45%
Stréptomycine	45%
Erythromycine	68%
Chloramphénicol	79%
Tétracyclines	80%

Dans ce but, nous avons déterminé l'antibiogramme des staphylocoques isolés. Le Tab. 3 rend les résultats cumulatifs; notre attitude thérapeutique a tenu compte de ces résultats, nous avons administré simultanément avec la griséofulvine, l'antibiotique trouvé le plus actif. Conjointement nous avons appliqué toujours des mesures thérapeutiques locales, que nous considérons absolument indispensables: décapage des croûtes, épilation des poils malades, ponction des pustules et des abcès, applications de compresses désinfectantes, suivies après quelques jours par d'onguents aux dérivés cortisoniques et antibiotiques (voir l'antibiogramme). De cette manière nous avons réduit la durée du traitement à 10 à 14 jours et de l'hospitalisation à 17 jours en moyenne.

Nous n'avons pas observé aucun cas de «sensibilisation croisée» entre les mycoses et l'antibiothérapie, ni l'apparition des trichophytides (lichen).

Bibliographie. 1. MEHNERT, B.: Arzneimittel-Forsch. **12**, 1166 (1962). — 2. RIMBAUD, P., J. A. RIOUX et S. RAVOIRE: Bull. Soc. franç. Derm. Syph. **70**, 43 (1963). — 3. BALOGH, E., and M. SIMON: Börgy. Ven. Szle (Budapest) **40**, 122 (1964). — 4. KAISER, L.: Dermatologica (Basel) **121**, 52 (1960).

Tratamiento de las tiñas on Griseofulvina

M. P. MIGUENS, Santiago de Compostela (Espagna)

En el año 1960 hemos publicado nuestras primeras experiencias en el tratamiento de las tiñas con Griseofulvina (PEREIRO, 1960). Despues de la aparición de preparados de Griseofulvina en microcristales (MCG), y de nuevas pautas establecidas por varios autores en el tratamiento de las tiñas (BLANK y col., 1959; COWAN, 1960; FREIEDNAN y col., 1960; GONZALEZ-OCHOA y col., 1960; IRANZO PRIETO y col., 1960; CONTRERAS DUEÑAS y col., 1962; NEVES y col., 1963; PEDRIQUE

ALVAREZ, 1964; etc.), hemos decidido disminuir la dosis total de medicamento de nuestros pacientes. En la mayoría de los enfermos administramos el medicamento durante 4 ó 5 días de cada semana, acompañado de un tratamiento local. En las tiñas del cuero cabelludo, este último consiste en lavado diario de cabeza, aplicación de preparados antifúngicos (ácido salicilico, yodo y alcohol al 1 ó $\frac{1}{2}$%, y una pomada antifúngica o Naftiomato-T). Cuando existen lesiones inflamatorias recurrimos además a la Penicilina y fomentaciones con sulfato de cobre.

Resultados obtenidos

a) *Tiñas del cuero cabelludo*. Tratamos en total 116 enfermos, de los cuales solo 72 vuelven a control. De ellos a un grupo de 42 pacientes, 2 adultos y los restantes niños de 1 a 12 años de edad, les administramos Griseofulvina MCG, oscilando la dosis de 125 a 500 mg diarios, durante 4 ó 5 dias a la semana (de 1 á 2 años, 125 mg; de 2 á 5, 250 mg de 5 á 10, 375 y 500 mg en sujetos mayores de 10 años). Los cultivos, antes de empezar el tratamiento, nos permitieron aislar: en 27 *M. canis*; en 1, *T. tonsurans*; en 3, *T. violaceum*; en 1, *T. mentagrophytes*; en 3, *T. schoenlein*; siendo en 7 el resultado de los cultivos negativo. El examen micológico directo con KOH (positivo en todos ellos antes de iniciar el tratamiento), se vuelve negativo en el 48% de los casos entre los 20 y 30 días, en el 82% entre los 30 y 60, y en el 96% entre los 60 y 90 días. Otros 30 pacientes fueron tratados con cristales normales (NCG). En 25 de ellos (13 por *M. canis*: 2 por *T. tonsurans*; 2 por *T. schoenlein*; y 8 con cultivo negativo) de 3 a 11 años de edad, administramos 500 a 750 mg diarios, todos los días de la semana. Entre los 20 y 30 días el examen directo fue negativo en el 52%; entre los 30 y 60 días en 93% y a partir de los 60 días negativo en un 100%. Otros 4 pacientes (3 tiñas por *M. canis* y 1 por *T. tonsurans*) recibieron de 500 á 750 mg diarios durante 3 á 5 días a la semana y 1000 mg diarios, 3 días a la semana, un enfermo de tiña favosa por *T. schoenlein*. El examen directo fue negativo en el 66% de los casos entre los 20 y 30 días y en un 75% entre los 30 y 60 días. Como podemos apreciar, los resultados han sido muy similares en todos los grupos, pues teniendo en cuenta el número de enfermos que han vuelto a control, las diferencias entre los tantos por ciento de negatividades en cada uno de ellos tiene poco valor.

b) *Dermatomicosis de la piel lampiña y barba*. En un total de 156 enfermos solo 78 han vuelto a control. En estos, comparando el grupo de los tratados simultáneamente con Griseofulvina y tratamiento local y aquellos en que utilizamos solo este último, no hemos podido apreciar diferencias muy manifiestas. De todas formas nos parece interesante recurrir al medicamento en dermatomicosis acompañadas de prurito intenso o localizadas en zonas en que es difícil la aplicación del tratamiento local (párpados, barba o micosis muy extensas).

c) *Onicomicosis tricofiticas*. En dos casos de onicomicosis de las manos (una ocasionada por *T. tonsurans* y la otra con cultivo negativo) tratados con MCG (500 mg diarios 5 días a la semana) a los 90 días era positivo el examen directo en uno y negativo en el otro. Igual resultado obtenemos en otros 2 pacientes (1 de ellos por *T. rubrum*) a los que administramos MCG. No logramos nunca negativizar las uñas de los pies en pacientes con onicomicosis de esta localización.

No observamos ninguna incompatibilidad medicamentosa en los casos tratados de tiñas del cuero cabelludo. Solamente dos pacientes con micosis de la piel lampiña se quejaron de cefalalgias, prurito, etc. que cedieron al suspenderle el medicamento.

Sporotrichosis Recurrens Cicatrisans
(Repeating Self-Healing Sporotrichosis)

R. N. MIRANDA, Dermatological Clinic of the Federal University of Paraná, Curitiba (Brazil)

From November 1961 to May 1967 15 cases of sporotrichosis were observed and studied in laborers who worked in a Pottery Industry localized near Curitiba.

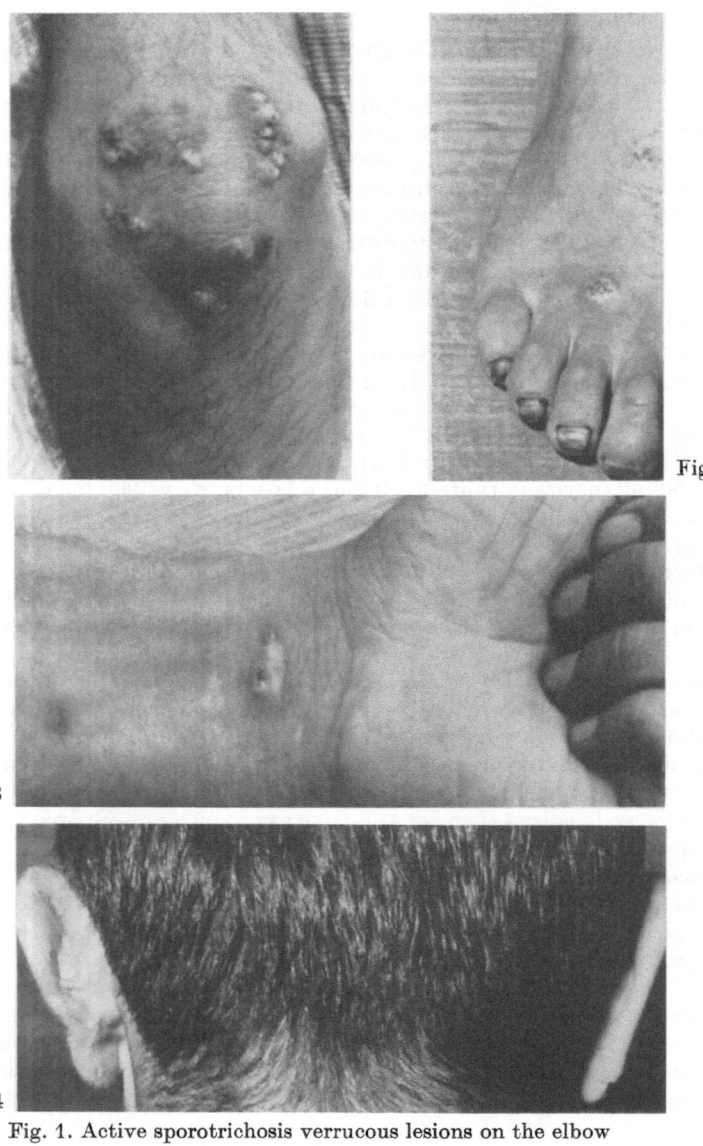

Fig. 1

Fig. 2

Fig. 3

Fig. 4

Fig. 1. Active sporotrichosis verrucous lesions on the elbow
Fig. 2. Active sporotrichosis furuncular lesion
Fig. 3. Scar of self-healed lesion on left and active lesion on right
Fig. 4. Scars of self-healed lesions on the ears

Table. *Studied Sporotrichosis Cases*

No	Name	Age	Sex	First examination	Active skin lesions	Scars	Mycologic diagnosis	Histopathology	Sporo-trichin-skin test	Treatment	Final cure
1	C. S.	33	♂	November, 1961	Verrucous and impetiginous		Sp. Schenkii		Positive	Iodine	October, 1962
2	M. N.	37	♂	December, 1961	Verrucous and impetiginous		Sp. Schenkii	Confirmatory	Positive	Iodine	Without follow-up
3	A. R.	59	♂	December, 1961	Verrucous		Sp. Schenkii				Without follow-up
4	A. C.	24	♂	December, 1961	Verrucous and impetiginous	Present	Sp. Schenkii		Positive		May, 1962
5	G. M.	24	♂	December, 1961	Verrucous	Present	Sp. Schenkii				October, 1962
6	M.E.V.L.	22	♀	December, 1961	Gummatous and verrucous		Sp. Schenkii		Negative	Iodine	October, 1962
7	O. P.	28	♂	December, 1961	Verrucous and impetiginous	Present	Sp. Schenkii				October, 1962
8	L. L. C.	27	♂	December, 1961	Furuncular	Present	Sp. Schenkii				Without follow-up
9	I. V. S.	18	♂	February, 1962	Furuncular and impetiginous	Present	Negative				October, 1962
10	T. B.	17	♀	February, 1962	Verrucous and papular	Present fourteen	Sp. Schenkii	Confirmatory	Positive	Iodine	December, 1963
11	J. C. P.	23	♂	February, 1962	Tubercular and impetiginous	Present	Negative	Confirmatory	Positive	None	October, 1962
12	B. R.	39	♂	October, 1962	None	Present	Sp. Schenkii		Positive	Iodine	December, 1960
13	A. J. M.	20	♂	November, 1962	Nodular with Lymphangitis	Present	Sp. Schenkii		Positive	Iodine	Without follow-up
14	J. G.	29	♂	November, 1965	Tubercular	Present			Positive	Iodine	May, 1967
15	C. B.	20	♂	November, 1965	Impetiginous	Present			Positive	None	May, 1967

13 of these patients presented the disease under special characteristics which led us to consider it being a different and until now undistinguished clinical form of sporotrichosis.

The main characteristics observed were as follows: 1. generally few superficial and small skin lesions of different ages and stages of growth and involution, together with scars of lesions already self-healed; 2. appearance of the disease owing to repeated and intermittent inoculations of the causal microorganism — *Sporotrichum Schenkii* — which introduces itself into the skin through the unclothed and traumatized regions of the body, where the lesions were present; 3. final and natural cure of the disease after an average space of time of two years, even if the individuals remain in the working environment, subject to sources of infection. It was not possible to isolate the causal microorganism from the straw (thought to be the reservoir of *Sporotrichum*) used to package the pottery, even after 600 attempts to obtain cultures.

The analysis of the table shows us the details of the cases studied. In this manner only two patients (n°s 6 and 13) presented deep lesions as most frequently seen in sporotrichosis. In all the other cases the skin lesions were small and superficial, either verrucous and impetiginous or papular, furuncular and tubercular, some of them almost healed without any treatment. Small scars were present in the majority of the patients, on the unclothed regions as well, reminding sometimes sequelae of small-pox or variola. Almost all individuals received iodic treatment after first clinical examinations, which certainly accelerated the cure. But the presence of self-healed lesions before the treatment and the two cases (n°s 11 and 15) finally cured without any medication show us the self-healing — and perhaps vaccinating — character of this sporotrichosis form now described.

Thanks are due to Drs. S. O. P. Costa, F. Schloegel and A. Elias for their aid in mycological examinations and to Drs. G. Kasting and A. Coelho for their histopathological contributions.

Notice: The latin name was given by Prof. F. E. Rabello (Rio de Janeiro).

Traitement expérimental des mycoses cutanées superficielles par l'Amphotéricine B

D. Peryassú et G. Löwy, Ecole de Médecine et Chirurgie de Rio de Janeiro (Brésil)

Une étude initiale réalisée en teignes avec des résultats satisfaisants sur la teigne microsporique nous a animés à essayer l'emploi de l'Amphotéricine B dans des lésions causées par des champignons. Le topique médicamenteux consistait d'une crème contenant de l'Amphotéricine B à une concentration de 1,25%. Comme antibiotique on avait associé le tétracycline à la dose de 2,5%. Dans tous les patients expérimentés même dans les cas de délai jusqu'à 45 jours, il y a eu une parfaite tolérance locale.

Matériel. Pour les recherches on avait utilisé: a) 1 cas de queratomycosis nigricans palmaris; b) 8 cas de pitiriasis versicolor; c) 4 cas de microsporides; d) 11 cas de dermatificie circinée. Le test thérapeutique dans l'application locale a consisté de l'usage trois fois par jour de la crème en question, en y faisant des massages. La méthode occlusive n'a pas été employée.

Résultats obtenus. 1. *Queratomycosis nigricans palmaris* (Tinea nigra palmaris). L'application du topique pendant 30 jours n'a pas réussi à detruire les lésions mais à peine à améliorer de 30% ce qui existait. Nous jugeons qu'elle a été inefficace dans le contrôle de la quératomycose en cause.

2. *Pitiriasis versicolor* (Tinea versicolor). Huit malades de l'âge de 4 à 30 ans ont été traités. Périodes de traitement de 10 à 45 jours. On a atteint les succès suivants: Un patient traité pendant 10 jours a amélioré de 80%. Abandon du contrôle. Deux malades avec des périodes de traitement de 20 à 28 jours ont amélioré de 90%. Abandon du contrôle. Cinq patients traités entre 30 et 45 jours. Deux cures ont été registrées avec 1 an de contrôle, après quoi un d'eux a présenté des lésions de nouveau (Nouvelle contamination?). Deux malades avec une amélioration de 80%, sans contrôle postérieur. Un malade traité pendant 34 jours n'a guère présenté d'améliorations significatives. En conclusion, succès de cure = 25%; résultats satisfaisants = 50% et sans succès = 25%.

3. *Dermatoficie circinée* (Tinea corporis). Ches les quatre patients porteurs de microsporides, la récupération totale a été obtenue dans des délais jusqu'à 40 jours. En face de la possibilité de la cure spontanée du procès, nous nous demandons si le succès que nous avons atteint n'a été dû à ce fait? Dans les onze cas de dermatoficie circinée on a enregistré les succès suivants: Cure clinique des lésions en 6, dans le délai de 30 jours. Contrôle des patients pendant 90 jours, sans avoir enregistré de la récidive. Chez les cinq malades restants il y a eu une amélioration jusqu'à 80% dans des périodes qui ont varié entre 25 et 45 jours de traitement. Il n'y a pas eu de contrôle postérieur parmi ce dernier groupe de malades. En guise d'un aperçu général de ce groupe, on conclue qu'il y a eu un succès satisfaisant de 54,5% des malades en expérience.

Conclusions finales. L'emploi de l'Amphotéricine B a été inefficace dans la queratomycosis nigricans palmaris. Elle a atteint 25% de cures dans la pitiriasis versicolor; 100% de cures dans la microsporide (cures spontanées?) et dans la dermatoficie circinée 54,5% de bons résultats. Parmi les 22 malades que nous avons étudiés dans la présente expérience thérapeutique, 14 sont parvenus à une cure ou à une amélioration de 90%, qui donne un index illusoire de 63,6% de récupération globale, ce qui ne traduit pas la vérité des faits, car dans l'étude séparée 25% de cure en pitiriasis versicolor, et 54,5% en dermatoficies circinées ne justifient point l'emploi de ce topique comme méthode usuelle de traitement.

Experimentelle Grundlagen der externen antimykotischen Therapie

W. Raab, Universitäts-Institut für medizinische Chemie Wien (Österreich)

Bei Anwendung von Kombinationspräparaten auf mikrobiellen Hautveränderungen erhebt sich immer die Frage, ob nicht die Anwesenheit anderer Wirkstoffe die Aktivität der antimikrobiellen Substanzen beeinträchtigt. Die Annahme, daß sich zwei verschiedenartige Wirkstoffe bei gemeinsamer Anwendung in ihren therapeutischen Effekten einfach summieren, erscheint ohne eingehendere experimentelle Prüfung nicht angängig. Im besonderen gilt dies bei Anwesenheit von Corticosteroiden in antimikrobiellen Präparationen, da Corticosteroide den Stoffwechsel von Pilzen aktivieren [1]. In den letzten Jahren wurden die Verhältnisse durch Kombination von fungistatischen Antibiotica, bakteriostatischen Antibiotica und Corticosteroiden noch weiter kompliziert. Im folgenden wird über Modellversuche berichtet, die sich mit der Veränderung antimykotischer Aktivitäten durch bakteriostatische Antibiotica und Corticosteroide befassen.

Die Untersuchungen erfolgten an Candida albicans und Saccharomyces cerevisiae im Warburg-Apparat. Die Verringerung der Sauerstoffaufnahme bei Ruhe-
atmung diente als Maß für die antimykotische Aktivität. Das Inkubationsmedium
bestand aus 2,8 ml Ringer-Lösung pH 7,4 mit 0,2 ml 5%iger Glucose (Temperatur
37 °C, Gasphase Luft). Wegen der schlechten Wasserlöslichkeit einiger untersuchter Wirkstoffe mußten die Untersuchungen zum Teil in einem Milieu mit 3% Alkohol durchgeführt werden; als Kontrollen dienten dann Versuchsansätze mit
gleicher Alkoholkonzentration. Es wurden ausschließlich Wirkstoffe und Wirkstoff-
kombinationen geprüft, die in der Lokalbehandlung von Hautveränderungen Anwendung finden.

Bei der Testung des Einflusses von Corticosteroiden auf den Stoffwechsel der
Hefen fand sich die klinische Erfahrung bestätigt, daß die alleinige Anwendung
von Corticosteroiden auf mykotischen Läsionen ungünstig ist. Sämtliche untersuchten Corticosteroide führten in Konzentrationen von 33 μg/ml zu einer deutlichen Erhöhung des Sauerstoffverbrauches der Testhefen. Die Zunahmen betrugen
zwischen 15 und 30% der Kontrollen. Untersucht wurden die Corticosteroide
Hydrocortison, Methylprednisolon, Triamcinolon und Dexamethason.

Verschiedene fungizide Substanzen (z. B. 4-Chlor-2-oxybenzoesäure-n-butyl-
amid, Dodecyl-triphenyl-phosphoniumbromid oder Dodecyl-dioxyäthyl-benzyl-
ammoniumchlorid) werden in Kombination mit Hydrocortison in der Lokalbehandlung von Mykosen eingesetzt. Die experimentelle Prüfung dieser Kombinationen ergab in Anwesenheit von Hydrocortison jeweils eine Verstärkung der antimykotischen Aktivität der fungiziden Substanzen [2].

Mit Hilfe der Warburg-Methode konnte auch die Zweckmäßigkeit der gleichzeitigen Anwendung zweier fungizider Substanzen überprüft werden. Die kombinierte Einwirkung von Dodecyl-triphenyl-phosphoniumbromid und von Dodecyl-
dioxyäthyl-benzylammoniumchlorid auf Suspensionen von Candida albicans führt
zu einer Steigerung des antimykotischen Effektes, der über das Maß einer einfachen
Summation hinausgeht.

In einer weiteren Untersuchungsreihe wurde die Wirksamkeit fungistatischer
Antibiotica in Gegenwart von Corticosteroiden geprüft. Nystatin (30 μg/ml) und
Pimaricin (30 μg/ml) zeigen in Gegenwart von Corticosteroiden (30 μg/ml) eine
verstärkte Hemmung der Sauerstoffaufnahme von C. albicans und Saccharomyces
cerevisiae. Bei den untersuchten Corticosteroiden handelte es sich um Hydrocortison und Triamcinolon, die auch klinisch mit den geprüften Antibiotica kombiniert
werden [3].

Deutsche Autoren konnten eine Beeinflussung der antimykotischen Wirksamkeit von Nystatin und Amphotericin B durch Aureomycin, Inamycin und Streptomycin nachweisen; je nach den Versuchsbedingungen erfolgt eine Verstärkung
oder Abschwächung der Aktivität der Fungistatica [4]. In der Praxis wird vor
allem Neomycin in Kombination mit fungistatischen Antibiotica angewendet. In
den eigenen manometrischen Untersuchungen war keine Beeinflussung der antimykotischen Aktivität von Pimaricin oder Nystatin durch Neomycin in Konzentrationen zwischen 0,2 und 200 μg/ml nachzuweisen. Zu gleichen Ergebnissen
führten Versuche mit einem anderen bakteriostatischen Antibioticum, Gramicidin.

Beträchtliche Unterschiede ergab die Prüfung von Präparationen, die ein fungi-
statisches Antibioticum, ein bakteriostatisches Antibioticum und ein Corticosteroid enthalten. Im Warburg-Versuch wurden die gleichen relativen Wirkstoff-
konzentrationen eingesetzt, wie sie im dermatologischen Externum vorliegen. Die
Testung einer Kombination von Nystatin, Neomycin und Triamcinolon im Verhältnis von 33:2,5:1 ergab keine Änderung der antimykotischen Aktivität des Nysta-
tins durch die Anwesenheit der anderen beiden Substanzen. Bei gleichzeitiger

Einwirkung von Pimaricin, Neomycin und Hydrocortison im Verhältnis von 2:1:2 erfolgte eine Verstärkung der antimykotischen Wirkung des Pimaricins; dieser Befund läßt sich mit der Anwesenheit relativ höherer Corticosterciddosen erklären.

Am Rande sei hier nur kurz darauf verwiesen, daß sich Warburg-Versuche auch zur Beurteilung kombinierter Wirkstoffeffekte auf Bakterien eignen. Zum Beispiel konnte in derartigen Versuchsserien eine Beeinträchtigung der bactericiden und bakteriostatischen Aktivität von Gentamycin durch Hydrocortison und Fluor-Methylenprednisolon ausgeschlossen werden [5].

Zusammenfassend läßt sich also aussagen, daß Untersuchungen der Zellatmung von Pilzstämmen ein ausgezeichnetes Modell darstellen für die Beurteilung kombinierter Effekte mehrerer Wirkstoffe. Es konnte festgestellt werden, daß Corticosteroide in Kombination mit fungiciden und fungistatischen Substanzen angewendet werden können, ohne daß eine Beeinträchtigung der antimykotischen Aktivität erfolgt. Die bakteriostatischen Antibiotica Neomycin und Gramioidin verursachen keine Veränderung der fungistatischen Wirksamkeit von Nystatin und Pimaricin und können deshalb unbedenklich in kombinierten Präparationen eingesetzt werden.

Literatur. 1. RAAB, W.: Symp. dermat. internat. Bratislava 1966. — 2. RAAB, W., u. R. WERNER: Int. Kongr. Chemother. Wien 1967. — 3. RAAB, W.: Arch. klin. exp. Derm. 228, 72 (1967). — 4. FEGELER, F., u. H. TILKORN: Symp. dermat. internat. Bratislava 1966. — 5. RAAB, W., u. J. WINDISCH: Int. Kongr. Chemother. Wien 1967.

Über den Einfluß von Moronal (-Nystatin) auf den Zellstoffwechsel von Candida albicans. (Autoradiographische Untersuchungen)*

M. RAHMANN-ESSER und F. FEGELER, Hautklinik der Westfälischen Wilhelms-Universität Münster (Deutschland)

Da in zunehmendem Maße therapeutische Erfolge mit Moronal beschrieben wurden, führten wir umfangreichere in vitro-Versuche durch, um die Wirkung von Moronal speziell auf den Zellstoffwechsel von Candida albicans zu prüfen. Mit der Warburg-Methode untersuchten wir den O_2-Verbrauch und gleichzeitig mit Hilfe des Einbaus radioaktiver Substanzen und der autoradiographischen Technik den Einfluß des Antimykotikums auf den DNS-, RNS-, Protein- und Kohlenhydratstoffwechsel. Einige der wichtigsten Ergebnisse seien hier mitgeteilt.

Um Veränderungen im Zellstoffwechsel unter Moronaleinfluß auch eindeutig beurteilen zu können, war es erforderlich, ein geeignetes Kulturmedium zu benutzen. Wir prüften hierzu das Wachstum einer jeweils gleichen, photometrisch ermittelten Menge von Candida-Pilzen in Nährbouillon, 10%igem Hammelserum und 1%iger Glucoselösung. Parallel dazu wurde die Wirkung von 65 γ Moronal/ml Kulturmedium auf die Atmung der Hefen untersucht (Abb. 1). In der Nährbouillon war der O_2-Verbrauch am stärksten. Die Moronaldosis brachte die Atmung fast zum Erliegen. Dagegen erlaubte das Serum als Substrat nur ein geringfügiges Wachstum. Verglichen mit der Kontrolle war die Hemmung nicht besonders deutlich. Erstaunlicherweise zeigten die Keime selbst in nur 1%iger Glucose einen regelmäßigen O_2-Verbrauch, der geringfügig über die Serumkurve anstieg. Erst nach etwa 4 Std zeigte sich die Hemmwirkung von Moronal auf die Atmung. Die

---

* Für wertvolle technische Hilfe sind wir Frl. MARGOT SCHMIDT zu Dank verpflichtet.

Glucoselösung stellte nach diesen Versuchen sicherlich kein optimales Nährsubstrat für Candida-Kulturen dar, was wir auch an einer verstärkten Chlamydosporenentwicklung feststellen konnten. Aber gerade dadurch, daß der Stoffwechsel nicht so lebhaft vor sich ging, konnten die Unterschiede innerhalb der Versuchszeit klarer verfolgt werden. Außerdem erwies sich die Glucose als Nährsubstrat für die Isotopenversuche als besonders günstig, da nur sie als einzige chemische Komponente neben den applizierten radioaktiven Verbindungen im Stoffwechselgeschehen zu berücksichtigen war.

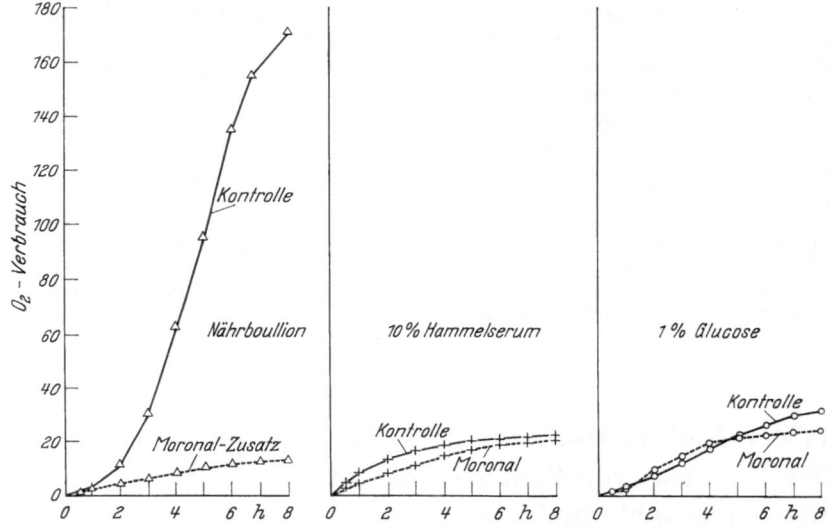

Abb. 1. Verminderung des in Warburg-Versuchen ermittelten O_2-Verbrauchs von Candida albicans in Nährbouillon, 1%igem Hammelserum und 1%iger Glucose als Kulturmedien bei Zugabe von 200 Moronal je Versuchsansatz

Um nun den Grundstoffwechsel von Candida albicans und seine Beeinflußbarkeit durch Moronal genauer zu untersuchen, wurden unter konstanten Warburg-Kulturbedingungen verschiedene radioaktive Vorstufen für hochmolekulare Zellverbindungen dem Glucosenährsubstrat zugesetzt und deren Einbau in die Zellen autoradiographisch nachgewiesen. Es handelte sich um folgende Substanzen: radioaktives 3H-Thymidin als DNS-Tracer, 3H-Uridin als RNS-Tracer, 3H-Histidin als Proteintracer und 3H-Glucose als Kohlenhydrattracer. Damit alle Versuche untereinander vergleichbar waren, wurden neben der jeweils zu testenden radioaktiven Substanz in gleicher Dosis die anderen Stoffe in unmarkierter Form der Glucoselösung zugesetzt, so daß stets die gleiche Menge an Thymidin, Uridin und Histidin zur Verfügung standen. Gegenüber einer Lösung ohne Zusätze führte diese Zugabe stets zu einer geringen Wachstumssteigerung der Candida-Zellen gemessen am O_2-Verbrauch.

Die mit Hilfe der Dipping-Filmtechnik hergestellten Autoradiographien ergaben bemerkenswerte Unterschiede sowohl im Einbau der einzelnen radioaktiven Substanzen in die Zellen als auch im Hinblick auf die Moronalwirkung innerhalb der 8 Std Versuchsdauer. Als Beispiel sind in Abb. 2 einige Autoradiographien über den Thymidin-, Uridin- und Histidin-Einbau in die Candida-Zellen mit und ohne Moronalzusatz zusammengestellt. Nach 8 Std Inkorporationszeit des radioaktiven Tracers hat ein starker Thymidineinbau in die Zellen der Kontrolle statt-

Kontrolle   Moronal-Zusatz

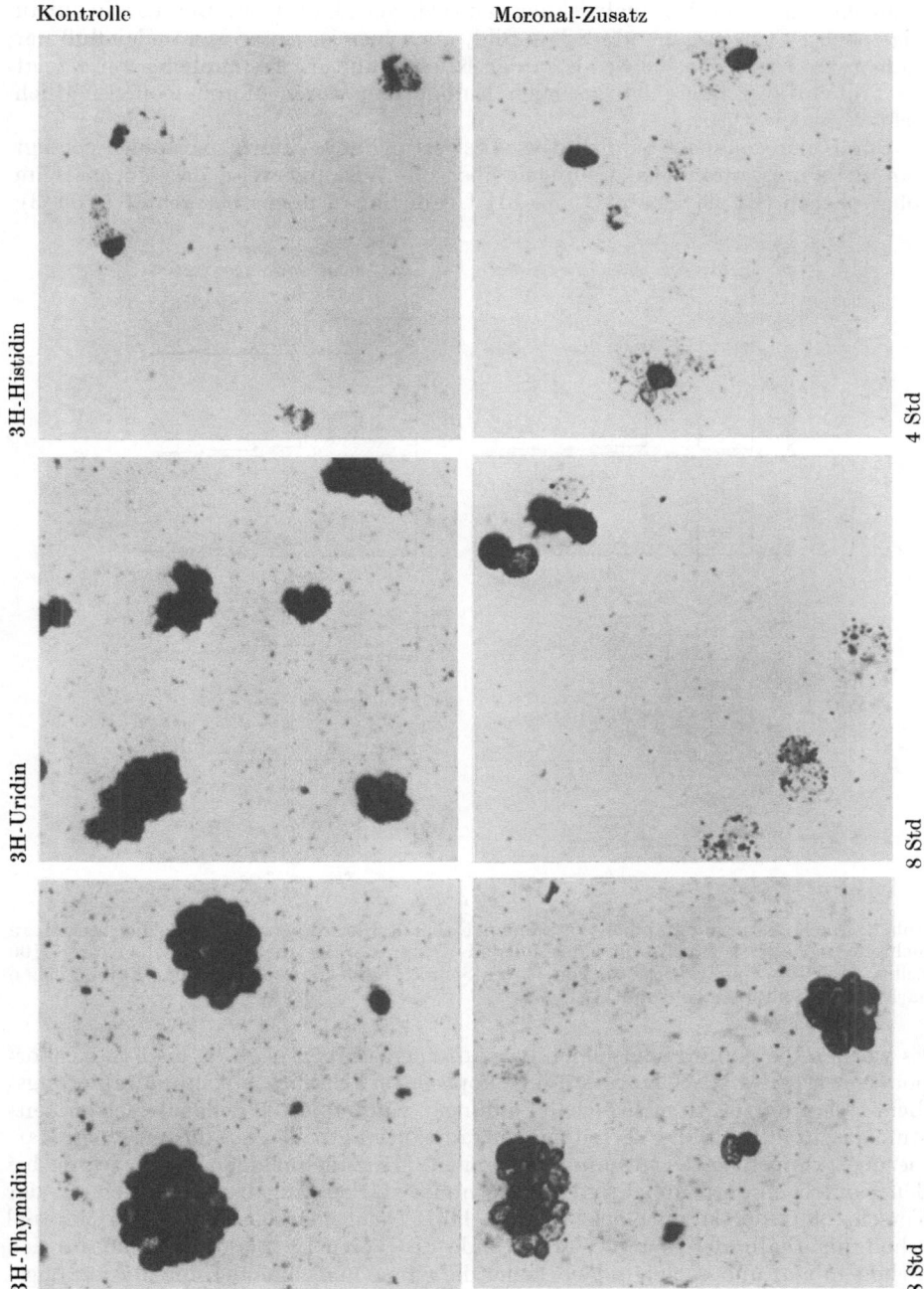

Abb. 2. Mikroautoradiographien des 3H-Thymidin-, 3 H-Uridin- und 3H-Histidineinbaus (25 μC/Versuchsansatz) in die Zellen von Candida albicans nach Inkorporationszeiten der radioaktiven Tracer von 8 bzw. 4 Std. Expositionszeit der Autoradiogramme 3 d. Durch Moronal bei Thymidin und Uridin verminderter Einbau, nicht bei Histidin

gefunden, der unter Moronalwirkung deutlich vermindert ist. Der Uridineinbau zeigt nach 8 Std ein ganz ähnliches Bild, auch hier ist unter Moronaleinfluß der Einbau des Tracers niedriger als in der Kontrollkultur. Erstaunlicherweise zeigt der Proteintracer nur einen geringen Einbau, der durch Moronal offensichtlich nicht verändert wird.

Durch eine genauere quantitative Auswertung der Autoradiographien gelangt man zu interessanten Feststellungen über die Wirkungsweise des Moronals im Zellgeschehen. Es sei hier z. B. der 3H-Uridineinbau näher betrachtet (Abb. 3).

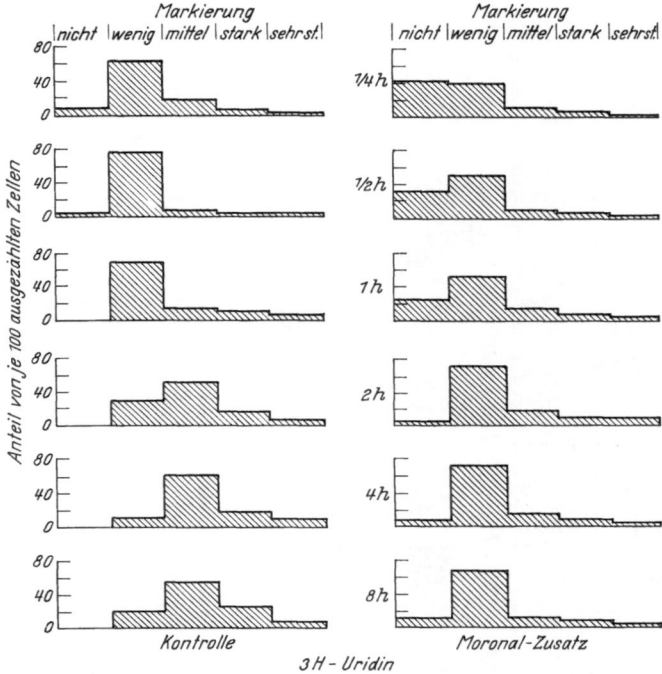

Abb. 3. Nach Autoradiographien zusammengestelltes Blockdiagramm über den Anteil an nicht, wenig, mittel, stark, sehr stark mit 3H-Uridin markierten Candida-Zellen für je 100 Zellen nach Inkorporationszeiten von $^1/_4$ bis 8 Std. Durch Moronal wird der Einbau schon nach kurzer Zeit stark gehemmt

Es wurden die Autoradiographien der einzelnen Proben nach $^1/_4$ bis 8 Std Inkorporationszeit des RNS-Tracers mikroskopisch im Hinblick auf ihre Markierungsdichte ausgewertet. In mehrfachen Zählungen wurden je 100 Zellen derselben Zeitstufe ausgezählt und die Verteilung der radioaktiven Zellen auf die einzelnen Markierungsgruppen im Diagramm aufgetragen. Mit zunehmenden Zeiten wurde bei den Kontrollen das radioaktive Uridin immer stärker eingebaut, wie sich aus der Verschiebung der Hauptblöcke ersehen läßt. Demgegenüber wirkte das Moronal schon innerhalb der ersten Viertelstunde des Versuchs stark hemmend auf den Uridineinbau, und es zeigte sich keine derartige Verschiebung der Markierungsintensitäten mit zunehmenden Zeiten wie bei der Kontrollkultur. Auch nach 8 Std gab es noch Zellen ohne jeden Tracereinbau und der Hauptblock blieb unverändert auf der Stufe „wenig", was bei den Kontrollen schon nach 2 Std nicht mehr der Fall war.

Dieser starke und sofort einsetzende hemmende Einfluß des Moronals auf den

RNS-Stoffwechsel scheint der wesentlichste Faktor in der Moronalwirkung überhaupt zu sein. Demgegenüber begann beim Thymidineinbau ein hemmender Einfluß erst nach 4 Std sichtbar zu werden, während beim Proteinstoffwechsel mit
dem Tracer Histidin während der 8-Std-Versuchsdauer überhaupt kein wesentlicher Unterschied gefunden wurde.

Vielleicht steht mit der RNS-Hemmung die von uns in den Moronalproben
festgestellte deutliche Tendenz zu verminderter Dauersporenbildung in enger Beziehung. Die hier mitgeteilten Ergebnisse sowie die, aus Zeitgründen nicht angeführten, ergänzenden Befunde über den Nachweis eines spezifischen Einbaus der
verwandten radioaktiven Tracer in hochmolekulare Zellverbindungen mit entsprechenden Enzymbehandlungen bringen uns in dem Verständnis um einen An-
satzpunkt des Moronals im molekularen Stoffwechselgeschehen der Candida albi-
cans-Zellen einen beträchtlichen Schritt weiter.

Literatur. FEGELER, F., u. M. RAHMANN-ESSER: Autoradiographische Untersuchungen
zum Stoffwechsel von Candidapilzen. (Im Druck).

Mechanism of Antifungal Action of Potassium Iodide on Sporotrichosis

H. URABE, T. NAGASHIMA and K. NAKASHIMA, Department of Dermatology,
Kurume University School of Medicine, Kurume (Japan)

It has long been known from experience that potassium iodide is highly effective in the treatment of sporotrichosis. GOUGEROT, DAVIS, BLOCH, LOCHER,
SHIBUYA, and others, carried out basic investigations into the therapeutic mechanism of this chemical, but their hypotheses have been based on their data obtained
with the mycelial phase of Sporotrichum schenckii. This fungus is one of those
pathogenic fungi which present dimorphism, and the infective form is the yeast
rather than the mycelial phase. We had felt that it was the yeast phase that was
to be investigated, and carried out studies comparing the two phases with respect
to susceptibility to iodide.

In vitro Studies

Sabouraud dextrose agar was used for the culture of the mycelial phase, and
brain heart infusion blood agar, for the culture of the yeast phase. According to
the fungistatic effect of potassium iodide in varying concentrations, it is clear that
the growth of the mycelial phase was suppressed only at iodide concentration of
20% or above, while a complete fungistatic effect was obtained at its concentration
of 6 to 7% for the yeast phase, indicating a greater susceptibility of the latter to
iodide. The study on the fungicidal effect yielded a similar result. Thus, the yeast
phase was found to be several times more susceptible to potassium iodide than the
mycelial phase, but the iodide concentrations necessary for the fungistatic or
fungicidal effect are too high in vitro, to explain the in vivo effect with its direct
action.

Our next approach to the problem was to study the fungicidal effect of molecular iodine and the result indicated that the mycelial phase was killed after
10 min in a 10 mg-% iodine solution while the yeast phase was killed in a 2 mg-%
solution after the same incubation period. A similar study was conducted using
iodine in potassium iodide solution in which the decrease of molecular iodine is
very small. The mycelial phase was killed after 1 h in a 10 mg-% iodine solution

or after 2 h in a 2 mg-% solution, and the yeast phase was killed after 1 h in a 1 mg-% solution.

Of particular interest was the finding in this study that the fungus remained viable in 10 ml of 1 mg-% solution but was killed if the amount of the same solution was increased to 50 ml or more, even though the iodine concentration and the time of reaction were the same. Similarly, in a 0.6 mg-% iodine solution, the fungus remained viable in the solution of less than 50 ml, and more than 100 ml was required for the fungicidal effect. At iodine concentration of 0.2 mg-%, 200 ml was necessary to kill the fungus, and at 0.1 mg-% or below, 200 ml was still insufficient to obtain the fungicidal effect. These results clearly suggested that the fungicidal effect was proportional to the volume of iodine solution at a given iodine concentration, if the amount of inoculum was kept constant. In fact, if the total iodine in the solution was calculated, the minimal amount of iodine necessary to kill the fungus was between 400 and 600 μg and was rather constant.

Human Study

Three grams of potassium iodide were given daily by mouth to healthy subject for a period of 7 days, and on the 8th day, 3 g was given in one dose and 2 h later, blood was taken which was immediately defibrinated. The defibrinated blood was inoculated with a known amount of the fungus in the yeast phase, incubated at 37 degrees Centigrade and the growth was measured using the Thoma's hemocytometer for cell count.

The starting cell count in the blood was about 1000/cmm, and the count was slightly reduced after 24 h in most instances, and increased thereafter. For the control, the blood withdrawn before the iodide administration was used. There was a definite fungistatic effect in the blood taken after the initiation of the iodide treatment, and the fungistatic effect was more pronounced in proportion to increasing doses of potassium iodide.

In conclusion, these results suggest that the therapeutic effect of potassium iodide for sporotrichosis is through the direct antifungal action of molecular iodine that is formed in the human body and exerts a fungicidal effect on the yeast phase of this fungus which is very susceptible to molecular iodine.

Fissured Nipples of Lactating Females and its Relation to Candida Infection

A. M. EL MOFTY, R. MEHAREB, H. M. EL KOMY and C. D. JEFFRIES, Department of Dermatology, Faculty of Medicine, Cairo University and Ministry of Health, Cairo (UAR)

Fissured nipples in lactating females is a common complaint in the crowded dermatological clinics of UAR. The aim of this work is to find out the role of candida albicans in causation of fissuring of the nipples of lactating females. In the present study 100 cases (50 lactating mothers and culturally). Fissured nipples were found in 34 out of the 50 cases (31 bilateral fissures and 3 unilateral). Most of the mothers suffered from mild to severe pain especially during suckling.

In most of the children clinical manifestations of Candidiasis in the form of napkin dermatitis, perleche and thrush with or without gastro intestinal symptoms were present.

Cultural Studies: Smears from fissures or skin of unaffected nipples were cultured on Sabauroud's Dextrose agar as well as nutrient agar for fungal and bacterial isolation and incubates at 37 °C. Smears from mouths and skin of napkin area of the children were similarly cultured.

Results: Out of the 34 cases of fissured nipples 13 (about 38%) revealed positive cultures of candida albicans. In about 77% of these cases (9) their children gave positive culture of candida albicans. Out of the remaining 21 cases 3 showed saprophytic fungi, 5 bacteria and 13 were culturally negative. Candida albicans was also found in 4 cases out of the 16 cases showing no fissuring of the nipples. In these 4 cases candida albicans was isolated from their children.

Discussion

From the results obtained in the present study it can be concluded that candida albicans is an important etiological factor in the causation of fissured nipples in lactating females. The repeated trauma of suckling, and the increased vascularity and soddeness of the nipples favour the process. Moisture and over cleanliness, disturbing the normal flora of the skin in the site, may be precipating factors. The infection is, most probably, transmitted to the mother from candidal infection of the suckling child as in about 77% of cases of fissured nipples candida albicans could be isolated from both the mother and the child. This proves that candida albicans can be a cause of fissuring of the nipples of lactating females.

Thrush was found to occur in 4% of the new born all over the world [1]. An increase in vaginal fungous diseases has been reported from various places [2, 5]. Rauramo [3] found candida in the vagina of 25% of a series of 305 pregnant women. Johnson and Mayne [4] found fungi in the vagina of 37% on routine examination of 667 pregnant women. Krupp and St. Romain [5] found positive vaginal cultures in 116 out of 232 pregnant women of which 99 (42%) were candida albicans. It has been also found that vaginal infestation with pathogenic monilia without clinical signs and symptoms is of frequent occurrence (i.e. carriers) [6]. Clinical manifestations only appear when a physiological disturbance occurs in the host or in the equilibrium of the flora [7].

This shows that candidal infection of the nipples of lactating mothers can also be a manifestation of auto inoculation from distant foci of candidiasis of the mothers themselves.

References. 1. Harris, L. J.: Amer. J. Obstet. Gynec. **80**, 30 (1960). — 2. Bjoro, K.: J. Norweg. Med. Ass. 13—14, July 1st (1956). — 3. Rauramo, L.: Acta Obstet. gynec. scand. Suppl. **XXX**, 484 (1950). — 4. Johnson, C. G., and R. Mayne: Amer. J. obstet. Gynec. **55**. 852 (1948). — 5. Krupp, P. J., and St. Romain: Vaginal Fungi during Pregnancy. J. Lowis, State Md. Soc. **112**, 5 May (1960). — 6. Garnier, G.: Year Book Dermat. and Syph. Ects, p. 307, 1956—1957. — 7. Dubos, R. J.: J. Amer. med. Ass. **1957**, 1477.

Symposium 8   **Malignant Melanomas**

Mélanomes malins

Melanomas malignos

Melanomalignom

Organizer

K. KITAMURA, Japan

Presidents

H. BEERMAN, USA

B. DUPERRAT, France

W. F. LEVER, USA

F. E. RABELLO, Brazil

Delegate of the Organization Committee

G. K. STEIGLEDER, Germany

Reports

Melanin Biosynthesis in Melanomas*

T. B. FITZPATRICK, Harvard Medical School, Massachusetts General Hospital, Boston, Massachusetts (USA)

The malignant melanoma continues to be a difficult and debatable problem in diagnosis and treatment. Now, however, new methods facilitating early diagnosis and some new approaches to the important problem of therapy are possible because of the rapid progress in our understanding of melanin biosynthesis during the past 10 years — more progress than in the previous 100 years.

This discussion will therefore begin with a précis of melanin biosynthesis and continue with applications of these facts to diagnosis and treatment.

The Tyrosine-to-Melanin Pathway in the Melanocyte

The structural basis of pigmentation in human skin and in neoplasms of pigment cells is the number and distribution of *melanosomes*. Melanosomes are specialized, structured, cytoplasmic particles (organelles) about the size of mitochondria, but completely distinct from mitochondria in nature and origin (MIYA-MOTO et al., 1967). The visibility of the internal structure, as seen in the electron microscope, varies with the density of the melanin content. Melanosomes are synthesized by ribosomes and probably consist of two parts: (1) a matrix or skeleton to which is attached, (2) the aerobic copper-enzyme, tyrosinase. The melanosome is composed of numerous (10 to 15) concentric sheets of a crystalline lattice; each sheet is formed by electron-opaque particles, the particles (80 Å × 30 Å) are arranged in rows, the rows being 85 Å apart (CLARK, 1967). The natural precursor, tyrosine, is transformed by the catalytic action of tyrosinase into an extremely dense amorphous polymer, melanin. Melanin comprises approximately 30% of the dry weight of a melanosome (DUCHON et al., 1967). The number of melanosomes produced and the fine structure of the melanosomes are regulated by (1) several genes, (2) by environmental factors, especially ultraviolet radiant energy, and, possibly, by (3) pituitary melanocyte-stimulating hormone and ACTH.

Established Applications in the Diagnosis of Malignant Melanoma

The unique feature of malignant melanocytes is the presence of melanosomes on which the specialized tyrosine-to-melanin pathway occurs. The presence of this specialized metabolic pathway is the basis for some established and some potential approaches to diagnosis and treatment of malignant melanoma.

1. *Histochemical tyrosinase test in amelanotic melanoma.* Melanoma without melanin can be identified by this simple, specific, and underutilized histochemical test, readily done in any laboratory. This reaction permits a specific diagnosis of melanoma in unpigmented undifferentiated tumors.

2. *Quantitative determination of intermediate metabolites in the tyrosine-melanin pathway.* In the urine of patients with metastatic melanoma there is an increased amount of dopa (TAKAHASHI and FITZPATRICK, 1964). The correlation of urinary dopa with the clinical course of melanoma has not been as extensively studied as has the determination of Thormählen-positive indole intermediates ("indole mela-nogens"). These indole-melanogens have been determined by quantitative colorimetric methods and chromatographic methods in 263 patients (DUCHON and

* Supported by United States Public Health Service, National Cancer Institute Grant Nr. CA-05010, and Damon Runyon Fund for Cancer Research.

PECHAN, 1965). The change in the amount of indole melanogens in the urine appears to have prognostic value, and a patient to be discussed showed a marked increase in indole melanogens one month before clinical dissemination.

3. *The quantity of dopa in malignant melanoma.* Dopa (probably as a peptide) is present in high concentrations in the melanosome (TAKAHASHI and FITZPATRICK, 1966). In an ingenious technique utilizing fluorescent microscopy, dopa or a dopa derivative can be shown to be present in neoplasms of pigment cells (FALCK et al., 1966). The fluorescence in malignant melanoma is more intense than it is in benign nevi.

Potential Applications in Diagnosis and Treatment

1. *Measurement of tyrosinase in serum.* This method depends on the formation of dopa from tyrosine by circulating serum tyrosinase (TAKAHASHI and FITZPATRICK, 1964). When purified human tyrosinase becomes available, sensitive and specific radio-immunoassay of tyrosinase will be possible.

2. *Variations in the fine structure of melanosomes.* Since the size and shape of melanosomes are probably regulated by genes, the fine structure of melanosomes in melanoma may be a genetic marker indicating malignant clones of cells. Recent studies (CLARK, 1967) have revealed that the number of concentric lattice sheets is reduced in the melanosomes of human malignant melanoma.

3. *Uptake of radioactive melanin precursors.* In 1952 at the Xe International Congress of Dermatology we proposed the hypothesis that there is a difference in the tyrosinase activity of benign and of malignant melanocytes; this was based on a histochemical radioautographic technique. We now know that this increased tyrosinase activity is related to the fact that a greater number of melanosomes are synthesized by the malignant cell. Nowhere, except in the expendable melanocytes of the hair bulb, is melanosome synthesis as rapid as it is in the melanoma cell. This permits selective localization of radioactive melanin precursors. Labeled precursors (tritiated and carbon[14]-labeled dopa) have been shown by BLOIS and KALLMAN (1964) and by HEMPEL and DEIMEL (1963, 1966) to be localized in melanomas of mice, the specific activity being much greater than that of any other tissue except the adrenal gland, which is expendable. An effort is now being made to synthesize melanin precursors containing gamma- or beta-emitting ions.

4. *Selective action of chemical agents on melanocytes.* Topical application of mercaptoamines and 4-isopropylcatechol has clearly shown (BLEEHEN et al., 1967) that these compounds have a selective action on mammalian melanocytes, leading to disappearance of melanocytes. Such agents may have a potential in the chemotherapeutic treatment of malignant melanoma.

Bibliography. BLEEHEN, S. S.: Clin. Res. **15**, 247 (1967). — BLOIS, jr., M. S., and R. F. KALLMAN: Cancer Res. **24**, 863 (1964). — CLARK, jr., W. H.: Unpublished studies, 1967. — DUCHON, J.: Unpublished studies, 1967. — DUCHON, J., and Z. PECHAN: Ann. N. Y. Acad. Sci. **100**, 1048 (1963). — FALCK, B.: Acta derm.-venereol. (Stockh.) **46**, 65 (1966). — HEMPEL, K.: In: Symposium on Structure and Control of the Melanocyte, pp. 162—175. Berlin-Heidelberg-New York: Springer 1966. — HEMPEL, K., and M. DEIMEL: Strahlentherapie **121**, 22 (1963). — MIYAMOTO, M.: Unpublished studies, 1967. — TAKAHASHI, H., and T. B. F. FITZPATRICK: J. invest. Derm. **42**, 161 (1964); — Nature (Lond.) **209**, 888 (1966).

Mélanoses neurocutanées of Touraine

T. KAWAMURA and S. IKEDA, Department of Dermatology; S. NODA, Department of Pathology, Faculty of Medicine, University of Tokyo; S. ISHIZU, Department of Dermatology; T. NAKAJIMA, Department of Pathology, School of Medicine, Tôhô University (Japan)

TOURAINE (1949) described the condition where growth of pigmented cells occurs in both of the skin and the central nerve organs, under the heading: Mélanoses neurocutanées. There are more than 30 cases reported outside of our country and seven (eight) cases reported in Japan (Table). The skin lesions in hitherto reported cases are nevus cell nevi.

The nevus cell nevi are explained to be caused by the origination of abnormal cells endowed with poor differentiating potency in the neural crest (T. KAWAMURA [1], 1956). PINKUS and MISHIMA [2] (1961) coined the term nevoblasts for such imaginary cells as mentioned. The nevoblasts which give rise to the nevus cell nevus are refered to here as ordinary nevoblast. Two polar types of cells namely the melanocytes and the Schwannian cells grow out from the normal neural crest. Ordinary nevoblast may give rise to a series of various intermediate cells in the spectrum between the both poler types. The ordinary and other nevoblasts tend to be distributed in the one or both of the cutaneous and perineural "Pigment-hülle" of WEIDENREICH.

Table. *Mélanoses neurocutanées reported in Japan*

Type	Reporters (year)	Age (Sex)	Skin (Histology)	Central Nerve Organ (Histology)	Autopsy
Nevus Cell Nevus	1. ABE et al. (1955)	21 years (♂)	Giant Nevus (Dermal)	Tumor & Melanose ? (+ Melanoma malignum)	Brain only
	2. ISHIZU, KATO[a] et al. (1959)	54 days (♂)	Giant Nevus (Dermal + j), Oral Mucosa (J)	Mélanose (Brain & Spinal Cord) (Nevoid ?)	+
	3. NAKAMURA et al. (1959)	12 years (♀)	Giant Nevus (No Histology)	Mélanose (+ Melanoma malignum)	Brain only
	4[b]. OKINAKA, KAWAMURA, IKEDA et al. (1963)	23 years (♂)	Giant Nevus (Dermal + j)	Infiltration & Mélanose (Brain & Spinal Cord) (+ Melanoma malignum)	+
	5. NISHIYAMA et al. (1963)	10 months (♀)	Disseminated Nevi (Dermal)	Mélanose (Brain) (Nevoid ?)	+
	6. FUKUDA, T. (1963)	31 years (♂)	Pigmented Nevi 10 Areas (Dermal)	Tumor & Mélanose (Brain & Spinal Cord) (+ Melanoma malignum)	+
	7. FUKUDA, Y. et al. (1964)	29 years (♂)	Giant Nevus (Dermal)	Tumor & Mélanose (Brain & Spinal Cord) (+ Melanoma (malignum)	+
N.Ota	8. KOJIMA et al. (1959)	37 years (♂)	N.Ota with Ocular Melanosis (No Histology)	Tumor & Mélanose (+ Melanoma malignum)	Living when reported

[a] present name: NAKAJIMA (one of the presenters)
[b] autopsied by NODA (one of the presenters)

In the central nerve organs, the cells originating from the neural crest are distributed in the soft meninges and their extensions namely perivascular tissue. Here again, they differentiate either to the melanocytes or to the Schwannian cells. In the mélanoses neurocutanées, nevus cells are distributed in the soft meninges and perivascular tissue. Because the mélanoses neurocutanées are the conditions where the nevus cells grow not only in the skin but also in the central nerve organ, they are to be classified in the category of the phalkomatosis. Thus the term Melanophakomatose coined by MUSGER is appropriate. The nevus Ota is a miniature of mélanoses neurocutanées (KAWAMURA [3], 1962; MUSGER [4], 1963). The question whether or not the nevoblast of Ota type may give rise to fully developed mélanoses neurocutanées might be open for further confirmation. However, the cases 8 of the table indicate that the simultaneous occurrence of nevus Ota and mélanose of the meninges with melanoma in the skull is possible.

The case 2 and 4 of the table were examined by us. In both of the cases, the skin lesions consist of extensive giant nevi and disseminated nevi. The histological findings taken from various portions of the nevi of both cases are revealed to be nevus cell nevus. As already shown by the table, it is common to all the Japanese cases that the nevus tissue is situated almost exclusively intradermal, even in two baby cases. This feature indicating the poor affinity of nevus cells to the epidermis is characteristic of this disorder in certain extent. In a specimen of case 2 in table, nevus cells push the epidermis upward instead of breaking into the latter. In another specimen of the same case, cordlike and globular structures are revealed in the deep dermis, while the superficial corium remains not invaded. The general structure of the nevus tissue is not unusual. Théques with pigmented nevus cells are found in the deep corium in the case 4. This finding is not unusual in giant nevi. The accumulation of cells on the inner surface of lymph vessel, the findings described by BOECKERS and their co-worker in the giant nevus, was found in the case 4. Because raticulin fibers are stained among the cells, they might be regarded as nevus cells. Théques are also found in the outer layer of vessels. Findings indicating conspicuous affinity of nevus cells to the vessels are found in the upper dermis in both cases. Neurinomatous nevus cell cords growing around blood vessels are revealed in the case 4.

The simplest and lowest grade finding in the central nerve organ in the cases 2 and 4 is a one layer growth of heavily pigmented nevus cells along blood vessels. They differ from the normal central nerve melanocytes by their lack of dendritic process. This finding is encountered in many areas in specimens of the case 2. The prevailing feature in the case 4 is the proliferation of less or not melanotic round cells with usually single nucleus but sometimes several nuclei. The pleomorphism of the latter series of cells have lead us to the diagnosis of malignant melanoma.

Conclusion. The mélanoses neurocutanées are disorders caused by the proliferation of the descendants of the ordinary nevoblasts in the skin, soft meninges and perivascular tissue of the central nerve organs. The possibility for the Ota type nevoblast to cause fully developed mélanoses neurocutanées was already suggested.

References. 1. KAWAMURA, T.: Hautarzt 7, 7 (1956). — 2. PINKUS, H., and Y. MISHIMA: Vth International Pigment Cell Conference, New York 1961. Ann. N.Y. Acad. Sci. **1963**, 256. — 3. KAWAMURA, T.: XII. International Congress of Dermatology, Washington D.C., USA 1962. — 4. MUSGER, A.: Hautarzt **14**, 106 (1963).

La mélanose circonscrite précancereuse de Hutchinson-Dubreuilh (M.H.D.)

B. Duperrat et J. M. Mascaro, Clinique Dermatologique Hôpital Saint-Louis, Paris (France)

Senile freckles Hutchinson, 1892,
Infective melanotic freckles Hutchinson, 1894,
Melanosis circumscripta precancerosa, Dubreuilh, 1912,
«Mélanose de Dubreuilh»,
«Melanotic freckles»,
«lentigo maligna» Becker (1954).

Définition: Chez les sujets de plus de 40 ans, apparition en un point quelconque du corps, d'une tache brunâtre, grisâtre ou noirâtre, plate, sans signes fonctionnels, polycirciné et polychrome, s'étendant progressivement, subissant des remaniements incessants, susceptible de dégénérer en mélanome malin.

Etiologie: Fréquence de plus en plus grande avec l'accroissement de la longévité humaine. Un peu plus fréquente chez les femmes. L'étude suivant les races est encore très incomplète. Age: en théorie apparaît après la 49ème année. Et il est exact que le nombre de M.H.D. augmente avec le nombre des vieillards. Mais à l'inverse, nombreux cas ayant débuté avant la 20e année. Siège: surtout la face, le front, les tempes, les joues, les paupières. En fait ubiquitaire car aussi les parties couvertes: le *tronc,* les paumes, les plantes, même les doigts, les parties génitales, les muqueuses: la bouche; localisation conjonctivale: la mélanose de Reese.

Histoire naturelle de la M.H.D.: Le début est totalement insidieux et souvent le malade, négligent, ne «montre» sa M.H.D. qu'après 15 ou 20 années d'évolution. La nappe pigmentée s'étend en tache d'huile et subit des remaniements perpétuels qui en modifient la forme, la superficie et surtout la *couleur.* Cette polychromie de brun, de gris et de noir est très particulière, allant du bistre pâle au noir-goudron. Parfois au contraire il se produit un éclaircissement spontané. Certaines plaques deviennent très étendues, couvrant par exemple l'hypochondre. La surface, le plus souvent glabre, est d'abord lisse puis tomenteuse, ou parfois même verruqueuse.

Dégénérescence: La dégénérescence n'est nullement obligatoire: «le nombre doit être fort grand de ceux qui arrivent à la fin de leurs jours porteurs d'un foyer de mélanose dont ils ne se sont jamais occupés» (Dubreuilh). Sa fréquence varie avec les statistiques: Dans 25 à 30% des cas pour la face. Par contre dans 90 à 100% des cas pour les extrémités. Cette dégénérescence survient dans les délais les plus variables: Friederich et Schneider rappellent les cas extrêmes: quatre semaines (Gartmann). 64 ans (Schuermann). Elle est, comme pour tous les naevi, annoncée par les symptomes ordinaires: hyperpigmentation (ou à l'inverse halo dépigmenté), prolifération, ulcération, saignement etc. Elle est *surtout non univoque* et l'examen des pièces opératoires, s'il montre surtout des *mélanomes malins,* peut aussi découvrir des papillomes, des botryomycomes, des épithéliomas, des épithéliosarcomes etc.

Pronostic vital: On admet communément que la M.H.D. dégénérée est un peu moins grave que le Mélanome Malin. C'est vrai dans l'ensemble, surtout sur la face. Par contre la M.H.D. des extrémités est toujours redoutable. En fait cette évolution ultérieure ne doit plus s'observer actuellement puisque la très lente évolution de l'affection donne une large possibilité d'intervenir avant le stade de dégénérescence.

Histologie: La M.H.D. passe par deux stades: d'abord un stade «éphélide» avec hyperpigmentation de la zone de jonction, sans thèques, puis un stade «lentigo», les thèques mélaniques «gonflant» les crêtes interpapillaires de l'épiderme comme des fruits lourds.

Il existe à ce moment *quatre composantes*: le lentigo respectant longtemps la vitrée; la mélanose remarquable par le volume et l'abondance des mottes pigmentaires; la réaction épidermique hyperplasique; la réaction conjonctive, lympho-plasmocytaire en nappe: celle-ci ne manque jamais et contraste avec l'aspect clinique non inflammatoire. Enfin, on note la présence de cellules mélaniques dans la paroi des poils et des glandes sudorales. Au stade de dégénérescence, rien ne distingue histologiquement, à notre avis, une M.H.D. dégénérée d'un Mélanome jonctionnel commun.

Histogénèse: La M.H.D. est traditionnellement considérée comme une forme «particulière de naevus pigmentaire tardif». Cependant, en 1960, MISHIMA faisant observer certains détails dont les trois plus frappants sont: la forme irrégulière des noyaux, la constance de la Dopa Réaction positive et surtout la «changeability» clinique, évoque l'hypothèse suivante: la M.H.D. serait un prémélanome non-naevique dérivant des mélanocytes matures.

Diagnostic: a) Le diagnostic clinique aidé de l'histologie est facile et on peut reconnaître la M.H.D. sur une coupe avec certitude. b) Par contre, en cas de M.H.D. dégénérée, la distinction avec le Mélanome de jonction peut être fort délicate. c) Après la cinquantaine, des «petites lésions» fréquentes apparaissent: «lentigo senilis» des mains, lentigos punctiformes tardifs des régions découvertes. Elles présentent les plus grandes analogies histologiques avec la M.H.D. d) Enfin, rappelons que, presque constamment, à l'inverse des autres naevi, *la M.H.D. est toujours unique.*

Traitement: 1. Il n'est plus question de «contempler» la M.H.D. pendant des années sans rien faire. Il faut, au contraire, la traiter dès qu'on la voit: soit par extirpation chirurgicale esthétique, soit tout simplement par *l'azote liquide.* 2. En cas de dégénérescence, même traitement que pour les M.M. mais possibilité, dans une forme très étendue, du visage par exemple, présentant un foyer de dégénérescence, d'extirper ce dernier sans enlever le reste de la mélanose, geste qui serait à proscrire dans toute autre variété de tumeur mélanique. 3. Enfin, dans les formes palpébro-conjonctivales dégénérées, possibilité d'utiliser les radiations ionisantes, en se rappelant que la M.H.D. devient de moins en moins sensible au fur et à mesure qu'on s'éloigne de l'oeil.

Spontaneous Regression of Malignant Melanoma

L. BOWDEN, Mixed Tumor Service, Memorial Sloan-Kettering Cancer Center, New York City (USA)

In a recent review of spontaneous regression of cancer, EVERSON [6] reported 130 documented instances of such regression. In this group there were twelve patients with malignant melanoma to which may be added three more instances reported in English medical journals [2, 3, 10] and one patient of my own. There appear to be at least 16 patients, therefore, with malignant melanoma observed and treated during the past 50 years who have shown well-documented spontaneous regression either of the primary lesion or of metastases, a few of whom have apparently remained permanently cured.

The purpose of this report is to present pathological and clinical data in support of the concept of spontaneous regression and to discuss briefly its nature.

The dynamic rather than static nature of skin is well-known. Lesions of the skin therefore understandably show change from time to time in response both to known stimuli as well as to unknown stimuli. Nevi of all types may show gross and microscopic change and may on occasion demonstrate complete resolution [1]. Such resolution or disappearance of nevi is usually totally unexplained and may occasionally be associated with loss of pigmentation in the skin immediately surrounding the lesion.

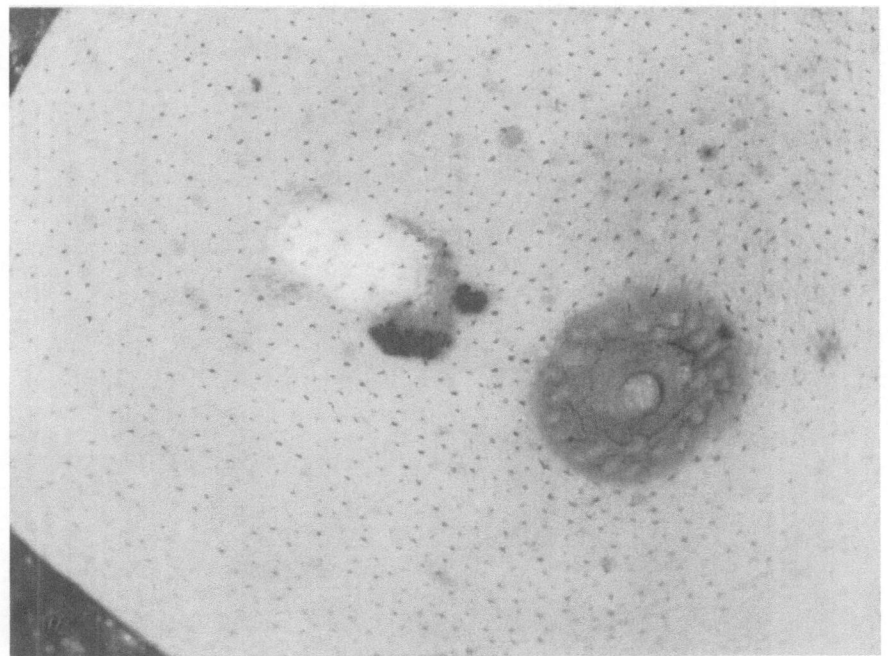

Fig. 1. J.S. 41-year old white male with malignant melanoma of skin of left breast showing central healing and depigmentation with peripheral growth of tumor

Malignant melanoma of the skin, whether arising *de novo* or on the basis of a previously existing nevus, characteristically pursues the course of a highly aggressive malignant tumor but may on occasion also show regressive changes at its primary site. Some melanomas will demonstrate peripheral spread with central clearing and loss of pigmentation in the central area of healing (Fig. 1). This characteristic, when present, appears to have no prognostic significance so long as actively proliferating melanoma persists in the periphery. Nevertheless, instances of such centrally healing melanoma have provided us with interesting specimens for study.

Histology of "Healing" Melanoma: Where melanoma is grossly visible the microscopic appearance is quite typical with anaplastic, polyhedral melanin-containing neoplastic cells obscuring and distorting normal structures and often destroying the overlying epidermis. A sharp demarcation is then noted both grossly and microscopically with reconstitution of the epidermis and infiltration of lymphocytes into dermis (Fig. 2). Study of the area of healing under higher magnification demonstrates some attenuation of the epidermis with quantitative diminution in the number of rete pegs and absence of pigmentation in the basal cells; the dermis is heavily infiltrated with lymphocytes and macrophages loaded with pigment. Scattered degenerating cells are thought to represent disintegrating melanoma cells (Fig. 3). Elsewhere in the area of gross healing the epidermis continues to show attenuation and absence of pigmentation in the basal layer but the dermis shows clearing of inflammatory infiltrate with early filmy fibrosis and telangiectasia (Fig. 4). The absence of pigment in the basal cells of the epidermis

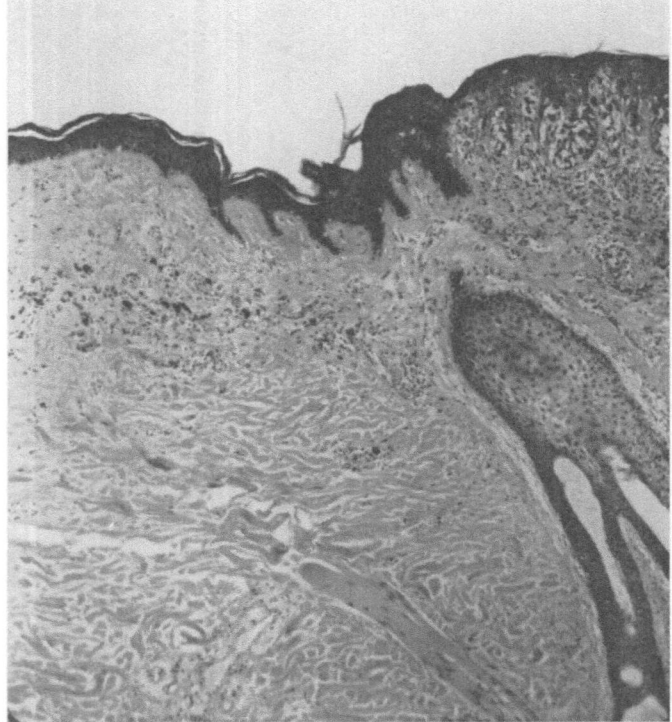

Fig. 2. J.S. Photomicrograph X 63 showing on the right active malignant melanoma invading epidermis with sharp demarcation and disappearance of melanoma on the left

and the small number of melanophores in the dermis account for the blanching or depigmentation noted grossly. It is believed that these histologic findings represent various stages in the spontaneous resolution of melanoma.

Melanoma of "Unknown" Primary Origin

On review of 992 histologically-proved cases of malignant melanoma treated at Memorial Hospital from 1935 through 1954 [4] we found 37 patients with metastatic melanoma in whom the primary could not be determined when subjected to critical analysis. Several other patients were studied, however, in whom either on the basis of past history or on the basis of physical findings the location of the primary lesion could be strongly suspected. Several of these patients described very adequately a previously existing pigmented lesion which they stated had in time "disappeared". Others showed on physical examination an area of skin, usually circular or oval and of small dimension, which was perceptibly paler than the surrounding integument and which lay in an area of the body consistent with the presentation of the metastases. One patient with metastatic melanoma in lymph nodes of the left groin stated that 12 years previously he had had a pigmented and ulcerated lesion in the skin of the left ankle which he had intermittently treated at home with an astringent and which after 2 or 3 years had disappeared. On physical examination the area where the lesion had been showed only an overall irregular area of depigmentation and atrophy of skin with four small flecks

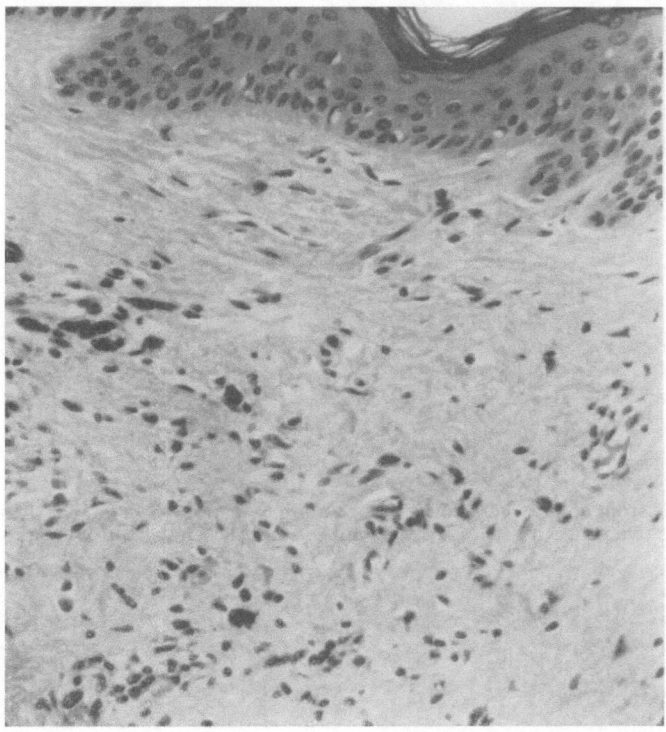

Fig. 3. J.S. Photomicrograph X 250 showing infiltration of leucocytes in dermis, macrophages filled with pigment and at least two degenerating cells possibly representing disintegrating melanoma cells

of pigmentation still evident (Fig. 5). Excision of this area was carried out with total embedding and representative sectioning and the microscopic appearance of these sections was entirely comparable to those obtained from areas of central healing in melanoma already described (Fig. 6 and 7). Similar microscopic findings were seen in other patients when the area of depigmentation suspected of being the site of primary melanoma was similarly excised, totally embedded and sectioned.

Although the microscopic appearance of areas of central healing in otherwise fully aggressive melanoma and the microscopic appearance of areas of depigmentation believed to represent the site of previously existing melanoma are generally non-descript, the similarity between the first which is obvious and the latter which is suspected is sufficient to justify, we believe, the conclusion that regression of melanoma has occurred in both instances, for reasons that at present are totally unknown.

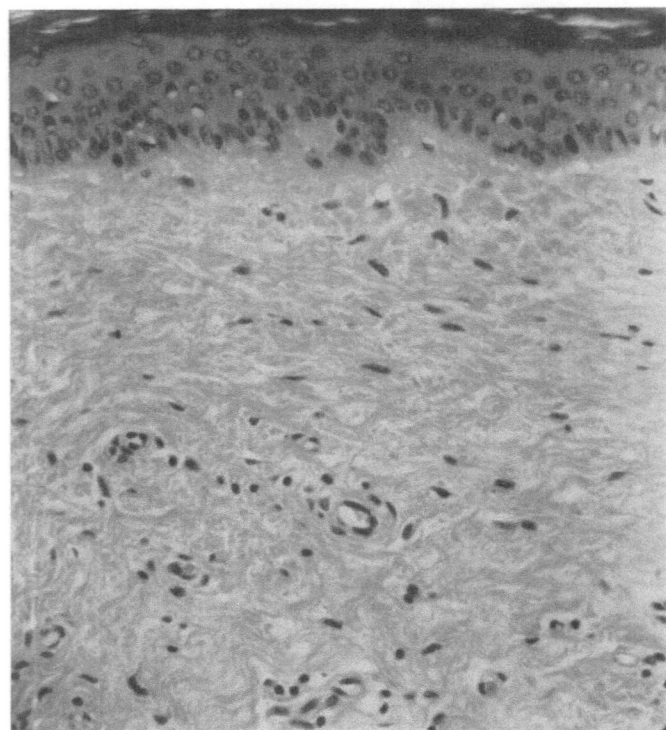

Fig. 4. J.S. Photomicrograph X 250 showing absence of rete pegs and lack of pigment in basal layer of epidermis with telangiectasis, fibrosis and clearing of leucocytes from the dermis

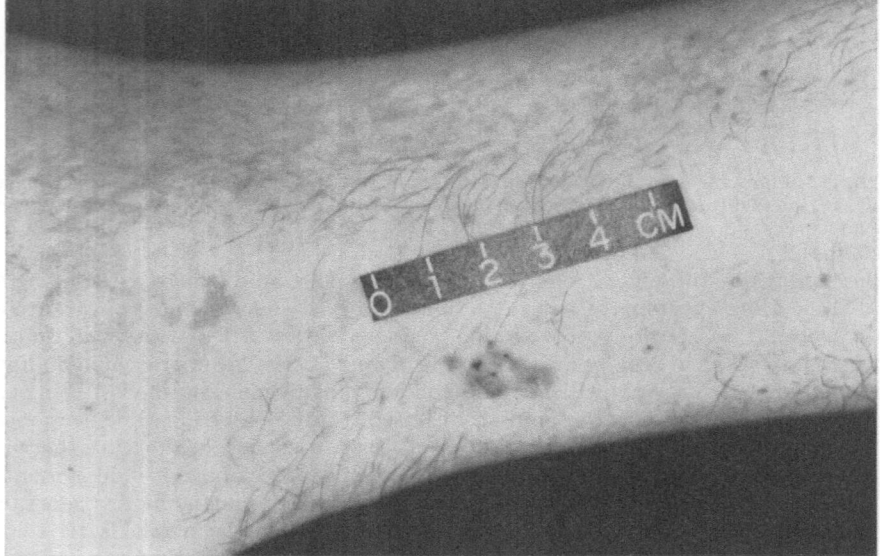

Fig. 5. F.B. 45-year old white male showing site of previously existing pigmented and ulcerated lesion of the skin of left ankle which had spontaneously healed some 8 to 9 years before this photograph

Discussion

Total, spontaneous and permanent resolution of malignant melanoma does, in all probability, occur rarely. The reported cases all presented evidence of sub-cutaneous and lymph node involvement and two were favorably associated with pregnancy but visceral involvement was infrequent and never histologically proved. All clinicians are familiar with an occasional patient who demonstrates long-term control of melanoma, sometimes for as long as 10 or even 15 years, ulti-mately showing further metastases and rapid decline. The cause for such long-term

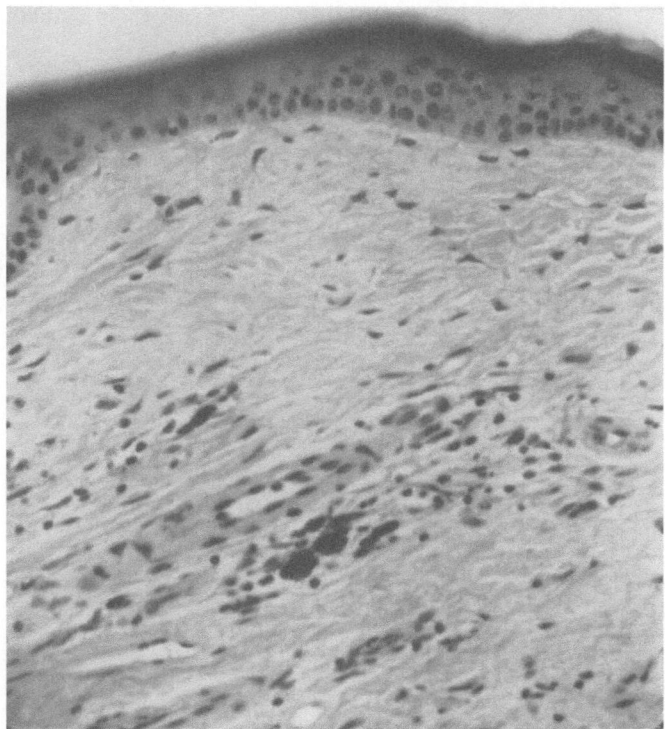

Fig. 6. F.B. Photomicrograph X 250 showing atrophy of epidermis with absence of pigmen-tation in basal layer and infrequent rete pegs. Telangiectasia, fibrosis and phagocytes contain-ing pigment are prominent features in the dermis

suspension of activity in these cases is equally unexplained. Both spontaneous permanent regression of melanomas as well as long-term suppression of melanoma is unpredictable.

The assumption is made that these fortunate individuals possess some type of circulating "antibody" against melanoma. In one human being temporary regres-sion of metastasis of melanoma was actually observed following administration of plasma secured from a patient with true spontaneous regression [9]. If circulating antibodies were the entire explanation, however, then the associated metastases in those patients showing local resolution of melanoma should have simultaneously resolved and all of these patients should have been cured. Such was not the case.

It is by no means certain that the mechanism of host resistance to neoplastic disease is comparable to that which is operative in host resistance to bacteria. When malignant melanoma is present, or has been recently resected, it has been noted that surrounding benign nevi assume histologic characteristics of "activation". Yet, the simultaneous occurrence of multiple primary melanomas in one individual is extremely rare, implying that, although there may be some systemic stimulus to junctional change in neval cells or in basal cells of the epidermis, some *local* change in environment accounts for the malignant lesion in that one location where it is found. The antithesis, by logical deduction, is that although metastasis of melanoma may be elsewhere fluorishing, the primary site must undergo regression or resolution, if it occurs at all, because of *local* change in environment.

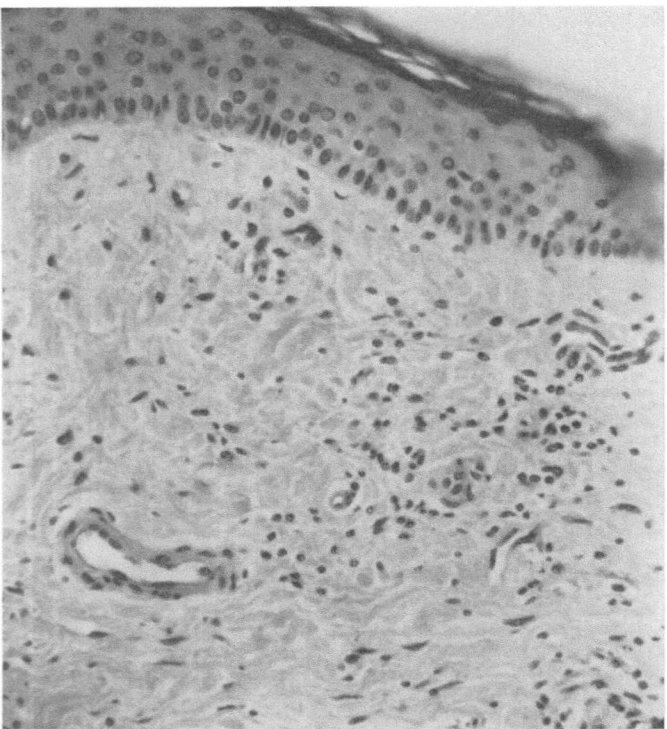

Fig. 7. F.B. Photomicrograph X 250 from another area in the healed lesion showing changes similar to those described in Fig. 6

Furthermore, the usual benign behavior of juvenile melanoma is unexplained unless one assumes that its local characteristics, namely, telangiectasia and delicate fibrosis of the superficial dermis and certain cellular differentiation which identifies it as different from adult melanoma, serve as a local restraint or barrier to an aggressive course.

Furthermore, when regression of melanoma is believed to have occurred, the frequently associated depigmentation of the skin is a local phenomenon. If it is possible to equate changes in pigmentation with changes in neoplastic potential of melanoma, then spontaneous resolution of melanoma should be associated with generalized changes in pigmentation if the mechanism of resolution were a systemic one. This is not the case.

For these reasons therefore we believe that the mechanism of human host-rejection of neoplastic tissue must be a local phenomenon, even if initiated or triggered by unknown systemic factors. In the case of malignant melanoma, when spontaneous regression does occur, the ultimate mechanism for such regression must reside in the skin and subcutaneous tissue alone.

References. 1. ALLEN, A. C.: The Skin. A clincopathologic treatise. St. LOUIS: C. V. Mosby Company 1954. — 2. ALLEN, E. P.: Brit. med. J. 1955, II, 1067. — 3. BAKER, H. W.: Amer. Surg. 30, 825 (1964). — 4. DAS GUPTA, T., L. BOWDEN, and J. W. BERG: S. G. & O. 117, 341 (1963). — 5. EVERSON, T. C., and W. H. COLE: Ann. Surg. 144, 366 (1956). — 6. EVERSON, T. C.: Ann. N.Y. Acad. Sci. 114, 721 (1964). — 7. SMITH, J. L., jr., and J. S. STEHLIN jr.: Cancer (Philad.) 18, 1399 (1965). — 8. SUMNER, W. C.: Cancer (Philad.) 6, 1040 (1953). — 9. SUMNER, W. C., and A. G. FORAKER: Cancer (Philad.) 13, 79 (1960). — 10. TODD, D. W., G. M. FARROW, R. K. WINKELMAN, and W. S. PAYNE: Proc. Mayo Clin. 41, 672 (1966).

Elektrometrie zur Früherkennung von malignanten Melanomen

N. MELCZER, Universitäts-Hautklinik Pécs (Ungarn)

Wird die lebende Haut mit Hilfe von unpolarisierbaren Elektroden von schwachem Gleichstrom durchströmt, so entstehen in der Haut unter den Elektroden infolge Elektrolysis chemische Veränderungen, und es kommt zur Induktion eines Polarisationsgegenstromes. Dieser ist dem primären Strom entgegengesetzt und ahmt einen Polarisationswiderstand oder Pseudoresistenz nach. Außer dieser Polarisationsfähigkeit verfügt die Haut über ein starkes Aufladungsvermögen.

Die Ursache der Polarisation der Haut und ihrer Polarisationskapazität ist zum Teil in der verschiedenen Ionendurchlässigkeit der Zellgrenzmembranen bzw. in der abweichenden Wanderungsfähigkeit dieser Ionen unter Gleichstromwirkung zu suchen. In der Ausbildung des Polarisationsstromes spielt jedoch die Aufladung der Helmholtzschen elektrischen Doppelschicht die Hauptrolle, die an allen polarisierbaren Gebilden und auch an den Epidermiszellen schon im Ruhezustand vorhanden ist.

Auf Grund der Untersuchungen von EBBECKE ist bekannt, daß die Polarisationsfähigkeit der Haut an Stellen von verschiedenen Reizungen und unbedeutenden Verletzungen reversibel auf eine kürzere Zeit abnehmen oder ganz verschwinden kann.

Es ist schon seit langem bekannt, daß die malignisierten Zellen eine erhöhte Permeabilität aufweisen. Diese Steigerung der Permeabilität ist nach WATERMANN die Ursache dafür, daß sich die infolge der Polarisation auftretende Pseudoresistenz bei exzidierten Geschwulstteilen in vitro und selbst die elektrische Kapazität des Geschwulstgewebes vermindern.

Bei unseren elektrometrischen Messungen menschlicher Melanomalignome ergab sich, daß sich der Polarisationswiderstand, die sog. Pseudoresistenz dieser malignen Wucherungen, in hohem Grade vermindert, und zwar auf permanente Weise, was mit einem einfachen Meßgerät leicht nachweisbar ist. Auf diese Weise kann man schon im Anfang der malignen Umwandlung — z. B. bei einem verdächtigen Pigmentnaevus — das Vorkommen der Malignität entscheiden.

Wir verwenden zur Messung der Pseudoresistenz der Melanomalignome ein Meßgerät mit direkter Potentiometerschaltung. Der Apparat besteht aus einer exosomatischen Gleichstromquelle (zwei Taschenlampenbatterien von je 4,5 Volt), einem Potentiometerwiderstand (10 Kiloohm) sowie einem Mikroampèremeter (50 uA) und einem Paar unpolarisierbarer Quecksilber-Kalomelelektroden nach OSTWALD.

Bei der Messung wird eine Elektrode auf die Handfläche und die andere ohne Druck auf das untersuchte Gebiet aufgelegt. Bei der Untersuchung wird der

Stromdurchfluß, d. h. also der Leitwert der normalen Haut bzw. von Melanomalignomen, ausgedrückt in Mikroampere, festgestellt. Wir bestimmen zuerst mehrmals
den Leitwert der normalen Umgebung der untersuchten Veränderung oder den der
symmetrischen Körperhälfte.

Das Verfahren läßt sich in erodiertem oder geschwürigem Gebiet nur mit der
nötigen Vorsicht anwenden. Da in solchen Fällen die Messung infolge des Ver-
letzungsstromes auch ohne bösartige Umwandlung eine Positivität nachahmen
kann, ist es notwendig, die Messung 2 bis 3 mm weit vom Rande des Substanz-
verlustes entfernt vorzunehmen. Ebenso muß man sich vor Augen halten, daß
schon nach unbedeutenden mechanischen Einwirkungen, z. B. nach Kratzen, sofort eine Positivität nachahmende Polarisationsverminderung entsteht, die stundenlang bestehen kann. In Zweifelsfällen ist es deshalb angezeigt, eventuell nach
Anwendung eines Okklusivverbands, nach 24 Std die Messung zu wiederholen.

Da vorherige Ionisationsbestrahlungen eine Verminderung der Permeabilität
der Haut verursachen, können wir bei bestrahlten Melanomalignomen trotz der
vorhandenen Malignität ein falsches negatives Resultat bekommen.

Da sekundäre Hautmetastasen von Melanomalignomen eine Zeitlang von unversehrter und deshalb gut polarisierbarer Haut bedeckt sind, sind dieselben für
elektrometrische Messungen im Anfang ungeeignet.

Das Verfahren übt auf den Patienten gar keine schädliche Nebenwirkung aus
und ergibt im Falle einer Malignität auch bei achromischen Melanoblastomen sowie bei Junction- und Compound-Naevi, juvenilen Melanomen und der Melanosis
circumscripta praecancerosa im Beginn einer bösartigen Umwandlung ein positives
Ergebnis.

Ich bin der Ansicht, daß diese elektrometrische Methode in der frühzeitigen
Erkenntnis der bösartigen Melanome eine besondere Stellung einnimmt.

The Surgical Treatment of Malignant Melanoma

R. W. RAVEN, Royal Marsden Hospital and Institute of Cancer Research, Royal
Cancer Hospital; Westminster Hospital, London (England)

The development of a malignant melanoma means certain death for many
patients, but this tragic consequence can be averted in a number of them by
adhering to certain principles of treatment. The tumour must be treated early
before dissemination occurs; it may be confused with other pigmented skin tumours
thus losing valuable time. Every excised skin tumour must be examined histologically; it is tragic to see patients with melanoma metastases who had skin tumours
removed without histology. When a skin tumour is a doubtful melanoma, it should
be widely excised and examined histologically, for partial removal is dangerous.

The cells comprising a malignant melanoma are loosely attached to each other,
so that individual cells are easily detached from the parent tumour and enter the
blood and lymphatic vessels to form metastases in other organs. Thus during the
excision the tumour must not be touched either by hand or instrument to avoid
disseminating cells into the wound, blood or lymphatic vessels. Adjuvant therapy
with systemic therapy or regional perfusion of extremities using Melphalan may
kill such disseminated cells.

Preventive Treatment

Malignant melanomas of the skin and mucous membranes arise from pre-existing junctional and compound naevi and rarely from a blue naevus. Such lesions are pre-malignant and these are the indications for surgical excision: a skin naevus subjected to repeated trauma; naevi coloured blue or black or showing signs of activity including increase in size or pigmentation, or bleeding and ulceration; and junctional naevi on the hands, feet, genitalia and mucous membranes. When excision is done, it includes an adequate margin of skin and deep fascia, or mucous membrane, so that all pigmented cells are removed.

Diagnostic Biopsy

A wrong diagnosis is not infrequently made, for a malignant melanoma can be confused with pigmented types of basal cell carcinoma, seborrhoeic wart and cellular naevus, in addition to pyogenic granuloma, cysts and whitlow. The diagnosis must be proved by excision-biopsy for histological examination before radical surgery is done. A biopsy that cuts through the tumour must not be done.

Radical Surgery

1. The Primary Skin Tumour

The tumour is excised with a wide skin margin making the encircling incision 5 cm from the tumour edge. The underlying deep fascia is more widely excised with an encircling incision 7.5 cm from the tumour edge. The skin defect is repaired with a split thickness skin graft from the unaffected thigh. The recipient and donor sites of the skin graft are measured, the graft being cut before excision of the tumour to avoid implanting tumour cells in the donor area.

Special skin sites. Interdigital cleft. Local wide excision is performed with a skin graft repair. Thus an amputation can usually be avoided. *Sole of foot.* Local wide excision is performed and a whole thickness skin graft is used to repair the skin defect, because of pressure effects. *Subungual.* Digital amputation at the meta-carpo- or metatarso-phalangeal joint is performed; a radical amputation is unnecessary. *Anus and Anal canal.* An abdomino-perineal excision of the rectum is performed. *Vulva.* A total vulvectomy is performed. *Lip.* A wide local excision of the tumour is performed.

2. The Regional Lymph Nodes

The majority of malignant melanomas occurs in the skin of the extremities, face, scalp and trunk and produce metastases in regional lymph nodes in situations amenable to radical block dissection. These are ilioinguinal, axillary and facio-cervical. No distinction is made between a prophylactic or elective block dissection; it is essential to do the operation in every patient whether or not the lymph nodes are palpable. I have excised lymph nodes which were not palpable and yet contained metastatic malignant melanoma cells on microscopical examination. It is stressed that lymph nodes should be excised with microscopical metastases, for it is often too late when they are clinically enlarged, the disease having spread more widely. Furthermore, large metastatic lymph nodes can be damaged during excision, implanting malignant cells in the wound.

The Monoblock Operation. When the primary tumour in the skin is situated at a distance of 7.5 cm or less from the regional lymph nodes, it is excised in continuity with the latter as a monoblock operation.

The Staged Operation. When the primary tumour in the skin is situated more than 7.5 cm from the regional lymph nodes, the block dissection of the regional lymph nodes is performed 2 weeks after the primary tumour is excised.

Principles of Lymph Node Block Dissection. Ilioinguinal Block Dissection. The femoral, inguinal, external and common iliac groups of lymph nodes are removed, using a skin incision commencing 5 cm above and internal to the anterior superior iliac spine curving downwards to the apex of Scarpa's triangle. Poupart's ligament is divided at the junction of the outer and middle thirds, so that the peritoneum can be reflected to the beginning of the common iliac artery. *Axillary Block Dissection.* The apical, central and pectoral lymph nodes are removed, using a curved skin incision over the anterior axillary wall. The axilla is opened up by dividing the tendons of the pectoralis major and minor muscles. *Facio-cervical Block Dissection.* The pre-auricular and cervical lymph nodes are removed using an incision from the zygomatic arch to the sterno-clavicular joint and along the clavicle to the trapezius muscle; another incision is made at right angles from the upper third to the submental region. The pre-auricular lymph nodes are excised with the superficial part of the parotid salivary gland and the cervical lymph nodes with the sternomastoid muscle and internal jugular vein.

Postoperative Radiotherapy. This is given to the regional lymph node area when histological examination shows metastases in the lymph nodes. The fields are placed so that adjacent groups of lymph nodes not excised are irradiated.

Adjuvant Chemotherapy. Part of the primary tumour is used for sensitivity tests to various carcinostatic drugs. The malignant melanoma cells are grown in tissue culture and usually Melphalan proves to be the best drug to kill the cells. The object is to rationalize chemotherapy which up to the present has been largely experimental. If we know the most potent carcinostatic drug for the particular tumour, this can be given later if recurrence or dissemination occurs. In the same way if the patient presents with disseminated disease, one or more superficial tumours are excised for organ tissue culture and sensitivity tests.

If the disease recurs in an extremity regional perfusion is carried out using an extra-corporeal pump-oxygenator apparatus to give the appropriate carcinostatic drug as proved by organ tissue culture. For other patients oral chemotherapy is used.

Adjuvant Vaccination. When a malignant melanoma recurs and it is possible to remove a small tumour, a vaccine is made of irradiated tumour cells. Several patients have been treated in this way, but it is too early to report any results. Special host-tumour relationships exist for malignant melanoma, because it is the tumour for which there are several reports of spontaneous regression.

Reference. RAVEN, R. W.: Ann. N.Y. Acad. Sci. **100**, 142 (1963).

Die Behandlung des malignen Melanoms mit schnellen Elektronen eines 15 MeV-Betatrons

G. F. KLOSTERMANN, Univ.-Hautklinik Göttingen (Deutschland)

Der Streit der Meinungen über die beste Therapie ist auf wenigen Gebieten so hart geführt worden wie auf dem Gebiet der Melanombehandlung. Die Überzeugungen speziell in der Alternative Operation oder Bestrahlung haben sich gelegentlich kompromißlos bis hart an den gegenseitigen Vorwurf des Kunstfehlers auseinandergelebt. Dabei hat es nicht an Versuchen gefehlt, die Überlegenheit des eigenen Vorgehens an Hand der Auswertung der Überlebensergebnisse zu belegen. Heute zeichnet sich vielfach eine gewisse Abmilderung und teilweise Annäherung

der Standpunkte ab. Die für verschiedene Behandlungsverfahren vorgelegten Er-
folgsstatistiken erscheinen auf Grund des relativ beschränkten Materialumfangs
der einzelnen Kliniken und der Heterogenität der Fälle mit einer Fehlerbreite behaftet, in der etwaige reale Unterschiede ausreichend durchgeführter chirurgischer
oder radiologischer Behandlungsverfahren untergehen.

Führende deutsche Kliniken haben sich daher zu einer von KALKOFF geleiteten
Arbeitsgemeinschaft zusammengeschlossen, in der die Fälle mehrerer Institute
nach gleichem Vorgehen dokumentationsgerecht erfaßt und bearbeitet werden,
so daß auf diese Weise endlich ein größeres, einheitlich gegliedertes, therapeutisch
jedoch verschieden behandeltes Material zusammengetragen wird, welches eines
Tages einen hoffentlich brauchbaren Vergleich der therapeutischen Methoden
liefern wird.

Unser eigenes Krankengut aus der Göttinger Klinik ist seit Beginn der Arbeitsgemeinschaft dieser zugeführt worden. Dieser Arbeitsgemeinschaft, in der jede
Klinik sich auf die Melanomtherapie ihrer eigenen Überzeugung festgelegt hat,
stellen wir als einzige Institution Melanomfälle zur Verfügung, deren Tumor mit
schnellen Elektronen eines Betatrons bestrahlt und in unmittelbarem Anschluß
daran in toto mit dem Bestrahlungsfeld operativ entfernt wird.

Wir würden es als verfrüht und dem Sinn der Arbeitsgemeinschaft widerspre-
chend betrachten, jetzt schon eine detaillierte Analyse unseres Materials vorzunehmen, um durch Vergleich unser Vorgehen mit anderen therapeutischen Verfahren zu messen und etwa auf diese Weise die Vorzüge der Behandlung mit
schnellen Elektronen darzutun. Wichtig ist es mir indessen, darauf hinzuweisen,
daß BODE an Hand vergleichender Auswertung unseres älteren, vor Gründung der
Arbeitsgemeinschaft, mit schnellen Elektronen behandelten Krankengutes bereits
gezeigt hat, daß die Ergebnisse reiner Elektronenbestrahlung, ohne Operation,
gemessen an den Überlebensergebnissen völlig im Bereich der Erfolgsquoten der
anderen schulmäßigen Behandlungsverfahren liegen, daß also im Hinblick auf die
Ausschaltung des Tumors die Elektronenbestrahlung keinesfalls schlechter als die
übrigen Verfahren abschneidet. Andere Autoren, wie HELLRIEGEL, ZUPPINGER,
haben diese Erfahrung bestätigt und sind wie wir von den Vorzügen der Elektronenbestrahlung überzeugt.

Faßt man die Bedingungen, unter denen die Ausschaltung des Tumors erfolgt,
näher ins Auge, so weist die Bestrahlung mit schnellen Elektronen geeigneter
Energie gegenüber der klassischen Strahlentherapie so wesentliche Vorteile auf,
daß wir sie als radiologische Methode der Wahl bei der Behandlung der primären
Melanome ansehen. Dieser Auffassung haben sich die übrigen Göttinger Kliniken
angeschlossen, so daß bei uns die Dermatologische Klinik mit dem Betatron sämtliche primären Melanome auch der Chirurgischen und Radiologischen Klinik zur
endgültigen Diagnostik und zum Behandlungsbeginn zugeführt bekommt. Die
Vorteile unseres Vorgehens beruhen auf den physikalischen Gesetzen der Energieabgabe der schnellen Elektronen des Betatrons im Gewebe, die zwar schlechthin
beim Einsatz dieses Gerätes gelten, aber vielleicht bei keiner Indikation so entscheidend zum Tragen kommen wie gerade bei der Melanombehandlung.

Wir überblicken die Vorzüge des Verfahrens seit nunmehr $18^1/_2$ Jahren an derjenigen Klinik, die unter BODE 1949 als erste Hauttumorbestrahlungen mit schnellen Elektronen eines Betatrons überhaupt vornahm, zur Entwicklung Wesentliches
beitragen konnte und inzwischen mehr als 30000 Bestrahlungen durchgeführt hat,
so daß wir uns auch auf Grund der klinischen Empirie für befugt halten, die Vorzüge des Verfahrens herauszustellen.

Schärfer als bei anderen Indikationsstellungen spitzt sich bei der Melanom-
bestrahlung die Frage der Dosierungsverteilung im Gewebe auf die Forderung nach

höchster Konzentration der Dosis im Tumorbereich und größter Schonung der Umgebung zu. Letzteres nicht nur relativ und im Hinblick darauf, daß eine Reihe von Autoren kaustische Dosen für das Melanom selbst empfiehlt, die bei mangelnder örtlicher Begrenzung der Strahlenwirkung zu weitreichenden Folgen in der Nachbarschaft des Tumors führen, sondern absolut, wenn man radiologisches und operatives Vorgehen am Primärherd kombinieren und den vorbestrahlten Tumor excidieren will und hierzu ein regenerationsfähiges Wundbett benötigt.

Kein anderes strahlentherapeutisches Verfahren bietet in bezug auf die Energieabsorption im Gewebe vergleichbar gute Bedingungen wie die Anwendung schneller Elektronen eines Betatrons geeigneter Energiebereiche. Dabei kann von der Voraussetzung ausgegangen werden, daß bei vorhandenen quantitativen Differenzen der biologischen Wirksamkeit die biologische Wirkungsart der corpusculären Elektronenstrahlung und der elektromagnetischen Röntgenstrahlung völlig gleich ist. Ist auch diese Gleichartigkeit wenigstens in groben Zügen als Basis für den medizinischen Einsatz der Methode immer angenommen worden, so sind doch eine größere selektive Wirksamkeit der schnellen Elektronen bei der Tumorbestrahlung schon seit SCHUBERT wiederholt erörtert worden und Unterschiede in der biologischen Wirkungsart auch auf Grund des verschiedenen Wellenablaufs der Röntgen- und Elektronenerytheme in drei bzw. zwei Wellen nicht abwegig erschienen. Nach zahlreichen Untersuchungen an andersartigen biologischen Objekten, deren Ergebnisse von MARKUS an der Göttinger Klinik mit subtilen Versuchsanordnungen überprüft und zum Teil korrigiert werden konnten, haben kürzlich MARQUARDT u. MARKUS bzw. MARKUS u. SCHLOTFELDT in weiteren Studien an Kulturen menschlicher Tumorzellen (HeLa-Zellen) und an Hand von Erythemmessungen des Strahlenerythems im Vergleich die Wirkung von schnellen Elektronen und Röntgenstrahlen unter Berücksichtigung eines Äquivalenzfaktors gleich gefunden. Für die Erythemstudien ist es dabei nur Voraussetzung, daß die Tiefendosiskurven im Gewebe für beide Strahlungen einander angeglichen werden, also die Dosisverteilung in den einzelnen Hautschichten sich in beiden Fällen entspricht, wodurch die von BODE schon früher geäußerte Auffassung des Wellenverlaufs des Strahlenerythems als Ausdruck der Reaktion der verschiedenen Gefäßplexus der Haut nachträglich belegt wird. Der Äquivalenzfaktor, ausgedrückt in der RBW (relative biologische Wirksamkeit verschiedener Strahlenarten), hat sich bei nur geringen Schwankungen in den Resultaten der verschiedenen Untersucher als für die überwiegende Zahl aller biologischen Objekte praktisch gleich und konstant erwiesen. Dies gilt nach subtilen klinischen Untersuchungen (BODE) auch für die Haut. Er ändert sich geringgradig in Abhängigkeit von der Energie der Strahlung. Die Schwankungen der RBW-Angaben für schnelle Elektronen bewegen sich etwa von 0,6 bis 0,8, meist 0,7 bis 0,8. In der Praxis der klinischen Dosierung erreichen wir daher biologische Äquivalenz bei einem Dosisverhältnis von 3 (Röntgen):4 (Elektronen).

Unter diesem Aspekt der Gleichheit der biologischen Wirkungsart von schnellen Elektronen und Röntgenstrahlen ist allein der Vergleich der räumlichen Dosisverteilung im Gewebe für die therapeutischen Belange von Interesse. Er ist aus den folgenden Abbildungen ersichtlich, deren Kurven von MARKUS in der Göttinger Klinik durchgeführte dosimetrische Untersuchungen zugrunde liegen. Abb. 1 zeigt die Tiefendosisverläufe schneller Elektronen verschiedener Energien. Infolge kontinuierlicher Abgabe eines nahezu gleichen Energiebetrages sinkt die Energie eines in das Gewebe eingeschossenen Elektrons in arithmetischer Progression bis auf Null ab. Das Elektron hat eine endliche Reichweite. In der Summation der Sekundäreffekte kommt es zu einem Dosisanstieg unter der Oberfläche. Die Dosis steigt also über 100% der Oberflächendosis an. Sie erreicht erst in einer, je nach Energie der eingeschossenen Elektronen unterschiedlichen, Tiefe des Gewebes, welche BODE als die „therapeutische Reichweite" definiert hat, wieder 100% der Oberflächendosis und fällt danach recht scharf auf Null ab.

Diese Schärfe des Abfalls ist eine Funktion der Homogenität der Elektronenenergie. Hierin ist das Betatron den Elektronen der Isotopen überlegen, die zwar auch eine endliche Reichweite, aber nicht so scharf ausgeprägte Verhältnisse von Dosismaximum und Dosisabfall zur Tiefe hin aufweisen.

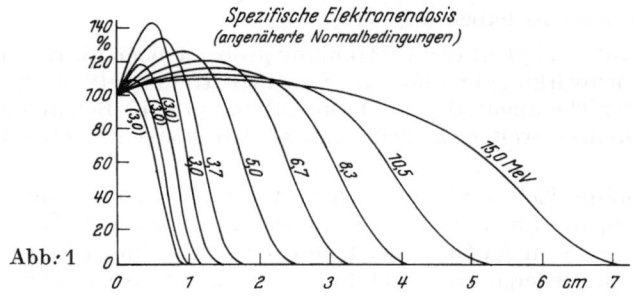

Abb. 1

Verlegung der „therapeutischen Reichweite" mit 100% Dosis an die Tumorunterfläche oder an die Grenze der bewußt mitgefaßten Sicherheitszone und praktisch völlig homogene Tumordurchstrahlung, oder sogar zusätzlicher Dosiszuwachs im Tumor selbst, kombiniert mit raschem Dosisabfall auf Null unterhalb der gewählten Tiefengrenze bei Anwendung der schnellen Elektronen — andererseits Dosisabfall (auf üblicherweise 50%) schon innerhalb des Tumors und die aus der prozentual gleichbleibenden Energieabgabe in geometrischer Progression folgende grundsätzliche Tiefenbelastung des Gewebes bei jeder Form von Röntgenbestrahlung — das ist das entscheidende Ergebnis des Vergleichs, welches schon vor der Analyse von Überlebensstatistiken für den Einsatz des Betatrons spricht, wo der damit ver-

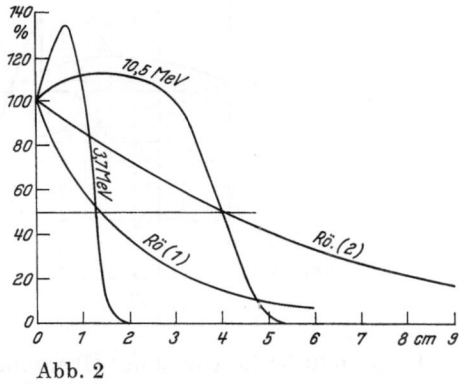

Abb. 2

bundene technische Aufwand ermöglicht werden kann. Abb. 2 zeigt den Vergleich kurvenmäßig an Hand der Tiefendosisverläufe je zweier Elektronen- und Röntgenstrahlungen gleicher Halbwerttiefen. Sowohl die weitaus größere Volumdosis im Herdgebiet als auch die praktisch absolute Tiefenschonung der schnellen Elektronen sind gegenüber der Röntgenstrahlung ganz evident.

Die Untersuchung ausreichend großer und vergleichbarer Patientenkollektive wird uns hoffentlich bald sichere Erkenntnisse über die Frage der dem Tumor zu applizierenden optimalen Dosis, über Sinn oder Sinnlosigkeit der zusätzlich durchgeführten Operation, über Fragen der Eigengesetzlichkeit des Krankheitsablaufes und andere bisher unklare Punkte liefern. Ob man aber eines Tages höheren Dosen sich zuwendet, welche aus der relativ geringeren Radiosensibilität der Melanomzellen gefolgert werden könnten, ob man sich zu dem von uns aus Sicherheitsbedürfnis gewählten kombinierten radiologisch-chirurgischen Vorgehen entschließt,

immer sind die Vorzüge der Betatronbestrahlung im Hinblick auf die Konzentration einer hohen Dosis im Tumor und die Gewebsschonung der Umgebung in
gleicher Weise zwingend. Wir können sogar sagen, daß unser Vorgehen der Operation im Anschluß an eine volle Tumordosis überhaupt erst durch die Elektronen-
anwendung befriedigend ermöglicht wurde, welche es durch die allseits, einschließlich zur Tiefe hin, scharfe Begrenzung des Strahleninsultes erlaubt, das gesamte
strahlenbelastete Gewebe mit dem darin enthaltenen Tumor als Block aus der
gesunden Umgebung herauszuschneiden, wobei wir gleichzeitig Wundverhältnisse
von guter Heilungstendenz haben.

Auch bei der Notwendigkeit der Bestrahlung großer Felder wirkt sich die Begrenzung der Strahlenwirkung im Sinne der Schichtbestrahlung (SCHREUS) segensreich aus, so daß der Therapeut, der den Lymphabfluß in seine Behandlung einbe-
ziehen will, die Grenzen weiter stecken kann als bei konventioneller Strahlentherapie.

Im Hinblick auf die Tiefendosen ist noch ein Wort zur Knochen- und Knorpel-
belastung zu sagen, die für viele Lokalisationen bedeutungsvoll ist. Phantommessungen von MARKUS an der Göttinger Klinik, deren Ergebnisse in der nächsten
Abbildung graphisch wiedergegeben sind, haben die nach physikalischen Gesetzen
zu erwartende, im Vergleich zur Röntgenbestrahlung weitaus geringere Knochen-
belastung beim Einsatz des Betatrons bestätigt.

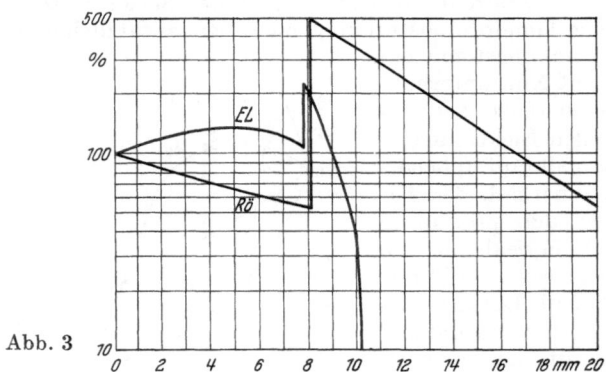

Abb. 3

Dargestellt ist in Abb. 3 der Übergang von Elektronen- und Röntgenstrahlung
aus einer Phantommasse für weiches Gewebe in eine solche mit den Absorptions-
verhältnissen von Knochen. Die spezielle Dosis springt an der Grenze bei der
Röntgenstrahlung auf den zehnfachen Wert, bei der Elektronenstrahlung nur auf
das Doppelte, steigt also für Röntgenenergie fünfmal stärker als für schnelle Elektronen an. Darüber hinaus sinkt die Elektronendosis im Knochen überaus steil ab,
affiziert also nur seine oberflächlichsten Partien. In dieser relativen Knochen-
schonung ist eine ganz entscheidende, praktisch höchst bedeutungsvolle Ergänzung
der Tiefenschonung zu erblicken.

Abschließend möchte ich unser Regelvorgehen bei der Behandlung kurz skiz-
zieren, wobei ich nochmals betonen möchte, daß wir meinen, bei kritischer Würdigung der bisherigen Statistiken seien mehrere Verfahren vertretbar. Wenn wir
Radiologie und Chirurgie zur Zeit kombinieren, so tun wir das, wie ich sagte, aus
Sicherheitsbedürfnis, ohne einen realen Gewinn bisher belegen zu können, ge-
schweige denn die Kombination zu einem Verfahren der Wahl erheben zu wollen.

Die Beobachtung unseres Krankengutes von 311 Fällen erlaubt uns aber die Feststellung, daß wir mit unserem Vorgehen das beim Melanom zu Erwartende leisten, und darüber hinaus, daß die funktionellen und meist auch die ästhetischen Ergebnisse am Ort des Primärtumors gut sind. Unter Berücksichtigung der RBW geben wir eine an 1000 R Röntgenstrahlen angeglichene Dosis schneller Elektronen als tägliche Fraktionierung an 8 aufeinander folgenden Tagen; die Eindringtiefe wählen wir so, daß möglichst auch zur Tiefe hin noch 1 cm gesunden Gewebes in die „therapeutische Reichweite" der schnellen Elektronen mit hineingefaßt wird. Im unmittelbaren Anschluß an die Strahlentherapie wird dann das gesamte Strahlenfeld einschließlich der mitbestrahlten Tiefe, also das gesamte durchstrahlte Volumen, mit dem darin enthaltenen Tumor entfernt und der Defekt vernäht oder durch Transplantation (gutes Anwachsen auf Grund radiologischer Entlastung der Unterlage) oder Verschiebeplastik gedeckt.

Es ist weder sinnvoll, noch kann es angezeigt sein, schon heute im Vorgriff auf die Tätigkeit der Freiburger Arbeitsgemeinschaft über das Melanom eine vergleichende Materialauswertung etwa zum Nachweis der Leistungen des Betatron zu versuchen. Es erschien aber vertretbar, im Rahmen eines Weltkongresses den Kollegen, die nach Ländern und Praxisgepflogenheiten unter zum Teil verschiedenen Voraussetzungen arbeiten, die Einsatzmöglichkeiten und Vorteile einer modernen strahlentherapeutischen Entwicklung auf Grund eigener, längerer Erfahrung aufzuzeigen und die in den letzten Jahren erarbeiteten allgemeinen Gesichtspunkte in den Vordergrund zu rücken, da sie unabhängig von den Irrtumsgefahren des Vergleichs unzulänglicher Therapiekollektive sind und die großen Vorteile des Verfahrens an sicheren Maßstäben und gerade im Hinblick auf den Einsatz am Melanom besonders eindeutig erkennen lassen.

Literatur. BODE, H. G.: 42. Kongress d. Nordwestdeutschen Dermatolog. Ges. Göttingen 27./28. 5. 61; — Arch. klin. exp. Derm. 219, 450 (1964). — HELLRIEGEL, W.: Disk. zu BODE 1964. — MARKUS, B.: Arch. klin. exp. Derm. 219, 509 (1964); — SWR-Nachrichten H. 17—19, (1962/63). — MARKUS, B., u. D. SCHLOTFELDT: Strahlentherapie 132, 206 (1967). — MARQUARDT, K., u. B. MARKUS: Dtsch. Röntgenkongress 1964, Teil B, 344. — SCHUBERT, G.: Strahlentherapie 1950. — ZUPPINGER, A.: Arch. klin. exp. Derm. 219, 437 (1964).

Histologische Diagnostik der Melanome

J. J. HERZBERG*, Dermatologische Klinik der Städt. Krankenanstalten Bremen (Deutschland)

„L'expérience nous enseignant constamment la modestie sur ce sujet, il est évident que toute tumeur foncée qu'elle que soit doit passer sous le microscope." B. DUPERRAT, 1966.

Das obige Zitat aus der meisterhaften Darstellung über die pathologische Anatomie der Melanome sowie die Feststellung von BECKER (1954), daß die Treffsicherheit der klinischen Diagnose beim dermatologisch nicht geschulten Arzt zwischen 45 und 48% liegt, unterstreichen die Bedeutung und die Schwierigkeit der feingeweblichen Diagnostik. Das Wissen um die schlechte Prognose oder die oft verstümmelnden, operativen Eingriffe lasten dem Histologen weiterhin eine Bürde an, der er sich nur durch die sorgfältigste Arbeitsweise entledigen kann. — Die Beurteilung der, wenn möglich auch Dopa-incubierten, wenigstens aber der

---

* Die Arbeit wurde durch die Deutsche Forschungsgemeinschaft dankenswerterweise unterstützt.

Tabelle 1. *Erscheinungen im Tumorbereich*

		primär	sekundär
I. Epi- dermis	1. Stratum corneum	Hyperpigmentierte, pyknoti- sche Melanomzellen oder Nester, Pigmentballen	Superortho-, und Para- keratose
	2. Stratum spinos.	Einzelelemente oder Nester epitheloider, globoider, blasiger Melanomzellen, Mitosen	Acanthose, pseudoepithe- liomatöse Wucherungen, lange schmale Keimleisten, Atrophie, Ulceration
	3. Stratum basale	Starke junktionale Aktivität, polymorphe, dicht gelagerte, große, meist epitheloide Melanomzellen, Mitosen	Reichlich „Klarzellen", überpigmentierte Basalzellen
	4. Basalmembran	durch- und unterbrochen	—
II. Cutis u. Subcutis	5. Wuchsform	⎰ oberflächen- superfiziell, ⎱ bündig exophytisch ⎫ oberflächen- ⎬ mit Tiefen- bündig ⎭ proliferation	Weitgehende Destruktion des präexistenten Gewebes, selten Nekrosen. Capillaren und pericapilläres Bindege- webe, argyrophile Fasern resistierend. Infiltrat: schwach ausgeprägt bis fehlend: Lymphoide, Histiocyten, Plasmazellen Eosinophile Leukocyten Mastzellen. Zahlreiche Melanophagen. Fakultative Erweiterung von Blut- und Lymphge- fäßen
	6. Zellverband	Nester, pseudoalveoläre Lagerung, Bündel endokriner Typ Zellregen (Auflösung des Verbandes) perithelialer Typ Neuroider Typ Anaplasie	
	7. Zelltyp	Epitheloide (große, kleine Z., globoide, naevoide, kuboide Z.) Spindelzellige (plumpe, schlanke Z.) Blasenzellen Riesenzellen (ein- und mehr- kernig) Dentritenzellen Anaplastische Elemente	
	8, a) Zellkern	Oval, rundlich, polycyclisch, groß, Strahlenkern, mehrere große Kernkörperchen.	—
	b) Zelleib	blaß-eosinophil, unterschied- lich dicht pigmentiert, meist scharf begrenzt, polycyclisch begrenzt.	
	c) Mitosen	Viele, wenig, fehlend, atypische	
	9. Pigmentierung	Stark (8%), mäßig (65%), schwach (23%), fehlend (4%)	Extra- und intracelluläres Pigment, meist perivascu- lär in Melanophagen
	10. Histochemie	Tyrosinase-Reaktion + Dopa-Oxydase-Reaktion + Unspezifische Cholinesterase —	

Tabelle 2. *Erscheinungen in der Geschwulstumgebung*

		primär	sekundär
	1. Stratum corneum —		—
	2. Stratum spinos.	Ganz vereinzelt eine polymorphe, epitheloide Melanomzelle	Angedeutete Acanthose
I. Epidermis	3. Stratum basale	Reichlich „Klarzellen". Kontinuierliche oder diskontinuierliche Proliferation einzelner Melanomzellen oder kleinerer Nester, wie präblastomatöse Melanose	Überpigmentierte Basalzellen
	4. Basalmembran	durchgehend intakt	—
II. Cutis	5. Stratum papillare: cutis	Kontinuierliche, meist diskontinuierliche Wucherung kleinerer Aggregate von Melanomzellen, epitheloid bis polymorphzellig	Oberflächenparalleles Infiltrat
	6. Stratum reticulare cutis	Melanomzellen, meist polymorph, in Haarfollikeln und in der Peripherie von Talgdrüsen. „Entlanggleiten" einzelner vielgestaltiger Melanomzellen am ekkrinen Schweißdrüsengang	Perifokales Infiltrat. Auffällige, *einzelne* Melanophagen pericapillär. Lymphgefäßektasie, fakultativ. Emboli in Lymphgefäßen
III. Subcutis	7. Oberflächliche Fettläppchen	Melanomzellen im Bereich der ekkrinen Schweißdrüsenschläuche	Mitosen an ekkrinen Schweißdrüsengangzellen, fokales Infiltrat, einzelne Melanophagen, Emboli in Lymphgefäßen, subintimale Tumorprogression in größeren Venen

Massonschen Silberimprägnierung und den üblichen Färbemethoden unterzogenen Gewebsstücke (ausgezeichnete Resultate liefert die kombinierte Incubations- und Imprägnationstechnik nach MISHIMA) soll eine dreidimensionale sein: sie erfaßt Zentrum sowie Rand der Geschwulst in je zwei zueinander senkrecht stehenden horizontalen Durchmessern und in der vertikalen Ebene. Der *heute* als wichtig herausgestellten Unterscheidung, ob ein malignes Melanom noch superfiziell ist oder bereits in die Tiefe proliferiert, wird das genaue Studium des peritumorösen Raumes an die Seite gestellt. Demgegenüber erscheint der Nachweis vom Einbruch der Geschwulstmassen in Gefäße, zumindestens im zentralen Tumorbereich, zweitrangig, weil die Entscheidung, ob wirklich eine Capillare vorliegt, oft nicht zu treffen ist. — Die Tumorzellabstriche ersetzen die feingewebliche Untersuchung nicht!

Die für ein malignes Melanom kennzeichnenden Merkmale sind in den Tab. 1 u. 2 enthalten.

Weniger für die feingewebliche Diagnose eines malignen Melanoms als für die Klassifikation und Prognose wichtig ist die Feststellung, welche verdächtigen Veränderungen in der *Geschwulstumgebung* vorliegen. Dazu zählen: die kontinuierliche oder diskontinuierliche, junktionale Aktivität im Sinne einer präblastomatösen

Melanose bzw. die Anwesenheit einer übernormalen Menge von „Klarzellen",
die Epidermisinvasion durch derartige Zellen, das bandförmig diese Erscheinungen begleitende Infiltrat, die subbasale, meist diskontinuierliche Tumor-
zellprogression, das „Absteigen" oder „Entlanggleiten" von Tumorzellen oder
kleineren Tumorzellaggregaten an den Hautanhangsgebilden, insbesondere an
ekkrinen Schweißdrüsenausführungsgängen, letztlich Mikroembolien von Ge-
schwulstelementen in dem lymphatischen Streubereich I. Sekundäre Erscheinungen
dazu sind: das nie fehlende Infiltrat, auffällige Melanophagen in perivasculärer
oder perifokaler Lokalisation, fakultativ Lymphgefäßektasie, Mitosen an den
ekkrinen Schweißdrüsengangzellen als Zeichen der Gewebsreizung.

Ähnlich bedeutungsvoll ist die oft schwierige Differenzierung von Primärtumor und Satellit, insbesondere, wenn letzterer Epidermotropie und Begleit-
infiltrat aufweist. Es fehlt zumeist die seitliche Tumorprogression als präblasto-
matöses Band, letztere als Zeichen der primär multiplen, ins Maligne ausgerichteten
junktionalen Aktivität in ein und demselben Hautfeld; auch die Epidermisinvasion ist nur begrenzt, fokal. Die „junktionale" Aktivität wird vorgetäuscht
durch große, polymorphe Melanomzellen, deren Zusammenhang mit intracanali-
culären Emboli durch die Tyrosinasereaktion dieser Zellen aufgedeckt werden
kann.

Zusammenfassend ist zu sagen: Je größer die persönliche Erfahrung des Histologen, desto vorsichtiger und bescheidener wird er in seiner Aussage, ob ein
gegebener pigmentierter Tumor ein malignes Melanom ist oder nicht.

Free Communications

Benign Juvenile Melanoma
Several Selected Aspects from a Study of 51 Lesions

R. ANDRADE, Laboratory of Skin Pathology, New York University Medical
Center, University Hospital, Skin and Cancer Unit, New York (USA)

This presentation deals with some unusual aspects of the clinico-pathological
entity of Benign Juvenile Melanoma (for details and literature on the subject see
review by KOPF and ANDRADE, 1965/1966). Since then eight more lesions have been
studied, making a total of 51 lesions in 48 patients. The youngest patient was
1 year old, and the oldest 45 years at the time of consultation (average 10.3 years).
There were 27 females, and 21 males all caucasians. The size of the lesions oscillated
between 2 and 19 mm (average 7.3 mm). The duration ranged between 2 months
and 22 years. 37 lesions were within the range of 2 months and 4 years (average
11.1 months); four were present since birth (patient ages 6, 10, 11 and 22 years);
seven lesions were of unknown duration. The distribution was 19 in the face,
2 in the neck, 10 in the upper and 10 in the lower extremities, 9 on the back and
1 on the buttock. Conservative excision was performed in 36 lesions, two of which
recurred and were reexcised; shave biopsy and electrodesiccation were applied to
eight lesions — two recurred and were excised. Two cases were left untreated
after biopsy and are under observation. The follow-up period ranges between
3 months and 11 years (average 3 years). There were no serious sequelae or metastases in any of these patients*.

---

* 11 of the 48 cases came from private physicians, Drs. G. POPKIN, S. BRODIE, A. SHAPIRO,
F. SCHELL, R. SCHER, R. STRITZLER, M. DANNENBERG, D. FISCHER, D. VERUT.

The following clinical and histological varieties of BJM will be presented:

1. The BJM "en plaque" and multinodular form (three cases, ages 1, 3, 16 years, all girls, on cheeks).

2. The multiple and agminated form on café-au-lait spot (one case, 2 year old girl, dorsum of wrist). Several red-brown nodules appear during the early years of life on a café-au-lait spot present since birth.

3. The granuloma telangiectaticum-like or angiomatous type: a bluish-red crusted and angiomatous pediculated lesion (one case, 7 year old boy, arm). This case had one associated unique feature not yet described: an increased number of sweat ducts (sweat duct nevus?), several of them dilated and cystic (hydro-cystoma?) and embedded in a markedly edematous and angiomatous stroma. The typical cells in the junction area and in the dermis were a minor component in the entire lesion. This stresses the hamartomatous nature of the benign juvenile melanoma.

4. The hard fibromatous type (two cases, ages 5 and 22 years, girls, big toe and dorsum of hand, duration 2 years and since birth, respectively). The stroma is predominantly formed by a fibrotic connective tissue with a moderate amount of connective tissue cells. When the typical BJM cells and nests are in a minority, a dermatofibroma may be misdiagnosed.These cases may also represent a regressive stage in the involution of a BJM, however.

5. A pure junctional type with typical BJM cells. This lesion is unusual (one case, 26 year old woman, flat, firm, pale-brown lesion of 1.0 × 0.5 cm on dorsum of foot, with the clinical diagnosis of dermatofibroma, but no fibrosis histologically).

6. The dark BJM lesions (variable shades from tan to brown). In this group, two types are of interest to us: a) a pigmented lesion with a pigmented, peri-lesional halo (one case, 2 year old boy cheek). This lesion began as a typical, tan-pink 0.5 cm nodule; and b) the deeply pigmented lesions (three cases, girls 3, 4 and 10 years, respectively, two on cheeks, one on side of neck). One of the lesions showed a marked pseudo-epitheliomatous hyperplasia with junctional activity, a few nests of large, round or oval cells with bizarre nuclei, and rare isolated cells with an abundant, well limited eosinophilic cytoplasm, and a dermal proliferation of spindle cells, which occur isolated or in bundles, and in some areas simulate a blue nevus.

7. The "round cell" type mentioned by GARTMANN (three cases, boys 5, 14 and 17 years old, two on back and one on earlobe). Typical BJM cells and/or giant cells are found in serial sections in the upper dermis, though only rare ones at times. Histologically, the lesions appear benign. Clinically, these three cases were typical. The hyperpigmented type (6 b, above) and the "round cell" type illustrate the relationship between BJM and the blue nevus and the group of nevus cell nevi, respectively.

8. Apparently, there are no recorded cases of familial BJM, and/or incidence in twins. Two patients in this series are identical twins (boys 11 years, with several BJMs of several years' duration on their backs). One had two lesions, both excised, the other had three lesions, two of which were excised. One of those, clinically typical, showed an alarming cellular pleomorphism and rare mitotic figures. In 4 years of follow-up there has been no recurrence. Without the clinical findings and a thorough knowledge of BJM this lesion could have been misdiagnosed as malignant melanoma. This case confirms that BJM is a clinico-pathological entity. It is also uncommon for the number of lesions.

The spontaneous natural history of BJMs ist not known. They may regress without traces or undergo fibrosis, pedunculation, lipidization and depigmentation or resorption, as in leukoderma acquisitum centrifugum, or become a common intradermal nevus. The so-called "Blasenzell"-nevus or "balloon-celled" nevus predominantly found on the head and neck in children (HORNSTEIN), but rare, may represent a regressive stage of BJM. In this series two lesions (25 year old woman and 6 year old girl) showed a marked and widespread vacuolization of the cellular cytoplasm. The child's lesion showed alcian blue and colloidal iron positive material, almost completely digested by hyaluronidase, in the vacuolated cells of some cellular nests.

There has been no undisputed evidence in the 20 years since the publication of SPITZ that a BJM has undergone malignant transformation (see also ECHAVARRIA and ACKERMAN). Therefore, the term "benign" should be added to the faulty but common term of Juvenile Melanoma.

Histochemical and electron microscopic studies have demonstrated the relationship of the BJM cells to the melanocyte (MISHIMA). For discussion of histochemical studies see KOPF and ANDRADE, WELLS and FARTHING; for electrometric studies see MELCZER and KISS.

References. ECHEVARRIA, R., and L. V. ACKERMAN: Cancer (Philad.) **20**, 175 (1967). — HORNSTEIN, O.: Arch. klin. exp. Derm. **226**, 97 (1966). — KOPF, A. W., and R. ANDRADE: Year Book of Dermatology, p. 7—52. 1965/1966. — MELCZER, N., and J. KISS: Dermatologica (Basel) **117**, 242 (1958). — MISHIMA, Y.: Arch. Derm. **91**, 519 (1965). — WELLS, G. C., and G. J. FARTHING: Brit. J. Derm. **78**, 380 (1966).

Über das Verhalten der Melanomzellen in vitro

B. ROHDE, Univ.-Haut- und Poliklinik Hamburg-Eppendorf (Deutschland)

Die auch in vitro nachgewiesene geringe Strahlenempfindlichkeit der Melanomzellen hat als Konsequenz die operative Entfernung des Primärtumors. Darüber hinaus haben jahrelange Versuche keinen Hinweis für das Ansprechen dieses Tumors auf eine Chemotherapie ergeben. Hierin stimmen die klinischen Ergebnisse mit den Untersuchungen in der Gewebekultur überein.

Im Gegensatz zu vielen in vitro permanent wachsenden Zellstämmen anderer Organe, stößt die Isolierung und Weiterzüchtung reiner Zellstämme von Melanocyten des Menschen auf Schwierigkeiten. Die Wachstumsbeobachtungen sind ausnahmslos an Hand von Mischzellkulturen des Melanoms gewonnen. In plasma-clot-Kulturen wandern nämlich neben den stark pigmentierten Melanocyten auch mehr oder weniger pigmentphagozitierende Bindegewebszellen aus. Die Unterscheidung der einzelnen Zellarten ist wegen des Pigmentgehaltes der Zellen, zumindest in den Erstkulturen, sehr schwierig.

Subkulturen können das Bild klären. Die wesentlich langsamer auswachsenden Melanocyten liegen in den folgenden Subkulturen oft nur in Einzelexemplaren vor und werden von den schneller wachsenden Bindegewebszellen verdrängt. Diese Situation läßt die Beantwortung spezieller Fragen in bezug auf das Verhalten der Melanocyten nicht zu.

Es wäre von großem Wert, wenn an Melanocyten-Reinzellkulturen z. B. das Verhalten dieser Zellart auch auf ionisierende Strahlen und Cytostatika näher studiert werden könnte. Es ist zwar zu erwarten, daß sich die isolierten Melanocyten ohne umgebendes Stromagewebe anders verhalten, doch überwiegen die Vorzüge der Kultur-Melanocyten. Derartige Reinkulturen würden die Beantwortung vieler Fragen erlauben, z. B.:

Wie läuft die Zellteilung der malignen Melanomzelle ab? Wie sieht der dynamische Ablauf der Pigmentbildung im Melanocyten aus? Durch welches biochemische Verhalten zeichnet sich der maligne Melanocyt aus ? Welche Beziehungen bestehen zwischen Form und Funktion des Melanocyten ? Verhalten sich die Zellen eines Melanoms gleichsinnig, ob melanotisch oder amelanotisch ?

Da die plasma-clot-Methode immer nur Mischzellkulturen ergeben kann, verwenden wir die Monolayer-Kulturtechnik, die nach bekanntem Verfahren durch Trypsinierung des Ausgangstumors erreicht wird. Durch unterschiedlich lange Trypsineinwirkung werden die Bindegewebszellen weitgehend ausgeschaltet. Schwierigkeiten stellen sich hier ein durch die oft relativ kleinen Gewebsstückchen bei Primärtumoren und durch das Fehlen einer optimalen Nährlösung.

Unter vielen Medien hat sich eine Mischung aus TCM 199 (PARKER und MORTON) unter Zusatz von 20% inaktiviertem Kälberserum als geeignet erwiesen. Serum vom Menschen, auch solches vom gleichen Patienten, hat sich bei uns nicht bewährt.

In der Monolayerkultur haften zunächst nur wenige, noch abgerundete pigmentierte Zellen an der Wand der Reagensgläser. Nach etwa 5 Std entwickeln sich zarte Zellausläufer. Frühestens nach 5 Tagen ist die Kultur zu einem Zellrasen ausgewachsen. Als Zelltyp herrscht die Spindelform vor. An den Rändern der Kulturen und in älteren Zellrasen treten bizarre Formen und gelegentlich mehrkernige Zellen auf.

Für Subkulturen eignen sich 5 bis 10 Tage alte dichtgewachsene Zellrasen. Die mechanisch gewonnene Zellsuspension zeigt gegenüber der mit Trypsin abgelösten ein schnelleres Anwachsen in den neuen Gefäßen. Es wird dabei der Nachteil, daß es sich mehr um Zellaggregate und weniger um Einzelzellen handelt, in Kauf genommen. Trypsinierte Subkulturen ließen sich nur unter großem Zellverlust und einer Wachstumsverzögerung anlegen.

Der Pigmentgehalt der Zellen nimmt in den Subkulturen ab.

Die besten Wachstumsbefunde, einschließlich guter Pigmentbildung in Subkulturen, lieferten Zellen von Melanommetastasen unter Cytostatikabehandlung. Es ist deshalb die Frage aufgeworfen, ob unter diesen Bedingungen die Wachstumstendenz der Melanomzellen angeregt werden kann.

Production of Melanomas in Hairless Mice with Ultraviolet Light

J. H. EPSTEIN, W. L. EPSTEIN and T. NAKAI, Division of Dermatology, Department of Medicine, University of California School of Medicine, San Francisco, California (USA), and The Chicago Medical School, Institute for Medical Research, Chicago, Illinois (USA)

Introduction. Though epidemiological studies suggest a relationship between sun exposure and malignant melanoma formation, experimental evaluation of this problem has been limited by the lack of a suitable model. Recent studies indicate that small benign pigmented growths in the skin of hairless mice can be stimulated to form invasive melanocytic tumors by repeated ultraviolet light exposures. In the present investigation we examined the development pattern of these ultraviolet induced melanomas. In order to accomplish this, benign pigmented blue nevi were produced on the posterior half of the backs of 63, 8 to 11 week old, pigmented hairless mice by a single application of 200 micrograms of 7,12-dimethyl-benz (a) anthracene (DMBA) in acetone. These blue nevi do not appear spontaneously in this strain of mice. 13 months later the mice were divided into two groups. Group 1 consisted of 18 mice with benign blue nevi less than 3 mm in diameter on the posterior half of their backs. At this time, tri-weekly, 5 sec ultraviolet light exposures were initiated and continued for 7 months utilizing a hot quartz contact lamp (which produced 2.44×10^5 ergs per sq. cm per second of mid-ultraviolet light energy at a distance of 3.4 cm).

Group 2 consisted of 45 mice with pigmented lesions as in Group 1. These animals received no ultraviolet light.

In addition 58, 15 to 16 month old pigmented hairless mice which had not received an application of DMBA were divided into two groups (Groups 3 and 4). These animals did not have any blue nevi at this time. Group 3 received ultraviolet light exposures as in Group 1 and Group 4 did not receive any ultraviolet light. The mice were observed regularly for 7 months.

Results

Melanoma formation. Only melanocytic tumors greater than 16 mm³ were tabulated. The first melanoma was noted in Group 1 by the 3rd week after initiation of the ultraviolet light exposures. By 18 weeks, 5 mice in Group 1 had developed melanomas. No further large melanocytic tumor formation appeared despite continued ultraviolet light applications. All of these tumors originated in the small benign pigmented lesions (blue nevi) and became larger than 40 mm³. Two of the growths reached proportions greater than 100 mm³. No similar pigmented tumors occurred in any of the control groups (2, 3, or 4).

Histology and Special Studies

Blue nevi. The blue nevi consisted of dense sub-epidermal accumulations of dermal melanocytes. The main component was a large polyhedral cell with a small eccentrically placed nucleus. The cytoplasm was distended with melanin granules and the nucleus had a darkly clumped chromatin pattern. The reticulum stain showed some supporting structure suggesting that these cells were not phagocytes.

Melanomas. The main component of the large melanotic tumor was an invasive pigment laden polyhedral cell similar to that seen in the benign blue nevus. However, the nucleus was abnormal in size, shape, and chromatin pattern, and invasion of the underlying musculature was a consistent feature.

Electron micrographs revealed that the main component of this tumor was a neoplastic cell filled with melanin granules measuring up to about one micron in diameter and appearing round to short oval in outline. Unlike the granules of dermal melanocytes in the blue nevi, many of these granules contained vessicles of varying electronopacity with a distinct substructure composed of finer granules. Only a few mitochondria were present in the tumor cells and their cristae often appeared indistinct. The cytoplasm contained numerous ribosome particles which were often free but sometimes attached to endoplasmic reticulum. The Golgi zone was infrequently seen but when present it was fairly well developed. Thus, the main component of the large melanotic tumors had the characteristics of neoplastic melanocytes rather than pigment laden macrophages.

Lymph nodes. The regional lymph nodes draining the melanomas consistently contained masses of large pigment laden polyhedral cells which appeared to be metastatic from the tumor. However, we were unable to determine the nuclear structure because of the decolorizing procedures necessary. No evidence of distant metastasis was noted.

Autoradiographs. 2 mm pieces of blue nevi and melanomas were studied by autoradiographic techniques. Incubation of these tissues with tritiated dopa and tritiated tyrosine showed a selective uptake of both dopa and tyrosine by the blue nevi and melanoma cells, thus indicating that the tumor cells produced melanin and were not simply macrophages.

Effects of Depigmenting Agents on Melanocytes and Melanogenesis

M. A. Pathak, G. Szabó, E. Frenk, S. S. Bleehen, Y. Hori and
T. B. Fitzpatrick, Harvard Medical School, Boston, Massachusetts (USA)*

The compounds that are presently used to produce cutaneous depigmentation when applied topically are hydroquinone and the monobenzyl, monomethyl, and monoethyl ethers of hydroquinone. N-(2-mercaptoethyl)-dimethylamine hydrochloride (MEDA) and beta-mercaptoethylamine hydrochloride (MEA) and sulfanilic acid, all of which are unrelated to known depigmenting agents of the hydroquinone group, also exert a depigmenting effect when injected intradermally into black goldfish. The hydroquinone groups of compounds do not consistently produce depigmentation, vary in their potency, and frequently irritate the skin. Ideally, depigmentation of skin by exogenous agents should involve selective action on melanocytes and melanogenesis without the induction of an inflammatory response in the epidermis. Experiments with various topically applied compounds have demonstrated that selective degeneration or loss of melanocytes in black guinea pigs can occur only in areas treated with mercaptoamines such as N-(2-mercaptoethyl) dimethylamine HCl (MEDA), 2-mercaptoethylamine HCl (MEA), and catechol derivatives such as 4-isopropylcatechol (4-IPC) and 4-methylcatechol.

33 compounds, some of them hitherto unrecognized as depigmenting agents, were evaluated on the epilated skin of the back and on the unepilated skin of the ear of pigmented guinea pigs. These compounds included some thiols and other mercaptoamines, catechol and several derivatives of catechol, several quinones, and other compounds. The compounds were applied once daily, five times a week, for periods up to one month, in concentrations ranging from 1 to 10 Gm-% in vanishing creams. The number of melanocytes and Langerhans' cells, and the tyrosinase activity of melanocytes and their reactivity with tyrosine and dopa were evaluated. Structural changes in melanocytes, Langerhans' cells, and keratinocytes were examined by electron microscopy.

MEDA and 4-IPC were potent depigmenting agents; 4-IPC was more potent than any compound yet tested. In areas treated with 5% 4-IPC and MEDA, depigmentation occurred in 1 to 2 weeks; with 1% and 3% preparations, in 2 to 3 weeks. Pigmentation of the hair was not affected. In MEDA-treated or 4-IPC; treated depigmented areas, almost no melanin granules were found in the epidermis, and the melanocyte count was significantly reduced (from 700 to 800 to 50 to 80 melanocytes/mm² with MEDA and 0 to 14 melanocytes/mm² with 4-IPC); The perikaryon and the dendrites of the epidermal melanocytes were markedly altered, and their tyrosinase activity and reactivity to dopa were also markedly decreased. The few remaining melanocytes appeared degenerative. Mild acanthosis due to epilation was seen in skin treated with 1 and 2 Gm-% MEDA and 4-IPC; 5% 4-IPC induced a mild inflammatory reaction; 5% MEDA, a more marked dermatitis. In epidermis treated with MEDA or 4-IPC, melanocytes could be detected only rarely by electron microscopy. Those that were found contained few melanized melanosomes. Some of them appeared as imperfectly melanized or malformed melanosomes. Evidence of cell degeneration could be detected in these rare melanocytes.

Depigmentation by any exogenous agent can result from 1. loss or degeneration of melanocytes; 2. interference with a) the biosynthesis of premelanosomes and

* Supported by United States Public Health Service Grants 5 R 01-CA-05003, CA-05010, and CA-05401 from the National Cancer Institute.

melanosomes, b) the conversion of tyrosine to dopa to melanin, c) the biosynthesis of tyrosinase or the active center of the enzyme, or d) the transfer of melanosomes to keratinocytes; and 3. chemical alteration of melanin present in melanosomes. Depigmentation by MEDA and 4-IPC appears to result from selective destruction and disappearance of melanocytes.

On the other hand, loss of pigment in the developing embryos of *Fundulus heteroclitus* maintained in sea water to which phenylthiourea (PTU) has been added (8×10^{-3} M) is brought about by a quite different mechanism. PTU arrested the melanization of melanosomes only and did not affect either melanosomal development or melanocytes. PTU caused depigmentation of the eye and body. Tyrosinase activity was inhibited. The uptake of tritiated dopa was reduced, but the incorporation of tritiated thymidine, valine, and leucine was not affected.

Dopa in Melanoma

H. RORSMAN, University of Lund (Sweden)

Some years ago when we were studying the adrenergic innervation of the skin using the fluorescence method of FALCK and HILLARP we found some fluorescent cells in the basal layer of the epidermis. These cells corresponded in their distribution and morphology to melanocytes.

The histochemical reaction used detects noradrenaline in the adrenergic nerves but also other catecholamines, serotonin and the immediate precursors of these compounds, DOPA and 5-hydroxytryptophane.

The essential feature of this method is a condensation of the compounds with formaldehyde which gives strongly fluorescent products easily detectable in fluorescence microscopy.

The induction of fluorescence in the melanocytes suggested that we had been able to detect DOPA as this substance is considered to be an intermediate in the melanin formation. In melanocytes where the melanin synthesis is rapid the fluorescence intensity was found to be increased. This is the case in the hair follicle melanocytes. After irradiation of the skin with UV or roentgen the fluorescence was also increased and could be detected in a larger number of melanocytes. In pathologic melanin-forming cells there is often a very strong fluorescence. In dermal nevi there is a strong fluorescence in the superficial portion, but in the deep parts the fluorescence is weak or absent. In the dermal nevi there is also an activation of the epidermal melanocytes. An interesting finding is that deep giant cells of dermal nevi have a strong fluorescence in contrast to the surrounding nevus cells. In junctional and compound nevi the fluorescence is much stronger in the junctional parts of the nevus. Malignant melanomas show a strong fluorescence in the tumour cells.

From the beginning we suspected that DOPA was the compound responsible for the fluorescence in the melaninforming cells. We have now together with Dr. ROSENGREN of theDepartment of Pharmacology, University of Lund, investigated the occurrence of fluorescence-inducing amines and DOPA in malignant melanomas. The content of catecholamines is very low and cannot explain the fluorescence observed.

However, with chromatographic and fluorometric methods a substance with the same characteristics as DOPA was detected and incubation with DOPA decarboxylase was followed by a formation of Dopamine proving the original presence of DOPA.

Until now we have examined 44 malignant melanomas of the skin and fluorescence has been found in all. Metastasis to the lymphnodes fluoresces also, but the intensity varies between cells.

Ocular melanomas differ in their fluorescence characteristics from skin melanomas. Thus out of eleven studied cases only four showed fluorescence. The background for this difference between skin melanomas and ocular melanomas has not yet been found.

Hamster skin melanomas and different mouse melanomas did not show fluorescence and there are thus interesting differences between species.

This fluorescence method, which seems to detect DOPA in melanin-forming cells, will give us new opportunities to study the metabolism of normal melanocytes and cells of melanomas and will perhaps also be of value in the diagnosis of these tumours.

Multiple Forms of Tyrosinase from Mammalian Melanoma

J. B. Burnett and H. Seiler, Harvard Medical School, Dept. of Dermatology Boston, Mass. (USA)

Tyrosinase (EC 1. 10. 3. 1) participates in the formation of natural tyrosine-melanin by catalyzing the conversion of tyrosine to 3,4-dihydroxyphenylalanine (DOPA) and, in turn, DOPA to DOPA-quinone. This paper is concerned with the isolation and characterization of multiple forms of tyrosinase from mouse and human melanomas.

Multiple forms of tyrosinase have been found in a number of plants and animals. By using a variety of physical and chemical techniques to isolate the tyrosinases from various organisms and organs, numerous characteristics of the enzymes have been established. Such data suggest that the composition or conformation of the active site of the tyrosinase molecule may be constant and that it is the inactive protein moiety of the enzyme that may undergo subtle change.

Harding-Passey, B-16, and Cloudman S-91 melanomas were grown and maintained by serial transplant in Swiss white, C 57 BL/6 J, and DBA/1 J mice, respectively. The tumors were grown to optimum size and quality for each strain, excised, quickly frozen, and stored at $-20\,^{\circ}\mathrm{C}$. Crude extracts of tyrosinase were prepared from tumor material by the method of Shimao which is a modification of the method of Brown and Ward. Due to differences in solubility, the tyrosinase was separated into two distinct fractions. The fractions are called "firmly bound tyrosinase" — the source of the associated or insoluble enzyme — and "freely extractable ('soluble') tyrosinase" — the source of the soluble enzyme.

Soluble tyrosinase is further fractionated into two distinct components, T^1 and T^2, by continuous-flow paper electrophoresis and this separation is confirmed by acrylamide-gel electrophoresis. Prior to continuous-flow paper electrophoresis, the two partially purified, soluble enzymes are present in a single solution; whereas following continuous-flow paper electrophoresis, each of these enzymes is isolated. The position of tyrosinase activity within each acrylamide gel is easily located by treating the gel with L-tyrosine or L-DOPA.

Associated or insoluble tyrosinase is released from the "firmly bound tyrosinase" precipitate by resuspending the precipitate and adding a non-ionic detergent. After 4 h with constant agitation at $5\,^{\circ}\mathrm{C}$, the suspension is centrifuged; the clear, light supernatant solution contains the solubilized enzyme, T^3. With acrylamide-gel electrophoresis, at least four bands of enzymic activity are easily discernible. The electrophoretic mobility of each of these forms of the enzyme is different from that of either of the soluble enzymes. It is not yet known whether these solubilized forms of the enzyme are attached to a non-enzymic, extraneous protein moiety or are aggregates of T^1, or of T^2, or of T^1 plus T^2.

Each form of tyrosinase has its characteristic R_x (position of migration) value. Each mouse-melanoma extract contains two soluble tyrosinases, T^1 and T^2, which migrate with characteristic R_x values of 0.62 and 0.51, respectively, and solubilized tyrosinases, T^3, which migrate with characteristic R_x values of 0.40, 0.28, 0.22, and 0.13.

Whereas the soluble forms of the enzyme, T^1 and T^2, are easily separated by continuous-flow paper electrophoresis, the solubilized forms of T^3 cannot be separated by this method, and further studies related to these forms of the enzyme are yet to be performed. Final purification of each soluble tyrosinase is achieved using a combination of ion-exchange and Sephadex columns. When the enzyme migrates as a single symmetric peak under conditions of ultracentrifugation and its specific activity has become constant, the corresponding acrylamide-gel pattern shows a single enzyme and a single protein band in corresponding positions of electrophoretic migration.

The tyrosinase in extracts from metastatic malignant human melanoma has also been examined by these techniques that have been developed for the separation and partial purification of tyrosinase in extracts from mouse melanomas. Enzyme extracts may be prepared from excised nodules, either fresh or fresh-frozen (—20 °C), since no differences can be discerned in the quality or quantity of enzyme obtained. Clear, distinct enzyme patterns are obtained in acrylamide-gel when the tyrosinase has been extracted from as little as 50 mg wet weight of human melanoma. When extracts of partially purified tyrosinase from human melanoma are subjected to acrylamide-gel electrophoresis and the mobilities of the active forms of this tyrosinase are compared with the tyrosinases from mouse melanoma (e.g., Harding-Passey melanoma), there is a unique 1:1 correspondence between the T^1, T^2, and T^3 positions of active enzymes from both mouse melanoma and human melanoma. Within the limitations of purification and enzymic assay described here, the extraneous protein present in the partially purified enzyme preparations does not influence or interfere with the electrophoretic mobilities of any of the active forms of tyrosinase.

Such data suggest that the major, outstanding active forms of both soluble and so-called "insoluble" tyrosinases present in enzyme extracts from human melanoma are probably the same as the tyrosinases from mouse-melanoma extracts with corresponding electrophoretic mobilities.

This investigation was supported by Public Health Service Research Grants CA-08292 and CA-05010 from the National Cancer Institute.

370 Mélanomes malins — Statistiques et pronostic

J. M. SIMONART, Clinique Dermatologique de l'Université de Bruxelles (Belgique)

Le naevocarcinome est un cancer au pronostic particulièrement sombre : 28,5% de survie au bout de 5 ans dans notre statistique portant sur 370 observations. Ce chiffre est inférieur à celui du cancer envisagé dans son ensemble (39%), à ceux du cancer du sein ou du col utérin (36,5%). La thérapeutique actuelle du mélanome malin comporte essentiellement une exérèse locale large et une thérapeutique ganglionnaire. Si la nécessité d'une exérèse locale très large est actuellement bien établie, l'intérêt du curage ganglionnaire est discuté. Aussi avons-nous comparé les délais de survie obtenus chez les patients qui ont subi un curage ganglionnaire et chez ceux qui ne l'ont pas subi.*

A. Statistique: Au stade I (pas de ganglions décelables), la comparaison a porté sur 64 cas, au stade II (ganglions cliniquement décelables) sur 119 cas.

Survie médiane	stade I	curage ganglionnaire pas de curage	21 mois 17 mois
	stade II	curage ganglionnaire pas de curage	12 mois 5 mois
Survie 5 ans	stade I	curage ganglionnaire pas de curage	62 % cas 59,5% cas
	stade II	curage ganglionnaire pas de curage	8,5% cas 0 % cas

La prolongation de survie obtenue par le curage est statistiquement valable au stade II, elle ne l'est pas au stade I.

B. Interprétation des résultats. Tous les patients dont les ganglions étaient envahis, mais aussi de nombreux patients dont les ganglions excisés n'avaient pas montré de cellules cancéreuses, sont morts de leur cancer à plus ou moins longue échéance. Le curage ne change donc rien au *pronostic final* du naevocarcinome.

L'étude de la physiologie du système lymphatique permet de comprendre pourquoi le curage ganglionnaire ne peut *guérir* un mélanome malin: lorsque les cellules cancéreuses se glissent dans les capillaires lymphatiques, elles ne sont pas automatiquement arrêtées au premier relais ganglionnaire. Des anastomoses existent en effet fréquemment entre des vaisseaux lymphatiques provenant de territoires distincts et se dirigeant vers des ganglions lymphatiques différents. De plus, il est actuellement démontré qu'il existe dans le naevocarcinome une dissémination précoce des cellules cancéreuses dans le sang. La précocité de cette dissémination sanguine doit sans doute être mise en rapport avec la riche vascularisation des naevi; cette riche vascularisation est la résultante d'un trouble embryologique mixte portant à la fois sur les crêtes neurales et les formations vasculaires. Les cellules cancéreuses peuvent donc sauter le barrage ganglionnaire tant par voie sanguine que par voie lymphatique; ainsi s'expliquent les observations de patients atteints de naevocarcinome au stade I, où le curage ganglionnaire montre l'absence de cellules cancéreuses, et qui néanmoins décèdent de leur cancer: les cellules malignes étaient déjà au-delà de ce premier relais ganglionnaire.

Il est donc capital de traiter le mélanome malin aussi précocement que possible, avant que les cellules malignes n'aient pu essaimer dans l'organisme par voie sanguine ou lymphatique. Les statistiques montrent d'ailleurs qu'une relation directe existe entre les chances de survie et la précocité du diagnostic: 50% de survie lorsque le patient consulte au cours des six premiers mois d'évolution, 30% de survie s'il consulte un an après les premiers symptômes, 1,5% si le délai est de 2 ans.

Lorsque le naevocarcinome a dépassé le stade de malignité locale, le curage ganglionnaire ne peut plus changer le pronostic final. Ce curage n'est néanmoins pas inutile: pratiqué sur des ganglions envahis par les cellules cancéreuses (stade II),

---

* Nous remercions Mlle le Prof. SIMON et Mle Prof. SMETS de l'Institut de Cancérologie de l'Université de Bruxelles d'avoir mis à notre disposition les dossiers des naevocarcinomes de l'Institut Bordet.

il prolonge la survie: 12 mois au lieu de cinq selon nos observations. Il s'agit là d'une survie moyenne: dans plus de 8% des cas, la survie dépasse 5 ans.

C. Conclusions. 1. Les moyens thérapeutiques actuels ne sont efficaces que sur des lésions au stade de malignité locale. Il est donc essentiel de pratiquer un diagnostic aussi précoce que possible. 2. Au stade II, le curage ganglionnaire donne un *coup de frein* à l'évolution de la maladie, mais il ne peut l'enrayer définitivement.

Bibliographie. ACHTEN, G., et J. M. SIMONART: Bull. Soc. franç. Derm. Syph. **73**, 698 (1966). — SIMONART, J. M.: Arch. belges. Derm. 1967 (sous presse).

A propos de 400 mélanomes malins cutanés

C. DUFOURMENTEL, R. MOULY et J. GLICENSTEIN, Hôpital Saint-Louis, Paris (France)

Nous avons exposé dans deux publications récentes [1, 2] notre statistique d'ensemble. Elle s'élève maintenant à 400 cas qui nous inspirent les conclusions suivantes:

I. Etiologie et clinique

1. Sexe. Approximativement deux femmes sont atteintes pour un homme.

2. Age. Chez l'homme, il existe un maximum à 60 ans, chez la femme il en existe deux à 30 ans et à 50 ans.

3. Siège. Chez l'homme la répartition est égale. Chez la femme, la fréquence est plus grande à la face (à cause de la mélanose de Dubreuilh) et la jambe.

4. Terrain: Nous n'avons pas rencontré de cas familiaux ni chez les noirs, un seul chez un Nord-Africain musulman.

5. Lésions pré-existantes: Dans 54% des cas seulement nous avons la certitude de l'existence préalable d'un naevus bénin existant depuis l'enfance. Dans 32% une lésion d'apparition tardive, mais cliniquement bénigne a précédé la dégénérescence (dans 7% des cas, il s'agissait d'une mélanose de Dubreuilh); dans 14% le mélanome est apparu en peau saine.

6. Rôle des Traumatismes: Le traumatisme accidentel a été manifeste dans un cas sur sept environ. Il a été discutable dans un cas sur trois, absent dans les autres. Les irritations chroniques n'ont pas semblé avoir la valeur qu'on leur attribue souvent.

7. Diagnostic: Le plus souvent, le diagnostic était fait cliniquement, mais c'est l'histologie seule qui ous a donné une certitude encore que dans certains cas, la malignité soit difficile à affirmer. Nous avons renoncé à l'examen histologique extemporané en raison de ses incertitudes.

8. Evolution: La tendance évolutive est extrêmement variable: *formes aigües* très rapidement mortelles (8%), *formes très lentes* ou à évolution bloquée. Nous avons même observé un cas de *guérison* (ou tout au moins de rémission complète) *spontanée* durant plus de 10 ans.

Les *adénopathies* n'existaient dès le Ier examen que dans 14% des cas; dans 20% des cas, elles sont apparues ultérieurement.

Malgré la très large exérèse que nous pratiquons, nous avons observé des *récidives* locales dans 12% des cas. Les *métastases viscérales* représentent la cause de mort habituelle; les *métastases cutanées* sont très fréquentes. Il faut insister sur les métastases «*in-transit*» qui surviennent entre la tumeur et le relai ganglionnaire

(14 cas). Favorisées par la stase lymphatique, elles surviennent surtout après curage ganglionnaire — même en l'absence d'envahissement.

II. Traitement

L'étude de nos cas nous a conduits à l'attitude thérapeutique suivante:

1. Sur la Lésion Elle-même

Exérèse au bistouri électrique, large mais non mutilante — Examen histologique soigneux après fixation et coloration. Si l'histologie confirme la malignité, nouvelle exérèse très large et allant jusqu'à l'aponévrose, excentrée par rapport à la lésion de façon à enlever plus dans le sens de la circulation lymphatique. Cette exérèse est menée au bistouri ordinaire. Une greffe de peau mince répare la brèche, soit dans le même temps, soit ultérieurement après avoir laissé bourgeonner. Cette technique comporte quelques exceptions, en particulier à la face chez la femme jeune où l'autoplastie est parfois préférée à la greffe pour des raisons esthétiques.

2. Sur les Ganglions

a) *Ganglions cliniquement envahis.* Si la lésion est proche du territoire ganglionnaire, opération monobloc enlevant simultanément le mélanome, les ganglions et tout le tissu intermédiaire susceptible de contenir des lymphatiques allant de l'un à l'autre. Si la lésion est distante, l'adénectomie n'est pratiquée que dans un second temps au moins trois semaines plus tard pour permettre aux cellules en cours de migration lymphatique d'avoir atteint le territoire ganglionnaire.

b) *Ganglions cliniquement sains.* Nous avons renoncé au curage de principe pour les raisons suivantes:

— La fréquence d'envahissement infra-clinique est faible (6 fois sur 38 curages de principe).

— les métastases migratrices dites «in-transit» ne sont pas exceptionelles après ces opérations.

— l'ablation de ganglions histologiquement envahis n'a pas amélioré le pronostic.

— l'ablation de ganglions histologiquement sains est parfois suivie d'une flambée de généralisation.

— l'ablation d'adénopathies apparues secondairement est d'un pronostic moins mauvais qu'on ne pourrait le croire (35% de survies de cinq ans) en tout cas meilleur que celui des curages de principe avec ganglions envahis.

— Le facteur moral est loin d'être négligeable. Or, le curage ganglionnaire signe pour le malade l'existence d'une lésion maligne.

— les séquelles d'un curage ganglionnaire (oedème de stase lymphatique, par exemple) ne sont pas exceptionnelles.

Au total, bien que toute statistique trop courte soit sujette à caution, nous pensons que les ganglions lymphatiques ne sont pas inutiles. Il n'est même pas impossible que les plus utiles soient ceux qui sont déjà histologiquement envahis. Si, en effet, il existe une lutte de l'organisme d'ordre immunologique c'est peut-être dans les ganglions où se trouvent en contact le tissu lymphoïde et quelques cellules cancéreuses que peuvent le mieux s'élaborer les anticorps salutaires.

Mais, bien entendu, à partir du moment où le ganglion est envahi au point d'être perceptible cliniquement, il n'est plus qu'un réservoir de cellules malignes qui peuvent essaimer ailleurs et il doit être extirpé à tout prix.

Bibliographie. 1. DUFOURMENTEL, C., R. MOULY et J. GLICENSTEIN: Bull. Soc. franç. Derm. Syph. **73**, 797 (1966). — 2. DUFOURMENTEL, C., R. MOULY et J. GLICENSTEIN: Mem. Acad. Chir. **93**, 410 (1967).

Zur Häufigkeit des malignen Melanoms. Ergebnis einer Umfrage

H. KÄSTNER, P. JORDAN und G. FORCK, Universitäts-Hautklinik Münster
(Deutschland)

Es interessierte die Häufigkeit des Vorkommens des malignen Melanoms. Das
Problem seiner Therapie ist bisher, wie man weiß, unbefriedigend gelöst. Wenn
auch nach eigenen Erfahrungen den Melanomkranken, wenn sie in Fachbehand-
lung treten, ein Weiterleben von einigen Jahren ohne Erscheinungen oft zuge-
sichert werden kann und einige Kranke endgültig ausgeheilt werden, so ist es doch
eine bei der Mehrzahl früher oder später tödlich endende Krankheit. Fehlt aber
eine befriedigende Therapie, so ist man bevorzugt an Frühbehandlung, Früherfas-
sung und Statistiken des Vorkommens interessiert. Sie versprechen in der Tat
bessere Behandlungsaussichten, und durch die Behandlung der Lentigo maligna
kennt man eine echte Prophylaxe des malignen Melanoms. Eindrucksmäßig würde
man sagen: Das maligne Melanom ist nicht so selten wie man oft glaubt. Es ist
aber gewiß nicht allzu häufig. In Kliniken mit speziellem Interesse dafür pflegen
sich verhältnismäßig mehr Fälle anzusammeln.

Über die Häufigkeit des Vorkommens des malignen Melanoms fanden sich folgende Angaben: Nach SPIER (1961/62) ist es „relativ selten". „Es stellt nur knapp
1% aller bösartigen Tumoren dar." Nach Erhebungen von MCDONALD müßte man
damit rechnen, daß jährlich 1,8 bis 2,5 neue m.M.-Fälle auf 100 000 Personen an-
fallen. Nach WILDNER (1963) bietet die Krebsmeldepflicht in der Deutschen Demokratischen Republik die Möglichkeit, verläßliche Angaben über die Morbidität
einzelner Geschwulstformen zu machen: 1953 bis 1956 wurden 1 629 Neuerkrankungen an malignen Melanomen registriert. Dabei entfielen von 1 570 1 230 = 78%
auf die Haut, 302 (19%) auf die Augen. 64% waren histologisch gesichert. Rund
98% waren demnach Melanome der Haut oder der Augen. 1959 fanden sich
553 Fälle von neuen Melanomen, gleich 1,2% der Neuerkrankungen an Krebs.

Die eigene Statistik beschränkt sich auf *Westfalen*, das eine der beiden Länder
von Nordrhein-Westfalen. Westfalen hatte 1966 7,8 Millionen Einwohner.

Die Univ.-Hautklinik veröffentlichte in einer Zeitschrift, dem Mitteilungsblatt der Ärzte-
kammer, das jedem Arzt und Facharzt in Westfalen zugestellt wird, einen Aufruf zur Zählung
aller Melanomfälle, soweit sie vom 1. Januar bis 31. Dezember 1966 neu in Behandlung oder
zur Kenntnis kamen. Kurze Angaben zu Vorgeschichte, Behandlung und Verlauf waren er-
wünscht. Es wurde jedoch nur um eine chiffrierte Mitteilung (Vornamen, Anfangsbuchstaben
des Zunamens und Geburtsdatum) gebeten. Die Ermittlung eines Melanomfalles wurde von
der Klinik mit 10,— DM honoriert. Die Fachkollegen wurden bei einem Colloquium durch
einen kurzen Vortrag mit Demonstration typischer Fälle von FORCK u. KÄSTNER besonders
aufmerksam gemacht.

Mitteilung gemacht wurde von:

68 Fällen.

30 Fälle stammten aus der Universitäts-Hautklinik,

11 Fälle aus der damit verbundenen Fachklinik Haus Hornheide.

Diese Zahlen, insgesamt 109 Fälle — rund 1,4 bezogen auf 100 000 Einwohner —
sind kleiner als die von MCDONALD errechneten 1,8 bis 2,5. Die Zahl MCDONALDS
ist vielleicht etwas zu hoch gegriffen. Andererseits dürfte die eigene zu niedrig
sein. Aus der *Stadt* Münster, die rund 200 000 Einwohner hat, wurden mindestens
drei Fälle bekannt. Ein Teil der Fälle Westfalens dürfte nicht mitgeteilt worden
sein, andere sind mit Sicherheit nicht *erfaßt* worden. Aus den Mitteilungen, die ja
nicht gesetzlich vorgeschrieben waren, sondern kollegial erbeten, war zu erkennen,

daß die Diagnose malignes Melanom oft erst am Befall der regionalen Lymph-knoten bzw. nach Auftreten generalisierter Metastasen erkannt worden ist.*

Das maligne Melanom ist als solches anzuerkennen, wenn die klinische Diagnose — früher oder später — histologisch bestätigt worden ist: Das war so gut wie aus-nahmslos der Fall für die 30 Fälle der Klinik, nicht unbedingt z. B. für die 68 mit-geteilten.

Bei den 29 Fällen, die von den Röntgenärzten gemeldet worden waren, sind eine Reihe von Fällen als maligne Melanome röntgenbestrahlt worden, ohne daß sie es völlig sicher waren. Zurückgewiesen wurden die histologisch als Naevuszell-naevi verifizierten Fälle.

Praktische Ärzte, Chirurgen, Internisten und Dermatologen haben etwa gleich viele Melanome gemeldet. Bei den Dermatologen ist zu berücksichtigen, daß von ihnen viele Fälle der Klinik oder Haus Hornheide direkt zugeschickt wurden. Auf weitere statistische Einzelheiten soll hier nicht eingegangen werden.

Folgende *Schlußfolgerungen* wären zu ziehen; sie bringen eine kräftige Bestäti-gung von vielem bisher schon Vermuteten:

1. Das maligne Melanom, im allgemeinen nicht sehr häufig, wird noch von der Ärzteschaft vielfach verkannt. Für die Bevölkerung gilt, daß ein Todesfall an malignem Melanom auf den Bekanntenkreis oft alarmierend wirkt und nicht so ganz selten zur Aufdeckung anderer Fälle führt.

2. Die Diagnose malignes Melanom ist schwierig. Den Dermatologen gehört die entscheidende Rolle. Größere Hautkliniken haben Behandlungszentren zu werden. Auch die histologische Untersuchung des malignen Melanoms ist schwierig. Nicht jede Pathologendiagnose ist richtig. Die Röntgenologen richten sich bisweilen zu gutgläubig nach der Einweisungsdiagnose, die besser von zwei Ärzten gestellt wird.

3. Die Statistik bedarf weiterer Pflege. Festlegung der Durchschnittsrate hat Interesse nicht zuletzt für einen internationalen Vergleich, insbesondere zwischen Völkern verschiedener Hautfarbe.

Lentigo Maligna and Malignant Melanoma

R. JACKSON, Ontario Cancer Foundation, Ottawa, Ontario (Canada)

Lentigo maligna is also known by the following names: la mélanose circonscrite précancéreuse (DUBREUILH), präcanceröse Melanose (MIESCHER), Hutchinson freckle, and melanotic freckle. From a study of 99 patients with malignant mela-noma of the skin [Canad. Med. Ass. J. 95, 846, (1966)], 21 of which arose in lentigo maligna, the following points are of interest:

1. Lentigo maligna itself is not a superficial malignant melanoma.

2. Approximately 25% (21 of 99) of all malignant melanoma arise from pre-existing lentigo maligna.

3. In certain cases it is very difficult, on the basis of the histopathological findings, to determine whether or not a particular lesion is benign or malignant. The inclusion of such borderline cases as malignant melanoma would favourably influence results of any treatment.

4. The long natural course (up to 40 years) of this lesion from freckle to malig-nant melanoma (Fig. 1) illustrates the biological stages from benignity to malig-nancy. No lentigo maligna develops into a malignant melanoma overnight.

---

* Die Lentigo maligna ist in der Statistik der hiesigen Fälle im allgemeinen nicht berück-sichtigt.

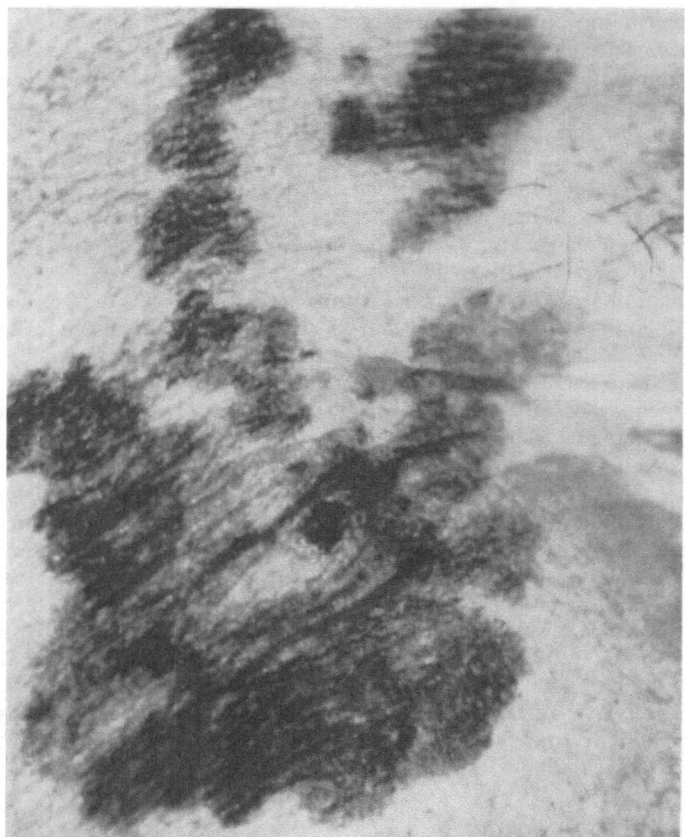

Fig. 1

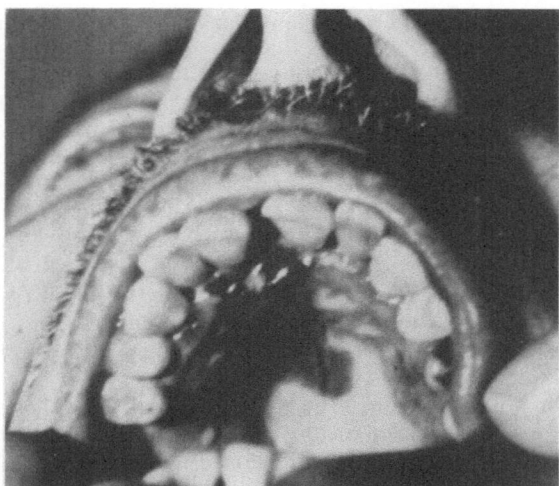

Fig. 2

5. Of 21 patients in whom a clinical and histopathological diagnosis of lentigo maligna was made as the origin of malignant melanoma, eight showed metastatic disease. Of 61 patients in whom malignant melanoma arose in other pigmented lesions, 22 showed metastatic disease. This seems to indicate that once malignant melanoma has developed, the prognosis is the same, no matter what the nature of the original lesion.

6. Multicentric malignant melanoma may arise in lentigo maligna.

7. Lentigo maligna may occur on the hard palate and there give rise to malignant melanoma (Fig. 2).

8. Malignant melanoma may be present in lentigo maligna without a nodule or ulcer.

Un diagnostic différentiel important des mélanomes. L'Angiokératome noir

G. E. Goetschel, Hôpital Saint-Louis, Paris (France)

Parmi les Angiokératomes (A.K.), les formes de Mibelli, de Fordyce et Sutton, de Fabry sont bien connues.

1. L'A.K. de Mibelli: Caractérisé par des petites formations rouges, de la taille d'une lentille ou davantage, recouvertes de squames kératosiques, adhérentes. Celles-ci siégeant électivement sur les faces dorsales des orteils, des genoux et des doigts, toujours chez des adultes jeunes, en général des filles.

2. L'A.K. de Fordyce et Sutton: Siégeant au niveau du scrotum chez des gens âgés.

3. L'A.K. de Fabry: Décrit par celui-ci en 1898 sous le nom de «Purpura hémorragique nodulaire»; puis, en 1915 sous le nom de «Angio-kératoma corporis diffusum», réalisant comme l'ont noté Ruitter et Pompen un syndrome cutanéo-cardio-vaso-rénal. Fabry divisa ensuite cette forme en deux types: la forme diffuse et la forme circonscrite.

Il faut noter que Lapierre en 1957 a présenté un cas associant A.K. de Fabry, A.K. du scrotum et de Mibelli.

Par contre, la forme solitaire bénigne que nous appelerons Angiokératome noir, n'a pas fait l'objet de publications très nombreuses si ce n'est la récente publication de D. O. Hayen: «Thrombosed Angiokeratoma simulating Malignant Melanoma» et surtout l'énorme travail sur les A.K. de R. Imperial et E. B. Helwig, dont nous avons eu connaissance alors que notre rapport était déjà rédigé.

En effet, nous nous interessons depuis plusieurs années à ce problème et nous avons réuni 20 cas qui peuvent s'ajouter aux 116 de Imperial et Helwig cas qui ont été vus soit en clientèle privée, soit dans le service du Prof. Duperrat à l'Hôpital Saint-Louis à Paris.

Le principal intérêt de ces malades, c'est que presque toujours ils nous ont été envoyés comme des mélanomes et bien souvent, nous nous sommes nous-mêmes mépris.

Clinique. L'A.K. noir apparait à n'importe quel endroit du corps. La distribution se fait à peu près équivalente sur la face antérieure et la face postérieure du corps, avec une nette prédominance pour le membre inférieur. Sur nos 20 malades, 16 avaient un A.K. noir localisé sur le membre inférieur, ce qui confirme les statistiques d'Imperial et Helwig. Cette lésion apparait à n'importe quel âge, même chez le vieillard mais surtout entre 15 et 35 ans.

Elle est en général indolore, ou à peine sensible.

Le sexe masculin est plus atteint que le sexe féminin, 70% pour nos cas.

C'est une lésion en général unique (Fig. 1), d'environ 2 à 8 mm de diamètre, plus ou moins saillante, verruqueuse, kératosique, dont la teinte varie du brun foncé, sur le violet, le gris foncé, le noir, le plus souvent d'ailleurs, franchement noir.

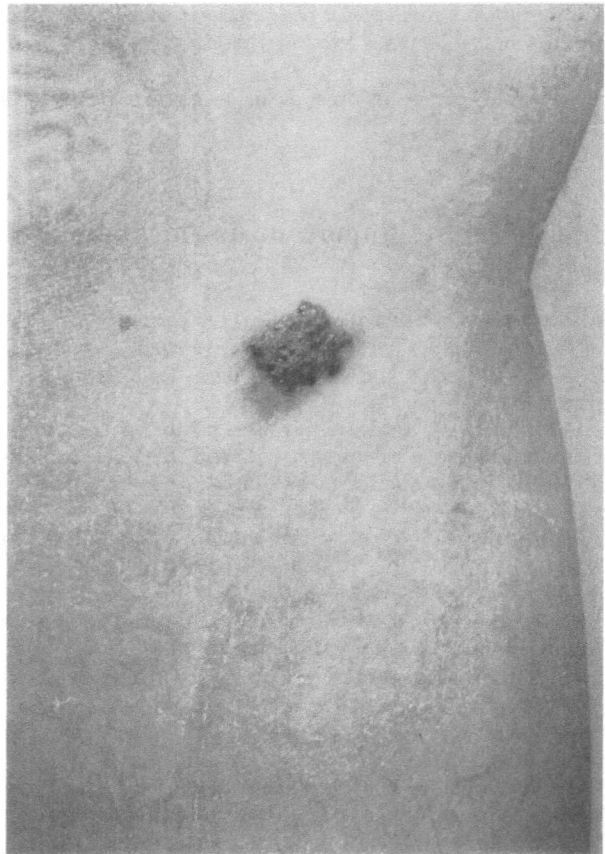

Fig. 1. Angiokératome de la face externe du coude considéré comme un mélano-carcinome rapidement évolutif

Cette prolifération noircit d'ailleurs progressivement, aussi, elle est presque toujours considérée à tort comme un mélanome.

Fait particulier: cette lésion qui est d'apparition récente, très noire d'emblée, s'accompagne souvent de petits nodules environnants eux aussi très noirs et parfois, la lésion unique est entourée d'une sorte de halo gris noirâtre.

Dans ces cas-là, la malignité semble ne faire aucun doute et ces malades nous sont toujours adressés avec le diagnostic de mélanomes malins; d'ailleurs, de nombreux patients ont été opérés très largement comme s'ils présentaient des mélanomes malins; c'est l'examen anatomo-pathologique de la pièce qui a rétabli le diagnostic exact.

Nous vous citerons pour exemple, la fille d'un de nos amis médecins, fille âgée de 25 ans:

L'apparition en un mois au niveau de la racine de la cuisse droite d'une tumeur noirâtre, extensive, légèrement kératosique, entourée d'un halo gris foncé, avait fait porter le diagnostic le plus sombre.

La biopsie de la pièce a montré un A.K. typique.

Histologie. En effet, l'histologie de ces lésions (Fig. 2) est assez caractéristique. Deux éléments essentiels: 1. En surface, l'hyperacanthose avec hyperkératose et papillomatose. 2. Ensuite, l'élément angiomateux, sous forme de cavités caverneuses qui sont parfois comme enchassées dans l'épiderme, signe pathognomonique et qui nous ont paru le plus souvent thrombosées d'une façon spontanée, ce qui

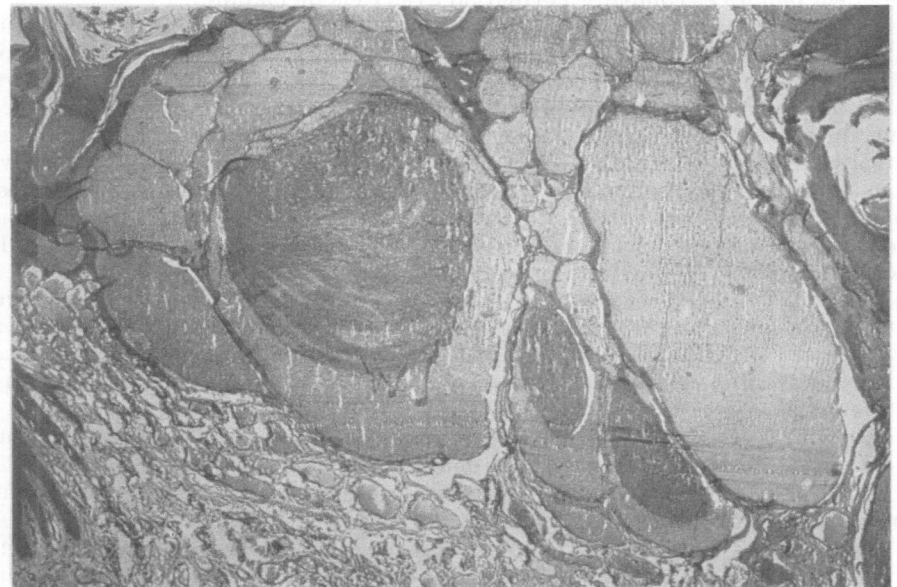

Fig. 2. Aspect typique de logettes cavernomateuses intriquées avec l'épiderme kératosique. Noter la présence de plusieurs thromboses en «grelots» qui sont si fréquentes dans cette lésion

expliquerait la couleur de la lésion. L'angiome est presque toujours de type caverneux, sans prolifération exubérante de l'endothélium.

Nos 20 coupes sont calquées les unes sur les autres et nous retrouvons les mêmes caractéristiques dans les deux articles américains.

Classification et etiologie. Les A.K. noirs n'ont rien de commun avec les A.K. diffus et systématisés.

Ils sont strictement localisés et presque toujours solitaires. S'agit il d'un noevus tardif? Nous aurions plutôt tendance à accepter une étiologie traumatique ou infectieuse qui les rapprocherait des papillomes infectieux. En faveur de cette hypothèse:

D'une part, la guérison très simple par simple excision.

D'autre part, la présence parfois d'un infiltrat inflammatoire non négligeable et enfin et surtout, l'interrogatoire des malades. En les interrogeant avec patience, on apprend très souvent qu'il y avait avant l'apparition de l'A.K. une minuscule croute qui a été grattée, exprimée, excoriée.

En Conclusion. Nous croyons utile de diffuser cette notion assez peu répandue d'une lésion très foncée, en général noire, qui peut parfaitement évoquer un mélanome de haute malignité et qui, en fait, est une tumeur absolument bénigne.

Les noevocarcinomes de l'enfant

R. Mouly, Cl. Dufourmentel et J. Glicenstein, Hôpital Saint-Louis, Chirurgie Plastique, Paris (France)

Il est classique de considérer que les mélanomes de l'enfant sont exceptionnels et que leur pronostic est meilleur que chez l'adulte. Cette notion est apparue encore plus nette depuis l'individualisation en 1948 par Sophie Spitz du «mélanome juvénile», variété de noevi bénins considérés à tort jusque là comme malins. Nous voudrions apporter huit nouveaux cas de noevocarcinomes chez l'enfant, rappeler ceux déjà publiés et comparer l'évolution avec celle de l'adulte.

Le premier cas rapporté semble être celui de Cazenave (1856), concernant un enfant mort à l'âge de 6 ans après 4 ans d'évolution d'un mélanome du membre inférieur disséminé. Dans la littérature, une certaine confusion est inévitable entre mélanome malin et mélanome juvénile bénin. Malgré les caractères histologiques différentiels, Allen et Spitz ne font eux-mêmes la distinction que dans 2/3 des cas. En prenant pour seul critère de malignité, l'apparition des métastases, Skov-Jensen et coll. (1966) relèvent 43 cas malins publiés authentiques de mélanomes. On peut distinguer trois variétés de mélanomes malins chez l'enfant: 1. le mélanome malin congénital, 2. le mélanome développé sur un grand naevus congénital, 3. le mélanome malin prépubertaire (variété habituelle).

1. Mélanome malin congénital. Il concerne la transmission de la mère à l'enfant d'un mélanome malin par voie transplacentaire. Cinq cas ont été publiés. Nous n'en avons jamais observé. Par contre, deux de nos malades ont présenté une dissémination massive d'un mélanome au cours d'une grossesse et sont mortes. L'enfant était normal.

Cas No. 1. Dissémination massive en cours de grossesse. Césarienne au 7ème mois, enfant normal, mort de la mère deux mois plus tard.

Cas No. 2. Généralisation au cours d'une grossesse, mort au 4ème mois. A l'autopsie, dissémination pelvienne, placenta et foetus indemnes.

2. Mélanome développé sur un grand noevus congénital. La dégénérescence d'un grand noevus congénital est une éventualité assez fréquente et elle peut se produire dès l'enfance. Pour Fish, sur 39 cas publiés de dégénérescence de noevi géants, 24 concernent des enfants avec un pronostic très sévère (14 morts, 5 disparus). Il est difficile de déceler cliniquement la transformation et elle est souvent révélée par une adénopathie métastatique. Nous avons rencontré dans trois cas l'apparition de bourgeons sur de grands noevi congénitaux, de siège variable: main, pied, région dorso-lombaire. Pour ce dernier, chez un nourrisson, un double noevocarcinome est apparu sur un vaste noevus pigmentaire et verruqueux (Bolgert). L'aspect clinique était pour ces trois cas celui d'un noevocarcinome. L'histologie ne put affirmer la malignité, sauf dans un cas. L'évolution s'est faite sans métastase. Nous ne retiendrons pas ces cas comme noevocarcinomes mais on doit connaitre la possibilité de bourgeons apparus sur de grands noevi pigmentaires dans l'enfance et les difficultés diagnostiques qu'ils soulèvent avec les mélanomes malins.

3. Mélanome malin prépubertaire. Ce groupe comprend les mélanomes malins chez les enfants de moins de 15 ans susceptibles de donner des métastases. Ils représentent dans notre statistique huit cas sur 400 soit 2% de l'ensemble de nos malades. Les caractères histologiques et évolutifs sont ceux des noevocarcinomes de l'adulte et ils ne peuvent être confondus avec un mélanome de Spitz. Sans détailler les observations, relevons les caractères suivants:

Sexe: 4 garçons et 4 filles.

Age: entre 2 et 13 ans avec une fréquence maximum autour de 10 ans (5 ont entre 8 et 11 ans).

Siège: surtout le membre inférieur — 5 dont 3 à la cuisse, 1 de l'aisselle, 1 de la main et 1 du dos.

L'évolution parait aussi grave sinon plus sévère que chez l'adulte. Deux ont seulement un recul d'un peu plus d'un an.

Six ont un recul de 5 ans ou plus; parmi eux:
— un a été perdu de vue,
— deux sont guéris sans récidive décelable,
— l'un depuis 5 ans et l'autre depuis 7 ans,
aucun de ces 2 cas, n'a présenté de métastase ganglionnaire.
— deux sont morts:

a) Fille de 8 ans = noevus de cuisse avec métastase ganglionnaire inguinale apparue un mois après l'exérèse-greffe de la lésion primaire, curage; 3 mois plus tard, métastase pulmonaire, décès.

b) Garçon de 6 ans = noevus de cheville, évolution mortelle en 3 ans après métastases ganglionnaires multiples et successives: inguinale, cervicale, sus-claviculaire puis métastase pulmonaire.

— Un peut être considéré comme disparu: garçon de 8 ans, noevus de main; 6 ans plus tard, métastase sous-cutanée du bras.

Il est difficile sur un nombre aussi réduit de cas d'apporter des conclusions statistiques. Nous devons cependant rappeler les points suivants, qui découlent de nos observations.

Le noevocarcinome de l'enfant existe étant entendu que le mélanome juvénile est considéré comme bénin et ne saurait lui être confondu. Il doit être divisé en trois formes:

Mélanome congénital. Très rare; la mère peut présenter une généralisation noevocarcinomateuse et l'enfant être indemne, comme dans nos deux cas.

Mélanome sur noevus géant. Très grave, pratiquement toujours mortel. Il peut exister des bourgeons sur de grands noevi qui seraient considérés comme des noevocarcinomes chez l'adulte et n'ont pas la même gravité chez l'enfant (trois cas).

Mélanome malin prépubertaire. Très analogue au mélanome malin de l'adulte dont il partage les principaux caractères. La mort par dissémination avec métastases ganglionnaires a été observée dans deux de nos huit cas.

Nevus y melanomas malignos

L. A. Rueda, Dermatopatólogo del Centro Dermatológico de Bogotá (Colombia)

I. Introducción

La aparición de francos Melanomas Malignos sobre lesiones pigmentarias preexistentes, es un hecho de común observación. Las estadísticas muestran historia de Nevus entre un 20 a 80% de Melanomas Malignos. Generalmente se admite la hipótesis de Allen y col. de que los Melanomas Malignos por su actividad junctural se originan en Nevus juncturales y compuestos de tipo premaligno. Viejos conceptos etiopatogénicos se han revaluado recientemente. Como no se ha demostrado la transformación de un nevus junctural histológicamente comprobado, en un Melanoma Maligno, hemos querido ocuparnos de este tema.

II. Material y metodos

Revisión clínica e histológica de 262 casos de Melanomas Malignos. 208 procedentes del Instituto Nacional de Cancerología de Colombia y 54 de la Cátedra de Dermatología de Barcelona. No se consideraron como Nevus las lesiones con evolución menor de 5 años ni aquellas manchas que eran evidentes Melanosis Precancerosas (HUTCHINSON, DUBREUILH). Los casos de Melanoma Maligno aparecidos sobre nevus, se dividieron en: a) aquellos sobre Nevus congénitos o de la infancia y b) sobre Nevus post-puberales.

III. Resultados

A. Generales. Destacamos los referentes a *Localización*: Notables diferencias porcentuales entre los casos estudiados en Colombia y los casos españoles. Las más sobresalientes son: *Pie:* Colombia 39,4%; Barcelona 11,1%; *Mano:* 6,2% y 1,8% y *Cabeza y Cuello:* 21,6% y 48,1%. Porcentajes similares para el *Tronco:* 12,5% y 11,1%. Diferencias no significativas en las demás regiones. La frecuencia de panadizos melánicos en Colombia fue alta: 9,5%.

B. Referentes a los casos sobre Nevus. 78 casos (30%) tenían antecedentes de "lunar" de variable duración. Se descartaron 10 manchas que eran evidentes Melanosis Precancerosas y 23 lesiones cuya evolución era menor de 5 años. Restan 45 casos (17,2%) clasificados así: Nevus congénitos 15, Nevus de la infancia 10, Nevus post-puberales 20.

1. Edad de transformación maligna. En todos los 25 casos sobre nevus congénitos y de la infancia, la transformación maligna ocurrió después de los 30 años de edad. De los 20 casos sobre Nevus post-puberales, solo en 2 el nevus apareció a los 15 y 18 años de edad, malignizándose 4 años más tarde en el primero y en fecha no determinada antes de los 25 años de edad en el segundo. En los 18 casos restantes el Nevus apareció después de los 25 años y se malignizó entre 5 y 30 años después, según los casos.

2. Menores de 30 años y Nevus. De 26 pacientes menores de 30 años, solo en 2 (casos citados) se estableció sobre nevus post-puberal. En los restantes casos de esta edad, en ninguno se instauró el Melanoma Maligno sobre Nevus.

3. Localización de nevus premalignos. Las regiones en que se registraron mayores porcentajes de Melanomas Malignos aparecidos sobre Nevus fueron: *Tronco:* (37,5%); *Brazo y antebrazo* (37,5%); *Muslo y pierna* (28,3%); *Dorso de pie* (25%) y *palma de la mano* (25%). Llama la atención la baja proporción de nevus como antecedente en los de planta del pie (9,2%) y en los panadizos melanóticos subungueales (3,8%). En los Melanomas de planta aparece más frecuentemente como antecedente un traumatismo sobre piel sana que un nevus pre-existente.

4. Tipo de nevus premaligno. Solo un caso sobre mancha plana. En los demás o no consta o era lesión sobreelevada.

5. Aspectos histológicos: La anatomía patológica de los 45 Melanomas Malignos aparecidos sobre Nevus, fué similar a la de los demás Melanomas.

IV. Comentario

Las publicaciones de diversos Autores muestran que los nevus son raros al nacimiento, poco frecuentes antes de los dos años y tan solo se observan en el 2,4% de los niños. Aunque la mayoría son juncturales, ya en la primera década existe un 17,9% de nevus celulares intradérmicos puros e inclusive nevus cerebriformes y neuroides.

En la pubertad ocurre un nuevo brote de nevus. En esta época el 50,4% de nevus son compuestos. Estos nevus disminuyen porcentualmente en la vida adulta, mientras permanece invariable el porcentaje de juncturales y aumenta el de intradérmicos. Estos hechos y sobre todo el que los nevus juncturales predominen en las extremidades y los nevus dérmicos en la cabeza, sugieren que las variaciones porcentuales de los nevus son debidas a la continua formación de nevus de distinto tipo. Por tanto, es probable que cada tipo de nevus se inicie como tal. La edad o el estado hormonal propio a dicha edad determinaría el tipo de nevus.

Nuestra casuística muestra que en ningún paciente menor de 30 años el Melanoma Maligno se originó sobre un Nevus congénito o de la infancia. Resulta pues, dudoso el dato suministrado por los pacientes mayores de 30 años de que su melanoma se instauró sobre nevus de este tipo. De otra parte, si en 24 pacientes menores de 30 años se trataba de Melanomas Malignos "d'emblée", es dudoso que en los otros dos pacientes de esta edad se originaran en nevus post-puberales, por el solo hecho de presentar un período de estabilización relativamente largo. En los Melanomas Malignos "d'emblée" es común observar períodos de estabilización de 2 y más años. Por tanto, es posible que los Melanomas Malignos aparecidos sobre supuestos nevus post-puberales, sean en realidad malignos desde su inicio y que por causas que desconocemos manifiestan un período de estabilización más o menos prolongado. En consecuencia, es posible que todos los Melanomas Malignos se inicien como tales.

En favor de esta tesis podemos aducir: a) El Melanoma Maligno predomina en los lugares en donde son más infrecuentes los nevus juncturales. b) La existencia de melanomas malignos primarios viscerales, en mucosas y semimucosas sin nevus previo. c) La existencia de melanomas malignos primarios múltiples, aparecidos solos o conjuntamente con nevus benignos, aún en niños. d) El bajo porcentaje de antecedentes de nevus de la planta, en nuestros casos lugar reportado como de mayor frecuencia de malignización de los nevus juncturales. e) Los casos de auténtico melanoma maligno aparecidos sobre nevus en calzón han sido en niños, lo que sugiere que el melanoma maligno aparece conjuntamente con el nevus y no sobre éste. f) Las diferencias porcentuales de localización del melanoma maligno entre Europa y Colombia indicarían que en la etiopatogenia del Melanoma Maligno influyen más los factores ambientales que la presencia de un nevus previo.

En conclusión, creemos que tanto los nevus benignos, cualquiera sea su tipo histológico, como los Melanomas Malignos se originan como tales, sin suceder transformación de unos en otros. La única precancerosis del melanoma es, a nuestro entender, la Melanosis precancerosa o Léntigo Maligno.

Early Diagnosis of Melanoblastoma with the Aid of Electrometric, Thermo-Differential and ^{32}P Uptake Test

A. GULBERT, National Oncological Institute, Budapest (Hungary)

It is generally known that in melanoblastoma an early diagnosis is decisive on the course of illness. Yet the biopsy usually applied is harmful on account of the danger of dissemination, on the other hand, biopsy associated with preoperative irradiation makes histological diagnosis difficult.

A number of tests has been applied to confirm the clinical diagnosis. The opinions of various authors on the value of these tests are contradictory.

We investigated the diagnostical value of the ^{32}P uptake test, the thermo-differential test and the Melczer and Kiss electrometric method. In the first group ^{32}P uptake test and thermo-differential test were applied simultaneously. For control purposes 50 cases of naevus pigmentosus have been examined where subsequently performed histological examinations did not show any malignancy. In this group low positive values were obtained in one case with thermo-differential test and in two cases with ^{32}P uptake test.

In the second group 167 cases of melanoblastoma in the 1st stage (primary tumour without metastasis) were subjected to ^{32}P uptake tests and thermo-differential tests. All 167 cases were histologically proved. Applying both tests positive results were obtained in 145 cases (87%). When using one test only positive results were obtained in 20 cases (11,9%). Negative results were obtained, by using both tests, only in two cases (1,1%). In the third group beside ^{32}P uptake and thermo-differential tests also Melczer and Kiss electrometry (Potenzial-differenzenmessungen) examinations were performed on 48 patients in the 1st stage of melanoblastoma. By using all three tests positive results were obtained in 35 cases (73,0%), in five cases (10,3%) positive results were obtained with two tests, in six cases (12,5%) positive results were obtained with one test only and in two cases (4,2%) results were negative with all three tests.

Conclusion. In the 1st stage of melanoblastoma the ^{32}P uptake and thermo-differential tests applied simultaneously proved to be of serious help in establishing the right diagnosis. Similar results were obtained by using these two biological tests plus the Melczer and Kiss method. The specificity of these biological tests seems to be proved by the fact that in naevus pigmentosus cases established clinically and confirmed histologically the results were negative in 98,0%.

Importance of the biological tests is shown by the fact that clinical diagnoses may, with their aid, be supported prior to histological examinations. By no means should it be considered that such biological tests are only sufficient in establishing a diagnosis without clinical and histological examinations.

Histologische Befunde beim transplantierten Melanom des Menschen

H. GARTMANN, Universitäts-Hautklinik Köln (Deutschland)

Wegen Aussichtslosigkeit konventioneller Behandlungsmaßnahmen wurden nach vorheriger Aufklärung bei einer 50jährigen Frau und einem 36jährigen Manne mit ausgedehnten Melanommetastasen in Anlehnung an das Verfahren von NADLER und MOORE zweimal wechselseitig ausgetauschte subcutane Metastasen in das Unterhautfettgewebe der Kranken eingepflanzt. 10 Tage nach der ersten Transplantation wurden Plasma-Leukocytenkonzentrate ausgetauscht, indem an 10 aufeinanderfolgenden Tagen täglich etwa 300 Millionen ungewaschene Leukocyten injiziert wurden. Bei der Frau erfolgte die erste Transplantation submammär rechts, die zweite nach 6 Wochen submammär links, 5 Wochen später starb sie. Beim Manne entwickelten sich nach der ersten Transplantation am Rücken weitere Hautmetastasen. 6 Wochen später wurde eine zweite Metastase der Frau in den linken Oberschenkel verpflanzt, die sich innerhalb von 5 Monaten völlig zurückbildete. Der Kranke starb 10 Monate später. Die transplantierten Metastasen ließen feingeweblich vor der Einpflanzung weitgehend gleichartiges globoid-zelliges, alveolär strukturiertes Melanomgewebe mit atypischen Mitosen und Melanin erkennen.

Histologische Befunde bei der Frau. Nach 6wöchiger Verweildauer wurden eine Hautmetastase sowie die submammär rechts transplantierte Metastase entfernt. Feingeweblich fand sich in ersterer kein Unterschied gegenüber dem Befund vor Beginn der Behandlung. Im Transplantat fanden sich mehrere verschieden große nekrotische Bezirke, die teils konfluiert, teils durch bindegewebige Septen getrennt waren, wobei es sich um Kolliquationsnekrosen mit reichlich sauren Mucopolysacchariden handelte. Sie enthielten ferner zahlreiche feinkörnige Melaningranula und im Randbereich Melanophagen. Manche Nekrosen wiesen Reststrukturen eines Netzwerkes auf, in dessen freien Maschen möglicherweise früher Zellen (Melanomzellen?) eingelagert gewesen waren. In den Netzfasern war reichlich Melanin vorhanden. Nach außen schloß sich zellreiches histiocytäres Granulationsgewebe mit einzelnen Fremdkörperriesenzellen an, das peripherwärts faser- und gefäßreicher wurde und kleine perivasale lymphocytäre Infiltrate mit Mastzellen in wechselnder Menge enthielt. In der weiteren Umgebung waren vermehrt Mastzellen und einzelne segmentkernige Leukocyten vorhanden. Melanomzellen waren nicht mehr erkennbar.

Histologische Befunde beim Manne. Die 6 Wochen nach der ersten Transplantation entnommene Hautmetastase ließ im Gegensatz zum Befund bei der Frau eine schwere nekrotisierende Entzündung erkennen. Im Bereich der Transplantation am Rücken entstand nach 7 Wochen eine Schwellung. Dort wurde 1 Woche später ein subcutaner tiefschwarzer Tumor von 8 cm Durchmesser exstirpiert, während das Transplantat nur knapp kirschgroß war. Der Gesamtaufbau war knotig und wurde lediglich von bindegewebigen Septen unterbrochen. Nach außen erfolgte Abgrenzung durch eine bindegewebige Kapsel. In der Peripherie zeigte die Geschwulst globoidzellige mitosenreiche, teils alveolär, teils endotheliomartig angeordnete Elemente mit lockerer Kernstruktur. Im Tumorparenchym lagen kleinste, nekrobiotische, von Leukocyten durchsetzte und um hyperämische Capillaren angeordnete Bezirke. Nach dem Geschwulstzentrum hin ließ der Zusammenhang der Tumorzellen nach, wobei es schließlich zu einer Lösung der Zellen aus ihrem Verband kam. In den Septen bestand unterschiedlich dichte, vornehmlich lymphocytäre Durchsetzung mit einzelnen Mastzellen. In der Nähe des Zentrums der Gesamtgeschwulst lag an einer Stelle ein kleinerer, relativ scharf abgesetzter Bezirk, dessen unregelmäßig geformte, plasmadichte, stark eosinophile Zellen mit pyknotischen, teilweise auch zerfallenden Kernen sich deutlich von den umgebenden Tumorzellverbänden unterschieden. Insgesamt erschien dieser Zellverband aufgelöst und ohne Verbindung der einzelnen Elemente untereinander. Ferner fanden sich darin weitgestellte thrombosierte Gefäße mit nekrotisch veränderten Wandungen sowie kleine Lymphocyteninfiltrate und Erythrocytenextravasate. Mastzellen fehlten. Entsprechende Untersuchungen ergaben, daß mit hoher Wahrscheinlichkeit ein Tumor mit männlichem Kerngeschlecht vorlag. Dies würde für die Entwicklung einer eigenen Metastase und gegen das An- und Weiterwachsen des Fremdtransplantates sprechen. Auch die histologischen Merkmale sprachen eher für das Vorliegen einer körpereigenen Metastase. Bei dem umschriebenen Bezirk dürfte es sich um den Rest des von der Frau stammenden Transplantates gehandelt haben.

Nach der Austauschtransplantation kam es weder zu auffälliger entzündlicher Reaktion am Orte der Einpflanzung noch zur Abstoßung der transplantierten Fremdmetastasen im eigentlichen Sinne, sondern zur — wenn auch bei Mann und Frau unterschiedlichen — Resorption. Es ist also nicht nur kein Erfolg, sondern sogar Wachstum von Metastasen aufgetreten, was das Ausbleiben einer Antigen-Antikörperreaktion vermuten läßt. Bei verschiedengeschlechtlichen Partnern kann der sog. Eichwald-Silmser-Effekt auftreten, der jede Homoiotransplantation mit dem Risiko des Nichtangehens belastet. Die „milde" Aufnahme des von der Frau stammenden Tumortransplantates durch den männlichen Organismus könnte möglicherweise auf Fehlen eines am Y-Chromosom lokalisierten starken Histokompatibilitätsgens („maleness antigen") zurückgeführt werden [vgl. GARTMANN und TRITSCH: Hautarzt **17**, 529 (1966)].

Veränderungen bei inoculierten Melanocyten

KH. WOEBER, Hautabteilung des Luisenhospitals, Aachen, und O. GRÜTZ †,
Universitäts-Hautklinik Bonn (Deutschland)

Bei subtilen dermato-histopathologischen Untersuchungen an menschlichen
malignen Melanomen konnte einer von uns (GRÜTZ) bereits 1953 darauf hinweisen,
daß berechtigte Zweifel an der üblichen Auffassung bestehen, wonach die Metastasierung allein durch celluläre Verschleppung zustande kommt. Beim Studium
histologischer Bilder wurden freie melanotische Granula in den Lymphspalten
beobachtet, die man nicht nur allein als „Abtransport von Pigment" deuten kann.
Sollten die Untersuchungen von MEIROWSKY, wonach melanotische Granula ein
Eigenleben führen und selbstvermehrungsfähig sind, zu Recht bestehen, so könnten
gegebenenfalls diese Befunde für das maligne Melanom an Bedeutung gewinnen.

In Erkenntnis dieser hier geschilderten histologischen und experimentellen
Befunde haben wir es seit etwa 10 Jahren als unsere Aufgabe angesehen, der
Bedeutung subcellulärer Elemente — in unserem Falle der Melanocyten des malig-
nen Melanoms — bei der experimentellen Forschung besondere Aufmerksamkeit zu
schenken. In enger Anlehnung an die Graffischen Untersuchungen bei der experi-
mentellen Leukämie der Maus haben wir zellfreie Filtrate des Harding-Passey-
Melanoms der Maus hergestellt, die wir unter verschiedenen Bedingungen und
Anordnungen in vivo beobachtet haben.

Es läßt sich an histologischen Serienschnitten bei größeren Versuchsreihen
ohne Schwierigkeit nachweisen, daß zellfrei subcutan injizierte Melanocyten
von dem tierischen Körper aufgenommen werden, indem sie nach kurzer Zeit
(einigen wenigen Tagen) in Bindegewebszellen eindringen und dort anscheinend
einen Vermehrungsvorgang erkennen lassen. Zum mindesten sind nach Ablauf
einiger Tage auch für die histologisch Geschulten keine Möglichkeiten mehr gegeben, Unterschiede zwischen subcellulär erzeugten melanotischen Geschwülsten
und den auf „klassische Weise" (d. h. durch Melanomzellen) erzeugten Tumoren
zu erbringen. Desgleichen lassen sich damit gut vergleichbare Bilder von menschlichen malignen Melanomgeschwülsten demonstrieren, die ähnliche histologische
Substrate zeigen.

Wenn es auch bisher noch nicht gelungen ist, die durch Melanocyten erzeugten
melanotischen Tumoren der Maus, bei denen im späteren Verlauf der Beobachtung
häufig Rückbildungsprozesse nachzuweisen sind, zum malignen Wachstum anzu-
regen, so dürfen diese Ergebnisse doch dahingehend interpretiert werden, daß

1. eine irgendwie geartete Traumatisierung von Melanomzellen zur Emigration
von Melanocyten führen kann, die ihrerseits Anlaß zu einer subcellulären und
später cellulären Metastasierung sein können, und

2. daß die relative Schwierigkeit einer chirurgischen oder strahlentherapeutischen Behandlung des malignen Melanoms darin zu suchen sein dürfte, daß einmal
bereits emigrierte Melanocyten nicht auszuschließen sind und zum anderen
durch die ionisierenden Strahlen nicht nur celluläre Elemente deletär beeinflußt
werden müssen, sondern Melanocyten als quasi „virus like bodies" vorhanden
sind, d. h. erfahrungsgemäß eine wesentlich höhere Dosis ionisierender Strahlen
benötigt wird als dies in der Strahlentherapie bekannt und üblich ist.

Literatur. GRÜTZ, O., u. KH. WOEBER: Krebsforsch. u. Krebsbekämpf. Bd. III, 43—47
(1959); — Arch. klin. exp. Derm. **214**, 346 (1962). — MEIROWSKY, E., and L. W. FREEMAN:
Docum. Med. geogr. trop. (Amst.) **6**, 112 (1954). — WOEBER, KH.: Radiobiol. Radiother. (Berl.)
6, 707 (1965).

Macromolecular Differentiation of Melanocytic and Nevocytic Malignant Melanomas*

Y. Mishima, Departments of Dermatology, Wayne State University School of Medicine, Detroit General Hospital, Detroit, Michigan, and Veterans Administration Hospital, Dearborn, Michigan (USA)

Unlike other cancers, particularly those of the internal organs, malignant melanoma of human skin can, theoretically, be virtually eradicated. The success of eradication depends on the precise recognition of the premalignant stages of the disease by clinical, biological and microscopic criteria.

In 1960 I suggested the possibility of non-nevoid tumors of the melanocyte, and found an example of a benign tumor of this type, the melanoacanthoma [1]. Since then I have reexamined the well established clinical entity, melanosis circumscripta praecancerosa Dubreuilh [2, 3, 4]. While Allen [5] has expressed the opinion that this lesion is a type of active junction nevus, its essential nature remains undetermined. Close examination has led to the conclusion that Dubreuilh's melanosis is not a type of active junction nevus, but instead represents premalignant stages of non-nevoid melanocytic tumors. Furthermore, I have described the histopathological criteria which have been used for the past 7 years by our department to separate these premelanomatous entities [6]. We have found these criteria to be effective for pathological diagnosis in most cases although light microscopic differentiation is often difficult after malignant transformation has occurred.

In addition, it has been found that the malignant melanomas developed from Dubreuilh's precancerous melanosis differ from those developed from junction nevus in regard to their malignancy as well as biological activity. The macromolecular and enzymic activities of these two types of malignant melanoma were therefore further studied. I would like to summarize here our recent findings on the separate ontogenies of these conditions.

Table 1. *Distinct Differentiating Features of · Malignant Melanomas Developing from Dubreuilh's Melanosis and Junction Nevus*

	Malignant Melanomas Developing from	
	Dubreuilh's Precancerous Melanosis	Junction Nevus
1. Growth rate	+	+++
2. Metastasis	+	+++
3. Invasiveness	+	+++
4. Radiosensitivity	++	±
5. Melanization	+++	+++ → —
Nature	Melanocytoma	Nevocytoma

Compared to the malignant melanoma developed from junction nevus, the melanoma developed from Dubreuilh's melanosis has a slower rate of growth, metastasis and invasiveness (Tab. 1). Furthermore, in contrast to the melanoma

* This investigation is supported in part by U.S. Public Health Service Research Grants CA-08891-01 and CA-05580-06 from the National Cancer Institute and AM-07981-04 from the National Institute of Arthritis and Metabolic Diseases, National Institutes of Health.

of junction nevus origin, melanoma from Dubreuilh's melanosis is radiosensitive and has not been found to assume the amelanotic form. The differences in the premalignant stages of the two tumors are seen in Tab. 2. Dubreuilh's precancerous melanosis, in contrast to junction nevus, is a condition which occurs during later life in exposed areas, is radiosensitive [7, 8] and has a high incidence of malignant transformation. The term "superficial melanoma" has been used loosely. It often refers to Dubreuilh's precancerous melanosis and malignant melanoma arising in it but in other cases to the early stages of melanoma arising from nevi. Typical Dubreuilh's melanosis (Fig. 1) exhibits the active proliferation of melanocytes having the appearance of atypical clear cells at the epidermal-dermal junction. The individual cells have a vacuolated cytoplasm and irregular shrunken nuclei. These atypical clear cells line up at the junction layer in a palisade fashion and in some areas exhibit a honey-combed appearance; however, no nevus cell nests are seen. In contrast, junction nevi (Fig. 2) have a tendency to form well-circumscribed massive cell nests in the lower epidermis. The cytoplasm of individual cells is homogeneous and their pericaryon is oval or cuboidal and distinctly outlined. Often these cells appear to form syncytial structures.

Table 2. *Distinct Differentiating Features of Dubreuilh's Melanosis and Junction Nevus*

	Dubreuilh's Precancerous Melanosis	Junction Nevus
1. Usual development	Old Age	Childhood
2. Solar exposure	Etiologic	Non-etiologic
3. Radiosensitivity	Sensitive	Non-sensitive
4. Malignant transformation	Frequent	Not frequent

Table 3. *Two Ontogenic Pathways Leading to the Malignant Melanomas, Malignant Melanocytoma and Malignant Nevocytoma*

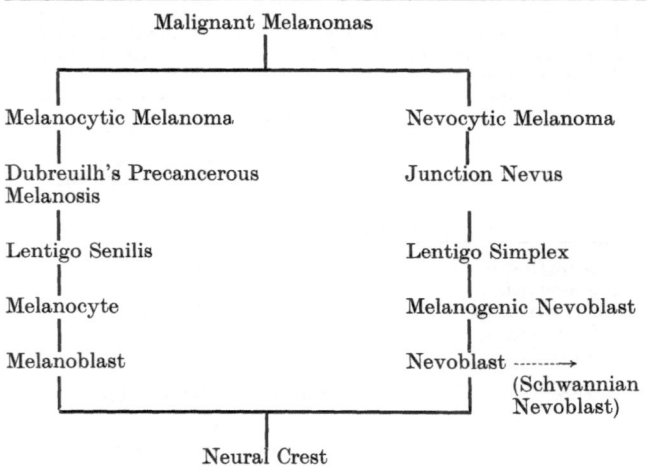

Dopa reaction of Dubreuilh's melanosis (Fig. 3) reveals the melanocytic nature of these cells by their intensely dopa-positive dendritic appearance and their proliferation without the formation of theques, in contrast to junction nevus (Fig. 4). The cells of Dubreuilh's melanosis can invade the dermis only after malignant transformation, acquiring intense tyrosinase synthesis (Fig. 5) whereas junctional nevus cells generally become intradermal nevus cells by the "dropping off" process, gradually losing their tyrosinase activity. Reciprocal to the decrease in tyrosinase activity, junction nevus cells show an increase in cholinesterase as they move downward in the epidermal-dermal structure acquiring a neuroid configuration [9].

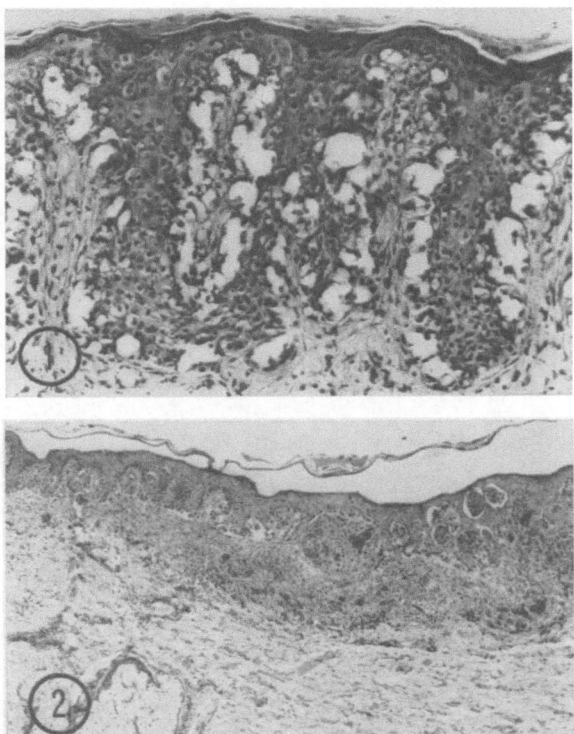

Fig. 1. Typical histological appearance of Dubreuilh's melanosis characterized by the proliferation of atypical clear cells at the epidermal-dermal junction which line up in a palisade fashion, exhibiting a honey combed appearance. Individual cells have a vacuolated cytoplasm and irregular shrunken nuclei. Hematoxylin eosin stain. × 120

Fig. 2. Junction nevus cells have a tendency to form well circumscribed massive cell nests. The cytoplasm of individual cells is homogeneous and distinctly outlined. Hematoxylin eosin stain. × 45

Electron microscopy further reveals the melanocytic rather than nevocytic nature of the cells of Dubreuilh's melanosis (Fig. 6). These cells proliferate in disorganized fashion among keratinocytes without the formation of distinct theques. The distinct dendritic nature of these cells is not seen at the light microscopic level without the aid of the dopa or premelanin reactions.

Another subcellular difference between Dubreuilh's melanosis and junction nevus is found in melanosome polymorphism. Dubreuilh's melanocytes can contain two types of melanosomes. Fig. 7 shows the type of melanosome which has characteristically been seen in cases of fully developed Dubreuilh's melanosis. These appear rod-shaped when sectioned along their short axis and round when cut parallel to their long axis. These rod-shaped granules average 600×200 mμ in maximum size with a range of 450 to 700 mμ × 150 to 250 mμ. When partially melanized and sectioned parallel to their long axis, they may exhibit a ring-like appearance. Since the examination of a large selection of these melanosomes cut at various angles reveals that the diameter of the round granules corresponds to the length of the rod-shaped granules, three dimensionally these melanosomes can be considered red cell shaped.

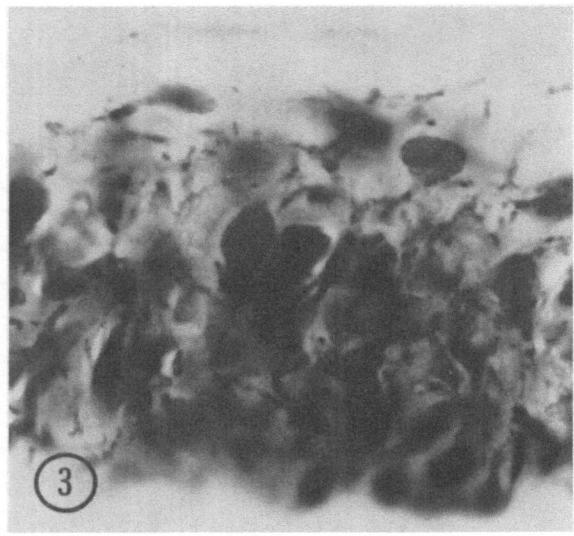

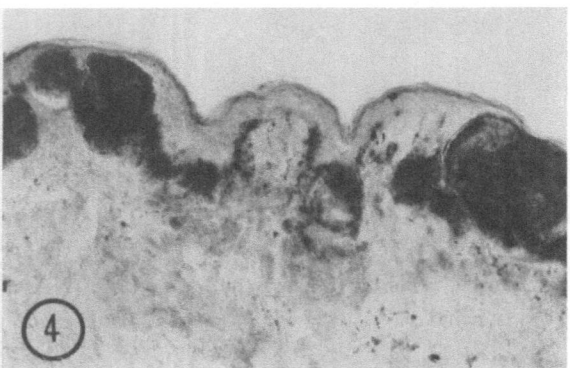

Fig. 3. Intensely dopa-positive atypical dendritic cells of Dubreuilh's melanosis show irregular proliferation without the formation of theques. Dopa reaction. × 920

Fig. 4. Dopa reaction of junction nevus revealing a distinct tendency to form enzymically active circumscribed nests. × 90

The other type of melanosome is more generally seen in earlier stages of Dubreuilh's melanosis and in the later stages may be seen among the red cell type melanosomes. These appear as elongated structures (Fig. 8) averaging 700 × 150 mμ in maximum size, with a range of 550 to 800 mμ × 100 to 250 mμ; they closely resemble normal melanosomes. Higher magnification (Fig. 9) demonstrates that these elongated melanosomes have internal structure exhibiting particle arrays with 300 Å longitudinal periodicity and 250 Å transverse periodicity. The internal structure is similar to normal melanosomes although the melanoprotein units appear to be larger. The carry over of melanosomes and/or the melanosome type synthesis from the preceeding stage is thus suggested.

In contrast to the melanosomes of Dubreuilh's melanosis, the melanosomes synthesized by junction nevus cells are short football-shaped (Rugby) bodies

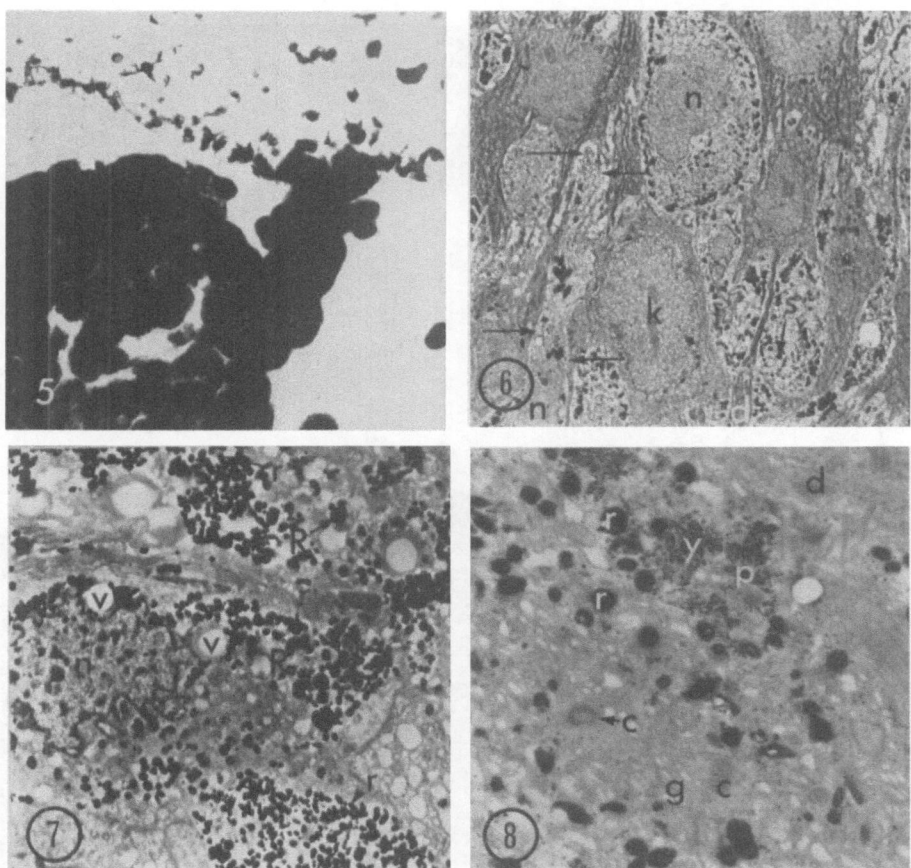

Fig. 5. In contrast to junction nevus the cells of Dubreuilh's melanosis can invade the dermis only after malignant changes have occurred, acquiring intense tyrosinase synthesis. Tyrosinase reaction. × 115

Fig. 6. Electron microscopy of Dubreuilh's melanosis indicates the melanocytic rather than nevocytic nature of these cells by the disorganized proliferation of dendritic cells (n) without the formation of theques. s melanosomes, d desmosomes, y glycogen, k keratinocytes arrows: dendrite. Fixed with OsO_4 and stained with phosphotungstic acid (PTA) and lead citrate. × 2,200

Fig. 7. The characteristic melanosomes synthesized by fully developed Dubreuilh's melanocytes appear rod-shaped (r) when sectioned along their short axis and as round bodies (R) when cut parallel to their long axis. Three dimensionally they can be considered red cell shaped. V Large vacuoles. Fixed with OsO_4 and stained with PTA and uranyl acetate (UrAc). × 3,650

Fig. 8. Elongated type of Dubreuilh's premelanosomes (P) and melanosomes may be seen more generally in earlier stages of Dubreuilh's melanosis and may occur along with the red cell-shaped bodies (r), the diameter of which is larger than the short axis of the elongated bodies. c centrioles, g Golgi apparatus, d desmosomes, y glycogen. Fixed with OsO_4 and stained with phosphotungstic acid and lead citrate. × 16,730

having a range of average maximum size of 500 × 150 mμ with a range of 400 to
600 mμ × 100 to 200 mμ. These melanosomes have a distinct internal structure
(Fig. 10) composed of a particle array which was seen in melanosomes studied as
distinct transverse lines having an 85 Å periodicity when sectioned along their
longitudinal axis.

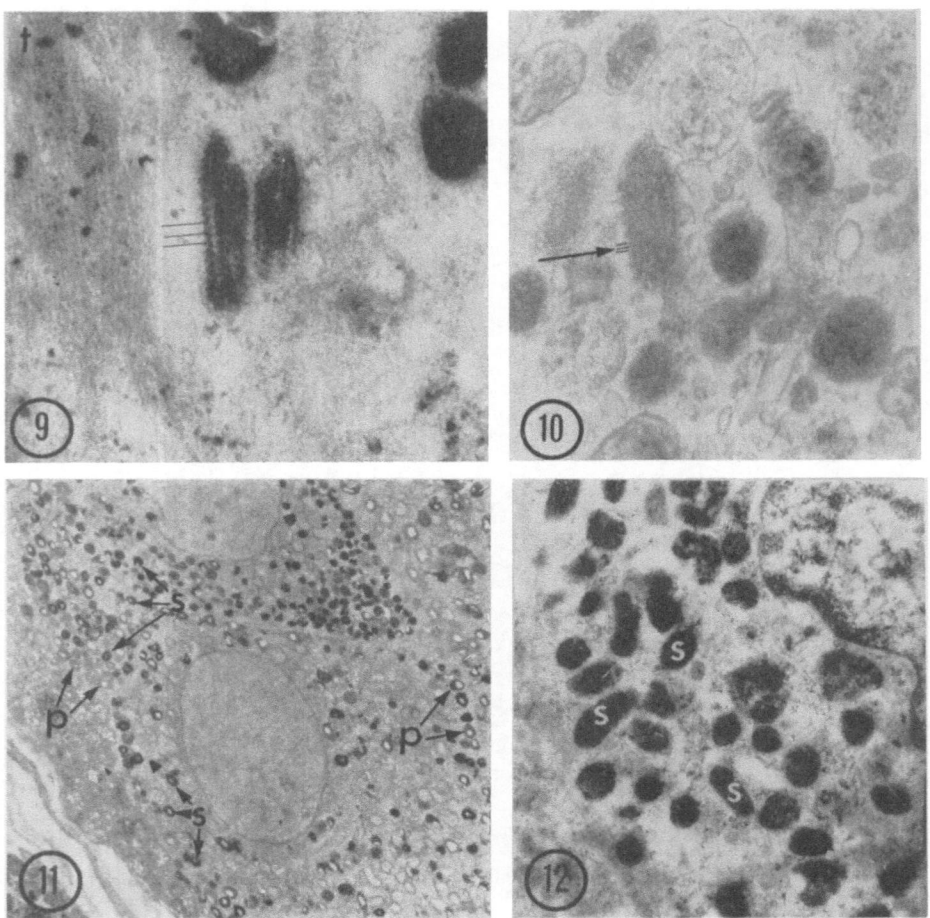

Fig. 9. Higher magnification of the elongated melanosomes seen in Dubreuilh's melanosis
showing internal structure which consists of particle arrays having 300 Å longitudinal periodicity and 250 Å transverse periodicity (arrows). Fixed with OsO₄ and stained with PTA and
lead citrate. × 45,400

Fig. 10. Characteristic premelanosomes synthesized by junction nevus cells are short foot-
ball shaped structures. High magnification shows a particle array appearing as distinct
transverse lines having 85 Å periodicity (arrow). Fixed with OsO₄ and stained with PTA and
lead citrate. × 59,800

Fig. 11. Premelanosomes (p) and melanosomes (s) seen in malignant melanoma from
Dubreuilh's melanosis are ellipsoid bodies often exhibiting a ring-like appearance, as exhibited by the melanosomes of Dubreuilh's melanosis. Fixed with OsO₄ and stained with PTA
and lead citrate. × 2,580

Fig. 12. Cigar shaped melanosomes (s) seen in malignant melanoma from junction nevus.
Fixed with OsO₄ and stained with PTA and uranyl acetate (UrAc). × 14,100

Furthermore, these melanosome differences can also be seen in the malignant melanomas resulting from these two conditions. Melanosomes (Fig. 11) observed in malignant melanoma developed from Dubreuilh's melanosis appear as ellipsoid bodies averaging 600×500 mμ in maximum diameter with a range of 450 to 800 mμ by 350 to 700 mμ. These bodies often exhibit a ring-like appearance as exhibited by the melanosomes of fully developed Dubreuilh's melanosis. On the other hand the studied melanosomes of melanotic melanoma developed from junction nevus are cigar-shaped bodies averaging 850×350 mμ in maximum size with a range of 650 to 950 mμ by 300 to 400 mμ (Fig. 12).

Another differentiating biological phenomenon is the spontaneous regression unique to Dubreuilh's melanosis. The area of spontaneous regression appears as a less pigmented, less indurated, somewhat atrophic region resulting in irregular

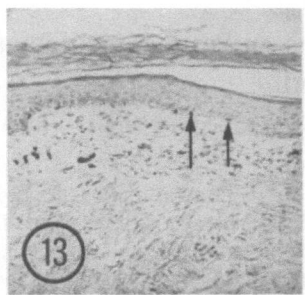 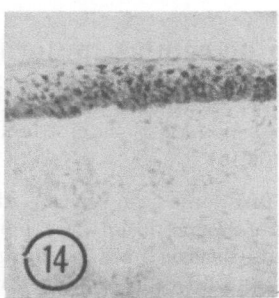

Fig. 13. Dopa reaction of the regressing area of Dubreuilh's melanosis reveals the disappearance of all high level atypical melanocytes, leaving only a normal number of junctional melanocytes (arrows). $\times$ 87

Fig. 14. Dopa reaction of an active area of Dubreuilh's melanosis reveals the proliferation of atypical melanocytes from the junctional to the granular layer in the epidermis. $\times$ 90

pigmentation. Stained by dopa reaction, the regressing area (Fig. 13) is characterized by the disappearance of proliferating atypical melanocytes which are seen in the active stage (Fig. 14). Electron microscopy confirms that all melanocytes seen in the high level in the active stage disappeared and are now limited to the junction layer [10].

Since we see the same decrease in number of melanocytes with electron microscopy as with the light microscopic dopa reaction, the possibility that the regression of Dubreuilh's melanosis is due to the transformation of dopa-positive to dopa-negative melanocytes is excluded. Furthermore the number of Langerhans cells does not show marked increase or abnormalities [10], thus ruling out the rapid turnover of Dubreuilh's melanocytes to Langerhans cells as the cause of regression. In contrast, regression of nevi at junction level does not normally occur although, after junction nevi have dropped into the dermis, regression by fibrosis can occur, as known in aged skin [11].

In the series of investigations of Dubreuilh's melanosis, it recently became apparent that Dubreuilh's melanosis can originate from lentigo senilis [12]. This is analogous to the development of junction nevi from lentigo simplex [9]. Recognition of the ontogeny of malignant melanocytoma can lead to adequate prophylaxis prior to the development of malignant melanoma.

On the basis of the present evidence, I would like to propose that in the future we consider human malignant melanoma to be not one but two diseases, melanocytic malignant melanoma and nevocytic malignant melanoma. which may be called malignant melanocytoma and malignant nevocytoma respectively. The differences in malignancy, radiosensitivity and prognosis, and differences in biological behavior may be explained by the separate ontogenies (Tab. 3) of these two conditions.

References. 1. MISHIMA, Y., and H. PINKUS: Arch. Derm. 81, 539 (1960). — 2. DUBREUILH, M. W.: Ann. Derm. Syph. (Paris) 3, 129, 205 (1912). — 3. DUPERRAT, B.: Ann. Derm. Syph. (Paris) 89, 319 (1962). — 4. GRINSPAN, D., y J. ABULAFIA: Arch. argent. Derm. 6, 351 (1956). — 5. ALLEN, A. C.: The skin: A clinicopathological treatise, 2nd Ed., p. 979. New York: Grune & Stratton, Inc. 1967. — 6. MISHIMA, Y.: J. invest. Derm. 34, 361 (1960). — MISHIMA, Y.: Cutis 2, 588 (1966). — 8. SCHIRREN, C. G.: Hautarzt 14, 493 (1963). — 9. MISHIMA, Y.: Arch. Derm. 91, 519; 92, 393 (1965). — 10. MISHIMA, Y.: Cancer (Philad.) 20, 632 (1967). — 11. STEGMAIER, O. C.: J. invest. Derm. 32, 413 (1959). — 12. MISHIMA, Y.: Melanotic tumors. In: Ultrastructure of normal und abnormal skin (ZELICKSON, A. S., ed.) p. 612. Philadelphia: Lea & Febiger 1967.

Investigación de células tumorales en sangre periférica en enfermos con melanoma maligno

A. ALIAGA y J. CALAP, Servicio de Dermatología, Facultad de Medicine, Valencia (España)

Uno de los problemas más serios de la dermatología es la aparición de un melanoma maligno. La conducta terapéutica varía según las escuelas. Los estudios futuros sobre estadísticas basadas en grupos grandes de enfermos, ayudarán al esclarecimiento de cual es la norma terapéutica a seguir. Ahora bien, en el momento actual de la investigación cancerológica, no podemos conformarnos con tomar normas puramente espectativas de tratamientos clásicos y por desgracia no siempre definitivamente efectivos. Siempre que estirpamos un melanoma, nos queda la duda de si recidivará. Este problema parece haber encontrado en parte, contestación con el estudio previo y posterior al tratamiento, de la existencia de células tumorales en sangre periférica. En efecto, como indican las publicaciones de HERRMANN 'y su escuela de Munich el estudio de células tumorales ofrece un medio de trabajo con distintas posibilidades: a) Como prueba de la actividad de los citostáticos y su aplicación individual según los casos. b) Como test de reconocimiento de las alteraciones que los citostáticos provocan en los organos hematopoyeticos, y c) Juicio pronóstico del tratamiento empleado. Planteadas las posibilidades de esta investigación, vemos su aplicación inmediata en el debatido problema de nuestra especialidad, si un melanoma debe ser tratado o no con radioterapia previamente a su estirpación. El estudio comprenderá varias etapas: 1°¿Se encuentran células tumorales en sangre periférica en el melanoma maligno de localización cutánea? 2° Caso de encontrarlas, en qué fase aparecen? 3° ¿Actúa la radioterapia local del tumor con disminución significativa de células tumorales en sangre periférica?

Nuestra presente comunicación no tiene como fin primordial sacar conclusiones definitivas al problema abordado, pues se basa en el estudio de un número reducido de enfermos. Mas bien lo que queremos intentar, es presentar las posibilidades de este trabajo que consideramos de gran utilidad en el momento actual de la investigación cancerológica.

Material y metodos

Hemos abordado la primera etapa del trabajo: ¿Se encuentran células tumorales en sangre periférica en el melanoma maligno? Para contestar a esta pregunta hemos realizado paralela e independientemente, investigaciones de células tumorales con dos técnicas distintas y dos grupos distintos de enfermos: 1- Grupo de enfermos procedentes de la clínica dermatológica universitaria de Valencia. 2- Grupo de enfermos procedentes de la clínica dermatológica universitaria de Munich.Todos los enfermos tenían como diagnóstico clínico e histológico: melanoma maligno.

Grupo 1. Hemos estudiado un grupo de enfermos afectos de melanoma maligno con la técnica de HERBEUBAL [7].

1. R. P. Mujer de 75 años. Presentaba un melanoma en palma y borde interno de mano izquierda. La toma de sangre periférica se hizo antes del tratamiento. Resultado: No se encontraron células tumorales.

2. T. B. Mujer de 60 años de edad: Presentando un melanoma maligno en cara anterior tercio inferior, de la pierna izquierda, presentaba metastasis a lo largo de dicho miembro. La toma se hizo antes de comenzar el tratamiento. Resultado: No se encontraron células tumorales.

3. E. S. Mujer de 56 años. Presentaba un melanoma maligno en la planta del pie derecho. La toma se hizo antes de comenzar el tratamiento. Resultado: No se encontraron células tumorales.

4. M. M. Mujer de 74 años. Presentaba un melanoma maligno en región fronto-temporal izquierda. La toma se hizo antes de comenzar el tratamiento. Resultado: No se encontraron células tumorales.

5. J. R. Muchacho de 18 años. Presenta un melanoma maligno en cara externa tercio medio de pierna derecha. La toma se hizo después del tratamiento quirúrgico, y una segunda toma se realizó al aparecer metastasis generalizadas. Resultado: Ambas tomas fueron negativas.

6. J. P. Hombre de 60 años. Presenta un melanoma maligno en mejilla izquierda. La toma se hizo antes del tratamiento. Resultado: No se encontraron células tumorales.

Grupo 2. En este grupo de enfermos procedentes de la clínica dermatológica universitaria de Munich, hemos utilizado la técnica de GASTPAR; modificación de la técnica de SEAL [8].

1. L. A. Mujer de 50 años. Melanoma maligno de mama izquierda. Tras recibir 12.400 r extirpación del tumor. La toma se hizo a mitad del tratamiento radio-terápico. Resultado: Se encontraron células activas tumorales aisladas.

2. M. P. Mujer de 60 años. No se encontraron células atípicas.

3. J. R. Hombre de 66 años. Melanoma maligno de mejilla. Hace 9 años se irradió y se extirpó posteriormente. El 30-3-67 recidiva y metástasis. La extración se hace el 7. 4. 67 estando el enfermo en tratamiento radioterápico de las lesiones matastasicas. Resultado: Se observan células tumorales (4 células tumorales entre tres preparaciones.

4. J. W. Hombre de 67 años. Melanoma maligno. Radioterapia y extirpación. El estudio se realiza tres días después de la extirpación del tumor. Resultado: Se observan abundantes células tumorales (12 células en 3 preparaciones).

5. A. G. Hombre de 55 años. Melanoma maligno en hombro derecho. La toma se realizó dos días después de la estirpación del tumor. Resultado: Existencia de células patológicas sin poder precisar su naturaleza tumoral.

6. J. H. Hombre de 52 años. Melanoma maligno en espalda. Se realiza la toma siete días después de la exeresis. Resultado: Abundantes células tumorales entre las que se encuentran dos mitosis (en dos preparaciones 12 células tumorales).

Conclusiones

En el grupo de enfermos estudiados en Valencia, todos los resultados fueron negativos. En contraste, el grupo de enfermos estudiados en Munich son significativamente positivos. No hemos podido establecer relaciones con el momento evolutivo del tumor, ya que en dos de los casos (2 y 5) estudiados en Valencia, la toma se realizó en pleno período metastásico, y en cambio en dos de los casos estudiados en Munich (4 y 5) el tumor estaba en una fase muy precoz y los resultados fueron positivos. Tal vez esta gran diferencia de resultados entre los dos grupos se deba a las diferentes técnicas empleadas, aunque a nuestro juicio la técnica de HERBEUBAL es la más perfecta.

Agradecemos el Prof. HERRMAN y Priv. Doz. GASTPAR su amabilidad al poner a nuestra disposición su laboratorio de investigación citológica.

Bibliografía. 1. HERRMAN, A.: Arch. Ohr-, Nas- u. Kehlk.-Heilk. **176**, 536 (1960). — 2. GASTPAR, H.: Münch. med. Wschr. **2**, 416 (1960). — 3. GRAEBER, F., H. GASTPAR und A. HERRMANN: Arch. Ohr-, Nas.- u. Kehlk.-Heilk. **176**, 802 (1960). — 4. HERRMANN, A.: Arch. Ohr-, Nas.- u. Kehlk.-Heilk. **178**, 263 (1961). — 5. GASTPAR, H., u. I. GRAEBER: Salzburg. Kongreßbericht 1961 (Krebsarzt). — 6. GASTPAR, H., u. A. HERRMANN: HNO. Wegw. f. gach. Prax. **12**, 97 (1964). — 7. HERBEUBAL: C. R. Soc. Biol. (Paris) **154**, 2 160, (1960). — 8. SEAL, S. H.: Cancer (Philad.) **12**, 590 (1960).

Some Mechanisms of Pox Virus Oncolysis in Malignant Melanoma. A Review of 50 Cases

G. W. MILTON and M. LANE BROWN, Department of Surgery, University of Sydney (Australia)

Trophism of viruses for specific cell types is well known. It seems possible that a virus could discriminate between normal and malignant cells. However, nearly all reported attempts at human cancer therapy have been unrewarding. Reviews by MOORE and SOUTHAM (1960) indicate that more understanding of the virus host-cell relationship is needed before predictability of selective destruction can be made.

50 patients, with disseminated malignant melanoma have been treated by injections of pox virus. An alteration in the expected course of the disease was observed in 15 patients following the intratumour injection of pox viruses. This is a preliminary report of some of the mechanisms detected so far in the virus-melanoma cell relation and a short review of our results.

Material and Methods

a) Method of virus injection. Except where lesions were specifically left uninoculated to be removed by excision biopsy later, all visible deposits of melanoma were directly injected with the virus. The optimal dose used was 4 to 600 times the normal vaccination dose of viruses.

b) Viruses. The viruses used have been (1) Smallpox vaccine, B. P. (2) Purified suspensions of vaccinia, (3) The Pasteur strain of neurovaccinia, (4) Rabbit pox.

c) Electromicroscopy. Specimens from the vaccinated and non-vaccinated lesions were routinely submitted to ultrastructural examination with a Philips 200 E. M.

Results

Of the 50 patients treated over the last 7 years, 21 are still alive. The duration of life compared with a similar set of non-virus treated patients with advanced multiple metastatic melanoma is increased in this series from 3 to 20 months.

Some localized tumour destruction occurred in practically all patients. However, generalised oncolysis is difficult to prove. One patient remained alive and well for 6 years and died of a cerebral haemorrhage; at autopsy small deposits of viable tumour were found in the ribs and vertebrae, but these had not caused her death. Three other patients are alive and well, and apparently free of all signs of diesase (Fig. 1 and 2).

The characteristic reaction followed in these patients is firstly the development of erythematous reaction and vesication in the vaccinated tumour deposits. As the inflammation subsides there is a residual blue-grey zone of pigmentation which over a period of months or years gradually disappears leaving small patches of vitiligo at the vaccination sites. Histological sections in the early phases show acute inflammatory response and later melanin loaded macrophages in the dermis, and later still considerable reduction in the number of epidermal melanocytes. This is not associated with an increase in Langerhans cells.

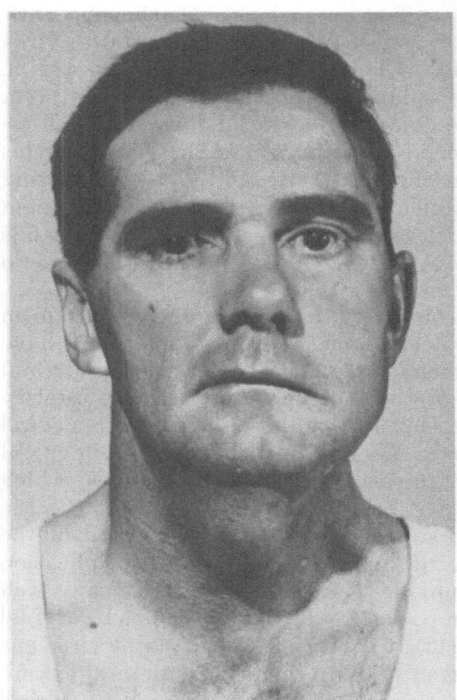 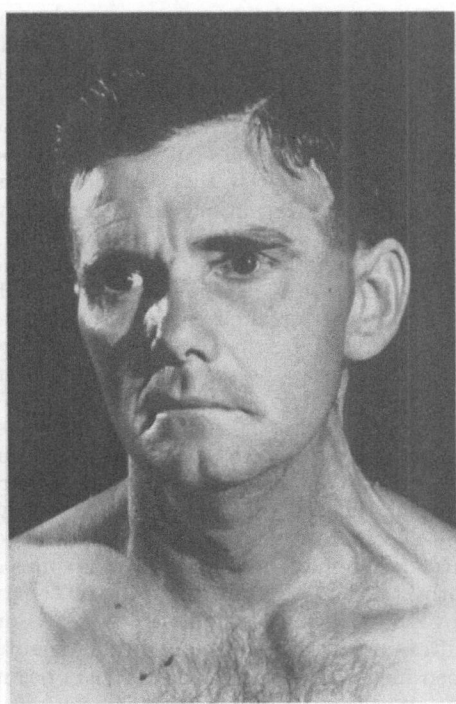

Fig. 1   Fig. 2

The most favourable response has been always in patients without visceral, cerebral or pulmonary metastases. The best results were obtained with skin metastases where the virus could be directly injected into the tumour. Systemic injection of viruses without the advantage of direct intratumour injection have been unsatisfactory. In one patient a round lung shadow, which may have been a metastasis, disappeared after virotherapy. No obvious improvement was attained in 32 patients who presented for this treatment with deep-seated metastases. The origin of the primary lesion, whether it arose from a pre-existing lesion or *de novo*, did not influence the result of treatment.

Electronmicrographs showed viral spread to nonvaccinated lesions only if there was some anatomical proximity. Viruses were found in all of the vaccinated lesions biopsied, and anti-vaccinia antibody levels as measured by haemagglutination inhibition rose in the expected fashion. No immune energy was observed. Three patients developed a generalized vaccinia reaction, but there were no untoward complications of the virus.

The results of cell culture on polyacrylamide gel of the patients' electrophoresed plasma proteins in two cases showed an inability of the melanoma cells to grow on the gamma-globulin fraction. This suggests that in these patients at least an antimelanoma antibody was produced (LANE BROWN, 1967).

Discussion

Spontaneous regression of recurrent malignant melanoma is a rare event, too unusual in fact to explain the regression produced in these cases (MILTON, LANE BROWN and GILDER, 1967).

The virus probably enhances anti-tumour factors, such as antimelanoma antibodies as demonstrated in two cases. It is suggested therefore that the virus allows enough tumour cell destruction for a large amount of tumour-specific antigen to be released, thus permitting a competent reticuloendothelial system to recognize this antigen as foreign. The tolerance to melanoma may well be related to the amount of melanoma-specific antigen which the immunocytes receive. An analogy to this situation is that of sympathetic ophthalmitis occurring after a penetrating injury to the eye, in which antigens protected from the main current of the body's milieu are suddenly released. The target cells over the bands separated by electrophoresis in continuous buffer are exposed in their micro environment to high concentrations of effector substances.

However with such variable results it is unlikely that this immune mechanism plays a large role in all cases. Other protective mechanisms, which may have played a role in the results are: (1) The melanocyte is a donor cell in its normal function and it is likely that the viruses of one cell could be passed on directly into neighbouring cells. The tumour cell specificity for the virus with direct viral multiplication in melanocytes alone has been observed ultrastructurally in one of the cases of general oncolysis. However, unvaccinated tumour nodules, which on later excision showed this effect, always had close anatomical proximity to the non-vaccinated metastasis and lead us to suppose that the direct spread of the viral lesion had occurred. (2) The fibrogenic properties of viral multiplication with scarring and incarceration of the tumour nodules in scar tissue may well have played a direct role in two of our patients who had prolonged survival with inoperable lymph node involvement. (3) It is possible that a latent virus has been initiated or that mutants have occurred. The routine ultrastructural examination of the pus from the vaccination reaction did not evince any morphological change in the viral structure. It has been suggested by HOLMES (1966) that morphological changes in pox viruses may indicate mutants, but the antigenic mutants of the rabbit poxes as determined by FENNER (1966) do not evidence ultrastructural changes.

Host survival has been a concomitant problem to experimental viral oncolysis. Often the viruses destroyed a tumour as well as the host. Pox viruses were chosen for these patients partly because of the low host toxicity.

Acknowledgements. We wish to thank the Commonwealth Serum Laboratories for their generous gift of smallpox vaccine. Professor F. FENNER, Professor P. DE BURGH and Professor J. LOEWENTHAL have been of great assistance. Dr. LANE BROWN has been supported by the N.S.W. State Cancer Council.

Richtlinien und unsere Erfahrungen in der Behandlung des malignomen Melanoms

Gy. Kárpáti, T. Venkei, Ö. Bihari, Gy. Németh und Anna Gulbert,
Budapest (Ungarn)

Im Staatlichen Onkologischen Institut und im Hauptstädtischen Onkoradiologischen Institut wurden in den Jahren 1950 bis 1960 insgesamt 537 histologisch bewiesene Melanomkranke behandelt.

Für die Melanoblastome sind dieselben allgemeinen Richtlinien maßgebend, wie für die Behandlung der anderen Malignome. Diese sind: Chirurgie, Radiologie oder die komplexe Anwendung dieser beiden, ev. Chemotherapie.

Unser Krankenmaterial wurde nach Sylven in drei Stadien eingeteilt: Stadium I sind die Fälle ohne Metastase; unter Stadium II verstehen wir Fälle, welche mit peritumoralen oder regionalen Metastasen auftreten. In Stadium III werden Kranke eingeteilt, welche bereits ferne Metastasen aufweisen.

I. St.	II. St.	III. St.	Insgesamt
413	99	25	537

Unsere Erfahrungen bezüglich der Behandlung der einzelnen Stadien sind die folgenden:

In Stadium I, also bei Melanoblastomen, welche keine Metastasen aufweisen, wird der Tumor meistens nach einer massiven Nahbestrahlung von 5000 R innerhalb 24 Std weit in das Gesundgewebe elektroexzendiert und nachher postoperativ bestrahlt.

Sollte die technische Durchführung der Excision zufolge der Lokalisation des Melanoms nicht möglich sein (Tumor um Mund, Auge, usw.), so wird von uns ausschließlich nur eine halbe Strahlenbehandlung angewendet. Es werden in zwei, eventuell in drei Serien insgesamt 10 bis 20000 R verabreicht — auch im Falle der Gefahr einer Radionekrose.

Bei Melanoblastomen im Stadium I wird die prophylaktische Bestrahlung der Regionen auch durchgeführt. Bezüglich deren Indikation besteht eine Meinungsverschiedenheit in der Fachliteratur.

Von unseren 413 Kranken im Stadium I erhielten auf Grund der obengenannten Prinzipien 90 nur eine chirurgische und 323 eine komplexe chirurgische und Strahlenbehandlung.

Eine prophylaktische Blockdissection haben wir nur in einigen wenigen ausgewählten Fällen durchgeführt.

Bei unserem Krankenmaterial haben wir bei den Melanomen im Stadium I in 65% eine Symptomfreiheit von 5 Jahren erzielt, welche den Angaben der Fachliteratur entspricht.

Im Stadium II, also in Fällen mit peritumoralen oder regionalen Metastasen, wird von uns bei dem primären Tumor dieselbe Methode angewendet, welche wir bei den Melanomen in Stadium I bekanntgegeben haben. Die regionalen Metastasen haben wir nach einer präoperativen Strahlenbehandlung auf dem Wege einer Blockdissection entfernt — und infolge der Gefahr einer Operationsdispersion — eine postoperative Bestrahlung der Operationsstelle durchgeführt. Die Versorgung des primären Tumors und seiner Metastasen wurde in einzelnen Fällen mit cytostatischer Behandlung durchgeführt.

Bei 99 unserer Melanomkranken im Stadium II haben wir auf Grund obiger Behandlungsprinzipien in 11,7% eine Symptomfreiheit von 5 Jahren erreicht.

In der Erzielung dieses Erfolges hat die Tätigkeit der Onkologischen Dispensaire-Organisation eine große Rolle gespielt, welche die organisierte posttherapeutische Kontrolle der Geschwulstkranken sichert.

Das Erkennen der frühen Rezidive oder Metastasen und eine adäquate therapeutische Versorgung derselben geben auch in der Perspektive der 5jährigen Überlebenszeit einige Möglichkeiten.

Die Tatsache, daß bei den Kranken mit Melanoblastomen in Stadium III — auch im Falle einer adäquaten Behandlung — mit einer 5jährigen Überlebenszeit praktisch nicht gerechnet werden kann und daß im Verhältnis die 3jährige Überlebenszeit — mit anderen Tumorarten verglichen — sehr niedrig ist, kann mit der extremen biologischen Malignität der malignen Melanome erklärt werden.

Observations concernant la prophylaxie et le traitment du mélanome maligne

E. Ujváry et I. Krepsz, Clinique de Dermatologie et de Radiologie de la Faculté de Médecin de Tg.-Mures (Roumanie)

Le mélanome maligne — l'une des tumeurs les plus graves — est généré dans la plupart des cas d'une lésion cutanée préexistente, d'habitude d'un nev pigmentaire et plus rarement d'un acromique, qui souffre une dégénérescence maligne, mais il peut apparaître aussi sur une peau d'aspect normal, sans être précédé d'une lésion cutanée préexistente. Le diagnostic clinique et histopathologique du mélanome maligne déjà installé, à l'exception des formes cliniques atypiques ou des localisations peu habituelles, ne pose pas de difficultés. En échange il est difficile a préciser le potentiel respectif du début de malignisation d'une lésion névique existente, qu'on pourrait dénommer mélanome «bénigne», ou reconnaître la nature névocellulaire d'une tumeur apparue sur une peau saine — nommée par Duperrat mélanome «d'emblée» dégénéré, ces aspects posent toute une série de problèmes vivement discutés sous rapport pathogénétique, diagnostic et de conduite thérapeutique. Ce sont ces problèmes qui appartiennent à l'ensemble de la prophylaxie du mélanome maligne et la prévention de cette affection très grave doit être posée au centre de notre attention. Ces lésions cutanées préexistentes, les cidits mélanomes bénignes, qui peuvent générer des mélanomes malignes, forment dans la plupart des cas des territoires de limites, qui intéressent plusieurs spécialités: la dermatologie, la cosmétologie, la chirurgie, l'oncologie etc.; ce fait contribue au manque d'une conduite unitaire et juste en ce qui concerne les cidits mélanomes bénignes.

Le problème la plus difficile de la prophylaxie c'est de préciser le potentiel de malignisation d'une lésion existente. Il faut reconnaître que nous ne disposons pas de critériums cliniques, histopathologiques et de tests biologiques, à l'aide desquels on pourrait constater avec certitude ce potentiel. Outre l'aspect clinique et évolutif de la lésion, les testes biologiques (l'activité de la thyrosinase tissulaire, la captation du ^{32}P, l'électrométrie, la thermodifférence, la dermatoscopie, etc). peuvent fournir des données informatives sur le potentiel de malignisation de la lésion respective. Nous nous sommes convaincus de l'utilité du teste de ^{32}P captation. Il faudrait utiliser ces preuves le plus souvent possible et corroborer leurs résultats avec l'aspect clinique et évolutif de la lésion. Dans la présence de n'importe quelle lésion cutanée qui provoquerait le plus petit doute sur le potentiel de malignisation, il faut intervenir de manière radicale, comme pour un mélanome maligne, par électrocoagulation, exérèse chirurgicale, qui ont comme but final la destruction aussi large et profonde que possible de la lésion, sans prendre en considération les conséquences cosmétiques.

Nous croyons que les possibilités offertes par la radiothérapie ne sont pas complètement utilisées dans la prophylaxie du mélanome bénigne. Dans la littérature nous rencontrons souvent la radiorésistance du mélanome maligne et des mélanomes bénignes. De même comme nous n'avons pas de critériums certains qui puissent déceler le potentiel de malignisation d'une lésion névique — pigmentaire ou acromique —, nous ne disposons pas de critériums qui pourraient démontrer la radiorésistance de la lésion en cause. Notre expérience paraît confirmer l'utilité de la radiothérapie dans la prévention du mélanome maligne. Souvent nous avons constaté la régression, c'est à dire la disparition du mélanome bénigne par suite de la radiothérapie. Nos observations ne confirment pas la validité absolue de la radiorésistance des mélanomes, tout au contraire, nous avons souvent constaté que justement ces lésions sont radiosensibles qui présentent des signes qui supposent un potentiel de malignisation ou d'irritation.

La radiothérapie n'est pas suivie par des destructions plus grandes que l'électrocoagulation radicale. En comparaison avec les autres méthodes, elle offre l'avantage de ne pas comporter les risques d'une intervention radicale, et même si elle n'est pas suivie par la disparition du mélanome bénin, elle peut être complétée par l'électrocoagulation ou par l'éxérèse chirurgicale des restes, en nous offrant la sureté d'effectuer ces interventions sur une lésion inactivée préalablement par des rayons X. Le seul inconvénient de la radiothérapie est présenté par le fait, qu'elle exclut le contrôle et la confirmation histopathologique de la nature de la lésion en cause. Nous considérons comme plus juste de renoncer à la confirmations histopathologique de la lésion, si cette dernière peut éviter au malade d'éventuels risques.

Données relatives au problème de la possibilité de dissémination après l'irradiation aux rayons X dans les cas du mélanome malin

T. VENKEI et Ö. BIHARI, Institut Oncologique National de Budapest (Hongrie)

Il est une question discutée souvent même de nos jours, si le traitement effectué aux rayons X du mélanoblastome favorise la dissémination ?

En vue de mettre au point la question, nous avons étudié les malades en deux groupes. Dans le premier groupe, à l'étape du mélanoblastome sans métastases, dans la première période, 238 malades ont reçu une thérapie adéquate, un traitement aux rayons X, chirurgical et complexe. Entre 1 et 6 mois, les métastases ont survenu dans 12,5% après le traitement aux rayons X, dans 10,0% après le traitement chirurgical et dans 6,7% après un traitement complexe. Dans l'autre groupe de 80 malades, étant également dans la première période, on a effectué, hors de l'Institut, une röntgenthérapie insuffisante, ou une intervention chirurgicale (biopsie, curetage, caustique), respectivement il arrivait une traumatisation équivalente à celle-ci, entraînant une hémorragie. Dans ce dernier groupe, des métastases se présentaient dans 50,0% à 57,1% entre 1 et 6 mois.

L'affirmation histologique des tableaux pathologiques se faisait, surtout au cours du traitement, par l'exérèse large et profonde de la tumeur primitive, tandis que, en cas d'une radiothérapie seule, à partir des métastases survenues ultérieurement.

Discussion et conclusion

Les résultats du premier groupe, vu la dissémination précoce, prouvent qu'entre la röntgenthérapie unique adéquate et le thérapie chirurgicale unique adéquate il n'y a pas une différence significative (12,5% : 10,0%). Dans le cadre du traitement complexe, on faisait irradiation et thérapie chirurgicale ou irradiation, thérapie chirurgicale ou irradiation, thérapie chirurgicale et l'administration des cytostatiques (dégranol, sarcolysin, SPG-SPI). Concernant la dissémination précoce (6,9% à 6,8%) les résultats des traitements complexes étaient meilleurs que ceux de la radiothérapie seule ou ceux de la thérapie chirurgicale seule.

Sur la base du deuxième groupe de malades, nous pouvons constater qu'après des interventions insuffisantes, la dissémination précoce se montre, comme il était à prévoir, dans un chiffre élevé du pourcentage (50,0% à 57,1%).

A la question posée dans l'introduction, si le traitement adéquat du mélanoblastome effectué par les rayons X favorise la dissémination, nous pouvons répondre, nous aussi, par un non catégorique, sur la base de nos examens.

The Uptake of Radioactively Labelled Compounds by Malignant Melanoma

M. S. BLOIS, Department of Dermatology, Stanford University School of Medicine, Stanford, California (USA)

The functioning melanocyte, whether normal or neoplastic, carries out a unique biochemical synthesis — the production of melanin pigment. This unique process should permit one to select appropriate, isotopically tagged compounds, which when administered to an experimental animal or a patient, will be selectively concentrated in the melanin of pigmented tissues — including melanoma. It has been shown [1] that such a selective uptake can be realized, and that it occurs by means of two different mechanisms.

First, if a biochemical precursor of melanin, in particular, dihydroxyphenylalanine (DOPA), is administered in labelled form it is found to be incorporated in the melanin pigment undergoing synthesis at the time of administration [2]. The radioactivity is thus selectively localized at sites of pigment synthesis. As a secondary result, since DOPA metabolism has a pathway in common with the synthesis of epinephrine, it is found that there is a concentration of radioactivity in the adrenal medulla. This mechanism leads to a selectivity of uptake which is proportional to the rate of melanin synthesis by the pigmented tissue.

A second totally different mechanism may lead to a generally similar result, and consists in the interaction of certain compounds with pre-existing melanin. Such compounds as chlorpromazine [3], and chloroquine [1, 4] are found to be reversibly adsorbed by melanin pigment *in vitro*, and thus to be selectively retained by pigmented tissues *in vivo*. This effect is proportional to the amount of melanin present in the tissue, and does not involve melanin synthesis itself since the compounds showing this binding are not chemically related to melanin and its precursors.

The differences between these two mechanisms is made more clear by considering the behavior of a specialized pigmented organ, the eye. The pigment of this organ seems to be synthesized mainly during prenatal life and proceeds very slowly, if at all, during adulthood. Administered DOPA therefore does not accumulate in this organ since melanin synthesis is low or non-existent. The systemic administration of chlorpromazine or chloroquine however results in a prompt and striking localization in the pigmented structures of the eye.

The action of this second mechanism in the case of melanoma is shown in the figure. The compound, iodoquine-[131]I (the iodine analogue of chloroquine, and a known melanin binding compound [1]) was administered to a melanoma bearing mouse by intraperitoneal injection. At various times after injection of this compound, the mouse was scanned by a clinical gamma ray scanning instrument which localizes the position of the bound iodoquine and shows the accumulation of radioactivity in the large pigmented melanoma. The accumulation of radioactivity in the liver is due to the detoxification of this compound in this organ and does not occur for example with chlorpromazine.

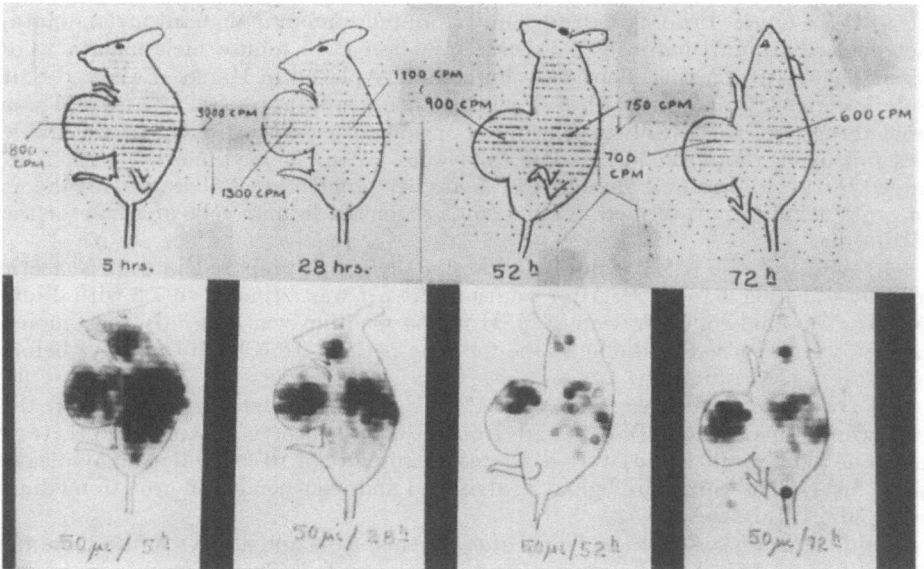

Fig. Gamma ray scans of a melanoma-mouse at various times after injection (I. P.) with 50 μc of iodoquine-I[131]

The clinical usefulness of these phenomena will depend first upon the degree of specificity for melanin shown by a particular compound, and secondly upon either the rate of melanin synthesis in the tissue or the amount of pre-existing melanin contained therein. Thus in a human case of metastatic malignant melanoma we found that the specific activity of a cutaneous metastasis (following administration of radio-iodoquine) was approximately four times that of the uninvolved whole skin, and that the latter had a specific activity some seventy times that of a blood sample drawn at the time of biopsy.

This research was supported in part by the U. S. Public Health Service under Grant CA-08064.

References. 1. BLOIS, M. S.: J. invest. Derm. (Submitted) 1967. — 2. BLOIS, M. S., and R. F. KALLMAN: Cancer Res. 24, 863 (1964). — 3. BLOIS, M. S.: J. invest. Derm. 45, 475 (1965). — 4. POTTS, A. M.: Invest. Ophthal. 3, 405 (1964).

Sensitization to X-Irradiation of Melanoma Cells Using Alpha-MSH

M. Lane Brown and G. W. Milton, Department of Surgery, University of Sydney, New South Wales (Australia)

Malignant melanoma is notoriously radio-insensitive. The mechanisms responsible for this lack of radio-sensitivity are not clear.

This report concerns the effect of synthetic alpha-melanocyte stimulating hormone (alpha-MSH; CIBA Basle) on the response to ionising radiation of mammalian melanoma (human and mouse) cells in vitro.

Materials and Methods

a) *Cell Culture*. Primary cultures only from ten human malignant melanomata, not derived from Hutchinson's Freckle, and ten B 16 mouse melanomata were used. The operation specimens were immediately placed in Hanks' Balanced Salt Solution at 37 °C and cut with fine scissors into 1 mm. cubes. 0.25% trypsin was used to prepare single cell suspensions. Concentration was adjusted to 10^6 viable cells/ml using the eosin index. The cells were grown in medium 199 with 20% added foetal calf serum. "Monolayers" (actually tangled sheets because of the loss of contact inhibition) formed in about 5 days for the human cells and less for the B 16 cells.

b) *Alpha-MSH*. A 2% solution of alpha-MSH was prepared in 0.02 N acetic acid by warming it to 40 °C. After solution, the pH was adjusted to 7.2 with dilute NaOH. The final concentration of MSH in the medium was 5 μg/ml. The "monolayers" were exposed to the hormone for time periods from 1/2 h to 2 days before exposure to X-irradiation.

c) *Irradiation*. After washing with Hanks' BSS and light trypsinisation, the cells were resuspended in BSS. 88 rads from a General Electric Maxima skin therapy machine (60 Kv, 100 r/min) were delivered to aliquote of 10 cells/ml in small plastic petri dishes. The cells were lightly centrifuged and resuspended in growth medium in Leighton tubes.

d) *Growth Rates Following Irradiation*. In each tube and always in the same ten microscopic fields, the cells were measured and counted. The differences in growth rate were analysed using the chi-squared test. The mean time to reform a "monolayer" was the simplest most definitive method of assessment of growth rate.

Results

Maximal cell death occured in those cells incubated with alpha-MSH and irradiated within 2 hr of exposure to the hormone. Control cells not incubated with MSH showed some cell death but recovered quickly to form monolayers within 5 days. Conversely irradiation to MSH exposed cells after 24 hr resulted in a high degree of radio-insensitivity. Cell morphology was not obviously affected by the hormone. However, surviving irradiated cells were larger and more bizarre and often amelanotic and multinucleate compared with those exposed to MSH.

Discussion

The mechanism of action of alpha-MSH on melanocytes is not definite. Calcium ions have been shown to be necessary for its action in amphibian melanophores and in some strains of melanoma cells. Cell culture studies indicate that its effect on human melanocytes is slow and melanogenesis may have to be mediated via cells of another lineage.

A mechanistic explanation for the early peak in cell death may be that of granule dispersion away from the nucleus. This would impede the possible interference of the melanin polymer and expose a vulnerable genome. However rapid granule dispersion was not observed under phase contrast in control monolayers.

Although serum protects cells from the tryptic effect, it is possible that the observed "radiosensitisation" is associated with trypsin to some degree. However all cells, controls and MSH-treated cells, were exposed to 0.25% trypsin for the same time.

Many claims for radio-sensitising drugs have been made. The clinically effective are few. Clinically a differential sensitisation, resulting in a more pronounced effect on the tumour cells than on normal tissues is required.

Some halogenated pyrimidines especially IDU (5-iodo deoxy uridine) have shown similar radiosensitisation in vitro. But this most likely sensitises normal tissues as well. Alpha-MSH is a more selective agent. Even so, normal melanocytes could be affected.

Most tissue-culture studies show that a smaller cell mass requires a smaller lethal x-ray dose than a larger cell mass. Perhaps the increase in total cell population which results in melanoma cell cultures after 48 hr exposure to the hormone explains the final radio-insensitivity. The mean lethal dose is exponential anyway. Cell anoxia is unlikely to explain this in-vitro protection.

MSH may predispose to a selected clone like methotrexate. BERRY showed that in culture, pre-treatment with methotrexate lead to a radio-sensitive clone.

Of course, the in-vitro situation is divorced greatly from the in-vivo. We intend now to try this in animals with melanomata.

Acknowledgements. This work was supported by the NSW State Cancer Council. It forms part of a thesis submitted for Ph. D. to University of Sydney (M. M. LANE BROWN). The help from Dr. V. BALMER (CIBA), Dr. ADRIAN JOHNSON, Dr. V. J. McGOVERN and Prof. J. LOEWENTHAL is greatly acknowledged.

Symposium 9   **Physiology of the Skin**

Physiologie de la peau

Fisiología de la piel

Physiologie der Haut

Organizer

G. B. MITCHELL-HEGGS, Great Britain

Presidents

S. W. MADDIN, Canada

M. K. POLANO, Netherlands

A. ROOK, Great Britain

H. THIERS, France

Delegate of the Organization Committee

K. WULF, Germany

Reports

Enzyme und Physiologie der Haut

G. K. STEIGLEDER, Universitäts-Hautklinik Köln (Deutschland)

Enzyme sind die „Katalysatoren der lebenden Zelle" (KARLSON) [15]. Sie steuern damit den Stoffwechsel in der Zelle und im Gewebe. Ihr Vorkommen und ihre Aktivität unter den in situ herrschenden Bedingungen gestatten daher Rückschlüsse auf funktionelle Vorgänge in den Organen. Die Isolierung und chemische Darstellung von Enzymen ist schwierig; daher wird ihr Vorkommen meist auf Grund der entsprechenden Aktivität, d. h. dem Grad der Aufspaltung des entsprechenden Substrates, vermutet. Die Aktivität hängt von zahlreichen Faktoren ab, die indirekt oder direkt die Aktivität eines Enzyms beeinflussen [4, 18, 26]. Erst neuerdings kann auf Grund der Eiweißstruktur mit Hilfe der Immunofluorescenz das Vorhandensein bestimmter Enzymmoleküle an Ort und Stelle nachgewiesen werden, also auch in inaktivem Zustand [29]. Ein großer Fortschritt auf dem Gebiet der Enzymforschung war im letzten Jahrzehnt vor allem durch Mikrobestimmungen möglich. In Anlehnung an Arbeiten von LOWRY am Gehirn wurden solche Verfahren vor allem von HERSHEY u. Mitarb. [14], ADACHI u. Mitarb. [1], GERSON u. Mitarb. [10] an Haut und Schleimhaut durchgeführt. Aus Nativschnitten isolierten diese Autoren einzelne Strukturen und Zellagen und analysierten in ihnen die Aktivität verschiedener Enzyme. Es zeigte sich, daß die mit solchen Verfahren gewonnenen Ergebnisse erstaunlich gut mit jenen übereinstimmen, die mit histochemischen Färbeverfahren erhalten wurden: Hatten doch manche Wissenschaftler befürchtet, daß beim Enzymnachweis mit Färbeverfahren weniger die Enzymaktivität als vielmehr andere Faktoren die Lokalisation des Farbstoffes im Gewebe bestimmen. Die Verläßlichkeit des Nachweises von Enzymaktivitäten mit Hilfe von Färbeverfahren gewinnt dadurch an Bedeutung, daß heute — vor allem mit Hilfe des Elektronenmikroskops — sogar Mikrostrukturen in der Zelle auf Grund von Farbstoffniederschlägen eine Enzymaktivität zugeschrieben wird [5].

Gewebe sind durch ein bestimmtes Enzymmuster gekennzeichnet, d. h. die Aktivitäten bestimmter Enzyme stehen in einem festen Verhältnis zueinander [14, 22, 23, 24]. Ferner unterscheiden sich Gewebe bei entsprechender Enzymaktivität durch das Vorkommen von Isoenzymen, d. h. Enzymen, die auf das gleiche Substrat wirken, aber einen anderen molekularen Aufbau haben [10, 28]. In der Haut findet man unterschiedliche Enzymmuster in Epidermis, Anhangsgebilden und Cutis; die Isoenzyme unterscheiden sich ebenfalls in den genannten Strukturen [7, 14, 19, 28].

Die Untersuchungsergebnisse der Enzymforschung lassen erkennen, daß der Energiestoffwechsel in der Epidermis dem anderer epithelialer Organe entspricht: Eine Energiegewinnung auf aerobem Wege über den Citronensäurestoffwechsel ist möglich; übereinstimmend wird von allen Autoren die hohe Glykolyserate der Epidermis hervorgehoben, also die Möglichkeit, aus Glykogen auf anaerobem Wege Energie zu gewinnen [6, 8, 9, 11, 12, 13, 14, 18, 20, 22, 23, 24, 25]. RASSNER bezeichnet die Epidermis als ein Gewebe mit hoher Glykolyserate bei starker Aktivität der Enzyme des Pentosephosphatcyclus und des Aminosäuremetabolismus [22, 23]. Mit zunehmendem Alter fällt nach SALFELD [24, 25] die Enzymaktivität in der Epidermis ab, aber nicht gleichmäßig: Die Enzyme des Citronensäurecyclus sind von diesem Aktivitätsabfall stärker betroffen als die der Glykolyse. Die Glykose-6-Phosphat-Dehydrogenase zeigt nicht nur keinen Aktivitätsverlust, ihre Aktivität ist im Alter sogar verstärkt [24]. Weitere Untersuchungen müssen klären, welche

Rolle dieses Enzym für die Keratinbildung und die Fettsäuresynthese in der Epidermis spielt. Neue Ergebnisse der Biochemie sprechen im Sinne älterer histochemischer Befunde, wonach in den tieferen gefäßnahen Schichten der verhornenden Epithelien vornehmlich Enzyme des aeroben Stoffwechsels aktiv sind, in den gefäßfernen Lagen dagegen die Energie vornehmlich durch Glykolyse anaerob gewonnen werden muß [9, 13, 14, 18, 20, 21]. So erklärt sich, daß die dickeren verhornenden Epithelien eine stärkere glykolytische Aktivität besitzen als eine dünne Epithelschicht [14]. Diese Situation ist von FERREIRA-MARQUES [8] durch die Unterteilung der Epidermis in ein Stratum oxybioticum und ein Stratum anoxybioticum veranschaulicht worden. Es wirft sich jedoch die Frage auf, ob die an Homogenaten gefundene hohe Glykolyserate der Epidermis wirklich genutzt wird.

HALPRIN u. OHKAWARA [12] ließen Epidermisschnitte auf einem Gewebskulturmedium schwimmen und versetzten damit das Gewebe in eine Situation, die der in vivo angenähert war. Solche Epidermisschnitte haben nur $^1/_{100}$ Teil an Milchsäure produziert wie unter optimalen Bedingungen gehaltene epidermale Homogenate [12]. Offenbar wird das verantwortliche Enzym, die Lactatdehydrogenase, in vivo durch Faktoren in der Zelle selbst gehemmt. Der Aktivitätsverlust ließ sich nicht durch einen Mangel an Substrat erklären. Wahrscheinlich ist eine solche Hemmung notwendig, um die irreversible Formation von Milchsäure zu bremsen und die Brenztraubensäure in der Zelle zu erhalten, die für andere Stoffwechselprozesse notwendig ist [12]. In der oberen Epidermis unmittelbar unter der Hornschicht findet man ein Lager von Enzymen, die offenbar als spezifische Funktion die Aufbereitung von Substanzen für die Hornschicht haben. Saure Phosphatase ist vielleicht an Keratohyalingranula gebunden [4]. Manche Enzyme gelangen anscheinend in die Hornschicht. Einige Befunde, darunter eigene Untersuchungen, weisen darauf hin, daß auch *auf* der Hornschicht die Aktivität mancher Enzyme nachzuweisen ist [26]. Es ist daran zu denken, daß sowohl durch die Aktivität als auch durch die Inaktivität oder durch das Fehlen von Enzymen das Vorkommen von Substanzen in der Hornschicht erklärt werden kann. Ein Beispiel ist die für den Strahlenschutz nützliche Anreicherung der Urocainsäure in der Epidermis durch eine Hemmung des Endabbaues des Histidins [2].

Auf die Enzymaktivität in den epithelialen Anhangsgebilden der Haut kann ich nur kurz hinweisen. Trotz gleicher Struktur können sich in ihnen die Enzymaktivitäten wesentlich unterscheiden [14]. Ein Beispiel sind die Befunde von BAELLIE, THOMSEN u. MILNE [3], daß nur in bestimmten Talgdrüsen eine Aktivität der 3-Alpha-, 3-Beta-, 11-Beta-, 16-Beta- und 17-Beta-Hydroxysteroid-Dehydrogenase nachzuweisen ist. Andererseits haben manche Strukturen ähnlicher embryonaler Herkunft einen verwandten Enzymsatz trotz verschiedenartiger morphologischer und funktioneller Differenzierung, z. B. die Milchdrüsen und die Talgdrüsen [14]. Nachdem nunmehr ein Verfahren beschrieben ist, um die Talgdrüsen aus der Haut zu isolieren, und bereits mikro-chemische Analysen isolierter Talgdrüsen veröffentlicht sind [16], dürfen wir auch auf wesentliche neue Erkenntnisse über den Fettstoffwechsel der Haut hoffen, die nicht ohne Folgerung für die Praxis bleiben werden. Bereits jetzt wurden histochemische, mit Färbemethoden gewonnene Befunde bestätigt, daß nämlich der Talg im Ausführungsgang der Talgdrüsen eine entscheidende Umwandlung erfährt [18, 26]. Auf die Gewichtseinheit bezogen, erweisen sich die Enzymaktivitäten in der Epidermis und in den epithelialen Anhängen der Haut meist mehrfach stärker als in der umgebenden Cutis [14, 28]. KLASCHKA [17] fand allerdings in Epidermis- und Cutisextrakten proteolytische Enzyme gleich aktiv. Es wirft sich die Frage auf, inwieweit epitheliale Anhangsgebilde aus der Cutis miterfaßt wurden und wie weit diese für die proteolytische

Aktivität verantwortlich sind. Bei anderen Enzymen der Proteolyse, nämlich den Leucinaminopeptidasen, ist erneut darauf hingewiesen worden, daß Isoenzyme in verschiedenem Maße löslich sind, also durch die Aufarbeitung und durch das Inkubationsmedium in verschiedenem Maße im Gewebe zurückgehalten und auch herausgelöst werden [7]. Bei der Beurteilung der Enzymaktivität in Epidermis. Cutis und Subcutis ist weiterhin folgendes zu berücksichtigen: In der Epidermis liegen die Gewebsbausteine vorwiegend intracellulär, in der Cutis vorwiegend extracellulär, die Cutis enthält vergleichsweise viel weniger Zellen. In der Subcutis hingegen liegt fast alles Material intracellulär, doch besteht dieses hochspezialisierte Gewebe vorwiegend aus Sonderbausteinen, den Fettzellen. Das Speicherprodukt Fett überwiegt mengenmäßig das Cytoplasma. Man muß also die Enzymaktivität auch in Beziehung zur Zellzahl setzen.

In der Cutis möchte ich nicht auf die Pigmentbildner, die Nerven und die Muskulatur mit ihren speziellen Enzymaktivitäten eingehen. Neben den Zellen der Gefäßwand, gekennzeichnet durch die Aktivität vieler Enzyme, finden sich im kollagenen Bindegewebe Zellen mit hohen Enzymaktivitäten. Hiervon haben uns vor allem die Esterasen und auch die proteolytische Aktivität in den letzten Jahren besonders beschäftigt [27]. Es hat sich gezeigt, daß die unterschiedliche Aktivität ein und derselben Zellart gerade im Bindegewebe funktionelle Besonderheiten manchmal leichter erkennen läßt als die Morphe. Die Mastzellen nehmen unter den Enzymträgern eine Sonderstellung ein. Sie sind durch die Fähigkeit ausgezeichnet, auch noch in fixierten Präparaten Naphthol-AS-D-Chloracetat zu spalten. Zahl und Enzymaktivität der Mastzellen in der Cutis werden offenbar von Vorgängen in den epithelialen Anhangsgebilden und in der Epidermis beeinflußt. Bei der Psoriasis haben wir gesehen, daß eine Vermehrung und eine Aktivitätssteigerung der Mastzellen in der oberen Cutis den psoriatischen Veränderungen der Epidermis parallel ging [27]. Unsere Ergebnisse legen nahe, daß funktionelle Veränderungen in den Epithelien von Veränderungen in der Cutis begleitet werden, die sich mit den üblichen morphologischen Methoden nicht erfassen lassen.

Hiermit möchte ich meine Ausführungen schließen, zumal in den kommenden Vorträgen eine Reihe von Fragen des Enzymstoffwechsels von Experten behandelt wird. Hoffentlich haben meine Hinweise deutlich gemacht, daß enzymatische Untersuchungen an der Haut in naher Zukunft Erkenntnisse erwarten lassen, die nicht nur von theoretischer Bedeutung sind, sondern sich auch in der Praxis auswirken werden.

Literatur. 1. ADACHI, K., and S. YAMASAWA: J. invest. Derm. 47, 293 (1966). — 2. BADEN. H. P., and M. A. PATHAK: J. invest. Derm. 48, 11 (1967). — 3. BAELLIE, A. H., J. THOMSON. and J. A. MILNE: Brit. J. Derm. 78, 451 (1966). — 4. BRAUN-FALCO, O., u. D. PETZOLDT: Arch. klin. exp. Derm. 223, 620 (1965). — 5. BRAUN-FALCO, O., u. M. RUPEC: Naturwissenschaften 52, 109 (1965). — 6. CRUICKSHANK, C. N. D.: Brit. J. Derm. 77, 603 (1965). — 7. DECKER, R. H., and C. H. DICKEN: J. invest. Derm. 48, 128 (1967). — 8. FERREIRA-MARQUES. J.: J. invest. Derm. 36, 63 (1961). — 9. FUKUI, K.: Jap. J. Derm. 75, 338 (1965). — 10. GERSON, ST. J., J. MEYER, and H. MATTENHEIMER: J. invest. Derm. 47, 526 (1966). — 11. HALPRIN, K. M.: Brit. J. Derm. 78, 541 (1966). — 12. HALPRIN, K. M., and A. OHKAWARA: J. invest. Derm. 47, 222 (1966). — 13. HASHIMOTO, T., and W. F. LEVER: J. invest. Derm. 47 421 (1966). — 14. HERSHEY, F. B.: Quantitative histochemistry of skin. In: The epidermis. hrsg. von MONTAGNA, W., u. W. C. LOBITZ. New York u. London: Academic Press 1964. — 15. KARLSON, P.: Kurzes Lehrbuch der Biochemie. Stuttgart: Thieme 1966. — 16. KELLUM. R. E.: Arch. Derm. Syph. (Chic.) 95, 218 (1967). — 17. KLASCHKA, F.: Arch. klin. exp. Derm. 215, 137 (1962). — 18. LEONHARDI, G., u. G. K. STEIGLEDER: Akt. Probl. Derm. 1, 47 (1959). — 19. LEWIS, CH., M. SCHMITT, and F. B. HERSHEY: J. invest. Derm. 48, 221 (1967). — 20. MIER, P. D., and D. W. K. COTTEN: Brit. J. Derm. 79, 170 (1967). — 21. NOGUCHI, Y., K. SEKI, T. SAITO, H. NAKAJIMA, Y. TAKANASHI, M. HIGUCHI, and H. KAWAMURA: Jap. J. Derm. 75, 168 (1965). — 22. RASSNER, G.: Arch. klin. exp. Derm. 222, 391 (1965). — 23. RASSNER, G.: Arch. klin. exp. Derm. 225, 398 (1966). — 24. SALFELD, K.: Arch. klin. exp. Derm. 225, 82

(1966). — 25. SALFELD, K.: Arch. klin. exp. Derm. **225**, 93 (1966). — 26. STEIGLEDER, G. K.: Arch. klin. exp. Derm. **219**, 585 (1964). — 27. STEIGLEDER, G. K.: Arch. klin. exp. Derm. **227**, 158 (1966). — 28. WEBER, G., and G. PFLEIDERER: Ann. N.Y. Acad. Sci. **94**, 933 (1961). — 29. YASUDA, K., and A. H. COONS: J. Histochim. Cytochem. **14**, 303 (1966).

Collagen Metabolism in Skin

CH. M. LAPIÈRE, Laboratory for Experimental Dermatology of the University, Hôpital de Bavière, Liège (Belgium)

The alteration of the collagen framework that arises from various pathological conditions in skin or any other connective tissue can be defined, on a morphological basis, only as a modification in amount or in organization. It is obvious that the static pictures seen in biopsies may result from many possibilities in terms of biochemical mechanisms. Any progress in the elucidation of their genesis requires investigations at the molecular level. Before defining such a molecular pathology, it is necessary to understand the various steps involved in the synthesis, the organization and the degradation of collagen in the tissues as well as in the control mechanisms that regulates them.

As seen by Ross (1965) with the aid of the electronmicroscope and autoradiography, labelled precursors of collagen injected into the animal are found to concentrate inside the fibroblasts on the endoplasmic reticulum. With the passage of time, the label migrates to the Golgi apparatus before being released in the extracellular fluid. With these observations, one visualizes the topography of the biochemical events leading to collagen synthesis in the fibroblasts. As for other proteins, it has been demonstrated that the synthesis of this large fibrous protein depends on an information transfer, a messenger-RNA copying the genetic material coded in the nuclear DNA. The formation of the two hydroxy-aminoacids, hydroxyproline and hydroxylysine, that are proper to collagen, is performed by an enzyme system requiring ascorbic acid as a cofactor (see UDENFRIEND, 1966, for review). Proline and lysine are hydroxylated after their incorporation in the growing peptide chain.

Collagen fibres are not seen inside of the fibroblasts but in their very close proximity. This observation and the fact that collagen in solution forms fibres *in vitro* upon heating to body temperature suggests that the collagen is released from the fibroblasts in a soluble form, the molecules polymerizing in fibres in the extracellular fluid. In skin, most if not all the collagen molecules are organized in fibres, the newly synthesized ones being extractable in isotonic saline at neutral pH, older molecules requiring increasing ionic strength or reduced pH to be solubilized (see GROSS, 1959). This maturation process that affects the intermolecular organization of the molecules in the fibres (JACKSON and BENTLEY, 1961) is accompanied by an intramolecular process of maturation, as the three coiled peptide chains forming the tropocollagen molecules are progressively linked by a covalent bond (MARTIN et al., 1963).

Under the fibrous form that is found in the tissues, collagen can be degraded only by a specific enzyme. The presence of such a collagenase has been demonstrated by GROSS and LAPIÈRE (1962) in several remodelling connective tissues. In dispersed form, the collagen is, however, susceptible to unspecific proteases at body temperature (LAPIÈRE, 1967).

In growing skin, a large proportion (50%) of the newly synthesized collagen is degraded before or soon after its polymerization while the rest of the molecules forming stable fibres, apparently are no longer removed in absence of remodelling (LAPIERE et al., 1966). During the process of remodelling, these collagen fibres loose their stability (the molecules become extractable in saline at 5 °C) before being degraded to peptides and free aminoacids. How the connective tissue maintains its function during the removal of the older framework is explained by the fact that a larger than normal proportion of the newly synthesized molecules are used to build up new stable fibres while the preexisting fibres are removed (LAPIERE et al., 1965).

One can postulate the existence of various control mechanisms that regulate the synthesis of the collagen in the fibroblast, its polymerization and organization in the tissues and its removal. The transport of aminoacids from the extracellular fluid to the interior of the cell, the translation of the genetic information, the activation of the aminoacids and maybe the release of the newly synthesized molecules represent possible controlled systems. According to *in vitro* experiments, the amount of newly synthesized collagen laid down in stable fibers could depend on the concentration of the molecules, on the rate of polymerization varying with the pH in the extracellular fluid and on the presence and concentration of pro-teolytic enzymes. The maturation of the collagen in the fibres can be influenced by the temperature and various compounds present in the extracellular fluid as well as by physical agents, ionizing radiation for instance (VAN CANEGHEM and LAPIÈRE, 1965). The removal of the fibres depends on the occurence and the concentration of a specific enzyme.

The various steps in collagen metabolism should therefore be understood as chemical or physicochemical reactions regulated by a number of factors, most of which are still unknown.

A detailed study of these parameters in various pathological conditions of the connective tissue should explain the mechanism by which they are produced. In some instance the basic principles of molecular biology have provided possible answers to some pathological disturbances. For example, the lack of Vit. C, affecting the hydroxylation of proline and lysine, is known to suppress the biosynthesis of collagen, inducing the alterations found in scurvy. The rapidly spreading infection by *Clostridium histolyticum* is possible thanks to a rapid destruction of the collagen by a specific bacterial collagenase. The abnormality of the collagen in the heritable disorders of the connective tissue, should be understood as an alteration of the genetic material leading therefore to the synthesis of abnormal molecules which demonstration awaits its proof.

In view of the complexity of the metabolism of collagen and of the lack of accurate knowledge about some reactions occuring even under normal conditions, it is not surprising that very few alterations of connective tissue have received an accurate diagnosis at the molecular level.

References. ROSS, R.: In: The use of radioautography in investigating protein synthesis. Symposium of the International Society for Cell Biology. LEBLOND, C. P., and L. B. WARREN, Ed. 4, 273 New York-London: Academic Press 1965. — UDENFRIEND, S.: Science 152, 1335 (1966). — JACKSON, D. S., and J. P. BENTLEY: J. biophys. biochem. Cytol. 7, 37 (1961). — GROSS, J.: In: Connective tissues, thrombosis and atherosclerosis, p. 77. I. H. PAGE. New York: Academic Press Inc. Publ. 1959. — GROSS, J., and CH. M. LAPIÈRE: Proc. nat. Acad. Sci. (Wash.) 48, 1014 (1962). — LAPIÈRE, CH. M.: Congrès International de Biochimie, Tokyo 1967. — LAPIÈRE, CH. M., A. BRUSCHI, M. L. TANZER, and J. GROSS: In: Calcified Tissues, Proceeding of the Second European Symposium, RICHELLE, L. J., et M. J. DALLEMAGNE, Collection des colloques de l'Université de Liège, p. 275, 1965. — MARTIN, G. R., K. A. PIEZ, and M. S. LEWIS: Biochim. biophys. Acta (Amst.) 69, 472 (1963). — LAPIÈRE, CH. M., C. ONKELINX et L. J. RICHELLE: In: Biochimie et Physiologie du Tissu Conjonctif, P. Comte Ed. Sté Orméco et Imprimeries du Sud-Est à Lyon Publ. 505, (1966). — VAN CANEGHEM, P., et CH. M. LAPIÈRE: C. R. Soc. Biol. (Paris) 159, 1250 (1965).

Physiological Response of Human Skin to Ultraviolet Light

M. A. Everett and R. L. Olson, Department of Dermatology, University of Oklahoma Medical Center, Oklahoma City, Oklahoma (USA)

Exposure of human skin to ultraviolet light (UV) results in the production of Vitamin D, melanin and cutaneous erythema. In addition, there are carcinogenic and bactericidal effects. These various responses are due principally to shorter wavelength UV. The characteristic erythema reaches maximum intensity 8 to 12 h following exposure and fades by 36 h. An increased thickness of keratin follows subsequently. With intense erythema, visible desquamation will appear at some time after 48 h. With less erythema, no visible desquamation will occur. The hyperpigmentation and hyperkeratosis will decrease as basal cells transverse the epidermis and are shed, usually within 14 to 40 days. The effects of a single exposure to sunlight may be evident for as long as 6 weeks, and residual pigmentation may persist even longer. This paper deals principally with the delayed erythema response.

Factors which determine the onset and degree of erythema include: 1. wavelength of the eliciting light; 2. anatomic site of exposure; 3. time; and 4. quantity of ultraviolet administered.

Time Relationships

It has been shown that there is variation in cutaneous susceptibility to ultraviolet throughout the year [1]. A maximum responsiveness is observed in the early spring and a minimum responsiveness is seen in the late summer. In our laboratory the minimal erythema dose for any given subject was not affected by the time of day at which the UV was administered.

We have demonstrated that the *length* of the latent period preceeding erythema is inversely proportional while the *intensity* and *duration* of erythema are directly proportional to the quantity of the ultraviolet administered.

Studies with monochromatic radiation [2] have revealed that the onset and duration of maximal erythema vary with wavelength (Fig. 1). Short wavelength erythema appears and fades more quickly. Maxima at longer

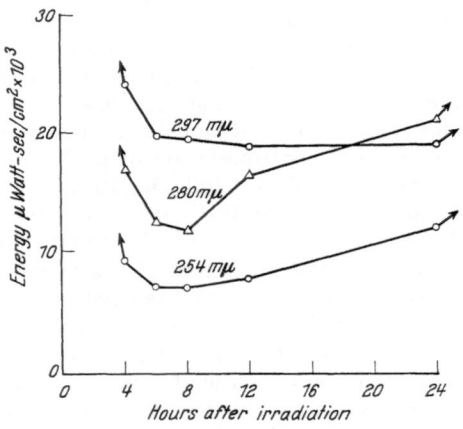

Fig. 1. Variations in MED by time following radiation at three wavelengths

wavelengths appear later and persist longer. At any given wavelength, the quantity of light required to produce erythema will differ depending on the time at which the subject is examined. The optimum time for *simultaneous* observation of erythema produced at several wavelengths has been determined to be approximately 8 h following exposure, since at this time short wavelength erythema has not yet begun to fade while long wavelength erythema is nearly fully developed.

Anatomic Relationships

(Fig. 2) The extremities are less sensitive to ultraviolet than the trunk, head and neck. Both the MED and the *relative* erythema effectiveness at different

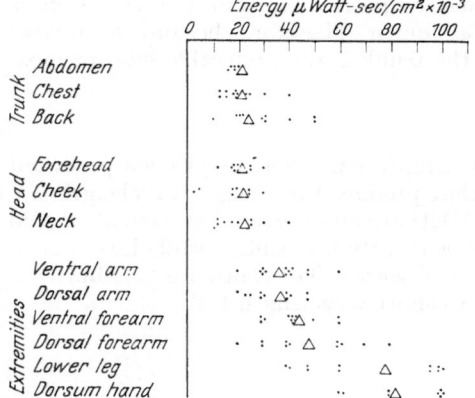

Fig. 2. Variation in MED by anatomic region

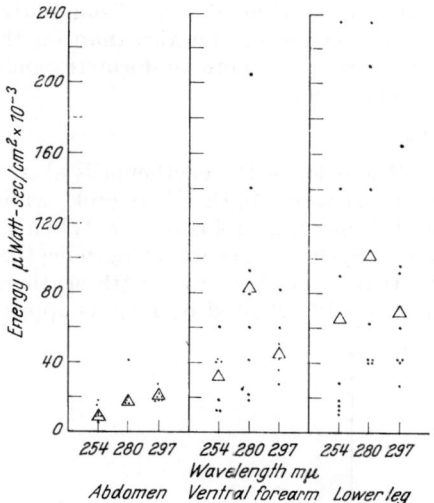

Fig. 3. Wavelength in anatomic region

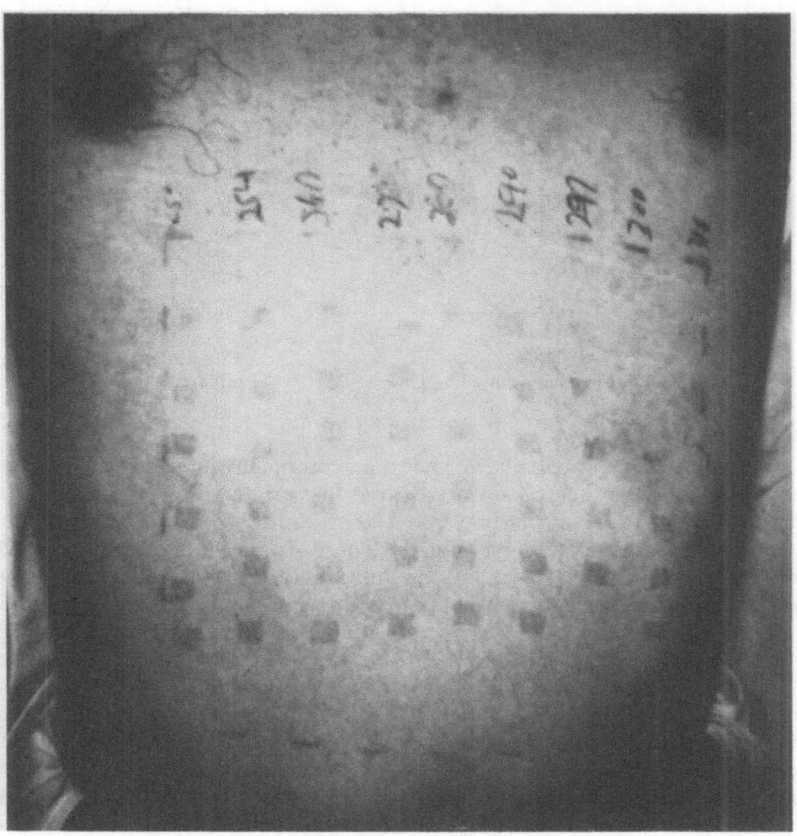

Fig. 4. Erythema response in typical patient

wavelengths (Fig. 3) vary from individual to individual, and the variation is greater on the extremities than on the abdomen. Therefore, because of greater sensitivity and more uniform response, the trunk is the preferable site for most of these studies.

Color

The color of the erythema is also wavelength dependent. Erythema produced by short wavelength UV is pink, while that produced by longer wavelength UV is of deeper hue and is redder. When ten MED are administered at each of several wavelengths, longer wavelength erythema is greatly intensified, while less intensification of shorter wavelength erythema is observed. Thus, intense "sunburn" is more readily elicited by long as opposed to short wavelength UV.

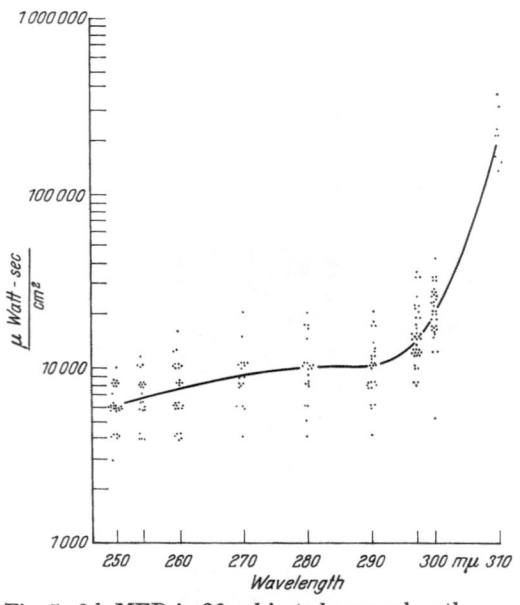

Fig. 5. 8 h MED in 36 subjects by wavelength

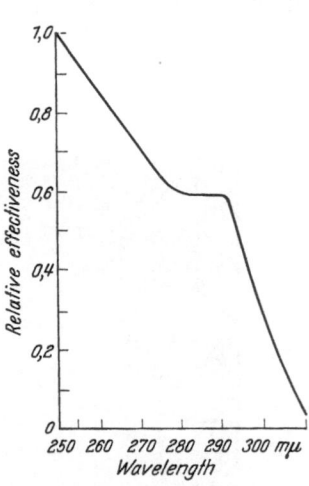

Fig. 6. Relative erythemal effectiveness

Quantitative Studies

In a series of studies utilizing a xenon arc monochromator [3], the erythema response of 36 subjects has been quantitated at various observation times. Eight intensities at nine wavelengths between 250 mμ and 310 mμ (a total of 72 tests) were administered to each subject (Fig. 4). These studies demonstrate (Fig. 5) that between the wavelengths 250 to 310 mμ, maximal erythema efficiency is seen at 250 mμ. A gradual decrease in erythema producing capacity obtains at successively longer wavelengths. This decrease in efficiency becomes marked at wavelengths longer than 300 mμ. When these quantitative data are plotted in terms of relative erythema effectiveness, the curve shown (Fig. 6) is obtained. The most efficient wavelength for producing erythema is 250 mμ. Larger amounts of energy are required to produce erythema when longer wavelengths are employed. In a more limited study (Fig. 7) of wavelengths shorter than 250 mμ, decreasing erythemal efficiency was observed. Likewise, in a study of the wavelengths 320 to 380 mμ, greatly increased quantities of radiation were required to produce minimal erythema. This energy curve differs considerably from the traditionally accepted curve. The quantitative erythemal energies reported in these studies agree substantially with *quantitative* measurements reported previously by BLUM and TERRUS [4], ROTTIER [5] and with the more extensive measurements by MAGNUS [6]. Findings similar to ours have been reported by FREEMAN and KNOX [7] (Fig. 8).

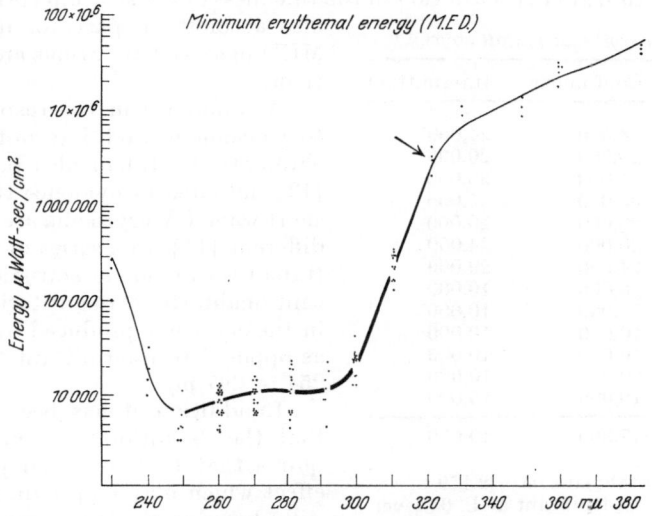

Fig. 7. MED at longer and shorter wavelengths

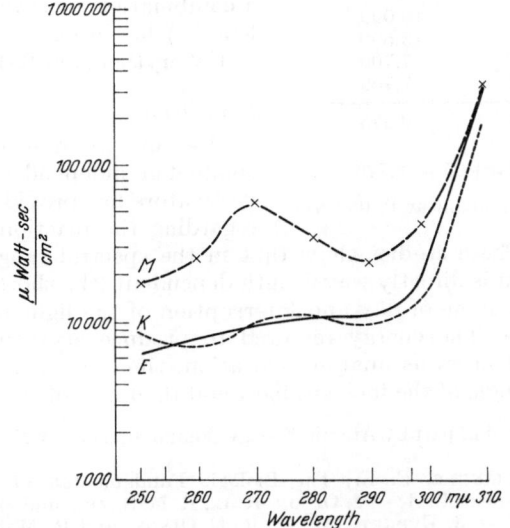

Fig. 8. MED's obtained by three investigators: M = MAGNUS; K = FREEMAN and KNOX; and E = EVERETT, OLSON and SAYRE

Some uncertainty exists regarding *relative* effectiveness in the *intermediate* UV range. Factors which may influence the MED produced by these wavelengths include: 1. thickness of the stratum corneum, and 2. the concentration of urocanic acid [8] a metabolic product of the epidermis present normally in significant concentrations [9, 10]. Both exhibit prominent UV absorption in the sunburn range. We have recently demonstrated [11] that whereas approximately 20% of the incident 250 mμ UV and 30 to 60% of 300 mμ UV penetrate the entire stratum corneum, only 4 to 15% of 270 to 280 mμ UV is transmitted. Additional studies have shown that removal of stratum corneum decreases the MED at every wavelength studied [12]. Variation in the thickness of the stratum corneum —may also account, in part, for differences in MED observed at various anatomic locations.

Table. 297 mμ erythema (μwatt sec/cm²)

Experiment	Continuous	Intermittant
1	24,000	24,000
2	20,000	20,000
3	24,000	35,000
4	35,000	35,000
5	20,000	20,000
6	20,000	24,000
7	24,000	29,000
8	8,000	10,000
9	10,000	10,000
10	10,000	10,000
11	10,000	10,000
12	10,000	10,000
13	10,000	10,000
Mean value	17,300	19,000

$t = \dfrac{d}{S_d} = 1.97$ tabular t.05 $= 2.179$
Insignificant at P. 05 level

254 mμ Erythema (μwatt-sec/cm²)

1	6,000	10,000
2	10,800	13,500
3	9,300	7,700
4	9,300	7,700
Mean value	8,850	9,575

$t = \dfrac{d}{S_d} = .472$ tabular t.05 $= 2.776$
Insignificant at P .05 level

A difference in the response of skin to continuous and intermittant monochromatic UVL had also been reported [13] and cited as evidence that long and short wave UV erythema are intrinsically different [14]. In a series of experiments (table) we found no statistically significant qualitative or quantitative difference in the erythema produced by continuous as opposed to intermittant UV at either 254 or 297 mμ.

In addition, it has been shown [15] that the "addition theorem" (which requires that for any given physiological effect which may be produced independently by several specific wavelengths of light, an equal effect can be produced by a combination of several of these wavelengths) has been verified as applicable to UV erythema at 254, 280 and 297 mμ.

Conclusion

Recent research on UV erythema conducted independently by several investigators has provided much new data regarding the reaction of human skin to ultraviolet light. These studies show that in the spectral range 250 to 310 mμ, cutaneous erythema is directly wavelength dependent (the shorter the wavelength the less the MED). Time of day and interruption of the light beam do not affect resultant erythema. The energy required to produce erythema is significantly modified by such factors as anatomic location, time of observation, size of the field of exposure, angle of the incident light and thickness of the stratum corneum.

This work supported in part by Atomic Energy Commission Grant Nr. AT—(40-1)—3578.

References. 1. ELLINGER, F. E.: The Biologic Fundamentals of Radiation Therapy, p. 193. New York: Elsevier 1941. — 2. OLSON, R. L., R. M. SAYRE, and M. A. EVERETT: Arch. Derm. **93**, 211 (1966). — 3. EVERETT, M. A., R. L. OLSON, and R. M. SAYRE: Arch. Derm. **92**, 713 (1965). — 4. BLUM, H. F., and W. S. TERUS: Amer. J. Physiol. **146**, 107 (1946). — 5. ROTTIER, P. B.: J. clin. Invest. **32**, 681 (1953). — 6. MAGNUS, I. A.: Brit. J. Derm. **76**, 245 (1964). — 7. FREEMAN, R. G., D. W. OWENS, J. M. KNOX, and H. T. HUDSON: J. invest. Derm. **47**, 586 (1966). — 8. EVERETT, M. A., J. H. ANGLIN jr., and A. T. BEVER: Arch. Derm. **84**, 717 (1961). — 9. ANGLIN, jr., J. H., A. T. BEVER, M. A. EVERETT, and J. H. LAMB: Biochim. biophys. Acta **53**, 408 (1961). — 10. EVERETT, M. A., J. H. ANGLIN jr., and A. T. BEVER: Arch. Derm. **84**, 717 (1961). — 11. EVERETT, M. A., E. YEARGERS, R. M. SAYRE, and R. L. OLSON: Photochem. Photobiol. **5**, 533 (1966). — 12. EVERETT, M. A., J. A. WALTERMIRE,

R. L. OLSON, and R. M. SAYRE: Nature (Lond.) **205**, 812 (1965). — 13. ROTTIER, P. B.: J. clin. Invest. **32**, 681 (1953). — 14. JILLSON, O. E.: In: EVERETT, M. A., R. L. OLSON, and R. M. SAYRE: Arch. Derm. **92**, 713 (1965). — 15. SAYRE, R. M., R. L. OLSON, and M. A. EVERETT: J. invest. Derm. **46**, 240 (1966).

The Clinical Significance of a Comparative Approach to the Physiology of Hair Growth

A. J. ROOK, Addenbrooke's Hospital, Cambridge (England)

Over a period of at least 50 years, and at a rapidly increasing rate, accurate knowledge of the processes of hair growth in many species of mammal has been accumulated by workers in different fields of biology. In the past 20 years a number of important conferences have encouraged greater collaboration and have related the findings in other species to the phenomena observed clinically in man, in whom hypotheses can less readily be subjected to experimental proof. With few exceptions the textbooks of clinical dermatology have followed a classical morphological approach and have not yet attempted to fit the very numerous disorders of human hair growth into any general biological scheme as an aid to logical classification, diagnosis and treatment and hence to more effective teaching and more rationally planned research.

The physiological and pathological changes in the hair coat in man as in any other mammal depend mainly on three interrelated but separable variables — the relative size of individual hair follicles, which determines the shaft diameter and hence the hair pattern; the alternation of periods of activity and rest, determining the moulting cycle, and the morphogenesis of the individual hair shaft, determining its physical and chemical properties.

Evolutionary Considerations

Hair has two main functions, protection and sexual display. Hair protects against cold and against ultraviolet light; the disastrous consequences of hairlessness can be observed in rare mutants of many species. A heavy hair coat is a handicap during the hotter months of the year. Seasonal moulting, allowing regular changes in the density and texture and sometimes the colour of the coat, was evolved to meet the hazards of a temperate climate. In such a climate with cold winters and warmer summers the spring is clearly the most opportune season in which to give birth to young. Studies on many species have established that the control of the moulting cycles is effected by the hormones of environmental adaptation, the thyroid and the suprarenal cortex, and that in some species the sexual cycles and moulting cycles have become closely linked.

ASHLEY MONTAGU (1964) has suggested that man lost the greater part of his protective hair coat when eccrine sweat glands were evolved to allow rapid but controlled loss of heat. Man no longer moults seasonally and, like other domesticated animals, has no regular mating season. Nevertheless the hormonal regulation of hair cycles in man betrays its origins, and the outstanding studies of CHASE, EBLING, JOHNSON and BOSSE of hair cycles in other mammals, provide the scaffolding on which has been fitted the more fragmentary facts available for man himself (BRAUN-FALCO, 1966). Conclusions based on observations in other species must be drawn with caution but the principle enunciated by BARRINGTON (1964), the comparative endocrinologist, provides a valuable guide. He points out that once an endocrine regulating mechanism has become established, evolutionary adaptations usually take the form of a quantitative change in end-organ response to a given hormone.

Hair Cycles

The disorders of hair cycles are characteristically potentially reversible for they involve no structural change in the follicle itself. If catagen is induced prematurely an increase in the relative proportion of follicles in telogen is inevitably followed by shedding of the resultant club hairs. This so-called telogen defluvium (KLIGMAN, 1961) has, as far as is known, no exact counterpart in other species, but has not yet been studied in other primates. In some rodents and in dogs hypothyroidism retards the initiation of a new anagen in resting follicles. Slowly progressive diffuse alopecia results. Hypothyroid alopecia in man may have a similar origin but has not been adequately investigated. Prolongation of anagen could results in an increase in the hair coat. Such a situation prevails in pregnancy in man and the guinea-pig the temporary synchronization of the follicles is reversed after parturition leading to a compensatory increase in the daily moult.

Hair Patterns

The hair concerned in sexual display in man, as in some other mammals, is the hair of the beard, the chest and abdomen and to a variable extent that of some areas of the back and limbs. Its development produces a conspicuous change in hair pattern and involves the enlargement of certain hair follicles which henceforth produce coarser hair of larger calibre. Functionally and hormonally the change is linked to sexual maturation, and is induced predominantly by androgen. The calibre of the hair present in each follicle at a given moment determines the hair pattern. The factors influencing hair pattern, are the genetically determined susceptibility of each follicle, the effect of ageing on the threshold of response, and the degree of endocrine stimulation to which the follicles are subjected. Disorders of hair pattern are characteristically not, or only partially reversible, since they involve a structural change in the size of the follicle.

The apparent simplicity of the relationship between the development of the sexual hair pattern and the degree of androgenic stimulation to which the follicles are subjected has led to unwarranted complacency in much of the clinical literature. Two rare syndromes demonstrate the complexity of the mechanisms controlling hair patterns and the extent of our ignorance. In premature pubarche, pubic and sometimes axillary hair appears in very early childhood, although breast development and the menarche occur at the normal age. It has often been cited as an example of abnormal end-organ response. However the fractionation of urinary C 19 steroids has shown increased androsterone and etiocholanolone (ZURBRUGG and GARDNER, 1963). In the testicular feminization syndrome, a male pseudo-hermaphrodite has a female phenotype with labial or intra-abdominal testes. At puberty feminine secondary sexual characters develop but paradoxically little or no sexual hair, although plasma testosterone approximates to normal male levels (FRENCH et al., 1965). This second syndrome may indeed represent a failure in end-organ response but it would be premature to make this assumption without further evidence.

Our concepts of the hormonal control of hair patterns are overwhelmed by acquired hypertrichosis lanuginosa, which contradicts the general rule that established patterns are not reversible. In its minor forms (FRETZIN, 1967) fine down appears on the face but in its extensive forms (ROOK, 1965) long lanúgo replaces vellus and terminal hair all over the body. No consistent endocrine abnormality has been discovered in these patients, but most of them were gravely ill.

The Structure of the Hair Shaft

A third variable determining the clinical state of the hair coat is the physical and chemical structure of the individual hair shaft. To the well known hereditary defects in shaft structure have recently been added the disturbances of keratinization in disorders of aminoacid metabolism and the interference with hair growth by ingested chemicals (ROOK, 1965). Of even wider clinical application is the demonstration by SIMS of Cambridge that the neglected and sometimes disputed observations recorded by PINKUS many years ago (PINKUS, 1928) are indeed correct. Severe systemic diseases of many types disturb protein synthesis by the follicle and produce distinct narrowing of the hair shaft analogous to Beau's lines in nails [SIMS, 1967 (1)]. SIMS' studies of hair growth in kwashiorkor [SIMS, 1967 (2)] have shown a gross reduction in shaft diameter and in rate of growth. Further quantitative studies of the hair shaft in systemic disease are badly needed. Meanwhile the many excellent investigations on wool growth in the sheep (RYDER, 1965) provide valuable and suggestive information which the dermatologist cannot afford to neglect.

In preparing this short review I have been very conscious of the quantity and quality of contemporary German contributions to our knowledge of hair growth and of the fact that I had no unpublished material to present. However most standard textbooks of dermatology still retain purely morphological classifications of diseases of the hair. Surely the time has come to insist on the importance to the clinician of differentiating disorders of hair pattern, of hair cycles and of shaft formation, as an aid to diagnosis and as a basis for logical investigation. And the clinician can interpret his findings only in the light of the steadily increasing studies of hair growth in other mammals.

References. BARRINGTON, E. J. W.: Hormones and Evolution. London: English Universities Press 1964. — BRAUN-FALCO, O.: Arch. klin. exp. Derm. **227**, 419 (1966). — FRENCH, F. S.: J. clin. Endocr. **25**, 661 (1965). — FRETZIN, D. F.: Arch. Derm. **95**, 294 (1967). — KLIGMAN, A. M.: Arch. Derm. **83**, 175 (1961). — MONTAGU, A.: J. Amer. med. Ass. **187**, 357 (1964). — PINKUS, F.: Die Einwirkung von Krankheiten auf das Kopfhaar des Menschen. 2nd Ed. Berlin: Karger 1928. — ROOK, A.: Brit. med. J. **1965, I**, 609; — Br. J. Derm. **77**, 115 (1965). — RYDER, M. L.: Wool Growth in Sheep. In: Comparative Physiology and Pathology of the Skin, p. 161 Edit. ROOK, A. J., and G. S. WALTON. Oxford: Blackwell 1965. — SIMS, R. T.: (1) Brit. J. Derm. **79**, 43 (1967); — (2) Arch. Dis. Childh. (1967) (In Press). — ZURBRUGG, R. P., and L. I. GARDNER: J. clin. Endocr. **23**, 704 (1963).

Physiologie der Hautoberfläche.
Die relative Bedeutung verschiedener Befunde

F. HERRMANN, Universitäts-Hautklinik Frankfurt a. M. (Deutschland)

Was ist *Hautoberfläche*? — Hier, ähnlich wie in Stockholm, verstehe man bitte darunter: Hautoberflächenfilm, Hornschicht und Intermediärzone. Allerdings werde ich fast ausschließlich Bemerkungen über den Film machen.

Die *Barrieren*funktion gehört zwar Herrn HORÁCEK, aber im Bestreben, Scheinwidersprüche zu beheben, möchte ich vorwegnehmen, daß sowohl diejenigen stichhaltige Gründe vertreten, die der gesamten Dicke der Hornschicht eine Sperrfunktion zuerkennen, der Basis allerdings eine — zufolge besonderer Abdichtung — verstärkte, wie auch alle Übergangszonenverteidiger und diejenigen, die in neuerer Zeit unter speziellen Bedingungen demonstrierten, daß sich innerhalb der Hornschicht ein Reservoir für exogen eingetroffenes Material bilden kann,

dessen Boden mehrere Male danach erneut durchbrochen werden kann, um wieder
Penetration zu erzeugen. Alle diese Befunde haben unsere Kenntnis von physiologischen Möglichkeiten gefördert. Jedoch wurden — wohl gemerkt — keine unter
natürlichen Bedingungen erhoben.

Nun muß ich zum *fettigen* Anteil* des *Oberflächenfilmes* übergehen, und zwar
zum *Spreiten.*

DVORKEN, MAGGIORA u. JADASSOHN teilten mit, daß sie keine Spreitung in
talgärmere Gebiete beobachten können. Dies steht im Gegensatz zu den Mitteilungen zahlreicher anderer, von denen ich wenigstens etliche nennen will, trotz des
1200 Worte-Limits: BUTCHER — direkte Demonstration auf der Haut; JAN WOLF,
— Abriß- und Adhäsionstechnik; SCHNEIDER u. Mitarb; KLEINE-NATROP und
LEJHANEC — indirekte Methodik; SULZBERGER u. Mitarb.; KVORNING, KLIGMANN
und SHELLEY — direkte gravimetrische Lipidbestimmungen, mit und ohne Behinderung der Ausbreitung.

SULZBERGERS Gruppe erklärte die Konstanz des Zufallsspiegels der Hautober-
flächenlipoide einerseits mit der Existenz einer Art von Oberflächenbehälter,
dessen Fassungsvermögen individuell und örtlich variiert, andererseits mit einer
Entfernung des Lipidüberschusses — zum Teil durch Zufallskontakte, zum anderen
durch Abwanderung, Spreitung von Material in umgebende Hautoberflächen-
gebiete.

Freilich ist hierfür eine normale Hautoberflächenbeschaffenheit zu postulieren.

JADASSOHNS Gruppe verfertigt Abdrucke, die in Osmiumsäuredämpfen ge-
schwärzt werden. Aber für Narben, zuvor Röntgenbehandelte, oder auch für
künstlich entfettete Haut zweifeln wir an normaler Oberflächenbeschaffenheit.

Zunächst können wir durch eigene Untersuchungen bestätigen, daß Abdrucke
von entfetteter Haut erstaunlich lange hell bleiben. Jedoch bestätigte sich unser
Verdacht, daß außer Aceton, Äther usw. auch die trockene Abdrucksbelastung
selbst — 600g, 2 min lang — die Hautoberfläche verändert: Abb. 1 zeigt in der
unteren Reihe Osmiumsäure-entwickelte Abdrucke sofort, $^1/_2$, 2 und 5 Std nach
dieser Belastung (über dünnem Cellophan), in der oberen die entsprechenden
Kontrollabdrucke nach Vorbelastung mit nur 60 g Belastung.

Auf Abb. 2 sieht man — unten — das mittels der Wolfschen Adhäsionstechnik dargestellte Relief der äußersten Hornschicht auf Tesa-Film ohne vorausgehende stärkere Druckbelastung; oben den jeweils kontralateralen Testbezirk,
sofort bis 8 Std nach der Kompressionsbelastung: Felderung und Sulci verwaschen!

C. G. SCHIRREN et al. veröffentlichten Serien ausgezeichneter Fettspreitungs-
bilder. Sie beschickten teils nicht entfettete, teils Petroläther-entfettete Bezirke
der Vorderarmbeugeseiten, deren Zufallsspiegel 30 γ/cm^2 = 0,3 mg pro 10 cm^2
betrug, mit Mengen von 58 bis 1130 γ Hautoberflächenfett. Abdrucke zur Os-
miumsäureentwicklung wurden pro Serie 1, 8 und 20 Std später genommen. Spreitung erfolgte entsprechend der aufgesetzten Fettmenge und der Zeitspanne bis zum
Abdruck. Ähnlich anderen folgern die Autoren, daß die Spreitungsgeschwindigkeit
wesentlich der aufgetragenen Fettmenge, dem Lipoidgefälle folgt. Jedoch negieren
sie, daß bei physiologischem Lipidspiegel eine nennenswerte Spreitung zu erwarten
sei. Wie ließe sich nun unter natürlichen Bedingungen feststellen, wo und wann
gerade ein wirksames Gefälle besteht ? Dieses schwindet wieder, ob man den Ausgleich als langsam oder schnell ansieht. SCHIRRENs aufgetragene „mittlere" Mengen
von Oberflächenfett befinden sich — ebenso wie auch eine der „Höchstmengen"

---

* Untersuchungen mit Unterstützung der Deutschen Forschungsgemeinschaft durchgeführt.

innerhalb physiologischer Größenordnung für Stirn- und Oberkörperhaut, wenn auch nicht für die Unterarmbeugeseiten mit ihrer überdies viel glatteren Oberfläche.

Um die Bedeutung der Spreitung für die relative Konstanz des Zufallsspiegels pro Hautstelle und Person zu manifestieren und in etwa mit dem Einfluß von Zufallsberührungen zu vergleichen, haben wir* wieder einmal — ähnlich wie früher

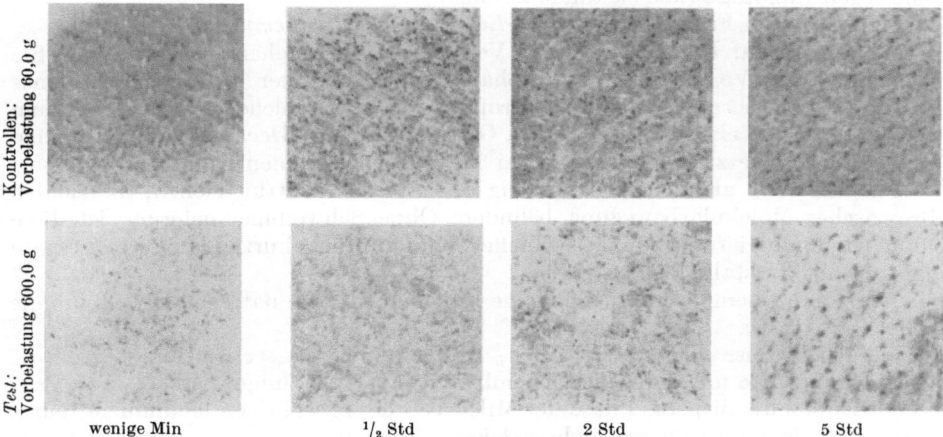

Kontrollen: Vorbelastung 60,0 g

Test: Vorbelastung 600,0 g

wenige Min   ¹/₂ Std   2 Std   5 Std
nach Vorbelastung

Abb. 1. Papierabdrucke mit je 60,0 g (entwickelt in OsO_4 Dämpfen)

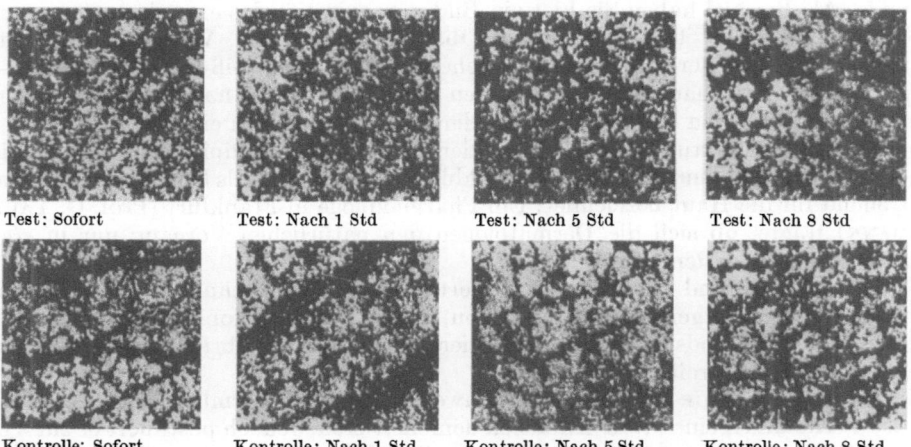

Test: Sofort   Test: Nach 1 Std   Test: Nach 5 Std   Test: Nach 8 Std

Kontrolle: Sofort   Kontrolle: Nach 1 Std   Kontrolle: Nach 5 Std   Kontrolle: Nach 8 Std

Abb. 2. Tesa-Film-Abdrucke im Dunkelfeld (re. und li. Oberarm). Obere Reihe = Testserie (li.): Sofort, 1 Std, 5 Std, 8 Std nach Belastung mit 600,0 g (300,0 gm an jedem der beiden Enden des Andruckbandes). Untere Reihe = Gleichzeitige Kontrollen von symmetr. gelegenen Bezirken (re.): Keine vorausgehende Belastung

und wie andere — das ätherlösliche Material von zwei symmetrisch gelegenen Bezirken gewogen, diesmal nach relativ kurzen Perioden. Der Testbezirk war durch einen flachen Hartgummiring abgedammt. In einem Teil der Untersuchungen war dessen Oberseite plastikvergittert, um Berührungen vorzubeugen. Der kontralaterale Bezirk diente Kontrollbestimmungen.

---

* S. Rust, P. Harth und F. Herrmann

Entsprechend allem Bekannten übertraf der unter Schutz gewonnene Spiegel den Kontrollwert. Waren Ausbreitung und Berührungen verhindert, übertraf der Testspiegel den Kontrollspiegel um etwa das Doppelte der Erhöhung, die nach Abdammung allein gefunden wurde. Die relative Konstanz des Zufallsspiegels dürfte also in ähnlichem Ausmaß durch Spreitung wie durch Abwischung überschüssigen Lipidmaterials zustande kommen.

Nun zur alten Frage, ob eine *natürliche Lipid-Schweißemulsion* vorkommt:

Aus einem auf Dr. SULZBERGERS Veranlassung entstehenden Film sehen Sie folgende kurze Vorschau. Zwecks phasenmikroskopischer Untersuchung eines unveränderten thermogenen Schweißtropfens wurde ein solcher behutsam mit dem verjüngten Ende eines geschmolzenen Glasstabs auf ein Deckgläschen oder einen Objektträger gesetzt. Beobachtung bei 33 °C in einer kleinen Kammer.

Sie sehen die ziemlich gleichförmig dispergierten Fettkügelchen, die sich in Brownscher Molekularbewegung befinden. Ohne Schweißnachlieferung ist diese Öl-/Wasseremulgierung zufolge schneller Verdampfung kurzlebig. Fettaggregate und oftmals Kristalle bleiben zurück.

Auch WOLF demonstrierte eine feine Lipidemulsion im nativen Schweiß um die Schweißduktostia.

Vergleichsweise zeigen wir Milch, 200fach mit Wasser verdünnt. Auf die Ähnlichkeit hatte uns der Kolloidchemiker ROLF JÄGER hingewiesen.

Ist einmal die disperse Phase der Milch von ihrem wäßrigen Medium getrennt, lassen sich die beiden Phasen nicht so leicht wieder in naturgetreuer Emulsion vereinigen. Ähnliches gilt für in-vitro-Bemühungen mit Schweiß und Ätherlösungsrückstand von der Haut. Trotzdem unternahmen wir weitere Mischversuche in vitro. Als Beispiel haben Sie hier ein Bild von agitationslos eingedrungenem, mit Fluorescein versetztem Schweiß im Oberflächenfett, bzw. W/O, bei 33 °C; als nächstes natürlicher, über 8 Std bestehender W/O (Schweiß-Oberflächenfett) — Bezug einer Stirnhaut (ähnliches fanden SPIER und SCHWARZ). Viele der Wassertröpfchen schließen hier ihrerseits wieder Lipidpartikelchen ein.

Die reichlich studierte Spreitung der Hautoberflächenlipide über Wasser ist doch wohl ein Beginn von Emulsionsbildung. Sie wird gern als belanglos oder unzutreffend für die Haut bezeichnet. Ein Pharmakologe in Frankfurt (Prof. G. TAUBMANN) fragte, ob sich die Dermatologen den natürlichen Vorgang nur in *einer* Dimension vorstellen.

SWANBECK und THYRESSON folgerten aus Untersuchungen von Hornlamellen mit Röntgenstrahlendiffraktion, Elektronmikroskopie und Infrarotabsorption, daß Lipidsubstanzen dispergiert an die Keratinfibrillen angelagert sind und auf diesen spreiten.

KLEINE-NATROP konnte auf den schweißarmen Vorderarmbeugeseiten lediglich das Vorkommen einer W/O-Emulsion demonstrieren. Jedoch postuliert er zur Vervollständigung des Griffinschen hydro-lipophilen Emulgator Balancesystems („H. L. B.") das Vorhandensein wirksamer Emulgatoren auf der Hautoberfläche. Kämen hier vielleicht auch fragmentierte Keratinfibrillen in Betracht (SWANBECK)?

Widerspruchsvolle Daten betreffen auch die natürliche Menge von *Glucose* auf der Hautoberfläche. Anwendungen des Glucoseteststreifens zufolge, welcher im wesentlichen Glucoseoxydase, Peroxydase und chromogenes O-Toluidin enthält, wurde Glucoseausscheidung auf Fingerhaut und andere Hautgebiete wiederholt beschrieben. Demgegenüber konnte mein Doktorand SEHR in ausgedehnten Prüfungen mit derselben Methode keinen positiven Befund erheben; auch nicht im Schweiß, in dem Laborvergleichsanalysen von Herrn LEONHARDI etwa 1 bis 2 mg-% ergaben. Freilich erzeugte exogener Transport zuckerhaltiger Kost, beispielsweise von Drops, anderen Süßigkeiten oder Früchten, mit der Hand zum

Mund, ausnahmlos Positivität auf Fingerbeeren und Handflächen, dann auch um den Mund herum; vom Mundgebiet oftmals Weiterverschleppung gesichtswärts. Bald danach war alles wieder hinweggefegt. Auch Glucosurieverunreinigung der Haut erzeugt „positive" Glucoteste.

Zum Verfolgen äußerer Verschleppung von Hautgebiet zu Hautgebiet genügte der Glucotest nicht. Da solche Untersuchungen dem Verständnis des „Springens" von Kontaktdermatitiden dienen können, ging Kollege SEHR einen bereits einmal in New York eingeschlagenen Weg. Er verfolgte nach Auftragung einer einfachen fluoresceinhaltigen Lotio deren Transport unter Woods Filter. War eine Zeigefingerbeere gepinselt, fluorescierten meist nach 1 Std Hände, Arme und Gesicht, nach 12 Std auch die Genital-, oft auch die Analgegend. Nach Pinselung von Fingernägeln, insbesondere des rechten Indexnagels, fluorescierten die Augenlider fast regelmäßig und selektiv innerhalb von 12 Std.

Some Remarks on the Barrier Function of the Epidermis

J. HORÁČEK, Trýb's Laboratory of the Skin Biochemistry, Brno (CSSR)

The adaptability of the organism during its development to the waterless milieu of the atmosphere of the earth was mainly due to the capacity of defense, protecting animals from drying up and from the biological noxious radiation. In fullfilling of the two fundamental conditions the development of the epidermal barrier of animals and human plays an important part [3].

Whereas the penetration of water through the integument in both directions always drew the attention of the research workers many other properties of the skin still remain a rather neglected field.

I should like to deal with some personal experimental experiences obtained in analysing a series of tangential microscopically controlled sections of the native human skin from the heel (Kryostat Dittes-Duspiva) [5].

In the thus made serial section we determined the whole nitrogen by micro-Kjeldahlisation [6] and the water content from the weight difference at standard drying of the slices. Further by extraction, hydrolysation and chromatography the lipids [1], proteins [2] and other components were determined.

The content of free water in the horny layer (Fig. 1) diminishes rapidly below the surface and then increases just as rapidly in the keratogenous zone to reach in the germinative parts of the epidermis the values constantly maintained in the corium. This distribution of molecularly not bound water in the horny layer is the result of an individual but constant passage of the epidermis and the keratogenous zone, which is rather abundantly hydrated. The hydratisation of the uppermost layers is moreover influenced by the imbibition of water from the surface of the skin which is constantly wettened by sweat. The basic conditions of hydratation are of course given by the chemical composition and the physical properties of the macromolecules of the fibrilary organized and non-organized keratin and many other hydrophil and hydrophob factors. The hydrating profile of the horny layer of the epidermis is under normal conditions not particularly influenced by the transductal diffusion of water from the intracorneal part of the sweat ducts. This manner of hydratation asserts itself only at abnormal, eventually pathological conditions about which will refer our collaborators [8].

The balance of hydratation of the horny layer of the epidermis is reacted by the supply of water from the deeper layers of the skin, its physical state and the chemical composition of the horny layer and the loss of water on the surface occasioned by the surrounding climate (or microclimate).

By measuring the permeability to the ultraviolet radiation of different wave length on series of tangentional sections proposed by the kryostat, we found a certain regularity of the nonhomogenity of the horny layer of the skin [4]. The skin of the sole prevents the influence of the melanin pigment absorption present in an absolutely unconstant quantity in the epidermis of other regions of the body.

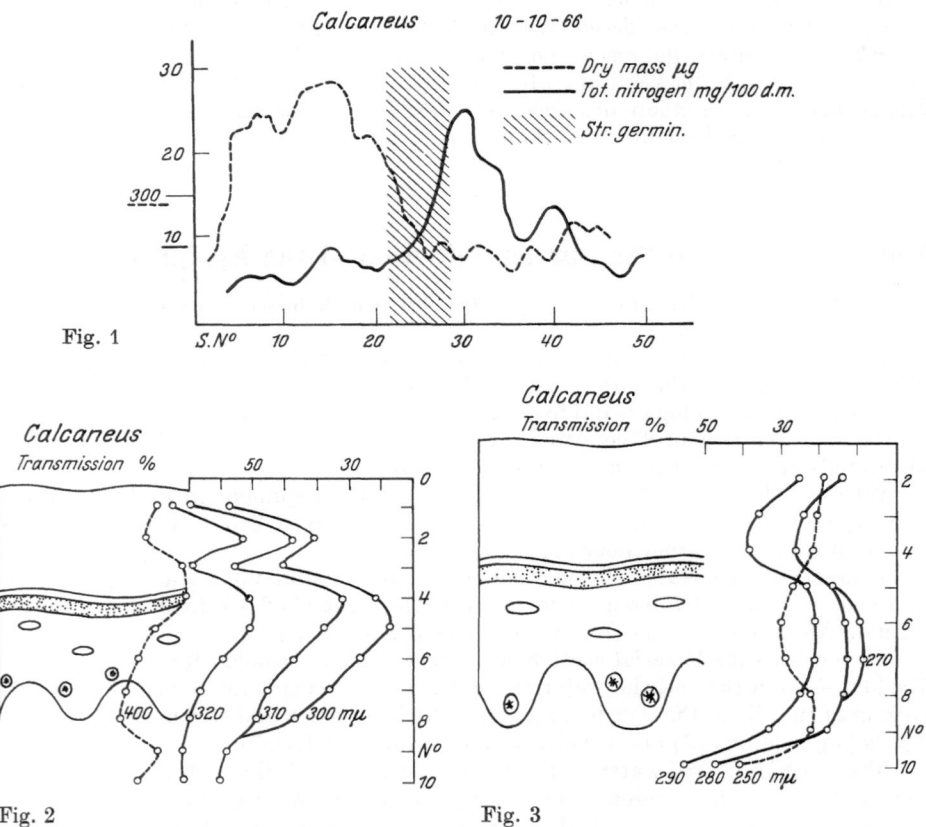

Fig. 1

Fig. 2   Fig. 3

Fig. 2 followes the permeability to rays having a length of 300, 310, 320 and 400 nm showing a slight diminution of the permeability in the middle of the thickness of the horny layer and a minimal permeability in the region of the keratogenous zone. The ultraviolet radiation in this region is most influenced by the wave length 300 nm, where the permeability diminishes by 8%. With the increasing wave length this diminution of the permeability is not so remarkable until at 400 nm the curve loses completely its characteristic course.

The laws of shorter wave lengths, which naturally do not exist now on the surface of the earth, are quite different (Fig. 3). The penetration of the wave lengths 290, 280, 270 and 250 nm do not show any striking changes in passing through the horny part of the epidermis. The minimum of permeability for the wave length 270 to 290 nm is limited on the stratum germinativum epidermis. Shorter wave lengths characterized in our graph 250 nm again show a noncharacteristical course with a marked minimum at the limit of the epidermis and the corium.

The non-homogenous hydratation and absorption of ultraviolet rays are the results of an integration of the particular properties of the material of the epidermal keratin. It may be said in general that the keratin originating in the keratogenous zone of the epidermis is not a stable matter but is *subject to a further individual development* of structure and properties in the course of ageing and the transfer

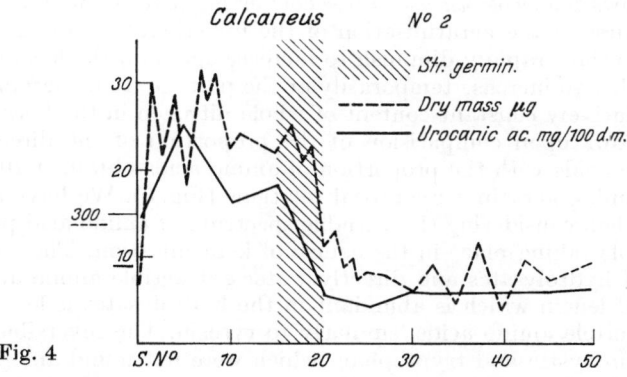

Fig. 4

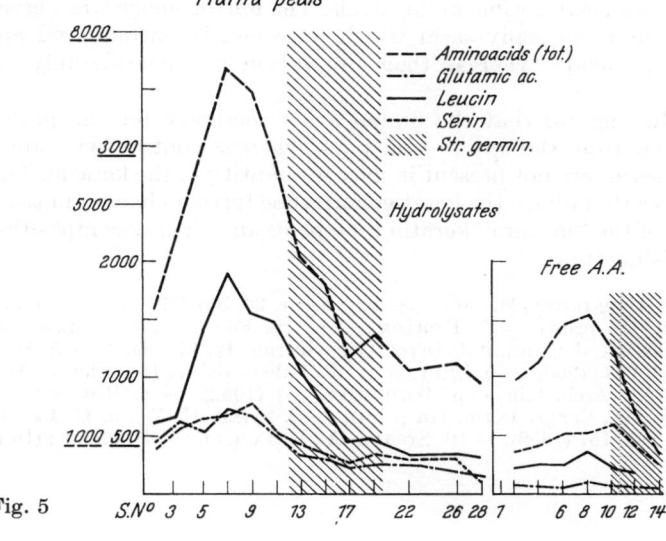

Fig. 5

towards the surface of the skin. This somewhat "passive" metabolism has up to now not been much studied. Not much attention has been given to further changes of the protein components of the horny layer except of partial observation to the urocanic acid. We ourselves [10] followed the distribution of the urocanic acid in the horny part of the epidermis as may be seen in the following Fig. 4. Its course confirms the former observations [9, 7] that the *quantity of urocanic acid* increases towards the depth of the horny layer.

Our analysis of tangential sections confirms in most of our examined specimens (3:2) that there was a double maximum in the horny part of the epidermis. The content of urocanic acid correspondend to the weight of the dry matter of the keratin except in the uppermost layer. Its content diminished rapidly down to zero in the germinative part of the epidermis.

We also tried [2] to elucidate some relations between the formation and the further fate of the keratin by studying *the amount of whole nitrogen* and the participation of the *different free and bound amino acids* in the different layers.

The Fig. 1 shows the *whole nitrogen* after converting it to the weight of the dry matter in the course of the keratinisation of the hyperkeratosis of the sole. The values from the surface rapidly diminish to increase again on the level of the str. lucidum and further to increase temporarily at the passage from the epidermis to the corium. A relatively constant content of whole nitrogen in the horny layer of the epidermis shows upon comparision of the proportion of the directly water extractible amino acids with the proportion of amino acids obtained after hydrolysis of the remaining keratin a reciprocal relations (Fig. 5). We have arrived at this conclusion when considering the variable spectrum of amino acid present the changes unvariable taking place in the course of keratinisation. The comparison of the content of hydrolysates and directly water extractible amino acids shows that the group of leucin which is abundant in the hydrolysates is less abundant among the extractible amino acids, similarly to tyrosin. The reversible relations are also evident in cystin and tryptophan, which were not found among the free acids of the keratin of the heel where as they are present in the hydrolysates. The same is also valid for the glutamic acid of which there are just traces in the part of the directly water-extractible amino acids. The mirror image was observed with alanin, glycine and especially serin which were chiefly encountered among the extractible amino acids, whereas their proportion was considerably smaller in hydrolysates.

These results suggest that the amino acids necessary for the production of keratin disappear from the amino acid pool, whereas contrarywise amino acids, as for instance serin, are not present in mayor quantity in the keratin. The quantitative data prove that above the keratigenous zone further changes in the structure and properties of the "mature" keratin take place and their decomposition ends in the stratum disjunctum.

References. 1. CERNIKOVÁ, M.: Fette, Seifen, Anstr. **62**, 587 (1960). — 2. CERNIKOVA, M., and J. HORÁČEK: (In print). — 3. HORÁČEK, J.: Acta Fac. med. Univ.-Brunnensis N° 16 (1965). — 4. HORÁČEK, J.: Ann. ital. Derm. Clin. Sperim. **19**, 87 (1965). — 5. HORÁČEK, J.: Derm. Wschr. **151**, 887 (1965). — 6. LEVY, M.: C. R. Lab. Carlsberg (Ser. chim.) **21**, 101 (1936). — 7. PASCHER, G.: Arch. klin. exp. Derm. **214**, 234 (1962). — 8. ROVENSKÝ, J., and J. ZÁHEJSKÝ: XIII. Int. Congr. Derm. (In print). — 9. SPIER, H. W., u. G. PASCHER: Arch. klin. exp. Derm. **209**, 181 (1959). — 10. ŠTRYCH, A., I. HAIS, and J. HORÁČEK: (In print).

Le pouvoir tampon de la peau

H. THIERS, Hôpital Edouard-Herriot, Lyon (France)

Ce que l'on dénomme le pouvoir tampon de la peau répond en réalité au pouvoir tampon: 1. du film hydrolipidique de la surface des téguments; 2. des fins débris cellulaires provenant de la desquamation permanente de la couche cornée; 3. du gaz carbonique qui s'échappe à travers les téguments. Donc la première notion est la complexité du système qui tend à s'opposer aux variations du pH de la surface cutanée sous l'influence d'une cause externe.

De ce fait, il est extrêmement invraisemblable que ce pouvoir tampon soit lié à l'activité d'un système unique. Il est légitime d'admettre qu'interviennent de multiples facteurs: 1. Les débris cellulaires provenant de la desquamation cornée représentent de fines granulations protéïques dont les pouvoirs d'absorption et de neutralisation ne sont pas négligeables — encore qu'on n'en ait pas étudié l'importance. 2. Les aminoacides (sueur, perspiration insensible) ont un rôle tampon classique: ils démasquent leur fonction basique en milieu acide, leur fonction acide en milieu basique (Zwitterion). 3. Le gaz carbonique forme avec les bicarbonates et les phosphates un système tampon également classique. 4. Par contre, les éléments du film qui interviennent dans l'élaboration du manteau acide de la peau ne jouent un rôle que dans une seule direction: la neutralisation de l'alcalinité en excès et c'est très probablement la raison pour laquelle la peau est mieux armée pour atténuer les réactions alcalinisantes que celles acidifiantes.

Diverses méthodes, toutes criticables, étudient le pouvoir tampon de la surface des téguments: 1. Variation du pH d'une solution titrée appliquée sur les téguments. 2. Appréciation (plutôt que mesure) d'un nombre de gouttes d'une solution alcaline nécessaires pour faire varier le pH local, ou apparaître une réaction érythémateuse d'alcalinocivité. 3. Mesure titrimétrique de la quantité d'une solution N/500 à N/1000 de soude ou d'acide chlorhydrique consommée par une surface cutanée connue pendant un laps de temps déterminé. C'est cette méthode que j'ai personnellement employée.

En fait, quelque soit la méthode, les résultats sont qualitativement convergents s'ils peuvent être quantitativement moins sûrs: 1. Les téguments sont mieux armés contre l'alcalinisation que contre l'acidification. 2. Normaux, ils rétablissent le pH initial après application d'une solution alcaline faible. 3. A l'état pathologique, ils tendent à perdre ce pouvoir spécialement au cours des dermatoses professionnelles. Il est possible, probablement mais non en toute certitude, dans un lot d'ouvriers encore normaux au moment de l'examen de prévoir d'avance ceux qui sont les plus aptes à présenter dans la suite une dermite: ce sont ceux qui résistent le moins à l'agression alcaline. 4. Nos recherches personnelles ont démontré que le nourrisson et le jeune enfant ont des téguments dont le pouvoir tampon est très faible: ce qui est à rapprocher de la grande fragilité de leur peau.

Free Communications

Studies of Some Glycolityc Pathways in the Skin of Rats Under Experimental Conditions*

G. Rabbiosi and A. Giannetti, University of Pavia, Dermatological Clinic, Pavia (Italy)

Considerable accumulation of data indicates that the carbohydrates in the epidermis may decompose along different pathways *in vitro*. The presence of enzymes of the Embden-Meyerhof cycle, of the Krebs cycle, and of the pentose

* Supported in part by C.N.R. (contract N. 115/633/461).

shunt has been histochemically and biochemically demonstrated. Moreover, investigations with glucose 1-C^{14} and glucose 6-C^{14} and with the respiratory activity of the skin support this view. However, adequate evidence of the activity of the various known metabolic pathways of carbohydrates in the epidermis *in vivo* is lacking.

The present study was undertaken to determine the glycogen, glucose, lactate and pyruvate values of the skin of rats under the following experimental conditions: 1. intravenous injection of glucose, 2. intravenous injection of insulin, 3. high carbohydrate diet, 4. starvation.

We emphasized the importance of the lactate to pyruvate ratio in order to assign quantitative dimensions to the glycolysis and the citric acid cycle in the skin *in vivo*. According to W. E. HUCKABEE (J. Clin. Invest. 37, 255, 1958) the excess lactate was used as an index of the extent of anaerobic metabolism. To our knowledge, this is not only the first application of this ratio to the study of the intermediate metabolism of the carbohydrates of the skin, but also the first utilization of enzymatic methods for the pyruvate and lactate of the skin.

The purposes of this report are: first, to demonstrate that both anaerobic glycolysis and cytric acid cycle operate in the skin. Secondly, to investigate whether anaerobic glycolysis is the predominant pathway in the skin in basic conditions equally as *in vivo* as *in vitro*. Finally, to investigate which glycolytic pathway is predominant under the influence of the different well known humoral and hormonal conditions.

Methods

77 rats of the Sprague Dawley strain weighing approximately 220 g were used. They were divided into five groups. A group of 15 rats was used to determine the basic values in the skin and in the blood. A second group was treated with a single intravenous injection of glucose (1 cc. sol. 33% per kg body weight). A third group of 15 rats was treated with a single intravenous injection of insulin (20 U. per kg). Another group of 17 rats was placed on a high carbohydrate diet for 20 days. The diet was composed as following: glucose 42%; saccarose 42%; casein 5%; hydrogenated oil 5%; cod liver oil 1%; dry leaven 1%; salts; vitamins. Finally, 15 rats were placed on starvation for 5 days. After a manual depilation of the anterior abdomen wall a specimen of skin (average weight 500 mg) was excised and homogenized. Lactate, pyruvate glucose and glycogen values were determined on the supernatant following the methods described in a previous report [G. RABBIOSI and A. GIANNETTI: Minerva derm. Atti S.I.D.E.S. 40, Suppl. 8, 424 (1965)].

Results

After intravenous injection of glucose (1 cc solut. 33% per kg body weight), no substantial change in the amount of glycogen in the skin was found. Lactate increases in a constant progressive rate, while glucose rises rapidly, reaching its maximum in half an hour. Pyruvate, after an increase at 15 min decreases slightly at 30 min (Fig. 1).

The level of glucose of the skin of rats decreases progressively after insulin injection but the value of cutaneous glycogen is not effected. There is an initial slight, non significant rise of the lactate after 15 min and interestingly a sharp and progressive decrease of the pyruvate level (Fig. 2).

A substantial increase in the glycogen, glucose and lactate content of the skin of rats on a high carbohydrate diet was found. However, there is no consistent increase in the cutaneous pyruvate of the skin (Tab. 1).

In rats starved for 5 days there was a significant decrease in the amounts of cutaneous glycogen, glucose and lactate; in addition the most outstanding result is the decrease in the level of the cutaneous pyruvate (Tab. 2).

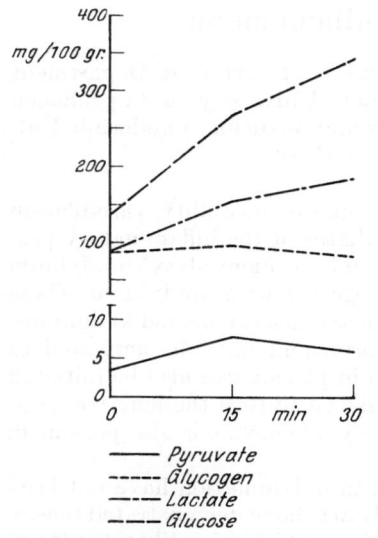

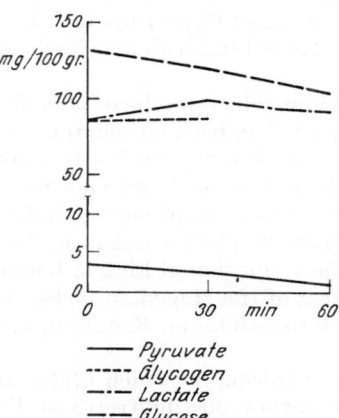

Fig. 1. Effect of intravenous injection of glucose (1 cc sol. 33% per kg body weight)

Fig. 2. Effect of intravenous injection of insulin (20 u. per kg body weight)

Table 1. *Effects of an High Carbohydrate diet on the Cutaneous Glycogen. Glucose, Lactate, Pyruvate Amounts in 17 Rats*

	Standard Diet	High Carbohydrate Diet
Glycogen	87,4	120,3
Glucose	132,9	165,0
Lactate	87,5	130,89
Pyruvate	3,6	4,2

The values are expressed in mg/100 g of fresh tissue.

Table 2. *Effects of Starvation on the Cutaneous Glycogen, Glucose, Lactate and Pyruvate Amounts in 15 Rats*

	Standard Diet	Starvation
Glycogen	87,4	65,4 (— 25%)
Glucose	132,9	45,2 (— 66%)
Lactate	87,5	49,5 (— 43%)
Pyruvate	3,6	2,8 (— 22%)

The values are expressed in mg/100 g of fresh tissue.

Conclusions

A careful analysis of the above results, was made in order to investigate the glycolytic pathways that the skin utilizes in each condition. The results of the analysis emphasized the importance of the behaviour of the lactate to pyruvate ratio. It shows that: 1. the skin may catabolyze the glucose both through the Embden-Meyerof cycle and the Krebs cycle; 2. under some conditions (i.e. induced hyperglycemia, high carbohydrate diet) anaerobic glycolysis is the predominant catabolic pathway in the skin; under other conditions (induced hyperinsulinemia) the Krebs cycle is utilized. It is suggested that the skin may take either route according to the particular hormonal and humoral condition present (i.e. the rate of glucose that is to be metabolized, the level of insulin, the need of energy ecc.).

Plasma Kinin Formation and Human Inflammation

H. Zachariae, J. Malmquist, J. A. Oates and W. Pettinger, Department
of Skin- and Venereal Diseases, Rigshospitalet, University of Copenhagen
(Denmark), and Departments of Pharmacology and Medicine, Vanderbilt University, School of Medicine, Nashville, Tennessee (USA)

Bradykinin, which produces pain, increased vascular permeability, vasodilation and leukotaxis has been considered a possible mediator of the inflammatory process. Two other kinin peptides, lysyl-bradykinin and methionyl-lysyl-bradykinin have also been identified and may be considered together with bradykinin. These peptides are split from plasma globulins by peptidases, usually named kallikreins. The kallikrein in plasma exists in an inactive form, and must be activated to catalyze the formation of kinins. Kinin formation in plasma can also be initiated by activation of the Hageman factor, which is believed to turn the inactive kallikreinogen into kallikrein. Kininase, or kinin destroying enzyme is also present in plasma.

The mechanisms by which kinins are released in inflammation have not been elucidated. Several possibilities exist. Edery and Lewis have demonstrated release of kinin forming enzyme into lymph after histamine, a histamine liberator (compound 48/80) or various forms of tissue injury. In initial studies we investigated if histamine, serotonin, niacin or endotoxin activated human plasma kallikrein.

The activating agents were incubated with 1.5 ml human plasma and 0.2 ml of Ca-EDTA-solution, acting as a kininase inhibitor, at 37 °C for 15 min. The incubations were stopped by adding three volumes of boiling absolute alcohol. The preparations were evaporated to dryness, taken up in saline and assayed on the estrus rat uterus for kinin activity. No direct activation of plasma kallikrein was demonstrated in this plasma system, which showed marked activation on addition of Celite, a diatomaceous silica product, which activates Hageman factor, acting in the same manner as glass.

So we assumed, therefore, that these inflammatory mediators rather than activating plasma kallikrein directly, create changes in vascular permeability, which permit plasma to enter the extravascular space, where conditions for activation could exist. Accordingly the following investigation was carried out to determine if kinins are formed, when plasma enters subcutaneous space.

Samples of 1 to 2 ml autologous human plasma was injected into human subcutaneous tissue. The injections were performed with siliconized syringes and siliconized hypodermic needles. The plasma was left in the tissue for exactly 5 min, and then withdrawn through the same needles by negative pressure maintained from the syringes and gentle massage of the tissue. The recovered fluid was assayed for kinin activity.

Fig. 1 shows that in all cases kinin was formed, when plasma was injected, while no kinins were formed, when physiological saline was injected as a control, or when the same amount of plasma was incubated *in vitro* for 5 min at 37 °C. A slightly acid pH favors the accumulation of kinins in the subcutaneous space. When buffered plasma (pH 6.3) with a plasma buffer ratio of five to two was injected, it was shown (Fig. 1) that approximately 10 times as much kinin was formed. Also here little or no kinin was produced by injections of saline and buffer into the subcutaneous tissue or by incubating buffered plasma (pH 6.3) *in vitro*. A slightly acid pH decreases kininase activity. This decrease may account for the increased accumulation of kinins.

Human plasma is not the only plasma, which may form kinins by injection into the subcutaneous space. The result of injections of buffered homologous rat, dog and guinea-pig plasma was also investigated. On the table you will note that in all cases kinins were formed, although less than in the human experiment.

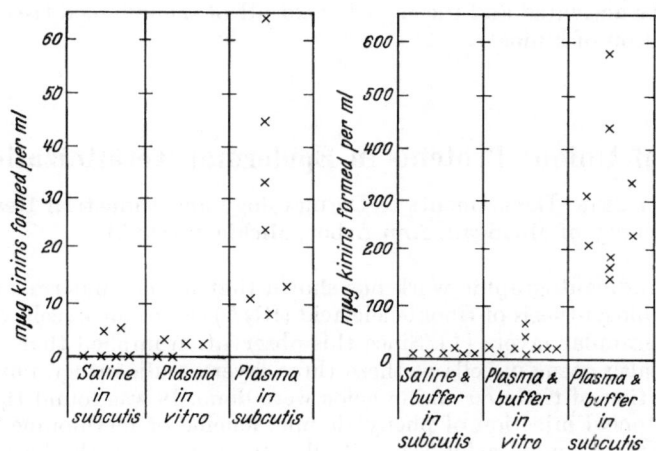

Fig. 1

Table. *Average amounts of kinins withdrawn from subcutaneous tissues of various species 5 min after injections of 0.5 to 1.5 ml of homologous buffered plasma (pH 6.3) or saline and 0.5 m phosphate buffer pH 6.3. Plasma: buffer volume ratio = 5:2*

Species	No. of Experiments	$m\mu g$ Klinins per ml $\pm$ S.E.	
		Buffered Plasma	Buffer and Saline
Man[a]	9	285 ± 16	1.3 ± 1.2
Rat	7	146 ± 10	2.1 ± 1.1
Dog	7	39 ± 6	2.6 ± 2.6
Guinea-Pig	4	32 ± 8	0 ± 0

[a] In man, autologous plasma and 0.25 M phosphate buffer.

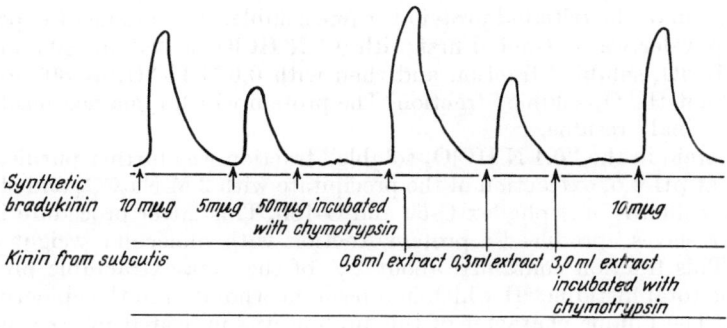

Fig. 2

Fig. 2 shows that kinin from human subcutis was completely inactivated by chymotrypsin and that the type of contraction induced by kinin from subcutis on the estrus rat uterus was similar to that induced by synthetic bradykinin.

In summary, our data show that histamine, serotonin, nicotinic acid and endo-toxin do not directly activate plasma kallikrein. The results of our study suggest that in inflammation, mechanical injury or primary mediators, such as histamine may permit the plasma protein to enter the tissues. In the extravascular space plasma may be activated and the slightly acid pH of the inflamed tissue will favor the accumulation of kinins.

Synthesis of Unique Proteins in Epidermal Keratinization

I. A. BERNSTEIN, Departments of Dermatology and Industrial Health,
The University of Michigan, Ann Arbor, Michigan (USA)

Previous radioautographic work has shown that in the epidermis of the new-born rat, the biosynthesis of ribonucleic acid (RNA) can occur in cells of the basal, spinous and granular layers [1]. Since this observation implied that protein synthesis might also occur in cells of these three layers, radioautographic studies of the incorporation of tritiated amino acids were done. It was found that 1 h after the intraperitoneal injection of phenylalanine, leucine or methionine to newborn rats, each of these amino acids was initially incorporated in the basal and lower spinous layers of the epidermis, whereas, tritiated histidine, as well as glycine, first appeared mainly in the granular and upper spinous layers [2]. One possible explanation for this differential initial localization of labeled histidine and glycine, is the synthesis in the upper viable cellular layers of protein containing an unusually high level of these two amino acids and little or none of the other three. To test this hypothesis, an attempt was made to isolate epidermal protein which contained a major portion of the epidermal tritium 1 h after the intraperitoneal injection of tritiated histidine [3].

Epidermis, separated from dermis by treatment with 0.24 M NH_4Cl, pH 9.5 at 0° for 15 min, was homogenized in 8 M urea-0.2 M Tris, pH 8.5. The urea-extract, treated with ribonuclease to degrade RNA, was dialyzed against dilute NH_4OH and the dialyzed solution, containing the extracted protein, was dried *in vacuo*. In preliminary experiments, this dried powder was extracted with dilute $HClO_4$ to remove any residual nucleic acids from the insoluble protein. Surprisingly, a large portion of the tritiated protein became soluble. In subsequent experiments, the dried powder was extracted first with 0.1 N $HClO_4$ at 24° for 30 min to yield a "0.1 N $HClO_4$-soluble" fraction and then with 0.6 N $HClO_4$ at 80° for 30 min to give a "hot-$HClO_4$-soluble" fraction. The protein which remained insoluble was called the "final" residue.

The protein in the "0.1 N $HClO_4$-soluble" fraction was further purified by precipitation at pH 4.5, extraction of the precipitate with 2 M Na_2CO_3 and chromatography on columns of Sephadex G-50 and G-100. This latter procedure involving "molecular sieves" produced a protein fraction with molecular weight of about 3×10^4. This fraction contained about 2% of the urea-extractable protein and 28% of the total histidine-^{3}H which had been incorporated in the epidermis in the first hour. The unique character of this protein was indicated by its solubility in dilute $HClO_4$ and by its amino acid composition (table). There was an 8-fold greater concentration of histidine in the "0.1 N $HClO_4$-soluble" fraction than in the "final" residue. Of the nine amino acids present, seven had reactive groups on their side chains. Phenylalanine, leucine and methionine were not included. Cysteine-residues were absent.

Table: *Amino Acid Composition (in amino acid residues/100 residues) of Three Protein Fractions*

Amino acid	0.1 N HClO$_4$-soluble[b]	Hot-HClO$_4$-soluble[c]	Final residue[c]
Glutamic acid	14.1	11.6	12.4
Serine	11.5	19.2	7.2
Glycine	15.3	33.8	15.6
Arginine	9.0	6.9	4.3
Alanine	11.8	5.9	7.3
Tyrosine	9.4	2.7	3.7
Histidine	6.9	3.2	0.8
Threonine	6.8	3.8	5.4
Aspartic acid	5.6	3.9	8.6
Lysine	a	2.1	3.7
Leucine	a	1.0	8.1
Isoleucine	a	1.0	4.3
Phenylalanine	a	1.7	2.7
Proline	a	a	1.4
Valine	a	1.7	6.3
1/2 Cystine	a	a	0.5
Methionine	a	a	1.4
(NH$_3$)	(6.8)	—	(11.0)

a not detected; b CHAKRABARTI and BERNSTEIN [4]; c HOOBER and BERNSTEIN [3].

The "hot-HClO$_4$-soluble" fraction, after chromatography on Sephadex G-50, also had an unusual amino acid composition (table). One-third of the residues were glycine. Serine, glutamic acid and glycine, together, constituted 64% of the protein. Because of the technique employed in the isolation, its molecular weight was considerably smaller than that of the "0.1 N HClO$_4$-soluble" fraction. The "hot-HClO$_4$-soluble" fraction also had no cysteine-residues.

Support for the concept that the "0.1 N HClO$_4$-soluble" protein was responsible for the initial localization of histidine-^{3}H in the upper viable cellular layers as seen by radioautography, has been provided by the successful recovery of this protein from the isolated granular layer [5]. Also, more recent radioautographic studies [6] have shown that serine and arginine were initially more highly localized in the granular layer, whereas, valine and lysine initially labeled the basal and lower spinous layers.

It seems likely that the "histidine-rich" protein is a subunit of a larger protein *in situ* [4]. Prior to treatment with HClO$_4$, the protein labeled with histidine-^{3}H had a molecular weight of about 2×10^5-approximately 6-times greater than that of the "0.1 N HClO$_4$-soluble" protein.

Although the function of these unusual proteins are at present unknown, their localization in the epidermal granular layer and their content of polar amino acids suggest that they play a vital role in keratinization-perhaps, in the organization of the keratin fibers.

Bibliography. 1. FUKUYAMA, K., and I. A. BERNSTEIN: J. invest. Derm. 41, 47 (1963). — 2. FUKUYAMA, K., T. NAKAMURA, and I. A. BERNSTEIN: Anat. Rec. 152, 525 (1965). — 3. HOOBER, J. K., and I. A. BERNSTEIN: Proc. nat. Acad. Sci. (Wash.) 56, 594 (1966). — 4. CHAKRABARTI, S., and I. A. BERNSTEIN: Fed. Proc. 26, 369 (1967). — 5. GUMUCIO, J., C. FELDKAMP, and I. A. BERNSTEIN: J. invest. Derm. 49, 545 (1967). — 6. FUKUYAMA, K., and W. L. EPSTEIN: J. invest. Derm. 47, 551 (1966).

Mechanism of Water Binding in Stratum Corneum

J. D. MIDDLETON, Unilever Research Laboratory, Colworth House, Sharnbrook Bedford (England)

When human callus is extracted with polar organic solvents followed by water, BLANK (1953) showed that the amount of water which the corneum can hold in a humid atmosphere is reduced. Neither solvent nor water alone has this effect. Very little material is extracted from callus by solvent or water alone but after solvent and water treatments considerable quantities of water soluble substances can be extracted. The properties of these water soluble substances have been reviewed by JACOBI (1959). They are hygroscopic and have been held responsible for the water binding properties of corneum.

The most probable action of organic solvents on callus is to remove lipid and it has been suggested (BLANK, 1953) that the water soluble substances are protected from dissolution by a coating of lipid. We undertook the work reported here in an attempt to discover how the lipids were protecting the water soluble substances and to gain a greater understanding of the mechanism of water binding in stratum corneum.

In most of our work we have used corneum from the footpads of guinea pigs. This was separated by incubating the skin in trypsin and urea. Water binding capacity was measured by comparing the dry weight with the weight after equilibration in an atmosphere of constant relative humidity. The more important results were confirmed on human callus.

Tab. 1 shows the effect of extracting with solvents and water on the water binding capacity of guinea pig footpad corneum.

Table 1. *Effect of solvent and water extractions on water binding of guinea pig footpad corneum*
Water bound at 93% R.H. (mg/100 mg dry wt corneum)

	solvent + water	water control
ether	28.9	42.2
n-hexane	23.8	43.6
tetrahydrofuran	19.3	43.6
chloroform/methanol (2:1 v/v)	26.8	43.8

In each case solvent and water extraction significantly reduced water binding. This suggests that the water binding properties of guinea pig footpad are similar to those of the human callus investigated by BLANK (1953) and to the newborn rat and guinea pig back skin corneum studied by SINGER and VINSON (1966).

Examination by thin layer chromatography of the lipids extracted from guinea pig footpad corneum by ether showed that the major lipids are cholesterol and phospholipid. These are the normal constituents of cell membranes (NICOLAIDES, 1964). Our hypothesis is that the lipids of the corneum cell membranes protect the water soluble substances from dissolution in water. According to this hypothesis the water soluble substances are intra-cellular and the cell membranes are permeable to water but not to the water-soluble substances so that water is held within the corneum cells by the process of osmosis.

In order to see whether corneum can take up and lose water by osmosis pieces of guinea pig footpad corneum were equilibrated in 2% sodium chloride solution, weighed, and transferred to salt solutions of different concentrations. After a further period of equilibration the weight changes were recorded. The whole experiment was repeated on corneum which had been extracted with chloroform/methanol to remove lipids. Tab. 2 shows the results.

Table 2. *Per cent weight changes of corneum transferred from 2% NaCl to different NaCl concentrations*

		Treatment	
NaCl conc^n (% w/v)	untreated	chloroform/methanol extraction	
0	+ 27	− 14	
1	+ 13	+ 3	
2	− 4	+ 8	
5	− 25	+ 10	
10	− 37	+ 11	

Intact corneum gained weight on transferring to more dilute solutions and lost weight in more concentrated solutions. This is to be expected from the laws of osmosis. After removal of lipid with chloroform/methanol these changes did not occur and the changes that were observed could be accounted for by the different densities of the salt solutions permeating the corneum. The removal of lipid by chloroform/methanol allowed the escape of the water-soluble substances into the salt solution so that the corneum no longer responded to changes in the osmotic pressure of the surrounding solution.

Tab. 3 shows the weight changes which occurred when pieces of full thickness corneum from the human palm and sole were transferred from 2 to 10% sodium chloride solution.

Table 3. *Per cent weight changes of human callus transferred from 2% to 10% NaCl solution*

	untreated	chloroform/methanol extracted
sole (female)	− 43.6	+ 4.3
palm (female)	− 50.3	+ 1.9
sole (male)	− 49.5	+ 5.4
palm (male)	− 54.0	+ 7.6

The human material behaves in the same way as guinea pig corneum and loses water to more concentrated salt solution. Extraction with chloroform/methanol prevents this.

Further evidence that it is the corneum cell membrane lipids which retain the water-soluble substances comes from the following experiment. When guinea pig footpad corneum is ground in liquid nitrogen a fine powder can be obtained. Examination of this powder under the electron microscope shows that the cellular structure has been completely broken compared to the normal structure seen in sections of untreated stratum corneum. We compared the effects of extracting with water and with ether followed by water on the water binding capacity of this powder and of intact corneum. Small pieces of corneum about 1 to 2 mm across were also included in this experiment to expose as large a surface area as possible without breaking too many cells so that the effects of any lipid layer on the natural surface of the corneum could be investigated. Tab. 4 shows the results.

Table 4. *Effect of solvent and water extractions on the water binding capacity of powdered and intact corneum*

Treatment	water bound at 90% R.H. (mg/100 mg dry wt corneum)		
	intact corneum	small pieces	powdered corneum
none	40.8	—	—
liquid nitrogen	40.2	40.3	43.2
liquid nitrogen and water extraction	42.9	37.4	24.4
liquid nitrogen and ether and water extractions	26.3	23.6	24.2

The data show that dipping in liquid nitrogen did not affect the water binding of intact corneum. As expected extractions with solvent and water significantly reduced the water binding of all three groups of corneum. The effect of water alone was not significant either on intact corneum or on the small pieces, and suggests that a surface lipid layer is not involved. Breaking the cell structure by powdering in liquid nitrogen resulted in water extraction alone reducing water binding capacity to the same extent as extractions with ether and water.

In a separate experiment we measured the quantity of water-soluble substances escaping from the corneum during water extraction by measuring extracted amino acids with the ninhydrin method. Water extracted more than ten times as much water soluble material from the powdered corneum as from intact corneum.

These experiments indicate that powdering the corneum has the same effect as solvent extraction in that the water-soluble substances become accessible to water extraction. This suggests that the lipids which prevent the dissolution of the water soluble substances and which are removed by solvents, are present in the cell membranes.

In summary, the water-soluble substances of the corneum hold water by a process of osmosis. For their activity they depend upon the presence of a surrounding lipid-containing membrane. Evidence has been put forward to suggest that this membrane is the cell membrane of the corneum cells.

References. BLANK, I. H.: J. invest. Derm. **21**, 259 (1953). — JACOBI, O. K.: Proc. Sci. Sect. Toilet Goods Ass. **31**, 22 (1959). — NICOLAIDES, N.: Lipids, membranes and the human epidermis. Chapter in: The Epidermis, p. 511. New York: Academic Press 1964. — SINGER, E. J., and L. J. VINSON: Proc. Sci. Sect. Toilet Goods Ass. **46**, 29 (1966).

Studies on the Epidermal Keratinization of the Human Fetus in vitro with Special References to the Electron Microscopic and Autoradiographic Observation

K. OKAMURA, K. IWASHITA and K. UEDA, Department of Dermatology, Kyoto Prefectural University of Medicine, Kyoto (Japan)

The organ culture of the isolated fragment from embryonic skin is the very helpful experimental method to understand various mechanisms of development of the skin such as proliferation and differentiation of the epidermal cells. Electron microscopic and autoradiographic studies were done on the epidermal keratinization in vitro of human fetus.

The skin fragments from thigh of the human fetus at the age of 3 months were cultivated by Leighton's sponge matrix method using roller tube with nutrient composed of Eagle's minimal essential medium, cow serum and chick embryonic extract. For electron microscopic study, cultured specimen was fixed in 2% OsO_4, dehydrated by alcohol, embeded in epon and cut by Porter Blum's microtom. The sections were stained by uranyl acetate and examined under the Hitachi electron microscope, model HS-7. For microautographic study (stripping-film method), specimens were incubated in 1 ml of Eagle's medium with 1 μC ^{3}H-thymidine for 2 h, and 20 to 50 μC ^{3}H-amino acids and 5 μC ^{35}S-cystine for 3 h. The labeling index of ^{3}H-thymidine was calculated by following formula: number of labeled cells / total number of cells able to proliferate $\times$ 100.

On the 5 or 6th day of cultivation, the keratinization first appeared light microscopically as a bandlike zone reactive to sulfhydral and disulfide between the periderm and the intermediate layer.

Electron microscopic study of the specimen on the 8 or 9th day of cultivation revealed germinative cells to have large nucleus with abundant mitochondria, endoplasmic reticulum and ribosome. In the deeper layer of stratum spinosum endoplasmic reticulum, mitochondria and ribosomes were also observed, but they were not so abundant as in the germinative layer. The microvilli were clearly recognized. The desmosome with attached tonofilament was observed in some cells. Tonofibrils were occasionally noted. In the upper layer tonofibrils were arranged in bundles or speckled pattern. Both nuclei and nucleoli were rather large. Over this area the spindle-shaped cells seldom had nucleus but tonofibril and fusiformed keratohyalin granules were noted in the cytoplasma. In the zone of the flat cells the nuclei were deformed or absent. The tonofilaments were thick and vesicles were scattered between filaments. In some areas of the same zone the tonofilaments were rather scarce and scanty microvilli were preserved between the cells. In the peridermal layer nucleoplasm was concentrated. There was no organelle in the cytoplasm. The cell wall was not visible in some areas and degenerated.

On the 8 to 9th day of cultivation, glycogen accumulated through the entire epidermal layer prior to the culture, reduced dramatically leaving only traces in the lower layer. Thus, in the 11th day explant, the bandlike zone that will be refered to as a cornified layer, thickened conspicuously showing parakeratosis.

Under the autoradiography, labeling from ^{3}H-thymidine was observed in the epidermal cells of the lowest two to four layers during the culture period of 3 to 8 days, and its labeling index showed the maximum on the 2nd to 3rd day (about 60%), followed by rapid decrease. The life-span of epidermal cells traced in the 3rd day explant was approximately 4 to 5 days. As to incorporation from ^{3}H-amino acids in the 5th day explant, glycine, methionine and tyrosine were mainly noted over the upper layer, and valine as well as leucine over the entire layer of the epidermis except the periderm and flat layer after 1 to 3 h incubation. Moreover, RNA synthesis examined using ^{3}H-uridine occurred in the viable cells of the entire epidermal layer in the 5th explant, and ^{35}-S-cystine labeled most heavily the uppermost epidermal layer except the periderm.

It may be concluded from the findings that the keratinization process of the epidermis cultured here was not the same as that of normal epidermis in vivo, but rather resembled that of parakeratotic epidermis in vivo, and indicated an active evidence of the progressive differentiation to cornification as PELC and FELL observed previously in the explant of embryonic chicken skin.

The Envelope of Epidermal Horny Cells*

A. G. Matoltsy, Department of Dermatology, Boston University School of Medicine, Boston, Mass. (USA)

The stratum corneum of the epidermis is in direct contact with the environment and is the primary protective cover of the organism. This layer of the skin consists of hardened horny cells which interdigitate at several points. In the electron microscope the horny cells can be seen to be enveloped by a thick (150 A)

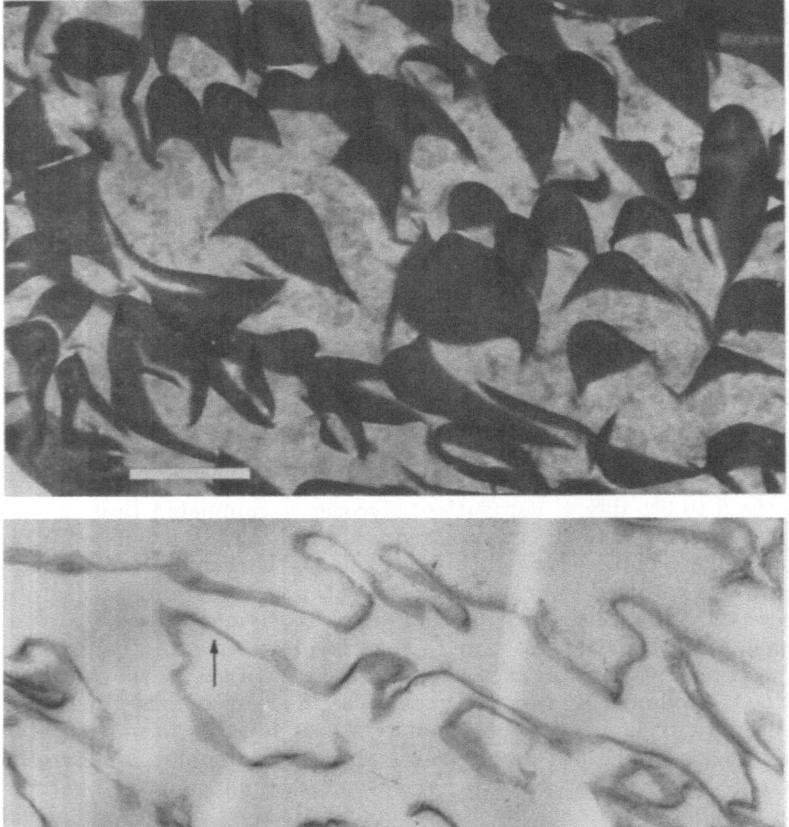

and folded membrane and to be filled with numerous filaments and an amorphous matrix [1, 2, 3]. The content of the horny cell (keratin) has been extensively studied and is commonly regarded as the main protective substance of the skin. The horny cell envelope so far has received little attention and generally is not considered as a part of the protective system. In order to learn more about the function of epidermal horny cell envelopes, we isolated them and studied their structure and composition. Our results are presented here briefly as follows:

* This work was supported by research grants AM 05924 and AM 05779 National Institute of Arthritis and Metabolic Diseases, United States Public Health Service.

Pure preparations of horny cell envelopes were obtained from both human epidermis and the epidermis of the cow's nose by our previously published technic [3]. This technic consists of repeated extraction of tissues with 0.1 N sodium hydroxide solutions and collection of the resistant material by centrifugation at 600 RPM. In the figure electron micrographs of epidermal horny cell envelopes are shown obtained by this isolation method. The upper picture shows an envelope fragment which was spread on the surface of a carbon coated grid and subsequently stained with PTA. The lower one shows a thin section of a pellet which was embedded into oxy resin and the section stained with lead hydroxide. Spread envelope fragments, as shown in the upper picture, appear as thin sheets with numerous finger-like projections lying flat over smooth parts of the envelope. The finger-like projections appear dark on the electron micrograph because in these regions the projecting portion of the envelope is superimposed upon the smooth portion and the specimen is much thicker. These envelope projections correspond to the interdigitations of horny cells seen in vivo. In thin sections, such as shown in the lower picture, finger-like projections as well as smooth portions of the horny cell envelope can be seen. In these preparations the envelope fragments appear twisted which is related to the direction of sectioning. Regions of the membrane cut at right angles (arrow) appear narrow and dense whereas regions cut at oblique angles appear wider and less dense. These findings thus show that the horny cell envelope is not a smooth membrane but a characteristically folded one. It is remarkable that the envelopes resemble their original structure after isolation; this fact alone is indicative that they consist of highly consolidated material having a high degree of physical strength and chemical resistance.

Chemical analyses showed that the envelopes consist of about two-thirds protein, and one-third lipid. A small amount of carbohydrate (1.4%) was also found to be present. Amino acid analyses of the protein component revealed that it contains proline (7.7 to 12.9%) and cystine (4.6 to 7.3%) in relatively large proportions [4]. The large amount of proline is incompatible with alpha-helical structure suggesting that the envelope protein is amorphous in nature. The large amount of cytine on the other hand indicates that it is well stabilized by disulfide bonds. The chemical resistance of the horny cell envelope, however, can not be fully explained by attributing it to -S-S- linkages because it resists the action of many reagents which split these bonds. We found that isolated envelopes resist the action of reducing and oxidizing agents such as sodium sulfide, thioglycolic acid and peracetic acid. We also noted that they are not digestible with trypsin or pronase.

The structural and chemical properties of the envelope which have been described indicate that this cell constituent has the highest degree of stabilization among the components of the horny cell. In view of this it seems appropriate to broaden our concept of the protective system of the organism and in addition to keratin to consider the envelope of the horny cell as part of the protective system.

References. 1. BRODY. I. J.: Ultrastruct. Res. **2**, 482 (1959). — 2. RHODIN, J. A. G., and E. J. REITH: In: Fundamentals of Keratinization. Washington: D. C. A.A.A.S. Publ. 70, 61 (1962). — 3. MATOLTSY, A. G., and P. F. PARAKKAL: J. Cell. Biol. **24**, 297 (1965). — 4. MATOLTSY, A. G., and M. N. MATOLTSY: J. Invest. Derm. **46**, 127 (1966).

Follicular Hyperkeratinization Induced in the Rabbit Ear by Human Skin Surface Lipids*

A. L. Lorincz, H. Krizek and S. Brown, Department of Medicine of the
University, Section of Dermatology, Chicago, Illinois (USA)

A characteristic, very early feature of the lesions of both acne vulgaris and
chloracne is hyperkeratinization of the sebaceous glandular duct and upper
follicular canal which leads to comedo formation [1]. Because chloracnegenic
chemicals applied to the inner surface of the rabbit ear can induce striking follicular
hyperkeratosis in its sebaceous follicles [2, 3, 4], we investigated the application
to this structure of human skin surface lipids and various fractions derived from
them for similar effects.

Skin surface lipids were obtained from young, adult male volunteers by
immersion of the scalp in a bowl of solvent [5] consisting of one volume of 95%
ethanol per three volumes of ether. Precautions were taken to avoid contamination
by hair grooming materials. Insoluble materials such as scales, hairs, etc. were first
removed by filtration and then solvent was removed partially by distillation and
finally by vacuum in a rotary evaporator. Lipid residues were pooled by transfer
with hexane and a little methanol. Control tests using the same kinds and amounts
of solvents and procedures were done with a simulated lipid specimen consisting
of 250 mgms of a tripalmitin petrolatum mixture in 1800 mls of solvent mixture to
demonstrate that the effects observed were not caused by possible trace impurities
in the solvents.

Tests were carried out with the whole scalp surface lipids as well as with the
following fractions derived from it: neutral fats [6], unsaponifiable matter [7],
and free fatty acids [6]. The materials were dissolved in acetone containing 10% of
95% ethanol and a number of one-ml volumes were applied on regulated schedules
to the inner surfaces of one epilated ear of adult male albino rabbits over periods
of 1 to 2 weeks. As controls, solvent alone or solution of simulated lipid was similarly applied to the other epilated ear of each animal. Total amounts ranging
between 250 to 1900 mgms of whole surface lipid were applied per animal in
various experiments. The various lipid fractions tested were applied in total
amounts calculated to be equivalent to the fraction they represented in the whole
lipid.

Activity in promoting follicular hyperkeratosis was judged from the stereomicroscopic appearance of the keratinous follicular casts observed on the under-
side of keratin disc preparations obtained from 20 mm punch biopsy specimens
taken from the base of the inner side of the ear [8]. The biopsy specimens were
first carefully digested in 0.1% pepsin and 0.012 N hydrochloric acid in physiologic
saline for about four hours to remove all except the keratinized portions of each
specimen. The keratin discs were then further processed, dehydrated and defatted
sequentially with saline, 1:1 ethanol-ether, and ether. In discs prepared from
control and untreated ears, follicular casts appeared as little more than small
nubs while in specimens showing follicular hyperkeratosis the follicular casts
were much enlarged and showed branch-like extensions into the ducts of the multi-
lobulated sebaceous glands.

Applications of whole scalp surface lipid and of its neutral fat, unsaponifiable
and free fatty acid fractions were capable of inducing follicular hyperkeratosis
in the rabbit ear. About 250 mgms of whole lipid represented the least amount

* This work was supported by U.S. Army Contract No. DA-49-193-MD-2341.

applied to one ear which produced a readily detectable response under the conditions of these experiments while amounts of unsaponifiables equivalent to six to
eight times this amount of whole lipid produced comparable effects. With the free
fatty acid fraction, amounts equivalent to 450 mgms of whole lipid were similarly
active. The keratogenic effect of the neutral fat derived from 300 mgms of whole
lipid was clearly less than that of this amount of the whole lipid. It was also noted
that the follicular hyperkeratosis evoked by the neutral fat fraction was accompanied by very little erythema in contrast to the results with the other fractions,
especially the free fatty acids.

Several individual fatty acids were also comparably tested. Oleic acid was
more active than palmitic acid and had minimally detectable effect at a dose
of approximately 70 mgms per rabbit ear. Linoleic and isostearic acid had about
the same follicular keratogenic activity whereas capric acid was distinctly less
active.

Although human skin surface lipid components and especially free fatty acids
were shown in these experiments to have follicular keratinization promoting
effects, much further work remains to be done before the possible significance of
these observations to the problem of the pathogenesis of acne can be determined.

References. 1. van Scott, E. J., and R. C. MacCardle: J. invest. Derm. 27, 405 (1956). —
2. Adams, E. M., D. D. Irish, H. C. Spencer, and J. K. Rowe: Indian Med. J. Hyg. Sect.
2, 1 (1941). — 3. Hofmann, H. T., and W. Neumann: Zbl. Arbeitsmed. 2, 169 (1952). —
4. Hambrick, jr., G. W.: J. invest. Derm. 28, 89 (1957). — 5. Bloom, R. E., S. Woods, and
N. Nicolaides: J. invest. Derm. 24, 97 (1955). — 6. Nicolaides, N., and R. C. Foster jr.:
J. Amer. Oil Chem. Soc. 33, 404 (1956). — 7. Cocks, L. V.: Analyst. 58, 203 (1933). — 8. Jones,
E. L., and H. Krizek: J. invest. Derm. 39, 511 (1962).

The Influence of Dimethyl Sulphoxide, Dimethyl Acetamide and Dimethyl Formamide on the Epidermal Barrier to Water

H. Baker, Institute of Dermatology, London (England)

The reasons for this study were twofold. The experiments were performed to
provide insight into the nature of the epidermal barrier and to evaluate the behaviour of these substances in the light of their potential usefulness as pharmaceutical
vehicles.

It is accepted that the stratum corneum is the principal barrier to the movement of all molecules across the epidermis. This barrier is not absolute and under
normal conditions small but measurable amounts of water are lost from the body
by trans-corneal diffusion. This loss depends mainly upon the environmental
humidity, and the skin surface temperature.

This transepidermal loss can be used as a parameter of barrier function, if
eccrine sweating is suppressed and the stratum corneum is at a constant degree of
hydration. The units in which the water lost is expressed are mg cm^{-2} hr $^{-1}$ and the
normal range for skin on the flexor aspect of the mid-forearm is 0.1 to 0.3.

Dried air or nitrogen is passed through a chamber strapped to the skin and the
humidity and temperature of the gas stream are monitored simultaneously by
sensitive electrical resistance hygrometers interposed in its pathway.

Anhidrosis was induced by the application of poldine methosulphate and the
sweat suppression checked by the starch-iodine test under thermal stress.

When the skin had been allowed to dry out in a stream of dry nitrogen the
basal reading was taken. Two ml of DMSO or other solvent under study were

then applied on lint for 30 min, removed, the skin wiped dry and dry air passed for a further 60 min. Readings were taken at intervals subsequently.

Fig. 1 shows what happened with DMSO in three subjects. All had normal basal readings. 90 min after first application the diffusive losses were respectively 8, 11 and 17 fold increased but this effect was rapidly reversed. Within $6^1/_2$ h the loss was reduced to within three-fold to four-fold normal. Subsequently it took about 2 weeks for the area to return to complete normality.

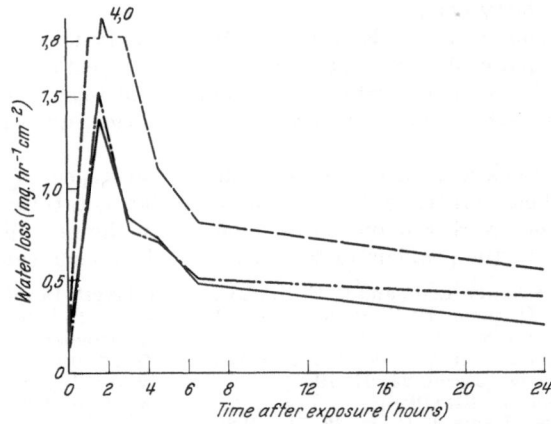

Fig. 1. Effect of dimethylsulphoxide on trans-epidermal water loss. Flexor aspect of mid-forearm, normal anhidrotic skin, three subjects

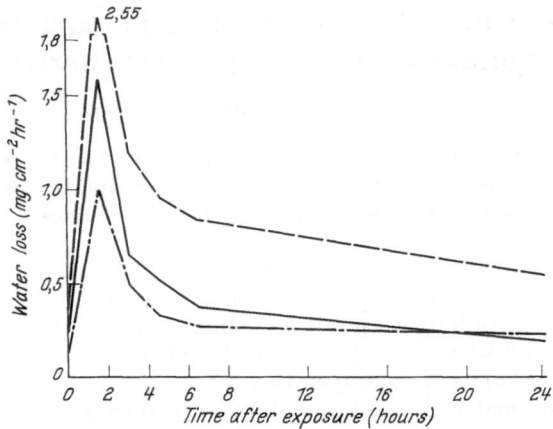

Fig. 2. Effect of dimethylformamide on trans-epidermal water loss. Flexor aspect of mid-forearm, normal anhidrotic skin, three subjects

Two other substances, dimethylformamide and dimethylacetamide have been shown to enhance percutaneous absorption and they were therefore investigated in the same way.

Dimethylformamide proved to be almost as potent as DMSO in increasing water loss but recovery was much more rapid. In two of the three subjects the skin had almost returned to normal in 24 h (Fig. 2).

Fig. 3 shows the same experiments with dimethylacetamide. It can be seen that this has a weaker effect the peak loss being increased only three-fold but restoration of barrier function is rapid and almost complete in 6 to 8 h.

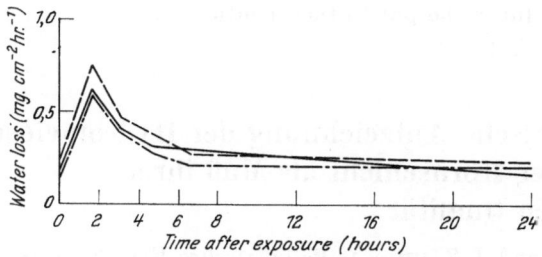

Fig. 3. Effect of dimethylacetamide on trans-epidermal water loss. Flexor aspect of mid-forearm, normal anhidrotic skin, three subjects

Table lists some of the desirable properties of a barrier suppressant. The barrier suppression should be marked but of short duration. The suppressant should be safe and not damaging to the skin.

Of the three substances studied here DMSO is the most irritant, producing whealing and erythema at high concentration. DMA is the least irritating but the weakest suppressant. Fig. 4 compares the three substances. It would appear that DMF combines high suppression with rapid recovery and, if uniformly safe, it will probable be a better vehicle than DMSO.

Table. *Ideal Properties of Barrier Suppressant*

1. High degree of suppression
2. Short Duration of suppression
3. Return of barrier function to normal
4. Not toxic if absorbed
5. Not irritant to skin
6. Good solvent

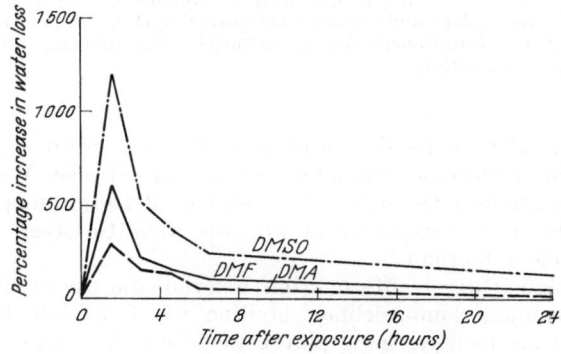

Fig. 4. Effect of DMSO, DMF and DMA on water loss expressed as percentage increases over pretreatment readings

What is the mode of action of these substances? Certainly they do not act simply by dissolving superficial lipid. Other powerful lipid solvents such as ether and acetone applied in vivo for an hour or more have no effect on diffusive water loss. DMSO, DMF and DMA are strongly hygroscopic and by holding water may greatly hydrate the stratum corneum thus enhancing penetration of various molecules including water itself.

On the basis of in-vitro experiments on mouse skin, SWEENY and colleagues have claimed that the effect of DMSO on the water barrier is irreversible. In summary, we have demonstrated that DMSO and the two related compounds DMF and DMA have a profound but reversible influence on the cutaneous barrier to water which may in the future be put to therapeutic use.

Die hygrometrische Aufzeichnung der Hydromeiose und das Abtrocknen der Hornschicht als Maß ihrer physiologischen Qualität

J. ROVENSKÝ und J. ZÁHEJSKÝ, Pädiatrisches Forschungsinstitut, Brünn, und Dermatologische Universitätsklinik, Brünn (Tschechoslowakei)

Wasser ist unter normalen Bedingungen der einzige bekannte natürliche „Plastifikator" der Hornschicht [1, 4, 5, 6]. Übermäßige Hydratation der Hornschicht führt zu physiologischer Unterdrückung der sensiblen Perspiration, also zu einem Zustand vorübergehender Hypo- bis Anidrose, welche als Hydromeiose bezeichnet wird [2, 3, 7, 8, 9, 10]. Aus dem Trocknungsablauf der hydratierten Hornschicht und aus der Erneuerung der unterdrückten Schweißaktivität können wir auf den Hydratationszustand der Hornschicht und damit auf ihre grundlegenden physiologischen Qualitäten schließen [3].

Material und Methodik

Es wurden kontinuell registrierende Widerstandshygrometer mit geringer Zeitkonstante (unter 0,5 sec) verwendet, welchen Feuchtigkeit von der Hautoberfläche durch einen Strom trockener Luft zugeführt wurde (Fläche der Abnahmekapsel 1,5 bis 3,5 cm²). Die Versuche wurden an 66 Schulkindern durchgeführt. Es wurde der Ablauf der Wasserabgabe durch Austrocknen und Schwitzen der Haut auf dem Handteller und auf dem Vorderarm unter normalen physiologischen Bedingungen und nach 30 min bis 72 Std dauernder Maceration durch destilliertes Wasser (oder Okklusivfolie) bei normaler Hauttemperatur registriert. Das Schwitzen wurde auf den Handtellern durch psychische Stimulation, auf dem Vorderarm durch thermalen Anreiz ausgelöst.

Ergebnisse

Nach dem Logarithmieren der primitiven Kurven sehen wir, daß das Abtrocknen der Hornschicht einen zweiphasigen Ablauf aufweist. Während die erste Phase einer unkonstanten Quantität des „freien" Wassers entspricht, läuft die zweite allmähliche Phase exponential ab, was den Gesetzen des einseitigen Trocknens der Folie entspricht.

Bei der Verfolgung der tranformierten Kurven, die die zweite exponentiale Phase der Abtrocknung kennzeichnen, stellten wir fest, daß die linearisierten Abschnitte von demselben Ausgangspunkt ausgehen, das heißt, daß der Grenzwert der Wasserkonzentration in der Hornschicht unabhängig von der Macerationszeit gleich ist. Nach einer länger als 24 Std dauernden Maceration beginnen die Kurven einen anomalen Verlauf zu nehmen. Der Grenzwert für die Sättigung verschiebt sich (Abb. 1). Bei Betrachtung des Abtrocknungsverlaufes auf der normalen schwitzenden Haut stellten wir fest, daß sich nach einer bestimmten Macerationszeit die Schweißaktivität verringert oder vollkommen aufhört. Die Zeit, die zur Erreichung dieser vorübergehenden Anidrose (Hydromeiose) benötigt wird, ist hauptsächlich von der Masse der Hornschicht abhängig. Die starke Hornschicht des Handtellers mit ihrer großen Quellungsfähigkeit verschließt die

Schweißdrüsenausgänge schon nach einer 30 min dauernden Maceration, wogegen die dünne Hornhautschicht auf dem Vorderarm dazu 4 bis 5 Std benötigt (Abb. 2).

Mit allmählicher Normalisation der Hydratationsverhältnisse treten größere Schweißabgaben auf, die eine jähe Anstiegswelle und einen langsamer ablaufenden Abstieg aufweisen. Dieser ist wahrscheinlich der Ausdruck des Eindringens von Wasser und des neuerlichen Austrocknens des periporalen Gebietes (Mikrozirkulation des Wassers). *Auf den Handtellern* registrierten wir nach 30 min Maceration (die geringste Zeit zum Erreichen der Hydromeiose) die erste Schweißabgabe zwischen der 2. bis 5. min. Zur vollständigen Regeneration der Schweißtätigkeit kam es zwischen der 40. bis 80. min, obwohl die basale Wasserabgabe nach der Maceration niedriger war als im unmacerierten Kontrollbezirk.

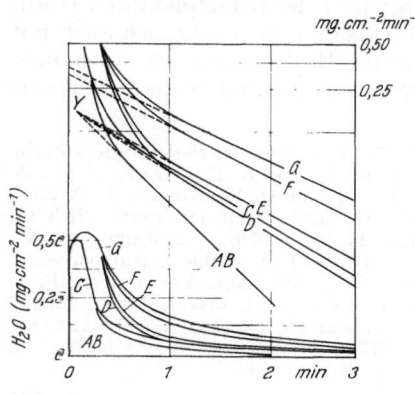

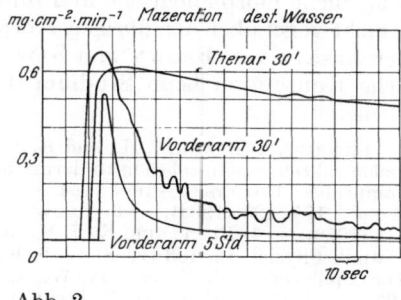

Abb. 2

Abb. 1

Abb. 1. Kurve *AB* Trocknungsablauf nativer Haut nach 90 bis 150 min Maceration (Wasser), Kurve *D* Trocknungsablauf nativer Haut nach 24 Std Okklusion (Folie), Kurve *C* Trocknungsablauf nativer Haut nach 24 Std Maceration (Wasser), Kurve *E* Trocknungsablauf nativer Haut nach 48 Std Okklusion (Folie), Kurve *F* Trocknungsablauf nativer Haut nach 72 Std Maceration (Wasser), Kurve *G* Trocknungsablauf nativer Haut nach 96 Std Okklusion (Folie). Die linearisierten Kurven schneiden sich in Punkt *Y*, die Kurven *F*, *G* schneiden sich nicht.

An dem Vorderarm hatte eine 30 min bis 3 Std lange Maceration keinen Einfluß auf das Schwinden der Schweißtätigkeit. Die absolute Hydromeiose entsteht nach einer 4 bis 5 Std dauernden Maceration. Das erste, durch thermalen Reiz hervorgerufene Schwitzen registrierten wir zwischen der 10. bis 30. min. Die vollkommene Wiederherstellung der Schweißtätigkeit dauerte 2 und mehr Std. Mit der Verlängerung der Maceration verlängert sich auch die Zeit, die zur Wiederherstellung der Schweißaktivität benötigt wird.

Diskussion

Durch die Verfolgung des Trocknungsverlaufes und der Veränderungen der Schweißaktivität auf der macerierten Epidermis ist es möglich, einige Details der Hydratationsmechanismen der Hornschicht näher zu analysieren. Während die erste Trocknungsphase vollkommen unregelmäßig verläuft, können wir nach der zweiten Phase, in der die Hornschicht mit Exponentialzeit trocknet, die Typen der Hornschicht nach der Regel der Logarithmuskurve klassifizieren. Da die Regel nach mathematischen Ableitungen dem Ausdruck D/L^2 entspricht (D = Koeffizient der Diffusion, L = die Dicke der Hornschicht), ist dieser Faktor eher ein Maß für die Hornschichtdicke als für die spezifische Struktur, die den Koeffizient für die Diffusion bestimmt.

Der Schweißdurchtritt durch die hydratierte Hornschicht hängt vor allem von ihrer Dicke ab. Während z. B. die ungefähr zehnmal stärkere Hornschicht des Handtellers die Schweißausgänge schon nach 30 min Maceration schließt, erzielen wir denselben Effekt auf der dünnen Hornschicht des Vorderarmes erst in 4 bis 5 Std (Abb. 2).

Die paradoxe Tatsache, daß die vollständige Erneuerung der physiologischen Schweißaktivität im Trockenluftstrom auf dem Vorderarm zwei- bis dreimal länger dauert als auf den Handtellern, spricht für einen anderen Mechanismus der Wasserbindung in diesen Gebieten und so für grundsätzlich verschiedene Zustände der Wassermikrozirkulation.

Unsere Schlüsse stimmen mit der Ansicht von KLIGMAN [6] über die unterschiedliche morphologische und funktionelle Spezifität der palmoplantaren Hornschicht gegenüber der übrigen Körperoberfläche überein. Sie deckt sich auch mit der Ansicht von BROWN und SARGENT [3] über die Hydromeiose als zweckdienliche Konzeption beim Studium der physiologischen Qualitäten der Hautoberfläche.

Literatur. 1. BLANK, I. H., and R. J. SCHEUPLEIN: The epidermal barrier. Progress in the biological sciences in relation to dermatology. 2. Ed. ROOK, A., and R. H. CHAMPION, p. 245. Cambridge: University Press 1964. — 2. BREBNER, D. F., and D. KERSLAKE: J. Physiol. (Lond.) 175, 295 (1964). — 3. BROWN, W. K., and F. SARGENT: Arch. environm. Hlth 11, 442 (1958). — 4. BUETTNER, K. J. K.: J. Appl. Physiol. 14, 261 (1959). — 5. JACOBI, O. K.: J. appl. Physiol. 12, 403 (1958). — 6. KLIGMAN, A. M.: The biology of the stratumcorneum. The Epidermis. Ed. MONTAGNA, W., and W. C. LOBITZ jr. p. 387. New York: Acad. Press 1964. — 7. PEISS, C. N., W. C. RANDALL, and A. B. HERTZMANN: J. invest. Derm. 26, 459 (1956). — 8. RANDALL‘ W. C., and C. N. PEISS: J. invest. Derm. 28, 435 (1957). — 9. SARKANY, I., S. SHUSTER, and M. C. STAMMERS: Brit. J. Derm. 77, 101 (1965). — 10. ZÁHEJSKÝ, J., J. ROVENSKÝ e A. PREIS: Ann. ital. Derm. Sif. (Palermo) 3, 430 (1965).

Physiologische Antiperspirants

H. P. FIEDLER, Wiss. Abt. C. H. Boehringer Sohn, Ingelheim am Rhein (Deutschland)

Jeder Wissenschaftler, der sich mit Problemen der Körperpflege beschäftigt, weiß, daß es heute keine Schwierigkeit mehr bedeutet, Bildung von Körpergeruch weitgehend zu vermeiden. Dank einer mustergültigen Zusammenarbeit zwischen Dermatologen, Bakteriologen und Kosmetikchemikern ist es gelungen, innerhalb kurzer Zeit Präparate zu entwickeln, die jeder Dermatologe ohne Bedenken auch für die Dauerbehandlung der Prädilektionsstellen der Körpergeruchbildung empfehlen kann.

Anders liegen die Verhältnisse bei der Behandlung der zumindest ebenso häufig auftretenden Hyperhidrosis localis. Es ist hinreichend bekannt, daß die lokale Hyperhidrosis insbesondere im palmoplantaren und axillaren Bereich nicht nur ein ästhetisches Problem ist, sondern in vielen Fällen auch zu einer erheblichen Belastung der Psyche führen kann. Es ist ferner bekannt, daß es nicht an Versuchen gefehlt hat, auch für die Behandlung der lokalen Hyperhidrosis zweckentsprechende Präparate zu entwickeln. Doch befinden wir uns hier nach unserem Dafürhalten trotz allem noch in den Anfangsstadien der eigentlichen Entwicklung. Denn die Masse der für die Körperpflege geeigneten Antiperspirants enthält nach wie vor als wesentliche Wirkstoffe adstringierend wirkende Metallverbindungen, insbesondere Aluminiumverbindungen, von denen mit ausreichender Sicherheit nur bekannt ist, daß sie lediglich eine Obstruktion der Schweißdrüsenpori bewirken und in vielen Fällen die Hyperhidrosis selbst nur in bescheidenem Umfang zu reduzieren wissen [1, 2, 3].

Zwar gelingt es, insbesondere bei vegetativ labilen Personen, durch orale Verabreichung von ataraktisch wirkenden Tranquilizern in vielen Fällen auch die bestehende palmoplantare und/oder axillare Hyperhidrosis günstig zu beeinflussen, doch sollte man derartige Präparate nur in besonders schweren oder kritischen Fällen vorsehen. Man sollte vielmehr bemüht sein, sich intensiver mit der Entwicklung solcher Präparate zu beschäftigen, die auch bei örtlicher Applikation die Schweißdrüsen gegebenenfalls direkt ansprechen, also physiologisch wirksam werden.

Daß die Entwicklung solcher Antiperspirants möglich ist, beweisen bereits 1951 von W. B. SHELLEY und P. N. HORVATH [4] mit Atropin und Scopolamin durchgeführte Versuche, ferner aber vor allem die ausgedehnten Untersuchungen der Jadassohnschen Klinik [5], die zeigen konnten, daß die Schweißdrüse an sich sehr empfindlich auf Substanzen von außen her — hier allerdings iontophorisierte — anspricht.

Wir möchten weiter erwähnen, daß auch topisch applizierte, anticholinergisch wirksame Substanzen transpirationshemmend wirken [6], daß das Hexopyrronium-bromid (Substanz AHR-483) nach topischer Applikation auch die axillare Transpiration deutlich hemmt [7] und daß schließlich Ester des Scopolamins, ferner Ester des 1-Methyl-4-hydroxypiperidins nach topischer Applikation eine gute transpirationshemmende, jedoch keine systemische Wirkung erkennen ließen [8].

Wir möchten es nicht versäumen, hier auch darauf hinzuweisen, daß M. B. SULZBERGER und F. HERRMANN [9] ein elektrophysiologisches Potential entlang den Schweißdrüsengängen und ferner feststellten, daß es deshalb möglich ist, die Schweißsekretion durch topische Applikation elektropositiver Substanzen zu beeinflussen. Wir haben diese Erfahrungen unter Anwendung der von der Jadassohnschen Schule entwickelten Testmethoden bestätigen und zeigen können, daß sich hierfür u. a. auch das N-(Beta-Oxyäthyl)-N-(Beta, Gamma-dioxypropyl)-dodecylamin, aber auch verschiedene andere Substanzen eignen.

Offensichtlich bestehen aber noch andere Möglichkeiten der Entwicklung wirksamer physiologischer Antiperspirants. Es ist bekannt, daß der Gehalt an Bernsteinsäuredehydrogenase während der Transpiration in den Schweißdrüsenzellen ansteigt, daß Malonationen das genannte Enzym hemmen und daß schließlich die topische Applikation von Natriummalonat zu einer Schweißhemmung führt. Schließlich ist hinreichend bekannt, daß für die Auslösung der Schweißsekretion im wesentlichen das Acetylcholin verantwortlich ist und daß das Acetylcholin durch Cholinesterase inaktiviert wird. Es ist bereits vermutet worden, daß bei insbesondere lokaler Hyperhidrosis die Acetylcholinspaltung und damit -inaktivierung infolge Cholinesterasemangels gestört ist, weshalb es sich lohnen würde zu prüfen, ob nicht auch topische Applikation von Cholinesterase ein direktes Ansprechen der Schweißdrüsen ermöglicht und damit zu einem Erfolg in der Behandlung der Hyperhidrosis führt.

Wir meinen, daß es bei dem Stand unserer Kenntnisse durch intensivere Zusammenarbeit zwischen insbesondere dem Dermatologen und dem mit der Entwicklung entsprechender Präparate vertrauten Chemiker möglich sein müßte, wirksame physiologische Antiperspirants zu entwickeln, Arzneimittel, die nach unserem Dafürhalten vor allem in der hautfachärztlichen Praxis dringend benötigt werden.

Literatur. 1. KALISH, J.: Drug, Cosmet. Ind. **77**, 614 (1955). — 2. KLARMANN, E. G.: Acta derm-venereol. (Stockh.) **37**, 59 (1957), — 3. PAPA, C. M., and A. M. KLIGMAN: J. invest. Derm. **47**, 1 (1966). — 4. SHELLEY, W. B., and P. N. HORVATH: J. invest. Derm. **16**, 267

(1951). — 5. vgl. u. a. KERNEN, R.. u. R. BRUN: Dermatologica (Basel) **106**, 1 (1953); —
R. BRUN: Amer. Perfumer Cosmetics **73**, 22 (1959); — W. JADASSOHN; Arch. klin. exp.
Derm. **219**, 63 (1964). — 6. HACKBORTH, D. E., and L. S. MARKSON: Arch. Derm. **83**, 659
(1961); — KNUDSON, E. A., and C. H. KONSTMANN-MEIER: Acta derm.-venereol. (Stockh.)
43, 154 (1963). — 7. STOUGHTON, R. B., F. CHIU, W. FRITSCH, and D. NURSE: J. invest.
Derm. **42**, 169 (1964). — 8. McMILLAN, F. S. K., H. H. HELLER and F. H. SNYDER: J.
invest. Derm. **43**, 363 (1964). — 9. SULZBERGER, M. B., F. HERRMANN, R. KELLER, and
B. V. PISHA: J. invest. Derm. **14**, 91 (1950); — SULZBERGER, M. B., and F. HERRMANN:
The clinical significance of disturbances in the delivery of sweat. Springfield, Ill.: Charles C.
Thomas Publisher 1954. — 10. ROSTENBERG, jr., A., and E. L. GONZALEZ: J. invest. Derm.
29, 251 (1957).

Sodium Secretion and Reabsorption by the Eccrine Sweat Gland

R. L. DOBSON, University of Oregon Medical School, Portland, Oregon (USA)

Sweat is essentially a dilute aqueous salt solution. The mechanism of its
elaboration and an attempt to define "normal" sweating in man will be the
subject of his presentation.

Functionally, the eccrine sweat gland consists of two major portions, the
secretory coil and the duct. The former elaborates a precursor fluid with a constant
content of sodium, while the latter is responsible for the ultimate concentration of
sodium in the sweat. The secretory cells actively transport sodium. Presumably,
the membranes of these cells are freely permeable to water since the concentration
of sodium in the precursor fluid is equal to its concentration in the extracellular
fluid, i.c., C. 140 mEq/L. As this fluid traverses the duct sodium is removed again
by a process of active transport but, in contrast to the secretory cells, the ductal
cells are relatively impermeable to water. Thus, the final secretory product, since it
results from reabsorption of sodium in excess of water, has a sodium concentration
invariably less than that of extracellular fluid. It seems likely that the ability to
change the composition of sweat resides solely within the duct. This regulatory
mechanism is sensitive to mineralocorticoids which produce an increase in sodium
reabsorption.

The function of the sweat gland is reputedly abnormal in a variety of systemic
diseases, but lack of definition of the normal range of expression of sweat gland
function has precluded a precise evaluation of the problem with the sole exception
of cystic fibrosis in children. This uncertainty stems from a basic attribute of the
sweat duct which has a limited capacity to reabsorb sodium. Thus, the concentration of sodium in the sweat is dependent in great part on sweat rate. This
means that normal sweat gland function cannot be defined in terms of the sodium
concentration of the sweat.

A slide shows a series of plots of sweat rate vs. sodium concentration obtained
in studies on normal young men. The extent with which sodium concentration will
vary with sweat rate is apparent.

However, if the same data are plotted in a different way, a linear relation
results. Here the rate of sodium excretion, that is, the actual amount of sodium
produced per unit time is plotted against sweat rate. Once the limited capacity
of the sweat duct to reabsorb sodium is exceeded, a straight line results which is
independent of sweat rate. This provides a potential means to define normal sweat
gland function since it can be shown that the slope of this line is equal to the sodium
concentration of the precursor fluid. By extrapolation the "x" intercept equals the
maximum free water clearance of the sweat duct and the negative "y" intercept is
equal to the maximum sodium reabsorption of the duct.

In plots obtained from a study of normal men, there is always a linear relation between sweat rate and the rate of sodium excretion at high sweat rates.

An analysis shows that the sodium concentration of the precursor or secretory fluid is roughly isotomic. Also note the range of sodium reabsorption and free water clearance which define the function of the duct.

The results of these preliminary studies suggested that this method of analysis would provide a simple means of attempting to define the limits of normal of human sweat gland function. There are, however, a number of factors which have to be considered. As I mentioned previously, the sweat duct is very sensitive to adrenal corticosteroids.

A slide shows the effect of the corticosteroid, 9 alpha fluorohydrocortisone and the diuretic, spironolactone on sweat gland function. The precursor fluid remains constant but both drugs exert a major effect on sweat duct function.

Another factor is salt intake. A high salt intake decreases sweat duct function; a low salt intake increases it.

Fortunately the menstrual cycle does not seem to exert much effect on sweating. Here are the results in a young woman studied at weekly intervals. The function of the sweat duct remains fairly constant.

From these studies it appears clear that it is possible to define the limits of normal function of the human eccrine sweat gland. It is also clear that considerable work will be necessary before this is accomplished. However, unless these data are obtained, studies which purport to show sweating abnormalities in a variety of systemic diseases will have limited value.

The Insensible Water Loss and Skin Temperature

F. A. J. THIELE and K. G. VAN SENDEN, Unilever Research Laboratorium, Vlaardingen (Netherlands)

Quantitative measurements of the insensible water loss of the human skin, for example at different sites on the forearm and on the palm of the hand show wide variations: 3 to 60 micrograms of water. $cm^{-2} \cdot min^{-1}$ on the forearm, and 30 to 150 micrograms of water $cm^{-2} \cdot min^{-1}$ on the palm of the hand.

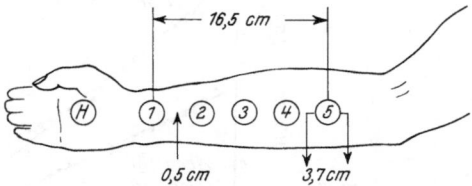

Fig. 1. Measuring areas on forearm ③ is midpoint between wrist and elbow

These experimental data suggest that external factors contribute considerably to these differences. Factors responsible for these differences have been investigated. Continuous measurements of water loss and skin temperature at constant contact pressure showed a striking relationship between both parameters.

These measurements have to be carried out in a temperature controlled room ($\pm$ 0.25 °C), the subjects being allowed to relax during a pre-conditioning period of 1 h. Emotional influences (e.g. mental stress) must be excluded. In all cases skin temperature and water loss tend to attain equilibrium values. In a stationary condition heat production and heat loss are in equilibrium. Climatic factors, such as temperature change, local heating and cooling, air turbulence, covered and uncovered state of the measuring sites, and the like, determine the degree of water

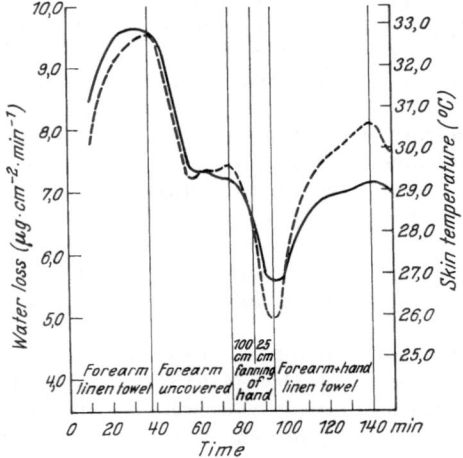

Fig. 2. Influence of cooling and heating on water loss (———) and skin temperature (- - - -) subject 12 (♀), measuring area ③

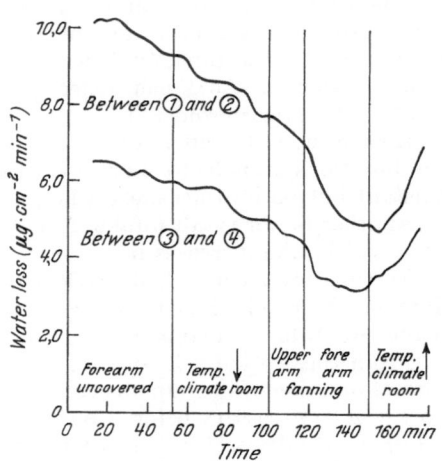

Fig. 3. Influence of cooling on water loss at two measuring areas of right forearm subject 4 (♂)

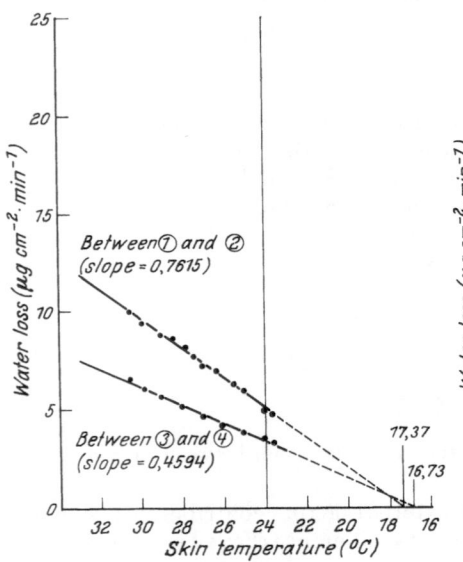

Fig. 4. Relationship between water loss and skin temperature at two measuring areas (cooling by temperature drop in climate room, fanning of upper and forearm) subject 4 (♂)

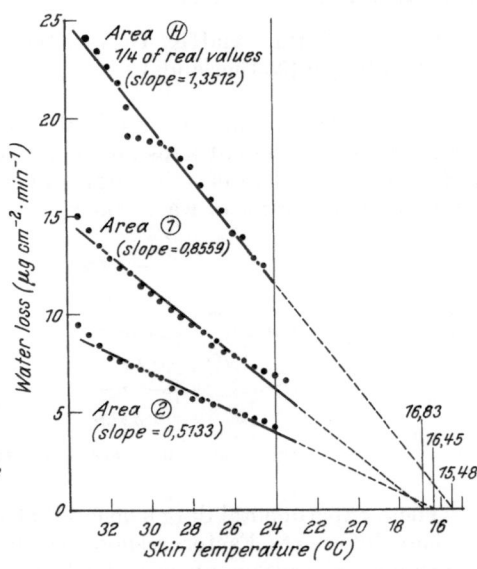

Fig. 5. Relationship between waterloss and skin temperature at three measuring areas subject 12 (♀)

loss. If water loss and skin temperature are plotted, we obtain straight lines. The reaction patterns of the forearm and the palm of the hand are basically equal in spite of the differences in anatomical structure and sweat gland population.

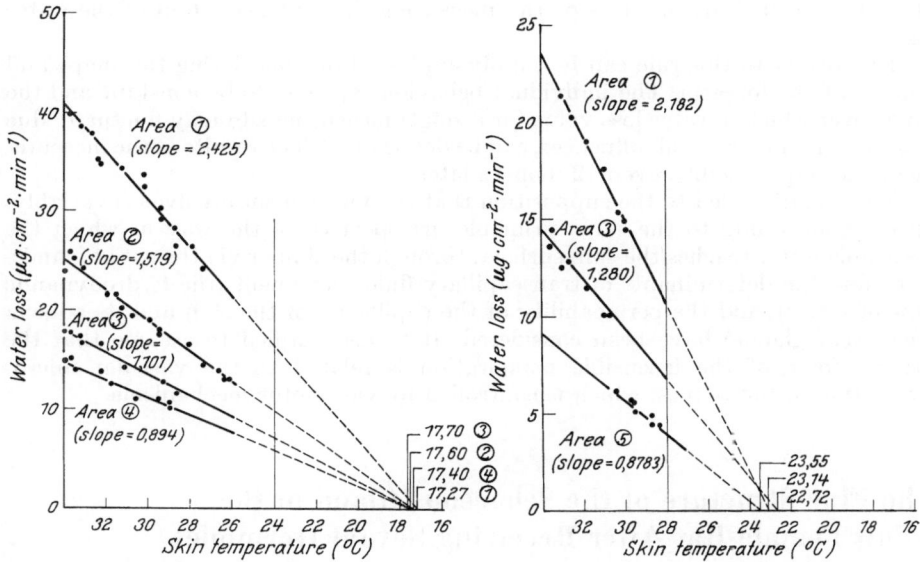

Fig. 6. Relationship between water loss and skin temperature at four measuring areas of an adipose subject, whose waterlosses are extremely high subject 13 (♀)

Fig. 7. Relationship between water loss and skin temperature at three measuring areas of a subject with long and meagre arms subject 2 (♀)

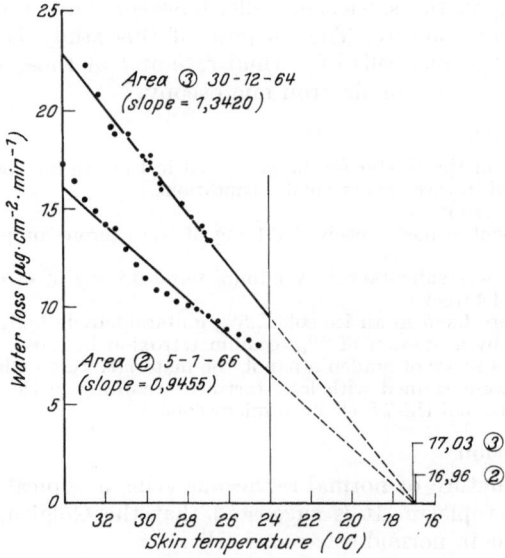

Fig. 8. Relationship between water loss and skin temperature at two adjacent measuring areas determined a year after one another [subject 14 (♂)]

Measurements on both skin areas invariably confirm that these water losses decrease or increase proportionally per degree Centigrade.

The straight lines which represent this relation all intersect the temperature axis at the same point. This point, calculated by means of the least squares, lies at 17.0 °C ($\pm$ 0.5), irrespective of the measuring site and the extent of the water loss.

Exceptions to this rule can be simply explained on considering the shape and volume of the forearm. The individual behaviour appears to be constant and the range over which a water loss value for a single measuring site may fluctuate, due to several minor external influences, can be determined. The results of the measurements are reproducible, even 12 months later.

These findings led to the supposition that the mechanism involved invariably, operates according to the same principle, irrespective of the way in which the insensible water reaches the skin surface: through the skin or via the sweat glands. Therefore the determinants of transcapillary fluid movement (the hydrodynamic flow of water), and the permeability of the capillaries of the skin and its adnexa (the sweat glands) have been considered. It seems justified to assume that the driving force of the insensible perspiration is related to the vascular microcirculation in the tissues, which is controlled by vasomotor mechanisms.

The Fine Structure of the Sebaceous Gland of the Adult Female Rat After Receiving Sexual Hormones

Y. SATO and M. MOROHASHI, Department of Dermatology, Niigata University School of Medicine, Niigata (Japan)

It is well known, both light-microscopically and clinically, that the activity of the sebaceous glands is controlled by the sexual hormones. These effects of sexual hormones upon the sebaceous cells, however, have not yet been studied at the level of ultrastructure. The purpose of this study is to reveal the fine structure of the sebaceous cells of normal rats and of those that have received sexual hormones by means of electron microscopy.

Materials and Methods

Female adult rats of the Wistar strain were used in this study. The sebaceous glands of these rats were studied in three experimental conditions.

1. The first group was intact.

2. This group subcutaneously received 0.1 mg of testosterone propionate daily during a 4-week period.

3. The last group was subcutaneously administered 0.1 mg of estradiol benzoate daily, also during a period of 4 weeks.

The specimens were fixed in an ice-cold 2.5% glutaraldehyde buffered at pH 7.4 sodium cacodylate, followed by a fixation of 2% osmium tetroxide buffered at pH 7.4 s-collidine. After dehydration in a series of graded ethanol, the materials were embedded in Epon-epoxy resin. Thin sections were stained with lead tartrate according to the methods of Millonig, then examined in a Hitachi HS-7 S electron microscope.

Results and Conclusion

On the fine structure of normal sebaceous cells, a typical Golgi apparatus is observed in the cytoplasm. It is suggested that the Golgi apparatus is a focal point for lipogenesis in normal sebaceous cells.

The sebaceous glands are enlarged and proliferated by the administration of androgen. The conspicuous changes of fine structure are observed in both the peripheral cells and in the partially differentiated cells. In the mature sebaceous cells, no apparent ultrastructural differences may be found. In the peripheral cells, however, the appearance of small lipid vacuoles may be observed, though they are not found in the normal cells.

The most striking feature of the peripheral cell is the development of agranular endoplasmic reticulum; that is, there is a marked increase in the amount of agranular vesicular and cisternal elements of the endoplasmic reticula. The characteristic structures, such as myelin-figured, concentric paired, agranular endoplasmic reticula, are observed. The endoplasmic reticula in irregular profiles containing lipid-like materials are found dispersed in the cytoplasm.

The transitional form of endoplasmic reticula, in which their membranes are partially attached with RNP granules, may also be recognized. Moreover, in addition to the RNP granules associated with endoplasmic reticula, a large number of RNP granules are found freely distributed in the cytoplasm. At several points, the cisterns of the agranular endoplasmic reticula are often continuous with the surface membranes of the lipid vacuoles.

It is postulated that the agranular endoplasmic reticulum is of prime importance in lipogenesis, similar in importance to that of the Golgi apparatus in normal sebaceous cells.

After an administration of estrogen, the sebaceous glands are reduced in size in contrast to the cases receiving androgen. The peripheral cells show the tendency to be similar in appearance to those of the epidermal cells. The partially differentiated cells, located inside the peripheral cells, show the dark stained cytoplasm filled with vesicular types of agranular endoplasmic reticula, and also the increase in the amount of wavy tonofilaments. But the lipid vacuoles are decreased in number.

This study reveals that there are some differences in both the structural features and the distribution of agranular endoplasmic reticula, assumed to be mainly involved in lipogenesis, between normal sebaceous cells and those treated with sexual hormones, such as androgen and estrogen. It is suggested that androgen causes a marked increase in the amount of agranular endoplasmic reticula, within which rapid lipid formation will occur, and, on the other hand, that estrogen suppresses the lipid formation because of a contrary action to androgen.

The in vivo Study of Cutaneous Lipogenesis

G. Lipkin and V. R. Wheatley, Department of Dermatology, New York University School of Medicine, New York (USA)

Introduction: The use of *in vitro* techniques for study of cutaneous lipogenesis, while possessing the advantages of convenience and reproducibility, nevertheless has certain disadvantages. It is known that lipogenesis varies with changes in temperature, pH, and oxygen tension [1]. Furthermore, availability of substrates will be dependent partly on the status of various intervening membrane barriers, including those of blood vessels and basement membranes of skin. Thus, *in vitro* findings may not accurately reflect physiologically determined events. It is therefore desirable to correlate *in vitro* data with that obtained from *in vivo* models. For this reason, we have used a physiologic *in vivo* perfusion technique, that of ADACHI and CHOW [2], to study incorporation of a variety of precursors into lipids of dog skin [3, 4, 5].

Experimental: In each experiment the skin flap on the medial aspect of the dog's thigh was isolated, with its blood supply, and perfused in situ for a 30 min period with 10 μc of a ^{14}C-labelled precursor. The skin was excised, the lipids extracted and fractionated, and the distribution of radioactivity in each fraction was measured.

Results: Data obtained are shown in Tab. 1 to 4.

Table 1. *Incorporation of various precursors into the lipids of dog skin*

Precursor	Number of Dogs	Total Lipid Incorporation as Percentage of Total Tissue incorporation	Specific Activity of Total Lipids	Specific Activity of Non-Lipids	Ratio of Specific Activity of Total Lipid to Total Non-Lipid
			(μc./gm.)		
Acetate	6	21.4%	0.138	0.146	0.94
Pyruvate	5	2.0	0.013	0.205	0.06
Isobutyrate	2	5.2	0.017	0.093	0.18

Table 2. *Incorporation of perfused amino acids into cutaneous lipids*

Amino Acid	No. of Perfusions	Lipid Total	Incorporation as % Tissue Activity		Efficiency of Lipogenesis[a]
					%
Glycine-1,2-^{14}C	2	0.30	0.95		2.9
Glycine-1-^{14}C	2	0.43	0.41		2.0
Glycine-2-^{14}C	2	0.78	0.75		3.6
Alanine-U-^{14}C	2	0.23	0.38		1.4
Isoleucine-U-^{14}C	3	1.10	4.80	2.20	12.6
Leucine-U-^{14}C	2	2.25	3.95		14.0
Valine-U-^{14}C	3	1.50	3.50	0.50	8.4
Phenylalanine-U-^{14}C	3	1.24	1.36	0.46	4.8

Amount perfused standardized at 10 μc

[a] Expressed in terms of acetate incorporation (Tab. 1, Column 3) as 100% efficiency.

Table 3. *Distribution of incorporated radioactivity in lipids derived from acetate, pyruvate, and amino acids*

	Acetate	Pyruvate	Glycine	Alanine	Isoleucine	Leucine	Valine	Phenylalanine
	% total lipid activity							
Free fatty acids	12.8	26.1	16.8	36.0	15.8	4.7	26.3	11.4
Hydrocarbons	0.1	0.3	0.2	0.3	0.7	0.2	0.3	0.2
Sterol esters	0.8	4.5	2.1	2.6	22.4	4.7	11.3	0.4
Waxes	0.7	1.9	1.9	1.7	4.9	4.5	3.5	1.0
Methyl esters of fatty acids	17.5	6.4	10.9	4.7	15.3	29.8	25.6	1.2
Triglycerides	28.4	21.8	17.4	22.3	25.8	36.8	10.2	5.9
Unidentified band	2.1	6.2	3.8	2.3	4.0	8.2	5.3	4.8
Free sterols	20.2	8.2	12.9	12.9	3.6	2.1	9.1	10.3
Polar lipids	17.4	24.6	33.1	17.1	7.5	9.2	8.5	64.9

Table 4. *Incorporation of perfused lipids into cutaneous lipids*

Precursor	Lipid Incorporation as % of Total Perfused Activity	Distribution		
		Epidermis	Dermis	Subcutaneous
Palmitic Acid	27.3	0.9	20.6	5.8
Triolein	30.0	0.7	18.3	11.0
Cholesterol	14.2	0.3	6.6	7.3
Cholesterol Oleate	4.4	0.1	2.0	2.3

Discussion

A. *Acetate, pyruvate, isobutyrate.* Acetate is very actively incorporated into free and esterified fatty acids, free sterols, and polar lipids, but not into hydrocarbons, sterol esters, or waxes. Pyruvate, though less readily incorporated than acetate, is more readily utilized than are several amino acids (including, as expected, one of its own precursors, alanine). Isobutyrate, a fatty acid, is incorporated significantly.

B. *Amino Acids.* Amino acids are much less readily incorporated than acetate, yet significant incorporation of the former does occur into all major lipid fractions. Both straight-chain (alanine and glycine) and branched-chain (leucine, isoleucine, and valine) amino acids are incorporated, but the branched type much more readily. This is of interest because branched-chain amino acids, unlike straight chain types, give rise both to branched- and straight-chain fatty acids, and may be utilized in more diverse ways. Furthermore, the sterol esters of human surface lipids have a predominance of branched and unsaturated fatty acids [6], so that the finding that the three branched-chain amino acids are most readily incorporated into sterol esters of dog skin suggests a similarity between the two species in this respect. The incorporation of amino acids into free sterols is noteworthy. Presumably alanine and isoleucine can be incorporated by way of their known catabolic product, acetyl CoA, but the high incorporation of valine, which forms propionyl CoA, rather than acetyl CoA, suggests the possibility of an alternate pathway of sterol biogenesis. The greater incorporation of isobutyrate than valine is consistent with the fact that the former is a known intermediate in the catabolism of the latter during lipogenesis.

C. *Lipids.* Significant uptake of a neutral fat, a fatty acid, a sterol, and sterol esters is observed into the lipids of epidermis, dermis and subcutaneous adipose tissue. Neutral fat shows little metabolic alteration, and hence may presumably reach the skin surface unchanged. However, in the epidermis, fatty acid shows up to 10% incorporation into neutral fats, and cholesterol up to 10% esterification. Cholesterol esters are unchanged in epidermis. In the adipose layer, fatty acids show up to 50% incorporation into neutral fats, while cholesterol esters show up to 15% liberation of their fatty acids.

Conclusion: It is hoped that sufficient data will be obtained under these physiologic conditions to provide a reference standard for future *in vitro* work in both dog and man.

References. 1. ERWIN, J., and K. BLOCH: Science **143**, 1006 (1964). — 2. ADACHI, K., and D. C. CHOW: J. invest. Derm. **39**, 299 (1962). — 3. LIPKIN, G., V. R. WHEATLEY, and C. MARCH: J. invest. Derm. **45**, 356 (1965). — 4. WHEATLEY, V. R., G. LIPKIN, and T. H. Woo: J. Lipid Res. 8, 84 (1967). — 5. LIPKIN, G., V. R. WHEATLEY, T. H. Woo, and C. MARCH: Studies of the lipids of dog skin IV: The *in vivo* incorporation of blood lipids into the lipids of isolated perfused dog skin. (To be published). — 6. NICOLAIDES, N.: Advances in Biology of the Skin, Vol. 4, Chapter XI. Ed. by MONTAGNA, W., R. A. ELLIS, and A. F. SILVER: New York: Macmillan Co. 1963.

Physiology of Human Sebaceous Glands-Hormonal Control Mechanisms

J. S. STRAUSS, Boston University School of Medicine, Boston, Mass. (USA)

In the short period of time available, I can only summarize our findings on the hormonal control of the large sebaceous follicles found on the human face. The data is based on microscopic observation and sebum production measurements.

Androgen is the prime and possibly the sole hormone reponsible for sebaceous gland development. Before puberty there is very little lipid differentiation, and the glands are very small. During adolescence the glands enlarge and there is a resulting increase in sebum production. The sebaceous glands are very sensitive to androgen, and small amounts, i.e. 5 mg of orally administered methyl testosterone, can stimulate the sebaceous glands in a prepuberal child. This response takes 1 to 3 weeks. It is a direct effect on the sebaceous glands that can be restricted to a local area under appropriate conditions when testosterone is applied topically. In addition to testosterone, we have shown that physiologic amounts of Δ4-androstenedione and dehydroepiandrosterone also may produce sebaceous gland stimulation. However, I wish to emphasize that *physiologic* amounts of progesterone do not stimulate human sebaceous glands.

How then do the gonads and the adrenal glands play a role in sebaceous gland function ? First it should be realized that the sebaceous glands vary in size and function at various ages. The prepuberal glands are very small. In both males and females glandular enlargement occurs at puberty. In the male, sebaceous gland function does not start to decrease until a very old age. In women, by contrast, sebaceous gland secretion, which is always less than in the male in adult life, decreases sharply after menopause. In the intact male, it would appear that testicular androgen maintains sebum production at high levels, even into old age. This is supported by the finding that sebum production drops significantly in elderly males when castration is performed. In the intact male, the adrenal gland probably plays no role in the support of the sebaceous gland, but if the testes are absent or non-functioning, adrenal androgens, such as dehydroepiandrosterone, maintain sebum production at levels higher than those of prepuberal subjects. In fact, sebum production can be decreased in the castrated male by the administration of adrenal-suppressive doses of prednisone.

There is ample evidence that the ovaries secrete androgenic steroids, and therefore ovarian androgens, but not progesterone, are probably responsible for sebaceous gland stimulation. The fall of glandular activity at menopause is undoubtedly due to the decrease in ovarian function at this time. The adrenal glands probably also play a role in the female since adrenal suppression with prednisone decreases sebum production significantly.

Estrogens, in sufficient doses, inhibit sebaceous gland function. The sebum-suppressive effect of estrogen does not appear to be dependent on peripheral competitive inhibition of androgens as the decrease can be reversed by the administration of exogenous androgen despite continued administration of the estrogen. In the male, it is known that doses of estrogen which decrease sebaceous gland function decrease circulating levels of plasma testosterone. Therefore, the administration of estrogens to decrease sebaceous gland function is of little practical value in males.

In contrast, in the female estrogen therapy is useful. Approximately 100 micrograms of ethynyl estradiol, or its equivalent are required. However, because of a variability in the response, some patients may require more estrogen. Estrogen administration is most practical with the use of the estrogen-progestin compounds now available for ovulation-suppression, which are administered for three weeks each month. It should be emphasized, however, that it is the estrogen and not the progestin, which causes the decrease, and any estrogen in equivalent amounts will be equally effective.

While estrogen administration is currently used in clinical practice for the treatment of acne, the administration of anti-androgens is purely experimental. We have studied two such anti-androgenic steroids in detail. Chlormadinone acetate, a progestin, has produced a decrease in sebum production when administered in high doses (40 to 60 mg/day). In the male subjects used in this study, a decrease in plasma testosterone was noted. Another steroid, 17-alpha-methyl-B-nortestosterone, also has produced a decrease in sebum production in some subjects. With this compound, sebaceous gland function has been most consistently decreased in females administered the drug orally, although a variable decrease of sebum production has also been observed in men given the drug both orally and topically.

Le contrôle hormonal de la glande sébacée chez l'homme

M. Bonelli, E. Alessi, C. Tomasini et S. Piccinini, Clinique Dermatologique de l'Université de Milan (Italie)

La glande sébacée est un target-organ très sensible à différents hormones. Dans l'espèce humaine, et dans les deux sexes, la testostérone et les hormones androgènes stimulent la glande sébacée, les oestrogènes l'inhibent. Les données histologiques et cliniques et les déterminations du sébum montrent une bonne

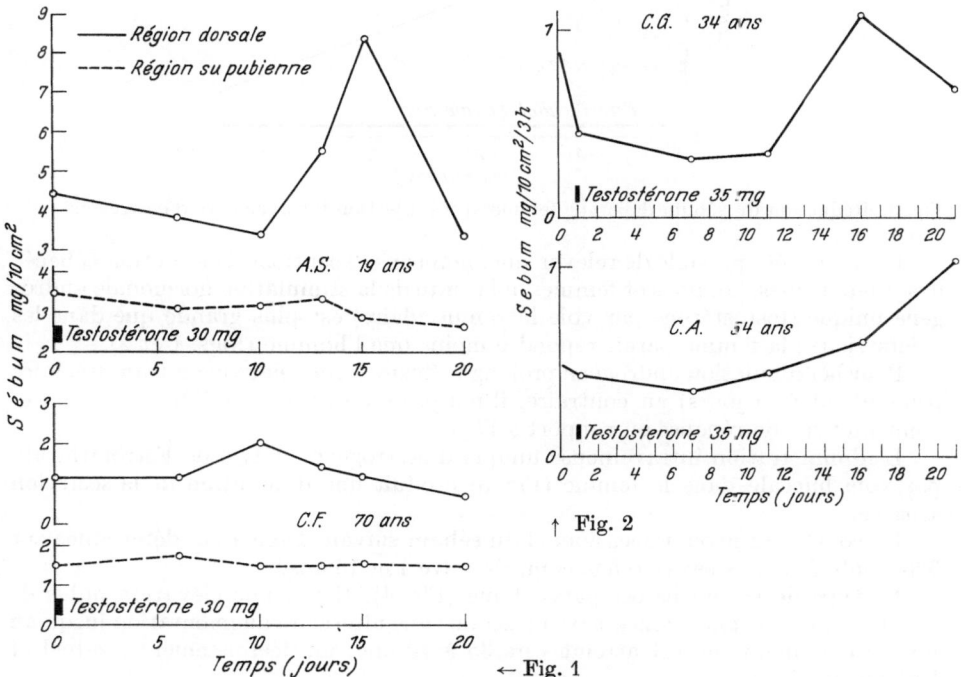

Fig. 1 et 2. Différences de la sécretion sébacée dans les deux sexes (masculin: sujets A. S. et C. F., féminin: sujets C. G. et C. A.) en rapport avec l'âge, après injection intramusculaire de testostérone

concordance à ce sujet. Des nombreuses recherches expérimentales sur les animaux (rat, souris, cobaye) ont donné des conclusions superposables. Les gonadotrophines et la progestérone, à des doses thérapeutiques même élevées, ne modifient pas appréciablement la fonction et l'histologie de la glande sébacée dans l'espèce humaine.

Pendant des recherches personnelles, des déterminations du sébum (niveau occasionnel et sécretion) ont été conduites parallèlement dans des sièges différents de peau (région dorsale et supra-pubienne, front), dans les deux sexes, en condition basale et après stimulation avec la testostérone. Le sébum n'a pas révélé un comportement différent, même en comparant des régions de peau particulièrement dépendantes des hormones (région supra-pubienne) avec des régions neutres (région dorsale). On a observé seulement un niveau plus haut dans les régions plus riches des glandes sébacées, comme le dos. Des remarquables variations d'un sujet à l'autre, après la même stimulation hormonale, sont attribuables aux différents niveaux hormonaux et à la diverse sensibilité des glandes sébacées dans chaque sujet.

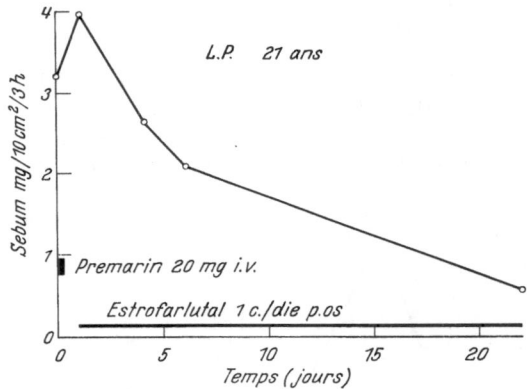

Fig. 3. Réduction du sébum dans une femme après injection intraveineuse d'oestrogène

Il a même été possible de relever que, non sans exceptions, la sécrétion sébacée des sujets jeunes, hommes et femmes, à la suite de la stimulation hormonale androgène unique (testostérone par voie intramusculaire) est plus grande que dans les sujets vieux; la femme paraît répondre moins que l'homme (Figs. 1 et 2).

Pour la stimulation androgène prolongée (testostérone par voie intramusculaire pendant 30 à 40 jours) au contraire, il n'a pas été possible de différencier clairement un type de réponse en rapport à l'âge.

L'administration intraveineuse unique d'oestrogènes suivie de Estrofarlutal* par voie buccale dans la femme (Fig. 3) produit une diminution de la sécretion sébacée.

La courbe du niveau occasionnel du sébum suivant l'âge a été déterminée sur 325 sujets des deux sexes, d'âge compris entre 1 et 75 ans.

Le type de la courbe est parabolique (Fig. 4). Il y a une élévation pubérale plus brusque et rapide dans le sexe masculin; une ultérieure augmentation jusqu'au niveau culminant qui est atteint vers 35 à 40 ans; un décroissement graduel et lent jusqu'à 75 ans.

A la région intrascapulaire, le sébum est plus abondant chez l'homme au dessus de 20 ans; plus élevé au contraire chez la femme au dessous de 20 ans.

A la région supra-pubienne le niveau sébacé de l'homme est toujours supérieur, sauf dans la première décade, dans laquelle les valeurs pour les deux sexes sont à peu près les mêmes.

* Estrofarlutal (Farmitalia) = éthinyl œstradiol 75 mg médroxyprogestérone acétate 2 mg.

Le comportement du sébum suivant l'âge peut être approximativement comparé à l'élimination urinaire des 17-kétosteroïdes totaux.

L'analyse du sébum par la chromatographie en couche mince permet de presenter quelques différences qualitatives individuelles par rapport à l'âge.

L'administration de prèparations anti-ovulatoires (éthinyl œstradiol 50 mg + médroxyprogestérone, acétate 5 mg*; éthinyl œstradiol 75 mg + médroxy-

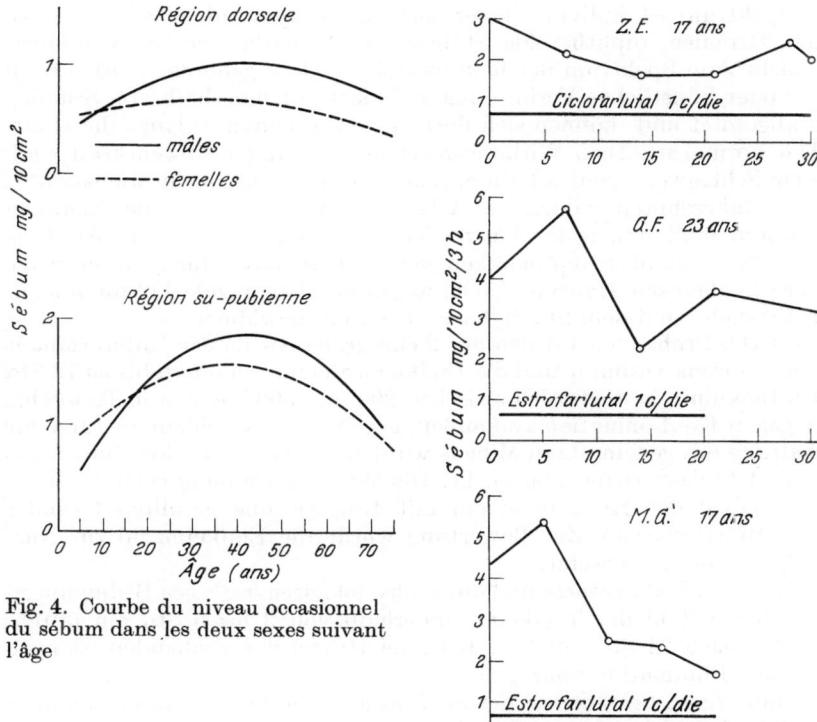

Fig. 4. Courbe du niveau occasionnel du sébum dans les deux sexes suivant l'âge

Fig. 5. Réduction du sébum dans l'homme jeune après traitement avec une préparation antiovulatoire (Estrofarlutal Farmitalia)

progestérone acétate 2 mg**) réduit le niveau sébacé dans les deux sexes. (Voire Fig. 5 chez l'homme.)

Elle constitue une thérapeutique très efficace et bien tolérée dans l'acné de la femme.

L'activité inhibitoire des oestrogènes sur la glande sébacée semble indirecte, probablement à travers l'inhibition hypophisaire des gonadotrophines, et peut-être des corticotrophines; au contraire la testostérone joue un rôle stimulant direct sur la glande sébacée.

---

* Ciclofarlutal Farmitalias
** Estrofarlutal Farmitalias

Der Einfluß des Hautoberflächenmilieus auf Staphylococcus aureus

E. Müller, Dermatologische Klinik und Poliklinik der Universität Würzburg (Deutschland)

Jeder Mensch beherbergt bekanntlich an seiner Hautoberfläche zahlreiche Keime. Ihr Spektrum ist individuell verschieden. Hauptsächlich gehören dazu Mikrokokken, Sarcinen, diphtheroide Stäbchen und apathogene Sporenbildner. Keime, die nicht zum Spektrum der hautansässigen Flora gehören, werden nach unfreiwilliger oder künstlicher Verimpfung auf die Haut innerhalb von Stunden oder Tagen abgetötet und können sich dort nicht vermehren, solange die Hautbeschaffenheit normal ist. Dem Wirkungsmechanismus dieser Abwehrkraft sind, teils unter dem Schlagwort „Selbstdesinfektions-" oder „Selbststerilisationskraft", seit mehreren Jahrzehnten zahlreiche Arbeiten gewidmet. Auf die Nennung einzelner Autoren muß wegen der Kürze der Zeit verzichtet werden. Als feststehend darf gelten, daß für Streptokokken gewisse Fettsäuren, für gram-negative Keime die Trockenheit der Hautoberfläche wesentlich hemmende Faktoren sind. Die eigenen Versuche sind dem Staphylococcus aureus gewidmet.

Bei nahezu 200 Probanden wurden auf 2 cm² große Areale der Unterarmhaut Staphylococcus aureus verimpft und die Endkeimzahlen nach 5 min bis zu 72 Std verfolgt. Das Inokulum bewegte sich zwischen 200 und 500 Keimen je Teststelle. Zum Schutz gegen Kontamination von außen, gegen Keimverschleppung und zur Aufrechterhaltung des gewünschten Milieus wurden die Versuchsfelder luftdurchlässig oder mit Uhrglasverband abgedeckt. Die Wiedergewinnung erfolgte durch gründliches Schaben der Haut in einem mit Ringerlösung gefüllten Cylinder (Methode von Burtenshaw). Zur Bewertung wurde die Endkeimzahl zur Ausgangskeimzahl in Relation gesetzt.

Auf der *normalen Hautoberfläche* und unter physiologisch *trockenen* Bedingungen vermindert sich die Zahl der Testkeime innerhalb von 2 bis 5 Std auf durchschnittlich 40%, nach 24 Std auf 5%. Bei zwei Drittel der Probanden ist nach 72 Std die völlige Elimination vollzogen.

Wird die Haut *durch Behinderung der Verdunstung feucht* gehalten, so kommt es nur bei etwa 50% der Probanden zur Elimination des Staphylococcus aureus. Beim Rest der Versuchspersonen setzt im Laufe des zweiten Halbtages eine kontinuierliche Vermehrung ein, die nach mehreren Tagen mit geröteten flachen Knötchen verknüpft sein kann.

Ein 5 min dauerndes *Ätherbad* der Haut vor der Beimpfung bewirkt unter der nachfolgenden Uhrglasbedeckung beim überwiegenden Teil der Probanden eine Begünstigung der Vermehrung des Staphylococcus aureus — auch in Fällen, bei denen auf der nicht vorbehandelten Gegenseite die Elimination des Staphylococcus aureus stattfindet. Offenbar beruht der Effekt des Ätherbades also auf einer Entfernung von keimhemmenden Substanzen von der Hautoberfläche. Jedoch muß es sich hierbei nicht unbedingt um Lipide handeln, da mit Äther auch andere Stoffe extrahiert werden.

Vergleichende Untersuchungen an *Körperregionen mit unterschiedlichen pH-Werten*, aber naturgemäß auch unterschiedlichem Drüsengehalt, nämlich Handinnenfläche, Unterarm, Ellenbeuge, Achselhöhle, Interscapularbereich, zeigen, daß der pH für sich allein nicht die ausschlaggebende Rolle spielt, die ihm früher zugeschrieben wurde.

Wird die *Hornschicht mittels Abriß* vor der Beimpfung weitgehend *entfernt*, so resultiert im *feuchten* Milieu ausnahmslos Vermehrung. Sie setzt schon kurz nach der Inoculation ein. Nach 24 bis 72 Std zeigen sich klinisch Veränderungen im Sinne einer oberflächlichen Pyodermie oder eines mikrobiellen Ekzems. Die ermittelten Endkeimzahlen sind die höchsten unter allen geprüften Versuchsmodifikationen.

Beläßt man hingegen die der Hornschicht beraubte und beimpfte Teststelle unter *luftdurchlässiger* Bedeckung, so kommt es zwar im Endeffekt auch zur Elimination des Staphylococcus aureus wie auf der unversehrten Haut. Jedoch erfolgt sie wesentlich langsamer, und bei etwa ein Drittel der Probanden geht ihr eine transitorische, am 24-Std-Wert ersichtliche Vermehrung voraus.

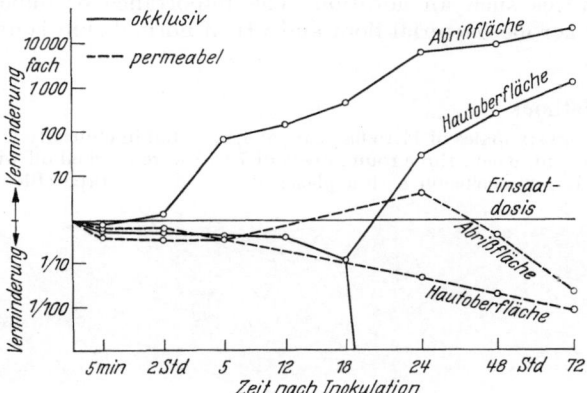

Auf entzündlich oder atrophisch *stärker schuppenden Herden* von Patienten mit Psoriasis, Narben und Pityriasis tabescentium wird der Staphylococcus aureus langsamer eliminiert als bei gesunden Probanden. Unter dem Uhrglasverband vermehren sich auf den schuppenden Herden die Staphylokokken stärker als auf normaler Haut.

Aus den Ergebnissen können folgende *Schlußfolgerungen* gezogen werden: Den cellulären und humoralen Abwehrkräften der Cutis ist das Stratum corneum als hochwertige Abwehrschranke vorgeschaltet. Fehlt die Hornschicht, so resultiert, ausreichende Feuchtigkeit vorausgesetzt, in jedem Fall eine fortschreitende Keimvermehrung, die mit entsprechenden klinischen Veränderungen kombiniert ist. Auf der normalen Hautoberfläche kann der Staphylococcus aureus nicht zum hautansässigen Keim werden. Entgegen den Anschauungen früherer Autoren ist die Austrocknung hierfür allenfalls zusätzlich wirksam, jedoch nicht der alleinige oder hauptsächliche Faktor. Auch im feuchten Milieu erfolgt bei etwa 50% der Probanden die Elimination des Staphylococcus aureus. Durch Ätherextraktion können hemmende Substanzen von der Hautoberfläche entfernt werden. Der pH-Wert für sich allein genommen spielt für die Vermehrung des Staphylococcus aureus keine wesentliche Rolle.

The pH and the Bacterial Flora of Normal Skin Under Fluocinolone*-Plastic Occlusion Treatment

E. A. KNUDSEN, Finseninstitute, Dept. of Dermatology, Copenhagen (Denmark)

It is generally accepted that systemic treatment with corticosteroids reduces the host's resistance to infections. Even if no significant change in bacterial and fungal skin flora from topically applied steroids has been shown [2] addition of antibiotics is often used. It is maintained that supplementary plastic occlusion especially motivates such an addition. The importance of fluocinolone-plastic occlusion to the aerobe bacterial flora and pH of normal skin is examined in the following study.

Materials and Methods

The subjects were six males of 11 to 68 years of age, tested in clinically normal skin on the inside of the upper arm, where three round areas of 7 cm² were marked off with adhesive tape (Leukoplast) Fig. 1. For occlusion a thin plasticfilm fixed with tape (Blenderm) was used

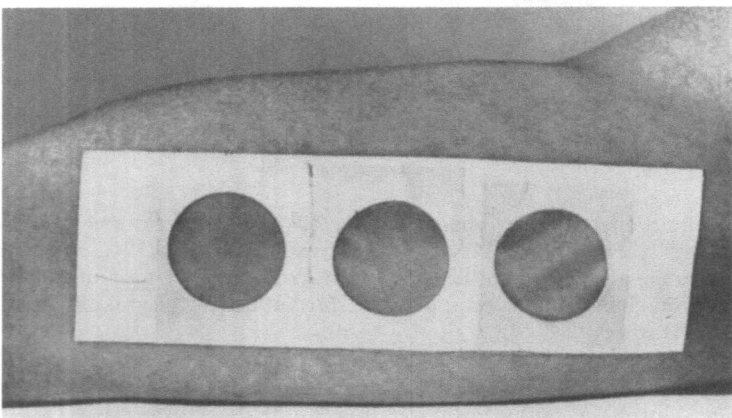

Fig. 1.

The pH-meter (Radiometer, Copenhagen) fitted up with skinelectrode was adjusted before and after each reading. Area I (table) was treated with fluocinolone acetonide cream (subject 1, 2 and 3) or ointment under plastic, area II with the corresponding base + plastic and area III with plastic alone. The creams and ointments were applied in a quantity of 1.5 to 3 mg/cm², at intervals of 1 to 2 days after preceding pH measuring. For collection of material for bacteriological** and mycological examination (Sabouraud's dextrose agar) a sterile swab was used. No cleaning of the skin was undertaken, and swabbing and pH reading only implied airexposition for 5 min altogether at each measuring.

Results

The pH rose from the average of about five to six during the experimental period (Fig. 2). The table shows which bacteria, classified according to international nomenclature [5] were found. Growth of up to ten colonies is marked by +, growth of 11 to 100 by ++, of more than 100 colonies by +++. Heavy growth of normal skin micrococci occured. Other nonpathogenic or usually nonpathogenic bacteria such as alpha and gamma hemol. streptococci, normal skin diphtheroids,

---

* Synalar, I.C.I.
** Undertaken by the State Serum Institute, Copenhagen.

Table. The pH the Bacterial Flora of Normal Skin under Fluocinolone-Plastic Treatment

Organism	Subject number	0			2–3			4–5			6–7		
		I	II	III	I	II	III	I	II	III	I	II	III
Normal Skin Micrococci	1	+++	+++	+++	—	++++	++++	+++	+++	+++	+++	+++	+++
	2	+++	+++	+++	++	++++	++++	+++	+++	+++	+++	+++	+++
	3	±	+	—	++	++++	+++	++	++	+	++	++	++
	4	+++	++	++	—	—	—	++	++	+	++	++	++
	5	—	+	+	0	0	0	0	0	0	0	0	0
	6	+++	+++	+	0	0	0	++	++	++	+++	+++	+++
Mean pH		4,9	4,9	5,0	5,2	5,6	5,7	5,9	5,9	6,1	5,6	5,8	5,9
Various Non-Pathogenic Bacteria	1	+	+	++	—	—	—	+	—	—	+	+	+
	2	++	+	±	—	—	+	—	+	++	—	±	±
	3	—	—	+	±	—	±	—	+	+	—	0	0
	4	±	—	—	+	0	—	0	0	—	0	0	0
	5	—	—	—	0	0	0	+	++	+	—	+	++
	6												
Mean pH		4,9	4,9	5,0	5,2	5,6	5,7	5,9	5,9	6,1	5,6	5,8	5,9
Staph. Aureus	1	—	—	—	++	++	—	+	++	—	±	+	±
	2	—	—	—	—	—	—	++	++	—	+	++	+
	3	—	±	+	—	—	—	—	—	—	—	—	—
	4	—	—	—	—	—	—	0	0	0	0	0	0
	5	—	—	—	0	0	0	0	0	0	0	0	0
	6	!	—	—	0	0	0	—	—	—	—	—	—
Mean pH		4,9	4,9	5,0	5,2	5,6	5,7	5,9	5,9	6,1	5,6	5,8	5,9
Gram-Negative Rods	1	—	—	—	—	—	—	—	—	—	—	—	—
	2	—	—	—	—	—	—	—	—	—	—	—	—
	3	—	—	—	++	—	—	++	—	—	0	0	—
	4	—	—	—	+	—	—	+	—	—	0	0	0
	5	—	—	—	0	0	0	0	0	0	0	0	0
	6	—	—	—	0	0	0	—	—	—	—	—	—
Mean pH		4,9	4,9	5,0	5,2	5,6	5,7	5,9	5,9	6,1	5,6	5,8	5,9

I: Fluocinolone Ointment or Cream under Plastic-Occlusion, II: Ointment or Cream Base under Plastic-Occlusion, III: Plastic-Occlusion alone.
+ / ++ / +++ : Scorings of Growth, ±: Only Growth on Subculture, —: No Growth, 0: No Test.

bac. subtilis-like gram-pos. rods, and bact. anitratum were found quite unsyste-
matically in the three testareas at different times.

Pathogens were represented by staph. aureus of four different strains, in four
of the six subjects (who otherwise had no clinical signs of infection with these),
and gram-neg. rods (E. coli and unidentified gram-neg. rods) were found on two
persons in a single culture. In one case (no 4) staph. aureus disappeared again
during the treatment. In the other three cases several thousand colonies were
cultured. As for apathogenics there was no difference of the growth in the three
testareas, while pathogenic bacteria were less frequent in the untreated area III.
In patient no 6, who had no clinical signs of infection, candida albicans was
cultured from area II after 6 days, otherwise fungi were never found. A slight

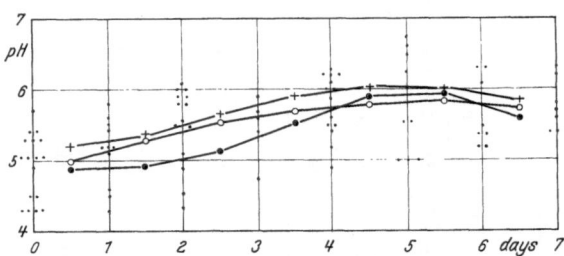

Fig. 2. The pH of normal skin under fluocinolone-plastic treatment. ●——● Mean Curve for
Fluocinolone Ointment or Cream under Plastic-Occlusion (Area I), O——O Mean Curve for
Ointment or Cream Base under Plastic-Occlusion (Area II), +——+ Mean Curve for Plastic-
Occlusion alone (Area III), · Single Scorings

erythema appeared in areas II and III in three cases, in one case in area I, towards
the end of the treatment. Staph. aureus was found in two of these cases, but not
pustules or other signs of clinical infection.

Discussion

The bacterial flora of the skin is influenced by many factors [1, 5. 6]. Among
these the humidity and pH of the skin. By plastic occlusion hydration and softening of the horny layer occur, which must be the main cause of the bacterial
growth. The rise of pH to values found in flexures has scarcely been of importance
however, as most skin bacteria, normal as well as pathogenic, grow well in the
whole pH range five to six [6]. Neither are the steroid and its vehicles seen to have
had any direct effect on the bacterial growth. On the other hand cream/ointment
under the present experimental conditions seem to have acted as "protector" for
areas I and II against bacteriostatics such as colophony and antioxydants in the
plaster templet [3, 4, 7]. The bacteriostatic effect, especially concerning staph.
aureus [3, 4] may be the cause of the fact that staph. aureus was only found in
two cases (table) in the cream/ointment-free area III.

References. 1. EVANS, J. A. ,W. M. SMITH, E. A. JOHNSTON, and E. R. GIBLETT: J. invest.
Derm. 15, 305 (1950). — 2. FRITSCH, C. J., and W. C. FRITSCH: Arch. Derm. 90, 604 (1964). —
3. HENRIKSEN, S. D., and O. GILJE: Acta derm. venereol. (Stockh.) 45, 471 (1965). —
4. HOUGHTON, R. H., and J. W. MAY: Nature (Lond.) 203, 100 (1964). — 5. MEYER-ROHN, J.:
Saprophytische und pathogene Bakterien der Haut. In: JADASSOHN: Handb. d. Haut- u.
Geschlechtskr. IV/1 A, Berlin-Heidelberg-New York: Springer 1965. — 6. PILLSBURY, D. M.,
and G. REBELL: J. invest. Derm. 18, 173 (1952). — 7. UPDEGRAFF, D. M.: J. invest. Derm.
43, 129 (1964).

The Alkali Neutralization Capacity of Human Skin in vivo

K. Schutter, Unilever Research Laboratorium, Vlardingen (Netherlands)

All neutralization experiments on human skin are based on measuring the rate at which the skin is able to change the pH-value of an aqueous solution. The pH-value can be measured in various ways, either by one or more indicators or by a system of electrodes in the solution. pH-registration by means of electrodes can be used to maintain an adjusted pH against the neutralizing influence of the skin. The quantity of acid or alkali needed to keep the pH constant against interfering influences can be dosed and recorded by appropriate instruments, in our case the Radiometer ex Copenhagen. The difference between the meter setting and the pH value measured by the electrodes in the solution is amplified and actuates the dosing unit which then adds so much alkali or acid that the difference is levelled out. If in the determination of the neutralization capacity we work according to this method then:

a) the amount of liquid is no longer important;

b) the titre of the acid or the alkali may vary provided it is known;

c) the experiment can be prolonged at will so that also exhaustion phenomena can be studied;

d) the neutralization capacity can be determined as a function of the pH-value to which the skin is exposed.

After the skin has been exposed to a sufficiently high pH for a sufficiently long time, a reasonably concentrated solution of the neutralized acids involved is obtained. By analysis of this solution it is then possible to gain an insight not only into the quantity but also into the quality of the acid valencies.

The cup which is placed on the skin is made of perspex with an interchangeable Teflon foot. The cup is provided with openings for the insertion of a combined glass/calomel electrode and a temperature compensator as well as with a water/nitrogen inlet and a connection for the syringe dosing burette.

Dependent on the desired pH the first contents of the burette will be needed to attain this pH-value. Once the liquid has reached the required pH, the curve described by the recorder will soon proceed linearly. By dividing the amount of alkali or acid dosed during the linear course of the curve by the time required and the surface area of the skin surface measured, the neutralization capacity in μeq/cm$^2 \cdot$ min is obtained.

Relationship between pH and alkali consumption

According to the same pH-stat method likewise without further pretreatment of the skin, the alkali neutralization capacity at various pH-values was measured. The pH-values were adjusted between 8.5 and 10.5. The increase in alkali consumption with the rise in pH of the contact liquid is distinct. However, the previously found great variation between the individual observations made it as yet speculative to speak of a rectilinear relationship. From the position of the points found so far the impression is gained that if there would ever be any question of a rectilinear relationship, this would only hold for a limited pH-range. At high pH-values ($>$ 10.25) the alkali consumption increases at an accelerated rate, whereas at pH-values ($<$ 9.5) the alkali consumption decreases only slowly.

Acid neutralization

On the analogy of the alkali neutralization capacity attempts were made to express the acid neutralization capacity of human skin in a numerical value.

So far it has been tried to determine the acid consumption necessary to keep the contact liquid on the skin at pH = 3.5. In general an amount of 0.6 to 0.8 μeq/cm^2 acid was required to attain this pH, i.e. 6 to 8 μeq for the total amount of 15 ml contact liquid on 10 cm^2 skin surface. After dosing this amount, hardly any acid was needed to keep the pH at 3.5, i.e. the acid consumption by the skin was extremely low and not comparable with the alkali neutralization capacity. The acid neutralization capacity becomes even lower than the above values, if it is realized, that to bring 15 ml pure water at pH 3.5 5 μeq acid is required. For the acid neutralization capacity of the skin so little remains that there is hardly any question of an acid neutralization capacity. Also at lower pH-values the total amount of acid required does not exceed the amount necessary to bring the water at the desired pH-value: also at pH 3 no acid is neutralized by the skin.

Titration

If after an alkali neutralization experiment part of the neutralization liquid is titrated with 0.01 N HCl, a curve with two equivalence points is obtained. Back titration with 0.01 N NaOH results in a curve with only oneequivalence point. The double transition of the first curve has disappeared. A curve similar to the first can be obtained by titration of a solution the pH-value of which has been kept constant at ten by means of the titrator during passing through air-(CO$_2$!). The latter solution contains therefore exclusively sodium carbonate. In both cases a value of 6.4 is found for the pK of the first proton split off, which is in correspondence with the literature values for the pK$_1$ of H$_2$CO$_3^5$.

The section of the titration curve between the two equivalence points is a measure of the amount of acid necessary to bring about the transition of NaHCO$_3$ (first equivalence point) to H$_2$CO$_3$ (second equivalence point). By calculating this amount for the total volume of the neutralization liquid and multiplying it by two the amount of alkali necessary for compensating the amount of CO$_2$ involved in the neutralization is found. This amount can be expressed as a percentage of the total amount of alkali required for the neutralization.

In the case of six test subjects (all measured on the fore-arm) values were found which varied between 60 and 98%. Naturally the part of the neutralization liquid used for the HCl back-titration was brought into the titration vessel under the exclusion of air contact.

To this end towards the end of the neutralization experiment on the skin, the nitrogen passed through was already let into this vessel in order to expel the air (CO$_2$). After determining the neutralization capacity part of the liquid was pressed into the titration vessel by means of nitrogen pressure. After titration the volume of this liquid and that of the liquid which had not been used for the titration were determined in order to calculate the titrated carbonate for the total amount of liquid. In general 2 to 3 cm^3 of the total amount of liquid (16 to 18 cm^3) was used for the titration.

Discussion

So far the alkali neutralization capacity of six persons has been determined over a period of some months. In order to come a standardization of the experimental conditions, the skin was in all experiments wiped off with 70% alcohol before the alkali was applied: subsequently pure water in the cup was brought onto the skin and brought to pH 3.5 with 0.01 N HCl. As soon as this pH-value had been attained, hardly any acid was used. After some minutes (4 to 5) the cup with liquid was removed from the skin, and the alkali neutralization capacity was determined after ca. 1 h.

Because of this pretreatment the starting point was the same for all; any skin impurities, particularly those originating from tap water in combination with soap rests, were removed beforehand. This method gives indeed an increase in reproducibility in the case of repeated measurements on one test subject.

The previous treatment with the acid solution has no consequences for the mean value of the alkali neutralization capacity but brings the variation within narrower limits as appeared from a large number of comparative experiments. The reduction of the variation is probably a result of cleaning the skin surface to be measured so that the starting point in the alkali neutralization is the same for all test subjects. The fact that the mean value is not influenced is probably connected with the incapacity of the skin to neutralize acid. We have no explanation for this absence of acid neutralization capacity: it is possible that under the influence of the H-ion concentration on the skin surface, changes take place owing to which the supply of neutralizing substances is blocked.

The influence of the adjusted pH-value on the alkali neutralization capacity is in itself not surprising. One is forced to the conclusion of a flux of acid valencies induced by a decrease in concentration. However, the course of the curve which indicates the relationship between pH and neutralization capacity is in conflict with this. It could sooner be supposed that on changing the pH the origin of the neutralizing acid valencies changes likewise. An indication in this direction was obtained from the fact that when the adjusted pH rises the contribution of CO_2 to the neutralization becomes relatively considerably smaller. The fact that in the case of a rise in pH to twelve serious skin damage occurs also points in this direction. Only on applying rather high alkali concentrations to the skin (in the order of 0.001 to 0.01 N) does the skin keratin itself begin to play a role in the alkali neutralization. Lower alkali concentrations are mainly neutralized by the buffer system $H_2CO_2 \cdot NaHCO_3$. Also in the case of measurements of the so-called skin pH this buffer system will play an important if not decisive role.

Über ultraviolett-absorbierende Verbindungen im Wasserlöslichen epidermaler Verhornungsprodukte

E. Schwarz, Hautklinik der Freien Universität Berlin (Deutschland)

Die wasserlöslichen Substanzen epidermaler Verhornungsprodukte stellen Überbleibsel diverser Keratinisationsprozesse dar. Als praktisch einzige ultraviolett-absorbierende, wasserlösliche Substanz findet sich in normaler menschlicher Hornschicht nur Urocaninsäure als cis- und trans-Isomere. Diese Imidazolverbindung ist ein Katabolit der Aminosäure Histidin. Sie kann als Repräsentant orthokeratotischer Prozesse gelten. Ihre Entstehung ist offensichtlich mit dem Auftreten von Keratohyalin verbunden. Urocaninsäure fehlt daher bei parakeratotischen Verhornungsstörungen, wie z. B. bei Psoriasis. Stattdessen treten im Wasserlöslichen parakeratotischer Verhornungsprodukte *andere* ultraviolett-absorbierende Verbindungen auf wie Uracil, Uridin, Hypoxanthin und angeblich auch Xanthin. Diese N-Basen scheinen nur prima vista aus dem Abbau von Nucleinsäuren zu stammen, wobei dann auch offen bliebe, welches Schicksal sie eigentlich bei Orthokeratose erleiden. Mengenmäßig entsprechen die im Schuppenmaterial nachweisbaren N-Basen auch keineswegs ihrer quantitativen Verteilung in den dort gefundenen Nucleinsäuren. Es hat sich ferner gezeigt, daß die als Xanthin angesprochene Substanz anderer Natur ist. Ihre UV-Charakteristik ist deutlich von Xanthin oder Xanthosin verschieden. Diese Substanz, die wir aus arbeitstechnischen Gründen „c" nennen, ist bislang nicht identifiziert worden. Sie verhält sich an Sephadex resp. BIO-Gel wie eine kleinmolekulare Verbindung.

Gegenstand der vorliegenden Untersuchung war das Verhalten der UV-absorbierenden Verbindungen in täglich gesammelten Schuppen eines Patienten mit erythrodermatischer Psoriasis während cytostatischer Behandlung mit dem Folinsäureantagonisten Methotrexat. Die auf der Abszisse angegebenen Zeitperioden umfassen anfänglich 2, später mit zunehmend geringer werdender Schuppung 3 Tage. Um einen quantitativen Vergleich mit den anderen UV-absorbierenden Substanzen zu ermöglichen, wurde für die unbekannte Substanz „c" eine molare Extinktion von 10000 zugrunde gelegt.

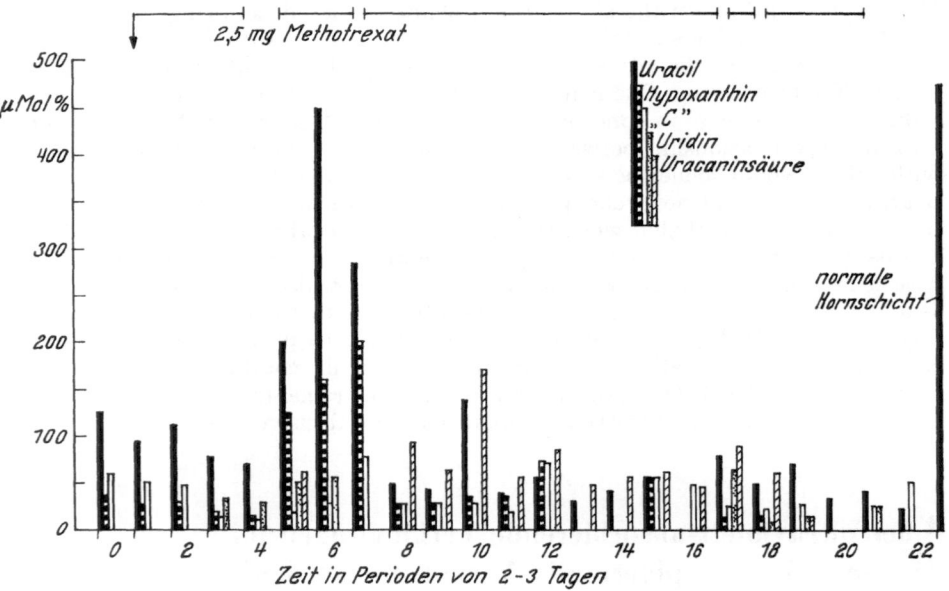

Abb. Psoriasis während der Therapie

Das Schema läßt erkennen, daß Uracil mengenmäßig prävaliert und daß unter dem Einfluß des Cytostatikums zunächst sogar eine weitere Vermehrung zu verzeichnen ist, ein Verhalten, das auch Hypoxanthin aufweist. Im Zuge der klinischen Besserung kommt es anschließend im Rahmen einer allgemeinen Reduzierung auch zu einer dieser beiden Substanzen. „c" wird unter Methotrexateinwirkung ebenfalls vermindert, es läßt aber die interkurrente Vermehrung wie bei den Vorgenannten vermissen. In Perioden der Verminderung von „c" tritt meist Uridin als weitere UV-absorbierende Substanz auf, als ob sie den Verlust ausgleichen würde.

Urocaninsäure als Repräsentant orthokeratotischer Prozesse fehlte anfänglich vollständig und trat erst während der Therapie etwa in zeitlichem Zusammenhang mit der interkurrenten Uracil- und Hypoxanthinvermehrung auf. Bei einer Restitutio ad integrum hätte schließlich eine Zunahme der UCS bis auf etwa 500 μMol-% (im Mittel), normaler Hornschicht entsprechend, und gleichzeitig ein Verschwinden der anderen UV-absorbierenden Verbindungen erwartet werden können. Ansätze dazu sind unter der Therapie erkennbar, verlieren sich aber schließlich wieder. Die analytischen Daten zeigen, daß trotz klinischer Besserung des Hautbefundes keine

„*echte*" Normalisierung erzielt worden ist. In der Tat fand sich sehr bald nach Absetzen des Cytostatikums eine Exacerbation.

Die vorgelegten biochemischen Befunde bieten demnach anscheinend die Möglichkeit einer objektiven Beurteilung des effektiv erzielten Behandlungserfolges. Unter Umständen ließe sich auch eine optimale Zeitspanne der cytostatischen Therapie erkennen, die in unserem Falle wahrscheinlich schon überschritten war.

Ultraviolettes Licht als Stimulus für Kininbildung in menschlicher Haut

R. K. WINKELMANN, J. EPSTEIN und K. WOLFF, Mayo Clinic und Mayo Foundation, Rochester, Minn. (USA), Division of Dermatology, University of California, San Francisco, Calif. (USA) und I. Univ.-Hautklinik Wien (Österreich)

Das durch entsprechende Wellenlängen ultravioletten Lichtes in menschlicher Haut ausgelöste Erythem erscheint gewöhnlich erst nach einer Latenzperiode. Diese verzögerte Antwort des Integuments auf die zugeführte Strahlenenergie stellt eine konstante Reaktionsform dar, wenn auch die Dauer einer derartigen Latenzzeit, in Abhängigkeit von Wellenlänge und Strahlenintensität, einigen Schwankungen unterworfen ist.

Im Gegensatz zu den Verhältnissen bei gewissen Labortieren, die einen biphasischen Reaktionsablauf nach UV-Exposition erkennen lassen [2], ist über diesen Zeitabschnitt beim Menschen wenig bekannt. Im folgenden soll daher über unsere Versuche, mittels der cutanen Perfusionsmethode in menschlicher Haut Histamin und Kinine während der UV-Latenzperiode nachzuweisen, berichtet werden.

Methoden

Es wurden insgesamt 22 Untersuchungen an sechs gesunden männlichen Versuchspersonen durchgeführt. Als Strahlenquellen dienten eine Bausch- und Lomb-Kohlenbogenlampe (National Therapeutic C Carbons), sowie eine Birtcher-Spot-Quarzlampe (Wellenlänge kleiner als 2550 Å), zur Gewinnung von Gewebsflüssigkeit wurde die cutane Perfusionsmethode [3] verwendet. Zu Beginn eines jeden Versuches wurde zunächst die Perfusion am Vorderarm der Testperson in Gang gebracht (physiologische Kochsalzlösung, Perfusionsgeschwindigkeit acht bis zwölf Tropfen/min), und nach einer Wartezeit von 10 bis 20 min (zur Ausschaltung spontaner und traumatischer Kinin- bzw. Histaminausschüttung) mit der Bestrahlung des perfundierten Areals begonnen. Mit der Kohlenbogenlampe wurden 10 bis 20 MED (= 20 bis 22 min), mit der Quarzlampe 30 MED (= 6 min) verabreicht; die Perfusate wurden während der gesamten Bestrahlungszeit, Latenzzeit und bei schon bestehendem Erythem bis zu $7^3/_4$ Std alle 5 min gesammelt und am isolierten Meerschweinchenileum und Rattenuterus auf das Vorliegen von Histamin bzw. Kininen untersucht.

Ergebnisse

Da sich die mit der Kohlenbogenlampe und Spot Quarzlampe erzielten Ergebnisse beträchtlich unterscheiden, werden sie gesondert besprochen.

Kohlenbogenlampe: Unter den angegebenen Bedingungen traten UV-Erytheme zwischen 29 und 76 min nach Beendigung der UV-Exposition auf und nahmen innerhalb der nächsten 24 Std an Intensität zu. Histamin konnte bei keinem der Bestrahlungsversuche im Perfusat nachgewiesen werden, und zwar weder während der Latenzperiode noch bei bereits bestehendem Erythem. Lokale 48/80 Injektion führte jedoch regelmäßig zur Freisetzung dieser Substanz.

Im Gegensatz dazu kam es nach Kohlenbogenbestrahlung regelmäßig zur Ausschüttung von Kininen. Die Kininproduktion begann 5 bis 20 min nach Beendigung der Bestrahlung und fiel daher in jedem Fall noch in die Latenzperiode, d. h.

es konnten diese Polypeptide immer 40 bis 100 min vor dem Auftreten des Erythems beobachtet werden. Bei kontinuierlicher Perfusion waren Kinine noch bis
zu 6¹/₂ Std nach Abschluß der Bestrahlung in den Perfusaten nachweisbar;
wurde mit der Perfusion jedoch erst nach der Bestrahlung begonnen, waren diese
Substanzen nur 20 min und 1 Std, jedoch nicht mehr nach 3 oder 24 Std zu erfassen. Eine Kininausschüttung konnte auch dann ausgelöst werden, wenn statt
der üblichen 10 bis 20 MED nur 1 MED verabreicht wurde, doch waren die
Amplituden der Uteruskontraktionen in diesen Fällen wesentlich schwächer.

Bei Fensterglasfilterung blieb die Kininproduktion aus, ebenso das nachfolgende UV-Erythem. Wurde das perfundierte Areal statt der UV-Strahlung einer
Wärmequelle ausgesetzt (150 W Glühbirne), die zu einer Erhöhung der Hauttemperatur bis zu 40 °C führte, kam es ebenfalls zu keiner Kininbildung. Um die
Kininausschüttung mit einer eventuell auftretenden gröberen Vasopermeabilitätsstörung zu korrelieren, wurde bei drei Versuchspersonen vor der UV-Bestrahlung
25 mg Evans-Blue intravenös injiziert. Doch kam es weder zum Zeitpunkt der
Kininfreisetzung noch nachher zu einer Bläuung des Testareals, obwohl sich eine
derartige Blaufärbung regelmäßig durch lokale 48/80 Injektion erfassen ließ.

Ergebnisse mit der Spot-Quarzlampe: Nach Bestrahlung mit dieser UV-Quelle,
die Wellenlängen bis zu 2550 Å aussendet (Gesamtdosis 30 MED), trat das UV-
Erythem nach 60 bis 120 min auf, doch waren in keinem Fall, weder während der
Latenzperiode noch nachher, Kinine im Perfusat nachweisbar. Während also
Wellenlängen bis zu 3150 Å regelmäßig zu Kininfreisetzung führten, blieb die
Ausschüttung dieser Substanzen bei Verabreichung von UV-Strahlen unter 2550 A
aus.

Diskussion

Die vor dem Auftreten des UV-Erythems, also während der Latenzperiode,
beobachtete Kininfreisetzung kann mit größter Sicherheit als direkter UV-Effekt
aufgefaßt werden. Eine Ausfilterung der Wellenlängen unter 3150 Å konnte die
Ausschüttung dieser Substanzen verhindern, ebenso kam es zu keiner Kininproduktion nach Einwirkung von Wärme. Wellenlängen von 2800 bis 3000 Å haben
sich im Tierversuch zur Erzielung eines UV-Erythems als wesentlich effektvoller als
kürzere Wellenlängenbereiche erwiesen, da erstere die Epidermis offenbar leichter
durchdringen können [1].

Eine Parallele dazu findet sich in unseren Versuchen, in denen es in keinem
Fall gelang, mit der Quarzlampe, die Wellenlängen von 2550 Å und darunter aussendet, Kinine freizusetzen. Da es auch hier nach einer Latenzperiode zur Ery-
thembildung kam, muß angenommen werden, daß die im längeren UV-Bereich ausgelöste Kininproduktion nicht als Ursache des Erythems aufzufassen ist. Dafür
spricht auch die Tatsache, daß nach der Bestrahlung mit Wellenlängen von 2550
bis 3150 Å Kinine wohl ausgeschüttet, aber nicht während der gesamten Dauer des
Erythems nachgewiesen werden können.

Über die Herkunft der beobachteten Kinine können wir derzeit keine Aussage
machen. Eine direkte Einwirkung der erythemauslösenden Strahlen auf das
cutane Gefäßsystem der Haut könnte zu einer Vasopermeabilitätsstörung und zu
einem Austritt von Alpha-2-Globulinen oder Kallikrein ins Gewebe führen. Doch
scheint es in der Latenzperiode zu keinen hochgradigen Permeabilitätsstörungen
zu kommen, wie unsere Versuche mit Evans-Blue zeigen. Andererseits könnte die
Kininproduktion auch auf eine Aktivierung des Gewebskallikreinsystems oder
eine Hemmung der Kininase zurückzuführen sein. Die früher postulierte Kininausschüttung durch neurale Faktoren oder die Schweißdrüsen scheint nach neueren
Befunden etwas in Frage gestellt [4].

Auch die Möglichkeit einer Kininbildung nach Freisetzung von Histamin ist relativ schwer zu akzeptieren, da Histamin in keinem unserer Versuche während der Latenzperiode nachgewiesen werden konnte.

Immerhin zeigen unsere Befunde, daß während der einem UV-Erythem vorausgehenden Latenzperiode Substanzen von Kinincharakter im Gewebe gebildet werden, womit auch beim Menschen der Hinweis auf eine vom Tierversuch bekannte biphasige UV-Reaktion vorliegt. Die Kininausschüttung ist vorübergehender Natur und unabhängig vom und sicher nicht verantwortlich für das UV-Erythem.

Literatur. 1. Everett, M. A., E. Yeargers, R. M. Sayre, and R. L. Olson: Photochem. Photobiol. **5**, 533 (1966). — 2. Logan, G., and D. L. Wilhelm: Brit. J. exp. Path. **47**, 286 (1966). — 3. Winkelmann, R. K.: J. invest. Derm. **46**, 220 (1966). — 4. Winkelmann, R. K.: Kinins from human skin. Medicina Cutanea (Im Druck).

Sur la réponse vasculaire biphasique au siège de l'érythème dû aux radiations ultraviolettes. Existe-t-il une réponse plus élémentaire que l'érythème?

G. Zina et A. Benedetto, Clinique Dermatologique de l'Université de Turin (Italie)

Avant-propos

1. Au XXXIXe Congrès Sides, consacré à la physiopathologie de l'inflammation cutanée, Flarer et Rabito ont conclu leur étude sur l'érythème, en envisageant la possibilité que la «latence» soit un phénomène complexe, l'expression d'une réponse plus élémentaire que l'érythème même.

2. Moyennant l'étude de la clearance cutanée du P 32, Zina et Bossi [Minerva derm **37**, 130 (1962)] ont constaté qu'au siège de l'érythème dû aux RUV de 2e degré interviennent des variations biphasiques de la clearance, qui s'expriment par un ralentissement de la vitesse d'épuration dans la phase de latence et par une accélération dans la phase d'érythème déclaré.

But de la présente recherche

Partant des points un et deux de notre avant-propos, nous avons examiné, de façon plus exhaustive, les conclusions de Zina et Bossi, afin de déterminer la reproductibilité réelle des constatations au siège de l'érythème dû aux RUV de 1er degré (E 1) et de 2e degré (E 2) et, dans la suite, d'étudier l'existence d'éventuelles variations, provoquées dans des zones cutanées stimulées par des doses subérythémigènes de RUV.

Notes sur la technique employée

Comme générateur de RUV, nous avons utilisé une lampe de quartz de 300 Watt à une distance foyer-peau de 50 cm. Comme traceuse, nous avons employé une solution de P 32 sous forme d'orthophosphate, à activé de 0,5 microcurie par mL, par injection intradermique à la dose de 0,10 mL. Les détections ont été effectuées par un compteur de Geiger-Muller, collimaté à une distance fixe de 3 cm et relié, par l'intermédiaire d'un ratemeter, à un enregistreur électromagnétique. Une fois déterminé le T $^1/_2$ nous avons calculé la clearance selon l'équation:

$$K \equiv \frac{0,693}{T\,^1/_2}.$$

Les valeurs, obtenues au siège de la stimulation des R UV, ont été mises en rapport avec celles de contrôle selon la formule

$$R = \frac{K \, RUV}{K \, Contrôle} \cdot$$

Chez huit sujets, la stimulation par RUV a été faite à des doses E 1 et E 2 et ensuite nous avons déterminé K à des distances de temps variables, depuis le moment de la stimulation, entre 30 min et 6 à 7 h. Chez quatre sujets, au contraire, nous avons déterminé K à des intervalles de temps compris entre 30 min et 6 h, au siège de la stimulation RUV par des doses nettement subérythémigènes. Chez tous les sujets, nous avons réalisé le K de contrôle dans un siège contro-latéral analogue.

Résultats

Nous avons résumé, en synthèse graphique, les données obtenues. Dans la figure, la ligne horizontale en correspondance de la valeur 1 en ordonnée correspond au point où le K au siège de la stimulation par RUV est égal à celui de contrôle. Les lignes verticales représentent les variations du rapport entre K RUV et K Contrôle aux différents temps de détermination au siège de E 1 et E 2. La bande hachurée représente les variations de la clearance au siège de la stimulation subérythémigène en fonction du temps entre stimulation et détermination de la clearance.

Il en résulte qu'au siège de la stimulation E 1 et E 2, en phase de latence, la clearance subit un ralentissement évident: s'approchant de E 1, les valeurs tendent à se reporter à proximité des valeurs de base et les dépassent ensuite, lorsque la réponse atteint, mais ne dépasse pas E 1. Au contraire, lorsque la réactivité atteint E 2, on assiste à une accélération très rapide de la clearance.

Au siège de la stimulation subérythémigène, la phase du ralentissement de la clearance apparaît prolongée et touche des valeurs fréquemment plus basses par rapport à celles au siège de E 1 et E 2, pour remonter ensuite lentement à la vitesse d'épuration de base.

Commentaire

Réserves à part sur le mécanisme, réel et intime, pathogénique des variations de la clearance, provoquées par les dommages causés par les RUV et qui peut entre autres, être attribué à un ensemble de modifications du courant hémato-lymphatique, de la perméabilité endothéliale, de l'inhibition des interstices conjonctivaux, il nous semble, de façon suffisamment fondée, pouvoir confirmer le point de vue de FLARER et RABITO. En effet, il résulte clairement, par nos recherches, que la stimulation subérythémigène due aux RUV provoque des altérations fonctionnelles évidentes, qui peuvent être considérées non plus comme un moment préparant la phase érythémateuse suivante, mais comme l'expression d'une réponse au dommage, plus simple que l'érythème lui-même.

A Cutaneous Role in the Regulation of the Body's Carbohydrate Milieu*

R. M. FUSARO and J. A. JOHNSON, Division of Dermatology, University of Minnesota Medical School, Minneapolis, Minn. (USA)

The skin constitutes about 10% of the body weight. The epidermis which has essentially no intercellular space accounts for most of the metabolic activity of the skin. The dermis is an extracellular fluid with little metabolic activity. The fluid

* Supported in part by USPHS Research Grant No. AM 03964.

volume of the dermal compartment is almost equal to that of blood plasma and is 5% of the body weight. In contrast, the dermal vascular tree accounts for less than 2% of the fluid volume of the skin. The skin can be visualized as a system of three associated compartments: 1. a small intravascular extracellular blood space, 2. a larger intracellular epidermal volume and, 3. a large fluid compartment — the "dermal ground substance sea".

Before examining the cutaneous role in the regulation of the carbohydrate milieu of the body, a few basic facts should be noted: 1. The enzymes of the EMBDEN-MEYERHOF pathway, of the hexose monophosphate (HMP) shunt, and of the Krebs cycle are present in epithelial tissue. 2. In vitro utilization of radioactive glucose by the epidermis demonstrates that 70% of glucose is converted to lactate, less than 30% is utilized via the HMP shunt, and less than 2% enters the Krebs cycle. 3. Lactate concentration of the skin of the resting animal is considerably higher than that of blood.

The metabolic activities of skeletal muscle and liver should be reviewed to evaluate their role in the body's utilization of glucose and lactate. Muscle cells exhibit a high degree of Krebs cycle activity. Muscle tissue during moderate to severe exercise utilizes glucose and releases lactate into the blood. However, resting or minimally active muscle utilizes lactate (venous levels are lower than arterial). In any case adenosine triphosphate (ATP) is required by muscle to perform contraction and synthesis of protein, and is obtainable from the oxidative phosphorylation of reduced nicotinamide adenine dinucleotide NADH (DPNH) arising from Krebs cycle activity. The muscle's ATP-producing capacity is exceeded only during periods of more than moderate muscular activity.

The liver performs not only the important functions of storing and releasing glucose according to the body's needs but also removes excess blood lactate by converting it to glucose. This conversion, coupled with the formation of lactate from glucose as a result of muscular contraction, forms the basis of the Cori lactic acid cycle.

We have developed a technique for examining rise and fall of skin glucose concentration after intravenous administration of dextrose to fasting humans. After a postinjection lag of 30 to 35 min skin glucose concentration reaches a maximum and thereafter decreases in a first-order decay manner. Assuming that skin mass is 10% of body weight and using the maximum skin glucose levels attained after injection of a known amount of glucose, we have found that approximately 20% of the injected dextrose (over a range of 35 to 45 g) is absorbed by the skin. Our data therefore indicate that the skin performs an important physiologic function as a temporary reservoir for excess blood glucose.

There are three possible fates for excess dermal glucose: 1. diffuse back into the blood; 2. flow back to the blood via the lymphatic system; 3. enter the epithelial intracellular compartment (see illustration). With respect to the first route, postinjection blood glucose normally decreases more rapidly than skin glucose levels; a point is reached during the test when skin glucose concentration is greater than blood glucose concentration. Our experimental data show that dermal extracellular glucose and dermal lymphatic glucose reach maximum concentration at the same time. Both take several (3 to 4) hours to return to normal prefasting levels. In contrast excess blood glucose levels return to fasting levels within $1^1/_2$ h. The second route in the skin thus balances the blood glucose levels also, as does the first route, but the second is out of phase with the first and occurs later.

The third possible route of excess skin glucose (entrance into the cell and conversion to lactate) has not to our knowledge been studied in vivo. The epidermis exfoliates at such a rate that it reproduces itself in less than 3 weeks. This energyrequiring synthesis necessitates the production of large quantities of ATP. Since the Krebs cycle is largely inoperative in skin, the efficient mechanism involving oxidative phosphorylation of NADH is not available for ATP production. The skin must rely on the substrate-level phosphorylation steps of the EMBDEN-MEYERHOF pathway for ATP production. Therefore it is likely that the skin converts large quantities of glucose to lactate in order to provide the necessary energy for its epidermal regeneration. A natural extension of this hypothesis is that skin lactate diffuses freely into the blood and is converted back to glucose by the liver. Thus one postulates a continuous "skin Cori cycle" (see illustration — Cycle II) which offers the concept that skin is provided not only with an adequate means of producing ATP, but with an additional mechanism for control of elevated blood glucose; that is, the conversion to lactate in the skin and transformation of the lactate to glucose in the liver where it can be stored as glycogen. Consideration of the "Skin Glucose-Lactic Acid Cycle (II)" (see illustration), suggests a mechanism whereby skin can play an active role in the removal of excess blood glucose. This concept also provides an economical means for skin to produce ATP via an otherwise inefficient glycolytic sequence. The illustration demonstrates our concepts of the role of skin in glucose and lactate homeostasis.

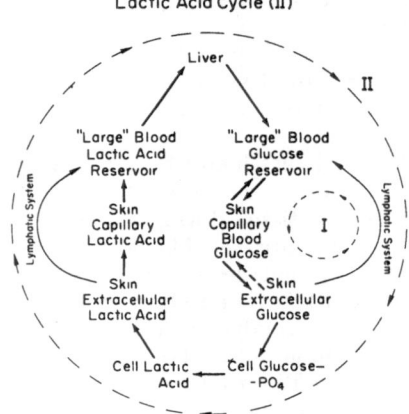

Skin Glucose Cycle (I) and Skin Glucose-Lactic Acid Cycle (II)

In conclusion, the skin has long been ignored as a factor in the maintenance of the carbohydrate milieu of the body. The size of this organ, the amount of a blood glucose load which it absorbs, and the necessity of the skin to produce ATP by an inefficient, nonoxidative mechanism suggest that the skin is of major importance in the maintenance of blood carbohydrate levels.

Research on Sialic Acid in the Human Skin*

A. GIANNETTI and G. RABBIOSI, University of Pavia, Dermatological Clinic, Pavia (Italy)

It is a well known fact that sialic acid is a component of various mucoproteins in higher animals. This has been shown in organic liquids [1, 2, 3, 4], in different secretions [5, 6, 7], parenchymas [8, 9, 10] and connective tissues. Among the last, its presence has been noted in the epiphyseal cartilage of young rabbits and pigs, in the costal cartilage of the rabbit, and in the aorta, cornea, bone, bovine dentine and pulp tissue [11]. From some of these tissues (aorta [12, 13], human cartilage [14], bovine bone [15]), the glycoprotein, containing sialic acid, has also been isolated.

* Supported in part by C.N.R. (contract 115/633/461).

As regards the skin, the only data so far published refer to glycoproteins isolated in the dermis of higher animals [16, 17, 18]. No research has been conduced, to our knowledge, on the sialo-proteins of the human dermis.

Since sialic acid is always present in the glucidic part in all glycoprotein extracted from the connective tissues, we thought that by demonstrating the presence of sialic acid in the dermis, we would have been able to prove the presence of a glycoprotein there also. With the Svennerholm method [8] executed on the homogenate of skin taken from different areas (abdomen, back of hand, nape, scalp) of individuals of varying ages, we showed that sialic acid is present in all the regions of skin examined, and that its quantity varies in direct relation to region and age.

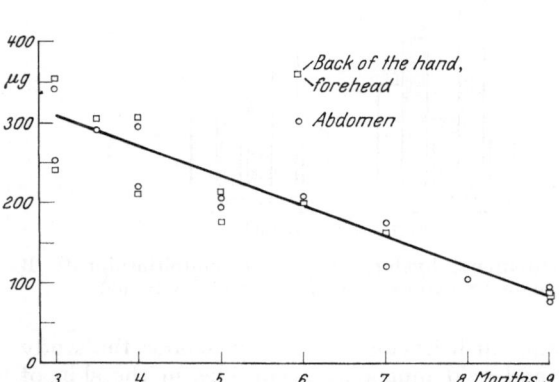

Fig. 1. Sialic acid content decrease in foetal skin with age. (The data are expressed in γ/100 mg of dry tissue)

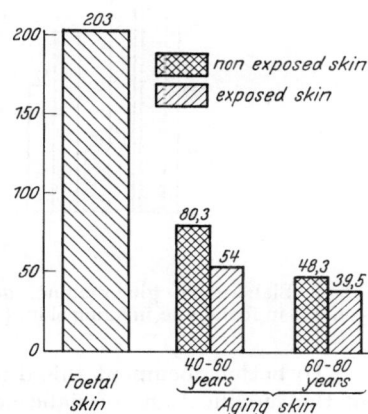

Fig. 2. Sialic acid content in foetal and in aging skin. (The data are expressed in γ/100 mg of dry tissue)

To be more precise about the entity of these differences and to study, analogously to our studies on the acid mucopolysaccharides, the importance of ecological factors (excluding those constitutional ones), we extended our research to the skin of the fetus and the adult of different ages, comparing, in each case studied, data obtained on skin taken from the abdomen, forehead, and back of hand and nape.

In Fig. 1 results are illustrated of observations made on twelve fetuses varying on age from 3 to 9 months. While there exists a certain variability from case to case, a higher concentration of sialic acid is evident in fetuses of 3 and 4 months of age, with a progressive reduction up until the 9th month. Comparing data obtained in the fetuses from 3 to 5 months of age with those of from 6 to 9 months, we encountered, in the skin of the abdomen, a significant difference ($P = 0.001$); in the skin of the back of the hand and forehead, the value is $P = 0.02$. It is important to take careful note of the fact that comparison between data of the different skin regions did not reveal any significant differences.

The study of cutaneous sialic acid, in the postnatal age covered subjects varying in age from 40 to 80 years (Fig. 2). Whether in areas where the skin is unexposed or exposed, the sialic acid content diminishes with the advancing of age. This phenomenon is well-documented and significant as regards the unexposed skin. For the areas of exposed skin, results are equally clear, even though our data are presently insufficient to illustrate their true significance. It is interesting to note that the determination of sialic acid in the exposed and unexposed areas in all subjects examined in which comparison was made, shows that the quantity of sialic acid is distinctly lower in the regions of exposed skin. This fact is in contrast with what has been noted regarding the behavior of the acid mucopolysaccharides that are present in higher concentration in exposed skin with respect to unexposed skin [19, 20, 21, 22, 23, 24] (see Fig. 3).

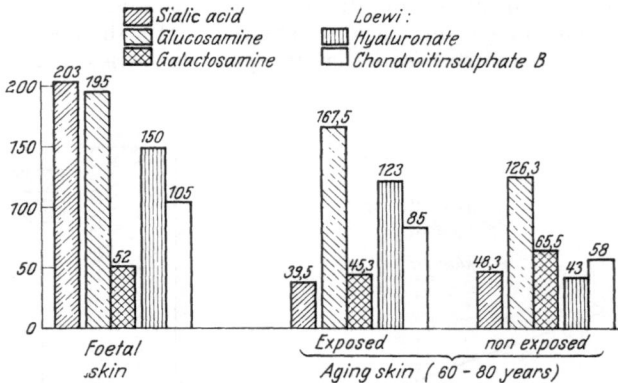

Fig. 3. Sialic acid, glucosamine, galactosamine, hyaluronate and chondroitinsulphate B content in foetal and in aging skin. (The data are expressed in γ/100 mg of dry tissue)

To better document this difference in behavior, we have in course the study of the modifications of sialic acid and acid mucopolysaccharides in the skin of animals when exposed to various types of radiation.

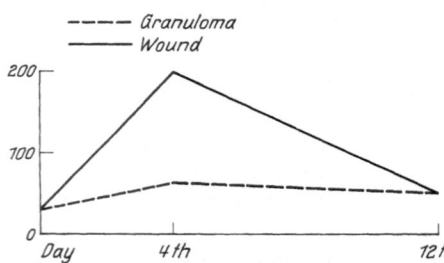

Fig. 4. Sialic acid content in skin wound healing and in the granulation tissue of cottongranuloma at the 4th and the 12th day in 1 year old rats. (The data are expressed in γ/100 mg of dry tissue)

The results of the research on the fetus confirm that the differences encountered in the adult's unexposed and exposed skin are not tied to a constitutional factor, but depend on ecological factors. The reduction of sialic acid with the advancement of fetal age would not verify itself only in the dermic tissue (25). The higher concentrations in the first months of fetal life could be justified by a greater metabolic requirement of youthful tissue with respect to that of the adult and the aged, where said tissue has reached its definitive structure.

In attempting to confirm this hypothesis, we studied the behavior of sialic acid in two tissues with extremely rapid metabolic exchange: the cotton-granuloma and the skin-wound healing tissue. Research was carried out on 1 year-old rats, taking the granulation tissue on the 4th and 12th days to pick up, in their most typical manifestations, the exudative-proliferative phase and the regenerative phase of the wound-healing tissue, and respectively, the most active metabolic moment, and the moment of the definitive balance of the granuloma. Results obtained are shown in Fig. 4. The increase of sialic acid is evident in both experimental conditions on the 4th day, as well as its fall on the 12th day, though at this point remaining in greater concentration than during basal conditions. In the wound-healing tissue, the increase of sialic acid on the 4th day is much greater than that observed in the granuloma and consequently, its fall on the 12th day is that much more evident. The distinct increase in sialic acid content in both experimental conditions shows that the connective tissues in rapid metabolic transformation, such as those of granulation, are characterized by an elevated concentration of sialic acid. In can be allowed, therefore, to consider exact the interpretation we put forth justifying the high sialic acid values in the skin of the fetus.

To demonstrate the validity of the aforesaid concept, on which all our observations are based, and that is that sialic acid in the dermis is an indicator of the presence of glycoproteins, it was indispensable to advance to the extraction of the sialoprotein of the human skin.

For this scope, we preferred to utilize the skin of the fetus, due to its greater richness in sialic acid with respect to that of the adult. Availing ourselves of the method that FISHKIN and BERENSON [26] used to isolate the glycoprotein from the turpentine granuloma, we succeeded in precipitating a substance from the skin homogenate that, at first analyses, results to be rich in sialic acid and in hexosamine and poor in uronic acids. We think, therefore, that it is actually a glycoprotein. We have in course purification procedures by means of starch gel electrophoresis, and expect to effect the analyses for characterizing it in the briefest time possible.

Bibliography. 1. WINZLER, R. J.: In: The Plasma Proteins (F. W. PUTNAM, ed.) Vol. 1, p. 309. New York: Academic Press 1960. — 2. ODIN, L.: Nature (Lond.) **170**, 663 (1952). — 3. BALAZS, E. A., and L. SUNDBLAD: J. biol. Chem. **235**, 1973 (1960). — 4. BALAZS, E. A., and R. W. JEANLOZ: The Amino Sugars. Vol. II/A. New York and London: Academic Press 1965. — 5. DISCHE, Z., P. DI SANT'AGNESE, C. PALLAVICINI, and J. YOULOS: Arch. Biochem. **84**, 205 (1959). — 6. GIBBONS, R. A.: Biochem. J. **73**, 209 (1959). — 7. MANDEL, I. D., and S. A. ELLISON: Ann. N.Y. Acad. Sci. **106**, 271 (1963). — 8. SVENNERHOLM, L.: Acta chem. scand. **12**, 547 (1958). — 9. ODIN, L., and N. TÖRNBLOM: Acta Soc. Med. upsalien **64**, 313 (1959). — 10. DISCHE, Z., G. ZELMENIS, and N. LARYS: Invest. Ophthal. **2**, 630 (1963). — 11. CASTELLANI, A.: Boll. Soc. ital. Biol. sper. **35**, 2145 (1959). — 12. BERTELSEN, S.: Nature (Lond.) **187**, 411 (1960). — 13. BUDDECKE, E.: Z. physiol. Chem. **318**, 33 (1960). — 14. ANDERSON, A. J.: Biochem. J. **82**, 372 (1962). — 15. HERRING, G. M., and P. M. KENT: Biochem. J. **89**, 405 (1963). — 16. BOSE, S. M.: Biochim. biophys. Acta (Amst.) **74**, 265 (1963). — 17. BOURRILLON, R., and R. GOTT: Biochim. biophys. Acta (Amst.) **58**, 63 (1962). — 18. BERENSON, G. S., and A. F. FISHKIN: Arch. Biochem. **97**, 18 (1962). — 19. SERRI, F., H. L. SPERANZA e H. MESCON: Boll. Soc. ital. Biol. sper. **38**, 1390 (1962). — 20. LOEWI, G.: Biochim. biophys. Acta (Amst.) **52**, 435 (1961). — 21. SOBEL, H.: J. Geront. **14**, 496 (1959). — 22. CLAUSEN, B.: Lab. Invest. **2**, 229 (1962). — 23. SWITH, J. G.: J. Soc. Cosmetic Chemists **16**, 527 (1965). — 24. RABBIOSI, G., e. A. GIANNETTI: Atti Convegni Farmitalia Ed. Minerva med. **1967**, 115. — 25. BOLOGNANI, L., R. CALDERA, and A. DE LUIGI: Exc. Med. Internat. Congr. — Series N. 120 — Fourth European Symposium on Calcified Tissues, Leiden 1966. — 26. FISHKIN, A. F., and G. S. BERENSON: Arch. Biochem. **95**, 130 (1961).

Mepyramine and Adrenergic Neurone

B. S. VERMA and O. D. GULATI, Departments of Dermatology and Pharmacology, Medical College and S.S.G. Hospital, Baroda (India)

Both an inhibition and a potentiation of the peripheral actions of adrenaline and noradrenaline have been described following the administration of antihistaminics [1, 2, 3, 4, 5, 6, 7]. Of particular interest however, are the observations of STONE et al. [8] and GOKHALE et al. [9] who reported that antihistaminics partially reversed the sympathetic nerve blocking action of guanethidine. In view of the frequent and common use of antihistaminics and of guanethidine in therapeutics it was of interest to examine this relationship in animal experiments and in human subjects. In this paper the adrenergic neurone blocking action of mepyramine and its antagonism of guanethidine was investigated in dogs and human subjects.

Methods

Experimental: Femoral arterial blood pressure of pentobarbitalized mongrel dogs weighing 8 to 18 kg was recorded by means of a mercury manometer. For eliciting response of blood pressure to carotid occlusion common carotid arteries were occluded simultaneously by means of artery clips for a period of 40 sec (CO_1) and 2 min (CO_2). Responses of retractor penis in situ were recorded in pentobarbitalized dogs according to the method described by LUDUENA [10]. The peripheral and of the cut lumbar sympathetic nerve was stimulated with rectangular pulses by means of bipolar electrodes (10 v, 0.3 msec duration and 20/sec frequency).

Human: 45 patients of both sexes (19 to 62 years) who attended the Dermatology Clinic of Shree Sayaji General Hospital for allergic skin conditions but whose routine clinical examination revealed no other abnormality were subjected to cold pressor test before any treatment was instituted. They immersed both hands in ice cold water at 6 °C for 1 min. Blood pressure in the sitting position was recorded before and thrice during the period of immersion. The mean of the three readings was taken as the cold pressor effect. Subjects who showed a rise of diastolic pressure of 20 mm Hg or more were selected for the study.

Results and Discussion

Experimental: In dogs intravenous injection of 5 mg/kg guanethidine caused a brief initial fall of blood pressure followed by a marked and sustained rise. 40 min after the administration of guanethidine, the blood pressure had returned to its original level, the pressor responses to bilateral carotid occlusion were

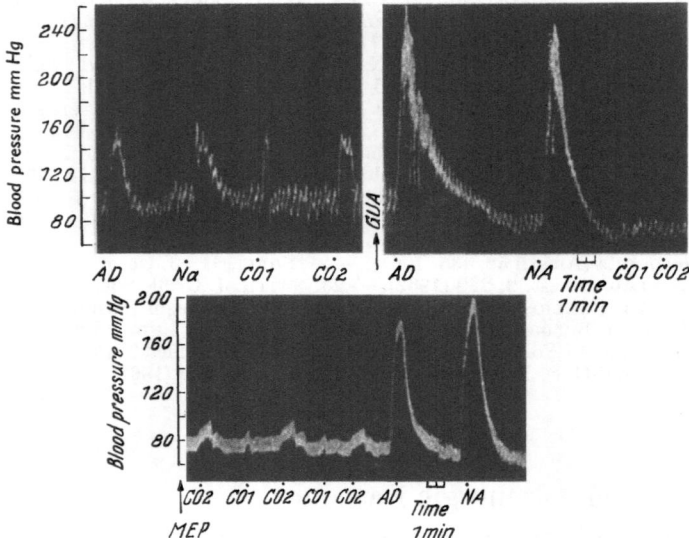

Fig. 1. Partial reversal of the blocking action of guanethidine (GUA) by mepyramine (MEP)

almost totally abolished (for 3 to 4 h) and pressor effects of adrenaline and noradrenaline were potentiated (for 3 to 4 h). Mepyramine (5 mg/kg) produced a brief depressor effect. 40 to 60 min after the injection of mepyramine the pressor effects of bilateral carotid occlusion were partially restored and potentiation of amine responses by guanethidine was somewhat reduced (Fig. 1). Mepyramine (5 mg/kg and 10 mg/kg) inhibited the response of the dog retractor penis to indirect stimulation (Fig. 2) in five of seven experiments. In the other two preparations the responses to indirect stimulation were slightly potentiated. This preparation was almost invariably more sensitive to exogenously administered adrenaline than to noradrenaline (Fig. 3). The responses to amines (1 μg/kg, 2 μg/kg, 4 μg/kg and 6 μg/kg) were potentiated by mepyramine in six of seven

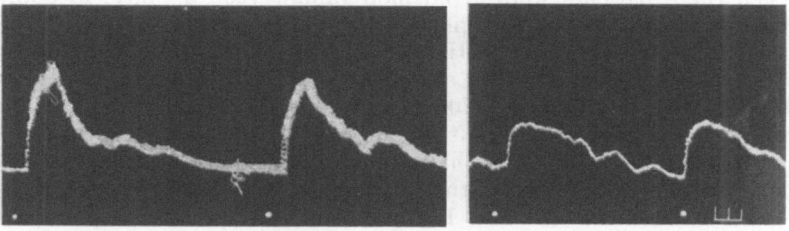

Fig. 2. Partial blockade by mepyramine of the responses of dog retractor penis to indirect stimulation (at dots). Left panel-control responses and right panel-responses after mepyramine. Time mark — 1 min

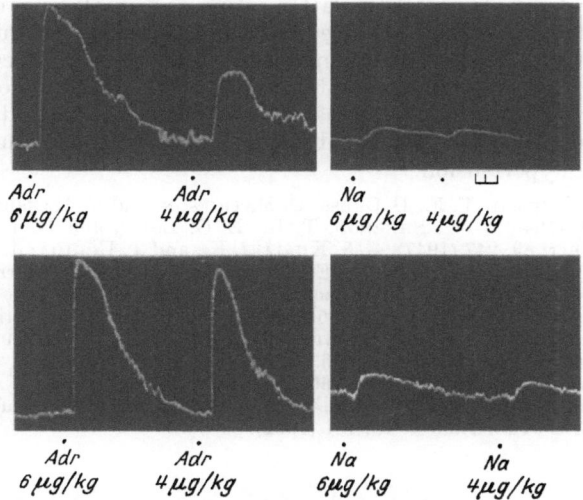

Fig. 3. Potentiation of pressor responses to adrenaline and noradrenaline by mepyramine. Upper panel — control responses and lower panel — responses after mepyramine. Time mark — 1 min

preparations. Responses to adrenaline were potentiated more than those to noradrenaline (Fig. 3). The blocking action of mepyramine could, therefore, be due to a possible bretylium-like adrenergic neurone blocking action of mepyramine.

Human: In 20 cases the mean cold pressor response before mepyramine was 20.6 ± 0.32 mm Hg. After a 2 week course of mepyramine (200 mg/day) the cold pressor response was significantly (p < 0.01) reduced; the mean value after treatment was 13.0 ± 0.8 mm Hg. As in the case of dog experiments the block was not complete indicating that in man and dog mepyramine exerts only a mild adrenergic neurone blocking action. In the five patients who received mepyramine (200 mg/day) for 2 weeks the pressor response to an intravenous infusion of noradrenaline

(4 μg/min) was not altered. Thus the effect of mepyramine in blocking cold pressor response could not have been due to interference with the action of the released adrenergic transmitter. Mepyramine could both prevent and reverse the blocking action of guanethidine on the cold pressor response. In ten patients the mean cold pressor response before treatment with guanethidine was 22.1 ± 0.7 mm Hg. A 2 week course of guanethidine (10 mg/day) resulted in an almost total blockade of the cold pressor effect. The mean value after guanethidine being 1.3 ± 0.35 mm Hg. When these patients were given mepyramine (200 mg/day) in addition to guanethidine for 7 days the cold pressor effect was partially restored; the mean value now being 8.4 ± 0.65 mm Hg. In a group of ten patients the mean cold pressor response at the start of the study was 22.8 ± 1.08 mm Hg. These patients were treated with mepyramine (200 mg/day) for 7 days. This was followed by guanethidine (10 mg/kg) for 2 weeks. Redetermination of the cold pressor response at the end of this period showed that guanethidine had not exerted its usual full blocking effect. The mean value of the cold pressor response at this time was 10.6 ± 1.1 mm Hg. The almost total block of the cold pressor response followed guanethidine observed in human subjects accords well with results of dog experiments. In view of the mild adrenergic nerve blocking action of mepyramine in dog and man the antagonism of the blocking action of guanethidine by mepyramine could be interpreted in terms of the latter acting as a weak or partial agonist. A similar explanation has been advanced for the antagonism of guanethidine by dexamphetamine [9, 11]. Antihistaminics are perhaps the most commonly used drugs in therapeutics. Interference by these drugs with the action of guanethidine which is a well established and valuable antihypertensive agent would enjoin caution in the use of mepyramine like drugs in patients who are being treated with guanethidine for hypertension.

References. 1. YONKMAN, F. F., D. CHESS, D. MATHIESON, and N. HANSEN: J. Pharmacol. exp. Ther. 87, 256 (1946). — 2. SHERROD, T. R., E. G. LOEW, and H. F. SCHLOEMER: J. Pharmacol. exp. Ther. 89, 247 (1947). — 3. KURIAKI, K., and T. UCHIDA: J. Pharmacol. exp. Ther. 113, 228 (1955). — 4. CHEN, G., R. C. ENSOR, and I. G. CLARK: J. Pharmacol. exp. Ther. 92, 90 (1948). — 5. LEHMAN, G.: J. Pharmacol. exp. Ther. 92, 249 (1948). — 6. BURN, J. H., and N. K. DUTTA: Brit. J. Pharmacol. 3, 354 (1948). — 7. INNES, I. R.: Brit. J. Pharmacol. 13, 6 (1958). — 8. STONE, C. A., C. C. PORTER, J. M. STAVORSKI, C. T. LUDDEN, and J. A. TORARO: J. Pharmacol. exp. Ther. 144, 196 (1964). — 9. GOKHALE, S. D., O. D. GULATI et B. P. UDWADIA: Arch. int. Pharmacodyn. 160, 32 (1966). — 10. LUDUENA, F. P.: In: Methods in Medical Research, ed. by H. D. BRUNER, p. 169. Chicago: Year Book Publishers 1960. — 11. DAY, M. D.: Brit. J. Pharmacol. 18, 421 (1962).

Lysosomes and the Skin

R. L. OLSON, R. NORDQUIST, J. NORDQUIST and M. A. EVERETT, Department of Dermatology, University of Oklahoma Medical Center, Oklahoma City, Oklahoma (USA)

Lysosomes are single membrane-bound intracytoplasmic organelles containing many acid-active enzymes [1, 2]. One of these enzymes, acid phosphatase, is used to identify lysosomes histochemically [3]. Lysosomal function is related to cellular

Fig. 1. Epidermal cell in tissue culture containing ferritin. Pinocytotic vesicles (P) containing ferritin enter epidermal cell and merge to form multivesicular body (MV)

Fig. 2. Epidermal cells 1 h after intradermal injection of ferritin. Pinocytotic vesicles (P) containing ferritin entering epidermal cell through intercellular space

Fig. 3. Epidermal cell 1 h after intradermal injection of ferritin. Phagosomes containing ferritin and melanosomes (M)

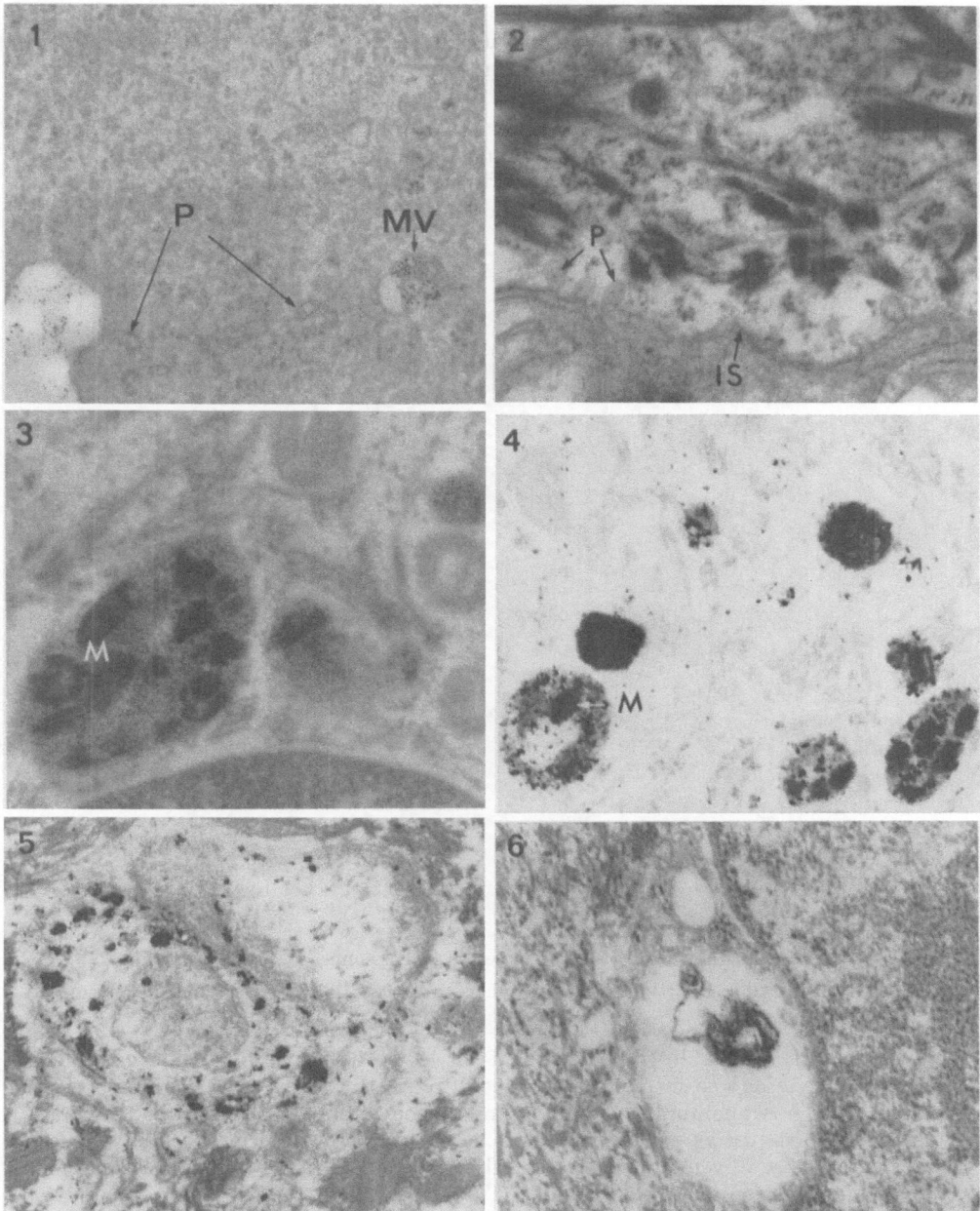

Fig. 1—3 (for Legends see page 1056)

Fig. 4. Acid phosphatase reaction normal skin. Reaction product is present on phagosomes containing melanosomes (M)

Fig. 5. Acid phosphatase reaction 24 h after ultraviolet light exposure. Reaction product is present on cytolysosome containing a degenerating mitochondrion

Fig. 6. Acid phosphatase reaction 24 h after ultraviolet light. Residual body

ingestion (pinocytosis and phagocytosis) digestion, and autolysis. The cell is ordinarily protected from lysosomal enzymes by a surrounding, semi-impermeable, lipoprotein membrane. If the cell is injured however, labilization of these membranes and release of enzymes may occur resulting in inflammation.

Several types of lysosomes are observed within epidermal cells. When substances enter the cell, they may be engulfed by infolding of the cell membrane. This process is known as *pinocytosis*. Within 1 h after intradermal injection of ferritin, the particles are seen throughout the intercellular circulation [4]. Ferritin

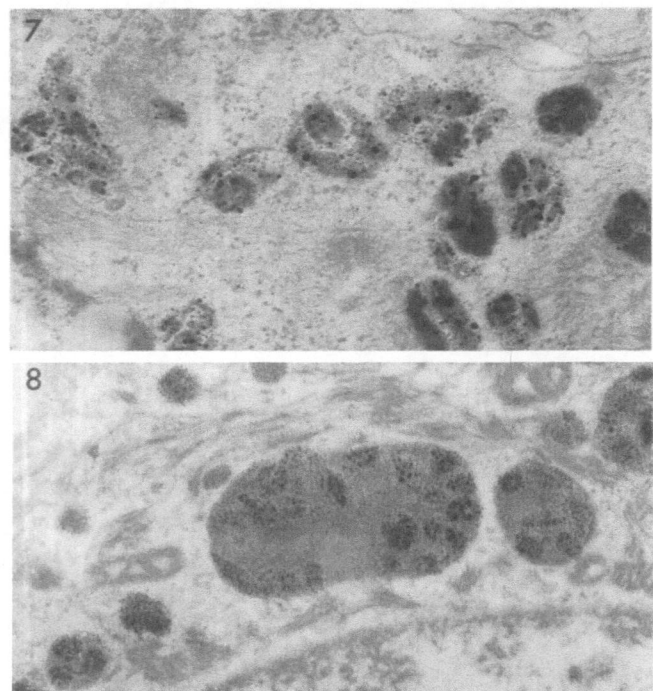

Fig. 7. PASM reaction. Reaction product is present in lysosomes containing melanin

Fig. 8. PASM reaction. Reaction product in phagosome containing ferritin and melanosomes

enters epidermal cells by pinocytosis at all levels of the living epidermis. The pinocytotic vesicles so formed merge, resulting in the formation of larger bodies (Figs. 1, 2). Those membrane bound organelles containing aggregates of exogenous material are known as *phagosomes* (Figs. 3, 4). When normal intracellular structures are enclosed by membranes and subjected to acid hydrolase digestion, *cytolysomes* (autophagic vacuoles) result. This type of organelle is prominent in tissues undergoing rapid differentiation, during starvation or following sublethal cell injury. *Residual bodies* result from the accumulation of materials not degraded by the acid hydrolases present within lysosomes (Figs. 5, 6).

By light microscopy, periodic acid-Schiff (PAS) positive granules appear in basal cell cytoplasm 12 h following UV [5]. These granules, presumed to be glycogen, are found principally in a supranuclear location — as is melanin. 72 h following UV, PAS positive granules are found predominately in the mid-

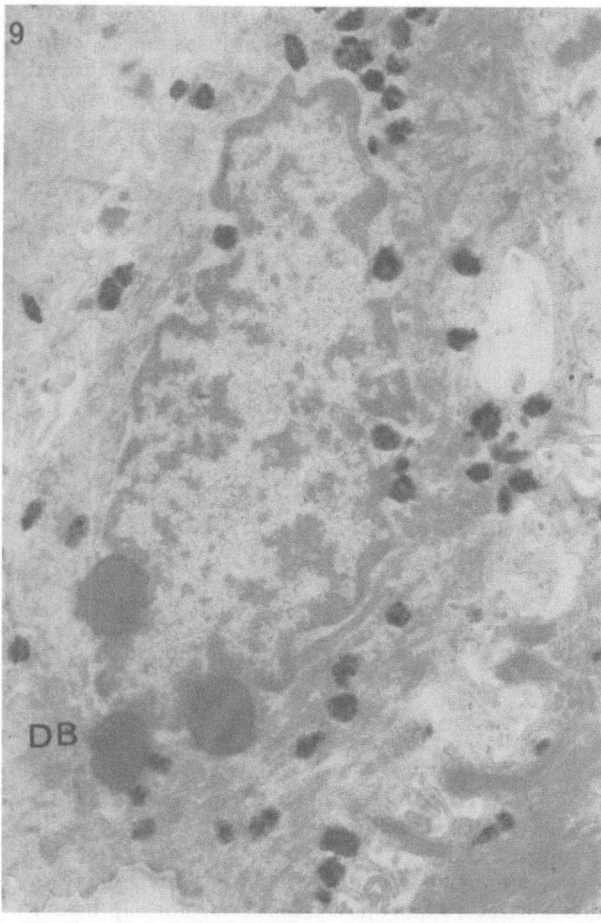

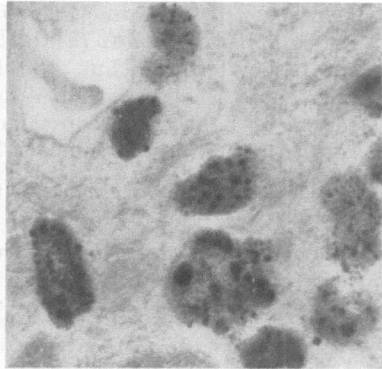

Fig. 9a. Higher magnification of supranuclear cap

Fig. 9. PASM reaction 12 h after ultraviolet light. Basal cell with many PASM positive granules. Dense body (DB)

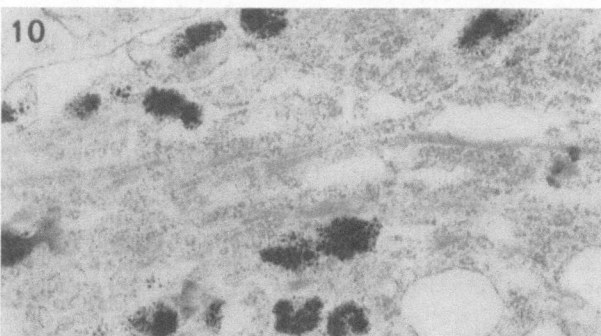

Fig. 10. PASM reaction 72 h after ultraviolet light. PASM granules are predominately within the mid-epidermis

spinous layer. A variant of the PAS reaction — periodic acid silver methenamine [6] (PASM) — may be employed for the identification of glycogen and neutral polysaccharides by electron microscopy. However, PASM stains melanin as well as glycogen and neutral polysaccharides. PASM material occurs within lysosomes together with melanin (Figs. 7, 8). 12 h after UV, PASM granules are predominately in basal cells. At 72 h PASM granules are predominately in lysosomes within the midepidermis. Thus, the PASM response to UV observed by the electron microscope is anatomically and temporarily analogous to the PAS response observed by light microscopy. However, by electron microscopy these granules are seen to be within lysosomes (Figs. 9, 9a, 10).

This work supported in part by the Atomic Energy Commission Grant No. AT — (40-1) — 3578 and American Cancer Society Grant No. E-450.

References. 1. DE REUCK, A. V. S., and M. P. ČAMERON: (eds.): Lysosomes. Boston: Little, Brown and Co. 1963. — 2. WEISSMAN, G.: New Engl. J. Med. **273**, 1084 (1965). — 3. OLSON, R. L., and R. E. NORDQUIST: J. invest. Derm. **46**, 431 (1966). — 4. NORDQUIST, R. E., R. L. OLSON, and M. A. EVERETT: Arch. Derm. **94**, 482 (1966). — 5. DANIELS, jr., F., D. BROPHY, and W. C. LOBITZ jr.: J. invest. Derm. **37**, 351 (1961). — 6. MOVAT, H. Z.: Amer. J. clin. Path. **35**, 528 (1961).

Modificaciones clínicas e histológicas de la reacción tuberculínica bajo la acción local del valerato de betametasona en cura oclusiva

A. CASALÁ, C. BIANCHI, O. BIANCHI, S. STRINGA y O. ROQUÉ, Policlin. Avellaneda, Buenos Aires (Argentina)

Se ha demostrado que los corticoides administrados por vía general o local provocan modificaciones en el tejido conectivo. Estas alteraciones han sido observadas en el tejido conectivo adulto normal, en el conectivo embrionario y en distintos procesos patológicos tales como los queloides, tejido de granulación y la fibrohialinosis de la esclerodermia [1, 2]. Dichas modificaciones consisten en una acción regresiva sobre las células y demás componentes del tejido conectivo. Además es conocida la acción vasoconstrictora que ejercen los corticoides aplicados sobre la piel [3] y los efectos inhibitorios que provocan sobre los fenómenos de hipersensibilidad inmediata [4]. Basados en estos hechos, se estudió la acción del valerato de betametasona sobre una reacción de hipersensibilidad retardada.

Material y métodos

Se estudiaron 15 enfermas mujeres entre 30 y 50 años de edad sensibles a la tuberculina a las cuales se les inyectó $^1/_{20}$ ml de solución de tuberculina bruta al $^1/_{10.000}$ en suero fisiológico en tres sitios del antebrazo (A.B.C). En el sitio A se aplicó una crema de valerato de betametasona al 0.1%; en el sitio B la misma crema al 0,05% y el sitio C se lo utilizó como control. Las enfermas se dividieron en tres grupos. En el grupo 1 se aplicó la medicación durante cinco días previos a la inyección de tuberculina; en el grupo 2 el corticoide se aplicó después de la inyección. La crema de valerato betametasona fué colocada bajo cura oclusiva con polietileno, siendo renovada la medicación cada 12 horas.

Como control del efecto del polietileno en otras cinco enfermas se lo aplicó directamente sobre la reacción tuberculínica realizándose el estudio histológico correspondiente.

Resultados

En todos los casos pudo apreciarse una neta disminución de la intensidad de la reacción tuberculínica en los sitios tratados con valerato de betametasona. Comparativamente con los controles se observó macroscópicamente:

1. Desaparición del eritema periférico.
2. Menor diámetro de la pápula.
3. Disminución de la infiltración.
4. Ausencia de vesiculización.

La histología evidenció:
1. Disminución de la congestión vascular.
2. Disminución de los infiltrados dérmicos en particular de los polimorfo-
   nucleares neutrófilos.
3. Desaparición de los fenómenos purpúricos.
4. Desaparición del edema dérmico e hipodérmico superficial.
5. Ausencia de vesiculización.
6. No hubo modificaciones en los fenómenos histológicos de la hipodermis
   profunda.

Los resultados fueron semejantes en los tres grupos de enfermas. Tampoco
se notó diferencia entre la acción de las dos concentraciones usadas (0,1 y 0,05%).
El polietileno aplicado directamente sobre la reacción de Mantoux no la modificó.

Comentarios

Numerosos trabajos han demostrado que los esteroides administrados por
boca o aplicados localmente disminuyen los infiltrados celulares y el edema [5]
de las lesiones inflamatorias. Además, Juhlin nota inhibición de las respuestas
vasculares de la piel a la histamina, serotonina, metacolina y trafuril que atribuye
a un efecto vasoconstrictor del corticoide en aplicación local [6].

MANCINI y col. [4] estudiaron el efecto que estas substancias producen sobre
las reacciones de hipersensibilidad inmediata. Histológicamente observaron
disminución de la congestión vascular, del edema y de los infiltrados. En cuanto a
los fenómenos de hipersensibilidad retardada, nuestros resultados demuestran que
el valerato de betametasona es capaz de inhibir el eritema periférico, disminuir el
diámetro de la reacción y de su infiltración y evitar la vesiculización.

Desde el punto de vista histológico es evidente la acción inhibitoria de la
congestión vascular, edema, vesiculización, infiltrados celulares y leucocitarios y de
los fenómenos purpúricos. Este efecto se observó especialmente en la dermis y en la
hipodermis superior lo que evidencia que el corticoide penetra hasta este nivel.

Bibliografía. 1. MANCINI, R. E., S. G. STRINGA and L. CANEPA: J. invest. Derm. **34**, 393
(1960). — 2. TAUBENHAUS, M.: Ann. N.Y. Acad. Sci. **56**, 666 (1953). — 3. McKENZIE, A. W.,
and R. B. STOUGHTON: Arch. Derm. **86**, 608 (1962). — 4. MANCINI, R. E., P. A. COLOMBI,
H. GALLI and L. ORCIUOLI: J. Allergy **32**, 471 (1961). — 5. MOON, V. H., and G. A. TERSHA-
KOVEC: Proc. Soc. exp. Biol. (N.Y.) **79**, 63 (1952). — 6. JUHLIN, L.: Acta derm.-venereol
(Stockh.) **44**, 322 (1964).

The Significance of Low Serum Iron Levels in the Causation of Itching

I. B. SNEDDON, Sheffield, and M. GARRETTS, Manchester (England)

Following the suggestion by one of us (Dr. I. B. S), that pruritus might be
related to low serum iron levels, a group of patients have been studied in whom the
association between the low serum Iron level and cutaneous itching seems to be
causal. These cases are characterised by the occurrence of itching, widespread or
localised, in patients who on estimation show a low serum Iron Level. The haemoglobin levels found in this group have been low in some, normal in others, while in

an interesting pair of patients with Polycythaemia RUBRA VERA, the haemoglobin has been abnormally high. In all, the response to treatment designed to
raise the serum Iron Level has been uniformly good. The response to treatment
has been too rapid for the raising of the haemoglobin level, where this has been low
initially, to be responsible for the disappearance of the itching. The level of serum
iron at which itching has been present has been in all cases below that recognised
as the usual normal level. The serum Iron Level at which itching has disappeared
has not been constant. In very low initial levels, itching has disappeared when the
serum Iron Level has been raised to levels which have been low enough to produce
itching in other cases, these latter cases seemingly requiring even greater raising of
the serum Iron Levels to effect relief of symptoms.

Except for some two cases of Infantile Eczema in Jamaican children, and a
young woman with anaemia of pregnancy, all the patients have been over 50 years
of age.

Table of Clinical Data

Case No.	Initials.	Sex	Age	Clinical state and cause if known	Initial Serum Fe.	Post Treatment Serum Fe.	Initial Hb-%
1	C. L.	♀	18	Pregnancy — Diffuse itching.	32	—	69
2	W. E.	♂	66	Post Gastrectomy Generalised pruritus	40	—	81
3	M. F.	♀	76	Anaemia Gen. pruritus	60	—	86
4	J. M.	♂	69	Peptic ulcer + Haematemesis + Generalised Pruritus	54	—	64
5	D. S.	♀	68	Hiatus hernia + Melaena	30	—	64
6	P. G.	♂	76	Post gastrectomy + Gen. Pruritus	35	—	93
7	F. G.	♂	62	Generalised Pruritus	52	116	89
8	A. L. P.	♂	64	Psoriasis + Itching	45	92	116
9	G. D.	♀♂	72	Generalised Pruritus	40	150	72
10	J. W.	♂	75	Itching of legs	58	90	110
11	W. P.	♂	62	Itching of shoulders	68	120	98
12	E. P.	♂	82	Itching of legs + Eczema	60	135	98
13	I. F.	♀	53	Lichen sclerosus + itching and anaemia	10	70	68
14	M. M.	♀	53	Neurotic excoriations	70	124	114
15	L. R.	♂	64	Gastrectomy + Megaloblastic anaemia + Generalised itching	40	126	60
16	D. B.	♀	86	Senile Pruritus	45	112	96
17	A. 1.	♂	63	Polycythaemia Rubra Vera	35	78	118
18	A. 2.	♂	58	Polycythaemia Rubra Vera	24	64	128
19	B. 1.	♂	1½	Infantile eczema	35	70	62
20	B. 2.	♂	3	Infantile eczema	25	78	58

Discussion. 20 cases are described in whom the relief of itching was related to a
rise in the serum iron level. Iron deficiency without anaemia has been described by
FIELDING, O'SHAUGHNESSY, and BRUNSTROM (1965). TSUCHIDA (1964) has shown
a correlation between the serum Iron Level and the health of the duodenal mucosa.
TURNBULL (1965) has demonstrated the decreased adsorbtion of radio iron after
Polya gastrectomy. HARD (1963) has shown non anaemic iron deficiency to be a
factor in diffuse loss of hair in young women. Patients have been described in
whom Psoriasis seemed to be related to a lowering of the serum calcium level
(SNEDDON, 1958), and in whom generalised eczema was related to lowering of
serum calcium level, (GARRETTS, and DENT, 1960). This communication suggests
that in certain patients, a lowering of the serum Iron level is responsible for the

onset of pruritus. Various itching states have been associated with low serum Iron levels from a variety of causes. All have shown a remarkable clinical response to treatment designed to raise the serum Iron Level.

Conclusion. Whereas the onset of itching in a patient over 50 years of age may have serious significance such as the occurrence of a neoplasia or reticulosis, some such cases may be suffering from a low serum Iron Level. This should be considered in cases with known Iron deficiency anaemia, and looked for in patients who have scars on the abdomen showing past gastric surgery. Treatment is successful, though in cases where malabsorption is the cause, treatment may have to be lifelong and the parenteral routes may be necessary for administration.

Bibliography. FIELDING, J., M. C. O'SHAUGHNESSY, and G. M. BRUNSTROM: Lancet **1965**, II, 7401. — GARRETTS, M., and C. E. DENT: Lancet **1960**, I, 1142. — HARD, S.: Acta. derm.-venereol. (Stockh.) **43**, 562 (1963). — SNEDDON, I. B.: Proc. roy. Soc. Med. 1958. — TSUCHIDA, J.: J. Okla. med. Ass. **76**, 655 (1964). — TURNBULL, A. L.: Clin. Sci. **28**, 499 (1965).

Comparatively Study on the Effects of Corticosteroids, Resochine and Synopene on the Arthus's Phenomenon in Rabbits

B. BAJDEKOV, K. BERTCHEV, B. BOJKOV and I. ISMIROV, Dermatological Clinic of the University of Sofia (Bulgaria)

With regard to the contradictory data existing in the Literature concerning the action of corticosteroids, resochine and synopene on Arthus's phenomenon, we undertook by means of biochemical, histological, histochemical and immuno-electrophoretical Methods, to study the changes induced with these drugs in rabbits with Arthus phenomenon.

This study was carried out on 48 rabbits chinchilla breed. Arthus phenomenon was produced in the animals in the following way: Every 4th day 1 ml horseserum for 1 kg body weight was injected all six injections.

The animals were divided in to the following groups: 1. control animals injected with horseserum s.c. only; 2. animals treated with urbasone — 4 mg kg weight 2 h before injections with horseserum; 3. treated on the same pattern with synopene (2 mg/kg); 4. treated on the same pattern with 10 mg/kg resochine. after the 6th injection all animals were killed by means of air embolism. Skin and subcutaneous tissue taken from the site of injection was fixed to 10% (v v) Formaldehyde solution, Carnau's mixture and freezed on dry ice. The following histochemical methods were used: PAS-reaction, treatment with salivary amylase, acetylation, deacetylation, esterification by Libie (1954), Staining with to Iuidine blue (by pH 2.0, 4.0, 6.0), alziane blue after STEEDMAN, LISON and method of HALL, sulfatization after method of MOORB-SCHOENBERG, methylation after method of LISON, VAN GISON, WEIGERTH (elastics and fibrin), BRASHE, FEULGEN; G-6-PDH, LDH, SDH after method of Nachlas HESS, PEARS, SKARPELLR.

Electrophoretically studied were — G-6-PDH and LDH isoenzymes in liens on experimental animals after VAN DER HELM. Immunoelectrophoretically study was carried out after Grabar. Histamine content in serum and skin was determined after Code's method.

Results and Discussion

Arthus phenomenon in the animals from the I group consisted in the formation of nodules (fa size 3 × 3 cm) the histopathological and histochemical examinations show central necrosis obliterated blood vessels and a great number of neutrophylic, leucocytes, histiocytes, fibroblasts, angioblasts, plasma cells lymphocytes and neo formation of blood vessels.

PAS-positive substances were found in increased quantity in the periphery of the nodules. DNH and RNA reactions were more intense in the same areas. G-6-PDH and LDH are to be found mainly in the histocytes, fibroblasts, plasma cells and angioblasts.

The histamine content of the nodules is almost the same as in control animals. The immunoelectrophoretic investigation of the serum shows 14 precipitation streaks. Through the G-6-PDH-test three isoenzymes were dicovered in the spleen LDH showed five isoenzymes fractions.

The animals from the IIud group had no skin changes. Histological and histo-chemical examinations show a moderate inflamatory infiltration consisting of neutrophylic leucocytes, fibroblasts, histiocytes, plasmocytes, rarely eosinophyles and lymphocytes. The content of RNA and DNA in plasmocytes, histiocytes and fibroblasts is clearly visible while in the other cells these enzymes are in a smaller quantity. Histamine content is considerably reduced. Immunoelectrophoretical precipitation streaks are reduced in the zones of albumins and beta-globulins while in the zone of globulins no precipitation was observed. The G-6-PDH test evi-denced the existance of only one isoenzyme. There are no changes in the LDH-test.

The examination of the animals from the IIIrd group demonstrated formations of nodules of a size 1 × 1.5 cm with inflammatory infiltrates and central necrosis. The remaining changes are similar to that of the I group. The histamine content is reduced. Immunoelectrophoretical and enzymatic characteristics are equal to these of the control group.

The animals of IVth group demonstrated histological and histochemical changes similar to that of the controls: large nodules with distinct pricipitation streaks in β_1 and β_2-globulin zones and high Histamine content.

This comparative study shows, that, there are distinct differences in the effect of the antiallergic drugs on the Arthus phenomenon: the urbason inhibits immuno-genesis changes G-6-PDH isoenzymes reduces histamine content in the nodules and inhibits strongly the local inflamatory reaction. On the contrary resochine has no influence (on the immunogenesis) as well as on the local inflamatory reaction and increases the histamine content. The changes in the animals treated with syn-pene in comparison with resochin treated and control animals, are less expressed.

Die Adenosintriphosphatase der normalen menschlichen Haut

C. ENE-POPESCU, II. Dermatologische Klinik, Bukarest (Rumänien)

Die ATP-ase ist ein Enzym der Esterasengruppe. Das Enzym spaltet das ATP in Adenosindiphosphat und anorganisches Phosphat, wodurch die für verschiedene Stoffwechselprozesse notwendige Energie frei wird. Dieses Enzym spielt eine besondere Rolle im Zwischenstoffwechsel, da zahlreiche chemische Zellstoffe (Kern-säuren, Phosphatide und andere Zwischenprodukte) Ester der Phosphorsäure sind.

Das Adenosintriphosphat, das Substrat, auf welches das Enzym wirkt, ist die unmittelbare Energiequelle der meisten chemischen Zellreaktionen. Es ist das Endprodukt der energieerzeugenden Systeme und findet sich in den contractilen Proteinsubstanzen (z. B. Cilien, Mitochondrien, Myofibrillen, Basalciliarkörper-chen usw.), siehe ESSNER, FABRICIO u. FOGH, 1962.

Die ATP-ase wurde das Objekt zahlreicher histochemischer Studien und be-

sonders bei Nierenzellen, Leberparenchym, Bauchspeicheldrüse und querge-
streiften, glatten Herzmuskelfasern beschrieben. Studien über das Vorhandensein
in der Haut sind spärlich. So untersuchten BRADSHAW, WACHSTEIN, SPENCE u.
ELIAS (1963) die Haut-ATP-ase und beschrieben sie in Epidermiszellen, Melanocyten und Coriongefäßen. Sie fanden, daß die kleinen Körnchen im Cytoplasma der
Melanocyten eine formalinresistente ATP-ase-Wirkung haben. Diese Körnchen
sind die Melanosomen, in welchen das Melanin gebildet wird. — RENATE WEHR-
MANN (1963) beschreibt die Hautenzyme und erwähnt die ATP-ase nur hinsichtlich ihrer Rolle im Zwischenstoffwechsel und bei der oxydativen Phosphorilierung.
CORMANE, DORTMOND u. KALSBEEK (1963) beschreiben fünf Enzyme in der menschlichen Haut, die alle das ATP spalten und darunter auch die ATP-ase. Unsere
Ergebnisse über die ATP-ase stimmen mit ihren überein.

In dieser Arbeit wollen wir das Vorhandensein der ATP-ase in den verschiedenen Strukturen der normalen menschlichen Haut untersuchen.

I. Material und Methode

Wir verwendeten excidierte Hautstücke vom Rücken bei 12- bis 68jährigen Personen. Die
Hautstücke wurden im Kryostat bei −20° zu einer Dicke von 15 bis 25 geschnitten.
Die von uns verwendeten histochemischen Methoden waren:
    1. Methode Padykula-Herman für die ATP-ase bei pH 9,4 (Calciummethode);
    2. Methode Wachstein-Meise für die ATP-ase bei pH 7,2 (Bleimethode).
    In der Calciummethode wurden als Aktivatoren Cystein (0,0025 M) und als Inhibitoren
PCMB (0,0025 M) für die Kontrolle der Reaktionsspezifität benutzt. Wir haben gleichzeitig
Kontrollschnitte im Inkubationsmilieu ohne ATP-Substrat gemacht.

II. Ergebnisse der Untersuchungen

Epidermis. Mit der Methode Padykula-Herman ergab es keine Reaktion,
mit der Methode Wachstein-Meisel konnte man eine schwache enzymatische
Reaktion in der Basalschicht beobachten.

Corium. Die Blutgefäße aller Kaliber in Corium und Subcutis zeigen bei beiden
Methoden eine intensive Enzymreaktion. Durch Hinzufügen des Aktivators
(Cystein) bzw. des Inhibitors (PCMB) tritt keine Änderung der Enzymreaktion
ein. Die Bindegewebszellen in Corium und Subcutis zeigen bei beiden Methoden
eine gleich schwache ATP-ase-Aktivität. Der Haarfollikel, tangential, longitudinal
und quergeschnitten, zeigt mit beiden Methoden eine starke ATP-ase-Aktivität.
Die Reaktion findet sich in der äußeren Scheide sowie in den Blutgefäßen des
fibrösen Sacks. Die innere Scheide zeigt keine Reaktion, ebenso das eigentliche
Haar. Das hinzugefügte Cystein führt zu einer kräftigeren Reaktion in der äußeren
Haarscheide, und man kann eine Diffusion des Enzyms in die Umgebung des
Follikels beobachten. Die Hinzufügung des Inhibitors hingegen führt zu einer Verminderung der Enzymreaktion. Die glatten Muskelfasern des Musc. arrector pilli
zeigen eine starke ATP-ase-Aktivität mit beiden Methoden. Mit Padykula-
Herman bringt der Aktivator eine Intensivierung der Reaktion, der Inhibitor
eine Verminderung. Im Bereich der Talgdrüsen weisen die umliegenden Blutgefäße bei beiden Methoden eine intensive ATP-ase-Aktivität auf. In der Zellschicht
der Außenseite der Drüse erscheint mit der Wachstein-Meisel-Methode die ATP-
ase-Aktivität stark, nimmt aber dann allmählich ab und ist in den mittleren Talg-
zellen nicht mehr zu finden. Im Bereich der Schweißdrüsen sieht man in den
Drüsenschläuchen (Schweißglomus) ein reiches Capillarnetz, das eine starke
Enzymreaktion bei beiden Methoden aufweist. Auch die sekretorischen Zellen
zeigen nach der Wachstein-Meisel-Methode eine starke ATP-ase-Aktivität. Mit
der Padykula-Herman-Methode ist die Enzymaktivität schwächer. Der Aktivator
verstärkt etwas, und der Inhibitor vermindert die Enzymaktivität in den sekretorischen Zellen. Die Epithelzellen des Schweißdrüsenausführungsganges weisen

mit beiden Methoden keine Enzymreaktion auf. Die begleitenden Blutgefäße haben dagegen eine starke Enzymaktivität.

Fettgewebe. Starke Enzymreaktion zeigen die Blutgefäße aller Kaliber im Interstitium und eine schwache Reaktion das äußere Cytoplasma der Adipocyten. Aktivator und Inhibitor verändern diese Reaktionen nicht. Die Nerven weisen eine starke ATP-ase-Reaktion in den Myelinscheiden der Neurofibrillen auf.

Alle Kontrollschnitte, die ohne Substrat inkubiert wurden, blieben reaktionslos.

III. Diskussion und Schlußfolgerung

Die Blutgefäße aller Kaliber in Corium und Subcutis, im fibrösen Sack des Haarfollikels, an der Außenseite der Talgdrüsen, in der Umgebung des Glomus und der Schweißdrüsenausführungsgänge zeigen eine intensive ATP-ase-Reaktion mit beiden Methoden. Die starken Reaktionen im Bereich des Gefäßendothels, die von Aktivatoren und Inhibitoren unbeeinflußt blieben, können dem Vorhandensein einer Polyphosphatase oder einer membran-spezifischen ATP-ase zugeschrieben werden. Die Untersuchungen von CSAKY (1965) zeigen im Bereich der Pinocytenbläschen der Capillarendothelien eine ATP-ase, die eine gewisse Rolle für den Kationentransport durch die Zellmembran spielt. McCLURKIN (1964) hat die durch Natrium aktivierte ATP-ase studiert, die die gleiche Bedeutung für die Natrium-Kationenübertragung durch die Zellmembran hat. Die Arteriolen und größeren Arterien in Corium und Subcutis haben wegen ihres Muskelanteils eine große ATP-ase-Aktivität. Der Zusatz des Inhibitors (PCMB) ruft bei der Padykula-Herman-Methode eine mäßig verminderte Reaktion in der Muskelschicht der Arterienwand hervor. Das spricht neben dem Vorhandensein der myofibrillären ATP-ase für das Vorhandensein einer anderen Polyphosphatase, die durch den Inhibitor unbeeinflußt bleibt.

In unseren Untersuchungen kommt zum Ausdruck, daß der Inhibitor PCMB in allen Hautstrukturen allgemein eine mäßige Inhibitorenwirkung bei pH 9,4 entfaltet, und daß der Aktivator Cystein auch nur eine mäßig verstärkte Wirkung auf die Enzymreaktion hat.

Hinsichtlich der ATP-ase-Aktivität in der Epidermis können wir sagen, daß wir in den von uns untersuchten Schnitten nach der Wachstein-Meisel-Methode im Vergleich zu den Untersuchungen von BRADSHAW, WACHSTEIN, SPENCE u. ELIAS eine deutliche Reaktion in der Basalschicht und nur eine sehr schwache Reaktion in der granulösen Schicht beobachtet haben.

Literatur. BARDEN, L.: J. Histochem. Cytochem. **9**, 621 (1961). — BERTELESSEN: Acta path. scand. microbiol. **48**, 303 (1960). — BRADSHAW, M., M. WACHSTEIN, J. SPENCE, and J. ELIAS: Histochem. Cytochem. **11**, 465 (1963); **10**, 731 (1962). — CASPERSSON, T.: II. Int. Kongr. J. Histoch. Berlin-Göttingen-Heidelberg: Springer 1964. — CORMANE, R. H., G. L. KALSBEEK und H. DORTMOND: Dermatologica (Basel) **127**, 381 (1963). — BRAUN-FALCO, O.: II. Int. Kongr. Histoch. 1964. — ESSNER, F. J., and P. FABRIZIO: J. Histochem. Cytochem. **13**, 647 (1965). — FREIMAN, C.: J. Histochem. Cytochem. **8**, 159 (1960). — GAUTHIER, G., and H. PADYKULA: J. Histochem. Cytochem. **10**, 661 (1962). — HORI, S., and J. GHARGH: J. Histochem. Cytochem. **11**, 71 (1963). — MONTAGNA, W.: Structure and Fonction of Skin-Ed-II. New York: Pergamon Press 1962. — MONTAGNA, W., and ELLIS: Advances in Biology of the Skin, Bd. 1. II: Cutaneous Blood Vessels and Circulation. New York: Pergamon Press 1961. — OLCKER, R., and R. ANDERSEN: J. invest. Derm. **45**, 168 (1965). — PADYKULA, H.: J. Histochem. Cytochem. **3**, 161, 170 (1955). — RASSNER, G.: Arch. klin. exp. Derm. **222**, 383, 391 (1965). — SANDLER, and BOURNE: J. Histochem. Cytochem. **10**, 636 (1962). — SELIGMAN, A.: II. Int. Kongr. Histoch. Berlin-Göttingen-Heidelberg: Springer 1964. — STEFĂNESCU, V., and A. HAGI-PARASCHIV: Simp. Histoch. Bukarest 1966. — SYUN HOSODA, and K. NAKAMURA: J. Histochem. Cytochem. **8**, 72 (1960). — WACHSTEIN, M., and LANGE: Amer. J. Path. **34**, 835 (1958). — WACHSTEIN, M., and E. MEISEL: J. Histochem. Cytochem. **4**, 424 (1956). — WACHSTEIN, M., E. MEISEL, and NIEDZWIEDZ: J. Histochem. Cytochem. **8**, 387 (1960). — WACHSTEIN, M., M. BRADSHAW, and ORTIZ: J. Histochem. Cytochem. **9**, 625 (1961). — WEHRMANN, R.: Gottron Bd. V/T I, 169. Stuttgart: Thieme 1963.

XIII. Congressus Internationalis Dermatologiae

XIII. Congressus Internationalis

Dermatologiae

31.7. – 5. 8. 1967 / München

Editors: W. Jadassohn and C. G. Schirren

Volume 4

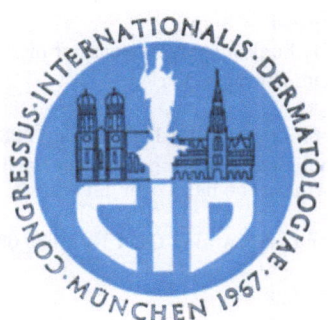

Springer-Verlag Berlin Heidelberg GmbH 1968

Additional material to this book can be downloaded from http://extras.springer.com

ISBN 978-3-642-49455-0   ISBN 978-3-642-49735-3 (eBook)
DOI 10.1007/978-3-642-49735-3

All rights reserved
No part of this book may be translated or reproduced in any form without written
permission from Springer-Verlag

© by Springer-Verlag Berlin Heidelberg 1968
Originally published by Springer-Verlag Berlin-Heidelberg New York in 1968
Softcover reprint of the hardcover 1st edition 1968

Library of Congress Catalog Card Number 68-8552

Title Number 1523

The reproduction of general descriptive names, trade names, trade marks, etc. in this
publication, even when there is no special identification mark, is not to be taken as a sign
that such names, as understood by the Trade Marks and Merchandise Marks Law,
may accordingly be freely used by anyone

Photos: pages *1—128:* L. HEIGL, H. GIESSNER, R. PRÖHL and W. GERSTENBREY

Volume 1   page
Preface . . . .   VII—X
Congressus Internationales Dermatologiae   XII
Contents . . . . XIII—XXXIX
Organization, Addresses and Course of the Congress . . . .   *1—128*
Main-Theme I—VII . . . .   1—525
Symposium 1—4 . . . .   527—703

Volume 2
Symposium 5—15 . . . .   705—1375
Case Presentations and Fundamentals on Film . . . .   1377—1382
Scientific Exhibition . . . .   1385—1591
Authors Index . . . .   1592—1598

Contents   Volume 2

Symposium 5: Malignant Reticuloses and Lymphomas

Reports

Histopathologic and Hematologic Changes in Malignant Lymphomas and Reticuloses.
 H. MONTGOMERY and R. K. WINKELMANN   707
Zur Nosologie und Einteilung der Reticulosen, Reticulosarkomatosen und verwandter
 Krankheitsbilder unter Berücksichtigung cytophotometrischer Untersuchungen.
 W. KNOTH   712
Patología y clínica de los reticulolinfomas óculopalpebrales. P. H. MAGNIN, M. C.
 MORGENFELD and R. L. CABRINI   714
The Identity and Treatment of the Lymphoma Mycosis fungoides. M. A. LUTZNER .   720

Free Communications

Klinik und Histopathologie der malignen Reticulosen. K. W. MACH   721
Cytological Studies on Lymphoma with Electronmicroscopy. H. FUJITA   724
Cutaneous Lymphoblastoma, Spontaneous Involution of Tumours. D. MAJCAN, D.
 STEVANOVIĆ and B. LALEVIĆ   725
Blood Vessel Morphology in the Reticuloses. T. J. RYAN   727
Generalized Giant-Cell Reticulohistiocytosis (Lipoid Dermatoarthritis) — Clinical and
 Histopathological Study of two Cases. P. NAZZARO, U. GRANELLI and A. BIGNAMI .   728
Malignant Development in Mastocytosis. F. SAGHER and Z. EVEN-PAZ   729
Sézary Syndrome. G. L. ROCHA, F. SANTOS, R. AZULAY and A. PETRARCA DE MESQUITA   731
Mycosis Fungoides. — Mode of Presentation of 55 Cases. P. D. SAMMAN   733
Cytological Diagnosis in Mycosis Fungoides. E. BREHMER-ANDERSSON and U. BRUNK   735
Triacetyl 6-Azauridine in Mycosis Fungoides. CH. J. MCDONALD, P. CALABRESI and
 R. C. DE CONTI   739
Ultrastructure de l'angio-réticulo-sarcomatose cutanée: Maladie de Kaposi. E. CALAS,
 H. BONNEAU and J. P. CESARINI   741
Zur Entität des sog. Morbus Kaposi. G. OEHLSCHLAEGEL   745
Les localisations cutanées spécifiques de la maladie de Waldenstroem. H. BARRIERE, P.
 LITOUX and B. BUREAU   747
Esquisse de la physionomie de l'angio-sarcomatose de Kaposi en Algérie (A propos de
 25 observations personelles). F. G. MARILL, E. HADIDA and J. SAYAG   748
Intérêt de la lymphographie dans les hématodermies. M. DANA, R. BOURDON, V. BISMUTH
 and J. P. DESPREZ-CURELY   750
Radiothérapie des hémoréticulopathies malignes. R. BOURDON and M. DANA   752

page

Symposium 6: Cosmetology; Biology and Pathology of the Hair

Cosmetology

Reports

Recherches sur le mécanisme d'action des antiperspirants. R. BRUN, N. HUNZIKER and
P. EVDOS 755

Hair Dyes. A. ROSTENBERG and G. KASS 758

Free Communications

International Dermatology and the World of Cosmetics. E. W. BRAUER 761

Hormonal and Microbial Influences on the Sebaceous Follicles in Acne. P. E. POCHI . . 762

Biology and Pathology of the Human Hair

Reports

Development of the Human Hair Follicle. — Biology and Pathology of the Human
Hair. F. SERRI 763

Alopecia areata, Basic Notions. G. MORETTI, A. REBORA, E. RAMPINI, F. CROVATO and
C. CIPRIANI 765

Klinik und Therapie der Alopecia areata. R. SCHUPPLI 769

Causes actuelles des alopécies féminines diffuses. E. SIDI †, J. BOURGEOIS-SPINASSE
and J. AROUÈTE 771

Free Communications

Propiedades depilatoria y citotóxica de la seleno-cistationina. F. KERDEL-VEGAS. . . 775

Control of Mammalian Hair Growth: Studies with a Cell-Free Protein Synthesizing
System. I. M. FREEDBERG 776

The Effects of Various Pathologic Conditions of the Scalp upon Hair Melanogenesis and
Hair Growth. W. KOSTANECKI 780

The Histological Changes in Idiopathic Premature Vertex Baldness in Women.
I. MARTIN-SCOTT 781

The Normal Trichogram of People Beyond 50 Years but Apparently not Bald.
J. M. BARMAN, I. ASTORE and V. PECORARO 783

Microscopic Studies of Pili Annulati. V. H. PRICE, R. S. THOMAS and F. T. JONES . . 786

Rate of Hair Growth. M. SAITOH, M. UZUKA, M. SAKAMOTO and T. KOBORI 788

Chronical Female Alopecia. M. BINAZZI 791

Le problème des états pseudopeladiques ou pseudopeladoïdes dans le cadre des alopécies
cicatricielles. M. JUON 793

La pelade, maladie psychosomatique. S. LAMBERGEON 795

Biological Depth Dose Studies in Electron Beam Therapy: Effects on Anagen Mouse
Hairs. L. H. LANZL and F. D. MALKINSON 796

Elektronenmikroskopische Befunde an den peritrichialen Nervenfasern des menschlichen Haarfollikels. C. ORFANOS 798

Die Behandlung der Alopecia areata im Kindesalter. J. TOMÁŠKOVÁ 801

Untersuchungen über die Veränderungen des Haares der Augenbrauen bei endogenem
Ekzem. H. LANGHOF† and M. MUNTEANU 803

Symposium 7: Mycoses (Superficial and Deep)

Reports

Untersuchungen über die Zuverlässigkeit eines „in vitro"-Lymphocytentests zwecks
Nachweises einer Dermatophyteninfektion. H. GÖTZ 807

Effects of Human Body Fluids on Candida albicans. V. D. NEWCOMER, J. W. LANDAU,
N. DABROWA and M. L. FENSTER 813

page

Histoplasmose Africaine. R. Vanbreuseghem 817

Micetomas y actinomicosis. A. González Ochoa 819

Pathogenesis of South American Blastomycosis (Lutz's Mycosis). A. Padilha-Gonçalves 824

Nouvelles acquisitions sur le mécanisme d'action de la Griséofulvine. P. Pinetti . . 826

Free Communications

Les onychomycoses. G. Achten 828

Aspects particuliers de l'épidermomycose causée par epidermophyton floccosum. I. Alteras and I. Cojocaru 830

Ultraestructura y citoquímica de la Candida albicans. L. F. Montes and V. S. Constantine. 831

Keloidal Blastomycosis (Jorge Lobo's Disease). S. Fraga and J. Lisbôa Miranda . . 831

A Look at Mycetoma in India. B. B. Gokhale, A. A. Padhye and M. J. Thirumalachar 833

Esporotricosis, estudio clínico epidemiológico. V. C. Jaramillo, G. C. Vélez, A. R. Moreno, I. R. Pizano and A. C. Cortés 835

Favus Infection in Iraq. G. F. Rahim 837

La macrocheilite de la blastomycose Sud-Américaine. J. Ramos-Silva and A. Padilha-Gonçalves 839

Experiencias en cuatro casos de cromoblastomicosis y su tratamiento. F. A. Ocampo, R. T. Perez and R. V. Victoria 841

Quelques aspects de la mycose de Lane-Pedroso (chromoblastomycose ou chromomycose) dans la région Amazonique (Brésil). D. Silva 842

Survey of the Mycoses in U.A.R. K. el Zawahry and M. el Zawahry 847

Main Transmission Routes of Spread of Trichophyton Mentagrophytes var. gran.-Infection from a Natural Focus to Man in a Foothill Region. L. Chmel, J. Buchvald and M. Valentová 851

Beitrag zum Problem tiefer anorectaler Mykosen. O. Male 852

Flore dermatomycosique actuelle dans la région d'Athènes et sensibilité des souches isolées à la griséofulvine. C. Kanitakis, U. Marcelou-Kinti and Chr. Georgiadis . . 854

Biological, Sanitarian and Environmental Factors in Dermatomycoses. D. Triceopoulos, O. Marselou-Kinti and A. Polychronopoulou 856

New Experiments on Culture, Immunology and Inoculation. J. de Azevedo Carneiro, R. D. Azulay and L. M. C. de Andrade 858

Sensibilisations de la peau par les dermatophytes. I. Cojocaru, I. Alteras and L. Dulamitǎ 859

La valeur du milieu Gluzman modifié par Condrea dans la préparation de la trichophytine. V. Costea, M. Carniol, M. Lazar and M. Ilies 861

Onychomycose due à alternaria tenuis. J. Delacrétaz and D. Grigoriou 863

Fungus-Allergy and its Skin Manifestations. E. Fejér 864

The Mycologic Laboratory Specimen. The Collection, Inoculation, and Culture Methods. H. C. Goldberg 866

Tinea Versicolor: The Electron Microscopic Morphology of the Genera Malassezia and Pityrosporum. F. M. Keddie 867

Effect of the Immunosuppressive Agent, Cyclophosphamide, on Experimental Systemic Coccidioidomycosis. J. W. Landau, L. Indianer and V. D. Newcomer 872

Enzyme des Kohlenhydratstoffwechsels bei Dermatophyten. W. Meinhof and G. Rassner 876

Microsporum Nanum as a Cause of Human Infections. J. F. Mullins and C. J. Willis 877

Les dermatophytes du sol en Bulgarie. P. Popchristov, V. Balabanoff, T. Filkov and P. Usunov 879

L'ultrastructure des grains dans les maduromycoses provoquée par Monosporium apiospermum. M. Stoian and A. Avram 881

page

On the Mycomimetic Pictures Found in Mycologic Examinations. P. SBERNA 883

Zur fermentativen Leistung von Fadenpilzen. W. ADAM 884

Parenté antigénique et localisation des antigènes dans le genre Candida: Etude par
immunofluorescence. P. RIMBAUD, J.-M. BASTIDE, M. BASTIDE and J. ALLEGRINI . 886

Essais de marquage de Candida albicans par radioisotopes. Etude de leur distribution
dans l'organisme du lapin. S. ANTONESCU 892

Observations of the Treatment of Superficial Mycosis in South-East Europe with CO_2
Snow (Method Haxthausen). M. BRNIČEVIĆ 893

La contamination staphylococcique des trichophyties suppurées. Résultats d'une thérapie combinée: Griséofulvine, antibiotiques antimicrobiennes et traitement local.
I. CAPUSAN, P. BALOSU and N. MAIER 895

Tratamiento de las tiñas on Griseofulvina. M. P. MIGUENS 896

Sporotrichosis Recurrens Cicatrisans (Repeating Self-Healing Sporotrichosis).
R. N. MIRANDA 898

Traitement expérimental des mycoses cutanées superficielles par l'Amphotéricine B.
D. PERYASSÚ and G. LÖWY 900

Experimentelle Grundlagen der externen antimykotischen Therapie. W. RAAB . . . 901

Über den Einfluß von Moronal (-Nystatin) auf den Zellstoffwechsel von Candida albicans
(Autoradiographische Untersuchungen). M. RAHMANN-ESSER and F. FEGELER . . 903

Mechanism of Antifungal Action of Potassium Iodide on Sporotrichosis. H. URABE,
T. NAGASHIMA and K. NAKASHIMA 907

Fissured Nipples of Lactating Females and its Relation to Candida Infection.
A. M. EL MOFTY, R. MEHAREB, H. M. EL KOMY and C. D. JEFFRIES 908

Symposium 8: Malignant Melanomas

Reports

Melanin Biosynthesis in Melanomas. T. B. FITZPATRICK 913

Mélanoses neurocutanées of Touraine. T. KAWAMURA, S. IKEDA, S. NODA, S. ISHIZU and
T. NAKAJIMA 915

La mélanose circonscrite précancereuse de Hutchinson-Dubreuilh (M.H.D.).
B. DUPERRAT and J. M. MASCARO 917

Spontaneous Regression of Malignant Melanoma. L. BOWDEN 918

Elektrometrie zur Früherkennung von malignanten Melanomen. N. MELCZER 925

The Surgical Treatment of Malignant Melanoma. R. W. RAVEN 926

Die Behandlung des malignen Melanoms mit schnellen Elektronen eines 15 MeV-
Betatrons. G. F. KLOSTERMANN 928

Histologische Diagnostik der Melanome. J. J. HERZBERG 933

Free Communications

Benign Juvenile Melanoma. — Several Selected Aspects from a Study of 51 Lesions.
R. ANDRADE 936

Über das Verhalten der Melanomzellen in vitro. B. ROHDE 938

Production of Melanomas in Hairless Mice with Ultraviolet Light. J. H. EPSTEIN,
W. L. EPSTEIN and T. NAKAI 939

Effects of Depigmenting Agents on Melanocytes and Melanogenesis. M. A. PATHAK,
G. SZABÓ, E. FRENK, S. S. BLEEHEN, Y. HORI and T. B. FITZPATRICK 941

Dopa in Melanoma. H. RORSMAN 942

Multiple Forms of Tyrosinase from Mammalian Melanoma. J. B. BURNETT and H.
SEILER 943

370 Mélanomes malins. — Statistiques et pronostic. J. M. SIMONART 944

A propos de 400 mélanomes malins cutanés. C. DUFOURMENTEL, R. MOULY and J.
GLICENSTEIN 946

page

Zur Häufigkeit des malignen Melanoms. Ergebnis einer Umfrage. H. Kästner, P. Jordan and G. Forck 948

Lentigo Maligna and Malignant Melanoma. R. Jackson 949

Un diagnostic différentiel important des mélanomes. L'Angiokératome noir.
G. E. Goetschel 951

Les noevocarcinomes de l'enfant. R. Mouly, Cl. Dufourmentel and J. Glicenstein 954

Nevus y melanomas malignos. L. A. Rueda 955

Early Diagnosis of Melanoblastoma with the Aid of Electrometric, Thermo-Differential and ^{32}P Uptake Test. A. Gulbert 957

Histologische Befunde beim transplantierten Melanom des Menschen. H. Gartmann 958

Veränderungen bei inoculierten Melanocyten. Kh. Woeber and O. Grütz † 960

Macromolecular Differentiation of Melanocytic and Nevocytic Malignant Melanomas.
Y. Mishima 961

Investigación de células tumorales en sangre periférica en enfermos con melanoma maligno. A. Aliaga and J. Calap 968

Some Mechanisms of Pox Virus Oncolysis in Malignant Melanoma. A Review of 50 Cases.
G. W. Milton and M. Lane Brown 970

Richtlinien und unsere Erfahrungen in der Behandlung des malignen Melanoms.
Gy. Kárpáti, T. Venkei, Ö. Bihari, Gy. Németh and A. Gulbert 973

Observations concernant la prophylaxie et le traitement du mélanome malin.
E. Ujváry and I. Krepsz 974

Données relatives au problème de la possibilité de dissémination après l'irradiation aux rayons X dans les cas du mélanome malin. T. Venkei and Ö. Bihari 975

The Uptake of Radioactively Labelled Compounds by Malignant Melanoma. M. S. Blois 976

Sensitization to X-Irradiation of Melanoma Cells Using Alpha-MSH. M. Lane Brown ·and G. W. Milton 978

Symposium 9: Physiology of the Skin

Reports

Enzyme und Physiologie der Haut. G. K. Steigleder 983

Collagen Metabolism in Skin. Ch. M. Lapière 986

Physiological Response of Human Skin to Ultraviolet Light. M. A. Everett and R. L. Olson 988

The Clinical Significance of a Comparative Approach to the Physiology of Hair Growth.
A. J. Rook 993

Physiologie der Hautoberfläche. Die relative Bedeutung verschiedener Befunde.
F. Herrmann 995

Some Remarks on the Barrier Function of the Epidermis. J. Horáček 999

Le pouvoir tampon de la peau. H. Thiers 1002

Free Communications

Studies of Some Glycolytic Pathways in the Skin of Rats Under Experimental Conditions. G. Rabbiosi and A. Giannetti 1003

Plasma Kinin Formation and Human Inflammation. H. Zachariae, J. Malmquist, J. A. Oates and W. Pettinger 1006

Synthesis of Unique Proteins in Epidermal Keratinization. I. A. Bernstein 1008

Mechanism of Water Binding in Stratum Corneum. J. D. Middleton 1010

Studies on the Epidermal Keratinization of the Human Fetus in vitro with Special References to the Electron Microscopic and Autoradiographic Observation.
K. Okamura, K. Iwashita and K. Ueda 1012

page

The Envelope of Epidermal Horny Cells. A. G. MATOLTSY 1014

Follicular Hyperkeratinization Induced in the Rabbit Ear by Human Skin Surface Lipids. A. L. LORINCZ, H. KRIZEK and S. BROWN 1016

The Influence of Dimethyl Sulphoxide, Dimethyl Acetamide and Dimethyl Formamide on the Epidermal Barrier to Water. H. BAKER 1017

Die hygrometrische Aufzeichnung der Hydromeiose und das Abtrocknen der Hornschicht als Maß ihrer physiologischen Qualität. J. ROVENSKÝ and J. ZÁHEJSKÝ . . 1020

Physiologische Antiperspirants. H. P. FIEDLER 1022

Sodium Secretion and Reabsorption by the Eccrine Sweat Gland. R. L. DOBSON . . 1024

The Insensible Water Loss and Skin Temperature. F. A. J. THIELE and K. G. VAN SENDEN 1025

The Fine Structure of the Sebaceous Gland of the Adult Female Rat After Receiving Sexual Hormones. Y. SATO and M. MOROHASHI 1028

The in vivo Study of Cutaneous Lipogenesis. G. LIPKIN and V. R. WHEATLEY 1029

Physiology of Human Sebaceous Glands-Hormonal Control Mechanisms. J. S. STRAUSS 1031

Le contrôle hormonal de la glande sébacée chez l'homme. M. BONELLI, E. ALESSI, C. TOMASINI and S. PICCININI 1033

Der Einfluß des Hautoberflächenmilieus auf Staphylococcus aureus. E. MÜLLER . . . 1036

The pH and the Bacterial Flora of Normal Skin Under Fluocinolone-Plastic Occlusion Treatment. E. A. KNUDSEN 1038

The Alkali Neutralization Capacity of Human Skin in vivo. K. SCHUTTER 1041

Über ultraviolett-absorbierende Verbindungen im Wasserlöslichen epidermaler Verhornungsprodukte. E. SCHWARZ 1043

Ultraviolettes Licht als Stimulus für Kininbildung in menschlicher Haut. R. K. WINKELMANN, J. EPSTEIN and K. WOLFF 1045

Sur la réponse vasculaire biphasique au siège de l'érythème dû aux radiations ultraviolettes. Existe-t-il une réponse plus élémentaire que l'érythème ? G. ZINA and A. BENEDETTO 1047

A Cutaneous Role in the Regulation of the Body's Carbohydrate Milieu. R. M. FUSARO and J. A. JOHNSON 1048

Research on Sialic Acid in the Human Skin. A. GIANNETTI and G. RABBIOSI 1050

Mepyramine and Adrenergic Neurone. B. S. VERMA and O. D. GULATI 1053

Lysosomes and the Skin. R. L. OLSON, R. NORDQUIST, J. NORDQUIST and M. A. EVERETT 1056

Modificaciones clínicas e histológicas de la reacción tuberculínica bajo la acción local del valerato de betametasona en cura oclusiva. A. CASALÁ, C. BIANCHI, O. BIANCHI, S. STRINGA and O. ROQUÉ 1060

The Significance of Low Serum Iron Levels in the Causation of Itching. I. B. SNEDDON and M. GARRETTS 1061

Comparatively Study on the Effects of Corticosteroids, Resochine and Synopene on the Arthus's Phenomenon in Rabbits. B. BAJDEKOV, K. BERTCHEV, B. BOJKOV and I. ISMIROV 1063

Die Adenosintriphosphatase der normalen menschlichen Haut. C. ENE-POPESCU . . 1064

Symposium 10: Effects of Radiation on the Skin

Reports

Radiobiologie cutanée. P. VAN CANEGHEM 1069

Strahlenwirkung im Hautbereich in Abhängigkeit von der verwendeten Strahlenqualität. A. PROPPE 1070

Strahlenwirkung im Hautbereich in Abhängigkeit von der verwendeten Strahlenqualität. F. WACHSMANN 1074

Indications dermatologiques du traitement ionisant. Traitement ionisant des épithéliomas et des mélanomes malins à l'aide de techniques de radio-sensibilisation nouvelles. E. G. Scolari 1078

Indications thérapeutiques des substances radioactives en dermatologie. B. Pierquin 1081

Algunos rasgos ultraestructurales de las radiolesiones. J. Cabré 1083

Preliminary Investigative Studies of the Laser Treatment of Angiomas. L. Goldman, R. J. Rockwell jr. and R. Meyer 1084

Free Communications

The Treatment of Skin Tumours with Radium and Hyperbaric Oxygen. C. Vallecchi and G. Mantellassi 1087

Nouvelle technique de Radiumthérapie en oxygène hyperbaryque. M. Nannelli and G. Mantellassi 1088

Acute Effects of Irradiation on the Skin. — A Histochemical and Chemical Study. A. K. Kurban and F. S. Farah. 1090

Biochemische Untersuchungen an Serum und Hauteiweißen von Ratten nach Röntgenbestrahlung. O.-E. Rodermund 1091

Radiations et tissu élastique cutané. M. Ledoux-Corbusier 1093

Problemas del uso de los rayos grenz en los negros y en los mulatos. M. A. Contreras 1094

Tierexperimentelles zur Röntgenfernbestrahlung der Haut. M. Betetto 1096

Dermatological Observations in the A-Bomb Survivors of Hiroshima and Nagasaki, Japan. M.-L. T. Johnson, T. Taura and P. B. Gregory 1097

Studies on Induction, Persistence and Recovery of Radiation Damage in Proliferative (Anagen) and Non-proliferative (Telogen) Rodent Hair Cell Populations. F. D. Malkinson and M. L. Griem 1099

Autoradiographische Untersuchungen zur epidermalen Proliferation unter physiologischen, pathologischen und experimentellen Bedingungen mit Tritium-markierten Nucleosiden. W. Born 1101

Histochimie des enzymes des follicules irradiés du cobaye. A. Kint and J. de Bersaques 1103

Untersuchungen zur experimentellen Photosensibilisierung mit Sulfanilamid und Phenothiazinen. K. Schwarz, J. Rothenstein and M. Schwarz-Speck 1106

Light is an Aetiological Factor for Certain Dermatoses in U.A.R. M. el Zawahry . . 1107

Heliotherapie und ihr Einfluß auf die Aktivität mancher Enzyme bei Psoriasiskranken. N. Balevska, J. Petkov, G. Mustakov, S. Jowev, N. Zlatkov and G. Tomov . . 1110

The Action Spectrum of Erythema Induced by Ultraviolet Radiation. Preliminary Report. D. Berger, F. Urbach and R. E. Davies 1112

The Absorption Spectrum of the Stratum Corneum as the Natural Sunscreen of Human Skin. A. R. H. B. Verhagen 1118

Prurigo actínico. F. Londoño 1122

Psoralen Therapy of Vitiligo in the Tropics. T. L. Fleisher 1124

Zur Kombinationsbehandlung der Mycosis fungoides mit Röntgenstrahlen und Spindelgiften. A. Wiskemann 1125

Photochemical Movement of Cholesterol in Skin. E. W. Rauschkolb and J. M. Knox 1126

Symposium 11: Immunology in Dermatology

Reports

Aetiology of Some Autoimmune Diseases. N. R. Rowell 1131

Aspects immunologiques du lupus érythémateux aigu disséminé. J. Thivolet . . . 1134

Autoimmunity in Pemphigus. T. Chorzelski 1135

Immunology of Acne Vulgaris. Dermal Hypersensitivity and Circulating Antibody Levels to Corynbacterium Acnes. S. M. Puhvel, T. H. Sternberg and R. M. Reisner 1136

page

Zur Immunologie in der Dermatologie. J. KIMMIG 1139

The Role of the Basophil in the Immune Response. W. B. SHELLEY 1143

Free Communications

Classes of Immunoglobulins Associated with Skin Sensitizing Properties. M. J. FELLNER and R. L. BAER 1144

Patterns of Skin Fluorescence in Lupus Erythematosus. R. H. CORMANE 1146

Delayed Hypersensitivity Responses in Immunologic Deficiency States. W. L. EPSTEIN 1148

Antikörpermangelsyndrome und Hautveränderungen. G. BREHM 1149

Zur Frage der Antigenspezifität von 2,4-Dinitrochlorbenzol-Epidermis-Conjugaten im Meerschweinchenversuch. F. KLASCHKA 1151

Antinuclear Factors in Clinical Dermatology. J. S. BECK, N. R. ROWELL and T. E. ANDERSON 1153

Vasoactive Substances at Sites of Cutaneous Allergies. TH. M. INDERBITZIN and P. J. GROB 1154

Application de la technique d'immunofluorescence en dermatologie. Y. MONTET, J. DUHEILLE and J. BEUREY 1156

Experimental Studies on the Pathogenesis of Acantholysis in Pemphigus. P. J. GROB and TH. M. INDERBITZIN 1158

Autoantibodies in Pemphigus Foliaceus. T. A. FURTADO, A. O. LIMA, G. O. ANDRADE and O. SEABRA 1159

L'apport de l'immuno-fluorescence dans la mise en évidence du rôle de l'allergie à Candida albicans dans certaines dermatoses communes. P. TEMIME, M. BENNE, M. LEBEUF, J. P. MARCHAND and PH. LATOURELLE 1162

Recherches électrophorétiques et immunophorétiques en moyens gélifiés sur protéines de muscle strié dans différentes collagénoses d'intérêt dermatologique. G. MARTINA and A. MIDANA 1168

Immunoelektrophorese der Serumproteine bei akuten und chronischen Formen des Erythematodes. T. BIELICKÝ, L. MALINA and J. OPPLT 1170

Immunologic Defect of the Skin in Lymphadenopathy. Y. NOGUCHI, K. ISHIWARA, M. HIGUCHI and S. YOSHIDA 1171

Immunologische Untersuchungen von Lymphocytenkulturen. Eine diagnostische Methode in der Dermatologie. H. J. HEITMANN 1174

Mechanisms of Anaphylaxis. M. W. GREAVES 1176

The Immunochemical Basis of the Urticarial Reaction. F. S. FARAH and A. K. KURBAN 1176

The Release of Serotonin in Hypersensitivity States. J. S. COMAISH 1179

Réactions sérologiques et terrain d'allergie humorale en dermatologie. CL. MIKOL and M. RENOUX 1180

Experimentelle Untersuchungen zur Desensibilisierung und Immunotoleranz gegen niedermolekulare Allergene. K. H. SCHULZ 1181

Experimentelle Sensibilisierung mit drei- und sechswertigem Chrom. M. SCHWARZ-SPECK 1183

Zur Frage autoallergischer Reaktionen bei der Neurodermitis. B. KOPECKÁ, E. SORKIN, S. BORELLI and A. FJELDE 1185

Delayed Reactivity to Bacterial, Mold and Viral Allergens in Atopic Dermatitis. G. RAJKA 1187

Das Shwartzman-Phänomen, eine dem Arthus-Phänomen ähnliche, pseudo-immuno-logische Reaktion der Haut auf Endotoxin. I. KUNICK and L. ILLIG 1187

Immunological Aspects of the Aldrich's Syndrome. G. IACOVACCI, S. UNGARI and F. AIUTI 1189

Mise en évidence d'anticorps circulants dans les manifestations cutanées de l'allergie à la pénicilline. J. PAUPE and CL. MIKOL 1190

Heutige Diagnostik der Penicillinallergie. P. MICHAILOV and N. BEROWA 1191

page

Symposium 12: The Skin and Internal Disease

Reports

Erythropoietic Protoporphyria. I. A. MAGNUS 1195
Xanthomatoses et maladies systémiques. A. BAZEX, A. DUPRÉ and B. CHRISTOL . . 1197
Skin Disorders in Relation to Malabsorption. G. C. WELLS 1200
Further Studies on Acrodermatitis Enteropathica. N. DANBOLT 1202
A New Classification for Lupus Erythematosus. J. R. HASERICK 1204
Angiokeratoma Corporis Diffusum. H. J. WALLACE 1207
Consideration of the Etiology of Pyoderma Gangrenosum. H. O. PERRY and P. DIDIS-
HEIM 1208

Free Communications

A Cutaneous Affection from Malabsorption. A. BACCAREDDA-BOY and F. CROVATO . . 1212
Hauterscheinungen bei Colitis ulcerosa. H. REICH 1214
Crohn's Disease Associated with Cutaneous Lesions. G. A. GRANT PETERKIN 1214
Lung Function in Patients with Cutaneous Vasculitis. M. CATTERALL 1215
Atteinte du rein au cours des allergides nodulaires dermiques de Gougerot. ST. BOULLE
and J. GUILAINE 1217
Therapie der Porphyria cutanea tarda (Ergebnisse in 9 Jahren). H. IPPEN 1218
Hautreaktionen bei rheumatischen Erkrankungen. E. WOHLSTEIN 1219
Studies on Iron Metabolism in the Porphyria Cutanea Tarda (P.C.T.). L. LEVI, C. L.
MENEGHINI, F. SPINELLI-RESSI and C. A. BETTINELLI 1222
Krankhafte Zusammenhänge zwischen Leber und Haut in "Porphyria cutanea tarda".
P. TÎRLEA and I. CĂPUSAN 1222
Schistosomiasis (Bilharziasis) der Haut. C. M. HASSELMANN 1224
Schistosomal Infestation of the Skin. A. M. EL MOFTY 1224
The Hepatitis Associated with Infantile Papular Acrodermatitis. V. A. PUCCINELLI . . 1228
Zum Krankheitsbild des Myxoedema circumscriptum praetibiale. CHR. EBERHARTINGER 1229
Natural Course of Various Types of Scleroderma. A. Follow-up-Study over a Period of
20 Years. Z. STAVA 1230
Preparation and Application of Lesional Casts in the Study of Cutaneous Disease.
D. A. ROE 1231
Perorale Kreatinbelastung bei Haut- und Muskelerkrankungen. H. W. KREYSEL and
M. JÄNNER 1232
Liquen rojo plano de la mucosa bucal. Su asociación con diabetes. Nuevas observaciones.
D. GRINSPAN, J. DÍAZ, L. O. VILLAPOL, J. SCHNEIDERMAN, R. BERDICHESKY, D.
PALESE and J. FAERMAN 1234
Sarcoidosis with Cicatricial Alopecia Resembling Generalized Discoid Lupus Erythema-
tosus. L. S. SAUTER 1235
Dermatological Aspects of Crohn's Disease. D. I. MCCALLUM and P. D. C. KINMONT 1237
A propos du syndrôme de Winterbauer (Syndrôme C.R.S.T.). A. PUISSANT, R. LECLERCQ
and F. VANBREMEERSCH 1238
Acanthosis Nigricans. — A Clinical Manifestation of Internal Disorders. T. YASUDA,
SH. NISHIYAMA and SH. TSUYUKI 1240
Glucorrhoea. Is this Pre-diabetes? J. R. G. AGIUS 1241
Hormonelle Untersuchungen und Behandlungsmethoden bei Acne vulgaris. F. TÓTH
and L. NÉKÁM 1243
Vorkommen von Paraproteinämie bei Pyoderma gangraenosum. H. RÖCKL 1244
Zur Problematik der Arthropathia psoriatica. F. VLČEK, M. ZBOJANOVA, G. NIEPEL
and Z. SITAY 1246

page

Quelques observations sur l'élimination urinaire des cétostéroïdes dans l'acnée féminine.
R. DUMITRIU, M. HAISUC, L. REITER, M. HONTARU and A. COSER 1248

The Seborrhoic Symptom Complex.— The Expression of a Disturbed Intestinal Malutilization of Vitamin B 12 as Proven by Measuring the Radioactivity after Administration of Co 60 Vitamin B 12. W. A. CASPER 1249

Diabetes and Impetigo Contagiosa (Passage from one Diabetic Family to Another
Diabetic Family Via a Related Cousin Carrier). B. R. HEARST 1251

Dermatitis uraemica Rössle. H. FISCHER 1252

Symposium 13: Bullous Dermatoses

Reports

Zur Klinik bullöser Eruptionen (Exklusive bullöse Genodermatosen). J. TAPPEINER   1257

Herpes Zoster and Nonmalignant Disease. L. H. WINER and E. T. WRIGHT   1259

Producción experimental de ampollas; su correlacción con los cambios estructurales en
las dermatosis ampollosas. D. J. GÓMEZ ORBANEJA   1262

La maladie de Duhring-Brocq à grosses bulles dite «pemphigoïde de Brocq», après la
cinquantaine. P. LE COULANT, L. TEXIER and P. BORAUD   1264

Subcorneal Pustular Dermatosis. A review after 10 years. D. S. WILKINSON   1266

Bullous Lesions in Patients with Internal Disorders. E. SKOG   1267

Corticosteroid Treatment of Pemphigus. C. T. NELSON   1270

Friction Blisters Produced under Controlled Conditions. TH. A. CORTESE jr., T. B.
GRIFFIN and M. B. SULZBERGER   1273

Free Communications

Experimental Investigations on the Acantholysis Induced by Staphylococcus pyogens.
Comparative Study with the Acantholysis on Pemphigus. B. ZILBERBERG   1275

An Electron Microscopic Study of Cutaneous and Oral Pemphigus Vulgaris. K. HASHI-
MOTO   1278

Localización de gamma globulina IgG y complemento (C'3) en la epidermis de enfermos
de Pénfigo vulgar. S. STRINGA, C. BIANCHI, A. CASALA, C. INGLESINI and O. BIANCHI   1283

Dermatite Bulleuse Mucosynéchante et Atrophiante. A. G. BELLONE, M. F. HOFMANN
and G. CAPUTO   1285

Experimental Friction Blisters: Histological Investigation. K. FUKUYAMA and TH. A.
CORTESE jr.   1288

Etude de la composition protéique du liquide des bulles dans les dermatoses bulleuses.
G. MOULIN and Y. MANUEL   1289

Nouvelles observations sur le phénomène citochémiotatique dans la bulle du pemphigus.
P. SERTOLI   1291

Hepatische Porphyrien: Veränderungen der Serumenzymaktivitäten und hämatologischen Befunde beim Menschen und bei der Ratte. H. PIETSCHMANN and W. RAAB .   1293

Interessante, bei den an bullösen Dermatosen leidenden Kranken erhobene hämatologische und gastroenterologische Befunde. V. ROZSÍVALOVÁ, F. MATĚJA, B. FIXA
and O. KOMÁRKOVÁ   1294

The Treatment of Porphyria Cutanea Tarda by Chelation. G. A. HUNTER and G. F.
DONALD   1296

Toxic Epidermal Necrolysis. M. B. LEWIS   1297

Acute Epidermal Necrolysis (Ritter-Lyell). — The Scalded Skin Syndrome.
P. J. KOBLENZER   1298

The Ultrastructure of Acantholysis in Lichen Planus. L. FRY and F. R. JOHNSON . .   1301

page

Symposium 14: Mycobacterial Infections of the Skin

Reports

Etude biologique récente dans la lèpre: Analogies antigéniques et séro-diagnostic de la lèpre par immunofluorescence sur bacille de Stefansky. F.-P. MERKLEN and F. COTTENOT 1305

Las formas submicroscópicas del m. leprae. J. GAY PRIETO and G. GABINO 1306

Die gegenwärtige Epidemologie und Bakteriologie der Hauttuberkulose in der Bundesrepublik Deutschland. F. EHRING 1308

Mykobakterienbefunde bei den sog. Tuberkuliden. N. SIMON 1312

Thalidomide in Lepra Reaction and in Hansen's Disease. J. SHESKIN, F. SAGHER, M. DORFMAN and J. CONVIT 1314

Free Communications

Geographical Distribution of Skin Tuberkulosis, Leprosy and Sarcoidosis in Japan. K. KITAMURA 1316

A propos des tuberculoses cutanées — leur classification — leur diagnostic biologique — leur traitement. M. BOLGERT and P. L. DELAIRE 1317

Lupus Vulgaris Gigantea Caused by Mycobacterium Avium. J. V. CHRISTIANSEN . . 1319

Atypical Acid fast Micro-Organisms in Scleroderma. A. R. CANTWELL, E. CRAGGS, J. W. WILSON and F. SWATEK 1320

Nature of the Antigen Responsible for the Kveim Reaction in Sarcoidosis. R. KOOIJ and J. W. VAN WAVEREN HOGERVORST 1322

Present Position of BCG Vaccination against Leprosy. L. M. BECHELLI 1323

Über die pigmentierten Naevi bei lepromatösen Leprakranken. Y. ISHIBASHI and T. KAWAMURA 1325

Mise en évidence du bacille de Hansen dans les lèpres apparemment abacillaires. F. COTTENOT, F.-P. MERKLEN and TRINH THI KIM MONG DON 1326

The Frequency of Intracellular Lipid in the Several Structureal Types of Leprosy. R. D. AZULAY and L. C. DE ANDRADE 1328

Cutaneous Response of Leprosy Patients to Living and Heated Mycobacterium Leprae Cultures on the Olitzki-Gershon Medium. M. DORFMAN, F. SAGHER, J. SHESKIN and A. L. OLITZKI 1329

Serum Immunoglobulin Changes in Leprosy and Tuberculosis. SOO DUK LIM and R. M. FUSARO 1332

Nuevos avances terapéuticos en lepra. J. C. GATTI, J. E. CARDAMA and L. M. BALINA 1334

Double Reversal of the Tuberculin Reaction in Sarcoidosis. S. H. SILVERS and F. S. GLICKMAN 1335

Clinical Applications of Shepard's Mouse Foot Pad Technique. P. FASAL and L. LEVY 1337

Impétigo herpétiforme Hébra Kaposi ou Psoriasis pustuleux généralisé (chez une femme âgée de 22 ans, apparu au cours de 5e mois de sa 2e grossesse). R. SAMII 1339

Symposium 15: Iatrogenic Diseases in Dermatology

Reports

Dermatosis iatrogénicas. Definición, patogénia, clasificación. M. I. QUIROGA 1343

The Aetiology of Toxic Epidermal Necrolysis. A. LYELL 1346

Iatrogenic Disease Due to Physical Treatment. A. N. DOMONKOS 1347

Eruptions du type L. E. et syndromes lupiques provoqués par des médicaments. CH. GRUPPER and G. A. C. MARCEL 1349

Dermatoses des traitements antidiabétiques. J. BEUREY, P. JEANDIDIER and A. BERMONT 1352

Iatrogenic Dyschromies. H. MÖLLER 1355

page

Free Communications

Photosensitive Dermatitis as an Iatrogenic Disease. T. KOBORI and H. ARAKI 1357

Les accidents cutanés de l'allergie humorale médicamenteuse. Intérêt du test de Shelley. J. MALEVILLE, H. BERGOEND and A. BASSET 1359

La thésaurismose cutanée par polyvinylpyrrolidone (PVP). J. M. LACHAPELLE . . . 1362

Mascaras pigmentarias como expresión iatrogénica a dosis altas y prolongadas de feniotiacina y derivados en el control de afecciones psiquiatricas. E. B. MOLINA LEGUIZAMÓN, A. A. CORDERO and E. FOLLMANN 1363

Necrolisis Epidermica Toxica. — Observaciones sobre 12 Casos. A. CORTÉS CORTÉS and V. CÁRDENAS JARAMILLO 1371

Dermatosis por anovulatorios. Y. ORTIZ 1373

Case Presentations and Fundamentals on Film

Second International Film Presentation of the Institute for Dermatologic Communication and Education

Keratosis Follicularis (Darier's Disease). N. KARLTORP and ST. FLODERUS 1379

Congenital Ichthyosiform Erythroderma. K. REHTIJÄRVI, K. KUOKKANEN and P. KARMA 1379

Xeroderma Pigmentosum. H. EL HEFNAWI 1379

Metastasizing Basal Cell Carcinoma. C. CH. THOMAS 1380

The Nevoid Basal Cell Carcinoma Syndrome. J. B. HOWELL and D. E. ANDERSON . . 1380

Gold Leaf Treatment of Cutaneous Ulcers. N. M. KANOF 1380

Diagnosis of Latent Psoriasis. G. HOLTI 1380

Surgical Treatment of Benign Acanthosis Nigricans. H. OLLENDORFF CURTH 1380

Pellagra and other Avitaminoses in the Bantu. M. ROSE 1381

Lupus Erythematosus. D. L. TUFFANELLI and W. B. REED 1381

Lipoid Proteinosis. R. M. CAPLAN 1381

Acrodermatitis Chronica Atrophicans (Herxheimer). F. HERRMANN and O. SCHULTKA . 1381

Granulomatous Dermo-Hypodermitis with Progressive Atrophy. J. CONVIT, FR. KERDEL-VEGAS and M. F. ALLENDE 1381

Report of the Institute for Dermatologic Communication and Education to the International Committee of Dermatology 1382

Scientific Exhibition

Clinical Dermatology

Die spontane Heilungsquote der Blutschwämme und die daraus zu ziehenden Schlüsse für die Prognose und Therapie. G. F. KLOSTERMANN 1387

Spontanverlauf der Säuglingshämangiome. A. PROPPE and H. HAUSS 1387

Laser Surgery of Angiomas with Special Reference to Port-Wine Angiomas. L. GOLDMAN, E. J. RITTER, R. J. ROCKWELL jr., R. MEYER, B. HENDERSON and K. WM. KITZMILLER 1388

Therapie hypercholesterinämischer Xanthomatosen. N. ZÖLLNER, M. GUDENZI and G. WOLFRAM 1390

Proteolytic Enzyme Treatment of Skin Ulcers. M. C. SPENCER 1393

Chemosurgery for the Microscopically Controlled Excision of Skin Cancer. FR. E. MOHS 1393

Multiple Punch Autografts for the Alopecias. D. B. STOUGH 1394

Evaluation of Parental Methotrexate for Intractable Psoriasis. CH. P. DEFEO, A. ALLYN and S. EISENBERG 1394

Zur Wirkung des hochalpinen Klimas in der atopischen konstitutionellen Neurodermitis. S. BORELLI, H. BRENN, ST. CHLEBAROV, C. ENE-POPESCU, H. GEHRKEN, B. KOPECKA, P. MICHAILOV and H. VOSSIECK. 1395

Klimatherapie von Hautkrankheiten an der Nordsee. W. PÜRSCHEL 1397

page

Die Verbrennung — ein dermatologisches Problem. Komplikationen, Therapie und Prophylaxe. G. WEBER and H. JURSCH 1400

A New Principle in Topical Corticosteroid Treatment. G. HAGERMAN 1406

Casus rari muco-cutanei. A. GREITHER and O. HORNSTEIN 1408

Visualization in Dermatology. K. K. MUSTAKALLIO 1409

Examen radiographique des tissus cutanés et sous-cutanés normaux et pathologiques. CH. GROS, A. BASSET, S. SCHRAUB, J. MALEVILLE, E. GROSSHANS and E. HEID . . 1409

Klassifizierung der Ichthyosen. U. W. SCHNYDER and B. KONRÁD 1411

Andrologie in Klinik und Praxis. C. SCHIRREN and H. GRELL 1413

Papulonecrotic and Acneiform Tuberculids. C. E. SONCK 1413

Exhibit on Genodermatoses. L. ZIPRKOWSKI 1418

A Case of Congenital Erythropoietic Porphyria. K. YAMAMOTO 1420

Contact Allergy in Scandinavia. B. MAGNUSSON, S.-G. BLOHM, S. FREGERT, N. HJORTH, G. HØVDING, V. PIRILÄ and E. SKOG 1421

Klinische Pharmakologie des neuen Histaminblockers Tavegil. L. KERP and H. KASEMIR 1425

Hautveränderungen und Antikörper-Mangelsyndrome. G. BREHM 1426

L'allergie de contact. J. FOUSSEREAU 1429

Chamber Test Method. V. PIRILÄ and L. FÖRSTRÖM 1430

Erythropoietic Protoporphyria. R. M. FUSARO, W. J. RUNGE, E. S. PETERKA. M. O. JAFFE, E. W. GOLTZ and C. J. WATSON 1432

Gegenüberstellung von Angiomatosis Kaposi (Sarcoma idiopathicum haemorrhagicum multiplex) und Stewart-Treves-Syndrom (Sarcoma angioplasticum in elephantiasi). H. TELLER and H. KRÜGER 1435

Une affection liée au sexe: la gérodermie ostéodysplasique. D. KLEIN, F. BAMATTER, A. FRANCESCHETTI, G. BOREUX, J. E. W. BROCHER and P. HOLENSTEIN 1443

Elektronenmikroskopische, histochemische und polarisationsoptische Untersuchungen bei Pemphigus familiaris benignus (Hailey u. Hailey). F. NÜRNBERGER and G. MÜLLER 1444

Pemphigus Benignus Chronicus and Keratosis Palmo-plantaris in a Finnish Family. C. E. SONCK 1444

Shibi-Gatchaki-Syndrome. Y. KATABIRA 1447

Cas Cliniques. A. BASSET 1448

Gnathostomiasis Cutis. Yangtze Edema in China and Similar Migrating Intermittent Swellings of the Skin in Japan, Both Due to Gnathostoma Spinigerum Owen, 1836. K. KITAMURA 1449

Plusieures dermatoses. G. SAKELLARIOU 1450

Seltene Hautkrankheiten. G. HARGITA 1451

Angiokeratoma corporis diffusum Fabry. R. DENK 1459

Die primäre Hautreaktion nach infektiösem Tsetsefliegenstich bei der afrikanischen Schlafkrankheit. H. E. KRAMPITZ 1459

Amoebiasis Skin Manifestations. TH. DOXIADES and J. CAPETANAKIS 1462

Skin Diseases in Arabian Countries: Certain Notes and Comments. M. EL ZAWAHRY . 1464

Die Tumormetastasierung von der Haut und in die Haut. H. DREPPER and F. EHRING 1465

Zur Pathologie cutaner Lymphgefäße. J. TAPPEINER and L. PFLEGER 1467

Neuere Aspekte zur Histopathologie der Alopecia areata. W. THIES and CH. FISCHER 1469

Befund Langerhans-ähnlicher Zellen in den Hauterscheinungen der Reticuloendotheliose von Letterer-Siwe. V. PUCCINELLI, F. GIANOTTI and R. CAPUTO 1472

Tetracycline Fluorescence in Squamous Cell Carcinoma. H. J. DONSKY and G. R. MIKHAIL 1474

Concept of the Molecular Cause of Albinism. G. F. WILGRAM 1475

Xeroderma pigmentosum. H. EL HEFNAWI 1476

Skin Tuberculosis, Leprosy, Cutaneous Leishmanosis, Favus. M. A. MALEKI 1476

page

Experimental Dermatology

A Cutaneous Rôle in the Regulation of the Body's Carbohydrate Milieu. R. M. Fusaro and J. A. Johnson 1477

The Interplay of Opposites. Immunological Reactions in the Skin. Th. M. Inderbitzin and P. J. Grob 1480

Autoradiographic Studies on Psoriatic Epidermis. S. Sotomatsu, Y. Igarashi and Y. Ooshima 1481

Die Mastzelle. A. Schauer 1483

Electronmicroscopy of Merkel's Tastzelle. K. K. Mustakallio and U. Kiistala . . . 1493

Bilddemonstration zur mikroskopischen Anatomie des Haarfollikels im Verlauf des Haarcyclus. H.-J. Bandmann and K. Bosse 1493

Zur Ultrastruktur des menschlichen Haarfollikels. V. Puccinelli and R. Caputo . . . 1494

Zur licht- und elektronenoptischen Struktur der Nerven am Haar. E. Hagen and G. Niebauer. 1495

Neuere Entwicklung der dermatologischen Virusforschung. Th. Nasemann 1499

Recent Observations on Langerhans Cells. K. Wolff, R. K. Winkelmann and K. Holubar 1502

Malignant Melanomas: Subcellular Differentiation of Nevocytic and Melanocytic Ontogeny. Y. Mishima. 1505

Epidermal Melanin Unit. M. A. Pathak, G. Szabó, T. B. Fitzpatrick, Y. Hori, S. S. Bleehen, E. Frenk, M. Miyamoto, M. Seiji and A. Breathnach 1506

Dermo-Epidermal Separation by Suction. N. Kiistala and K. K. Mustakallio . . 1513

Comparative Study with the Acantholysis in Pemphigus. Experimental Investigations on the Acantholysis Induced by the Staphylococcus pyogenes. B. Zilberberg . . 1513

Pathophysiologie allergischer Dermatosen. G. Stüttgen, I. Gigli and F. Herrmann 1514

Das mikrobielle Ekzem. H. Röckl, F. Schröpl, E. Müller and G. Peter 1516

Experimental Eczema of the Guinea Pig. N. Hunziker 1518

Terpentinöl-Intoxikation bei Arbeitern einer Schuhcreme-Fabrik verursacht durch d-Alpha-Pinen. F. Nürnberger 1522

Enzymaktivitätsmuster im Serum und in Erythrozyten bei verschiedenen Hautkrankheiten. H. Holzmann, B. Morsches, G. W. Korting and R. Denk 1524

Immunofluorescence Studies of the Skin. R. H. Cormane, E. H. Baart de la Faille, J. B. van der Meer, A. A. W. ten Have-Opbroek and W. W. Muijs van de Moer 1524

Herkunft der mononucleären Entzündungszellen (Makrophagen) bei der unspezifischen Entzündung (Untersuchungen am Rebuck'schen Hautfenster bei der Ratte). M. Begemann 1531

Unspezifische und spezifische Wirkstoffe bei allergischen Reaktionen der Cutis. G. Stüttgen, J. Gigli and F. Herrmann 1531

Allergens of Quinone Structure. K. H. Schulz, P. Schmidt and H. Grell 1531

Methode zur Hornschichtdickenmessung in vivo. F. Klaschka and R. A. Krause . . 1533

Dermatological and Immunological Aspects of Cryoglobulinaemia. K. K. Mustakallio and O. Wagner 1534

R.U.V., X-Ray and Alpha-particles Micrography of the Skin. A. Tosti 1535

L'Exploration thermographique en dermatologie. Ch. Gros, C. Vrousos, J. Alt and A. Basset 1539

The History of the Dermatological Section of the Royal Society of Medicine. T. J. Ryan, Y. M. Clayton, E. J. Moynahan, J. F. Kennedy, P. Polani and I. A. Magnus . . 1541

Zellphysiologische Aspekte der Psoriasis vulgaris. O. Braun-Falco, E. Christophers, S. Marghescu, D. Petzoldt, G. Rassner and M. Rupec 1546

Mycology

Mikroskopische Demonstration von Fadenpilzen und Hefen. H. Braun and C. Schönborn 1550

page

Faserzerstörung durch Dermatophyten und keratinophile Pilze. L. KREMPL-LAMPRECHT   1550

Dermatophyten und ihre Hauptfruchtformen. G. A. DEVRIES and L. KREMPL-LAMPRECHT   1555

Serological Relationship of the Dermatophytes of Emmons-Conant-System. H. PALDROK
and K. R. SUNDSTRÖM   1556

Adaptationsphasen der Dermatophyten in Zusammenhang mit ihrer Klassifikation.
V. A. BALABANOFF   1556

Epidemiologische Analyse des Vorkommens von Dermatophyten in der Slowakei.
L. CHMEL.   1560

Einige biochemische Eigenschaften der Isothiocyanate. A. BOJANOVSKÁ   1560

Trichofytocid Spofa® (5% p-bromphenylisothiocyanat) bei der Behandlung von
Trichophytosis. L. CHMEL, M. VALENTOVÁ and J. BUCHVALD   1561

Histopathomorphologische Befunde der Haut nach der Applikation von Trichophytocid.
L. CHMEL and A. BOJANOVSKÁ   1561

Chromomycosis Caused by a New Species Chmelia slovaca. L. CHMEL, I. KOCHOVÁ and
A. BOJANOVSKÁ   1562

The Third Case of Chromomycosis in the Territory of Czechoslovakia. L. CHMEL, I.
KOCHOVÁ, A. BOJANOVSKÁ and B. KONRÁD   1563

Pilzerkrankungen innerer Organe. T. WEGMANN   1563

Survey of Mycoses in U.A.R.   M. EL ZAWAHRY   1564

Clinical Diagnosis of Onychotrichophytosis. J. ALKIEWICZ and W. SOWINSKI   1564

Favic Infections in the Surroundings of Göttingen. M. KIRSCH-NIETZKI   1566

Pilzinfektionen im Bereich des Auges. D. H. HOFFMANN   1566

Parasitic Forms of the Causative Fungi in the Cutaneous and Visceral Lesions of Chromoblastomycosis. R. FUKUSHIRO and S. KAGAWA   1568

Chromomycosis (in the World and in Finland). T. PUTKONEN   1570

Relations entre formes cliniques et espèces mycologiques. A. BASSET et M. BASSET   .   1570

Dermatomykosen bei Säugetieren. H. KRAFT   1570

Mykosen bei Tieren (Befall durch Aspergillus, verschiedene Dermatophyten und
Alternaria). H. KRAFT   1572

Maduromykose beim Pferd. B. SCHIEFER and B. GEDEK   1573

Beitrag zur Mykologie der Systemmykosen: Histoplasmose und Kryptokokkose.
H. KARUGA.   1574

Vorkommen von Dermatophyten im Boden und bei Tieren als mögliche Infektionsquellen. D. JANKE   1577

Trichophytie und Blastomykose. Zs. HERPAY   1580

Ultrastructure of Dermatophytes. W. MEINHOF and W. VOGELL   1581

Infektionen durch Candida albicans. J. THURNER   1584

Quantitative Methoden der Antimykotikaprüfung. W. DITTMAR   1586

Enzymhistochemische Untersuchungen an Dermatophyten. K. HOLUBAR and O. MALE   1590

Dermatophyten und Schimmelpilze. B. BRAUN, H. RIETH and C. FINGER   1590

Additional Demonstrations

Kollegheft der Vorlesung von F. VON HEBRA, geschrieben von F. CURTI, zur Verfügung
gestellt von O. GRUMBACH unter Vermittlung von O. GANS   1590

Histopathology of Leprosy. M. L. BRUBAKER and P. FASAL   1590

Antibiotics and the Placebo Reaction in Acne. R. C. SAVIN and M. CHANCO-TURNER .   1590

Authors Index   1592

Symposium 10   **Effects of Radiation on the Skin**

Effets des radiations sur la peau

Efecto de las radiaciones en la piel

Strahlenwirkungen auf die Haut

Organizer

Fr. Flarer, Italy

Presidents

M. A. Everett, USA

L. Goldman, USA

J. Konopik, Czechoslovakia

E. G. Scolari. Italy

Delegate of the Organization Committee

A. Proppe, Germany

Reports

Radiobiologie cutanée

P. VAN CANEGHEM, Laboratoire de Radiobiologie, Université de Liège (Belgique)

Nous aborderons quelques problèmes ayant fait l'objet de recherches durant ces dernières années, en nous limitant aux effets de doses de radiations ionisantes ne dépassant pas quelques milliers de rads ($\pm \leq$ 3000 rads).

A. Erythème précoce

JOLLES et HARRISON ont particulièrement étudié la pathogénie des réactions cutanéo-vasculaires précoces chez le lapin après injection de bleu de pontamine. Elles débutent 30 min après administration locale d'environ 1000 R et disparaissent après 24 h. Puisque des inhibiteurs enzymatiques tels que l'acide ε-aminocaproïque et l'inhibiteur de la trypsine du soya sont actifs, il y a probablement une libération ou activation de protéases. Les auteurs estiment qu'il n'y a pas de rapport entre l'érythème précoce chez l'homme et la réaction qu'ils ont mise en évidence chez le lapin. Cette assertion paraît pour le moins prématurée. Ce genre de recherches est rendu d'autant plus difficile qu'il est dangereux d'extrapoler d'une espèce animale à l'homme parce que la réactivité cutanée précoce semble être très variable suivant l'espèce animale considérée. L'image histologique de l'érythème précoce correspond à celle due à une action protéolytique discrète. Si l'on se base sur les recherches de MARKUS et SCHLOTFELDT sur l'érythème cutané après irradiation chez le lapin, la réaction vasculaire de JOLLES et HARRISON paraît se superposer du moins en partie à l'érythème précoce.

B. Le poil en tant que réactif radiobiologique

Le poil peut être considéré comme un organe se prêtant admirablement, tant à des études de radioprotection, qu'à des recherches dosimétriques biologiques. Ses réponses aux rayons X sont multiples et permettent de faire des études aussi bien qualitatives que quantitatives. Sous l'influence des radiations ionisantes 1. sa vitesse de croissance peut être ralentie, 2. sa morphologie s'altère, le poil devient dysplasique, 3. si la dose est suffisante, il tombe et le seuil épilatoire est à peu près constant chez une race pure, 4. par irradiation locale on peut observer un déphasage de la pousse chez des animaux à cycle pilaire synchrone, 5. le poil peut perdre son pigment. Alors que le seuil épilatoire est plus bas en phase anagène qu'en phase télogène, le poil grisonne plus facilement quand il est au repos. On peut aussi étudier certaines modifications biochimiques du poil.

C. Irradiation superficielle

Quand elle est suffisamment intense pour provoquer une radioépidermite exsudative étendue, une irradiation superficielle peut causer la mort de l'animal, de même qu'une brûlure étendue. Sur 60 souris chauves ayant reçu sur leur face dorsale 2500 R à 16 kV; filtre 0; C.D.A. 0,5 mm cellon, quatre seulement ont survécu. La cause de la mort n'est pas exactement connue chez le mammifère, pas plus du reste qu'en cas de brûlure où elle paraît être complexe. Chez la grenouille où la peau joue un rôle dans les échanges électrolytiques et gazeux, la mort coïncide avec la chute de l'épithélium.

D. Protection

a) par substances endogènes. Certaines substances possédant des propriétés radioprotectrices peuvent être produites ou libérées dans l'organisme (Tab. 1).

Des agressions et des traumatismes, même relativement bénins, peuvent modifier
la radiorésistance de l'organisme et ceci d'une façon positive ou négative suivant
le laps de temps qui s'écoule entre l'agression et l'irradiation. Il semble que la
radiosensibilité corresponde à la phase catabolique et l'augmentation de la
résistance à la phase anabolique compensatrice consécutive à l'agression.

Tableau 1. *Quantités équivalentes de différentes substances injectées dans la peau (γ dans 0,1 ml
de NaCl 9⁰//₀₀), protégeant localement le pelage du souriceau après administration générale de 550 R*

Substances	γ/0,1 ml	μM
Cystéamine	30	0,39
Mercaptoéthanol	30	0,39
Bradykinine	3,5	0,0028
Histamine	0,5	0,0045
Sérotonine	0,1	0,00057
Adrénaline	00,5	0,00027

Tableau 2. *Action comparative de la cystéamine et de la cystamine sur le système pileux du rat*

	Injection locale	Injection i. p.
Cystamine	—	+
Cystéamine	+	± ou —

   b) Actions comparées de la cystéamine et de la cystamine. On admet que dans
l'organisme ces deux substances peuvent se transformer l'une dans l'autre. Elles
pourraient donc être utilisées plus ou moins indifféremment. Si cette assertion se
vérifie quand on prend comme critère la survie au trentième jour après irradiation
totale au moyen de rayons pénétrants, ce n'est plus le cas quand on prend l'épilation ou la dysplasie pilaire comme critère (Tab. 2). Cette différence entre l'action
de la cystamine et de la cystéamine se retrouve quand on prend comme critère
la radioépidermite exsudative chez la souris chauve. Il semble que pour ce· qui est
de la protection locale dans la peau, la cystamine ne puisse pas se transformer en
cystéamine comme c'est le cas quand elle est injectée par voie i.p. La protection
locale après injection i.d. de cystéamine paraît être due à l'anoxie causée par la
présence de groupements SH, d'autres substances thiolées dépourvues de propriétés
radioprotectrices par voie générale ayant la même action que la cystéamine quand
elles sont injectées localement. Quand on compare chez la souris les modifications
du taux des groupements sulfhydryles et disulfures combinés aux protéines dans la
rate, organe hématopoïétique, et dans la peau après injection de cystamine ou de
cystéamine, ce taux s'élève plus dans la rate; pour la cystéamine il est même
négligeable dans la peau.

Strahlenwirkung im Hautbereich in Abhängigkeit
von der verwendeten Strahlenqualität

A. PROPPE, Hautklinik der Christian Albrechts-Universität Kiel (Deutschland)

   In der dermatologischen Bestrahlungstherapie kommt es darauf an, die kranken oberflächlichen Gewebsschichten vergleichsweise möglichst hoch, die tiefer
gelegenen gesunden Regionen dagegen möglichst niedrig zu belasten. Die Auf-

gabe der optimalen Dosisverteilung läßt sich dabei am einfachsten durch die geeignete Wahl einer langwelligen Röntgenstrahlenqualität erfüllen. Beim bisherigen Stand unserer Kenntnisse ist die im individuellen Fall jeweils günstigste Weise dieser Strahlenverteilung jedoch vorerst nur in sehr grober. Annäherung zu erreichen.

Eine Voraussetzung dazu bestünde in der Bestimmung der relativen Tiefendosiskurven im Gewebe. Im langwelligen Röntgenstrahlenbereich gibt es dazu noch keine befriedigende Methode. Wie stark die bisher veröffentlichten Ergebnisse der Messungen voneinander abweichen, zeigt die Abb. Die Gründe für die ungenügende Übereinstimmung liegen einerseits im Mangel an einer geeigneten, in der Praxis zu verwendenden Meßkammer und andererseits in der Schwierigkeit, ein gewebsäquivalentes Phantommaterial zu finden. Die jüngst von MARKUS erstellten Dosisabfallkurven für einige langwelligen Strahlenqualitäten dürften bisher den Verhältnissen im Gewebe am nächsten kommen (vgl. Abb.). MARKUS hat eine eigens dazu konstruierte Meßkammer und die von ihm entwickelte Phantommasse M 3 benutzt.

Dennoch bleibt die Beurteilung der quantitativen Beziehungen zwischen der Strahlenwirkung im Hautbereich und der Strahlenqualität unsicher.. Die Bedenken entstehen zunächst aus Vorstellungen, die sich auf die selektive Absorption der Elemente im Gewebe beziehen. Hinzu kommt, daß die Absorptionsgröße der Röntgenstrahlen, nämlich die dritte Potenz ihrer Wellenlänge, im langwelligen Bereich besonders stark ins Gewicht fällt. Die theoretischen Bedenken erscheinen durch klinische Erfahrungen sehr gestützt. Aus der eigenen Klinik haben WAGNER, STUTZER und HELL Beispiele dazu vorgelegt. Aber an der Eindeutig-

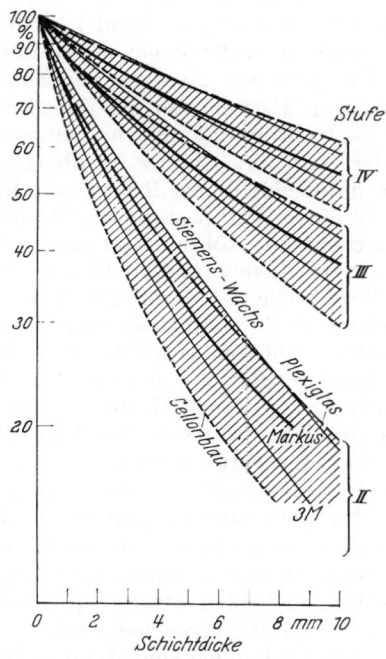

Abb. Fehlerbreite der relativen Tiefendosen in Abhängigkeit von verschiedenartigen Phantomsubstanzen bei den Dermopan-Stufen II, III und IV

keit der Zusammenhänge sind immer noch Zweifel offen. So empfehlen sich weitere Anstrengungen, um den Sachverhalt aufzuhellen.

Einen Fortschritt für das Verständnis der biologischen Strahlenreaktion im Hautbereich hat die These BODES gebracht: Die Verlaufsweise des Erythems hängt von der Etage der Hautschicht ab, die von der Strahlung getroffen wird; die Strahlenempfindlichkeit der unterscheidbaren Hautschichten ist verschieden groß; in den verschiedenen Etagen der Hautschichten läuft die Strahlenreaktion zeitlich verschieden schnell ab. Die Mehrwelligkeit eines Strahlenerythems ist folglich als die Integration voneinander unabhängiger, zeitlich unterschiedlich schnell verlaufender Etagenreaktionen aufzufassen. BODE hat seine These auf Experimente mit schnellen Elektronen gegründet. Er hat dabei das Dosismaximum wahlweise in die kritischen Hautschichten gelegt. In der Folge hat MARKUS (1967) aus dem Vergleich der Erythemwirkungen von langwelligen Röntgenstrahlen mit solchen von schnellen Elektronen nachweisen können, daß die Bodesche These auch für die Röntgenstrahlen gilt. In seinen Experimenten sind — mittels des Tests an der Phantommasse M 3 — die prozentualen Tiefendosiskurven beider Strahlenarten einander angeglichen worden. Die kritische Schicht für die erste Erythemwelle liegt weniger als 1 mm unterhalb der Oberfläche; die Schichten für die zweite und dritte Erythemwelle liegen deutlich tiefer.

Eine Röntgenstrahlung besteht nun aus einem breiten Bündel von Strahlen sehr unterschiedlicher Wellenlängen. Im langwelligen Bereich macht sich diese Inhomogenität in der unterschiedlichen Eindringtiefe der jeweils wirksamen Dosisanteile sehr bemerkbar. Daher ergibt sich aus der Bodeschen These, daß für die biologische Wirkung im Hautbereich die spektrale Verteilung des Röntgenstrahlenbündels maßgebend ist. Die Kennzeichnung der Strahlenqualität durch eine mittlere Wellenlänge, die Halbwertschicht, ist hierbei nicht mehr ausreichend.

Die genauere Analyse der Zusammenhänge in klinischen Beispielen bleibt schwierig. Fast hätten die jüngst veröffentlichten Nachuntersuchungsergebnisse bei bestrahlten Säuglingshämangiomen von LUGER einerseits und KLOSTERMANN andererseits eine Chance für überraschende Einblicke in die biologischen Reaktionen unterschiedlicher Röntgenstrahlenqualitäten geboten.

In einem Fall bestand die Strahlenquelle in einem Philipsgerät: 20 mm Focus-Hautabstand, Röhrenspannung 50 kV, Halbwertschicht 0,28 mm Al; im anderen in einem Siemensgerät: 15 mm Focus-Hautabstand, Röhrenspannung 60 kV, Halbwertschicht 4,3 mm Al. Erwartungsgemäß hat bei ungefährem Überblick die härtere Strahlung des Siemensgerätes bei den Gruppen gleicher Gesamtdosis jeweils zu höheren Anteilen von Bestrahlungsfolgen — Teleangiektasien, Atrophien, Pigmentstörungen — geführt als die weichere Strahlung des Philipsgerätes. Beim Versuch, den Vergleich im einzelnen durchzuführen, deutet sich jedoch an, daß der Häufigkeitsgang der Strahlenrelikte mit Zunahme der Gesamtdosis bei beiden Bestrahlungsverfahren verschieden ist: Die Häufigkeit der Teleangiektasien geht erheblich strammer mit der zunehmenden Dosis der weicheren Strahlung parallel, die Atrophie dagegen sehr viel mehr mit der Dosis der härteren. Der Zuwachs der Pigmentstörungen mit der Dosis — nicht die absolute Häufigkeit, die bei der härteren Strahlung immer etwa doppelt so hoch wie bei der weicheren ausfällt — scheint bei beiden Strahlenqualitäten von gleicher Größe zu sein. Es ist offenkundig, daß die verschiedenartigen Relikte an unterschiedliche Etagen der Hautschichten gebunden sind. Bedauerlicherweise aber verhindert der Mangel an einer einheitlichen, zum Vergleich geeigneten Befunddokumentation, den Beweis dafür in stichhaltiger Weise zu führen.

Noch gemeinsam mit WAGNER hatte ich es unternommen, am Modell der Psoriasis vulgaris das Verhältnis der luft-ionometrisch bestimmten Dosen zur biologischen Wirkung bei den wichtigsten in der Dermatologie therapeutisch verwendeten weichen Strahlenqualitäten zu testen. Als Kriterium wählten wir für alle Strahlenqualitäten die gleiche absolute Tiefendosis in 1 oder 2 mm Hauttiefe, wie sie aus den relativen Tiefendosen der Phantommessungen jeweils zu errechnen ist. Die Methodik führte die Ergebnisse allerdings vor das „non liquet" der Fragestellung. Es bleibt dabei nämlich unsicher, ob — was vorausgesetzt war — die relativen Tiefendosen der Phantomsubstanz auch den absorbierten Dosen in den kritischen Hautschichten entsprechen.

Solche Vergleichsuntersuchungen lassen sich bei Hautkrankheiten offenbar nur auf der Grundlage der auf die Hautfläche aufgestrahlten Standardionendosis durchführen. Neben anderen Gründen haben auch diese Erfahrungen meine Meinung bestärkt, daß es in der dermatologischen Strahlentherapie wenig sinnvoll ist, mit der hier bis jetzt nicht realisierbaren Größe der im Gewebe absorbierten Dosis, der Einheit Rad, zu rechnen.

Endlich bietet es sich an, aus histologischen Befunden Schlüsse auf die Bedeutung der Strahlenqualitäten für die Strahlenwirkung im Hautbereich zu ziehen. Wir pflegen Melanome mit den Stufen II (29 kV, 0,3 mm Al), III (43 kV, 0,6 mm Al) oder IV (50 kV, 1,0 mm Al) des Dermopan zu bestrahlen. Etwa 3 bis 4 Monate später, nach Abklingen der Strahlenreaktion, wird der Herd excidiert. Der histologische Schnitt zeigt dann in der Regel im bestrahlten Bereich eine nach der Tiefe zu scharf begrenzte, parallel zur Oberfläche verlaufende Schicht des Papillarkörpers, die von elastischen Fasern entblößt ist. Wir haben 24 Präparate ausgewertet: 2, die mit Stufe IV, 15, die mit Stufe III, und 7, die mit Stufe II bestrahlt worden waren. Dabei sind die Dosen der unterschiedlichen Strahlenqualitäten mit der gemessenen Entfernung von der Hautoberfläche zur beschriebenen Grenzschicht korreliert worden. Man darf dabei nicht zuviel erwarten. Eine Reihe von Faktoren beeinträchtigt das Fundament der Aussage: Die unkontrollierbare Schrumpfung der Präparate, Infiltrate im Papillarkörper, die Streuung des Zeitraumes zwischen Bestrahlung und Excision des Herdes, die topographischen Unterschiede, die Verschiedenheit des Alters und des Geschlechts. Dennoch erscheint es bemerkenswert, daß die Grenzschicht für die Elastikaschädigung bei Stufe IV durchschnittlich 0,26 mm, bei Stufe III 0,27 mm und bei Stufe II 0,30 mm unterhalb der Hautoberfläche gefunden wird. Sind die Differenzen in statistischer Sicht keineswegs signifikant, so ist es erstaunlich genug, daß die Maße gleich sein sollen, während die umgekehrte Tendenz ihrer Größenordnungen zu erwarten gewesen wäre. Die entsprechenden Durchschnittswerte für die Dosen betragen 6600, 6530 und 6470 R, für die Intervalle nach der Bestrahlung 3 Monate 13 Tage, 3 Monate 17 Tage und 3 Monate 26 Tage.

Mein Mentor, WALTHER GAHLEN, hat mich meiner Idee über biologisch wirksame Isodosen in den Hautschichten wegen — gewiß mit Recht — getadelt. Aber er möge verzeihen, daß — was auch immer ich zur Klärung des Sachverhaltes unternehme — die Variation der langwelligen Strahlenqualitäten unter meinen Händen zu quantitativ unerwarteten Strahlenwirkungen in den Hautschichten führt. Ich bin daher glücklich, von DREXLER und PERZL aus dem Wachsmannschen Institut für Strahlenschutz erfahren zu haben, daß die Meßtechnik für niederenergetische Quantenstrahlung durch den Einsatz von Halbleiterdetektoren, wie sie in der Kernphysik verwendet werden, erheblich verbessert worden ist. Es ist zu erwarten, daß die Darstellung der spektralen relativen Dosisleistung der in der Dermatologie verwendeten Strahlenqualitäten im Verein mit einer topographisch differenzierteren Elementaranalyse der Hautschichten hilft, die biologischen Reaktionen der Haut auf Röntgenstrahlen besser zu verstehen.

Literatur. BODE, H. G.: Hautarzt 1, 15 (1950). — DREXLER, G., u. F. PERZL: Spektren diagnostischer Röntgenstrahlen. Deutscher Röntgenkongreß, Baden-Baden, 20.—23. April 1967. — KLOSTERMANN, G. F.: Z. Haut- u. Geschl.-Kr. **41**, 132 (1966). — LUGER, A.: Z. Haut- u. Geschl.-Kr. **40**, 421 (1966). — MARKUS, B.: Strahlentherapie **101**, 111 (1956); — Die Messung von Tiefendosiskurven im Weichstrahlbereich (Im Druck). — MARKUS, B., u. D. SCHLOTFELDT: Strahlentherapie **132**, 206 (1967). — Symposium VIII: Radiobiology and Dermatological Radiation Therapy. Proc. XII. Int. Congr. Dermat. Sept. 1962. Washington D.C. I, Excerpta med. (Amst.), Sect. XIII, 615 (963).

Strahlenwirkung im Hautbereich in Abhängigkeit von der verwendeten Strahlenqualität

F. WACHSMANN, Institut für Strahlenschutz der Gesellschaft für Strahlenforschung, München (Deutschland)

Lange Zeit galt in der Strahlentherapie und besonders auch bei der dermatologischen Strahlenanwendung, daß weiche Strahlungen, angeblich „weil sie stärker absorbiert werden", biologisch wirksamer seien als harte (vgl. u. a. SCHREUS u.

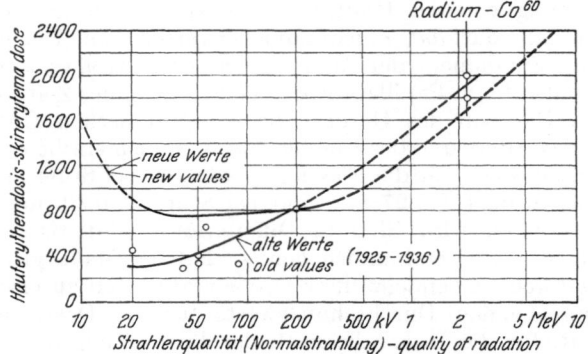

Abb. 1. Hauterythemdosen nach alten und neuen Quellen

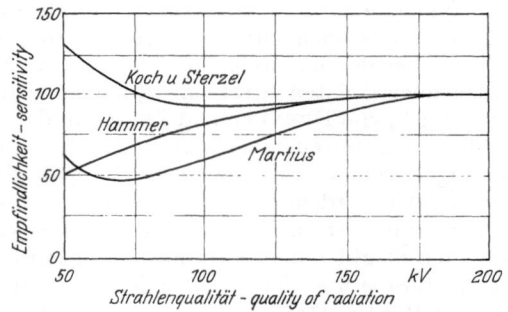

Abb. 2. Energieabhängigkeit alter Dosimeter

SCHÖNHOLZ [1] oder HALBERSTAEDTER [2]). So wurde z. B. von GLAUNER und LANGENDORFF [3] noch 1949 angegeben, daß die zur Erzeugung eines Erythems erforderliche Dosis bei 50 kV Röhrenspannung 400 R betrage, während bei den in der Tiefentherapie verwendeten harten Strahlungen die „Hauteinheitsdosis" bekanntlich etwa 800 R beträgt (WINTZ u. WITTENBECK [4]). In Abb. 1 sind die von verschiedenen älteren Autoren angegebenen Erythemdosen bei Röntgenstrahlen verschiedener Härte durch kleine Kreise angegeben. Daß diese im Gebiet weicher Strahlungen mit den heute als richtig erachteten Werten nicht übereinstimmen, mag zum Teil wenigstens auch daran liegen, daß die alten Dosimeter alles andere als energieunabhängig waren (Abb. 2). Von HOLTHUSEN und seinen Mitarbeitern [5, 6] wissen wir, daß die biologische Wirkung von Röntgenstrahlen im ganzen Bereich der „konventionellen Strahlentherapie", d. h. also von etwa 20 bis 300 kV Röhrenspannung, praktisch unabhängig von der Strahlenenergie ist.

GRÀU [7] bestätigt diese Auffassung bis herunter zu 10 kV. Sie gilt allerdings natürlich nur unter der Bedingung, daß die Dosis bis zum Erfolgsorgan — in unserem Fall das Stratum germinativum der Haut — auch tatsächlich hingelangt (SEAMAN u. Mitarb. [8]). Das heißt, daß bei sehr weichen Strahlungen höhere Oberflächendosen verabreicht werden müssen, um einen bestimmten Effekt zu erzielen, nicht aber, daß ihre biologische Wirksamkeit kleiner ist. Tiefendosen weicher Strahlungen zeigt Abb. 3.

Auch bei sehr energiereichen Strahlungen ist „die Toleranz der Haut" aber größer als bei den konventionellen Strahlungen. Dies kann zwei Gründe haben: einen sehr gut erfaßbaren physikalischen, nämlich den „Aufbaueffekt" (DREXLER

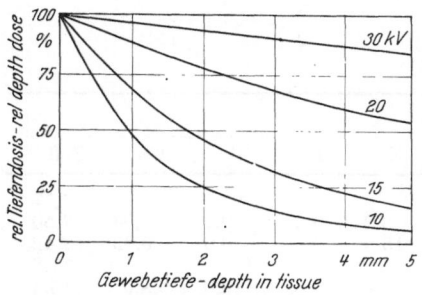

Abb. 3. Dosisabfall weicher Strahlungen   Abb. 4. Aufbaueffekt harter Strahlungen

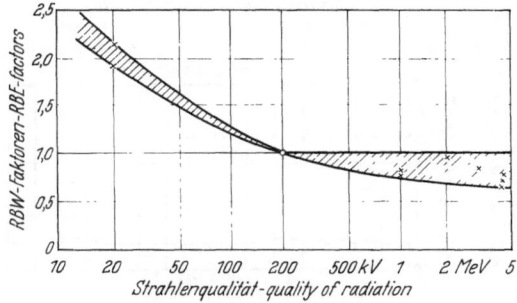

Abb. 5. RBW-Faktoren der Haut (nach verschiedenen Autoren)

u. WACHSMANN [9]), der zu einer Entlastung der Oberfläche führt (Abb. 4), und einen weniger gut geklärten, der mit der „relativen biologischen Wirksamkeit" der sog. RBW oder englisch RBE zusammenhängt. Für die Haut von verschiedenen Autoren ermittelte RBW-Werte sind in Abb. 5 wiedergegeben (nach WACHSMANN u. PINI [10]).

Dies wären die Verhältnisse roh betrachtet! Berücksichtigt man aber die Absorptionsgesetze der Strahlung (Tab. 1), so erkennt man, daß die Absorption weicher Strahlungen in starkem Maße, nämlich mit der vierten Potenz, von der Ordnungszahl der absorbierenden Stoffe abhängt. Die Ordnungszahl der verschiedenen Gewebe ist aber keineswegs stets dieselbe. Außer Knochen (SPIERS [11]) können die effektiven Ordnungszahlen auch anderer Gewebe, besonders der Haut und ihrer Anhanggebilde, die zum Teil Elemente höherer Ordnungszahl enthalten, von der von Luft oder Wasser abweichen (Tab. 2). Die aus der Literatur entnommenen Werte über die atomare Zusammensetzung der verschiedenen Gewebe schwanken allerdings stark. Aus der Abweichung von der Wasseräquivalenz ergibt sich z. B.

eine starke Dosisentlastung für Fettgewebe, aber möglicherweise auch eine Dosiserhöhung bei der Einstrahlung energiearmer Strahlungen z. B. in der Hornhaut, im Haar und in starkem Maße in Cystin (MAYNEORD [12]) und Knochen (Abb. 6).

Tabelle 1. *Absorptionsgesetze für Röntgenstrahlung*

Prozeß	Energiebereich	Abhängigkeit von Z und A
Photoprozeß	< 100 keV	$\dfrac{\tau}{\varrho} = C_1 \cdot \dfrac{Z^4}{E^3}$
Compton — Absorption	50 keV — 100 MeV	$\dfrac{\sigma}{\varrho} = C_2 \cdot \sigma_e \cdot \dfrac{L \cdot Z}{A}$
Paarbildung	> 1,02 MeV	$\dfrac{\pi}{\varrho} = C_3 \cdot E \cdot Z^2$

Tabelle 2. *Zusammensetzung verschiedener Gewebe*

Element (Gewichts-%)

Gewebe	C	H	O	S	N	K	P	Ca	Zeff
H_2O		11	89						7,57
Muskel	10,4	10,1	75,38	0,51	3,2	0,2	0,1	0,04	7,50
Haar	51	10	20	4	15	0,1	0,07	0,05	7,42
Cystin	33,9	5,7	30,2	30,2					11,8
Knochen	37,3	4,2	37,3	∼0	∼0		0,08	18,0	38,0	15,4
Hornhaut									∼8.0

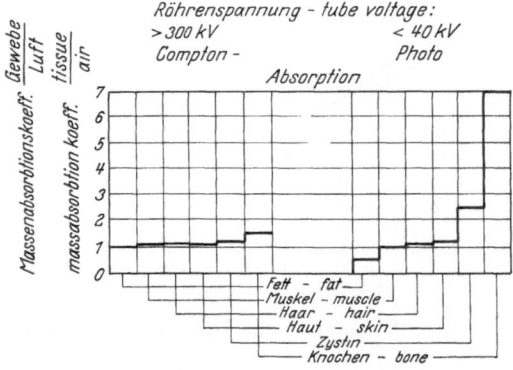

Abb. 6. Absorption von Röntgenstrahlen in verschiedenen Geweben

Von verschiedenen Autoren — so z. B. auch von meinem Vorredner — wurde unter der Annahme einer Anhäufung schwerer Elemente in gewissen Mikrostrukturen der Haut, wie z. B. den Papillen oder Zellkernen, die Möglichkeit einer selektiven Absorption gewisser Wellenlängen erörtert. Dies ist in Anbetracht der in der Dermatologie benützten meist schwach gefilterten Strahlungen, z. B. von Berylliumfensterröhren, durchaus nicht abwegig. Die Spektren dieser Strahlungen können wir erst in neuerer Zeit mit Hilfe von Halbleitern genauer analysieren (DREXLER [13]). Sie zeigen den großen Anteil weicher Strahlen der Dosis besonders bei schwacher Filterung (Abb. 7). Mit diesen Spektren werden wir uns in Zukunft sicher noch beschäftigen müssen. Hier seien zunächst nur die Spektren der Strahlungen der vier Stufen des Siemens-Dermopans gezeigt (Abb. 8).

Trotzdem glaube ich aber, daß der Effekt einer selektiven Absorption in der Hauttherapie praktisch eine nicht allzu große Rolle spielen dürfte. Einerseits liegen die Absorptionskanten der Stoffe, aus denen unser Körper und die Haut aufgebaut sind, in der Regel so niedrig, daß die zu ihrer Anregung erforderlichen weichen Strahlungen nur stark geschwächt bis in die biologisch wirksame Tiefe der Haut gelangen. Dann darf man aber auch nicht vergessen, daß, selbst wenn es

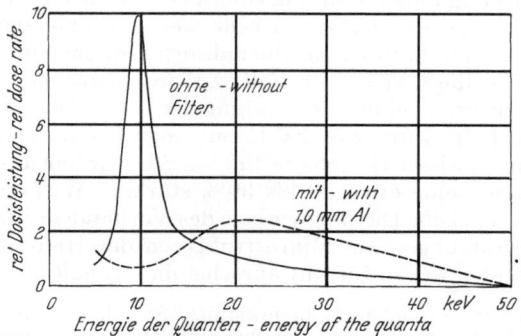

Abb. 7. Bremsspektren von zwei verschieden stark gefilterten 50-kV-Strahlungen

in der Haut Mikrostrukturen gibt, in denen Stoffe höherer Ordnungszahl signifikant angereichert sind, die Dosis in diesen Mikrogebilden des „Grenz-schichteffektes" (WACHSMANN u. DREXLER [14]) wegen nicht den Wert erreicht, den sie der effektiven Ord-nungszahl des Gewebes entsprechend erreichen würde, wenn das Gebilde ausgedehnter wäre (Abb. 9). Dies ist einfach darauf zurückzuführen, daß die z. B. von einer Bremsstrahlung von 50 kV Röhrenspannung gebildeten Photoelektronen eine mittlere Reich-

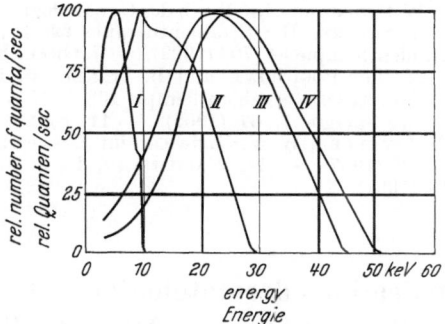

Abb. 8. Vorläufige Bremsspektren der vier Stufen des Siemens-Dermopans

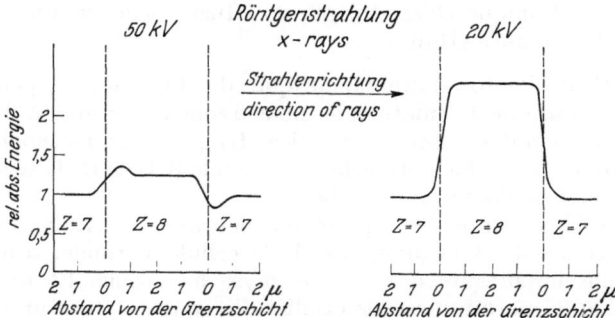

Abb. 9. Grenzschichteffekt bei weicher Strahlung

weite von 8 μ und die einer 20 kV-Strahlung von nur 1 μ besitzen, und somit der größte Teil der Energie der Sekundärelektronen nicht im Mikrogebilde selbst, sondern außerhalb dieses absorbiert wird.

Wenn man von Röntgenbremsstrahlungen verschiedene biologische Wirkungen erwartet, muß man schließlich aber auch daran denken, daß diese alles andere als monochromatisch sind (Abb. 7 u. 8). Eventuell in Frage kommende selektive Absorptionen werden also weitgehend verwischt.

Zusammengefaßt kann also festgestellt werden, daß nach heutiger Auffassung harte und weiche Röntgenstrahlen, vom physikalischen Standpunkt aus betrachtet, etwa gleiche Wirkung haben müßten, sofern sie das Erfolgsorgan nur homogen durchsetzen. Dies ist bei der Haut bei sehr weichen und sehr energiereichen Strahlungen — im ersten Fall der Strahlenabsorption, im zweiten des Aufbaueffektes wegen — allerdings nicht der Fall. Außerdem machen sich in der Haut und ihren Mikrostrukturen bei der Anwendung der in der Dermatologie gebräuchlichen weichen Strahlungen unter 50 kV Erzeugungsspannung auch die durch die nicht Luftäquivalenz gewisser Gewebe bedingten Absorptionsunterschiede stärker bemerkbar. Sie können eine etwa 20 bis 30% stärkere Wirkung weicher Strahlungen verständlich machen. Die Möglichkeit des Vorhandenseins einer selektiven Wirkung weicher Strahlungen auf Mikrostrukturen der Haut wird jedoch schon des Grenzschichteffektes wegen für unwahrscheinlich gehalten.

Literatur. 1. Schreus, H. Th., u. L. Schoenholz: Strahlentherapie **24**, 485 (1927). — 2. Halberstaedter, L.: In: Jadassohn, Handbuch der Haut- und Geschlechtskrankheiten, Bd. V/2. Berlin: Springer 1929. — 3. Glauner, G., u. H. Langendorff: In: Jüngling, Allgemeine Strahlentherapie. Stuttgart: Enke 1949. — 4. Wintz, H., u. F. Wittenbeck: In: W. Stoeckel, Handbuch der Gynäkologie, Bd. IX/2, München: J. F. Bergmann 1933/35. — 5. Holthusen, H.: Strahlentherapie **22**, 1 (1926). — 6. Braun, R., u. H. Holthusen: Strahlentherapie **34**, 707 (1929). — 7. Grau, E.: Hautarzt **6**, 82 (1955). — 8. Seaman, W. B., M. M. Ter-Pogossian, and B. Ittner: Radiology **65**, 260 (1955). — 9. Drexler, G., u. F. Wachsmann: Strahlentherapie **132**, 1 (1967). — 10. Wachsmann, F., e M. Pini: Radiazione de alte energia **1**, 67 (1962). — 11. Spiers. F. W.: Brit. J. Radiol. **22**, 521 (1949). — 12. Mayneord, W. V.: Acta Un. int. Cancer **11**, 271 (1937). — 13. Drexler, G.: Atompraxis **13**, 185 (1967). — 14. Wachsmann, F., u. G. Drexler: Strahlentherapie, Sonderband **66**, 287 (1967).

Indications dermatologiques du traitement ionisant.
Traitement ionisant des épithéliomas et des mélanomes malins à l'aide de techniques de radio-sensibilisation nouvelles

E. G. Scolari, Clinique Dermatologique et Institut de Photoradiothérapie, Université de Florence (Italie)

Dans l'Institut Photoradiothérapeutique de Florence, dépendance de la Clinique Universitaire de Dermatologie, nous avons expérimenté deux méthodes de radiosensibilisation des cellules tumorales. La première méthode emploie une substance chimique, le cyclohexilsuccinate de soude (CESNa); la seconde méthode est basée sur l'effet de l'oxigène hyperbare.

Le point de départ de notre expérimentation avec le CESNa est l'hypothèse que la cellule tumorale, à la différence de la cellule normale, trouve sa source d'énergie la plus importante dans la glycolyse anaérobie. Et nous avons constaté que le CESNa, parmi une série étudiée d'analogues structuraux du glucose, est le meilleur inhibiteur de la glycolyse. Cette propriété, démontrée par une série de recherches convénables, porte à une souffrance métabolique de la cellule tumorale et des cellules qui, en raison de leurs exigences énergétiques très élévées, ont recours aussi à la source glycolytique. Ces cellules en souffrance succombent par suite de doses de radiations inférieures aux doses létales ordinaires [1].

Notre expérience clinique sur l'activité radiosensibilisante du CESNa date de 9 ans et concerne 827 cas [2, 3, 4]. En employant les doses radiologiques de routine:

Le pourcentage des insuccès diminue de 7% à zéro pour les épithéliomas baso-cellulaires, et de 10% à zéro pour les épithéliomas spinocellulaires cutanés. On obtient une augmentation du 20% des résultats positifs dans les épithéliomas de la cavité orale, des premières voies respiratoires et des génitaux. Les résultats sont meilleurs sur les localisations ganglionnaires aussi. L'effet des radiations a été amélioré aussi sur les mélanomes malins. A mentionner la régression obtenue quelquefois des métastases ganglionnaires dans ces cas.

Le traitement par des doses de routine résout $^2/_3$ des épithéliomas résultés radio-résistants, ou récidivés après l'application de doses identiques non associées au radio-sensibilisateur [5]. La roentgendépilation temporaire des teigneux a été obtenue avec 166 r seulement pour champ, et avec diminution de $2 \div 5$ jours du temps de latence [6].

Notre emploi de l'oxygène hyperbare dans la radiothérapie des épithéliomas et des mélanomes malins est basé sur des principes déjà largement appliqués en oncologie.

On sait depuis plusieurs années que la radio-résistance augmente dans les tissus normaux rendus anoxiques même par simple compression. Les tumeurs ont certainement des zones anoxiques, surtout quand elles s'accroissent rapidement et en masses solides éloignées des vaisseaux du stroma, ce qu'il arrive dans les épithéliomas spinocellulaires. Mais indépendamment de sa structure histologique, une tumeur est aisément atteinte de l'anoxie, surtout quand elle croît parmi des tissus rigides, lesquels conditionnent une stase péritumorale.

En tout cas, l'oxygène doit atteindre des vaisseaux, par diffusion, les zones pro-fondes de la tumeur. Et l'on peut démontrer à l'aide de mesures polarographiques (Cater et Silver, [7]) et de modèles (Thomlinson et Gray, [8]) que la tension de l'oxygène dans les cellules descend à zéro dans l'espace d'une ou deux cen-taines de microns. On constate un gradient analogue de la souffrance cellulaire, à partir des éléments bien oxygénés à proximité du stroma jusqu'aux éléments presque dépourvus d'oxygène en contact avec le «coeur nécrosique» de la tumeur, complètement anoxique (Back et Ambrus [9]). La radio-sensibilité diminue parallèlement, des cellules oxygénées à celles qui sont presque anoxyques, suivant un rapport de $3:1$.

Ce qui est accepté en général c'est que la nouvelle prolifération de cellules radio-résistantes, en tant qu'hypoxyques, conditionne les insuccès de la radio-thérapie des tumeurs. La possibilité d'une nouvelle croissance semble dépendre de l'augmentation de l'oxygène ambiant disponible (Cater et Silver, [7]) et de l'hyperémie inflammatoire promues par les nécroses cellulaires: deux phénomènes provoqués par la radiothérapie elle-même. D'autre côté, la destruction des cellules hypoxiques au maximum, demanderait une dose triple de radiations, ce qui serait incompatible avec la survivance nécessaire du tissu péritumoral normal.

Parmi les nombreuses techniques conçues dans le but d'augmenter la radio-sensibilité des cellules tumorales anoxiques, celle qui a prévalu c'est la technique consistant à faire respirer au patient de l'oxygène comprimé à plusieurs atmos-phères (Churchill-Davidson [10]).

Le mécanisme de l'effet-oxygène n'est pas bien connu. On a parlé de l'alté-ration certaine provoqué par l'oxigène hyperbare dans quelques systèmes enzy-matiques, en particulier dans les systèmes contenant des groupes thioliques. Toutefois, on n'a découvert jusqu'à présent ni la localisation exacte du dommage, ni son étendue, ni son rôle dans un phénomène qui semble être, vraisemblable-ment, déterminé par plusieurs facteurs. Les études sur les radicaux libres ont appuyé l'hypothèse affirmant que l'effet indirect des radiations est intensifié par une disponibilité d'oxygène plus élevé. Cela diminue les probabilités d'une recombination des radicaux produits par la radiolyse de l'eau; en effet, ils peuvent se combiner avec l'oxigène moléculaire pour former des radicaux-péroxydes, ou bien des radicaux organiques par déhydrogénation. D'autre part, des radicaux libres et des peroxydes se forment aussi pour l'effet de l'oxygène hyperbare lui seul, suivant la théorie de GERSCHMAN [11]. Toutefois, on ne peut affirmer que ce-mécanismes soient exclusifs ou prédominants pour l'effet-oxigène. ALPERN et FLANDERS (cités par WOOTTON) et d'autres Auteurs, suivant la théorie de la cible, avancent l'hypothèse que l'oxygénation joue un rôle dans les réactions méthioniques. Un lien rompu peut se rétablir dans une molécule protéique-cible, mais l'oxygène présent peut s'opposer à la réconstruction en considant le dommage. De ce point de vue, les peroxydes organiques dérivant de l'irradiation, prennent la signification de refus, au lieu de médiateurs du dommage cellulaire.

D'autre côté, les caractéristiques physiques de l'oxygène nous permettent de supposer que la production d'ions par les radiations porte à la constitution de champs électriques locaux intenses, lesquels sont à même de rompre les liens de molécules polaires telles que les molécules protéiques. L'oxigène, un gaz para-magnétique, serait en mesure de modifier les champs mentionnés (WOOTTON [12]), avec des effets finals considérables au point de vue biologique. En tout cas, il est certain, que la nature des effets chimiques est différente dans l'état d'anoxie et d'oxygénation; et une telle différence entraîne une amélioration des résultats de l'irradiation thérapeutique des tumeurs, ainsi qu'une expérimentation toujours réconfirmée l'a révélé.

Un problème qui nous a beaucoup intéressé c'est celui qui concernait l'opportunité d'associer les deux techniques de radio-sensibilisation des tumeurs que nous connaissons de façon plus approfondie, à savoir: l'oxygénation hyperbare et l'emploi du cyclohexylsuccinate de sodium.

Etant donné la diminution de son patrimoine enzymatique, la cellule tumorale doit toujours avoir recours à la glycolyse anaérobie comme source d'énergie, quelle que soit sa teneur en oxygène. D'autre part, l'hyperoxygénation baisse la glycolyse anaérobie de la cellule cancéreuse. Cet «effet Pasteur» s'ajoute, donc, à l'action d'inhibition parallèle, exercée sur la glycolyse par le CESNa. En outre, comme M. NANNELLI et G. GABRIELLI [13] l'ont démontré, les rayons X, bêta et gamma en présence du CESNa déclenchent la production de radicaux libres, dont l'action synergique avec l'action des radicaux oxydants intensifiée par l'oxygénation est vraisemblable. Et donc nous avons employé le CESNa de façon constante chez nos patients irradiés en oxygénation hyperbare.

La source radiogène que nous avons choisie est le Radium, que le patient porte sur lui sous forme de moulages. Le patient peut alors être admis avec son moulage dans une grande chambre hyperbaryque de 5 m³ de volume, où il peut rester pendant 2 h à 3 athm. abs. d'oxygène pur, à son aise et sans danger. Mes collaborateurs M. NANNELLI et G. MANTELLASSI expliqueront l'emploi et les avantages de la grande chambre au cours de cette séance.

Jusqu'à présent nous avons traité de 75 patients atteints d'épithéliomas baso-cellulaires, d'épithéliomas épino-cellulaires cutanés et des muqueuses orales et génitales, en partie avec métastases gauglionnaires, ou de mélanomes malins. Le nombre des cas et la période d'expérimentation ne nous permettent pas encore de donner des conclusions définitives ou d'élaborer des statistiques. Mais nous pouvons affirmer que l'expérimentation de cette technique a marqué un progrès, par rapport à la radiothérapie commune, surtout en ce qui concerne les résultats obtenus en matière de métastases ganglionnaires. Mes collaborateurs C. VALLECCHI et G. MANTELLASSI rapporteront au cours de cette séance les détails de la technique thérapeutique et les résultats obtenus.

Bibliographie. 1. Scolari, E. G., M. Nannelli, and C. Vallecchi: Progr. biochem. Pharmacol. **1**, 681 (1965). — 2. Scolari, E. G., D. Boiti, C. Vallecchi und M. Nannelli: Hautarzt **15**, 285 (1964). — 3. Scolari, E. G., C. Vallecchi e M. Nannelli: Ital. gen. Rev. Derm. **5**, No. 4 (1964). — 4. Scolari, E. G., C. Vallecchi, and M. Nannelli: Progr. biochem. Pharmacol. **1**, 707 (1965). — 5. Scolari, E. G., M. Nannelli e C. Vallecchi: Ital. gen. Rev. Derm. **3**, 1 (1962). — 6. Scolari, E. G., e D. Boiti: VI. Congr. Naz. Radiobiol. Med. Trieste 1962, Atti pp. 429—433, vol. 2 (CNEN 1962). — 7. Cater, D. B., and I. A. Silver: Acta radiol. (Stockh.) **53**, 233 (1960). — 8. Thomlinson, R. H., and L. H. Gray: Histological structure of some human lung cancers and possible implications for radiotherapie. Brit. J. Cancer **9**, 539 (1955). — 9. Back, and Ambrus: J. nat. Cancer Inst. **30**, 17 (1963). — 10. Churchill Davidson, I.: Modern Trends in Radiotherapy. Ed. Deely, and Wood. London: Butterworth 1967. — 11. Gerschman: Science **119**, 623 (1954). — 12. Wootton, P.: Oxygen as a radiotherapeutic adjuvant. In: Progress in Radiation Therapy Vol. II, ed. F. Buschke. New York: Grune and Stratton 1962. — 13. Nannelli, M., e G. Gabrielli: Ital. gen. Rev. Derm. **4**, No. 4 (1965).

Indications thérapeutiques des substances radioactives en dermatologie

B. Pierquin, Institut Gustave Roussy, Villejuif (France)

La radiothérapie en dermatologie a été considérablement renouvelée depuis ces dernières années par l'utilisation des substances radio-actives artificielles, à la fois en endo et en plésio-radiothérapie.

1. Le matériel radio-actif

On dispose de plusieurs émetteurs béta pur ou béta gamma. *Phosphore 32*, émetteur béta pur utilisé essentiellement dans les applicateurs cutanés de contact (plésiocuriethérapie). *Strontium 90*, émetteur béta pur également utilisé en applicateur de contact (plésiocuriethérapie). *Yttrium 90*, émetteur béta pur utilisé en puncture par aiguilles (endocuriethérapie). *Césium 137*, émetteur béta gamma, utilisé en puncture sous forme d'aiguilles (endocuriethérapie). *Iridium 192*, emetteur béta gamma, utilisé en puncture sous forme de fils ou d'épigles (endocuriethérapie).

L'intérêt de ces radio-éléments est double: sur le plan clinique, il permet une meilleure adaptation du matériel radio-actif au volume-cible, sur le plan technique, il permet une meilleure protection pour le personnel médical.

2. Les indications thérapeutiques

A. Lésions bénignes. a) Il s'agit avant tout des *angiomes* que l'on peut décolorer par applicateurs (Phosphore 32, strontium 90): 1500 à 2000 rads par applicateur, ou que l'on peut réduire par endocuriethérapie (Yttrium 90): 1500 à 2000 rads par applicateur. Dans ces indications, il s'agit de bétathérapie pure. b) *Chéloïdes:* Immédiatement après l'excision de la tumeur chéloïdienne, une irradiation par fil d'Iridium 192 (technique par tubes plastiques) peut être réalisée au niveau de la ligne d'incision. Dose: 1500 rads. Gamma-thérapie.

B. Tumeurs malignes. Il s'agit avant tout des cancers primitifs de la peau, baso- ou spino-cellulaires: a) *dyskératoses pré-néoplasiques:* plésio-curiethérapie par applicateurs de Phosphore 32 ou de Strontium 90: 20000 rads. Béta-thérapie pure. b) *petits cancers T-1, T-2:* endocuriethérapie par aiguilles de Césium 137: 7500 rads Gamma-thérapie. c) *cancers étendus de la peau T-3, T-4:* endocuriethérapie avec technique de préparation non radio-active avec Iridium 192: 7500 rads Gamma-thérapie.

Nous voulons particulièrement insister sur ce dernier chapitre où l'endocurie-thérapie a permis de réaliser de grands progrès dans le traitement de ces larges cancers.

3. L'endocuriethérapie des cancers étendus de la peau

Trois techniques avec préparation non radio-active sont utilisables : technique par tubes plastiques avec fils radio-actifs, technique par aiguilles hypodermiques avec mandrin radio-actif, technique par gouttières vectrices avec épingles radio-actives. Toutes trois utilisent l'Iridium 192.

De ces trois techniques de préparation non radio-active, les deux les plus utilisées au niveau des cancers étendus de la peau, sont d'une part, la technique par tubes plastiques et, d'autre part, la technique par aiguilles hypodermiques.

En effet, l'une et l'autre peuvent être utilisées en entrée et sortie en réservant une zone inactive au niveau du point d'entrée et du point de sortie de la peau, ce qui permet d'éviter tout surdosage à ce niveau, donc toute cicatrice inesthétique. Il n'en est pas de même pour la technique par gouttières vectrices, dont la tête, soit sous forme d'un petit oeillet en aiguille simple, soit sous forme d'une branche transversale en épingle double, reste à la surface de la peau et entraîne par conséquent un surdosage sur l'épiderme donnant lieu à une cicatrice inesthétique.

Schématiquement, on peut reconnaître à chacune de ces techniques les indications cliniques suivantes :

1. Pour les tubes plastiques, les indications cliniques sont celles avant tout, de larges lésions dépassant 50 mm de diamètre et couvrant des zones cutanées relativement planes, avec un tissu cellulaire sous cutané épais. C'est le cas en particulier de la peau jugale et, d'une façon générale, de celle des membres et du tronc.

2. Les aiguilles hypodermiques avec mandrin radioactif, sont plutôt réservées à des lésions de dimensions inférieures (35 à 40 mm), plus particulièrement au niveau de zones cutanées de recouvrement osseux ou cartilagineux (front, nez, oreille).

3. Quant à la technique par gouttières vectrices avec épingles, elle est surtout réservée aux indications de lesions péri-orificielles où l'opérateur ne peut utiliser qu'une technique à entrée simple : lésions de la marge de l'anus par exemple ou encore des orifices narinaires.

Nous utilisons ces techniques de préparation non radio-active avec l'Iridium 192 au niveau de la peau depuis 5 ans. Les quelques figures commentées dans ce travail permettent de se rendre compte des résultats obtenus auprès de lésions de diverses localisations. Sur une centaine de malades ainsi irradiés, nous pouvons reconnaître :

1. une bonne cicatrisation au niveau de lésions largement étendues de 3 à 7 cm de diamètre, dans la mesure où l'ulceration céntrale n'a pas détruit totalement la couche de Malpighi. On assiste alors à une réépidermisation rapide dans les semaines qui suivent la fine de l'application avec des doses tumorales de l'ordre de 7500 R dans le plan de l'irradiation.

2. pour des lésions de très large extension et particulièrement pour des lésions profondément ulcérées, avec destruction complète des plans épidermiques et dermiques sur plusieurs centimètres de diamètre, on ne peut évidemment espérer une cicatrisation rapide et complète. Mais ce que l'on peut constater, c'est une stérilisation de lésions même très largement étendues, jusqu'à 10 cm de diamètre au besoin, donnant lieu à une ulcération centrale propre, qui se réépidermisera très lentement dans les mois et années suivants.

Une chirurgie réparatrice post-curiethérapique mériterait d'ailleurs d'être discutée sous forme de greffes épidermiques, voire de plasties.

Algunos rasgos ultraestructurales de las radiolesiones

J. Cabré, Clinica Dermatologica Universitaria, Cadiz (España)

Clásico es el hecho de que el carácter *clinico* primordial de las radiolesiones consiste en un manifiesto polimorfismo, resultante de toda la serie de factores causales que las desencadenan. Los elementos esenciales de tan variada sintomatología son: eritema, hiperpigmentación,. vesiculación, formación de ampollas, ulceración. escaras y necrosis, asi como formación de teleangiectasias, atrofia y esclerosis, Signos clinicos que han permitido distinguir ciertas formas clinicas (v. pej. Du-courtioux y Civatte, o Lepennetier y Rabeau).

Los autores clásicos disntinguen desde el punto de vista *histológico* entre lesiones agudas y lesiones tardías (comp. con Gans y Steigleder, J. Civatte, H. Z. Lund, W. Lever). Los elementos fisulares esenciales de las mismas pueden resumirse del modo siguiente: degeneración hidrópica de las células epiteliales, alteraciones nucleares de las mismas, infiltrado inflamatorio perianexial, dilatación vascular acompañada de edema parietal y de proliferación endotelial, edema y homo-geneización de la colágena. Puede completar este cuadro microscópico la necrosis de la epidermis y del dermis superior, acompañada de una reacción de leucocitos polinucleares. En las formas tardias la imagen tisular viene constituída por alte-raciones en el espesor de la banda epidermica, cuyas células muestran numerosas imagenes de mitosis y de disqueratosis individual, presencia de papilomatosis fenómenos de esclerosis conjuntiva con marcada basofilia, neoformación conectiva distribuida perivascularmente, espesamiento de las paredes vasculares en dermis profundo con imagenes de trombosis y recanalización, y ausencia de anejos cutáneos respetandose en parte las glándulas sudoriparas.

Puede resumirse diciendo que la acción de las radiaciones ionizantes sobre la piel acarrea un cese en la actividad mitótica, un aumento irregular de la talla nuclear, fenomenos de multinucleación, edema del endotelio vascular y dilatación capilar afectándose la componente fibrilar conjuntiva.

Nuestra intención es la de sistematizar los hechos observados al microscopio electrónico estudiando piezas procedentes de sujetos que presentaban radio-lesiones terapeuticas. Se estudiaron fragmentos obtenidos mediante biopsia practicada con punzón en cinco sujetos irradiados por carcinoma espinocelular, y en dos sujetos radiados con finalidad terapeutica complementaria (uno caso de castración terapeutica, y uno caso de depilación por tiña).

Metodo: fijación de primera intención en formol tamponado al 4% durante una hora. Lavado en tampon fosfato a pH 7,2 durante media hora. Refijación en tetraoxido de osmio al 1% durante dos horas. Deshidratación en acetona. Inclusión en Durcupan ACM (Fluka). Cortes ultrafinos en microtomo tipo Porter-Blum. Contraste con acetato de uranilo y citrato de plomo según Reynolds. Observación en microscopio electrónico Elmiskop I Siemens a tensiones de 60 y 80 kV.

Resultados. Distinguimos en nuestra serie de investigación dos categorias de resultados morfologicos. Una la constituida por las piezas obtenidas de radio-lesiones motivadas por tratamiento anticanceroso, y otra representada por las radiodermitis consecuentes a tratamientos coadyuvantes.

En el primer grupo hemos recogido los detalles siguientes. Las modificaciones ultraestructurales más manifiestas asientan en el cuerpo mucoso de Malpighio. Las células espinosas presentan anomalías nucleares consistentes en numero exagerado de nucleos voluminosos provistos de varios nucleolos gigantes, de configuración irregular y en número de dos o tres. Menos frecuentes son las imágenes de picnosis nuclear, con desaparición de la membrana nuclear. En el reticulo endoplasmico de numerosas células se aprecian dilataciones de las cisternas, provistas de una superficie granular. Estas formaciones "seudo-vacuolares" rechazan las tonofibrillas que aparecen constituyendo haces mucho más densos. No se observan las mitocondrias. Los desmosomas son muy numerosos, aparecen más alargados y más anchos, presentando con regularidad 13 bandas. No se observan células pigmentarias ni granulos de melanina. La mebrana basal presenta en algunas zonas características normales, en otros puntos falta. En el dermis se distinguen la gran cantidad de células plasmáticas dotadas de cisternas muy dilatadas, linfocitos sin alteraciones morfologicas, algun mastocito con manifiestos fenómenos de liberación granular. Los histiocitos muestran grandes y enormes lisosomas. Escaso numero de fibroblastos de estructura normal rodeados de numerosas fibras colágenas. Estas últimas presentan una configuración, unas dimensiones y una periodicidad absolutamente normales. El endotelio vascular aparece en algunas zonas muy adelgazado, en otros puntos el citoplasma celular está edematoso.

En las piezas del segundo grupo las células del cuerpo mucoso de Malpighio presentan una morfología casi normal. Los desmosomas ofrecen una estructura normal. Se observan mitocondrias mal conservadas. Las células dendriticas de la capa basal aparecen con absoluta normalidad. Presencia abundante de granulos de melanina dentro de las células epiteliales circundantes. La membrana basal está conservada. Los nucleos de las células espinosas estan provistos de nucleolos de tamaño considerable no excediendo en numero a uno o dos. En el dermis destacan por una parte el numero aumentado de capilares con engrosamiento parietal, con notable edema del citoplasma celular, y por otra la presencia de abundantes leucocitos polinucleares.

Concluyendo diremos que esta serie de imagenes vienen a confirmar los datos obtenidos mediante la investigación histologica con el microscopio fotónico.

Preliminary Investigative Studies of the Laser Treatment of Angiomas*

L. GOLDMAN, R. J. ROCKWELL jr. and R. MEYER, Laser Laboratory, The Children's Hospital Research Foundation, Cincinnati, Ohio (U.S.A.)

One of the challenges in dermatology is the treatment of angiomas, the progressive forms and especially the resistant port-wine lesion. Angiomas have been treated with many diverse therapies, including surgery, excisional grafting, dermabrasion, electrosurgery, cryosurgery, radiation, injections and covering tattoos [1, 2]. Controls are necessary, especially with the cavernous angiomas because of the natural course of events in the spontaneous clearing of many, not all, of these lesions. However, the port-wine lesion is resistant to all forms of treatment. At present, tattooing with zinc oxide and titanium dioxide is done. It is of interest that studies of MIESCHER [3] and others have emphasized the fact that the resistance to therapy of the port-wine lesion is associated with the maturity and hamartomatous character of the cellular, vascular elements of this lesion. The other significant feature of the port-wine lesion is the extent and depth of many of the vascular structures. Occasionally, there may be mixtures of portwine and cavernous angiomas and the cavernous phase of this may be progressive even in adults. We have reported previously acquired angiomas and the laser

* Supported by a grant from The John A. Hartford Foundation.

treatment of some of these lesions [4]. An acquired, truly port-wine spot is rare. We have observed three such lesions in adults, two in males. The vascular reactions from the oral ovulation suppressive medications produced a port-wine lesion on the leg of a young woman.

One of the features of the biomedical applications of the laser is the evidence that some lasers are absorbed by color and the color of the angioma lends itself to absorption by certain lasers.

Laser Instruments

For 4 years, we have used the laser systems in the treatment of angiomas [7]. These include the ruby laser, 6943 A°; the neodymium laser, 10,600 A°; the argon laser, 4480 to 5145 A° with specific wavelengths at 4880 A° blue, 4765 A° light-blue, and 5145 A° green; and the varbon dioxide laser, 106,000 A°. As yet, we have had no experience with the ultraviolet laser [8].

We have used animal test models to attempt to work out some of the parameters of the laser reaction in angiomas. These test models have included red tattoo in the rabbit and miniature pig skin [5] and the use of the comb and wattle of the chicken [6]. Experience has shown that tattoo models in the rabbit and also in the skin of the miniature pig have not been effective since these tattoo masses do not simulate in optical properties or vascular dynamics of blood vessel systems. The comb and wattle are adequate in spite of certain anatomical features such as hyperkeratosis, nucleated red cells, mucoid connective tissue, and hormonal control of vascular structures. The comb, although it has a thicker stratum corneum, is easier to use than the wattle.

Testing Techniques

For the patient, the test areas are given as small test spots in selected areas. These test areas vary according to the target area, the location of the lesion and the general goal of the treatment. For the ruby lasers, the average treatment is 55 to 65 joules/cm^2, target areas of 1.76 cm^2 with the pulse duration of 2 to 3 milliseconds. In the neodymium laser, the outputs are between 55 to 65 joules/cm^2 with target area of 2 cm^2. Q-switched giant pulsed laser systems, just under study, with 35 to 100 megawatts power output and argon lasers vary from 0.5 to 1.5 watts. There is initial charring. These areas are then observed for a period of 4 to 6 weeks. During this period, the crust peels off and the redness fades gradually. At this time, additional tests may be done or extensive treatments may be started. A total of some 64 benign and malignant vascular lesions have been treated. Four patients who have had previous tattooing for the treatment of port-wine lesions have also been studied [9, 10] (Tab. 1). In brief, the histopathological studies of the laser reaction in angiomas is that of a nonspecific coagulation necrosis of the collagen and elastic fibers and vascular elements followed by cicatrix formation.

Table 1. *Laser Treatment of Vascular Lesions*

Lesion	Number	Improved	No Improvement
Port-wine	60	42	18
Cavernous Angiomas	4	4	
"Senile" Angiomas	4	4	
Spider Angiomas	2	2	
Mafucci's Syndrome	1	1	
Lymphangioma	1		1
Kaposi Hemorrhagic Sarcoma (small selected nodules)	3	3	
Angiosarcoma	1	1	

The reactions which have occurred following treatment have been increased redness for a brief period of time, superficial transient atrophy, some superficial scarring and occasional revascularization, and in one adult with mixed port-wine and cavernous nodules an occasional small cavernous nodule after laser therapy. Hemorrhage has not been a significant feature of the laser treatments except in this same patient with mixed port-wine and cavernous angiomas. It has been said by WAISMAN [12] that there are more residual radiation damages than persistent angiomas. In more than 4 years of laser treatments, then, radiation sequela similar to those of X-ray or radium have not been observed.

Table 2. *Reactions in Laser Treated Areas of Port-wine Lesions in 60 Patients*

Superficial Scarring	3
Revascularization After Lightening	4
Minor Telangiectasia	1
Cavernous Nodule (Patient with Mixed Port-wine + Cavernous)	1

Transillumination of the eyes from passage of laser beam through soft tissues of the face has to be considered. Studies at the present time with the use of photodetectors photography, including color infrared about the face and neck, have not shown any significant findings. A type of reflectant plastic eye shield is being developed to permit laser treatments over the eyelids.

Results of Treatment

We have not been able to increase the energy output without the avoidance of significant scarring. In brief, as with tattooing, the more superficial type, the less the response. The darker and thicker lesions show a greater response.

It is emphasized that this treatment is investigative and, perhaps, not even practical for the patient with an extensive type of lesion. Yet, the lightening in color even for a small area is persistent and usually cosmetically acceptable, one diffulty is the reticular pattern produced by the circular pattern of the impact areas. The results in the port-wine lesions are of considerable interest. Obviously, it is difficult to evaluate the effects in the capillary and cavernous types except in selected patients or when they are progressive.

The treatment of malignant lesions in the form of angiosarcomas and Kaposi's sarcomas have been of interest since high output ruby lasers have succeeded in destroying the small lesions, 0.5 to 1.5 cm in diameter When these nodules are large or extensive, the laser treatments are scarcely practicable. Angiosarcomas have also been treated and here, too, significant destruction of small lesions was accomplished. As a test model for the malignant vascular tumors, the transplant of malignant vascular tumors produced by SWARM with thorium in the albino mouse was used to study the parameters of laser reactions in malignant vascular lesions.

Conclusions. The laser treatment of angiomas is a form of investigative surgery and should not supplant conventional therapy when such conventional treatment is required and is available. The general rule at present is that if you do not need the laser, do not use it. Preliminary studies over the past 4 years have shown significant results which warrant continued investigative studies for resistant vascular lesions, such as the port-wine spots, and for those progressive capillary and cavernous accessible angiomas.

References. 1. MARTIN, L. W.: Amer. J. Surg. 107, 511 (1964). — 2. CONWAY, H., and R. E. MONTROY: N. Y. J. med. 65, 876 (1965). — 3. MIESCHER, G.: Dermatologica (Basel) 106, 176 (1953). — 4. GOLDMAN, L., and D. RICHFIELD: Acta derm.-venereol. (Stockh.) 46, 177 (1966). — 5. MONTAGNA, W., and S. JUN JEUNG: J. invest. Derm. 43, 11 (1964). — 6. RITTER, E.: Life Sci. 5, 1903 (1966). — 7. GOLDMAN, L., R. WILSON, and K. W. KITZMILLER: Investigative studies of the laser treatment of angiomas. Meeting of the Noah Worcester Dermatological Society, West Palm Beach, Florida, USA, April 1, 1966. — 8. GOLDMAN, L., and R. J. ROCKWELL jr.: J. Amer. med. Ass. 198, 641 (1966). — 9. GOLDMAN, L., E. RITTER, R. J. ROCKWELL jr., R. G. WILSON, K. W. KITZMILLER, R. MEYER, and J. A. EHA: Investigative studies of laser therapy of angiomas. American Academy of Dermatology, Meeting in Bal Harbour, Florida, USA, December 3—8, 1966. — 10. GOLDMAN, L., E. J. RITTER, R. J. ROCKWELL jr., R. MEYER, B. HENDERSON, and K. W. KITZMILLER: Laser surgery of angiomas with special reference to the port-wine lesions. American Medical Association, Meeting in Atlantic City, New Jersey, USA, June 18—22, 1967. — 11. SOLOMON, H., L. GOLDMAN, B. HENDERSON, D. RICHFIELD, and M. FRANZEN: Histopathology of the laser treatment of port-wine lesions. In press. — 12. WAISMAN, M.: Pers. communications. — 13. SWARM, R. L.: Pers. communications.

Free Communrcations

The Treatment of Skin Tumours with Radium and Hyperbaric Oxygen

C. Vallecchi and G. Mantellassi, Photoradiotherapic Institute, University of Florence (Italy)

Tumoral tissue has a mainly anaerobic metabolism together with a low oxygen concentration. It is then possible to irradiate a malignancy with better results when we correct at the same time its peculiar physiopathology, the prevailing anaerobic glycolysis and hypoxia.

For many years at the Photoradiotherapic Institute of Florence the possibility has been demonstrated of interfering with anaerobic glycolysis with an inhibitor, Sodium cyclohexylsuccinate (CESNa) associated with radiotherapy.

The "oxygen effect" is well known: in radiotherapy, pressurized chambers are used in order to furnish to the neoplastic cells the oxygen which they are missing owing to the insufficient blood flow, thus increasing their radiosensitivity.

The originality of our method of radiotherapy consists in having joined these two different methods of radiosensitization, which are synergistic and selective for neoplastic tissues; and in particular in the creation of a new technique of hyperbaric oxygen therapy (H.P.O.). The latter is based on the use of Radium with a large high pressure chamber (particulars are reported by E. G. Scolari and by M. Nannelli and G. Mantellassi in this session).

75 malignancies were treated with the tumour dose given in a "continual", "fractional" or "alternated" method, the irradiation being administered by a Radium mould applied to the region to be treated. The radium preparation, their technical characteristics and the calculations of the dose correspond to classical radium therapy. The H.P.O. was applied daily or every other day in a variable number of sittings where the patient received pure oxygen for 2 h at 3 ata.

The *continual* irradiation was given to 33 basal cell epitheliomas; 3000 r were given on the surface of which only about one tenth in H.P.O. This was the first dosage plan in our prudent preliminary experience.

The *alternated* irradiation consisted in applying a low intensity mould constantly while the patients is at normal atmospheric pressure. A higher intensity mould is applied during the session of H.P.O.

This technique was applied in twelve cases of squamous cell epitheliomas of the skin, lower lip or external genitalia and in nine malignant melanomas. The total dose was 4000 r on the surface for the epitheliomas and 8000 r for melanoblastomas. Of the latter dose about two thirds was administered under pressurized oxygen.

With the *fractional* irradiation the tumour dose was totally administered under pressurized oxygen. The dose varied on the surface from 3500 to 6000 r. Five cases of carcinoma of the lower lip or oral cavity, 14 cases of limph gland metastases due to skin or .oropharingeal carcinomas (9) and melanoblastomas (5), 1 metastatic lymphosarcoma and a case of mycosis fungoides were treated with this technique. For the whole duration of radiotherapy CESNa was administered to all, at the average dose of 2 g a day, by mouth. For a clinical comparison of the effect of the combined Radium/H.P.O./CESNa efficacy we have used the case reports of the Institute, with conventional treatments. Since it is impossible to consider survival time, we can only emphasize an increased rate of favourable results in respect to analogous situations where ordinary radiological measures where used alone. In particular, after 1 year of observation, we obtained regression of 33 basal cell epitheliomas with lower doses than ordinarily used. More significant is the response of highly malignant tumours, total clinical regression in 12 out of 17 squamous cell epitheliomas in advanced stages. Surprising are the observations on the response of melanomas and lymph gland metastases of varied primary tumours. Of 24 of these, notoriously radioresistant, 8 had a complete involution, 11 a partial regression followed by a persistent clinical quiescence, and only 5 were insensitive to the treatment.

The radiation reactions were intense, but their duration was short. No necrosis, not even in cartilage, was observed, but, on the contrary, repair was prompt.

The satisfactory response of our H.P.O. technique to clinical needs, was revealed in our previous report. It should be emphasized that the use of Radium with a hyperbaric chamber like ours allows us to maintain simultaneous exposures to H.P.O. and radiations for a prolonged period of time.

There is also a double advantage. It is possible to irradiate with the principle of chronological fractioning of the dose, and with the normal method of continuous curietherapy. Now-a-days we prefer the "alternated" irradiation. Finally we should not ignore the possibility of treating at the same time two patients, when their tumours are small and the radium load is small and screened so as to avoid significant total-body exposures to the patients.

Nouvelle technique de Radiumthérapie en oxygène hyperbaryque

M. NANNELLI et G. MANTELLASSI, Institut de Photoradiotherapie, Université de Florence (Italie)

Dans le but d'augmenter la radio-sensibilité des tumeurs, on emploie depuis quelques années la technique de les irradier au moyen de chambres spéciales où les patients respirent de l'oxygène hyperbare.

Dans l'Institut de Photoradiothérapie de l'Université de Florence, nous avons effectué des modifications essentielles à la méthode en question, visant à réduire au minimum quelques inconvénients considérables. En ce qui concerne les techniques employées jusqu'à présent, l'impossibilité de placer dans une chambre hyperbaryque les grandes unités radiothérapeutiques, et la nécessité du centrage des champs, imposaient l'emploi de petites chambres tubulaires à une seule place. La constriction dans un milieu si peu confortable est une expérience qui provoque un tel «stress» qu'il faut quelquefois avoir recours à l'anesthésie générale, aussi pour diminuer les risques d'intoxication par oxygène qui sont augmentés de façon considérable par les troubles émotifs.

Nous avons employé — pour la première fois en ce domaine — le Radium appliqué au patient comme moulage: de cette façon la source des radiations est placée à l'intérieur de la chambre hyperbaryque. Cela a permis d'employer une grande chambre Galeazzi (mod. 35/e modifié: volume $5\,m^3$, dimensions $2 \times 2 \times 2\,m$). A l'intérieur, qui est bien éclairé, des bancs confortables, une table avec des magazines, etc., rendent le séjour tout à fait supportable aussi aux patients émotifs ou atteints de claustrophobie. Un appareil interphonique assure la communication constante avec l'extérieur; un ventilateur et deux filtres de chaux sodée pourvoient à la fixation du bioxyde de carbone. Un nouveau système de dépuration, que nous avons conçu avec la Firme Galeazzi, est en cours d'installation; ce dernier permet une climatisation complète de la chambre, éliminant des températures et des niveaux d'humidité excessifs lesquels, outre créer une sensation de malaise, constituent d'autres motifs de "stress". Ces derniers doivent toujours être évités car ils participent certainement au mécanisme complexe de l'intoxication par oxygène. Avant la pressurisation la chambre, alimentée avec des évaporateurs d'oxygène liquide, est lavée jusqu'à ce que le pourcentage d'oxygène mesuré atteigne presque 100%. La vitesse de pressurisation est ensuite réglée sur la base de l'aptitude des patients à compenser la pression sur la membrane tympanique par les moyens classiques, sur lesquels ils sont opportunément instruits; en général, la pression standard de 3 atmosphères absolues (ata) est atteinte en 15 min, et cette dernière est maintenue pendant 2 h.

Un des objectifs principaux de notre technique est l'exploitation maxima dans le temps de la synergie oxygène-radiations, exploitation qui d'habitude est entravée considérablement par la toxicité de l'oxygène hyperbare; à 3 ata, les symptômes d'intoxication sont assez fréquents et précoces, comme le démontrent les casuistiques des Marines Militaires et celles des différents radiothérapistes, qui, toutefois, ne dépassent presque jamais 15 min d'exposition à 3 ata.

Nous avons prolongé l'exposition jusqu'à plus de 2 h entières par jour, éliminant au maximum les facteurs stressants, en particulier les facteurs émotifs. Nous avons atteint de but à l'aide d'un milieu confortable, et surtout par l'emploi d'un nouvel anxiolithique (3-hydroxibenzodiazepinone, ou ADUMBRAN). Cette préparation au début expérimentée sur les animaux, nous a révélé des propriétés protectrices excellentes par rapport aux phénomènes causés par l'hyperoxie. Dans l'application clinique, sur 390 traitements nous avons enregistré un seul cas de faible intoxication, qui pouvait être attribuée à l'administration arbitraire d'un remède sympathomimétique. L'action de l'Adumbran—dépourvue, en apparence, des effets d'augmentation du trouble nerveux irréversible décrits pour les barbituriques, — semble être plus que symptomatique: mais si ce n'était que cela, son utilité pratique ne changerait pas, car le symptôme "convulsions" est très précoce et très lointain de l'apparition de lésions irréversibles. En outre, la crise convulsive, inoffensive en elle-même, crée des problèmes très sérieux dans une chambre hyperbaryque, à cause du risque de traumatismes et de l'attention extrême nécessaire à la décompression du patient qui peut, la glotte fermée, être atteint de lésions pulmonaires même mortelles par suite d'une décompression faite à la hâte; en tout cas, cette dernière, avec l'oxygène, n'entraîne pas le danger d'embolies.

En ce qui concerne le traitement ionisant, décrit dans les détails par C. VALLECCHI et G. MANTELLASSI au cours de cette séance, on doit souligner que la proximité de la source et du tissu élimine toute contamination "de paroi" et les variations dosimétriques d'hyperpression.

Le traitement hyperbaryque, bien qu'il soit exécuté aux limites de la tolérance, a été supporté de façon excellente par tous les patients, même s'il s'agissait de vieillards et de patients affaiblis. Les seuls inconvénients consistent en de rares et faibles baro-traumatismes de l'oreille moyenne (hémotympane).

Acute Effects of Irradiation on the Skin
A Histochemical and Chemical Study*

A. K. KURBAN and F. S. FARAH, Division of Dermatology (Department of Medicine) of the American University of Beirut and the American University Hospital, Beirut (Lebanon)

The past couple of decades have witnessed marked interest in the biologic effects of irradiation because of the increasing use of, and exposure to radioactive substances. The skin is accessible to accidental as well as intentional irradiation from a variety of sources. It is also readily available for observation and study and thus lends itself well to the evaluation of the effects of irradiation.

Over 70 years ago, STEFENS described an erythematous eruption in an X-ray technician [1]. SCHOLTZ [2] in 1902 was the first to make a thorough clinical and histological study of the skin following X-irradiation. The contributions of MIESCHER, JADASSOHN and others in this field are well known and need no comment [3].

The purpose of this communication is to present a brief review of our knowledge of the acute cellular and enzymatic changes in the epidermis and the chemical alterations in the dermis following X-irradiation. The changes described are those following a single exposure of 4000 to 6000 r (40 to 60 KV H.V.L. around 1 mm Al).

The Epidermal Alterations

The epithelial structures of the skin are quite susceptible to the effects of ionizing radiation. Within a few hours, there is arrest of mitotic activity in the basal cell layer. This is followed by progressive changes in the epidermal cells which exhibit abnormal mitoses, pyknotic nuclei, micronuclei and dispersed chromatin; and later, the appearance of giant cells [4]. The cytoplasm becomes swollen. These changes progress during the subsequent 2 to 3 weeks culminating in superficial ulceration of the epidermis [5].

During this period other changes take place in the desoxy- and ribonucleic acids, the disulfide (SS) and sulfhydryl bonds (SH) and in various cellular enzymatic reactions.

The changes in the DNA-RNA make-up of epidermal cells are evidenced by fluorochrome staining, specific histochemical reactions and the effects of desoxyribonuclease (DNase). The normal nuclear fluorescence is quenched with Thioflavine T (TT) and lost with Acridine Orange. These changes in the DNA are further exhibited by the diminution of the Feulgen reaction and more so by the fact that DNase fails to digest completely the nuclear material. All these reactions confirm the susceptibility of nuclei to the effects of ionizing irradiation. The inability of DNase to act on the nuclear DNA may signify a major alteration in the DNA molecular structure and/or configuration.

Coincident with the nuclear changes described, there is a decrease in SH bonds and a milder decrease in SS bonds. BARRON et al. [6] reported similar findings. The change in the SH bonds may be due to their being masked, blocked, or oxidized to SS bonds. The ultimate effect is the production of hyperkeratosis in which the keratin is different from the normal keratin as shown by the altered fluorescence with Acridine Orange.

Few investigators have reported on the effects of irradiation on enzyme systems in different tissues. In the skin, varied results have been reported. KARCHER [7] demonstrated a decrease in the activity of succinic dehydrogenase,

* Supported by The International Atomic Energy Agency, Contract No. 219/RB.

DNP diaphorase and non-specific esterases in the rabbit skin. BRUNI and MAZZA [8], working with guinea pig skin, showed increased activity of alkaline phosphatase and alphanaphthyl and Tween esterases. Our investigations in the guinea pig skin demonstrate that various enzyme systems respond differently. Alkaline phosphatase activity in the guinea pig sebaceous gland shows an initial increase following irradiation, followed by a decrease and eventual disappearance as the glands degenerate [9]. Beta Glucoronidase activity in epidermal cells is greatly decreased 48 h following irradiation. Of the different dehydrogenases, TPN- and DPN-specific Glutamate Dehydrogenases (Glu DH/TPN and Glu DH/DPN), Glycerine-1-phosphate Dehydrogenase (GDH/DPN), DPN-specific Isocitrate Dehydrogenase (IDH/DPN) and Lactate Dehydrogenase (LDH) exhibit marked decrease in activity 1 week after irradiation; whereas Glucose-6-phosphate Dehydrogenase (G 6 PDH), TPN-specific Isocitrate Dehydronegase (IDH/TPN) and others do not show consistent changes. The interpretation of the effects of irradiation on enzymatic activity remains obscure as it is not clear whether the irradiation affects the enzyme directly or indirectly.

The Dermal Alterations

The most striking early macroscopic change is the erythema. Microscopically there is edema of the dermis with an infiltrate of neutrophils, lymphocytes and plasma cells. The endothelial cells are swollen and their nuclei are vesicular, irregular or even granulated and multiple. The fibroblasts also display nuclear deformities and cytoplasmic swelling. There are changes in the collagen fibers which are described as swollen and hyalinized.

It became evident to us that the changes in the dermal components in response to irradiation as seen by light microscopy may not reveal all the alterations taking place.. A chemical determination of the hexosamine and hydroxyproline content of the guinea pig skin following irradiation was undertaken. The results show no statistically significant change at p = 0.01.

References. 1. DANIEL, J.: Science **3**, 562 (1896). — 2. SCHOLTZ, W.: Arch. Derm. Syph. (Berl.) **59**, 87 (1902). — 3. LACASSAGNE, A., and G. GRICOUROFF: Action of Radiation on Tissues. An Introduction to Radiotherapy. New York and London: Grune and Stratton 1958. — 4. BRUNST, V. V.: Amer. J. Roentgenol. **89**, 624 (1963). — 5. MELLETT, P. G.: Brit. J. exp. Path. **41**, 160 (1960). — 6. BARRON, E. S. G.: J. gen. Physiol. **32**, 537 (1949). — 7. KARCHER, K. H.: Strahlentherapie **116**, 70 (1961). — 8. a BRUNI, L., e A. MAZZA: Minerva derm. **37**, 104 (1962). — 8b. MAZZA, A., e L. BRUNI: Minerva derm. **37**, 134 (1962). — 9. KURBAN, A. K.: J. invest. Derm. **39**, 1 (1962).

Biochemische Untersuchungen an Serum und Hauteiweißen von Ratten nach Röntgenbestrahlung

O.-E. RODERMUND, Univ.-Hautklinik Bonn (Deutschland)

Mit der von RODERMUND, FASOLD, TURBA und LEINBROCK entwickelten Methode der Fraktionierung und Charakterisierung von Rattenhauteiweißen sollte untersucht werden, ob und welche Veränderungen nach Röntgenbestrahlung an diesen Eiweißen sich nachweisen lassen. Enthaarte Bauchhaut von Ratten wurde nach hochdosierter Röntgenbestrahlung geringer Energie (12 bis 20000 R Dermopan 29 kV, 0,3 Al-Filter) homogenisiert und zunächst mit Ammonacetatpuffer vom pH 7,0, dann mit 0,5 m Essigsäure, sodann mit einem 6 m harnstoffhaltigen

Na-Boratpuffer vom pH 8,0, zuletzt mit gleichem Puffer unter Zusatz von Natriumborhydrid extrahiert, die vier Fraktionen anschließend dialysiert und lyophilisiert.

Die Untersuchung erfolgte für alle Fraktionen mit der CAF-Elektrophorese nach KOHN und der Immunelektrophorese nach SCHEIDEGGER, wobei zur Präcipitation das Antirattenserum der Behringwerke zur Anwendung kam. Die Fraktionen II bis IV wurden chromatographisch mit einer CMC-Säule von 7 cm Länge und 0,9 cm Durchmesser (Kapazität 0,7 meq/g) aufgetrennt und in 2 ml-Portionen/4 min geschnitten, anschließend mit Folinreagens im Zeiss-Spektralphotometer ausgewertet.

Bei der *CAF-Elektrophorese* zeigte die sog. Fraktion I ein dem Serumeiweißdiagramm ähnliches Bild. Es ließ sich dabei nach Röntgenbestrahlung ein Absinken des Gamma-Globulinanteils feststellen. Ein Absinken des Albumins und ein Anstieg des Alpha-2- und Beta-Globulins, wie er in den entsprechenden Untersuchungen des Serums zu erkennen war, ließ sich nicht konstatieren. Die sog. Fraktionen II und III ergaben jeweils nur eine Bande, zum Teil mit Abgrenzung einer farblich unterschiedenen Vorbande; Unterschiede zwischen bestrahlter und nichtbestrahlter Haut konnten daran nicht erkannt werden. Die Wanderung von Fraktion IV war nicht einheitlich.

Bei der *Immunelektrophorese* ließ sich im Serum nach Röntgenbestrahlung deutlich die Verminderung des Gamma-Globulinanteils, insbesondere des 7-S-Gammaglobulins, sowie auch eine Verminderung des Albumins erkennen. Eine Alpha-Globulinvermehrung dagegen ließ sich nicht sicher abschätzen.

Die *immunelektrophoretische Untersuchung der Fraktion I* ergab dem Serum entsprechende Präcipitatlinien. Es ließ sich bei einem Vergleich zwischen unbestrahlter Haut und Serum erkennen, daß die Verteilung der Plasmaeiweiße in der Haut nicht gleich der Verteilung im Blut ist. Es zeigte sich in der Hautfraktion ein deutliches Zurücktreten des Gamma-Globulinanteils gegenüber dem Albumin, während andererseits auch kleinere Eiweißanteile, z. B. einer, dessen Präcipitatlinie etwa dem Transferrin oder dem Beta-1c-Globulin entsprechen dürfte, in einer dem Serum nicht nachstehenden Stärke ausgebildet waren.

Alpha-1-Lipoprotein und Alpha-1-Antitrypsin stellten sich erheblich schwächer dar als im Serum, während sich eine wohl als Alpha-1x-Glykoprotein anzusehende Linie in ihrer Intensität vom Serum nicht unterschied. Bei bestrahlten Tieren läßt sich bei der immunelektrophoretischen Darstellung der Fraktion I kein sicherer Unterschied qualitativ oder quantitativ abschätzen, zumal die etwa zu erwartenden Veränderungen in den bei der Hautfraktion gegenüber dem Serum bereits gleichsinnig veränderten Bereichen liegen.

Bei der *säulenchromatographischen Trennung des Kollagens* zeigten sich bei Fraktion II bei unbestrahlter Haut zwei deutliche peaks nach durchschnittlich 72 und 104 min sowie ein angedeuteter dritter peak nach 168 min bei einem nur schwach ausgeprägten anfänglichen Austritt folinpositiver Substanzen. Bei Fraktion III ließen sich zwei dicht nebeneinander stehende peaks darstellen bei gleichfalls nur geringem anfänglichen Austritt folinpositiver Substanz. Bei Fraktion IV folgte meist einem anfänglichen schmalen steil ausgeprägten peak ein zweiter kleinerer nach 24 min, dann ein breiter hoher nach 72 min.

Bei bestrahlter Haut zeigten sich charakteristische Veränderungen. Fraktion II wies nach einem stärkeren anfänglichen Austritt folinpositiver Substanzen eine flachere, plateauartige, eben eingekerbte Kurve auf. Bei Fraktion III fiel ein anfänglicher relativ schmalbasiger steilgipfliger Austritt folinpositiver Substanz auf, die zweigipflige Kurve war zu einem flacheren Plateau reduziert.

Bei Fraktion IV waren ebenfalls ein vermehrtes anfängliches Austreten folin-

positiver Substanz und eine Verringerung und Verflachung der peaks, insbesondere des dritten peak, zu erkennen.

Diese Befunde entsprechen somit hinsichtlich des Serums den in der Literatur
dargestellten. Es geht weiter daraus hervor, daß bei den applizierten Strahlen-
dosen eine rasch zur Wirksamkeit kommende Schädigung des leicht- und des
schwerlöslichen Kollagens auftritt.

Fräulein HILDEGARD HÖNIG D'ORVILLE danke ich für technische Assistenz.

Radiations et tissu élastique cutané

M. LEDOUX-CORBUSIER, Clinique Dermatologique de l'Université de Bruxelles
(Belgique)

Dans le domaine de la pathologie du tissu élastique cutané, il nous a paru
intéressant d'établir un parallèle entre *les radiodermites chroniques* provenant de
régions couvertes du corps et *l'élastose sénile*, autre dermatose causée par les
radiations électromagnétiques. Trois questions ont été posées:

1. Y a-t-il hypertrophie élastique dans les radiodermites chroniques?

Comme divers auteurs, nous avons en effet constaté dans les radiodermites
chroniques une nette augmentation de fibres se colorant comme les fibres élastiques normales.

Deux *conditions* sont cependant nécessaires à cette observation: la dose ionisante (nr), appliquée sous une tension de 85 à 200 KV, doit être suffisante
(> 2.500 r) mais non excessive (< 6.000 r); le temps de latence entre l'irradiation et l'examen anatomo-pathologique doit être suffisamment long. Ce temps
dépend de la dose ionisante administrée et nécessite un minimum de plusieurs
mois.

C'est la *meilleure pénétration* tissulaire des radiations ionisantes par rapport à
celle des rayons ultra-violets qui doit vraisemblablement être rendue responsable
de ce que dans les radiodermites chroniques les lésions s'étendent à tout le derme et
entreprennent les vaisseaux profonds tandis que dans l'élastose sénile l'hypertrophie élastotique se cantonne au derme supérieur. L'image d'une élastose sénile
montre les fibres élastotiques épaissies, circonvoluées, agglomérées à hauteur du
derme supérieur. Par contre dans les radiodermites chroniques, l'hypertrophie
élastotique qui se retrouve sur toute la hauteur du derme prend en profondeur une
disposition ondulatoire très particulière ou bien se dispose en tous sens.

2. Cette hypertrophie est-elle constituée de fibres élastiques?

Nous inspirant des travaux de BRAUN-FALCO sur l'élastose sénile (1956, 1957)
et d'études concernant le pseudo-xanthome élastique (FISHER et coll., 1958) nous
avons procédé à des investigations similaires:

L'absence de biréfringence de ces fibres élastotiques tant dans l'élastose sénile
que dans les radiodermites chroniques permet d'éliminer leur nature collagène.

Les premiers résultats de leur observation faite au microscope électronique
par le Professeur PIERARD et Mr. KINT (1965) montre que leur texture est analogue à celle des fibres élastiques normales.

L'étude comparative de la fluorescence spontanée et de la fluorescence induite
de ces fibres montre une analogie remarquable entre les fibres élastiques normales,
les fibres de l'élastose sénile et celles des radiodermites chroniques.

Enfin la digestion par l'élastase de ces mêmes fibres est un argument en faveur de leur *nature élastique*.

Quelques clichés démontrent la fluorescence des fines fibres élastiques normales, celle très importante des fibres agglomérées de l'élastose sénile et celle des longues fibres des radiodermites chroniques. D'autres images permettent de constater qu'après 60 min d'action d'une solution à 1 % d'élastase, les fibres élastiques ne sont plus mises en évidence par la fuchsine résorcine.

3. Quelle est l'origine de ces fibres élastiques?

De même que pour l'élastose sénile, on ne peut encore répondre à cette question. S'agit-il de fibres provenant de la transformation de fibres collagènes en fibres élastiques ou s'agit-il de fibres élastiques néoformées ?

La néoformation des fibres élastiques semble actuellement l'hypothèse la plus probable. En effet jamais on n'a pu mettre en évidence de stade intermédiaire entre les fibres collagènes et les fibres élastiques. De plus, JELLINEK (1962) irradiant des lapins, a observé de nouvelles fibres dermiques colorées par les colorants des fibres élastiques.

En conclusion: Il existe donc dans les radiodermites chroniques une *élastose radiodermitique* qui occupe toute la hauteur du derme à l'inverse de celle de l'élastose sénile. Cette différence doit vraisemblablement être attribuée à la plus grande pénétration des radiations ionisantes. Un faisceau d'arguments histo-physico-enzymatique plaide en faveur de la nature élastique de ces fibres néo-formées. Nous poursuivons actuellement nos études expérimentales par des irradiations de peau de porc et espérons percer ainsi plus avant le mystère de ces élastoses.

Bibliographie. Les principales références sont reprises dans les publications suivantes: LEDOUX-CORBUSIER, M.: Arch. belges Derm. 18, 81 (1962). — ACHTEN, G., et M. LEDOUX-CORBUSIER: Elastose sénile et élastose radiodermitique. XIIe Congr. des derm. de lang. franç. Paris 1965 (sous presse).

Problemas del uso de los rayos grenz en los negros y en los mulatos

M. A. CONTRERAS, Universidad Nacional Pedro Henriquez Ureña y Clínica de la Piel Dr. M. Contreras, Santo Domingo (República Dominicana)

Durante los últimos años ha habido una tendencia marcada hacia el uso de radiaciones cutáneas ionizantes blandas. Los dermatólogos cada día evitan más el uso de las llamadas radiaciones convencionales, de suerte que en las últimas dos décadas ha habido un incremento notable en el uso de los rayos grenz o rayos intermediarios. Estos rayos son ondas electromagnéticas de alrededor de dos unidades angstrom con una capa hemireductora de 15 a 35 micras de aluminio. Son rayos X blandos producidos por un aparato de rayos X de poca potencia, de 6 a 15 KV y que producen efectos clínicos y biológicos especiales. Con su uso no hay proliferación epitelial, ni hiperplasia, ni neoplasia, ni alteraciones vasculares, como secuela. Prácticamente no tienen efecto acumulativo. La relación tera-péutica entre ellos y los rayos X convencionales es de diez a uno. Su mayor virtud consiste en que producen rara vez radiodermatitis, a menos que no se usen dosis excesivas [1, 2, 3].

En los individuos de piel blanca se uso está sustituyendo paulatinamente a los rayos X convencionales, en el tratamiento de las afecciones cutáneas benignas. Cuando dichos rayos se aplican a individuos de piel hiperpigmentáda [4], especialmente de la raza negra y en los mulatos, se presentan hipercromías residuales, que producen un efecto cosmético desagradable que muchas veces dura semanas o meses para desaparecer. Aún con dosis mínimas de 200 r se presentan estos fenómenos. Si se usan dosis altas, de 1000 r en adelante el fenómeno se acentúa aún más.

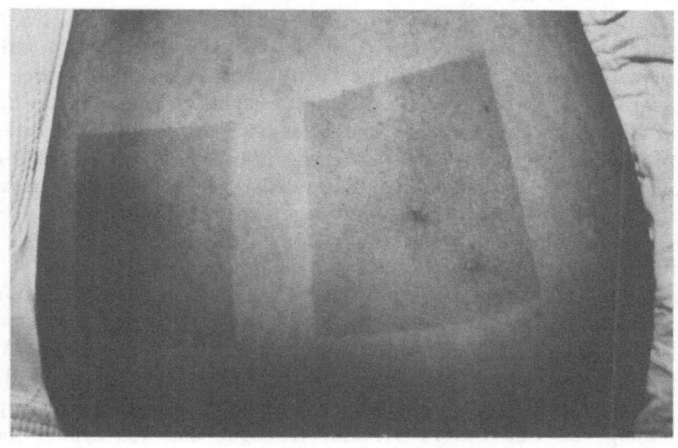

Metodo Usado

En nuestra clínica usamos un aparato Dermopan, que tiene 4 escalones. El primer escalón trabaja con 10 KV 25 MA con una capa hemireductora de 0.025 mm, de aluminio y que corresponde a los rayos grenz. Se aplica con un cono de 10 cm de diámetro a una distancia foco piel de 10 cm.

Nuestra población es mayormente de piel hiperpigmentada, negros, mulatos y blancos de piel obscura [5]. Con el uso de estas radiaciones vemos muy corrientemente molestas hipercromías. A medida que las dosís aumentan se acentúa la hipercromía. La hiperpigmentación se acompaña de eritema en dosís por encima de 1000 r. Puede haber ligera vesiculación. Luego la piel se descama con desprendimiento de la capa córnea que a veces deja hipocromía residual por un tiempo.

Vamos a mostrar una serie de fotografías en que se usaron dichos rayos en pacientes negros y mulatos. Los casos tratados incluían psoriasis, neurodermatitis circunscrita, dermatitis por contacto, eczema de las manos, etc. A algunas de ellas se le aplicaron dosís elevadas con el fin de resaltar el efecto pigmentogénico de los rayos grenz.

Resultados

Es evidente el problema cosmético a que hacemos alusión, de tal suerte que casi constituye una contraindicación el uso de estos rayos en los pacientes de estas razas, especialmente, si la afección para la cual se usan, está situada en las áreas descubiertas, y más aún si la afección se localiza en la cara.

Referencias. 1. BUCKY, G., and F. G. COMBES: Grenz Ray Therapy. New York: Springer 1954. — 2. MAC KEE, G. M., and A. C. CIPOLLARO: X Rays and Radium in the Treatment of Deseases of the Skin. Philadelphia: Lea & Febiger 1946. — 3. GLASSER, O.: Physical Foundation of Radiology, ed. 2. New York: Hoeber 1952. — 4. WRIGHT, L. W.: Arch. Derm. 89, 417 (1964). — 5. CONTRERAS, M. A.: Dermatología Int. 4, 130 (1965).

Tierexperimentelles zur Röntgenfernbestrahlung der Haut

M. BETETTO, Dermatologische Klinik, Ljubljana, (Jugoslawien)

Mit der Entwicklung der Weichstrahltherapie mittels Be-Röhre hat sich auch die Röntgenfernbestrahlung der Haut mit ungefilterter weicher Strahlung aus Entfernungen von 50 cm (GREEN, JENNINGS und HENDTLASS, 1951), 80 cm (WISKEMANN, 1951), 90 cm (PROPPE, 1954, WAGNER, 1955) und 2 m (SCHIRREN, 1954) mit hohen Dosen durchgesetzt.

Selbstverständlich ist man sich der Differentheit solcher Methodik für den Organismus voll bewußt, es werden doch auch bei solcher Bestrahlung, trotz größter Absorption der Strahlen in der Haut, kleine Dosen auf das Innere des Organismus verabreicht. Die Wirkung auf kritische Organe wurde deshalb eingehend durch die Untersuchung des Blutbildes während der Therapie (vor allem SCHIRREN, WAGNER, PROPPE) und durch die Messungen der Gonadenbelastung kontrolliert (SCHIRREN, HAUMAYR und DITTMAR). Bei den Blutuntersuchungen konnten keine strahlenbedingten Abweichungen von der Norm festgestellt werden. Lediglich die Messungen der Gonadenbelastung ließen die Vorstellung der Keimepithelschädigung ohne einen sinnvollen Strahlenschutz zu.

Experimentelles ist dabei unseres Wissens nichts geleistet worden, weshalb wir folgende Tierversuche durchführten. Es handelt sich um die Bestrahlung von 20 Meerschweinchen zählenden Gruppen und um das Vergleichen der Wirkung am Blutbild und an den Gonaden mit den unbestrahlten Kontrollgruppen.

Es wurde mit ungefilterter weicher Strahlung (50 kV) unter therapieähnlichen Bedingungen aus der Entfernung von 1 m (GHWT 1,4 mm) von oben und von beiden Seiten dreimal wöchentlich durch 40 bzw. 24 Wochen bestrahlt.

Somit wurde bei den hämatologischen Versuchen durch dreimal 50 r Oberflächendosis (OD) pro Tag in 40 Wochen eine OD von 18 000 r (dreimal 6000 r) erreicht, was einer Dosis von etwa 720 r in der Bauchhöhle des Tierphantoms entspricht. Bei den Versuchen über die Keimschädigung wurde in 24 Wochen eine OD von 10 800 r (dreimal 3600 r), bzw. von etwa 360 r an die Gonaden (gemessen am Tierphantom) eingestrahlt.

Vergleicht man eine Durchschnittskurve der absoluten Blutzellenzahlen der unbestrahlten Kontrollgruppe mit der analogen Kurve der bestrahlten Tiere durch 40 Wochen, so sieht man ein langsames Abfallen der letzteren, besonders bezüglich der Leukocyten und Lymphocyten. In beiden Kurven sind beträchtliche Amplituden zu verzeichnen, doch in keiner sinken sie unter ein normales Minimum. Kein einziges Hämogram an sich ist also abnormal bzw. für die Röntgenschädigung bezeichnend. Diese offenbart sich erst, wenn die Durchschnittskurven der bestrahlten und unbestrahlten Tiere untereinander verglichen werden.

Somit kann man auch beim viel größeren Menschen, dessen blutbildendes System der weichen Strahlung bedeutend schwerer erreichbar ist als beim Meerschweinchen, unter üblicher therapeutischer Dosierung eine im Blutbild festzustellende Schädigung, trotz an das Innere des Organismus gelangender Dosis, nicht erwarten.

Außerdem beweisen die Experimente auch, daß das Blutbild durch die Bestrahlung des peripheren Blutes in der Haut gewiß nur unbedeutend beeinflußt wird.

Die Wirkung auf das Keimepithel wurde durch den histologischen Befund des Hodens untersucht. Es wurden dazu in regelmäßigen Abständen immer drei Tiere aus der bestrahlten und ein Tier aus der unbestrahlten Kontrollgruppe genommen. Sichtbare Strahlenschäden traten in der 12. Bestrahlungswoche, nach der OD von 5400 r (dreimal 1800 r) bzw. von etwa 180 r an den Gonaden, auf. Die Keimzellen wurden je nach ihrer Reife entsprechenden Strahlenempfindlichkeit und mit der steigenden Gesamtdosis in folgender Reihenfolge seltener: Spermatogonien, Spermatocyten, Spermatiden, Spermien. In der 24. Versuchswoche, nach einer gesamten OD von 10800 r (dreimal 3600 r) bzw. von etwa 360 r an den Gonaden, konnte man keine spermatogenen Elemente mehr finden, womit das Experiment beendet war.

Die Beeinflussung des Keimepithels durch die ungefilterte weiche Strahlung ist also recht groß. Diese Feststellung ist nach den Ergebnissen unserer Versuche um so mehr von praktischer Bedeutung, da der menschliche Hoden der weichen Strahlung leichter zugänglich ist als der des Meerschweinchens, dessen Hoden in der Tiefe liegt.

Werden die Ergebnisse unserer hämatologischen Versuche mit denjenigen am Hoden verglichen, so kann man nicht übersehen, daß das einzelne Blutbild nach den Dosen, die das Keimepithel aufs schwerste geschädigt haben, noch als normal anzusehen war. Danach muß man das Blutbild als praktisch wichtigsten Indikator des Strahlenschadens auch bei Röntgenfernbestrahlung der Haut nur mit Resignation betrachten.

Die Übertragung dieser Versuchsergebnisse auf den Menschen ist wegen der sehr ähnlichen Reaktivität des Meerschweinchens gegenüber der ionisierenden Strahlung bis zu einem gewissen Grade möglich.

Dermatological Observations in the A-Bomb Survivors of Hiroshima and Nagasaki, Japan

M.-L. T. Johnson, T. Taura and P. B. Gregory, Hiroshima (Japan)

The search for the late effects of radiation in the survivors of Hiroshima and Nagasaki has been extended to the skin. Over a two-year interval the biennial routine examination of survivors and their controls, matched for age and sex, has included a complete dermatological evaluation. The design of the study was to record specific dermatological pathology plus a wide range of variations in texture and appearance of the epidermis and its appendages. Semiquantitative evaluations were attempted on skin color, temperature, number of nevi, and the changes which are commonly associated with aging, with exposure to actinic radiation, with injury and response to injury, and with X-irradiation, in an effort to define the dermatological stigmata of the A-Bomb experience.

In our adult study sample of 10,650 the common signs of aging; wrinkling, atrophy, and elastosis of the skin; graying of the hair; arcus senilis; and the appearance of lentigines, seborrheic keratoses, epithelial tags, senile hemangiomata, etc., were all increased in relation to age. So, too, was the spotty depigmentation of the skin we associate with the elderly; in fact, skin color generally lightened with age, especially in females where the data confirmed by reflectance studies reached extremely high significance levels. Ephelides and junctional nevi were less prevalent in the older groups.

Among the exposed, the pattern of appearance of age-related phenomena and their increased prevalence with each 5-year increase in age was not remarkably different. The trend, however, was for them to appear earlier. To elaborate further the role of exposure, the frequencies of age-related observations in people known to have been at varying distances from the hypocenters of the bombs were examined statistically using the chi-square test of exposure group differences. Three sets of comparisons were made, based on ground distance and estimations of radiation sustained. All three yielded equivalent results:

1. < 1400 meters   — > 1400 meters plus nonexposed
2. < 1400 meters   — > 3000 meters plus nonexposed
3. 100 rads or more   — > 3000 meters plus nonexposed

At 1400 m in Hiroshima the adjudged gamma dose to the unshielded was 35 rads, the neutron dose 18; at a comparable point in Nagasaki it was 176 and 3 rads, respectively. The data presented compare those exposed at less than 1400 m with the group that combines those at 3000 m and beyond with the nonexposed. Further analyses concern sex and age, contrasting those under and over age 20 at the time of the bomb (ATB) — meaning an age break of about 40 at dermatological examination.

Graying of the hair, senile depigmentation of the skin, lentigines, arcus senilis and scleral changes of the eye, including thickening and injection, were found to be increased in the < 1400-m-group in both sexes and both age groups, those less than and those over 20 years old in August 1945. Lightened eye color showed a significantly increased prevalence in exposed males who were less than 20 years ATP; so, too, lightened skin color in the exposed of both sexes and at all ages. Lentigines were also found excessively in the exposed and to greater significance levels in those under 20 years old when exposed. Junctional nevi, noted previously to disappear with advancing years, were more prevalent among patients exposed at a younger age.

Pigmentary changes not considered age related, such as perifollicular hyperpigmentation, were significantly increased in prevalence among the exposed. So, too, was melasma unassociated with pregnancy. By contrast, the prevalence of telangiectasia and keratoses, both regarded as radiation related, were increased among the controls reflecting perhaps the higher percentage of farmers in that population.

As to neoplastic changes, certain benign lesions were more common among the exposed. For example, neurofibromata, fibroepitheliomata, dermatofibroma, and hypertrophic scars and keloids unrelated to bomb injury were present in a significantly increased number. Scars of all types related to the bomb, including flash burn and glass cuts, were present in 1418 exposed patients; 249 (17.5%) were considered cosmetically significant. Malignant neoplastic changes was most rare, diagnosed in only two of the 10,650 patients. One was a squamous cell carcinoma occurring in chronic X-ray dermatitis; the other a Bowen's squamous cell carcinoma in an elderly farmer.

A curious finding of increased prevalence among the exposed was that of certain vascular aberrations, such as cutis marmorata, coldness of the extremities, and Raynaud's phenomenon.

In summary, the dermatological imprint of one instantaneous exposure to ionizing radiation as experienced in Hiroshima and Nagasaki includes the increased prevalence among the exposed of various recognized signs of aging, of pigmentary changes, of benign neoplastic lesions and of certain vascular aberrations. Malignant neoplasm was not a significant finding.

Studies on Induction, Persistence, and Recovery of Radiation Damage in Proliferative (Anagen) and Non-proliferative (Telogen) Rodent Hair Cell Populations*

F. D. Malkinson and M. L. Griem**, Department of Medicine (Section of Dermatology), Department of Radiology and Argonne Cancer Research Hospital***, Chicago, Illinois (USA)

For some time it has been widely accepted that the magnitude of cellular radiosensitivity is related to proliferative activity. In the mouse, anagen hair matrix cells undergo division every 12 to 13 h, but no mitosis occurs in telogen hairs. Consequently, resting and growing hairs provide good material for comparisons of intensity of radiation injury as well as rates of subsequent recovery in resting and actively dividing cell populations.

Materials and Methods

Experiments were carried out in young female Carworth Farms No. 1 mice, in which anagen lasts 17 to 20 days. All animals were plucked on both haunches, and those animals treated in telogen received radiation to the right haunch 24 days later. At post-radiation intervals up to 12 days, single groups of 6 to 31 animals were plucked again. 4 days after plucking, all mice received 3 to 5 uCi of ³H-DL-serine injected intravenously. 20 days later the "second generation" hair was removed from irradiated and control sites for study.

Animals irradiated in anagen were replucked 24 days after initial plucking. 12 days later groups of 12 to 19 animals received single doses of radiation to the right haunch. 2 days after irradiation all animals were given 3 to 5 uCi of ³H-DL-serine intravenously. On the 24th day all hairs from the irradiated and control sides of each mouse were plucked for study.

Hair samples were weighed and then placed in a combustion apparatus in the presence of oxygen. Volatile substances were removed and radioactivity in the remaining material was assayed as tritiated water in a liquid scintillation spectrometer. Throughout the study control and irradiated sites were compared directly in the same animal.

Radiation was administered with a Machlett OEG-60 tube at 45 kv and 30 ma with 2 mm Al added filtration. The dose rate was 387 rads/min at a focal skin distance of 11 cm.

Results and Discussion

Serine is incorporated into hair keratin and into nuclear and cytoplasmic proteins. Since protein synthesis is a radiosensitive process, radiation damage in hair can be measured by reduced serine incorporation into protein.

All animals treated in anagen showed decreased uptake of serine into hair 48 h after irradiation (Tab. 1). Reduction of serine incorporation into anagen hair after the preceding telogen hairs were irradiated revealed that telogen damage also occurs and is similarly dose-dependent (Tab. 2). Equal reductions in serine uptake required an approximately two-fold higher dose for telogen than for anagen hair. When telogen hairs were irradiated and allowed to remain in telogen, no recovery from injury was observed for periods up to 12 days (Tab. 3). In anagen hairs, however, or in telogen hairs plucked immediately after irradiation, complete recovery with normal serine uptake was found after the same 10 to 12 day period (Tab. 4).

The two-fold greater radiosensitivity of anagen, compared to telogen, hairs may partly reflect higher metabolic activity and greater vascularity with higher

* This work was supported in part by United States Public Health Service Grant No. RH 00280-04, Division of Radiological Health.
** United States Public Health Service Career Research Development Awardee No. 1 K 3-C A 19, 415-01.
*** Operated by The University of Chicago for the United States Atomic Energy Commission.

oxygen tension. Increased radiosensitivity may also depend upon the presence in anagen matrices of cells in all phases of the cell cycle, including highly sensitive stages such as G_2 and M. By contrast, telogen hair cells are presumably in prolonged G_1 stage, a less radiosensitive phase of the cycle.

Table 1. *Reduced Levels of* ^{3}*H-DL-Serine in Mouse Hair Following Irradiation in Anagen*

Dose (rads)	Animals	DPM/mgC (control side)	DPM/mgX (irrad. side)	X/C %	Standard error of the mean
100	19	982	866	84.6	3.97
250	13	1,153	980	79.1	4.80
500	12	3,268	2,027	62.9	4.24
600	18	687	330	45.6	4.27

Percentages are expressed as an average ratio of DPM/mg of the irradiated side to the control side (X/C).

Table 2. *Reduced Levels of* ^{3}*H-DL-Serine in Subsequent "Generation" of Mouse Hair Following Irradiation in Telogen*

Dose (rads)	Animals	Interval between irradiation and plucking	DPM/mgC (control side)	DPM/mgX (irrad. side)	X/C %	Standard error of the mean
500	8	Nil	236	192	86.0	7.16
1,000	9	Nil	246	130	57.1	5.75
1,500	6	Nil	268	83	39.1	7.07

All animals were plucked immediately after irradiation. Percentages are expressed as an average ratio of DPM/mg of the irradiated side to the control side (X/C).

Table 3. *Reduced Levels of* ^{3}*H-DL-Serine in Subsequent "Generation" of Mouse Hair Following Irradiation with* 1000 *Rads in Telogen*

Animals	Interval between irradiation and plucking	DPM/mgC (control side)	DPM/mgX (irrad. side)	X/C %	Standard of the mean
20	6 h	209	149	71.3	3.80
20	12 h	154	116	75.2	3.80
17	24 h	76	50	65.8	2.33
8	4 days	117	89	76.0	7.16
13	8 days	286	186	65.0	3.46
19	12 days	239	160	66.9	4.01

Percentages are expressed as an average ratio of DPM/mg of the irradiated side to the control side (X/C).

Table 4. ^{3}*H-DL-Serine Uptake in Anagen Mouse Hair Following Irradiation Earlier in Anagen or in Preceding Telogen*

Dose (rads)	Animals	Hair cycle at irradiation	Interval between irradiation and injection ^{3}H-serine	DPM/mgC (control side)	DPM/mgX (irrad. side)	X/C %	Standard error of the mean
500	15	Anagen (3rd day)	10 days	233	248	105	7.10
1,000	31	Telogen	8 days	438	243	56	3.93
1,000	16	Telogen	12 days	1141	1097	96	3.12

Irradiated telogen hairs were plucked immediately after exposure to X-ray; ^{3}H-serine uptake was determined for the succeeding generation of hair. Percentages are expressed as an average ratio of DPM/mg of the irradiated side to the control side (X/C).

While telogen hair damage was unchanged 12 days after radiation, anagen hairs completely recovered during the same time period. Probably the increased metabolic rate in anagen matrix cells favors repair processes. In addition, many damaged cells may have been eliminated from the matrix by incorporation into the hair shaft.

The establishment of radiation-induced, dose-dependent changes in the incorporation of serine into hair provides a simple, non-destructive in vivo method for evaluating a number of diverse radiobiological phenomena.

Autoradiographische Untersuchungen zur epidermalen Proliferation unter physiologischen, pathologischen und experimentellen Bedingungen mit Tritium-markierten Nucleosiden

W. Born, Univ.-Hautklinik Freiburg i. Br. (Deutschland)

Einführung

Die Epidermis mit ihrem ständigen peripheren Substanzverlust infolge von Abschuppung, kompensiert durch Zellregeneration aus der Keimschicht, kann als ein physiologisch gesteuertes Funktionsmodell gesehen werden. Im einfachsten Falle des harmonischen Zusammenspiels entspricht einem vermehrten oder verminderten Verbrauch ein vermehrter oder verminderter Zellnachschub. Beide unterliegen individuellen, topographischen, tageszeitlichen, jahreszeitlichen, altersabhängigen und anderen Schwankungen, welche innerhalb gewisser Grenzen als normal anzusehen sind. Das System gleicht einem Regelkreis mit der offenbaren Tendenz, Störeinflüsse auszugleichen. Maximale Ausgleichsreaktionen können pathologisch erscheinende Formen annehmen, oder das System kann quantitativ überfordert werden und dekompensieren. Eine qualitative Überforderung läßt es entgleisen, beispielsweise in carcinomatös enthemmtes Zellwachstum. Experimentelle Eingriffe von außen können ebenfalls das Regelsystem stören oder es stützen und vor Dekompensation bzw. weiterer Entgleisung bewahren.

Methodik

Die Technik der Autoradiographie mit Nucleinsäurebausteinen ermöglicht neue Einblicke in diese Zusammenhänge. Den zu prüfenden Zellverbänden haben wir daher für ihre Nucleinsäuresynthese vor allem das Nucleosid Thymidin angeboten, welches zuvor durch Ersatz von Wasserstoffatomen an seiner Methylgruppe mit sog. schwerem Wasserstoff oder Tritium radioaktiv markiert worden war. Mit diesem Tritium-Thymidin reichern sich diejenigen Zellen an und werden so ihrerseits markiert, die innerhalb des Generationscyclus gerade ihre Synthesephase durchlaufen. Sie können im histoautoradiographischen Bild u. a. gezählt und topographisch zugeordnet werden. Durch ihre Markierung sind sie leicht zu erkennen. Ferner sind sie allgemein viel zahlreicher zu finden als Mitosen, da die DNA-Synthese um ein vielfaches länger dauert als die Mitose, und somit innerhalb eines gleichen Zeitraums entsprechend mehr Zellen in der DNA-Synthese als in der Mitose stehen müssen.

Tierversuche

Nicht immer erlaubt die Beobachtung vermehrter Generationsphasenbilder unter dem Mikroskop ein sicheres Urteil darüber, ob diese Folge eines gesteigerten Zellumsatzes sind oder ob sie einer Verlangsamung des normalen Ablaufs der betreffenden Phase entsprechen. Besonders bei Kurzzeitinkubationen von Gewebestückchen in vitro entstehen relative Momentaufnahmen, die einer weiteren

Analyse bedürfen. Wie wir an Versuchen mit Mäuseohren in vitro sehen konnten, ist eine solche möglich durch gleichzeitige Bestimmung des Mitoseindex und des DNA-Synthese- bzw. Markierungsindex. Dabei fanden wir spezifische Beziehungen von allgemeiner Gültigkeit: So entsprechen vermehrte DNA-Synthesen bei unveränderten Mitosezahlen als Antwort auf einen hemmenden Einfluß einem längeren Verweilen der Zellen in der DNA-Synthesephase, also einer primären DNA-Synthesestörung; nach einem Proliferationsreiz ist derselbe Befund Ausdruck einer beginnenden Umsatzsteigerung durch Verkürzung der ersten Zellruhephase (G 1-Phase), es konnten also mehr Zellen in die DNA-Synthese eintreten. *In Abhängigkeit vom Langzeiteffekt eines Einflusses kann im zugeordneten Kurzzeitversuch mit dieser Methode für jede denkbare Kombination der Mitose- und DNA-Synthesezahlen der primäre Angriffsort im Generationscyclus bestimmt werden.*

Als Beispiel seien unsere Befunde nach *Extraktion einer wasserlöslichen thermolabilen Substanz aus den Hautschuppen gesunder Versuchspersonen* und deren Einfluß auf die Epidermisproliferation von Mäuseohren in vitro angeführt. Nach zweistündiger Inkubation der Gewebeproben mit der Testflüssigkeit fanden wir jeweils weniger Zellen in Mitose und mehr Zellen in DNA-Synthese als bei den Kontrollen, die mit der gleichen Testlösung — jedoch nach halbstündiger Erhitzung auf 90 °C — inkubiert worden waren. *Der Befund beweist nicht nur die Einwirkung, sondern zeigt erstmalig auch den Angriffspunkt eines epidermiseigenen Hemmstoffs,* welcher demnach störend in die DNA-Synthese eingreift und die Zellen hierin länger festhält, so daß nur wenige von ihnen über eine etwa 20 min andauernde prämitotische sog. zweite Ruhephase (G 2-Phase) in die Mitose eintreten konnten. Bereits begonnene Mitosen kamen während der Versuchszeit zum Abschluß, d. h., daß dieser epidermiseigene und wohl der physiologischen Regulation dienende Hemmstoff jedenfalls nicht an der gleichen besonders empfindlichen Stelle wie z. B. bestimmte Infektionen, ionisierende Strahlen oder sog. Mitosegifte in den Generationscyclus der Zellen eingreift. Er verlangsamt vielmehr die DNA-Synthese, ohne sie offensichtlich qualitativ zu verändern.

Klinische Versuche

Wir glauben, auf Grund unserer tierexperimentellen Studien das Instrument der DNA-Synthesemarkierung auch im klinischen Experiment gezielter einsetzen und erhaltene Ergebnisse besser interpretieren zu können.

Bei den klinischen Fragestellungen kommen gewöhnlich nur in-vitro-Untersuchungen in Betracht, da mit einer Personengefährdung durch Tritium-Thymidin schon bei Aufnahme von wenigen Mikrocurie zu rechnen ist. Es werden daher frischen Gewebeproben radioaktiv markierte Nucleoside in körperwarmen Inkubationslösungen zum Einbau in die Zelle während der Nucleinsäuresynthese angeboten, wobei Gewebescheiben bis zu 1 mm Dicke eine vollständige Durchtränkung ermöglichen. An Biopsien mit einer hierzu von uns konstruierten Scheibenstanze konnten so die Einbauverhältnisse an normaler Haut und bei dermatologischen Veränderungen geprüft werden. Gemeinsam mit KALKOFF wurde darüber hinaus gezeigt, daß durch lokale Einwirkung von fluorierten Corticosteroiden unter Plastikfolie für 48 bis 96 Std die normale DNA-Synthese in der menschlichen Epidermis ebenso wie die gesteigerte DNA-Synthese bei Psoriasis vulgaris fast schlagartig und nahezu vollständig zum Erliegen kommt. Ferner konnten wir gemeinsam mit KALKOFF u. REINHARD feststellen, daß Cignolin eine ähnliche Wirkung nicht entfaltet. Aufschlußreich ist die Beobachtung, daß beim *Keratoakanthom* im Gegensatz zum Stachelzellcarcinom und zu anderen Tumoren sowie Präcancerosen die *DNA-Synthesen streng auf eine basale bis unmittelbar parabasale Zellschicht beschränkt* sind. Zeitweilig verminderte und später vermehrte DNA-

Synthesen in der menschlichen Epidermis nach Einwirkung von Röntgenstrahlen oder von Ultraviolettstrahlen entsprachen den im Tierversuch beobachteten Reaktionen. Vermehrte DNA-Synthesebilder fanden sich ferner u. a. beim Lichen ruber und beim akuten Ekzem, jeweils durch fluorierte Corticosteroide prompt unterdrückbar. Besondere diagnostische Bedeutung könnte ferner der Beobachtung zukommen, daß *beim Psoriatiker offenbar in typischer Weise auch klinisch nicht veränderte Haut mehr Zellen in DNA-Synthese zeigt als die Haut gesunder Kontrollen* an topographisch vergleichbaren Stellen.

Solche und zahlreiche andere Ergebnisse unserer autoradiographischen Untersuchungen mit markierten Nucleinsäurebausteinen, auf die hier nicht mehr eingegangen werden kann, lassen den Wert dieser in unserem Fach bisher nur vereinzelt angewandten histologischen Spezialuntersuchungsmethode für die Bearbeitung dermatologischer Fragestellungen deutlich werden.

Literatur. KALKOFF, K. W., u. W. BORN: Hautarzt **16**, 534 (1965) — Klin. Wschr. **43**, 1335 (1965). — KALKOFF, K. W., W. BORN und W. REINHARD: Arch. klin. exp. Derm. **227**, 857 (1966).

Histochimie des enzymes des follicules irradiés du cobaye

A. KINT et J. DE BERSAQUES, Clinique Dermatologique de l'Université de Gand (Belgique)

Les premières altérations histologiques du follicule anagène irradié s'observent au niveau du bulbe 24 h environ après l'exposition aux rayons X. Les autres parties du follicule ne présentent aucune altération avant 3 ou 4 jours (GEARY, 1952; MONTAGNA et CHASE, 1956). Des constatations semblables ont été faites par l'un de nous (DE BERSAQUES, 1965) après épilation de poils irradiés et au cours d'études portant sur l'incorporation d'acides aminés marqués dans la kératine de follicules exposés aux rayons ionisants. Les troubles du métabolisme des acides nucléiques sont cependant précoces, ainsi que CATTANEO et coll. (1960) ont pu le démontrer dans leurs travaux autoradiographiques après injection de thymidine marquée.

S'il est acquis qu'au cours du cycle pilaire normal ou pathologique l'intensité de certaines réactions enzymatiques évolue (BRAUN-FALCO, 1958, 1961; MONTAGNA, 1962; BRAUN-FALCO et THIANPRASIT, 1963; KINT, 1966; PETZOLDT, 1966), la littérature ne contient que de rares données concernant l'évolution de l'activité enzymatique du follicule irradié. Seuls MONTAGNA et CHASE (1956) décrivent une diminution de la phosphatase alcaline dans les papilles dès le 3e jour suivant l'irradiation. L'étude des variations enzymatiques provoquées par les rayons ionisants pourrait cependant nous fournir des indications utiles au sujet du mécanisme de leur action. C'est pourquoi nous avons étudié dans ce travail l'histochimie de quelques enzymes dans des follicules soumis à l'action des rayons X.

Matériel et méthodes

L'étude a été effectuée sur quatre séries de cinq cobayes. Les follicules anagènes ont été obtenus par épilation du dos. Dans les zones ainsi traitées, plusieurs endroits ont ensuite été irradiés simultanément avec l'appareil de contact de Philips (50 KV, 0,5 mm Al, 6 cm DFP, 1.020 r). Des biopsies ont été prélevées journalièrement pendant huit jours.

Après congélation à la neige carbonique, les pièces on été traitées d'après les techniques permettant la mise en évidence de la phosphatase alcaline, de la phosphatase acide, des estérases aspécifiques, des enzymes protéolytiques, de la cytochromeoxydase, de la succinodéshydrogénase et des réductases de tétrazolium liées au NAD et au NADP.

Tableau. *Altérations enzymatiques observées dans les follicules irradiés du cobaye: biopsies, prélevées, entre 0 et 8 jours*

		0	1	2	3	4	5	6	7	8
Phosphatase alcaline	Capillaires	++	++	++	++	+|+	+|+	+|+		
Phosphatase acide	Papille	++	++	++	++	+|+	+|+	+|+	+|+	
	Epiderme (c. basale)	+	+	+	+	+	+	+	+	+
	Gaine follic. interne	++	++	++	+|+	+|+	+|+	+|+	+|+	+|+
	Gaine follic. externe	+	+	+	+|+	+|+	+|+	+|+	+|+	+|+
	Bulbe	+	++	++	+|+	+|+	+|+	+|+	+|+	+|+
Estérases aspécifiques	Epiderme (c. basale)	+	+	++	++	+|+	+|+	+|+	+|+	+|+
	Gaine follic. interne	+|+	+|+	+|+	+|+	+|+	+|+	+|+	+|+	+|+
	Gaine follic. externe	+	+	++	+|+	+|+	+|+	+	+	
	Bulbe	++	+	++	+					
	Glande sébacée	+	+	+	+	+	+	+	+	+
Enzymes protéolytiques (substrat: LNA)	Epiderme (c. basale)	+	+	+	+	+	+	+	+	+
	Bulbe			++	+|+	++	++			
	Papille	+	++	++	++	++	++	++	++	++
	Follicule en régression	+	+	++	++	+|+	+|+	+|+	+|+	+|+
Cytochromeoxydase	Epiderme (c. basale)	++	++	++	++	++	+	+	+|+	+|+
	Gaine follic. externe	+	+	+	+	+	+	+	+	+
	Bulbe	++	++	++	++	+|+	+|+	+|+	+|+	+|+
	Glande sébacée	+	+	+	+	+	+	+	+	+
Succinodéshydrogénase	Epiderme (c. basale)	++	++	++	++	+|+	+|+	+|+	+|+	+|+
	Gaine follic. externe	+	+	+	+	+	+	+	+	+
	Bulbe	++	++	++	++	++	++	++	++	++
	Glande sébacée	++	++	++	++	+|+	+|+	+|+	+|+	+|+
Réductases de tétrazolium liées au NAD	Epiderme (c. basale)	++	++	++	++	++	+	+	+|+	+|+
	Gaine follic. externe	+	+	+	+	+	+	+	+	+
	Bulbe	++	++	++	++	++	++	++	++	++
	Glande sébacée	++	++	++	++	+|+	+|+	+|+	+|+	+|+
Réductases de tétrazolium liées au NADP	Epiderme (c. basale)	++	++	++	++	++	++	++	++	++
	Gaine follic. externe	+	+	+	+	+	+	+	+	+
	Bulbe	++	++	++	++	++	++	++	++	++
	Glande sébacée	+	+	+	+	+	+	+|+	+|+	+|+

Résultats

Nous ne décrirons pas ici les · localisations normales des enzymes étudiés, celles-ci étant bien connues (BRAUN-FALCO, 1958, 1961; HASHIMOTO, OGAWA et LEVER, 1962; HASHIMOTO et OGAWA, 1963). Nous nous bornerons donc à la description des altérations enzymatiques observées dans les follicules irradiés (voir tableau).

La phosphatase alcaline mise à part, dont l'activité dans la papille des follicules s'atténue après l'irradiation, les enzymes hydrolytiques (phosphatase acide, estérases aspécifiques) ne présentent pas d'altérations histochimiques durant les 3 premiers jours suivant l'exposition aux rayons ionisants. A.partir du 4e jour on observe une diminution progressive de l'activité de toutes les réactions hydrolytiques et la coloration est quasi négative à la fin de la phase de régression.

Les enzymes protéolytiques se comportent différemment et la méthode de BURSTONE et FOLK nous révèle une augmentation modérée de leur activité à partir du 4e jour suivant l'irradiation.

La cytochromeoxydase, la succinodéshydrogénase et les réductases du tétrazolium liées au NAD et au NADP restent inchangées durant les 4 premiers jours et leur activité diminue ensuite rapidement.

Discussion

Il apparaît d'après nos observations, que les rayons ionisants n'ont pas un effet immédiat sur la répartition et l'activité histochimique des enzymes étudiés. Cette constatation indique que l'irradiation n'influence pas directement le métabolisme du cytoplasme. Les premières altérations métaboliques consistent, ainsi que l'ont démontré CATTANEO et coll. (1960), dans le blocage de la synthèse de l'ADN, blocage qui est réalisé $1/_2$ h après l'irradiation; la formation de l'ADN peut reprendre éventuellement après environ 24 h. Les altérations morphologiques et histochimiques observées après 3. ou 4 jours pourraient être dues à une anomalie dans la synthèse de l'ADN ou à la perturbation des rapports ADN-ARN, l'ARN messager ne pouvant plus transmettre les informations nucléaires au cytoplasme. La présence dans les cellules d'enzymes histochimiquement décelables ne signifie toutefois pas nécessairement que le métabolisme cellulaire évolue normalement; les réserves enzymatiques du cytoplasme dépassent en effet largement ses besoins et peuvent à elles seules entretenir l'activité métabolique de la cellule durant quelque temps. Ainsi s'expliquerait le décalage observé entre l'apparition des premières lésions métaboliques et celle des premières altérations histochimiques.

Au cours du cycle pilaire normal ou pathologique (pelade) les altérations enzymatiques accompagnent l'involution folliculaire et s'observent à partir du début de la phase catagène (KINT, 1966). Il est en outre démontré que l'activité mitotique du follicule diminue nettement au cours de la seconde moitié de la phase anagène (BRAUN-FALCO, 1962) et la détermination histophotométrique de l'ADN nous a révélé moins d'ADN dans les noyaux du bulbe à la fin de la phase active, que dans la période anagène précoce. Une diminution de l'ADN nucléaire semble donc précéder les altérations morphologiques de la phase catagène.

Le mécanisme de régression folliculaire provoquée par les rayons ionisants est donc fort semblable à celui du cycle pilaire normal ou à celui que l'on observe dans la pelade. Il s'agit dans chaque cas d'un arrêt ou d'une altération primaire de la synthèse de l'ADN, suivie à distance d'altérations cytoplasmiques.

Bibliographie. BRAUN-FALCO, O.: Dans: MONTAGNA, W., and R. A. ELLIS: The biology of hair growth, p. 65—90. New York: Acad. Press 1958; — Arch. klin. exp. Derm. **214**, 176 (1961); **215**, 63 (1962). — BRAUN-FALCO, O., e R. THIANPRASIT: Minerva derm. **38**, (suppl. al N 1) 252 (1963). — CATTANEO, S. M., H. QUASTLER, and F. G. SHERMAN: Radiat. Res. **12**,

587 (1960). — DE BERSAQUES, J.: Over de synthese van keratine. Thèse Gand, 236 p. Bruxelles: Arscia 1965. — GEARY, J. R.: Amer. J. Anat. **91**, 51 (1952). — HASHIMOTO, K., and K. OGAWA: Amer. J. Anat. **113**, 35 (1963). — HASHIMOTO, K., K. OGAWA, and W. F. LEVER: J. invest. Derm. **39**, 21 (1962). — KINT, A.: Histogenetische studie van het basocellulair epithelioma. Thèse Gand, 402 p. Bruxelles: Arscia 1966. — MONTAGNA, W.: The structure and function of skin. IIe Ed. New York: Academic Press 1962. — MONTAGNA, W., and H. B. CHASE: Amer. J. Anat. **99**, 415 (1956). — PETZOLDT, D.: Arch. klin. exp. Derm. **227**, 513 (1966).

Untersuchungen zur experimentellen Photosensibilisierung mit Sulfanilamid und Phenothiazinen

K. SCHWARZ, J. ROTHENSTEIN und M. SCHWARZ-SPECK, Dermatologische Univ.-Klinik Zürich (Schweiz)

Tierexperimentelle Untersuchungen und die klinischen Befunde an 57 Patienten mit lichtabhängigen Dermatosen durch Sulfonamide und Phenothiazine hatten gezeigt, daß zwischen den beiden Gruppen bedeutende Unterschiede bestehen. Während die Sulfonamidfälle praktisch immer der strengen Definition der Photoallergie von EPSTEIN, BURCKHARDT, BAER und HARBER genügten, ergaben sich für die Phenothiazinfälle recht viele Übergangsformen von photoallergisch und photosensitiv zu kontaktallergisch. Wir haben uns gefragt, ob ein Zusammenhang zwischen den klinischen Differenzen und dem photochemischen Verhalten des Sulfanilamids bzw. Chlorpromazins bestehen könnte.

Wir wußten, daß in vitro die Bestrahlung mit ungefiltertem Licht der Quarzlampe das Sulfanilamid spektrophotometrisch fast schlagartig in einen blauen, sich nicht mehr weiter verändernden Stoff umsetzt, wobei sich die Absorption weit in das Sichtbare hinein verschiebt und das Maximum im UV C verschwindet.

Im Gegensatz dazu wird Chlorpromazin durch die Bestrahlung nur langsam und spektrophotometrisch über *mehrere* Intermediärprodukte verändert. Dabei verschieben sich Minima und Maxima graduell, und die Absorption erstreckt sich ebenfalls ins Sichtbare hinein.

Das photochemische Wirkspektrum und der Energiebedarf von monochromatischer Strahlung wurde am Xenon-Lampen-Monochromator bestimmt. Davon zeige ich Ihnen einige representative Beispiele:

Im Absorptionsmaximum des Sulfanilamids um 259 nm genügen 444 mW/cm² · sec zum Verschwinden des Maximums und zur Verlängerung der Absorption ins Sichtbare.

Die doppelte Energiemenge erzeugt bei Einstrahlung am Ende der Absorption um 310 nm gleichsinnige Veränderungen, jedoch ist die Umsatzzahl bedeutend kleiner.

Im kleineren zweiten Absorptionsmaximum des Chlorpromazin führen 783 bis 3142 mW/cm² · sec der 307 nm-Strahlung zum allmählichen Verschwinden dieses Maximums, Verschiebungen am ersten Maximum und zur Verlängerung der Absorption ins Sichtbare.

Dieselben Erscheinungen werden durch Bestrahlung im Absorptionsminimum von 280 nm erhalten, doch braucht es naturgemäß bedeutend höhere Energien.

Die erwähnten Unterschiede der Phenothiazin- und Sulfanilamidphotoallergie mögen sehr wohl mit der verschiedenen Anzahl der photochemisch aus den Haptenen entstehenden Übergangszustände und Umsetzungsprodukte zusammenhängen: Beim Chlorpromazin stehen zur Bildung des Vollantigens viel mehr Intermediärprodukte zur Verfügung als beim Sulfanilamid. Da das natürliche Sonnenlicht die Wellenlängen 290 bis 310 nm ebenfalls enthält, darf man wohl auch in der Haut bei Isolation und Abwesenheit dieser Substanzen mit ähnlichen photochemischen Umsetzungen rechnen wie in vitro. So stehen für EPSTEINS „primary reaction" das Absorptionsspektrum der Substanzen und das photochemische Wirkspektrum in guter Übereinstimmung. Für den Typus der fakultativ sich anschließenden Sensibilisierung stehen jedoch beim Chlorpromazin viel mehr

Möglichkeiten offen als beim Sulfanilamid. In diesem Sinne sprechen die nachfolgenden Untersuchungen über die experimentelle Chlorpromazinsensibilisierung.
Darin sollte die pathogenetische Rolle des Lichtes näher abgeklärt werden:

Etwa 100 Albinomeerschweinchen wurden in drei Gruppen eingeteilt. Die *Sensibilisierung*
erfolgte auf drei verschiedene Arten:
1. Pinselung mit 5% Chlorpromazin, täglich über 3 Wochen.
2. Chlorpromazinpinselung und anschließende Bestrahlung mit Erythemdosen der unge-
filterten Quarzlampe.
3. Zuerst Bestrahlung und anschließende Chlorpromazinpinselung.
Die Art der Auslösung und die Anzahl der positiven Testresultate sind im Dia dargestellt.
Sie entnehmen daraus, daß das Licht für den Erfolg der Sensibilisierung zwar essentiell ist, daß
es jedoch keinen Unterschied macht, ob die Bestrahlung vor oder nach der Chlorpromazin-
applikation erfolgte. Die Sensibilisierungsraten unterscheiden sich in den Gruppen 2 und 3 nur
wenig, wenn auch in der dritten Gruppe etwas mehr photoallergische Reaktionen zur Beobachtung kamen. In beiden Gruppen waren zudem 20 bis 25% der Tiere lichtempfindlich geworden!

Zweifellos haben wir es hier mit einem besonderen Typus einer lichtabhängigen
„photoallergischen" Sensibilisierung zu tun. Die direkte Entstehung des eigentlichen „Photoallergens" aus dem Hapten Chlorpromazin unter der Bestrahlung
scheint dabei nicht entscheidend zu sein, weil die der Hapten-Applikation vorausgehende Bestrahlung zum gleichen Resultat führt! Wir möchten die pathogenetische Rolle des Lichtes nicht nur als unspezifisches Adjuvans auffassen. Die
Versuche lassen vermuten, daß die Haut die Fähigkeit zur Bildung des Vollantigens erst durch die UV-Bestrahlung erlangt, sei es, daß das Hapten Chlorpromazin in der bestrahlen Haut anders metabolisiert wird als in der nicht bestrahlten, sei es, daß nicht nur das Hapten, sondern bevorzugt ein Carrier durch das
Licht so aktiviert wird, daß die Kupplung zum (Photo-)Allergen erst erfolgen
kann.

Sollte diese Auffassung durch weitere Untersuchungen gestützt werden können,
fallen auch die Diskrepanzen zwischen dem Absorptionsspektrum der zur Photoallergie führenden Substanzen und dem bei der Testung verwendeten Wirkspektrum im langwelligen UV dahin. Selbstverständlich müssen Energietransfers
von Hautstrukturen auf das Hapten und Verschiebungen des Absorptions-
spektrums des Haptens in der Haut beachtet werden.

Light is an Aetiological Factor for Certain Dermatoses in U.A.R.

M. el Zawahry, Kasr-el-Aini, Faculty of Medicine, Cairo University (U.A.R.)

In our countries, the Arabian zone, light is a provocative factor for certain
dermatoses met within that area and particularly in U.A.R. The most important
of these are the following:

Lichen Planus Tropicus (L.P.T.)

Is a form of lichen planus which occurs on the exposed parts of the body when
these are exposed to sun and light (Fig. 1). The lesions are commonly annular but
may be papular or even plaques, itchy violaceous, shiny, scaly and leave long
lasting post-lichen pigmentation. Itching is more intense during summer and
with light and sun exposure and during that season the lesions are more active
and infilterated, they subside during winter and recur next summer. The favourite

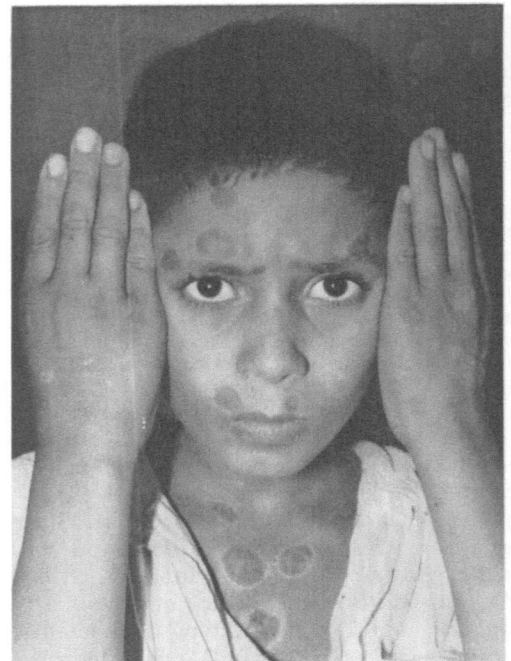

Fig. 1. Lichen planus tropicus

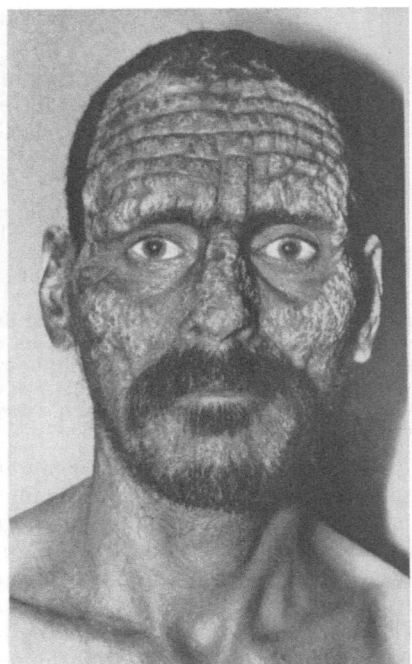

Fig. 2. Psoriasis of the face

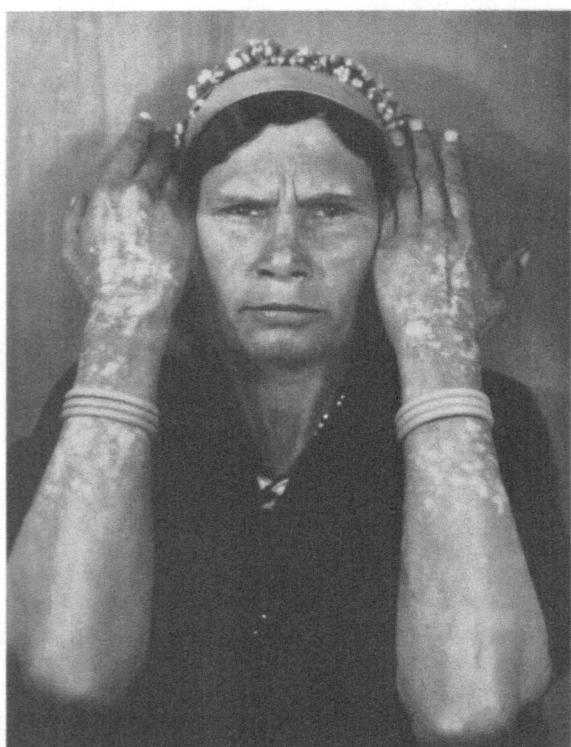

Fig. 3. Vitiligo on exposed parts

sites are the face especially forehead, cheeks and lips, also the V-shaped area of the chest and dorsum of the hands. Heat is also a factor in L.P.T. and patients sitting in front of fire especially bakers, may get it. The patients are usually children young adults and mostly peasants and those living in the village. Nutritional deficiency state is manifest in most of the cases. Histologically the lesions of L.P.T. are the same as those seen in ordinary lichen planus. The treatment is better when patients are protected from further light and sun exposure, and they benefit when given antimalarial drugs, nicotinic acid and other elements of the Vitamin B complex. In a statistical report out of 220 lichen planus cases 88 i.e. 40% of them had the clinical variety of L.P.T.

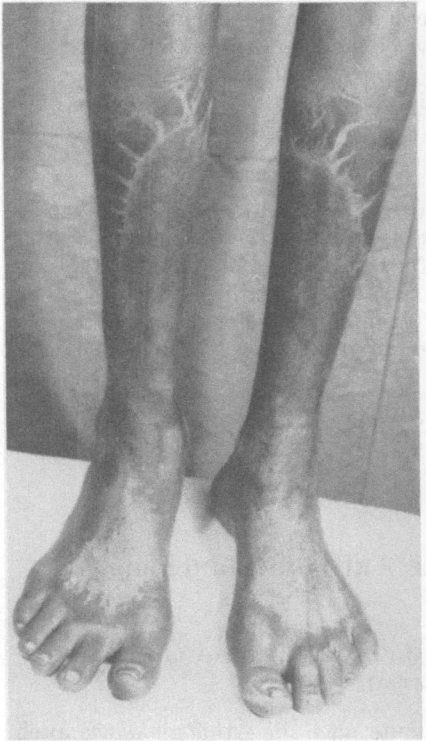
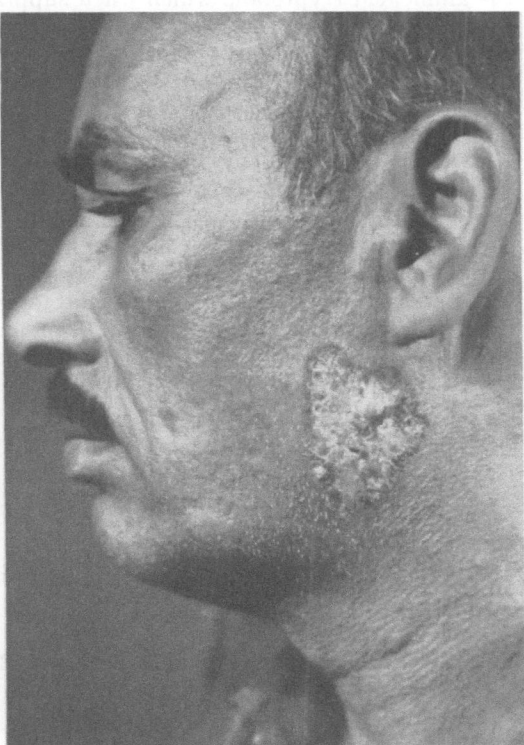

Fig. 4. Pellagra   Fig. 5. Ulcerated L.E.

Psoriasis

Psoriasis in U.A.R. constitutes 3% of the whole dermatoses and the exposed parts of the body are affected in 3% of the cases (Fig. 2). Light is an aetiological factor for these cases and the face, V-shaped area of the chest and dorsum of the hands are the sites more visited. The lips are frequently affected in these cases (2%) especially the lower lip and the lesions are more intense during summer and even may itch. I saw a case of psoriasis having a butterfly distribution on the face.

Vitiligo

It is not rare to get vitiligo on the exposed parts of the body (Fig. 3) and after over exposure to sun and light in our patients especially those spending the summer vacation near the sea shore or having an out-door position. Light is a definite factor for these cases and the lesions spread on further light or ultra-violet exposure. Antimalarial drugs are helpful for such cases and sun screening is the wise procedure. The patients by time learn that their behaviour assists a lot in the management of such cases.

Pellagra

Pellagra was prevalent in our countries in the past, nowadays the incidence of pellagra came down and it constitutes 0.2% of our dermatoses. Pellagrens suffer from light and their dermatitis is initiated and augmented by light exposure. Deficiency of the diet especially in the vitamin concerned, i.e., nicotinic acid or the aminoacid tryptofane which when supplied could be converted into nicotinic acid in the body is the causative factor. Increased demand during certain age periods as in adolescence or during pregnancy, or lactation results in partial deprivation and latent or manifest pellagra may happen. Such latent cases are made manifest by light exposure. The characteristic of our cases is the presence of a double border, one of scaleness and the other of pigmentation (Fig. 4).

Ulcerated Lupus Erythematosus (L.E.)

The incidence of discoid L.E. is rising in our people. Light is a definite provocative factor and our sunny countries favour that relation. We do meet ulcerated L.E. on the face and scalp although rare (Fig. 5). During the last year (1966) I saw three cases of ulcerated L.E. and the biopsy was typical of L.E. Certain other dermatoses depend on light exposure ranging from simple solar dermatitis up to frank malignancy, but the above mentioned are outstanding clinical entities nowadays commonly seen in our people.

References. ZAWAHRY, M. EL.: Skin Diseases in Arabian Countries, vol. 1, 2 and 3, 1963, 1964 and 1967; — Excerpta med. (Amst.) Sect. XIII, **1964**, 313; — Dermatologia Int. **4**, 2, 92 (1965); — Derm. Digest. **5**, 95 (1966).

Heliotherapie und ihr Einfluß auf die Aktivität mancher Enzyme bei Psoriasiskranken

N. BALEVSKA, J. PETKOV, G. MUSTAKOV, S. JOWEV, N. ZLATKOV und G. TOMOV, Hohes Medizinisches Institut, Sofia (Bulgarien)

Trotz zahlreicher Untersuchungen bleibt heute noch die Ätiologie sowie auch die Pathogenese der Psoriasis vulgaris ungeklärt und stellt eines von den großen Problemen der Dermatologie vor. Immer mehr und mehr wird heute die Auffassung angenommen, daß bei der Psoriasis eine Überproduktion von epidermalen Zellen — eine Hyperepidermopoese — im Vordergrund steht (KREBS). Die Psoriasis kann man also als eine abnorm starke Regeneration der Epidermis auffassen. Bei den erhöhten regenerativen Prozessen ist die Erforschung des Enzyminhaltes der psoriatischen Epidermis von großem Interesse. Histochemische Untersuchungen bei Psoriasis zeigen eine erhöhte oder herabgesetzte Aktivität mancher Enzyme, so daß auf Grund dieser Resultate die Psoriasis von manchen Autoren als eine Enzymopathie genetischen Ursprungs aufgefaßt wird (GRÜNEBERG). Die Untersuchung der histochemischen Veränderungen in den psoriatischen Läsionen, besonders die Verfolgung der Dynamik des Prozesses und der Veränderungen in der Enzymaktivität während der verschiedenen Phasen der Erkrankung, ist mit großen Schwierigkeiten verbunden. Deswegen ist die Erforschung der Serumenzyme bei Psoriasiskranken und die Verfolgung ihrer Dynamik von großem Interesse.

Wie bekannt ist, hat BÜCHER vorgeschlagen, die Enzyme in Zellen und Sekretionen einzuteilen. Es wird angenommen, daß die einzelnen Organe ein quantitativ verschiedenes Sortiment von den sog. Hauptkettenenzymen haben, die den wesentlichen Teil der Zellenenzyme bilden. Unter diesem Standpunkt stellt die Erforschung der Serumenzyme bei Psoriasis besonders die Veränderungen der Enzymdynamik im Krankheitsverlauf und während des Heilungsprozesses dar.

Von dieser Auffassung ausgehend, haben wir uns die Aufgabe gestellt, die Dynamik der Aktivität mancher Serumenzyme im Laufe der Heilung zu verfolgen. Die Heliotherapie wurde bei Kranken mit Psoriasis an der Meeresküste durchgeführt. Unsere Beobachtungen wurden an Psoriatikern (800 Personen) durchgeführt, und wir haben in 98,7% der Fälle therapeutische Beeinflussung. Während der Behandlung wurden alle Kranken nur der Aktino- und Tallasotherapie — ohne gleichzeitige Anwendung irgendwelcher Medikamente — unterzogen.

Unsere Experimente wurden in den Jahren 1960 bis 1966 an der bulgarischen Küste am Schwarzen Meer durchgeführt.

Wir haben die Serumenzyme Asparagin Transaminase, Alanin Transaminase, Cholinesterase, Fructose-diphosphat Aldolase und Leuzinamino-Peptidase bei Kranken mit Psoriasis vulgaris vor und nach 30tägiger Behandlung am Schwarzen Meer untersucht.

Die Resultate dieser Untersuchungen sind in der nachstehenden Tabelle angegeben.

Tabelle. *Der Stand einiger Enzyme vor und nach der Behandlung am Meer bei Kranken mit Psoriasis vulgaris*

	N	Vor der Behandlung	N	Nach der Behandlung
Asparagin Transaminase (AsT-SGOT)	59	$31,18 \pm 12.48$	50	$29,00 \pm 8,59$
Alanin Transaminase (AlT-SGOT)	59	$21,24 \pm 9,83$	50	$26,00 \pm 7,21$
Cholinesterase	59	$38,86 \pm 14,16$	50	$34,20 \pm 8,39$
Fructose-diphosphat Aldolase ALD	65	$5,3 \pm 2,33$	61	$5,7 \pm 2,44$
Leuzinamino-Peptidase (LAP)	64	$9,4 \pm 5,52$	64	$8,00 \pm 4,38$

Die Ergebnisse der Aktivität dieser Enzyme im Blutserum bei Kranken mit Psoriasis vulgaris stehen im Widerspruch mit den Literaturangaben. WEBER u. WÜRST finden keine Abweichung von den normalen Werten, SALFELD u. VOGELSBERG geben erhöhte Werte an. Unsere Untersuchungen erlauben uns, folgende Schlußfolgerungen zu ziehen.

1. Die Asparagin Transaminase zeigt während der Heliotherapie allmähliche Verminderung ihrer Aktivität, ja unmittelbar nach ihr sind die erhaltenen Werte niedriger als die Ausgangswerte.

2. Die Alanin Transaminase zeigte aber während der Heliotherapie eine Erhöhung der Aktivität, die auch unmittelbar nach ihrer Beendigung hoch bleibt.

3. Bei der Cholinesterase, die bei Kranken mit Psoriasis niedrigere Werte ergab als bei der Kontrollgruppe, wurde eine allmähliche Verminderung der Aktivität auch nach der Heliotherapie festgestellt.

4. Die Fructose-diphosphat Aldolase, die beinahe zweimal höhere Werte bei den Psoriatikern als bei der Kontrollgruppe aufwies, zeigte nach der Behandlung, wenn auch unbedeutend, eine Erhöhung der Aktivität.

5. Die Leucinamino-Peptidase zeigte auch eine verminderte Aktivität nach der Heliotherapie.

6. Die Heliotherapie wirkt sicher auf die Aktivität einer Reihe von Serumenzymen bei Kranken mit Psoriasis. Darauf beruht wahrscheinlich die gute Beeinflussung der Erkrankung mit dieser Behandlung.

7. Zur weiteren Aufklärung der pathogenetischen Mechanismen bei der Heliotherapie der Psoriasis sind vergleichende histochemische Untersuchungen der psoriatischen Plaques und der Serumenzyme notwendig. Solche Untersuchungen sind in unserer Klinik schon im Gang.

The Action Spectrum of Erythema Induced by Ultraviolet Radiation. Preliminary Report*

D. BERGER, F. URBACH and R. E. DAVIES, Skin and Cancer Hospital, Department of Dermatology, Temple University School of Medicine, Philadelphia, Pa. (U.S.A.)

In recent years, considerable uncertainty has arisen concerning the action spectrum of the human skin [1, 2]. Furthermore, there is much disagreement about the interpretation of the classic work of HAUSSER in this field, each investigator choosing to select those statements which fit his particular observations and interpretations [3].

At a recent conference [4], details of the design of high intensity spectral instruments used for action spectra studies were described, and it became apparent that significant errors could have been introduced by the high stray light characteristics of single monochromators. There was little uniformity about just what was considered "minimal erythema", and about the time course of the events studied by different investigators.

In order to critically restudy these phenomena, a high intensity spectral instrument with excellent stray light characteristics was designed and assembled in our laboratories. The following components were used: A Spex model 1400 grating double monochromator, each grating ruled at 1200 lines per mm, and blazed for 300 nm. (The size of each grating is 102 × 102 mm, Czerny-Turner mount. Relative aperture f/6.8. Dispersion: 1.08 nm/mm at the first exit slit and 0.54 nm/mm at the second exit slit.) The light path thru the system is schematically outlined in Fig. 1. Slits were designed and built by the Regulus Corporation, San Diego, California. (Maximum opening 6.5 mm, maximum height 20 mm, bilateral jaw movement, micrometer controlled to 0.01 mm.) The monochromtora is nitrogen purged to minimize damage to the gratings.

The light source consists of an Osram XBO 2500 watt xenon compact arc lamp in a gas tight, explosion proof housing supplied by Schoeffel Instrument Company, Westwood, New Jersey. The lamp housing is forced air cooled, the circulating air being further cooled by a cold water heat exchanger. The light is focussed by means of a quartz condensing lens 2.4 inches clear diameter with a nominal focal length of 3 inches. The focussed beam is reflected by means of a UV reflecting, IR transmitting ("cold") dichroic mirror (Optical Coating Laboratories, Incorporated) onto the entrance slit. Measurements of energy output were made with a thermopile (Eppley Corporation, Newport, Rhode Island), stray light measurements were made with a photo multiplier assembly (tube type R 106) supplied by Spex.

* Supported by the JOHN A. HARTFORD Foundation and USPHS Grant ES 00269.

Performance characteristics of the high intensity double monochromator are as follows:

Bandwidth (50%): At first exit slit, 6.5 mm maximum slit opening, 1.08 nm/mm, maximum bandwidth 7 nm; at second exit slit, 6.5 mm maximum slit opening, 3.5 nm maximal bandwidth. *Transmission:* First half of the monochromator—43%, second half of the monochromator—35%, overall transmission entrance slit to second exit slit—15%.

Stray light characteristics: Less than 0.04% intensity of the primary peak radiation at first exit slit, less than 0.00001% at the second exit slit. (Stray light includes all wavelengths 2.5 bandwidths away from the center of the primary radiation.)

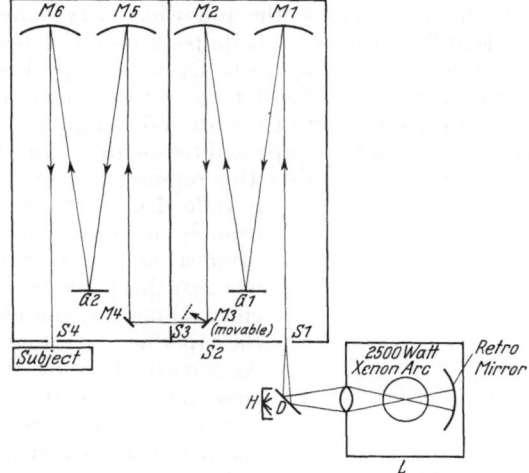

Fig. 1. Schematic top view of high intensity spectral instrument. *L* Lamp housing containing 2500 watt XBO Osram xenon compact arc lamp. *D* Ultraviolet reflecting, infra-red transmitting dichroic mirror. *H* Heat sink. *M* First surface mirrors. S_1 Entrance slit. S_2 First exit slit, single monochromator mode. S_3 Intermediate slit. S_4 Second exit slit, double monochromator mode. *G* Gratings, 102×102 mm, blazed for 300 nm, 1200 lines per mm

Power output: First exit slit: 254 nm: 0.45 mw/cm²/nm; 300 nm: 1.95 mw/cm²/nm; 320 nm: 2.3 mw/cm²/nm. *Second exit slit:* 254 nm: 0.15 mw/cm²/nm; 300 nm: 0.6 mw/cm²/nm; 320 nm: 0.7 mw/cm²/nm.

Maximum power output: First exit slit: 254 nm: 3 mw/cm²; 300 nm: 11 mw per cm²; 315 nm: 12 mw/cm²; 320 nm: 13 mw/cm². *Second exit slit:* 254 nm: 0.52 mw/cm²; 300 nm: 2 mw/cm²; 315 nm: 2.3 mw/cm²; 320 nm: 2.5 mw/cm².

Thus, with a bandwidth of 3.5 nm, it is possible to deliver a dose of radiation from the second exit slit sufficient to cause a "mild" (i.e. slightly above minimal) erythema in 84 sec at 254 nm, in 9 sec at 300 nm, in 13 min at 315 nm and in 25 min at 320 nm.

Preliminary results of action spectra studies

Utilizing the second exit slit of the high intensity spectral instrument described above, 6 mm diameter circular areas of skin on the abdomen of five male white subjects, ranging in age from 22 to 46 years, were irradiated with carefully measured doses of ultraviolet radiation. The 50% bandwidth in all cases was 2.16 nm, the stray light was less than 10^{-5} of the primary waveband. All irradiations were performed in the morning during a 3 week period in June and July of 1967, in an air-conditioned room (about 72 °F.). Output measurements were made immediately before and after each series of radiations at any one wavelength in any one subject and varied no more than 5%. Erythema measurements were made at 4, 8, 24 and 48 h, by visual inspection by the same observer under a Macbeth Examolite light source in a darkened room, and thru a series of Kodak red Color Balancing gelatin filters. The disappearance of the sharp outlines of the erythematous spots on observation thru the red filters was used as a criterion for grading erythema.

General comments

Our preliminary results confirm the major observations of HAUSSER in all respects [3]. Worth singling out are the following: Erythema due to 254 nm radiation appears within 3 to 4 h, reaches its peak intensity between 8 and 12 h, and has begun to subside markedly by 24 h. Even at its peak intensity the color is a pale pink-red, and it is very difficult to be certain of the minimal erythema dose. At very low doses (of the order of less than 5 millijoules) something can be seen which is clearly (because of the shape and reasonably sharp borders) produced by the radiation. Yet it is not clear that this represents true erythema; the color is yellowish brown and seems to be extremely superficial, almost "on" the skin. Studies are in progress to determine whether this phenomenon represents vascular change, or some chemical reaction in the superficial (stratum corneum ?) layers. As remarked on by HAUSSER, even five times minimal erythema doses produce no severe erythema with 254 nm. In contrast, the MED for wavelengths from 280 to 313 nm is quite sharply defined. The erythema produced by wavelengths 297, 303 and 313 nm is deep red-purple and peaks in 24 to 28 h. It persists 3 to 5 days and imperceptibly changes into pigmentation.

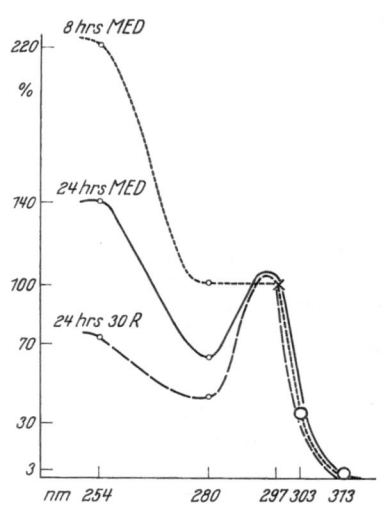

Fig. 2. "Action Spectrum" of Human Skin. Averages of values for five subjects, abdominal skin, second exit slit. Note great similarity for wavelength from 297 to 313 nm, and marked differences for 8 h MED, 24 h MED and a curve constructed by using values for moderate erythema (Kodak Color Balancing filter 30 R)

A striking, and as far as we know hitherto, unreported observation is the effect of body position on erythema. Examination in the sitting and the lying positions showed that all erythematous areas fade significantly and within 3 to 10 sec on assuming the horizontal position. This effect is significant enough to shift the MED point by 40 to 80%. Because of this phenomenon, all our readings were taken with subjects in the sitting position.

Averages and limits, minimal and slightly more than minimal erythema doses

The great effect of time after irradiation and of choice of degree of redness on the "action spectrum" of human skin is shown in the table and Fig. 2. For comparison, Hausser's figures for slightly more than MED's are shown (Fig. 3). Preliminary experiments suggest that the true sensitivity peak lies between 290 and 294 nm.

From 297 nm on, there appears to be a remarkably good agreement between most published figures. The disagreement at shorter wavelengths clearly is due to differences in time of evaluation and the difficulties inherent in the delineation of "minimal erythema".

Furthermore, if an erythema grade slightly above minimal is used as reference point (30 R) the resultant action spectrum closely approaches that originally described by HAUSSER (table). This is not at all surprising, since HAUSSER used a "moderate" erythema for construction of his action spectrum and specifically points out the difficulties and uncertainties inherent in "minimal erythema" measurements [3].

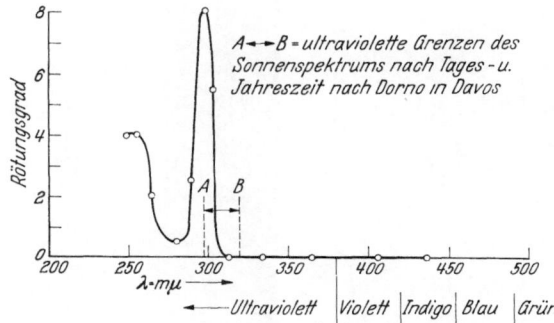

Fig. 3. Action spectrum for "moderate erythema" produced by giving a *constant* dose of ultraviolet radiation and measuring erythema grade observed at 24 h. This is *not* a minimal erythema dose action spectrum. Data of HAUSSER [3]

Table. *Averages and limits (in millijoules) for minimal erythema doses read at 8 and 24 h, and for a "moderate" erythema dose (read thru a 30 R Kodak Color Balancing filter) at 24 h. All radiation given at the second exit slit, bandwidth 2.16 nm. See also Fig. 2*

nm	MED 8 h (millijoules)	MED 24 h (millijoules)	30 R 24 h (millijoules)
254	6.3 (3.5— 8.4)	10.0 (6.0—17.0)	19.4 (10—40)
280	14.0 (5.0—24.0)	22.0 (12.0—33.6)	32.0 (23—48)
297	14.0 (6.0—24.0)	14.0 (6.0—24.0)	14.0 (7.0—20.0)
303	39.0 (28.0—48.0)	41.0 (34.0—48.0)	45.0 (40.0—48.0)
313	632 (450—770)	630 (540—770)	724 (540—770)

Effects of "stray" light

As has been pointed out before, single monochromators are bedeviled by "stray" light, i.e. radiation passing the exit slit other than the band desired. In many monochromators, this stray light can amount to 1% of the primary wavelength intensity. The need to consider this radiation is most critical at longer wavelengths where total irradiation time is very long, and where small quantities of highly erythema effective short wavelengths "stray" radiation are passed thru the instrument. This is a particularly serious problem when high intensity continuous spectrum light sources (such as compact xenon arcs) are used as energy sources.

To demonstrate the need for consideration of "stray" light, the arms of two subjects were given identical doses of UV (with the same bandwidth) from the first and second exit slit at wavelengths 297 and 313 nm. As can be seen in Fig. 4, there is no difference at the highly effective wavelength 297 nm (Fig. 4a), but a

significant difference in minimal erythema dose was found between the first and
second exit slit at wavelength 313 nm (Fig. 4b). (313 nm: Subject 1—first
exit—MED 540 millijoules, second exit—1280 millijoules; Subject 2—first exit—
MED 540 millijoules, second exit—900 millijoules.) In this case, stray light accounted for about 50 to 65% of the total effective dose at 313 nm!

The absence of a noticeable plateau or dip in the vicinity of 280 nm reported
by some observers may very well be due to stray light, and the reports of erythema
produced by wavelengths longer than 330 nm are almost certainly due to this
phenomenon.

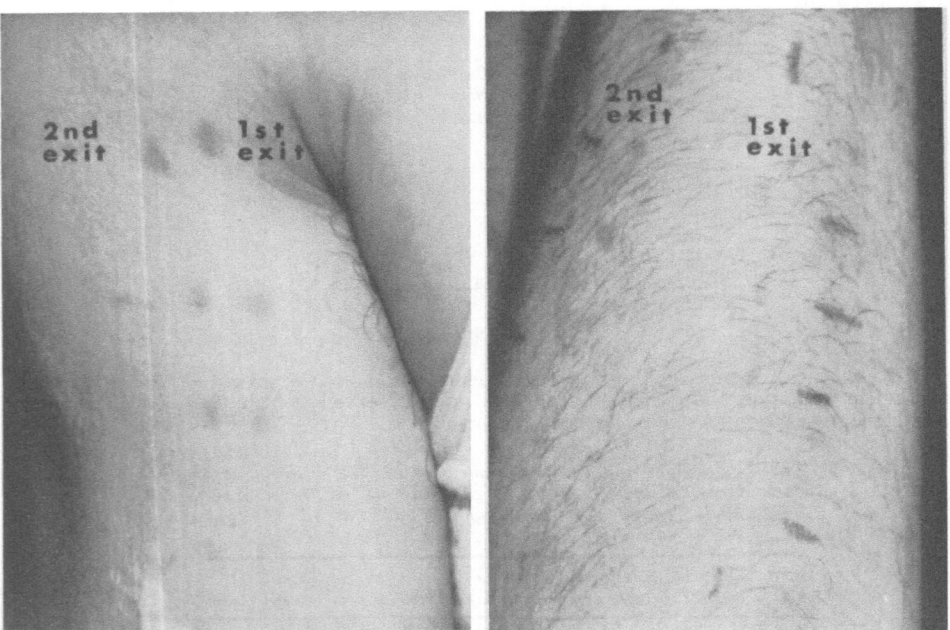

Fig. 4. Effect of "stray" light. Erythema produced by equal doses of energy from the first and
second exit slit of the Skin and Cancer Hospital high intensity spectral instrument. a) at
297 nm note no difference between single and double monochromator mode. b) at 313 nm
note much greater effect of lesser energy at the single monochromator mode

The "erythema range" effect

One of the most fascinating observations of KARL HAUSSER was that there
appears to be a significant difference between the dose needed to produce slight
and maximal erythema by different wavelengths. This concept is of great potential
significance for the prevention of sunburn and the understanding of diseases due
to light. To reproduce Hausser's experiments, it is necessary to have a reasonably
reliable means of quantitatively measuring erythema. For this purpose, we used
the Kodak Color Balancing filters which are readily available, although not of an
ideal shade of red. The disappearance of the sharp outlines of the erythematous
spots when viewed thru the filters under a Macbeth Examolite lamp was used as
a criterion for grading.

The results of five such investigations are shown in Fig. 5. The 10 R filter was
arbitrarily assigned the value of 1; this blanked out slightly more than minimal
erythema at 254 nm.

Considering the crude system used, the similarity to Hausser's data is striking (Fig. 6). In essence, Fig. 5 shows that five times the minimal erythema dose produces nowhere near maximal erythema at 254 nm, while 2.5 times the minimal erythema dose produces maximal erythema dose at 303 nm. Thus, while it takes much more energy to produce any erythema at 303 nm than at 254 nm, proportionately not much more than the threshold dose produces a significant burn.

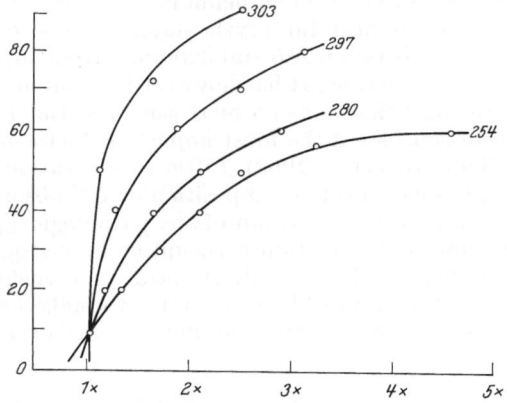

Fig. 5. The "erythema range" effect. Data from experiments of five subjects plotted to show degree of erythema produced by increasing doses of ultraviolet radiation (second exit slit, bandwidth 2.16 nm, erythema measured with Kodak Color Balancing filters). The points are expressed as multiples of the dose needed to develop erythema slightly above minimal (10 R filter).

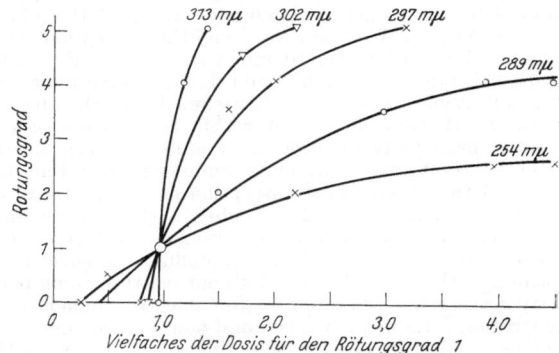

Fig. 6. The "erythema range" effect. Data of HAUSSER [3] plotted as in Fig. 5

We are in the process of designing better quantitative measuring systems for erythema measurements so as to repeat these studies more accurately. Under any circumstances, it appears quite clear that direct summation of the biologic effects of various wavelengths of ultraviolet radiation is not appropriate, a fact which has recently been pointed out very nicely by GEORGE FINDLAY of South Africa [5].

References. 1. EVERETT, M. A., R. L. OLSON, and R. M. SAYRE: Arch. Derm. **92**, 713 (1965). — 2. SAYRE, R. M., R. L. OLSON, and M. A. EVERETT: J. invest. Derm. **46**, 240 (1966). — 3. HAUSSER, K. W., u. W. VAHLE: Wiss. Veröff. Siemens **6**, 102 (1927). — 4. URBACH, F. (Editor): The Biologic Effects of Ultraviolet Radiation. Oxford: Pergamon Press (In press). — 5. FINDLAY, G. H.: Brit. J. Derm. **79**, 148 (1967).

The Absorption Spectrum of the Stratum Corneum as the Natural Sunscreen of Human Skin

A. R. H. B. Verhagen, Dutch Medical Research Centre, Nairobi (Kenya)

In the development of the physical theory concerning light protection, it is generally recognised that the stratum corneum is protecting the living underlying tissue against the potentially harmful, erythematogenic and carcinogenic rays of the short wave ultraviolet: between 285 and 320 nm*. Keratin, like most proteins, has a high absorption of these rays. It has however been often implied or assumed that the stratum corneum behaves as an inert screen in this respect: only variations in thickness were considered the most important factor in the sensitivity of human skin to UV light (Rottier, 1962). Little consideration has been given to the possibility, that photochemical decomposition of UV absorbing substances or any other biochemical alteration as a result of any pathological process might alter the absorption spectrum of the stratum corneum and consequently transmission through this layer. Most methods to isolate the stratum corneum have been developed for normal skin: It is impossible for example to make cantharidine blisters both in irradiated skin and in eczematized skin of chronic polymorphous light eruptions (CPLE).

Methods and Materials

Vermeer et al have designed a simple apparatus for investigation of soluble substances of the stratum corneum dysiunctum, the upper part of the horny layer. It consists of a brass cylinder, 4 cm in diameter, open at the bottom, which can be placed upon the skin and filled with fluid (solvent). Two tapering teflon rollers are attached to a central rotating spindle in the cylinder; the skin is gently "washed" during a certain period, being softly rubbed by the rollers and soaked by the fluid. After a routine period of 6 min "washing" the solution is poured from the cylinder, filtered twice through Whatman No. 1 and the absorption spectrum is measured in the spectrophotometer (Zeiss PMQ II. 10 mm curvettes) in the wavelengths between 600 nm (where absorption is always negligible) and 225 nm. Five nanometer intervals were used in the short wave ultraviolet. It is generally assumed that the absorption curve of the stratum corneum in the short wave ultraviolet within the sunspectrum (UV-B) is due to protein or its metabolites, principally the aromatic aminoacids tryptophan and tyrosin and to urocanic acid, a metabolite of another aromatic aminoacid, histidine. In accordance with this assumption, we found that the corneal absorption curve, as it had been described by many authors, was very adequately reproduced when a strongly alkaline solution, e.g. a sodium hydroxide-boric acid buffer of pH 10,75 was used as a solvent in the "washing apparatus". Neutral or weakly alkaline buffers did not reproduce the curve (Fig. 1). Neither was this the case after washing with fatty solvents. With our usual washing period of 6 min, only the most superficial layer was removed: often no difference was demonstrable in histological sections between the stratum corneum of washed and non-washed skin.

In the graphs demonstrated in this paper the extinction values (E) of the solution will be given and not the transmission in percentage (T). (E = 2 — log T.).

An example of a normal extinction curve is shown in Fig. 1. It bears a striking resemblance to the absorption curve described by other authors for the stratum corneum or epidermis as a whole.

1. The first series of experiments were mostly carried out in Europeans. Part of the skin of the back or arm was irradiated with a xenonlamp (Osram OXBF 6000) with a ultraviolet filter (Schott WG 6, 2 mm) to exclude wavelengths which are not present in natural sunlight (shorter than 285 nm). The subjects were irradiated with several (usually about 5) times their previously determined minimal erythema dose (M.E.D.). The skin was "washed" in the irradiated area and in the adjoining non-irradiated area, between 24 and 48 h after the irradiation, when an erythema was present.

2. The second series of experiments consisted of washing and determining the extinction curves of the solution in patients with the dermatitis type or plaque type of C.P.L.E. Specimens were taken both from the exposed eczematized areas as well as from the adjacent apparently

---

* nm = nanometer = millimicron.

normal skin which had been covered by the clothes. In the neck or on the upper arm the disease is often sharply marginated. These experiments were done in 11 Europeans and 13 Africans. It should be noted that C.P.L.E. is fairly common among Africans in the Kenya Highlands.

3. A third experiment consisted of irradiating the skin of the back of patients with C.P.L.E. with several times the M.E.D. and determining the extinction curve after 24 h and after several days.

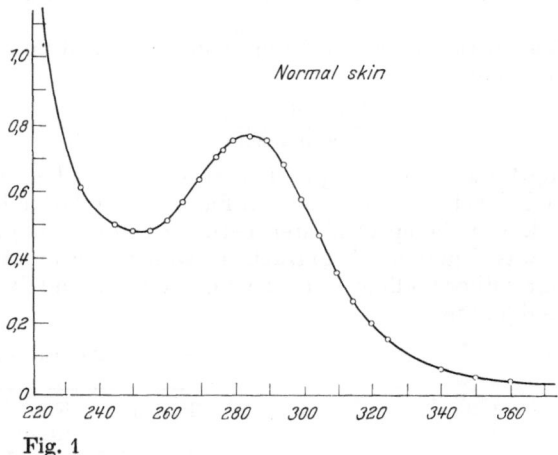

Fig. 1

Results

Ad 1. Fig. 2 shows an example of the effect on the extinction curve in normal European subjects. One finds a loss of extinction and accordingly a much higher transmission in wavelengths between 250 and 305 nm, the spectral area which corresponds in normal skin with the base of an absorption top at about 280 nm. In ten subjects, this was a fairly constant phenomenon, but the absorption top is more distinct in normal skin in one subject than in the other and changes are most outspoken in subjects with a high top. In three West-Indian negroes the M.E.D. and consequently the irradiation time was much higher; accordingly the above mentioned changes were even more outspoken.

A drawback of our rather crude method of collecting specimens of the disjunct part consists in the slight differences in concentration of the two solutions: in one specimen the whole curve may be at a slightly higher level than in the other.

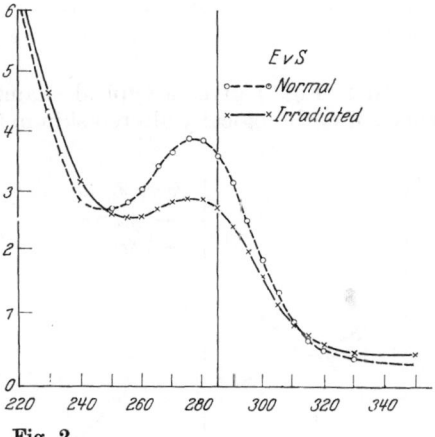

Fig. 2

Absolute comparisons of extinction values were excluded for this reason. However, it is possible to demonstrate that the absorption top at 280 nm becomes less distinct by comparing the E-values at the top (280 nm) with other values in the same sample outside the spectral area of the absorption top. The short wave ultraviolet especially can be used for this purpose, as light absorption is caused in these wavelengths by a multitude of epidermal constituents, including most amino acids.

It is clear for example that the quotient:

$$\frac{E\ 280}{E\ 250}$$

is representative for the relative height of the extinction top (see Fig. 2). In Tab. 1 this quotient is compared for the irradiated and non-irradiated skin in these normal white subjects.

Another method to circumvent differences in concentration of the solution is to calculate the quotient:

$$\frac{E\ \text{irradiated skin}}{E\ \text{normal skin}}$$

for every wavelength an make a graph of these values. In Fig. 3 this diagram is given for the same extracts as were shown in Fig. 2. The relative loss in extinction in the irradiated skin in the spectral area between 250 and 300 nm is apparent; this phenomenon was found in all extracts in which a clear absorption top at 280 nm was present. Other findings were the high values found for this quotient at wavelengths around 320 nm.

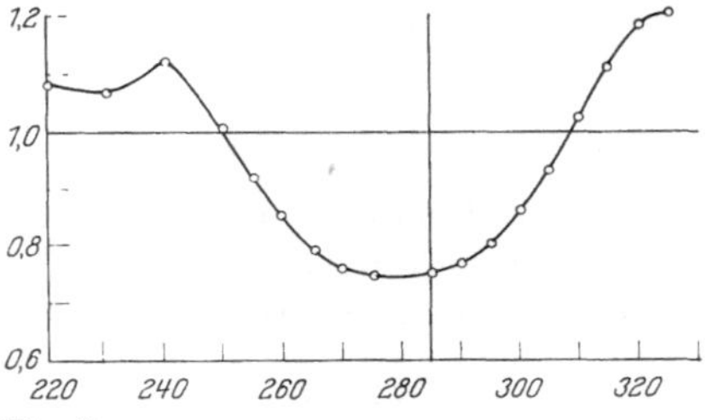

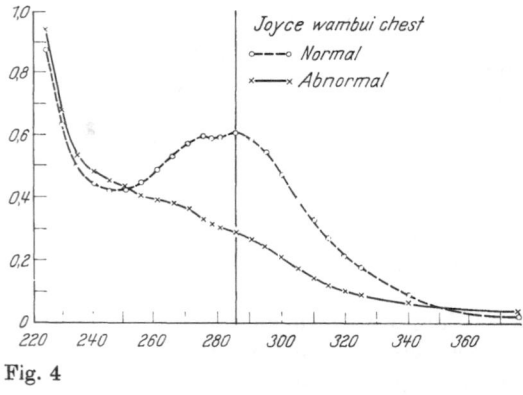

Fig. 3

Table 1. *Normal Subjects* $\frac{E\ 280}{E\ 250}$

Patient no.	Non irradiated	Irradiated
1	1,43	1,07
2	1,76	1,43
3	1,10	1,03
4	1.05	1,05
5	1,57	1,55
6	1,51	1,25
7	1,44	1,27
8	1,44	1,12
9	1,49	1,24

Ad 2. Fig. 4 gives a typical example of the changes found in the extinction curve of pathologically altered skin in C.P.L.E. The loss in absorption includes the

Fig. 4

Joyce wambui chest
o---o *Normal*
x——x *Abnormal*

Table 2. *C.P.L.E. Europeans* $\frac{E\ 280}{E\ 250}$

Patient no.	Non irradiated	Irradiated
1	1,58	1,04
2	1,43	0,88
3	1,47	0,90
4	1,27	0,80
5	1,36	1,02
6	1,30	0,83
7	1,30	0,77
8	1,45	1,40
9	1,44	0,84
10	1,05	0,93
11	1,23	1,10

spectral area between 250 and 320 nm: the relative increase in absorption at 320 nm, which was found in irradiated skin of normal subjects in the first series of experiments, was not found in this group.

Tab. 2 illustrates the differences in the quotient $\dfrac{E\,280}{E\,250}$ between normal and irradiated skin in the European group; in the African group the same changes were present, though to a lesser extent. The relative decrease in absorption extends however into the sunburn spectrum (285 to 320 nm) and to demonstrate this, we have given in Tab. 3 the quotient $\dfrac{E\,300}{E\,235}$: the extinction in a highly erythemato-genous area of the spectrum (E 300) is compared to another wavelength in the short wave ultraviolet. Similar relative diminutions in extinction could be calculated for all wavelengths between 260 and 320 nm, when these extinction values are divided by values obtained in spectral areas outside these limits, both in short wave (225 to 260 nm) and long wave (320 to 375 nm) ultraviolet.

Table 3. *C.P.L.E. Africans* $\dfrac{E\,300}{E\,235}$

Patient no.	Non irradiated	Irradiated
1	0,54	0,52
2	0,81	0,73
3	0,48	0,41
4	0,57	0,53
5	0,28	0,24
6	0,48	0,40
7	0,56	0,43
8	0,61	0,44
9	1,06	0,71
10	0,52	0,29
11	0,94	0,40
12	0,59	0,29
13	0,82	0,30

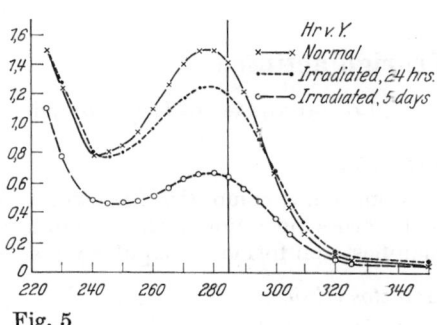

Fig. 5

It is probable that the stratum corneum dysiunctum may lose up to 50% of its light absorbing capacity in the 260 to 320 nm area.

Ad 3. Fig. 5 shows an example of the changes after artificial irradiation of the skin of the back of a patient with C.P.L.E. (xenonlamp). Changes found 24 h after irradiation, bear much similarity to changes mentioned in normal subjects in the first series of experiments; but changes after 5 days resemble the curve in the eczematized skin of C.P.L.E. and parakeratosis could be found histologically.

Discussion

The alkali solvable substances of the dysiunctum have an almost identical absorption curve with the stratum corneum as a whole and are mostly debris of the keratinisation process.

Further investigations are needed to show whether these changes are also present in the keratin as a solid structure. The changes found in the first series in normal subjects after irradiation seem to have little practical importance for protection against sunlight, as the area of decreased absorption extends only slightly into the spectrum of natural terrestrial sunlight (wavelengths longer than 285 nm); the higher absorption around 320 nm might even represent a protective action in this spectral area. But the changes in eczematized skin of C.P.L.E. are certainly of practical importance. They do not provide any explanation in regard to the cause of C.P.L.E. as the extinction curves in these patients in non-irradiated areas proved to be normal; but I would like to advance the hypothesis that once the exposed skin has become eczematized, the diminished absorption of short wave ultraviolet in the dysiunct part might start a vicious circle: the light protective function of the corneum must be further impaired in the pathologically altered skin.

This might provide an explanation for the fact that some patients have such an impressive hypersensitivity clinically in the exposed skin, whereas diagnostic investigation on the normal skin gives only slight abnormalities.

It should be stressed that the disappearance of the absorption top at 280 nm is not only present in C.P.L.E., but is found in all parakeratotic skin in psoriasis, dermatitis or dermatitis exfoliativa. However, in these other diseases this seems to be due more often to ,,filling up" (increase) of the 250 nm minimum than to the outspoken decrease in longer wavelengths, which might be characteristic for light sensitivity. It is impossible to discuss in the short paper other findings in normal skin, other diseases and the biochemical explanation of the changes; we hope to publish these in another publication.

Prurigo actinico

F. Londoño, Centro Dermatológico Federico Lleras Acosta, Bogota (Colombia)

Definición

Conocemos como *Prurigo actinico* a un *tipo epidemiológico, clínico y evolutivo* de las erupciones Polimorfas Lumínicas, que se presenta en las grandes alturas, se manifiesta en forma de pápulas y placas de infiltración y es de duración indefinida.

Aspectos clínicos

1. *Tipos de lesiones.* Las lesiones principales en las formas no complicadas de la dermatosis son manchas hipocrómico-escamosas (forma de comienzo); pápulas aisladas (principalmente en los miembros) y placas de infiltración (principalmente en el rostro). A estos elementos pueden sumarse liquenificación, eczematización, impetiginización y forúnculos, todo lo cual lo consideramos como complicaciones.

2. *Topografía.* La dermatosis afecta exclusivamente los sitios descubiertos; predomina en los sitios prominentes y no afecta las áreas protegidas de los sitios descubiertos. En el rostro las lesiones se localizan principalmente en las regiones malares, en el dorso de la nariz, en la frente, en los pabellones auriculares, en los labios y en el mentón. Puede haber compromiso conjuntival. En el cuello los elementos predominan en sus caras laterales. La cara posterior está afectada principalmente en los hombres. En el tronco las lesiones asientan casi exclusiva- mente en la "V" del escote; sin embargo, en las mujeres, pueden apreciarse lesiones en la región superior del dorso. En las extremidades superiores están afectados el dorso de las manos y la cara posterior de los antebrazos. Las extremi- dades inferiores son asiento de lesiones únicamente en las mujeres y los niños.

Aspectos epidemiologicos

1. *Relativos a las personas.* a) Sexo: La enfermedad predomina netamente en el sexo femenino en cuanto se refiere a sujetos adultos. En la niñez y en la senectud la frecuencia por sexos es similar. b) Edad: Las edades mas afectadas son las com- prendidas entre los 7 y los 14 años y después de los 50 años. En la primera infancia y en la edad adulta, la dermatosis es poco frecuente. c) Biotipo: No existe ningún biotipo especialmente afectado. La dermatosis afecta indistintamente a personas morenas y blancas. d) Situaciones fisiológicas: La dermatosis tiene preferencia por

las edades prepuberal y postclimatérica. Dos de nuestros casos, ambos del sexo masculino, curaron al llegar a la pubertad. El embarazo parece tener efecto favorable en la evolución de la dermatosis.

2. *Relativas al medio ambiente.* a) Altitud: El Prurigo Actínico se presenta de manera casi exclusiva en personas qué viven por encima de los 2.000 m de altura. Sin embargo la enfermedad no tiene tendencia a regresar cuando los pacientes se sitúan al nivel del mar. b) Condiciones sociales: Practicamente todos los pacientes pertenecen a las clases sociales con menores recursos económicos. c) Ocupación: Las ocupaciones son muy diversas pero predominan aquellas que exigen prolongada exposición a la luz.

Aspectos histológicos

Los hallazgos constantes en este aspecto son la acantosis, el edema intercelular, la exocitosis, los infiltrados inflamatorios polimorfos netamente delimitados en manchones perivasculares y la proliferación y dilatación de los capilares.

Laboratorio

Los hallazgos positivos en este aspecto parecen ser de poca significación. Solo merecen mención la disminución del índice de saturación y el aumento del índice de volúmen en los eritrocitos y la frecuente ausencia de bacilo Coli en los coprocultivos. Como hechos negativos destacamos la ausencia de uroporfirinas y porfobilinógeno en la orina de los enfermos y el no aumento de coproporfirinas. Por otra parte la investigación de protoporfirina eritrocítica libre por el método indirecto descrito por PETERCA, RUNGE y FUSARO, fue negativa en todos los casos.

Tratamiento

Hasta el momento no hemos encontrado ningún medicamento francamente útil en el Prurigo Actínico. Sin embargo, llamamos la atención sobre los efectos parcialmente favorables obtenidos con la Piridoxina a altas dosis y con los suplementos alimenticios a base de aminoácidos.

Aspectos etiopatológicos

Los anteriores conocimientos nos permiten concluír que el Prurigo Actínico es producido por la acción de los rayos ultravioleta que se encuentran notoriamente aumentados en las grandes alturas, actuando sobre personas que consumen mínimas cantidades de proteínas y que posiblemente por situaciones hormonales especiales las anabolizan defectuosamente. Pensamos que el déficit en ácido urocánico como consecuencia de una dieta pobre en proteínas y en ácido fólico puede ser la causa de menor capacidad defensiva frente a los rayos ultravioleta. No creemos que exista un mecanismo de fotosensibilización puesto que hemos demostrado que una dosis suficiente de rayos ultravioleta es capaz de producir, en cualquier persona, lesiones similares a las que caracterizan al Prurigo Actínico. Es decir que en este cuadro existiría una disminución de la capacidad defensiva de las personas frente a los rayos ultravioleta y no una respuesta cualitativamente anormal.

Comentarios

Consideramos que el siguiente paso en relación al estudio de los mecanismos etiopatogénicos del Prurigo Actínico, debe consistir en la verificación de la hipótesis propuesta mediante estudios sobre la bioquímica de la histidina, el ácido urocánico, el ácido fólico, el ácido forminiminoglutámico, la histamina y la piridoxina, comparativamente en individuos enfermos y en personas sanas.

Psoralen Therapy of Vitiligo in the Tropics

T. L. Fleisher, Ashford Medical Center, Santurce, Puerto Rico (USA)

Introduction. Since the natural history of vitiligo is a gradual and variable one, the efficacy of any therapy is difficult to measure. The purpose of this study was to evaluate the treatment of vitiligo with trimethylpsoralen und subsequent midday, tropical sun exposure.

Methods

Otherwise healthy, consecutive, private vitiligo patients were utilized as subjects in San Juan, Puerto Rico. Histories and physical axeminations were performed. Prospective subjects were eliminated if any systemic disease was present or suspected. Lack of motivation, extreme youth or previous treatment with eight methoxypsoralen were also considered cause for withholding therapy. Trimethylpsoralen was administered in initial doses of 10 or 20 milligrams daily, 2 h prior to sun exposure at noon. Sun exposure was initiated for 2 to 5 min and gradually increased to 30 min daily. Depending upon the response of the subject, the dose of the drug was increased up to 50 milligrams daily. All subjects were photographed at each visit.

Results

Of 161 subjects 53 were observed without treatment. 81 subjects were followed at least 6 months. Seven Subjects who were followed for more than 6 months were found to be incapable of utilizing the medication as prescribed. Of those subjects apparently treated as previously outlined, 68 showed improvement, 6 showed none. The remainder were not observed for sufficient time to permit conclusions for several reasons. These include their recent inclusion in the group, the cost of medication, the inaccessibility of the sun at the desired hour and moving away from Puerto Rico. The ages, sexes and duration of the disease prior to treatment are illustrated in the following tables.

Table 1
Sex Distribution

Sex	Number
Male	58
Female	103

Table 2. *Age Distribution*

Sex	Median Age	Average Age
Male	30	$30^1/_2$
Female	$27^1/_2$	$27^1/_2$

Table 3. *Duration*

Sex	Average Number of Years
Male	7
Female	$7^1/_2$

A well defined sequence of improvement was seen in those subjects who repigmented. This sequence is illustrated in the following table. In only four subjects was this sequence not observed; two subjects improved on the hands first and one on the feet and one on the malleoli first.

Complete repigmentation was achieved on the sites comprising the first three groups listed in Tab. 4. The face usually repigmented during the 1. year of treatment. The areas listed in the fourth and fifth orders of response have not been observed to completely repigment although treatment and observation continue.

Table 4. *Sequence of Repigmentation*

Order of Response	Site of Repigmentation
First	Face except lips and angles of mouth
Second	Neck, ears, hairy areas of extremities
Third	Trunk, elbows, knees, lips, angles of mouth
Fourth	Hands, nape, feet, medial aspects wrists
Fifth	Malleoli, perjungual areas

Table 5. *High Dose Therapy*

	Milligrams of Trimethylpsoralen/Dose		
	30	40	50
Number of Subjects	24	12	18

Repigmentation was first discernible at the poral orifices. The small primary areas of pigment enlarged and coalesced. Variations in the shade of the new pigment gradually faded. A temporary darkening of normal skin also occurred. This darkening blended with the adjacent skin. These variations were more easily identified with a Wood's Lamp (3660 A° UVL).

In 53 treated subjects repigmentation on the initial dose slowed or stopped. In these subjects the trimethylpsoralen dose was increased as charted in Tab. 5. Sun exposure time remained unchanged, never exceeding 30 min. Several subjects used a high dose on more than one occasion.

There was no relation between the duration of the disease and the response to treatment. In the oldest subject, age 78, the disease of more than 50 years duration started to respond on the face during the 1. month of treatment.

Undesirable side effects were few. One patient presented increased pigmentation of a melanocytic nevus. Another who was also taking birth control pills developed chloasma, a not uncommon occurrence when trimethylpsoralen is not used.

Two subjects reported the onset of tingling or mild pruritus which was relieved by the administration of 50 mg of vitamin C daily.

Generalized partial depigmentation occurred in two subjects who remained in the sun for several hours following the ingestion of 20 mg of trimethylpsoralen. This depigmentation responded to trimethylpsoralen therapy when sun was taken in the previously prescribed doses.

In conclusion the results of this study of the treatment of vitiligo with trimethylpsoralen and sunlight in the tropics, as illustrated by color transparencies, induces repigmentation. Facial repigmentation occurred first and was usually complete in less than a year. The hairy trunk and extremity areas repigmented slower. The distal extremities repigmented more slowly and partially. Repigmentation was not related to the duration of disease.

Zur Kombinationsbehandlung der Mycosis fungoides mit Röntgenstrahlen und Spindelgiften

A. WISKEMANN, Univ.-Hautklinik Hamburg (Deutschland)

Röntgenstrahlen bewähren sich seit Jahrzehnten zur palliativen Behandlung der Mycosis fungoides. Nach längerer Strahleneinwirkung kommt es nicht selten zu einer Minderung der Strahlenempfindlichkeit. In derartigen Fällen kann die Chemotherapie mit Cytostatica versucht werden. Die primäre und ausschließliche cytostatische Behandlung ist jedoch weniger wirksam als die Röntgenstrahlenbehandlung. Darüber hinaus ist sie mit unangenehmen Nebenwirkungen wie Leukocytendepression und Durchfällen belastet.

MALKINSON, GRIEM u. MORSE berichteten 1961 über die synergistische Wirkung von Colchizin und Röntgenstrahlen auf Mäusehaare in Abhängigkeit vom Zeitintervall zwischen Injektion des Cytostaticums und Bestrahlung. Bei einem Intervall von 16 Std sahen sie den größten Prozentsatz dysplastischer Haare, d. h. einen maximalen Effekt, und bei einem Intervall von 4 bzw. 8 Std keinen Effekt. In eigenen Versuchen konnten wir diesen Befund für Colzemide Ciba bezüglich der Epilation von Meerschweinchenhaaren bestätigen. Das Podophyllinderivat Proresid Sandoz zeigt gleiche Ergebnisse.

In Analogie zu den Tierversuchen konnten MALKINSON u. Mitarb. Mycosis-fungoides-Infiltrate, die auf 600 r nicht mehr ansprachen, durch i.v. Injektionen von 3 mg Colchizin und Bestrahlung nach 16 Std mit 600 r wieder zur Einschmelzung bringen. Inzwischen verfügen sie über Beobachtungen an fünf Mycosis-fungoides-Patienten, von denen vier auf die kombinierte Behandlung gut ansprachen.

Seit 1962 behandeln wir solche Mycosis-fungoides-Patienten, welche auf eine Dosis von 300 r bei adäquater Strahlenqualität nicht mehr deutlich reagieren, kombiniert mit 4 mg Colzemide oder in jüngster Zeit auch mit 400 mg Proresid und 300 r Röntgenstrahlen. Dabei wird das Spindelgift 16 Std vor einmaliger Bestrahlung i.v. injiziert. Von 15 Patienten mit histologisch verifizierter Diagnose reagieren 12 wieder in befriedigender Weise auf die Dosis von 300 r. Die kombinierte Behandlung wird in zwei- bis dreiwöchigen Abständen bis zur Erscheinungsfreiheit wiederholt.

Die klinische Beurteilung der Bestrahlungserfolge ist wegen der unzureichenden Meßbarkeit des Effektes, der Möglichkeit spontaner Regressionen und der Einwirkung zusätzlicher Faktoren angreifbar. Dennoch sind wir von den Vorteilen einer kombinierten Behandlung in der geschilderten Weise überzeugt. Bei nachlassender Strahlenempfindlichkeit muß die Strahlendosis nicht erhöht werden. Bei normaler Strahlenempfindlichkeit kann sie wahrscheinlich erniedrigt werden. Unangenehme oder gar riskante Nebenwirkungen wie bei längerer ausschließlicher cytostatischer Therapie sind nicht zu befürchten.

Literatur. MALKINSON, F. D., M. L. GRIEM, and P. H. MORSE: J. invest. Derm. **37**, 337 (1961). — GRIEM, M. L., and F. D. MALKINSON: Amer. J. Roentgenol. **47**, 1003 (1966).

Photochemical Movement of Cholesterol in Skin

E. W. RAUSCHKOLB and J. M. KNOX, Department of Dermatology, Baylor University College of Medicine, Texas Medical Center, Houston, Texas (USA)

In earlier work, our laboratory demonstrated that a significant reduction in the level of freely extractable cholesterol in the skin occurs on exposure to sunlight. Skin punch biopsies were obtained from male caucasians before and 24 h after exposure to the midday sun. The cholesterol content was determined by chloroform extraction of the biopsies and by isolation on thin layer chromatography. A striking reduction was consistently seen.

To learn more about this phenomenon, we repeated the experiments in such a way that skin specimens were isolated from the circulatory system and freed from the effects of any other physiological system. Skin specimens removed 1 to 2 h after death were suspended in an environmental chamber constructed to permit control of temperature, humidity, and oxygenation, and equipped with a silica lens which was optically flat and transmitted virtually all wave lengths of visible and ultraviolet light. The skin specimen was then exposed to a full erythema dose of broadspectrum ultraviolet light from a mercury arc source or to natural sunlight. Analysis of the skin specimens showed that both sunlight and ultraviolet light induced a highly significant reduction in the freely extractable cholesterol in the absence of any other physiological mechanisms. The freely extractable cholesterol content in six control specimens of caucasian skin was on the average 69.08 μg/gm. After 2 min irradiation with ultraviolet light, a reduction of 47.5% of the resting level had occurred. It was evident that this phenomenon was the result of a promptly occurring photodynamic reaction *in situ*.

On further study of the problem, we discovered that cholesterol exists in the skin in three physically or chemically distinct forms: one obtained with ease by extraction with chloroform, which was the form studied in the experiments described above, a second, released by potassium hydroxide hydrolysis (7.5% in 50% ethanol, refluxed 30 min) and a third form which remains firmly associated with the non-hydrolyzable fraction of skin and is not released even by prolonged digestion with KOH.

We are now in a position to state that the reduction of freely extractable skin cholesterol by ultraviolet light actually represents the transposition of sterol from the free to the non-hydrolyzable bound form. A typical experiment illustrating the phenomenon is as follows:

Human skin, epidermis and dermis, was placed in Ringer's solution containing 10 microcuries of cholesterol 4-C-14. The highly radioactive solution and skin specimens were in contact for 18 h at 3 °C. Labeled cholesterol entered the skin by passive diffusion. The tissue was thoroughly rinsed to remove surface contamination; contiguous specimens served as control or irradiated samples. Extraction of the skin before and after hydrolysis revealed that C-14 cholesterol did diffuse into the skin and mix with the cholesterol pools. The specific activity of the free and KOH hydrolyzable forms of cholesterol was distinctly different, indicating absence of equilibrium and confirming the existence of separate pools. The total C-14 content of the skin was determined by combustion. The results indicate that upon irradiation there were:

1. about a 50% drop in the C-14 cholesterol in the freely extractable pool as anticipated (vide supra);

2. no significant change in the KOH hydrolyzable fractions;

3. a sharp increase in radioactivity, calculated by the difference method, in the non-hydrolyzable fraction.

It was concluded that the photodynamic effect on cholesterol is to convert the free form into a sterol firmly associated with a non-hydrolyzable, water soluble moiety. The chemical nature of the sterol conversion product and of the binding substance are presently under study.

Immunology in Dermatology

Immunologie en dermatologie

Immunología en dermatología

Immunologie in der Dermatologie

Organizer

ST. JABLONSKA, Poland

Presidents

F. FÖLDVARI, Hungary

F. P. MERKLEN, France

W. B. SHELLEY, USA

Delegate of the Organization Committee

C. M. HASSELMANN, Germany

Reports

Aetiology of Some Autoimmune Diseases

N. R. ROWELL, Department of Dermatology of the University,
Leeds (England)

It is well known that certain connective tissue diseases, and other diseases such as psoriasis, have a characteristic age and sex distribution. These features cannot be ignored when any aetiological theory is considered. Mathematical study of the age- and sex-specific onset rates, viewed as a function of age, together with other genetic, immunological and clinical evidence, suggests that they are disturbed-tolerance autoimmune diseases and that genetic factors and somatic mutations are implicated in their aetiology [BURCH and ROWELL, 1963, 1965 (1) and (2)]. Two groups of autoimmune diseases appear to occur. Where tissues can be freely infiltrated by small lymphocytes as in discoid lupus erythematosus, systemic lupus erythematosus and systemic sclerosis, the primary pathogens are lymphocytes carrying cellular autoantibodies, whereas in diseases affecting tissues behind a blood-tissue barrier, such as in psoriasis, the primary pathogen is humoral and may migrate with the α_2 macroglobulin fraction.

Spontaneous disturbed-tolerance lymphocytic autoimmune disease

The mathematical and theoretical analysis of this work is complicated but briefly, when the age-specific onset rates for each sex are plotted against the age at onset on log-log scales, curves are obtained in which there is a rise to a peak followed by a steep fall. In the case of systemic lupus erythematosus, discoid lupus erythematosus and systemic sclerosis the onset is later in males than in females. Curves of this type are consistent with the view that such diseases are confined to genetically-predisposed individuals. More individuals develop the disease as the population ages, until all the predisposed individuals have developed the disease and the onset rate falls to zero. Moreover, it can be shown that diseases of this type are restricted to particular sub-populations, characterized by specific genotypes. Few would doubt that patients with systemic lupus erythematosus and systemic sclerosis have a genetic background in view of the higher incidence of connective tissue diseases, of antinuclear factors, complement fixing antibodies and disturbances of serum proteins in the families of patients as compared with control groups. Moreover, both systemic and discoid lupus erythematosus have been reported in monozygotic twins.

Where a dominant X-linked inheritance factor occurs there will always be more predisposed females than males because females have two X-chromosomes whereas males have only one. Dominant X-linked alleles account for the characteristic female sex predominance in discoid and systemic lupus erythematosus and in systemic sclerosis, although the position is complicated in discoid lupus erythematosus as there appear to be three distinctive, but not necessarily unrelated, genotypes in this disorder (BURCH and ROWELL, 1968). The fact that the same disease has not been reported as occurring in father and son is in favour of X-chromosome linkage. It is not yet possible to assess autosomal inheritance factors, although they undoubtedly make an essential contribution.

The *initiation* of disease in predisposed individuals results from the occurrence of one or more specific random events, the average rate of which in a given genotype and for a given disease is constant throughout life and is independent of secular or geographical factors. These random events, we believe, are somatic mutations. Burnet's forbidden clone hypothesis (BURNET, 1959) provides an explanation as to how a small number of somatic mutations can cause widespread disease. The mutations occur in lymphoid stem cells. As a result forbidden clones of lymphocytes, synthesizing cellular autoantibodies, occur. There follows a latent period, between the time of the last mutation and the development of overt symptoms and signs of the disease, during which the clone or clones proliferate and attack target tissues carrying complementary antigens. The average duration of this latent period depends on environmental factors, but for a given environment and for this class of disease, is twice as long in females as in males. It varies from less than 1 year to 30 years, according to the disease.

Fortunately there is an endogenous defence mechanism against the development of forbidden clones and autoimmune disease, and this is probably mediated by immunoglobulins. (Lack of immunoglobulins would account for the high incidence of autoimmune disease in agammaglobulinaemia.) Environmental factors such as trauma, viral and bacterial infections, drugs, physical and mental stress may compete for this defence mechanism, thus precipitating the disease within the latent period or exacerbating the clinical course of the disease once it has developed. This defence mechanism is more efficient in females as the synthesis of immunoglobulins depends, in part, on genetic factors involving the X-chromosome. Clinically this is supported by the observations of KELLUM and HASERICK (1964) that the prognosis in systemic lupus erythematosus is better in females and my own similar observations in systemic sclerosis.

The distribution of organ involvement may be associated with specific forbidden clones, or be due to genetic differences in the antigenicity of the target tissues or to local vascular factors. The latter could also account for patchy distribution of lesions within a single organ.

There is no evidence that immunoglobulin autoantibodies, such as the antinuclear factors, are pathogenic (ROWELL and BECK, 1967). They arise as the result of damage to tissues releasing material to which the body is intolerant. Their absence in some patients is probably due to genetic differences in the capacity of individuals to produce these antibodies. On the other hand, there is evidence for the pathogenicity of cellular autoantibodies in this type of disease. TRAYANOVA and her colleagues (1966) have shown that lymphocytes from patients with systemic lupus erythematosus and systemic sclerosis may destroy cells in tissue culture and STASTNY et al. (1963) have reported that cellular autoantibodies may cause sclerodermatous skin changes in homologous disease in rats.

The known clinical, immunological and familial overlap between autoimmune diseases suggests that a single gene may be involved in more than one, multifactorial, predisposing genotype.

This concept of disturbed-tolerance lymphocytic autoimmunity may apply to other disorders not previously considered autoimmune. For example, the age- and sex-distribution of lichen planus is consistent with this type of aetiology and, of course, in this condition dense dermal lymphocytic infiltration is a prominent histological feature. Lichen planus appears to be a disorder in which there are two genotypes associated with early and later onset.

Spontaneous disturbed-tolerance humoral autoimmune disease

Not all autoimmune disease concerns cellular autoantibodies. In those disorders where the immediate target tissue lies behind a blood-tissue barrier, as in psoriasis, the autoantibodies are humoral. They are not immunoglobulins, but may circulate with the α_2 macroglobulins. In this type of autoimmunity the defence mechanism is equally effective in males and females and may involve phagocytic cells.

It is well recognised that psoriasis is a genetically determined disorder but most authors admit its genetics are complicated. It is widely assumed that the observed peak modes of onset of 11 and 45 years in females and 15 and 45 years in males are due to hormonal influences, but our analyses [BURCH and ROWELL, 1965(2)] are consistent with the interpretation that these modes represent two distinct, but related, subpopulations at risk. Somatic mutations in stem cells in predisposed individuals lead to the development of forbidden clones of cells secreting humoral autoantibodies and these are the attacking agents promoting hyperplasia of epidermal basal cells and other changes.

The latent period is of equal duration in males and females in this type of autoimmunity. In some cases infections, particularly streptococcal, may compete for the body's defence resources causing precipitation or exacerbation of the disease.

These controversial concepts, the details of which will be found in the original papers, are compatible with the known facts of age, sex and familial distribution, the spontaneous onset in some patients and precipitating factors in others. They may also apply to diseases whose aetiology is at present considered to be "idiopathic" as well as such processes as the control of organ size (BURWELL, 1963), neoplasia and ageing.

Proposed Outline of Pathogenesis of Spontaneous Disturbance-Tolerance Autoimmune Disease

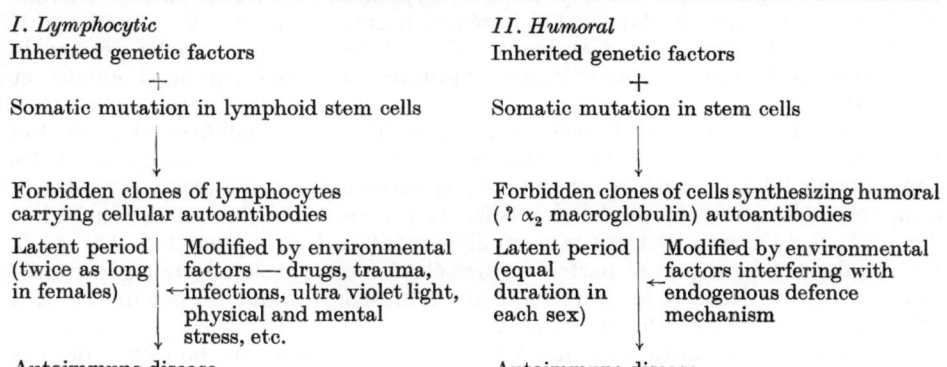

References. BURCH, P. R. J., and N. R. ROWELL: Lancet 1963 II, 507; — (1) Amer. J. Med. 38, 793 (1965); — (2) Acta derm.-venereol. (Stockh.) 45, 366 (1965); — Acta derm.-venereol. (Stockh.) 48. 33 (1968). — BURNET, F. M.: The clonal selection theory of acquired immunity. London: Cambridge University Press 1959. — BURWELL, R. G.: Lancet 1963 II, 69. — KELLUM, R. E., and J. R. HASERICK: Arch. intern. Med. 113, 200 (1964). — ROWELL, N. R., and J. S. BECK: Arch. Derm. 96, 290 (1967). — STASTNY, P., V. A. STEMBRIDGE, and M. ZIFF: J. exp. Med. 118, 635 (1963). — TRAYANOVA, T. G., V. V. SURA, and G. J. SVET-MOLDAVSKY: Lancet 1966 I, 452.

I would like to acknowledge my debt to Dr. P. R. J. BURCH whose work on the analysis and interpretation of age- and sex specific onset rates forms the basis for this paper.

Aspects immunologiques du lupus érythémateux aigu disséminé

J. Thivolet, Faculté Mixte de Médecine et de Pharmacie, Lyon (France)

La découverte du phénomène L.E. par Hargraves a marqué une étape capitale d'une part, en apportant un moyen de diagnostic biologique du L.E.A.D. dont l'emploi a entrainé de profondes modifications dans l'étude clinique et d'autre part en révélant l'existence de phénomènes d'auto-immunisation au cours du L.E.A.D. qui apparait ainsi actuellement comme l'une des maladies humaines où l'auto-immunisation joue le plus constamment un rôle.

Comment se présente cette auto-immunisation?

Bien que des auto-anticorps très variés puissent être décelés chez certains malades, l'auto-immunisation dans le L.E.A.D. est avant tout antinucléaire. Parmi les nombreuses méthodes de détection des anticorps antinucléaires, la réaction d'I.F. sur noyaux, de technique simple et de grande sensibilité, a suscité de nombreux travaux. Après avoir vérifié la réactivité de noyaux et d'espèces animales de tissus très variés (hommes, mammifères, oiseaux, poissons etc., leucocytes, foie, thyroïde, muscle, thymus, etc.), nous avons adopté les frottis de sang de souris apportant des noyaux leucocytaires et révélant les anticorps antinucléaires par une fluorescence homogène et exécuté ainsi plus de 8000 réactions. Beck ayant signalé que les noyaux des trypanosomes étaient formés surtout d'A.N.D. nous avons dès lors réalisé la réaction avec des frottis de sang de souris infectées par Trypanosoma Gambiense. Cette technique personnelle permet la recherche qualitative et quantitative simultanée des anticorps anti-noyaux et anti A.D.N.

Nos résultats, en accord avec ceux de la littérature, confirment pour 138 L.E.A.D. examinés, la présence pratiquement constante des anticorps et les titres élevés (89% à 1/64 et au dessus); la meilleure sensibilité de la méthode comparée à la recherche de cellules L.E.; la présence d'anticorps antinucléaires dans 28% des cas mais à titres rarement élevés (15% à 1/64 et plus) dans 200 cas de P.C.R.; dans 12% des cas et parfois à titres élevés dans la sclérodermie généralisée progressive; la découverte peu fréquente d'anticorps dans beaucoup d'autres affections et même chez des sujets sains.

Parallèlement les anticorps anti A.D.N. présents seulement dans 43% des cas de L.E.A.D. ne sont pas spécifiques non plus de cette maladie.

Ainsi, les auto-anticorps antinucléaires ne sont pas «spécifiques» du L.E.A.D. mais bien que le phénomène d'auto-immunisation antinucléaire semble être très largement distribué, c'est dans le L.E.A.D. qu'il est, de loin, le plus constant et le plus intense.

En pratique, bien qu'aucune réaction biologique ne soit pathognomonique du L.E.A.D., la technique d'I.F. quantitative sur noyaux, en permettant d'apprécier avec une grande précision l'intensité de l'auto-immunisation antinucléaire, apporte les renseignements les plus utiles au diagnostic biologique. Elle permet en outre, de suivre l'évolution des malades traités, de mieux adapter les doses de corticoïdes et apporte quelques renseignements pronostiques.

La signification physio-pathologique et pathogénique de cette auto-immunisation antinucléaire n'est pas encore très claire.

Les anticorps antinucléaires sont-ils directement pathogènes? Rien ne permet de l'affirmer bien qu'on ait pu démontrer récemment leur fixation in vivo en particulier au niveau des lésions cutanées.

Quelle est l'origine de l'auto-immunisation du L.E.A.D. ? De tels phénomènes peuvent résulter essentiellement soit de l'altération d'antigènes tissulaires sous l'effet d'aggressions exogènes (virales ou autres) soit, pour des antigènes se trouvant normalement en état de ségrégation, d'une fuite accidentelle en dehors de leur site normal soit enfin d'un dérèglement acquis mais surtout héréditaire des mécanismes normaux d'immunorégulation et d'immunotolérance. C'est cette dernière hypothèse qui est essentiellement valable par élimination des deux premières et surtout parce que les arguments en faveur d'altérations héréditaires de l'immunotolérance sont tirés de l'étude des cas humains de L.E.A.D. familiaux, des «modèles animaux» de L.E.A.D. et des effets de la thymectomie néonatale.

Nos études ont porté sur deux familles comportant chacune un frère et une soeur atteints d'un L.E.A.D. à forme polyviscérale grave. Ces cas viennent s'ajouter aux nombreuses observations analogues déjà rapportées dans la littérature (près de 100). Une enquête sérologique systématique sur 69 sujets consanguins normaux de 19 malades nous a montré la fréquence de l'hyper-gammaglobulinémie et le faible pourcentage d'anticorps antinucléaires (4/69) à titres bas.

La maladie «lupus-like» des souris NZB et hybrides est bien connue maintenant et dans ce «modèle» animal, le rôle de l'hérédité dans la genèse de la maladie a été démontré par transferts spléniques. D'autres «modèles» existent probablement chez les chiens atteints de diathèse rhumatismale où nous avons trouvé des taux assez élevés d'anticorps antinucléaires.

Expérimentalement il est difficile d'obtenir une immunisation antinucléaire. Aussi nous avons étudié les effets de la thymectomie néonatale chez des souris Swiss et recherché en particulier l'apparition des auto-anticorps antinucléaires chez ces animaux. A partir de la 15ème semaine ces auto-anticorps apparaissent et sont retrouvés chez plus de 70% des animaux survivants à 25 semaines. Des anticorps anti A.D.N. ont également été rencontrés. Des expériences complémentaires semblent indiquer que la thymectomie néonatale joue surtout en altérant les capacités d'identification et de reconnaissance des antigènes. Il resterait à établir que de telles anomalies existent chez les malades atteints de L.E.A.D. Des études récentes ont attiré aussi l'attention sur les anomalies radiologiques du thymus chez ces malades et sur les associations morbides entre cette maladie et les tumeurs thymiques. Cette hypothèse n'exclue pas le rôle de certains médicaments qui pourraient jouer seulement un rôle révélateur de l'anomalie héréditaire plus ou moins accentuée selon les individus et pouvant même rester latente en l'absence d'aggression médicamenteuse ou autre.

On peut enfin discuter des rapports entre le L.E.A.D. et le lupus érythémateux chronique qui ne semblent pas présenter les mêmes anomalies immunologiques.

Autoimmunity in Pemphigus

T. CHORZELSKI, Department of Dermatology, School of Medicine, Warsaw (Poland)

The finding of auto-antibodies directed against intercellular substance of the epidermis in the sera of patients with pemphigus by means of immunofluorescent technique began a new ere in the investigations of autoimmune pathogenesis of the disease.

Our own studies covering 84 cases have proved that the "pemphigus" autoantibodies are pathognomonic for this disease and their titre strictly depends upon the extent and severity of skin lesions. The controls consisting of 1300 patients including 35 cases of dermatitis herpetiformis and 33 of pemphigoid were negative, except this last condition in some cases of which we did find auto-antibodies directed against the basement membrane. It is yet unknown against which epidermal antigens the "pemphigus" auto-antibodies are directed. The results of immunoelectrophoresis and immunodiffusion with epidermal extracts prepared by several different methods were negative. Only two sera of patients with extensive skin lesions showed repeated precipitation with a saline extract of epidermal antigens (mixture of extract and pemphigus sera in capillary tubes incubated at 4°).

In order to demonstrate the exact localisation of "pemphigus" auto-antibodies we have employed immuno-electron-microscopic technique using ferritin labelled pemphigus globulin. We demonstrated that "pemphigus" auto-antibodies react not only with the intercellular substance but also with antigens present at the site of cell membrane. Immunofluorescent staining of skin biopsies from the vicinity of pemphigus blisters showed immunoglobulins of the IgG type bound in vivo. A concomitant in vivo binding of human complement (C_3, C_4) showed with specific anti $\beta_1 C'$ immune serum is a further proof of an antigen-antibody reaction taking place in vivo at these sites. The pathogenetic role of "pemphigus" auto-antibodies is completely obscure.

Extremely interesting are in this respect cases of our own in which pemphigus co-existed with myasthenia gravis. In one of them pemphigus erythematosus developed after thymectomy and the skin lesions of lupus erythematosus type after exposure to sunlight. This patient's serum contained circulating auto-antibodies directed against intercellular substance, striated muscles and antinuclear antibodies. The appearance in one patient of all these allegedly autoimmune conditions and particularly thymoma, which is believed to play a key role in autoimmune mechanisms is in favour of immunological background of pemphigus.

Immunology of Acne Vulgaris. Dermal Hypersensitivity and Circulating Antibody Levels to Corynbacterium Acnes[*]

S. M. Puhvel, T. H. Sternberg and R. M. Reisner, Department of Medicine, Division of Dermatology, UCLA School of Medicine, Los Angeles, California (USA), and Division of Dermatology, Harbor General Hospital, Torrance, California (USA)

Evidence published in the past 15 years [1, 2, 3, 4] has indicated that *Corynebacterium acnes* is the organism found most frequently in lesions of acne vulgaris. This anaerobic gram positive rod whose predominant habitat is the sebaceous follicles of human skin is found in great numbers in the initial stages of acne lesions. It can be cultured with ease from comedones, and it is not until the later pustular stages of acne, that the organisms gradually disappear from the lesions.

Based on the well documented observation that cortisone can be used successfully in the treatment of some cases of acne vulgaris [5], we carried out a study to determine the dermal hypersensitivity of patients with acne vulgaris to *C. acnes*

* This study was supported in part by USPHS Grants Al-06048-03 and TI-AM 5265-07 and by a grant from the Elliott and Ruth Handler Foundation.

[6]. Two different antigens from *C. acnes* were used to test for immediate and delayed dermal hypersensitivity. The first, designated as the disrupted antigen, was prepared from mechanically ruptured cultures of *C. acnes*, and was similar to the antigen described for the complement fixation test for *C. acnes* [7]. The other antigen, designated as the extracellular antigen, contained only non-dialysable, extracellular products of *C. acnes* but no whole organisms. It was prepared from filtrates of the organisms grown in saline solution in dialysis bags immersed in peptone-thioglycollate broth. Both antigens reacted strongly in *in vitro* serologic tests with hyperimmune serum to *C. acnes*.

Subjects for skin testing were volunteers from a prison population at the California Institution for Women, Frontera, California. 46 subjects had varying degrees of acne, and 46 were controls without acne. Results of the skin tests were read for immediate hypersensitivity 20 min, and for delayed hypersensitivity 24 and 48 h after inoculation. Levels of circulating antibody to *C. acnes* in the sera of all subjects were determined prior to skin testing by the bacterial agglutination and the complement-fixation tests. Results of the immediate and delayed hypersensitivity tests are shown in Tabs. 1 and 2, and the relationship of the strength of the immediate hypersensitivity reaction to circulating antibody levels in Tab. 3.

Table 1. *Immediate sensitivity to C. acnes antigens in patients with acne, and in controls*

Antigen	Dosage	Acne			Controls		
		No. tested	No. positive	%	No. tested	No. positive	%
Disrupted[a]	1/1000,000	46	8	17.3	46	5	10.8
	1/10,000	39	31	79.5	43	14	32.5
Extra-cellular[b]	1/1000	46	22	48.8	46	1	2.1
	1/100	43	34	79.0	44	10	22.7

[a] gms of lyophilized disrupted *C. acnes*/ml buffered saline.
[b] mg of antigen protein/ml buffered saline.

Table 2. *Delayed sensitivity to C. acnes antigens in patients with acne and in controls*

Antigen	Dosage	Acne			Controls		
		No. tested	No. positive	%	No. tested	No. positive	%
Disrupted	1/100,000	46	2	4.3	46	0	0
	1/10,000	39	4	10.2	43	3	7.0
Extra-cellular	1/1000	46	2	4.3	46	0	0
	1/100	43	9	20.9	44	4	9.1

Table 3. *Relationship between the agglutinating antibody titers to C. acnes and the strength of the immediate sensitivity reaction to the extra-cellular antigen from C. acnes*

Agglutinating titer	Strong positive	Doubtful positive	Negative
40 or less	0	2	25
80—160	3	3	9
320—640	9	10	13
over 640	12	5	1

The following conclusions could be drawn from this study:

1. Patients with acne vulgaris showed a significantly greater degree of immediate hypersensitivity to *C. acnes* than controls without acne. With the 1:1000 dilution of extracellular antigen 48.8% of the patients with acne gave positive immediate reactions compared to 2.1% of the controls.

2. The immediate hypersensitivity was shown particularly to the soluble extracellular antigen from *C. acnes*.

3. If patients were further categorized according to the severity of their acne, the group with severe scarring showed the highest frequency of immediate sensitivity response.

4. The delayed hypersensitivity to *C. acnes* antigens in patients with acne did not differ significantly from the response in controls without acne.

5. There was no clear cut correlation between the strength of the immediate hypersensitivity response and the level of circulating antibodies to *C. acnes*.

These findings suggest that an extracellular antigen from *C. acnes* produces immediate dermal sensitivity in the patients with acne. The chemical nature of this antigen has not been fully analysed yet, but standardization was carried out by nitrogen content, which was assumed to represent the protein content of the antigen.

It is puzzling that hypersensitivity could not be correlated with the circulating antibody levels, but similar results were reported by RUDZKI et al. when they demonstrated that anti-streptolysin titers in patients with skin diseases did not correspond to the immediate dermal sensitivity to streptolysin.

We have previously demonstrated using bacterial agglutination and complement fixation tests that circulating antibody levels to *C. acnes* are higher in patients with acne than in controls without acne [7, 9]. It has also been shown that this elevation in antibody levels in acne vulgaris is found only with *C. acnes*, and not with *Staphylococcus epidermidis*, the other organism frequently isolated from lesions in acne [10].

Preliminary studies in our laboratory have demonstrated that inoculation of suspensions of *C. acnes* intradermally in rabbits produces localized abscess-like lesions at the site of inoculation. These lesions drain large amounts of pus from which *C. acnes* can be re-cultured. This ability to produce abscesses in rabbit skin on intradermal inoculation has been found with a number of organisms, including *Odontomyces viscosus*, streptococci, and staphylococci [11, 12]. SCHUSTER et al. link this toxic property of the bacteria to the mucopeptide fraction of the cell wall of gram positive bacteria. Immunization of rabbits against the specific organism may reduce the production of abscesses in the rabbit skin on further intradermal challenge by the same organism [12, 13, 14]. Preliminary results from our studies with *C. acnes* have indicated that some rabbits can be protected from abscess production by hyperimmunization against *C. acnes*. Hyperimmunity in such instances is measured by the level of circulating antibodies to *C. acnes* in the rabbit serum.

It has been demonstrated that inoculation of live cultures of *C. acnes* into cysts of steatocystoma multiplex produces inflammation and rupture of the cysts [15]. It would be interesting to know whether one could protect the patient from *C. acnes* induced inflammation by hyperimmunization against the organism.

Acknowledgements: The authors wish to express their thanks to Drs. A. F. PEREYRA and M. W. MODISHER, at the California Institution for Women, Frontera, California, for their interest and cooperation in this project.

References. 1. SMITH, M. A., and P. M. WATERWORTH: Brit. J. Derm. **73**, 152 (1961). — 2. SHEHADEH, N. H., and A. M. KLIGMAN: Arch. Derm. **88**, 829 (1963). — 3. POCHI, P. E., and

J. S. STRUASS: J. invest. Derm. **36**, 423 (1961). — 4. MEYER-ROHN, J.: Arch. Derm. Syph. (Berl.) **197**, 542 (1954). — 5. BLINSTRUB, R. S., R. LEHMAN, T. H. STERNBERG, and D. L. STRAUB: Curr. ther. Res. **5**, 414 (1963). — 6. PUHVEL, S. M., I. K. HOFFMAN, R. M. REISNER, and T. H. STERNBERG: J. invest. Derm. (In press) 1967. — 7. PUHVEL, S. M., I. K. HOFFMANN, and T. H. STERNBERG: Arch. Derm. **93**, 364 (1966). — 8. RUDZKI, E., K. MOSKALEWSKA, E. MACIEJOWSKA und M. BLASZYZYK: Arch. klin. exp. Derm. **220**, 535 (1964). — 9. PUHVEL, S. M., M. BARFATANI, M. A. WARNICK, and T. H. STERNBERG: Arch. Derm. **90**, 421 (1964). — 10. PUHVEL, S. M., M. A. WARNICK, and T. H. STERNBERG: Arch. Derm. **92**, 88 (1965). — 11. SCHUSTER, G. S., J. A. HAYASHI, and A. N. BAHN: J. Bact. **93**, 47 (1967). — 12. SCHWAB, J. H., and W. J. CROMARTIE: J. exp. Med. **111**, 295 (1960). — 13. ABDULLA, E. M., and J. H. SCHWAB: Proc. Soc. exp. Biol. (N.Y.) **118**, 359 (1965). — 14. SCHWAB, J. H., and W. J. CROMARTIE: J. Bact. **74**, 673 (1957). — 15. KIRSCHBAUM, J. O., and A. M. KLIGMAN: Arch. Derm. **88**, 832 (1963).

Zur Immunologie in der Dermatologie

J. KIMMIG, Univ. Hautklinik Hamburg (Deutschland)

Der Begriff Immunologie umspannt zweifellos auch alle jene Reaktionen des Organismus, die unter dem Begriff der Allergie zusammengefaßt werden. Die sog. „Ide", d. h. allergische Reaktionen, die dem Spätreaktionstypus zuzuordnen sind, etwa Tuberkulide, Mykrobide, Mykide, sind für das Verständnis vom molekular-pathologischen Denken her gesehen heute noch am schwierigsten zu deuten. Am ehesten gelingt es bei den Tuberkuliden, einen Zusammenhang zwischen den klinischen Erscheinungen und Produkten, die als Stoffwechselprodukte der Mykobakterien aufzufassen sind, zu beweisen. Im Rahmen einer Tagung über Allergie und Tuberkulose haben wir 1961 diese Zusammenhänge folgendermaßen formuliert: „Die exanthematischen Formen der Hauttuberkulose, die Tuberkulide, der Lichen skrofulosorum, das papulo-nekrotische Tuberkulid und die indurativen Formen des Erythema induratum Bazin und das Erythema nodosum (ausgelöst durch Mycobacterium tuberculosis) unterscheiden sich wesentlich im Verhalten von den übrigen Hauttuberkulosen, indem sie gegenüber Proteinen aus Mykobakterien bereits auf Verdünnungen von 1:1000000 bis 1:10000000 positiv reagieren." Diese Reaktionen sind nicht ganz einfach als Antigen-Antikörperreaktionen zu deuten. Mit reinen Proteinen aus Mykobakterien ist eine echte Sensibilisierung des Organismus nicht möglich. Jedenfalls sind Antikörper, wie das bei den allergischen Reaktionen beim sog. Frühtypus der Fall ist, nicht nachweisbar. Die Reaktionen, die wir bei intracutaner Applikation an der Haut beobachten, gehören klinisch und histologisch zum Spättypus. Das Fehlen der humoral nachweisbaren Antikörper veranlaßte LETTERER dazu, die Allergieformen des Spättypus von der Antigen-Antikörperallergie zu trennen; er prägte dafür den Begriff der dysregulativen Allergie. Bei der Spätreaktion sind folgende Kriterien der Allergie noch erfüllt:

1. Voraussetzung für die Spätreaktion ist die Sensibilisierung, d. h. der Organismus muß mit dem Allergen in Kontakt gekommen sein.

2. Die Reaktion ist spezifisch.

3. Die Auslösbarkeit der Erscheinungen ist abhängig von der chemischen Struktur des Allergens.

4. Das anatomische Substrat bedingt das klinische und histologische Bild, das von der Norm abweicht.

Das Allergen, das in den reinen Tuberkelproteinen vorliegt, ist kein echtes Antigen. Die Tuberkelproteine können aber im Organismus, wie RAFFEL gezeigt hat, zu Vollantigenen werden. Sobald die Proteine aus Mykobakterien mit den D-Wachsen bzw. dem Cordfaktor zusammen dem Organismus injiziert werden, werden sie zu Vollantigenen. Die chemische Konstitution der D-Wachse und des Cordfaktors wurde von LEDERER am Pasteur-Institut Paris aufgeklärt. Die chemische Konstitution ist aus den folgenden Formeln ersichtlich:

Cordfaktor

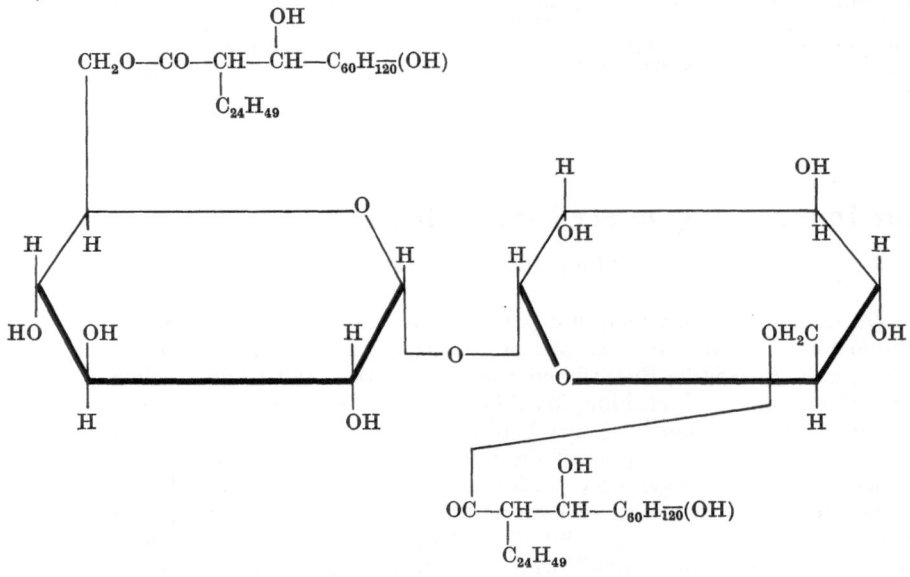

Chemische Struktur des D-Wachses aus dem virulenten humanen Stamm Brèvannes von Mycobacterium tuberculosis

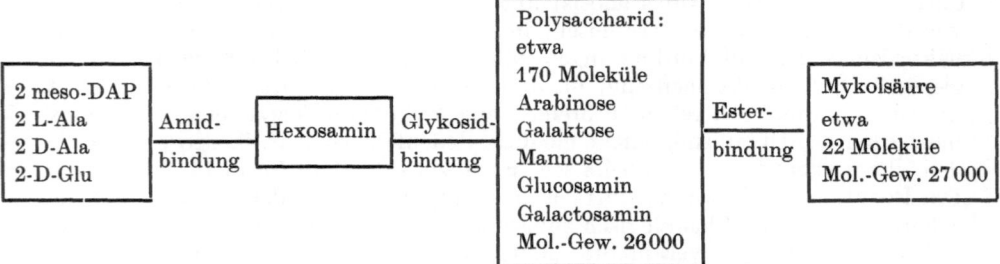

Mit der Kombination Tuberkelproteine und Cord-Faktor bzw. D-Wachs sind Reaktionen vom Frühtypus, also anaphylaktische Schockreaktionen, auslösbar. Ebenso ist der Spätreaktionstypus möglich. Echte Antigene haben hochmolekulare Träger mit spezifischer Gruppe. Dieses Bauprinzip wäre bei Komplexen aus Mykobakterienproteinen mit Cord-Faktor bzw. D-Wachsen erfüllt. Es wäre demnach nur noch die Frage nach dem spezifischen Antikörper zu klären. Die Tuberkulinallergie läßt sich passiv übertragen, aber nur, wenn man Lymphocyten bzw. Leukocyten überträgt. Das Gelingen der Übertragung ist abhängig vom Sensibilisierungsgrad des Spenders. Die Erfolgsreaktion ist schon nach 10 bis 24 Std beim Empfänger auslösbar; damit ist der Einwand entkräftet, daß es sich hierbei um eine aktive Sensibilisierung handeln würde, denn dies würde mindestens

6 bis 10 Tage erfordern. Die Übertragung der Tuberkulinallergie ist nicht an intakte Zellen gebunden, sie gelingt auch mit Extrakten und zerstörten Zellen. Die allergischen Spätreaktionen lassen sich auch bei A-Gamma-Globulinämien übertragen, der Antikörper kann also kein Gamma-Globulin sein.

Die chemische Natur des „Übertragungsfaktors" aus Lymphocyten ist unbekannt. Das spezifische Granulom kann, was seinen epitheloidzelligen Anteil betrifft, erklärt werden durch die in Mykobakterien vorhandenen Lipide, die aus verzweigten Fettsäuren aufgebaut sind. Mit diesen Substanzen lassen sich im Tierexperiment epitheloidzellige Granulome erzeugen. Die chemische Natur solcher Substanzen ist bekannt. Es handelt sich im wesentlichen um Mykolsäure und deren Ester, die auch beim Abbau der D-Wachse eine Rolle spielen. Die biologischen bzw. pathologischen Eigenschaften der Mykoside sind noch ungeklärt. Die chemische Konstitution des Mykosids B ist bekannt. Nach SMID u. a. handelt es sich bei diesem Stoff um ein Glykolipoid, das ein Molekül 2-0-Methylrhamnose und zwei Moleküle Mykocerosinsäure in Verbindung mit einem aromatischen Analogen des Innosits enthält. Von den Phospholipoiden weiß man seit den Arbeiten von ANDERSEN, daß sie stickstoffarm sind und Inosit sowie D-Mannose enthalten. Sie spielen eine wichtige Rolle im Aufbau der B.C.G.-Stämme Die Immunisierungsvorgänge im Zusammenhang mit Phosphoglykolipoiden sind noch weitgehend ungeklärt.

In der Theorie von LAWRENCE, die sich auf jahrelang durchgeführte Untersuchungen stützt (PAPPENHEIMER und GOOD), wird ein sog. Transferfaktor postuliert, der sich in wesentlichen Eigenschaften von einem echten Antikörper unterscheidet, der aber doch noch einen reaktiven Faktor darstellt, der in der Zelle gebildet wird. Zu dieser Theorie soll hier nur gesagt werden, daß sie einige Eigenschaften der Tuberkulinreaktion zu erklären vermag, daß aber eine genaue Deutung nicht möglich ist, solange die Chemie des Transferfaktors noch unbekannt ist. Die Fraktionen, mit denen LAWRENCE experimentiert, sind damit nicht einheitlich.

In diesem Zusammenhang soll auf die nahe Verwandtschaft zwischen Tuberkulin und Ekzemreaktionen hingewiesen werden.

1. Sowohl Tuberkulin als auch niedermolekulare Ekzematogene mit bekannter chemischer Struktur führen bei epicutaner Applikation zu einer ekzematischen Reaktion.

2. Die intracutane Zufuhr von Ekzematogenen bewirkt eine papulöse Reaktion (eventuell bis zur Nekrose), die dem Bild der Tuberkulinreaktion entsprechen kann.

3. Beide Reaktionstypen haben eine Latenzzeit von 12 bis 24 Std.

4. Beide Reaktionen können bei Patienten mit A-Gamma-Globulinämie ausgelöst werden. Ein wichtiger Unterschied besteht darin, daß ein cytotoxischer Effekt von niedermolekularen Ekzemallergenen auf isolierte Gewebszellen von sensibilisierten Spendern bisher nicht nachgewiesen werden konnte.

Das Verhalten von Lymphocyten von Tieren, die gegen Mykobakterien bzw. Proteine aus pathologischen Mykobakterien sensibilisiert sind, ist hierbei besonders aufschlußreich. Solche Lymphocyten verändern in der Kultur bei Zugabe von Tuberkulin völlig ihre Struktur. Es kommt zur vacuoligen Degeneration im Plasma und zur Auslösung von Mitosen.

Aus den angeführten Gründen möchten wir die Tuberkulinreaktion zu den allergischen Reaktionen des Spättypus zählen, bei der das ganze Geschehen sich als echte Antigen-Antikörperreaktion mit zellständig fixierter Antikörperbildung erklären läßt.

Die Genese des mikrobiellen Ekzems, die besonders von ROBERT, MIESCHER und STORCK, MEYER-ROHN, RÖCKL u. a. bearbeitet wurde, ist auch heute noch

Muraminsäure

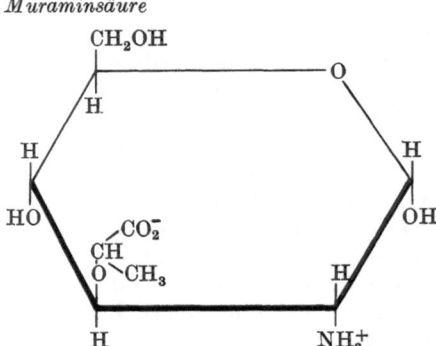

umstritten. Die „ekzematöse Streu-
reaktion", ausgehend von einem isolierten Herd an der Haut, die man als
Mikrobid ansprechen kann, ist für das
mikrobielle Ekzem besonders charakteristisch. MIESCHER war der Ansicht,
daß es sich bei diesem Mikrobid um
ein Phänomen handelt, das durch un-
belebte Stoffe aus den Membranen der
Bakterien (Staphylokokken) zustande
kommt, oder an dem deren Stoffwechselprodukte beteiligt sind. RÖCKL u.
Mitarb. fanden bis zu 40% positive
Reaktionen schon auf die erste epicutane Applikation von Staphylokok-
keninfiltraten. Der serologische Nachweis von spezifischen Antikörpern
beim mikrobiellen Ekzem, etwa durch
Agglutination, Präcipitation, Komple-
mentbindung, Imunoadherenz, ist
nicht spezifisch genug, um bezüglich
der allergischen Genese im Sinne einer
Antigen-Antikörperreaktion bindende
Schlüsse ziehen zu können. Schon vor
65 Jahren haben SCHOLZ und RAAB
die Behauptung aufgestellt, daß Kul-
turfiltrate aus Staphylokokken eine
dem Ekzem ähnliche Reaktion an der
Haut auslösen würden, Bakterienleiber würden dagegen eine Impetigo erzeugen. MIESCHER und STORCK glaub-
ten, daß es sich um Albumine handeln
könnte. Die von WESTPHAL angegebenen Methoden zur Isolierung von bakteriellen Pyrogenen (Staphylokokken,
Sarcinen, Corynebakterien) wurden
von MEYER-ROHN übernommen. Die
mit diesen Methoden dargestellten

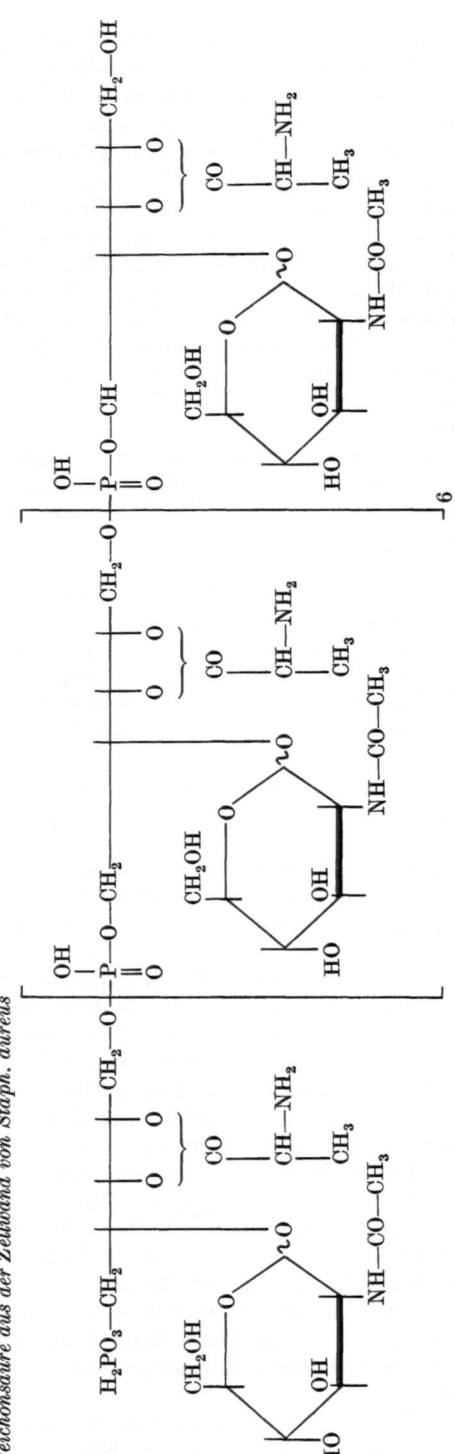

Teichonsäure aus der Zellwand von Staph. aureus

Extrakte können zwar entzündliche Reaktionen auslösen, haben aber keine ekzematogene Wirkung. Die von Röckl untersuchten Fraktionen sind damit noch nicht einwandfrei identifiziert. Die Substanzen, die bisher aus Staphylokokken isoliert wurden und die chemisch aufgeklärt sind, sind die Muramin- und Teichonsäure. Diesen Verbindungen kommt die folgende chemische Konstitution zu (Baddiley).

Baddiley hat 100 g lyophilisierte Staphylokokken für uns aufgearbeitet. Die Staphylokokken wurden von einem mikrobiellen Ekzem gezüchtet. Die beiden wasserlöslichen Fraktionen, von denen eine aus den Zellwänden stammte und Teichonsäure war, und eine aus dem Cytoplasma, deren chemische Natur unbekannt ist, wurden von uns an einem geeigneten Krankengut durchgetestet. Die Reaktionen waren unspezifisch und für die Erklärung des mikrobiellen Ekzems als Antigen-Antikörperreaktion im Sinne einer Spätreaktion nicht verwertbar. Von Gunnar Haukenes (Institut für Mikrobiologie in Norwegen) liegt bisher eine große Zahl von Veröffentlichungen vor über immunchemische Studien von Polysaccharid A aus Staphylococcus aureus. Über die biologischen bzw. pathologischen Eigenschaften dieser Substanz im Hinblick auf das mikrobielle Ekzem ist bisher nichts bekannt geworden. Zusammenfassend kann festgestellt werden, daß es sehr wahrscheinlich ist, daß Glykoproteide oder ähnliche Verbindungen beim Zustandekommen der Spätreaktion die Ursache sein können, daß aber mit dem bisherigen Ergebnis kein exakter Beweis möglich ist.

Es ist bekannt, daß Pilzinfektionen die Bildung humoraler Antikörper auslösen können, ebenso können sie die Ursache sein für allergische Reaktionen vom verzögerten Typus. Die Trichophytinreaktion ist als allergische Reaktion mit der Tuberkulinreaktion verwandt. Sie hat ähnlich wie die Tuberkulinreaktion ihr Reaktionsoptimum nach 24 bis 48 Std. Sofortreaktionen durch freie Antikörper vom Reagintyp kommen ebenfalls vor (Sulzberger u. Kerr, 1930; Markussen, 1937; Jadassohn u. Suter, 1951; Lindemeyer u. Lerger, 1962).

Die serologisch nachweisbaren Antigene sind hochmolekulare Polysaccharide mit sehr geringem Gehalt an Stickstoff, vermutlich Aminozucker (Seeliger 1963/65). Die Verbindungen, die für die Spätreaktionen ursächlich in Frage kommen, sind noch unbekannt. Barker, Cruickshank, Morris und Wood haben aus Trichophyton mentagrophytes ein Glykopeptid isoliert, das am Meerschweinchen Früh- und Spätreaktionen auszulösen vermag. Die Abspaltung des Kohlenhydratanteils schwächte die Sofortreaktion ab. Die Entfernung der Peptide hat den Verlust der Spätreaktion zur Folge. Die Biochemie der Stoffe, die allergische Reaktionen vom Früh- und Spättypus auszulösen vermögen, ist für Mykobakterien am besten bekannt, für Staphylokokken und hautpathogene Pilze aber erst im Beginn einer Aufklärung. Die chemische Konstitution dieser sehr beachtenswerten Verbindung wird uns einen sehr wesentlichen Schritt in der Molekularpathologie der allergischen Spätreaktionen vorwärtsbringen.

The Role of the Basophil in the Immune Response

W. B. Shelley, Department of Dermatology, University of Pennsylvania, School of Medicine, Philadelphia, Pennsylvania (USA)

It is becoming increasingly evident that the basophil leucocyte participates actively in the immune response. In all generalized urticarial or anaphylactic reactions of the immediate allergic type, there is a dramatic and sustained drop in the total number of circulating basophils. This in part reflects basophil degranulation and release of histamine. Significantly, such an immune phenomenon can be reproduced *in vitro* by exposing the sensitized individual's blood to an appropriate antigen in the proper concentration.

We have found the enumeration of circulating basophil leucocytes to be of especial diagnostic importance in studying patients with allergic reactions. Experimentally it has been shown in animals and in man that, as one becomes sensitized to an antigen, the basophil count begins to rise as a result of increased production by the bone marrow. Therefore, while sensitization is occurring, the absolute basophil count rises. Once sensitization has occurred the absolute basophil count remains at an elevated level and, if the patient is not challenged with the appropriate antigen, the count gradually falls to lower levels. However, if the patient is challenged with the sensitizing antigen, the absolute basophil count falls rapidly (resulting in anaphylaxis), or slowly (resulting in urticaria, flushing, or headache). We have used this information in the past as a research tool in identifying the sensitizing antigen in various allergic problems.

The *in vitro* technique of identifying offending allergens, whether they be drugs, foods, or other chemicals, consists of exposing the patient's blood to a dilute non-toxic concentration of the compound in question. After a 15 min room temperature incubation period, the basophils are viewed with a new neutral red staining technique. This permits demonstration of immediate hypersensitivity states by virtue of the fact that in sensitized patients the basophils undergo degranulation and granulolysis.

In the event that the patient has no basophils, an indirect test may be performed using rabbit basophil leucocytes as the test object since these basophils may be passively sensitized by the addition of the patient's blood containing circulating antibodies.

Interestingly, basophils accumulate at the site of delayed allergic reactions as, for example, contact dermatitis. This would appear to be a specific immune response since it does not occur in primary irritant reactions, nor is it limited to the skin. Possibly such local basophilia should make us aware of the fundamentally close relationship of the immediate and delayed reactions.

Free Communications

Classes of Immunoglobulins Associated with Skin Sensitizing Properties*

M. J. FELLNER and R. L. BAER, Department of Dermatology, New York University School of Medicine, New York, N. Y. (USA)

Since the last International Congress, significant advances have been made in the knowledge of skin sensitizing antibodies and of their role in various forms of cutaneous reactions. Reaginic activity indicating the presence of skin sensitizing antibodies has been reported to be associated with the gamma G 7 S and gamma M 19 S and gamma A globulin fractions in different publications [1, 2, 3].

More recently, ISHIZAKA and ISHIZAKA [4] working with serum, predominantly from ragweed-sensitive, atopic patients, have localized skin sensitizing activity in a separate fraction, distinct from the other previously described immunoglobulin

* This work was supported by grants AI 07728 and TI-AM-5326 from the United States Public Health Service.

fractions IgG, IgA, IgM and IgD. They have used the term immunoglobulin E for the fraction containing the antibody presumed to be responsible for skin sensitization. These observations still do not rule out the possibility that skin sensitizing antibodies may also be contained in other fractions of immunoglobulins. The table shows a classification of the presently known immunoglobulins and lists their principal characteristics.

Table. *The Immunoglobulins in man*

	IgG	IgA	IgM	IgD	IgE
Sedimentation	7 S	8—11 S	19 S	7 S	8—11 S
MW	150.000	150.000	900.000		> 150.000
Human skin-sen.	?	?	?		yes
Normal level MG/ML	12	4	1.2	0.3	?

Recently, we have studied the role of skin sensitizing antibodies in various clinical forms of allergic reactions associated with urticaria in penicillin sensitivity [5, 6]. We have used direct skin tests for wheal-and-flare reactivity with penicillin G and with penicilloyl-polylysine, as well as hemagglutination tests for IgG and IgM penicilloyl-specific antibodies. The evidence now available from the studies of others and from our own studies suggests that *all* urticarial reactions due to penicillin are mediated by skin sensitizing antibodies, whether the urticaria occurs alone or in association with manifestations in other organs. Thus skin tests either with penicillin itself or with penicilloyl-polylsine almost invariably elicit wheal reactions in penicillin urticaria.

"Immediate" urticarias with anaphylactic reactions in most instances are mediated by skin sensitizing antibodies specific for the determinants other than the penicilloyl grouping and are associated with positive skin tests to penicillin G. However, such urticarial reactions can occur also in patients who have positive skin tests to penicilloyl-polylysine and negative skin tests to penicillin G, particularly in that small proportion of patients with highly avid skin sensitizing antibodies of penicilloyl specificity and unusually low titers of IgG blocking antibodies.

"Accelerated" urticarias occurring within 2 to 72 h after penicillin therapy is given usually are mediated by skin sensitizing antibodies of benzylpenicilloyl haptenic specificity. Thus they are associated with positive skin tests to penicilloyl-polylysine, while skin tests with penicillin G are usually negative.

In urticarias associated with serum sickness-like reactions, usually occurring approximately 1 to 3 weeks following initiation of penicillin therapy, skin tests are always positive during the acute or convalescent phase either to penicillin G or to penicilloyl-polylysine.

If the conclusion is correct that all these different clinical varieties of penicillin urticarias are mediated by skin sensitizing antibodies, then the pronounced differences in the *clinical* manifestations associated with these urticarias must depend on other factors such as antibody specificity, tissue fixation of antibodies, blocking IgG antibody titer, dose of drug, formation and location of antigen-antibody complexes as well as other specific and non-specific factors.

Bibliography. 1. TERR, A. I., and J. D. BENTZ: J. Allergy **36**, 443 (1965). — 2. HEREMANS, J. F., and J. P. VAERMAN: Nature (Lond.) **193**, 1091 (1962). — 3. FIREMAN, P., W. E. VANNIER, and H. P. GOODMAN: J. exp. Med. **117**, 603 (1963). — 4. ISHIZAKA, K., T. ISHIZAKA, and M. M. HORNBROOK: J. Immunol. **97**, 840 (1966). — 5. FELLNER, M. J., and R. L. BAER: J. invest. Derm. **48**, 384 (1967). — 6. LEVINE, B. B., A. P. REDMOND, M. J. FELLNER, H. E. VOSS, and V. LEVYTSKA: J. clin. Invest. **45**, 1895 (1966).

Patterns of Skin Fluorescence in Lupus Erythematosus

R. H. Cormane, Dept. of Dermatology of the University, Binnen Gasthuis Hospital, Amsterdam (Netherlands)

The occurrence of different classes of immunoglobulins (Ig) whether or not in combination with complement, in the region of the dermal-epidermal junction is a characteristic diagnostic criterion for lupus erythematosus (LE), in patients without history of pemphigoid or dermatitis herpetiformis [1, 2, 3, 4, 7, 8, 10, 11].

Different patterns of fluorescence of the *dermal-epidermal junction* have been seen in a great number of biopsies from skin of patients with LE after the direct staining method, using commercially available horse anti-human globulin* antisera.

Two main patterns can be distinguished: a) homogeneous staining of the "junctional" region; b) fine or coarse granular deposits in this region.

Each of these patterns may occur in the whole dermal-epidermal region of a section or only in areas of it, otherwise respectively as a continuous or discontinuous zone. The impression was gained that the aspect of fluorescence of the "junctional" region depends for a great deal on the duration, activity and form of the disease (LE) [1]. Moreover, it is for this study of considerable importance to know if therapy (i.e. corticosteroids or anti-malarial drugs) was given to the patients before immunofluorescent examination [4]. During therapy with corticosteroids, for example, a homogeneous staining of the dermal-epidermal junction can shade off into the granular pattern of fluorescence. One may argue therefore that a homogeneous staining of the "junctional" region is the result of closely packed deposits of immunoglobulins in this region.

In the "junctional" region of the uninvolved skin of patients with (Systemic) LE (with and without skin lesions) and of those with C(hronic) D(iscoid) LE with systemic involvement, immunoglobulins can also be located, mostly as granular deposits [1, 2, 11].

Further investigations have shown that in some cases of CDLE without systemic involvement Ig could also be detected in the dermal-epidermal region of the uninvolved skin [1, 2, 4, 11]. According to our experiences these cases show a tendency for transition to the form of CDLE with systemic involvement [1, 4].

Therefore, I think it useful to introduce the name "transistory type of CDLE" to classify this form.

Besides fluorescence of the region of the dermal-epidermal junction in LE other patterns of skin fluorescence can be distinguished.

In a paper concerning an immunofluorescent study of the skin lesions in systemic LE some authors [15] confirm our findings in LE with respect to the occurrence of gamma-globulins (IgG) in the region of the dermal-epidermal junction. Moreover, they mentioned localization of Ig and complement (beta-1c-globulin) in the walls of bloodvessels and in hematoxylin bodies subjacent to the dermal-epidermal junction and in the nuclei of cells in the epidermis as well as in the cutis in skin lesions of three out of nine patients with SLE.

In this context should also be mentioned that the presence of IgG and complement in the walls of the bloodsvessel of the dermis in eight cases with nodular vasculitis was reported [14], and considered as characteristic for this disease.

The occurrence of Ig and their classification in the walls of *cutaneous bloodvessels* has been extensively studied [1]. From these studies it can be concluded

---

* Progressive Laboratories Inc., Distributed by Roboz Surgical Instrument Co. Inc., Washington 6, D.C.

that the localization of Ig in the walls of cutaneous bloodvessels is not specific for any disease. It can even be seen in skin of healthy individuals. In LE, however, fluorescence of cutaneous vessels must have some meaning judging from the frequent occurrence of this phenomenon. Apparently there seems to exist a correlation between the frequency of the localization of Ig in vessel walls in the uninvolved skin of patients with various forms of SLE and the severity of the disease process. Moreover, we [1] got the impression that in LE skin lesions fluorescence of vessel walls may also depend on the local activity of the disease process.

As to the staining reaction of bloodvessels, also different types of fluorescence have been observed: a) a rather homogeneous staining of entire vessel walls, which is the most frequent finding; b) a staining restricted to the cell "enveloppes" of the endothelium sometimes surrounded by a less intensely staining halo; c) a finely stippled staining in, and sometimes also around, vessel walls.

Another pattern of skin fluorescence is that of deposits of staining material mainly localized subjacent to the dermalepidermal junction. In their size, shape and anatomic location these structures correspond to the so-called "hematoxylin bodies".

It was demonstrated that the aggregates consist of DNA complexed with IgG [6, 16]. Some authors [13] described them as: "elastic globes", due to the fact that they are stainable by all methods for the demonstration of elastic fibres and digested by all the enzymes that attack elastic tissues. At any rate their occurrence in the upper part of the dermis is not related to any particular disease.

Staining of *nuclei*, homogeneous or speckled, is reported to occur only in the epidermis of the skin at the site of LE lesions, while neighbouring areas of skin treated in the same way did not show this type of staining [15].

Judging from recent results [12] there seems to exist a correlation between the presence of ANF in the serum and nuclear fluorescence of skin sections from the same patient after staining by the direct immunofluorescent method. This was observed in some patients with systemic lupus erythematosus. Investigations are in progress to find out whether this is specific for LE or not.

The *dermis* in sections of skin lesions and normal controls may show a diffuse fluorescence, as already has been reported [5]. This is a nonspecific fluorescence due to the presence of Ig as well as other serum proteins. It can be weakened by thoroughly washing of the sections before staining.

If, however, the collagen bundles are swollen and the interfibrillary ground substance may be present as homogeneous "fibrinoid" clumps, as can be seen in various forms of LE, these areas show a yellow-green fluorescence. This is caused by the presence of different serum proteins in these areas, which can easily be demonstrated with conjugates directed against these proteins.

The *m. arrector pili* is in general barely stained; however, sometimes a bright staining of this smooth muscle was observed. The meaning of this phenomenon is up to now obscure.

The fluorescence of the *granular layer* should also be considered as nonspecific, which can be demonstrated by specificity tests. Depending on the titer of the antisera and the methods used, various patterns of fluorescence of the skin can be seen. For these reasons it is necessary to be quite circumspect when interpreting the results of immunofluorescent studies of skin. Although the method appears to be simple, several pitfalls can undermine its usefulness. It is apparent from the published accounts that most of the authors have been mindful of these limitations.

Literature. 1. BAART DE LA FAILLE-KUYPER, E. H., and R. H. CORMANE: 177th meeting of the Dutch Society of Dermatologists, Nijmegen, March 11, 1967. — 2. CORMANE, R. H.: Lancet 1964 I, 534. — 3. CORMANE, R. H., R. E. BALLIEUX, G. L. KALSBEEK, and W. HYMANS:

Clin. Exp. Immunol. 1, 207 (1966). — 4. CORMANE, R. H. (1967): Pathologia Europaea 2, 170 (1967). — 5. GITLIN, D., B. H. LANDING, and A. WHIPPLE: J. exp. Med. 97, 163 (1963). — 6. GODMAN, G. C., A. D. DEITCH, and P. KLEMRERPE: Amer. J. Path. 34, 1 (1958). — 7. HAVE-OPBROEK, A. A. W. TEN: Acta derm.-venereol. (Stockh.) 46, 68(1966); — 8. HAVE-OPBROECK, A. A. W. TEN: Dermatologica (Basel) 132, 109 (1966). — 9. JOHNSON, G. D., E. J. HOLBORROW, and C. E. GLYNN: Lancet1965 II, 878. — 10. KALSBEEK, G. L., and R. H. CORMANE: Lancet 1964 II, 178. — 11. KALSBEEK, G. L., and R. H. CORMANE: Dermatologica (Basel) 134, (1957). — 12. MEER, J. B. V. D., and R. H. CORMANE: To be published. — 13. PINKUS, H., A. H. MEHREGAN, and R. G. STARRICO: J. invest. Derm. 45, 81 (1965). — 14. STRINGA, S. G., C.B IANCHI, and Z. B. ZINGALE: J. invest. Derm. 46, 1 (1966). — 15. TAN, E. M., and H. G. KUNKEL: Arthr. and Rheum. 9, 37 (1963). — 16. WILSON, R. M., R. R. ABBOTT, and D. K. MILLER: Amer. J. med. Sci. 241, 31 (1961).

Delayed Hypersensitivity Responses in Immunologic Deficiency States*

W. L. EPSTEIN, Division of Dermatology, Department of Medicine, University of California, School of Medicine, San Francisco, California (USA)

In recent years the concept of immunologic deficiency associated with systemic illness has gained currency. We previously demonstrated that a sensitive measure of delayed sensitivity in man was *induction* of contact-type delayed sensitivity to simple chemicals, 2,4-dinitrochlorobenzene (DNCB) and paranitrosodimethyl aniline (NDMA) [1]. We have used this method to assess cellular sensitivity in patients with a number of diverse diseases, known or suspected to be associated with immunological deficiency, such as hypo-gamma-globulinemia, lymphoreticular malignancies, ataxia-telangiectasia, sarcoidosis, rheumatoid arthritis, cirrhosis, and psoriasis (treated and untreated with immunosuppressive drugs). In each experiment, suitable controls also were tested, such as patients with other forms of cancer, neurologic defects, osteoarthritis, acute and chronic hepatitis, and infectious mononucleosis with liver involvement, as well as healthy volunteers. For convenience, these subjects are listed together as chronic disease controls. No terminal, toxic, or bedridden patients were included as a previous unreported study indicated such patients show a nonspecific, markedly reduced response to simple chemicals. As an additional investigation, some groups were tested for pre-existing contact sensitivity to poison oakpoison ivy allergens by topical exposure to pentadecyl catechol (PDC), a commonly acquired sensitivity in the United States. The concentrations, method of application, and patch test interpretations have been described elsewhere [1, 2].

Results and Discussion

The findings are detailed in the table. They indicate two clearcut and expected classes of hyporeactors; namely: 1. a group composed of patients with sarcoidosis and rheumatoid arthritis who have a moderate degree of depressed delayed reactivity; and 2. a group with much more limited capacity to react, namely patients with hypo-gammaglobulinemia, lymphoreticular malignancies and ataxia-telangiectasia. A surprise was the depressed reactivity of patients with cirrhosis which was not seen in patients with acute and chronic infectious hepatitis, excluding lupoid hepatitis. Alcoholic cirrhosis is not generally considered a disease of immunologic deficiency. Yet it is conceivable the disease results in a

* This study was supported in part by State of California, Special State Appropriation 1966, CHZ-110, Psoriasis Research.

defect in phagocytosis which is reflected by a ineffectual processing of delayed allergens. Clearly, further work in this area is indicated.

Table. *Frequency of Sensitization to DNCB and NDMA and Reactivity to PDC*

Disease Category	DNCB	NDMA	PDC
Healthy controls	502/732 (69%)	375/692 (54%)	80—90% (2)
Chronic disease controls	90/148 (60%)	47/149 (31%)	
Adult-type hypo-gamma-globulinemia	1/11	0/11	5/11
Lymphoreticular malignancy			
([3] and unpublished data)	9/39	4/39	14/26
Ataxia-telangiectasia [4]	2/19	1/19	NT[a]
Sarcoidosis [5]	8/23	3/23	18/22
Rheumatoid arthritis [6]	24/55	17/56	NT[a]
Cirrhosis	8/35	7/35	NT[a]
Psoriasis [7]			
Treated with immunosuppresive			
therapy	4/26	1/25	21/25
Not treated	8/16	5/16	NT[a]

[a] Not tested.

The data in patients with psoriasis has been published [7]; a few more untreated psoriatics have been tested. The findings support the conclusions of others that untreated psoriatics have borderline normal delayed responses. The findings further suggest that psoriatics are on the verge of "immunologic bankruptcy" and immunosuppressive therapy pushes them over the brink.

The findings with PDC skin tests, although far from complete, are consonant with the idea that patients with severe involvement of the delayed sensitivity system also have a limited ability to react to presumably pre-existing sensitivities.

Conclusions

Induction of delayed contact sensitivity to simple chemicals presents a simple and very sensitive method to assess the immunological status of the delayed sensitivity system in various disease states. NDMA is perhaps more sensitive than DNCB in detecting borderline immunologic deficiency. The method is not a useful diagnostic or prognostic tool in individual patients.

References. 1. EPSTEIN, and KLIGMAN: J. invest. Derm. 31, 103 (1958). — 2. KLIGMAN: Arch. Derm. 77, 149 (1958). — 3. EPSTEIN: J. invest. Derm. 30, 39 (1958). — 4. EPSTEIN: Int. Arch. Allergy 30, 15 (1966). — 5. EPSTEIN, and MAYOCK: Proc. Soc. exp. Biol. (N.Y.) 96, 786 (1957). — 6. EPSTEIN, and JESSAR: Arth. and Rheum. 2, 178 (1959). — 7. EPSTEIN, and MAIBACH: Arch. Derm. 91, 599 (1965).

Antikörpermangelsyndrome und Hautveränderungen

G. BREHM, Univ.-Hautklinik Mainz (Deutschland)

Seit der Beschreibung von BRUTON (1952) über einen Fall von A-Gamma-Globulinämie begann man sich intensiv mit Krankheitsbildern zu beschäftigen, die heute am besten nach BARANDUN, BÜCHLER und HÄSSIG als Antikörper-mangelsyndrom bezeichnet werden. Die zahlreichen hierbei zu findenden Hautveränderungen können nicht selten als Leitsymptom bzw. Verdachtsmoment für die Diagnose gelten. Die Antikörpermangelsyndrome zeigen meist eine Störung des humoralen Abwehrsystems, wie es sich in den Immunglobulinen darbietet, zum

Teil aber auch Störungen der cellulären Abwehr im Sinne der allergischen Spätreaktionen und schließlich auch in einigen Fällen Veränderungen im Bereich
beider Systeme. Die Antikörpermangelsyndrome kann man einteilen erstens in die
idiopathischen isolierten Formen. Dazu gehören kongenitale AMS der Knaben,
(BRUTON), die AMS mit schwerer Lymphopenie (sog. Schweizer Form), die AMS
mit lymphatischer Hyperplasie, die AMS ohne lymphoreticuläre Dysplasie, die
Dys-Gamma-Globulinämie vom Typ II und die erworbenen AMS-Formen, zum
Beispiel bei chronisch lymphatischer Leukämie, Thymom, Myelom, Makroglobulinämie Waldenström, Morbus Hodgkin, nach Splenektomie, bei verschiedenen endokrinen und metabolischen Krankheiten, Amyloidose, Vaccinia gangränosa.
Anzuschließen wären hier das Louis-Bar-Syndrom, das Wiskott-Aldrich-Syndrom
und die idiopathische familiäre Dyproteinämie. Als dritte Hauptform wären die
frühkindlichen transitorischen AMS zu nennen.

Die fehlende oder mangelhafte immunologische Abwehr äußert sich von seiten
der Haut vor allem im Auftreten von Pyodermien und Mykosen. Je stärker der
Ausfall der Immunglobuline, desto stärker im allgemeinen auch der Befall der
Haut. Die kongenitalen Formen weisen im allgemeinen mehr dermatologische
Veränderungen auf als die erworbenen oder Begleit-AMS. Pyodermien, hervorgerufen durch Staphylokokken, seltener Streptokokken, Enterokokken, Pyocea-
neus und andere Erreger, zeigen klinisch das Bild von multiplen Abscessen,
Furunkeln, Schweißdrüsenabscessen, Mastitis, Pyoderma gangränosum, Impetigo,
Erysipel, schlechtheilenden Wunden und Nekrosen nach Operationen und intra-
muskulären Injektionen. Die mykotischen Infektionen sind vor allem Soorin-
fektionen mit Beteiligung von Haut, Schleimhaut und inneren Organen, aber auch
therapieresistente Tricho- und Epidermophytien. Wenn auch im allgemeinen die
Abwehr gegen Virusinfektionen kaum gestört ist, werden gehäuft Herpes zoster-
Infektionen beobachtet.

Durch eine äußerste Resistenzschwäche ohne Abheilungstendenz zeichnet sich
die seltene, letal endende Vaccinia gangränosa aus, während Eccema herpetica-
tum-Fälle ebenfalls vorkommen. Milchschorf, endogenes Ekzem, bzw. atopische
Dermatitis werden bei kongenitalen Formen der AMS vermehrt gefunden. Asthma
bronchiale und Pollinosis als Allergien vom Frühreaktionstyp werden dagegen nur
selten beobachtet. Prick- und Intracutantests, d. h. eine Allergie vom Frühreaktionstyp auf verschiedene Antigene, sind bei den AMS meist negativ, während
die Spätreaktionsallergie vom Ekzemtyp meist nicht gestört ist, was positive
Sensibilisierungsversuche mit Dinitrochlorbenzol bzw. Dinitrofluorbenzol zeigen.
Dagegen ist die Spätreaktionsallergie vom Tuberkulintyp uneinheitlich; neben stets
negativen Reaktionen finden sich auch Fälle, bei denen nach BCG-Impfung ein
Positivwerden der Tuberkulinreaktion zu verzeichnen ist. Je stärker der immunologische Defekt, um so größer ist die Immunotoleranz gegenüber Haut- und Lymph-
knoten-Transplantaten beim kranken Empfänger ausgeprägt. Es hat den Anschein, als ob bei einigen AMS eine pleiotrope Wirkung der Gene vorliegt, was
das Vorkommen von verschiedensten Erkrankungen, wie Lupus erythematodes,
rheumatischer Arthritis, Paltauf-Sternberg in der Familie von AMS-Kranken,
zeigt. Einzelne Fälle von AMS vergesellschaftet mit Lupus Erythematodes,
Sklerodermie und Dermatomyositis sind beschrieben worden. Ein dermatologisch
bemerkenswertes Krankheitsbild ist das Louis-Bar-Syndrom, welches eine cerebellare Ataxie, Telangiektasien der Augenbindehaut, der Gesichts- und Körperhaut, Hyperpigmentierungen, Depigmentierungen, varioliforme Narben und
ichthyosiforme Hautveränderungen aufweist.

AMS zeigen nicht selten auch uncharakteristische Exantheme urticarieller,
maculöser oder nodöser Morphe. Erythema nodosum nach Medikamentenein-

nahme, ebenso wie Auftreten von urticariellen Erscheinungen nach Gamma-Globulin oder Penicillin weisen darauf hin, daß nicht immer sämtliche immunologischen Abwehrmechanismen defekt sind. Uhrglasnägel- und Trommelschlägelfinger weisen auf die häufig vorkommenden kardio-pulmonalen Störungen sowohl bei der kongenitalen als auch bei der erworbenen AMS hin. Wir konnten an seltenen Hautveränderungen bei einem Brüderpaar Ichthyosis vulgaris beobachten, wobei ein Junge eine ausgeprägte A-Gamma-Globulinämie im Sinne der AMS der Knaben, der zweite eine Hypo-Gamma-Globulinämie mit Ichthyosis vulgaris aufwies. An Begleit-AMS beobachteten wir eine solche bei einem Gamma-G-Plasmacytom mit Siebfurunkel an der Unterlippe, eine Hypo-Gamma-Globulinämie bei einem Melanom mit Tonsillenmetastase, ein isoliertes Fehlen von Gamma-A-Globulinen bei Psoriasis arthropathica und eine Gamma-M-Hypoglobulinämie bei einem Franceschetti-Zwahlen-Syndrom.

Diese Ausführungen sollten Ihnen zeigen, daß ausgehend von bestimmten Hautveränderungen bei entsprechender Anamnese an ein Antikörpermangelsyndrom gedacht werden sollte. Mit Hilfe der Immunelektrophorese, quantitativer Immunglobulinbestimmung und der Prüfung der natürlichen und experimentell erzeugten Antikörper wie Iso-Agglutininen, Antistreptolysintiter, Tuberkulintestung und Sensibilisierungsversuchen mit DNCB ist ein objektiver Nachweis eines Antikörpermangelsyndroms möglich. In diesem Zusammenhang möchte ich auf die ausführliche Darstellung in der Zeitschrift „Hautarzt" und auf die Ausstellung auf diesem Kongreß verweisen.

Zur Frage der Antigenspezifität von 2,4-Dinitrochlorbenzol-Epidermis-Conjugaten im Meerschweinchenversuch

F. Klaschka, Hautklinik der Freien Universität Berlin im Rudolf-Virchow-Krankenhaus, Berlin (Deutschland)

In Sensibilisierungsstudien mit 2,4-Dinitrochlorbenzol (DNCB) wurden Meerschweinchen (MS) mit freiem Hapten oder DNB-Conjugaten in systematisch variierter Form epi- und intracutan sowie intraperitoneal und intravenös behandelt. Die nach 2- bis 3wöchiger Latenzperiode mit stets gleicher atoxischer DNCB-Flächenkonzentration, d. h. mit 60 γ DNCB auf 4 cm² Flankenhaut ausgelösten Epicutantestreaktionen zeigten bei regelmäßiger *makro-* und *mikroskopischer* Analyse unterschiedliche Formen der Kontaktallergie: Bei epicutan wie auch bei intracutan sensibilisierten Tieren fanden sich bevorzugt *epidermo-*cutane Reaktionsbilder, entsprechend dem „klassischen" allergischen Kontaktekzem. Extracutan, d. h. intraperitoneal und intravenös vorbehandelte MS zeigten dagegen fast ausschließlich *cutane* Reaktionen. Durch anschließende epicutane DNCB-Applikation ließ sich hier sekundär eine zusätzliche epidermo-cutane Reaktivität induzieren.

Angesichts dieser Befunde konnte als klassisches Ekzemantigen ein *epidermis*-spezifisches Haptenconjugat vermutet werden. Bei den mit in-vitro-Conjugaten aus DNCB und autologer bzw. homologer Gesamtepidermis sensibilisierten Versuchstieren traten jedoch nach Erstauslösung nicht — wie erwartet — epidermo-cutane, sondern allenfalls cutane Reaktionen auf. Nach Zweitauslösung innerhalb von 3 bis 4 Tagen reagierten die Tiere makroskopisch zum Teil außerordentlich verstärkt. Sie zeigten histologisch das mit DNCB erstmals beobachtete Bild der Epidermolyse, charakterisiert durch Achromasie, Auflösung des Epidermiszellgefüges,

Ablösung der Epidermis vom Corium, Ansammlung von Serum in den Epidermis-
lücken und dichte Immigration von Lympho- und zahlreichen Granulocyten.
Vergleichbare Lyse-Phänomene am Ort des primär sicher atoxischen Epicutan-
tests sahen wir auch bei intracutan mit DNCB und Freundschem Adjuvans
nebeneinander vorbehandelten MS, die während der Sensibilisierungsphase im
Bereiche der Adjuvansinjektion eine ausgedehnte Epidermisnekrose aufwiesen.

Die histologisch nach einheitlichem Beurteilungsschema gut abgrenzbaren Reaktionen vom epidermo-cutanen, cutanen und epidermolytischen Typ lassen sich
tierexperimentell regelmäßig reproduzieren. Sie werden in erster Linie geprägt von
dem in freier oder konjugierter Form angewendeten Allergen bzw. dessen Applika-
tionsmodus und sind demnach Ausdruck einer unterschiedlichen Antigenspezifität.
Den im Cutisbereich persistierenden Reaktionen mit einem wahrscheinlich aus
Hapten und *Corium*anteilen gebildeten Antigenmotiv stehen epidermal betonte
Ekzemreaktionen und Epidermolysephänomene gegenüber, deren Epidermotropie
sich zwanglos als Organotropie epidermaler Carrier-Substanzen erklären läßt. Da
wir von der chemischen Natur der epidermalen Conjugatpartner aber vorerst
keine experimentell gesicherten Vorstellungen besitzen, liegt es nahe zu fragen,
ob sich Ekzemreaktion und Epidermolysephänomen hinsichtlich ihrer *Qualität*,
d. h. durch besondere Antigen-Antikörper-Spezifität, unterscheiden oder lediglich
quantitative Abweichungen ein und desselben Reaktionstyps darstellen.

In dieser Studie wird an DNCB-vorbehandelten MS mittels histologischer Epi-
cutantestanalyse eine Klärung dieser Frage angestrebt. Zwei, aus größeren Versuchsreihen ausgewählte Gruppen von sechs bzw. acht Albino-MS wurden zunächst
in Wiederholungsversuchen mit DNCB sensibilisiert und zeigten bei epicutaner
Auslösung mit 15 γ DNCB/cm^2 makroskopisch annähernd gleiche Testreaktionen.
Mikroskopisch fand sich bei den Tieren der ersten Gruppe eine Epidermolyse, bei
der zweiten Gruppe dagegen eine Ekzemreaktion. Sämtliche Tiere wurden nun
gleichzeitig und nebeneinander mit DNCB-Flächenkonzentrationen von 6, 9, 12
und 15 γ/cm^2 auf je 4 cm^2 Flankenhaut nachgepinselt. 24 Std später wurden aus
den vier Testarealen eines jeden Tieres nach makroskopischer Beurteilung repräsentative Proben für die histologische Analyse entnommen.

Die *Ergebnisse* der makro- und mikroskopischen Untersuchungen sind in der
Tabelle zusammengefaßt. Bei den Tieren der ersten Gruppe nimmt die Intensität
der makroskopischen Reaktionen mit den zur Auslösung stufenweise erhöhten
DNCB-Flächenkonzentrationen eindeutig zu. Das histologische Reaktionsbild
zeigt dagegen sehr einheitlich das Phänomen der Epidermolyse, und zwar weitgehend unabhängig von der Höhe der verwendeten Testkonzentration. Trotz der
zum Teil deutlichen Quantitätsunterschiede sprechen die insgesamt auffallend
gleichförmigen Histobefunde in erster Linie für die qualitative Eigenständigkeit
der Epidermolysereaktion. Hinsichtlich ihrer Auslösbarkeit mit niedrigen Aller-
gendosen gilt sozusagen das Alles-oder-Nichts-Gesetz.

Bei den Tieren der zweiten Gruppe, die makroskopisch insgesamt etwas
schwächer reagieren als die der ersten, finden sich ausschließlich Ekzemreaktionen,
und zwar auch bei den vier stark positiven MS der Ekzemgruppe. Von gleicher Bedeutung sind die bei Tieren der zweiten Gruppe regelmäßig auftretenden Ekzemreaktionen entweder vom epidermo-cutanen *oder* cutanen Typ, wiederum weitgehend unabhängig von den zur Auslösung verwendeten DNCB-Konzentrationen.
Nicht der Sensibilisierungsgrad, sondern die Qualität der Kontaktreaktion, d. h.
die Antigen-Antikörper-Spezifität ist demnach ausschlaggebend für die Ausbildung eines bestimmten Reaktionstyps. Die vorliegenden Ergebnisse sprechen eindeutig für die unterschiedliche Antigenspezifität bei den epidermal betonten
Ekzem- und Epidermolysereaktionen.

Tabelle. *Ergebnisse makro- und mikroskopischer Epicutantestanalysen bei zwei Versuchstier-gruppen nach Auslösung mit abgestuften DNCB-Flächenkonzentrationen. Histologisch werden Lyse-Reaktionen und Ekzeme vom epidermo-cutanen ((ep > cut) und cutanen (cut) Typ, ferner nicht sicher einzuordnende Zwischenformen (ep-cut) unterschieden.* Beurteilungskriterien s. Arch. klin. exp. Derm. **224**, 216 (1966)

Versuchstiere	Test mit γDNCB. pro cm²	Epicutantestergebnisse								
		makroskopisch					mikroskopisch			
		?	(+)	+	+/ ++	++	ep > cut	ep cut	cut	Lyse
1. Gruppe mit	6	—	2	4	—	—	2	—	—	4
Epidermolyse:	9	—	1	2	3	—	—	1	—	5
6 Tiere	12	—	—	1	4	1	—	—	—	6
	15	—	—	—	3	3	—	—	—	6
2. Gruppe mit	6	5	3	—	—	—	3	2	3	—
Ekzemreaktionen:	9	—	5	3	—	—	3	2	3	—
8 Tiere	12	—	2	6	—	—	4	2	2	—
	15	—	—	4	4	—	5	2	1	—

Vorstellbar als epidermisspezifisches *Ekzem*antigen wäre eine Verbindung zwischen dem Hapten und einem Carrier aus der Sphäre der Epidermiszell*membran*. Letztere bietet dem epicutan applizierten Ekzemallergen auf seinem überwiegend intercellulären Resorptionsweg jedenfalls eine bevorzugte Conjugationsgelegenheit. Nach der Testauslösung entbrennt die epidermo-cutane Ekzemreaktion vorwiegend an der Zellmembran. Bei der Epidermolysereaktion richtet sich die Antigen-Antikörperreaktion offenbar gegen das Zellinnere, möglicherweise gegen ein Antigenconjugat aus Hapten und *cytoplasmatischem* Epidermismaterial. Noch fehlen strukturanalytische Beweise für die Existenz derartiger epidermisspezifischer Antigenconjugate. Die vorliegenden Versuchsergebnisse erscheinen aber richtungweisend für weitere rationelle Analysen des Ekzemantigens in vivo und in vitro.

Antinuclear Factors in Clinical Dermatology

J. S. BECK, N. R. ROWELL and T. E. ANDERSON, The Royal Infirmary, Aberdeen, and The General Infirmary, Leeds (Great Britain)

Since their introduction 8 years ago, tests for antinuclear factor have become widely used and they have virtually replaced the L.E. cell test in clinical practice. From the laboratory point of view the ANF has the great advantage of being a reproducible serological test that does not require great skill in interpretation. Over the years many techniques have been introduced; these vary greatly in their sensitivity so that the findings in one centre need not necessarily apply to another. Recently a subcommittee of the British Medical Research Council have recommended one technique, and we shall describe our findings with this test.

This is an indirect immunofluorescence test in which cryostat sections of rat liver are used as substrate. The patient's serum is applied at 1 in 16 dilution in saline for 30 min at room temperature. After washing in saline, the section is stained with a fluorescein conjugated antiserum to human γ-globulin. The section is washed in saline, mounted in buffered glycerol and examined with ultra violet/blue violet light under darkground illumination.

We have examined serum from 559 patients attending the skin clinics of the Royal Infirmary, Aberdeen, and the General Infirmary, Leeds. The ANF tests were performed without knowledge of the clinical diagnosis.

Lupus erythematosus. ANF tests were positive in 86% of patients with systemic disease and in 33% of patients with discoid lesions.

Scleroderma. ANF was present in 68% of patients with progressive systemic sclerosis, in 40% of patients with generalised scleroderma and in 7% of patients with morphoea.

Arthritis and related disease. ANF was present in two of six patients with rheumatoid arthritis; it was also found in one patient with nodular vasculitis and one with Raynaud's disease but both were siblings of patients with discoid L.E. High titre ANF was found in one patient who presented with nodular vasculitis, one patient with chilblains and one with Raynaud's disease; these three patients subsequently developed S.L.E. and are included in the previous table. Rather surprisingly, ANF tests were negative in all our patients with polyarthritis nodosa and other forms of arthritis. Only one of twelve patients with dermatomyositis had ANF.

Controls. ANF tests were negative in 121 patients with a variety of dermatological conditions selected because of some clinical similarity to the connective tissue disease or because their aetiology was completely unknown. It is of interest that 18 patients with erythema multiforme were negative in view of the known syndrome of episodes of erythema multiforme in discoid lupus erythematosus.

Temporal changes in ANF patients with S.L.E. and P.S.S. 20 patients have been followed over periods of 2 to 10 years. All have shown fluctuations in titre, but these have not been sufficiently clearly related to changes in the clinical conditions to be of value in predicting the course of the disease. We have found that E.S.R. values are of more value in this respect.

Conclusions. In this trial of the ANF test recommended by the subcommittee of the M.R.C. we have found in dermatological practice that it is very rarely positive (and always weak) in patients with diseases other than the connective tissue diseases. It is frequently positive in patients with L.E. and scleroderma, and the incidence (and titres) are related to the extent of the disease. We have found that this test is rarely positive in polyarthritis nodosa and dermatomyositis (and we wonder whether these diseases are basically different from L.E. and scleroderma). The titre of ANF test is of little value as a guide for the immediate prognosis in the individual patient.

Vasoactive Substances at Sites of Cutaneous Allergies

Th. M. Inderbitzin and P. J. Grob, Department of Dermatology, Tufts University School of Medicine, Boston, Mass. (USA)

A constant feature of all types of cutaneous hypersensitivity reactions are vascular changes, namely vasodilatation and increased permeability for plasma.

The following mediators are of importance in mediating the vascular changes at sites of the immediate type of hypersensitivity reactions: histamine, serotonine, plasma kinins, slow reacting substances, components of complement as well as proteolytic enzymes and cationic proteins derived from polymorphonuclear white blood cells. The latter play a major role in the mediation of the vascular damages occurring at the site of an Arthus lesion [1].

Delayed type hypersensitivity reactions also show increased vascular permeability. On comparison with the acute urticarial wheal the vascular leakage is less intense and, instead of being of short duration, it occurs over a long period of time. In delayed hypersensitivity reactions, such as allergic contact dermatitis, the vascular reaction responsible for the erytheme and edema occurs in the venules predominantly [2]. It has been claimed by some [3] and denied by others [4] that the vascular changes at the site of delayed cutaneous hypersensitivity reactions are diminished by antihistamines. In our experiments, edema formation, at least at the sites of an allergic contact dermatitis in guinea pigs was greatly reduced when the animals were treated prior to the challenge and after the challenge with an antihistamine [5]. This treatment, however, in no way interfered with the extravasation and the tissue infiltration with lymphocytes, a process which initiates the tissue lesions of allergic contact dermatitis, such as the formation of intraepidermal vesicles.

In 1964 we reported on the presence of a vasoactive factor in extracts of various organs [6]. This factor, which differed from all hitherto known vasoactive substances was termed permeability increasing factor (P.I.F.). At the present stage of purification 60% of the P.I.F. consists of an acidic (anionic) protein and 40% of an as yet unidentified component.

Upon intradermal injection into laboratory animals the P.I.F. enhances the vascular permeability in doses of 1γ and below, thus leading to local edema formation. Both in vivo and in vitro the P.I.F. is a powerful histamine releaser. Its ability to release histamine from isolated rat mast cells is inhibited by serum [7]. Its histamine releasing activity in vivo is neither affected by sodium salicylate, the soy bean trypsin inhibitor, 2-deoxyglucose nor significantly affected by serum. The P.I.F. resists heat (100 °C), digestion with trypsin and alkaline hydrolysis. P.I.F. obtained from extracts of rat and guinea pig skin was not antigenic when rabbits were used for sensitization.

Since the P.I.F. is also a constituent of lymph node cells, i.e., of lymphocytes, we determined the concentration of the P.I.F. and the extent of the changes in vascular permeability at the site of a delayed type allergic contact dermatitis in guinea pigs. Our studies showed that the concentration of the P.I.F. as well as that of histamine rose and fell in parallel with the waxing and waning not only of the dermatitis but also of the vascular permeability changes [5, 8]. The concentration of the two vasoactive substances reached a maximum within 24 to 36 h after the epidermal challenge of the sensitized animals with the antigen.

Both the increased levels of the P.I.F. and of histamine seem to be due mainly to an influx of these two substances with the infiltrating lymphocytes, since their accumulation was suppressed in lymphopenic or panleukopenic animals. But also the edema formation was diminished in the leukopenic animals. The latter observation is in contrast to that of MAIBACH and MAGUIRE [9] who reported that the vascular response is independent from the infiltrative cellular response at the site of an allergic contact dermatitis in guinea pigs.

It is likely that the histamine and the P.I.F. following their release from the invading lymphocytes cause the change in venous permeability. The simultaneous onset of the lymphocytic extravasation and of the vascular permeability changes, as well as the increased levels of histamine and of P.I.F. in the reacting area favor a relationship between the vascular response and the lymphocytic extravasation.

Thus far, very little is known about the activities of lymphocytes in areas of delayed hypersensitivity reactions; nor is the mechanism known which determines the migration of lymphocytes to areas containing the antigen. It has been postulated that the antigen first provokes the extravasation of a few "committed"

73*

lymphocytes which are specifically able to recognize and to interact with the antigen. This interaction then leads to the activation and to the release of mediators which attract "non-committed" lymphocytes which make up the major part of the lymphocytic tissue infiltration at sites of delayed hypersensitivity reactions. The studies of SCHILD and WILLOUGHBY [10] seem to favor this view. They obtained from lymph node cells a factor (lymph node permeability factor) which not only increased the cutaneous vascular permeability but also led to an infiltration of the skin with lymphocytes when injected intradermally into laboratory animals. Our studies [11] have shown that this lymph node permeability factor contains two vasoactive components, namely ribonucleic acid (RNA) and the P.I.F. Whether or not these two vasoactive substances are capable to attract lymphocytes is as yet not known.

References. 1. COCHRANE, CH. G., and B. S. AIKIN: J. exp. Med. 124, 733 (1966). — JANOFF, A., and B. W. ZWEIFACH: J. exp. Med. 120, 747 (1964). — 2. FLAX, M. H., and J. B. CAULFIELD: Amer. J. Path. 43, 1031 (1963). — 3. MAYER, R. L.: Ann. Allergy 5, 113 (1947). — 4. VOISIN, G. A., and F. TOULLET: Foundation Symposium: Cellular Aspects of Immunity, p. 373. Ciba J. A. Churchill Ltd. 1960. — 5. OHTAKI, N., and T. M. INDERBITZIN: Delayed Hypersensitivity (DNCB) Contact Dermatitis in Panleukopenic Guinea Pigs (In preparation). — 6. INDERBITZIN, T. M., F. MAAG, and T. CHORZELSKI: Int. Arch. Allergy 26, 181 (1965); 29, 213 (1966). — 7. KELLER, R.: Pers. communication. — 8. INDERBITZIN, T. M.: Int. Arch. Allergy 8, 150 (1956); — Mechanism of Hypersensitivity. Boston: Little Brown 1959. — 9. MAIBACH, H. I., and H. C. MAGUIRE: J. invest. Derm. 41, 123 (1963). — 10. SCHILD, H. O., and D. A. WILLOUGHBY: Brit. med. Bull. 23, 46 (1967). — 11. INDERBITZIN, T. M., A. KELL, and G. BLUMENTAL: Int. Arch. Allergy 29, 417 (1966).

Application de la technique d'immunofluorescence en dermatologie

Y. MONTET, J. DUHEILLE et J. BEUREY, Hôpital Fournier, Nancy (France)

Depuis leur découverte par COONS et Col. les techniques d'immunofluorescence ont trouvé de nombreuses applications en Dermatologie. Les unes concernent la détection directe d'agents pathogènes bactériens, viraux, mycosiques ou parasitaires dans les lésions cutanées. Elles ont un intérêt pratique immédiat en facilitant le diagnostic étiologique. D'autres ont eu pour but de démontrer le. mécanisme pathogénique de processus allergiques dont des méthodes différentes avaient déjà permis de soupçonner l'existence. Mais nous voudrions surtout insister sur l'apport le plus original de ces techniques: la découverte de phénomènes auto-immuns au cours de certaines dermatoses. Après les travaux de RAPPAPORT, RASKIN, PARISH, NEWCOMER, BEUTNER, nous avons personnellement employé cette technique selon des modalités décrites par ailleurs [5], pour étudier les sérums de 60 malades. Chez cinq d'entre eux, nous avons également étudié par immunofluorescence directe et indirecte des biopsies cutanées prélevées en zone saine ou au niveau des lésions.

Pemphigus

Sur neuf malades atteints de pemphigus vulgaire ou végétant, sept possédaient des anticorps sériques se fixant sur les limites cytoplasmiques des cellules de l'épiderme et de ses annexes, ainsi que sur tous les épithéliums de type malpighien kératinisés ou non. Nous avons été frappé par le fait que l'épithélium antérieur de la cornée reste négatif alors que l'épithélium conjonctival voisin réagit fortement. De même les canaux excréteurs des glandes sudoripares et les galactophores mammaires retiennent les anticorps alors que la portion secrétrice des tubes sudoripares

et les acini mammaires ne se marquent pas. Les épithéliums cubiques ou cylindriques unis ou pseudostratifiés muqueux ne retiennent pas ces anticorps. De même
la totalité des parenchymes tissulaires testés sont restés négatifs avec la plupart
des sérums sauf deux qui se fixaient l'un sur le myocarde, l'autre sur le cytoplasme
des cellules thyroïdiennes. Nous pensons que dans ces deux cas il s'agit d'anticorps
antiorganes surajoutés aux anticorps antipeau. Enfin, ces anticorps réagissent non
seulement avec l'épiderme humain, mais aussi avec des téguments d'origine
animale. Ils sont dépourvus de spécificité d'espèce. En cela, notre expérience personnelle confirme entièrement les observations de BEUTNER [1]. Nous estimons
néanmoins que la recherche des anticorps doit être faite sur de l'épiderme humain
ou à la rigueur de primates mais non sur la peau provenant d'autres espèces, en

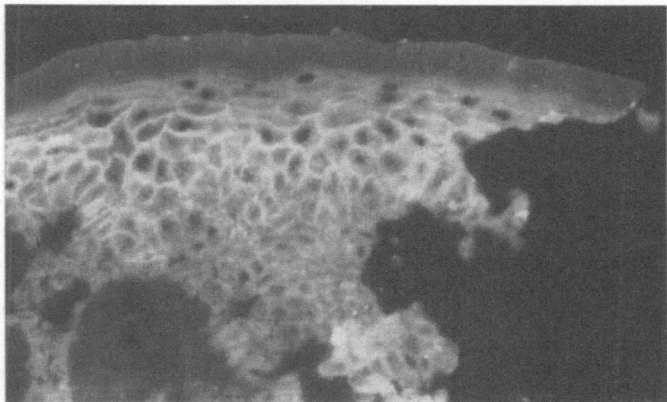

Fig. Angle de décollement d'une bulle de pemphigus. Technique de fluorescence directe:
au contact du sérum antigammaglobuline fluorescent apparaît une fluorescence à la périphérie des cellules des corps muqueux de Malpighi dans l'épiderme bordant la bulle de pemphigus

raison de nombreuses interférences immunologiques qui risquent d'entraîner des
réactions faussement positives. Les titres de ces anticorps sont variables: le maximum observé est de 1/512. Chez deux malades en rémission thérapeutique, nous
n'avons pas trouvé d'anticorps. Dans cinq cas, les sérums des malades ont pu être
testés sur leur propre peau, confirmant qu'il s'agit bien d'autoanticorps. L'examen
des lésions par immunofluorescence directe a montré dans ces cinq cas que des
gamma-G-globulines s'étaient fixées in vivo sur les limites cellulaires de l'épiderme
avoisinant les lésions et sur les cellules acantholytiques.

Maladie de Duhring-Brocq

Nous avons observé trois cas de maladie de Duhring-Brocq. Par immunofluorescence indirecte, nous avons retrouvé chaque fois des anticorps se fixant sur
la jonction dermo-épidermique sous forme d'un fin liseré fluorescent, qu'il s'agisse
ou non de la propre peau du malade, ces anticorps réagissent également avec la
basale d'autres épithéliums malpighiens.

Maladie lupique et affections apparentées

A côté de ces auto-anticorps dirigés contre l'épiderme, on peut observer au
cours des affections cutanées, des anticorps réagissant avec d'autres tissus. Notons
en premier lieu la maladie lupique et les affections apparentées au cours desquelles des facteurs antinucléaires sont détectés avec une très grande fréquence. La

similitude des perturbations immunologiques rencontrées dans le lupus érythémateux disséminé et dans le lupus chronique discoïde tend à confirmer l'étroite
parenté de ces deux affections.

Autres affections auto-immunes

Nous voudrions également signaler le cas du myxoedème cutané prétibial où
des anticorps antithyroïdiens sont observés non seulement dans le sérum mais au
sein même du tissu myxoedémateux (KRISS et PLESHAKOV). Ces faits sont à rapprocher des données fournies par l'immunofluorescence dans les cas d'amylose.
Cette technique permet de retrouver dans les dépôts amyloïdes la présence de
gamma-globulines associées à du fibrinogène. Pour certains auteurs, la substance
amyloïde ne serait que le témoin de conflits prolongés entre des anticorps, parfois
des auto-anticorps, et les antigènes éventuellement tissulaires, correspondants
(WALFORD et LEE).

Conclusion

De nombreux autres domaines offrent encore à l'immunofluorescence un champs
d'application prometteur : processus tumoraux et paranéoplasiques, purpuras et
vascularites, hypodermites nodulaires etc. Cependant, l'acquisition la plus importante que l'on doive à cette technique reste la découverte des autoanticorps
antiépiderme. Leur rôle dans la production ou l'entretien des lésions reste encore
incertain en dépit des nombreux travaux qui ont tenté de l'élucider.

Bibliographie. 1. BEUTNER, E. H., E. RHODES, and E. J. HOLBOROW: Clin. exp. immunol.
2, 141 (1967). — 2. CHORZELSKI, T., S. JABLONSKA, and M. BLASZCZYK: Acta derm.-venereol,
(Stockh.) **26**, (1966). — 3. CHORZELSKI, T. P., V. WEISS, and W. F. LEVER: Arch. derm. **93**,
570 (1966). — 4. CHORZELSKI, T. P., J. F. VON WEISS, and W. L. LEVER: Path. Europ. **1**,
268 (1966). — 5. MONTET, Y.: Thèse médecine, Nancy 1966, n° 125.

Experimental Studies on the Pathogenesis of Acantholysis in Pemphigus

P. J. GROB and TH. M. INDERBITZIN, Department of Dermatology, Tufts
University, School of Medicine, Boston, Mass. (USA)

The bullae of patients with pemphigus form due to acantholysis. Acantholysis
denotes a loss of coherence between stratified squamous cells.

The detection in the serum of patients with pemphigus of antiepithelial antibodies that are tissue specific but not species specific has led to the question as to
whether the acantholysis in pemphigus is an immunologic phenomenon.

Recent experiments in our laboratories have demonstrated that acantholysis
can be induced by an immunologic mechanism. The water soluble proteins were
extracted from rabbit esophagus mucosa with a 6% solution of KCl. The residual
tissue was washed with distilled water and then lyophilized. The lyophilized
material when suspended in the serum of patients with pemphigus absorbed the
antiepithelial antibodies present in the serum. That all the antiepithelial antibodies
had been absorbed could be proven by the fact that the previously positive indirect
immunofluorescent test had become negative.

The tissue fraction of rabbit esophagus to which the pemphigus antibodies
were bound was designated as epithelial antigen and was used for the homologous
immunization of rabbits after incorporation into complete Freund's adjuvant.

Rabbits, when repeatedly injected with the antigen, produced in their serum antiepithelial antibodies. These antibodies were bound *in vitro* to autologous, homologous and heterologous stratified squamous epithelium, but not to non-stratified epithelium, such as ileal mucosa. On indirect immunofluorescent testing, the antibodies were bound to the stratified epithelium in such a way that the immunofluorescence either outlined the boundaries of all squamous epithelial cells or merely of the basal cell layer.

Thus, the antiepithelial antibodies and the pemphigus antibodies reacted both in the immunofluorescent test and in the absorption tests with the same tissue component of stratified epithelium or at least with a component having common antigenic reacting sites.

Although the autoantibodies were present in high titers in the serum of the immunized rabbits, direct immunofluorescent tests revealed in these rabbits *in vivo* the absence of autoantibodies. This observation suggested the existence of an efficient barrier between the epidermis and the plasma preventing any possible damaging effects that the antiepithelial antibodies could have exerted *in vivo*. In further experiments *in vivo* penetration of the epithelial antibodies into the antigen-containing epidermis took place and intraepidermal acantholysis occurred, thus establishing the acantholysis can be triggered by an immunological mechanism.

In order to obtain *in vivo* pentration of the serum antibodies into the epidermis of rabbits, the epidermis was first made moderately acanthotic by daily applications for 10 days of sodium lauryl sulfonate to the skin surface. Then the cutaneous vascular permeability was increased by the local application of dry ice for 20 sec, thus initiating the extravasation of plasma into the subepidermal tissue. It was hoped that the application of both sodium lauryl sulfonate and of dry ice to the skin would alter the permeability of the dermal-subepidermal junction sufficiently to allow the passage of subepidermally accumulated plasma. Thus, if the plasma contained antiepithelial antibodies, they would then be able to react with the epithelial antigen.

In normal animals, the application of sodium lauryl sulfonate and of dry ice led only to minor epidermal changes that in no instance were suggestive of acantholysis. The intraepidermal acantholytic cleft that were produced, in animals with high titers of antiepithelial antibodies showed in the center detached acantholytic epidermal cells and at the margin partial acantholysis.

In conclusion, our observations support the view that acantholysis in pemphigus represents an immunologic phenomenon.

References. GROB, P. J., and T. M. INDERBITZIN: J. invest. Derm. (In print). — INDERBITZIN, T. M., and P. J. GROB: J. invest. Derm. (In print).

Autoantibodies in Pemphigus Foliaceus

T. A. FURTADO, A. O. LIMA, G. O. ANDRADE and O. SEABRA, Dermatologic Clinic, Faculty of Medical Sciences, Catholic University of Minas Gerais, Belo Horizonte (Brazil). First Chair of Internal Medicine, Faculty of Medicine, Federal University of Rio de Janeiro (Brazil)

BEUTNER and JORDON [1] were the first to demonstrate the presence of autoantibodies to the intercellular substance of epithelial tissues in sera of patients with pemphigus vulgaris using indirect immunofluorescent technique. The autoantibody nature of these antibodies could be demonstrated by testing the patient's skin with patient's own serum. These results were confirmed by Waldorf et al. [2] and by Chorzelski et al. [3] who found a decrease in antibody titers following treatment with corticosteroids. In this paper we present the results of our investigation carried out in patients with pemphigus foliaceus in whom serologic studies were made with different methods.

Material and Methods

Sera of patients. Samples of blood were collected from 27 patients with pemphigus foliaceus whose diagnosis were established by histological and clinical criteria.

Antigens. Two antigens were employed: crude saline extract from whole human skin and polysaccharide obtained by the phenol-water technique of Westphal et al. [4]. The following methods were used:

1. *Indirect immunofluorescent testing* (Dedmon et al. [5]).
2. *Hemagglutination:* direct hemagglutination reaction with polysaccharide from human skin (Middlebrook and Dubos [6]) and passive hemagglutination reaction with crude saline extract from human skin (Boyden [7] and Stavitsky [8]).
3. *Conglutinating complement fixation* test according to Bier et al. [9].
4. *Agar-gel diffusion precipitation* by means of Oakley and Fulthorpe's [10] method.
5. *Passive cutaneous anaphylaxis* was attempted by the method of Ovary [11].

Controls: The sera of 20 normal individuals were tested as controls.

Results and Comments

In single determinations, antibodies in the sera of 21 out of 27 patients with pemphigus foliaceus were shown to combine with an intercellular substance of the prickle-cell layer of the epidermis of normal human skin (Tab. 1). No antibodies

Table 1. *Indirect Immunofluorescent Reaction of Normal Human Skin with Sera from Patients with Pemphigus Foliaceus*
Highest Serum Dilution Giving Positive Reaction

Patient n° Sex, Age	Intracellular Substance of the Prickle cell layer	Basement zone	Cyto- plasmic	Extent of disease	Duration of disease
1 ♂ 49	1:10	—	—	slight	30 mo
2 ♂ 48	1:10	—	—	slight	2 yr
3 ♂ 30	—	—	—	none	3 mo
4 ♂ 18	—	—··	—	none	6 mo
5 ♂ 22	1:10	—	—	slight	1 yr
6 ♂ 51	1:20	—	—	moderate	15 mo
7 ♂ 48	1:10	—	—	slight	5 mo
8 ♂ 30	1:10	—	—	slight	3 yr
9 ♂ 14	1:20	—	—	slight	8 mo
10 ♂ 71	1:20	—	—	moderate	11 yr
11 ♂ 16	—	—	—·—	none	54 mo
12 ♂ 42	1:80	—	1:80	extensive	3 mo
13 ♂ 16	—	—	—	none	6 yr
14 ♂ 31	1:40	—	—	moderate	1 yr
15 ♂ 58	—	—	—	none	3 yr
16 ♂ 19	1:80	—	1:80	extensive	5 mo
17 ♀ 41	1:40	—	—	moderate	16 mo
18 ♀ 14	1:80	—	—	moderate	4 yr
19 ♀ 11	1:80	—	—	extensive	30 mo
20 ♀ 9	1:20	—	—	moderate	2 yr
21 ♀ 11	1:40	—	—	moderate	1 yr
22 ♀ 8	1:80	—	—	extensive	10 mo
23 ♀ 18	1:80	—	—	moderate	30 mo
24 ♀ 34	—	—	—	none	17 mo
25 ♀ 50	1:80	—	—	extensive	5 yr
26 ♀ 33	1:20	—	—	moderate	3 yr
27 ♀ 40	1:80	—	—	extensive	31 mo

against the basement zone of the epidermis could be demonstrated and immunofluorescent antibodies to the cytoplasm of epidermal cells were found only in the
sera of two patients. All the 20 sera of normal individuals were negative. The
six patients in whom no antibodies were found had no active disease: five were

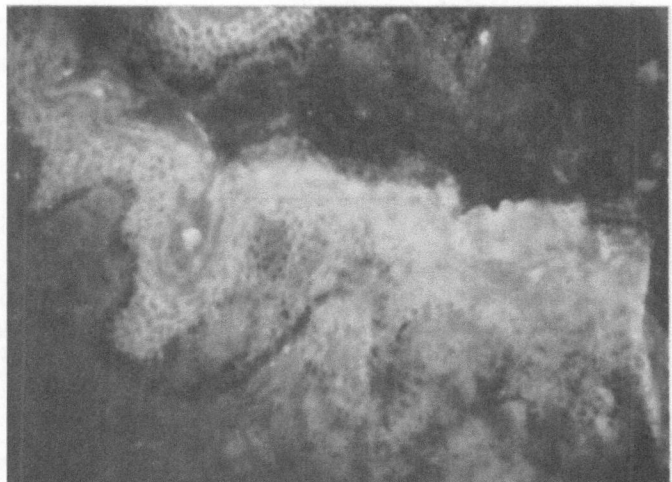

Fig. 1. Immunofluorescence of the intercellular substance of the
prickle-cell layer of the epidermis

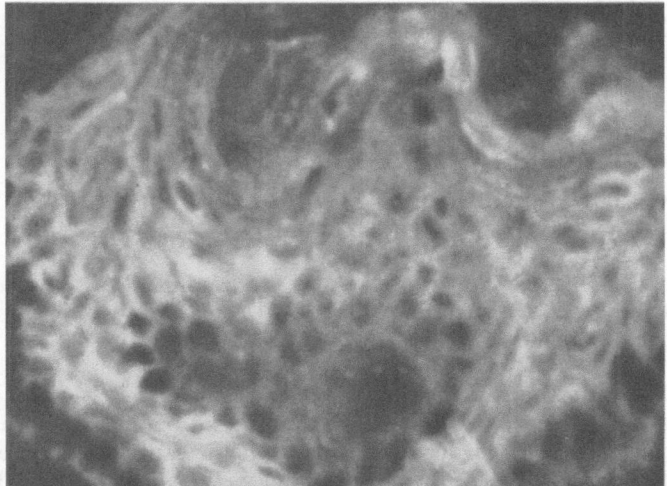

Fig. 2. Immunofluorescence limited to the intercellular substance
of the prickle-cell layer of the epidermis

under control with corticosteroids and one had discontinued therapy 1 month
before. On the contrary, in the group of 21 patients with antibodies all had skin
lesions. The serum titers of antibodies were higher (1:80) in the six patients who
had more extensive involvment of the skin. The nine patients with moderate extent
had titers ranging from 1:80 to 1:20. The lowest reactivity (1:10) was observed
in the patients with discrete skin lesions. There is, then, a correlation between the

Table 2. *Comparison of Extent of Lesions of Patients with Pemphigus Foliaceus and Serum Titers of indirect Immunofluorescent Staining of Intercellular Substance of the Prickle Cell Layer of Human Skin*

Extent of Lesions	Total n° of Cases	Titers of indirect immunofluorescent reactions				
		1:80	1:40	1:20	1:10	Neg.
Extensive	6	6	—	—	—	—
Moderate	9	2	3	4	—	—
Slight	6	—	—	1	5	—
No lesion	6	—	—	—	—	6
Total	27	8	3	5	5	6

level of antibody titers and the activity of the disease (Tab. 2). The research of antibodies to total extract of human skin and to polysaccharides isolated from human skin was negative with the methods of hemagglutination, conglutinating complement fixation, agar-gel diffusion precipitation and passive cutaneous anaphylaxis (PCA).

References. 1. Beutner, E. H., and R. E. Jordon: Proc. Soc. exp. Biol. (N.Y.) **117**, 505 (1964). — 2. Waldorf, D. S., A. J. L. Strauss, and C. W. Smith: Arch. Derm. **93**, 28 (1966). — 3. Chorzelski, T. P., J. F. von Weiss, and W. E. Lever: Arch. Derm. **93**, 570 (1966). — 4. Westphal, O., O. Luderitz und F. Bister: Z. Naturforsch. **7b**, 148 (1952). — 5. Dedmon, R. E., A. W. Holmes, and F. Deihardt,: J. Bact. **89**, 734 (1965). — 6. Middlebrook, G., and R. Dubos: J. exp. Med. **88**, 521 (1948). — 7. Boyden, S. V.: J. exp. Med. **93**, 107 (1951). — 8. Stavitsky, A. B.: J. Immunol. **72**, 360 (1954). — 9. Bier, O., R. Furtado, and E. Cisalpino: Proc. Soc. exp. Biol. (N.Y.) **95**, 335 (1957). — 10. Oakley, C. L., and A. J. Fulthorpe: J. Path. Bact. **65**, 49 (1953). — 11. Ovary, Z.: Progr. Allergy **5**, 459 (1958).

L'apport de l'immuno-fluorescence dans la mise en évidence du rôle de l'allergie à Candida albicans dans certaines dermatoses communes

P. Temime, M. Benne, M. Lebeuf et J. P. Marchand (avec la collaboration technique de Ph. Latourelle), Service de Dermatologie et de Syphiligraphie, Hôtel-Dieu, Marseille (France)

Les méthodes destinées à mettre en évidence un ou des facteurs étiologiques sont toujours accueillies avec faveur dans toutes les disciplines médicales. Il en va ainsi en Dermatologie. Aussi dès que la recherche des anticorps fluorescents anti-Candida albicans a été techniquement possible, avons-nous essayé de confirmer ou d'infirmer le rôle de l'allergie au Candida albicans dans quelques dermatoses, en confrontant les résultats obtenus avec cette méthode immunologique et ceux obtenus avec les réponses des intradermoréactions de Candidine à différentes concentrations, méthode dont l'intérêt mais aussi les limites, sont connus de tous. Qu'il nous soit permis de rappeler, à ce propos, notre travail portant sur 502 cas, rapporté à Montpellier, en Juin 1960, aux Journées Nationales des Dermatologie [1].

Ainsi, avons-nous utilisé parallèlement et conjointement ces deux techniques immuno-allergologiques chez 90 patients: *75 malades présentaient une dermatose de type allergique* où le rôle du Candida albicans pouvait, en principe, être soulevé en raison du contexte clinique et biologique; *15 autres malades, pris comme témoins,* étaient atteints d'une affection cutanée de type non allergique ou vénérienne, où le rôle du Candida albicans n'était pas concevable, si ce n'est que comme agent non pathogène ou de surinfestation.

Chez certains de ces patients, nous avons tenté de nous livrer à une étude dynamique de l'I.F., en recherchant des mouvements possibles des anticorps fluorescents avant et après les I.D.R. de Candidine, comme nous l'avons fait pour les antistreptolysines (après I.D. d'antigènes streptococciques) [2] ou pour les réagines syphilitiques (après I.D. de suspension aux tréponèmes tués) [3].

Principes des méthodes utilisées

1. Recherche des anticorps fluorescents anti-Candida albicans

La technique d'immuno-fluorescence découverte par Coons [4] dès 1941, est actuellement très largement utilisée. Des différentes modalités d'applications de celle-ci, la plus couramment utilisée est la recherche directe des anticorps, et c'est cette réaction que nous pratiquons pour mettre en évidence les anticorps anti-Candida albicans*. Nous résumons ici très sommairement cette technique que nous n'exposerons pas.

Un antigène donné est mis en contact avec le sérum suspect de contenir des anticorps spécifiques, ceux-ci vont alors se fixer sur l'antigène. Ce premier complexe antigène — anticorps ainsi formé pourra se comporter lui-même comme un antigène vis-à-vis d'un sérum anti-gamma-globuline humaine préparé expérimentalement et conjugué à de l'iso-thiocyanate de fluorescéine. Le nouveau complexe ainsi formé examiné en lumière ultra-violette, émet une fluorescence jaune caractéristique. C'est GORDON [5] qui en 1958 réussit à différencier à l'aide de cette méthode plusieurs souches de levures du genre Candida mais d'espèce différente. Ses observations devaient être confirmées plus tard par KAPLAN et KAUFMANN. L'antigène utilisé est de souche Candida albicans dont on a fixé sur lame une goutte de suspension. Les sérums à tester sont au préalable décomplémentés 15 min à 56°, puis dilués en tampon pH 7,2.

On dépose sur la suspension de levures, une goutte des dilutions sériques que l'on porte ensuite à 37°, pendant 30 min en atmosphère humide. Les lames sont alors lavées soigneusement, égouttées et reçoivent une solution d'anti-gamma-globuline humaine fluorescente. On porte à nouveau à 37° pendant une $1/2$ h en atmosphère humide, puis après lavage soigneux, les préparations sont montées entre lame et lamelle dans une goutte de glycérine tamponnée. On examine alors en lumière ultra-violette. Au cours de chaque série, on aura pris soin de préparer un sérum témoin négatif connu et un sérum témoin positif connu. Les réactions positives donnent une fluorescence jaune très franche alors que les réactions négatives ne donnent qu'une fluorescence jaunâtre ou légèrementbleutée.

Les sérums étudiés ont tous été testés qualitativement d'abord puis quantitativement ensuite.

Nous avons seulement admis comme positives les I.F. à partir du titre d'1/200; pour nous mettre à l'abri d'erreurs possibles, nous avons considéré, peut-être à tort, comme négatives les réactions au 1/100 et au 1/50 pour éliminer d'éventuelles fluorescences non spécifiques.

2. Intradermo-réactions à la candidine (I.D.R.)

Nous avons pratiqué des injections intradermiques des dilutions de Candidine de l'Institut Pasteur en solution de Coca au 5000ème, 10000ème, 50000ème, 100000ème, 500000ème et millionième. Une intradermique témoin était toujours faite avec de la solution de Coca. La lecture a été effectuée à la 48ème heure, avec recherche systématique d'une réaction focale ou syndromique (R.F.). Nous n'insisterons pas sur ces notions devenues routinières.

---

* Pour une plus grande commodité de la rédaction de notre travail, cette recherche sera désignée I.F. ou appelée «immuno-fluorescence».

Résultats

1. Globaux

    Statiques: I.F. positives depuis 1/200 jusqu'à 1/1 600   43 cas,
                I.F. négatives   47 cas.
    Comparatifs: I.F./I.D.R.

Concordances:	I.F. (+) I.D.R. (+)	37 cas (9.R.F)
	I.F. (—) I.D.R. (—)	11 cas
Discordances:	I.F. (+) l.D.R. (—)	6 cas
	I.F. (—) I.D.R. (+)	36 cas

2. Selon les dermatoses (90 cas)

    A — de type allergique (75 cas)

7 kératodermies palmaires et/ou plantaires	4 I.F. (+)
7 intertrigos (grands plis et/ou inter-orteils)	5 I.F. (+)
35 eczémas et dysidroses	13 I.F. (+)
9 urticaires chroniques	5 I.F. (+)
4 onyxis de type mycosique (1 associé à des levurides secondes, 1 associé à une colite chronique à candida)	3 I.F. (+)
3 érythèmes de type noueux ou A.N.D.	2 I.F. (+)
1 érythème polymorphe	1 I.F. (+)
2 prurits vulvaires	2 I.F. (+)
3 balanites	2 I.F. (+)
1 blépharo-conjonctivite	1 I.F. (—)
1 glossite à candida	1 I.F. (—)
1 érythrodermie	1 I.F. (+)
1 prurit anal	1 I.F. (+)

    B — de type non allergique (15 cas)

6 psoriasis	3 I.F. (+)
1 ulcère de jambe	1 I.F. (—)
1 phlébite superficielle	1 I.F. (—)
2 syphilis primo-secondaires	2 l.F. (—)
1 paraphimosis	1 I.F. (—)
1 acné	1 I.F. (—)
1 érythème prémycosique	1 I.F. (—)
1 syndrome de Reiter	1 I.F. (—)
1 urétrite amicrobienne	1 I.F. (—)

Commentaires

A. Des résultats globaux

1. *Dermatoses de type allergique.* La recherche d'anticorps fluorescents anti-Candida albicans donne globalement 39 I.F. (+) chez 75 malades atteints de dermatoses de type allergique où le rôle de Candida albicans peut être soulevé ou envisagé, en particulier dans les eczémasvésiculeux ou cornés, les intertrigos, les balanites, les prurits vulvaires, les onychoses avec paronychies et les urticaires.

Dans ce même groupe de 75 malades, les I.D.R. à la Candidine se montrent positives dans 66 cas. On constate ainsi un nombre tellement grand de réponses positives aux I.D.R., qu'il est permis de mettre en doute leur valeur spécifique, lorsqu'on les considère isolément: les réponses à caractère anamnestique témoignant d'une atteinte moniliasique antérieure doivent constituer une part non négligeable de ces nombres élevés.

2. *Dermatoses de type non-allergique.* Chez 15 malades atteints d'affections cutanées ou vénériennes de type bon allergique, l'I.F. a été trouvée quatre fois positive. Dans trois cas, il s'est agi de psoriasis comportant des lésions des plis: un psoriasis interverti et un psoriasis érythrodermique. Dans ce même groupe, les I.D.R. se sont montrées neuf fois positives, donc deux fois plus souvent que les I.F.

B. *Confrontation de concordances et discordances*

Un dicton français dit: «Une hirondelle ne fait pas le printemps». En Médecine, un seul signe clinique ou biologique ne fait pas le diagnostic. Il est donc important pour étayer un diagnostic étiologique de disposer de plusieurs éléments aussi bien dans le domaine clinique que paraclinique. C'est ainsi qu'il nous a semblé important de confronter:

1. le parallélisme des I.F. et des réponses aux I.D.R./CA
2. les R.F.
3. les I.F. effectuées avant et après I.D.R. à la CA
4. la présence ou l'absence de CA dans les lésions.

1. *Parallélisme entre I.F. et I.D.R.*

1. *Dermatoses de type allergique.* Chez 36 malades, nous avons noté une concordance entre les I.F. (+) et les I.D.R. (+):
dans 4 kératodermies ou eczémas cornés sur 7 cas:
dans 4 intertrigos divers sur 7 cas;
dans 13 eczémas et dysidroses sur 35 cas;
dans 5 urticaires sur 9 cas;
dans 3 onychoses sur 4 cas;
dans 1 érythème polymorphe sur 1 cas;
dans 2 érythèmes noueux ou apparentés sur 3 cas;
dans 2 prurits vulvaires sur 2 cas;
dans 2 balanites sur 3 cas.
Chez de tels malades, la concordance des I.F. (+) et des I.D.R. (+) est très en faveur d'une allergie à Candida Albicans.

2. *Dermatoses de type non allergique.* Parmi les 15 malades, on trouve chez l'un deux seulement une concordance entre I.F. (+) et I.D.R. (+): il s'agit d'un psoriasis érythrodermique ayant comporté différentes lésions des plis qui peuvent constituer un focal sepsis moniliasique. Le parallélisme entre la positivité des I.F. et des I.D.R. est donc particulièrement restreinte, ce qui constitue un argument d'élimination du rôle de l'allergie à Candida.

2. *Les R.F. après I.D.R./CA*

Les R.F. ou réactions syndrômiques ne sont pas tellement fréquentes, dans notre série de malades puisqu'elles ont été notées seulement neuf fois et cela uniquement chez des malades atteints de dermatoses de type allergique et, ce qui plus est, seulement chez des malades où I.F. (+) et I.D.R. (+) étaient concordantes: dans un cas de kératodermie sur sept, et un intertrigo sur sept. Dans deux dysidroses palmo-plantaires et un eczéma (sur 35) dans une onychose (sur 3); dans une balanite (sur 3) et sur deux urticaires (sur 9 cas). Il est à souligner que dans aucun des cas de dermatoses non allergiques, il n'a été observé de R.F. et cela même quand les I.D.R. étaient fortement positives.

3. *Les I.F. avant et après I.D.R./CA*

Dans un trop petit nombre de cas, nous avons pu nous livrer à une sorte d'étude dynamique des I.F. Nous avons noté une ascension du taux des anticorps fluorescents anti-candida albicans dans quatre cas seulement: 1 dysidrose, où le taux est passé de 1/200 à 1/400, puis à 1/800; 1 eczéma papulovésiculeux où l'I.F. négative avant est devenue positive au 1/400è après les I.D.R.; 1 urticaire avait un taux initial de 1/400è qui est devenu 1/800è, dans une autre urticaire l'I.F. est passée du 1/50è au 1/200è. Parcontre, dans un intertrigo, un psoriasis interverti et dans un cas de diabétides génitales, le taux est resté identique (1/800—1/800; 1/400—

Tableau 1

Dermatoses	Résultats globaux		Concordances et discordances IF/I.D.R.			
	IF (+)	I.D.R. (+)	IF (+) IDR (+)	IF (−) IDR (−)	IF (+) IDR (−)	IF (−) IDR (+)
1. Type allergique						
7 Kératodermies — ecz. cornés	4	7	4 (1 R.F.)	0	0	3
7 Intertrigos	5	6	4 (1 R.F.)	0	1	2
35 Eczémas et dysidroses	13	32	13 (3 R.F.)	3	0	19
9 Urticaires et prurigos	5	8	5 (2 R.F.)	1	0	3
4 Onychoses et paronychies	3	3	3 (1 R.F.)	1	0	0
1 Erythème polymorphe	1	1	1	0	0	0
3 Erythèmes noueux ou appar.	2	3	2	0	0	1
2 Prurits vulvaires	2	2	2	0	0	0
3 Balanites	2	2	2 (1 R.F.)	1	0	0
1 Blépharo-conjonctivite	0	1	0	0	0	1
1 Glossite	0	1	0	0	0	1
1 Erythrodermie	1	0	0	0	1	0
1 Prurit anal	1	0	0	0	1	0
75	39	66	36	6	3	30
2. Type non allergique						
6 Psoriasis	3	3	1	3	2	0
1 Ulcère de jambe	0	0	0	1	0	0
1 Phlébite superficielle	1	0	0	0	1	0
2 Syphilis primo-secondaires	0	2	0	0	0	2
1 Paraphimosis	0	0	0	1	0	0
1 Acné	0	1	0	0	0	0
1 Syndrome de Reiter	0	1	0	0	0	1
1 Erythème pré-mycosique	0	1	0	0	0	1
1 Urétrite avec méatite	0	1	0	0	0	1
15	4	9	1	5	3	6

1/400; 1/800—1/800). Il faut souligner que parmi ces quatre cas où l'on a observé une ascension de l'I.F., deux (une dysidrose et une intertrigo) avaient montré une R.F. Ces deux derniers cas, nous paraissent répondre formellement à une allergie à Candida albicans car ils ont montré: concordance I.F: (+) I.D.R. (+), R.F. et I.F. ascensionnelle après I.D.R.

4. A présence ou l'absence de Candida albicans dans les lésions

Elle nous parait être seulement un argument d'approche. La présence de Candida albicans peut étre constatée au titre de saprophyte, elle n'implique pas son rôle antigénique dans la dermatose en cours. Nous avons noté la présence de Candida albicans dans les ongles chez un kératodermique, dans les squames d'un intertrigo, dans les ongles de trois onychoses, dans les selles d'un urticarien, dans le vagin de deux prurits vulvaires, sur la langue dans une glossite, que l'on peut considérer comme des manifestations allergiques à des levures, mais aussi dans le vagin d'une acnéique après antibiothérapie récente. Le C.A. ne peut pas être considéré comme antigénique dans un tel cas. A l'opposé, la recherche négative de C.A. dans les lésions ne peut faire éliminer son rôle comme allergène à partir d'un focal sepsis méconnu.

A la suite de notre travail, il nous apparait que: *l'association de trois ou mieux de quatre critères immuno-allergologiques: concordance I.F. (+)/I.D.R. (+), R.F. et augmentation de l'I.F. après I.D.R. de Candidine* constitue une preuve de la réalité du rôle de l'allergie à Candida albicans dans les dermatoses où l'on les constate. Il en a été ainsi dans certains eczémas et dans les urticaires. *L'association de deux critères: I.F. (+) et I.D.R. (+) constitue pour nous un faisceau d'arguments très probants en faveur de l'étiologie allergique moniliasique dans les dermatoses inflammatoires communes: eczémas, intertrigos, prurits ano-génitaux, paronychies et aussi urticaires.*

Considérés séparément, les résultats des I.F. et des I.D.R. (sans R.F.) sont beaucoup plus discutables. Les tests positifs isolés, immunologiques ou allergologiques ont peu de valeur spécifique pour mettre en évidence une allergie «actuelle» an cours, à candida albicans.

Tableau 2. *Concordances*

Affections	IF (+) IDR (+)	R.F.	I.F. ↗
Kératodermies	4 s/ 7 cas	1	
Intert igos	4 s/ 7 cas	1	
Eczémas et dysidroses	13 s/35 cas	3	2
Urticaires	5 s/ 9 cas	2	2
Onycho-paronychies	3 s/ 4 cas	1	
Erythèmes noueux ou apparentes	2 s/ 3 cas		
Prurits vulvaires	2 s/ 2 cas		
Balanites	2 s/ 3 cas	1	

Conclusions

L'intérêt de la recherche des anticorps fluorescents anti-candida albicans nous apparaît d'emblée comme devant être souligné dans l'étude étiologique des dermatoses inflammatoires où le rôle de l'allergie à Candida albicans peut être suspecté ou avancé d'après les signes cliniques et les examens de laboratoire. Cet intérêt est d'autant plus grand que le taux de la dilution sérique est plus élevé et que les réponses positives aux I.D.R. de Candidine s'accompagnant d'une réaction focale ou syndromique.

Ainsi, certains résultats de l'enquête allergologique peuvent être confirmés par les données de cette technique immunologique qui mérite de figurer dans les examens biologiques, systématiques, pratiqués pour la *mise en évidence de l'allergie au Candida albicans dans certaines affections cutanées communes: eczémas, inter-trigos, prurits ano-génitaux, paronychies* et aussi *urticaires*. Chez de tels malades, la concordance en positivité des résultats des méthodes immuno-allergologiques, forme un faisceau d'arguments en faveur de la réalité de l'allergie moniliasique en Dermatologie qui, on le sait, n'est pas encore admise sans discussion, ni scepticisme.

Bibliographie. 1. Temime, P., P. Y. Castelain, J. Besson, Y. Privat et M.Benne: Bull. Soc. franç. Derm. Syph. **1960**, 738. — 2. Temime, P., M. Benne et Ph. Santini: Bull. Soc. franç. Derm. Syph. **1962**, 238. — 3. Ranque, J., G. Tramier et P. Temime: Presse méd. **1963**, 413. — 4. Coons, A. H., H. J. Creech, R. N. Jones et Berliner: J. Immunol. **45**, 159 (1942). — 5. Gordon, M. A.: Proc. Soc. exp. Biol. (N.Y.) **97**, 684 (1958).

Recherches électrophorétiques et immunophorétiques en moyens gélifiés sur protéines de muscle strié dans différentes collagénoses d'intérêt dermatologique

G. Martina et A. Midana, Clinique Dermatologique de l'Université de Turin (Italie)

Il y a quelques années, dans une note préalable, nous avons signalé les résultats de nos premières recherches, effectuées sur gel d'agar, sur les propriétés électro-cinétiques des protéines extractibles à basse force ionique des muscles humains normaux.

Dans la suite, toute une série de recherches sur d'autres moyens gélifiés, nous ont permis de confirmer l'existence d'un profil électromyographique, qui est caractéristique et constant pour les deux types de muscles humains normaux: lisse et strié.

Quoique difficiles, ces recherches préliminaires étaient, en rapport au caractère fragmentaire des données bibliographiques à notre disposition, base indispensable dans la suite pour un étude des protéines musculaires pathologiques.

Deux ordres de considération peuvent justifier le fait de s'être engagés dans ces recherches: d'une part si l'on considère qu'à côté de la dermatomyosite, dont le tableau clinique est dominé par la lésion musculaire, d'autres graves dermatoses, telles que l'érythématode et la sclérodermie, peuvent présenter en outre des lésions cutanées caractéristiques une participation musculaire, bien que l'extension et la précocité d'apparition puissent en être différentes; d'autre part si on considère que les dosages cortisoniques élevés et prolongés, qui peuvent être indispensables dans certaines dermatoses ou dans périodes évolutives particulières, intéressent certainement le métabolisme musculaire.

A la suite de ces considérations et, en plus, intéressés par des indications d'auteurs concernant les recherches effectuées dans myopathies neurologiques sur la base de nos données obtenues par l'étude électrophorétique sur moyens gélifiés, nous avons pensé qu'il serait intéressant étudier les muscles striés de malades dermatologiques.

Dans ce but, nous avons préparé des extraits à basse force ionique de muscles squelettiques, prélevés sous anesthésie locale, chez 6 sujets atteints de dermato-myosite, chez 3 malades d'érythématode chronique, chez 2 cas d'érythématode subaigu et enfin dans 2 cas de sclérodermie diffuse. Ces extraits ont été soumis, selon modalités que nous avons illustrées précédemment, à l'électrophorèse sur agar et sur acétate de cellulose, comparant naturellement les «profils» avec ceux qui sont caractéristiques des muscles striés humains normaux.

Cette brève note préalable expose les résultats que nous avons obtenus: *modifications des muscles striés chez les malades atteints de dermatomyosite*. Il est clairement visible, soit sur l'acétate, soit sur agar, que le profil électromyophorétique,

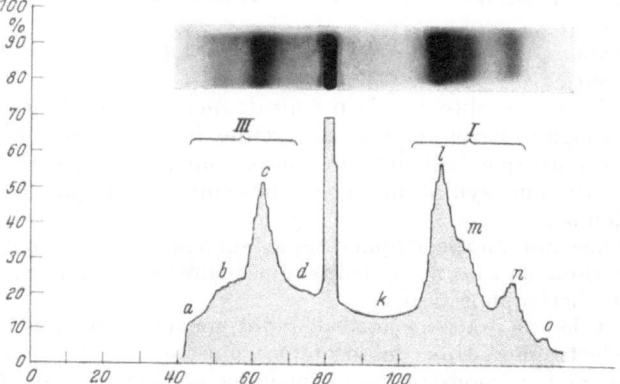

Fig. 1. Electromyophérogramme striée humaine normale

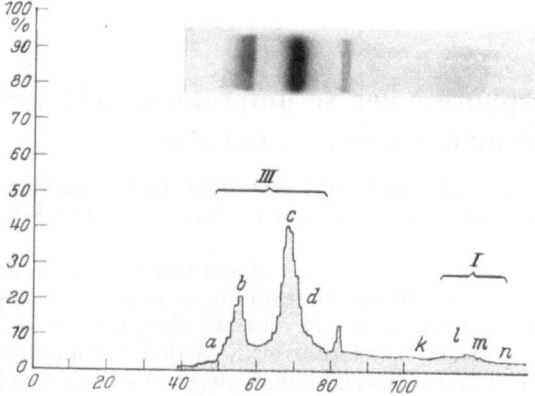

Fig. 2. Electromyophérogramme striée dans la phase finale de la dermatomyosite

déjà dans la phase du début de la dermatose, se modifie à cause d'une diminution considérable du pourcentage des myogènes et d'un accroissement relatif des myoalbumines; la fraction myogène la plus atteinte semble peut-être la «l», alors que l'accroissement des myoalbumines s'observe surtout pour les fractions «b» et ‹d».

Dans les stades plus avancés de la dermatose le tableau myophorétique démontre une ultérieure diminution imposante du groupe des myogènes qui peut arriver jusqu'à une disparition totale de différentes fractions, tandis que le pourcentage des myoalbumines demeure toujours élevé.

Le fait que le tableau électrophorétique du muscle strié dans la dermatomyosite semble présenter des analogies évidentes avec celui du muscle lisse humain normal, est suggestif. Recherches ultérieures et approfondies sont souhaitables. Pour le

moment, qu'il nous suffise d'avoir pu démontrer que déjà dàns le *stade initial* de la
dermatomyosite, tout le profil électromyographique est altéré, surtout à la charge
des myogènes.

Au stade suivant ou plus grave de la dermatose, tandis que les myogènes conti-
nuent à se réduire, il ne semble pas y avoir d'autres modifications à la charge des
myoalbumines, fait qui — si confirmé — peut présenter un certain intérêt s'opposant à la théorie de FISCHER selon laquelle les myoalbumines tireraient leur
origine de la décomposition ou de la synthèse manquée des autres protéines
musculaires.

*Modifications des muscles striés dans l'érythématodes subaigu et chronique et dans
la sclérodermie.*

Aucun des tracés obtenus n'a permis de mettre en évidence des modifications
certaines et significatives pour les différentes fractions protéiniques musculaires,
démontrant ainsi que, soit dans la sclérodermie, soit dans l'érythématode tout
étant présente une symptomatologie musculaire clinique, le tissu musculaire
résulte indemne.

Recherches immunoélectrophorétiques sur agar ont pu démontrer que la contamination sérique de tous nos extraits musculaires est rare et ne peut pas infirmer
les résultats électrophorétiques.

Au point de vue pratique nous pouvons conclure que dans la dermatomyosite
l'examen électrophorétique des protéines musculaires, étant donné la difficulté
bien connue de la démonstration histologique de l'existence de lésions précoces de
la fibre musculaire, peut représenter un élément diagnostique très ·important et
précoce.

Immunoelektrophorese der Serumproteine bei akuten und chronischen Formen des Erythematodes

T. BIELICKÝ, L. MALINA und J. OPPLT, Dermatologische Klinik der Medizinisch-
Hygienischen Fakultät der Karls-Universität Prag (Tschechoslowakei)

Da die Immunoelektrophorese einen tieferen Einblick in die Veränderungen der
Serumproteine ermöglicht, hielten wir es für angebracht, eine Gruppe von 45 Kranken mit verschiedenen Formen des Erythematodes (E.) von diesem Standpunkt
aus zu untersuchen. Vorausgesetzt, daß der E. zu den Autoimmunitätskrankheiten
gehört, ist zu erwarten, daß Abweichungen insbesondere in den Immunoglobulin-
fraktionen vorhanden sein werden. Nicht weniger wichtig sind auch die Unterschiede zwischen den einzelnen Formen des E., welche eventuell über ihre gegenseitigen Beziehungen informieren könnten.

Wie in unseren früheren Mitteilungen, teilten wir unsere E.-Patienten in vier
Gruppen ein: akuter E. 9 Fälle, chronischer disseminierter E. 10 Fälle, chronischer
diskoider E. 14 Fälle und chronischer nichtvernarbender E. 12 Fälle. Über diese
letzte Gruppe besteht keine Einigkeit über ihre Zugehörigkeit zum E., und sie
wird auch als „Lymphocytic infiltration" von JESSNER und KANOFF bezeichnet.

Die Untersuchungen wurden in zwei Phasen durchgeführt. In der ersten wurde
die klassische Immunoelektrophorese benutzt. Auf diese Weise wurden die Konzentrationsänderungen und semiquantitativen Abweichungen der Fraktionskon-
zentrationen bewertet. Die zweite Phase folgte etwa nach 4 Monaten. Dabei wurden
einerseits die Ergebnisse der ersten Phase neu überprüft, andererseits wurden
die Immunoglobuline und andere wichtige Fraktionen mit der quantitativen

Immunodiffusionsmethode von OPPLT durchgeführt. Das Prinzip beruht in der Messung der radialen Diffusion des aufgelösten Proteins in einem 1,5% Agar-Gel. Die Diffusion der Proteine steht im direkten Verhältnis zu dem Logarithmus deren Konzentration.

Die Ergebnisse der klassischen Immunoelektrophorese zeigten, daß Konfigurations- und Konzentrationsänderungen oder beide in 25 der 45 Fälle, d. h. in 55%, vorhanden sind. Beim akuten E. sind diese Änderungen in allen Fällen zu beobachten. Bei den chronischen Formen sind die Änderungen am häufigsten beim chronischen nichtvernarbenden E. (75%), weiter folgten der chronische diskoide E. mit 35% und der chronische disseminierte E. überraschenderweise nur in 20% der Fälle.

In der zweiten Phase wurden nur diejenigen Fälle untersucht, welche in der ersten Phase Abweichungen zeigten. Quantitativ wurden insbesondere die IgG-, IgA-, IgM-, Beta-$_{1A}$- und Beta-$_{1C}$-Fraktionen untersucht. Die Frequenz und Art der Abweichungen beim akuten und beim chronischen diskoiden E. blieben während der 4 Monate unverändert. Eindeutig ist die Vermehrung der IgA-Fraktion bei dem akuten E. Dies steht im Einklang mit den Beobachtungen von JABLONSKA, SELIGMAN, HERMANN und SCHULZ u. a. Gleich häufig waren die Konzentrationsänderungen der IgM-Fraktion, doch in verschiedener Richtung. Die IgG- und Beta-$_{1C}$-Fraktionen waren nur in einem Drittel der Fälle vermindert. Konfigurationsänderungen sind fast in allen Fällen vorhanden gewesen.

Eine ähnliche Stabilität der Immunoglobuline wurde auch beim chronischen diskoiden E. gefunden. Im Gegensatz zum akuten E. kommt hier regelmäßig eine Konzentrationsverminderung der IgG-Fraktion vor. In den IgA- und IgM-Fraktionen sind Abweichungen nur in der Hälfte der Fälle zu finden. Auch hier sind die Konfigurationsänderungen regelmäßig. Unerwartet waren die mäßigen Veränderungen bei dem chronischen disseminierten E. mit Fraktionsänderungen nur bei zwei der zehn Kranken, und zwar in einem Fall Konfigurationsänderungen, im zweiten in der Konzentration der IgA-Fraktion.

Am wenigsten stabil waren die Änderungen bei dem nichtvernarbenden chronischen E., und zwar nicht in der Häufigkeit der Abweichungen, sondern im Befall der einzelnen Fraktionen. Die Ergebnisse bei dieser Gruppe ermöglichen keine Schlußfolgerungen.

Unsere Befunde sind teilweise nicht im Einklang mit den bisherigen Beobachtungen. Es steht fest, daß die Immunoglobuline beim akuten E. im höchsten Maße verändert sind. Die Veränderungen bei den chronischen Formen des E. stellen die Frage, ob die bisherige Auffassung über die Reihenfolge der Krankheitsintensitäten der einzelnen Formen des chronischen E. richtig ist. Die Änderungen bei dem nichtvernarbenden chronischen E. scheinen dafür zu sprechen, daß hier eine auffällige Immunitätsstörung vorliegt.

Immunologic Defect of the Skin in Lymphadenopathy

Y. NOGUCHI, K. ISHIWARA, M. HIGUCHI and S. YOSHIDA, Department of Dermatology, University School of Medicine, Yokohama (Japan)

Reviewing a large number of literatures on inadequacies of the specific immunologic defenses, GOOD et al. [1] described three major categories of immunological deficiency diseases. These are agammaglobulinemia-hypogammaglobulinemia, Hodgkin's disease including a lymphoma-leukemia disease and sarcoidosis, where the latter two diseases are usually associated with lymphadenopathy, and they have a tendency to suppress tuberculin reaction. While a complication with lymphoma and herpes zoster is frequently observed. In order to make a study of relationships between skin reactions to a group of delayed reacting antigens and lymphadenopathy, those patients with lymphoma-leukemia group, sarcoidosis and herpes zoster were examined.

Methods and Materials

As a group of delayed reacting antigens, 1:2000 and 1:100 old tuberculin, purified staphylotoxoid and purified vaccine lymph were employed, and they were given intracutaneously. The tests were read after 48 h for tuberculin and purified vaccine lymph and after 24 h for purified staphylotoxoid respectively. Patients with a lymphoma-leukemia disease (40 cases), sarcoidosis (7 cases) and herpes zoster (104 cases) were tested, however, cellular transfer of tuberculin hypersensitivity originated by LAWRENCE [2, 3] was tried in a small number of cases with or without lymphoma. Further, immunoelectrophoretic analysis of sera from the selected cases has been made in this study.

Results

Skin tests revealed that a general depression of the delayed type of allergic reactivity in patients with a lymphoma-leukemia disease exclusive of myelogenous leukemia which is lacking in lymphadenopathy. However, such a cutaneous anergy to tuberculin was conspicuous as compared with other delayed reacting antigens

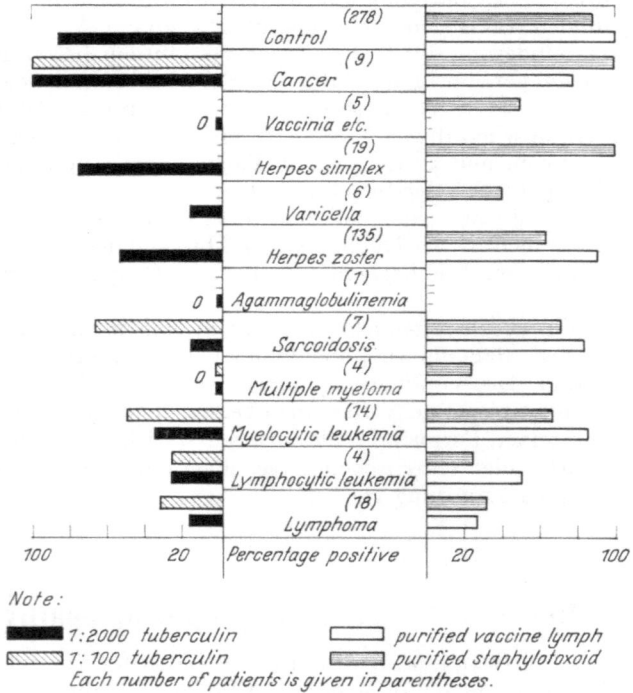

Fig. Incidence of positive skin reaction to delayed reacting antigens

(figure). Also, anergy to tuberculin was observed in both multiple myeloma and agammaglobulinemia. Suppressed tuberculin reaction in patients with sarcoidosis seemed rather unsteady, as their negative reaction to 1:2000 tuberculin was readily converted to positive reaction by using 1:100 tuberculin, while the reaction in lymphoma was usually unchanged. Relatively high incidence of tuberculin anergy in herpes zoster is worthy of notice in comparison with normal response in herpes simplex, however, the conversion to positive reaction was common as herpes zoster improved. Of 104 cases with herpes zoster, 50 showed attenuated reaction to tuberculin, where 37 (74%) including 4 cases of the disseminated type were associated with lymphadenopathy, while 24 (44.4%) out of 54 cases with positive tuberculin reaction had lymphadenopathy (Table). This suggests that lymphadenopathy may play a significant role in anergy to tuberculin. In the meantime, normal response to delayed reacting antigens was observed in herpes simplex, however, low incidence of tuberculin hypersensitivity in both varicella and vaccinia may due to lack of experience in tuberculous infection.

Table. *Relationship between Lymphadenopathy and Tuberculin Reaction*

	No. of cases	(A) Result of tuberculin reaction[a]	(B) Associated with lymphadenopathy	Percentage (B/A)
Herpes zoster	104	+ 54	24	44.4 (%)
		− 50	37	74.0 (%)
Herpes simplex	16	+ 12	3	25.0 (%)
		− 4	2	50.0 (%)

[a] 1:2000 Old tuberculin was employed.

Selected cases with anergy to tuberculin, including a lymphoma-leukemia disease 3, multiple myeloma 2, sarcoidosis 1, herpes zoster 2 and varicella 1, were given the intracutaneous injection of peripheral blood leukocytes from a tuberculinpositive donor 24, 48, or 78 h before tuberculin injection. By this passive cellular transfer those patients with sarcoidosis, herpes zoster and varicella readily converted to a positive tuberculin reaction, while one case with multiple myeloma got a tuberculin hypersensitivity by this procedure. This indicates that the nature of an immunologic defect in these diseases are different, however, the anergic patients with malignant lymphadenopathy seem to resist such conversion.

Immunoelectrophoretic analysis of 35 sera from the patients mentioned above revealed that the conversion of tuberculin hypersensitivity is not correlate with a change in patterns of major immunoglobulins, such as IgG, IgA and IgM.

Comment

Since 1952, when BRUTON [4] originally described a child with congenital agammaglobulinemia, special attention has been drawn to the inadequacies of the specific immunologic defenses. The concept of immunological deficiency diseases (GOOD et al.) [1] and that of Antikörpermangelsyndrom (BARANDUN et al.) [5] make a great contribution to understand this unique phenomenon "immunologic defect" in man, which is classified into three major categories, such as agammaglobulinemia-hypogammaglobulinemia, a lymphoma-leukemia disease and sarcoidosis.

Regardless of the first category, main cause of which is a deficit in immunoglobulins, an attention should be drawn to the lymphadenopathy which is fairly common to both Hodgkin's disease and sarcoidosis, while both are anergic to tuberculin and suffer from pathologic processes which involve the lymphoid and reticuloendothelial system. However, major difference is that the conversion to positive tuberculin reaction by cellular transfer is successful in sarcoidosis as URBACH et al. [6] reported already, while it is unsuccessful in Hodgkin's disease. Another point concerning a deficit in allergy of the delayed type may be a frequent

occurrence of herpes zoster in a lymphoma-leukemia disease [7 to 11], though most
of them had been presumably previously exposed to varicella-zoster virus.

These findings suggest that an involvement of lymphoid and reticuloendothelial
system disturbs a production of cellular antibodies which may cause immunologic
defect, particularly cause a general depression of the delayed hypersensitivity.

References. 1. GOOD, R. A., W. D. KELLY, J. RÖSTEIN, and R. L. VARCO: Progr. Allergy
6, 187 (1962). — 2. LAWRENCE, H. S.: Proc. Soc. exp. Biol. (N.Y.) 71, 516 (1949). — 3. LAWRENCE,
H. S.: J. clin. Invest. 34, 219 (1955). — 4. BRUTON, O. C.: Pediatrics 9, 722 (1952). —
5. BARANDUN, S. VON, H. J. HUSER und A. HÄSSIG: Schweiz. med. Wschr. 88, 78 (1958). —
6. URBACH, F., M. SONES, and H. L. ISRAEL: New. Engl. J. Med. 247, 794 (1952). — 7. WRIGHT,
E. T., and L. H. WINER: Arch. Derm. 84, 242 (1961). — 8. DE MORGANS, J. M., and R. R.
KIELAND: Arch. Derm. 75, 193 (1957). — 9. BLUEFARB, S. M.: Arch. Derm. Syph. (Chic.) 57,
319 (1948). — 10. RODNAN, G. P., and G. W. RAKE: New Engl. J. Med. 254, 472 (1956). —
11. MERSELIS, jr., J. G., D. KAYE, and E. W. HOOK: Arch. intern. Med. 113, 679 (1964).

Immunologische Untersuchungen von Lymphocytenkulturen*
Eine diagnostische Methode in der Dermatologie

H. J. HEITMANN, Klinik und Poliklinik für Hautkrankheiten, Klinikum Essen
der Universität Bochum (Deutschland)

Kultiviert man Lymphocyten des Blutes in einem Nährmedium bestimmter
Zusammensetzung, so hat sich gezeigt, daß diese Zellen unter „in vitro" Bedingungen nicht nur am Leben erhalten werden können, sondern daß die Lymphocyten in Gegenwart bestimmter Stimulantien zu proliferativen Reaktionen und
mitotischen Teilungen veranlaßt werden können. PEARMAIN (1963), HIRSCHHORN
u. Mitarb. gelang es vor 4 Jahren, immunologisch kompetente Lymphocyten von
tuberkulinpositiven Patienten durch das spezifische Antigen (Tuberkulin) zu zahlreichen Mitosen zu stimulieren. Ferner konnten dabei Transformationen der
kleinen mononucleären Elemente in große, unreif erscheinende, basophile lymphoblastenähnliche Zellen mit nucleoliartigen Chromatinverdichtungen der Kerne beobachtet werden.

Nach Kenntnis von diesen Untersuchungen lag es nahe, aus dem dargelegten
immunbiologischen Verhalten der Lymphocyten eine Versuchsanordnung zu entwickeln, um fraglich antigene Substanzen zu testen (HEITMANN, 1967). Dabei
interessierte uns die Penicillinallergie in ganz besonderem Maße. Es standen uns
Patienten zur Verfügung, die urticarielle, exanthematische und ekzematöse Hautveränderungen nach Penicillin geboten hatten. Zur Kontrolle untersuchten wir
gleichzeitig gesunde Personen, bei denen eine Penicillinallergie zuvor sicher ausgeschlossen wurde.

Die Methodik war zunächst relativ kompliziert. Jetzt gelang es uns jedoch,
eine wesentlich einfachere Mikro-Vollblutmethode zu entwickeln, die sich nicht
nur für wissenschaftliche, sondern auch für routinemäßige Untersuchungen eignet.
Es werden Testkulturen angelegt, denen das zu untersuchende Antigen hinzugefügt wird. Ferner werden sog. negative und positive Kontrollkulturen durchgeführt. In den negativen Kontrollkulturen wird auf den Zusatz von Stimulantien
verzichtet. In ihnen findet man nach erfolgter Inkubation überwiegend kleine,
mononucleäre Elemente und keine Mitosen. In den positiven Kontrollkulturen
kommt es unter dem Einfluß von einem unspezifischen pflanzlichen Stimulans
(Phytohämagglutinin) regelmäßig zur Transformation der Lymphocyten in große,

* Mit Unterstützung der Deutschen Forschungsgemeinschaft.

unreif erscheinende, basophile lymphoblastenähnliche Zellen mit nucleoliartigen Chromatinverdichtungen der Kerne und zu zahlreichen Mitosen. In den Testkulturen schließlich kann man beobachten, daß die immunologisch kompetenten Lymphocyten von sensibilisierten Patienten (positiver Allergietest) unter dem Einfluß des spezifischen Antigens (Penicillin) ein Zellbild zeigen, das mit den positiven Kontrollkulturen vergleichbar ist, während bei den gesunden Personen (negativer Allergietest) dieser Befund vermißt wird. Ihr Zellbild läßt sich vielmehr mit den negativen Kontrollkulturen vergleichen.

Zur Untersuchung der Zellkulturen eignet sich die Fluorescenzmikroskopie in hervorragendem Maße. Als Farbstoff wird Acridinorange von uns verwandt. Auf Grund seiner metachromatischen Fähigkeit lassen sich damit nicht nur Zellstrukturen, sondern auch histochemische Besonderheiten demonstrieren. Bei Anwendung in einem bestimmten pH-Bereich stellt sich die Desoxyribonucleinsäure grün dar, während die Ribonucleinsäure eine rote Fluorescenz aufweist. Ein Nachteil der Analyse besteht darin, daß die optische Auflösung geringer sein kann als bei der Hellfeldmikroskopie, da das Licht vom fluorescierenden Objekt nach allen Richtungen ausgestrahlt wird. Der unbestreitbare Vorteil der Methode besteht aber in der überaus einfachen und raschen Handhabung sowie in der Möglichkeit, detaillierte Kenntnisse an lebenden Zellen zu gewinnen. Freilich verlieren die Objekte nach längerer UV-Bestrahlung ihre Vitalität und Leuchtkraft. In dem Fall kann jedoch die Mikrophotographie helfend einspringen, um einmal erhobene Befunde sogleich zu dokumentieren.

Auf den dann gezeigten Diapositiven weisen die Kerne der Leukocyten eine leuchtend grüne Fluorescenz auf. Einzeln liegende kleine Zellen charakterisieren ein „negatives" Resultat. Demgegenüber sind die „positiven" Ergebnisse besonders bemerkenswert. Die Zellen finden sich nicht mehr einzeln, sondern zu kleineren und größeren Gruppen vereint. Der Durchmesser der Kerne ist erheblich vergrößert. Ferner erkennt man in ihnen nucleolitartige Verdichtungen und in einer ganzen Reihe von Zellen rot fluorescierende Granula im Cytoplasma. Zahlreiche Mitosen, bei denen die Chromosomen besonders bei mikroskopischer Betrachtung deutlich zur Darstellung kommen, sind der Ausdruck lebhafter proliferativer Zellreaktionen und zugleich das Resultat einer spezifischen Stimulation im Falle einer Penicillinallergie.

Zusammenfassend läßt sich folgendes über die „in vitro" Kultivierung von Lymphocyten sagen: Handelt es sich um immunologisch kompetente Zellen von Patienten, die gegenüber Penicillin sensibilisiert sind, so kommt es nach Zusatz des spezifischen Antigens (Penicillin) zum Kulturmedium zur Transformation der kleinen mononucleären Elemente. Nach 4 bis 5 Tagen werden zahlreiche Mitosen und überwiegend große, lymphoblastenartig erscheinende Zellen mit nucleoliartigen Chromatinverdichtungen der Kerne beobachtet. Dieses immunbiologische Verhalten eröffnet die Möglichkeit zu einem neuartigen „in vitro" Allergietest. Wir sind bemüht, unsere Untersuchungen nicht nur bei der Penicillinallergie durchzuführen, sondern diese auch auf andere fraglich allergene Substanzen auszudehnen.

Literatur. HEITMANN, H. J.: Hautarzt 18, 152 (1967); — Hautarzt 18, 459 (1967). — HIRSCHHORN, K., F. BACH, R. L. KOLODNY, I. FIRSCHEIN, and N. HASHEM: Science 142. 1185 (1963). — PEARMAIN, E., R. R. LYCETTE, and P. H. FITZGERALD: Lancet 1963, I, 637,

Mechanisms of Anaphylaxis

M. W. GREAVES, University Department of Dermatology, Newcastle upon Tyne (England)

Characterisation of anaphylactic histamine release from basophil leucocytes has been carried out using a new in vitro system derived from the rabbit, and the results have enabled comparisons to be made with mechanisms of anaphylaxis in three other species: man, the guinea pig and the rat.

A method has been devised for obtaining a cell suspension rich in basophils but free of platelets from rabbit blood using differential and density gradient centrifugation. 25 ml samples of blood yield basophil suspensions containing 2 to 3μg histamine, the amount correlating significantly with the basophil count in the suspension. The estimated histamine content (ng) of 10^3 rabbit basophils is 1.3 ± 0.3 S.D. Sustained active sensitisation of rabbit basophils was readily achieved by use of adjuvant, and basophil suspensions from sensitised animals released 40 to 80% of their histamine on challenge with antigen in vitro at 37 °C. Histamine release was measured by bioassay.

Rate of histamine release from rabbit basophils (50% in $2\frac{1}{2}$ min) is slower than from rat or guinea pig mast cells, but faster than from human leucocytes (50% in 10 min). Temperature sensitivity in the rabbit basophil system resembles that seen in the guinea pig and rat. Release is abolished below 30 °C and markedly reduced above 43 °C, maximum release occurring at 37 to 40 °C. Omission of calcium from the system abolishes histamine release from rabbit basophils, human leucocytes and rat mast cells. In the guinea pig inhibition is incomplete unless a chelating agent is added. Sulphydryl blocking agents (Iodoacetate, N-ethylmaleimide and parachloromercuribenzoate) inhibit anaphylactic histamine release from rabbit basophils and rat and guinea pig mast cells in low concentration (0.1 to 2 mM). Inhibition is also produced by disulphide reducing agents (thioglycollate, cysteine, reduced glutathione and sulphite) in rabbit basophils and rat and guinea pig mast cells, but with low concentrations potentiation of histamine release occurs in guinea pig and rat systems presumably owing to increase in free-SH-groups.

The evidence indicates that anaphylaxis in rabbit basophils is activated by an intracellular temperature dependent, short-lived, calcium-requiring, -SH enzyme-like system, which in a way as yet unknown leads to histamine release. Comparative studies in the four species reveal similarities as well as differences in this biochemical mechanism which presumably reflect variation in the basic biochemical pattern.

The Immunochemical Basis of the Urticarial Reaction*

F. S. FARAH and A. K. KURBAN, Department of Medicine, Division of Dermatology of the American University of Beirut and the American University Hospital, Beirut (Lebanon)

Urticarial reactions result from direct effects of histamine, released from the mast cells of the skin. This histamine release is brought about by a variety of factors, one of which is an antigen-antibody interaction.

* Supported by a P.H.S. research grant (AI-2910) from the National Institute of Health, Institute of Allergy and Infectious Diseases P.H.S., Bethesda, Md., USA.

The first recognition of the allergic or immunologic basis of "some" of the urticarial reactions was pointed out in 1905 by the careful observations of VON PIRQUET who associated urticarial reactions with serum sickness. This association was supported and confirmed by the passive transfer of urticarial reactions by PRAUSNITZ and KÜSTNER (1920).

The Prausnitz-Küstner (P-K) reaction has eversince been widely used for the demonstration of the wheal and erythema or urticarial antibodies, and may still be one of the better means for testing for and evaluating some of them [1].

The antibodies responsible for mediating the urticarial (Wheal and Erythema) reactions have been cause for controversy in the literature. It has been thought by some workers [2, 3] that these are unique monovalent non-precipitating antibodies, demonstrable by the P-K reaction. They were heat labile and did not fix complement. Others, however, did not attach as much significance to the uniqueness of the antibody and believed that technical difficulties of measurement of the Wheal and Erythema antibodies had been a handicap in their understanding and their study [4, 5].

It is advantageous to consider the antibodies responsible for the Wheal and Erythema reactions as belonging to two classes of immunoglobulins. There are those that belong to the spontaneously occuring reaginic type of antibody (IgA) formed in Atopic Individuals and there are those that belong to the induced bivalent and precipitating antibody that belong to the IgG class. These may be formed against purified antigens or even haptens.

The purpose of this communication is to show that induced, classical (IgG) precipitating antibodies are capable of eliciting wheal and erythema skin responses whether occupied at one or at both active sites.

We have been able to obtain purified antibodies (directed against 2,4-dinitrophenyl group) from rabbits and guinea pigs, and have studied their properties [6]. They were found to specifically precipitate to more than 90% with dinitrophenyl antigens, and when injected into the human skin, the precipitating antibodies elicited a wheal and erythema response [7].

The purified antibodies were then subjected to heating at various degrees and were made to complex with albumin. This complex was shown to behave like a monovalent antibody as evidenced by the decreased precipitating power and the inhibition of precipitation [8]. Yet this complex was found capable of eliciting a wheal and erythema response in the human skin [8]. To clarify the role of valence further, it was sought to determine the smallest amount of antibody that could elicit a reaction in the human skin — and it was found to be about 4 ugN. Utilizing this value — a constant amount of antibody was titrated with varying amounts of antigen. It was found, that a positive wheal and erythema response was obtained with various antigen/antibody ratios. Ratio of Ag/Ab of 1/1 elicited a response (Tab. 1). In other words, positive responses were obtained when one DNP occupied one antibody active site. No responses were obtained with ratios of less than 1/1.

The importance of the ratio (Ag/Ab of 1/1) as a limiting factor for the elicitation of a positive wheal and erythema response was further established when antigens and antibodies were mixed in the desired proportions and then injected into the skin. Here again a ratio of Ag/Ab of 1/1 still holds (Tab. 2).

These findings confirmed the hypothesis that precipitating antibodies occupied at one or both sites could elicit a wheal and erythema response. A final proof for this hypothesis comes from the results of experiments of antibody fractionation. Here — antibodies were reduced with 2-Mercaptoethylamine [9, 10] to yield two half molecules each with one antibody active site. These half molecules could be reconjugated to reform the original antibody or could be reconjugated with half molecules obtained in a similar manner from normal, gamma globulin. There results then an antibody molecule which has *one* active antibody site only with respect to DNP.

Table 1. *Influence of Decreasing Amounts of Antigen on the Wheal and Erythema Response*

Subject	Test No.	Skin Sites Prepared with ugN	Tested with DNP-HSA		Response Grade	Ratio[a] Ag:Ab
			as DNP muM	Protein ugN		
IV.	1.	Guineapig Purified Ab 48.76	19.8	10.0	+	
	2.	Guineapig Purified Ab 48.76	1.98	1.0	+	1:1
	3.	Guineapig Purified Ab 48.76	0.99	0.5	0	
V.	1.	Rabbit Purified Ab 4.93	87.2	25.9	++	
	2.	Rabbit Purified Ab 4.93	8.72	2.59	++	
	3.	Rabbit Purified Ab 4.93	0.87	0.259	++	
	4.	Rabbit Purified Ab 4.93	0.218	0.0648	+	0.88:1
	5.	Rabbit Purified Ab 4.93	0.109	0.032	0	
VI.	1.	Rabbit Purified Ab 4.93	87.2	25.9	++	
	2.	Rabbit Purified Ab 4.93	8.72	2.59	+	
	3.	Rabbit Purified Ab 4.93	0.872	0.259	+	
	4.	Rabbit Purified Ab 4.93	0.218	0.0648	+	0.88:1
	5.	Rabbit Purified Ab 4.93	0.109	0.0324	0	
	6.	Rabbit Purified Ab 4.93	0.872 + 248[b]	0.259	0	

[a] Ratio of antigen: Antibody calculated as ratio of uM DNP to uM antibody protein. The ratios shown are the lowest at which a response occurred.

[b] Added 2,4-Dinitrophenyllysine (DNP-lys). All duplicate reactions similarly inhibited.

Table 2. *Wheal and Erythema Responses with Predetermined Antigen-Antibody Ratios*

Subject[a]	Test No.	Material Injected	Ratio Ag:Ab	Response Grade
VII.	1.	Rabbit Purified Ab 4.7 ugN + DNP + HSA	1:2	±
	2.	Rabbit Purified Ab 4.7 ugN + DNP + HSA	1:1	++
	3.	Rabbit Purified Ab 4.7 ugN + DNP + HSA	2:1	+
	4.	Rabbit Purified Ab 4.7 ugN + DNP + HSA	4:1	++

[a] Similar test done on five other subjects and showed similar results.

[b] Other ratios in this experiment of Ag:Ab of 10:1, 20:1, 52:1 gave positive response. All responses were inhibited with 320 muM of DNP-lys.

Table 3. *Wheal and Erythema Responses with Reconjugated Antibodies*

Subject	Reconjugated antibody	Total amount per[a] skin site	Response		Abbreviations
	PB	42.8	++		PB = Purified antibody
	PB	7.36	+		PB-PB = reconjugated antibody where each half molecule originated from purified antibody.
	PB-PB	3.8	++		
		7.13	+		PB-GG = reconjugated antibody where half molecules came from purified antibody and the other from normal gamma-globulin.
	PB-GG	4.05	++		
		7.1	+		
	PB-GG (abs)	7.1	+		PB-GG *absorbed* = similar to above, but where it was incubated with antigen and streptomycin — the supernate being used for the skin tests.

[a] Challenged with antigen DNP-HSA as 4.88 muM of DNP and 1.76 ugN as HSA.

This reconjugated but monovalent antibody was found capable of eliciting a wheal and erythema skin response (Tab. 3).

It is concluded from the above, that antibodies occupied at either one or both active sites are capable of eliciting the wheal and erythema skin response.

References. 1. KUHUS, W. T., and A. M. PAPPENHEIMER jr.: J. exp. Med. **95**, 363, 375 (1952). — 2. SHERMAN, W. B., A. E. O. MENZEL, and P. B. SEEBOHM: J. exp. Med. **92**, 191 (1950). — 3. KABAT, E. A.: Proc. 3rd Internat. Congress of Allergy 1958, p. 167. — 4. VAUGHAN, J. H., and E. A. KABAT: J. exp. Med. **97**, 821 (1953). — 5. FARAH, F. S., M. KERN, and H. N. EISEN: J. exp. Med. **112**, 1195 (1960). — 6. FARAH, F. S., M. KERN, and H. N. EISEN: J. exp. Med. **112**, 1211 (1960). — 7. FARAH, F. S., and A. K. KURBAN: J. Immunol. **11**, 507 (1966). — 8. FARAH, F. S., A. K. KURBAN, and H. T. CHAGLASSIAN: J. Immunol. **93**, 300 (1964). — 9. PALMAR, J. L., A. NISONOFF, and K. E. VAN HOLDE: Proc. nat. Acad. Sci. (Wash.) **50**, 314 (1963). — 10. STEIN, S. R., J. L. PALMER, and A. NISONOFF: J. biol. Chem. **239**, 2872 (1964).

The Release of Serotonin in Hypersensitivity States

J. S. COMAISH, University Department of Dermatology and The Royal Victoria Infirmary, Newcastle upon Tyne (England)

It has been known for a long time that histamine may be released from blood platelets and/or basophils during the course of antigen-antibody reactions in man and this phenomenon has been used for the in vitro diagnosis of clinical hypersensitivity. In vivo studies of anaphylaxis in the rabbit have shown that there is an increase not only in plasma histamine but also serotonin levels following challenge, accompanied by a fall in the number of circulating platelets (WAALKES et al., 1957). So far however there has been no convincing evidence that serotonin plays any part in human hypersensitivity, nor is it clear that it is released during the course of antigen-antibody reactions in vitro.

We have investigated this problem using ^{14}C-labelled serotonin. When incubated in vitro with an appropriate amount of ^{14}C-labelled 5-HT human platelets rapidly absorb activity until as much as 70 to 90% of that available in the medium is concentrated in the tiny volume of platelets. Once absorbed the 5-HT is retained for long periods without significant loss if a source of energy such as glucose is available. These facts render platelet labelling with ^{14}C-5-HT a comparatively simple task. A particular feature of the technique used is the avoidance of washing after labelling which is permitted by this great avidity of platelets for serotonin. This offers considerable advantages not only in time saved but more importantly in the reduced manipulation of the platelets which are very sensitive to even mild mechanical trauma.

Methods

Glassware, needles and syringes were siliconized. Platelet rich plasma was obtained by centrifuging heparinised rabbit arterial or human blood (venous) diluted (1:2) in ice-cold Tyrode's solution at 120 g at 4 °C for 15 min. The platelet count was adjusted to 100,000/mm³ and 0.1 μc of 14C-labelled 5-hydroxytryptamine of specific activity 79 μc/mg was added to each 20 ml platelet-rich plasma. This was incubated at 37 °C for 20 min and then divided into aliquots. The first two aliquots were controls and to the remaining tubes were added increasing amounts of antigen. In experiments involving passive transfer of serum antibody duplicate serum controls were included. In using the passive transfer or indirect method it is essential to dilute the human serum up to a hundred-fold to avoid non-specific 5-HT release from rabbit platelets. All tubes were incubated at 37° for 30 min. At the end of this period the amount of serotonin released was estimated by scintillation counting of the supernatants obtained after centrifuging the tubes at 9,000 g for 20 min. The activity of the supernatants used as controls subtracted from that of the tubes containing antigen gave the amount of activity released by antigen during incubation. The amount of 5-HT released was then expressed as a percentage of that taken up during incubation by the controls.

Results

a) *Some substances* can be shown to release 5-HT from normal human platelets. Thus quinine caused 25% release even at 5×10^{-5} M. Tetanus toxoid (fluid, 40 Lf/ml) also caused as much as 53% release in dilutions up to 1:960.

b) *Antigen-antibody* reactions may also release 5-HT. 20 patients have been studied who reacted adversely to equine anti-tetanus serum, penicillin, tetracycline, bacitracin and other drugs. In twelve of these it was possible to show that the patients' own platelets or sometimes normal rabbit platelets released significant quantities of 5-HT when incubated with antigen and the patient's serum or plasma (COMAISH and CUNLIFFE, 1967; CASPARY and COMAISH, 1967). Heating the serum at 56 °C for 60 min abolished its serotonin — releasing capacity. So also did prolonged storage at —10 °C. There is a limited range of antigen dilutions over which this reaction occurs so that as wide a range as practicable has been employed in attempts to detect peak serotonin release. For a period after a severe clinical reaction (eg. anaphylaxis) there may be no detectable serotonin release, but thereafter a peak is achieved which then declines at a variable rate. This phenomenon has also been observed with release of histamine in animal and human hypersensitivity.

It is of interest to note that rabbit platelets have provided a more sensitive indicator of an antigen-antibody reaction than human platelets in a number of cases. Elucidation of the correct haptenic determinants in penicillin and other drug hypersensitivity might increase the value of this technique.

References. CASPARY, E. A., and J. S. COMAISH: Nature (Lond.) **214**, 286 (1967). — COMAISH, J. S., and W. J. CUNLIFFE: Brit. J. clin. Pract. **21**, 97 (1967). — WAALKES, T. P., H. WEISSBACH, J. BOZICEVICH, and S. UDENFRIEND: J. clin. Invest. **36**, 1115 (1957).

Réactions sérologiques et terrain d'allergie humorale en dermatologie

CL. MIKOL et M. RENOUX, Faculté de Médecine, Paris (France)

Depuis H. DALE, qui a montré le rôle fondamental de *l'histamine*, de nombreuses tentatives ont été faites pour mettre en évidence chez les sujets atopiques une réactivité particulière de l'organisme vis-à-vis de cette substance. D'après R. BENDA, certains sérums humains protègent le cobaye contre l'action toxique de l'histamine administrée en aérosols: ce pouvoir *histamino-protecteur* répond à une résistance anti-histaminique naturelle et manque chez les allergiques. En 1952, J. L. PARROT a décrit la propriété de certains sérums humains de fixer in vitro une fraction de l'histamine qui leur est ajoutée: ce *pouvoir histaminopexique* est d'environ 30% chez le sujet normal et s'annule chez l'allergique.

Technique des réactions au latex

En 1961, nous avons proposé l'emploi de particules de polystyrène comme support de l'histamine dans une réaction de séro-agglutination. Des dilutions croissantes de sérum sont mises en présence d'une suspension de *latex* et *d'histamine*, incubées à 56 °C pendant 2 h et examinées le lendemain après centrifugation. En 1965, nous avons proposé une réaction analogue utilisant la *sérotonine*. Le sérum d'un sujet normal donne une séro-agglutination nette, supérieure à 1/80. Le sérum d'un sujet atteint d'allergie atopique (urticaire, eczéma constitutionnel) ne donne pas d'agglutination ou donne une agglutination de titre faible; la réaction au latex permet donc d'opposer deux types de sérums. Nos premiers résultats, publiés à la Société Médicale des Hôpitaux de Paris en 1961, ont été confirmés depuis, notamment par ceux de J. L. PARROT et ceux de C. HURIEZ en France, par ceux de A.G. PALMA-CARLOS au Portugal, par ceux de E. PISANI en Italie.

Résultats

Sur 772 réactions à l'*histamine-latex*, figurent 171 urticaires et oedèmes de Quincke, 549 eczémas (161 eczémas constitutionnels, 180 eczémas de contact, 208 eczémas microbiens) et 52 prurigos. Des réponses normales ne se voient que pour 68 urticaires (40%) et pour 42 eczémas constitutionnels (26%); au contraire, elles se voient dans 95 eczémas de contact (53%) et dans 100 eczémas microbiens (48%); elles se voient aussi dans 20 prurigos (38%). Sur 440 réactions à la *sérotonine-latex* figurent 107 urticaires et oedèmes de Quincke, 301 eczémas (99 eczémas constitutionnels, 87 eczémas de contact, 115 eczémas microbiens) et 32 prurigos. Des réponses normales ne se voient que pour 36 urticaires (34%) et pour 38 eczémas atopiques (38%); au contraire elles se voient dans 44 eczémas de contact (51%) et dans 65 eczémas microbiens (57%); elles se voient aussi dans 17 prurigos (53%).

Commentaires

L'absence d'agglutination du latex en présence d'histamine ou de sérotonine apparaît comme un témoin du terrain d'allergie humorale, au même titre que l'absence d'histaminopexie plastique mesurée par la méthode pharmacologique: elle est retrouvée très généralement dans les eczémas constitutionnels et les urticaires; au contraire une séro-agglutination normale se voit assez souvent dans les eczémas par contact et les eczémas microbiens où la part de l'agent externe de sensibilisation est prépondérante. Ces réactions au latex sont de technique facile et méritent d'être associées aux tests cutanés lors de l'exploration des dermatoses allergiques.

Experimentelle Untersuchungen zur Desensibilisierung und Immuntoleranz gegen niedermolekulare Allergene

K. H. SCHULZ, Univ.-Hautklinik Hamburg (Deutschland)

Durch Antigene hervorgerufene spezifische Herabsetzung immunologischer Reaktionen kann sich sowohl auf die Allergie vom verzögerten Typ als auch auf andere, durch humorale Antikörper induzierte Reaktionsformen (Übersichten s. DE WECK und FREY; ASHERSON u. a.) erstrecken. Unsere Untersuchungen, über die hier zusammenfassend berichtet werden soll, betrafen lediglich die durch niedermolekulare Allergene hervorgerufene Kontaktallergie, und zwar wurde der Einfluß einmaliger oder wiederholter Zufuhr der spezifischen Allergene auf den Sensibliisierungsgrad untersucht. Als Versuchstiere dienten Albino-Meerschweinchen eines einheitlichen Inzuchtstammes. Die verwendeten Allergene (Haptene) bzw. Haptenconjugate waren folgende: 2,4-Dinitrochlorbenzol (DNCB), Thioglykolsäurehydrazid (Th-Sre-Hydrazid), 4-Fluor-3-nitroacetophenon (FNA) und verschiedene Aminosäureconjugate des FNA, Chlormethylimidazolin (CMJ).

Die Sensibilisierung der Tiere erfolgte durch epicutane Applikation der Allergene. Zum Zwecke der Erzielung einer Desensibilisierung oder Toleranz wurden die Substanzen epicutan, oral oder intravenös verabfolgt.

1. *Epicutane Applikation:* In einer Versuchsreihe wurde der Frage nachgegangen, ob wiederholte epicutane Applikationen des spezifischen Allergens einen Einfluß auf den Sensibilisierungsgrad der Tiere hatten. Für diese Experimente wurden DNCB und das schwächer wirksame Th-Sre-Hydrazid verwendet. Nach erfolgter Sensibilisierung, die durch mehrtägige Vorbehandlung mit 1% DNCB bzw. 5% Th-Sre-Hydrazid erreicht wurde, wurden die Meerschweinchen etwa 3 Monate lang täglich am gleichen Hautbezirk mit einer nicht toxischen Allergendosis behandelt (DNCB 0,1%, Th-Sre-Hydrazid 1%). In mehrwöchigen Abständen an nicht vorbehandelter Haut (gegenüberliegende Flanke) vorgenommene Teste gaben Aufschluß über den Sensibilisierungsgrad. Die gesamte Beobachtungszeit erstreckte sich über 9 Monate.

Im Vergleich zu nicht vorbehandelten Kontrolltieren zeigte sich, daß durch die langfristige epicutane Einwirkung der Allergene DNCB und Th-Sre-Hydrazid eine deutliche Abschwächung der Reaktionsfähigkeit, d. h. eine Desensibilisierung erreicht werden kann, die noch mehrere Monate nach Beendigung der epicutanen Behandlung nachweisbar war. Daß es sich dabei um ein spezifisches Phänomen handelt, geht aus weiteren Experimenten mit Doppelsensibilisierungen gegen zwei chemisch verschiedene Allergene hervor.

Insgesamt stehen die Befunde in guter Übereinstimmung mit den von JADASSOHN und BRUN sowie HUNZIKER erzielten Ergebnissen.

2. *Orale Zufuhr:* In einer zweiten Versuchsreihe wurde DNCB über einen Zeitraum von 100 Tagen täglich in einer Dosis von 3 mg/die oral gegeben. Mit oralen Zufuhren wurde zu verschiedenen Zeiten vor und nach der Sensibilisierung begonnen: bei einer Gruppe von zehn Tieren 6 Wochen, bei einer zweiten Gruppe 3 Wochen vor der Sensibilisierung; die dritte Tiergruppe erhielt die erste orale Dosis mit Beginn und die vierte Gruppe 3 Wochen nach der Sensibilisierung.

Es zeigte sich, daß auch auf diese Weise eine Abschwächung der Reaktionsfähigkeit zu erreichen war, jedoch waren deutliche Unterschiede in Abhängigkeit vom Beginn der Fütterung zu verzeichnen. Während der Sensibilisierungsgrad der Kontrolltiere über die ganze Versuchsdauer von 137 Tagen etwa gleichmäßig hoch blieb, sank er bei den anderen Gruppen in unterschiedlichem Maße ab. Die am längsten vorgefütterten Tiere der ersten Gruppe verloren ihre Reaktionsfähigkeit am schnellsten und fast vollständig. Dieser Befund bestätigt das von CHASE erstmalig beschriebene Phänomen, das als eine besondere Art von Immuntoleranz angesprochen werden kann (s. auch CHASE und BATTISTO). Wurde mit der Allergenfütterung jedoch erst 3 Wochen nach der Sensibilisierung begonnen, so war der Erfolg wesentlich geringer. Eine leichte Herabsetzung der Reaktionsfähigkeit war aber auch hier festzustellen.

3. *Intravenöse Injektion:* In Analogie zu den Untersuchungen von FREY, DE WECK und GELEICK wurde weiterhin untersucht, ob die intravenöse Injektion von Allergenen zu einer Beeinflussung der Sensibilisierung führt. Für diese Experimente wurden 3-Fluor-4-nitroacetophenon (FNA) und verschiedene Aminosäureconjugate benutzt. Mehrere Gruppen von Meerschweinchen, die mit FNA sensibilisiert worden waren, erhielten einmal 20 mg FNA intravenös injiziert. 6, 12, 24, 48 Std sowie 1 Woche nach der Injektion wurden epicutane Teste mit verschiedenen Konzentrationen von FNA vorgenommen, um die allergische Reizschwelle zu ermitteln. Dabei ergab sich bei den Tieren, die 6, 12 und 24 Std nach der Injektion von FNA getestet wurden, eine deutliche Herabsetzung der Empfindlichkeit. Dieser Hemmeffekt war aber schon nach 48 Std sowie auch später nicht mehr vorhanden. Diese Befunde entsprechen denen von FREY und DE WECK und weisen auf eine nur kurzdauernde vorübergehende Hemmung hin.

Wurden an Stelle des freien FNA dessen Aminosäureconjugate wie FNA-

Glycin, FNA-Aminocaproat, FNA-Prolin und FNA-Phenylalanin gleichzeitig mit der epicutanen Applikation von FNA bei vorher sensibilisierten Tieren injiziert, so war keine Hemmwirkung festzustellen.

Mit Chlormethylimidazolin (CMJ), dessen starke sensibilisierende Wirkung wir kürzlich nachweisen konnten und das den Vorteil weitgehender Wasserlöslichkeit hat, wurden Versuche zur Immuntoleranz durchgeführt. Zweimal im Abstand von 2 Wochen mit Dosen von 20 bis 30 mg/kg intravenös vorbehandelte Meerschweinchen waren durch eine nachfolgende epicutane Behandlung wesentlich schlechter epicutan zu sensibilisieren als unvorbehandelte Tiere. Es war eine partielle Immuntoleranz eingetreten.

Experimentelle Sensibilisierung mit drei- und sechswertigem Chrom

M. SCHWARZ-SPECK, Dermatologische Universitätsklinik Zürich (Schweiz)

Frühere Versuche hatten gezeigt, daß beim Meerschweinchen eine Sensibilisierung gegen dreiwertiges Chrom auf epicutanem Weg mit Hilfe des Netzmittels Triton X-100 erzeugt werden kann. Die derart sensibilisierten Tiere reagierten in einem hohen Prozentsatz auch gegen sechswertiges Chrom in Form von Kaliumbichromat. Dies warf die Frage auf, ob man es dabei mit einer echten Kreuzreaktion zu tun hat, oder ob das dreiwertige Chrom als eigentlicher Sensibilisator beim Chromekzem betrachtet werden muß, indem die sechswertige Stufe in der Haut zur dreiwertigen reduziert wird.

In einer neuen Versuchsreihe sensibilisierten wir deshalb nochmals eine Gruppe von 29 Meerschweinchen epicutan mit dreiwertigem Chrom (Chromsulfat = CrIII) unter Verwendung von Triton X-100 als Netzmittel (Gruppe A) und eine Kontrollgruppe von 19 Tieren nur mit Triton allein (Gruppe B). Weitere 27 Meerschweinchen wurden mit sechswertigem Chrom in Form von wäßrigem Kaliumbichromat (CrVI) auf vorher mit Äther entfetteter Haut sensibilisiert (Gruppe C). Der Sensibilisierungserfolg ist auf Tab. 1 ersichtlich: Von den 29 Tieren der Gruppe A (Sensibilisierung mit CrIII + Triton) reagierten 27 Tiere positiv auf 0,5%ige CrIII-Sulfatlösung in Triton, wobei es zu recht starken Hautreaktionen auf das dreiwertige Chrom kam. Die Kontrollgruppe B gab bei einer kleinen Zahl von Tieren schwach positive Hautreizungen bei der Auslösung mit dem Netzmittel allein. 20 von 27 Tieren der Gruppe C (Sensibilisierung mit CrVI) reagierten positiv auf sechswertiges Chrom, wobei aber die Intensität der Sensibilisierung gegen die sechswertige Stufe des Chroms schwächer ausfiel als die Sensibilisierung auf dreiwertiges Chrom der Gruppe A.

In der Erwartung, daß die in der Literatur beschriebene experimentelle Sensibilisierung gegen Bichromat (CrVI) mit Hilfe von Natriumlaurylsulfat eine bessere Sensibilisierung ergeben würde, haben wir auch noch eine solche Versuchsreihe durchgeführt. Aus Tab. 2 geht hervor, daß bei diesem Sensibilisierungsverfahren mit dem Netzmittel Natriumlaurylsulfat 14 von 20 Meerschweinchen, ohne Verwendung des Netzmittels jedoch nur 10 von 20 Tieren gegen sechswertiges Chrom positiv reagierten. Dies bedeutet eine eher schlechtere Sensibilisierungsrate als bei der oben erwähnten Methode. In einer weiteren Kontrollgruppe E wurde nur mit Natriumlaurylsulfat behandelt; es ergaben sich bei wenigen Tieren schwache Hautreaktionen auf das Netzmittel. Die Prüfung der verschieden sensibilisierten Tiergruppen auf Kreuzreaktionen gegen dreiwertiges Chrom bzw.

sechswertiges Chrom sind in der Tab. 1 zusammengefaßt. In der Gruppe A reagierten die mit CrIII + Triton sensibilisierten Tiere gegen CrIII und CrVI vergleichbar stark, ebenfalls in der Gruppe C die mit CrVI sensibilisierten Tiere
gegen CrVI und CrIII. Hingegen fielen die Reaktionen in der Gruppe D, welche
mit CrVI + Natriumlaurylsulfat sensibilisiert worden war, schwächer aus mit
CrIII als mit CrVI.

Einen noch besseren Vergleich gibt die prozentuale Auswertung der positiven,
schwach positiven und negativen Hautreaktionen, wie sie in Fig. 1 für die einzelnen Tiergruppen graphisch dargestellt ist. Daraus sind wiederum die fast identisch
starken Reaktionen der Gruppen A und C gegenüber drei- und sechswertigem
Chrom ersichtlich.

Aus der Tatsache, daß sechswertiges Chrom in der Haut zu dreiwertigem
reduziert werden kann und aus den bisher erwähnten eigenen Versuchen könnte der
Schluß gezogen werden, daß das dreiwertige Chrom das eigentliche Ekzematogen
beim Chromekzem darstellt.

Im Gegensatz zu diesen eindeutigen Resultaten steht das Ergebnis des Sensibili-
sierungsversuches mit sechswertigem Chrom unter Verwendung von Natriumlaurylsulfat, bei welchen die Sensibilisierungsrate auf sechswertiges Chrom gegenüber der dreiwertigen Stufe beträchtlich überwiegt. Die Widersprüche können
meines Erachtens nur in den verschiedenen Netzmitteln, welche in den Versuchen
verwendet wurden, gesucht werden. Vermutungen über deren differente pathogenetische Bedeutung für die experimentellen Chromsensibilisierungen wären
natürlich sehr verlockend, doch muß ich mich an dieser Stelle darauf beschränken,
deren Wichtigkeit für die gegensätzlichen Untersuchungsresultate mit den verschiedenen Methoden hervorzuheben.

In den in vitro-Versuchen haben wir die zeitliche Abnahme von sechswertigem
Chrom bei Inkubation mit 10 μ dicken Hautschnitten von sensibilisierten und
nicht sensibilisierten Meerschweinchen der Gruppe A (Sensibilisierung mit CrIII +
Triton), der Gruppe B (Sensibilisierung mit Triton) und der Gruppe C (Sensibilisierung mit CrVI) bestimmt. In Abb. 3 sind die Mittelwerte aller Versuche, die in
verschiedenen Puffersystemen bei pH 5,4, pH 7,0 und pH 8,0 durchgeführt
wurden, aufgetragen. Daraus geht hervor, daß die zeitliche Abnahme insbesondere
im sauren pH-Bereich am stärksten ist und bis auf 40% des Ausgangswertes
sinken kann. Aber auch gewisse Unterschiede in der Abnahme des CrVI-Gehaltes
je nach Puffersystem sind ersichtlich.

Vergleicht man die zeitliche Abnahme des sechswertigen Chroms bei stark
sensibilisierten Tieren gegenüber schwach sensibilisierten oder negativ reagierenden Tieren, so zeigt sich nur bei Phosphatpuffer pH 5,4 und pH 7,0 sowie bei
Citronensäurepuffer pH 5,4 eine etwas stärkere Abnahme bei den stark sensibilisierten.

Die naheliegende Annahme, daß bei stark sensibilisierbaren Meerschweinchen
ein stärkeres Reduktionsvermögen von sechswertigem Chrom zur dreiwertigen
Stufe vorliegen müßte, ließ sich nicht überzeugend bestätigen. Der Unterschied
zwischen Sensibilisierten und Nicht-Sensibilisierten scheint also offensichtlich
nicht vorwiegend in der reduktiven Umwandlung des sechswertigen Chroms zur
dreiwertigen Stufe zu liegen.

Auch in unseren in-vitro-Untersuchungen zeigt sich, daß das Problem des
experimentellen Chromekzems nicht einfach zu lösen ist.

Zur Frage autoallergischer Reaktionen bei der Neurodermitis

B. Kopecká, E. Sorkin, S. Borelli und A. Fjelde, Dermatologische Abteilung des Sanatoriums Valbella, Davos-Dorf (Schweiz), und Schweizerisches Forschungsinstitut, Medizinische Abteilung, Davos-Platz (Schweiz)

Trotz zahlreicher Untersuchungen sind die Ätiologie und Pathogenese der Neurodermitis noch immer unbekannt. Whitfield und Storm van Lauwen haben bereits postuliert, daß ein Individuum gegen seine eigene Haut sensibilisiert werden kann. Positive Hautreaktionen vom Soforttypus bei Atopikern nach Injektion von homologen Schuppenextrakten wurden als Beweis für einen Prozeß der Autosensibilisierung angesehen. Eindeutige Beweise am experimentellen Tier für eine Autosensibilisierung gegen Haut wurden in der Folge von zahlreichen Autoren erbracht. Die Hauptschwierigkeiten, eine Autoallergie gegen Haut als Ursache einer menschlichen Erkrankung, z.B. der Neurodermitis, zu beweisen, liegen in der Isolierung und Charakterisierung der Antigene der Haut und sodann in der nur schwer auszuschließenden Anwesenheit von exogenen mikrobiellen Antigenen. Ferner stellt sich die Frage, ob selbst bei einem gelungenen Nachweis von Autoantikörpern gegen Hautkomponenten diese unbedingt für die pathogene Rolle in Frage kommen.

Um als Beweis für eine Autosensibilisierung gegenüber Haut gelten zu können, müssen folgende strikte Kriterien erfüllt sein:

1. Haut- oder Schuppenextrakte sollten eine Hautreaktion erzeugen.

2. Serumantikörper sollen nach intracutaner Verabreichung deutliche Hautreaktionen erzeugen.

3. Intracutane Verabreichung von autologen (sensibilisierten?) Blutleukocyten sollte eine Hautreaktion erzeugen.

4. Antikörper gegen Hautkomponenten müssen bei allen Erkrankten nachweisbar sein.

Hinzu käme noch

5. die Fähigkeit autologer Hautkomponenten, morphologische Veränderungen und mitogene Effekte an Blutleukocyten von Erkrankten zu erzeugen.

Wir möchten im folgenden über die Ergebnisse unserer experimentellen Untersuchungen bei Neurodermitikern berichten.

Versuche mit autologen Hautextrakten

Sämtliche 32 Neurodermitiker zeigten eine positive Hautreaktion, 23 von 32 reagierten mit einer ++ oder +++ Reaktion. Bei den acht getesteten gesunden Versuchspersonen zeigten sich keine ++ oder +++ Reaktionen. Die Reaktionen bei den Neurodermitikern erreichten binnen 20 bis 50 min ihr Maximum, bei Patienten dauerten die Reaktionen länger als 1 Std. Bei sieben Patienten waren noch nach 48 Std schwache Restreaktionen sichtbar. Einige der Patienten zeigten nach intracutaner Verabreichung von autologem Hautextrakt Maximum Diameter bis zu 22 × 25 mm (Kontrollösungen bis höchstens 11 × 13 mm). Histamin als mögliche Ursache von falsch positiven Reaktionen konnte durch eine Reihe von Kontrollversuchen ausgeschlossen werden. Nach Dialyse von Hautextrakten waren dieselben unverändert hautaktiv. Quantitative Histaminbestimmungen in den Hautextrakten ergaben zwar eindeutig die Gegenwart von Histamin, die Menge war aber um das vier- bis zehnfache kleiner, als sie zur Auslösung einer typischen Histaminreaktion notwendig ist. Auch sind die Reaktionszeiten und der Charakter der Reaktionen total verschieden.

Intracutanteste mit autologen Schuppenextrakten

Bei den 20 geprüften Patienten wurde in 15 Fällen eine stark positive Reaktion (+++) beobachtet. Die Reaktion trat zwar wie mit Hautextrakten sofort ein, war aber in der Regel viel stärker und von längerer Dauer. Oft zog sich die Reaktion über mehrere Tage hin, was auf eine Spätallergiekomponente hinweist. Nur eine der acht gesunden Kontrollen reagierte stark (+++).

Intracutanteste mit Eigenserum

Diesen Versuchen lag die Arbeitshypothese zugrunde, daß Autoantikörper nach Wechselwirkung mit Komponenten der Haut eine Hautreaktion auszulösen vermögen. 28 von 29 Neurodermitikern reagierten lediglich leicht positiv oder negativ auf Eigenserum, alle Gesunden negativ. Von Interesse sind aber die Befunde bei sechs Patienten, die mit Eigenserum an kranker Stelle stark positiv (++ oder +++) und an gesunder Stelle negativ oder schwächer positiv reagierten.

Intracutanteste mit autologen Blutleukocyten

Es war zu untersuchen, ob die neurodermitischen Erscheinungen durch eine Reaktion der Blutleukocyten mit hauteigenen Stoffen mitbedingt oder ausgelöst wurden. 2 bis 5×10^6 Blutleukocyten wurden injiziert. Von 16 Neurodermitikern reagierten fünf mäßig bis stark positiv, fünf weitere zeigten eine leicht positive Reaktion. Die gesunden Probanden zeigten negative oder + Reaktionen.

Der Test für Antikörper gegen autologe Haut- und Schuppenkomponenten wurde mit der Gerbsäure-Hämagglutinationsreaktion ausgeführt. Die Seren von normalen Kontrollen und einem Drittel der Neurodermitiker zeigten negative Hämagglutinationsteste. 65% der Neurodermitiker zeigten schwache Antikörperaktivität gegen Haut- und Schuppenextrakt (Titer $^1/_2$ bis $^1/_{32}$).

Die Vorstellung einer Autosensibilisierung als Ursache der Neurodermitis wurde auch in Gewebskulturversuchen getestet. Morphologische Veränderungen und mitotische Wirkungen von autologen Hautextrakten auf Blutleukocyten wurden festgestellt. Salzwasserkontrollen hatten keine Wirkung, und bei Gesunden war der Hautextrakt fast wirkungslos.

Versuchen wir die hier nur auszugsweise gewonnenen Ergebnisse dieser Untersuchungen zu überblicken, so ergibt sich folgendes Bild:

1. Der Antikörpernachweis gegen Hautkomponenten ist nicht bei allen Neurodermitikern gelungen.

2. Serumantikörper induzierten nur vorübergehende schwache Hautreaktionen.

3. Autologe Blutleukocyten gaben ebenfalls nur schwache Reaktionen.

4. Autologe Haut- und Schuppenextrakte gaben gute bis sehr starke Reaktionen vom sofortigen bzw. verzögerten Typ, in einigen Fällen zeigte auch das Serum- und Hautextraktgemisch starke Reaktionen. Hautextrakte zeigen eine mitogene Wirkung auf autologe Blutlymphocyten des Neurodermitikers.

Aus diesen Untersuchungen kann der Schluß gezogen werden, daß zwar Hinweise für eine Autoallergie bei Neurodermitis vorliegen, aber eine strenge Beweisführung noch aussteht. Es darf erwartet werden, daß durch verbesserte Extraktionsmethoden der Antigene, speziell aus der erkrankten Haut, weitere Einblicke gewonnen werden können.

Delayed Reactivity to Bacterial, Mold and Viral Allergens in Atopic Dermatitis

G. RAJKA, Karolinska Sjukhuset, Stockholm (Sweden)

The aim of the study was to investigate delayed reactivity in patients with atopic dermatitis. Controls were patients with various dermatoses (chiefly with eczemas) and, in part, patients with respiratory atopies. The allergens used were:

PPD second strength	Mumps vaccine 1:10
Tuberculin 0.1 mg	Schick test
Streptococcal extract	Trichophytin 1:50
Staphylococcal extract	Saline control

The results are summarized in the table. From this table it is evident that the delayed reactivity was significantly lower in atopic dermatitis than in controls.

Table. *Positive Delayed Reactions in Atopic Dermatitis and Control Groups*

Allergens	I Atopic Dermatitis Patients	II Controls with Skin Diseases	III Respiratory Atopics
Streptococcal extract	3/50	27/50	15/25
Staphylococcal extract	5/50	29/50	14/25
Tuberculin 0.1 mg	0/50	13/50	5/25
PPD 0.002 mg/ml	11/16	16/16	
Mumps vaccine 1:10	8/16	15/16	
Schick-Test	6/16	10/16	
Trichophytin 1:505	1/30	7/20	

Das Shwartzman-Phänomen, eine dem Arthus-Phänomen ähnliche, pseudo-immunologische Reaktion der Haut auf Endotoxin*

I. KUNICK und L. ILLIG, Universitäts-Hautklinik Freiburg (Deutschland)

Das lokale Shwartzman-Phänomen der Haut erscheint als intensive hämorrhagische Nekrose auf entzündlicher Basis; klinisch und histologisch ähnelt es außerordentlich dem Arthus-Phänomen. Man weiß aber seit vielen Jahren sicher, daß es *nicht* auf einer Antigen-Antikörperreaktion beruht. Leider ist es am Menschen schwer diagnostizierbar, obwohl es sicher ein wichtiges und interessantes Modell für einen Purpuramechanismus darstellt. Seit bekannt wurde, daß das *generalisierte* Sanarelli-Shwartzman-Phänomen auf einer komplexen Gerinnungsstörung mit intravasculären Fibrinablagerungen beruht, wurde eine Überprüfung auch des lokalen Shwartzman-Phänomens auf pathogenetische Faktoren systemischer Natur notwendig.

Hämatologische Untersuchungen während des Zeitintervalls zwischen intracutaner Präparation und intravenöser Auslösung mit Coliendotoxin ergaben beim Kaninchen einen eindeutigen Leukocytensturz mit Tiefpunkt in der 2. Std, einen

---

* Mit freundlicher Unterstützung der Deutschen Forschungsgemeinschaft.

75*

Anstieg der Beta-Lipoproteide im Serum mit Gipfel nach 18 bzw. 24 Std (also kurz vor der Auslösung) und leichte Gerinnungsstörungen mit Verzögerung der Gerinnselbildung und Verbreiterung des Thrombelastogrammes. Obwohl der präparative Vorgang bekanntlich streng auf das Hautorgan und auf das injizierte Areal begrenzt bleibt, mußte also doch ein Teil des Endotoxins aus der Haut rasch in die Blutbahn gelangt sein. Statistisch signifikant waren die gefundenen Blutveränderungen aber nur bei relativ hohen intracutanen Endotoxindosen, und zwar im Hinblick auf den Gerinnungsmechanismus und im Hinblick auf die Serumlipoproteide bis zu einer Dosis von etwa 50 γ herab; für den Leukocytensturz konnte die Grenzdosis nicht sicher ermittelt werden. Für die Vorbereitung zum Shwartzman-Phänomen lag die Grenzdosis aber auf jeden Fall wesentlich niedriger als für die Erzeugung von Gerinnungsänderungen und Fettspiegeländerungen, nämlich bei 0,5 μg/kg. Solche niedrigen intracutanen Endotoxindosen haben keine sicher nachweisbaren Blutveränderungen mehr zur Folge. Deren Beteiligung am Präparationsvorgang erscheint also schon aus diesem Grund unwahrscheinlich. Hinzu kommt, daß wir inzwischen in noch nicht abgeschlossenen Untersuchungen mit K. SCHNEIDER die Angabe einiger Autoren bestätigen konnten, daß das lokale Shwartzman-Phänomen bei Verwendung hoher Toxindosen auch *intracutan* ausgelöst werden kann, *und zwar unter sicherem Ausschluß des Blutweges*. Schließlich muß noch einmal hervorgehoben werden, daß der Präparationsvorgang stets streng auf das Injektionsareal begrenzt bleibt, was ebenfalls gegen die entscheidende Mitbeteiligung hämatologischer bzw. systematischer Faktoren spricht.

Unter Berücksichtigung der wichtigen Untersuchungen von STORCK u. Mitarb. (1951) wurden wir daher weitgehend auf die alte Ansicht von APITZ zurückgeführt, nach welcher der präparative Vorgang des lokalen Shwartzman-Phänomens in erster Linie an den *Gefäßen* der Haut stattfindet (sog. endotheliale Umstimmung), im Gegensatz zum generalisierten Phänomen.

STORCK u. Mitarb. hatten bekanntlich am Ort der Präparation eine hochgradige *Verminderung der Capillarresistenz* nachgewiesen, und wir konnten ihren Befund bestätigen. Jedoch fiel uns schon bei den ersten Stichproben eine mangelnde topographische Übereinstimmung der präparativen Blutungsneigung im Saugglockentest und der nachfolgenden Shwartzman-Reaktion auf. Bei systematischen Nachuntersuchungen mit zwei Shwartzman-aktiven und einem Shwartzman-inaktiven Endotoxin* an 62 Tieren fanden wir inzwischen zusammen mit E. PAUL leider, daß die von STORCK u. Mitarb. entdeckte Verminderung der Capillarresistenz nach intracutaner Toxininjektion Shwartzman-*unspezifisch* ist. Sie hing nämlich von der Höhe der Endotoxindosis und von der Art des Endotoxins ab, jedoch *nicht* von seiner Shwartzman-Aktivität. So reagierten z. B. bei Präparationsdosen von 100 μg Coliendotoxin von sechs Tieren alle sechs mit einer stark erhöhten Blutungsneigung, während es bei einer Dosis von 10 μg nur noch sechs von zwölf Tieren waren, wobei aber *alle* ein Shwartzman-Phänomen bekamen. Wurde die Haut dagegen mit dem Shwartzman-inaktiven Streptolysin 0 präpariert, so wiesen die Injektionsstellen bei 100 μg Toxin nur an einem von sieben Tieren, bei 1000 μg jedoch an fünf von sieben Tieren eine starke Blutungsneigung auf, *ohne* daß aber ein Shwartzman-Phänomen auslösbar war.

Somit kann also die auffallende Verminderung der Capillarresistenz nach intracutaner Endotoxinverabreichung wider Erwarten *nicht* als ein für die Shwartzman-

---

* 1. E. Coli; 2. Serratia marcescens (detoxifiziert); 3. Streptolysin 0. Für die Überlassung bzw. Herstellung der Endotoxine danken wir Herrn Dr. O. LÜDERITZ, Max Planck-Institut Freiburg, Herrn Dr. B. URBASCHEK, Krebsforschungsinstitut Heidelberg, und Herrn Prof. A. H. NOWOTNY, Temple Univ. School of Medicine, Dept. of Microbiol., Philadelphia, Pensilvania, USA.

Präparation entscheidender Faktor angesehen werden. Die Natur des Präparations-vorganges bleibt weiterhin im Dunkel, und neue Untersuchungen müssen abklären, welche örtlichen oder systemischen Faktoren für das Zustandekommen der eigen-artigen pseudo-immunologischen, hämorrhagischen Reaktion tatsächlich verant-wortlich sind.

(Ausführliche Veröffentlichung erfolgt in Kürze im Arch. klin. exp. Derm.)

Literatur. HOIGNÉ, R., F. KOLLER und H. STORCK: Dermatologica (Basel) **103**, 234 (1951)

Immunological Aspects of the Aldrich's Syndrome

G. IACOVACCI, S. UNGARI and F. AIUTI, Clinica Pediatrica, Clinica Malattie Infettive dell'Università, Istituto Dermatologico S. Gallicano, Rome (Italy)

The Aldrich's syndrome is generally characterized by a particular dysgamma-globulinemia as well as by a symptomatological triad represented by thrombocyto-penic purpura, atopic eczema and decreased resistance to infections.

We have carried out an immunological study of a young patient, 10 years old, who came to our hospital. Since his first months of life, thrombocytopenic purpura was noticed as well as repeated haemorrhagic enterocolitis, eczematic eruptions and continuous infections represented by sinusitis, middle otitis, bronchitis, pyo-dermitis.

The results of the immunological analysis effected are shown hereunder:

Blood group	O Rh +
Natural alpha and beta isoagglutinins	none
Immunoelectrophoresis (qualitative method according to SCHEIDEGGER)	
G and A immunoglobulin	normal
M immunoglobulin	none
Immunodiffusion (semiquantitative method according to OUCHTERLONY)	
G and A immunoglobulin	normal
M immunoglobulins	less than 1/4
Radial simple immunodiffusion (according to MANCINI)	
Ig G 750 mg-%	(norm. 750 to 1500 mg-%)
Ig A 240 mg-%	(norm. 130 to 250 mg-%)
Ig M 7 mg-%	(norm. 60 to 150 mg-%)

Our researches have emphasized the absence of the natural isoagglutinins and a strong decrease of the M immunoglobulin. And this is also in accordance with what is frequently pointed out in the recent literature. That is why, in accordance with WEST and coll., the Aldrich's syndrome may be included among the forms of dysgammaglobulinemia.

In the literature have been mentioned: by GIEDON, a case presenting, together with the susceptibility to infections and absence of A gamma and M gamma glo-bulins, an eczematous dermatitis. By BARANDUM and coll. a case with repeated infections, eosinophilia, low A gamma, M gamma isoagglutinins and thrombocyto-penia. These clinical symptoms may be considered as uncomplete forms of Aldrich's syndrome, lacking in the former case, the thrombocytopenia and in the latter the eczema.

In all these forms, however, the most important immunological characteristic is the decrease of the Ig M. The quantitative dosage of this fraction, as it was made in our case, seems particularly important to us. In fact this globulin constitutes the first anticorpal reply both in the newborn and in the adult, and then its absence may explain easy infections. In these patients a systematic therapy with gamma-globulins may be particularly useful.

Mise en évidence d'anticorps circulants dans les manifestations cutanées de l'allergie à la pénicilline

J. Paupe et Cl. Mikol, Hôpital Beaujon, Clichy (France)

La recherche des anticorps circulants par une méthode simple et reproductible permet de démontrer avec certitude l'existence d'une allergie à la pénicilline. La fréquence de cette dernière et le risque qu'elle représente justifient le développement des méthodes qui permettent de la détecter in vitro.

Le test de Shelley, basé sur la dégranulation des basophiles de lapin par la réaction antigène-anticorps, donne des résultats assez difficiles à interpréter.

Le test de transformation lymphoblastique des lymphocytes peut servir à la détection de la sensibilisation à la pénicilline mais il exige une installation pour culture de cellules.

L'anaphylaxie passive in vitro de l'iléon de cobaye ne nécessite qu'un appareillage pour organes isolés. Il nous a permis de détecter des anticorps antipénicilline en cas d'urticaire ou de choc anaphylactique.

La réaction d'hémagglutination est de technique facile. Elle avait été proposée par C. Huriez qui utilisait la fixation de la pénicilline sur les hématies par diazotation. A la suite de A. B. Ley et de A. H. DeWeck, nous utilisons une technique par simple adsorption de la pénicilline sur des hématies humaines du groupe 0 en milieux alcalin (pH 9).

Ont été étudiés selon cette méthode les sérums de 77 sujets cliniquement allergiques à la pénicilline et de 47 témoins apparemment non allergiques. Ces malades étaient atteints d'urticaire ou d'œdème de Quincke (41 cas), de réaction anaphylactique (7 cas), d'érythème tardif (19 cas), ou d'eczéma (10 cas).

L'hémagglutination a été positive dans 24 cas d'urticaire-œdème de Quincke, 4 cas de choc anaphylactique, 4 cas d'érythème tardif et 2 cas d'eczéma.

En groupant les sujets qui ont fait des accidents d'hypersensibilité humorale se trouvent 28 positivités sur 48 sérums examinés. Par contre sur les 27 cas évoquant une hypersensibilité cellulaire, les réactions d'hémagglutination n'ont été positives que dans 6 cas. Dans la série témoin, dont certains sérums provenaient de malades ayant reçu antérieurement de la pénicilline, il n'y eut que trois positivités.

Ainsi, la réaction d'hémagglutination ne met généralement en évidence d'anticorps que dans les accidents d'allergie humorale. Dans ce cas, le prélèvement ne doit être fait que 8 jours après l'accident initial en raison de la disparition des anticorps circulants lors du conflit immunologique.

En conclusion, la réaction d'hémagglutination semble d'un appoint utile pour le diagnostic d'une allergie à la pénicilline qui ne saurait cependant être éliminé devant une réaction négative.

Heutige Diagnostik der Penicillinallergie

P. Michailov und N. Berowa, Universitäts-Hautklinik Sofia (Bulgarien)

Die Penicillinallergie stellt heutzutage in der Medizin ein aktuelles Problem dar. Verschiedenen Autoren nach schwankt ihre Häufigkeit zwischen 1 bis 15%. Besonders alarmierend sind die schweren Reaktionen vom Frühtyp (allergischer Schock, Urticaria, Ödema Quincke, Asthma bronchiale u. a.), die immer wieder zur Beobachtung kommen, dramatisch verlaufen und zuweilen letal enden können.

Die objektive Diagnostik der Penicillinallergie ist sehr schwierig, weil noch immer Methoden fehlen, die sie mit absoluter Sicherheit bestimmen. Das Vorhandensein verschiedener Arten von Penicillinantikörpern, die Unspezifität der klinischen Reaktionen sowie das Risiko, mit dem die direkten diagnostischen Methoden (verschiedene cutane Proben) verbunden sind, stellen wesentliche Schwierigkeiten zur Entwicklung einer spezifischen Diagnostik dar.

Die ausführliche Anamnese vor dem Beginn der Penicillinbehandlung, in bezug auf allgemeine allergische Reaktivität (Asthma, Heuschnupfen, Ekzem), medikamentöse Allergie, Kontakt und Verträglichkeit des Penicillins usw., bleibt immer noch eine der hauptsächlichsten diagnostischen Maßnahmen. Die zur Zeit angewandten diagnostischen Methoden gehen davon aus, daß bei der Penicillinallergie drei Hauptarten allergischer Antikörper vorhanden sind: 19s γ_1- und 7s γ_2-hämagglutinierende und 7s γ_1-hautsensibilisierende (de Weck, Lewin).

In vorliegender Arbeit haben wir versucht, unsere Ergebnisse aus der Anwendung der verschiedenen direkten und indirekten diagnostischen Methoden zu vergleichen, um ihren Anwendungsbereich und diagnostischen Wert zu präzisieren. Wir haben 736 Kranke mit verschiedenen klinischen Formen der Penicillinallergie untersucht.

Von den direkten diagnostischen Methoden, die als Objekt den Kranken selbst haben, verwendeten wir: die epicutanen Proben, die Scarifikation und die intracutane Probe. Von den indirekten (serologischen) Methoden verwendeten wir: den nephelometrischen Test, die Immunodiffusion nach Ochterlony, den Basophylendegranulationstest nach Shelly und die passive Hämagglutination nach Boyden.

Ergebnisse

Die epicutane Probe beweist die Penicillinallergie in 79% der Fälle mit aktiver Kontaktallergie; in 23,2% der Fälle mit aktiver Reaktion vom Frühtyp und nur in 1,7% der Fälle mit Latentallergie, d. h. solche Fälle, die nur anamnestische Angaben für eine durchgemachte aktive Penicillinallergie vom Früh- oder Spättyp geben, ohne momentan klinische Symptome aufzuweisen.

Der Scarifikation- und der Prick-Test beweisen die Penicillinallergie in 70% der Fälle mit aktiven allergischen Reaktionen vom Frühtyp, in 87,8% der Fälle aktiver Kontaktallergie und in 26,5% der Fälle mit Latentallergie.

Die intracutane Probe mit Penicillin-G haben wir bei verhältnismäßig wenig Kranken (78) angewandt. Wir haben sie schnell aufgegeben, da sie bei den Kranken schwere allergische Reaktionen vom Frühtyp auslösen kann. Dabei soll auch die Möglichkeit einer aktiven Sensibilisierung in Betracht gezogen werden, Komplikationen, die vielleicht mit PPL oder anderen neuen Penicillinderivaten vermieden werden könnten.

Mit der indirekten Probe haben wir folgende Ergebnisse erhalten: Nephelometrische Tests nach Hoine ergaben bei 67% der Kranken mit Allergie vom Frühtyp positive Ergebnisse. Leider gab es auch viele positive Ergebnisse bei

Kontrollpersonen. Seiner Unspezifität wegen haben wir diesen Test bald aufgegeben. Immunodiffusion nach OUCHTERLONY gab nur ausnahmsweise positive Ergebnisse (1 bis 2%), demzufolge ist sie unzuverlässig für die Diagnostik der Penicillinallergie. Der Basophyllendegranulationstest nach SHELLY gab uns bei 52% der Fälle mit aktiven allergischen Erscheinungen vom Frühtyp positive Resultate. Bei den Fällen mit Latent- oder Kontaktallergie blieb er immer negativ. Die passive Hämagglutination nach BOYDEN gab bei 54% der Fälle mit frühallergischen Reaktionen positive Ergebnisse; bei 8,7% der Fälle mit Kontaktallergie und in 5% bei Latentallergie. Nach den Ergebnissen erwies sich diese Probe als die empfindlichste und zuverlässigste von den indirekten Methoden.

Zusammenfassend kann gesagt werden, daß die indirekten Methoden, obwohl neuer und harmloser, weniger empfindlich als die direkten sind. Ihre richtigen Anwendungsbereiche sind die manifesten allergischen Reaktionen vom Frühtyp.

Der diagnostische Wert der verschiedenen Methoden hängt direkt von der allergischen Reaktion ab. Die Indikationen der Anwendung verschiedener Methoden sind unserer Erfahrung nach folgende: bei den aktiven allergischen Reaktionen vom Frühtyp — die passive Hämagglutination und der Basophyllendegranulationstest sind zuverlässig; bei den aktiven kontaktallergischen Reaktionen — die Läppchenprobe und der Scarifikationstest; bei der Latentallergie — der Scarifikationstest und Läppchenprobe. Man kann wohl sagen, daß bis jetzt keine Methode besteht, die auf eine sichere Weise die Penicillinallergie beweisen kann. Die positiven Proben nach der einen oder anderen Methode objektivieren nur einige Penicillinantikörper. Das bedeutet leider nicht, daß gerade diese Antikörper verantwortlich für die klinischen Erscheinungen sind. Es ist wohl bekannt, daß bei der Penicillinallergie sog. „begleitende" Antikörper oft zu finden sind, ohne einen pathogenetischen Wert zu besitzen. Es ist möglich, daß die Anwendung von Penicillin bei Kranken mit starken positiven Reaktionen ohne Folgen verläuft. Diese Tatsache konnte mit dem „begleitenden" Charakter der Antikörper, sowie mit der menschlichen Reaktivität überhaupt, erklärt werden. Es ist bekannt, daß letztere nicht nur von imunologischen sondern auch von hormonalen und neurogenen Einflüssen bestimmt wird.

Auch die negativen Ergebnisse der Proben schließen mit Sicherheit das Vorhandensein einer Penicillinallergie nicht aus. Es ist wohl möglich, daß die Antikörper einen geringen Titer während der Zeit der Untersuchung haben, oder die Allergie von anderen Arten von Antikörpern bedingt ist als jenen, die mit der verwendeten Methode zu entdecken sind.

Zum Schluß möchten wir sagen, daß trotz der Unvollkommenheit der verschiedenen diagnostischen Methoden die breite Penicillinanwendung sowie die Häufigkeit der allergischen Reaktionen, mit der sie verbunden ist, die vorläufigen Untersuchungen zur Penicillinallergie absolut notwendig machen.

Symposium 12   **The Skin and Internal Disease**

Peau et maladies internes

Piel y enfermedades internas

Hauterscheinungen bei inneren Krankheiten

Organizer

L. A. BRUNSTING, USA

Presidents

A. BACCAREDDA-BOY, Italy

A. BAZEX, France

M. SEIJI, Japan

H. J. WALLACE, Great Britain

Delegate of the Organization Committee

R. M. BOHNSTEDT, Germany

Reports

Erythropoietic Protoporphyria

I. A. Magnus, Institute of Dermatology, St. John's Hospital for Diseases of the Skin, London (England)

Erythropoietic protoporphyria (EPP) is a quite common cause of photosensitivity of the skin that is often familial. What seems to have been the first published case, was a baby under the care of Sir Archibald Gray (1926). The case was neither properly documented nor a final diagnosis arrived at at that time, but I was able to have access to private notes made by Sir Archibald; he characterized the case as "hydroa aestivale" with photosensitivity, without "haematoporphyrinuria", but with excess stool porphyrin. Blood porphyrin chemical assay was not done at that time and indeed it is difficult to see how it could have been with methods then available. The same patient, now an adult, was correctly diagnosed and very thoroughly investigated, including extensive isotope studies, nearly 40 years later (Gray et al., 1964).

Credit is due to Treibs for first pointing out the increase of protoporphyrin in red cells and stool in this disease (Kosenow and Treibs, 1953). The biochemical and photobiological background was worked out quantitatively by Prof. Rimington and others (Magnus et al., 1961; Holti et al., 1963) simultaneously but independently of Langhof et al. (1961) in Germany. Since then there have been numerous published cases, and I know of as many again that have not been published, from a number of different countries, mostly in North Europe and the USA. Spanish, Latin American, Japanese and Chinese cases are also known.

Of our 23 personal cases that have been fully studied clinically, photobiologically, biochemically and histochemically, twelve were familial (six different families). Nearly all present a characteristic clinical picture. Of the acute manifestations the most striking are subjective, i.e. a burning sensation whilst being exposed to sun. Symptoms may be produced either directly by sun, sometimes through window glass or occasionally even through thin clothing. The burning sensation may start during exposure or soon afterwards, and last hours, days, even weeks. This may be the only notable manifestation, though most patients also show erythema or swelling, less often urticaria, ecchymoses, vesicles. Later there may be small bullae, crusts and superficial scarring. The last feature, in our cases in England at least, is so trivial as to be easily overlooked.

For most purposes these patients are under the care of the dermatologist only. However some have to see surgeons who have removed gall stones and gall bladder. The relatively high incidence of cholelithiasis in young males is presumably due to a high concentration of protoporphyrin, insoluble in the bile (Cripps and Scheuer, 1965).

Although primarily a dermatological disease, some cases through misdiagnosis, were labelled malingerers or strayed into the hands of psychiatrists; these were cases with severe subjective sensations of burning in the skin with minimal objective changes. Others have been confused with lipoid proteinosis where the skin histology has close similarities (Rimington et al., 1967).

The diagnosis of EPP is in principle very easy, the history distinctive, the biochemistry and photobiology highly characteristic. Red cell protoporphyrin and, to a lesser extent, coproporphyrin are raised; the stool protoporphyrin is usually high also, but the urinary porphyrin normal. Red cells show the characteristic orange-red fluorescence of porphyrins when illuminated by violet light; but this fluorescence is unstable.

Why was this disease, in our experience common, overlooked for so long? We only stumbled on this condition through doing action spectroscopy on the skin. We knew what the action spectrum for porphyria cutanea tarda was; when we came across patients with the same action spectrum that did *not* have urinary porphyrin in excess, we suspected a "new" kind of porphyria. But it required the collaboration of porphyrin biochemists, haematologists and histochemists, for the picture to be finally clarified.

I think there are two reasons why EPP was overlooked. Firstly the notion of a porphyria *without* excess urinary porphyrin was somewhat startling. 10 years ago a negative urine for porphyrin was considered enough to dismiss this diagnosis. Secondly I think we must lay a little blame at the feet of HANS FISCHER. This man, a giant in porphyrin chemistry, with a world wide influence, is of course one of Munich's most famous men of science. Not wishing to be ungracious, I do this with hesitation. But he was far too great a man to worry about being reproached over what is a quite small matter, when one considers his life's achievements. I refer to the matter of the photosensitizing properties of protoporphyrin. In a paper by FISCHER and SCHNELLER of 1923 it is stated that protoporphyrin has *no* photosensitizing effect in Man. This statement was made, one can now see with hind sight, on slender evidence. For FISCHER, himself, and independent workers showed that protoporphyrin photosensitizes paramecia or laboratory animals *in vivo* and chemical reactions *in vitro*. That protoporphyrin is the porphyrin in the skin in EPP which causes photosensitivity seems more or less proven by the microfluorospectrophotometric work of RUNGE (PETERKA et al., 1965).

The basic cause of EPP is genetic. What exactly this lesion is remains unknown. There is the evidence of abnormal porphyrin metabolism in the bone marrow and, from isotope and histological studies, of some kind of liver dysfunction (GRAY et al., 1964; CRIPPS and SCHEUER, 1965). Yet, in contrast to Gunther's disease, red cell and haemoglobin production is virtually always normal. Also conventional liver function tests, where they have been done, have proved, in contrast to porphyria cutanea tarda, to be normal.

I would like to end by mentioning the rôle we believe lysosomes play in the production of skin lesions in EPP and indeed probably in other types of photosensitization. We believe that the photosensitizing agent, which in the case of EPP is protoporphyrin, damages the lysosome wall by photo-oxidation and that this liberates lytic enzymes that lead to the release of chemical mediators that cause the observed skin lesion. Perhaps it is here, at the level of the initial photochemical reaction, rather than in the seemingly formidable area of the molecular biology of genetics that a quick and easy future lies for combating the symptoms of this disease and porphyria in general. But we must not be too short sighted; who knows how long it will be before specific drugs are available with, let us say, an anti-operon activity?

References. CRIPPS, D. J., and P. J. SCHEUER: Arch. Path. 80, 500 (1965). — GRAY, A. M. H.: Quart. J. Med. 19, 381 (1926). — GRAY, C. H., A. KULCZYCKA, D. C. NICHOLSON, I. A. MAGNUS, and C. RIMINGTON: Clin. Sci. 26, 7 (1964). — HOLTI, G., I. A. MAGNUS, and C. RIMINGTON: Brit. J. Derm. 75, 225 (1963). — KOSENOW, W., u. A. TREIBS: Z. Kinderheilk. 73, 82 (1953). — LANGHOF, H., H. MUELLER und L. RIETSCHEL: Arch. klin. exp. Derm. 212, 506 (1961). — MAGNUS, I. A., A. JARRETT, T. A. J. PRANKERD, and C. RIMINGTON: Lancet 1961 II, 448. — PETERKA, E. S., R. M. FUSARO, W. J. RUNGE, M. O. JAFFE, and C. J. WATSON: J. Amer. med. Ass. 193, 1036 (1965). — RIMINGTON, C., I. A. MAGNUS, E. A. RYAN, and D. J. CRIPPS: Quart. J. Med. 36, 29 (1967).

Xanthomatoses et maladies systémiques

A. Bazex, A. Dupré et B. Christol, Clinique Dermatologique, Hôpital La Grave, Toulouse (France)

Généralités

Dans ce court exposé nous ne pouvons envisager que les principales maladies systémiques susceptibles de se compliquer de Xanthome (X.): myxoedème, néphrose lipoïdique, pancréatites, affections résultant d'une erreur du métabolisme du glucose, affections hépatiques et hématopoïétiques.

Comme dans toute xanthomatose, surviennent sur les téguments et les muqueuses, un ou plusieurs des trois types de X.: X. éruptifs, X. tubéreux, X. plans.

Suivant l'absence ou la présence de modifications portant au niveau du sang sur la lipémie, les triglycérides (T.G.), le cholestérol total (C.T.) et estérifié (C.E.), les phospholipides (P.L.) et la migration des lipoprotéines (L.P.), on rattache les X. à plusieurs syndromes parfois isolés, parfois associés chez un même malade, différents non seulement sur le plan biologique mais encore sur les plans clinique et pronostique.

Dans les X. normolipidémiques: il n'existe aucune anomalie dans le dosage des lipides et le lipidogramme. Cliniquement se développent surtout des X. plans. Le pronostic dépend de l'étiologie.

Dans les X. hyperlipidémiques: suivant le lipide de taux le plus élevé on distingue: 1. *Les X. hyper C.T.:* le taux du C.T. est très élevé ainsi que celui des P.L., par contre le taux des T.G. est voisin de la normale. Au lipidogramme il existe une *hyperbétalipoprotéinémie*. Ces anomalies biologiques s'accompagnent de X. tubéreux et plans et, à la longue, d'altérations vasculaires diverses de pronostic grave. 2. *Les X. hyper T.G.:* le phénomène capital est l'augmentation du taux de T.G. Lorsque ce taux est très élevé le sérum est lactescent; on les divise suivant l'aspect du lipidogramme en deux catégories: *X. hyperchylomicronémiques:* le taux des T.G. dépasse toujours $3 \text{ g-}^0/_{00}$. Le C.T. et les P.L. sont légèrement en dessus de la normale. L'injection d'héparine ne fait pas disparaître la lactescence du sérum. Des X. éruptifs apparaissent lorsque l'hyperlipidémie dépasse un taux variable pour chaque malade. Des manifestations douloureuses abdominales, d'origine splénique ou pancréatique sont susceptibles de survenir. Un régime pauvre en graisse abaisse le taux des lipides sanguins et fait disparaître les xanthomes. *X. hyperprébéta L.P.* Le taux des T.G. est moins élevé que dans la forme X. précédente: le C.T. et les P.L. ne s'élèvent que si l'hyperlipidémie est massive. Les trois types cliniques de X. peuvent s'observer. Ils s'associent parfois à une hyperglycémie de degré variable. Des complications vasculaires, spléniques, hépatiques, oculaires peuvent survenir. Seule une restriction des hydrates de carbone peut réduire l'hyperlipidémie.

Principales maladies internes s'accompagnant de xanthomatoses

Myxoedème: bien que cette maladie s'accompagne toujours d'une hyperlipidémie, l'apparition des X. est l'exception et ne survient que chez les adultes. Le C.T. est à un taux élevé, et le lipidogramme signale une hyperbéta L.P. Parfois s'associe une augmentation du taux des T.G. se traduisant par une hyperprébéta L.P. Les X. sont de type tubéreux ou plans. Des X. éruptifs surviennent parfois. Le traitement par les hormones thyroïdiennes fait chuter le taux des lipides sanguins et atténue ou fait disparaître les X.

Néphrose lipoïdique. Bien que la lipémie soit toujours élevée la présence de X. est assez exceptionnelle: le taux des lipides est très élevé et porte essentiellement sur les T.G. L'examen du lipidogramme met en évidence une altération complexe caractérisée par une hyperchylomicronémie associée à une hyperprébéta L.P. Les X. sont toujours de type éruptif et les poussées sont passagères. Leur disparition ainsi que la chute de la lipémie sont obtenues par des traitements qui suppriment l'hypoprotidémie. Dans les formes secondaires où un traitement est impossible, peuvent apparaître des X. tubéreux ou plans ainsi que les complications inhérentes à l'hyperbéta L.P.

Pancréatites. P. aiguë. La cause principale en est l'intoxication alcoolique. Les manifestations biologiques et cliniques apparaissent dans les heures ou les semaines qui suivent l'intoxication. La lipémie est très élevée et cette élévation est en rapport avec l'augmentation des T.G., le C.T. et les P.L. étant à un taux voisin de la normale. Au lipidogramme on aperçoit une augmentation des prébéta L.P. La glycémie est toujours élevée. Les X. sont de type éruptif et au fur et à mesure que s'atténuent les signes pancréatiques la lipémie revient à un taux normal et les X. disparaissent. *P. chronique calcifiante:* la lipémie n'est que modérément élevée. Au cours des poussées aiguës le tableau clinique et biologique réalisé est celui des pancréatites aiguës. Mais les phénomènes ne s'atténuent que lentement. Si les poussées se répètent la lipémie reste constamment très élevée et des X. tubéreux et plans peuvent apparaître.

Erreur portant sur le métabolisme du glucose

1. *Diabète:* seuls les diabètes insulino-résistants ou mal soignés ainsi que ceux qui apparaissent au cours d'acromégalies sont susceptibles de se compliquer d'hyperlipidémie. L'hyperlipidémie est très élevée. L'augmentation porte avant tout sur les T.G. mais le C.T. et les P.L. sont à un taux normal ou modérément élevé. Au lipidogramme les anomalies se traduisent par une prébéta L.P. associée tantôt à une hyperchylomicronémie, tantôt à une béta L.P. Il existe toujours des X. éruptifs localisés sur la peau et la muqueuse buccale pouvant s'infecter secondairement et se surmonter de pustules. Des X. tubéreux et plans peuvent apparaître, le foie est augmenté de volume et les complications inhérentes à l'hyperprébéta L.P. surviennent précocement. L'hyperlipidémie et les manifestations cliniques qui en découlent ne disparaissent que si le diabète peut être traité

2. *Maladie de Von Gierke.* Les caractères biologiques et cliniques des X. qui surviennent dans un nombre assez élevé de cas, sont identiques à ceux du diabète, bien que parfois le lipidogramme indique seulement une élévation des prébéta L.P.

Affections hépatiques. Exceptionnellement peut survenir une xanthomatose au cours de cancer du foie. En pratique une seule affection peut être retenue: *c'est la cirrhose biliaire xanthomateuse.* Elle résulte soit d'une oblitération des canaux biliaires extrahépatiques (congénitale ou acquise), soit d'une obstruction des canaux biliaires intrahépatiques (primitive ou secondaire à une infection, à une intoxication). La cirrhose évolue lentement, débute par un ictère de type rétentionnel avec gros foie et manifestations prurigineuses intenses, puis surviennent l'hyperlipidémie et les X. Les P.L. se trouvent à un taux très élevé, le C.T. est modérément accru, mais le C.E. est fortement abaissé. Les T.G. sont normaux, sauf chez l'enfant où ils sont légèrement augmentés. Le lipidogramme est tout à fait particulier: les alpha L.P. sont diminuées, la majorité des L.P. migrent autour de la zone béta et prébéta et la partie protéique serait surtout formée de polypeptides. L'éruption débute par des X. plans se transformant en X. tubéreux: ils peuvent survenir en tous points des téguments mais tout spécialement sur le siège des excoriations et les paumes. Mis à part les cas exceptionnels où il est possible de rétablir la perméabilité des canaux biliaires, l'hyperlipémie et les X. persistent indéfiniment.

Affections hématopoïétiques

1. *Myélomes multiples.* Depuis ces dernières années les observations de X. se sont multipliées. Leur apparition peut coexister avec celle du myélome ou lui succéder (ce qui est le plus fréquent) ou la précéder (ce qui est exceptionnel). On peut observer des *X. hyperlipidémiques.* Ce sont les plus rares, les T.G. sont toujours très élevés, le C.T. à un taux normal ou peu élevé. Au lipidogramme, on aperçoit un précipité des L.P. sur la zone correspondant à la protéine anormale (prébéta le plus souvent). Cliniquement les xanthomes se présentent, au début sous l'aspect de xanthomes éruptifs et se transforment par la suite en xanthomes plans ou tubéreux. *Les X. normolipidémiques:* Sur le plan clinique il s'agit de X. plans qui ont comme caractéristique d'être très étendus, plusieurs centimètres de diamètre, et d'être parsemés de stries et de taches hémorragiques ou brunâtres. Ils ne s'étendent que très lentement et ne disparaissent jamais.

2. *Histiocytosis X.* Dans la maladie de Letterer-Sive et dans la maladie de Schuller-Christian il a été signalé des X. Il s'agit de X. normocholestérolémiques

Tableau 1. *Tableaux récapitulatifs*

Type de xanthomatose	Aspect du lipidogramme	Taux des lipides dans le sang	Aspect clinique des xanthomes	Pronostic inhérent à la xanthomatose
Normo-lipidémique	Normal	Cholestérol: normal Phospholipides: normales Triglycérides: normales	Plans	Bon
Hyper-lipidémiques	Hyperbétalipo-protéinémie	Cholestérol $+++$ Phospholipides $+++$ Triglycérides $+$	Tubéreux, plans.	Possibilité d'accident vasculaire
	Hyperchylo-micronémie	Cholestérol $+$ Phospholipides $+$ Triglycérides $+++$	Eruptifs	Bon
	Hyperprébéta-lipoprotéinémie	Cholestérol $+$ Phospholipides $+$ Triglycérides $+++$	Eruptifs surtout tubé-reux, plans	Possibilité d'accident vasculaire

Tableau 2

Affection en cause	Type biologique des xanthomatoses	Particularités de la xanthomatose
Myxoedème	Hyperbéta associée parfois à hyper-prébétalipoprotéinémie	Guérit par disparition du myxoedème
Néphrose lipoïdique	Hyperchylomicronémie associée à hyperprébétalipoprotéinémie	Ne guérit que par la disparition de la néphrose
Pancréatite	Hyperprébéta	Guérit par la disparition de la pancréatite
Diabète et maladie de Von Gierke	Hyperprébéta parfois associée à une hyperchylomicronémie ou à une hyperbétalipoprotéinémie	Ne guérit que par la disparition des troubles glucidiques
Cirrhose biliaire xanthomateuse	Hyperprébéta lipoprotéinémie avec très forte élévation des phospholipides	Ne guérit que si la cirrhose peut être traitée

Affections hématopoïétiques	1er type:
	    hyperprébétalipoprotéinémie
	2ème type:
	    normocholestérolémie
		Peut s'améliorer par traitement de l'affection hématopoïétique, ne disparaît jamais.

pouvant se présenter sous l'aspect de X. plans ou de X. tubéreux susceptibles de simuler les naevo-xanthoendothéliomes.

3. Il a été publié des observations de X. au cours de *macroglobulinémies* (la xanthomatose a les mêmes caractères cliniques et biologiques que dans les myélomes multiples), de *leucose myéloïde ou lymphoïde* où les X. sont de type normolipidémique plan.

Skin Disorders in Relation to Malabsorption

G. C. WELLS, St. Thomas's Hospital, London (England)

Defective absorption from the small intestine may become manifest at any age, and the clinical picture varies widely. Steatorrhoea is usually obvious, but important malabsorption can exist in the absence of diarrhoea and with normal faecal fat. We now use the term "coeliac syndrome" to cover a large complex of symptoms and signs which includes childhood coeliac disease, adult coeliac disease, idiopathic steatorrhoea, gluten enteropathy, and enteropathy secondary to other illness. Essential to the coeliac syndrome is marked villous atrophy (flat mucosa) on jejunal biopsy (PINK and CREAMER, 1967). Elimination of gluten from the diet is usually, but not always, decisive in correcting the malabsorption; the success rate being about 70%.

Reviews of large groups of patients with coeliac syndrome reveal a rather high incidence (10 to 20%) of skin disorders (COOKE et al., 1953), and this has been the experience of Dr. CREAMER and myself with patients investigated at St. Thomas's Hospital. Some of these skin disorders are common to malabsorption states and to other wasting diseases, some are related to deficiency of essential food factors, and others (pruriginous and eczematous) have a relationship with the coeliac syndrome that is unexplained.

Skin disorders in coeliac syndrome

Pigmentation (melanosis). Minor degrees of general melanosis are common in coeliac syndrome, and patchy facial pigmentation (chloasma) may be seen. Occasionally the general melanosis is so striking as to suggest Addison's disease, from which distinction may be difficult (McBRIEN et al., 1963). In cases where eczema is present there may be associated lesional pigmentation.

Acquired ichthyosis. Mild ichthyosis is quite common in coeliac syndrome, as in other long-term wasting diseases. Sometimes this may provide the starting point for eczema craquelé. Rapid onset of more severe general ichthyosis, especially if disproportionate to the wasting, may suggest lymphoma involving the small intestine, a sequence that is known to complicate the coeliac syndrome (GOUGH et al., 1962).

Defective hair and nails. Sparseness and dryness of the hair, and defective nail growth are seen in the more severe cases of coeliac syndrome. They are usually associated with low serum calcium (SIMPSON, 1954) or with anaemia.

Mouth lesions. Sore tongue with atrophy of the filiform papillae and oral ulcers are common in coeliac syndrome, and are related to deficiency of iron, of folate, and occasionally of vitamin B 12. Oral ulcers are sometimes the presenting symptom in coeliac syndrome.

Purpura. Failure to absorb vitamin K may lead to prolonged prothrombin time with resultant purpura and bruising. In this situation dangerous bleeding may occur (SHAW, 1960).

Rosacea. MARKS et al. (1967) made a detailed study of gastrointestinal findings in 62 patients with rosacea in comparison with 62 patients with other skin diseases. No greater incidence of gastrointestinal abnormality was found in patients with rosacea, in whom gastric and jejunal biopsies showed no consistent abnormality. This contrasts with the report of WATSON et al. (1965) of a rather high incidence of small intestine malabsorption in their group of patients with rosacea. Our patients with coeliac syndrome have not shown an undue incidence of rosacea.

Psoriasis. In our patients with coeliac syndrome the incidence of psoriasis has been no greater than that of the normal population. It is possible that exacerbations of malabsorption may aggravate the psoriasis (COOKE et al., 1953), though a severe extension of psoriasis may adversely affect the small intestine (COPEMAN and BOLD, 1965).

Eczema and pruritus. Recalcitrant eczema has been noted in patients with coeliac syndrome, and occasionally eczema has been the first symptom (WELLS, 1962). However, in most of the patients whom we have studied there has been some evidence, in retrospect, to suggest latent coeliac syndrome. The eczema has no specific features. Itching is severe and lichenification is usual. Seborrhoeic, discoid and papulovesicular patterns are seen, and sometimes general exfoliative dermatitis. An unusual degree of pigmentation in relation to the lesions may draw attention to the possibility of malabsorption. The importance of the association lies in the response of the eczema to treatment of the coeliac syndrome. However, no single factor is mandatory. A gluten-free diet may be essential to recovery (FRIEDMAN and HARE, 1965). Correction of low serum calcium alone may be effective (DENT and GARRETTS, 1960), and some patients have responded well to correction of folate deficiency.

On the other hand patients with poorly controlled coeliac syndrome may have severe wasting and multiple deficiencies without necessarily showing any signs of skin disease. Furthermore, investigation of patients with eczema will only rarely reveal evidence of coeliac syndrome (FRY et al., 1966; DORAN et al., 1966). Another difficulty has been demonstrated by MARKS et al. (1966) who find that widespread eczema or psoriasis may lead to secondary steatorrhoea, with some reduction of villous pattern on jejunal biopsy; and this is reversible through effective topical skin therapy. It seems possible that widespread eczema or psoriasis, with their increased epidermal mitotic activity may deplete the body of folate (KNOWLES et al., 1963) and this in turn might interfere with jejunal function. Some other explanation is needed, however, for the high incidence of jejunal abnormality in dermatitis herpetiformis.

Dermatitis herpetiformis. MARKS et al. (1966) investigated twelve patients with dermatitis herpetiformis, two of whom had symptoms of malabsorption. Jejunal biopsies in these twelve patients revealed a high incidence of histological abnormality with five cases showing marked villous atrophy (flat jejunal mucosa). In one case no treatment had been given for the dermatitis herpetiformis so that medication was not responsible for the jejunal changes. These findings have been confirmed by TONGEREN et al. (1967) who report subtotal villous atrophy in three of nine jejunal biopsies in patients with dermatitis herpetiformis. This finding is surprising since patients with dermatitis herpetiformis usually continue under observation for many years without ill health. However, SMITH (1966), in a review of 96 cases of dermatitis herpetiformis noted that 2 diamino-diphenyl-sulphone-dependent patients had frank gluten enteropathy. In some cases there was evidence of coeliac syndrome before the onset of dermatitis herpetiformis.

Comment

Our main concern has been with patients with obstinate eczema or pruriginous conditions in whom there is latent coeliac syndrome which is difficult to diagnose. While this condition is certainly rare, relative to the problem of eczema in general, it is important in that management of the coeliac syndrome may benefit the patient in all respects. We have insufficent data on other malabsorption states to allow comparison though the impression at present is that other conditions such as pancreatic steatorrhoea are not associated with eczema or pruriginous skin eruptions.

References. COOKE, W. T., A. L. P. PEENEY, and C. F. HAWKINS: Quart. J. Med. **22**, 59 (1953). — COPEMAN, P. W. M., and A. M. BOLD: Proc. roy. Soc. Med. **58**, 425 (1965). — DENT, C. E., and M. GARRETTS: Lancet **1960 I**, 142. — DORAN, C. K., M. A. EVERETT, and J. D. WELSH: Arch. Derm. **94**, 574 (1966). — FRIEDMAN, M., and P. J. HARE: Lancet **1965 I**, 521. — FRY, L., R. M. H. MCMINN, and S. SHUSTER: Arch. Derm. **93**, 647 (1966). — GOUGH, K. R., A. E. READ, and J. M. NAISH: Gut **3**, 232 (1962). — KNOWLES, J. P., S. SHUSTER, and G. C. WELLS: Lancet **1963 I**, 1138. — MARKS, J., S. SHUSTER, and A. J. WATSON: Lancet **1966 II**, 1280. — MARKS, R., R. J. BEARD, M. L. CLARK, M. KWOK, and W. B. ROBERTSON: Lancet **1967 I**, 739. — MCBRIEN, D. J., R. V. JONES, and B. CREAMER: Lancet **1963 I**, 25. — PINK, I. J., and B. CREAMER: Lancet **1967 I**, 300. — SHAW, S.: Brit. med. J. **1960 II**, 647. — SIMPSON, J. A.: Brit. J. Derm. **66**, 1 (1954). — SMITH, E. L.: Trans. St. John's Hosp. derm. Soc. (Lond.) **52**, 176 (1966). — TONGEREN, J. M. H., W. J. B. M. STAAK, and P. H. M. SCHILLINGS: Lancet **1967 I**, 218. — WATSON, W. C., E. PATON, and D. MURRAY: Lancet **1965 II**, 47. — WELLS, G. C.: Brit. med. J. **1962 II**, 937.

Further Studies on Acrodermatitis Enteropathica

N. DANBOLT, Oslo (Norway)

Acrodermatitis enteropathica (Ae) is a condition with characteristic cutaneous manifestations which is attributed to certain metabolic disturbances in the intestinal tract. Hydroxyquinoline derivates give remarkably good symptomatic relief, and this clinical fact provides the basis for certain theories concerning the pathogenesis of this condition. The syndrome was first described as a clinical entity by Dr. CLOSS and myself in 1942 [3].

I have subsequently had the opportunity to observe a girl with Ae from the age of 2½ until now, when she has reached the age of 21 [2]. During this time I have undertaken a series of special studies to evaluate my own view and the views of others on the pathogenesis of the condition. A short account of these studies forms the substance of this paper.

1. The effect upon the clinical symptoms of chemotherapeutic "disinfection" of the intestinal tract

At the time of this trial the patient was 20 years old [2]. She had been treated for a long time with sub-curative doses of hydroxyquinoline and her symptoms could be described as moderate. The treatment consisted of alternating courses of Bacimycin* two tablets 5 times a day for 3 days followed by Phthalylsulphatiazole 1 g 5 times a day for 7 days, the treatment being continued for 5 weeks in all. Bacteriological examination of the faeces during this time showed varying growth of E. coli, Proteus, Enterococci and Candida, but by the end of the course of treatment culture gave no growth of pathogenic organisms. No therapeutic effect was observed from this treatment.

---

* One Bacimycin tablet contains 15.000 Units of Bacitracin and 0.3 g of Neomycin.

2. Does Ae result from a defect in the metabolism of essential fatty acids?

In 1965, Dr. RALPH CASH [1], Southfield, Mich. USA, informed me that his observation during the treatment of a case of Ae led him to the belief that the cause of the condition could be a defect in the metabolism of unsaturated fatty acids. He pointed to the similarity between Ae and the effect of a deficiency of essential fatty acids which in puppies, can produce diarrhoea, alopecia, seborrhoeic, dermatitis and itching. In a child with Ae, who subsequently died, he had observed some therapeutic effect from large doses of linoleic acid. Dr. CASH advanced the theory that patients with Ae are unable to synthesise certain unsaturated fatty acids and suggested that parenteral supply of linoleic acid should have a therapeutic effect. For 10 days, my patient was given a daily infusion of 500 ml Infonutrol which is rich in linoleic acid, but no therapeutic effect was observed. Examination of the blood and urine were carried out during this time at the Institute of Clinical Biochemistry (Prof. ELDJARN) at the Rikshospital, Oslo, to ascertain if there were any changes in the unsaturated fatty acids, but no pathological changes could be demonstrated. This trial gave no evidence to support the theory that Ae is caused by a deficiency of essential fatty acids.

3. Is Acrodermatitis enteropathica due to an enzyme deficiency in the mucosa of the intestinal tract?

In 1963, E. J. MOYNAHAN [5] put forward the view "that there may be an enzyme defect in the intestinal mucosa, as a result of which a substance, probably a protein present in the diet, is not being broken down completely into its constituent amino acids, and as a result of which a toxic substance is being absorbed, which is responsible for the characteristic skin lesion and also for malabsorbtion by the intestinal mucosa". Histochemical examination of histological sections from the jejunal mucosa in a girl aged 18 months with the typical picture of Ae showed a reduction in succinic dehydrogenase reaction. A biopsy was taken from the mucosa in the small intestine of my patient, when she was 20 years old. She had then only scattered skin lesions as she was under treatment with hydroxyquinolines. Histological and histochemical analyses were carried out by Prof. OLAV H. IVERSEN at the Institute of General and Experimental Pathology (University of Oslo). The histological picture revealed no abnormality and the succinic dehydrogenase activity showed no deviation from normal.

4. Is a disturbance of tryptophane metabolism responsible for Ae?

In my first publication in 1942, an account was given of a trial of tryptophane loading in one of the patients with Ae and an increase in symptoms was noticed when 2.500 mg L.-tryptophane was administered. In 1963, Dr. OLLE HANSSON, Uppsala, Sweden [4], put forward the following theory:

"It is suggested that the disease is due to an alteration in the normal tryptophane metabolism. Through a deviation to "the Quinoline pathway", an enzymatic failure results in a production of a metabolite with toxic effects on the cutaneous and intestinal epithelium. It is suggested that the chemical configuration of the metabolite is so similar to that of the halogen-substituted 8 — OH quinolines that the latter will prevent the toxic effect by "competition" or, will obviate the metabolic production by enzyme — blocking."

On the basis of this theory, a trial of loading with L.-tryptophane was carried out, the patient was then taking chlorquinaldon (Siosteran) orally and was practically symptom-free. She took 4 g L.-tryptophane by month, but no increase in her symptoms was observed. Before the ingestion of the tryptophane, two-dimensional paper chromatografy was carried out, on a 24 h-urine specimen at the Institute of Clinical Biochemistry (Prof. ELDJARN), and showed a normal amino-acid pattern. An identical pattern was found in the 24 h-urine collected after trypto-phane medication. It was then, however, possible to demonstrate tryptophane in amounts less than 300 mg measured semi-quantitatively. Repeated examina-tions of the urine for xanthurenic acid and 5 hydroxy-indolacetic acid gave nega-tive results. These trials gave no support to the theory that an alteration of tryptophane metabolism is the cause of Ae.

Conclusion: Although all the trials have failed to shed any light on the patho-genesis of Ae, it is the authors opinion that continued study should be concentrated particularly both on the theory that there is an enzyme defect in the mucosa of the intestinale tract and a disturbance of tryptophane metabolism, since Ae must be considered to be an "inborn error of metabolism".

References. 1. CASH, R.: Pers. communication. — 2. DANBOLT, N.: Hautarzt **15**, 25 (1964). — 3. DANBOLT, N., and K. CLOSS: Acta derm.-venereol. (Stockh.) **23**, 127 (1942). — 4. HANSSON, O.: Acta derm.-venereol. (Stockh.) **43**, 465 (1963). — 5. MOYNAHAN, E. J.: Proc. roy Soc. Med. **56**, 300 (1963).

A New Classification for Lupus Erythematosus

J. R. HASERICK, Division of Dermatology, Case Western Reserve University, Cleveland, Ohio (USA)

Lupus erythematosus (L.E.), with its capacity for involving every organ and tissue, is a disease that is not easy to classify. Because of a dermatologic heritage that goes back to the first descriptions of the skin lesions by BIETT [1] in 1838, the naming of the disease by another French dermatologist CAZENAVE [2] in 1850, and the linkage with visceral disease by the Viennese dermatologist KAPOSI [3] in 1872, previous classifications have been quite understandably based upon derma-tologic changes. These are now obsolete.

The description of the L.E. phenomenon [4], and the later discovery of the blood factor [5] responsible both for the L.E. phenomenon and for the recent anti-nuclear fluorescent technics, led to diagnostic tests which in turn proved the disease to be masquerading behind many hitherto unsuspected clinical entities. Thus, previous classifications of L.E., admittedly inadequate even for the dermatologic changes were totally insufficient for the newer visceral or systemic syndromes that have become generally acceptable aspects of lupus erythematosus.

Clearly a new, broader organizational classification of the disease is indicated. Without universal understanding and agreement, definitive and comparative studies on the disease are not possible. Valuable information on the geographic distribution of L.E. is not available at present. Neither is it possible to evaluate the incidence of the disease, and we are thus denied the important information of an increase or a decrease in incidence. Most importantly, it is not possible to evaluate treatment programs utilized by various world wide medical centers, because one group is not sure exactly what another group means, either by degree of type, from the ambiguous, descriptive terms used in older classifications.

Two terms or phrases were used which have double meanings, easily misinter-preted because of ambiguity. The words *acute, subacute,* or *chronic* can be and are interpreted as either indicating: 1. severity of illness and organ involvement, or 2. of duration. In the classification proposed herewith, these vague terms are replaced by concepts of severity, i.e., *mild, moderate,* or *severe.* The terms acute, subacute, and chronic are replaced with *old, new,* and *recurrent.* The other term with a double meaning is *disseminated*. Dermatologists have always used this word in the superficial, scattered sense. It stems from the Latin word "disseminare" meaning seeded (-semin) afar (dis-, apart) or "to sow seed" and thus has a superficial quality of clear meaning to dermatologists. Unfortunately, other medical disciplines have ignored the background of the word and have employed it to mean systemic or visceral. In the new classification the word *disseminated* is used only in the original sense, namely to designate scattered skin lesions. The term *systemic* will replace the word *disseminated* in its visceral meaning. In the English language *systemic* has been accepted over *visceral* though they are accepted as having identical meanings by most clinicians.

In the classification proposed here the term *systemic* is used exclusively when there are *no* specific skin lesions; whereas, disseminated diagnostic dermatologic lesions may or may not be associated with visceral manifestations. There are a different incidence, prognosis, and perhaps even a different geographic distribution in regard to patients who have *systemic* L.E. (Group IV) and those with *disseminated* L.E. (Groups II and III).

There are four groups in the new classification.

Group I. The L.E. diathesis is included for the patient who has no dermatologic or visceral symptoms, but who has either laboratory evidence of systemic involvement or a history suggestive of L.E. manifestations.

Group I. *L.E. Diathesis*
(must Total Five or More Points)

A. *Laboratory*	Points	B. *History of*	Points
1. L.E. test + ...	3	1. Pleurisy	2
2. Antinuclear factor (> 1:80)	3	2. Photosensitivity	2
3. S.T.S. (BFP) + ...	2	3. Discoid L.E.	2
4. Coombs + ...	1	4. Purpura	1
5. Low WBC (< 3,000)	1	5. Hemolytic anemia	1
6. High globulin	1	6. Rheumatic fever, chorea	1
7. High sedimentation rate	1	7. Arthritis	1
8. Unexplained anemia...........	1	8. L.E. in family	1
(Hb. 9 g-% or less)			
9. Latex fixation	1		

Group II. Nonsystemic L.E. with specific dermatologic lesions of L.E. To the experienced dermatologic clinician the skin lesions in patients in this group are diagnostic, and dermatopathologic support, while not absolutely necessary, is easily obtained. Type A. Lymphocytic, is a controversial type and is included for completeness rather than as an absolute category. For our purposes this is considered to be identical with Jessner's lymphocytosis cutis and chronic polymorphic light eruption when it is limited to the temporal regions. The absence of liquefaction degeneration of the basal layer separates this group from Type B, Discoidal and Type C, Erythematous.

Group II. *Nonsystemic L.E.*
(Specific Dermatologic)
(O.R.N.-old, recurrent, new)

A. *Lymphocytic*

B. *Discoidal*
    1. Localized
    2. Disseminated
    3. Hypertrophic
    4. Profundus
    5. Bullous

C. *Erythematous*

Group III. Systemic (or visceral) L.E. with specific dermatologic lesions of L.E. Note the absence of Type A: Lymphocytic from this group. This is omitted because of the absence of evidence for conversion of this type to Group III or IV with systemic involvement. Types B to O (see Group IV) may be added for more specific identification of the kind of visceral involvement.

Group III. *Systemic L.E.*
(Specific Dermatologic)
(O.R.N.-old, recurrent, new)

A. Dermatologic (Specific)

I. *Discoidal*   II. *Erythematous*
1. Localized   1. Mild
2. Disseminated   2. Moderate
3. Hypertrophic   3. Severe
4. Profundus
5. Bullous

(B to O, see Group IV)

Group IV. Systemic (or visceral) L.E. with nonspecific or nondiagnostic dermatologic manifestation. Type B dermatologic lesions, while commonly seen in systemic L.E. are also seen in other non-L.E. conditions.

Group IV. *Systemic L.E.*
(Nondiagnostic Dermatologic)
(O.R.N.-old, recurrent, new)

B. Dermatologic (nonspecific)
1. Photosensitivity
2. Urticaria
3. Alopecia
4. Vasculitis (ulcers, lupus pernio)
5. Miscellaneous (e.g. flame hemorrhages)
C. Hematologic
1. Idiopathic thrombocytopenic purpura
2. Anemia
3. Dysproteinemia
D. Neurologic
1. Epilepsy
2. Peripheral neuropathy
E. Psychiatric

F. Gastrointestinal
1. Chronic ulcerative colitis
2. Lupoid hepatitis
3. Miscellaneous
G. Musculoskeletal
H. Renal
I. Pulmonary
J. SLE with negative L.E. tests
K. Mixed collagen
(e.g. scleroderma with + L.E. tests)
L. Cardiovascular
M. Ophth. — Otolaryng.
N. Endocrine
O. Miscellaneous

The author acknowledges and borrows from the excellent dermatologic classifications of O'LEARY [6], of URBACH and THOMAS [7], and of DUPERRAT [8]. In addition, the efforts of RUPE and NICKEL [9] to diagnose systemic lupus erythematosus by a point system are appreciated. In a sense, the proposed classification is a combination of all of the above classifications, with an attempt to widen the spectrum of factors by encompassing the subclinical state known as the *L.E. diathesis* and the most severe systemic varieties.

References. 1. BIETT, T.: quoted in: Abrégé pratique des maladies de la peau, by CASENAVE, A., et H. E. SCHEDEL: p. 386. Paris 1828. — 2. (Erythème Centrifuge) Ann. Mal. Peau Syph. **3**, 297 (1850—1851). — 3. KAPOSI, M.: Arch. Derm. Syph. (Berl.) **4**, 36 (1872). — 4. HARGRAVES, M. M., H. RICHMOND, and R. MORTON: Proc. Mayo Clin. **23**, 25 (1948). — 5. HASERICK, J. R., and D. W. BORTZ: J. invest. Derm. **13**, 47 (1949). — 6. O'LEARY, P. A.: Proc. Mayo Clin. XV, 675 (1940). — 7. URBACH, E., and C. C. THOMAS: Brit. J. Derm. **51**, 343 (1939). — 8. DUPERRAT, B.: L.E. Lupus Erythémateux Disseminé. Paris: Flammarion 1958. — 9. RUPE, C. E., and S. N. NICKEL: Henry Ford Hosp. Bull. **12**, (1964).

Angiokeratoma Corporis Diffusum

H. J. WALLACE, London (England)

I report here the clinical history and necropsy of a man with A.K.C.D. with particular reference to the neurological symptoms. H.W. died at the age of 31. At the age of 8, attacks of excruciating pain began in the toes and were followed a few months later by similar pains in the fingers and penis. As in other patients with A.K.C.D. he had great difficulty in describing the pain which had a burning quality located between skin and bone. The pains were essentially peripheral, lasting from a few hours to several days. Most attacks appeared to occur spontaneously although a few were caused by trauma and extremes of temperature. Initially the pains occurred at intervals of several weeks but later increased in severity and frequency often accompanied by fever and a raised ESR. At the age of 19 vertigo, nystagmus and proteinuria were noted with mild impairment of renal function. An intravenous pyelogram showed a right-sided hydronephrosis and megaloureter, which at operation was shown to have been caused by a persistently contracted segment of the lower end of the ureter.

The diagnosis of A.K.C.D. was not made until he was 20 years of age when he had characteristic signs in the skin, superficial layers of the cornea and on muscle biopsy. By this time 700 mgm pethidine daily were required to control the pain, but with this dosage he was able to stay at his work.

A year before his death he had attacks of myoclonus, the cause of which was not determined. During one of these attacks he sustained a fractured femur and later died from a pulmonary embolus.

His family history is in keeping with the concept of A.K.C.D. as a sex linked recessive disorder with partial expression in the female. His brother three years younger also has A.K.C.D. of equal severity complicated by a contracture of the iliopelvic colon. An elder brother is unaffected. The mother has a few skin lesions typical corneal dystrophy but no other abnormality.

Studies were carried out in order to try to determine the cause of the pain, but with inconclusive results. Investigations of the central nervous system including cutaneous sensibility, biopsy of a digital nerve, and nerve endings and an electro encephelogram were all normal. Serum creatine kinase, aldolase and an electromyogram were also normal. Vascular flow studies during and in between attacks were inconclusive. The pain was unaffected, except on rare occasions, by full doses both orally and parenterally of antihistamines, autonomic mimetic agents, vasoconstrictors, vasodilators and corticosteroids. It was also unaffected by stellate ganglion block. The effect of the pethidine is unlikely to have been caused by its action on smooth muscle since pure muscle relaxants gave no relief. Other centrally acting preparations such as chlorpromazine were largely ineffective. The pain was relieved when the arterial supply was occluded, until the disappearance of all cutaneous sensation except to deep and repeated pinprick.

The indescribable nature and site of the pain usually unaccompanied by other physical signs appear to set it apart from acroparaesthesia, neuropathies, ischaemia, thalamic syndromes and causalgia.

The effects of peripheral provocation and blockade suggest that the origin of the pain, in part at least, is likely to be at the periphery, possibly by way of a chemical mediator. An experimental approach is proposed to test this hypothesis in another patient with A.K.C.D.

Many other neurological manifestations have been reported in A.K.C.D. including headaches, dizziness, cerebrovascular accidents, paraplegias and epilepsy.

Abnormalities of the myenteric plexus of the viscera have also been described and examination of the contracted ureter in this patient also showed vacuolation of the myenteric ganglia. I have however been unable to discover any other comparable record of myoclonus in A.K.C.D. in the ebsence of true epilepsy.

At the necropsy particular attention was paid to the findings in the central nervous system and for which I am indebted to my collaegue, Dr. V. STEWARD. In addition to ordinary microscopy electronmicroscopy and biochemical analyses were also carried out but will not be described here. The tissues were stained with H. & E. Luxol Fast Blue, SPIELMEYER, NISSL and P.A.S.

In addition to the characteristic A.K.C.D. reaction in vessels and macrophages, the most striking changes were seen in cellular distension and vacuolation of the ganglia of the lateral column containing the cellular relay of the sympathetic system. Similar changes were also seen in the dorsal efferent nucleus of the vagus, in the supra optic nucleus, in the dorsal root ganglia and substantia nigra.

Since similar changes have been reported in the absence of A.K.C.D. their exact significance must await investigation with newer techniques now being conducted. Preliminary results obtained by Dr. STEWARD both in this and other necropsies of A.K.C.D. suggest that the essential constituent of these changes in the ganglia is the sphingo-lipid of A.K.C.D.

Even if these reactions prove to be specific their relation to the neurological symptoms are at present ill defined. The changes in the autonomic nervous system centrally and peripherally suggest that this should be a particularly fruitful field for research.

Consideration of the Etiology of Pyoderma Gangrenosum*

H. O. PERRY and P. DIDISHEIM, Mayo Clinic and Mayo Foundation, Section of Dermatology and of Clinical Pathology, Rochester, Minnesota (USA)

Pyoderma gangrenosum (PG) is a rare cutaneous disorder that has been recognized clinically because of its distinctive morphologic features [1]. The ulcerated, frequently painful lesions occur predominantly on the lower part of the legs. They are recognized from their liquefying and necrotic characteristics which produce rapid peripheral extension and central necrosis of tissue, sometimes with sphacelus formation. Marked pus formation accompanies the reaction. A band of bright erythema surrounds the ulcer, which indicates extension of the disease.

The earliest description by BRUNSTING, GOECKERMAN, and O'LEARY [1] emphasized the presence of an underlying systemic disease, most often chronic ulcerative colitis, and the skin lesions were causally related to these. Subsequently, ROSTENBERG [2] proposed that PG may be a Shwartzman reaction, and more recently McKAY [3] has suggested this phenomenon with disseminated intravascular coagulation and diffuse thrombus formation in small vessels as the cause of the skin lesions. PG has been considered an immunologic disease because some patients have altered levels of serum proteins [4] and because some reject autogenous skin grafts [5]. Failure to recover the same bacterial or fungal organism from lesions of PG would seem to discount the lesion's being primarily infectious [6].

Because the etiology of this disease remains obscure [4], it was decided to study a group of these patients in greater detail. Included among the standard and

* This investigation was supported in part by Research Grant HE-5008 from the National Institutes of Health, Public Health Service.

special laboratory examinations performed on these patients for underlying systemic or bowel disease were a number of tests of coagulation and hemostasis. These included bleeding time (Duke's method), platelet count (Brecher-Cronkite method), clot retraction, Lee-White coagulation time, recalcified plasma clotting time [7], prothrombin time, Stypven time [8], whole-blood clot lysis time, urea-solubility test for factor XIII (fibrin-stabilizing factor) [9], and "retarded" thromboplastin-generation test [10]. Biopsy specimens from the lesions of PG were evaluated especially for evidence of thrombosis of vessels. Serum-protein electrophoretic patterns were determined on all patients. Serum immunoglobulins IgA, IgG, and IgM were measured by a radial immunodiffusion method [11] employing Immunoplates (Hyland Laboratories). Anti-DNA and anti-DNP were measured by the fluorescent spot tests of FRIOU [12] and CASALS and coll. [13] to assess possible autoantibody production.

Eight patients seen during the past year were studied. Each had fulfilled the clinical characteristics for the diagnosis of PG as previously outlined. Of the eight patients, one (case 5) had chronic ulcerative colitis, one (case 6) had regional ileitis, one (case 8) had diarrhea concomitantly with skin lesions but no bowel disease could be detected, and one (case 1) had had inflammatory disease of the lungs 6 months before the onset of the skin disease (Tab. 1). These findings would tend to confirm past experience [6] that fewer patients now are recognized as having underlying bowel or other disease, especially chronic ulcerative colitis, in association with PG. That the bowel acts as a focus of gram-negative bacteria for cutaneous sensitivity [14] seems lacking in many of the patients.

Table 1. *Clinical Data on eight Patients with Pyoderma Gangrenosum*

Case	Age, sex	Distribution of lesions	Gastrointestinal complaints	Proctoscopic findings	X-ray examination	Treatment	Outcome
1	30 ♀	Left leg	No	Neg.	ND[a]	Systemic steroids	Healed, 6 mo[b]
2	31 ♂	Feet	No	Neg.	Colon neg.	Sulfapyridine	Healed, 2 mo
3	19 ♂	Generalized	No	ND[a]	ND	Systemic steroids	Death, septicemia
4	19 ♂	Legs, feet	No	Neg.	Colon neg.	Sulfapyridine, topical wet dressings	Healed, 4 mo
5	17 ♀	Legs, feet	Yes	CUC	Colon CUC	Sulfapyridine	Under care, healing
6	17 ♀	Lower part of legs	Yes	Neg.	Colon neg.; small bowel: regional ileitis	Sulfapyridine	Observed 5 days
7	54 ♂	Ankles	No	Neg.	Colon neg.	Sulfapyridine	Under care, healing
8	58 ♀	Left leg	Yes	Neg.	Stomach, small bowel, and colon neg.	Sulfapyridine	Healing

[a] ND = not done; CUC = chronic ulcerative colitis.
[b] Patient had pulmonary infection 6 months before pyoderma gangrenosum.

Salicylazosulfapyridine used systemically has been of benefit in the treatment of many patients with PG even though disease of the bowel was not present. Sulfapyridine [15], because it is the active degradation product of salicylazosulfapyridine, is now frequently given as the primary systemic treatment. Systemic use of corticosteroids proved of value in the treatment of patients with especially destructive skin lesions.

The results of the tests of coagulation and hemostasis in seven patients (1 to 7) were compared with the clinical activity of the PG (Tab. 1 and 2). Results of all of these tests were within normal limits except for slight prolongation of the prothrombin time (21 to 22 sec, controls 17 to 18 sec) in patients 2 and 5, and accelerated thromboplastin generation in patients 2, 3, and 5. This finding in patient 5 is not surprising since evidence of accelerated thromboplastin generation and venous thrombosis has been observed in association with chronic ulcerative colitis [16, 17]. The reason for the accelerated reactions in patients 2 and 3 is unexplained.

Table 2. *Coagulation Data on seven Patients with Pyoderma Gangrenosum*

Case	Platelets per mm³	Coagulation time, min	Bleeding time, min	Clot retraction, hr	Prothrombin time, sec	Plasma clot time, sec	Prothrombin consumption, sec	Stypven time, sec	Thromboplastin generation acceleration, grade
1	378,000	6	4	2	18	77	50	10	0
2	271,000	8	2	2	21	80	25	14	3
3	230,000	4	1	1	19	75	51	10	4
4	320,000	7	2	2	19	84	26	13	0
5	373,000	10	3	1	22	76	29	13	3
6	182,000	6	2	2	19	75	24	14	0
7	218,000	8	3	2	19	82	31	9	0
Normal range	175,000 to 375,000	6—10	1—6	1—2	17—19	70—105	>22	8—17	0—1

The principal laboratory features of the intravascular coagulation syndrome [3] are thrombocytopenia and significant deficiencies of prothrombin, fibrinogen, and factors V and VIII. Thrombocytopenia was not present in any of the patients studied here. Had any of the other defects mentioned been present, they should have been evident in a prolongation of the prothrombin, Stypven, or plasma clot time or in reduced activity in the retarded thromboplastin-generation test. Instead, the results of these tests were normal or near-normal, or indicated increased rather than decreased clotting-factor activity. Hence intravascular coagulation with "consumption coagulopathy" either is absent in these patients or, if present, probably does not play a consistent or prominent part.

The histopathology of PG is not specific but consists of necrosis of tissue with a marked acute and chronic inflammatory reaction and an increase in the number of vessels present. Endothelial proliferative changes have been reported [18]. However, scrutiny of biopsy material from four patients (1, 6, 7, and 8) failed to show evidence of thrombosis of vessels, which indirectly speaks against hypercoagulability with thrombosis as a mechanism in the production of the skin lesions (figure).

Electrophoresis of the serum proteins showed a decrease of serum albumin as the most consistent abnormality, with four patients (1, 2, 3, and 5) possessing less than normal levels of albumin. Both decreased and increased levels of gammaglobulin have been reported [4], but in these eight patients the levels were normal.

Levels of serum immunoglobulin IgA, IgG, and IgM* presented no consistent pattern of alteration (Tab. 3). Thus, no direct evidence for an immunologic basis for PG was uncovered. Though immunoglobulin levels are frequently elevated in such diseases as lupus erythematosus and rheumatoid arthritis, which may have an immunologic origin, these levels are usually normal in such diseases of proven hypersensitivity as systemic drug reactions, autoimmune hemolytic anemia, and allergic rhinitis.

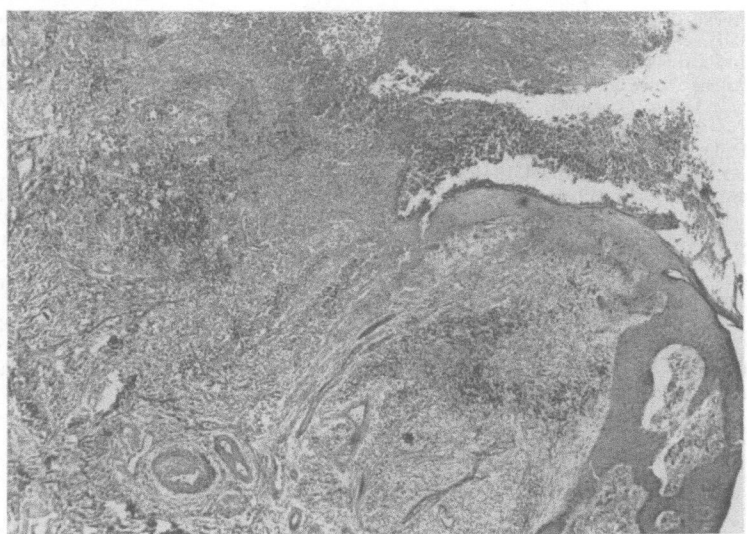

Fig. Pyoderma gangrenosum. Vessels underlying inflamed and necrotic areas are free of thrombosis. Vessels are considered to be involved only secondarily. (Hematoxylin and eosin; × 40)

In all eight patients, tests for anti-DNA and anti-DNP autoantibodies gave negative results. Also, the results of LE clot tests in seven patients (not done in patient 2) were negative. Similarly, though the absence of antinuclear antibodies in the serum of these does not support an immunologic hypothesis for the etiology of PG, it cannot be taken as very strong evidence against it.

The study of these eight patients with PG failed to substantiate any of the commonly accepted theories of the etiology of the disease.

Only four of the eight patients had associated disease, which was either proved by laboratory means (three patients) or suggested by the history. The remaining four patients were apparently otherwise healthy; in these the belief that PG

Table 3. *Immunoglobulin Levels (mg/ml) in eight Patients with Pyoderma Gangrenosum*

Case	IgA	IgM	IgG
1	4.3	1.0	12.5
2	3.05	0.83	13.5
3	1.95	0.33	7.0
4	3.1	1.0	16.0
5	0.43	0.64	17.7
6	4.6	1.6	22.0
7	3.9	1.4	10.5
8	2.05	1.5	13.0
Normal[a]	2.8±0.7	1.2±0.35	12.4±2.2

[a] Normal mean ± standard deviation.

is the cutaneous reflection of underlying disease was not substantiated. Although some abnormal results occurred in the test methods employed, no consistent

* Studies of serum immunoglobulins and anti-DNA and anti-DNP antibodies were done in the laboratory of F. C. McDuffie, M.D.

pattern of findings emerged that would permit classification of patients with PG as possessing a characteristic coagulation defect. If the phenomenon of intravascular coagulation is important etiologically in PG, test methods other than those employed will be required to elucidate these defects. Immunologic mechanisms may be involved in the production of PG, but evidence of these as reflected by altered immunoglobulin levels or the presence of unusual antibodies is lacking. The cause of PG has yet to be established.

References. Brunsting, L. A., W. H. Goeckerman, and P. A. O'Leary: Arch. Derm. **22**, 655 (1930). — 2. Rostenberg, jr., A.: Brit. J. Derm. **65**, 389 (1953). — 3. McKay, D. G.: Disseminated Intravascular Coagulation: An Intermediary Mechanism of Disease. New York: Hoeber Medical Division, Harper & Row, Publishers, 1965. — 4. van der Sluis, I.: Dermatologica (Basel) **132**, 409 (1966). — 5. Long, P. I., and C. T. Uesu: J. Amer. med. Ass. **187**, 336 (1964). — 6. Perry, H. O., and L. A. Brunsting: Arch. Derm. **75**, 380 (1957). — 7. Owen, jr., C. A., F. D. Mann, M. D. Hurn, and J. M. Stickney: Amer. J. clin. Path. **25**, 1417 (1955). — 8. Fullerton, H. W.: Lancet **1940 II**, 195. — 9. Duckert, F., E. Jung, und D. H. Shmerling: Thrombos. Diathes. haemorrh. (Stuttg.) **5**, 179 (1960). — 10. Thompson jr., J. H., C. A. Owen jr., J. A. Spittell jr., and C. A. Pascuzzi: Amer. J. clin. Path. **37**, 63 (1962). — 11. Fahey, J. L., and E. M. McKelvey: J. Immunol. **94**, 84 (1965). — 12. Friou, G. J.: Arthr. and Rheum. **5**, 407 (1962). — 13. Casals, S. P., G. J. Friou, and L. L. Myers: Arthr. and Rheum. **7**, 379 (1964). — 14. Jablónska, S.: Hautarzt **15**, 584 (1964). — 15. Schoch, jr.. E. P., and C. H. McCuistion: J. invest. Derm. **25**, 123 (1955). — 16. Spittell, jr., J. A., C. A. Owen jr., J. H. Thompson jr., and W. G. Sauer: Coll. Papers Mayo Clin, **55**, 53 (1963/64). — 17. Graef, V., A. H. Baggenstoss, W. G. Sauer, and J. A. Spittell jr.: Arch. intern. Med: **117**, 377 (1966). — 18. Lever, W. F.: Histopathology of the Skin, Ed. 3, p. 653. Philadelphia: J. B. Lippincott Company 1961.

Free Communications

A Cutaneous Affection from Malabsorption

A. Baccaredda-Boy and F. Crovato, University of Genoa, School of Medicine, Department of Dermatology, Genoa (Italy)

The origin of the term "malabsorption syndrome" goes back as far as 1953, when Cross used it to indicate an alteration in the reabsorption of foods, particularly of fats.

At the beginning the syndrome included any kind of steatorrhea, both primitive and secondary, then it was limited by Lambling only to assimilation disorders of the intestine and referred to as "intestinal malabsorption".

A consequence of the altered reabsorption is the qualitative and quantitative deficit of hematochemical components which results in a clinical picture.

Some tests are indispensable for both the diagnosis. Other organs and apparatusses are involved, among which the skin. Rhagades, hyperkeratosis, desquamation and pigmentation were noticed. The same malabsorption origin may account for cases of psoriasis, enteropathic acrodermatitis, atopic eczema, erythrodermic and Duhring syndromes.

Among skin disorders of the vasomotory and micro-angiopathic types, rosacea was particulary investigated and recently a particular measleslike exanthema which we called "microangiosis erythemato-teleangectasica eruptiva perstans" was studied.

This case concerned a girl of 18 years of age with negative physiological and pathological anamnesis, except steatorrhea dating from her childhood and a slight but progressive thinning in last years. About 2 years ago without any subjective symptom, a rash was observed. The patient was covered with erythematous-lenticular little spots, among which fine telangiectases could be seen. The exanthema was considerably stronger after meals. The histologic examination showed considerable capillary ectasia in the papillary and medium dermis with slight perithelial reaction. The tests showed an "intestinal malabsorption syndrome", which was supported, particularly, by the high percentage of fats in the feces (excreted fats pro/die 5.8 g) and the D-xylose positive test (after 5 h the excreta with urine reached 1.9 g). A diet without gluten produced considerable improvement in the cutaneous rash; the improvement was increased by excluding carbohydrates, and then only telangiectases were present. The interruption of the diet without gluten and carbohydrates was followed by relapse.

Treatments with steroids, antibiotics and dihydroxiquinoline did not give any results. Dihydroxiquinoline was administered because it is efficacious in enteropathic acrodermatitis, which, according to some Authors, may be connected with intestinal malabsorption. The effectiveness of this compound in enteropathic acrodermatitis was explained by HANSONN with is competitive action on the chinurenic derivatives produced by an altered turnover of tryptophan, which are toxic on intestinal villi.

Apart from the clear responsability of chinurenic derivatives and their mode of action, Hansonn's statement seems generically right, above all for what concerns tryptophan.

DANBOLT and CLOSS, however, noticed that the oral administration of L-tryptophan in cases of enteropathic acrodermatitis was followed by clinical aggravation and high indicanuria.

In our too, the administration of tryptophan caused the relapse of cutaneous disorders. A considerable increase of 5-oxyndolacetic acid (together with the presence of small amounts of 5-hydroxytryptamine) corresponded to the absence of hyperindicanuria. The amount of 5-oxyndolacetic acid was high, under basal conditions, in the case of "microangiosis".

These results can help in the pathochemical interpretation of enterocutaneous symptomatology.

We know that the forerunner of serotonin was tryptophan, which is first oxidized to 5-hydroxytryptophan and then, by losing the carboxyl group, forms 5-hydroxytryptamine and is eliminated in the form of 5-oxyndolacetic acid. In normal metabolism of tryptophan, only 1% of the acid introduced with the diet follows this route, while, according to SIOERDSMA, in patients affected by "carcinoid syndrome" it reaches even 60%.

According to the Author, the vasomotory troubles noticed in these patients must be ascribed to this metabolism deviation. The increased production of serotonine at the expense of nicotinic acid may be responsible for disorders of the pellagroid type. These data, together with clinical analogies with carcinoidomatosis (vasomotory alterations, diarrhea, etc.) suggest that vasal cutaneous troubles may depend in hyperserotoninemia also in cases of abnormal absorption. This theory can be confirmed by the therapeutical results produced by cyproheptadine; in fact doses of 8 mg pro/die of the latter were administered to our patients and produced not only the resolution of the cutaneous disorders, but also regulated the abdomen.

Concluding, according to our experience, cutaneous manifestations of intestinal malabsorption may consist of a temporary or permanent dilatation of the tiny vessels of the skin; the high amount of 5-oxyndolacetic acid in urine suggest the hypothesis that the manifestations may depend on serotonin, which, in some cases probably derives from an altered metabolism of tryptophan.

Bibliography. BACCAREDDA-BOY, A., J. CROVATO: Eritrosi, teleangectasie nelle gastropatie e nel malassorbrimento intestinale. Atti della Accademia Medica Lombarda. Scinposio su: Medicina Interna e Dermatologia, 1966.

Hauterscheinungen bei Colitis ulcerosa

H. REICH, Universitäts-Hautklinik Münster (Deutschland)

Die häufigsten cutanen Begleiterscheinungen der Colitis ulcerosa sind:
1. das Erythema exsudativum multiforme (einschließlich seiner Varianten);
2. Erytheme, die teils an die der Papulo-nekrotischen Tuberkulide, teils an die des Erythema nodosum bzw. der „Nodularen Vasculitis" erinnern;
3. Dermatitis-herpetiformis-ähnliche vesiculöse Hautausschläge;
4. psoriasiforme Exantheme;
5. die Pyodermite végétante (HALLOPEAU);
6. das Pyoderma gangraenosum (BRUNSTING u. Mitarb.).

Seltener werden simultan mit der Colitis ulcerosa lichenoide (namentlich folli-culär-lichenoide) Exantheme — wie beispielsweise der Lichen sclerosus — beobachtet. Gelegentlich trat gemeinsam mit der Colitis ulcerosa eine Alopecia areata auf. Auch akneiforme Efflorescenzen wurden hin und wieder beobachtet.

Den Dermatologen interessiert darüber hinaus die Syntropie der Colitis ulcerosa mit rheumatischen bzw. rheumatoiden Symptomen; im Vordergrund steht hier die Spondylarthritis ankylopoetica.

Crohns's Disease Associated with Cutaneous Lesions

G. A. GRANT PETERKIN, Skin Department, Royal Infirmary, Edinburgh (Great Britain)

Variously known as Crohn's disease, Regional Ileitis, Regional Enteritis, or Granulomatous Proctitis, this is yet another condition which presents non-caseating foci with foreign-body giant cells, such as occur in sarcoidosis, pseudo-tuberculoma silicoticum, giant-cell arteritis, etc., in which we dermatologists have been so interested in recent years.

This disease was first fully described by CROHN and his colleagues (1932), although EDWARDS (1964) points out that it was first mentioned many years ago by Sir WATSON CHEYNE as "non-tuberculous enteritis". It has been described by CARD (1964) as being characterised by non-specific chronic inflammation of the small, or sometimes the large bowel. The etiology is quite obscure; some have suggested that it is a type of sarcoidosis; some a form of tuberculosis due to unusual strains; some that it is related to silicotic granuloma. PHEAR (1960), after a full investigation of 40 cases, found no evidence of sarcoidosis, although the Mantoux test gave no reaction in 70%; JAMES (1958) found the Kveim test negative in ten patients.

Although often mistaken for each other, Ulcerative Colitis and Crohn's disease are not related, and the skin lesions of the former are very different from those of CROHN's. So far, in dermatological literature, there has been little mention of Crohn's disease, but reference to skin involvement can be found in some surgical and medical papers. LOCKHART-MUMMERY and MORSON (1964) mention sinus formation in 8% of 311 cases. NEVIN (1961) described a chronic granuloma associated with the disease, and SCOTT (1961), and HUNTER-CRAIG (1961) both demonstrated single cases with ulceration and fissuring of the genito-crural areas. Here is a picture of this type of ulcer in a woman originally diagnosed as having ulcerative colitis, but sections taken from the margins of ulcers showed the typical "sarcoid-like" reaction. The early stage shows as a small indolent granuloma, such as occurred in a young man with granulomatous proctitis. PARKES, MORSON and PEGUM (1965) showed at the Royal Society of Medicine a woman with Crohn's disease with a granuloma of the perianal region, intertrigo of the crural and submammary folds, eczematides of the feet, and a large ulcer under the right breast showing the characteristic histological picture. In the discussion on this case, SNEDDON (1965) referred to a patient with this granulomatous reaction of the ano-genital region who also had Acne Conglobata. Another picture shows a severe Acne in a young man with Crohn's disease; the Acne healed with treatment, but he has now developed a perianal sinus.

An Allergic Vasculitis was confirmed histologically. In a man who was operated on for acute obstruction due to CROHN'S. Periarteritis, erythema nodosum and other allergic reactions have been reported on rare occasions e.g. 2 out of 222 cases, and various vitamin deficiencies have been recorded. A child with Crohn's disease and malabsorption syndrome, showed acquired xeroderma and follicular hyperkeratosis.

It is suggested that we dermatologists should be alert for cutaneous manifestations which may be associated with Crohn's disease, and which may in fact lead to its diagnosis. These may be classified as follows:

1. Malabsorption syndrome.
2. Allergic reactions, such as vasculitis, periarteritis, nodosa, erythema nodosum, eczematides.
3. Sudden severe and indurated Acne of the trunk and face.
4. Perianal granulomata.
5. Deep fissured ulcers especially of the ano-genital area.
6. Sinus formation, usually perianal.

References. CARD, W. I.: Chapter on Crohn's disease. In: The Principles and Practive of Medicine, ed. Sir STANLEY DAVIDSON. Edinburgh: E. & S. Livingstone 1964. — CROHN, B. B., L. GINZBURG, and G. D. OPPENHEIMER: J. Amer. med. Ass. **99**, 1323 (1932). — EDWARDS, H.: J. roy. Coll. Surg. Edinb. **9**, 115 (1964). — HUNTER-CRAIG, C. J.: Proc. roy. Soc. Med. **54**, 1019 (1961). — JAMES, D. G.: Pers. Communication to PHEAR (vide infra.) (1958). — LOCKHART MUMMERY, H. E., and B. C. MORSON: Gut **5**, 493 (1964). — NEVIN, R. W.: Proc. roy. Soc. Med. **54**, 137 (1961). — PARKS, A. G., B. C. MORSON, and J. S. PEGUM: Proc. roy. Soc. Med. **58**, 241 (1965). — PHEAR, D. N.: Lancet **1958** II, 1250. — SCOTT, O. L. S.: Proc. roy. Soc. Med. **54**, 1019 (1961). — SNEDDON, I. B.: Proc. roy. Soc. Med. **58**, 241 (1965).

Lung Function in Patients with Cutaneous Vasculitis

M. CATTERALL, Respiratory Function Unit, The Middlesex Hospital, London (England)

The ten patients, whose lung function was studied, suffered from allergic vasculitis, cutaneous polyarteritis nodosa of the livedo reticularis type and necrotising arteriolitis. The disease was restricted to the skin and comprehensive clinical and laboratory investigations failed, with two exceptions, to reveal any other systemic involvement. The two exceptions were patients whose chest x-rays showed slight changes of cystic formation at the bases.

There were seven women and three men and their ages varied from 61 to 20 years. The cutaneous manifestations varied from a reticular livedo to frank necroses with subsequent development of black scabs which separated to form ulcers.

Two patients, both men in their 50's suffered from very severe skin lesions with multiple small red areas with black scabs over the face, trunk, arms and legs.

Slide I shows the legs of one of them. He had been in and out of hospital for 3 years and had been treated with steroids with no success. These lesions caused considerable pain and distress.

In the eight other cases, the lesions formed nodules in the dermis, a variety of the disease sometimes called nodular vasculitis. Only one patient complained of breathlessness.

The lung function of the patients was tested by measurements of the components of the lung volumes, resting and forced ventilation and the transfer factor (or diffusing capacity) by the single breath method. It will be remembered that small lung volumes suggest a restrictive (or fibrotic) process and large volumes characterise emphysema. Maximum voluntary ventilation is a test of the overall function of the thoracic cage, the elasticity of the lung parenchyma and the cardiac output. The transfer factor measures the rate at which inhaled carbon monoxide passes across the alveolar capillary membrane into the pulmonary capillary blood. This region, where gas exchange takes place, consists of the alveoli, the connective tissue and the vasculature of the pulmonary capillaries.

A low result is expected if: 1. The capillaries are involved in pathological changes which render their walls less permeable to the diffusion of gas. 2. The blood flow through them is interrupted by abnormalities in the arterioles supplying them. 3. Any diffuse fibrotic process in the lungs. In anaemia, with reduced red blood corpuscles, the transfer factor is also low and in such patients, the test was repeated after the anaemia had been treated.

Results. The respiratory systems of six of the ten patients were entirely normal. In the remaining four, which included both men with the very severe skin lesions, the transfer factor was reduced to less than 57% of predicted normal. The other two patients with a low transfer factor were women, with much less severe skin lesions, one of whom had suffered from malaise and pyrexia for 2 years. In two of these four patients, there were slight radiological changes suggestive of cystic formation and confined to the bases. Lung volumes and resting and forced ventilation were normal in all ten cases.

Discussion. It has been recognised by several workers that histological changes occur in many organs, even in cases of apparently cutaneous disease, and involvement of the lungs has been recognised radiologically. But as WINKLEMAN (1964) showed, these radiological changes were not consistent nor diagnostic. The interest of the lung function results was that they revealed one consistent abnormality in four of the ten cases tested. This was the impaired transfer factor (or diffusing capacity), tests of ventilation and lung volumes being normal. This abnormal lung function was to be expected, if the cutaneous changes of vasculitis were present also in the blood vasculature of the lungs. Histological evidence of disease has obvious advantages, but lung biopsy presents difficulties in that only a tiny part of an enormous surface is examined and the investigation is sometimes dangerous. Post mortem examinations may be blurred by terminal respiratory illness. Skin lesions and malaise restricted activity and so only one patient complained of dyspnoea, in spite of significant lung dysfunction.

It is concluded that tests of lung function are required for the full investigation of patients with cutaneous vasculitis and these tests frequently provide useful additional information.

References. WINKELMANN, R. K., and W. B. DITTO: Medicine (Baltimore) **43**, 59 (1964).

Atteinte du rein au cours des allergides nodulaires dermiques de Gougerot

St. Boulle et J. Guilaine, Paris (France)

Les allergides nodulaires dermiques de Gougerot, dont l'expression clinique est habituellement trisymptomatique (nodules-purpura — micro-cocardes) peuvent s'associer à des signes d'atteinte viscérale. La plus fréquente est l'atteinte rénale dont de nombreux cas ont déjà été publiés. Les caractères qui se dégagent de ces observations (protéinurie franche, très forte tendance hématurique, peu de tendance à l'oedème et moins encore à l'hypertension artérielle, altérations peu importantes des épreuves fonctionnelles, évolution par poussées parallèles aux signes cutanés et articulaires) rapprochent cette néphropathie de celle du syndrome de Schönlein-Henoch.

Les deux observations que nous résumons ci-après nous ont paru intéressantes car elles sont plus complètes que celles qui ont été jusqu'alors rapportées, en particulier sous l'angle anatomique.

Obs. I. (avec B. Antoine, M. Miroux et Mlle H. de Montera). Homme de 50 ans ayant fait un abcès du poumon à staphylocoques. 8 mois plus tard, apparition d'une maladie trisymptomatique typique confirmée par biopsie (il existe une hypersensibilité très accentuée au vaccin antistaphylococcique, avec réaction focale). En même temps, apparaît une protéinurie avec hématurie microscopique à 425.000 hématies/min, urée sanguine à 0,67 g, P.S.P. à 31% en 70 min, ébauche de syndrome néphrotique humoral. La V.S. est très accélérée, mais on ne trouve ni oedème ni H.T.A.

La biopsie rénale montre une image de glomérulo-néphrite segmentaire avec blocs fibreux occupant une partie du floculus et synéchiées avec la capsule de Bowman. L'atteinte varie d'un glomérule à l'autre dans son intensité. L'évolution est favorable. Les épreuves rénales s'améliorent, se stabilisent et se maintiennent sans récidive après un recul de 2 ans.

Obs. II. (avec G. Richert, P. Amiel et Morel-Maroger). Femme de 50 ans, porteuse depuis 6 mois d'une néphropathie, avec oedème, protéinurie à 5 g, azotémie à 0,70 g et H.T.A. à 19/10. Un traitement de streptomycine I.M. améliore le syndrome rénal mais fait apparaître une éruption faite de nodules dermiques, de purpura et de placards urticariens s'associant à des arthralgies. Le diagnostic d'allergides de Gougerot est confirmé par biopsie.

Les examens complémentaires montrent une ébauche de syndrome néphrotique humoral, une hématurie à 42.000 hématies/min, une clearance de la créatinine à 53 cc/min.

La biopsie rénale montre une image de glomérulo-néphrite focale avec prolifération endo-capillaire, dépôts hyalins intercapillaires et image en double contour des basales. Aucun foyer infectieux ne peut être découvert chez cette malade qui garde, après 2 ans, d'importantes séquelles rénales. La plupart des médicaments qui lui ont été administrés, en particulier l'érythromycine, ont déclenché des nouvelles poussées cutanées et rénales.

La confrontation de ces deux observations appelle quelques commentaires.

Sur le plan dermatologique, si la première reproduit un aspect trisymptomatique typique et reconnaît une origine infectieuse (staphylococcique), la seconde est moins pure sur le plan clinique puisque les cocardes d'érythème polymorphe manquent et sont remplacées par des placards urticariens et qu'on n'a pas pu démontrer un mécanisme de sensibilisation bactérienne. Néanmoins, l'évolution par poussées arthralgiques, l'aspect histologique spécifique, la sensibilité à divers médicaments ainsi que la tendance à la chronicité permettent sans discussion d'intégrer notre second cas dans le groupe des allergides de Gougerot dont seules les lésions nodulaires dermiques sont constantes.

Sur le plan néphrologique, le problème est infiniment plus complexe. Malgré l'évolution par poussées, la tendance à la chronicité et l'existence d'un syndrome néphrotique, les deux cas ne sont nullement superposables ni cliniquement, ni anatomiquement. Cliniquement, si la première observation reproduit les grandes lignes du schéma de la néphrite purpurique, il en va différemment dans la seconde

où existent des oedèmes, une H.T.A. passagère et une très faible tendance hématurique.

Anatomiquement, le premier cas correspond à une glomérulo-néphrite de type
franchement segmentaire avec nécrose puis transformation en un bloc fibreux et
tendance synéchiante d'une partie du floculus. Dans le second cas, la glomérulo-
néphrite prend le type focal touchant certains glomérules mais alors globalement
et respectant les autres. De plus, les lésions non nécrosantes sont membrano-
prolifératives avec dépôts hyalins inter-capillaires. On doit donc les opposer.

La confrontation de ces faits avec les données actuelles concernant les néphro-
pathies du purpura rhumatoïde montre que si la première observation se rapproche
de ce groupe, la seconde, en revanche, s'en écarte totalement. Lorsqu'on relit
l'histoire de cette malade, on s'aperçoit que le syndrome cutané évocateur n'est
survenu que *secondairement*. On peut donc se demander, et c'est là notre interprétation, s'il ne s'agit pas en réalité d'allergides nodulaires d'*origine médicamenteuse* (streptomycine en particulier) chez une femme porteuse d'une néphropathie
pré-existante et d'autre nature. Dans cette optique, la disparité de nos deux
observations s'explique parfaitement.

Therapie der Porphyria cutanea tarda
(Ergebnisse in 9 Jahren)

H. Ippen, Univ.-Hautklinik Düsseldorf (Deutschland)

Vor 9 Jahren begann ich Patienten mit Porphyria cutanea tarda durch
wiederholte Aderlässe zu behandeln. Nach den notwendigen Voruntersuchungen
des Porphyrin-Stoffwechsels, der Erythropoese und der Leberfunktion wurde
unter regelmäßiger Kontrolle von Blut und Urin zunächst wöchentlich, später
monatlich, je ein halber Liter Blut entzogen. Die Behandlung wurde beendet,
wenn der Porphyringehalt des Urins unter 50 γ-% abgesunken war. Bei einem Wie-
deransteigen der Porphyrinausscheidung über 100 γ-% wurden erneut monatliche
Aderlässe so lange durchgeführt, bis die Urinausscheidung wieder unter 50 γ-% lag.
Die Auswertung der Therapie bei 101 Patienten hatte folgende Ergebnisse:

1. Bei 69 Patienten sank die Porphyrinausscheidung durch die Behandlung
um 80% oder mehr ab, bei 14 Patienten betrug der Abfall 60 bis 80%. Bei 18
Patienten, die die Behandlung abbrachen oder noch behandelt werden, betrug
der Abfall der Porphyrinausscheidung weniger als 60%.

2. 36 Patienten brachen die Behandlung ab, und zwar 30, nachdem bei einem
Absinken der Porphyrinausscheidung auf 60% oder weniger die klinischen
Symptome verschwunden waren.

3. Von 47 Patienten waren 22 bisher bis 3, 25 4 bis 8 Jahre erscheinungsfrei.

4. Unter den 47 Patienten, die mit Porphyrinkonzentrationen unter 50 γ-%
klinisch symptomfrei wurden, stieg die Porphyrinausscheidung bei 13 nach 1 bis
8 Jahren wieder an. Solche Rezidive treten vor allem dann auf, wenn die Porphyrin-
konzentration im Urin vorher nicht auf unter 50 γ-% gesenkt worden war.

5. Bis zum Verschwinden der Hautsymptome mußten meist 2 bis 3 l Blut, bis
zur Normalisierung der Porphyrinausscheidung 2 bis 12 l (im Mittel etwa 4,5 l) Blut
entzogen werden.

6. Das Charakteristikum der Porphyrie, die überwiegende Ausscheidung
Äther-unlöslicher Porphyrine, bleibt bei den meisten Patienten auch bei quantitativ völlig normaler Prophyrinausscheidung nachweisbar.

7. Unter den klinischen Symptomen verschwinden Blasenbildung und Verletzlichkeit als erste. Hypertrichose und Hyperpigmentierung verringern sich erst gegen Ende der Behandlung oder im ersten Jahr danach. Auch die verstärkte Faltung der Gesichtshaut und die sklerodermoiden Veränderungen bilden sich fast immer weitgehend oder vollständig zurück. Beides sind also echte Symptome der Porphyria cutanea tarda.

8. Dagegen läßt der Diabetes, der bei ungefähr 20% der Patienten nachweisbar ist, keine Beeinflussung durch die Therapie erkennen.

9. Pathologische Leberfunktionstests, insbesondere die Bromthaleinexkretion, normalisierten sich unter der Behandlung. Leberbiopsien sprechen für eine Verringerung der morphologischen Veränderungen.

10. Der meist erhöhte Eisengehalt des Serums sank unter den Aderlässen unter die Norm ab, kehrte aber einige Monate nach Ende der Behandlung auf normale Werte zurück.

11. Weder der Hämoglobingehalt noch der Proteingehalt des Blutes sanken während der Aderlässe unter die Norm ab. Die Serumproteine stiegen sogar häufig über Werte von 7,5 g-% und zeigten eine Verschiebung zu den niedermolekularen Fraktionen.

12. Subjektiv fühlten sich alle Patienten nach der Behandlung völlig gesund und voll arbeitsfähig. Außer Alkoholabstinenz, die jedoch von etwa der Hälfte der Patienten sicher oder wahrscheinlich nicht eingehalten wird, wurden keine diätetischen oder medikamentösen Maßnahmen durchgeführt.

Die einzige Kontraindikation der Aderlaßtherapie besteht in einer stärkeren Anämie, wenn sich diese nach dem ersten Aderlaß nicht bessert. Sie wurde bisher in drei Fällen beobachtet und erwies sich als refraktär gegen alle bekannten hämatopoetischen Faktoren einschließlich des Adermins. Weitere von den bei der Tarda bekannten abweichende Symptome sprechen dafür, daß es sich hierbei um eine eigene Krankheit handelt. Erwähnenswerte Zwischenfälle wurden bei mehr als 1000 Aderlässen nie beobachtet.

Damit sprechen meine Beobachtungen insgesamt dafür, daß Aderlässe eine wirksame und gefahrlose Behandlungsmethode für die Porphyria cutanea tarda darstellen. Mit ihrer Hilfe können nahezu alle Patienten mit dieser häufigen Porphyrie auf Jahre beschwerdefrei gehalten und etwaige Rezidive bereits beherrscht werden, bevor erneut Hautveränderungen auftreten.

Hautreaktionen bei rheumatischen Erkrankungen

E. Wohlstein, Derm. Abteilung des Krankenhauses in Bad Piešťany (Tschechoslowakei)

Es ist fraglich, ob der „Rheumatismus" ein genügend scharf begrenzter Krankheitsbegriff ist und ob die anatomisch-histologisch erfaßbaren Merkmale der Hautreaktionen genügen, von „rheumatischen Reaktionen der Haut" überhaupt zu sprechen. Wenn wir diese Frage bejahen können, sind drei Möglichkeiten gegeben.

1. Hautreaktionen können in kausalem Zusammenhang mit der rheumatischen Erkrankung stehen;

2. die rheumatische Erkrankung kann ein nichtspezifischer Kofaktor bei der Entstehung der Hautreaktion sein;

3. es kann eine zufällige, synchrone Koincidenz zwischen der rheumatischen Erkrankung und der Hautreaktion bestehen.

Das entscheidende Kriterium der Klassifikation der rheumatischen Erkrankung ist der vorwiegend entzündliche und nichtentzündliche Charakter der Erkrankung. Arthritis urica und Arthropathia alcaptonurica werden neuerdings als pararheumatische Krankheiten bezeichnet. Durch Störungen im Metabolismus, inkretorisch, neurogen oder durch Zirkulationsstörungen bedingte sog. ,,Rheumatoide'' (GEBHARDT, 1896) sollen als unechter Gelenkrheumatismus vom echten Rheumatismus abgegrenzt werden.

Der echte Gelenkrheumatismus ist histologisch durch fibrinoide Nekrosen und Anwesenheit von Aschoffschen Knötchen charakterisiert. Auf dieser Basis kann die Zugehörigkeit zum echten Rheumatismus hauptsächlich der Febris rheumatica und der Polyarthritis chronica progressiva zuerkannt werden, welche Krankheitsbilder konventionell in die Gruppe der diffusen Erkrankungen des Kollagens (Kollagenopathien) eingereiht werden.

Die verhältnismäßig große Anzahl der bekannten diagnostischen Methoden zur Feststellung des echten Rheumatismus und zur speziellen Abgrenzung von den übrigen heterogenen rheumatischen Krankheitsbildern hat vorläufig nur fakultativ-orientierenden Wert.

Bei rheumatischen Personen erleidet das Hautorgan Störungen in der Innervation, Thermoregulation, im vasomotorischen Gleichgewicht, in der Strömungsgeschwindigkeit des Blutes und in der allergischen Bereitschaft, was zu dysfunktionellen Zuständen im Organismus führt, welche für die Haut des Rheumatikers pathognomonisch sind. Die elektrodermatometrische Kurve (WOHLSTEIN) ist für die Polyarthritis chronica progressiva elektiv kennzeichnend und leistet in unklaren Fällen gute Dienste.

Bei progressiven chronischen Polyarthritiden ist der Glutathionspiegel im Blute herabgesetzt, wodurch die bekannte hemmende Wirkung der Sulfhydrylverbindungen auf die Melanogenese wegfällt, was auch die Tendenz zu Hyperpigmentationen verständlich macht. Die Blockade des normalen Abbaues des Tyrosins dürfte für die Pigmentstörungen verantwortlich sein (Dyscoloratio tyrosinurica, WOHLSTEIN).

Bei Störungen des Schwefelmetabolismus im Sinne von gesteigertem Bedarf oder bei herabgesetzter Produktion (Polyarthritis chronica progressiva) wird Schwefel aus seinen Depotorganen ausgeschwemmt, um den Detoxikationsprozeß in lebenswichtigen Organen zu ermöglichen. Hierbei kommt es zur Destruktion in den Vorratskammern des Schwefels (Epidermis, Haare, Nägel, Knorpel der Gelenke). Bei progressiven Polyarthritiden beobachtet man tatsächlich destruktive Veränderungen an diesen Organen. An der Haut melden sich Symptome des herabgesetzten Widerstandes gegen äußerliche und innerliche Reize.

Erythema anulare rheumaticum (LEHNDORFF-LEINER) repräsentiert in reinster Form das spezifische rheumatische Exanthem, und die Majorität der Autoren akzeptiert auch den Rheumatismus nodosus (HILLIER-JACCAUT) als echte, adäquate rheumatische Erkrankung der Haut. Problematisch ist die Stellung des Erythema exsudativum multiforme et nodosum. Diskutiert wird auch die Zugehörigkeit einiger Formen von Periarteriitis, Panarteriitis nodosa, Panvasculitis zu den hyperergisch-rheumatischen Erkrankungen. Strittig ist auch die Frage der Zugehörigkeit zum rheumatischen Formenkreis der Apoplexia cutanea (GOTTRON), nodular disease amerikanischer Autoren, der Behçetschen Krankheit, wenn diese von Gelenkschwellungen und Erythema nodosum begleitet sind. Ungeklärt ist ferner die Stellung der thrombocytopenischen thrombotischen Purpura von MOSCHCOWITZ im Rahmen der Kollagenosen und des Rheumatismus. Es soll noch versucht werden, eine übersichtliche Darstellung der Hautreaktionen bei Polyarthritis chronica progressiva zu geben.

I. Hautreaktionen, welche in kausalem Zusammenhang mit rheumatischen Erkrankungen stehen:

1. Nagelveränderungen: Keratosis subungualis, Cera guttans, Striae transversae, Onychorrhexis, Onychia destruens.
2. Trophische Störungen, leichte Atrophie der Haut, glatte, glänzende, gespannte Haut mit Schwinden des subcutanen Fettgewebes.
3. Trophische Störungen der Haare, Defluvium capillitii, besonders in fortgeschrittenen Fällen.
4. Hyperpigmentierungen der Handrücken und der dorsalen Seite des Vorderarmes, persistierende, dunkelpigmentierte Narben nach Furunkeln und Pyodermatosen, Dyscoloratio tyrosinurica (WOHLSTEIN).
5. Hämorrhagische Veränderungen der Haut (Leukopenie, Thrombocytopenie), Acrocyanosis, Livedo racemosa et reticularis, Haemorrhagiae subunguales, Teleangiectasiae, Erythrosis palmaris (WOHLSTEIN), Erythrosis paraungualis (FREUND).
6. Akrosklerotische Veränderungen vorwiegend an den Händen (Pseudoskleroderma), Keratodermien hauptsächlich an den Füßen, Raynaudsches Syndrom, spontane und sekundäre Keloide (WOHLSTEIN), interstitielle Calcinosen.
7. Pachy-spondyl-osteoarthritis französischer Autoren — Cutis gyrata et plicata (WOHLSTEIN).
8. Necrosis in rheumatismo chronico (LICHTWITZ).

II. Hautreaktionen als nichtspezifischer Kofaktor bei progressiver Polyarthritis:

1. Dupuytrensche Kontraktur — auf den direkten Zusammenhang mit der humeroskapularen Periarthritis und Arthrosis habe ich schon im Jahre 1943 hingewiesen.
2. Pseudo-Dupuytrensche Kontrakturen (tendogene, myogene, dermogene).
3. Striae distensae über Gelenkschwellungen der chronischen Arthritis.
4. Xanthomatosis tuberosum multiplex, eventuell auch andere benigne Tumoren.

III. Synchrone Koincidenz der rheumatischen Erkrankung mit der Hautreaktion:

1. Dysidrotische, intertriginöse und mykotische Ekzeme.
2. Sudamina, Miliaria.
3. Pyodermien und mikrobiale Ekzeme.
4. Dermatomykosen und Kandidosen.
5. Pruritus, Urticaria und andere pruriginöse Dermatosen.

Die Aufgabe, über Rheumatismus und Hautreaktionen in ihrem gegenseitigen Zusammenhang zu sprechen, ist keine leichte, insbesondere, wenn wir bedenken, daß man leicht verführt wird, mehr oder minder ungeklärte Krankheitszustände auf der Grundlage von hyperergischen Reaktionen und nichtüberzeugenden histologischen Befunden mit echtem Rheumatismus zu identifizieren. Diese und ähnliche Voraussetzungen dürfen uns nicht verleiten, dem einzig richtigen Weg der objektiven Beobachtung der kausalen Zusammenhänge zu folgen.

Literatur. GOTTRON, H. A.: Beiträge zur modernen Therapie, 401—408, Jena: Gustav Fischer 1959. — LEJHANEC, G., P. PROCHÁZKA, and P. HYBÁŠEK: Čs. Derm. **37**, 77 (1962). — TRAPL, J., and B. BEDNÁŘ: Histologie kožních chorob, 1957, Štátní zdravotnícké nakladatelství. — WOHLSTEIN, E.: Čs. Derm. **26**, 261 (1951); **29**, 342 (1954); **32**, 81 (1957); — Derm. Wschr. **143**, 548 (1961).

Studies on Iron Metabolism in the Porphyria Cutanea Tarda (P.C.T.)

L. LEVI, C. L. MENEGHINI, F. SPINELLI-RESSI and C. A. BETTINELLI, Dermatological Clinic, Milan (Italy)

From the clinical point of view P.C.T. and haemochromatosis show several analogies. Both are more frequent in male and according to numerous Authors, seem to be a familiar disease; alcoholism is often involved. In both diseases cutaneous pigmentary disturbances are seen and deposits of iron in the hepatic and Kupfer cells and in the stroma are found. For these reasons it seemed useful to study the iron metabolism in patients affected by P.C.T. In 16 patients the sideraemia, the coefficient of saturation of transferrin, the clearance rate from the plasma of radioiron, the incorporation of radioiron by the cells and the hepatic and bone marrow uptake have been evaluated.

In most cases the sideraemia and the coefficient of saturation were increased. In eight patients the clearance rate of radioiron was found lower than normal. The hepatic uptake was higher in eleven patients, the bone marrow uptake lower in 15 patients. The incorporation of radioiron by the red cells was within the normal limits in twelve cases and decreased in four. Several liver function tests (bromosulphalein and transaminase tests and prothrombine time) were positive. On the basis of studies we may suggest that the modifications of iron metabolism in P.C.T. are analogous to those found in haemochromatosis and can be demonstrated even when cutaneous alterations are not important. As the result of these modification the deposition of iron in the liver is increased. The hypothesis is suggested that the hepatic dysfunction is responsible of the photosensitive cutaneous alterations, which become evident when the patients are exposed to the sunlight. We are not able to say if modifications of iron metabolism in P.C.T. are the cause or the consequence of the hepatic disfunction.

Krankhafte Zusammenhänge zwischen Leber und Haut in „Porphyria cutanea tarda"

P. ȚÎRLEA und I. CĂPUȘAN, Dermatologische Klinik, Cluj (Rumänien)

Unter den Zusammenhängen zwischen Haut und Gesamtorganismus nehmen die metabolischen eine besondere Stelle ein, nicht nur wegen ihrer Häufigkeit, sondern auch wegen der Komplexität ihrer Erscheinungen am Tegument. Im Rahmen dieser Zusammenhänge nimmt der zwischen Leber und Haut eine bedeutende Stelle ein.

Lange Zeit blieb die Feststellung dieser Zusammenhänge auf den Rahmen der Registrierung klinischer Fälle beschränkt. Man stellte die gleichzeitige Existenz von Hauterscheinungen und Leberschaden fest. So wurden beschrieben Ikterus und Pruritus bei Hepatitiden oder bei Verschluß der Gallenwege, Fragilität der Gefäße, Veränderungen des Haarwuchses, eventuell mit Gynekomastie, Angioma stellatum oder Pigmentierung des Gesichtes bei Cyrrhosen usw.

Dank der Entwicklung der klinischen Biochemie wurden in den letzten Jahrzehnten neue Erkenntnisse über Zusammenhänge zwischen Leber und Haut erzielt. In pathologischer Hinsicht bezieht sich eine dieser in die Augen stechenden

Leber-Hautverbindungen metabolischen Charakters auf Leberporphyrien. Ein Prototyp ist die Porphyrie cutanea tarda.

Ohne auf Einzelheiten der Hautsymptomatologie einzugehen, erwähnen wir die aktinomechanische Fragilität der Epidermis mit Blasen, Erosionen, oberflächlichen Narben mit Cysten, Hyperpigmentierung oder vitiligo-ähnlichen Flecken, an offenen Stellen lokalisiert, mit relativer Hypertrichose dieser Stellen, Konsistenzänderung der Unterhaut. Dies sind die wichtigsten pathognomonischen Elemente der Hautveränderungen.

In bezug auf Leberstörungen sei erwähnt, daß sie bei dieser Krankheit schon 1935 festgestellt wurden. Seither findet man sie in konstanter Weise wieder.

Die Beteiligung der Leber wird schon in der Vorgeschichte der Krankheit gefunden durch Feststellung von hepatotropen Noxen, wie Alkoholmißbrauch, langdauernde Behandlung mit Arsenpräparaten, Mißbrauch von Barbiturpräparaten, Hepatitis epidemica, zufällige oder Berufsintoxikationen (Pb, Hexachlorbenzen, u. a.). Klinisch findet man eine diskrete Vergrößerung der Leber mit vermehrter Konsistenz beim Palpieren. Die bioptische Punktion ergibt fettige Degeneration, ziemlich diskrete Veränderungen vom Typus der chronischen Hepatitis sowie hämosiderotische Ablagerungen, durch welche sich das Krankheitsbild der Hämochromatose nähert. In den Leberzellen findet man 30- bis 100mal mehr Porphyrine gegenüber der normalen Leber. Diese Substanz bildet sich und findet sich dann im Parenchym. Die kolloidalen Labilitätsproben überschreiten selten die normalen Grenzen, aber die Ausscheidung des Bromsulfaleins ist in den meisten Fällen gestört. Nach unseren Feststellungen, die mit denen anderer Forscher übereinstimmen (IPPEN, WALDENSTRÖM), deuten die Mittelwerte auf 5 bis 10% Retention hin. Die Transaminasen — wichtige Indikatoren des biologischen Zustandes der Leberzelle — wachsen gleichfalls zu pathologischen Werten an. Nach unseren Untersuchungen wurde TGO im Blute auf 60 bis 170 Karmen-Wroblewsky-Einheiten angewachsen gefunden, TGP auf 40 bis 316 Einheiten.

Im Laufe unserer Untersuchungen über Beteiligung der Leber fanden wir, in Übereinstimmung mit TEODORESCU, IPPEN u. a., auch ein Absinken der Ausscheidung von 17-Ketosteroiden im Harn auf Werte zwischen 3,5 bis 4,5 mg/24 h. Da der Blutdruck dieser Kranken normal war, klagten sie nicht über Asthenie, auch war ihr eosinopenischer Index (Thorn-Test) normal. Da die geringere Ketosteroidurie auch bei evolutiver Hepatitis und in Cyrrhose feststellbar ist, haben wir die verringerte Ausscheidung der 17-Ketosteroide nicht als den Ausdruck einer Corticosuprarenalinsuffizienz gedeutet, sondern als Folge einer Störung in der Leber. In diesem Sinne findet man auch eine größere Anzahl von experimentellen Befunden. Die Beziehungen zwischen Störung des Steroidstoffwechsels und Störung der Leber vom Porphyrietypus ergeben sich auch aus den Beobachtungen, welche auf eine Porphyrie von verspätetem Typus nach andauernder Verabreichung von Oestrogenen hinweisen.

Aus unseren Ausführungen ergibt sich in überzeugender Weise, daß die Porphyria cutanea tarda ein Modell der Leber-Hautkorrelation darstellt, bei welcher die humorale gegenseitige Abhängigkeit im Rahmen des Porphyriestoffwechsels offenbar ist. Beide sind von Bedeutung, sowohl in der Pathologie der Leber als auch der Haut.

Wir glauben, daß die treffendste Benennung für dieses Leiden „Chronische Leber-Haut-Porphyrie" wäre. Sie enthält die vier grundlegenden Charakteristiken des klinischen Bildes: die Gegenwart der Porphyrine in pathologischen Mengen, Hautveränderungen, Leberleiden sowie chronischer Verlauf der Erkrankung.

Schistosomiasis (Bilharziasis) der Haut

C. M. HASSELMANN, Universitäts-Hautklinik Erlangen (Deutschland)

Die starke Zunahme der Schistosomiasis in den meisten tropischen und sub-
tropischen Ländern ist vor allem eine Folge der außerordentlichen Entwicklung
der Landwirtschaft mit dem Bau von großen Staubecken und Bewässerungskanä-
len, wodurch das dauernde Fortbestehen der Zwischenwirtsschnecken sehr be-
günstigt wird. Infolge der dadurch bedingten hohen Morbidität von Schistosomiasis
kann der Arzt in warmen Ländern zunehmend kleine Hautpapeln sehen, die
Schistosomeneier enthalten, meistens von Schist. haematobium. Wenn die Ablage
im Bereich des kleinen Beckens, insbesondere der Submucosa von Blase und Darm,
oder auch in den Labien, entweder direkt per continuitatem oder aber auch durch
die bestehenden arterio-venösen Anastomosen der Hämorrhoidal- und Blasenvenen
(GELFANT, BLACK) unter Umständen erklärt werden kann, so ist der Verschlep-
pungsweg in entfernte Hautbereiche wie z. B. des Bauches, der Kopfschwarte oder
sogar ins Gehirn noch nicht völlig geklärt; abgesehen vom eventuellen Vorhandensein eines offenen Foramen ovale, könnte unter Umständen eine solche Verschleppung von Schistosomeneiern aus den zuführenden Venen vom Becken, Darm und
Leber durch "intrapulmonary arterio-venous communications" (MARCHAND,
DE FARIA u. a.) in arterielle Gefäße zur Haut ermöglicht werden.

Diese verhältnismäßig kleinen Hautpapeln sollten nicht mit den viel größeren
Tumoren bei Onchocerciasis verwechselt werden. (Demonstration von Farbdias
mit der Infektionskette bei Schistosomiasis, kopulierende männliche und weibliche
Schistosomen, Eier in der Blasenschleimhaut, Labia minor, Leber, Kopfhaut,
Onchoceriasis-Tumoren.)

Schistosomal Infestation of the Skin

A. M. EL MOFTY, Kasr el Aini University, Cairo (U.A.R.)

Schistosomiasis was recognized by the Ancient Egyptians and was known as
âaâ disease. It was only in 1851 [1] that THEODOR BILHARZ discovered the worms
responsible for the disease. S. japonicum was discovered 54 years after the discovery of BILHARZ.

Geographical Distribution: S. haematobium is found in Africa, Mediterranean
countries and India, S. mansoni in Africa and Latin America. S. Japonicum is
confined to the Far East.

Life Cycle. *In the definitive host:* Cercariae penetrate the skin, reach the lymphatics, and then the blood stream, to the lungs, left side of the heart, to the
arterial circulation, get distributed to all organs of the body. Those which reach
the liver, get mature, copulate and then migrate against the blood stream to their
final habitat where they lay ova. S. haematobium inhabit mainly the urinary tract,
S. mansoni the segmoido-rectal part of the colon, while S. japonicum the terminal
part of the ilieum, the caecum and ascending colon.

In the intermediate host: Ova reaching small canals, drains and lakes hatch and
meracidia are liberated. The latter enter the specific snail host (Bulinus species for
S. haematobium, Planorbis for S. mansoni and Oncomelania for S. japonicum)
where they develop into cercariae.

Cutaneous manifestations of schistosomiasis can be due to both human and non-human schistosomes [2, 3, 4], and at any stage of the life cycle in the human body from the time of entry of cercariae into the skin to the stage of oviposition. Accordingly, these manifestations can be divided into two principal categories:

1. Those in the invasive stage; include:

1. Shortly after penetration of the skin by human cercariae, there is mild irritation of the skin with allergic cutaneous eruptions including urticarial reaction, itchy papules or multiform erythemata. Non-human cercariae; as avian, murine, and mammalian schistosomes produce severer reactions mounting to dermatitis (Swimmer's itch, and Clam digger's itch).

2. After 2 to 4 weeks, symptoms of anaphylactoid reaction may appear. These include: a) urticaria, b) mild pyrexia with marked urticaria, c) prolonged pyrexia without urticaria.

2. Stage of oviposition; include:

1. Genital and perigenital granulomata. These begin as symptomless infiltrated papules and nodules which slowly but steadily enlarge in size, fuse and ultimately produce warty and cauliflower-like masses. These lesions are due to deposition of ova reaching the location through various portocaval anastomoses that usually exist, or through anastomoses created by an operation in the site, e.g. suprapubic cystostomy.

2. Extragenital cutaneous granulomata occurring in sites away from portocaval anastomoses. These begin as solid infiltrated skin-coloured or slightly darker papules which are discrete at first, but later fuse and form irregular plaques with mulberry-like surfaces and satellites around them.

3. Periumbilical lesions may be due to ova which reach the site through a patent urachus.

Report of Cases: 14 cases of schistosomal granulomata of the skin are included.

I. Perigenital and Genital Granulomata: This included four cases, three males and one female. Their ages were 12 to 22 years. The lesions were in the form of cauliflower-like masses or irregularly- shaped plaques, with satellite papules or nodules (Fig. 1). S. haematobium ova were found in the urine in three cases, and S. mansoni in faeces in one case.

II. Extra-genital Granulomata: This included ten cases, nine males and one female. Their ages varied from 8 to 22 years. The lesions were found on the periumblical area (three cases), anterior abdominal wall (one case), sides of the trunk (one case), the presternal region (one case), back and shoulders (two cases), nape of the neck (one case). Sometimes more than one site in the same patient were involved (Figs. 2, 3, 4). S. haematobium ova were found in the urine in nine cases, and S. mansoni in faeces in one case. The lesions were discrete papules or nodules, tumourlike masses and plaques having mulberry-like surfaces with satellite lesions at the periphery, or cauliflower-like growths.

The Pathology: The pathology of genital and extragenital schistosomial granulomata is identical to that evoked by infiltration by schistosomal ova in other organs. There are tubercle-like nodules 1 to 2 mm in diameter, which consist of one or more ova surrounded by several layers of epitheloid histiocytes, together with foreign body giant cells. Eosinophils and fibroblasts accumulate at the periphery. Diffuse schistosomal infiltration may be also found, particularly in cases with plaque formation (Figs. 5 and 6).

Comment: Perigenital and genital schistosomal granulomata are more common in females and usually consult gynaecologists. Extragenital cutaneous granulomata are more commonly seen in males; out of ten cases, only one female was encountered. Ectopic schistosomiasis is known to be caused by S. haematobium. However S. mansoni infection was found in two cases.

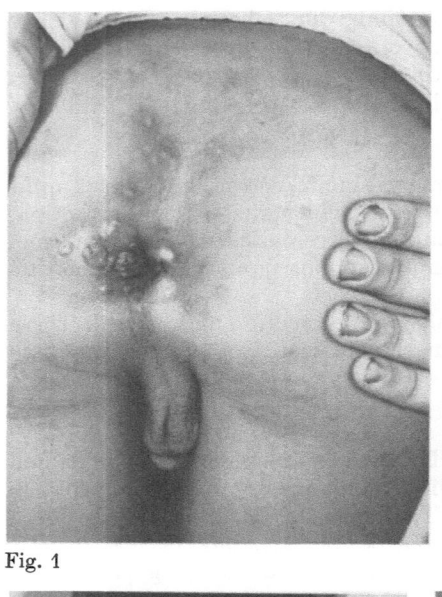

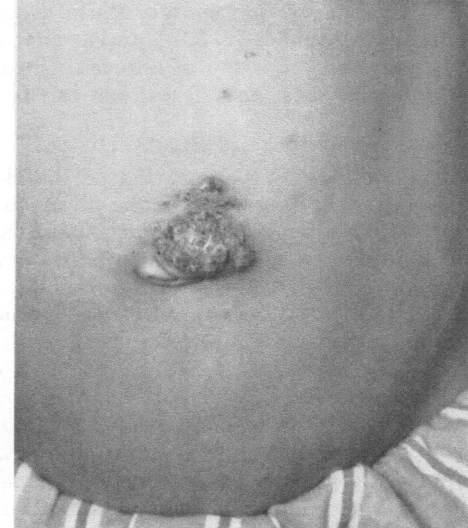

Fig. 1   Fig. 2

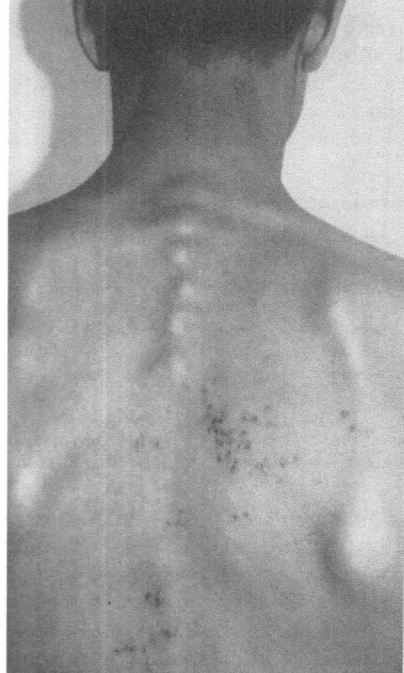

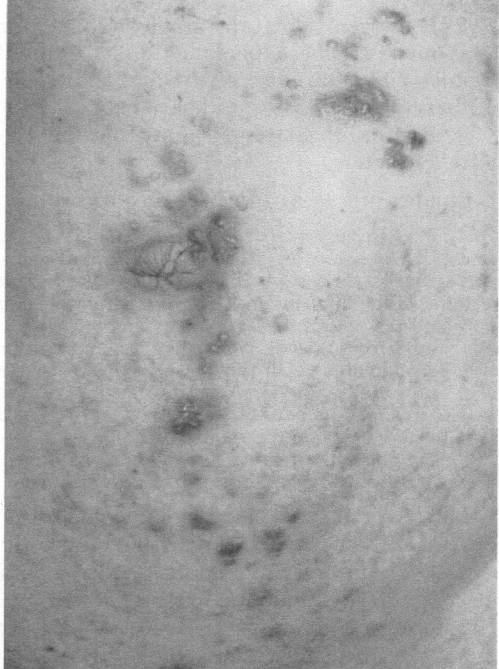

Fig. 3   Fig. 4

Cutaneous granulomata respond to antibilharzial treatment. One or two courses are usually sufficient to cause involution of the lesions, and their complete disappearance in 1.5 to 3 months, leaving slightly hyperpigmented macules. Tartar emmetic is the most effective drug.

The occurrence of extragenital granulomata may be explained by: 1. The maturation of the cercariae in the skin without the necessity of passing to the liver. 2. The presence of patent foramen ovale. 3. The passage of ova or worms from

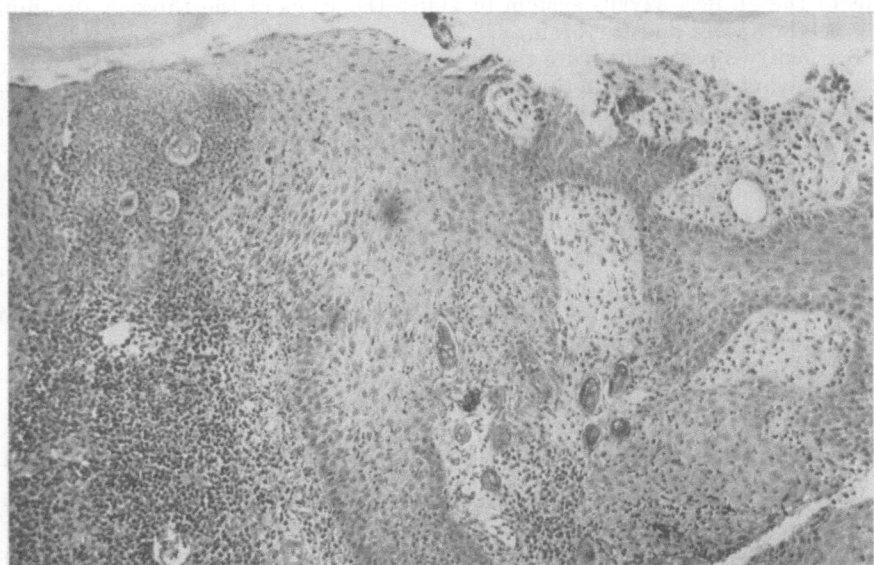

Fig. 5

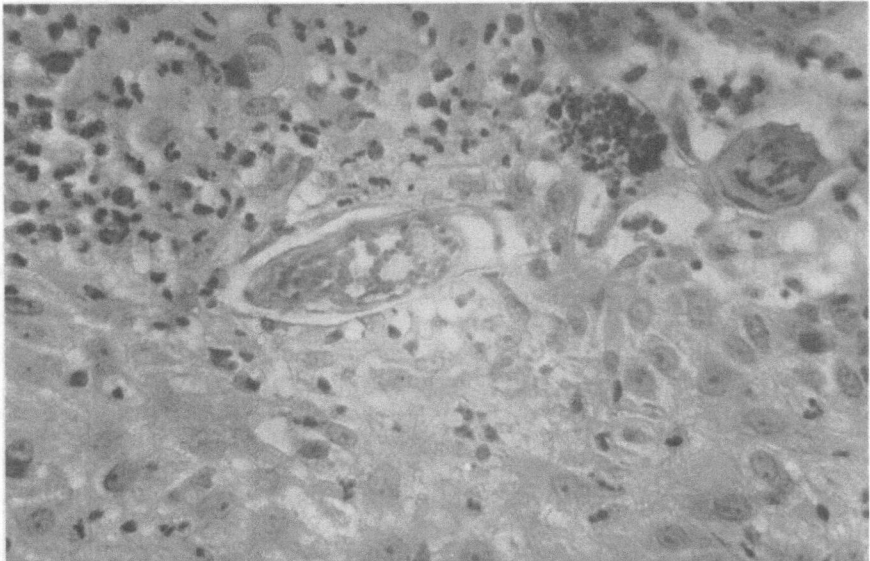

Fig. 6

their habitat, through the capillaries of the liver, to the lungs, to the general circulation through pulmonary arterio-venous shunts. 4. The migration of worms from the usual habitat against the blood stream; from the iliac veins and vena

cava, they proceed to the communications between lumbar and epigastric veins.
5. The ova may make use of the vertebral venous system which has connections
with the veins of the body cavities as well as with the veins of the spinal canal,
veins of the girdles, azygos system of veins, the veins of the thoraco-abdominal
wall, pelvic viscera and the brain.

The last two possibilities are the most acceptable. No patent foramen ovale or
patent urachus were found in this series or in previously reported cases. Maturation
of cercariae in the skin is unlikely to occur as intrahepatic maturation is essential.
Moreover, no worms have been found in the skin lesions in this series or previously
reported ones. That ova are carried to the skin by the arterial blood whereby the
ova have passed through pulmonary arterio-venous shunts, is also unlikely as ova
are found mainly surrounding the veins.

References. 1. BILHARZ, T.: Z. Wissen, Zool. IV, 53 (1852). — 2. EL MOFTY, A. M.: Gaz.
Kasr-El-Aini Fac. Med. 9, 107 (1941). — 3. EL MOFTY, A. M.: Brit. J. Derm. 68, 252 (1956). —
4. EL MOFTY, A. M., and K. M. CAHILL: Dermatology Trop. 8, 157 (1964). — 5. CORT, W.:
Amer. J. Hyg. 52, 251 (1950).

The Hepatitis Associated with Infantile Papular Acrodermatitis

V. A. PUCCINELLI, Dermatological Clinic of the University of Milan (Italy)

Infantile papular acrodermatitis has an onset characterized by a lentiform
erythemato-papular cutaneous eruption, often purpuric, on the face, neck, buttocks and limbs. The trunk is almost always spared. There is no itching and the
illness lasts 20 to 40 days and does not relapse. The disease appears in children
from 6 months to 15 years of age and in some instances may be contagious.

The dermatitis is always associated with: 1. lymphadenopathy of the principal
subcutaneous districts produced by hyperplastic reticulo-histiocytary lymphadenitis, and 2. anicteric hepatitis (rarely icteric —5% of cases) lasting several
months. This hepatitis usually is not clinically evident but presents the whole
series of serum enzyme and liver-function alterations characteristic of the type
defined viral.

Histologic studies carried out on liver biopsy specimens obtained from children
affected by the dermatitis presented the alterations characteristics of so-called
viral hepatitis, i.e. cellular polymorphism, balloon-cells, glycogen depletion and
acidophile necrotic areas as far as the hepatocytes are concerned; round-cell infiltration, increased eosinophils and Kupffer's cells and intense fibrillogenesis were
instead present in the portal spaces and lobules.

Liver biopsies performed many months (more than 30) after the acute phase
showed in some cases structural disorder of liver parenchyma characterized by
formation of sclerotic bands tending to surround and infiltrate the hepatic lobules.
The new formed connective tissue was shown to be rich in mononucleated cells
and eosinophils.

Ultrastructural study of the liver biopsy material revealed "cellular transpar-
ency", vacuolization, normal mitochondria, absence of intrahepatic lipidic inclusions, presence of lamellar degeneration of the endoplasmic reticulum, thickening
of the cell-membrane, increased lysosomes, lesions in Disse's space and precocious
fibrillogenesis. In the acute phase of the hepatitis, hepatocyte alterations prevail,
whereas later intense fibrosis is prevalent.

The reporting of the above findings is thought to be useful for the following reasons: 1. Onset of the hepatic involvement in a phase shortly preceding the dermatitis permits the study of extremely precocious hepatic alterations. 2. The complex of clinical and histopathological findings, principally represented by an activation of the reticulo-endothelial system, tends to support the hypothesis of a viral etiology of the acrodermatitis.

Zum Krankheitsbild des Myxoedema circumscriptum praetibiale

Chr. Eberhartinger, II. Universitäts-Hautklinik in Wien (Österreich)

Das Myxoedema circumscriptum praetibiale ist ein besonders in den letzten Jahren häufig kasuistisch beschriebenes Krankheitsbild. Es tritt im Rahmen der Hyperthyreose, speziell nach Schilddrüsenausschaltung (chirurgisch, medikamentös, strahlentherapeutisch) und nur in Ausnahmefällen spontan auf. Pathogenetisch wurde angenommen — zahlreiche diesbezügliche Publikationen liegen vor —, daß die prätibial gelegenen Hautveränderungen nicht direkt durch die Schilddrüsenfunktionsstörung, sondern — unterschiedlich vom hypothyreotischen Myxödem — hypophysär bedingt sein sollen. Durch den Ausfall der Schilddrüse soll es zu einer vermehrten Ausschüttung von thyreotropem Hormon kommen, dem nach Meinung vieler Autoren neben dem schilddrüsenstimulierenden Effekt auch unter anderem eine Bindegewebswirkung zukommt. Allerdings blieben diese Ansichten über die Bedeutung dieses Hormons nicht unwidersprochen. Vor allem die Tatsache, daß das thyreotrope Hormon bei solchen Patienten nicht vermehrt gefunden wurde, war auffällig. Bonnyns wies beim diesjährigen Kongreß der Gesellschaft für Thyreoideaforschung im Juni in Louvain auf diese Befunde hin und konnte bestätigen, daß auch bei Komplikationen der Hyperthyreose, wie Exophthalmus und prätibialem Myxödem, der Blutspiegel des thyreotropen Hormons subnormal ist. Dabei wurde auch auf die auffälligen Befunde des hohen Titers von LATS (long acting thyroid stimulator) bei diesen Erkrankungen hingewiesen, Befunde, die noch weiterer Klärung bedürfen.

Die Hautveränderungen des prätibialen Myxödems bestehen bekanntlich in platten- oder knotenförmigen Infiltrationen am Unterschenkel, manchmal von beträchtlichem Ausmaß, so daß der ganze Unterschenkel und Fußrücken beidseits ergriffen sein können. Feingeweblich bestehen diese Infiltrate aus Mucinablagerungen. Oft — aber nicht immer — ist gleichzeitig ein Exophthalmus vorhanden, wobei bemerkenswert ist, daß die histologischen und histochemischen Gewebsbefunde in den Augenhöhlen und am Unterschenkel ähnlich sind. Asboe Hansen machte vor kurzem eine, nach seinen Angaben erstmalige, Beobachtung des Auftretens von Mucinablagerungen in bestehenden Narben bei Patienten mit prätibialem Myxödem. Schon früher war ja die Tatsache, daß Narben innerhalb des prätibialen Myxödems bei diesen Patienten oft Keloidbildung und in diesen Schleimablagerungen zeigten, bekannt.

Auch wir konnten in den letzten Jahren bei verschiedenen Patienten mit prätibialem Myxödem feststellen, daß sich die Schleimablagerungen nicht nur auf die klassische Lokalisation beschränkten, sondern auch in schon bestehenden oder im Zeitraum der Schilddrüsenausschaltung oder nach derselben gesetzten Narben auftraten. So zeigte ein 32jähriger Patient, der 1963 wegen Hyperthyreose strumektomiert wurde, nach 3 Monaten ein massives prätibiales Myxödem, gleichzeitig trat Keloidbildung mit Schleimablagerung in der Strumektomienarbe und eine Vergrößerung schon bestehender Impfnarbenkeloide am Oberarm auf. Auch in letzterer

Lokalisation wurde Mucin gefunden. Ein anderer Fall betraf eine 54jährige Patientin, bei der seit 6 Jahren ein prätibiales Myxödem bestand. Es kam bei dieser nach einer Hallux valgus Operation im Narbenbereich zu starker Keloidbildung mit den ganzen Zehenrücken einnehmenden massiven Schwellungen. Feingewebliche Untersuchungen aus diesem Areal ergaben ebenfalls Schleimablagerungen.

Histologisch und histochemisch sind die Mucinablagerungen an den klassischen Stellen und in den Narbenbereichen im wesentlichen gleich; auffällig ist nur, daß innerhalb der zum Teil hypertrophischen Narben die Schleimablagerungen herdförmig sind, während prätibial praktisch die gesamte Cutis diffus durchzogen ist.

Das Auftreten von Mucin in jüngeren oder älteren Narben bei Patienten mit prätibialem Myxödem scheint unserer bisherigen Erfahrung nach nicht häufig zu sein. Warum einige Patienten an bestimmten Lokalisationen und zu gewissen Zeiten dieses Phänomen zeigen, ist ungeklärt und bedarf noch weiterer Beobachtung.

Natural Course of Various Types of Scleroderma.
A Follow-up-Study over a Period of 20 Years

Z. STAVA, 2nd Dermatological Clinic, Charles' University, Prague (Czechoslovakia)

Between 1946 and 1966 we dealt with a total of 157 cases of diffuse scleroderma who were examined and/or hospitalized. The majority returned for regular follow-ups. In the spring of 1967 questionnaires were sent out enquiring into the progress of the disease, or the cause of death. The 136 replies were then tabulated. The time, onset (i.e. Raynaud's phenomenon, hardening of the skin, joint pains), mode of progress, involvement of oesophagus, lungs and heart, time of death and its cause were evaluated. The entire work was carried out by the same observer who examined the 136 patients over the last 20 years.

Results

Our series has been divided into four major groups according to the degree and the type of involvement at the time of admission.

The first group, acrosclerosis 1, often imitates Raynaud's disease with only slight signs of scleroderma on fingers and face. We had 33 patients, all females. The disease started with Raynaud's phenomenon. Sclerodermatous changes set on after an interval of, on the average, 8 years. In the majority of patients there was only slow impairement; nine remained stationary; six died from various causes. What is remarkable, is that there are twelve patients within this group who, over the period of 11 to 48 years, could be diagnosed as having simply Raynaud's disease. All the same, half of these complained of difficulties in swallowing. This observation points to a close relationship between acroscleroderma and Raynaud's disease.

Within the second group, acrosclerosis 2, there were 30 patients, once more all females. Sclerodermatous changes on the hands were more pronounced, there were trophic lesions on finger tips, mask-like faces. The interval between Raynaud's phenomenon and the actual scleroderma was shorter, 6 years. The majority worsened slowly, seven rapidly, ten died.

Acrosclerosis 3 presented further sclerodermatous changes on arms and neck, mutilations of fingers, loss of weight, marked involvement of inner organs.

We examined 33 patients, all females. The interval between the Raynaud's phenomenon and hardening of the skin was the shortest, 5 years on the average. More than one third of the patients died.

The fourth group was that of diffuse generalized scleroderma (malignant variety). Its characters are: sudden onset, hardening edema of the skin without or with slight secondary Raynaud's phenomenon on hands; involvement of large areas of the skin; rapid progress..We had 18 cases, eleven women and eight men. Only seven are still alive, mostly bed ridden. All others died within the period of 4 months to 6 years. There were signs reminiscent of progressive rheumatoid arthritis with acute onset, of dermatomyositis, of acute systemic lupus erythematosus.

Outside the groups remain six chronic cases in which diffuse scleroderma and progressive rheumatoid arthritis could not be distinguished; nine cases which could not be easily classified; they will be analyzed elsewhere.

Does acroscleroderma affect men? Out of 15 men in our series seven suffered from generalized malignant scleroderma. Three had sclerodactylia in connection with rheumatoid arthritis, four with pneumatic hammer disease; one man only could be classified as having acrosclerosis.

Conclusions

1. Acrosclerosis or acroscleroderma predominantly affects females. It usually starts with Raynaud's phenomenon. At the time of onset it cannot be distinguished from the Raynaud's disease. But even cases of typical Raynaud's disease of long duration may show involvement of oesophagus, lungs and heart similar to that in progressive scleroderma.

2. The course of acroclerosis very often is the more severe the earlier in life the disease starts, the shorter the interval between the Raynaud's phenomenon and the sclerodermatous changes, the earlier and the more marked the joint pains are. This rule does not apply generally. It is virtually impossible to make a prognosis for any particular case.

3. The life expectancy in acroscleroderma is shorter than in normal individuals. Acute heart failure seems to be the main cause of death in elderly acrosclerosis patients. Contrary to previous reports, there does not seem to be a special tendency to carcinoma.

4. In severe acroscleroderma periods of impairement may alternate with periods of no progression at all and even of relative improvement.

5. Rare diffuse generalized scleroderma seems to be a distinct entity apart from acrosclerosis. It affects both men and women and has a very poor prognosis.

Preparation and Application of Lesional Casts in the Study of Cutaneous Disease

D. A. ROE, Graduate School of Nutrition, Savage Hall, Cornell University, Ithaca, New York (USA)

It is frequently necessary in dermatology to obtain permanent records which allow evaluation of the size of three dimensional skin lesions. Measurement of these lesions is important in determining therapy as well as the results of therapy. In the past clinical photographs, scale drawings and wax moulages have been used as recording media, but their usefulness in precise mensuration depends on the availability of skilled technicians or medical artists. On the other hand, plaster casts of lesions can be easily prepared by physicians in research or clinical practice. Widescale production and distribution of orthodontic impression compounds and gypsum plasters have made this possible. Molds can be prepared from alginate pastes which preserve the fine detail of the lesions and this detail is then maintained in the casts. Circumferential or area measurements of single or grouped lesions, reproduced on the cast, can be made by the use of a planimeter.

In practice, two elastic impression powders have been used, which differ only slightly in their physical characteristics*. The alginate powder is rapidly mixed with water at room temperature and the resultant paste is either transferred to a porcelain container, large enough to cover the entire area to be reproduced or spread on a plastic sheet. The container or sheet is then applied to the lesions and firm pressure is exerted for 3 to 4 min or until the paste has set and permits easy detachment from the skin. Fixation is not necessary but casts are immediately prepared in gypsum plaster which sets in 25 min. If immediate casting is not possible, the impression must be covered with a plastic sheet to prevent drying, which causes loss of detail. Appropriate dating and coding of the casts is absolutely necessary when these are to be used as records in therapeutic trials or other clinical studies.

This technique has recently been used in studies of hypocholesterolemic agents and it has been shown that in patients with hyperlipoproteinemias, the resolution of cutaneous xanthomata parallels the rate of fall of the serum cholesterol. Since resolution of the xanthomata may be very slow, it is difficult to demonstrate by simple clinical photographs, but the casts provide direct evidence of small changes in the size and number of the lesions in any one area of the body. Similarly casts are used to demonstrate therapeutic response and change in size of keloids, sarcoidal nodules and primary or metastatic carcinoma, as well as of other papular, nodular or ulcerative lesions. Whereas at present, preparation of casts has found special application in the measurement of cutaneous lesions associated with metabolic or neoplastic disease, the teaching potential of these records should be emphasized. Casts may be used to supplement study collections of clinical photographs especially where it is desirable to show the evolution of specific dermatoses or other lesional change with time.

The impression powders used in the present study were Coe-Alginate (Coe Laboratories, Inc., Chicago 21, Illinois) and Jelset Impression Powder (Opotow Dental Manufacturing Corporation, Brooklyn, N.Y.). The gypsum plaster used in the casts was obtained from Modern Materials, St. Louis, Missouri.

Perorale Kreatinbelastung bei Haut- und Muskelerkrankungen

H. W. KREYSEL und M. JÄNNER, Univ.-Hautklinik Hamburg (Deutschland)

Die Erkrankungen der Skeletmuskulatur werden von den Klinikern als Myopathien bezeichnet. Dieser Determination aber kommt nur eine allgemeine Bedeutung zu. Sie bezieht sich sowohl auf Fehlbildungen als auch auf entzündliche Veränderungen der Muskelfaser selbst. Diese entzündlichen Muskelveränderungen bei der Dermatomyositis, dem hautständigen, chronischen und visceralen Erythematodes, der progressiven Sklerodermie, der Panarteriitis nodosa und als Vergleich hierzu der perikollagenen Amyloidose sollen Gegenstand unserer Betrachtung im Rahmen einer unter standardisierten Versuchsbedingungen durchgeführten peroralen Kreatinbelastung sein. Hierbei wurden 1,32 g Kreatin-Monohydrat in

Wasser gelöst, nach 3tägiger Standarddiät peroral appliziert. Richtungweisend für unsere Überlegungen waren die Beobachtungen bei der Muskeldystrophie, die durch eine verminderte Kreatininelimination und eine gesteigerte Kreatinausscheidung gekennzeichnet ist. Unsere Untersuchungen basieren auf Ergebnissen, die wir bei muskelgesunden Männern und Frauen im Alter von 18 bis 55 Jahren erhoben haben, die die perorale Zufuhr von Kreatin ohne Anstieg der Serumkonzentrationen, unabhängig von Geschlecht und Alter, durch eine verstärkte Kreatininausscheidung beantworteten.

An einem Krankengut von 24 Dermatomyositis-Patienten, 15 progressiven Sklerodermien, 6 Panarteriitiden, 2 perikollagenen Amyloidosen, 10 chronisch discoiden und 4 visceralen Erythematodesfällen wurden perorale Kreatinbelastungen durchgeführt und die ermittelten Werte mit dem Zeichen- und Wilcoxen-Test auf Signifikanzbedingungen geprüft. Hierbei kamen wir zu folgenden Ergebnissen:
Die Werte vor der Belastung lassen keine signifikanten Differenzen erkennen. Unter der Belastung werden die Unterschiede deutlicher. Verminderte Kreatinin- und erhöhte Kreatinausscheidungen sind bei der Dermatomyositis als typische Zeichen der Muskelparenchymschädigung anzusprechen, während bei der progressiven Sklerodermie als Ausdruck einer Herdmyositis diese aufgezeigten Veränderungen nicht so deutlich in Erscheinung treten. Bei der Panarteriitis nodosa, dem visceralen Erythematodes, der perikollagenen Amyloidose zeigten die Kreatinkonzentrationen im Urin im Wilcoxen- und Zeichentest bezogen auf den Mittelwertsvergleich keine eindeutigen Veränderungen, obwohl unter der Belastung bei allen Fällen eine Zunahme beobachtet wurde. Die relativ kleine Zahl der uns zur Verfügung stehenden Patienten dürfte hierfür eine Erklärung liefern.

Eindrucksvoll und signifikant gesichert dagegen erscheinen die Kreatinkonzentrationen bei allen untersuchten Krankheitsbildern im Serum und lassen bei einem Mittelwertsvergleich graduelle Unterschiede erkennen. Die Belastungsergebnisse bei den chronischen, hautständigen Erythematodesfällen ergaben keine Hinweise für eine muskuläre Kreatinstoffwechselstörung.

Im Zusammenhang mit unseren Kreatinbelastungen haben wir EMG-Untersuchungen durchgeführt. Unser Dank gilt den Herren Dr. PUFF und Dr. SCHOCKE (Neurolog. Univ.-Klinik, UKE). Pathologische Ableitungen der angeführten Krankheitsbilder korrelieren sowohl mit signifikanten von der Norm abweichenden Kreatinbelastungsergebnissen als auch mit dem Grad der morphologischen Besonderheiten. Früh- und Restzustände lassen sich vor allen Dingen bei der Dermatomyositis durch die perorale Kreatinbelastung abgrenzen. Bei den anderen Krankheitsbildern ergeben die aufgezeigten Kreatin/Kreatininveränderungen Anhaltspunkte für eine graduelle Muskelschädigung, die einer Herdmyositis entspricht.

Die Bedeutung dieser zum Teil aufwendigen und sehr empfindlichen Untersuchungen glauben wir darin zu sehen, daß bei klinisch verdächtigen Personen mit einer nur einmalig ermittelten Kreatinbestimmung nicht verwertbare Zufallsergebnisse im Urin und Serum registriert werden, während die unter standardisierten Versuchsbedingungen durchgeführte perorale Kreatinbelastung im Hinblick auf die Aussagefähigkeit einer echten Myopathie zu diagnostisch reproduzierbaren Werten führt. Damit könnte bereits in einem möglichst frühzeitigen Stadium durch die Störung im Kreatinhaushalt eine Muskelbeteiligung erfaßt werden, wo Elektromyographie und Histologie zunächst noch keine typischen Veränderungen erkennen lassen. Die perorale Kreatinbelastung kann somit nach unserer Auffassung als weiteres Hilfsmittel im Rahmen der Diagnostik den anderen Untersuchungsmethoden gleichwertig an die Seite gestellt werden.

Liquen rojo plano de la mucosa bucal.
Su asociación con diabetes. Nuevas observaciones

D. Grinspan, J. Díaz, L. O. Villapol, J. Schneiderman, R. Berdichesky, D. Palese y J. Faerman, 2da. Cátedra de Dermatología de la Facultad de Ciencias Médicas y Centro Municipal de Blastomas de Piel, Buenos Aires, y Boca-Hospital, Rawson (Argentina)

Queremos destacar en esta comunicación el hallazgo de un hecho clínico de particular interés: la frecuencia significativa de diabetes en los enfermos con liquen rojo plano de la mucosa bucal, en especial en sus formas atípicas.

Métodos usados

El diagnóstico de diabetes se hizo clínicamente, completado con el estudio de la glucemia, la glucosuria y las pruebas de sobrecarga del aparato glucorregulador. Para la determinación de la glucemia se usaron los métodos de Somogyi Nelson y Folin Wu. En las pruebas de sobrecarga el de Conn y Fajans. En doce líquenes se buscó histológicamente en biopsias de la piel del dorso de manos con coloración de PAS el engrosamiento de la membrana basal de los vasos del plexo subpapilar, hallazgo corriente en diabéticos. El diagnóstico de Liquen Rojo Plano se hizo por la clínica y la histopatología.

Nuestros hallazgos

Sobre 76 casos en los cuales buscamos alteraciones del metabolismo hidrocarbonado hallamos 26 diabéticos (34,21%) (Cuadro 1).

De los 26 enfermos diabéticos, 9 tenían liquen típico y 17 atípico. Para estos últimos el porcentaje de diabetes asociada se eleva a 65,3% (Cuadro 2).

Cuadro 1

N° de pacientes estudiados con liquen	Diabéticos	
	N° de pacientes	%
76	26	34,21

Cuadro 2

Total Diabéticos y liquen	Formas típicas de liquen		Formas atípicas	
	N°	%	N°	%
26	9	34,6	17	65,3

De los 26 diabéticos 14 eran mujeres y 12 hombres. Doce casos fueron rotulados de diabéticos por sus datos clínicos y curvas patológicas, algunas halladas reiterando la búsqueda. Los 14 restantes porque presentaban la diabetes clásica.

En doce casos de líquenes tomados al azar, en los que se buscó histopatológicamente el engrosamiento de la membrana basal de los vasos del plexo subpapilar de la piel del dorso de manos se halló en tres enfermos un grado III (presunción de diabetes). Estos tres casos resultaron ser los únicos diabéticos de la serie.

Realizamos además una búsqueda de Liquen Rojo Plano en un grupo de 70 enfermos diabéticos del Servicio de Nutrición del Hospital Rawson. Su enfermedad tenía un tiempo de evolución entre 1 mes y 35 años. La mayor parte de los pacientes (65) estaban en tratamiento. En este grupo encontramos tres líquenes típicos (4,61%). Entre cinco diabéticos sin tratamiento se halló un liquen erosivo. Total: cuatro líquenes en 70 diabéticos (5,71%).

Consideraciones

Entendemos por formas típicas de liquen, las manchas blancas en red o arboriformes o punteadas, en especial del tercio posterior de la mucosa yugal o con ese mismo aspecto en otras localizaciones (labio, lengua, etc.).

Llamamos formas atípicas a aspectos ampollares, penfigoides, erosivos, vegetantes, queratósicos, etc. 13 de los 17 casos de líquenes atípicos asociados a diabetes eran erosivos predominantemente.

Otro hecho a destacar es que de los 26 casos de liquen en asociación con diabetes, 22 de ellos estaban localizados exclusivamente en la boca, 2 en la boca y glande y 2 en la boca y piel. Esto indicaría que la mayor frecuencia de diabetes y liquen se vería en los casos de localización bucal exclusiva.

Queremos señalar también la frecuencia con que hemos hallado, en estos casos de asociación de liquen y diabetes, hipertensión arterial, ya que siete de estos enfermos la tenían.

Otro hecho de valor es que de los 26 enfermos con liquen y diabetes, solo doce conocían su alteración metabólica, por lo que resulta que en 14 de ellos, el diagnóstico de diabetes se hizo como consecuencia del diagnóstico de liquen.

Por último una observación de gran interés terapéutico, es que el tratamiento de la diabetes y de la hipertensión, fueron suficientes, por si solos, para controlar las lesiones de liquen bucal y especialmente transformar las formas erosivas en típicas. Unicamente en cinco casos no se obtuvieron mejorías evidentes del liquen. Estos hechos terapéuticos pudieron confirmarse, ya que cuando los enfermos descontrolaban su diabetes o su hipertensión, desmejoraban sus lesiones. Estos resultados terapéuticos acrecientan el valor del hallazgo por ser bien conocida la dificultad del tratamiento de los líquenes atípicos de la boca y de sus manifestaciones objetivas y subjetivas, con las terapéuticas corrientes para el liquen rojo plano.

Esta comunicación realizada con un mayor número de casos confirma nuestros primeros hallazgos efectuados como comunicación previa al V° Congreso Ibero Latino Americano de Dermatología realizado en Buenos Aires en Noviembre de 1963.

No hemos hallado otra bibliografía.

Sarcoidosis with Cicatricial Alopecia Resembling Generalized Discoid Lupus Erythematosus

L. S. Sauter, Division of Dermatology, Department of Medicine, New York Medical College, and Department of Medicine, St. Clare's Hospital, New York, N.Y. (USA)

The clinical appearance of the cutaneous lesions in sarcoidosis takes a great variety of forms. It is not uncommon in sarcoidosis to see different types of skin lesions in the same patient, particularly if the eruption is extensive. Clinically, the skin lesions of sarcoidosis can imitate those seen in several internal diseases such as tuberculosis, leprosy, lymphoma and deep mycoses. They may also resemble granuloma annulare, necrobiosis lipoidica diabeticorum and discoid lupus erythematosus.

The purpose of this report is to call attention to those cutaneous manifestations of sarcoidosis which simulate discoid lupus erythematosus (DLE).

Recently a 43 year old Negro man was presented [1] with an extensive eruption which mainly consisted of many discoid scaly and crusted patches involving the extremities and the trunk. Many of the skin lesions showed atrophy and telangiectasia. Similar scaly atrophic lesions were present around and in the external ear canal; these types of lesions are usually seen in DLE. The most striking finding was

a scarring alopecia of the scalp showing hyper- and hypopigmentation and telangiectatic vessels and resembling DLE.

The abnormal laboratory data included increased serum gamma globulins, an
elevated bromsulfalein dye retention test and an elevated erythrocyte sedimentation rate.

Multiple lupus erythematosus cell preparations, rheumatoid factor, cryo-
globulins, and deoxyribonucleic acid agar precipitation were negative. Acid- fast
organisms were not found in sputum or gastric washings, and cultures for acid
fast bacilli and fungi showed no growth. Intradermal tests with purified protein
derivative of tuberculin in first, intermediate, and second strength were repeatedly
negative. Intracutaneous injections with histoplasmin, coccidioidin, and blastomycin did not show any abnormal reaction.

Chest x-rays showed increase in the bronchial-vascular markings of both hilar
and para-hilar areas. Nodular infiltrates were seen in the lower two-thirds of both
lung fields. Pleural effusions were noted in both basal lung fields. There was prominence of lymph nodes in both hilar areas, with marked calcification. Pulmonary
function studies showed highly abnormal values, suggestive of interstitial pulmonary fibrosis.

Skeletal survey revealed radiolucent changes of the left ulna, the middle
phalanx of the left ring finger, and the left clavicle.

The initial histopathological findings* of the first biopsy were not diagnostic. The
examination of the histological sections of the second biopsy showed scattered small
granulomas composed of epithelioid cells together with a lesser number of small
round cells and an occasional multinucleated giant cell. The histopathological examination of the lung biopsy revealed sarcoidal granulomas. No microorganisms were
found in histological sections of the skin or lung biopsy with Fite's and PAS stain.

The clinical appearance of this case strongly resembled DLE. Jörgensen [2]
reviewed numerous reports of patients stated to have DLE and sarcoidosis simultaneously or subsequently. In addition, he described three patients with sarcoidosis
who were thought to have DLE. By evaluating the clinical course and the histopathological findings in both the reported and his own cases, Jörgensen came to
the conclusion that all these patients had only sarcoidosis. The erroneous diagnosis
of DLE was made in those patients because too much reliance was put upon the
clinical appearance. A scarring baldness of the scalp was a striking finding in
our patient. Alopecia of the scalp was mentioned by Atwood and Nelson as a
rare finding in sarcoidosis [3]. Very few reports of histopathologically proven
cases of sarcoidosis with atrophic alopecia were found in the literature. One
patient was described by Ronchese [4], who pointed out the strong resemblance
of the scalp lesions to DLE. Baker [5] reported another case. His patient had
erythematous infiltrated plaques with atrophic changes which clinically did not
suggest sarcoidosis. It was strongly suggestive that the patient's pleuropulmonary
disease was due solely to sarcoidosis. However, because of the bilateral pleural
effusions, which are very rarely seen in patients with sarcoidosis [6], a lung biopsy
was performed to eliminate any doubts as to the nature of the pleuropulmonary
findings. Specifically, elimination of tuberculosis from consideration was of great
importance, in view of contemplated corticosteroid therapy. The histopathological examination of the lung biopsy confirmed the diagnosis of sarcoidosis.

In closing, among the many variations of skin lesions which may occur in
sarcoidosis, emphasis was placed on the close resemblance that may occur between
sarcoidosis and DLE.

---

* I am indebted to Dr. Victor de Luccia for performing the lung biopsy.

References. 1. SAUTER, L. S.: Arch. Derm. **94**, 670 (1966). — 2. JÖRGENSEN, G.: Arch. klin. exp. Derm. **214**, 445 (1962). — 3. ATWOOD, W. A., and C. T. NELSON: Med. Clin. N. Amer. **49**, 783 (1965). — 4. RONCHESE, F.: Arch. Derm. **64**, 806 (1951). — 5. BAKER, H.: Proc. roy. Soc. Med. **58**, 243 (1965). — 6. KOVNAT, P.: Ann. intern. Med. **62**, 120 (1965).

Dermatological Aspects of Crohn's Disease

D. I. McCALLUM, Nottingham General Hospital, and P. D. C. KINMONT, Derbyshire Royal Infirmary, Derby (England)

Crohn's disease, first described in 1932 as a disorder of the terminal ileum, is now recognised as a condition of unknown aetiology which may attack any part of the gastro-intestinal tract from the stomach to the anus (regional enteritis). It seems probable that the primary pathological change is in the lymphatics of the gut and mesentery; this results in gross thickening of the affected areas of the bowel wall and of the adjacent mesentery and lymph nodes. The mucosal surface of the gut becomes ulcerated and fistulae are particularly liable to occur, both internally, and externally in the perianal region, in relation to laparotomy scars and elsewhere on the anterior abdominal wall, groins or genitalia. The histopathological picture is one of dilatation and tortuosity of the lymph vessels, and of aggregations of epithelioid cells, lymphocytes and occasional giant cells — a characteristic but not a diagnostic one.

The clinical findings in Crohn's disease may be acute or chronic. In the acute condition it simulates acute appendicitis, causing cramp-like pain in the right lower quadrant of the anterior abdomen, or in the periumbilical region. In the chronic phase there is vague abdominal pain and diarrhoea with watery stools. Occult blood is usually demonstrable in the stool. The patient becomes anaemic, loses weight and may be pyrexial. Fistula formation is particularly liable to occur. Obstructive symptoms are present in 10% of cases. While lengthy remissions may occur, the disease tends to progress relentlessly. Diagnosis depends primarily on recognition of the clinical features, and partly on X-ray investigation, although 5% of cases show no radiological abnormality.

The differential diagnosis includes acute and chronic appendicitis, ulcerative colitis, tuberculous enteritis, and carcinoma of lower bowel.

Complications

Haemorrhage may be so severe on occasion as to cause a profound anaemia and even to endanger life. Subacute obstruction occurs in 10% of cases, arthralgia and iritis in less than 5%, whilst carcinoma and amyloid change are very rare. Stunting of growth and of sexual development in children may result. Of particular interest to the dermatologist are perianal fistulae and abscesses and fistulae and abscesses on the anterior abdominal wall, in the groins and submammary regions. Erythema nodosum, pyoderma gangrenosum, palmar erythema in the absence of demonstrable liver disease, and thrombophlebitis of thighs and legs may also occur.

In a series of eight cases seen by the authors there were six in whom extensive perianal ulceration was the main feature; one of these also suffered from erythema nodosum. A seventh patient had pyoderma gangrenosum, and the eight had an ulcer in the ano-rectal region and a diffuse mauve intensely hard infiltration of the buttocks which was thought clinically to be sarcomatous, but on histopathological examination showed features of Crohn's disease in both sites. A review of the casenotes of 137 patients suffering from Crohn's disease seen by medical and surgical colleagues in the Nottingham and Derby areas in recent years (including the cases mentioned above) has been carried out, and the following skin complications noted:

1. Those due to direct extension of the disease process
   a) Perianal ulceration, ischio-rectal abscesses, fistula-in-ano 24
   b) Ulceration or fistulae on anterior abdominal wall, especially in relation to
      laparotomy scars, and to the umbilicus and vulva 28
   c) Involvement of the groin and submammary regions 2
   d) Granuloma of buttock 1
2. Vascular reaction
   Erythema nodosum.. 1
   Pyoderma gangrenosum 1
3. Those resulting from interference with bowel function and from resultant asthenia,
   malabsorption syndrome, glossitis, pharyngeal ulceration and furunculosis 19
4. Unexplained and possibly unrelated conditions, e.g., pigmentary anomalies 4

Total   80

These eighty complications occurred in fifty-eight patients; in the present series there is, therefore, an incidence of dermatological complications in 42,4%.

General medical and surgical textbooks state that approximately 20% of cases of Crohn's disease are complicated by skin involvement of one sort or another. It is surprising that no reference is made to this disease process in dermatological textbooks, nor in those books which deal with skin manifestations of internal disease.

Four cases in the present series of eight were diagnosed initially as ulcerative colitis; in several other cases which have been reviewed the ischio-rectal abscesses and fistulae-in-ano were thought to be tuberculous in origin. No ischio-rectal abscess investigated pathologically and bacteriologically in the Nottingham-Derby area in recent years had been proved to be due to tuberculosis; there seems to be little doubt that the great majority of these abscesses and fistulae are due to Crohn's disease. Referring to perianal and perirectal fistulae Bockus concludes "If fistulae occur in a patient with diarrhoea, study must be carried out to exclude the presence of regional enteritis".

A propos du syndrôme de Winterbauer (Syndrôme C.R.S.T.)

A. PUISSANT, R. LECLERCQ et F. VANBREMEERSCH, Paris (France)

En 1964 WINTERBAUER décrivait un groupement morbide associant télangiectasies, syndrôme de Raynaud, sclérodactylie, calcinose cutanée et sous-cutanée; il concluait son important travail en suggérant que ce syndrôme «C.R.S.T.» était une entité parmi le groupe des maladies du collagène; il le distinguait de la sclérodermie généralisée.

Nous suivons depuis 1965, sept malades présentant l'ensemble des symptômes tenus pour caractéristiques du syndrôme «C.R.S.T» = cinq femmes de 26 à 56 ans et 2 hommes de 34 ans; le syndrôme de Raynaud, signe initial est apparu de 7 à 25 ans plus tôt; la sclérodactylie, la calcinose et les télangiectiasies sont évidentes dans tous les cas; une de nos malades a été hospitalisée avec le diagnostic d'angiomatose de RENDU-OSLER pour des hémoptysies dues à des dilatations vasculaires bronchiques visibles en bronchoscopie.

Rapprochant les observations de WINTERBAUER (1964), DE CARR, HEISEL, STEVENSON (1965), DE VEREL (1956) cité par WINTERBAUER, le travail original publié par THIBIERGE et WEISSENBACH en 1911 dans les Annales Françaises de Dermatologie, et nos constatations, nous pensons pouvoir faire les cinq remarques suivantes:

Première remarque: *L'observation princes de* THIBIERGE et WEISSENBACH *est la plus belle description qu'on puisse trouver du syndrôme «C.R.S.T.».*: chez leur malade de 44 ans l'affection évoluait depuis la 28° année, avait débuté par un syndrôme de Raynaud compliqué trois mois plus tard de sclérodactylie puis d'ulcérations digitales avec expulsion de «caillou»; progressivement s'étaient constituées des télangiectasies sur le visage, le cou et le thorax.

Deuxième remarque: Il faut toutefois noter que le travail de THIBIERGE et WEISSENBACH était consacré aux «concrétions calcaires sous-cutanées» au cours de la sclérodermie. WINTERBAUER a eu le mérite d'insister sur l'importance des télangiectasies ou cours de certaines sclérodermies, de souligner la ressemblance de ce genre de sclérodermie avec l'angiomatose hémorragique familiale de RENDU-OSLER et de démontrer par l'enquête clinique et généalogique de ses sept cas les différences fondamentales qui séparaient les deux affections; la toute récente observation d'association des deux maladies par HADIDA et coll. semble être unique. Cependant la possibilité d'un problème diagnostique difficile entre ces maladies avait déjà fait l'objet de publications, dont celle de BAUMGARTNER dans «Dermatologica» en 1959.

Troisième remarque: WINTERBAUER *a cependant replacé dans l'actualité une notion importante: l'apparition parfois très précoce des télangiectasies dans la sclérodermie.* A. TOURAINE avait signalé ce fait en 1941; il pensait qu'on pouvait y voir le témoignage du rôle des lésions vasculaires dans la constitution de la scléro-atrophie cutanée. D'autres auteurs sont ensuite revenus sur cet argument: DUPERRAT et coll. en 1959, BAZEX et coll. en 1964, DUPERRAT et coll. en 1965.

Quatrième remarque: *Le syndrôme «C.R.S.T.» ne doit pas être distingué de la sclérodermie généralisée.* L'étude de TUFFANELLI et WINKELMANN sur 727 cas de sclérodermies généralisées observées de 1935 à 1958 à la Mayo Clinic le montre bien: ces auteurs ont noté une maladie de Raynaud ou des troubles vasculaires divers dans 90% des cas, des télangiectasies dans 13,8% des cas, une calcinose dans 18,9% des cas. THIERS, MOULIN, ROUHANI, dans un travail récent, retrouvent même angiome et télangiectasies dans la moitié de leurs sclérodermies généralisées. L'apport de WINTERBAUER trouve sa justification et ses limites dans la remarque faite par TUFFANELLI et WINKELMANN que «les télangiectasies sont surtout fréquentés chez les malades présentant le syndrôme de THIBIERGE-WEISSENBACH».

Cinquième remarque: *Le début de la sclérodermie par l'association dite syndrome «C.R.S.T.» est loin d'avoir la signification favorable que lui a donné* WINTERBAUER. Déjà parmi les sept cas publiés en 1965 par CARR, HEISEL, STEVENSON, l'autopsie d'un malade a montré que des lésions «sclérodermiques» oesophagiennes et pulmonaires avaient été responsables de la mort. Dans nos sept cas personnels, si l'évolution est relativement lente comme le souligne WINTERBAUER, les examens complets ont toujours prouvé la nature systémique et gravement évolutive de la maladie: troubles oesophagiens cliniques et radiocinématiques dans trois cas; dyspnée d'effort dans quatre cas; signes radiologiques d'atteinte pulmonaire dans deux cas; altérations des épreuves fonctionnelles respiratories (diminution de la capacité respiratoire, bloc alvéolo-capillaire, augmentation des volumes statiques et diminution du volume expiratoire maximum seconde) dans trois cas; anomalies électrocardiographiques importantes dans trois cas; insuffisance rénale avec hypertension artérielle grave dans un cas; forte accélération de la V.S.G. dans trois cas. Ces troubles s'associaient de différentes manières selon les cas, mais aucun de nos sept malades n'en était exempt.

Conclusion: *Le syndrôme de* WINTERBAUER *est une forme clinique de la scléro-dermie;* s'il fallait l'individualiser, c'est à THIBIERGE et WEISSENBACH qu'il conviendrait de l'attribuer puisque ces auteurs l'ont décrite en 1911.

Bibliographie. VON BAUMGARTNER, P.: Dermatologica (Basel) 118, 279 (1959). — BAZEX, A., R. SALVADOR, A. DUPRE, A. FOURNIE, M. PARANT et B. CHRISTOL: Bull. Soc. franc. Derm. Syph. 71, 206 (1964). — CARR, R. D., E. HEISEL, and TH. STEVENSON: Arch. Derm. 92, 519 (1965). — DUPERRAT, B., L. GOLE, A. PUISSANT, J. MONTFORT et D. LEROY: Bull. Soc. franç. Derm. Syph. 72, 126 (1965). — HADIDA, E., H. SARLES, J. SAYAG et F. TASSOM: Bull. Soc. franç. Derm. Syph. 73, 514 (1966). — PUISSANT, A., R. FISCHER et P. L. DELAIRE: Rev. Méd. (Paris) 7, 961 (1966). — TOURAINE, A.: Bull. Soc. franç. Derm. Syph. 48, 355 (1941). — THIBIERGE, G., and R. J. WEISSENBACH: Ann. Derm. Syph. (Chic.) 42, 129 (1911). THIERS, H., G. MOULIN et A. ROUHANI: Bull. Soc. franç. Derm. Syph. 73, 528 (1966). — TUFFANELLI, D., and R. K. WINKELMANN: Arch. Derm. 84, 359 (1961). — VEREL, D.: Lancet 67, 914 (1956). — WINTERBAUER, R. H.: Bull. Johns Hopk. Hosp. 114, 361 (1964).

Acanthosis Nigricans — A Clinical Manifestation of Internal Disorders

T. YASUDA, SH. NISHIYAMA and SH. TSUYUKI, Department of Dermatology, Kanto Teishin Hospital, Tokyo (Japan)

Acanthosis nigricans is a symmetric, hyperpigmented, papillary and hyper-keratotic reaction of the folds of the skin. This is seen in the flexural areas of the body, particularly the axilla, neck, groin, antecubital and perigenital region, and in some cases also on the exposed areas of the skin such as the face and the back of the hands and feet.

However, it is a well recognized fact that approximately half of the reported cases of this disease are associated with malignant diseases of the internal viscera, particularly of the stomach. Most commonly the tumor is an adenocarcinoma. This is true in Japan also.

The terms malignant and benign acanthosis nigricans have been used to separate those cases associated with malignancy from those cases which do not demonstrate this relationship but are rather caused by some internal disorders.

The term pseudoacanthosis nigricans was introduced by CURTH to discribe those cases presumed to be the local effect of obesity. He further stated that this may be considered a phenotype of benign acanthosis nigricans.

At present it is recognized that acanthosis nigricans may be caused by the following factors: 1. genetic factor, 2. endocrinopathy, 3. obesity, 4. drugs, 5. hepatic diseases and 6. malignant tumor.

However, it is very difficult to distinguish all these forms clinically and histologically. This means that some common etiologic factors must play a rôle in the pathogenesis of this skin manifestation.

Histologically, in typical acanthosis nigricans, papilla projects upward as a fingerlike projection and is covered with the thickened stratum malpighii with hyperkeratosis, that is papillomatosis. In this histological picture the primary change is in the papilla; those in the epidermis are secondary to this. Such histo-logical changes are produced by the peripheral circulatory disturbance, which may be seen in capillary microaneurisma with edema in the papilla, and by the changes of the collagen and its ground substance in the subpapillary layer, which is seen in perivascular fibroblast infiltration without inflammation.

These changes result from some metabolic fault or endocrinopathy. In fact, acanthosis nigricans may also be produced by some drugs, such as niacin, dimethylstilbesterol and corticosteroid (TROMOVITCH, KATZENELLENBOGEN, PAPA). Other authors have also reported the association of benign acanthosis nigricans with endocrinologic disturbances and hepatic diseases (WINKELLMAN, BROWN, TUFFANELLI, SCHWARTZ). We may further postulate that the same process, that is to say a metabolic or endocrinologic fault resulting from malignant disease, would participate in the production of acanthosis nigricans maligna.

In addition to this metabolic or endocrinologic factor, some irritation from outside and congenital basis may play a role in the manifestation of acanthosis nigricans. This idea is supported by the following facts.

1. Most of the cases of acanthosis nigricans, especially those of benign type, are accompanied by striae atrophicae. It may be supposed that hormonal factors, especially the hyperactivity of the pituitary gland, are mainly responsible for this skin change, while mechanical factors determine the direction of this striae formation. This is also suggested by the fact that Cushing's syndrome-like state is produced by the administration of corticotropin and that this striae occurs in the period of increased pituitary activity, such as puberty and pregnancy.

2. Both acanthosis nigricans and striae atrophicae are seen in the same collagen tissue diseases, such as Marfan's syndrome and Ehlers-Danlos' disease. This show that the collagen tissue changes play an important role in the production of acanthosis nigricans.

As stated above, it is difficult to distinguish all forms clinically and histologically, but some authors state that cutaneous changes of benign type be less severe and more extensive than those of malignant type. This might depend on the degree and extent of the above mentioned pathogenetic process. If the process is localized, there occur verrucous papules as often seen in and around acanthosis nigricans. And surely we know that in some cases the verrucous papules are so prominent that they are sometimes mistaken for another disease, such as Verrucosa generalisata or Lewandowsky's disease. We have observed a case of such a skin manifestation and it had the predilection for that of acanthosis nigricans including mucous membrane of the mouth. The patient was 71 years old and was found to have gastric cancer by gastroscope. Histologically it was adenocarcinoma. And the skin manifestation regressed after the resection of the tumor.

In conclusion, we would like stress the following facts: 1. Acanthosis nigricans is the rare skin manifestation caused from various kinds of the etiologic factors. 2. In all clinical forms they show the common skin changes indistinguishable from each other. 3. Its primary change lies in the papilla as shown by the peripheral circulatory disturbance in the papilla and the collagen tissue change in the sub-papillary layer. 4. The change in the epidermis is secondary to this. 5. The degree and extent of the skin manifestation depend on how these primary changes occur. 6. If the change is localized, verrucous papules may be the main skin change in acanthotic nigricans.

Glucorrhoea. Is this Pre-diabetes?

J. R. G. AGIUS, Dermatological Clinic, King Georges V Hospital, Valetta (Malta)

Certain persons secrete glucose in their sweat in detectable amounts, a state which may be termed "glucorrhoea" (or "dermoglucorrhoea"). MILLER and RIDOLFO [1] were the first to appreciate the importance of this, and they evolved a "skin-surface-glucose" test, from which they concluded that a positive reaction indicated a recently elevated blood sugar. These and other authors [2, 3], however, could not harness this test to the early diagnosis of diabetes because of the number of positive reactions in non-diabetics and negative reactions in known diabetics. Unaware of this work, in 1963, I developed a similar test, suitable as a bedside test (DE BONO [4]), which can be considered as a modification of that of MILLER and RIDOLFO.

Glucorrhoea test

Method. The active end of Clinistix* is moistened in tap water and held for 8 sec between the (unwashed) thumb and each of the opposing fingers successively, first of one hand and then of the other, for a total of about 1 min (64 sec). No change of colour was taken as a negative reaction. A minimal intensity of blue (a similary arbitrary) classification of intensity of colour was used by HUNT et al. [5]) was interpreted as an immediate positive reaction, while if the same intensity was reached within 5 min of the end of the test, it was interpreted as a delayed positive reaction. The urine was tested for glucose immediately after. A discrepancy in the results had been observed between the two hands [1, 6], but this difficulty was overcome in the glucorrhoea test.

Results

The glucorrhoea test was carried out by me on 2984 subjects over a period of 4 years. Each subject was tested at the time he presented for examination. Of this total, 822 gave an immediate positive reaction and 478 a delayed positive reaction.

Chlorpropamide tolerance.* It is well known that diabetic patients in general tolerate oral anti-diabetic agents well. These have been given by FAJANS and CONN [7, 8] to "asymptomatic diabetics" to stimulate endogenous secretion of insulin. It was argued, therefore, that oral anti-diabetic agents might be tolerated also by non-diabetic subjects with a positive glucorrhoea test. Their exhibition might even stimulate endogenous insulin production. Chlorpropamide* was chosen for this study because of its prolonged action, because it may be administered in a single dose, and because it is relatively cheap. The dose of chlorpropamide administered was calculated according to: 1. degree of positivity of the glucorrhoea test, 2. age, 3. bodyweight. The dose was somewhat reduced if the subject undertook much physical exertion.

A normal adult giving an immediate positive reaction was given 250 mg in a single morning dose [10]. This was halved in cases with a delayed positive reaction. Adolescents and children were only treated if they gave an immediate positive reaction. The former received a maximum of 100 mg daily, but the dose was reduced if the bodyweight was low. The dose for children above the age of 6 months was calculated on the following formula:

$$\frac{\text{age in years}}{2\ (\text{age in years} + 12)} \text{ of 250 mg .}$$

Chlorpropamide was administered to all subjects giving a positive glucorrhoea test, but excluding pregnant women. This treatment was continued for periods ranging from a few weeks to several months, and was given in addition to the treatment usually prescribed for the particular disease for which the subject had attended.

Eight subjects with a negative glucorrhoea test were used as controls and given chlorpropamide. All of them rapidly developed alarming symptoms of hypoglycaemia even though they were receiving a reduced dose. Because of this studies on controls were not considered justified. None of the subjects with a

---

* Clinistix an enzyme glucose oxidase test paper made by Ames Co. My thanks are due to Pfizer Ltd for a generous supple of "Diabenese" brand of chlorpropamide.

positive glucorrhoea test complained of serious hypoglycaemic symptoms while on chlorpropamide, even when, in the latter part of the study carbohydrate intake was restricted very much. Only twelve subjects complained of headaches, nausea or emptyheadedness, which were eliminated by reduction in the dose of chlorpropamide. During the treatment with chlorpropamide glucorrhoea sometimes diminished or even diasppeared, but this did not necessarily produce side effects.

Discussion

The tolerance of subjects with glucorrhoea to chlorpropamide even after a severe reduction in the intake of carbohydrates contrasts with the lack of tolerance in controls receiving a much smaller dose. It confirms the findings of MILLER and RIDOLFO that glucorrhoea indicates a disturbance of carbohydrate metabolism. Many authors [11 to 19] in the past have used oral anti-diabetic agents empirically in the treatment of various skin diseases. A certain percentage of these cases developed side effects thus rendering the treatment hazardous. Since the glucorrhoea test distinguishes those who are tolerant to oral anti-diabetic agents (at least to chlorpropamide) from those who are not, this hazard is now eliminated.

References. 1. MILLER, D. I., and A. S. RIDOLFO: Diabetes 9, 48 (1960). — 2. WEST, K. M., D. R. ROCKWELL, and J. A. WULFF: Diabetes 12, 58 (1963). — 3. GOADBY, H. K.: Medical Annu. 1965, 164. — 4. DE BONO, E. F.: Brit. med. J. 2, 1040 (1965). — 5. HUNT, J. A., C. H. GRAY, and D. E. THOROGOOD: Brit. med. J. 2, 586 (1956). — 6. Physician's Bull. 25, 34 (1960). — 7. FAJANS, S., and J. W. CONN: Diabetes 9, 83 (1960). — 8. FAJANS, S., and J. W. CONN: Quoted by 9 (1964). — 9. PFEIFFER, E. F., and R. ZIEGLER: Triangle (En) 7, 1 (1965). — 10. Current practice, Brit. med. J. 1, 521 (1963). — 11. ANDREWS, G. C.: Arch. Derm. 84, 711 (1961). — 12. SPOOR, H. J.: Clin. Med. 70, 911 (1963). — 13. SINGH, I.: Brit. J. Derm. 73, 362 (1961). — 14. COHEN, J. L., and A. D. COHEN: Canad. med. Ass. J. 80, 629 (1959). — 15. DEPAOLI, M., e G. MARTINA: Minerva med. 51, 3505 (1960). — 16. FREDRIKSSON, T., and E. SKOG: Acta derm.-venereol. (Stockh.) 39, 327 (1959). — 17. BAUER, G.: Medico 2, 35 (1964). — 18. NEUMANN, E.: Dermatologica (Basel) 117, 172 (1958). — 19. WOLFRAM, VON ST.: Hautarzt 10, 471 (1959).

Hormonelle Untersuchungen und Behandlungsmethoden bei Acne vulgaris

F. TÓTH und L. NÉKÁM, I. Frauenklinik und Haut- und Venerologische Klinik der Medizinischen Universität Budapest (Ungarn)

Die gesteigerte Talgabsonderungswirkung der Androgene beweisen zahlreiche tierexperimentelle Untersuchungen und an Menschen durchgeführte Beobachtungen, ebenso bekräftigen viele Beobachtungen und Untersuchungen die Hemmwirkung der Oestrogene auf die Talgdrüsen. Wir führten hormonelle Investigationen an 60 an Acne leidenden Frauen und zehn Männern durch. Das Alter ersterer war zwischen 15 und 34, mit einem Durchschnitt von 23,4 Jahren, letzterer zwischen 15 und 21, mit einem Durchschnittsalter von 19 Jahren. Vor und während der Behandlung bestimmten wir die Ausscheidung von hypophysengonadotropem Hormon, Pregnandiol, Total-Oestrogen und 17-KS. Die Bestimmungen führten wir immer in der gleichen Phase des Menstruationscyclus durch. Neben den Hormonbestimmungen führten wir bei jedem Patienten routinemäßig Leberfunktions- und Magensäuresekretionsuntersuchungen durch. In unserem Laboratorium war die tägliche 17-KS-Ausscheidung der gesunden Frauen 9,2 mg. Die Durchschnittswerte der an Acne leidenden Patienten sind 13,6 mg. Das sind

4,4 mg mehr als der normale Wert. Die Normalwerte des hypophysengonadotropen Hormons schwankten zwischen 20 bis 40 IU. Bei den an Acne leidenden Patienten war der Durchschnittswert 63,7 IU. Die normalen Werte der totalen Oestrogenausscheidung sind 20 bis 40 γ pro Tag, bei Patienten mit Acne 30,9 pro Tag. Wenn wir die Oestrogen- und Androgenration in Betracht ziehen, finden wir das absolute und relative Androgenübergewicht bei 42 Patienten. Im Laufe der Behandlung verabreichten wir ungarische Oestrogenprodukte und von der Organonfabrik hergestelltes Orgametril und Gestyl. Nach MAUVAIS-JARVIS u. Mitarb. hemmt das Lynoestrenol die Produktion von Testosteron, Etiocholamon und Androsteron, welche die Funktion der Talgdrüsen steigern. Während der Behandlung verabreichten wir den Patienten vom 1. bis 15. Tag des Menstruationscyclus — dem Oestrogenmangel entsprechend — 40 bis 60 mg Oestrogen und dreimal 400 IU Gestyl intramuskulär. Vom 15. bis 24. Tag des Menstruationscyclus gaben wir täglich eine Tablette Orgametril (5 ml Lynoestrenol) und 1 mg Oestradiol per os. Dieses Behandlungsschema wandten wir je nach der Besserung 3 bis 4 Monate lang an. Im weiteren, vom 5. Tag des Menstruationscyclus an bis zum 15. Tag zweimal 0,5 mg Oestradiol, danach 10 Tage lang eine Tablette Orgametil und 0,5 mg Oestradiol per os. So erreichten wir einen hohen Oestrogenspiegel in der ersten Phase des Menstruationscyclus und dadurch hemmten wir die Wirkung der Androgene. In der zweiten Phase des Menstruationscyclus dagegen hemmten wir mit Lynoestrenol die Produktion der Androgene und Progesterone, gleichzeitig kompensierten wir mit Oestrogenen die Antioestrogenwirkung des Lynoestrenol. Unsere männlichen Patienten bekamen täglich eine Tablette Orgamitril und zweimal 0,5 mg Oestradiol.

Mit obiger Behandlungsmethode gelang es uns, die Hautveränderungen und die vorgefundenen hormonellen Störungen vorteilhaft zu beeinflussen. Trotz der großen Dosis von Oestrogenen kamen in keinem einzigen Fall Blutungsstörungen oder bei den Männern Gynokomastia vor. Unsere Therapieergebnisse können wir wie folgt zusammenfassen:

12 Fälle wurden symptomlos,
21 besserten sich stark,
12 besserten sich mäßig,
 7 besserten sich kaum,
 8 blieben unverändert.

Unsere Ergebnisse hängen von der Quantität der Medikamente ab, weil diejenigen Patienten, welche das meiste Oestrogen und Lyoestrenol erhielten, am schnellsten heilten.

Vorkommen von Paraproteinämie bei Pyoderma gangraenosum

H. RÖCKL, Dermatologische Klinik und Poliklinik der Universität Würzburg (Deutschland)

Das offenbar erstmals 1903 von BOSELLINI (Granuloma herpetiforme ,,exoticum''), im Jahre 1930 von BRUNSTING, GOECKERMAN und O'LEARY unter dem Namen Pyoderma gangraenosum beschriebene, charakteristische Krankheitsbild ist *keine* Pyodermie, das heißt keine Krankheit, die durch Staphylokokken oder Streptokokken hervorgerufen wird. In Anbetracht der noch unbekannten Ätiologie ist es deshalb besser, die Bezeichnung *Dermatitis ulcerosa* (D.u.) (KRESBACH, 1959) zu verwenden. Dies auch deshalb, weil bekanntlich in einem relativ hohen Prozentsatz der Fälle gleichzeitig eine *Colitis ulcerosa* vorkommt (nach Perry und Brunsting in 60%, Röckl in etwa 30 bis 40%).

Tabelle 1. *Befunde bei den bisher bekannten Fällen von Dermatitis ulcerosa mit Paraproteinämie* (Schröpl)

Fall Nr.	Autoren	Jahr	Verhalten der pathologischen Eiweißfraktion bei der elektrophoretischen Untersuchung		Knochenmarkpunktat	Bence-Jones-Protein
			Papier-E.	Immuno-E[a].		
1	Duperrat, Goguel u. Galy	1962	β	γA	o.B.	$\varnothing$
2	Röckl, Knedel und Schröpl	1964	γ^1	γA	o.B.	$\varnothing$
3		1964	β	γA	überwiegend atypische Plasmazellen[b]	+
4		1964	β	γA		$\varnothing$
5		1964	γ_1	γA	geringe Vermehrung von Plasmazellen	$\varnothing$
6	Thivolet, Pellerat, Hermier und Durano	1964	β	γA	90% Plasmazellen	$\varnothing$
7	van der Sluis	1966	β	γA	o.B.	+
8		1966	β	γA	Vermehrung von Plasmazellen	(+)
9	Schröpl	1967	α_2	γA	Vermehrung von Plasmazellen	$\varnothing$

[a] γA = γ_1A = β_2A.
[b] Sektionsbefund: plasmacelluläre Infiltration in Knochenmark, Milz, Leber, Lymphknoten und Niere.

Die Hauterscheinungen der D.u. sind so charakteristisch, daß auf eine Beschreibung hier verzichtet werden kann. Hingewiesen sei lediglich auf die typische wie gestrickt aussehende Narbenbildung nach Abheilung, weil durch sie sehr häufig eine Diagnose noch retrospektiv möglich ist. — Wir wissen heute, daß Antibiotica gleich welcher Art die D.u. nicht beeinflussen können. Dagegen ist eine prompte günstige Beeinflussung nur durch Corticosteroide möglich (Röckl, 1965). Die Histopathologie ist uncharakteristisch. Laboratoriumsuntersuchungen gleich welcher Art haben lange Zeit keine für diese Krankheit spezifischen oder immer wieder zu beobachtenden Befunde erbracht. Auffallend jedoch war, daß gelegentlich eine stark bis extrem beschleunigte BSG besonders erwähnt wurde. Nachdem von mir 1957 erstmals bei einem Fall von D.u. mittels Serum-Eiweißelektrophorese eine zweifache Gamma-Fraktion nachgewiesen wurde, konnte ich — gemeinsam mit Schröpl und Knedel (1964) — bei vier von sechs D.u.-Fällen das Vorliegen einer Gamma-A (β_2A, γ_1A = Synonyma!)-Paraproteinämie nachweisen. Die Bestimmung erfolgte mittels Ultrazentrifuge und Immunoelektrophorese. Diese Befunde konnten inzwischen auch von anderen Autoren bestätigt werden (Tab. 1).

Schon früher wurde über D.u.-Fälle berichtet, bei denen wahrscheinlich eine Paraproteinämie vorlag. Diese wurde allerdings meist nicht genau charakterisiert, bzw. die Befunde wurden fälschlich als Hypo-Gamma-Globulinämie gedeutet (Tab. 2).

Tabelle 2. *Fallbeschreibungen von Dermatitis ulcerosa, bei denen wahrscheinlich eine Paraproteinämie vorlag* (SCHRÖPL)

Autoren	Jahr	Befunde, die für eine Paraproteinämie sprechen
MARCUSSEN	1955	Beta-Globuline 29,2 bis 38,5 rel.-%, Gamma-Globuline vermindert bis fehlend
WRIGHT u. GRECO	1956	Beta-Globulin 23,8 rel.-%, Gamma-Globulinverminderung
BOLTON, HEWITT,		Zwischen β_2 und γ_1 liegende, nicht näher charakterisierte
YEOMAN und WARIN	1959	pathologische Eiweißfraktion
SOLTA	1961	Beta-Globuline 20,2 rel.-%
COWAN	1961	α_2-Globuline 34 rel.-%, Bence-Jones-Protein im Urin, starke vermehrung von Plasmazellen im Knochenmark, röntgenologische Untersuchung o.B.

Bedeutungsvoll erscheint es uns, daß im Sternalmarkpunktat gelegentlich eine Vermehrung von typischen oder auch atypischen Plasmazellen beobachtet werden kann.

Welche ätiopathogenische Bedeutung diese Paraproteinämie, die bislang immer vom Typus der Gamma-A-Paraproteinämie war, hat, kann vorerst nicht gesagt werden. Ein zufälliges Zusammentreffen scheint in Anbetracht des relativ seltenen Vorkommens der Gamma-A-Paraproteinämie nicht wahrscheinlich. Nach MÄRKI und WUHRMANN dürften diese Befunde bei D.u. zur Gruppe der sog. rudimentären Paraproteinämie gehören, bei denen eine Erkrankung des lympho-plasmo-reticulären Systems (noch) nicht faßbar ist. Die Autoren sprechen von einem Frühsymptom eines Plasmocytoms. Diese Auffassung könnte eine Bestätigung erhalten durch einen unserer Fälle, bei dem sich im Laufe der mehrjährigen Beobachtung ein autoptisch gesichertes Plasmocytom entwickelt hatte.

Literatur. COWAN, M. A.: Brit. J. Derm. **73**, 415 (1961). — MÄRKI, H. H., u. F. WUHRMANN: Klin. Wschr. **43**, 85 (1965). — RÖCKL, H.: Fortschritte der praktischen Dermatologie und Venerologie. 5. Band, S. 93. Berlin-Göttingen-Heidelberg: Springer 1965. — RÖCKL, H., M. KNEDEL und F. SCHRÖPL: Hautarzt **15**, 165 (1964). — SCHRÖPL, F.: Arch. klin. exp. Derm. — SLUIS, I. v. D.: Dermatologica (Basel) **132**, 409 (1966). — THIVOLET, I., B. PELLERAT, CL. HERMIER et B. DURANT: Lyon méd. **30**, 107 (1964). — Weitere Literaturangaben finden sich bei H. RÖCKL: Pyodermien. In: Handbuch d. Haut- u. Geschl.-Kr. von J. JADASSOHN, Ergänzungswerk, hrsg. v. MARCHIONINI, A., u. H. GÖTZ, IV, 1 A, p. 79. Berlin-Heidelberg-New York: Springer 1965.

Zur Problematik der Arthropathia psoriatica

F. VLČEK, M. ZBOJANOVA, G. NIEPEL und Z. SITAY, Forschungsinstitut für Rheumakrankheiten in Piešťany (Tschechoslowakei)

Die psoriasische Arthropathie leidet an dem Schicksal derjenigen Krankheiten, die ins Grenzgebiet zweier medizinischer Disziplinen gehören. Die Problematik dieses Krankheitsbildes trat doch besonders in den letzten Jahren hervor, seit die chronisch verlaufenden Rheumaerkrankungen den Charakter einer Sozialkrankheit erworben haben.

Das simultane Auftreten der Psoriasis und der Gelenksveränderungen ist keine genau begrenzte nosologische Einheit, denn die Alteration der Gelenke kann in Form einer progressiven chronischen Polyarthritis, einer typischen Arthropathie, einer Bechterewschen Krankheit oder verschiedener diagnostisch unklarer Deform-polyarthritiden erscheinen.

Im allgemeinen sind die Gelenksveränderungen bei Psoriasis schwerer, und es entstehen relativ frühzeitig sekundäre arthrotische Veränderungen, besonders im Bereiche der zwischenphalangealen Gelenke. Eine typische psoriasische Arthro-pathie beginnt auf den terminalen Phalangen der Hände bzw. der Füße [6].

Das röntgenologische Bild ist in einzelnen Stadien der Krankheit verschieden. Verhältnismäßig oft haben wir atrophische Knochenveränderungen, periartikuläre Exostosen und eine Verkürzung der distalen Phalangealknochen gefunden (Arthritis mutilans [4]).

Unser Bericht stellt ein therapeutisches, nicht kontrolliertes Experiment bei Patienten mit Psoriasis und Gelenkerkrankungen dar, bei denen eine Standardkur in Schwefelthermen (eine isolierte Badetherapie) durchgeführt wurde.

Die Häufigkeit der Psoriasis arthropathica im Verhältnis zur Psoriasis vulgaris wird unterschiedlich beziffert [2, 3]. In unserem Krankengut wurden 2,4% Pso-riatiker mit Gelenksschädigung aufgefunden. Alle — es waren 38 Fälle — wurden im Forschungsinstitut für Rheumakrankheiten während 5 Wochen hospitalisiert und nach der Entlassung in 3- und 6monatigen Zeitabständen rheumatologisch und dermatologisch kontrolliert.

Tab. 1 zeigt die Verteilung der Gelenksveränderungen:

	Zahl	Poly-arthritis chron. progress.	Typische Arthro-pathie	M. Bechterew
Männer	18	10	7	1
Frauen	20	14	6	—
	38	24	13	1

Bei drei Männern wurde noch eine Sacroileitis diagnostiziert. Mit anderen Autoren übereinstimmend sind wir der Ansicht, daß diese Veränderungen der ileo-sakralen Gelenke als besondere Lokalisation der psoriasischen Arthritis zu betrachten sind [5].

Tab. 2 stellt die Altersverteilung der Patienten dar:

	Alter der Patienten	Dauer der Psoriasis	Dauer der Gelenkser-krankung
Männer	51,8 (16—69 J.)	16,4 (1—51 J.)	8,5 (2—21 J.)
Frauen	46,5 (34—69 J.)	14,3 (1—38 J.)	10,7 (1—36 J.)

Es wurde kein Zusammenhang zwischen der Zeit des Auftretens von Psoriasis und Gelenkserkrankungen festgestellt. Bloß bei drei unserer Fälle kam es zur gleichzeitigen Schädigung der Haut und der Gelenke. In einem Drittel unserer Fälle kam es zur gleichzeitigen Verschlechterung der Dermatose und der Gelenksschä-digung.

Von den Laborbefunden waren Latex- und Hellers Test bei zwei Männern und drei Frauen positiv. Die Urikämie wurde bei fünf Männern (6,5 bis 10,3 mg-%) und zwei Frauen (6,5 mg-% und 8,7 mg-%) erhöht.

Bis auf eine 16jährige Patientin wurde in allen Fällen eine Nagelbeteiligung festgestellt, wobei schwere Formen von Psoriasis mehr Veränderungen als die leichteren aufwiesen. Es wurden keine Geschlechtsunterschiede im Sinne der Nagelbeschädigung beobachtet [1].

Tab. 3 zeigt die Ergebnisse der Badekur:

	Wesentliche Verbesserung	Mittlere Verbesserung	Nichtbeein- flußt
Männer	11	6	1
Frauen	9	8	3
Gesamtzahl	20	14	4

Zusammenfassend wurde ein besserer Effekt der Badekur bei weniger fort-geschrittenen Arthritiden mit kleinerer Hautbeteiligung festgestellt.

Diese Arbeit soll zu einer objektiven Wertung der Ergebnisse der Balneo-therapie in Schwefelthermen bei Patienten mit einer psoriasischen Arthropathie, zur Ermittlung der Unterlagen für ein kontrolliertes Experiment und schließlich zur Vereinigung der therapeutischen Verfahren dienen.

Literatur. 1. CALVERT, H. T., M. A. SMITH, and R. S. WELLS: Brit. J. Derm. **75**, 11 (1963). — 2. HOLZEGEL, K., u. CH. MÜLLER: Derm. Wschr. **12**, 324 (1967). — 3. LOMHOLT, G.: Psoriasis, Prevalence course and genetics. A census study on the prevalence of skin diseases on the Faroe Islands. Copenhagen 1963. — 4. LUTZ, W.: Lehrbuch der Haut- und Geschlechtskrank-heiten. Basel-New York: Karger 1957. — 5. ROBECCHI, A., e S. DI VITTORIO: Minerva derm. **4**, 129 (1965). — 6. SITAJ, Z., and G. NIEPEL: Progresívna polyartritída. Bratislava 1963.

Quelques observations sur l'élimination urinaire des cétostéroïdes dans l'acnée féminine

R. DUMITRIU, M. HAISUC, L. REITER, M. HONTARU et A. COSER, Centre Dermato-Vénérologique, Bucarest (Roumanie)

Des observations cliniques ont pu établir l'influence de certaines glandes endocrines dans l'apparition et l'évolution de l'acnée vulgaire, mais le mécanisme physio-pathologique de ces états présente encore bien des inconnues. Etant connue l'action excitante des hormones andronènes sur la sécretion des glandes sébacées, on a été tenté de leur accorder un rôle important parmi les mécanismes en question, mais cette supposition n'a pas été confirmée par les dosages des céto-stéroïdes urinaires qui ont montré des chiffres très différents d'un cas à l'autre. Dans cette situation, on peut se demander si les chiffres globaux normaux, ou même abaissés de ces produits ne pourraient masquer un accroissement des fractions androgéniques isolées des cétostéroïdes urinaires.

Pour élucider ce problème nous avons fractionné par la cromatographie sur la colonne d'oxyde d'aluminium les cétostéroïdes urinaires, en séparant trois fractions (le déhidro-épiandrostérone (DHA) dans la première fraction, l'androstérone (A) et l'éthyocolonolone (E) dans la deuxième et les 11-oxi-stéroïdes (11-oxi) dans la troisième).

Ces dosages ont été pratiqués chez 34 femmes atteintes d'acnée vulgaire et chez dix femmes normales. Les témoins ont montré une élimination urinaire totale des 17-cétostéroïdes variant entre 5,95 et 11,77 mg par jour, avec une moyenne de 9 mg et une déviation standard de (σ) = 2,03, tandis que chez les femmes malades les chiffres variaient entre 5,90 et 17,91 mg par jour, avec une moyenne de 10,51 mg (σ = 2,94). La première et la dernière fraction (DHA et 11-oxi) ont présenté des variations non-significatives: pour le DHA la moyenne étant de 1,40 g par jour (σ = 1,07) chez les malades et de 1,32 mg (σ = 1,16) chez les témoins; pour l'11-oxi, la moyenne a été de 3,09 mg par jour (σ = 1,31) chez les malades et de 2,98 mg par jour (σ = 1,28) chez les témoins. La seule différence que nous avons notée c'est dans l'élimination de la seconde fraction (A + E), qui était de 6,01 mg par jour (σ = 2,38) chez les malades et de 4,69 mg par jour (σ = 1,59) chez les femmes normales. Le rapport entre les cétostéroïdes d'origine ovarienne (A + E) et ceux d'origine surrénale (DHA et 11-oxi) était donc de 1,66 chez les malades et de 1,20 chez les femmes normales. Basés sur ces chiffres, nous pouvons affirmer une certaine augmentation des cétostéroïdes d'origine ovarienne, chez les malades atteintes d'acnée vulgaire.

Parmi nos malades, 20 présentaient une hyperpilosité d'intensité variable, mais sans rapport avec la quantité des androgènes ou avec l'intensité des lésions cutanées. Dans 29 cas, l'acnée s'était installée à la puberté, tandis que dans les cinq autres, l'apparition des lésions coïncidait dans un cas avec une grossesse, dans un cas avec une délivrance anormale (avortement) et dans deux avec la régularisation du cycle menstruel. Les lésions cutanées présentaient des accerbations prémenstruelles et parfois intermenstruelles dans 19 cas. L'examen·cyto-hormonal, pratiqué dans 17 cas montrait une hypofolliculinémie dans 13 cas, une hyperfolliculinémie dans deux cas et une situation normale dans deux. Seulement neuf de nos malades présentaient des troubles cliniques du cycle menstruel. Toutes ces données plaident en faveur d'une influence de la fonctionnalité ovarienne dans l'apparition et les poussées évolutives de l'acnée vulgaire des femmes et des jeunes filles.

L'inconstance des signes cliniques ainsi que la variabilité des chiffres de l'élimination urinaire des cétostéroïdes font penser à une origine primitive hypophysaire avec participation secondaire gonadique et parfois surrénale.

The Seborrhoic Symptom Complex —
The Expression of a Disturbed Intestinal Malutilization of Vitamin B 12 as Proven by Measuring the Radioactivity after Administration of Co 60 Vitamin B 12

W. A. CASPER, St. Vincent's Medical Center and Sea View Hospital, Staten Island, New York (USA)

In the whole dermatological field there is probably no more common condition which involves the whole man and his environment more than what we call Seborrhea.

The disorder may start in utero when maternal hormones are active and produce the vernix caseosa. A defect may result in the birth of a baby with a cradle-cap. In later years a great number of these infants throughout their life manifest varied conditions as heavy dandruff, early alopecia, blepharitis, otitis

externa, submammillary dermatitis, and pruritus ani. To all these skin-eruptions
I would like to apply the term: Seborrhoic Symptom Complex.

The seborrhoic disorders have been attributed to a variety of causes among
which climate, hormonal disorders, race, and stress are most often mentioned.

Another important influence in producing these conditions is diet. Nutritional
defects, particularly those relating to the deficiency of the Vitamin B Complex,
which are all essential constituents of an epidermal enzyme system, have been
described as a causative factor.

Based on the concept that this skin disorder may be due to a defective absorption phenomenon and a faulty carbohydrate metabolism, we have given
initially to more than 100 patients with one or all of these symptoms intramuscular
injections of Vitamin B 12, 1000 mcg for periods of 6 to 8 weeks with the most
gratifying results.

In as much as this disease is manifested by periods of remissions and exacerbations evaluation of this therapy would be difficult. However, from this group
28 patients, male and female, with the clinical picture of Seborrhea were selected
for the study of B 12 absorption by means of urinary excretion of Cobalt 60
Vitamin B 12.

Presently, available data indicate that in normal subjects a major portion of
dietary or orally administered Vitamin B 12 is absorbed in the distal part of the
small intestines.

We excluded therefore from our study conditions which normally interfere
with absorption of Vitamin B 12 such as diverticulosis of the small bowel, sprue,
multiple strictures, blind loop syndrome, pernicious and macrocytic anemias.

While the study with Cobalt 60 B 12 is not a diagnostic test of the mal-ab-
sorption syndrome in itself, it indicates that there is a defect in Vitamin B 12
absorption and in conjunction with our clinical results may serve as conclusive
evidence of the beneficial influence of Vitamin B 12 on the many facets of the
seborrhoic symptom complex.

The normal range of urinary excretion of Cobalt 60 B 12 in the Radioisotope
section of St. Vincent's Hospital is from 7 to 22% of the ingested dose.

The range of urinary excretion of Cobalt 60 B 12 of patients in this study was:

Number of Patients	Range %
19	0—5
4	6—10
5	11—15

None reached the upper level of urinary excretion of Cobalt 60 Vitamin B 12 of 22% or higher which we would usually find in normal non-seborrhoic individuals.

Furthermore, it is known that B 12 absorption in diabetes mellitus is decreased. Our clinical observation confirms the fact that a high carbohydrate diet especially sweets and sucrose in patients with normal fasting bloodsugar values,
may aggravate the seborrhoic skin eruptions.

13 patients were selected for examinations of post-prandial bloodsugar determinations. Nine of these patients were found to have a disturbed carbohydrate
metabolism and would be defined as suffering from "Chemical Diabetes".

There was no definite relationship established between the degree of malabsorption as judged by urinary excretion of tagged B 12 and remission of the skin
eruption. The presence of chemical diabetes had no influence upon the remission of
Seborrhea.

We are usually inclined to associate the therapeutic effect of Vitamin B 12
with B 12 deficiency of Pernicious Anemia. However, more recently, nonspecific
enzymatic function of B 12 in catalizing Thio oxydation was reported. It is quite
possible that this nonspecific oxidation property causes an additional oxidation of

fatty substances resulting in amelioration of the seborrhoic symptom complex, just achieving what the faulty carbohydrate metabolism failed to do.

This concept needs further investigation. However, in view of the remarkable clinical results with injections of Vitamin B 12, nutritional defect and specifically intestinal malabsorption or malutilization has to be strongly considered as an etiological factor of the seborrhoic symptom complex.

Diabetes and Impetigo Contagiosa
(Passage from one Diabetic Family to Another Diabetic Family Via a Related Cousin Carrier)

B. R. HEARST, Microbiology Dept., Loyola University, Stritch School of Medicine, Hines, Illinois (USA)

Passage of impetigo contagiosa from one diabetic family to another, maritally-related, diabetic family through a paternal cousin, was incidentally noted, in the course of therapy for an 11 year old patient, a known diabetic for 2 years with a chronic ulcer of the left foot. On her first visit, Kitty was accompanied by her mother, who had characteristic acnoid lesions, and by her 10 year old paternal cousin, who had visible impetigo contagiosa of his face. Her 9 year old brother, also present, had no visible skin lesions. Nor did her father, who came later to take home his family. Within several weeks, the cousinly impetigo spread to Kitty's brother and father. Though Kitty and her mother were equally exposed, none of these two females contracted the infection.

Kitty's maternal and paternal diabetic history reveals that the women were involved in the metabolic disease. Kitty's maternal grandmother was diagnosed as a diabetic when aged 60 years. This maternal grandmother had six children; three non-diabetic males and three females of which two were diabetic. The third daughter, Kitty's mother, did not have any diabetic history. However, all these six children had recurrent boils, acne and "styes on their eyes", since childhood. Kitty's mother was sixteen years old when she had a staphylococcus osteomyelitis of the right shin bone. Kitty's paternal grandmother was a known diabetic of many years. All her male children never had any diabetic history. These male children did have a history of recurrent boils and acne since childhood. Kitty's paternal cousin and her father (paternal uncle to the paternal cousin) had no diabetic histories. Within the past week, the paternal cousin had come for a summer's to his uncle's family. At that time, he had the impetigo lesions on his face. This disease had originated in the left axilla.

Kitty and her entire family were tested for diabetes during the first office visit. All, except Kitty, were negative. Microbiological studies revealed that all were literally covered with staphylococcus aureus from head to foot. In addition this micro-organism was also recovered from Kitty's chronic ulcer of the foot as well as from her cousin's impetigo (from which streptococci were also obtained).

In the course of several weeks, the impetigo spread from the paternal cousin to the maternal cousin (Kitty's brother) and finally to Kitty's father, who was the target from the maternal cousin (his son) and the paternal cousin (his nephew). Though the son developed a facial lesion, the father's involvement was more extensive; first appearing in the external ear canal, then the left eyebrow and finally the face.

At the time of these observations, the author was studying an extensive animal sample, in order to determine in incidence of S. aureus to coincidental pyodermia. Several thousand cold and warm-blooded animals were tested according to standard procedure but though there was almost 100% S. aureus incidence yet there was a negligible incidence of staphylococcal pyodermia. Indeed, S. aureus was normally found in all animals both in health and in disease. However further study seems necessary to correctly interpret the presence of these micro-organisms. An interesting observation is that though the maternal and paternal women of Kitty's family do have diabetic histories, yet, it is the men and boys who acquire impetigo contagiosa by passage from the paternal diabetic family to the maternal diabetic family via a paternal cousin.

In summary, though the paternal and maternal diabetic familial histories seem to implicate females yet the non-diabetic males are attacked by impetigo contagiosa.

Dermatitis uraemica Rössle

H. Fischer, Univ.-Hautklinik Tübingen (Deutschland)

Hautveränderungen bei Urämiekranken können mechanisch durch Kratzeffekte bedingt sein, toxisch — analog der nekrotisierenden Gastroenterokolitis und der fibrinösen Polyserositis — oder hyperergisch-vaskulitisch auf Grund einer Harnwegsinfektion bzw. einer Drogenallergie bei gleichzeitiger Ausscheidungsinsuffizienz.

Wir haben an der Univ.-Hautklinik Tübingen im Laufe der letzten 10 Jahre 251 Hautkranke behandelt, bei denen der Harnstoffspiegel im Blutserum auf mehr als 60 mg-% erhöht war. Davon litten 69 an ekzematösen Hautaffektionen, 55 wiesen irgendwelche hyperergische Hautreaktionen (einschließlich Urticaria) auf und 50 bakterielle Hautinfektionen einschließlich varicösem Symptomenkomplex.

Von 22 Kranken lag eine Probeexcision vor: Bei zwölf war ein koordiniertes Krankheitsgeschehen an Haut und Nieren anzunehmen, davon bei acht auf Grund eines vasculitischen Geschehens. Vier Kranke wiesen Hyperplasien des reticulohistiocytären Systems auf. Bei dem Rest bestand kein erkennbarer innerer Zusammenhang. Nur bei drei Kranken mit einem Harnstoffspiegel von 63 bis 72 mg-% fanden sich die perivasculären Rundzellinfiltrate, eventuell in Kombination mit fleckigen Ödemen in der oberen Cutis, wie sie Rössle für die urämische Dermatitis als kennzeichnend herausgestellt hat. Eine 65 Jahre alte Kranke mit pyelonephritischer Schrumpfniere und ausgedehnten, kleinpapulösen, zum Teil ulzerierten Erythemen wies darüber hinaus nekrotisierende Epitheldefekte auf mit starker fibrinoider Verquellung am Grund ohne wesentliche entzündliche Begleitreaktion, lediglich mit einer umschriebenen Blutung in der Tiefe. Der Harnstoffspiegel im Serum betrug 120 mg-%, Kreatinin 6,1 mg-%.

Bei den Kranken, bei denen sich die Hautveränderungen als vasculitisch erwiesen, enthielt der Urin regelmäßig auch Erythrocyten. Die folgende Hautexcision stammt von einem 69 Jahre alten Mann mit extrarenaler Niereninsuffizienz und Harnstoffwerten bis 225 mg-%. Bei einem anderen Kranken mit drogenallergischer Vasculitis und Hämaturie ergab die Nierenbiopsie eine Glomerulitis.

Unabhängig davon, ob ein koordiniertes Krankheitsgeschehen vorlag oder innere Zusammenhänge nicht bestanden, waren bei 14 Kranken im histologischen

Präparat mehr oder weniger schwere degenerative Veränderungen an den Schweiß- und Talgdrüsen nachweisbar, wie sie ähnlich auch RössLE und CAWLEY beobachtet haben.

Zusammenfassend wird festgestellt: Die von RössLE beschriebenen urämischen Hautveränderungen bei chronischer Niereninsuffizienz sind auch in unserem Beobachtungsgut die Ausnahme. Weitaus im Vordergrund stehen aufgepfropfte vasculitische Erscheinungsbilder, die meistens mit einer Hämaturie einhergehen. Der hohe Anteil infektiöser und ekzematöser Hautaffektionen im gesamten Beobachtungsgut spricht ebenfalls für die große Bedeutung der Harnwegsinfektion, welche hyperergische Hautreaktionen im Sinne einer superfiziellen Vasculitis bzw. eines hämorrhagischen Mikrobids im Gefolge hat. Möglicherweise besteht ein Zusammenhang mit dem immundepressiven Effekt der Urämie und der Beeinträchtigung des Komplements sowie einer eventuellen Begleitcoagulopathie. Kompensatorisch müßte dann die celluläre Abwehr vermehrt beansprucht werden, ein Vorgang, der auch das relativ häufige Auftreten reticulohistiocytärer Reaktionen in dem vorliegenden Beobachtungsgut erklären würde.

Bullous Dermatoses

Dermatoses bulleuses

Dermatosis con formación de ampollas

Bullöse Dermatosen

Organizer

F. Sagher, Israel

Presidents

J. Gomez Orbaneja, Spain

W. C. Lobitz, USA

D. S. Wilkinson, Great Britain

L. H. Winer, USA

Delegate of the Organization Committee

K. W. Kalkoff, Germany

Reports

Zur Klinik bullöser Eruptionen
(Exklusive bullöse Genodermatosen)

J. Tappeiner, I. Univ.-Hautklinik Wien (Österreich)

Die bullösen Dermatosen im engeren Sinne — Pemphigusgruppe und klinisch
ähnliche Hauteruptionen unbekannter Ätiologie — stehen heute, wie vor
100 Jahren, im Mittelpunkt dermatologischer Diskussion. Die auf Grund klinischer
und histologischer Merkmale getroffene Unterteilung in
  a) die Pemphigusgruppe (P.),
  b) die Dermatitis herpetiformis Duhring (D.h.),
  c) das bullöse Pemphigoid (b.P.) und
  d) das narbenbildende Schleimhautpemphigoid
ist derzeit wohl allgemein anerkannt. Diese nosologische Ordnung wird aber zunehmend durch Einzelbeobachtungen gestört, bei denen das klinische Bild mit dem
histologischen Befund nicht übereinstimmt.

Im Gegensatz zur Auffassung von Lever ist nach unserer Erfahrung im mikroskopischen Präparat die verschiedene Lokalisation des Hohlraumes bei intra-
epithelialen Blasen — suprabasal, subcorneal resp. innerhalb des Stratum granulosum — nicht unbedingt für eine bestimmte P.-Form pathognomonisch. Ferner
kann eine Pathomorphose, d. h. die klinische und histologische Umwandlung
einer P.-Variante in eine andere, (P. vulg. — P. erythematosus) vorkommen.
Zum Beweis seien zwei Fälle angeführt:

40jährige Beamtin aus Griechenland mit den typischen Veränderungen eines P. erythematodes, der seit 3 Jahren besteht und auswärts erfolglos behandelt wurde.
Aufnahmebefund: im Gesicht, am Capillitium und am Stamm, insbesondere an der
vorderen Brustpartie fingernagel- bis kindhandtellergroße, von Schuppenkrusten bedeckte
Areale. Nikolski in der unmittelbaren Umgebung der Herde positiv. Schleimhäute frei. Histol.:
suprabasale akantholytische Blase. Tzanck-Test pos.

Für dieses klinische Bild eines P. erythematodes wäre eine in den oberen
Epidermislagen lokalisierte Blase typisch und nicht wie im vorliegenden Fall eine
suprabasale Blase.

Die zweite Patientin erkrankte im 44. Lebensjahr an einem P. vulg. mit Schleimhautbeteiligung. Neben schwerer Beeinträchtigung des Allgemeinbefindens häufige Fieberattacken
bis zu 40 Grad. Nikolski positiv. Jodkaliprobe negativ. Tzanck-Test positiv. Zwei in Intervallen entnommene Biopsien ergaben suprabasale Blasen. Nach Cortisontherapie rasch einsetzende Besserung. Mit geringer Erhaltungsdosis war Pat. wieder arbeitsfähig, jedoch nie
völlig erscheinungsfrei. Rezidive in Form schlaffer Blasen auf unveränderter Haut konnten
durch zeitweise Erhöhung der Cortisondosen beherrscht werden. 4 Jahre nach Krankheitsbeginn, nach einer Gesamtdosis von 60000 mg Cortison, neuerliche Eruption, vorwiegend an
Brust und Rücken mit etwa fingernagelgroßen, teils konfluierenden, mit gelblichgrauen
Schuppenkrusten bedeckten Plaques ohne vorausgehende wahrnehmbare Blasenbildung.
Nikolski auch in der Nachbarschaft der Krankheitsherde positiv. Histol.: Spaltbildung mit
akantholytischen Zellen nur innerhalb des Stratum granulosum.

Es hatte sich also das klinische Krankheitsbild des P. vulg. mit der suprabasalen Blase in einen klinischen P. erythematosus mit einer im Stratum granulosum lokalisierten Blase umgewandelt. Möglicherweise ist diese Pathomorphose
auf die langdauernde Cortisontherapie zurückzuführen.

Die von einigen Autoren beschriebene Umwandlung subepithelialer in intra-
epitheliale Blasen, also einen histol. Übergang einer D.h. in eine Erkrankung der
P. Gruppe, haben wir niemals feststellen können. Wohl aber wurden in den letzten
Jahren häufiger Erkrankungen beobachtet, bei denen klinisch die Diagnose

D.h. gestellt wurde und die auf Grund des histologischen Befundes der P. Gruppe zuzurechnen sind.

Zwei solcher Fälle seien zur Diskussion gestellt:

43jährige Patientin; Beginn der Erkrankung vor 3 Jahren. Wiederholt traten morphologisch gleichartige, jedoch an Extensität zunehmende Eruptionen in nahezu symmetrischer Anordnung an Stamm und Extremitäten auf. Es bestanden münzen- bis handflächengroße, kreisrunde oder polycyclisch begrenzte erythemato-urticarielle Herde, die verschieden dicht von stecknadelkopf- bis kleinerbsengroßen, überwiegend prallen, zum Teil unregelmäßig gestalteten Bläschen besetzt waren. Vereinzelt auch Bläschen auf nicht veränderter Haut. An Mundschleimhaut und Genitale Erosionen. Bluteosinophilie zwischen 1 bis 7%. Jodkaliprobe negativ. Tzanck-Test positiv. Wiederholte Biopsien zeigten einheitlich eine suprabasale Blase.

Diese Erkrankung, die klinisch seit 3 Jahren unverändert das Bild einer D.h. aufweist, gehört histologisch zum P.v.

Den analogen histologischen Befund einer suprabasalen akantholytischen Blase mit positivem Tzanck-Test fanden wir in einer Blase vom Unterbauch eines 43jährigen Patienten, bei dem seit einem Jahr an Stamm und Extremitäten eine rezidivierende Aussaat papulokrustöser Efflorescenzen mit einzelnen intakten kleinerbsengroßen Bläschen besteht. Pat. ist Epileptiker und nimmt Hydantoinpräparate.

Unserer Meinung nach sind es solche Beobachtungen wie die eben geschilderten, die wiederholt in der Literatur als Beweis angeführt werden, daß ihre klinische Interpretation nicht in das derzeit gültige Konzept paßt.

Häufigen Anlaß zu diagnostischen Unklarheiten geben bullöse Erkrankungen, die ausschließlich — oder fast ausschließlich — die Schleimhäute befallen, da der P.v. der Schleimhaut und das narbenbildende Schleimhautpemphigoid anfänglich klinisch identische Erscheinungen aufweisen.

Zwei Beobachtungen eines histologisch verifizierten P.v. mucosae, bei dem jahrelang nur die Lippen- und Mundschleimhaut ergriffen waren, seien erwähnt.

34jährige Patientin mit seit 2 Jahren bestehenden schmerzhaften Erosionen der Zunge, der Lippen-, Wangen-, Gaumen- und Pharynxschleimhaut. Haut frei. Tzanck-Test positiv. Histol. aus der Unterlippenschleimhaut: suprabasale Epidermisabhebung mit akantholytischen Zellen. Auch sehr hoch dosierte Cortisontherapie über Monate ohne wesentlichen Erfolg. Nach Reduzierung der Cortisondosis plötzliche Aussaat erythemato-urticarieller bullöser Herde. Pat. hatte vorher Barbitursäurepräparate genommen.
Histologisch: suprabasale akantholytische Blase. Interkurrent Auftreten eines trotz Antibiotica schwer verlaufenden Erysipels. Daraufhin, sowie unter hohen Cortisondosen. rascher Rückgang der Haut- und Schleimhautveränderungen.
60jähriger Landwirt mit gleichartigen Schleimhautveränderungen und analogem histol. Befund. Erst 3 Jahre nach Beginn der Erkrankung traten vereinzelt schlaffe Blasen im Nabelbereich auf.

Auch die Definition des b.P. bietet Schwierigkeiten. Wir verstehen darunter eine blasige Eruption unbekannter Ätiologie von chronischem Verlauf, die von der P.-Gruppe histologisch, von der D.h. klinisch abgegrenzt werden kann. Allerdings ist die Unterscheidung gegenüber der D.h. oft schwierig, da sich das klinische Bild im Verlaufe der Erkrankung ändern kann:

Bei dem 66jährigen Pensionisten traten seit einigen Monaten wiederholte Schübe von prallen und schlaffen Blasen überwiegend auf normaler Haut auf. Schleimhäute frei. Jodkaliprobe negativ. Tzanck-Test negativ. Histol.: subepitheliale Blase. Es wurde die Diagnose eines Alterspemphigoids gestellt. Die anfänglich versuchte Sulfontherapie war wirkungslos. Die Cortisonbehandlung brachte fast völlige Abheilung. Nach Reduktion der Dosis Auftreten eines generalisierten erythemato-urticariellen Exanthems mit einzelnen Blasen, die ein positives Nikolski-Phänomen zeigten. In Unkenntnis der Vorgeschichte wäre dieser Ausbruch als D.h. gedeutet worden.

Beim Schleimhautpemphigoid, das mitunter auch mit vereinzelter Blasenbildung des Integumentes vergesellschaftet ist, kommt die Narbenbildung oft erst nach Monaten zustande. Es ist daher im Anfangsstadium der Erkrankung die Diagnose nur auf Grund des histologischen Befundes möglich.

Herpes Zoster and Nonmalignant Disease

L. H. WINER and E. T. WRIGHT, Dermatology Section, Medical Service,
Wadsworth Hospital, Veterans Administration Center, Los Angeles, and
Department of Medicine, Division of Dermatology, UCLA School of Medicine,
Los Angeles, California (USA), Dermatologic Research Foundation of
California, Inc.

In a previous paper the authors studied the association of herpes zoster and
malignancy as it occurred during a 5-year period in a 1500-bed Veterans Administration General Medical and Surgical Hospital [1]. The primary purpose was to
determine the incidence of zoster in all types of malignancy. The study encompass-
ed the years 1954 to 1958 inclusive. During this period there were 55,279 hospital
admissions; 147 (0.26%) of these had zoster. 34 of the 147 patients had an associated malignancy and in the remaining 113, no associated malignancy was found.

In the present study we have reviewed the records of 48 of the 113 patients
who had zoster not associated with malignancy. The records of 65 of the 113
patients were unavailable for study. It was our purpose to determine if zoster was
associated with any particular disease or diseases belonging to a particular system.
In addition to the associated diseases, the following data were recorded: age (at
time of onset of zoster), sex, duration of the zoster, location of the zoster skin
lesions, and the cause of death (if death occurred in the hospital or at a later date
if this information was available). The associated diseases were classified into seven
categories; cardiovascular, urinary, gastrointestinal, pulmonary, skin, central
nervous system, and genital.

The results are summarized in Tabs. 1 to 5, Tab. 1 presents the age distribution.
Age groups were divided into 21 to 40, 41 to 50, 51 to 60, 61 to 70, 71 to 80, and
81 to plus. The largest number of patients were in the 61 to 70 year age group.
In addition, five patients were in the 71 to 80 year age group, and five patients
were in the 81—plus age group. Since the mean age for the total of 48 patients
was 49 years, and considering the relatively smaller percentage of population in
the age groups of 71 to 80 and 81—plus, it can be seen that zoster is a disease
of older people.

Table 1. *Age Distribution*

Age Group	21—40	41—50	51—60	61—70	71—80	81+
No. of Pts.	7	8	9	14	5	5
Mean Age	49					

Tab. 2 summarizes the number of patients and number of associated systems
involved. Six patients had no associ-
ated disease. The mean age of this
group was 41 years, which is less than
the mean age for the total of 48 patients, or 49 years. The largest number of patients had only one associated
system involvement, but as the mean
age increased so did the number of
associated system involvements. There were six patients with three or more associated systems involved and the mean age for this group was 77 years.

Table 2. *Systems Involvement*

No. of Systems	None	One	Two	Three or more
No. of Patients	6	24	11	6
Mean Age	41	57	62	77

Tab. 3 records the frequency of associated systems involved. The reader will
note that there were 20 patients who had some type of cardiovascular disease, or

42% of the total; 15 patients who had some type of urinary tract disease, or 31% of the total, etc. This table demonstrates that the most frequently associated diseases were those belonging to the cardiovascular, urinary, and gastrointestinal systems. Several patients had more than one system involved as noted in Tab. 2; hence in Tab. 3 the number of patients totals more than 48 and the total of the individual percentages listed is greater than 100.

Table 3. *Frequency of Systems Involved*

	CV	URY	GI	PUL	Skin	CNS	Genital
No. of Pts.	20	15	15	7	5	5	2
Percent of total No. Pts.	42	31	31	14.6	10.4	10.4	4

Table 4. *Systems Involvement in Order of Frequency*

System(s)	No. Pts.	System (s)	No. Pts.
Cardiovascular	7	Genital	1
Urinary	6	GI-Pulmonary	1
GI	4	GI-CNS	1
CV-URY	3	GI-Skin	1
Pulmonary	2	CV-Pulmonary	1
CNS	2	CV-GI	1
Skin	2	CV-GI-URY	1
CV-CNS	2	CV-PUL-Genital	1
GI-URY	2	CV-PUL-GI-URY	1
CV-GI-URY	2	CV-GI-URY-Skin	1
		None	6

Tab. 4 records the systems involved in order of frequency and the number of patients studied. Thus there were seven patients with associated disease of the urinary system; four patients with associated disease of the gastrointestinal system; three patients with combined associated diseases of the cardiovascular-urinary systems, the cardiovascular-central nervous system and the gastrointestinal-urinary systems; two patients each with associated disease of the pulmonary system only, the central nervous system only, and the skin only. Six patients had no associated disease, one patient had an associated disease of the genital system, and nine patients each had a variety of one-only to four-combined associated systems diseases.

Table 5. *Age Category Percentages*

	Age in Years		
	up to 45	45 to 64	65 and up
Herpes zoster unassociated with malignancy	% 21	% 52	% 27
CV Disease	16	47	37
GU Disease	21	41	38

Tab. 5 shows the number of patients by percentage in the various age categories. The groups include patients with herpes zoster (unassociated with malignancy), patients with cardiovascular disease and patients with genitourinary disease in the total hospital population for the 5 year period included in the study. It will be noted that herpes zoster, cardiovascular diseases, and genitourinary diseases were not common under the age of 45. The diagnosis of herpes zoster unassociated with malignancy was made most frequently between the ages of 45 to 64. This was also true for diseases of the cardiovascular and genitourinary systems. After the age of 65, the diagnosis of herpes zoster was made much less frequently, however this was not true for diseases of the cardiovascular and genitourinary systems.

The most common disease noted involving the cardiovascular system was arteriosclerotic heart disease. This accounted for almost half of the 20 patients. The remaining diseases in order of frequency were hypertensive heart disease, rheumatic heart disease, cor pulmonale, and single cases of pericarditis, luetic aortitis, angina pectoris and myocardial infarction.

Disorders of the prostate were the most commonly noted diseases of the genitourinary system. Benign prostatic hypertrophy was found in seven patients, prostatic adenoma in one and prostatitis in one. The next most common disorder was pyelonephritis, being noted in three patients, followed by isolated examples of nephrocalcinosis, urethritis, epididymitis, ureteral calculi, and spermatocele.

Duodenal ulcer was the most common disorder of the gastrointestinal system and accounted for one-third of the 15 patients. This was followed in order of frequency by cirrhosis of the liver, pancreatitis and single cases of cholecystitis, diverticulitis, and esophageal hiatus hernia.

Emphysema was the most common disorder involving the pulmonary system. Six of the seven patients had emphysema and three of the six had an associated pneumonia. The seventh patient had pulmonary tuberculosis.

Disorders of the skin were relatively simple and included the following: dermatophytosis, carbuncle, pruritus ani, and discoid lupus erythematosus.

The same was true for disorders of the central nervous system. Although the presence of neuralgia due to herpes zoster is well known [3], no other neurological diseases occurred predominately. Diseases noted were multiple sclerosis, encephalomalacia with hemiparesis and asymptomatic neurosyphilis.

Discussion

The number of patients obtained for this study is too small from which to derive statistical significance, but the data seems to give some meaningful information. Examination of Tabs. 3 and 4 would seem to indicate that herpes zoster was commonly associated with diseases of the cardiovascular and genitourinary systems. However examination of Tab. 5 demonstrates that this merely reflects prevalence of these diseases in this general hospital population.

In this study herpes zoster was a disease of the middle and older age groups but not of the extremes of age; i.e., the very young and the very old. This was in marked contrast to our previous findings of herpes zoster associated with malignancy in which the average age of patients with zoster associated with various types of carcinoma was 69. A striking exception was the average age of zoster associated with Hodgkins disease; i.e., 30.

The present study deals with a selected group with respect to age and sex. Of the 48 patients, only one was a female and none was under the age of 20 years. During the period of time of this study (1954 to 1958 inclusive) females accounted for only 0.03% of hospital discharges; thus the present data does not include children or young people and is restricted to an almost all male population. Due to these restrictions, definite statements cannot be made. After comparing the information of our previous study and the present one, it would seem useful to consider the possibility of an associated malignancy in an elderly male patient whenever a diagnosis of herpes zoster is made. The exception to this is the young age group of patients with zoster and Hodgkins disease. In this situation the presence of zoster was primarily a poor prognostic sign with respect to longevity.

Our findings with respect to severity, duration, and results of treatment will not be discussed since they in no way differ from other published papers on herpes zoster. In no instance was zoster a cause of death nor did it appear to contribute to the cause of death. The onset of zoster in patients with nonmalignant disease was not an unfavorable sign. This is in contrast to the findings reported with regard to the appearance of zoster in patients with internal malignancy.

Bibliography. 1. WRIGHT, E. T., and L. H. WINER: Arch. Derm. **84**, 242 (1961). — 2. Annual Classification of Discharges — 1959, Veterans Administration Center, GMHS Hospital, Medical Record Library Service, August 1960. — 3. BLANK, H., and G. RAKE: Viral and Rickettsial Diseases of the Skin, Eye and Mucous Membranes of Man, Boston: Little Brown & Co 1955.

Producción experimental de ampollas; su correlacción con los cambios estructurales en las dermatosis ampollosas

D. J. GÓMEZ ORBANEJA, Hospital Clinico de la Facultad de Medicina, Madrid (España)

En las enfermedades con manifestaciones ampollosas la estructura histológica nos permite establecer diferencias, haciendo posible su separación cuando la clínica no aporta datos suficientes para ello. Esas diferencias estructurales de la lesión ampollosa nos dice además que el mecanismo de su producción es distinto en cada una de ellas. Según el sitio en que tiene lugar la acumulación del líquido, serán diferentes los elementos que se alteran y que de manera normal mantienen unidos y resistentes a su separación, los componentes de las capas de la piel, epidermis y dermis. Por eso el lugar en que se rompe esa conexión normal, supone una alteración patológica de una cierta calidad.

Habria una relación entre morfología alterada y función modificada. Conocida una podría deducirse la otra, lo que podría permitir actuar sobre el mecanismo alterado y constituir al tratamiento del proceso morboso.

Así la morfología patológica, microscópica, de la ampolla, diferente en los distintos procesos morbosos, lleva a su diagnóstico bien definido en muchos casos. En el pénfigo, un fenómeno de acantolisis, separación de unas células epidérmicas de otras, nos dice que, pese a las semejanzas clínicas que puedan tener, es muy distinto de la separación dermo-epidérmica del Duhring y del Penfigoide. Por otra parte cabe establecer diferencias entre estos y la ampolla del eritema exudativo multiforme, o entre este y la Necrolisis epidérmica tóxica de Lyell. Añádase la diferente estructura, bien definida de las ampollas de la Epidermolisis congenita ampollosa, en sus formas simples y distrofica. Y ténganse en cuenta, tambien, las ampollas y sus diferencias, en las manifestaciones con ese caracter, del eczema, o de la urticaria; el eczema ampolloso o la urticaria ampollosa.

Así sirvan como ejemplos estos que expresamos a continuación de nuestra experiencia:

La acantolisis masiva, separación de casi la totalidad de unas células de otras, en el pénfigo vulgar, con sus alteraciones celulares; el aspecto "degenerativo" de las células acantolíticas del pénfigo foliáceo, con alteraciones nucleares y la presencia de "granos" de DARIER, incluso en la capa córnea, o la afectación más limitada a la zona inferior del cuerpo de malpigio en el pénfigo vegetante, sin que estas alteraciones repercutan sensiblemente sobre las capas superiores. Habría sin duda diferencias estructurales en los diferentes tipos de pénfigo.

Bien definida es la estructura de la ampolla del Duhring, con sus infiltrados papilares, la presencia de una necrosis papilar, y el despegamiento de la epidermis, sin alteraciones de la dermis en el Penfigoide, lo que explica el mayor tamaño de la ampolla, por lo común.En cambio en el Eritema exudativo multiforme, la epidermis desplazada presenta una necrosis de las capas profundas de la misma (como el fuego que avanza en el bosque). Cuadros clínicos bien definidos, o al menos distintos, presentan alteraciones estructurales distintas.

Mencionemos por último, para completar los ejemplos, la alteración necrótica (en las fases precoces del proceso) de las capas superiores del cuerpo mucoso de malpigio, por debajo de la capa granulosa, en la Necrolisis epidermica tóxica y la acantolisis con sus células malpigianas apenas alteradas, en el Pénfigo benigno familiar; otras veces son células bien conservadas con nucleos mostruosos.

Parecería evidente que a cada cuadro histológico (consiguientemente clínico), correspondiera un mecanismo distinto. Sería el conocimiento de esos mecanismos lo que nos podría aclarar su patogenia. Como esos mecanismos no son bien conocidos, debemos recurrir para ponerlos en evidencia a la acción de distintas substancias, de conocida composición, que determinasen alteraciones iguales o similares, es decir la provocación experimental de las distintas modalidades estructurales de las ampollas. Algunas substancias nos son ya conocidas, aunque su acción ampollosa se ha considerado en conjunto: por ejemplo, la cantaridina, el calor, la cisteina, las soluciones con Ph extremos, el bromuro de litio, etc.

En la provocación experimental de las ampollas, con distintos agentes físicos y químicos, hemos encontrado alteraciones que pueden compararse o identificarse, con las que observamos en la patología.

Así la cantaridina determina una acantolisis, con separación de las células epidérmicas, que aparecen alteradas como en el Pénfigo, en contraste con lo que sucede en la acción del borato sódico en que las células acantolíticas aisladas unas de otras, mantienen su estructura poligonal (como si fuera simplemente una afectación de la substancia cementante similar a la visto en el Pénfigo benigno familiar).

La acción del Clh., parece determinar una alteración del citoplasma, conservándose las membranas celulares y los nucleos algun tiempo, situación similar a la producida por acción de agente virasicos, o a la forma ampollosa de la eritrodermia ictiosiforme congenita. Por el calor, es el despegamiento dermoepidermico el fundamental, con alteración de las células de la capa basal, proximas (semejanza con el Duhring). En la acción de la Cisteina, seria la lesion preferente una necrosis de la zona superior del cuerpo de malpigio, por debajo de la capa granulosa, como lo hemos visto en nuestros casos de necrolisis epidermica tóxica de Lyell, en su fase precoz.

Semejanzas que nos dicen que los mecanismos son distintos, y que ampliando nuestro conocimiento y analizando el modo de acción de los distintos agentes sobre las funciones cutaneas que mantienen la estructura normal, podamos precisar cual es funcionalmente lo alterado. En este sentido continuamos nuestros estudios de relacionar en el campo experimental, las alteraciones morfológicas similares a las clínicas, con la acción de substancias de composición conocida, que actúan sobre mecanismos biológicos solo hasta ahora parcialmente aclarados.

La maladie de Duhring-Brocq à grosses bulles dite «pemphigoïde de Brocq», après la cinquantaine

P. le Coulant, L. Texier et P. Boraud, Clinique Dermatologique del'Université Bordeaux (France)

La maladie de Duhring-Brocq semble avoir changé d'aspect et son pronostic s'être aggravé dans ces vingt dernières années. On dit et on a écrit que la forme à petites bulles décrite par Duhring (variété herpétiforme) est plus rare alors que la variété à grosses bulles que Brocq avait déjà dénommée «pemphigoïde» est plus habituelle après la cinquantaine. Enfin, certains voient dans l'apparition de ce syndrome éruptif l'annonce d'une manifestation néoplasique viscérale. Pour avoir une idée personnelle sur la justification de ces faits, nous avons consulté le dossier des maladies de Duhring-Brocq observées dans le service de la Clinique Dermatologique de Bordeaux, ces 12 dernières années. Dans cette étude, volontairement succinte, nous conserverons la classification clinique de Brocq, qui semple correspondre parfaitement à l'observation des faits:

1. Variété à grosses bulles pemphigoïdes (Brocq),
2. Variété polymorphe,
3. Variété herpétiforme (Duhring).

Etude numérique

En 12 ans, nous avons observé des maladies de Duhring-Brocq, qui suivant le sexe, se répartissent ainsi: 58,5% de femmes, 42,5% d'hommes. 80,4% des cas apparurent après 50 ans, 51,2% apparurent après 70 ans. Sur 41 cas, nous avons observé:

a) 14 formes à grosses bulles   (34,1%)   { 9 après 70 ans, / 0 avant 50 ans.

b) 21 variétés polymorphes   (51,2%)   { 8 après 70 ans, / 7 entre 50 et 70 ans, / 6 avant 50 ans.

c) 6 dermatites herpétiformes (14,5%)   { 4 après 70 ans, / 2 avant 50 ans.

Ces chiffres montrent clairement que la «pemphigoïde» survient surtout chez le sujet âgé, à partir de 50 ans, avec la même fréquence d'ailleurs que la variété polymorphe.

Pronostic

41 dossiers comportent: 8 décès rapides après une seule poussée évolutive, dont 7 après 70 ans et 1 entre 50 et 70 (une forme polymorphe) 3 décès sur 14 pemphigoïdes, 5 décès sur 15 polymorphes.

Il apparaît donc que la forme bulleuse (pemphigoïde) n'est pas de pronostic plus grave que la variété polymorphe. Après 70 ans, le pronostic de maladie de Duhring-Brocq doit donc être très réservé puisque nous avons noté dans les deux variétés (pemphigoïde et polymorphe) sept décès sur 17 cas, soit 41,1%, alors qu'avant 70 ans, nous n'avions avec ces mêmes variétés qu'un décès sur douze cas, soit 8,3%. La variété herpétiforme qui est nettement moins fréquente est aussi d'un pronostic moins sévère. Nous n'avons pas constaté de décès parmi les porteurs de cette variété, même après 70 ans.

La maladie de Duhring-Brocq. Syndrome paranéoplasique

Sur les 41 malades qui font l'object de cette étude, trois qui avaient dépassé 70 ans et présentaient la forme pemphigoïde étaient très probablement atteints de *néoplasie viscérale.*

1. Moelena isolé chez un cachectique décédé, sans possibilité de vérification anatomique.

2. Lésions vertébrales radiologiques de type métastasique, décès rapide.

3. Masse pulmonaire refoulant le diaphragme, découverte à l'examen radiologique. Malade perdu de vue. Deux malades (soit 4,8%) étaient atteints de néoplasmes vérifiés.

a) Chorio-épithéliome chez une femme de 24 ans, atteinte de variété polymorphe. b) Cancer de la vessie chez une femme de 70 ans, atteinte de variété polymorphe et morte des suites de l'intervention.

Clinique

Il ne semble pas qu'on puisse ajouter quoi que ce soit à la description magistrale que Brocq avait brossée, il y a 60 ans, de cette forme pemphigoïde. Lever a voulu en faire une forme voisine du pemphigus, en raison de son pronostic plus grave, peut-être de son apparition en peau saine, dans quelques cas. Le signe de Nikolsky est parfois positif au voisinage des lésions. Mais cette forme se différencie du pemphigus par l'absence d'acantholyse et c'est pour nous un signe différentiel majeur. On ne saurait revenir sur cette question, ailleurs fort bien étudiée.

Notre statistique, peu importante sans doute, montre cependant que la forme pemphigoïde n'est pas plus grave que la variété polymorphe chez le vieillard.

Histologie

Nous n'avons pu pratiquer que 26 vérifications histologiques sur les 41 cas étudiés. Si la clinique peut entraîner un doute sur l'unicité de la maladie de Duhring-Brocq, devant ces trois tableaux différents, l'histologie nous permet de rétablir l'unité, et de n'en faire que des variétés éruptives d'une même maladie. C'est en effet grâce aux travaux de A. Civatte, qui fournirent un critère histologique, que l'on a pu distinguer les différentes affections bulleuses entre elles, et particulièrement les pemphigus caractérisés par la bulle acantholytique. Par la suite, Dupont, Pierard et Fontaine, puis J. Civatte montrèrent les différentes images permettant de diagnostiquer la maladie de Duhring-Brocq.

Commentaires et conclusions

41 cas, bien sûr, n'est pas un chiffre qui permette des conclusions définitives, mais ce chiffre permet peut-être de résumer ce que l'observation soigneuse de ces malades a pu évoquer:

1. Il n'est pas douteux que la maladie de Duhring-Brocq correspond à un ensemble histologique toujours semblable à lui-même et une allure clinique où trois variétés éruptives se juxtaposent:

a) la variété herpétiforme: rare chez les gens âgés;

b) la variété polymorphe;

c) la variété pemphigoïde habituelle chez les gens ayant dépassé la cinquantaine, numériquement égale, d'un pronostic aussi sérieux qu'il s'agisse de l'une ou l'autre de ces deux variétés.

Nous ne suivrons pas Lever qui voudrait faire de la pemphigoïde une forme bâtarde du pemphigus chronique. Histologiquement, c'est une maladie de Duhring-Brocq; cliniquement, elle peut être bénigne ou grave, mais pas plus inquiétante que la variété polymorphe.

2. Quant à la nature paranéoplasique de cette affection, conception soutenue par de nombreux auteurs, il semble bien que cette notion mérite d'être retenue. Car chez les 41 malades de notre statistique, nous comptons 4,8% de néoplasmes vérifiés, sans tenir compte des présomptions, ce qui porterait ce chiffre à plus de 8%. Ces chiffres parlent et n'exigent aucun commentaire.

Subcorneal Pustular Dermatosis
A review after 10 years

D. S. WILKINSON, Whitecroft, Amersham (Great Britain)

In 1956 SNEDDON and I [10] described seven cases of a pustular dermatosis with features that seemed to us to be characteristic and different from those seen in other pustular diseases. We little realized at the time how much interest and controversy would be arroused by this uncommon and rather unimportant disease. In 1962 I [13] was able to find references to 54 further cases of which only fulfilled exactly the original criteria — notably those described by BOLGAERT [1], DUPERRAT [3], GRACIANSKY [4], STEVANOVIC [11], and SUURMOND [12]. Other cases had atypical features, for instance those of DOGLIOTTI [2], and SAR-KANY [9], but were acceptable if the borders of the disease were somewhat widened. Others were very different from the original cases.

Now that nearly 100 cases have been described through the world it is pertinent to ask three questions: does the disease still exist as an entity? what limits may be set to its variations? with what conditions is it most likely to be confused?

In describing this condition SNEDDON and I merely wished to separate off from the difficult and confused group of indeterminate pustuloses a particular variety in which a subcorneal unilocular pustule was associated with an eruption of rather large flaccid pustules rapidly rupturing to form circinate and arcuate erythematosquamous lesions which extended irregularly, leaving normal or slightly pigmented skin in the centre. We did not imply that all pustular eruptions which at any one time might show a subcorneal histology or a peripherally extending pattern were examples of this disease. But the diagnosis had sometimes been made on that basis. The conformity of the disease must, therefore, be stressed; isolated pustules rupturing to form circinate erythematosquamous lesions and then resolution; reiteration of this pattern over a long period; absence of marked constitutional upset; little or no itching. Of the patients originally described none have died of the disease and in none has the pattern changed into that of typical dermatitis herpetiformis, psoriasis or pemphigus. A close personal observation of a later patient enabled me to study the earlier histological features: congestion of the upper dermal vessels with neutrophil polymorphs, rapid migration of these through the epidermis to the subcorneal position, and the formation of a purely subcorneal pustule. I have not seen a Munro microabscess in any typical case and the epidermis itself is remarkably unaffected by this explosive invasion. Though acantholysis has been notably absent and would always arouse suspicion I see no reason why a few cells should not show this change, as in impetigo.

These features and their persistence in this pattern over a very long period confirm us in the belief that whatever its nature, this pustular dermatosis should be retained, for the present at least, as an entity [5].

It is only to be expected that the first delineation of a disease should be redrawn in the light of further cases. But the cardinal features must be present.

To those cases reported may be added another 18, the details of which have kindly been supplied to me by colleagues in the U.K. and elsewhere. I have seen several of these personally. The same difficulties have occurred as in the published material. In some the histological features are atypical, in others the pustules are pin-point or the erythematosquamous phase diffuse and sheet-like. In a few there were features of psoriasis or marked constitutional symptoms. These are, I think, inadmissable. In striking contrast are those patients in whom both the lesions and the histology are typical and remain so. The response to dapsone or to sulpha-pyridine appears to have some diagnostic value, typical cases responding more readily than those with atypical features.

Three diseases must especially be mentioned in the differential diagnosis; dermatitis herpetiformis, pemphigus foliaceus and pustular psoriasis. Impetigo herpetiformis is a far more severe disease with clinical and histological [6, 7] features that distinguish it. The distinction from dermatitis herpetiformis has been much discussed [5, 10, 13]. The arguments against the identity of the two diseases are, I think, more valid than those in favour. Pemphigus foliaceus can be a cause of difficulty, especially in the early stages. Sheet-like involvement of the skin, lack of a clear circinate margin and of central clearing, persistent scaling and the histology sooner or later confirm the diagnosis. Psoriasis is, I think, the disease most likely to be confused. But here also the pustules are smaller and less flaccid than in S.P.D.: other stigmata of psoriasis may be present or appear in time and there is no response to dapsone. The histology, especially if examined serially, shows other changes, notably small microabscesses or a multilocular "spongiform" pustule [6, 7].

Whenever doubt exists repeated biopsies must be undertaken and examined most carefully. The patient may have to be observed on several occasions before a decision is reached.

Whatever the relation of this syndrome to other pustular diseases, this extra-ordinary rapid subcorneal accumulation of neutrophil polymorphs presents an obvious model for the further study of this phenomenon. Immunoelectrophoretic [8] und similar investigation on future patients may throw some light on the mechanism by which this cell is attracted to the epidermis in the amicrobial pustuloses.

References. 1. BOLGAERT, M.: Bull. Soc. franç. Derm. Syph. **64**, 695 (1957). — 2. DOGLIOTTI, M.: Minerva derm. **33**, 73 (1958). — 3. DUPERRAT, B.: Ann. Derm. Syph. (Paris) **84**, 574 (1957). — 4. GRACIANSKY, P. DE.: Bull. Soc. franç. Derm. Syph. **67**, 434 (1960). — 5. GRACIANSKY, P., et S. BOULE: Presse méd. **71**, 779 (1963). — 6. KOGOJ, M. F.: Bull. Soc. franç. Derm. Syph. **69**, 661 (1962). — 7. LAPIERE, M. S.: Bull. Soc. franç. Derm. Syph. **69**, 670 (1962). — 8. PETERSON, jr., W. C.: Acta derm.-venereol. (Stockh.) **45**, 203 (1965). — 9. SARKANY, I.: Brit. J. Derm. **70**, 307 (1958). — 10. SNEDDON, I. B., and D. S. WILKINSON: Brit. J. Derm. **68**, 385 (1956). — 11. STEVANOVIC, D. V.: Dermatologica (Basel) **119**, 223 (1959). — 12. SUURMOND, D.: Dermatologica (Basel) **116**, 114 (1958). — 13. WILKINSON, D. S.: Bull. Soc. franç. Derm. Syph. **69**, 674 (1962).

Bullous Lesions in Patients with Internal Disorders

E. SKOG, Karolinska Sjukhuset, Dermatologiska Kliniken, Stockholm (Sweden)

Bullous lesions of the skin and mucous membranes may coexist with a number of widely differing internal disorders. No common denominator for these disorders is demonstrable in the light of present knowledge. The bullous lesions thus may accompany malignant diseases of a variety of organs, neurologic conditions [23, 28] of many types, disorders of the liver and intestines and endocrinologic disturbances (Tab. 1).

Table 1. *Internal Disorders sometimes Associated with Bullous Lesions of the Skin*

Malignant neoplasms	
Liver disorders	hepatic porphyria
Neurologic disorders	prefrontal leucotomy, subdural haematoma, spinal cord lesions, Parkinsonian encephalitis, carbon monoxide poisoning, tumours
Gastrointestinal disorders ?	acrodermatitis enteropathica
Endocrine disorders ?	impetigo herpetiformis, herpes gestationis

The connexion between an internal disorder and bullous lesions of the skin is often obscure. In some cases an association can only be assumed, for example that in acrodermatitis enteropathica the primary factor is an intestinal disease or that a parathyroid disturbance causes impetigo herpetiformis.

The ideal proof of a causal connexion is of course that healing of the internal disorder is accompanied by healing of the bullous lesions which flare up again if the internal disease recurs. Radical removal of malignant tumours has been followed by disappearance — very rapid in some cases [36] — of coexistent cutaneous bullae, which reappeared when metastases subsequently developed. Proof of this kind is only seldom obtainable, however, since many of the internal disorders, notably malignant tumours, are steadily progressive. In such cases it may be extremely difficult to exclude the possibility of an independent coexistent bullous dermatosis such as dermatitis herpetiformis or a bullous erythema multiforme evoked by drugs.

Why the skin should react with formation of bullae in certain internal disorders has been a subject of considerable speculation. As early as 1925 ROTHMAN [29] suggested two possible causal mechanisms when the underlying disease was neoplastic. The first was that tumour cells reach the skin and are destroyed there, thus producing a reaction corresponding to that underlying the formation of tuberculids and mycids. According to the second theory, toxic substances which form in the tumour have special affinity for the skin and give rise to the bullae. More than 40 years after ROTHMAN's report, no better explanation is available, and no proof has been obtained of one or the other of the causal mechanisms. Experiments have been published [2] in which tumour cells were traced to the skin, where they were destroyed and then gave rise to capillary dilatation and lymphocytic infiltration. In one case an extract was prepared from the tumour and was intracutaneously injected into the same patient, but no reaction followed [36].

Own observations

The relationship between internal disorders and the cutaneous symptoms may be exemplified by 15 cases of concomitant malignant disease and bullous lesions of the skin. These cases were seen at the Department of Dermatology at Karolinska sjukhuset, Stockholm, during the past 15 years (Tab. 2). The malignant conditions affected many organs. The appearance of the cutaneous lesions resembled in most cases dermatitis herpetiformis or bullous pemphigoid, and less often erythema multiforme.

In five cases the skin lesions appeared less than 1 month after the malignant disease was diagnosed: In two of these cases the skin lesions actually preceded the tumour symptoms. The other patients had had a malignant disease for varying periods before the bullae appeared. In five cases the skin lesions occurred late in the course of the neoplastic disease — 2 to 8 months before death.

Table 2. *15 Cases of Malignant Internal Disease Associated with Bullous Skin Lesions*

Malignancy	No. of cases ♂	♀	Age range (years)	Clinical Skin Picture bullous lesions only	poly- morphic lesions	erythema multi- forme type
Carcinoma of breast		3	65—71	2		1
Carcinoma of uterus		2	44—65	1	1	
Carcinoma of prostata	3		60—77	1	1	1
Carcinoma of rectum	2	1	48—83	1	2	
Carcinoma of bladder		1	62	1		
Leukaemia (lymphatic, myeloid)	1	1	56—61		2	
Lymphosarcoma	1		63			1
Total	7	8	44—83	6	6	3

Four patients are now asymptomatic. In one of them the skin lesions disappeared shortly after radical extirpation of mammary cancer. The three other patients in this group are receiving Stilbestrol treatment for prostatic cancer and their bullous lesions have gradually subsided.

Histologic studies of the skin showed in all cases but one subepidermal bullae with more or less abundant eosinophil leukocytes in the bullous contents, around the blood vessels and in the dermis. In the single case of intraepidermal bullae there were no signs of acantholysis, but the blisters contained eosinophil leukocytes. Between the three clinically distinguishable groups shown in Tab. 2 no definite microscopical differences were found.

These observations are in agreement with data obtained from a survey of the approximately 50 cases in the available literature [1 to 22, 24 to 27, 29 to 41]. In about half of these cases the skin lesions had a polymorphic appearance resembling dermatitis herpetiformis, whereas the other cases were of bullous pemphigoid or relatively rarely, erythema multiforme type. In a few reported cases also lichen ruber bullous has appeared [21]. Biopsy was performed in about one-third of these cases and with very few exceptions [11, 35] the bullae were subepidermal.

Conclusions

Bullous lesions of the skin or mucous membranes in patients with internal disorders are not common. The internal disorders may be of widely varying type, but the commonest probably are malignant tumours. The skin lesions are in most cases compatible with dermatitis herpetiformis, bullous pemphigoid or, more rarely, bullous erythema multiforme. Microscopy shows the bullae to be subepidermal in most cases.

References. 1. ARNOLD, H. L.: Arch. Derm. **60**, 143 (1949). — 2. BALABANOV, K., u. V. C. ANDREEV: Dermatologica (Basel) **129**, 461 (1964). — 3. BLOCH, B.: Arch. Derm. Syph. (Chic.) **87**, 287 (1907). — 4. BLUEFARB, S. M.: Arch. Derm. **72**, 506 (1955). — 5. BOGROW, S. L.: Arch. Derm. Syph. (Chic.) **98**, 327 (1909). — 6. BUREAU, Y., A. JARRY et H. BARRIERE: Bull. Soc. franç. Derm. Syph. **62**, 238 (1955). — 7. CANIZARES, O., and M. J. COSTELLO: Arch. Derm. **70**, 379 (1954). — 8. CORBEILLE, C.: Minn. med. **11**, 678 (1928). — 9. COSTELLO, M. J., O. CANIZARES, M. MONTAGNA, and C. M. BUNCKE: Arch. Derm. **71**, 605 (1955). — 10. DAVIS, H.: Brit. J. Derm. **34**, 12 (1922). — 11. DEGOS, R., E. LORTAT-JACOB et J. DURAND: Bull. Soc. franç. Derm. Syph. **61**, 121 (1954). — 12. DEGOS, R., R. ROURAINE et A. LECLERCQ:

Bull. Soc. franç. Derm. Syph. **68**, 863 (1961). — 13. ELLIOTT, J. A.: Arch. Derm. **37**, 219 (1938). — 14. EPSTEIN, E., and K. MAC EACHERN: Arch. intern. Med. **60**, 867 (1937). — 15. GONZÁLES, J. L., u. S. ZIZZIUS: Zbl. Haut- u. Geschl.-Kr. **105**, 34 (1959). — 16. HAUF, A.: Zbl. Chir. **52**, 2699 (1925). — 17. KINGERY, F. A. J., and L. F. MONTES: Arch. Derm. **78**, 293 (1958). — 18. KREIBISCH, C.: Arch. Derm. Syph. (Chic.) **122**, 3 (1923). — 19. KRINER, J., y S. BRAUN-STEIN: Arch. argent. Derm. **9**, 335 (1959); — Zbl. Haut- u. Geschl.-Kr. **108**, 140 (1960). — 20. KÖNIGSTEIN, H.: Arch. Derm. Syph. (Chic.) **119**, 107 (1913). — 21. MAGNUSSON, B.: Dermatologica (Basel) **134**, 166 (1967). — 22. MARKS, J. M.: Proc. roy. Soc. Med. **54**, 225 (1961). — 23. McLUDY, T.: J. Neurol. Neurosurg. Psychiat. **13**, 106 (1950). — 24. MILBRADT, W.: Derm. Wschr. **105**, 1586 (1937). — 25. MILIAN, M.: Bull. Soc. franç. Derm. Syph. **33**, 2 (1926). — 26. NORMAN, T.: Urol. cutan. Rev. **55**, 352 (1951). — 27. OPPENHEIM, M.: Arch. Derm. Syph. (Chic.) **101**, 379 (1910). — 28. ROBERTSON, E. E.: Brit. med. J. **1953** I, 291. — 29. ROSENTHAL, S. K.: Arch. Derm. Syph. (Chic.) **150**, 304 (1926). — 30. ROTHMAN, S.: Arch. Derm. Syph. (Chic.) **149**, 99 (1925). — 31. SACHS, O.: Wien. klin. Wschr. **34**, 317 (1921). — 32. SCUTT, R.: Brit. med. J. **1952** I, 139 .— 33. SIEGEL, J. M.: Arch. Derm. Syph. (Chic.) **59**, 659 (1949). — 34. SJÖGREN, G.: Acta derm.-venereol. (Stockh.) **33**, 518 (1953). — 35. SKOG, E.: Acta derm.-venereol. (Stockh.) **44**, 114 (1964). — 36. SNEDDON, I. B.: Brit. med. J. **1966** II, 405. — 37. THIERS, H., P. LABEZE, J. FAYOLLE et PELLOUX: Lyon méd. **33**, 126 (1956). — 38. TRANTS, E. F.: Arch. Derm. Syph. (Chic.) **38**, 974 (1938). — 39. USLAND, O.: Med. Rev. **44**, 13 (1927). — 40. WEBER, F. P.: Proc. roy. Soc. Med. **20**, 1057 (1927). — 41. Case records of the Massachusetts General Hospital. New Engl. J. Med. **214**, 213 (1936).

Corticosteroid Treatment of Pemphigus

C. T. NELSON, Department of Dermatology, College of Physicians and Surgeons, Columbia University; The Presbyterian Hospital, New York, N.Y. (USA)

Clinical results obtained during the past 18 years have amply confirmed the fact that internally administered corticosteroids are the only really effective agents now available for controlling pemphigus. I say this despite the many well-recognized risks inherent in long-term corticosteroid therapy.

Our experience with pemphigus at the Columbia-Presbyterian Medical Center during the corticosteroid era now consists of 85 patients. The first 75 of these will afford the basis for my remarks today.

Table 1. *Mortality in 75 Cases of Pemphigus*

Diagnosis	Number of Patients	Living	Dead
Vulgaris	58	31	27[a]
Erythematosus	9	7	2
Foliaceus	5	3	2
Vegetans	3	2	1
Totals	75	43	32

[a] Three died from unrelated causes at a time when pemphigus was under complete control.

The distribution of these patients according to the type of pemphigus is shown in Tab. 1. These data indicate that 32 of the first 75 patients with all forms of pemphigus seen at Columbia-Presbyterian since 1949 are dead — 29 from disease-related causes. This is an overall mortality of about 40% due to the disease or the complications of its treatment. The salvage rate (60%) has been stationary, that is, has not improved appreciably during the past 10 years.

The most common single cause of death remains uncontrolled pemphigus (eight patients). This is true despite the relatively enormous dosages of corticosteroids employed in treatment (often up to 1 or 2 g of cortisone equivalents per day). Most of our patients who died, however, succumbed to the toxic effects of corticosteroid treatment, bacteremia (six patients) and thromboembolic phenomena (eight patients), being the most frequent precipitating causes of death.

Although pemphigus occurs more frequently in males, sex does not appear to influence prognosis. Age, however, is a significant factor in the mortality rate. Tab. 2 shows the distribution of our cases by age at onset of the disease. Of the 14 patients who had the onset of their disease after the age of 60 years, only three survive. Contrast this with the 21 to 40 year age group wherein only three of 17 have died.

Another rather striking finding is that most patients in our pemphigus vulgaris group who died from the disease or its treatment, did so during the first 3 years. This is shown in Tab. 3. 21 of the 24 disease-related deaths occurred within the first 3 years. No patient in our series died of the disease or the complications of its therapy after the 5th year. In other words, if we can keep our patients with pemphigus vulgaris alive during the first 3 years of their disease, the prognosis becomes rather good.

Table 2. *Age of Onset Vs. Survival — 75 Cases of Pemphigus*

Age (Yrs.)	Number	Living	Dead
21—40	17	14	3
41—60	44	26	18
61—80	14	3	11
	75	43	32

Table 3. *Mortality* in 55 Patients with Pemphigus Vulgaris Related to Duration of Disease*

Duration (Yrs.)	Number of Patients	
	Alive	Dead
0—3	9	21
4—6	7	3
7 and over	15	0

* Disease-Related Deaths Only

Table 4. *Mortality in 58 Patients with Pemphigus Vulgaris Related to Maximum Daily Dose of Steroid*

Mg. Cortisone Equiv.	Number of Patients	
	Lived	Died
Less than 1000	28	8
Over 1000	6	16

The mortality rate in patients with pemphigus vulgaris is also related to the initial dosage of corticosteroids needed to bring about control of the disease process. As shown in Tab. 4, 16 of 22 patients receiving more than 1 g of cortisone equivalents per day died from the disease or its treatment. On the other hand, only eight of the 36 patients requiring a daily dose of less than 1 g of cortisone equivalents to control their pemphigus have died.

These data suggest that the severest cases of pemphigus vulgaris progress rapidly, require very high initial corticosteroid dosage, and carry a high fatality rate. However, once the patient has survived for 3 years, the prognosis becomes good, regardless of age, and regardless of the maximum dosage of corticosteroids needed to bring the disease under control.

The disease appears to lose some of its virulence as time goes on and the amount of corticosteroid necessary for both maintenance and control of exacerbations decreases. Although others have reported a significant number of patients in whom corticosteroid therapy can be discontinued completely and a permanent remission maintained, we have only seven patients out of 43 survivors who have reached this happy situation. Moreover, all seven of these had the disease more than 10 years before this permanent remission (without therapy) was attained.

Just as the prognosis of pemphigus improves greatly if we are able to keep the patient alive during the first 3 years of his illness, so, too, is the prognosis greatly improved if the patient's pemphigus is sufficiently mild to go for a period of several months without requiring corticosteroid therapy. Therefore, when one is confronted with a fresh case of pemphigus it is good practice to observe the patient, perhaps once weekly for several weeks, to learn just how rapidly the disease is progressing. There are certain mild cases of true pemphigus vulgaris whose disease is not severe enough to seek medical attention for several months after onset. We know that these will require less corticosteroid for treatment and will do better in the long run.

However, once it becomes clear that corticosteroid treatment must be started, then one must treat in massive enough dosage to control and prevent all cutaneous lesions. In other words, once one is committed to treat a case of pemphigus vulgaris with corticosteroids, the dosage required is that which is sufficient to control all cutaneous manifestations.

Because of the high dosage and prolonged corticosteroid therapy required to control this disease, extensive baseline laboratory and radiological data are needed before starting treatment. In addition to the usual laboratory procedures, roentgenograms of the chest and vertebral column and an upper gastrointestinal series are obtained. While these patients are on initial high-dosage corticosteroid therapy, low salt, high protein bland diets, potassium chloride, antacids, antibiotics, anticoagulants, anticholinergics, insulin and psychomimetics should be used when indicated.

The prophylactic use of antibiotics is contraindicated because of the emergence of masked and resistant microbial infections. The use of estrogen-androgen treatment for its anabolic effect in the face of prolonged corticosteroid therapy, and of calcium supplements in an effort to retard osteoporosis, are felt by some to be worthwhile additions to the therapeutic regimen.

In the cases included in this report, corticotropin, cortisone, and its derivatives prednisone, methyl prednisolone, triamcinolone and dexamethasone were used in various patients at different dosage schedules and at different times. Since these drugs may be used interchangeably, we calculate their dosage in cortisone equivalents. Although some of these compounds as evaluated by the patients may seem more satisfactory than others, all appear to be equally effective in controlling the disease when given in equivalent amounts. In the large dosage we employ, the various compounds show similar untoward effects, except that weakness seems to be more pronounced in the patients who receive triamcinolone and dexamethasone. On the other hand, these compounds appear to cause fewer electrolyte disturbances and less fluid retention.

The initial dosage required in the treatment of pemphigus will usually be 300 to 400 mg of cortisone equivalents per day in mild cases and up to 800 mg of cortisone equivalents per day in the more severe ones. If the disease is not controlled by the original dosage (that is, if new cutaneous blebs continue to develop) after 7 to 10 days, then the daily amount of corticosteroid is doubled.

Once the disease is brought under control, as evidenced by the absence of new cutaneous lesions for 7 days and the healing of the lesions already present, the daily dosage may be reduced over a period of several weeks to 150 to 200 mg of cortisone equivalents. Thereafter, further reduction is very gradual and usually many months will be required before a daily maintenance dose of 50 to 100 mg of cortisone equivalents can be achieved. During this period, if an exacerbation of the pemphigus occurs, the daily dose of corticosteroid should be increased to twice that in effect when the flare-up was noted.

In the last analysis, the criterion for the adequate suppression of this disease by corticosteroids is the absence of all cutaneous manifestations. This is not to say, however, that an occasional bullous lesion with apparent spontaneous healing may not occur. Under such circumstances, an increase in corticosteroid dosage would not be warranted. The mouth is almost always involved in pemphigus vulgaris and in five of six patients the disease starts there. The response of oral lesions to corticosteroid therapy, however, is a poor indication of degree of control because erosions of the mouth are the last to heal and often persist for many months after all cutaneous lesions have cleared. Therefore, only if oral erosions are the sole lesions present should any attempt be made to use their response as a measure of adequacy of treatment.

Friction Blisters Produced under Controlled Conditions

Th. A. Cortese jr., T. B. Griffin and M. B. Sulzberger, Dermatology Research Program, U. S. Army Medical Research Unit, Presidio of San Francisco, San Francisco, California (USA)

This report will review our work of the past 3 years during which we have systematically studied experimental friction blisters in search of those factors which enhance or decrease the skin's susceptibility to frictional injury.

Methods

Friction blisters on the palms and soles of male subjects have been mechanically produced by linear and twist rubbing technics [1]. Linear rubbing in a to-and-fro direction was accomplished at selected skin sites under controlled conditions of moisture, stroke rate, stroke

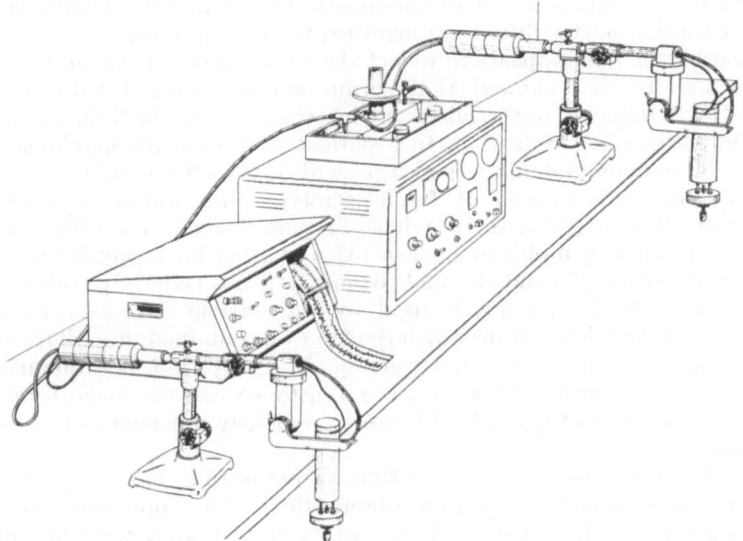

Fig. A drawing of our newest Twist Blistering Apparatus (U.S. Navy Photograph)

length, rubbing pressure and with different rubbing materials. Twist rubbing could be carried out simply by using the eraser on the end of an ordinary lead pencil rotated alternately in a clockwise and counter-clockwise direction while pressing downward against the skin. This method was used in our studies which did not require quantitation of the frictional forces. A new twist blistering apparatus still under construction* (see Fig.) will be able to rub two selected skin sites simultaneously at any angle under controlled conditions of rotational speed, arc excursion, rubbing pressure, and with different rubbing materials. The unique features of this instrument are: 1. a pneumatic pressure system which maintains a constant load against the rubbed site, and 2. minimal internal mechanical friction to permit the accurrate quantitation of the torque skin frictional resistance.

Findings

Blister Formation: Several prerequisites of skin are essential for the clinical and experimental production of friction blisters. The stratum corneum must be sufficiently thick and resistant to withstand the superficial frictional forces which are being transmitted downward into the epidermis. Otherwise an abrasion results. Moreover, the skin must be relatively immovable and supported by the underlying structures. It is for these reasons that friction blisters can be readily produced on the palms and soles and not on "thin" or "loose" skin.

When skin possesses the essential prerequisites, friction blister formation will proceed in two stages: 1. the production of an intraepidermal cleft which is the product of a shearing effect resulting from the frictional forces at the surface being transmitted to the deeper layers; and 2. the influx of fluid into the blister compartment. An adequate hemodynamic pressure is required for the latter and complete filling usually takes place within 1 to 2 h.

Blister Fluid: The constituents of the fluid in friction blisters are qualitatively identical to those of serum, but differ quantitatively [2]. The sodium, potassium, and chloride levels in friction blister fluid corresponded to those in the serum. Calcium, however, was significantly less, with an average level of 7.1 mg-% as compared to an average serum concentration of 9.1 mg-%.

At various intervals after blistering trauma the mean total protein concentration varied somewhat. At 1 h it was approximately one-third that of the serum and at 20 h it was slightly less than one-fourth the serum level. Qualitatively, the proteins of friction blister fluid were identical to those in serum.

Friction blister fluid appears to reflect the composition of serum, both normal and abnormal. Studies showed that serum albumin tagged with radioactive iodine (^{131}I) was detected in the blister compartment when the fluid was aspirated at 3 h after intravenous injection. In a patient with multiple myeloma, the abnormal serum gamma globulin was also present in the blister fluid.

A meaningful comparison of the electrolyte and protein constituents of friction blister fluid [2] with the previously reported data on the fluid of blisters from disease (such as pemphigus vulgaris [3], and other blistering dermatoses [4]) and from cantharidin [5] and thermal [6] injury is not strictly possible owing to the different methods of analysis used by the various investigators and the different ages of the blisters from which the fluid was obtained. For all the different blisters studied, the fluid contents were qualitatively, but not quantitatively, identical to those of serum. However, in no instance was the mean total protein concentration of any of the kinds of blisters previously reported as low as that of friction blisters.

Blister Healing: The course of friction blister healing has been recorded by clinical, histologic and photographic observations [7]. Approximately 70% of blisters which were either aspirated once at 24 or 36 h after their production or drained three times during the first 24 h, showed adherence of their tops to the blister base by 48 h after blistering trauma. This differed significantly from the figure of only 16% of blisters showing adherence of the blister tops at 48 h when

---

* Constructed by the Biomechanical Department at the Naval Radiological Defense Laboratory, San Francisco, California.

they were not aspirated and their fluid underwent natural resorption. (Blisters protected from rupture could remain fluid-filled and intact for as long as 2 weeks.) In those blisters whose tops reattached to the blister base, the appearance of the blistered site was similar to that of the surrounding normal skin except for a slight brown discoloration. The blister top may remain permanently fixed to its base, or it may become detached following additional injury or upon hydration of the site with water or sweat.

References. 1. SULZBERGER, M. B., T. A. CORTESE jr., L. FISHMAN, and H. S. WILEY: J. invest. Derm. 47, 456 (1966). — 2. CORTESE, jr., T. A., M. W. SAMS jr., and M. B. SULZBERGER: (Submitted for publication). — 3. KANDHARI, K. D., and J. S. PASRICHA: J. invest. Derm. 44, 246 (1965). — 4. EL-HEFNAWI, H., Z. A. GAWAD, and M. K. EL-MARSAFY: Proc. XII Int. Cong. Derm. Vol. II, pp. 1323—1328. New York: Excerpta Medica Foundation 1962. — 5. LEWIS jr., E. L.: (Submitted for publication). — 6. NÄNTÖ, V., and J. VILJANTO: Acta chir. scand. 124, 19 (1962). — 7. CORTESE jr., T. A., K. FUKUYAMA, W. EPSTEIN, and M. B. SULZBERGER: (Submitted for publication).

Free Communications

Experimental Investigations on the Acantholysis Induced by Staphylococcus pyogens. Comparative Study with the Acantholysis on Pemphigus

B. ZILBERBERG, Faculty of Medicine, University of S. Paulo (Brazil)

Since 1949, the majority of the authors agreed that acantholysis is the essential alteration in pemphigus. These same authors also called attention to the fact that other diseases may show acantholysis, like Familial Benign Chronic Pemphigus, Dyskeratosis Follicularis, and sometimes, Epitheliomas, Keratosis Senilis and Impetigo. In Impetigo, I found in some cases, by the smear Tzanck's test, acantholytic cells not distinguishable from those of Pemphigus and STEIGLEDER [1] describes similar findings in a case of reccurrent pyodermatitis.

In the other hand, LOWENTHAL [2] studying some cases of Familial Benign Chronic Pemphigus, by experimental inoculation of cultures of Staphilococcus pyogenes on the skin of a patient, succeeded to induce acantholysis peculiar to this disease. In 1960, ZILBERBERG [3] in successful experiments in many volunteers with cultures of Staphylococcus pyogenes, demonstrated that this bacteria may induce on the skin alterations on the epidermal cells similar to the acantholysis in Pemphigus. Though it is known that in pyodermatitis in general there may be acantholytic cells similar to those of Pemphigus, nevertheless, no experimental study has been carried out before my researches in 1960, and later, to prove that the pyogenic bacterias are responsible for this acantholysis.

Some authors, STORCK [4] in 1948, and later SCHRÖPL et al. [5] in 1963, dealing with allergic microbian eczema, made several patch tests in this condition and in the biopsies the only histologic findings they described is spongiosis.

It is not mentioned in these papers other alteration like acantholysis in the vesicles or in epidermis.

During the past few months, new findings in 20 experimental inoculations of volunteers, led me to more precise conclusions. I feel that these results are interesting enough for presentation at the International Congress of Dermatology in Munich.

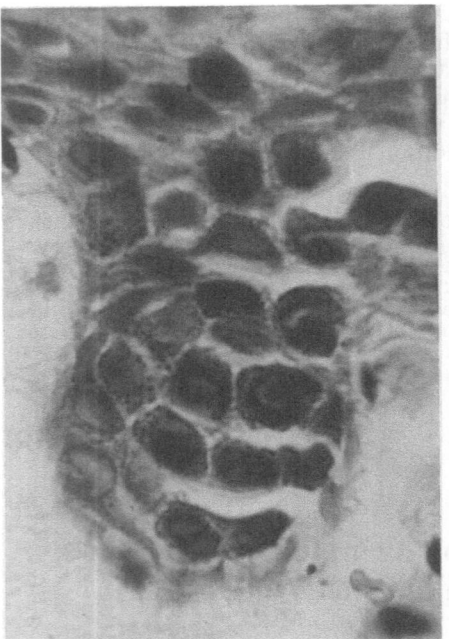

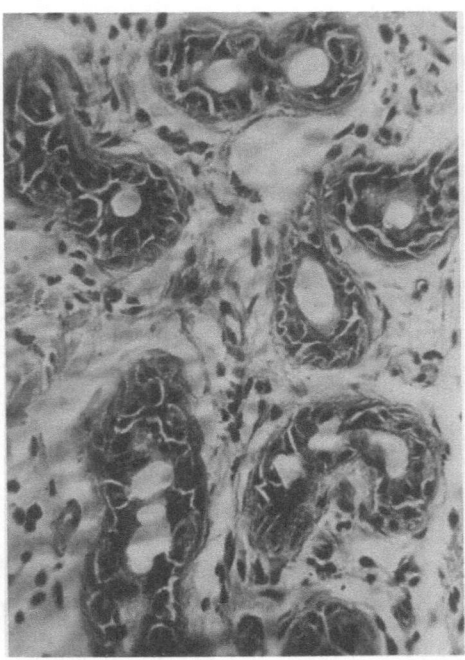

Fig. 1. Experimental inoculation with staphylococcus. A rete ridge with several acantholytic cells (H. & E. 1200 ×)

Fig. 2. Experimental inoculation with staphylococcus. Secretory portion of ecrines glands. Dissociation of the epithelial cells (H. & E. 240 ×)

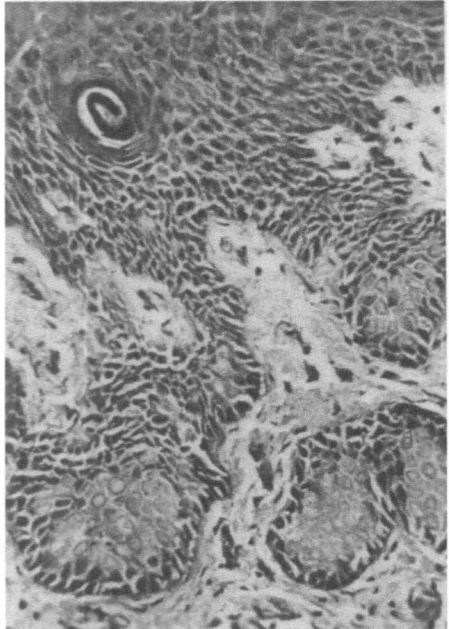

Fig. 3. Pemphigus vegetans. Several clefts and pycnotic nuclei in a irregularly acanthotic epidermis (H. & E. 480 ×)

Material and Methods: 62 volunteers free from pyodermatitis and allergic eczema, were inoculated with cultures of *Staphylococcus pyogenes* coagulase positive. Some of them were exclusively inoculated with a filtrate toxin of the bacteria. The skin was rubbed with sandpaper after washed many times with 70° of alcohol and ether before patch tests. Simultaneous controls were made with distilled water, physiologic serum and steril culture medium. In a few cases, toxin and a bacterial suspension were administered through superficial intradermic injections. Biopsies were taken after 24 and 48 h, fixed in 10% formalin and stained with H. & E. and Gram. Cultures from inoculated areas always showed *Staphylococcus pyogenes aureus* coagulase positive, while cultures from control areas were steril.

A comparative study of acantholytic changes in Pemphigus and those in experimental Staphylococcic inoculations led to the following *conclusions:* in Pemphigus, two types of acantholysis may be present, one which occurs exclusively in Pemphigus, and one produced by secondary staphylococcic infection of pemphigus lesions. These two acantholytic patterns are clearly distinguishable and may be found together in the same area.

It is known, that of the many bacteria found in the skin, Staphylococcus is the most frequent. Liquid from Pemphigus bullae and excoriated areas is a good culture medium. In the past litterature about the bullae dermatoses, one find frequently mentioned that cultures from pemphigus bullae show *staphylococcus aureus* in a majority of cases.

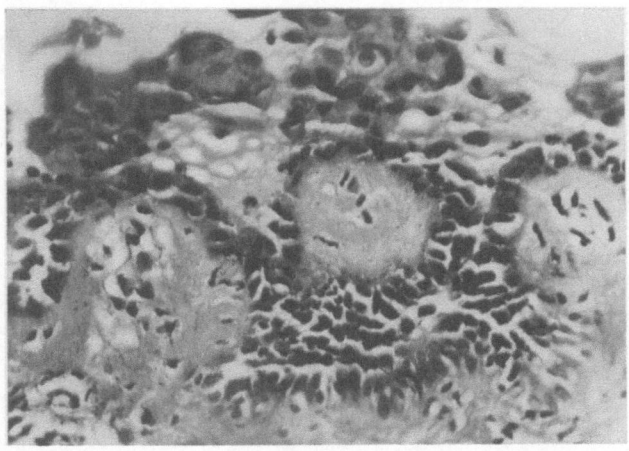

Fig. 4. Pemphigus vulgaris. The upper portion represents the floor of the bulla, with several typical pemphigus cells. The lower portion correspondend to the rete ridges show typical staphylococci acantholysis with pycnotic hyperchromatic and irregular nuclei (H. & E. 320 ×)

Staphylococcic alterations of the skin show four different forms: 1.acantholytic cells floating in pustules which are rich in polymorphonuclear leucocytes; 2-clefts, formed by rupture of the desmosomes; 3.alterations of epidermal cells, which consist of shrinkage of nuclei or disappearence of the cytoplasm after rupture of the desmosomes; there is pycnosis and hyperchromatism of the nuclei, which are irregular and frequently elongated, filiform; 4. a peculiar alteration of the secretory portion of the sweat glands: the epithelial cells are dissociated, with clear spaces between them.

It is generally known that not the bacteria but the toxin causes the lesions in the organism. The present study has confirmed this point of view. The sweat glands alterations mentioned above, when found in pemphigus or other dermatoses, suggest a secondary staphylococcic infection.

References. 1. Steigleder, G. K.; Aust. J. Derm. **3**, 11 (1955). — 2. Löwenthal, L. J. A.: Arch. Derm. **80**, 318 (1959). — 3. Zilberberg, B.: Piodermite Vegetante de Hallopeau e Penfigo Vegetante. Pesquisas experimentais sobre a etiologia da Piodermite Vegetante de Hallopeau. S. Paulo: Revista dos Tribunais 1960. — 4. Storck, H.: Dermatologica (Basel) **96**, 117 (1948). — 5. Schröpl, F., E. Müller und H. Röckl: Arch. klin. exp. Derm. **215**, 523 (1963)

An Electron Microscopic Study of Cutaneous and Oral Pemphigus Vulgaris

K. Hashimoto, Department of Dermatology, Tufts University School of Medicine, Boston, Massachusetts (USA)

The adhesion among epidermal cells and among the cells of the oral epithelium is brought about: 1. by desmosomes; 2. by the interlocking of the villous

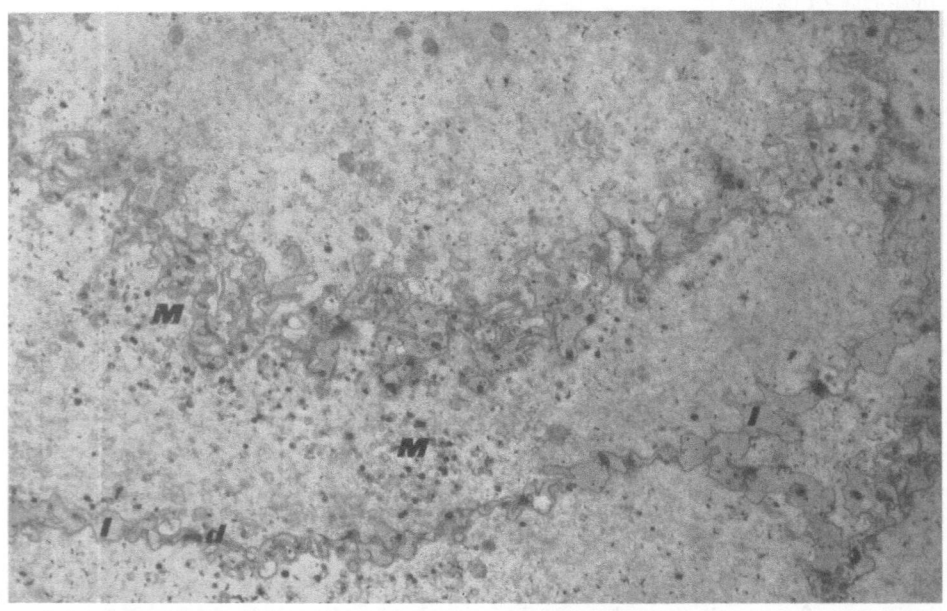

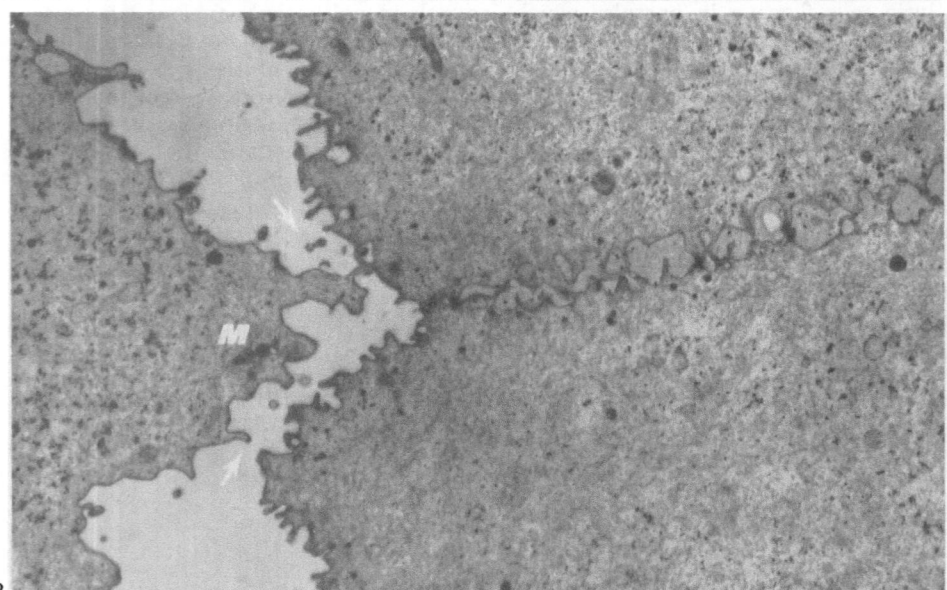

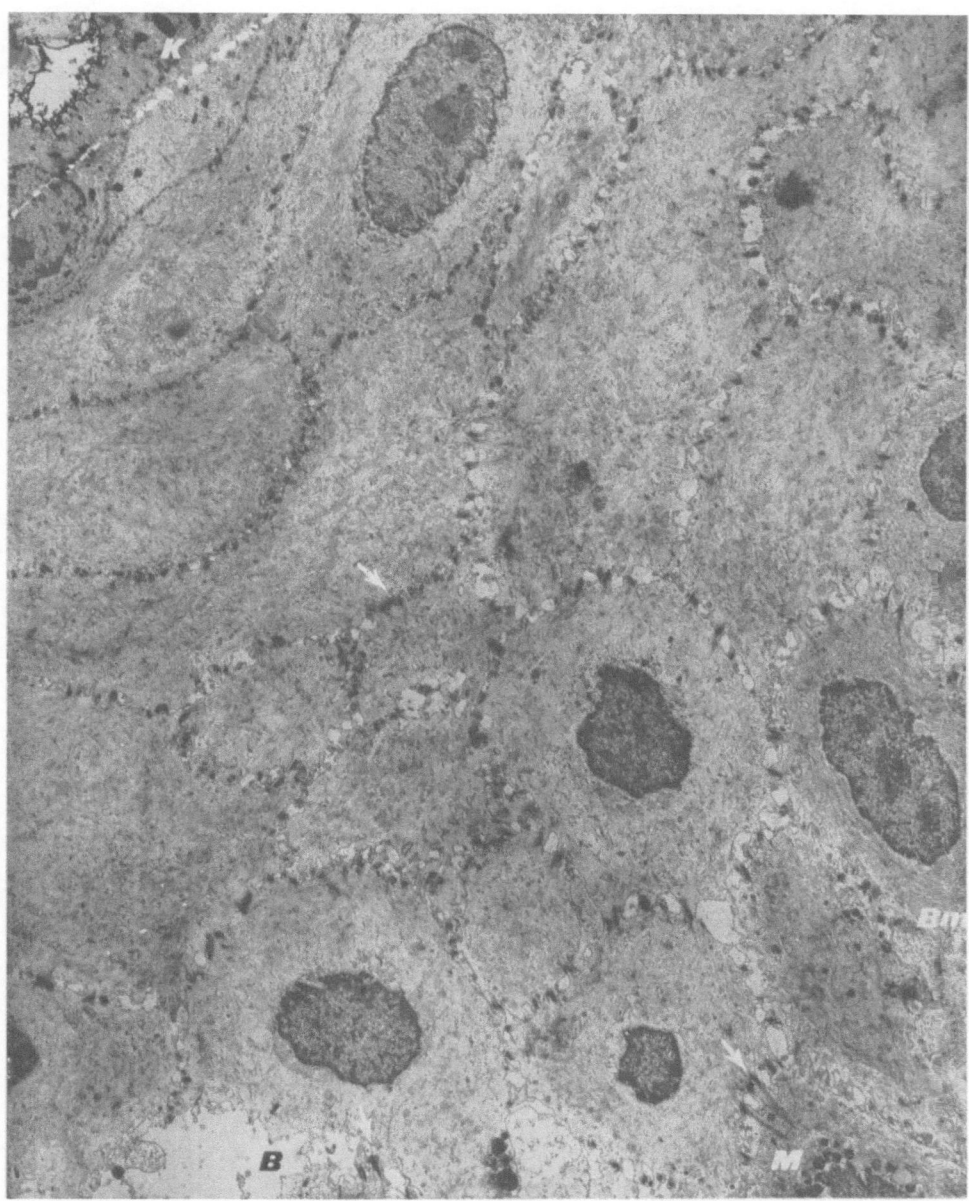

Fig. 3. *Intact desmosomes* (arrows) still connect severely damaged cells in which practically all tonofilaments have disappeared. The intercellular spaces are widened. *B* acantholytic bulla. *K* keratohyaline granules. *M* melanin granulea in a basal cell. *Bm* basement membrane. × 4,250

←

Fig. 1. *Non-acantholytic cells* in a lesion of oral pemphigus vulgaris. Note the intact intercellular cement substance (*I*), and the increased number of abnormal membrane-coating granules (*M*). Desmosomes (*d*) are not well developed. × 8,500

Fig. 2. *The cement is dissolved* and the left cell has separated by acantholysis (arrows), while the two cells on the right are still connected by cement and are intact. *M* membrane-coating granule. × 8,500

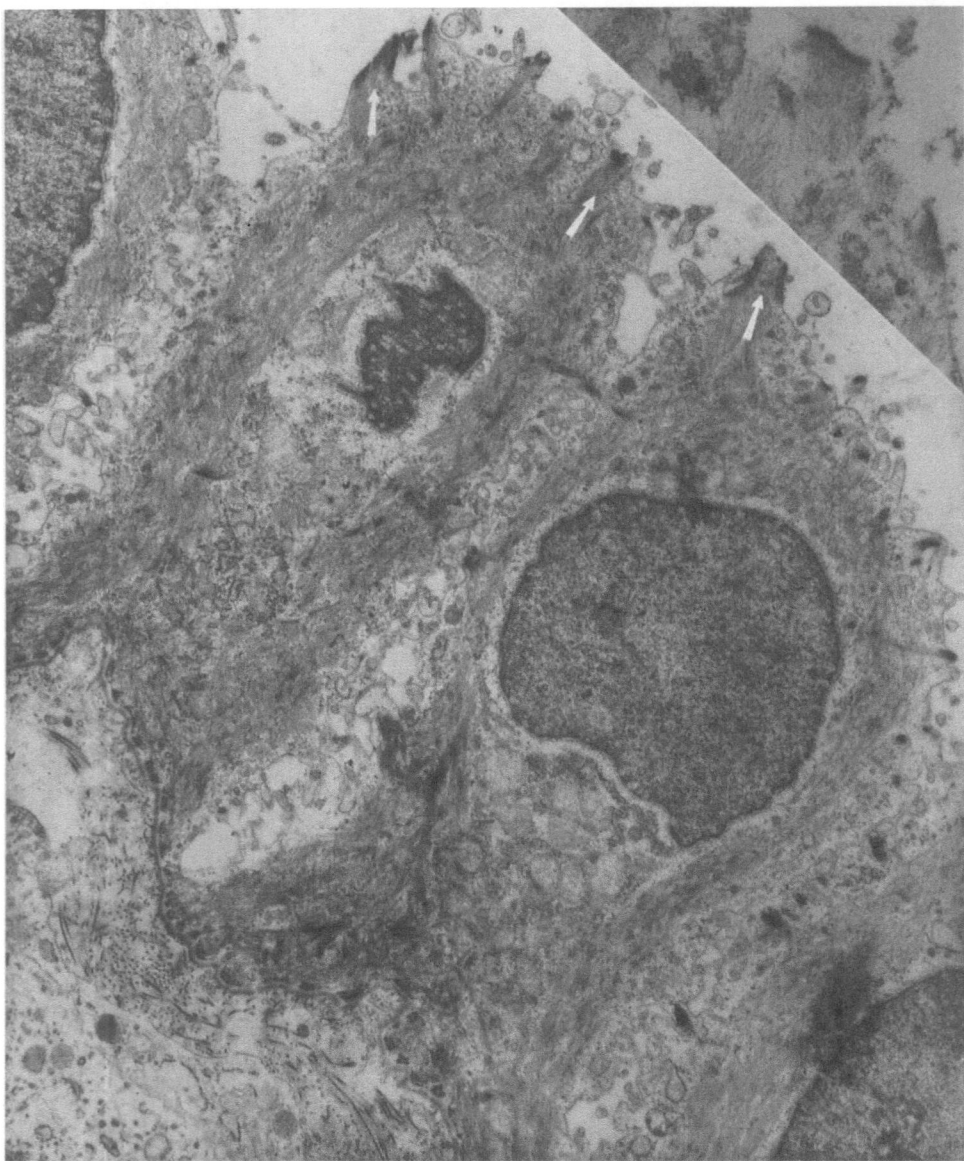

Fig. 4. *Intact attachment plaques with attached tonofilaments* are seen in two acantholytic basal cells (arrows). This picture indicates that the cement was primarily affected and not the desmosomes or the desmosome-tonofilament complex. Insert: Enlargement of separated desmosomes. × 44,000, × 14,500

projections of adjoining cells; and 3. by the intercellular cement substance (Fig. 1). In the upper layers of the normal epidermis and of the normal oral mucous membrane, desmosomes tend to disappear, whereas intercellular cement increases. This cement apparently is supplied by the membrane-coating granules which are discharged from cells in the upper layers.

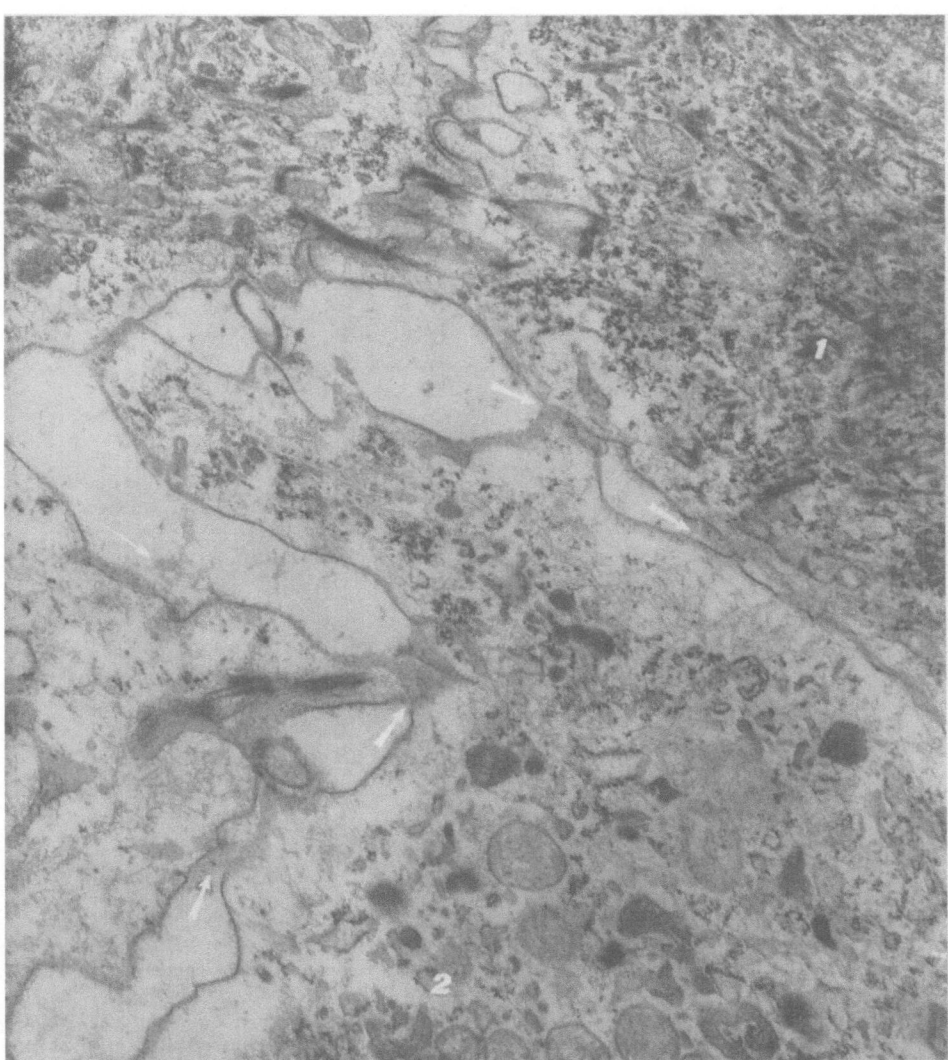

Fig. 5. *In spite of a complete disappearance of desmosomes* in two apposing cells (1, 2) and the disappearance of tonofilaments in one of these cells (2), the two cells are still attached to one another by intact cement (thick arrows). Thin arrow: disolved cement floating in the intercellular spaces. × 30,000

In pemphigus vulgaris of the skin and particularly of the buccal mucosa, it was found that dissolution of the intercellular cement substance and widening of the intercellular spaces was the primary event (Fig. 2). Because the cells of the normal buccal mucosa are mainly connected by the cement and their desmosomes are not well developed, dissolution of the cement as a result of pemphigus resulted in separation of the cells from one another. Abnormal membrane-coating granules were present. Tonofilaments often appeared clumped or were even absent, while the attachment plaques of desmosomes were still intact (Fig. 3). Many cells in the epidermis appeared clear because most of their tonofilaments had disappeared.

Although separated from one another in most areas, these cells were still connected by a few intact desmosomes (arrows). Thus, separation of cells ensued when dissolution occurred in the intercellular cement that was located either between the desmosomes of neighboring cells or between two neighboring cells independently of the desmosomes (Fig. 4). Not infrequently, intact attachment plaques with attached tonofilaments were still seen between basal cells otherwise separated by acantholysis (Fig. 5). It was concluded that the cement present between either desmosomal attachment plaques or other portions of apposed plasma membranes is the substance which was primarily affected and not the desmosomes

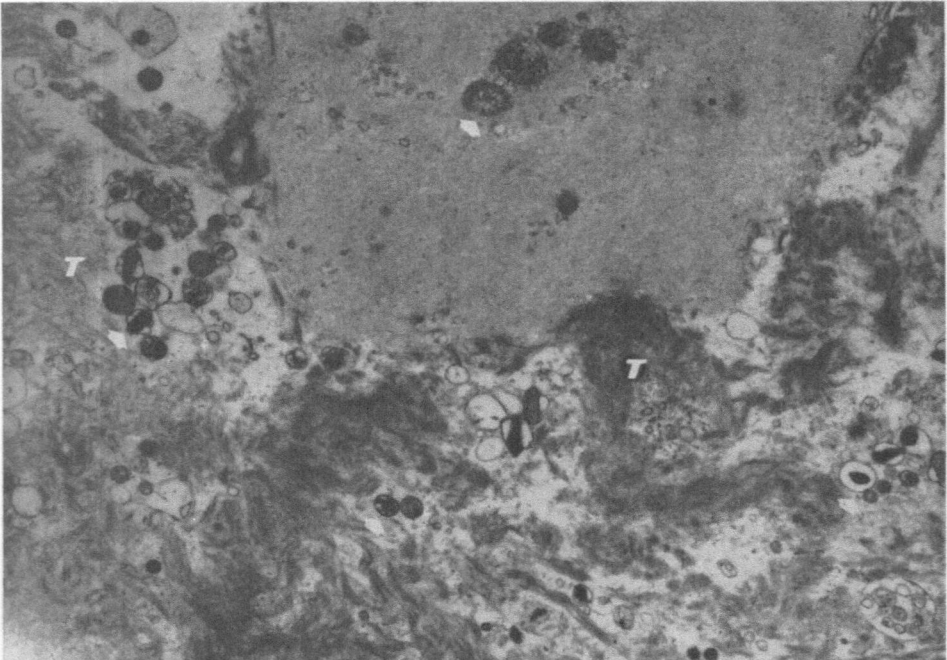

Fig. 6. Numerous *lysosome-like dense bodies* are present in an acantholytic degenerated cell and within an acantholytic blister (arrows). *T* degenerated tonofilaments. × 14,500

or the demosome-tonofilament complex. Not infrequently, one could see that in spite of a complete disappearance of desmosomes in two apposing cells and a great reduction in the amount of tonofilaments, cells were still adhering to each other by means of areas where the cement was still intact. Dissolved cement floating in the intercellular spaces was also seen.

The membrane-coating granules which produce the intercellular cement were found to be abnormal in some lesions, and numerous lysosome-like organelles were present. Lysosome-like dense bodies were present in great numbers in acantholysed and degenerating cells and also within blisters formed by acantholysis. The cohesion between the basement membrane and the basal cells was maintained even in a very advanced stage of acantholysis (Fig. 4). These observations correspond well with the immunofluorescence findings.

These reported findings indicate that alteration in the intercellular cement, which is present both between desmosomal attachment plaques and between neighboring plasma membranes, is responsible for the initiation of acantholysis in pemphigus vulgaris. It is interesting that in pemphigus foliaceus acantholysis occurs only in the granular layer where desmosomes even under normal circumstances have largely disappeared and the cement is largely responsible for holding apposing cells together. The frequent appearance of initial lesions in the mouth in pemphigus vulgaris may also be related to the fact that the epithelial cells of the oral mucosa have poorly developed desmosomes but are surrounded by a large amount of cement, especially in the upper layers.

References. HASHIMOTO, K., u. W. F. LEVER: Dermatologica (Basel) **135**, 27 (1967). — J. invest. Derm. **48**, No. 6 (1967). — BEUTNER: J. Amer. med. Ass. **192**, 682 (1965).

Localización de gamma globulina IgG y complemento (C'3) en la epidermis de enfermos de Pénfigo vulgar

S. STRINGA, C. BIANCHI, A. CASALA, C. INGLESINI y O. BIANCHI, Instituto de Investigaciones Medicas, Hosp. Tornu., Buenos Aires (Argentina)

En recientes estudios se ha puesto en evidencia que en la patogenia del pénfigo interviene un mecanismo inmunológico. Mediante el empleo del método indirecto de inmunofluorescencia se demostró en el suero de enfermos de pénfigo la existencia de anticuerpos que se fijan en las zonas periféricas de las células epidérmicas y de algunas mucosas de epitelío estratificado. Además utilizando el método directo en biopsias de piel sana y ampollada se encontraron depósitos de gamma globulina en las mismas zonas [1, 2, 3, 4]. El presente trabajo fué efectuado para: 1. determinar en la piel de los enfermos de pénfigo el tipo de gammaglobulina fijada a la célula epidérmica; 2. investigar la presencia de complemento en esos mismos lugares.

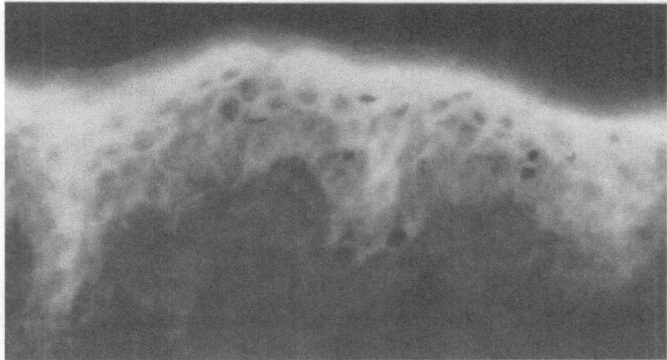

Fig. 1. Microfotografía de piel no ampollada de penfigo vulgar, incubada con suero anti-IgG marcado con isotiocianato de fluoresceina. Se aprecia intensa fluorescencia en la periferia de las células espinosas. Identica imagen se obtuvo al incubar con anti-C'3 humano

Material y métodos

Se efectuaron biopsias con "punch" de piel sana y de pequeñas ampollas en cuatro enfermos de pénfigo vulgar sin tratamiento y cuyo diagnóstico habia sido confirmado histológicamente. Cada biopsia fué dividida en dos partes; una ellas fué utilizada para estudio histológico (Hematoxilina y eosina) y la otra inmediatamente cortada por congelación en secciones de cuatro micrones. Estos cortes fueron incubados con los siguientes antisueros: anti-IgG, anti-IgA, anti-IgM y anti C'3. Los antisueros se obtuvieron en conejos y se marcaron para su uso con

isotiocianato de fluoresceina. La especificidad de los mismos fue controlada por inmuno-
electroforesis y antes de ser usados fueron absorbidos con polvo de hígado y convenientemente
diluidos para evitar la fluorescencia inespecífica.

Se realizaron los controles correspondientes al método directo de inmunofluorescencia y
además se efectuaron incubaciones con suero antialbúmina humana, anti-fibrinogeno humano y
anti-C'3 de rata marcados con isotiocianato de fluoresceina.

Resultados

Las tinciones con hematoxilina y eosina revelaron, en las lesiones ampollares
de todos los casos estudiados, la típica acantolisis suprabasal del pénfigo vulgar
mientras que las biopsias de piel normal no revelaron alteraciones histológicas.

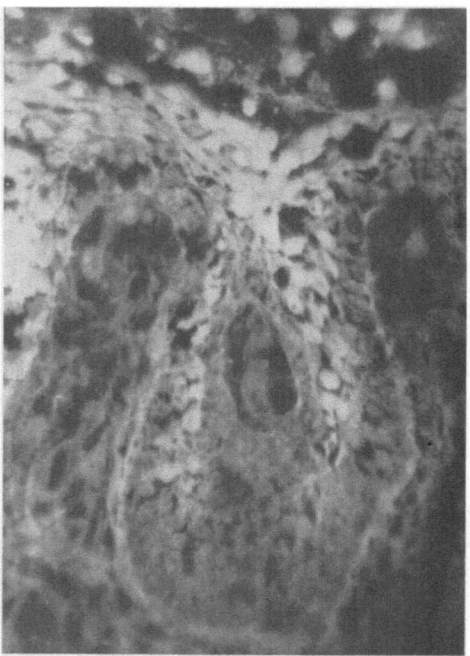

Fig. 2. Microfotografía de una ampolla de pénfigo ubicada sobre un folículo pilosebaceo
incubada con suero anti-IgG marcada. Las células acantolíticas desprendidas presentan
intensa fluorescencia uniforme de su citoplasma, mientras que las más profundas muestran
imágenes similares a las de la Fig. 1

El método directo de inmunofluorescencia demostró, tanto en la piel normal
como en la ampollada, fluorescencia brillante en la periferia de las células mal-
pighianas solamente en las secciones incubadas con anti-IgG y anti-C'3. Esta
positividad disminuía claramente con los bloqueos correspondientes. Las células
acantolíticas desprendidas mostraban fluorescencia uniforme en todo su citoplasma
aún en aquellos preparados no incubados con antisueros, es decir que estas células
presentan fluorescencia espontánea acentuada.

Comentarios

El pénfigo, entidad de patogenia desconocida, ha sido estudiado desde el
punto de vista inmunológico poniéndose de manifiesto la existencia de anticuerpos circulantes contra determinadas estructuras epidérmicas. El título de
estos autoanticuerpos parece aumentar con la gravedad del proceso y disminuye

con la administración de corticoides al mejorar los pacientes. Además en la piel de estos enfermos se encontró depósitos de gamma globulina que representarían el anticuerpo fijado a las células epidérmicas. Nuestros hallazgos demuestran que la única globulina que es posible detectar en la epidermis aparentemente sana o ampollada es del tipo IgG, no existiendo otras proteinas séricas. Además hemos podido comprobar depósitos de C'3 en los mismos sitios que se deposita IgG. Si bien es cierto que los métodos de inmunofluorescencia no permiten afirmar que una gammaglobulina fijada a un tejido representa un anticuerpo, sin embargo el hecho de que esté unida al complemento, refuerza la posibilidad de la existencia de un mecanismo antigeno-anticuerpo a ese nivel. En síntesis, la presencia de IgG y C'3 en ausencia de otras proteinas séricas parece confirmar que una reacción inmunológica tendría lugar a nivel de la periferia de las células espinosas de la epidermis penfigosa.

References. 1. BEUTNER, E. H., W. F. LEVER, E. WITEBSKY, R. JORDON, and B. CHERTOCK: J. Amer. med. Ass. 192 (1965). — 2. WALDORF, S. D., C. W. SMITH, and A. STRAUSS: Arch. Derm. **93**, 28 (1966). — 3. WRIGHT, E. T., R. L. EPPS, and V. D. NEWCOMER: Arch. Derm. **93**, 562 (1966). — 4. CHORZELSKI, T. P., J. F. VON WEISS, and W. F. LEVER: Arch. Derm. **93**, 570 (1966).

Dermatite Bulleuse Mucosynéchante et Atrophiante

A. G. BELLONE, M. F. HOFMANN und G. CAPUTO, Univ.-Hautklinik Mailand (Italien)

Unter den bekannten Definitionen dieses Krankheitsbildes haben wir die von LORTAT-JAKOB geprägte vorgezogen, d. h. „Dermatite Bulleuse Mucosynéchante et Atrophiante (D.B.M.S.A.)", da sie das klinische Bild am besten charakterisiert.

Auf Grund unserer 15jährigen Erfahrung an nunmehr 27 Fällen möchten wir das Krankheitsbild folgendermaßen umreißen:

in mehr oder weniger langen Zeitabständen auftretende Bildung von Blasen auf beschränkten Haut- oder Schleimhautarealen;
ständige Rezidive in situ;
vorwiegender Schleimhautbefall, hauptsächlich in Mund und Auge, mit Beteiligung mehrerer Schleimhäute im weiteren Verlauf;
verzögerte Heilung der einzelnen Läsionen, besonders an den Schleimhäuten, so daß die älteren Läsionen einen erosiv-ulcerativen Aspekt annehmen;
vorübergehender, ev. episodischer Befall der Haut im Gegensatz zur Kontinuität und Progredienz der Schleimhauterscheinungen;
häufige Narbenbildung an Haut und Schleimhäuten;
chronischer progressiver Verlauf;
günstige Prognose quoad vitam, ungünstige quoad functionem, zumal bei Schleimhautbeteiligung;
vorwiegend gutes Allgemeinbefinden; Resultate der Laborprüfungen ohne besondere Bedeutung;
dermo-epidermale Blasenbildung, nie Acantholyse (Differentialdiagnose zum Pemphigus); Plasmazellenanreicherung in der oberen Cutis an Blasengrund und unterer Narbengrenze;
starke Veränderungen der Ultrastruktur der Basalmembran bis zum völligen Verschwinden sowohl am Blasengrund und dessen unmittelbarer Nähe wie auch in den atrophischen Narbenbildungen. In einem der sechs ultramikroskopisch untersuchten Fälle waren im Epithelzellkern Mikrokörper unbekannter Natur sichtbar;
in Serien übertragbare cytopathogene Wirkung des Blutserums bei 14 der 20 daraufhin untersuchten Fälle. Dieses Phänomen hat die D.B.M.S.A. mit der Gruppe der großen bulleusen Dermatosen gemein;
starke Therapieresistenz (Corticosteroide, ACTH, Chloroquin, Griseofulvin, Sulphone).

Zur Progredienz der Lokalisationen (Tab. 1) ist vor allen Dingen zu sagen, daß man nicht auf die Bindehautbeteiligung warten sollte, um die Diagnose zu stellen. Der Augenbefall war nur in sieben unserer Fälle die erste Lokalisation; in vielen Fällen wurde die Bindehaut erst sehr spät befallen und in manchen nach 10 und mehr Jahren noch gar nicht. Das Alter bei Krankheitsbeginn ist sehr verschieden und lag bei keinem unserer Fälle vor dem 20. Lebensjahr.

Tabelle 1. *Dermatite Bulleuse Mucosinéchante et Atrophiante (D.B.M.S.A.)* Krankengut geordnet nach Augenbeteiligung

Geschl.	Alter bei Beginn Jahre	Beobach- tungsdauer Monate	Erster- scheinung	Augen- beteiligung	Krank- heitsdauer Jahre
♀	57	2	Augen	sofort	5
♀	56	1	Augen	sofort	$2^1/_2$
♀	40	36	Augen	sofort	14
♀	55	1	Augen	sofort	7
♀	40	$^1/_2$	Augen	sofort	21
♀	55	$1^1/_2$	Augen	sofort	20
♀	71	6	Augen	sofort	3
♀	60	34	Augen	sofort	3
♀	85	14	Schlundkopf	nach $^1/_2$ J.	$1^1/_2$
♀	32	3	Haut	nach $^1/_2$ J.	3
♀	66	6	Mundhöhle	nach $^1/_2$ J.	$3^1/_2$
♀	64	18	Genitalien	nach 2 J.	$4^1/_2$
♀	43	2	Haut	nach $2^1/_2$ J.	15
♀	57	2	Mundhöhle	nach 3 J.	5
♂	64	36	Haut	nach 5 J.	8
♀	62	$1^1/_2$	Haut	keine	3
♀	45	10	Haut	keine	2
♀	66	1	Haut	keine	$^1/_6$
♂	75	6	Haut	keine	$^1/_3$
♀	45	42	Haut	keine	4
♂	74	2	Haut	keine	$^1/_4$
♂	39	96	Haut	keine	15
♀	27	$1^1/_2$	Genitalien	keine	$2^1/_2$
♀	54	34	Mundhöhle	keine	4
♀	46	5	Mundhöhle	keine	10
♂	48	9	Mundhöhle	keine	$1^1/_2$
♀	51	$5^1/_2$	Haut	keine	$1^1/_3$

Die Multiplizität (Tab. 2) der Haut- und Schleimhautlokalisationen zeigte sich im Verlauf der Zeit in 24 unserer 27 Fälle, kann aber auch jahrelang fehlen. Beim Bestehen einer einzigen Lokalisation ist dann die Diagnose beim Fehlen von skleroatrophischen Narbenbildungen fast unmöglich. Die Wahrscheinlichkeits- diagnose beginnt beim Bestehen folgender Erscheinungen:

relativ monomorphe Blasenbildung;
häufige Rezidive in Situ;
Blasengrund erosiv-ulcerativ;
kontinuatives Bestehen der Schleimhautläsionen bei vorübergehender oder fehlender Hautbeteiligung.

Die Diagnose ist gesichert, wenn hinzukommt:

Beteiligung mehrerer Schleimhäute, nacheinander oder gleichzeitig;
Bindehautläsionen mit Synechien;
skleroatrophische oder sklerotische Narbenbildung an der Haut und an den Schleimhäuten.

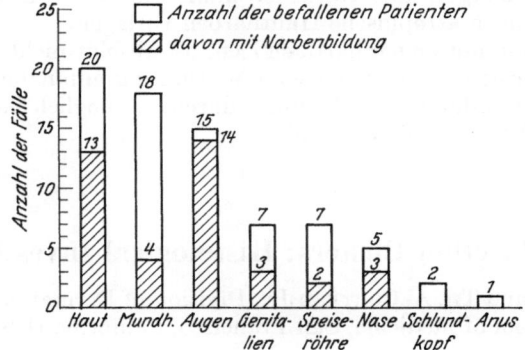

Lokalisation der D.B.M.S.A. im Verlauf der Erkrankung bei 27 Patienten

Anzahl der befallenen Patienten
davon mit Narbenbildung

Tabelle 2. *Dermatite Bulleuse Mucosinéchante et Atrophiante (D.B.M.S.A.)*
Lokalisation im Verlauf der Krankheit mit (×) und ohne (●) Narbenbildung

Fall	Dauer der Krankheit Jahre	Schleimhäute								
		Auge	Mund-höhle	Schlund-kopf	Kehl-kopf	Speise-röhre	Nase	Genit.	Anus	Haut
1	5	×	●		●					
2	2½	×	●							●
3	14	×	×							×
4	7	●	●	●		●	×	×		
5	21	×								
6	20	×					●			
7	3	×	●							×
8	4½	×	×		●	●		×		●
9	5	×	●							
10	8	×	×		×	×	×	×		×
11	1½	×	●	●				●	●	●
12	3		●							●
13	2		●					●		×
14	2 M.									×
15	4 M.		●							×
16	2½							●		
17	4		●			×	×			×
18	3	×	×					●		●
19	4									×
20	10		●							×
21	3	×	●			●				×
22	15	×	●		●	●				●
23	3 M.									×
24	3½	×	●							
25	1½					●	●			×
26	15									×
27	1⅓		●							●

Die höchste Incidenz von Narben und Synechien kommt bekanntlich der Bindehaut zu. Wir möchten jedoch betonen, daß, obwohl die Hautbeteiligung scheinbar stets vorübergehender Natur ist, immerhin bei 13 unserer 20 Patienten mit Hauterscheinungen atrophische Hautnarben vorlagen.

Wir haben es also mit einem hartnäckigen, oft absolut nicht benignen Krankheitsbild zu tun, dessen Abgrenzung vom M. Duhring anfänglich schwierig, aber im Verlauf der Erkrankung dem Kliniker durchaus möglich ist, auch wenn die charakteristische Augenbeteiligung fehlt.

Experimental Friction Blisters: Histological Investigation

K. Fukuyama and Th. A. Cortese Jr., Division of Dermatology, University of California, School of Medicine, San Francisco, California (USA)

Friction blisters are among the common lesions of human skin. Despite their frequent occurrence, clinical and histological studies of the natural course of friction blister healing are still lacking. Recently the clinical course was followed on experimentally produced friction blisters [1]. This paper reports the histopathology of the blisters at various stages of healing.

Materials and Methods

16 adult civilian volunteers participated in this study. Two friction blisters were produced on the hypothenar eminence of each palm using the pencil eraser twist rubbing technic [2]. Punch biopsies (4 mm) of 34 intact blisters were obtained immediately at 1, 24, 48, 72 and 96 h; and at 5 and 14 days after the blister trauma, Specimens were fixed in buffered-neutral 10% formalin, cut at 4 microns and stained with hematoxylin and eosin.

Results and Discussion

Biopsy immediately after the blistering trauma always revealed the blister cleft within the Malpighian layer of the epidermis. The horny layer and the granular layer of the blister top did not show significant alteration. The Malpighian cells were, however, elongated as though mechanically stretched. The cytoplasm had lost its homogeneity and appeared thready and eosinophilic. These changes were more striking in the upper portions of the Malpighian layer than in the lower level and in the basal layer, and closely resembled the effects of mild thermal injury. However, the other changes reported for thermal injury such as acantholysis, subepidermal bullae, and dermal inflammatory infiltrate were not observed. Both thermal and mechanical factors may be involved in the basic pathogenesis of friction blisters.

1 h after the blistering the changes were more pronounced in the upper Malpighian cells, but cells in the lower level of the epidermis appeared rounded and seemed to have recovered somewhat from the frictional damage. The blister base consisted of two different cellular types: damaged cells and those preserved.

By 24 h the granular cells of the blister top appeared the same. The blister base showed an increase of normal-appearing cells consisting of basal and Malpighian cells. Mitotic figures were not particularly increased, but it is conceivable that these cells resulted from the rapid multiplication of the recovered cells.

Keratohyalin granules were observed by 48 h in the cells located just below the damaged Malpighian cells. This finding suggests the newly formed cells were differentiating at a much faster rate than that of normal. Since the granular cells of the blister top remained unchanged, two granular layers were seen at this time.

In contrast to the cells below the blister cavity which were dividing and differentiating rapidly, those in the blister roof seemed to have stopped differentiating any further. This possibility was well illustrated in specimens taken at 14 days after blistering injury. The granular cells still retained their morphology between the old and newly formed horny layers.

Conclusion. Experimentally produced friction blisters were studied histologically. The blister cleft always formed within the Malpighian layer. Malpighian and basal cells were injured and appeared mechanically stretched. Epidermal cell regeneration at the blister base proceeded rapidly with new cell formation and cell differentiation. New granular cells appeared within 48 h. Granular cells at the blister top remained morphologically unchanged following the onset of blister formation, suggesting a cessation in their further differentiation.

References. 1. CORTESE, T. A.: Presented at the American Medical Association meeting, Section of Dermatology, June 1967. — 2. SULZBERGER, M. B.: J. invest. Derm. 47, 456 (1966).

Etude de la composition protéique du liquide des bulles dans les dermatoses bulleuses

G. MOULIN et Y. MANUEL, Clinique Dermatologique et Institut Pasteur de Lyon, Hôpital E. Herriot, Lyon (France)

Nous désirons présenter les résultats de l'étude électrophorétique du liquide de bulles pratiquée chez 114 malades porteurs de dermatoses bulleuses. Cette étude a comporté une électrophorèse sur papier, une immuno-électrophorèse et une électrophorèse en gel d'amidon. Les immun-sérums utilisés ont été l'immun-sérum antisérum humain standard n° 223 de l'Institut Pasteur de Paris et l'immun-sérum antisérum humain du Laboratoire Central de Transfusion Sanguine d'Amsterdam. Chaque fois que cela a été possible, l'étude électrophorétique a été réalisée simultanément sur le sérum correspondant.

Résultats

1. Toutes les protéines identifiées dans le sérum sont retrouvées dans les liquides de bulles des différentes dermatoses bulleuses chaque fois que la concentration de ceux-ci est suffisante.

2. Dans un cas de zona généralisé au cours d'un myélome osseux multiple, nous avons retrouvé dans le liquide de bulle la protéine myélomateuse du sérum, comme le fait avait été signalé par B. POTTER et D. MERRILL.

3. Il n'a pas été possible de mettre en évidence dans les liquides de bulles des protéines absentes normalement dans le sérum telles que les protéines dites tissulaires qui ont été décrites dans le liquide céphalo-rachidien.

4. Le rapport alpha-1/alpha-2-globulines est toujours supérieur à celui du sérum correspondant en cas de brulûres thermiques et de manière moins nette au cours de la maladie de Duhring-Brocq. Dans ces deux types de bulles, les macroglobulines, en particulier l'alpha 2 macroglobuline, se trouvent à une concentration inférieure à celle du sérum. Cette constatation s'inscrit en faveur d'un processus de filtration alors que dans les autres affections bulleuses la composition protéique est identique à celle du sérum tant quantitativement que qualitativement, à la concentration près dans certains cas.

5. Sur 114 liquides de bulles, nous avons trouvé 32 fois à l'immuno-électrophorèse une ligne de précipitation extérieure à la zone béta 2 globulines qui

n'existait pas sur le tracé immuno-électrophorétique du sérum. Cette ligne nous semble correspondre à la présence de produits de fibrinolyse. En effet, nous avons retrouvé une ligne identique dans certains sérums présentant une fibrinolyse pathologique, dans le sérum de femmes en période menstruelle, dans certains liquides pathologiques (en particulier le liquide céphalo-rachidien au cours des hématomes sous-duraux) et enfin dans des sérums et du fibrinogène traités par la streptase streptococcique. Cette ligne semble correspondre d'ailleurs à la fraction externe de la ligne de précipitation anormale du fibrinogène qu'ont trouvée dans certains liquides de bulles HERMANN et SCHULTZ, SCHULTZ et SCHWICK avec un immun-sérum antifibrinogène. La présence de ces produits de fibrinolyse dans les bulles de diverses dermatoses ne semble pas le fait du hasard:

Présence de Produits de Fibrinolyse (+)

Bulles de cause infectieuse			*Bulles de cause physique*	
Zonas	9— 0		Brulûres thermiques	13— 0
Bulles microbiennes	5— 4 +		Traumatiques	5— 3 +
Bulles de cause allergique			Porphyries	5— 0
Eczémas de contact	7— 0		Gelures	2— 1 +
Dysidroses	16—12 +		*Divers*	
Toxidermies bulleuses	7— 2 +		Purpura bulleux	2— 1 +
Dermatoses bulleuses			Erythema elevatum	2— 1 +
Erythème polymorphe	12— 1 +		Inclassé	5— 0
Duhring-Brocq	21— 7 +			
Pemphigus	3— 0		Total	114—32 +

Nous les avons retrouvés par exemple, spécialement intenses quatre fois sur cinq dans des liquides de bulles microbiennes et aucune fois sur neuf liquides de bulles de zona (où le liquide très peu abondant, présentait une composition protéique identique à celle du sérum). Dans les bulles de dysidroses, la ligne extérieure aux béta 2 est présente 12 fois sur 16 alors qu'elle est absente dans les sept liquides provenant d'eczéma de contact. Nous avons un seul résultat positif sur douze erythèmes polymorphes bulleux recidivants alors que dans la maladie de Duhring-Brocq nous la retrouvons 7 fois sur 21. Cette fibrinolyse anormale, toujours absente dans les sérums correspondants, s'observe donc avec une fréquence significative dans les liquides de bulles microbiennes ou traumatiques, dans les dysidroses et la maladie de Duhring-Brocq alors que nous ne l'avons retrouvée ni dans les brulûres thermiques ni dans les eczémas de cause externe ni dans les zonas et les porphyries. Il ne semble pas exister de rapports entre la présence de produits d'activité fibrinolytique d'une part et le rapport alpha 1/alpha 2 globulines d'autre part.

Discussion

Cette étude électrophorétique montre donc que la composition protéique du liquide de bulles est qualitativement très comparable à celle du sérum et comporte peu de différences selon le genre d'affection bulleuse. Le liquide de bulle est identique à celui du sérum dans la plupart des cas: dans les zonas, les eczémas et les toxidermies bulleuses par exemple. Par contre dans les brulûres thermiques et la maladie de Duhring-Brocq, la plus faible concentration en macroglobulines indique un processus de filtration qui rapproche la composition de ces bulles de celle du liquide interstitiel. Dans ces cas, la concentration protéique étant plus forte que celle du liquide interstitiel, on peut envisager soit qu'il s'agit d'un mélange de sérum et de liquide interstitiel, soit qu'il se produit une résorption de la partie aqueuse du liquide interstitiel de la bulle pour rétablir l'équilibre oncotique.

La présence de produits de fibrinolyse n'est mise en évidence que dans certaines dermatoses bulleuses. Elle s'explique aisément dans les bulles hémorragiques (traumatisme, purpura bulleux) et dans les bulles microbiennes par la présence d'enzymes microbiennes. Sa présence dans les dysidroses par opposition à son absence dans les eczémas de contact peut s'expliquer par des altérations vasculaires libératrices d'enzymes protéolytiques, mais cette hypothèse que pourraient étayer les résultats obtenus dans la maladie de Duhring-Brocq n'est pas confirmée par la négativité habituelle dans les érythèmes polymorphes bulleux, affection où les lésions vasculaires sont les plus importantes.

Nous n'avons pas encore étudié le type de gamma A globuline présente dans ces bulles et nous ne pouvons affirmer si les immuno-globulines trouvés dans ces liquides de bulles tirent toutes leurs origines du sérum ou si certaines ont une origine locale.

Nouvelles observations sur le phénomène citochémiotatique dans la bulle du pemphigus

P. SERTOLI, Primario Reparto Dermatologico, Osp. S. Carlo, Genova-Voltri (Italie)

Après nos précédentes observations (1966) dans lesquelles nous avons, pour la première fois, mis en évidence dans le liquide de bulle dans deux cas de pemphigus

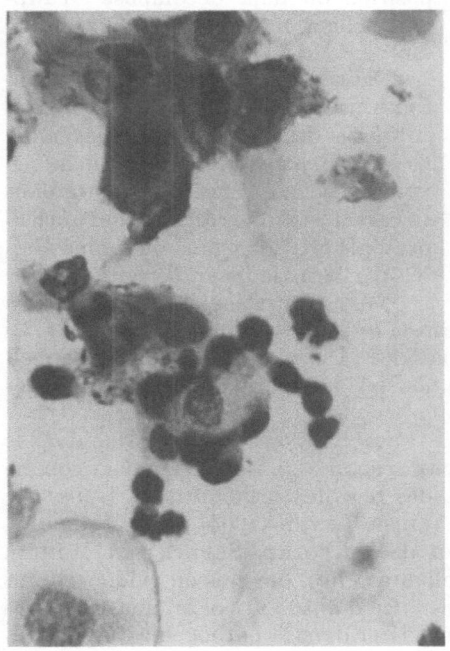 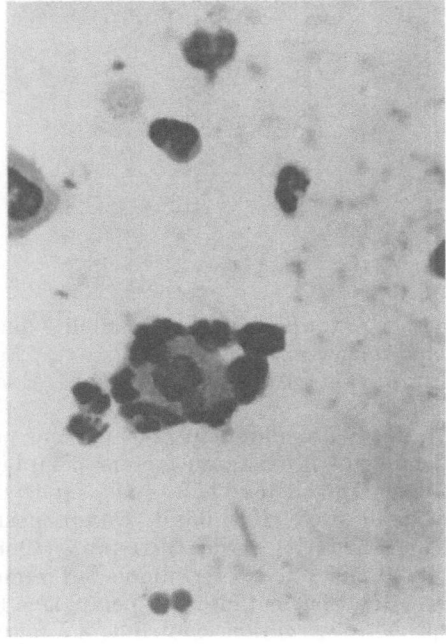

Fig. 1   Fig. 2

la présence de cellules acantolitiques entourées d'une couronne de neutrofilés comme une rosette, nous avons ou la possibilité de poursuivre les recherches dans d'autres deux cas de pemphigus: un homme âgé de 73 ans, avec p. chronique (muqueux-cutané) décédé pour infarctus mycardiaque et une femme âgée de 58 ans avec pemf. chronique cutané-muqueux (oral et vaginal) remise en bonnes et persistantes conditions après un traitement adéquat antibotique cortico-steroidé.

Dans les deux cas l'examen du liquide, du fond et du toit de bulle colorés avec May-Grundwald-Giemsa, avec le P.A.S. et avec le Feulgen, a permis de mettre en évidence les cellules acantolitiques entourées de neutrofiles et de éosinofiles identiques à celles que nous avons déjà observées dans les premiers deux cas. De telles images que nous ne sommes pas arrivés à mettre en evidence dans d'autres dermatoses vésicules-bulleuses (sans esclure avec cela la possibilité éventuelle de leur présence) comme aussi dans les vésicules d'un Zoster brachial apparu dans le p. de pemphigus durant son séjour dans notre département, nous font admettre le caractère de constance dans nos quatre cas.

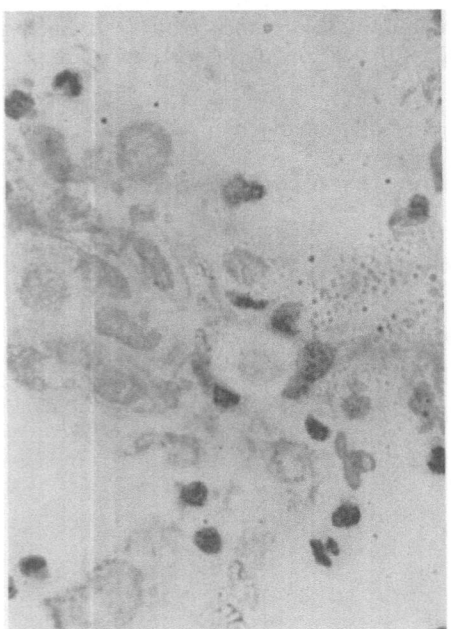

Fig. 3

Les formations que nous avons observées peuvent rappeler les formations obtenues par LEONI (1952) et par JASINSKY-STIEFEL (1953) en liquide de bulle par la cantaridine.

Dans celles-ci, cependant, les neutrofiles entourent un matériel nucleoprotoplasmatique en phase de décomposition ou déjà décomposé en rapport à l'action lésive par la cantaridine.

Dans nos cas c'est la cellule acantolitique du pemphigus qui apparait entourée des neutro-eosinofiles indépendamment de n'importe quelle noxa-artificielle et encore évidente dans sa caractéristique constitution nucleoprotoplasmatique plus ou moins altérée par la maladie en activité.

Nos observations nous engagent à admettre toujours plus la possibilité que dans la bulle du pemphigus il advient des phénomènes cito-chemiotactique responsables des formations à rosette qui rappellent davantage les formations du L.E. que non pas un commun phénomène fagocitaire.

Jusqu'à maintenant nous n'avons pas les éléments pour admettre que dans le pemphigus il existe un facteur pemphigueux responsable du phénomène comme il existe un facteur L.E. mais, sur la base des récentes recherches de BEUTNER, et de JORDON (1964/65) de CHRORZELSHI, WEISS, LEVER (1965) et de WALDORF, SMITH-STRAUSS et de BETHSEDA (1966) et de THIVOLET, SEPETDJIAN MONIER (1966), qui, avec la technique de l'immunofluorescence, ont mis en évidence dans les altérations cutanées du pemphigus l'existence d'auto anticorps, nous retenons que nos observations contribuent à faire considérer dans la pathogénie du pemphigus l'intervention aussi d'un mécanisme auto-immunitaire.

Bibliographie. CHORZELSKI, T. P., F. VON WEISS, and F. W. LEVER: Path. Europ. I, 268 (1966); — Arch. Derm. **93**, 570 (1966). — LEONI, A.: Minerva. derm. **27**, 5 (1952). — SERTOLI, P.: Minerva. derm. **41**, 160 (1966). — THIVOLET, J., M. SEPETDJIAN e S. C. MONIER: (In corso di pubblicazione). — WALDORF, D. S., C. SMITH, and A. STRAUSS: Arch. Derm. **93**, 28 (1966).

Hepatische Porphyrien: Veränderungen der Serumenzymaktivitäten und hämatologischen Befunde beim Menschen und bei der Ratte

H. PIETSCHMANN und W. RAAB, Univ.-Institut für med. Chemie, Wien (Österreich)

Wie schon der Name sagt, nimmt die Leberfunktion eine zentrale Stellung für das Zustandekommen der hepatischen Porphyrien ein. Bei Porphyria cutanea tarda gestatten jedoch die klassischen Leberfunktionsprüfungen nur in den seltensten Fällen das Ausmaß der Leberstoffwechselstörung zu erfassen. Im Krankengut der II. Medizinischen Klinik (Vorstand Prof. Dr. K. FELLINGER) und der II. Hautklinik (Vorstand Prof. Dr. A. WIEDMANN) fand sich unter 35 Patienten mit Porphyria cutanea tarda in zehn Fällen das Vorliegen völlig normaler klassischer Leberfunktionsproben.

Die moderne Leberdiagnostik stützt sich auf die Bestimmung von Enzymaktivitäten im Serum; mit diesen Methoden kann eine wesentlich genauere Erfassung von Leberstoffwechselstörungen erfolgen. Die Bestimmung der Transaminasen im Serum (GOT und GPT) ergab bei 32 von 35 Patienten mit Porphyria cutanea tarda pathologische Aktivitäten; auch die Aktivitäten der SDH und der ALD waren in der Mehrzahl der Fälle außerhalb der Norm. Nur die Aktivitäten der LDH und der alkalischen Phosphatase im Serum zeigten sich meist unverändert.

Diese Ergebnisse erlauben die Schlußfolgerung, daß die Bestimmung leberfunktionsabhängiger Serumenzymaktivitäten bei Porphyria cutanea tarda ein wichtiges Hilfsmittel zur Beurteilung der Schwere des Krankheitsbildes und zur Verlaufsbeurteilung darstellt. — Die hämatologischen Untersuchungen bei 35 Patienten mit Porphyria cutanea tarda ergaben mit Ausnahme der Eisenspiegel praktisch keine Auffälligkeiten [1].

Bei der Ratte bewirkt die Vergiftung mit Hexachlorbenzol das Auftreten einer Porphyropathie; die toxische hepatische Porphyrie der Ratte wurde häufig als Versuchsmodell für die Porphyria cutanea tarda des Menschen herangezogen, da beim Menschen ebenfalls durch Hexachlorbenzol eine toxische hepatische Porphyrie ausgelöst werden kann [1]. Um die Vergleichbarkeit des Versuchsmodelles zu prüfen, wurden nun auch bei Ratten mit toxischer Porphyrie die mit der Leberfunktion im Zusammenhang stehenden Serumenzymaktivitäten untersucht. Ferner erfolgten Untersuchungen des Blutes und des Knochenmarkes der Ratten mit toxischer hepatischer Porphyrie, um auch vom hämatologischen Gesichtspunkt aus eine Vergleichsmöglichkeit zu schaffen. 40 Albinoratten von 150 g Körpergewicht erhielten durch 10 Wochen 0,2% Hexachlorbenzol zur Nahrung zugesetzt; am Ende dieser Periode wurden die Tiere getötet und für die enzymatischen und hämatologischen Untersuchungen herangezogen.

Bei sämtlichen Ratten lag im Serum eine erhöhte Aktivität der SDH vor (durchschnittliche Erhöhung auf 1220%). 39 von 40 Ratten zeigten eine erhöhte Aktivität der Transaminasen im Serum (GOT und GPT). Bei 37 der 40 Ratten fand sich eine erhöhte Aktivität der LDH im Serum. Die Aktivitäten der ALD und der alkalischen Phosphatase im Serum waren fast immer normal. Das Blutbild der porphyropathischen Ratten zeigte deutliche pathologische Veränderungen: der Hämoglobinwert lag signifikant niedriger als bei normalen Ratten (10,6g-% gegenüber 13,2 g-%; $P < 0,005$!), und im Differentialblutbild fanden sich zahlreiche unreife Zellen der myeloischen Reihe sowie lymphocytäre Reizformen. Im Knochenmark lagen Zeichen einer toxischen Schädigung vor. Enzymhistochemisch

(alkalische Phosphatase, Esterase, ATP-ase) fanden sich an Blut- und Knochen-
markszellen keine Auffälligkeiten.

Das gleichsinnige Verhalten der leberfunktionsabhängigen Serumenzymaktivitäten bei Patienten mit Porphyria cutanea tarda und bei Ratten mit
toxischer hepatischer Porphyrie läßt sich als Hinweis dafür werten, daß in beiden
Fällen eine ähnliche Leberstoffwechselstörung vorliegt. Die Verschiedenheiten
im Verhalten der LDH und SDH liegen nur in der prozentualen Aktivitätssteigerung, was sich auf die unterschiedliche Akuität der beiden Prozesse zurückführen
läßt. Diese Annahme findet sich durch die hämatologischen Befunde bestätigt:
bei den Patienten mit Porphyria cutanea tarda liegt ein normales Blutbild und
Knochenmark vor, während bei den Ratten mit toxischer hepatischer Porphyrie
deutliche, auf ein akutes toxisches Geschehen hinweisende Veränderungen im
strömenden Blut und im Knochenmark bestehen.

Zusammenfassend läßt sich aussagen, daß die Hexachlorbenzolporphyrie der
Ratte hinsichtlich der *Art* der Leberstoffwechselstörung ein gut geeignetes Modell
für die Porphyria cutanea tarda des Menschen darstellt. Bezüglich der *Akuität*
der Leberstoffwechselstörung unterscheiden sich die beiden verglichenen hepatischen Porphyrien ganz wesentlich voneinander. Diese Tatsache sollte bei Übertragung der am Versuchsmodell gewonnenen Ergebnisse Berücksichtigung finden.

Literatur. 1. PIETSCHMANN, H., W. RAAB und O. HARTL: Wien. Z. inn. Med. **47**, 349
(1966). — 2. OCKNER, R. K., and R. SCHMID: Nature (Lond.) **189**, 499 (1961).

Interessante, bei den an bullösen Dermatosen leidenden Kranken erhobene hämatologische und gastroenterologische Befunde

V. ROZSÍVALOVÁ, F. MATĚJA, B. FIXA und O. KOMÁRKOVÁ, Univ.-Hautklinik
Hradec Králové (Tschechoslowakei)

Ein zufälligerweise bei einer Pemphigoidkranken festgestelltes pathologisches
Myelogramm führte zur Untersuchung einer größeren Krankenzahl. Gleichzeitig
versuchten wir, die Ursache der festgestellten Änderungen unter Benutzung weiterer Untersuchungsmethoden zu erklären.

Material und Methodik

Wir untersuchten 36 Kranke (davon 14 Fälle von M. Duhring, 14 Pemphigoid- und
8 Pemphigusfälle). Es wurden folgende Untersuchungen durchgeführt: Untersuchung des
Sternalpunktates, elektrophoretische und immunoelektrophoretische Analyse der Bluteiweiß-
stoffe, 2stündige Analyse des Magensaftes mit 0,5 mg Histaminchlorid, Magenbiopsie mittels
einer bioptischen Saugsonde, Schilling-Test mit Vitamin B_{12} ^{58}Co.

Tabelle 1. *Immunoelektrophoretische Analyse der Bluteiweißkörper*

	Morbus Duhring	Pemphigoid	Pemphigus
Vermehrung sämtlicher Immunoglobuline	2	4	—
Defizit sämtlicher Immunoglobuline	1	—	—
Defizit IgM	6	2	5
Defizit IgA	7	3	5
Normal	—	2	2

Tabelle 2

	Hämomyelogramm		Magensaft		Magenbiopsie			Schilling-Test	
	P	N	P*	N	P		N	P	N
	A	B			AG	SG		< 10%	> 10%
Morbus Duhring	8	7	—	7	2	5	1	3	8	6
Pemphigoid	8	7	3	8	2	4	1	3	3	5
Pemphigus	3	3	2	7	1	2	2	2	—	2
Summe	19	17	5	22	5	11	4	8	11	13

Erläuterungen: A: Vermehrung der roten Reihe. B: Vermehrung der Lymphoreticulären Reihe mit Eosinophilie. AG: Atrophische Gastritis mit ev. Darmmetaplasie. SG: Oberflächengastritis. P*: Erniedrigte Werte der HCL-Ausscheidung entweder die histaminores. Achlorhydrie.

Diskussion

Von 36 an bullösen Dermatosen leidenden Kranken wurde bei 19 eine Vermehrung der Erythropoese mit megaloblastoiden Elementen und mit einer Linksverschiebung festgestellt (davon achtmal bei M. Duhring, achtmal beim Pemphigoid und dreimal beim Pemphigus, Tab. 2). Bei den meisten Kranken wurden histaminoresistente Achlorhydrie, eventuell eine verminderte Gesamtausscheidung von HCl, atrophische Gastritis, eventuell auch mit einer intestinalen Metaplasie der Magenschleimhaut, sowie auch herabgesetzte Werte des Schilling-Testes festgestellt. Es war keine Differenz zwischen den behandelten und nicht behandelten Kranken zu beobachten. Ein größerer Unterschied dürfte sich bei den an M. Duhring leidenden Kranken ergeben. In dieser Gruppe wurde atrophische Gastritis in 42% gegenüber 25,5% der Kontrollgruppe festgestellt. Bei der statistischen Auswertung müßte eine größere Krankengruppe untersucht werden. Der gleichzeitige Befund von Achlorhydrie, atrophischer Gastritis sowie einer Vitamin B 12-Resorptionsstörung wird nunmehr als ein präperniziöser Zustand angesehen. Wir können daher entsprechend unseren Ergebnissen darauf schließen, daß die bei unseren Kranken festgestellten pathologischen Myelogramme mit der primären Läsion der Magenschleimhaut, und zwar mit der atrophischen Gastritis, die zu der histaminoresistenten Achlorhydrie und Resorptionsstörung des Vitamin B 12 führt, zusammenhängen. Durch die erwähnte Beobachtung werden die in einigen Arbeiten wiederholt beschriebenen gleichzeitigen pathologischen Befunde des gastrointestinalen Traktes, insbesondere der Schleimhaut, deren Folge eine Resorptionsstörung ist, bestätigt.

Das Eiweißspektrum wurde mit der Papierelektrophorese verfolgt, die erhobenen Befunde erwiesen sich als vollkommen uncharakteristisch. Zu einer näheren Analyse hauptsächlich der Immunoglobulingruppe wurde auch die immunoelektrophoretische Analyse durchgeführt (Tab. 1). Bei den meisten Kranken wurde ein Defizit von sowohl IgA- als auch von IgM-Globulinen gleichzeitig oder isoliert festgestellt. Bei sechs Kranken wurde eine Vermehrung, bei einem Kranken ein Defizit sämtlicher Immunoglobuline festgestellt. Bei vier Kranken wurden normale Befunde erhoben. Die Befunde sehen wir als vollkommen uncharakteristisch für einige der untersuchten Erkrankungen an.

The Treatment of Porphyria Cutanea Tarda by Chelation

G. A. HUNTER and G. F. DONALD, Adelaide (South Australia)

PETERS (1957) reported favourable results in cases of acute intermittent porphyria treated by chelation with sodium calciumedetate. When our biochemists brought this to our notice, we began a trial of this treatment in cases of porphyria cutanea tarda. Since 1960 we have treated most of our cases of cutaneous porphyria by this method and our biochemists have extensively investigated these patients before, during, and after treatment, in an attempt to explain the effectiveness of this treatment (ROMAN, 1967).

In the past 8 years 34 patients with cutaneous porphyria have been seen in South Australia, which has a population of just over one million, so that not less than one person in 30,000 suffers from cutaneous porphyria. The incidence may in fact be much higher, as these cases are being recognised at an increasing rate as clinicians other than our dermatological colleagues become increasingly aware of the condition. Six (18%) of our 34 patients were born in Poland; five more (15%) in adjacent areas of Eastern Europe. 0.72% of the population of South Australia were born in Poland, and just under 2.0% in Poland and adjacent Eastern Europe. This suggests a high comparative incidence of cutaneous porphyria amongst Slavonic peoples who have come to our sunny climate.

25 of our 34 patients have been treated by chelation with sodium calciumedetate. At first we treated our patients by intravenous infusions, followed by oral maintenance therapy. Recently we have relied mainly on oral therapy alone, and the results have still been good in most cases. We would now reserve intravenous therapy for cases failing to respond to adequate oral dosage and for the commencement of treatment in patients showing very high urinary porphyrin excretions.

Oral doses have been about 4 g daily, increasing to maximum tolerated doses when response has been slow, and reducing as the skin lesions cleared. Diarrhoea has been the limiting factor in oral dosage, but has been the only toxic effect. Doses as high as 12 g daily have been tolerated. Doses of only 2 g daily have not been tolerated in a few cases and at this dose the treatment has usually been ineffective. Intravenously we have given 4 g to 8 g daily for 5 days, divided in two daily infusions, and no toxic effects were seen.

Clinically it was soon evident that although all patients obtained some benefit with treatment, the most dramatic improvement was seen in cases with sclerodermiform lesions, the more common bullous cases showing a slower response.

Biochemically our patients have shown high pretreatment excretion of both uroporphyrin and coproporphyrin in the urine, contrary to the usual statement that only uroporphyrin excretion is raised in porphyria cutanea tarda.

Large rises in excretion of uroporphyrin, coproporphyrin and zinc in the urine, were produced by intravenous chelation, also high serum zinc levels. The significance of zinc levels requires further investigation.

Patients with initial levels of urinary porphyrins not over ten times normal usually responded very well. Most of the cases with sclerodermiform lesions were in this range. The cases with very high porphyrin excretions, up to 50 or 100 times normal responded slowly. There was, however no strict correlation between initial urine levels and clinical response, nor did we find any fixed level above which symptoms occurred and below which they did not.

STATHERS (1966) has reported good results from cholestyramine treatment in cutaneous porphyria, again the most dramatic effects being in sclerodermiform cases. Cholestyramine binds porphyrins in the bowel, but this does not account for the marked rise in urinary excretion of porphyrins it produces in these cases.

The only two cases we have so far treated with cholestyramine confirm its usefulness. It is a much more expensive drug than sodium calciumedetate, and we still regard oral sodium calciumedetate as our first line of treatment in porphyria cutanea tarda. Cholestyramine offers an alternative in those cases which are unable to tolerate oral edetate or who may fail to respond completely after adequate trial of this treatment.

References. DONALD, G. F., G. A. HUNTER, and A. E. J. TAYLOR: Aust. J. Derm. 8, 97 (1965). — ROMAN, W.: Enzymologia **32**, 37 (1967). — STATHERS, G.: Lancet **1966**, **2**, 780.

Toxic Epidermal Necrolysis

M. B. LEWIS, Sydney (Australia)

In 1956, LANG and WALKER described an unusual bullous eruption followed by desquamation and death. LYELL, in the same year, reported four similar cases. All instances described a clinical resemblance to scalding, skin tenderness, pain, disinclination to move the limbs followed by vesiculation and on recovery, healing without scarring. Since 1956, POTTER, AUERBACH and LORINCZ, BAIRD and REICHELDERFER have provided further communications on this unusual syndrome. In early reports, death occurred in many instances. This paper deals with a report of eight infants treated at the Royal Alexandra Hospital for Children, Sydney, Australia, varying in age from 7 weeks to 10 years. A full description of a typical case is as follows:

A male child, aged 2 years, was admitted with the following history. 10 days prior to admission, he was treated for Impetigo with Mysteclin V. and Neosporin. 3 days prior to admission, blistering had occurred on the face. This was treated with Tetracyclines. When examined, he exhibited acute erythema of the face, with flaccid bullae occurring over large areas of both cheeks. At the same time, although there was no general erythema of the skin, marked local general tenderness of the body was evident. The following day, a generalised erythema occurred within the tender areas. Gradually, the temperature rose to 38.4 °C with gross desquamation and large areas of denuded epithelium, leaving raw, tender areas. Irritation and pain on handling was gross. Treatment with Solucortef 550 mg, Prednisone 10 mg was given and Chloromycetin 125 mg sixth hourly. The child was treated as for burns with open therapy. No clothes under a bed cradle. Haemotological examination was normal and swabbings of the skin showed no pathogenic bacteria. Gradually the erythema spread from the face to cover the entire trunk and both upper and lower limbs were affected. In daily examinations, the skin came away in folds. Nikolsky's sign was present. After several days of gross toxicity during which the temperature rose to 40 °C, the pyrexia and toxicity slowly abated. The child made a slow but uneventful recovery.

The general features of all cases showed a marked clinical resemblance to scalding. Toxicity was constantly present. Nikolsky's sign was evident in all instances. Desquamation of the glabrous skin included the entire trunk and limbs in some cases, pyrexia with purulent conjunctivitis and extreme distress on movement was invariably found. Skin swabbings, haemotology, X-rays and microurine examinations were inconclusive.

In all case histories, with one exception, drug ingestion was noted from 3 days to 2 weeks prior to onset. In the 7 weeks old child, the mother was given Penicillin for a tonsillitis whilst breast feeding. In two children, there is a history of sunlight exposure prior to onset. All children survived except one case; a ninth child, aged 3 days, reported to me since this paper was written.

Treatment: This was varied, in most instances of acute severe toxicity, Prednisone or Solucortef was administered. The use of Telfa (polythene) was most useful in nursing. The local use of simple emollients, extreme care in handling, Barrier nursing as in the treatment of burns and antibiotics is recommended.

Etiology: This has not been established but it may represent an unusual hypersensitivity to drug, bacterial viral or immunisation factors.

Micro-pathology revealed these features: A detachment of the epidermis at the dermo-epidermal junction. Diffuse separation of the stratum corneum along the planes of cleavage, necrosis of the epidermal cells and acantholysis. WOLF states that a review of the literature revealed that only 50% of biopsied cases showed epidermal necrosis, also the combination of epidermal necrosis and dermo-epidermal cleavage seems to be a poor prognostic sign.

Differential diagnosis: LYELL states that the primary difference between toxic epidermal necrolysis, erythema multiforme, dermatitis herpetiformis and pemphigus vulgaris is that in the latter conditions definite dermal inflammatory changes are present. These are absent or minimal in toxic epidermal necrolysis. In some cases, acute semi-purulent reaction of eyes and mouth simulated Steven Johnson's syndrome. However, the ano-genital area was not affected.

References. BAIRD, R., and T. E. REICHELDERFER: Clin. Paediat. **2**, 16 (1963). — BEARE, M.: Arch. Derm. **86**, 638 (1962). — LANG, R., and J. WALKER: S. Afr. med. J. **30**, 97 (1956); **31**, 713 (1957). — LYELL, A.: Brit. J. Derm. **68**, 355 (1956). — POTTER, B., R. AUERBACH, and A. LORINCZ: Arch. Derm. **82**, 903 (1960). — WOLF, R. L.: Med. Tms. (N.Y.)**93**, 1350 (1965).

Acute Epidermal Necrolysis (Ritter-Lyell) The Scalded Skin Syndrome

P. J. KOBLENZER, The Children's Hospital of Philadelphia, Philadelphia, Pennsylvania (USA)

Historical. In July 1868 — 99 years ago — Professor VON RITTERSHAIN at the Foundling Institute in Prague saw his first case of dermatitis exfoliativa neonatorum — 10 years later he had seen 297 of them and published a report on his findings. His clinical description bears the hallmark of the great age of clinical observation and could not be bettered. He describes the onset as a circumscribed, harmless looking perioral erythema, followed by exudative lesions and crusting, as well as rhagades of the vermillion border. This is followed by loosening of the epidermis, without circumscribed bulla formation. The loosened epidermis peels off easily, denuding extensive areas of the body surface. "The suspicion of scalding is a very reasonable one". He and later authors describe a few deviations from this picture. He took a rigid stand on his belief that the disorder was confined to neonates and it was left to later authors to moot the possibility that the condition might occur in older children also. In 1957 Lyell published his well-known paper Toxic Epidermal Necrolysis: An eruption resembling scalding of the skin, and by now close on 200 similar cases have been reported. In 1955 the author saw a case of Ritters disease and in 1958 his first two cases of Lyell's syndrome. He was immediately struck by the similarity and in 1961 Frain-Bell and Koblenzer describing six cases of Toxic Epidermal Necrolysis mooted the possibility of the identity of Ritters disease and Lyell's syndrome. Since that paper the author has collected data on a further ten cases ranging in age from 1 month to 8 years occurring in a 3 year period at The Children's Hospital of Philadelphia. In addition, post mortem material from an epidemic of Ritters disease has been reviewed and data have been garnered from the extensive literature on both conditions.

Clinical Material. The author's cases fell into two distinct groups. In seven of them the disease was the reason for admission and the course was short, benign and absolutely characteristic displaying in turn all the phases described by RITTER. Three others developed the condition whilst under therapy and in hospital already. All three ended fatally and the evolution was atypical. One patient, a neonate suffering from hydrocephalus and other associated abnormalities, developed the condition following extensive surgery. Staphylococcus aureus was at no time recovered from any cultures.

In two other cases there was reasonable suspicion of extensive virus infection. One of them proved to be suffering from cytomegalic inclusion body disease and died within 24 h of the onset of generalized exfoliation at the age of 1 month. The other presented with extensive ulceration of the oral mucous membranes and wide spread cutaneous petechiae. A throat culture grew coagulase positive hemolytic staphylococcus aureus. Exfoliation was followed by death in 48 h. Post mortem examination showed ulceration of the esophagus, trachea and cardia of the stomach in addition to the oral mucosa. Extensive focal hepatic necrosis was also found. There is some histopathologic evidence of the presemce of a viral infection — possibly herpes simplex. Deviant cases such as this are frequently found in the literature of Ritters disease — particularly with involvement of mucous membranes.

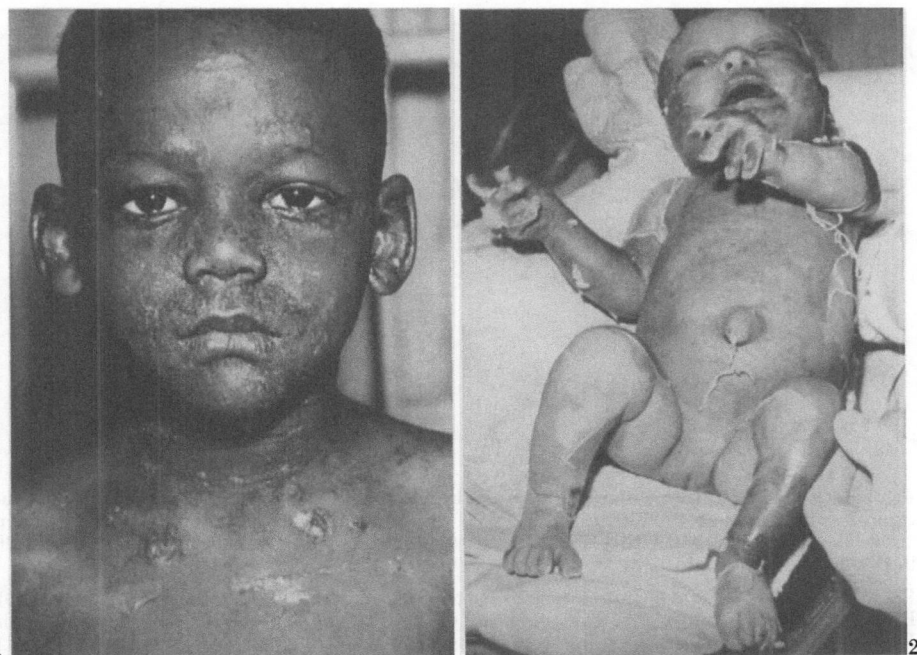

1   2

Fig. 1. Classical early lesions in acute epidermal necrolysis. There is periorbital and perioral crusting and rhadages of the vermillion border. Note the positive Nikolsky sign on the upper chest

Fig. 2. Severe involvement in a month old infant showing generalized exfoliation. The evolution was atypical and periorificial involvement was much less marked. The resemblance to scalding is very striking here

Pathology: Examination of many biopsies and post mortem material from Lyell's syndrome and Ritter's disease have left the author in no doubt that the changes seen are specific, characteristic and identical in the two conditions. They consist in essence in a reversal of the tinctorical properties of the stratum corneum and the affected parts of the stratum malpighii when stained with hematoxylin and eosin. A line of cleavage of varing depth but appearing as low as the dermo-epidermal junction separates affected from unaffected stratum malpighii. Only the former stains eosinophile. Initial lysis and pyknosis of nuclei is followed by a parakeratosis like change. The stratum corneum usually takes up a basophilic stain. The dermis is essentially unaffected, though two cases showed dilatation of the papillary capillaries and even extravasation of red blood cells. The upper $^1/_3$ of the hair follicles is similarly affected, but eccrine sweat ducts are spared. The bullae formed by separation of the necrotic layer are usually empty, though occasional acantholytic cells are seen. Material from cases of Ritter's disease showed identical changes.

Etiology: RITTER in his unique series could not find a shred of evidence that the disease might be engendered by some form of contagion. Since the beginning of the present century, however, incontrovertible evidence of staphylococcal etiology, specifically those belonging to Phage group two has become available. It is of outstanding interest that the same organisms have lately also been found in Lyell's syndrome including two cases in the authors own series.

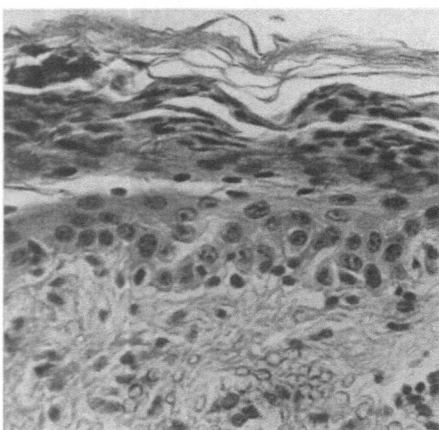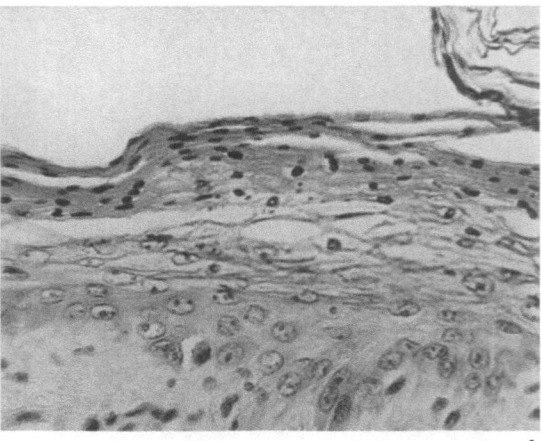

a   b

Fig. 3a. Case from author's own series. Hematoxylin and Eosin x 430. The section shows the typical appearance at 48 h after onset. Note deep staining and parakeratosis in the layer, above the transepidermal separation. The vascular ectasia and extravasation of red blood cells in the dermis are atypical

Fig. 3b. Autopsy specimen from a case of Ritters Disease (LEE, H. F., et al., J. Ped. 41, 159). Hematoxylin and Eosin x 430. The epidermal changes resemble in every respect those seen in Fig. 3a. Dermal changes are typically trivial in this case

In many cases of both Ritter's and Lyell's syndrome, however, a meticulous search failed to reveal any organism. In some of these good evidence exists that this may be a form of drug sensitivity. Recurrence of the syndrome following re-exposure to an offending drug would seem to provide irrefutable evidence in support of this hypothesis. In the authors series viral infection might also have played a part in at least two cases.

The condition then would appear to be a multietiologic symptom complex not confined to any age group. Infection with Phage group two staphylococcus aureus may well be the predominating etiologic factor in infancy and childhood. Drug sensitivity seems a frequent cause in the older age group.

The identity of Ritter's disease and Lyell's syndrome: In view of the identical clinical and histopathologic picture and the similarity of the etiologic factors it would appear reasonable to assume that Ritter's disease and Lyell's syndrome are identical, and the author proposes that the united syndrome be called acute epidermal necrolysis (RITTER-LYELL).

Reference. KOBLENZER, P. J.: Arch. Derm. **95**, 596 (1967). This contains all the references alluded to in this article.

The Ultrastructure of Acantholysis in Lichen Planus

L. Fry and F. R. Johnson, The London Hospital, London (Great Britain)

The aetiology of lichen planus is unknown and there has been very little fundamental work on the ultrastructural changes in this disease. In this investigation 1200 electron micrographs from 11 patients with lichen planus have been studied in different stages of the disease process. It was considered that the initial pathology was most likely to be in the stratum basale and/or the stratum spinosum and this report describes our findings in these layers.

In the early stages of the disease process there was slight dilatation of the intercellular space, and this increased progressively in the intermediate and late stages. As the intercellular space became more dilated the number of finger-like processes and desmosomes of the keratinocytes progressively decreased. In the initial stages of the breakdown of a desmosome there was a decrease in the density of the intercellular material and of the dense intermediate layer which bisects it. The tonofibril masses associated with the disintegrating desmosomes were less dense and contained fewer tonofilaments. The dense plaques of the desmosome, applied to the inner leaflet of the plasma membrane, were also less dense. It appeared that not all the desmosomes of any one cell underwent these degenerative changes simultaneously. Many desmosomes appeared structurally normal although there was a decrease in their total number.

The tonofibrils lost their orderly arrangement and distribution. They showed a progressive decrease in number and electron density. These changes were related to the dilatation of the intercellular space, loss of desmosomes, and loss of finger-like process. In the late stages all the desmosomes and tonofibrils had disappeared and the contour of the cells had a smooth appearance. In addition to the changes in the stratum basale and stratum spinosum breaks and reduplication of the basal lamina were frequently found.

These changes are similar to those reported in pemphigus vulgaris, but without detailed studies based on known time sequences it is not possible to be certain whether the initial changes occurred in the intercellular space, in the cell connections, or within the cell.

Two types of intranuclear structures were seen which were not present in the control material. The first was lamellar in appearance. In size it ranged from 260 to 1200 mμ. The second intranuclear structure was a membrane bound granular mass varying from 1200 to 1900 mμ. On morphological grounds alone neither of these structures could be considered to be viral in nature, but the second type was similar in structure to mycoplasma.

Mycobacterial Infections of the Skin

Infections mycobactériennes de la peau

Infecciones micobacterianas de la piel

Mykobakterielle Infektionen der Haut

Organizer

S. HELLERSTRÖM, Sweden

Presidents

L. M. BECHELLI, W. H. O. / O. M. S.

K. HIGUCHI, Japan

F. LATAPI, Mexico

I. B. SNEDDON, Great Britain

Delegate of the Organization Committee

P. JORDAN, Germany

Reports

Etude biologique récente dans la lèpre:
Analogies antigéniques et séro-diagnostic de la lèpre par immunofluorescence sur bacille de Stefansky

F.-P. Merklen et F. Cottenot, Hôpital St. Louis, Paris (France)

L'immunofluorescence révèle en microscopie de fluorescence l'antigène figuré, microbien ou non, sur lequel s'est fixé un anticorps spécifiquement correspondant auquel a été incorporé préalablement un fluorochrome. La technique dite indirecte, ou technique du sandwich, dépiste la fixation sur un antigène figuré d'un éventuel anticorps sérique par fixation secondaire de la fraction gamma-globulinique marquée par un fluorochrome d'un immunsérum antiglobulines humaines.

L'utilisation de ces techniques a permis de montrer sur des bacilles de Hansen de frottis spléniques l'existence d'anticorps sériques au cours de lèpres essentiellement lépromateuses (Morris et Audisio), existence que nous avons pu confirmer sur frottis de mucus nasal dans les sérums de formes tant lépromateuses que tuberculoïdes. L'immunofluorescence nous a permis de montrer l'existence d'analogies antigéniques entre bacille de Hansen, bacille de Calmette-Guérin et bacille de Stefansky de la lèpre murine, des frottis de l'un ou l'autre de ces bacilles permettant par réaction croisée de, dépister les anticorps sériques développés aussi bien dans la lèpre humaine que dans la lèpre murine, mais dans les seules tuberculoses cavitaires très évolutives (ce qui correspond à ce que l'on sait du développement d'anticorps circulants chez les tuberculeux).

La parenté antigénique entre bacilles de Hansen et de Stefansky permet de mettre facilement en évidence les anticorps circulants de la lèpre humaine et de procéder à leur étude quantitative sur un support antigénique qui n'est plus un bacille de Hansen d'origine diverse et de valeur antigénique variable, mais un bacille de Stefansky d'une même souche aisément entretenue sur l'animal et de constance antigénique plus satisfaisante. L'appréciation quantitative du taux d'anticorps est réalisée par dilutions successives des sérums étudiés.

Technique. Des frottis de bacilles de Stefansky, fixés 10 min dans l'acétone, sont recouverts du sérum à étudier aux dilutions successives de 1/8, 1/16, ... 1/1024. Après 20 min de contact, les frottis sont rincés abondamment à l'eau physiologique tamponnée à pH 7,2, puis recouverts de la fraction gamma-globulinique de l'immunsérum antiglobulines humaines conjuguées à l'isothiocyanate de fluorescéine. Après nouveau contact de 20 min, les lames sont rincées puis séchées. La lecture est faite en microscopie de fluorescence sur fond noir; les bacilles sur les lames positives apparaissent jaunes sur fond obscur et la dilution la plus élevée permettant encore de les voir donne le taux des anticorps. L'immunsérum antiglobulinique est obtenu à partir d'un pool de sérums de lapins immunisés avec des gamma-globulines humaines selon Kabath et Mayer. Sa fraction gamma-globulinique, précipitée par le sulfate d'ammonium, purifiée par dialyse, est redissoute en sérum physiologique à concentration de 12 à 13 mg de protéine par cc, puis conjuguée au sel de fluorescéine selon Nairn et enfin purifiée au charbon actif.

Résultats. La possibilité de fausses-négativités par phénomène de zone pour des sérums trop riches en anticorps a conduit à ne pratiquer ce séro-diagnostic *qu'avec des sérums dilués au $^1/_8$ et au-dessus.*

Totalement absente chez les 25 premiers témoins à réaction tuberculinique négative, une immunofluorescence sur bacille de Stefansky a été ultérieurement trouvée avec certains sérums apparemment normaux dilués à $^1/_2$, à $^1/_4$, voire même à $^1/_8$ et $^1/_{16}$; peuvent être en cause certains *facteurs non spécifiques de positivité,* ou *les réactions croisées avec une infection tuberculeuse latente.*

Des recherches d'anticorps sériques furent pratiquées sur 359 sérums provenant de 137 hanséniens et de 94 sujets suspects de lèpre. Le séro-diagnostic par immunofluorescence sur bacille de Stefansky semble de valeur certaine dans le diagnostic de la lèpre humaine.

Tous les sérums d'Hanséniens contenaient des taux élevés d'anticorps circulants, taux variables selon la forme de la lèpre et selon l'ancienneté et l'efficacité d'un traitement antihansénien : le taux des anticorps sériques décroît régulièrement à mesure que progresse l'amélioration biologique et clinique.

Les très fortes positivités observées dans les lèpres non antérieurement traitées, atteignant et dépassant généralement la dilution $^1/_{1024}$ dans les formes lépromateuses, $^1/_{512}$ dans les formes tuberculoïdes, restant encore de l'ordre de $^1/_{256}$ et de $^1/_{128}$ pour les lèpres lépromateuses négativées depuis 6 mois à 1 an et pour les lèpres tuberculoïdes blanchies récemment, conduisent à retenir comme *de valeur diagnostique certaine* les immunofluorescences encore positives pour les dilutions qui dépassent ou atteignent *le cent-vingt-huitième* ($^1/_{128}$),chiffre assez généralement atteint dans les formes indéterminées non traitées.

Les positivités-limites correspondant à des taux de dilution inférieurs au cent-vingt-huitième méritent d'être discutées et interprétées: il peut s'agir de lèpres anciennement traitées et blanchies, ou encore peut-être d'une contamination latente et non évolutive en pays d'endémie hansénienne; mais, en l'absence de traitement antihansénien antérieur, l'immunofluorescence semble *éliminer la possibilité d'un diagnostic initial de lèpre quand elle ne dépasse pas la dilution du huitième et même du seizième* du sérum étudié, tandis qu'une positivité limite à $^1/_{32}$ et même à $^1/_{64}$ ne semble pas permettre d'affirmer toujours avec certitude l'infection par le bacille de Hansen.

Las formas submicroscopicas del m. leprae

J. GAY PRIETO y G. GABINO, Escuela Profesional de Dermatologia y Venereologia, Madrid (España)

Desde 1963 hemos conseguido la transmisión en serie a la membrana corioalantoidea del embrion de pollo en el duodécimo día de su incubación de material procedente de distintas lesiones leprosas. Las lesiones pueden transmitirse en serie, utilizando la clásica técnica de inoculación en la membrana coriolantoidea de los virólogos y en algún caso hemos llegado al 14 pase.

Las lesiones macroscópicas se caracterizan por nódulos de 3 a 4 mm de diametro de color amarillento, ligeramente umbilicados en su centro. En los pases sucesivos estas lesiones son mas grandes y mas extensas. Los nódulos son iguales sea cual fuera el material inoculado inicialmente lepra lepromatosa con bacilos, lepra tuberculoide o indeterminada sin bacilos o material filtrado de lepromas.

Histológicamente los nódulos están formados por un denso acúmulo de células espumosas, vacuoladas, de aspecto histiocitoide. En la periferia desigualmente entremezcladas, aparecen células de aspecto linfoide y monocítico. Los vasos sanguineos están dilatados y repletos de los típicos hematíes de pollo, nucleados. Los infiltrados se disponen preferentemente en torno a estos vasos.

En los primeros pases con material procedente de lepra lepromatosa pueden observarse algunos bacilos acidorresistentes y a partir del tercer pase solamente gránulos acidorresistentes y algunos acúmulos de material parcialmente acidorresistente, que se tiñe en color rojopardusco con el método de Ziehl-Nielssen. A partir del 6° ó 7° pase la estructura lepromatoide con células espumosas vacuoladas, se va sustituyendo por células histioides de aspecto de fibrocitos, que recuerda las estructuras de los lepromas histiocitoides descritos por WADE. La ultraestructura de las lesiones alantoides se parece a la que se encuentra en la lepra lepromatosa humana. En las grandes zonas vacuoladas se observan figuras mielínicas, menos pronunciadas que las descritas en la lepra lepromatosa humana; las mitocondrias aparecen degeneradas y se forman lisosomas, en algunos de los cuales pueden verse restos bacilares. Estos citolisosomas, que parecen envueltos en una membrana, pueden contener restos de retículo endoplasmático, o restos de bacilos. A partir de 3° ó 4° pase aparecen unas formaciones, que nunca hemos observado fuera de las lesiones de lepra experimental, idénticas a las fotografiadas por CONVIT e IMAEDA en las lesiones leprosas experimentales del hámster. Son unos cuerpos ovalados de 500 Å a 1.000 Å, en los que claramente se percibe una membrana limitante, y en el interior, masas irregulares de diversa apetencia osmiófila. Para CONVIT e IMAEDA serían bacilos degenerados, porque el huésped no es favorable al desarrollo de típicas formas acidorresistentes.

En los primeros pases, pueden verse algunas formaciones bacilares típicas, en esta imagen aparecen en una invaginacion de protoplasma, que le da una falsa apariencia de situación intranuclear, un bacilo, con la característica zona clara, que corresponde a la cápsula cérea y encima del mismo una formacion lisosómica. En esta otra, se observa el protoplasma vacuolado de una típica célula espumosa en el que se ven formaciones idénticas, irregularmente esféricas u ovoides, claramente delimitadas por una doble membrana bien definida en la fotografía, en cuyo interior existen abundantes formaciones esféricas, mas densamente osmiófilas, en algunas de las cuales se adivina una zona periférica más clara y un nucleolo central mas densamente osmiofilo, que pudiera considerarse como formas L grandes. Al romperse la membrana de estas formas L grandes, liberan en el protoplasma unas partículas, que hemos bautizado con el nombre de "partículas virus like", en las que se percibe con mayor claridad una membrana o cápsula, una zona periférica mas clara y un nucléolo central intensamente osmiófilo, que tal vez correspondan a los "elementos bodies" o formas L pequeñas.

En otra imagen, procedente del quinto pase de una lepra lepromatosa se observan estas partículas "virus like", con su estructura típica, membrana limitante, una zona clara marginal y un nucleolo mas densamente osmiófilo. Existen algunas figuras mielínicas en forma de un filamento arrollado irregularmente en espiral.

No tenemos tiempo de ocuparnos de la ultraestructura de la lepra humana para lo que remitimos nuestros trabajos anteriores, únicamente queremos proyectarles a Vds una visión panorámica de una célula de Virchow, que muestra la notable alteracion de las mitocondrias que han perdido por completo las crestas y un globi de bacilo que estan yustapuestos al núcleo de una célula espumosa. La cubierta cérea de los bacilos "muerde" el límite del núcleo dándole un aspecto dentado. Aparentemente sobre el mismo, pero seguramente en realidad en una invaginacion protoplásmica, encontramos una formación, superponible a las que describíamos en la figura 6, correspondiente a las lesiones de alartoides, idénticas a las observadas en el hámster por CONVIT e IMAEDA.

En esta otra figura, puede observarse a gran aumento dos bacilos de Hansen que estan dividiéndose longitudinalmente y muestran la importancia de la cubierta cérea que es transparente electromicroscópicamente. En las microfotografias siguientes, procedente de una lepra tuberculoide sin bacilos, de solamente unas pocas semanas de existencia, se observan en la epidermis unas formaciones encapsuladas que recuerdan extraordinariamente las formas L grandes que hemos descrito en la lepra experimental. No es posible descartar completamente que se trate de gránulos de melanina completamente atípicos, aunque no recuerdan en absoluto ni su forma ni su estructura.

La falta de espacio nos impide extendernos en mas consideraciones. Creemos que la explicación de que el 80% de las formas de lepra no tienen bacilos se debe a que existe una forma no acidorresistente ni bacilar del bacilo de Hansen que probablemente tiene un ciclo evolutivo.

No puede sin embargo descartarse como lo prueban las recientes investigaciones del grupo de leprólogos de Cebú y las mas recientes del Profesor LANE BARSKDALE que se trate de unos gérmenes asociados al bacilo de Hansen y cuya presencia es imprescindible para el desarrollo del mismo.

Die gegenwärtige Epidemiologie und Bakteriologie der Hauttuberkulose in der Bundesrepublik Deutschland

F. EHRING, Fachklinik „Haus Hornheide" des Westfälischen Vereins für Krebs- und Lupusbekämpfung, Handorf bei Münster/Westfalen (Deutschland)

Welche Änderungen hat die Hauttuberkulose in den vergangenen Jahren durchgemacht? Neuerkrankungen werden kontinuierlich seltener. Dies gilt für alle Formen. Diese Abnahme betrifft besonders Kinder und Jugendliche. Im Gegensatz zu früher findet man bei ihnen kaum noch Tbc luposa und kaum noch Tuberkulose der peripheren Lymphknoten. Besonders stark zurückgegangen sind die exogenen Formen. Die hämatogenen und lymphogenen Formen haben heute das Übergewicht. So erkranken bei der Lymphknotentuberkulose die submandibulären Knoten heute nur noch selten. Sie gehören meist zu einem Primärkomplex. Relativ häufig geblieben ist die meist lymphogene oder hämatogene Tuberkulose in den caudalen Halspartien. Bei dieser Form sind häufig auch andere Lymphknotengruppen, Lunge und Knochen tuberkulös erkrankt [EHRING (1)].

Die Hauttuberkulose ist heute viel schneller zu heilen als früher. So ging vor allem bei der Tbc luposa die Zahl der aktiv Erkrankten noch wesentlich stärker zurück, als dem Rückgang der Neuerkrankungen entsprochen hätte. Nicht ganz so viel Gewinn brachten die modernen Behandlungsmethoden bei der Tuberkulose der peripheren Lymphknoten. Sie war schon früher dank der von BRÜGGER ausgearbeiteten Operationsmethode gut heilbar.

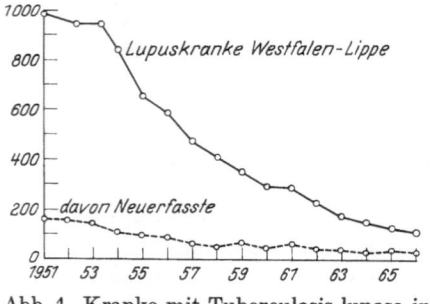

Abb. 1. Kranke mit Tuberculosis luposa in Westfalen-Lippe

Tabelle 1. *Neumeldungen in Westfalen-Lippe (7 Mill. Einwohner)*

Jahr der Meldung	Tuberculosis			
	luposa	verr.	indurat.	n. lymph.
1952—54	398	13	59	671
1955—57	242	17	38	548
1958—60	163	17	31	419
1961—63	136	10	29	383
1964—66	86	3	9	353
1952—66	1025	60	166	2374

Die Folgen der Hauttuberkulose sind heute viel weniger schwerwiegend als früher. Im westfälischen Krankengut fanden sich bei Tbc luposa Mutilationen und funktionelle Störungen 1935 bei 58%, 1950 bei 11%, 1963/65 nur noch bei 5% der neu erfaßten Kranken (BLEIDORN). Auch „Lupuscarcinome" sind heute viel seltener geworden.

Tab. 1 zeigt die Zahl der seit 1952 neu gemeldeten Kranken in Westfalen-Lippe. Der Rückgang ist evident, selbst wenn man berücksichtigt, daß heute vielleicht weniger Kranke gemeldet werden als früher. Hauttuberkulose und ihr Verdacht sind in der Bundesrepublik wie alle Tuberkulosen meldepflichtig. Westfalen-Lippe ist mit 7 Mill. Einwohnern der größte und der am längsten, schon seit 1927, vom sog. „Beauftragten für die Tuberkulose der Haut und hautnahen Lymphknoten" zentral überwachte Hauttuberkulosebezirk in Deutschland. Die Berichte aus den übrigen Bezirken, welche beim Zentralkomitee zur Bekämpfung der Tuberkulose von KALKOFF gesammelt werden, lassen grundsätzlich die gleiche Entwicklung erkennen.

Tab. 2 zeigt am gleichen Krankengut, daß die 1963/65 erfaßten Kranken oft erst als Erwachsene erkrankt sind. Die 1950 neu Gemeldeten waren dagegen zum großen Teil schon als Jugendliche von Tbc luposa befallen. Das Erkrankungsalter hat sich also zum Erwachsenen hin verschoben.

Tabelle 2. *Erkrankungsalter bei Tbc luposa*

Erkrankungs-alter	1950	1963/65
0—20	46 = 42,6%	9 = 15,8%
21—40	30 = 27,7%	24 = 42,1%
41—60	26 = 24,1%	14 = 24,6%
über 61	6 = 5,6%	10 = 17,5%
0 bis über 61	108	57
fehl. Ang.	41	1

Tabelle 3. *Erkrankungsalter an Halslymphknotentuberkulose*

Lebensalter	bis 30		ab 31	
Myco-bacterium	tuberc.	bov.	tuberc.	bov.
vor 1959	146	52	68	2
ab 1960	24	4	40	3

Tab. 3 zeigt den starken Rückgang der Halslymphknotentuberkulose und Tbc cutis colliquativa besonders bei Jugendlichen. Dies gilt für beide Erregerformen, besonders aber für das Mycobacterium bovis. Zugrunde gelegt sind der Tabelle 339 Kranke von 1963 Kranken mit Lymphknotentuberkulose der Klinik „Haus Hornheide", bei welchen der Erregernachweis gelang.

Die schnelle Heilbarkeit der Tbc luposa ergibt sich aus Abb. 1. Die Kurve der aktiv Erkrankten sinkt viel stärker ab als die der Neumeldungen. Betrachtet man die Tuberkulose der Haut und hautnahen Lymphknoten *bakteriologisch*, so fällt auf, daß das Mycobacterium bovis erheblich stärker zurückgegangen ist als das Mycobacterium tuberculosis. Bei Tbc luposa und verrucosa fanden sich bei den 1947 bis 1956 Erkrankten beide Mykobakterienarten noch etwa gleich häufig. Bei den 1957 bis 1966 Neuerkrankten fand sich das Mycobacterium bovis nur noch bei jedem vierten Kranken.

Noch stärker ist der Rückgang des Mycobacterium bovis bei der Tuberkulose der hautnahen Lymphknoten, wie Tab. 4 für das Krankengut von „Haus Hornheide" zeigt. Selten und nur bei Kindern fanden sich atypische Mykobakterien. Dort, wo Haut- und Lymphknotentuberkulose im Rahmen des Generalisationsstadiums erkrankten, liegt die tuberkulöse Erstinfektion oft um Jahre früher. Neuinfektionen mit Mycobacterium bovis sind heute noch viel seltener.

In der *Chemoresistenz* interessiert vor allem das Isoniazid. Hier ist eine Zunahme chemoresistenter Keime zu beobachten. Tab. 5 zeigt dies bei der Austestung mit 0,2 γ INH für die Tbc luposa und für die Lymphknotentuberkulose. Nach unseren Erfahrungen muß man aber auch schon bei einer Resistenz gegen 0,05 γ INH klinisch mit einem deutlich schlechteren Ansprechen rechnen. Etwa

20% der Keime waren in unserer Klinik 1966 gegen diese Konzentration bakteriologisch resistent.

Tabelle 4. *Lymphknotentuberkulose und Mykobakterienart*

Erkrankungs-jahr	Mycobacterium		
	tuberc.	bov.	atypic.
1952—56	97	36	—
1957—61	52	11	3
1962—66	47	5	1

Tabelle 5. *Resistenzzunahme gegen 0,2 Gamma-INH bei 265 bakteriologisch bestätigten Tuberkulosen*

Zahl der Untersuchungen	Tuberculosis	
	luposa	n. lymph.
1959—62	5%	2%
1963—66	13%	10%
Gesamtzahl	105	160

Tab. 6 und 7 zeigen die Restistenz bei Tbc luposa und Lymphknotentuberkulose gegen weitere Tuberkulostatika. Sehr häufig sind resistente Keime gegen
Äthioniamid, nicht ganz selten auch gegen Streptomycin. Fast vollkommen
fehlen sie gegen PAS und Conteben. Eine Zunahme der Resistenz gegenüber diesen
Tuberkulostaticis ist nicht eindeutig. Das Auffallende ist aber nicht die Zunahme
als solche. Erstaunlich ist, daß das Resistenzproblem bei der Hauttuberkulose
erst so spät auftaucht. Wahrscheinlich handelt es sich beim INH im wesentlichen
nur um eine Zunahme der *primären* Resistenz. Unter der Behandlung mit INH
konnten wir, wie SIMON u. BERENCSI in Ungarn, weder bei der Tbc luposa noch bei
der Tuberkulose der peripheren Lymphknoten ein Ansteigen der bakteriellen
Resistenz beobachten, wohl aber unter Streptomycin und Äthioniamid.

Tabelle 6. *Tbc luposa et verrucosa*

Medikament Dosis (Jahr der Untersuch.)	sensibel		resistent	
	tbc.	bov.	tbc.	bov.
INH 0,2 γ (1959—66)	52	42	3	8
Strepto. 5 γ (1959—66)	47	49	7	1
PAS 1 γ (1951—66)	110	64	3	8
Conteben 1 γ (1959—66)	52	50	3	0
Äthioniamid 10 γ (1962—66)	15	21	17	12

Tabelle 7. *Lymphknotentuberkulose*

Medikament Dosis (Jahr der Untersuch.)	sensibel		resistent	
	tbc.	bov.	tbc.	bov.
INH 0,2 γ (1959—66)	138	14	6	2
Strepto. 5 γ (1959—66)	124	16	17	0
PAS 1 γ (1959—66)	144	15	0	1
Conteben 1 γ (1959—66)	137	16	7	0
Äthioniamid 10 γ (1962—66)	32	3	24	2

Die bakteriologischen Untersuchungen verdanken wir in nun 15jähriger
Zusammenarbeit Frau Prof. Dr. MEISSNER vom Forschungsinstitut Borstel
(Direktor: Prof. Dr. Dr. E. FREERKSEN). Die Tabellen stützen sich auf das Krankengut von „Haus Hornheide". Dieser Wandel im Bild der Hauttuberkulose hat verschiedene Ursachen. Es gelang, in der BRD die Rindertuberkulose von 1951 bis
1961 von 40% auf 0,4% zu reduzieren (MEYN; EHRING u. PULICOTTIL). Dies ließ
die Tbc verrucosa und luposa bei Schlachtern und Tierärzten fast völlig wegfallen
und reduzierte die Neuerkrankungen bei Tbc luposa und Lymphknotentuberkulose.
Erheblich war der Einfluß der Chemotherapie. Sie begann 1947 mit den Thio-
semicarbazonen, dem späteren Conteben. KALKOFF konnte in „Haus Hornheide"
mit diesem Präparat 1947 eine schwere Tbc luposa und damit zum ersten Mal
eine Tuberkulose chemotherapeutisch heilen. Die Tbc luposa und verrucosa ge-

hören bis heute zu den Tuberkuloseformen, die besonders gut auf Chemotherapie ansprechen. Mit den weiter entwickelten Präparaten konnten dazu die Zahl der offen Lungentuberkulösen reduziert und so auch für die Hauttuberkulose viele Infektionsquellen verstopft werden. Ebenfalls von Bedeutung waren die Verbreitung der BCG-Schutzimpfung und die Hebung des Lebensstandardes in der BRD. Die zentrale Bekämpfung der Tuberkulose der Haut und hautnahen Lymphknoten durch Landesbeauftragte bewirkte, daß alle Fortschritte in der Therapie schnell dem Gros der Kranken zugute kamen. Diese Einrichtung, von STÜRMER 1927 in Westfalen geschaffen, wurde 1934 auf alle deutschen Länder ausgedehnt.

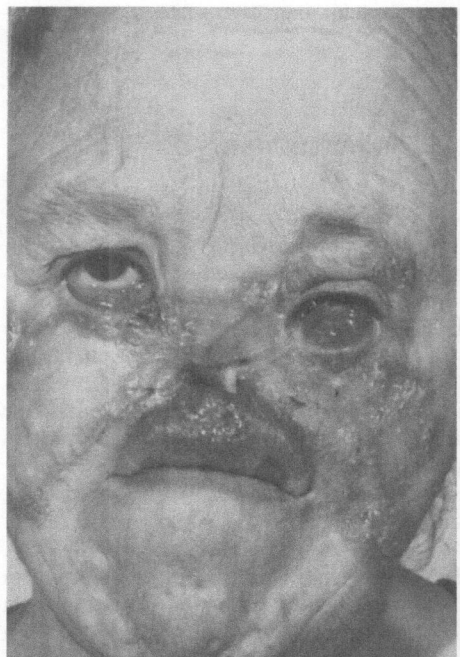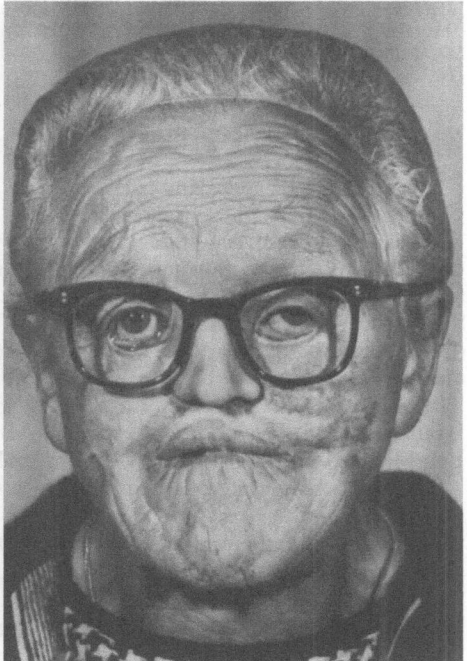

Abb. 2 und 3. F. K., vor der Behandlung und nach Wiederherstellung

Welchen Schwierigkeiten und Aufgaben steht die Bekämpfung der Hauttuberkulose heute gegenüber? Die Zunahme der Chemoresistenz gegen INH bedarf besonderer Beachtung. Am Anfang jeder Therapie sollte daher eine Resistenzbestimmung stehen. Bei Tbc luposa und sensiblen Keimen genügt nach wie vor die ambulante Monotherapie mit INH. Bei Sensibilitätsminderung und bei Lymphknotentuberkulose ist Kombination mehrerer Medikamente nötig, zusätzlich soweit eben möglich chirurgische Therapie. Es bleibt noch die Sorge um die alten Fälle. Viele Kranke haben aus der Zeit von 1940 Entstellungen und Röntgenschäden zurückbehalten. Sorgfältige Überwachung, wenn möglich plastische und epithetische Wiederherstellung und Ersatz der carcinomgefährdeten Haut machen derartige Menschen gesellschaftsfähig und vermeiden die Krebsgefahr. Das neue Bundessozialhilfegesetz schafft die finanzielle Basis, jedem Bedürftigen die Last seiner Krankheit zu erleichtern.

Abb. 2 und 3 zeigen eine Kranke mit Tbc luposa, nach der Literatur die erste chemotherapeutisch geheilte Tuberkulose vor der Behandlung mit TB I 698, dem späteren Conteben, und heute, wiederhergestellt.

Literatur. Bleidorn, H.: Inaug. Dissert., Münster (In Vorbereitung). — Brügger, H.:
Tuberkulose der peripheren Lymphknoten. In: Handbuch der Tuberkulose, IV, 57—109.
Stuttgart: Thieme 1964. — Ehring, F.: (1) Verhandlungsbericht der XXII. Dtsch. Tbc-Tag.
1966 (Im Druck); — (2) Dtsch. med. Wschr. 92, 62 (1967). — Ehring, F., u. H. J. Heite:
Tuberk.-Arzt 14, 487 (1960). — Ehring, F., u. M. Pulicottil: Prax. Pneumologie 20, 633
(1966). — Fabry, H.: Prax. Pneumologie 21, 35 (1967). — Kalkoff, K. W.: (1) Z. Haut- u.
Geschl.-Kr. 3, 280 (1947); — (2) Die Tuberkulose der Haut. Stuttgart: Thieme 1950; —
(3) Ergebn. ges. Tuberk.- u. Lung.-Forsch. XIII, 331 (1956). — Meissner, G.: (1) Tuberk.-
Arzt 15, 151 (1961); — (2) Beitr. Klin. Tuberk. 127, 170 (1963); — (3) Beitr. Klin. Tuberk.
132, 38, 82 (1965). — Meyn, A.: Mh. Tierheilk. 11, 71 (1962). — Meyer-Rohn, J.: Untersuchungen zur Chemotherapie der Hauttuberkulose. Stuttgart: Thieme 1956. — Moncorps, C.,
u. K. W. Kalkoff: Med. Klin. 42, (1947). — Proppe, A., u. G. Wagner: Z. Haut- u. Geschl.-
Kr. 21, 1 (1956). — Simon, W., u. C. Berencsi: Arch. klin. exp. Derm. 225, 123 (1966). —
Stühmer, A.: Strahlentherapie 35, 193 (1930).

Mykobakterienbefunde bei den sog. Tuberkuliden

N. Simon, Szeged (Ungarn)

Auf Grund der Arbeiten von Darier u. a. ist bekannt, daß die Tuberkulose in
der Haut über die mannigfachsten klinischen und histologischen Eigentümlich-
keiten verfügende Varianten hervorrufen kann, unter denen eine ganz besondere
Stelle die sog. Tuberkulide einnehmen. Diese wurden früher in jedem Falle als
durch hämatogene Streuung von Tuberkelbakterien ausgelöste Gewebsreaktionen
aufgefaßt. Heute wissen wir bereits, daß die Bezeichnung Tuberkulid eine Pro-
jektion vielfältiger und in ihrer Ätiologie verschiedener Erkrankungen auf der
Haut sein kann. Es ist auch bekannt, daß in Verbindung mit den Tuberkuliden das
Postulat Kochs heute keine Geltung mehr hat.

In einer früheren Arbeit haben wir zusammen mit Berencsi bereits mitgeteilt,
daß es uns gelang, aus den Läsionen der klassischen Krankheitsformen der Hauttuberkulose, dem Lupus, der Tuberculosis verrucosa, Mycobacterium tuberculosis,
allein mit Züchtungsmethoden in 75,3% Erreger nachzuweisen. Später versuchten
wir mit E. Szabó auch an einem größeren Tuberkulidkrankengut aus den einzelnen
Hautveränderungen die Tuberkelbakterien nachzuweisen, und zwar aus den
Läsionen von zwei Kranken mit histologisch identifizierter Tbc follicularis lichenoides, von 24 mit Tbc papulo-necrotica und 25 mit Tbc indurativa Bazin.

Zum Bakteriennachweis wurden möglichst die aus den frischesten Läsionen
stammenden Gewebsstückchen homogenisiert und die Homogenisate dann auf
Löwenstein-Jensen-Nährboden bzw. in Meerschweinchen verimpft. Die histologische Untersuchung der Gewebsschnitte erfolgte mit den Färbeverfahren von
Ziehl-Neelsen u. Aplas.

In den sich auf Jahre erstreckenden Untersuchungen konnten wir lediglich in
je einem Fall von Tbc indurativa Bazin und Darier-Roussy-Sarkoid ein positives
Züchtungsergebnis erhalten, aus den Hautläsionen von Tbc follicularis lichenoides
und Tbc papulo-necrotica konnten Tuberkelbakterien in keinem einzigen Falle
nachgewiesen werden. Die beiden positiven Züchtungsergebnisse zeigen, daß der
Nachweis der Tuberkelbakterien bei der Bazin-Krankheit vielleicht leichter
möglich ist und ferner, daß Gottron das Darier-Roussy-Sarkoid mit Recht der
Tbc indurativa zuzählte. Die Erklärung für die seltenen Bakterienfunde scheint
plausibel. Bei den Tuberkuliden erfolgen die sog. plauzibacillären Streuungen in
die bereits hyperergische Haut, und so wird verständlich, daß die in geringer Zahl
in die Haut gelangenden Tuberkelbakterien nach Letterer schnell peptisiert
werden. Positive bakterielle Befunde bei Tuberkuliden sind auch in der Literatur

ziemlich sporadisch erwähnt, und ein Teil derselben beruht nur auf histologischem Nachweis und nicht auf Kultur- oder Tierversuchen. Auf das Fehlen der Bakterien deutet z. B. bei der Bazin-Krankheit auch die Beobachtung hin, daß sich deren abscedierender Form nie der sog. Etagenlupus hinzugesellt. Die Antituberculotika sind auch meistens deshalb unwirksam, weil sie ausschließlich auf die lebenden Tuberkelbakterien wirken und einen direkten Effekt auf die tuberkulotischen Gewebe — wie wir in Modellversuchen nachwiesen — nicht besitzen.

In weiteren Versuchen haben wir den Nachweis der Tuberkelbakterien aus den Läsionen von 16 Lupus miliaris disseminatus- (im weiteren L.m.d.) Kranken versucht, deren klinische Symptome und Krankheitsverlauf wir seit Jahren kontinuierlich verfolgen. Überraschend war, daß es uns im Laufe langer Jahre nicht ein einziges Mal gelang — weder aus frischen, noch aus alten Papeln dieser Krankheit —, Tuberkelbakterien nachzuweisen.

Parallel mit den bakteriologischen Untersuchungen wurden bei sämtlichen Kranken auch diejenigen klinischen und Laboratoriumsuntersuchungen angestellt, die zur Bekräftigung — oder zum Ausschluß — der tuberkulotischen Genese der Krankheit nötig erscheinen.

L.m.d. wird heute in unseren meisten Hand- und Lehrbüchern als Folge der hämatogenen Streuung der Koch-Bacillen betrachtet, therapeutisch empfiehlt man — ebenso wie beim L. vulgaris — INH. Heute wird die tuberkulotische Herkunft der Erkrankung nur noch von wenigen, z. B. EHRING, bezweifelt, obzwar Literaturangaben über bakteriologische und pathogenetische Untersuchungen an einem größeren Krankengut nicht bekannt sind.

Wir haben die Erkrankung vorwiegend bei Männern im mittleren Alter mit gesundem Aussehen — seltener bei Frauen — beobachtet. Von unseren 16 Patienten wußten 15 nichts darüber, irgendwann an Tuberkulose gelitten zu haben. Bei keinem von ihnen wurde in der Lunge aktive Tbc gefunden, bei vieren fanden sich nur Spuren verkalkter Primärkomplexe. Kalkschatten in der Halsregion wurden nicht beobachtet. Während der langen Beobachtungszeit sahen wir kein einziges Mal, daß irgendeiner der Kranken an irgendeinem extrapulmonalen Prozeß gelitten hätte. Auch tuberculo-allergische Augensymptome — wie sie bekanntlich bei Tuberkuliden häufig sind — kamen bei keinem von ihnen zur Entstehung.

Die Tuberkulinempfindlichkeit der Kranken wurde wiederholt kontrolliert, und ferner mit Bencard-Antigenen nach Reaktionstypen gesucht, die für die L.m.d.-Krankheit charakteristisch sind. So hohe Tuberkulinempfindlichkeit bzw. hyperergische Reaktionen, wie sie bei zahlreichen Tuberkuliden vorkommen, haben wir bei unseren L.m.d.-Kranken in keinem einzigen Falle gesehen. Da ein beträchtlicher Teil der Bewohnerschaft tuberkulotische Infektionen durchgemacht hat, ist verständlich, daß wir bei 9 unserer 16 Patienten eine mittlere Mantoux-Reaktion erhielten, bei den übrigen 7 — d. h. in der anderen Hälfte der Fälle — fiel die Reaktion negativ aus. Eine derart hohe Mantoux-Negativität ist bei den Tuberkuliden unvorstellbar. In den Mantoux-positiven Fällen zeigte die Intensität der wiederholten Tuberkulinimpfungen später nur geringe Schwankunken, daher erscheint uns die Ansicht anderer Autoren über die sog. wechselnde Tuberkulinempfindlichkeit nicht erwiesen. Beim L.m.d. haben wir nach den Tuberkulinproben weder eine lokale Reaktion noch eine Dissemination der Papeln beobachtet. Die Westergreen-Werte wurden nie als pathologisch befunden, bei Tuberkuliden sind sie häufig erhöht.

Auf Grund unserer bisherigen klinischen und Laboratoriumsuntersuchungen glauben wir mit großer Wahrscheinlichkeit ausschließen zu dürfen, daß bei der überwiegenden Mehrheit der L.m.d.-Kranken den Tuberkelbakterien eine pathogenetische Rolle zukommt.

In einer früheren Mitteilung berichteten wir, daß in 15 bis 20% der Tuberkulide die tuberkulotischen Lymphknoten anamnestisch oder katamnestisch — mitunter zusammen mit anderen tuberkulotischen Erscheinungsformen — auffindbar sind. EBERHARTINGER fand ebenfalls bei 10 seiner 21 Bazin-Kranken verschiedene tuberkulotische Manifestationen vor, darunter in fünf Fällen Skrofuloderm. Beim L.m.d. gilt als literarische Rarität, wenn — sei es anamnestisch, sei es katamnestisch — einmal Skrofuloderm gefunden wird. Der Hamburger Dermatologe SCHULZ hat einen solchen Fall mitgeteilt. Wir sahen lediglich bei einem unserer 16 Patienten eine alte Skrofulodermnarbe. Aus den Papeln konnten — von einigen Staphylokokkenstämmen abgesehen — Krankheitserreger nicht ausgezüchtet werden. Die Ergebnisse unserer immunoelektrophoretischen Untersuchungen entbehren noch der Einheitlichkeit. In den histochemischen Untersuchungen wich die Aktivität einiger mitochondrialer Enzyme nicht von der des lupösen Gewebes ab. Elektronenmikroskopisch konnten wir in den Histiocyten des L.m.d. die erstmalig von APLAS beim Boeck-Sarkoid und von KALKOFF in den epitheloiden Zellen des lupösen Gewebes beschriebenen Cytosomen nachweisen.

Auf Grund einiger klinischer Beobachtungen messen wir gewissen Fokalinfektionen Bedeutung bei. Ein gutes Beispiel hierfür war ein Patient, in dessen Gesicht im Laufe der Jahre 16mal immer neue Schübe auftraten, und zwar stets ein paar Tage nach stattgehabten Mandelentzündungen.

Thalidomide in Lepra Reaction and in Hansen's Disease

J. SHESKIN, F. SAGHER and M. DORFMAN, Department of Dermatology and Venereology, Hadassah University Hospital and the affiliated Hospital for Hansen's Disease, Ministry of Health, Jerusalem (Israel) and
J. CONVIT, Department of Dermatology, Vargas University Hospital, Caracas (Venezuela)

Drugs used in the treatment of Hansen's disease are not effective in all patients. Moreover, some of the drugs cause anaemia and are capable of provoking a lepra-reaction or aggravating the existing one. Anti-reaction preparations of antimony may be toxic and long-term steroid therapy may cause side effects. In cases where pain is a prominent feature morphine must occasionally be added, and in neuritis perineural infiltration with novocaine.

All these problems stimulated the search for other effective anti-lepra-reaction drugs. In 1964 we tried out thalidomide in Israel in the lepra-reactions, attaining good results with dose of approximately 6 mg per kg of patient's weight. On this basis we made comparative trials with placebo. The results of the first trials can be seen in Tab. 1.

34 comparative trials were performed. In 22 lepra-reactions, where thalidomide was administered, either alone or with sulfones or sulfones and steroids, there was a rapid and sometimes dramatic regression. While in twelve reactions where placebo, with or without sulfone, was given, there was no alleviation of the symptoms whatsoever. In order to confirm these findings with a double-blind study on a larger number of patients, 173 trials were performed on 59 patients in Venezuela. The results obtained from this double-blind study were as follows:

Out of 85 reactions treated with thalidomide (Tab. 2) improvement was seen in 91.76% of cases and no change was found in 8.24%. No exacerbation of symptoms was seen. The following results were obtained in 88 reactions treated with a placebo: 27.26% showed an improvement, 50% had no change and 22.74% became worse. According to the law of probabilities, such a result could be due to coincidence, in only one case in more than a million. 105 biopsies were performed before and after treatment. In those patients where placebo was given, the histological picture remained invariable. However, where thalidomide has been given,

Table 1. *Immediate Effect of 34 Assorted Therapeutic Tests in 22 Lepra-Reactions*

Treatment	Number of Therapeutic Tests	Clinical Improvement within 48 h
Thalidomide alone	13	13
Thalidomide and DDS	8	8
Thalidomide and DDS and steroids	1	1
Total Thalidomide	22	22
Placebo alone	6	0
Placebo and DDS	6	0
Total Placebo	12	0

Table 2. *Comparison of Results of Treatment with Thalidomide and Placebo*

	Total		Improved		No change		Worsened	
	Number of Patients	%	Pat.	%	Pat.	%	Pat.	%
Thalidomide	85	100	78	91.76	7	8.24	0	0
Placebo	88	100	24	27.26	44	50	20	22.74

regression could be seen in the inflammatory infiltrate of the reactional lesion, but not in the leproma itself. Having seen the favourable clinical effect of thalidomide on lepra-reaction of the lepromatous leprosy type, we tried this drug in the disease itself. 24 patients received this drug alone, in doses of 200 to 400 mg/day, for periods of 3 to 19 months. The results can be seen in the following table:

Table 3. *Results of Treatment with Thalidomide in Hansen's Disease*

	Total Number of Patients	Improved	No change	Worsened
Clinical	24	5	8	11
Bacteriological	24	—	20	4
Immunological	24	—	24	—
Histological	24			

There was no change in the leproma component of the lesion; there was a reduction in the non specific inflammatory infiltrate.

Five patients showed an improvement and eight showed no change. In eleven patients the disease process became slightly worse. Bacteriological studies did not show any improvement, on the contrary, four patients turned positive. Immunological studies, including the Mitsuda test, did not show any change. Histological studies showed no change in the leproma component of the lesion;

however, there was a reduction in the non specific inflammatory infiltrate. Laboratory tests showed a tendency to normalization in the erythrocyte sedimentation rate and the leucocyte count. The liver function tests, erythrocyte count and urine constitution remained unchanged.

13 of the 24 patients showed an increase in weight of 3 to 15 kg. Various side effects were found; these include drowsiness, constipation, dryness of oral and nasal mucosa, unilateral peripheral edema, difficulty in erection and a vesicular or erythematous eruption. In most of the patients these symptoms, apart from constipation, became milder as treatment was continued.

As regards the dynamics of thalidomide, there are no definite conclusions yet. However, recent experiments suggest that it may have immuno-suppressive properties.

To conclude: thalidomide was found to be effective in lepra-reaction of the lepromatous type and disappointing in the dimorphous form. We had no opportunity of treating patients suffering from lepra-reaction in tuberculoid and indeterminate leprosy. In the treatment of Hansen's disease itself with thalidomide, no favourable results were seen in a therapeutical trial up to 19 months.

Thus, the combined administration of sulfone and thalidomide is being tried. This treatment, still in its early stages, seems to give promising results, especially in patients suffering from recurrent lepra-reactions, thus enabling to proceed with specific anti-leprosy treatment.

Free Communications

Geographical Distribution of Skin Tuberculosis, Leprosy and Sarcoidosis in Japan

K. KITAMURA, Tokyo Teishin Hospital, Tokyo (Japan)

Geographical distribution of skin tuberculosis in Japan, which was reported in the last Washington Congress 1962, is studied again, this time together with that of leprosy and sarcoidosis. For this it should be taken into consideration that Japan consists of a chain of islands extending from the northeast (45 °N, 145 °E) to the southwest (30 °N, 130 °E) and the climate varies considerably remarkably from the northern and cold to the southern and warm areas of the country in accordance with the descent of latitude. The average atmospheric temperature in eight cities representing one to one eight districts of the country ascends from the north to the south nearly gradually in such an order as 7.6 °C in Sapporo, 11.3 °C in Sendai, 14.7° C in Tokyo, 14.4 °C in Nagoya, 15.5 °C in Osaka, 14.7 °C in Hiroshima, 15.3 °C in Matsuyama and 15.7 °C in Kumamoto.

Statistics hitherto published from several dermatological university clinics indicate that the ratio of patients having *skin tuberculosis* to all patients as well as the frequency of *lupus vulgaris* among skin tuberculosis is generally higher in North Japan than in South Japan. This coincides with the generally affirmed more frequent occurrence of skin tuberculosis, especially of lupus vulgaris in the cold than in the warm areas of the world. The ratio of patients with skin tuberculosis to all patients is 0.92% in Sapporo in Hokkaido, the northernmost district of the country and 0.55 and 0.28% respectively in Fukuoka and Hurume, both in Kyushu, the southernmost district. The frequency of lupus vulgaris among skin tuberculosis is 35.8% in Sapporo, 5.3% in Fukuoka and 0.6% in Kurume. One thing to be pointed out here is that the frequency of *tuberculosis verrucosa cutis* among skin tuberculosis is contrary to that of lupus vulgaris much higher in South Japan than in North Japan, namely 20.0% in Fukuoka, 27.6% in Kurume and 8.8% in Sapporo. This leads us to such presumption that some climatic conditions in South Japan may probably have a part in the occurrence of this disease form, which is regarded as an inoculation tuberculosis and that — if we give further scope to our imagination — the same climatic conditions in South Japan also would play a rôle in the occurrence of *leprosy*, which is considered to develop by inoculation with lepra bacilli probably primarily in the skin. In fact, according to the examination made in 1960, 29,9% of all 9,937 leprosy patients received into eleven National and three private leprosaria is from Kyushu, the southernmost district of the country, while patients from each of other seven districts amount only 1.3 to 17.0%.

Sarcoidosis has become in Japan in recent years an object of general concern. As an etiologically not yet clarified, but independent systemic disease it is regarded now as having nothing to do with tuberculosis as well as with leprosy. The ratio of sarcoidosis patients per 100,000 population in each of eight districts of the country decreases from the north to the south from 1.25 in Hokkaido to 0.21 in Kyushu gradually and just contrary to the higher prevalence and mortality of pulmonary tuberculosis in South Japan than in North Japan. The ratio of all 700 sarcoidosis patients accumulated from the whole country up to the end of 1964 to the national population in 1960: 93,418,574 is 0.75 per 100,000.

All these coincidence and contradiction of geographical distribution observed among pulmonary and skin tuberculosis, especially lupus vulgaris and tuberculosis verrucosa cutis, leprosy and sarcoidosis are stated here merely as statistical facts. Further investigation should be made with due regard to the etiopathogenetic mechanism of each disease.

A propos des tuberculoses cutanées — leur classification, leur diagnostic biologique, leur traitement

M. Bolgert et P. L. Delaire, Hôpital St. Louis, Paris (France)

Il est classique depuis Darier (1896) de distinguer deux groupes de dermatoses tuberculeuses: les *tuberculoses cutanées dites vraies* et les *tuberculides*. Le premier, groupant ulcères, gommes, lupus et tuberculoses verruqueuses, est caractérisé par un aspect histologique spécifique, et la présence du bacille de Koch (décelé par examen direct, inoculation ou culture). Depuis les travaux de Civatte (1938) ne sont considérés comme appartenant légitimement au second groupe que le lichen scrofulosorum, l'acnitis de Barthélémy, les tuberculides papulo-nécrotiques et ulcéreuses, ainsi que certains érythèmes indurés et noueux. Histologiquement, ces dermatoses ont inconstamment un caractère tuberculoïde plus ou moins net; elles sont souvent banalement inflammatoires; on n'y décèle jamais le B.K. et leur nature n'est suspectée que par l'existence chez le malade d'antécédents tuberculeux ou de lésions extra-cutanées plus ou moins discrètes (pulmonaires, ganglionnaires, etc.). Darier soulignait l'action variable, curatrice ou aggravante des injections de tuberculine.

Nous avons montré dans des travaux antérieurs [1] que la conception de Darier ne se justifiait pas au triple point de vue bactériologique, histologique et pathogénique; de plus, les thérapeutiques antituberculeuses utilisées selon certaines règles, guérissent également les deux groupes de dermatoses. Aussi, nous paraît-il préférable de classer les tuberculoses cutanées de la façon suivante :

Tuberculose d'évolution caséeuse:

    1° Ulcéreuse   chaucre d'inoculation ; ulcère secondaire ; ulcère atypique
    2° Gommeuse   dermique (scrofuloderme) ; hypodermique ; lymphangitique
    3° Fongueuse et végétante

Tuberculose non caséeuse (Parfois nécrose ou caséification ébauchée) :

Tuberculoses dermiques	1. Structure épithélioïde		— lupus
		B.K. facile à mettre en évidence	— tuberculose verruqueuse
	2. Structure folliculaire nette ou ébauchée	B.K. difficile ou impossible à mettre en évidence	lichen scrofulosorum acnitis tuberculides papulonécrotiques ; tuberculoses dermiques ulcéreuses

Tuberculoses hypodermiques Erythème induré de Bazin,
                                   Erythème noueux tuberculeux.

Nous nous limiterons ici à rappeler les éléments de leur *diagnostic*, qui sont : 1° leur *aspect clinique* et l'existence inconstante de *signes généraux* («patraquerie» bacillaire de Burnand) ; 2° La fréquence des *antécédents* tuberculeux ; 3° La mise en évidence du *B.K.* : elle est, en fait, très rare dans les «tuberculides» ; 4° La *biopsie:* souvent assez évocatrice dans les tuberculides dermiques, elle l'est rarement dans les tuberculoses hypodermiques ; personnellement nous avions souligné [2] l'intérêt de la *répétition* des biopsies : après quelques semaines d'un traitement actif, les lésions primitives exsudatives banales prennent un aspect folliculaire, avant de s'effacer par la suite. 5° Les *arguments biologiques* sont de valeur inégale : formule sanguine sans intérêt ; vitesse de sédimentation variable, taux des antistreptolysines normal.

A la cuti-réaction tuberculinique, communément utilisée, souvent très positive, nous préférons *l'intradermo-réaction* (tuberculine IP 48 à trois unités) provoquant après 6 à 8 jours un nodule rouge de 5 mms de diamètre, parfois plus volumineux, pouvant reproduire en miniature les lésions spontanées, et s'accompagnant intconstamment de réactions focale et générale. Un signe de valeur, jusqu'ici méconnu, réside dans la *longue persistance* (parfois 1 à 2 mois) d'abord d'un nodule rosé, puis d'une macule érythémato-pigmentée.

Le *traitement* de la tuberculose cutanée, déjà transformée en ce qui concerne le lupus par la vitaminothérapie D 2 massive (Charpy) semble avoir reçu une solution définitive grâce aux antibiotiques antituberculeux majeurs : streptomycine, acide para-amino-salicylique (PAS) et isoniazide (I.N.H.). Mais, selon les périodes, les pays et les auteurs, ces médicaments furent utilisés de façon diverse, tantôt isolément, tantôt en association, soit entre eux, soit avec vitaminothérapie. La posologie et la durée du traitement furent généralement inférieures à celles conseillées par les phtisiologues. C'est ainsi que streptomycine et PAS, seuls ou associés, agissent favorablement dans les ulcères et les gommes, que l'I.N.H. détermina la guérison de nombreux lupus, mais dont certains récidivèrent. Dès 1955, il fut conseillé d'associer les trois antibiotiques et la vitaminothérapie (ACHTEN, HURIEZ) : des succès furent obtenus en proportion variable selon la forme de tuberculose. Depuis une dizaine d'années, nous considérons personnellement que l'association des trois antibiotiques majeurs peut guérir *toutes* les tuberculoses cutanées s'ils sont administrés à doses suffisantes pendant 18 mois à 2 ans ; l'adjonction de vitaminothérapie D 2 paraît préjudiciable.

Posologies: streptomycine pantothénique: trois injections hebdomadaires de 1 g, jusqu'à 50 à 80 g; isoniazide 10 à 15 mg/kg/jour, soit 600 mg à 900 mg par jour; PAS: 12 g par jour. Durant le premier mois: association des trois médicaments, puis I.N.H. et streptomycine, celle-ci relayée par PAS pendant 2 à 3 mois, puis I.N.H. seul. Ce schéma peut être modifié en cas d'intolérance mais l'un de nous dans sa thèse [3] a pu faire état de 37 tuberculoses, dont 15 lupus et 12 érythèmes indurés, revus après plusieurs années: 35 succès et deux échecs par traitement mal suivi.

Bibliographie. 1. BOLGERT, M., et G. LEVY: Sem. Hôp. Paris **30**, 1864 (1950). — BOLGERT, M.: Sem. Hôp. Paris **43**, 870 (1967). — 2. BOLGERT, M.: Bull. Soc. franç. Derm. Syph. **69**, 74 (1962). — 3. DELAIRE, P. L.: Thèse, Paris 1954.

Lupus Vulgaris Gigantea Caused by Mycobacterium Avium

J. V. CHRISTIANSEN, Department of Dermato-venerology, Marselisborg Hospital, University of Aarhus (Denmark)

Lupus vulgaris (l.v.) is now a rare disease in Denmark. Only few fresh cases are encountered. Mycobacterium humanum (M. humanum) is the organism which caused l.v. most frequently, but also cases caused by Mycobacterium bovinum (M. bovinum) are seen. In a series of 2903 cases of l.v. in which the tubercle bacillus was subjected to typing in 214 cases HORWITZ (1960) found 74% with M. humanum and 26% with M. bovinum. No cases of l.v. caused by Mycobacterium avium (M. avium) were identified.

In the following I will present an unusually great and resistent cases of l.v. caused by M. avium.

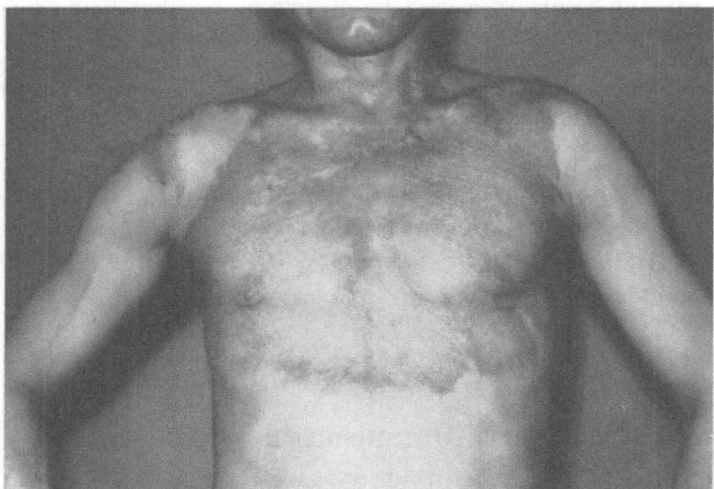

Fig. Lupus vulgaris

Case history

The patient, a farmer now 31 years old, has been followed for more than 10 years. In 1951, when he was 17 years old, he had an inflammation in the left clavicula, and Mycobacterium was proved by culture, but typing was not performed. Surgical treatment was followed by success.

In 1956 the patient was seen in the dermatological department for the first time. We found a typical l.v. over the left clavicula and manubrium sterni. The affected area was 70×45 mm. Characteristic granulomas of tuberculosis were found but Mycobacterium was then not proved. Treatment with isoniazid was started, but we lost contact with the patient after a month.

In 1958 the patient arrived again. The l.v. had grown to an area of 11×23 cm. Treatment with isoniazid was instituted again together with para-aminosalicylic acid (PAS). We also used the Finsen therapy, but a few months later the patient disappeared again.

In 1960 we saw the patient again. The l.v. area had now grown to 23×24 cm. The patient was taken into the ward for more than 6 months, and later followed in the clinic. In 1960 to 1961 he received a total amount of 190 g of isoniazid and 2000 g of PAS. Treatment with the Finsen method, streptomycin and calciferol was also attempted. Still all treatments were without convincing effect.

In 1961 a new skin biopsy was taken and now it was possible to find Mycobacterium, which proved to be M. avium, resistent to isoniazid, PAS and streptomycin. The culture and typing were performed by the department of pathology, University of Copenhagen. In addition the department of tuberculosis, Statens Seruminstitute, Copenhagen, also found M. avium in two different skin biosies taken in 1962 and 1965.

Since 1961 various further treatments had been tried, alone and in combinations. We have used different sulfonamids such as sulfathiazol and avlosufon. Also fucidin, cycloserin and erythromycin have been tried. In the last four months we have used a combination of cycloserin, erythromycin and rifamycin AMP (Ciba). In spite of this the affected area has still grown and the total area is in may 1967 about 2000 cm².

Tuberculin tests (Mantoux): 1. human tuberculin 1 TU: negative; 2. human tuberculin 10 TU: 12 mm; 3. avian tuberculin 5 TU: 15 mm; 4. xenopa tuberculin 5 TU: 18 mm; 5. scrofulaceum tuberculin 5 TU: 15 mm.

Roentgenograms: pulmones: calcified glands at hilus; columna: no processes; left clavicula: healed proces.

Examinations: SR 2 to 5 mm, Hb 90 to 95%; serumkreatinin 1.1 mg-%; serum-Ca: 4.2 to 4.8 meq/l.

Discussion

Infections caused by M. avium have until now been rather uncommon in Denmark. ENGBAEK (1964) has from 1935 to 1961 recorded the total number of registered cases in Denmark caused by M. avium, and has found nine patients with glandular tuberculosis and 15 cases with pulmonary processes. ENGBAEK (1964) writes: "The possibility of encountering avian tubercle bacilli is great in Denmark and the risk of both aerogenic, alimentary and contact infection exists. However, thanks to the high natural resistance of man to these bacteria, the number of manifest infections is small."

The present patient is the first case of lupus vulgaris in Denmark, and possibly in the world, caused by M. avium. All kinds of treatment have been without succes. The affected area has grown slowly for several years, but are now expanding more quickly. We are indeed most seriously worried as to the future of our patient.

References. HORWITZ, O.: Lupus vulgaris cutis in Denmark 1895—1954. Copenhagen 1960. — ENGBAEK, H. C.: Acta tuberc. scand. 44, 108 (1964).

Atypical Acid fast Micro-Organisms in Scleroderma

A. R. CANTWELL, E. CRAGGS, J. W. WILSON and F. SWATEK, Kaiser Hospital, Los Angeles, and Veterans Hospital, Long Beach, California (USA)

In recent years there has been increasing interest in the role of atypical mycobacteria in the production of human disease. The best known example is pulmonary "tuberculosis" due to *Mycobacterium kansasii*. Other reports, some of which have not been confirmed, implicate certain mycobacteria in the production of subcutaneous granulomas, panniculitis, skin ulcerations, bone and joint disease, blood disorders, and in collagen diseases.

We have been interested in searching for the presence of mycobacteria in the skin of patients with scleroderma. The first case report associating a mycobacterium in scleroderma was published by Wuerthele-Caspe Livingston in the United States in 1947. Delmotte in 1953 in Belgium reported nine additional cases in whom mycobacteria were demonstrated. The researchers in this field stress the extremely pleomorphic capabilities of the microbe, and emphasize that the agent has a "life cycle" which can *simulate* at certain stages micrococci, "diptheroids", intermittently acid-fast bacteria, and fungi resembling Nocardia. Some researchers also claim that the microbe has a "l" form and a virus-like phase.

In addition the organism may appear in tissue as "yeast-like" or "globoidal" forms.

Case 1. The first patient to be presented is a 37 year old Mexican man with scleroderma. He had had pulmonary tuberculosis 7 years prior to the development of his scleroderma. In addition to the typical sclerodermatous changes, he had multiple ulcerations of the trunk. Biopsy of the trunk lesions revealed scleroderma with non-specific ulceration. When carefully studied, smears of deep skin biopsy material revealed the presence of very rare acid-fast bacilli either in "granule" formation or singly. Fite-Faraco stained sections of these ulcerations showed rare acid-fast bacteria. Culture on LOWENSTEIN-JENSEN medium produced pin-point creamy colonies, which on smear, showed a peculiar Nocardia-like organism. Culture on blood agar revealed micrococcal-like forms with a tendency to produce true acid-fast bacilli. Peculiar yeast-like bodies were also noted in the panniculus underlying these ulcerations, which in our opinion are suggestive of the "globoidal" tissue forms described by LIVINGSTON. Several months before the patient's death, rare acid-fast bacilli, and numerous coccal forms of the organism were present in tissue section within the collagen bundles and within the endothelial wall of the blood vessels of the cutis. These findings were confirmed at the Carville Leprosarium in Louisiana. It is interesting to note that despite the past history of pulmonary tuberculosis and the presence of acid-fast bacilli in the lesions, the tuberculin test was not positive.

Case 2. The skin of a 33 year old Negro with typical skin changes of scleroderma was examined bacteriologically. A biopsy was taken from the forearm and also from the thigh, and careful study of smears revealed the presence of rare acid-fast bacteria. Culture from the forearm yielded orange-pigmented colonies in Lowenstein-Jensen medium which suggested *Nocardia*. Culture from the thigh yielded yellow colonies, more compatible with atypical mycobacteria. The patient was treated empirically with INH and PAS. Culture performed again 3 months later from the same areas revealed pin-point creamy colonies of bacilli, some of which were acid-fast. On another occasion the isolate resembled a non acid-fast bacterium with a tendency to filament like *Nocardia*. Dr. RUTH GORDON was unable to identify this organism precisely.

She did state that the microbe was compatible with a mycobacterium or a *Nocardia*, or a number of other genera. Careful review of Fite-Faraco stained sections revealed rare acid-fast bacteria. Some of the bacilli had a slight branching tendency in tissue.

Case 3. A 42 year old Caucasian man with typical scleroderma was also examined bacteriologically. Smears of skin biopsy material revealed very rare collections of acid-fast bacteria in "granular" formation. Culture was compatible with a mycobacterium. The species was undetermined. Stained sections showed several acid-fast bacteria which could be identified in the collagen.

It is hoped that these studies will stimulate others to undertake a thorough and painstaking bacteriologic investigation of the skin in scleroderma, in order to further clarify the precise cause of this disease of unknown etiology.

Nature of the Antigen Responsible for the Kveim Reaction in Sarcoidosis

R. Kooij and J. W. van Waveren Hogervorst, Department of Dermatology, Gemeenteziekenhuis, The Hague (Netherlands)

It has been shown that one can obtain sometimes positive "Kveim-reactions" in patients with sarcoidosis with suspensions of "normal" or at least with non-sarcoid tissue. Putkonen [1] has reported positive Kveim-reactions with a suspension of leukaemic lymphglands. Kooij [2] concluded in his paper on the third international conference on sarcoidosis that tissue breakdown products, which are both present in Kveim-antigen and other tissue suspensions, are chiefly responsible for the sarcoid reactions. This view finds support in an example out of the pathology, namely the occurrence of sarcoid reactions in regional lymphglands of malignant tumours. If this hypothesis is correct it might be possible to prepare a kind of Kveim-antigen from non-sarcoid tissue. This would have the advantage that the great drawback of the scarcity of Kveim-antigen could be overcome.

We are now trying to find the most suitable tissues to prepare such an antigen. Therefore many preparations have to be tested in human beings, which meets with practical difficulties. For this reason we have injected intracutaneously some preparations in guinea pigs and rabbits. In a few cases a sarcoid reaction comparable with a positive Kveim-reaction was evoked in a rabbit with a suspension of a non-sarcoid human spleen. With the same preparation occasionally a sarcoid reaction was obtained in a human being. With sarcoid reaction is meant a more or less nodulated granuloma of histiocytic-epithelioid cells with intermixture of round cells. We have also prepared preparations from animal tissues (spleen, liver) and obtained also in a few guinea pigs and rabbits a sarcoid reaction. Most of the cases however showed a non-sarcoid granuloma or nothing at all. With one animal spleen suspension we obtained a sarcoid reaction in a patient with a sarcoid cervical lymphnode of which a human tubercle bacillus was cultivated.

It was striking that some animals, especially one rabbit showed more often a sarcoid reaction on various preparations, than other animals. This rabbit had been injected very often with several tissue suspensions and also had at one time had intracutaneously Freund's adjuvant. Other animals which had been injected in the same way showed not or less frequently a sarcoid reaction. This points to some individual mode of reaction (terrain sarcoidique probably genetically determined just as in sarcoidosis). In the same rabbit a Kveim-antigen obtained from Putkonen evoked a granuloma resembling a positive Kveim-reaction. In a few cases we obtained with an intradermal injection of a mixture of a normal tissue suspension and Freund's adjuvant rather strong reactions in rabbits and guinea pigs.

The above results show that with homologeous and heterologeous tissues one can evoke in some human individuals and also in some animals a sarcoid reaction resembling a positive Kveim-reaction. The common tissue components of the tissue suspensions may act as antigen. It is now well known that tissue components, if sufficiently altered by infection, irradiation, or burn or by treatment with denaturating agents that they are regarded as foreign by the lymphatic apparatus, may induce a kind of autoimmunisation, in otherwise normal experimental animals and man as described by Waksman [3]. In this way, in a number of instances, cellular sensitivity has been produced against constituents of liver, spleen, skin and others. Injections of heterologeous tissue, which contains constituents cross-reactive with similar components of the host's tissue have been found to induce the formation of antibody capable of reacting both with the immunizing antigen and with the host's own tissue. This might also be the case in our experiments. This could be proved by the demonstration of hetero-cross-reactive (auto) antibodies. Interesting in this respect is that RACOVEANU et al. [4] found in seven out of eleven cases with pulmonary sarcoidosis anti-lung antibodies. The reaction of Kveim and the reaction to normal tissue suspension can be explained in this way and the normal tissue suspension might cross-react with the Kveim-antigen. These findings have a bearing on the nature of the Kveim-reaction. With Kveim-antigen one can detect probably certain immunological changes of individuals.

This concept is in agreement with the results reported by HART et al. [5], who found positive Kveim-reactions in a large proportion of clinically normal young adults who had failed to be converted to tuberculin sensitivity following two B.C.G. vaccinations.

The authors assume that these positive Kveim-reactions are not due to occult or clinical sarcoidosis, but are the results of some novel immunological change brought about by the B.C.G. vaccination itself. That B.C.G. vaccination can cause the conversion of negative (MITSUDA) lepromin reactions to positive is a well-known fact. This (MITSUDA) lepromin reaction resembles in its timing and gross appearance much the Kveim-reaction. Also "lepromin" prepared from normal healthy skin or liver without leprosy bacilli can evoke the same, though weaker, pattern of response, in patients with different types of leprosy and in healthy people as by lepromin itself.

In our experiments there is an indication that Freund's adjuvans might intensify the granulomatous respectively sarcoid reaction to suspensions of normal tissue. These findings are in support of the view of HART et al.

References. 1. PUTKONEN, T.: Acta derm. venereol. (Stockh.) **25**, 393 (1945). – 2. KOOIJ, R.: Acta med. scand. **176**, (Suppl. 425, 79 (1964). – 3. WAKSMAN, B. H.: Medicine (Baltimore) **41**, 93 (1962). – 4. RACOVEANU, C.: Proceedings 4th internat. conf. on Sarcoidosis, p. 291, Paris 1966. – 5. HART, P. D'ARCY, D. N. MITCHELL, and I. SUTHERLAND: Brit. med. J. **1964 I**, 795.

Present Position of BCG Vaccination against Leprosy

L. M. BECHELLI, World Health Organization, Geneva (Switzerland)

Only two items can be considered in this paper and the main data are summarized.

I. Effect of BCG vaccination on the lepromin test in healthy individuals

From the studies carried out it would appear that: 1. BCG may accelerate the conversion to positive of the lepromin test in children, particularly below 4 years; 2. there is a group of poor or slow responders in whom it would seem that lepromin reactivity cannot be achieved. Only field studies may determine whether this acceleration would be useful to individuals not yet exposed to M. leprae, and usefulness of BCG to contacts, to the child population probably exposed, or to those who are persistently lepromin negative.

II. Epidemiological studies on value of BCG in prevention of leprosy

To our knowledge, four trials are currently in progress:

1. First results of the Uganda trial are encouraging (KINNEAR BROWN, STONE and SUTHERLAND [1]). The average interval between intake and follow-up was

about 2 years. Considering children who were tuberculin-negative or tuberculin-positive in Grade I or II at intake (Heaf multipuncture technique), ,,there were 89 cases among the unvaccinated children, representing an incidence of 11.0 per 1000 children, and 18 among the vaccinated children, namely, 2.2 per 1000, which is one-fifth of the incidence in the unvaccinated group. The possibility of this difference having occurred by chance is remote (less than one in a million). The percentage reduction in incidence of leprosy in the vaccinated group, compared with the corresponding unvaccinated group, was 80%''. The lesions represented the early form of the disease and, in both vaccinated and unvaccinated groups, were nearly all tuberculoid; some may resolve spontaneously. It is therefore considered particularly important to follow-up the trial children for many years to see how the lesions evolve. It is concluded that BCG vaccination of children in Eastern Uganda has conferred considerable protection against the early form of leprosy for a period of 1 to 3 years. The percentage reduction in leprosy incidence is apparently independent of the child's age when vaccinated. Confirming Bechelli and Quagliato's data [2, 3], KINNEAR BROWN et al state: "there is a suggestion from the figures that in some individuals vaccination may even have stimulated the development of the disease". From this they infer that "if widespread BCG vaccination is being undertaken in an area where leprosy is endemic, it would therefore be wise to screen the older children and to withold vaccination from those with incipient leprosy lesions as well as those with obvious disease". The authors add that "Apart from the uncertainty attached to the short period of observation, it would be unwise to conclude that the present results will necessarily apply to other areas". The Uganda findings, where only 8% of leprosy patients are lepromatous, will not necessarily be valid in communities with different proportions of lepromatous cases or different total prevalences. "The present results are clearly only preliminary, and a longer period of observation will be needed before it is possible to make a full evaluation of the effects of BCG vaccination in leprosy".

2. In Karamui (Eastern New Guinea), RUSSELL, SCOTT and WIGLEY [4, 5], 8 ($3.45^0/_{00}$) and 18 ($7.84^0/_{00}$) cases were observed respectively among 2318 BCG-vaccinated and 2295 unvaccinated persons. According to the authors no definite conclusions can be reached from the preliminary findings, but results are encouraging.

3. In Malaya, MCFADZEAN and SINGH [6] are conducting a trial whose results are not yet known*.

4. Since August 1964, a field study conducted by WHO is under way in Burma [7], where the proportion of lepromatous patients is higher than in Uganda. At end May 1967, 44,803 inhabitants had been examined and 18,131 children allocated to the BCG-vaccinated and control groups. To now, there is no evidence of BCG action decreasing the incidence of leprosy or influencing the form of the disease in the new cases. BCG might also have stimulated the development of the disease. It is hoped to present preliminary results of this trial at the IX. International Congress of Leprology, 1968.

Conclusions: The controlled clinical trials are long-term studies and are aimed at determining the value of BCG in preventing the appearance of early forms of the disease and especially of lepromatous leprosy, the principal source of infection. Epidemiologically, it is essential to protect that part of the population (poor or slow reactors to lepromin) more prone to acquire leprosy and develop the infectious form of the disease. In this respect, it seems difficult to establish the prophylactic value of BCG, since the lepromatous type habitually starts as indeterminate

---

* According to Dr. PETTIT this trial has been terminated.

leprosy and untreated cases take many years to evolve; on the other hand, the treatment of indeterminate patient prevents the development of lepromatous leprosy. Notwithstanding, if BCG causes a decrease in the tuberculoid rate, this already represents important progress. In the light of the foregoing, we may conclude that the value of BCG vaccination in the control of leprosy has not yet been determined. At this stage it is unwise and premature for WHO to recommend BCG vaccination for the prevention of leprosy.

References. 1. KINNEAR BROWN, J. A., M. M. STONE, and I. SUTHERLAND: Brit. med. J. 1, 7 (1966). — 2. u. 3. BECHELLI, L. M., and R. QUAGLIATO: Abstracts of VI. Congreso Internacional de Leprologia Madrid 1963; — Rev. bras. Leprol. 24, 23 (1956). — 4. RUSSELL, D. A., G. C. SCOTT, and S. C. WIGLEY: Int. J. Leprosy 32, 235 (1964). — 5. RUSSELL, D. A.: Japan-US Leprosy Tuberculosis Conference, Abstracts (1966). — 6. McFADZEAN, J. A., and SINGH: Leprosy Rev. 31, 145 (1960). — 7. BECHELLI, L. M.: Japan-US Leprosy Tuberculosis Conference, Abstracts (1966).

Über die pigmentierten Naevi bei lepromatösen Leprakranken

Y. ISHIBASHI und T. KAWAMURA, Dermatologische Klinik der Universität Tokyo (Japan)

Für die Lepra ist charakteristisch, daß mit Vorliebe die peripheren Nerven befallen werden. Die besondere Affinität der Leprabakterien zu den peripheren Nervenelementen ist von vielen Autoren, schließlich auch von uns bestätigt worden. Neuerdings wurde nach submikroskopischen Befunden von IMAEDA u. CONVIT, dann nach neurohistologischen Untersuchungen von englischen Forschern die Bedeutung der Schwannschen Zellen bei leprösen Prozessen hervorgehoben. Da die Naevuszellen und die Zellen der blauen Naevi als Abkömmlinge der Neuralleiste aufgefaßt werden können, ergab sich die Frage, wie diese sich bei der Lepra verhalten. Diese Zellen werden von KAWAMURA als fehl differenzierte Neuralleistenzellen aufgefaßt, was später PINKUS u. MISHIMA mit dem Begriff der ,,Naevoblasten" ausgedrückt haben.

Wir haben jetzt das Verhalten der Leprabakterien bei vier Naevuszellnaevi und einem blauen Naevus von vier lepromatösen Leprakranken lichtmikroskopisch untersucht. Die Präparate wurden mit H.E., die Bakterien mit Hallbergs Nachtblau und als Gegenfärbung Massons Trichrom gefärbt.

Beobachtung 1: 43jähriger Mann. Seit etwa 1 Jahr am ganzen Körper infiltrierte Erytheme. Er hatte einen reiskorngroßen pigmentierten Naevus, in dessen Umgebung ein leichtes Erythem mit Infiltration zu erkennen war. *Histologie:* Dermaler Naevuszellnaevus, der nur vereinzelt Bakterien in einigen Naevuszellen enthielt. Im übrigen Korium Lepragranulom mit vielen Bakterien. Die Leprabakterien scheinen zu den Naevuszellen eine gewisse Affinität zu haben. Diese ist aber nur sehr gering.

Beobachtung 2: 73jähriger Mann, seit 6 Monaten bestehen lepröse Erytheme am ganzen Körper. Er hatte zusätzlich einen pigmentierten Naevus am linken Oberarm, dessen Rand nicht erythematös verändert war. *Histologie:* Epidermo-dermaler Naevuszellnaevus ohne Bakterien. In der direkten Umgebung dieses Naevus finden sich kaum lepröse Veränderungen und keine Bakterien. Dieser Befund spricht weder für noch gegen die Annahme einer Affinität der Bakterien zu den Naevuszellen.

Beobachtung 3: Gleicher Patient wie Beobachtung 2. Er hatte außerdem einen blauen Naevus am rechten Unterarm, der von Leprabakterien herdförmig befallen war. Einige pigment-haltige, vacuolisierte Zellen mit mehreren Bakterien waren als dermale Melanocyten anzusehen, weil sie für Chromatophoren zu ungewöhnlich gestaltet erschienen oder einen zu langen Zelleib aufwiesen. *Beurteilung:* Hier kann eine Affinität zu den blauen Naevuszellen angenommen werden.

Beobachtung 4: 23jähriger Mann. Seit 1¹/₂ Monaten hatte er am ganzen Körper rötliche Plaques, Infiltrierte Erytheme und Knötchen. In der Sacralgegend pigmentierter Naevus. In dessen Umgebung fanden sich klinisch keine leprösen Veränderungen. Das histologische Bild weist nur einen dermalen Naevuszellnaevus auf. Keine Bakterien und keine lepromatösen Prozesse. Die Frage einer Beziehung zwischen Bakterien und Naevuszellen bleibt offen.

Beobachtung 5: Ein 31jähriger Mann hatte seit $2^1/_2$ Jahren am ganzen Körper lepröse Efflorescenzen. Am Rücken hatte er einen erbsgroßen dermalen Naevuszellnaevus in einem leprösen Erythem. *Histologisch* fanden sich leprazellenartige Vacuolisierungen der Naevuszellen mit vielen Bakterien. Während im bindegewebigen Stroma des Naevusgewebes kaum lepröses Granulom vorhanden war, fand sich solches genügend in der weiteren Umgebung. Die Vacuolisierungen der Naevuszellen sind nicht nur im oberflächlichen Teil des Naevus, sondern auch in tieferen Schichten zu erkennen. An einer Stelle findet man in der Tiefe des Gewebes ein lepromatöses Granulom, das sich anscheinend nach dem Abbau der Naevuszellen durch Leprabakterien entwickelt hat. In Nervenbündeln des Naevus sind mehrere Bakterien nachweisbar. Hier ist aber nur eine unbedeutende Granulombildung zu erkennen.

Die erwähnten Befunde zeigen definitiv, daß eine deutliche Affinität der Leprabakterien zu den Naevuszellen vorkommt. Dieser ausgesprochene Tropismus der Leprabakterien zu den Naevuszellen und die bei den letzteren auftretenden Veränderungen sind schon 1938 von BERTELLOTTI beschrieben worden, ohne daß dabei die histogenetische Beziehung der Naevuszellen zu den Schwannschen Zellen erwähnt wurde. Wenn es sich bisher auch nur um einen Fall handelt, so ist dieser Befund doch genügend für eine Affinität der Leprabakterien zu den Naevuszellen beweisend. Die Naevuszellen scheinen sich durch ihren Bakterienreichtum und die Vacuolisierung zu Bausteinen des Leproms umzuwandeln.

Auf Grund der bisher bekannten Befunde lepromatöser Veränderungen an den Schwannschen Zellen und nun auch Naevuszellen möchten wir annehmen, daß die hämatogen in die Haut gestrandeten Leprabakterien sich primär in den Schwannschen Zellen der Nervenperipherie ansiedeln. Die wohlbekannte, nach dem leprösen oder tuberkuloiden Pol gerichtete Wucherung der histiocytären Elemente ist dagegen die sekundäre Reaktion gegenüber den primär veränderten Schwannschen Zellen.

Mise en évidence du bacille de Hansen dans les lèpres apparemment abacillaires

F. COTTENOT, F.-P. MERKLEN et TRINH THI KIM MONG DON, Hôpital St. Louis, Paris (France)

Le *bacille de Hansen* n'est généralement pas retrouvé dans les lésions cutanées des formes tuberculoides, voire borderline ou indéterminées. Sa disparition des lésions lépromateuses est généralement considérée comme test de blanchiement. Il est cependant intéressant dans de multiples cas de chercher à mettre en évidence la bacille de Hansen dans les lésions apparemment abacillaires.

I. *Détection des mycobactéries en microscopie de fluorescence*

La microscopie de fluorescence peut faciliter la découverte des mycobactéries fluorescentes à grossissement plus faible (objectif 40 X, oculaire 10 X), donc sur un champ plus étendu que la recherche des mêmes mycobactéries après coloration de Ziehl. La recherche du bacille de Hansen surchargé de substance fluorescente (fluorescence secondaire) fut proposé par RADNA (1938), peu après les travaux parallèles de HAGEMAN sur le bacille de Koch (1937); mais son intérêt pratique a été discuté: reconnu dans l'ensemble par HENDERSON et coll. (1942), CURBELLO, HERNANDEZ et coll. (1952), GOHAR (1952), VON HAEBLER (1954), NERURKAR et KHANOLKAR (1952), il est nié par DUBOIS, SWERTS (1950), COHEN (1953). Les études poursuivies au pavillon de Malte à l'Hôpital St. Louis ont conduit à une technique dérivée d'AUGIER et de BOY: après fixation alcoolique, les préparations sont mises 10 min dans une solution de fluorochrome (auramine lg, rhodamine B 0,10 g, tween 80 de 3 à 4 cc et eau distillée 1000 cc); puis différenciées par un mélange d'alcool absolu (deux parties) et d'acide acétique (une partie). Après lavage à l'eau distillée, la fluorescence de fond est éteinte par rinçage avec un mélange de trois parties d'une solution A et de deux parties d'une solution B, mélange dilué au $^1/_{10}$ avant emploi (Solution A: bleu de méthyle lg., alcool absolu 50 cc, acide acétique 50 cc et eau distillée 100 cc. Solution B: cristal violet lg, alcool absolu 10 cc et eau distillée 100 cc). Sur la préparation lavée et séchée, les bacilles apparaissent jaune orangé sur fond bleu noir. En décolorant rapidement la préparation par l'alcool acétique, on peut ensuite faire comparativement une coloration de Ziehl. Ont été ainsi comparées 150 lames correspondant à 54 étalements de mucus nasal et 96 frottis biopsiques provenant de lèpres humaines. Sur 54 prélèvements de *mucus nasal* 47 furent concordants négatifs, 2 concordants positifs, 3 ne furent positifs qu'au Ziehl, 2 qu'en fluorescence. Ainsi, en ce qui concerne la recherche de bacille de Hansen dans le mucus nasal, la microscopie de fluorescence est loin d'être toujours supérieure. Sur *96 frottis biopsiques*, 62 étaient négatifs par les 2 méthodes, 24 positifs par les 2 méthodes, 2 étaient positifs au seul Ziehl, 8 par la seule fluorescence. La méthode de fluorescence ne doit pas supplanter la coloration de Ziehl, à laquelle elle n'est pas toujours supérieure, même pour les frottis biopsiques.

II. Concentration des mycobactéries dans les broyats tissulaires

HENDERSON avait déjà obtenu des concentrations de bacilles de Hansen après broyage aqueux de tissu lépreux et extraction huileuse avec centrifugation. KHANOLKAR et RAJALAKSHMI ont ultérieurement broyé des prélèvements de moindre volume par laminage entre un corps de seringue métallique et un piston à vis, après macération du prélèvement pendant 4 à 8 h dans une solution d'acide acétique à 1%; les bacilles concentrés dans un surnageant d'éther de pétrole et d'éther sulfurique sont recherchés en microscopie de fluorescence. DHARMENDRA et MUKHERJE, FIGUEREDO et DESAI ont modifié la phase liposoluble. LEW et CARPENTER évitent les dilacérations tissulaires en faisant une macération trypsique. Enfin KAR, ELLISTON et TAYLOR ont mis au point une méthode parfaitement adaptée au très petit volume des biopsies cutanées et dont nous avons vérifié la valeur. Le fragment biopsique est mis à macérer 4 h à + 4° dans un faible volume (0,4 cc) d'une solution d'acide acétique à 2%, puis broyé à la main dans un microbroyeur de Potter pendant 10 min; après 20 min de repos, le surnageant est transvasé dans un tuve à hémolyse où l'on verse quatre gouttes de chloroforme. Après centrifugation de 5 minutes à 1500 t/m, un dépôt d'interface blanchâtre apparait entre le culot chloroformique et le surnageant acétique: ce dépôt est étalé en couche mince, puis coloré par la méthode de Ziehl.

Cette méthode a été utilisée parallèlement à la méthode classique de coloration des frottis biopsiques sans enrichissement chez 20 malades. Toutes 2 furent négatives chez 10 d'entre eux. Chez les 10 autres malades, 3 eurent des bacilles par les 2 techniques, 7 après enrichissement; or 6 d'entre eux étaient d'anciens lépromateux considérés comme blanchis et abactériens depuis de nombreuses années. Cette méthode d'enrichissement, particulièrement simple, permet de retrouver des mycobactéries intratissulaires dans les cas où les méthodes classiques échouent; elle a permis en particulier de retrouver des bacilles acido-résistants non seulement dans les formes classiquement abacillaires de lèpre, de diagnostic souvent délicat faute de preuve bactériologique, mais aussi chez d'anciens lépromateux semblant blanchis et bactériologiquement négativés.

The Frequency of Intracellular Lipid in the Several Structureal Types of Leprosy

R. D. Azulay, Federal Fluminense University (Brazil), and
L. C. de Andrade, Department of Pathology of the Institute of Leprology,
Rio de Janeiro (Brazil)

Leprocytes were described by Virchow as having vacuoles due to intracellular edema. Later on several writers pointed out that those vacuoles were only negatives signs observed in H.E. sections due to fat solvents treatment and that appropriately stained frozen sections showed intracellular lipid in the histiocytes. Recently Rath de Souza and Alayon [1], Portugal [2], Azulay and L. Andrade [2], emphasized the diagnostic value of the fat staining in the different histological types of leprosy. The present report is based on the examination of 7,357 specimens of skin biopsies, which were stained by H.E. procedure, by fat stainings (Sudan III and IV, Scharlach R, Fett-rot and other) and by Ziehl-Wade II technics. The results are condensed in the following table:

Table. *Results of the Examination for Intracellular Lipid in 7375 Cases of Leprosy*

Histological Structure	Lipid positive		Lipid negative		Lipid doubtful		Total
	N° of cases	%	N° of cases	%	N° of cases	%	
Active lepromatous	2234	98.89	22	0.98	3	0.13	2259
Regressive lepromatous	910	100.00	0	0.00	0	0.00	910
Residual lepromatous	117	100.00	0	0.00	0	0.00	117
Borderline	60	70.58	20	23.52	5	5.89	85
Indeterminate	0	0.00	3036	100.00	0	0.00	3306
Indeterminate to lepromatous	o	0.00	26	96.30	1	3.70	27
Indeterminate to tuberculoid	0	0.00	85	100.00	0	0.00	85
Quiescent tuberculoid	0	0.00	595	100.00	0	0.00	595
Reactional tuberculoid	0	0.00	261	100.00	0	0.00	261
Total							7375

This research has shown:

1. Intracellular lipid is a predominant feature in lepromatous leprosy (98.89% of positivity). A very few cases are either lipid-negative (0.98%) or lipid-doubtful (0.13%); the lipid negative are very recent cases of lepromatous leprosy—and they resemble histiocytomes. The lipids appears as either droplets whose periphery is deeper stained or granules inside the histiocytes and are entirely different from lipid of sebaceous gland and fat cells of hypoderm. *Regressive lepromatous* (cases under treatment which still present very few and degenerated bacilli) and *residual lepromatous* (cases under treatment which are bacelli-negative but still present some Virchow's cells) are 100% lipid-positive.

2. On the contrary tuberculoid and indeterminate form do not present at all intracellular lipid. Even the reactional tuberculoid cases which present vacuolated cells alike Virchow's cells are lipid-negative, for, those vacuoles are due to intracellular edema and not to presence of lipid.

3. The borderline cases (cases which present both lepromatous and tuberculoid features) are 70.58% lipid-positive; those lipid-positive cases show a tendency—towards lepromatous.

4. The presence of intracellular lipid is a sign of lack of resistence and shows a bad prognosis.

Bibliography. 1. Souza, P. R., y F. Alayon: Rev. bras. Leprol. **10**, 369 (1942). — 2. Portugal, H.: J. Leprosy **15**, 162 (1947). — 3. Azulay, R. D., y L. M. C. Andrade: O valor da pesquisa de lipídio no diagnóstico dos vários tipos estruturais, encontrados nalepra. Estudo realizado en 1053 casos. Terceira-Conferencia Panamericana de Leprología. Buenos Aires 1951.

Cutaneous Response of Leprosy Patients to Living and Heated Mycobacterium Leprae Cultures on the Olitzki-Gershon Medium

M. Dorfman, F. Sagher, J. Sheskin and A. L. Olitzki, Department of Dermatology and Venereology, Hadassah University Hospital, and Hospital for Hansen's Disease, Ministry of Health, and Department of Clinical Microbiology, Hadassah University Hospital, and Department of Bacteriology, Hebrew University-Hadassah Medical School, Jerusalem (Israel)

Olitzki and Gershon [1] have reported the growth of an acid-fast bacillus from human leproma material in Eagle's medium enriched with an extract of mycobacterial saprophytes. Laboratory evidence suggests that this bacillus may be identical with *M. leprae*. In accordance with the principles of the Koch phenomenon, differences in the reaction of leprosy patients to injections of living and heated preparations of this culture might be expected to provide indirect evidence that these are cultures of Hansen's bacillus.

Materials and Method

The cultures tested were from a lepromatous leprosy patient. The bacilli were separated from the medium and washed three times with normal saline, Suspensions were used of fifth, fourth and third sub-cultures in normal saline in a concentration of 1×10^8 bacilli per ml, the preparations being standardized with regard to optical density. Suspensions of killed bacilli were prepared by heating at 100 °C for 60 min. 0.1 ml of the test suspension was injected intracutaneously in the left upper arm, in an area apparently free of skin lesions. The sites of injection were examined every 2 days for 30 days. Results are reported at 48 h and at 21 days after injection. Biopsies were made from the site at 21 days. Three groups of patients were tested:

1. In an initial study (December, 1965), six leprosy patients were injected with live suspensions of fourth and fifth subcultures. Control tests in these patients were later made (February, 1966) with heated suspensions of fourth subculture. These patients were also tested with lepromin and tuberculin (Old Tuberculin, 1:50,000).

2. In the second group, eight leprosy patients were injected simultaneously (June, 1966) with live and heated suspensions of fifth subculture. These patients were tested with lepromin and PPD tuberculin, 5 units per 0.1 ml.

3. a) Live suspension could not be tested in non-leprosy patients. The heated suspension of fifth subculture was tested in eight non-leprosy volunteers. Simultaneous control injections were made in these patients with the culture medium, viz. Eagle's medium enriched with saprophytic mycobacteria. b) A further eight non-leprosy volunteers were tested with a heated suspension of third subculture. Simultaneous control injections were made in these patients with saline derived from the third washing of this bacillary suspension.

Results

The leprosy patients in the first group (Tab. 1) showed an infiltrated papule of at least 5 mm at 21 days after the injection of live bacilli, in three of them with marked central necrosis. All three patients in whom necrosis occurred suffered from active lepromatous leprosy and two of them were of reactional type. Injection of a heated suspension of bacilli in the same patients was followed at 21 days by the appearance of an infiltrated papule as before or somewhat smaller, but in no case was there a necrotic reaction. It should be noted that the heated suspension was prepared from an older subculture (fourth) than the living suspension (fifth), and that in addition it was used 2 months later than the living suspension. This age factor might partly account for the differences in reaction produced by the two suspensions. The live and the killed suspensions appeared to behave immunologically in a way related neither to tuberculin nor to lepromin, to both of which antigens the patients did not react.

Table 1. *Skin Reactions to Live and Killed Bacteria — (Group 1)*

Patient	Diagnosis	Dec. 1965 Live Bacteria 5th Subculture[a] (Papule mm)		Feb. 1966 Killed Bacteria 4th Subculture (Papule mm)		Tuberculin Reaction 1:50,000 (Papule mm)	Lepromin Reaction (Papule mm)	
		48 h	21 days	48 h	21 days		48 h	21 days
A. Y.	Lepromatous (inactive)	4	5	4	5	0	0	0
B. M.	Lepromatous (reactional)	15	10[b]	10	7	0	0	0
A. Y.	Lepromatous (reactional)	5	5	5	4	4[c]	0	0
O. Y.	Lepromatous (active)	2	6[b]	5	5	0	0	0
S. D.	Lepromatous (inactive)	6	6	2	4	0	3[c]	3[c]
P. Z.	Lepromatous (reactional)	20	15[b]	10	5	0	0	0

[a] In the first patient (A.Y.), 4th subculture was injected.
[b] Nodule with marked central necrotic ulcer. A pustule appeared on the 5th or 6th day, was covered by a crust, which gradually blackened and fell between the 9th and 13th day to reveal an ulcer of 4 to 6 mm in diameter.
[c] Flat papule with minimal infiltration.

Table 2. *Skin Reactions to Live and Killed Bacteria of Fifth Subculture (June 1966)*

Patient	Diagnosis	Live Bacteria (Papule mm)		Killed Bacteria (Papule mm)		5u. PPD/ 0.5 ml (Papule mm)		Lepromin (Papule mm)	
		48 h	21 days	48 h	21 days	48 h	21 days	48 h	21 days
O. M.	Lepromatous (reactional)	2	2	2	3	10	0	0	0
I. A.	Lepromatous (burnt-out)	2	5	2	2	4	0	2	2
B. M.	Lepromatous (reactional)	6	5	8	1	15	0[a]	0	0
B. G.	Tuberculoid	4	5	3	3	—	—	—	6
B. R.	Indeterminate (burnt-out)	3	4	2	3	25	0	—	4
L. S.	Lepromatous (active)	1	4	1	0	4	0	3	0
P. Z.	Lepromatous (reactional)	10	4	5	0	8	—	0	0
S. Y.	Lepromatous (inactive)	2	3	1	2	20	0	0	0

[a] No papule present, but 4 mm subcutaneous infiltration palpable.

In the second group (Tab. 2), the size of the papule resulting from the living injection (generally 4 to 5 mm) exceeded that from the heated (generally 1 to 3 mm). No necrotic lesions occurred. Two of the patients who showed necrotic reactions in December, 1965, did not do so when retested in June, 1966, with the same suspension. Since skin tests were performed in this second group 6 months later than the tests with live bacilli in the first group, again the storage period may partly explain the diminution in reaction seen after injecting live bacilli. It is difficult to explain, however, the diminution in reactions with killed bacilli. In this group were included two lepromin-positive patients. All the patients gave 48-h reactions to PPD in a concentration of 5 units per 0.1 ml, but at 21 days no papule was present although the site of injection was marked by redness, hyperpigmentation and/or scaling, and in one patient there was also a palpable subcutaneous infiltration.

Table 3a. *Reactions in Non-leprous Patients to Heated Bacteria of Fifth Subculture (August 1966)*

Patient	Diagnosis	Killed Bacteria (Papule mm)		Control[a] (Papule mm)	
		48 h	21 days	48 h	21 days
M. M.	Ulcus cruris	5	3	5	0
M. E.	Lymphocytic infiltration	7	5	6	2
A. S.	Keratosis follicularis	5	5	8	2
W. E.	Ulcus cruris	5	4	3	0
B. F.	Aph'thous stomatitis	3	5	5	2
S. S.	Psoriasis	7	5	12	0
B. M.	Eczema manum	6	7[b]	9	0
R. E.	Kaposi's sarcoma	3	4	0	0

[a] Control = Eagle's medium enriched with saprophytic mycobacterial extract.
[b] Necrotic ulcer of 4 mm diameter appeared after 7 days.

Table 3b. *Reactions in Non-leprous Patients to Heated Bacteria of Third Subculture (August 1966)*

Patient	Diagnosis	Killed Bacteria (Papule mm)		Control[a] (Papule mm)	
		48 h	21 days	48 h	21 days
W. G.	Erysipelas recidivans	4	4	1	2
K. Y.	Hydradenitis inguinalis	3	3	0	1
E. N.	Keratosis follicularis	3	3	1	0
I. C.	Xeroderma pigmentosum	2	2	0	0
S. M.	Post-sarcoidosis	3	4	0	2
G. R.	Ulcus cruris	3	2	0	0
U. Y.	Eczema manum	3	5	1	1
B. S.	Lupus miliaris facei	3	1	1	0

[a] Control = saline from third washing of killed bacteria.

The same heated suspension of fifth subculture produced papules of at least 4 mm in seven out of eight non-leprosy patients; and in one patient, with dermatitis of the hands in an actively eczematous stage, there was a necrotic reaction (Tab. 3a). In a further eight non-leprosy patients tested with suspensions of heated third subculture (Tab. 3b), a papule of at least 4 mm occurred in only three. Control injections of Eagle's medium enriched with saprophytic extract produced a 48-h, and not a 21-day reaction (Tab. 3a); while control injections of saline derived from the third washing of the bacillary suspension produced no significant reactions at 48 h nor at 21 days (Tab. 3b), thus excluding the possible effect of the saprophytic extract in the culture medium.

Regional lymphadenopathy and systemic reactions were not observed in any case. 38 biopsies were taken at 21 days and examined histologically. The papular lesions revealed a granulomatous structure similar to a leproma in most leprosy patients [2].

A scientific proof that the mycobacterium grown on the Olitzki-Gershon medium is myco-bacterium leprae is very difficult as long as no animal is found susceptible to this disease. Therefore suspensions of these cultures were injected into human leprous and non-leprous volunteers. It could be assumed that the injection of the living cultured bacillus in leprous patients will produce similar reactions as living tubercle bacilli injected into tuberculous animals or humans. The reactions of these cultures suspensions behaved different from reac-tions to lepromin and tuberculin. No clear difference could be found between the reaction of living and killed bacilli injected into human leprous volunteers. There were some necrotic reactions following the injection of living bacilli but the small number of these trials is not sufficient to draw definite conclusions.

References. 1. OLITZKI, A. L., and Z. GERSHON: Israel J. Med. Sci. 1, 1004 (1965). — 2. SAGHER, F., E. LIBAN, A. ZUCKERMAN, and E. KOCSARD: Int. J. Leprosy 21, 459 (1953).

Serum Immunoglobulin Changes in Leprosy and Tuberculosis*

Soo DUK LIM, Department of Dermatology, Seoul National University, Seoul (Korea), and R. M. FUSARO, Dermatology Clinic, University of Minnesota Hospitals, Minneapolis, Minn. (USA)

Because of the possibility of varying immune response to the complex anti-genic structure of Mycobacterium leprae, we studied the serums of 232 untreated leprosy patients with immunoelectrophoresis. We previously reported data (Tab. 1) which indicated that certain differences exist in the serum immuno-protein responses of patients with the three types of leprosy.

Table 1. *Number of Leprosy Patients with Prominent IgA and IgM Serum Arcs on Immunoelectrophoresis (IEP) Patterns*

Leprosy Type	Total No. in each type	Immunoproteins	
		IgA	IgM
		(Number and Percentage of Patients)	
Lepromatous "L"	86	44—(51%)	84—(94%)
Tuberculoid "T"	91	83—(91%)	56—(62%)
Indeterminate "I"	55	37—(67%)	27—(49%)

In a similar investigation of 50 patients with pulmonary tuberculosis, a majority had more prominent IgA arcs than the control group while only a small percentage had prominent IgM arcs. Differences remained similar when patients were subclassified with respect to the extent of their pulmonary tuberculosis.

Because these reports demonstrated semi-quantitative differences between the immune responses of patients with leprosy and patients with tuberculosis, we have now quantitated in the same patients IgG, IgA, and IgM serum proteins by a specific immuno-chemical method (Oudin capillary tube technique).

The results of studies of 216 patients with leprosy, 46 patients with pulmonary tuberculosis, and 153 normal subjects (controls) are summarized in Tab. 2. Because the patterns of statistically significant changes are difficult to visualize

* Supported in part by USPHS Research Grant No. AI 05565.

in Tab. 2, Tab. 3 graphically demonstrates the significant changes. The IgG levels are significantly elevated in both diseases but the highest elevations are found in the "L" type of leprosy and in the advanced stage of pulmonary tuberculosis.

Table 2. *Serum IgG, IgA and IgM Proteins Concentrations*

Subject or Patient	Number of	Immunoproteins		
		IgG	IgA	IgM
		(mg of serum protein $\pm$ S.D. [standard deviation] / 100 ml serum)		
Control	153	2035 $\pm$ 22.5	267 $\pm$ 5.1	94 $\pm$ 1.7
Leprosy	216	2498 $\pm$ 25.8 ↑	274 $\pm$ 5.3	110 $\pm$ 2.6 ↑
"L"	82	2598 $\pm$ 70.4 ↑	261 $\pm$ 8.6	131 $\pm$ 5.5 ↑
"T"	83	2410 $\pm$ 57.7 ↑	286 $\pm$ 7.3 ↑	55 $\pm$ 2.6
"I"	51	2306 $\pm$ 76.8 ↑	274 $\pm$ 3.4	98 $\pm$ 3.8
Tuberculosis	46	2422 $\pm$ 74.1 ↑	324 $\pm$ 14.3 ↑	84 $\pm$ 3.5 ↓
Advanced	15	2583 $\pm$ 133.5 ↑	361 $\pm$ 26.9 ↑	93 $\pm$ 7.5
Mod. Adv.	15	2339 $\pm$ 96.6 ↑	314 $\pm$ 19.4 ↑ *	85 $\pm$ 6.5
Minimal	16	2348 $\pm$ 117.6 ↑	298 $\pm$ 26.4	82 $\pm$ 4.5 ↓

Significantly evelated ↑ or decreased ↓ from normal values at p < 0.01 level unless indicated with asterisk ↑ * which indicates significance of p < 0.05.

IgA immunoproteins were significantly elevated in tuberculosis patients but especially in the patients with advanced pulmonary tuberculosis. With increased pulmonary involvement with tuberculosis, the IgA levels become more significantly elevated. Although the IgA proteins were not significantly elevated for the 216 patients with leprosy, analysis of the three types of leprosy patients' serums, showed that patients with the "T" type had significant elevation.

IgM proteins were significantly elevated in leprosy patients but were significantly decreased in tuberculous patients. The increase in leprosy patients occurred only in the "L" type while the decrease in the tuberculous patients was in those with minimal involvement. This contrast is interesting to note.

Table 3. *Statistically Significant Changes of Table 2*

	Immunoproteins		
	IgG	IgA	IgM
Leprosy	↑	—	↑
"L"	↑ ↑	—	↑
"T"	↑	↑	—
"I"	↑	—	—
Tuberculosis	↑	↑	↓
Advanced	↑ ↑	↑ ↑	—
Mod. Adv.	↑	↑	—
Minimal	↑	—	↓

Single arrow (↑ elevated or decreased ↓) indicates significant difference from normal values.
Double arrows (↑ ↑) indicated highest significant response in that serum immunoprotein.
— indicates no significant difference.

The immunoprotein changes in the three types of leprosy show distinctly different patterns. The pattern of changes in the tuberculous patient are somewhat similar to the pattern in the "T" type of leprosy but different from the "L" type of leprosy.

Nuevos avances terapeuticos en lepra

J. C. GATTI, J. E. CARDAMA y L. M. BALINA, Hospital Muniz y Servicio de Dermatología, Buenos Aires (Argentina)

Las sulfonas (FAGET, 1941) inician la terapéutica efectiva de la enfermedad. Constituyen las medicaciones de primera linea con el thiambutosine y sulfamidas de eliminación lenta. Referiremos solamente adelantos de algun valor real.

I. Quimioterapicos

Sulfonas. Insístese en dosis bajas (200 a 400 mg semanales) obteniéndose igual efecto terapéutico, menos toxicidad y menos estados reaccionales. Altas dosis perturbarían el mecanismo enzimático celular (especialmente lisozímico) que determina la eficacia terapéutica de las sulfonas. Por mecanismo similar, los corticoesteroides interferirían en forma más intensa ese mecanismo enzimático.

Thiambutosine (Ciba 1906). Suspensiones oleosas al 20% (1 g semanal) no aportan ventajas sobre la administración oral.

Sulfamidas de eliminación lenta. Igual efecto clínico y baciloscópico han mostrado las formas ultralentas. Entre ellas citamos: 4 sulfanilamida 5,6-dimetoxipirimidina (Fanasil). 1 a 1,50 g dosis unica semanal (oral o intramuscular). Sulfapirazinmetoxine (Kelfizina) por tener menor afinidad a las proteinas plasmáticas deja mayor cantidad de fármaco a disposición de la proteina tisular y bacilar (ataque al binomio bacilo-celula de Virchow). Administrase por via bucal, progresivamente, hasta llegar a 2,50 g en dosis unica semanal.

Derivados de Fenazina (B. 663 Geigy). Dosis de 100 a 300 mg diarios bucales, proporcionan buenos resultados clínicos y bacteriológicos; mostrando además efectos antiinflamatorios beneficiosos en reacción leprosa. Suele ocasionar eritemas e hiperpigmentación transitorias.

Oxidiazolonas: Vadrine (S 131). Acción leprostática especialmente en el primer año y de utilidad en asociación con sulfonas; vía oral.

Etionamida (Trecator). Resultados clínicos favorables; en dosis de 1 g diario, vía bucal. Puede ocasionar: anorexia, náuseas, adelgazamiento.

Isoxil. Manifiesta buenos resultados clínicos y baciloscópicos en dosis de 500 mg orales diarios.

II. Antibioticos

Han mostrado valor clinico y baciloscópicos:

Cicloserina: 750 mg a 1 g diarios oral. Puede ocasionar: náuseas, vómitos, brotes de reacción. Contraindicada en la epilepsia.

Rifamicina: Vía intramuscular, 1 g diario. Ambas alto precio.

Oxitetraciclina: Solo efectivo los primeros meses de administración (100 mg intramuscular cada 24 h).

Griseofulvin: Alguna utilidad en lepra reacción.

III. Asociacion de medicamentos

Fundamentado en que con la suma de bajas dosis de 2 ó 3 medicamentos parecería disminuir el número e intensidad de los fenómenos reaccionales, manteniendose igual efecto terapéutico. Hemos empleado: D.D.S. 0,025 g + sulfamidas de eliminación lenta (sulfametoxidiazina o sulfametoxipiridazina) 0,250 g (dosis diarias bucales).

Otras: Vadrine con Sulfonas; Thiambutosine, D.D.S. y Sulfametoxidiazina; Thiambutosine, D.D.S. y Cicloserina; Etisul y D.D.S.; etc.

IV. Tratamiento de la reaccion leprosa

Multiples medicaciones se citan en la literatura de utilidad para la reacción leprosa, mostrando la moderada efectividad de ellas y recordándonos además los factores que pueden determinar cada brote reaccional; hecho que se debe valorar para no indicar terapéuticas al azar.

Corticoesteroides y A.C.T.H., en dosis habituales y curas prolongadas, constituyen los medicamentos que más rapidamente yugulan el brote, no evitando su reaparición, al suspenderlos (pacientes corticoide-dependientes). Además: recordar su acción iatrogénica. Reservarlos para casos especiales en los que otras terapéuticas se hayan mostrado inefectivas o la intensidad del cuadro lo requieran. Dejamos de lado medicaciones clásicas, tales como derivados antimoniales, gluconato de calcio, antipalúdicos de sintesis, etc. citando unicamente las recientes y de utilidad:

Thalidomida: Recientes publicaciones la muestran en dosis de 400 a 500 mg diarios bucales, de gran efectividad. Empleada en aquellos casos en que no pueden presentarse efecto teratogénicos.

B 663 Geigy: Nos hemos ya referido a su efecto antiinflamatorio y especifico en la enfermedad.

Asociaciones enzimaticas. Lisozyma, oral o inyectable (200 a 600 mg diarios) y derivados de "carica papaya" y "ananas comosus" bucales. La medicación específica no debe ser suspendida sino en casos de brote intenso. Disminución de las dosis y agregado de alguno de los medicamentos antes enumerados.

En brotes prolongados y repetidos transfusiones sanguineas.

V. Prevencion de deformidades, rehabilitacion y educacion

El tratamiento no consiste unicamente en la administración de drogas. El enfoque moderno orientase además, a la prevención de deformidades (cuidado de extremidades anestésicas con medidas fisioterapéuticas) o su corrección una vez producidas estas (rehabilitación física y psicológica). El enfermo será cuidadosamente educado para el empleo prudente de manos y pies. 20 años atrás disponíamos de las sulfonas. Hoy, drogas de similar efecto terapéutico y tolerancia permiten superar intolerancias, resistencias o acostumbramientos a una droga, alternando o sumando dosis bajas de varios fármacos. Las nuevas terapéuticas mucho influyen para modificar el concepto de las campañas antileprosas: *"Tratamiento intensivo, profilaxis terapéutica, rehabilitacion en lugar de aislamiento compulsivo e indiscriminado".*

Double Reversal of the Tuberculin Reaction in Sarcoidosis

S. H. SILVERS and F. S. GLICKMAN, State University of New York, Downstate Medical Center Brooklyn, New York (USA)

Introduction

The significance of this report lies in the reversal and re-reversal of the tuberculin reaction in sarcoidosis, in association with the institution and discontinuance of steroid therapy in a patient who simultaneously received anti-tuberculosis therapy. The relationship between tuberculosis and sarcoidosis will be discussed in the light of reactivation of a tuberculin reaction and its suppression.

Case report

A 43 year old married, negro female was seen on March 4, 1966 for an eruption of 3 years' duration. She first noted a gradually enlarging, asymptomatic swelling above the outer margin of the left eye lid. This was biopsied on October 15, 1964. The report was sarcoidosis involving the lachrymal gland. Since then she has noted further enlargement of the swelling over the eye, swelling and discoloration over the right cheek, spots on the back and shoulders and lumps on the arms and legs. The patient was born in South Carolina and spent her childhood there. Her husband was hospitalized several days before her first visit because of active pulmonary tuberculosis.

On physical examination the patient was a well-developed, alert negro female. Her appearance was that of her stated age. Examination of the skin revealed a soft, egg-shaped swelling over the left lachrymal gland measuring $4 \times 2 \times 1.5$ cm. There was a large, hyperpigmented, tense, slightly raised plaque covering most of the right cheek, with central ulceration. Several similar but smaller, circular plaques without ulceration were present on the shoulders and back. Multiple deep, movable, subcutaneous nodules were palpable on the extremities, varying from 1 to 2 cm in diameter. Generalized lymphadenopathy was present. The liver was palpable two finger breadths below the costal margin. The remainder of the physical examination contained no significant findings.

The laboratory data were as follows: urine, straw colored, sp. g. 1.010, sugar negative, albumin negative; microscope showed occasional clumps of WBC in a voided specimen. CBC: hemaglobin 12.2 gm, hematocrit 36%, WBC 7,000, 60 polys, 7 stabs, 28 lymphs, 1 eo, 4 monos. VDRL negative. Total protein 6.9, albumin 3.8, globulin 3.1. Calcium 5.9 m. eq./l. The Tine test was negative. X-ray studies: chest plate negative, bone survey negative. A biopsy of the plaque on the right cheek confirmed the clinical diagnosis of generalized sarcoidosis.

In view of the intimate relationship with a patient suffering from active pulmonary tuberculosis the patient was started on treatment with INH (a) 100 mg t.i.d. simultaneously with steroid therapy consisting of prednisone 5 mg four times daily. Within 1 week after the onset of therapy some softening and flattening of all lesions was noted. By March 25, 1966 all lesions had flattened to a half to a quarter of their original thickness. The nodules noted on the extremities had completely disappeared. On April 22, 1966 a sputum was reported positive for acid fast bacilli and a (b) Tine test was positive. The finding of the acid fast bacilli proved to be a laboratory error, but at the time, (c) PAS 4.0 gm. t.i.d. was added to the therapeutic regime. The cutaneous lesions and nodules completely regressed by June of 1966, leaving only some hyperpigmentation. The dosage of prednisone was gradually diminished until on October 31, 1966, it was discontinued. PAS and INH were continued. Gradual recurrence of all nodules and plaques was noted, including that in the lachrymal gland area. A Tine test was done on December 14, 1966 and was negative. At this time all lesions had recurred. Antituberculosis therapy was continued.

Comment

There is a long and voluminous literature concerning the relationship between tuberculosis and sarcoidosis. The subject is still fraught with controversy. Many explanations regarding the etiology of sarcoidosis have been suggested in addition to M. tuberculosis. Pine pollen, beryllium, zirconium, Hansen's bacillus, fungi and mycobacteria have been implicated [1]. The present trend appears to be away from the consideration of M. tuberculosis as the culprit. Present day sarcoidosis research appears to be following either of two tracks. These can be described as epidemiological and immunological [2].

Epidemiologic research is based on the rather odd geographic distribution pattern for the disease. Although sarcoidosis is worldwide in incidence, some peculiar facts exist. The highest incidence of sarcoid in the world occurs in Sweden, yet the incidence for Finland is extremely low. Sarcoid is extremely common in the American female negro, particularly if she comes from the southeastern states, yet rare for the American caucasian.

There is evidence from the United States and Sweden that the distribution of the disease parallels the distribution of pine pollen. However, evidence from other parts of the world appears to refute this correlation [3—6]. It will be of interest to the epidemiologists to discover whether the offspring of migrant negroes from the southeastern United States persist in having a high incidence of sarcoid.

Immunologic research has unearthed some intriguing information. Tuberculosis carries with it a specific phage. Normally, the patient produces neutralizing antibody against this phage. MANKIEWICZ [7] has shown that patients with sarcoid produce little or no phage-neutralizing antibody. Yet if sarcoidal tissue is cultured in vitro along with phage-neutralizing antibody of rabbit origin, then, MANKIEWICZ reports, one can isolate an "anonymous mycobacterium" from the tissue culture. He suggests that in the absence of phage-neutralizing antibody there is an increased number of phage organisms present in the sarcoid patient, and thus few mycobacteria, even though the acid fast organism may be the etiologic agent. Other investigators have implicated the atypical mycobacteria.

KALLINGS and LÖFGREN [8] on the other hand, consider the absence of phage-neutralizing antibody to be simply part of the overall immunologic disturbance in sarcoidosis.

Tuberculosis, atypical mycobacteria, pine pollen: these have been the leading contenders for the distinction of being the etiologic agent in sarcoidosis. Other factors mentioned above have been considered, but the evidence for any of these is cartainly not overwhelming.

IRGANG [9] considered the specific question, "Is sarcoidosis in the negro synonymous with tuberculosis ?" His conclusion was no, based upon the reasoning that the co-incidence of the two diseases statistically should not be too unusual, the fact that it is possible for the sarcoidal reaction to suppress the immunologic evidence for pre-existing tuberculosis, and the fact that anti-tuberculosis therapy has no effect on sarcoid. He concludes that the "rare case of sarcoid terminating in tuberculosis" merely represents activation of pre-existing latent tuberculosis by sarcoid.

Our case would seem to support Irgang's conclusions.

References. 1. ATWOOD, W. G., and C. T. NELSON: Med. Clin. N. Amer. 49, 783 (1965). — 2. SILTZBACH, L. E.: Amer. J. Med. 39, 361 (1965). — 3. TERRIS, M., M. M. ZISKIND, C. McGILL, and E. STREET: Amer. Rev. resp. Dis. 87, 509 (1963). — 4. CUMMINGS, M. M., E. DUNNER, and J. H. WILLIAMS jr.: Ann. intern. Med. 50, 879 (1959). — 5. ISRAEL, H. L., and M. SONES: Bibl. tuberc. (Basel) 16, 214 (1961). — 6. NOBECHI, K.: Amer. Rev. resp. Dis. 84, 148 (1961). — 7. MANKIEWICZ, E.: Acta med. scand. Supp. 425, 68 (1964). — 8. KALLINGS, L. O., and S. LÖFGREN: Acta med. scand. Supp. 425, 33 (1964). — 9. IRGANG, S.: Skin 3, 247 (1964).

Clinical Applications of Shepard's Mouse Foot Pad Technique

P. FASAL and L. LEVY, United States Public Health Service Hospital, San Francisco, California (USA)

SHEPARD was the first to show that lepra bacilli obtained from human patients will multiply when inoculated into the foot pads of mice [1, 2]. His work has since been confirmed by REES [3] and others [4].

Changes in the staining quality of lepra bacilli observed by light and electron microscopy led REES and VALENTINE to postulate that bacilli which did not stain uniformly were not viable [5]. It was also found that the number of uniformly staining bacilli decreased in patients with lepromatous leprosy during successful treatment with dapsone [6]. Eventually, SHEPARD and McRAE [7] were able to show that there was a direct correlation between the proportion of solidly staining bacilli in the inoculum and the subsequent rate of multiplication in the mouse foot pad, thus confirming that non-solid bacilli are nonviable.

For the past 3 years, biopsy specimens from patients with lepromatous leprosy, from the Leprosy Service of the United States Public Health Service Hospital in San Francisco, were divided; one half was sent to Shepard's laboratory and inoculated into mouse foot pads, while the other half was kept in San Francisco. Here it was fixed in formalin, embedded in paraffin, sectioned and stained by a modification of the Fite-Faraco method [8]. The technique for the examination of the morphology of lepra bacilli in tissue sections, has been reported separately [9].

It was found that the morphological index (MI), i.e. the percent of solidly staining bacilli of all bacilli present, determined from the tissue sections in San Francisco, compared well with the M.I. determined in the tissue homogenates prepared in Shepard's laboratory. At this time, the results of the harvest in the mouse foot pads from 39 such specimens obtained from 26 patients, as well as the solid counts from the tissue sections are available. This report describes the application of this combined method in four groups of patients representing four different sets of circumstances.

1. Untreated patients. Seven specimens were obtained from patients with lepromatous leprosy who had never received specific treatment. In all cases, foot pad inoculation showed growth and the morphological index or solid ratio in the tissue sections was high.

2. Effect of successful therapy. Specimens from two patients with lepromatous leprosy were obtained before and several months after dapsone therapy was initiated. While the pretreatment specimens had shown multiplication in the foot pads and a high solid count in the tissue sections, the later specimens caused no growth in the foot pads and no solid bacilli were demonstrable in the tissue sections.

3. Resistance to dapsone treatment. In the biopsy specimens of one patient with lepromatous leprosy, the foot pad inoculations were consistently positive and the solid ratio in tissue sections remained high up to 12 months of continued administration of dapsone. That the bacilli were indeed dapsone resistant was proven when dapsone given to the mice, inoculated with tissue homogenate from the patient, failed to stop multiplication of bacilli in the foot pads.

4. Erythema nodosum leprosum. So far, specimens from six patients with erythema nodosum have been processed. In none of the six cases was growth demonstrable in the mouse foot pads. Although there were numerous bacilli in the tissue sections, in only one of the six cases were two solid staining bacilli found in 300 bacilli counted. These findings are compatible with the hypothesis that the presence of large numbers of nonviable bacilli in the tissues of patients with lepromatous leprosy is of etiologic significance in the production of erythema nodosum leprosum.

SHEPARD's successful transmission of human lepra bacilli to the foot pads of mice has greatly advanced our knowledge of the disease leprosy, and continues to stimulate research. The most spectacular of the recent research efforts is an extension of Shepard's method. REES and co-workers [10] recently succeeded in inducing experimentally a disease in mice which is identical with lepromatous leprosy in man. They used thymectomized mice, which were also irradiated to suppress the immune response and inoculated them intravenously. We have attempted to illustrate some of the practical applications of Shepard's mouse foot pad technique in this preliminary report, applications which are of importance to the practicing leprologist.

References. 1. Shepard, C. C.: Amer. J. Hyg. **71**, 147 (1960). — 2. Shepard, C. C.: J. exp. Med. **112**, 445 (1960). — 3. Rees, R. J. W.: Brit. J. exp. Path. **45**, 207 (1964). — 4. Janssens, P. G., and S. R. Pattyn: VIIIth Internat. Congress of Leprology. Rio de Janeiro, September 1963. — 5. Rees, R. J. W., and R. C. Valentine: Int. J. Leprosy **30**, 1 (1963). — 6. Waters, M. F. R., and R. J. W. Rees: Int. J. Leprosy **30**, 266 (1962). — 7. Shepard, C. C., and D. H. McRae: J. Bact. **89**, 365 (1965). — 8. Fite, G. L., P. J. Cambre, and M. H. Turner: Arch. Path. **43**, 624 (1949). — 9. Levy, L., P. Fasal, and L. P. Murray: Arch. Derm. **95**, 451 (1967). — 10. Rees, R. J. W., E. Palmer, M. F. R. Waters, and A. G. M. Weddell: Symposium on Sulfones, sponsored by the U.S.-Japan Cooperative Medical Science Program, Office of International Research, National Institutes of Health. San Francisco, May 10, 1967.

Impétigo herpétiforme Hébra Kaposi ou Psoriasis pustuleux généralisé

chez une femme âgée de 22 ans, apparu au cours du 5ᵉ mois de sa 2ᵉ grossesse

R. Samii, Université Melli, Téhéran (Iran)

Pour les pellicules du cuir chevelu, elle utilisait depuis 2 mois un schampoing à base de Sélénium. Les lésions érythémateuses squameuses et les pustules sont apparues au cours de ce traitement autour du cuir chevelu, vers le cou et les oreilles, le visage les bras et surtout les deux coudes. Les lésions pustuleuses se sont développées vers les aisselles, les seins, l'ombilic, les cuisses. Ensuite un soulèvement épidermique érosif de 10 à 20 cm de diamètre s'est présenté sur la cuisse gauche. Puis les pustules ont atteint les deux jambes, les deux pieds, les plantes de pieds et se sont presque généralisées sur tout le corps. Cela a présenté l'aspect d'une érythrodermie érythémateuse squameuse sèche. Au bout de trois semaines d'hospitalisation, les squames se sont détachées, la peau est devenue propre mais rouge; puis de nouvelles pustules sont apparues sur le bord latéral du thorax de côté droit et se sont développées vers l'abdomen. Pas de lésions des muqueuses, ni de prurit, ni de cuisson, ni de douleur mais des frissons, des tremblements, de la fièvre irrégulière qui montait surtout la nuit et disparaissait dans la matinée. La malade était très abattue et très constipée. Elle n'avait jamais eu aucune dermatose sauf un seul onyxis d'un gros orteil qui datait de 4 ans.

L'examen de laboratoire a montré un contenu de pustules négatif en examen direct, mais en culture peu de staphylocoques coagulase négatif. Hypocalcémie (88/1000), hypoglycémie (690 mg/1000) VS accélérée (63 à la 1ᵉʳᵉ h), hyperlococytose (16150).

Histologie: L'épiderme me paraît hyperkératosique et hyperachantosique, montrant des épines épithéliales plus ou moins prolongées. On peut remarquer l'oedème et l'infiltration des cellules neutrophiles dans la couche épithéliale formant pustule sous-cornée avec spongiose.

La couche dermique est infiltrée par des cellules inflammatoires à localisation périvasculaire. Il me semble qu'il s'agit d'un impétigo herpétiforme ou d'un psoriasis pustuleux généralisé.

Traitement: 60 mg prednisolon, 1 g, ¹/₂ ampiciline, 2 g érythromycine, androgène ordinaire 25 mg tous les 2 jours et androgène retard 50 mg tous les 5 jours. Chlorure de calcium qui a augmenté le calcium de la malade 15 jours après son hospitalisation jusqu'd 93/1000. C'est pourquoi on n'a pas utilisé A.T. 10 (calcamine, dihydrotachystérol).

Symposium 15   **Iatrogenic Diseases in Dermatology**

Maladies iatrogènes en dermatologie

Enfermedades iatrógenas en dermatología

Iatrogene Schäden in der Dermatologie

Organizer

M. I. QUIROGA, Argentina

Presidents

R. L. BAER, USA

J. GRANDBOIS, Canada

H. KUSKE, Switzerland

F. H. STERNBERG, USA

Delegate of the Organization Committee

W. GAHLEN, Germany

Reports

Dermatosis iatrogénicas. Definición, patogénia, clasificación

M. I. Quiroga, Academia Nacional de Medica, Buenos Aires (Argentina)

Si bien la literatura médica ha incorporado ya hace años el término iatrogénias como un capítulo de la patología general, es recién en el Congreso Internacional de Medicina Interna, reunido en Buenos Aires en 1964, que el mismo figura como uno de los temas principales en un certamen de esta naturaleza.

El Comité Organizador de este Congreso Internacional de Dermatología ha creído oportuno incluir tembién en sus simposios, el tema *dermatosis iatrogénicas* confiándome la organización del mismo. Por estas razones me ha parecido conveniente antes de escuchar las comunicaciones científicas, exponer el punto de vista personal sobre la definición, mecanismos patogénicos y límites de las *iatrogenias en dermatologia*.

Según T. R. Harrison, en su obra Medicina Interna, "las perturbaciones iatrogénicas serían aquellos efectos adversos inducidos por el médico al tratar a sus enfermos, e incluye, no solamente el daño directo que les causa durante la aplicación de medidas diagnósticas o terapéuticas sino las lesiones que pueden provocarles con actos o palabras. El término generalmente implica la aparición de un efecto perjudicial que puede evitarse si el médico es cuidadoso y razonable".

Por nuestra parte denominamos *dermopatías iatrogénicas* a las lesiones, erupciones a alteraciones orgánicas o funcionales de la piel y sus anexos, provocadas o desencadenadas por el médico como consecuencia de: a) *su acción terapéutica*, cualquiera sea la via empleada, interna o externa y la naturaleza de la medicación (biológica, química, física, quirúgica); b) de su *actuación para el diagnóstico*; y c) de su *comportamiento anímino frente al enfermo*.

En general puede decirse que si bien las alteraciones iatrogénicas son pasajeras y no ofrecen gravedad, no es menos cierto que, en determinades casos conducen a la muerte. Lorenzo Velazquez en el Congreso Internacional de Medicina Interna antes mencionado, cita a Landells, quien refiriéndose a Inglaterra ha podido señalar que de 4000 autopsias, sólo el 0,5% por ciento son atribuíbles a errores médicos de cualquier tipo, ó sea a enfermedades iatrogénicas.

En el registro general de muertes, en Inglaterra y en lo referente al año 1960, señala inculpando las muertes producidas por fármacos o agentes terapeúticos de causa iatrógena de la siguiente forma: 16 a consecuencia de la insulina, 13 por la cloromicetina ó cloranfenicol; 10 por sulfas; 8 por penicilina; cifras menores por otros fármacos y las siguientes por otros factores o agentes terapeúticos, tales como: 39 por radiaciones, 20 por transfusión, a 11 por electrochoque. Como vemos, agrega B. Lorenzo Velazquez, la proporción, en todo daso, de muerte es pequeña y, como es sabido no siempre debe culparse al médico en estos casos desgraciados. Refiriéndonos a la piel, las condiciones anatómicas y fisiopatológicas bien conocidas de este órgano justifican la frecuencia con que se observan, así como la variedad y su mayor o menor gravedad evolutiva.

La situación de "órgano de choque", u "órgano frontera", expuesto a la acción terapeútica no sólo tópica, sino también la que busca acción sobre las vísceras o medio interna a través de la piel (inyecciones, fricciones con principios activos, radiaciones, intervenciones quirúrgicas) y en muchas ocasiones la pérdida o deficit de los mecanismos de defensa y protección la frecuencia de estas manifestaciones que hoy nos ocupan y los diversos mecanismos por los cuales ellas pueden producirse y que pasamos a mencionar.

Mecanismos de acción de las iatrogénias en dermatología

Estos se producen por: 1. acción y efectos locales; 2. acción transcutánea con efectos secundarios viscerales o del medio interno y repercusión secundaria sobre la piel; 3. actuación anímica frente al enfermo.

1. La acción iatrogénica local puede ejercerse mediante agentes químicos, biológicos, físicos o quirúrgicos. Los agentes químicos producen estos efectos por acción cáustica o irritativa, intolerancia, idiosincrasia o hipersensibilidad, dando origen a manifestaciones agudas, inflamatorias, ampollares, eczematosas, necróticas, etc. Según su importancia podrán curar con restitución ad integrum, ó, como sucede a veces, dejando secuelas atróficas o cicatrizales que en algún caso han llegado a convertirse en un nuevo foco de iatrogénia definitiva. Son bien conocidas por todos las reacciones a los más diversos antisépticos, las sulfamidas, la penicilina y otros antibióticos, antihistamínicos, anestésicos, etc. adoptando por lo general el tipo de las dermatitis de contacto de mayor o menor intensidad y extensión. No son raras tampoco las hipercromias y las discromias paradojales. La aplicación de substancias o preparaciones queratolíticas o exfoliantes como la resorcina y en especial el ácido tricloroacético con fines de borrar pigmentaciones diversas (cloasma, efélides) puede, en ocasiones, ser seguida de una reacción pigmentaria de mayor intensidad aún que la que se deseaba tratar. Del mismo modo han sido observadas discromias provocadas por la aplicación de cremas con monobencileter de hidroquinona, quizá por su mala preparación o distribución en el excipiente, puntos blancos sobre el fondo hiperpigmentado, que puede observarse aún en sitios alejados de su aplicación. Entre los agentes de orden *físico*, son las radiaciones las que ocupan el primer lugar en cuanto a la frecuencia e importancia de los fenómenos iatrogénicos. Ellos pueden acontecer por tres motivos: a) aplicación incorrecta; b) mala indicación o contraindicación; c) como consecuencia inevitable de lesiones cutáneas por terapia profunda en la irradiación de tumores viscerales. Como veremos más adelante este distingo es de importancia grande ya que del mismo dependerá el grado de culpabilidad del médico. En cuanto a las dermatoiatrogénias por actos quirúrgicos, hemos tenido oportunidad de registrar en nuestra experiencia personal, alteraciones cutáneas de tipo *trofoneurótico* traducido por palidez, hiperhidrosis y enfriamiento perdurable después de un año, por la ligadura prolongada en la raíz de un dedo para mantener la anestesia por novocaína para una intervención en la extremidad distal. Hemos visto tembién producirse y mantenerse en forma crónica un eczema trófico y microbiano con los límites superior e inferior correspondiendo a una lipofasciectomia (operación de KONDOLEON) en el tratamiento del linfedema de las extremidades inferiores; estos y otros ejemplos podrían citarse como secuelas de actos quirúrgicos realizados sin las precauciones debidas que ellos exigían.

2. *La acción iatrogénica transcutánea con efectos viscerales o del medio interno y repercusión secundarias obre la piel*, es el segundo y tal vez el más interesante aspecto de este tema. La substancia incorporada por vía interna, es capaz de actuar por diversos mecanismos: tóxico, fotosensibilizante, intolerancia, idiosincrasia, hipersensibilidad, fenómeno de Sanarelli-Shwartzman, reacción de Jarisch-Herxheimer, desequilibrio ecológico, mecanismo biotrópico, embolia arterial, interferencia enzimática, etc. Las manifestaciones cutáneas en estos casos presentan una rica gama de matices que puede ir, desde un simple cambio de color circunscripto como la *mácula eritemato pigmentaria* producida por algunas drogas, hasta las dermatosis ampollares graves que pueden producir la muerte como la *necrolisis epidérmica toxica* o sindrome de Lyell (1956), cuadro sobreagudo al que nos referiremos más adelante.

Un mecanismo curioso que hemos tenido ocasión de observar en dos oportunidades es el que se presenta en forma indirecta o transmitida. Dos niñas, una de 1 año y otra de 8 meses de edad, presentaron hiperpigmentación de las areolas mamarias, estrias y pigmentación de axilas y edema, metrorragia y pigmentación de vulva, es decir signos de pubertad precoz inducida, debida a la absorción de estrógenos incorporados a cremas cosméticas que sus respectivas madres utilizaban en abundancia, para mejorar la piel de las manos. En una de ellas el diagnóstico correcto del dermatólogo evitó una iatrogenia mayor, ya que se había propuesto una solución quirúrgica interpretándolo como una manifestación de un grave trastorno endocrino. Como se ve, se trata de una verdadera iatrogenia transmitida sin participación médica. Hemos dicho más arriba que la dermatosis producida por medicación interna puede llegar a ser gravísima y mortal en muchos casos, como sucede en la *necrolisis epidérmica tóxica*.

Aunque de este cuadro se ocupará en este Simposio, el mismo doctor LYELL, a quien corresponde el mérito de haberla considerado por primera vez en 1956 como una entidad iatrogénica, deseo recordar que las manifestaciones de la necrolisis epidérmica tóxica, o *epidermolysis necroticans combustiforme* como la llamó SOLTERMANN en 1959, habían sido ya observadas y mencionadas aunque sin darle la importancia de una entidad como lo hizo el doctor LYELL. Así DEGOS menciona los casos descriptos por SUSKIND en 1948, JAEGER en 1952 y 1953, DEGOS, GARNIER, MALLARMÉ y OSSIPOVSKY en 1953, JAEGER y DELACRETAZ en 1955, KNEZEVIC y HIRTZLER en 1955 y LANG y WALKER en 1956.

Por nuestra parte hasta el año 1964 tuvimos oportunidad de observar cinco casos de diagnóstico clínico e histopatológico. En la encuesta bibliográfica que aquel año realizamos sobre el posible agente causal, y que sumamos a nuestros cinco pacientes, en total 28, surgieron los siguientes medicamentos: aceite de quinopodio (1); actinomicina (1), butazolidina (6), diaial (1), fenoftaleína (1), fenobarbital (2), neomicina (1), oro (1), penicilina (4), prometazina (1), pirazolona (1), salicilato (1), sulfonas (1), tetraciclina (2), sulfamidas (2), piramidon (2) e hidantoina (1). No insistiremos más sobre este asunto que será tratado con más extensión por otros relatores.

Clasificación de las dermatosis iatrogénicas. Como complemento al tema que tratamos me ha parecido conveniente clasificar estas dermatosis de acuerdo a la participación que corresponde al médico en su producción. En tal sentido podemos decir que existe la *iatrogénia culposa*, la *iatrogénia no culposa o imprevisible* y la *iatrogénia obligada y previsible*. En el primer grupo se agruparían aquellas producidas por error o falta de diagnóstico; por estudio incompleto del enfermo; por desconocimiento de la terapéutica o de la técnica de los exámenes complementarios empleados; errores de dosificación; desconocimiento de los efectos secundarios sobre la piel; contraindicaciones; comunicación anímica inadecuada y vulnerante para el enfermo. Las *iatrogénias no culposas* serían aquellas en que no se incurre en las fallas mencionadas. Ellas escapan a la previsión exigible al médico aunque no a su participación. Juegan en ellas el papel principal, por una parte el propio organismo de enfermo, sus condiciones particulares de intolerancia o labilidad o de padecimientos anteriores olvidados y omitidos en la anamnesis y por otra parte la medicación no suficientemente ensayada o con dosificación inadecuada o de efectos secundarios desconocidos. En el tercer grupo incluimos las *iatrogénias obligadas y previsibles*. En ellas el médico conoce previamente los efectos nocivos que desencadenará su actuación tal como sucede con las "pruebas de provocación" formando parte de un examen diagnóstico complementario, o la aparición de un sindrome de Cushing en la terapia por corticoides.

En esta introducción hemos tratado de aclarar algunas ideas sobre este simposio sobre *dermatosis iatrogénicas* cuya organización me ha sido confiada y cuyo éxito está asegurado por la cantidad y calidad de los relatos y comunicaciones anunciadas, que contribuirá al mejor conocimiento de este campo de la patología general aplicado a la dermatología.

The Aetiology of Toxic Epidermal Necrolysis

A. Lyell, Royal Infirmary, Glasgow (Scotland)

When I described the striking sequence of cutaneous events that I called "Toxic Epidermal Necrolysis" (T.E.N.) I suggested that a circulating toxin damaged the epidermis and resulted in its necrosis. It may be difficult at this point in time to look back and to define without bias exactly what was meant by toxic, but the general idea undoubtedly was that this form of disease fitted into the group of toxic erythemas among which scarlet fever, scarlatiniform eruptions, measles, rubella, erythema multiforme, the figurate erythemas and the erythematous drug eruptions would have been placed. The assumption underlying the whole group was that a circulating noxious substance damaged the skin. Whether it did so by a direct poisonous effect or through an allergic mechanism was immaterial, as also was its nature, whether an infectious agent, the product of infection, a drug or a metabolite of cancer. It seemed likely that the eruption of T.E.N. would have been described previously—indeed I referred to Lang and Walker's paper in my original communication—and this has proved to be so. For example there is quite a literature, particularly in German, on "Measles Pemphigoid" (Masernpemphigoid), the illustrations of which strongly resemble T.E.N.

Of my original four patients case 4 seemed to be fairly certainly a drug eruption, due to phenylbutazone. The lady of case 1 might haven taken a drug deliberately to provoke the reaction, though this is mere supposition based upon subsequent observations that she had a hysterical personality and that haematemesis and melaena followed Dover's powder (ipecac. and opium) with aspirin. Case 3 had severe heart disease and was shown at necropsy to have had a pyaemia. He had received drugs for both conditions, but it was felt unreasonable to incriminate any particular drug. But Case 2 had had no drugs whatever. I questioned her exhaustively, in the full knowledge of how difficult it can be to determine what drugs a patient has really been taking, whether at the recommendation of the doctor, the chemist, or on his own account, and whether the drugs have been given by mouth, by injection, by inhalation, by inunction or via any of the natural orifices. It seemed to me likely, then, that of my 4 patients 1 had almost certainly reacted to a drug, 1 had almost certainly not, and 2 might have done.

It came as something of a shock, therefore, to find that most authors assumed that T.E.N. was always a drug eruption. Naturally in a short time the list of drugs that was believed to precipitate T.E.N. was as long as your arm, since the majority of patients presenting themselves to a doctor with any illness get treated with some sort of drug, and it is easy to make a list of the main drugs that have been administered. One of the fallacies of this point of view is that symptoms such as fever, malaise, shivering and sore throat often precede the eruption of T.E.N. in the natural course of events, and yet the drugs that are used to treat the prodrome are blamed for the exanthem. It would be as logical to blame the rash of measles on the aspirin given for the prodromal catarrh. I do not wish to imply that T.E.N. cannot be caused by drugs. It obviously can. I would merely suggest that the drugs that the patient has received should be reviewed more critically, with particular reference to the time at which they were given and to the indications that prompted their use.

It has recently been my privilege to review case reports of T.E.N. supplied by my colleagues in Britain in response to a questionnaire that I had prepared. It appears that drugs can be strongly suspected in about one quarter of the cases. Another quarter seems to have no relationship to drugs, or, for that matter, to any other event, and it has been classified as idiopathic. Drugs given in the idiopathic group had been used to treat what I took to be prodromal symptoms of T.E.N. Some patients have had no drugs whatever, confirming my own observation that it is possible to suffer from T.E.N. in the absence of preceding drug therapy. It was notable that those cases attributed to drugs often had an eruption resembling erythema multiforme major (Stevens-Johnson syndrome), whereas the idiopathic group did not. That accounts for half of the cases but what about the remainder? In another quarter, mostly infants and children, the common factor appeared to be staphylococcal infection, usually impetigo contagiosa.

There is no sharp distinction between these cases and those that are reported in the U.S.A. as Ritter's disease. The final quarter suffered from a miscellany of conditions that may or may not have been related aetiologically. There were poisonings (carbon monoxide, barbiturates, colchicine), lymphoma, exfoliative dermatitis and sundry infections, for example of the urinary tract or gut. Of course most of these cases had been treated with a variety of drugs, and any investigator who was determined to find a drug as his scapegoat would be able to include these two groups of patients within his trophy bag, although he would be hard pressed to find any common pattern of therapy in the miscellaneous group.

The object of my paper is to state unequivocally that it is possible to suffer from T.E.N. without having taken any drugs. It is probable that only about one quarter of the cases is primarily due to the effects of drugs, although the proportion could conceivably be as high as three quarters. An eruption resembling erythema multiforme major is commonly seen in cases suspected of being due to drugs, but is not seen in idiopathic cases. It would be helpful and interesting to look at any future cases that we may see with these considerations in mind.

Iatrogenic Disease Due to Physical Treatment

A. N. Domonkos, New York (USA)

Perhaps nowhere is the saying, "For every action there is a reaction," more apt than in the field of dermatologic physical treatment. Only a brief outline of physical methods and their possible iatrogenic changes can be given in the time allotted to this subject.

The most frequent method of physical treatment is actinotherapy. This embraces ultraviolet rays, infrared rays, laser beams, ultrasonics and ionizing radiation. Ultraviolet radiation alone may produce burns varying from first to third degree, exfoliation, ulceration and scarring. Ultraviolet therapy in ordinary dosage may cause severe burns when used in conjunction with externally applied photosensitizing agents such as tar, oil of bergamot, sulfonamides and 8-methoxypsoralen. Photosensitizing medicinal agents taken internally may also cause severe reactions. These medications can be the phenothiazines, sulfonamides, demethylchlortetracyclines, griseofulvin and some of the hypoglycemic sulfonylurea agents.

The injudicious use of infrared rays therapeutically may produce burns. In rare instances coagulation necrosis may be produced.

Ultrasonic therapy is a form of sound vibration used in frequencies between 0.8 and 1 megacycle. There are thermal and non-thermal components of this type of therapy. Excessive dosage may produce muscle necrosis and gaseous cavitation in tissue overlying large airfilled spaces of the body.

Light Amplication by Stimulated Emission of Radiation, commonly known as Laser, is an extraordinary monochromatic high intensity, high energy form of light. Its dermatologic use is the experimental treatment of carcinomas of the skin, melanoma, sarcomas, nevus flammeus and other tumors. Its multiphasic reaction produces thermal effects with vaporization, coagulation necrosis and elastic stress. The skin changes are burns of various degrees, scarring or dehydration and cauterization.

Ionizing radiation in the form of radium, radioactive isotopes, roentgen rays, grenz rays or electron beams is still the most prevalent form of physical treatment. Numerous studies in bygone years have failed to yield means for the prevention of radiation damage to the human body. Excessive chronic radiation produces radiodermatitis, hyperpigmentation, ulceration and eventually carcinoma of the skin. Genetic changes may occur with only small radiation exposure.

Surgical diathermy is tissue destruction by heat production. The resistance of the tissue to the passage of high frequency circuit produces the therapeutic effect. The various forms are electrodesiccation, fulguration, electrosurgical knife, electrocoagulation, electrocautery and electrolysis by shortwave or galvanic currents. The improper use of these forms produces coagulation necrosis, ulceration and eventual scarring. Metal deposits in the skin may be caused by galvanic electrolysis when the positive pole is used as the electrode.

Cryotherapy, using refrigerants such as liquid nitrogen boiling at — 196 °C or solid carbon dioxide boiling at — 57 °C, is frequently used in removing neoplasms. The use of liquid nitrogen, especially over the palmar surfaces of the fingers, may result in liquid nitrogen neuropathy. Anesthesia to touch and pain of a persistent nature may result. Cryotherapy may also produce bullae with hemorrhagic fluid formation, ulceration, necrosis and scarring.

Dermabrasion or skin planing for removal of scars may produce miliae soon after the procedure. Persistent erythema may last for months. Pigmented streaks are seen when only the superficial layers of the skin are removed without the basal cell layer containing melanocytes. Permanent scarring is inevitable when dermabrasion is done on the neck and trunk. Extreme sensitivity to the sun may be permanent after dermabrasion.

Prolonged and constant pressure on the skin may produce decubitus ulcers. Alopecia of the scalp vertex may occur after long periods of general anesthesia when the head is kept in a stationary position. The initial changes of swelling and exudation are followed in about 28 days by alopecia at the site of prolonged pressure.

Occlusive polyethylene film dressings to the skin may produce folliculitis, especially when an ointment is used under the film. In addition, ulceration has been noted after prolonged application.

Intralesional therapy with suspensions of corticosteroids may produce emboli with blinding when injected near the eye. Hematomas and sloughing ulcerations may occur especially when air pressure injection is used, however, most frequent is the occurence of atrophy of the subcutaneous tissue causing cavitation at the site of injection. Currently the injection of silicone preparations for the removal of wrinkles, filling in of depressions on the skin and for increasing the size of the breast has produced infrequent granulomatous reactions with persistent erythema and swelling at the site of injection.

Tattooing for cosmetic blemishes and nevus flammeus may induce photo-sensitivity when cadmium or cinnabar is applied as the pigment. A marked erythema results whenever exposure to sunlight occurs.

Finally, ear piercing may produce keloids of the ear lobes, especially in those who have keloidal tendencies. These are some of the iatrogenic changes that may be induced by physical methods. It is evident that great care should be exercised when these methods of treatment are used.

Eruptions du type L.E. et syndromes lupiques provoqués par des médicaments

CH. GRUPPER et G. A. C. MARCEL, Hôpital Saint-Louis, Paris (France)

L'inflation des chimiothérapies les plus diverses, de plus en plus intenses et prolongées, dans un nombre croissant d'affections médicales, a conduit à une véritable explosion de manifestations pathologiques iatrogènes: alors qu'il y a 30 ans tout se limitait aux accidents dûs à l'arsenic, au bismuth, au mercure, à l'iode, au brome, à la quinine ou à la vaccinothérapie, on assiste actuellement, avec les médications modernes, à une prolifération extraordinaire d'effets secondaires post-thérapeutiques qui réalisent les tableaux les plus divers, isolés, associés ou dissociés: éruptions cutanées, viscérites, anomalies anatomo-pathologiques et surtout biologiques. C'est ainsi qu'est né dans les 15 dernières années, le concept de «lupus like syndrome» iatrogénique, qui simule à s'y méprendre le lupus idiopathique. La littérature médicale parue sur ce sujet au cours de ces dernières années est considérable et, sans vouloir faire un bilan exhaustif, à propos de nos observations personnelles portant sur 25 cas, nous commentons brièvement les données de la littérature et résumons les mécanismes physio-pathologiques invoqués par les divers auteurs.

Pratiquement, ces lupus iatrogéniques peuvent: simuler le L.E., avant tout sur le plan clinique; aggraver un L.E. antérieurement connu, provoquant soit une reprise évolutive, soit une symptomatologie additionnelle inhabituelle au cours d'un L.E. idiopathique; créer de novo un L.E. jusqu'alors latent ou en rémission prolongée: les sujets seraient atteints d'une diathèse lupique (HAZERICK, ALARCON-SEGOVIA) jusqu'alors muette, sans expression clinique, le médicament agissant alors comme un facteur révélateur de provocation.

En réalité, chacun des médicaments dits «lupogènes» peut réaliser ces trois types de tableaux: simulation, aggravation ou révélation d'un L.E.

I. Simulation d'un L.E. C'est le plus souvent l'aspect d'une lucite des parties découvertes, face et dos des mains, que réalisant avant tout, par le mécanisme de la photo-sensibilisation, les psychotropes, les sulfamides, les tétracyclines. Nous en avons vu quatre cas après imprégnation prolongée avec la phénothiazine et l'imipramine. Dans tous ces cas, le tableau ne comporte qu'une éruption simulant le L.E. de la face ou des mains, sans viscérite et sans anomalie biologique. L'éruption disparaît avec la suppression des drogues et réapparaît au moment de leur ré-introduction.

II. Aggravation d'un L.E. antérieurement connu, qu'il s'agisse d'un L.E. chronique ou d'un L.E. systémique en phase quiescente: sous l'influence de certaines médications isolées ou associées, telles que Pyramidon, antipyrine, phénolphtaléine, phénylbutazone, sulfamides, propylthiouracile, pénicilline, tétracyclines, transfusions sanguines. Nous avons assisté dans 14 cas, à un remaniement symptomatique d'aggravation clinique et biologique rentrant dans le cadre bien connu d'hypersensibilité aux médicaments des lupiques. Sous l'influence de ces médications, on notait: soit une activation d'un L.E. discoïde jusqu'alors quiescent; soit l'apparition d'une poussée évolutive d'un L.E. systémique jusqu'alors en rémission; soit l'installation de manifestations insolites telles que: urticaire, érythème polymorphe, manifestations vésiculo-bulleuses buccales ou cutanées, purpura ou simples toxinides érythémato-pigmentées.

La plupart de ces aggravations post-thérapeutiques s'accompagnent d'anomalies biologiques: apparition d'anticorps jusqu'alors non détectés, modifications hématologiques, leucopénie, poussée d'hémolyse, etc.

Ces accidents nous ont paru imprévisibles, cédant après la suppression du médicament que nous nous sommes gardés de ré-introduire, se produisant chez certains lupiques alors que d'autres malades supportent les mêmes drogues sans le moindre inconvénient.

III. Création de novo ou révélation d'un L.E. jusqu'alors méconnu. Nous l'avons notée dans sept cas, comme tous les auteurs après une imprégnation assez prolongée, plusieurs semaines, avec des médicaments dissemblables sur le plan de leur structure chimique ou de leur action biologique. a) Dans 2 cas il s'agissait de chlorpromazine, révélant un L.E. chez la mère et chez la fille; b) dans 2 cas il s'agissait de la phénylbutazone; c) dans 2 cas du propylthiouracile; d) dans 1 cas de la tétracycline.

Dans la totalité de ces observations, il s'agissait de sujets présentant des affections en apparence étrangères à un lupus (psychose, polyarthrite, hyperthyroïdie, dilatation des bronches). Après une imprégnation thérapeutique de quelques semaines ou de quelques mois, on a vu apparaître: des viscérites, isolées ou associées, avant tout myoarthralgies, pleurésie, adénopathies, accompagnées de fièvre: des anomalies biologiques, isolées ou associées, telles que: hyper-gammaglobulinémie, leucopénie, faux B.W., L.E. Cells, facteurs anti-nucléaires, qui authentifiaient un L.E. jusqu'alors insoupçonné.

L'évolution de ces lupus réalisés par les drogues a été variable: dans 3 cas, la simple suppression du médicament a entraîné une régression complète, en 3 à 12 mois; dans 2 cas cette évolution régressive n'a été obtenue qu'après adjonction de corticothérapie et d'anti-malariques; dans 2 autres cas enfins, (après phénylbutazone et tétracycline) le L.E.S. continue à évoluer compliqué actuellement d'une néphropathie.

On trouve dans la littérature actuellement plus de 200 cas de «lupus like syndrome» plus ou moins complets sur le plan clinique, anatomopathologique ou biologique. Nous avons groupé dans le tableau suivant les médicaments incriminés dans la littérature.

Ainsi on peut voir que de nombreuses médications ont été accusées, avec une fréquence très diverse, d'induire, d'aggraver ou de simuler un tableau de L.E. chronique, subaigu ou systémique. Les cas les plus authentiques et les mieux connus semblent être en rapport avec une chimiothérapie intensive et prolongée, prescrite pour des affections chroniques: l'hydralazine, les anti-convulsivants, la procaïnamide et l'I.N.H.

Le syndrome s'installe après une imprégnation thérapeutique toujours importante et prolongée, il est plus ou moins complet: soit multisystémique, soit, comme dans le L.E.S. idiopathique, frappant avec prédilection un viscère: manifestations pleuro-pulmonaires avec l'hydralazine, manifestations rénales avec les anti-comitiaux. Ce sont surtout les anomalies biologiques, associées ou isolées, d'apparition simultanée ou successive, qui donneraient l'authenticité du « lupus like syndrome » induit par les médicaments : hyper-gamma-globulinémie, L.E. cells, anticorps anti-nucléaires, anticorps anti-D.N.A. Parfois c'est l'argument familial qui est évoqué : présence chez les collatéraux d'un L.E. ou d'une collagénose voisine ; présence d'anticorps anti-nucléaires, faux B.W., ou simple hyper-gamma-globulinémie.

Médicaments et lupus érythémateux

			Si-mule	Ag-grave	Pro-voque	Nombre cas approx.
Anti-hypertensifs	Mono-hydralazine	Apressoline Hyphex.			+	> 131
Anti-épileptiques	Diphénylhydantoïnes Méphénytoine Diones	Dihydan, Solantyl Sédantoïnal Epidione, Paradione				
	Phénobarbital Primaclone Succinimide Azepine	Gardénal Mysoline Zarontin Tégretol	+		+	> 25
Procainamide		Pronestyl			+	> 14
Anti-tuberculeux	Isoniazide (I.N.H.) Streptomycine Ethionamide	Rimifon Streptomycine Trécator	+	+	+ +	> 10 > 10
Psychotropes	Glutéthimide Chlorpromazine Thioridazine Prochlorpémazine Perphénazine Chlorprotixène Chlordiazépoxide Méprobamate Imipramine	Doridène Largactil Melleril Témentil Trilifan Taractan Librium Procalmadiol Tofranil	+ + + + + +	+ + +	+	> 10
Antithyroidiens	Thiouraciles	Propylthiouracile Méthylthiouracile	+		+	> 5
Tétracyclines	Déméthylchlortétra-cycline Anhydrotétracycline Epianhydrotétra-cycline	Mexocine { Tétracyclines vieillies	+	+	+	> 6
Sulfamides	Sulfadiazine Sulfaméthoxy-pyridazine Chlorothiazide	Adiazine Sultirène Diurilix	+	+	+	
Phénylbutazone					+	+
Phénolphtaléine					+	
Pyramidon					+	
Antipyrine					+	
Anthiomaline					+	
Griséfuline				+	+	
Pénicilline				+	+	
Bismuth					+	
Sels d'or					+	
Vaccinations					+	
Transfusions					+	

Doit-on retenir ces derniers arguments comme suffisamment probants pour faire le départ entre une simple réaction médicamenteuse même prolongée et un authentique L.E. induit par la médication incriminée¿ Quelle est la fréquence de la diathèse lupique latente dans la population moyenne d'un pays ? Quels sont les rapports exacts entre l'affection initiale traitée par le médicament qui sera ultérieurement incriminé comme lupogène et la diathèse lupique ou le L.E.S. ? Ne s'agissait-il pas déjà d'un L.E.S. dont les manifestations inaugurales peuvent être protéiformes ? Par quels mécanismes un médicament peut-il induire un L.E. ? Différentes hypothèses ont été discutées:

a) *un mécanisme immunologique:* le médicament ou le produit de son métabolisme intermédiaire, se comporte comme un antigène complet ou incomplet, déclenchant une réaction d'hypersensibilité chez des sujets porteurs d'un système immunologique génétiquement perturbé par la présence de nombreuses globulines anticorps à orientations multiples.

b) *un mécanisme toxique:* soit toxicité directe, soit toxicité indirecte, par le biais d'une chélation: rôle possible du groupement diamine présent dans beaucoup de ces médicaments lupogènes et agissant sur l'équipement enzymatique; soit action sur la paroi lysosomique fragilisée directement ou indirectement par ces médicaments.

En réalité, questions et hypothèses posent plus de problèmes qu'elles n'expliquent les faits observés en clinique. Seules des études systématiques, à l'aide de paramètres biologiques et de techniques uniformes, admises par tous les observateurs, permettront une appréciation de la véritable responsabilité du médicament, de la fréquence et de l'importance du risque thérapeutique. En attendant un tel accord et de telles études systématiques: 1. toute notion de réaction d'intolérance précoce ou retardée à tout médicament doit faire proscrire l'usage de celui-ci chez un lupique connu; 2. avant l'institution de toute chimiothérapie prolongée un bilan clinique et biologique à la recherche d'une diathèse lupique s'avère indispensable, afin de préciser la part exacte qui incomberait éventuellement à ces médicaments.

Pour la bibliographie: voir thèse G.A.C. Marcel, Paris 1967.

Dermatoses des traitements antidiabétiques

J. Beurey, P. Jeandidier et A. Bermont, Centre Hospitalier Régional de Nancy (France)

Si nombreuses que soient les médications que l'on oppose au diabète, il n'en est pas une qui ne soit susceptible d'entraîner des complications dermatologiques.

I. Les *sulfamides hypoglycémiants* provoquent deux sortes de manifestations.

A. *Réactions allergiques.* Tous peuvent être en cause, mais plus particulièrement ceux dont la formule comporte une amine en position para sur le noyau benzénique (2259 R. P. ou glybuthiazol et surtout B.Z. 55 ou carbutamide: jusqu' à 5,4% d'accidents sur 7193 malades dans la statistique de Bradley en 1959), et reproduire n'importe quelle manifestation dermatologique de l'intolérance médicamenteuse (dans un délai de 1 à 3 semaines, mais en quelques heures seulement chez les sujets déjà sensibilisés). C'est souvent un simple prurit, une urticaire, une toxidermie fixe (érythémateuse, vésiculeuse, bulleuse ou pigmentée), un érythème du 9ème jour, un eczéma, une photo-dermatose; plus rarement un purpura (presque toujours non thrombopénique), un érythème polymorphe, une dermite bulleuse à type de Dühring ou de pemphigus, une toxidermie noueuse, une érythrodermie squameuse ou même vésiculo-oedémateuse; exceptionnellement un syndrome de Stevens-Johnson, une épidermolyse de Lyell, une réaction d'hypersensibilité généralisée plus ou moins grave, voire mortelle.

B. *Erubescence paroxystique ou syndrome vaso-moteur.* Décrit pour la première

fois en 1956 par BERTRAM, BENDFELDT et OTTO, ce syndrome s'observe assez fréquemment avec certains sulfamides hypoglycémiants mais surtout le P. 607 ou
chlorpropamide (16 fois sur les 160 malades de KISSEL, DEBRY et ROYER): intense et
brutale vaso-dilatation qui, pendant une heure en moyenne, empourpre le visage, le
cou et même la partie supérieure du thorax, pouvant s'accompagner de malaises
mais sans gravité. L'érubescence paroxystique survient à peu près toujours à l'issue
d'un repas comportant du vin ou toute autre boisson alcoolisée. Par leur expérimentation sur le rat, KISSEL et ses collaborateurs ont montré (thèse de ROYER,
1963) qu'au chlorpropamide est attachée une propriété «anti-alcool» identique
à celle qui dans le disulfirame (antabuse) est appliquée à la cure des éthyliques:
dans l'un comme dans l'autre cas, cette action s'exercerait grâce à une fonction
anti-oxydante qui bloque la dégradation de la sérotonine endogène, cette dernière
ayant en effet le pouvoir de reproduire le tableau du syndrome vaso-moteur.

II. Avec les *biguanides*, les incidences dermatologiques sont infiniment plus
rares: sur plus de 10000 malades, STERNE ne relève en 1959 que deux ou trois cas,
et seulement chez l'enfant; plus tard sont publiées des observations concernant
aussi des adultes, mais la proportion d'ensemble reste faible (0,40% selon ALBA-
HARY). Ce sont essentiellement de bénignes et fugaces manifestations d'intolérance,
surtout des urticaires et des eczémas.

III. Les complications dermatologiques dues à l'*insuline* sont au nombre de
quatre.

A. *Accidents d'intolérance.* En présence d'un mélange aussi complexe qu'une
préparation d'insuline, il n'est pas facile de préciser quels sont les facteurs responsables. On a incriminé surtout les impuretés ou résidus d'extraction, en particulier
des protéines d'origine pancréatique. Il est de fait que la fréquence des accidents,
d'abord élevée (de 3,2 à 13,8% dans la statistique générale d'ALLAN et SCHERER
en 1932, et jusqu'à 31 et même 55,8% dans certaines estimations), a très sensiblement diminué avec la purification plus poussée du médicament (entre 0,5 et 1%).
Toutefois, pour ceux que ne prévient pas la méthode des recristallisations successives, c'est la molécule d'insuline elle-même qui doit être considérée comme
responsable (PALEY). Il faut aussi tenir compte des agents antiseptiques ou
stabilisants qu'on associe à l'hormone, et surtout des substances-retard (sulfate
de protamine, surfène) qui augmentent sensiblement la fréquence des accidents
locaux (statistique de PALEY et TURNBRIDGE), alors que leur pouvoir antigénique
apparaît des plus douteux. En fait, il n'y a là contradiction que dans la mesure
où, conformément à l'opinion généralement admise, toutes ces manifestations
d'intolérance ressortiraient à la seule allergie, telle qu'elle a été démontrée par les
travaux de DÜNNER et DOHRN, de TUFT, puis de LOWELL, de BERSON, YALOW
et coll. Or, après les publications de GELFAND, FABRYKANT et ASHE (1954) et de
H. HAGEN, W. HAGEN, HEINSEN, OLTERS et SCHEFFLER (1958), on peut se
demander si n'intervient pas, pour nombre d'accidents locaux, une sensibilité
naturelle du derme, et l'étude que nous venons d'en faire (thèse de BERMONT)
semble nous autoriser à leur attribuer un substrat ortho-ergique, que nous avons
trouvé indifférent à l'origine animale mais non à la protamine, et surtout lié aux
impuretés et plus encore au pH.

1. *Accidents locaux.* Beaucoup d'entre eux, pensons-nous, relèvent exclusivement
de l'ortho-ergie: simple érythème circonscrit avec discrète infiltration, immédiat
ou précoce, et guérissant en 2 ou 3 jours. Mais le processus peut s'accentuer, s'aggravant même jusqu'à produire des indurations et des placards, voire pseudo-
phlegmoneux, et dont la résorption est difficile: c'est qu'intervient alors l'allergie,
dont la forme majeure est le phénomène d'Arthus, pouvant évoluer vers une
nécrose plus ou moins bien limitée, mais parfois plus étendue, exceptionnellement

délabrante. Dans quelques cas, en particulier quand les injections n'ont pas été strictement sous-cutanées, la nécrose est très superficielle et circonscrite, laissant des cicatrices varioliformes (PALEY et TURNBRIDGE, WHITTAKER, OAKLEY).

2. *Accidents généraux*. Rares (de 0,1 à 0,2% selon STONE, FRANKEL et BAKER), ils apparaissent généralement après plusieurs mois de cure: urticaire surtout, et plus rarement prurit étendu, érythème, eczéma, purpura, érythrodermie, choc anaphylactique.

B. *Oedèmes insuliniques*. Signalés pour la première fois en 1923 par L. BLUM et H. SCHWAB, ils s'observent toujours après d'assez fortes doses médicamenteuses, mais leur délai d'apparition varie d'une ou deux semaines (KLEIN, MARKS, ROLDAN, SHERMAN et FETTERMANN) à plusieurs mois (RAMBERT). D'aspect banal, ils vont du gonflement discret aux grosses infiltrations diffuses et même généralisées. La résorption se fait spontanément en une à quatre semaines sans qu'on suspende l'insulinothérapie. La cause en est peut-être une hydrophilie accrue des tissus par formation de glycogène due à l'insuline (inclusions de glycogène dans les cellules adipeuses des huit jeunes malades de KLEIN et coll.).

C. *Obésité insulinique*. Décrite par JOSLIN en 1930 puis par RATHERY, elle survient après des cures importantes et prolongées, et presque toujours chez des femmes, souvent mal réglées: elle est diffuse et modérée mais a pour particularité de donner au visage un aspect pseudo-myxoedémateux. Il s'agit d'une véritable *lipopexie tissulaire*, vérifiée au microscope par BLOTNER (1933).

D. *Lipodystrophies*. Décrites dès 1926 par DEPISCH et par BARBORKA, elles surviennent dans 2 ou 3% des cas (si l'on exclut les formes mineures), touchant enfants et adultes (surtout femmes en période d'activité génitale).

1. *Hypertrophies*. Habituellement isolées à l'état fruste, elles sont par contre presque toujours associées aux atrophies quand elles sont importantes. Leur siège est celui des injections: fessier et plus encore crural. Elles ressemblent à des lipomes (histologiquement aussi).

2. *Atrophies*. Isolées ou combinées aux hypertrophies, elles sont plus souvent fessières que crurales, se prolongeant alors souvent vers le bas. Ce sont des plaques affaissées, déprimées en cuvette, dont la surface va de la pièce de 1 franc à la paume de main et au-delà. La disparition du pannicule adipeux permet de palper les faisceaux musculaires, d'ailleurs indurés. Les atrophies sont généralement indolentes, parfois même de sensibilité diminuée, mais se prêtent mal aux injections (pénétration et résorption difficiles). Elles sont très souvent délimitées par un bourrelet de consistance ferme, qui est en faveur d'un stade préalable d'hypertrophie (JOSLIN, KEHRER, CHIMENES). Spontanée ou non, la réparation se fait souvent en partie, mais elle est exceptionnellement complète. L'*histologie* montre une atrophie de l'hypoderme. La *pathogénie* demeure obscure, et nous ne retiendrons que la théorie de l'action métabolique directe de l'insuline sur le tissu adipeux: elle a été démontrée par les expérimentations de FAWCETT, de RENOLD et coll., de CHIMENES, du moins en ce qui concerne l'hypertrophie (mais celle-ci est vraisemblablement le stade initial de l'atrophie, aboutissement dont le mécanisme resterait inexpliqué). De tout ceci a été tiré un utile enseignement pour la *thérapeutique*: plus important que celui des traitements proposés est le rôle de la prophylaxie, qui consiste surtout à répartir méthodiquement les injections d'insuline dans l'espace et dans le temps.

En conclusion, cette revue des incidences dermatologiques au cours des traitements antidiabétiques permet d'en mieux mesurer l'importance et la multiplicité. Il n'est pas douteux que leur connaissance est capitale pour le dermatologue autant que pour l'interniste.

Iatrogenic Dyschromies

H. MÖLLER, Dept. of Dermatology, University of Lund (Sweden)

Changes in skin color may be cáused by the physician, or rather, by the drugs prescribed by him. The most common offenders are shown in the first slide. There are the metallic drugs, chlorpromazine, antimalarials, busulfan, and hydantoins.

Metals, when used as drugs, have been known for decades as hyperpigmenting agents. Lead, silver, bismuth, mercury and many others may be mentioned. They are taken up and stored in both skin and mucous membranes. The clinical picture may vary somewhat, but the bluish-gray color is similar between the different metals. In the first place the hue is caused by the deep localization in the dermis of the metal, which gives rise to optic phenomena of refraction and scattering, the so-called Tyndall phenomenon. In these metallic hyperpigmentations there is, however, also a component of actual melanin formation. In fact, in hemochromatosis, with its metallic gray color, iron is taken up in small amounts by dermal phagocytes. The color itself, however, seems to be caused by newly formed melanin.

Chlorpromazine, for many years the predominant drug for schizophrenia, induces a characteristic dyscoloration. This was first reported in 1962 from France as a "visage mauve", and has since then been thoroughly studied, not the least in Canada. Only light-exposed areas are involved, i.e. mainly the face and dorsal aspects of hands. The color is usually a deep violaceous. For this complication to develop high daily doses and a prolonged therapy are required, and, of course, exposure to ultraviolet light. It should be pointed out that the hyperpigmentation is not a consequence of a dermatitis, eczematous or other. This is easily concluded from the histologic picture. There is an increased amount of melanin, mainly in the epidermal basal cell layer. Also, the drug itself may be taken up and stored in the dermal connective tissue. Experimental studies have shown that chlorpromazine is specifically taken up by melanin-containing tissues. Judging from electron-microscopic work a complex of melanin and some chlorpromazine metabolite is formed in the dermis. This complex with its deep location gives the violaceous color. If the drug is withdrawn or tapered down the color may disappear, but not necessarily. Since chlorpromazine is the only drug given in giant doses for long time we do not know if a chemically related compound also has this side-effect. It is most probable that it does. A chelating agent, penicillamine, together with a low copper diet to inhibit tyrosinase activity, has been tested with some benefit. A suitable sunscreen is probably the best way of avoiding chlorpromazine dyspigmentation.

The *antimalarial drugs* may induce a wide spectrum of dyscolorations of skin, hair and mucous membranes. *Quinacrine* was long used as a prophylactic and it was soon reported that patients acquired a disseminated yellow coloration, somewhat similar to carotenemia and even icterus. In World War II quite another dyschromia developed among soldiers on quinacrine. It occurred as bluish-green deposits localized mainly to cartilaginous structures, for instance, in the hard palate, tip of the nose and wings of the nose. It was called a pseudo-ochronosis because of the localization and the bluish hue. Deposits were, however, also formed in the conjunctiva as well as nail beds of fingers and toes. In the nail beds consumption of quinacrine could be disclosed by a bright yellow-green fluorescence in Wood's light. The nature of the pigment is not defined. With *chloroquine*, no diffuse yellowing has been noted and very few reports on bluish deposits may be found. A typical side-effect of chloroquine treatment, however, is a bleaching of hair, and this involves hair of all body areas. There is no simultaneous depigmentation of the skin. Only blonds seem to lose hair color. This hair whitening depends partly on loss of pigment but also on storing of the drug proper or a metabolite. The affected hair yields the same type of fluorescence as a chloroquine salt solution. With chloroquine dark patches of pigment deposits on pretibial areas have been reported and also a diffuse melanosis on light-exposed skin. *Hydroxychloroquine* is much more innocuous to skin and hair and no accumulated evidence on dyschromias induced by this drug exists. Finally, with *amodiaquine*, both bluish-green deposits in cartilaginous structures and nail beds, and a melanosis in light-exposed skin, have been reported. The different possible dyschromias following treatment with antimalarials are illustrated schematically in the next slide: Hair is bleached by chloroquine. The entire skin may become yellow from quinacrine. A melanosis on light-exposed areas is induced by chloroquine and amodiaquine. Cartilaginous structures may be the site of quinacrine and amodiaquine deposits.

Another drug inducing an interesting pigmentation is *busulfan*, or Myleran, which is an alkylating agent used in chronic myeloic leukemia. 5 to 10% of patients acquire a homogenous brown covering the whole body skin, i.e. not necessarily light-exposed areas. The color type, as well as histologic studies have indicated that a melanin synthesis has occurred. In a few cases brown patches have been observed in oral mucous membranes, and this, together with evidence of fatigue, weight loss and hypotension, has raised the question if busulfan pigmentation is part of an Addisonian syndrome. Laboratory tests have, however, never disclosed an adrenal insufficiency. Furthermore, pituitary melanocyte stimulating hormone is excreted in normal amounts in these cases; and busulfan is not a so-called darkening agent, i.e. a melanin granule dispersing factor. It is possible that busulfan inactivates epidermal sulfhydryl groups and thus activates tyrosinase.

Patches of increased melanin formation in the face, the so-called melasma or chloasma, is usually of hormonal origin, and especially related to a current or passed pregnancy. It may, however, also be drug-induced. Long-time treatment with *hydantoins* for epilepsy has been reported in several cases to provoke melasma of the forehead, cheeks, neck and arms. Mainly women are affected, and light is a contributing factor. The hydantoins are "darkening agents", i.e. melanin granule dispersing factors. This property, together with the female preponderance, and the chloasma type speak in favor of a hormonal pathogenesis.

A few reports on other iatrogenic dyschromias have been published. In connection with the hydantoin-induced melasma it is natural to mention the identical hyperpigmentation induced by *contraceptive pills*. This effect, however, may have been expected since the female hormones of "the pill" causes a condition very similar to a real pregnancy.

As earlier mentioned drugs may be stored in tissues and thereby discolor. *Tetracyclins* are thus taken up by calcifying structures. Brownish-gray streaks and patches develop on the teeth of children on long-term treatment with these drugs. The teeth fluoresce in Wood's light. The drugs pass the placenta barrier and if given to pregnant women the deciduous teeth of the fetus may be discolored. If given to a child of between 2 months and 2 years of age, also the permanent teeth take color.

The changes in skin pigment induced by the drugs mentioned do not threaten life. They are, however, often disfigurating and should therefore be recognized in time by the responsible physician.

Free Communications

Photosensitive Dermatitis as an Iatrogenic Disease

T. Kobori and H. Araki, Department of Dermatology, Teishin Hospital, Tokyo (Japan)

In recent years, the incidence of photosensitive dermatitis due to ingested and externally applied drugs is increasing in our country as a peculiar iatrogenic disease seen in the field of dermatology. These skin diseases have called our attention to the investigation of their causal drugs.

Method of Investigation

Toshiba Xenon Lamp which had been developed through the cooperation of our department was used as a light source. Various filters were interposed between skin and light source to determine the effective wave length. The amount of light energy irradiated was calculated in ERG at the same time. To determine the causal drugs, photopatch tests and phototests after ingestion of the drug were carried out.

Incidence at Our Clinic

Incidence of photosensitive dermatitis caused by drugs observed at Department of Dermatology, Tokyo Teishin Hospital, during 1963 to 1966 are shown in Tab. 1. The total number of patients were 104. Sulfonamides, benzothiadiazines, sulfonylurea hypoglycemics, phenothiazines, griseofulvin and sodium cyclohexylsulfamate were proved to be the causal drugs.

Some Causal Drugs of Photosensitive Dermatitis

We would like to mention here some causal drugs decided to be photoallergen through our investigation.

1. *Sodium Cyclohexylsulfamate*. We found that sodium cyclohexylsulfamate, which is one of the widely used artificial sweetening agents, might act as photoallergenic agent. We would like to show a typical case with photosensitive dermatitis due to this sweetening agent. A 35-year-old woman has

Table 1. *Incidence of solar dermatitis caused by drugs observed by the Department of Dermatology, Tokyo Teishin Hospital, during 1963 to 1966*

Causal drugs	No. of patients
Sulfonamides	24
Benzothiadiazines	31
Benzothiadiazines (photoleucomelanodermitis)	8
Sulfonylurea hypoglycemics	3
Phenothiazines	3
Griseofulvin	8
Sodium cyclohexylsulfamate	27
Total	104

had recurrent severe photodermatitis on the exposed area for the past 2 years. No considerable drugs were taken. As she had worked as a candy maker, various candy materials were tested until this sweetening agent was proved to be the causal chemical compound. Both photopatch tests and phototests following ingestion of this material were positive. Her skin lesions improved quite rapidly when she stopped taking this material. It was thought, therefore, that sodium cyclohexylsulfamate caused her skin condition. 17 similar cases have been seen so far at our OPD. We imagine that there will be more patients since this agent is very widely used in various candies, cans and juices. Some of these cases were also sensitive to sulfonamides. The chemical formula of sodium cyclohexylsulfamate is different from sulfonamides in the benzylring where no double bond is present. The photocross-reaction between sodium cyclohexylsulfamate and sulfonamides is very interesting to us. However, whether sodium cyclohexylsulfamate is a sensitizer or elicitor is not known at present.

2. *Griseofulvin*. We have seen eight cases with photosensitive dermatitis due to griseofulvin. In all of these cases, the photopatch tests and the phototests after ingestion of griseofulvin were positive. It was characteristic that most of these eight cases showed photosensitivity for the period of several years after stopping of griseofulvin. There were five cases which showed a photo-cross-reaction between griseofulvin and the other antibiotics such as penicillin, fradiomycin, kanamycin and streptomycin. There is, however, no relationship in chemical structure among griseofulvin and the other antibiotics in any respect. This type of photocross-sensitization might be considered an autologous photoallergic reaction in nature.

Table 2. *The summarized data of eight cases of photo-leucomelanodermatitis observed by our Dermatology Department*

age	sex	causative drugs	duration of administ.	period to onset of solar dermatitis after administ. of drugs	period to onset of photo leucomelanoderm. after administ. of drugs
38 to 82 years	male 7 female 1	chlorobenzene-2, 4-disulfon-amide 5 benzyl-hydrochloro-thiazide 1 hydroflume-thiazine 1 polythiazide 1	1.5 M. to 12 M.	0.5 M. to 12 M.	2 M. to 13 M.

3. *Benzothiadiazine Derivatives*. Benzothiadiazine derivatives caused photosensitive dermatitis followed by characteristic leucomelanodermatitis. In this type of photosensitive dermatitis, erythema and papules appeared on the exposed area in the beginning. When these skin eruptions faded, pigmented and depigmented macules developed. We have observed eight cases of such skin manifestation during the past 2 years. As shown in Tab. 2, it was noticed that five of these patients was induced by chlorobenzene-2,4-disulfonamide as causative drugs and that the duration of administration of these drugs, period to onset of skin manifestation varied case by case. The number of patients with this type of photosensitive dermatitis during the past 2 years at 41 hospitals in Japan was 195, therefore this type of iatrogenic disorder seems to occur rather frequently. It was quite interesting that dopa stain of the specimen taken from depigmented area was positive in many melanocytes, and we consider this finding to be postinflammatory leucoderma. All these patients have been revealed to be negative in both photopatch tests and phototests after ingestion of drugs. So far we have could not concluded whether this disorder would develope under the mechanisms of photoallergy or phototoxicity. We would like to call this type of photosensitive dermatitis "photoleucomelanodermatitis".

Les accidents cutanés de l'allergie humorale médicamenteuse. Intérêt du test de Shelley

J. Maleville, H. Bergoend et A. Basset, Clinique Dermatologique, Hospices Civils, Strasbourg (France)

Depuis 3 ans, nous nous sommes attachés à la Clinique Dermatologique de Strasbourg à l'étude des manifestations d'intolérance médicamenteuse par voie générale dont nous avons pu colliger 450 observations, ce qui représente 5% de nos nouveaux consultants externes.

Leur diagnostic étiologique nous a posé des difficultés: si l'anamnèse menée avec la rigueur d'une enquête policière garde une valeur primordiale, si l'aspect clinique fournit des indications d'orientation, l'étiologie ne bénéficie guère des apports paracliniques (tests épicutanés, intradermoréactions, éosinophilie entre autres). L'image histologiques avec les altérations de la basale, l'infiltrat en bandes horizontales péri vasculaire du derme superficiel, la migration pigmentaire, les altérations vasculaires nous a paru par contre fournir des renseignements valables. L'importance d'un diagnostic étiologique précis a cependant des applications prophylactiques et thérapeutiques telles, que nous avons tenté d'établir un parallèle entre la symptomatologie clinique et le test de Shelley in vitro dont nous avons déjà montré l'intérêt dans des travaux antérieurs [Bull. Soc. franç. Derm. Syph. **73**, 39 (1966). — Thèse H. Bergoend, Strasbourg 1966].

Considérations générales

Sexe: Il existe une légère prédominance masculine: 236 cas contre 214 cas féminins. *Ages:* Les accidents d'intolérance chez l'enfant sont rares: 2 cas, l'un à 18 mois, l'autre a 7 ans (urticaire dans les deux cas). Les sujets entre 10 et 19 ans représentent 4,22% de l'ensemble (19 cas). Accroissement progressif entre 20 et 60 ans puis diminution à partir de 60 ans.

Symptomatologie

Caractères généraux. Le caractère premier des manifestations cutanées d'intolérance est la *symétrie* des lésions. Si l'on excepte l'érythème pigmenté fixe on peut considérer qu'une éruption non symétrique est rarement une réaction d'intolérance par voie générale.

Le deuxième élément est le *prurit:* souvent discret, existant essentiellement au début de l'éruption, il peut parfois faire défaut. Le troisième élément d'orientation est le polymorphisme fréquent des lésions aboutissant à *simuler* une ou plusieurs affections à la fois: association de lésions séro-papuleuses, en cocarde, bulleuses. L'éruption médicamenteuse «singe» l'affection sans la reproduire exactement.

Aspect clinique des manifestations observées

Nous les avons groupées dans cinq cadres généraux dont le détail sera retrouvé dans la thèse déjà citée.

Manifestations anaphylactiques: choc anaphylactique, urticaire oedème, de Quincke qui groupent 191 cas, soit 42,5%.

Manifestations érythémateuses: érythrodermies, érythèmes morbiliformes papuleux, érythèmes divers, érythèmes solaires, érythèmes contusiformes, érythèmes pigmentés fixes, réunissant 164 cas soit 37%.

Manifestations bulleuses: érythème polymorphe, ectodermose pluri orificielle et syndrome de Stevens Johnson, syndrome de Lyell, maladie de Brocq-Duhring: 36 cas soit 8%.

Manifestations «*vasculaires*», purpura, purpura nécrotique des membres inférieurs, éruption papulo-nécrotique à type de parapsoriasis varioliforme, panartérites et périartérites noueuses, agranulocytoses: 44 cas soit 9,75%.

Affections divers: dysidrose, fièvre, prurit, bromides, éosinophilie etc. 15 cas soit 3,3%.

Tableau 1

Manifestations cliniques	Total	Mis en évidence d'un allergène	Pourcentage
Choc anaphylactique	26	26	100
Urticaire	151	119	79
Oedème de Quincke	14	14	100
Erythrodermie	55	42	71
Erythème morbiliforme papuleux	31	25	80
Erythème solaire	15	11	73
Erythèmes divers	45	27	60
Erythème contusiforme	8	7	87
Erythème pigmenté fixe	10	8	80
Erythème polymorphe	12	10	83
Ectodermose et syndrome de Stevens-Johnson	3	3	100
Syndrome de Lyell	13	13	100
Maladie de Brocq-Duhring	8	0	0
Purpura	10	5	50
Purpura nécrotique des membres inf.	20	16	75
Erythème papulo-nécrotique	9	7	77
PAN et Agranulocytose	5	5	100
Dysidroses	4	3	75
Affections diverses	11	2	18
	450	347	72%

Le pourcentage important de tests de Shelley trouve positif s'explique à notre avis par la sélection des malades: nous ne testons pas toutes les urticaires, un diagnostic d'orientation étant fait au paravant; il en est de même pour les érythrodermies et les différents érythèmes. Nous avons par contre testé tous les érythèmes pigmentés fixes, tous les syndromes de Lyell, toutes les éruptions papulonécrotiques à type de parapsoriasis varioliformes.

Particularités cliniques de certaines éruptions

L'urticaire médicamenteuse peut être aigue, survenant tout au début ou en cours d'un traitement, ou chronique. Toujours histaminique à son début elle peut dans certains cas se transformer au bout d'un certain temps d'évolution en urticaire cholinergique, en particulier dans l'urticaire à la Pénicilline. [R. SCHUPPLI: Schweiz. med. Wschr. 81, 589 (1951). — A. BASSET, H. BERGOEND et E. GROSS-HANS: Rev. Praticien 31, 4449 (1966)]. Cliniquement, l'éruption est très souvent figurée (avec à la limite des lésions en cocarde), l'atteinte palmo plantaire, précoce, est très évocatrice.

Les *érythrodermies médicamenteuses* sont le plus souvent aigues, bénignes ou subaigues, correspondant à la «dermatite exfoliante aigue bénigne» de BROCQ, évoluant vers la guérison en 10 à 15 jours. Mais la surinfection très fréquente peut entraîner la chronicité.

Le groupe des *maladies bulleuses* semble d'après nous très fréquemment lié à une intolérance médicamenteuse. Si ce fait est admis par la grande majorité pour le syndrome de Lyell, le syndrome de Stevens-Johnson et l'ectodermose érosive qui n'en seraient que des formes mineures [BAZEX, SALVADOR, DUPRÉ, PARANT et CRISTOL: Bull. Soc. franç. Derm. Syph. 69, 106 (1962)], cela est beaucoup plus discuté pour l'érythème polymorphe. Les éruptions que nous avons étiqueté ainsi sont en fait beaucoup plus des éruptions à type d'érythème polymorphe que des érythèmes polymorphes vrais avec leur symptomatologie et leur localisation si caractéristiques.

Nous avons testé huit *maladies de Brocq-Duhring* à l'iode. Tous les tests furent négatifs. Or certaines avaient subi des poussées après ingestion de ce médicament.

L'affection que nous appelons *purpura nécrotique des membres inférieurs* est faite d'ulcérations nécrotiques associées à un purpura, pétéchial parfois, plus souvent papuleux et bulleux. Le syndrome hématologique se réduit le plus souvent à une fragilité capillaire. Ce syndrome nous semble intéressant à connaître car évoluant indéfiniment si le médicament (salicylé le plus souvent) n'est pas supprimé. Or ces lésions, algiques, entraînent la prise de salicylés.

Les *éruptions papulonécrotiques* peuvent prendre l'aspect du parapsoriasis aigu en gouttes ou du parapsoriasis varioliforme de Mucha et nous posons la question de l'origine médicamenteuse de ce syndrome.

Enfin *certaines dysidroses* nous paraissent liées à une intolérance à l'iode. Le test de Shelley y est positif et des poussées de dysidrose, parfois accompagnees d'exanthème s'observent lors de l'absorption de produits iodés.

Tableau 2. *Essai de détermination du médicament en fonction de la symptomatologie (statistique établie avec les cas testés)*

	Pénicilline %	Procaïne %	Salicylés et antalgiques %	Iode %	Divers %
Choc anaphylactique	27	39	22	7,0	19
Urticaire	34	23	13	3,8	25
Oedème de Quincke	22	28	28		22
Erythrodermies	21	14			24 Strepto
Eruptions bulleuses et syndrome de Lyell	19	15	23		Sulfamides 38
Purpura nécrotique des membres inférieurs			87		13
Eruptions papulo-nécrotiques			57		43

Ainsi les manifestations anaphylactiques semblent essentiellement dues à la Pénicilline, à la Procaïne et aux antalgiques, les érythrodermies à la Pénicilline et surtout à la Streptomycine, les syndromes bulleux aux sulfamides et aux antalgiques; les manifestations vasculaires aux antalgiques.

Toutes ces données évidemment ne sont valables que si le test de Shelley permet la mise en évidence d'anticorps circulants dans les conflits immunologiques médicamenteux. Notre impression de la valeur du test repose sur la reproductibilité du test à des périodes variables, sur le concordance entre le laboratoire et la clinique (réintroduction d'un allergène, élimination de l'allergène en cause, réintroduction de tous les médicaments suspectés exception faite de l'allergène). Le test de Shelley est cependant l'object de nombreuses critiques: il est possible que ces critiques soient fondées si toutes les précautions de prélèvement, de conservation du sérum, de minutie dans l'exécution du test ne sont pas respectées. Notre expérience prouve que les résultats dans les tests qui nous sont demandés de l'extérieur, sont beaucoup plus sujets à caution que ceux exécutés dans notre clinique, en raison du non respect de certaines précautions fondamentales: intervalle d'une quinzaine de jours entre l'accident et la prise de sang, séjour aussi limité que possible du sang à la température ambiante.

La thésaurismose cutanée par polyvinylpyrrolidone (PVP)

J. M. Lachapelle, Clinique Dermatologique de l'Université de Louvain (Belgique)

En 1964, nous avons décrit avec le Prof. Dupont une dermatose d'un type inédit. Une femme de 36 ans, atteinte de diabète insipide et traitée par des injections de pituitrine liée à la polyvinylpyrrolidone (PVP), avait développé sur le thorax, le cou et les membres supérieurs un grand nombre de papules. L'examen histologique d'une d'entre elles révélait la présence d'importants dépôts d'une substance amorphe qu'une étude histochimique identifiait à la PVP.

Depuis lors trois cas tout à fait analogues ont été observés en France, l'un par Cabanne, Chapuis, Duperrat et Putelat, le deuxième par le Prof. Bazex et ses collaborateurs, le troisième, non encore publié, par Le Coulant, Texier. Leuret et Geniaux.

La parenté anatomo-clinique des trois premières observations nous autorise à préciser les caractères de cette nouvelle maladie iatrogène.

La polyvinylpyrrolidone (PVP) est une macromolécule inerte utilisée en thérapeutique par voie veineuse comme substitut du plasma et par voie sous-cutanée ou intramusculaire comme véhicule-retard, assurant la libération progressive de diverses médications. Elle n'est pas métabolisée par l'organisme et les molécules les plus lourdes (d'un poids moléculaire supérieur à 40.000) ne peuvent franchir le filtre rénal. Elles s'accumulent indéfiniment dans les cellules du système réticulo-endothélial. Il est classique de retrouver des dépôts de PVP dans le foie et dans la rate de sujet qui plusieurs années auparavent avaient reçu une perfusion unique de la substance.

Des manifestations cliniques liées à cette accumulation sont beaucoup plus rares. Elles surviennent après administration de doses considérables de PVP. Jusqu'à présent, tous les malades qui ont présenté de semblables manifestations sont atteints de diabète insipide et traités par des injections quotidiennes de pituitrine-PVP. Delbarre, Paolaggi et Basset ont suivi deux patients qui présentaient des douleurs ostéoarticulaires et chez lesquels la biopsie fémorale avait révélé une thésaurisation massive de PVP.

L'infiltration cutanée par PVP a une traduction clinique assez semblable chez notre malade et chez celle du Prof. Bazex. Il s'agit de papules arrondies, de 3 à 4 mm de diamètre, de coloration rouge-cuivrée, assez prurigineuses. A la base du cou et sur le haut du thorax, elles sont étroitement juxtaposées mais ne confluent pas. Dans le cas de Cabanne et coll., il s'agit au contraire d'un vaste placard unique de 10 à 15 cm de diamètre situé dans la région présternale, rouge-violacé, nettement infiltré, discrètement prurigineux.

Il faut noter qu'aux points d'injections de la substance, il n'existe aucune induration. C'est après résorption que la PVP se dépose secondairement dans le derme à distance des sites d'injection.

A l'examen histologique, on constate l'existence d'un infiltrat aux limites imprécises qui s'étale sur toute la hauteur du derme. Il est formé par des éléments histio-cytaires aux contours ovalaires et au noyau nucléolé ainsi que par quelques cellules géantes. Le cytoplasme des cellules est bourré de vacuoles contenant une substance amorphé basophile à coloration par l'hématéine-éosine. Certaines cellules géantes contiennent en outre un corps astéroïde. Des amas de cette substance basophile existent aussi à l'état libre dans les espaces interstitiels en particulier autour des glandes ou entre les cellules adipeuses de l'hypoderme.

Par une étude histochimique approfondie la substance est identifiée à la PVP.

Elle est en effet colorée en pourpre par le Chlorazol Fast Pink BK, en rouge-vif par le Rouge Congo selon la méthode de FREIMAN et GALL, en brun-acajou par le Lugol, en rose foncé par le Kernechtrot, en brun-noir par l'Orcéine, en violet par l'aldéhyde fuchsine de Gomori. Elle n'est pas colorée par les colorants des graisses, ni par le PAS. Elle est orthochromatique au Bleu de Toluidine et au Violet de Paris. Ces propriétés tinctoriales sont superposables à celles de la PVP thésaurisée dans le foie et la rate de cobayes, auxquels nous avions injecté la substance par voie sous-cutaneé.

Deux ans après l'interruption de la thérapeutique chez notre patiente et son remplacement par le tannate de pitressine, une nouvelle biopsie a été pratiqueé et a permis de constater la persistance d'importants dépôts de PVP sous forme de vacuoles à l'intérieur des histiocytes du derme. Cependant les affinités tinctoriales de certaines vacuoles se sont modifiées. Elles prennent toujours les colorants spécifiques de la PVP, mais en outre elles sont colorées par le mucicarmin, par le PAS et par les colorants des radicaux sulfhydrile (CHEVREMONT, DDD de BARRNETT et SELIGMAN). Ceci semble indiquer une combinaison de la PVP avec des protéines tissulaires, combinaison dont la nature intime nous échappe. Certaines de ces modifications avaient été signalées par HUBNER en pathologie expérimentale et par WIDGREN dans un cas de thésaurismose ganglionnaire.

Nous avons pratiqué dans notre cas personnel une étude au microscope électronique. Dans le cytoplasme des cellules, existent des vacuoles caractéristiques. De forme sphérique ou ovoïde, elles sont de taille très diverse, supérieure à celles des mitochondries, attaignant ou dépassant celle des noyaux. Elles semblent limitées par une simple membrane. Leur contenu est très clair (c'est à dire relativement perméable au flux électronique). Ces images — les premières à être décrites en pathologie — sont en accord avec les images de thésaurisation expérimentale de macromolécules dans le foie de la souris (GABLER, HUBNER, DE DUVE et WATTIAUX).

Chez les trois malades, il est presque certain que les organes nobles ont accumulé la PVP sans que cette thésaurisation n'ait eu — jusqu'à présent tout au moins — de traduction clinique.

En *conclusion*, il nous a paru intéressant de rapporter ces observations de connaissance toute récente afin de mettre en garde contre l'emploi à long terme de certaines médications-retard dont le véhicule est la polyvinylpyrrolidone.

Bibliographie. BAZEX, A., A. DUPRÉ, GÉRAUD, RASCOL, A. GUILHEM et P. CANTALA: Arch. belges Derm. **XXI** (1966) (A paraître). — CABANNE, F., J. L. CHAPUIS, B. DUPERRAT et R. PUTELAT: Ann. Anat. path. **11**, 385 (1966). — DUPONT, AD., et J. M. LACHAPELLE: Bull. Soc. franç. Derm. Syph. **71**, 508 (1964). — LACHAPELLE, J. M.: Dermatologica (Basel) **132**, 476 (1966). — LACHAPELLE, J. M., et A. BOURLOND: Bull. Soc. franç. Derm. Syph. **74**, (1967).

Mascaras pigmentarias como expresión iatrogénica a dosis altas y prolongadas de feniotiacina y derivados en el control de afecciones psiquiátricas

E. B. MOLINA LEGUIZAMÓN, A. A. CORDERO y E. FOLLMANN, Catedra de Dermatología de la Facultad de Ciencias Medicas de Buenos Aires (Argentina)

La cloropromacina es una droga derivada de la fenotiacina. Sintetizada por BERNTHESEN en 1883, permaneció relegada hasta 1934, en que se la utilizó como insecticida por sus cualidades tóxicas. 4 años más tarde, en 1938, fué empleada como antihelmíntica y en 1944 contra el paludismo y las tripanosomiasis. HALPERN la ensayó posteriormente como antihistamínico y SIGNALD, DUREL y PELLERAT en algunos casos de parkinsonismo. WINTER puso en evidencia su acción coadyuvante con los hipnóticos y LABORIT la incorporó en 1948 a sus cocktails para intervenciones quirúrgicas y la hibernación artificial. Los primeros ensayos farmacológicos se realizaron en Francia, en 1950, demostrando que la droga poseía importante acción neuroléptica, motivo de su promoción en psiquiatría y otras especialidades médicas. Composición química y propiedades:

La cloropromacina se presenta en forma de un polvo blanquecino, ligeramente granuloso, de sabor amargo y de acción anestésica local, especialmente en las mucosas. Muy soluble en agua, cloroformo y alcohol es insoluble en ésteres y benzenos; su ph es variable y oscila entre 4 y 5, con tendencia a la acidez.

Su fórmula química corresponde a un clorhidrato de cloro 3 (dimetilamino-3 propil) 10 fenotiacina; C 17 N 19. Sus principales propiedades son: neuropléjicas, sobre el sistema neuovegetativo periférico y central; simpaticolítica al comienzo, luego se vuelve vagolítica. De acción selectiva sobre los centros mesodiencefálicos y vegetativos, controla al sistema autónomo, inhibiendo los reflejos visceroviscerables.

Por su acción adrenolítica regula los mecanismos adrenérgicos y los efectos exitomotores de la adrenalina. Espasmolítica, antipirética, anticonvulsivante y potencializadora de los barbitúricos, es además anestésica e inhibidora de los reflejos condicionados, propiedades que le confieren su acción neuroléptica.

En el comercio se presenta para el consumo en comprimidos, supositorios, gotas, jarabe y ampollas.

En dermatología tiene indicaciones precisas en todos aquellos procesos cutáneos en los cuales los factores psicosomáticos juegan un papel definido o en afecciones tegumentarias que se acompañan de trastornos del carácter o de la emotividad (JUNTER) tales como dermatosis generalizadas eritrodermias, pénfigos y parapénfigos o en otras en que patología del tejido conjuntivo está comprometida.

La cloropromocina como otros derivados de la fenotiacina y drogas similares de su tipo puede originar en determinadas circunstancias y personas, manifestaciones cutáneas variadas y polimorfas, que al exteriorizarse producen dermatosis con características clínicas particulares que facilitan su diagnóstico. CONCALVES LEITAO, fue uno de los primeros en observarlas y señalarlas, agrupándolas bajo el común denominador de accidentes por la cloropromacina. En su mayoría estos accidentes son dermatitis por contacto, localizadas en áreas descubiertas y en las que el factor lumínico incide ostensiblemente, motivo de su relación con las fotodermatosis. Sus portadores son pacientes sometidos a la acción de la droga o personal de enfermeros y ayudantes encargados de distribuir el medicamento, en otras oportunidades personas de servicio, a los que estan confiados el lavado de las ropas de cama, prendas interiores, higiene de los orinales, encargados de preparar la droga y darle la forma comercial para su consumo o envasarla.

En 1953 PELLERAT, RIVES y MURAT estudiaron 8 casos de dermatitis de contacto por Ampliactil, en enfermeros de un hospital de salud mental, a las que se sumaron otros producdas por ingestión de derivados de la fenotiacina Terrier contemporáneamente infilteó la piel con cloropromacina con fines anestésicos locales, sin registrar accidentes alérgicos inmediatos. HURIEZ, GRAUX, FONTA, PRUVOT y PIERRE MARTIN, comunicaron en 1953, 9 casos de dermatitis venenata, que como en los casos anteriores eran enfermeros encargados de inyectar cloropromacina, además de estreptomicina; el fenómeno fué interpretado como una sensibilización de grupo.

En el mismo artículo dichos autores comentaban la intolerancia de los enfermos psoriásicos y eccematosos, a los gangliopléjicos, a dosis terapéuticas comunes. PINARD corre el telón del año 1953 con un par de pacientes sensibilizados al grupo fenetacínico. Al año siguiente LE COULANT, DONADIEU y GARCES comunicaron nuevos accidentes en 4 enfermeros, con lesiones en cara y manos y SIDI, KINCLY y LONQUEVILLE sus experiencias de sensibilización cruzadas con Ampliactil y Fenergan, llamando la atención sobre su elevada incidencia.

En nuestro país, en 1954, QUIROGA LEGUIZAMÓN y CASTILLO ensayan la droga por primera vez, en curas de sueño prolongado, en 10 internados en el servicio de piel del Hospital RAMOS MEJIA con el fin de controlar un grupo de dermatosis alérgicas muy pruriginosas e irreductibles a los tratamientos clásicos. Los resultados ínmediatos fueron alentadores y no se apreciaron fenómenos de intolerancia medicamentosa. CORDERO y BERARD, arribaron a las mismas conclusiones y coincidieron en reafirmar la bondad de la nueva terapéutica. En 1955 se realizaron dos reuniones de importancia mundial sobre beneficios y accidentes originados por la cloropromacina y drogas afines, en psiquiatría.

En 1956 WAINFEL y CASALÁ en la Argentina comunicaron los primeros casos de intolerancia al Ampliactil en enfermeros encargados de distribuir la droga. Dos años más tarde, CORDERO, MOLINA LEGUIZAMÓN y VIVOT, publicaron un trabajo de estadística realizado en el Hospital Nacional de Neuropsiquiatría de Varones, en el que llamaron la atención sobre la poca incidencia de casos encontrados en el examen practicado a 230 enfermeros de dicho nosocomio, registrando unicamente a 4 casos de eccema por contacto. Con posterioridad, CASALÁ y MENDOZA reactualizaron el tema y señalando que el número de sensibilizados a la cloropromacina suele ser variable, oscilando entre el 5 y el 85%; esta disparidad aparente según los autores estaría en relación directa con el lugar de trabajo, intensidad laboral, tiempo de exposición al medicamento, profilácticas, etc. Simultáneamente MOLINA LEGUIZAMÓN al encontrar 10 casos de dermatitis por Ampliactil en enfermos del Hospital de Neuropsiquiatría de Varones, enfocó el problema bajo el aspecto de una probable enfermedad profesional, haciendo las consideraciones correspondientes.

Pero a fines de 1958 el director del Hospital Provincial de Enfermedades Mentales de Essondale del Canadá, solicitó la colaboración de un grupo de dermatólogos por llamar la atención una curiosa pigmentación que observara en las zonas tegumentarias descubiertas de algunos de sus pacientes recluídos, a los que se les venía administrando dosis altas y prolongadas de cloropromacina o derivados compuestos de la fenotiacina, por sus trastornos mentales y de conducta, irreversibles a las dosis terapéuticas comunes de 50 a 200 mg. Las conclusiones de ese estudio probaron que estos pacientes pigmentados padecían una melanosis crónica accidental, consecutiva al uso de la droga o dosis masivas e indefinidas. Los comentarios sobre la presencia de una nueva modalidad de intolerancia cutánea al grupo neuroléptico, tan de moda y actualidad en psiquiatría y otras especialidades, despertó el interés de muchos colegas, que los aconsejaban como terapéutica coadyuvante y paralela en procesos clínicos diversos. El interés por esta discromia dió origen a una serie de estudios, pruebas de laboratorio, biológicas, etc., antes de reconocerla como tal. Sucesivamente a la primera observación, le siguieron muchas otras. PERROT y BOURIADA presentaron en la Sociedad francesa de dermatología y sifilografía una alienada con "visage mauve" atribuible a la cloropromacina. 2 años más tarde, (1964) ZELICKSON y ZELLER hallaron 8 casos de esta discromia, a los que se agregarían otros 70, encontrados por GREINER y BERRY al examinar un millar de alienados recluídos en una clínica de Columbia Británica, sometidos a tratamiento exclusivo con cloropromacina durante algo más de 1 año, con dosis de hasta 1500 mg diarios. Posteriormente estos mismos autores efectuaron un examen ocular a 131 pacientes a los también se les administraba

cloropromacina, pero en dosis inferiores, no mayores a los 300 mg diarios, durante
un lapso variable, entre 3 a 9 años. Con la lámpara de hendidura describieron
alteraciones muy características en el cristalino. En noviembre de 1964, HAYS,
LYLE y WHEELER encontraron 5 mujeres de tez blanca internadas en un hospital
psiquiátrico, con lesiones pigmentarias de cara, que les recordaba las producidas
por las argirias. En la actualidad se continúan describiendo y presentando nuevos
casos de este sindrome pigmentario recientemente incorporado a la dermatología
y privativo de pacientes psiquiátricos sometidos a dosis masivas de fenotiacina
y sus derivados, durante tiempo prolongado.

Dosis y tiempo mínimo necesario para la inciación de esta discromia

Según la opinión de algunos autores, la dosis mínima necesaria para que se
origine esta discromia, en ningún caso debe ser inferior a los 600 mg diarios de
cloropromacina. Las pruebas realizadas en un grupo de alienados sometidos a
cantidades menores a la señalada, no lograron producir la pigmentación de su piel.
Al elevarlas, aparecerían las primeras manifestaciones discrómicas, cuya gama
colorimétrica varía lentamente hasta alcanzar el color azul pizarra, con las süce-
sivas y correspondientes exposiciones al sol; en cuanto al tiempo de su administración consideraron la del año calendario como el mínimo necesario para la aparición
de las primeras variaciones.

Descripción del cuadro clínico de esta dermatosis

Las primeras manifestaciones de este proceso iatrogénico fueron observadas
en mujeres, interpretándose erróneamente como propias del sexo femenino y
vinculadas con trastornos endocrinos, ya que droga es capaz de alterar la función
hiposisaria, originando galactorrea, amenorrea y diabetes insípida. Su hallazgo
ulterior en varones sirvió para descartar esa interpretación. Localizadas en zonas
cutáneas descubiertas, particularmente en áreas que hacen relieve, tales como la
frente, la nariz, los pómulos, etc. es la cara, el cuello, el triángulo del escote, los
antebrazos, el dorso de las manos y de los pies y ocasionalmente las piernas,
los sitios mas frecuentemente afectados. Su generalización aunque rara, ha sido
descripta por algunos autores. Suele respetar la piel protegida por las ropas, como
así también a los enfermos gotosos que no exponen a la luz ni al sol. Generalmente se
presentan en placas, de forma variable y extensión progresiva, de matices diversos,
impresionan y recuerdan la piel bronceada por el sol. Las primeras manifestaciones
de esta pigmentación crónica y acumulativa se inician en primavera, para insensiblemente acentuarse durante el verano. Una vez establecida, es difícil que
desaparezca, aún en invierno; tampoco se atenúa con la reducción de la dosis de la
droga; su reemplazo por otros medicamentos o con prevención en estos pacientes
exposiciones solares. Algunos autores han sugerido y realizado encierro de estos
enfermos en habitaciones obscuras, durante lapsos variables, hasta de 4 semanas
consecutivas; la disminución de las dosis de cloropromacina, su administración con
queladores, suspensión de la droga, uso de D-penicilamina, etc.; en un solo caso,
logró la desaparición por completo de pigmentación cutánea; en otro se obtuvo
ligera mejoría, la que se perdió al exponerlo a la D-penicilamina con el objeto de
bloquear la tirosinasa, que interfiere en la producción de melanina.

Al inciarse la máscara pigmentaria su color es castaño obscuro, tonalidad que
pierde para virar insensiblemente a un marrón acentuado, gris azulado, azul pizarra
o al purpúreo. Esta gama colorimétrica tendría relación con el tipo de piel del
sujeto, sexo, tiempo de exposición a la luz, dosis de cloropromacina, período de
su administración, hábitos del enfermo, estación calendaria, etc.

Las áreas cutáneas cubiertas, los pliegues y las mucosas de estos pacientes suelen no estar afectados, no así las faneras que como sucede con los pelos, cambian de color, para volverse blanquecino pimienta, hasta en el 85% de los casos. Las uñas, en cambio, ocasionalmente suelen estar comprometidas y cuando ello sucede, es un signo de mal pronóstico.

También se han descripto lesiones oculares, que distan de ser constantes. GRIE-NER y col., DELONG, POLEY y MCFARLAINE han encontrado retinopatias pigmentarias, coriorretinitis centrales, opacidades en la córnea y el cristalino; depósitos de gránulos blancos y amarillentos, que con la lámpara de hendidura se los reconoce fácilmente por su aspecto estrellado. Para estos autores los cambios mas importantes, notorios y específicos, serían los del cristalino. Algunos oftalmólogos hablan de alteraciones en el humor acuoso y las consideran patonogmónicas de esta discromía. Hay quienes refieren haber observado crisis oculógiras, cicloplejias y miosis.

Las autopsias de algunos pacientes que fallecieron durante el tratamiento con cloropromacina, tal los 12 enfermos jóvenes asistidos por GREINER y NICHOLSON, revelaron lesiones pigmentarias viscerales. Los órganos mas comprometidos resultaron el hígado, corazón, riñones, glándulas endocrinas, sistema nervioso central y los vasos.

Estudios complementarios de esta dermatosis

A las observaciones clínicas estos pacientes pigmentados siguieron una serie de estudios e investigaciones con el fin de conocer su patogenia. Con la técnica de la ventana de piel se observó el desplazamiento de la melanina a los vasos sanguíneos de la dermis con lo cual se explicaba satisfactoriamente las melanosis generalizada encontrada en las autopsias. Su transporte o el de un material de apariencia similar como así también las células que toman parte normalmente en una reacción inflamatoria, fueron marcados. WASSERMANN observó con esta técnica que estas partículas pigmentarias eran tomados por los macrófagos en la dermis y luego depositadas en el corion, en las áreas perivasculares. El estudio metabólico de la cloropromacina realizado por PERRY y col. en 1964, en el hombre, permitió conocer una gran variedad de derivados de la misma y determinar al menos teóricamente su responsabilidad, acción farmacológica y efectos tóxicos. Uno de ellos, el 7 hidroxiclorpromacina sería excretado por la orina, la que expuesta a la luz solar adquiriría un color púrpureo casi inmediato. Su mutación colorimétrica sugirió la idea de que este metabolito podría ser el responsable de la coloración purpúrea de la piel. En las mismas se hallaron además otros conjugados fenólicos; uno de ellos en una concentración mayor que el 7-hidroxiclor-promacina y químicamente desmetilado.

PORTER efectuó algunas pruebas de espectrofotométricas comparativas de áreas cutáneas pigmentadas del brazo y de la cara, encontrando modificaciones melánicas acentuadas en las curvas logradas a favor de la segunda, resultado que le sugirió la posibilidad de que existieron otras sustancias colorantes, además de las melaninas.

PERRY, CULLING, BERRY y HANSEN, completaron sus investigaciones realizando el estudio histológico comparativo de piel normal y de piel pigmentada. Las diferencias encontradas consistieron en depósito importante de pigmento amarillo castaño en las células adyacentes de los capilares de la dermis superficial y una acentuada disminución de las mismas a nivel de la hilera basal, con el método de la hematoxilina eosina. Con la coloración de Masson Fontana, localizaron un depósito de granos negros muy finos a nivel de dichas capas y una intensa actividad tirosinásica en la basal, la que disminuía en los depósitos pigmentarios dérmicos, llegando a ser mínima o nula en la piel normal. Con las reacciones de

Lillie se lograron resultados similares; en cambio con la reacción de Schmorl se
pudo identificar a la melanina y a la premelanina. La prueba de Perl del azul de
prusia les permitió descartar la presencia de hemosiderina, por falta de hierro. Los
resultados de todas estas pruebas histoquímicas demostraron la casi imposibilidad
de diferenciar la ·melanina del pigmento perivascular dérmico. Los depósitos
pigmentarios parecerían localizarse en los macrófagos vecinos a los capilares y a
los de la capa basal. Las conclusiones a que llegaron estos autores después de sus
pruebas fueron que la 7-hidroxiclorpromacina u otros metabolitos se acumularían
en la piel y en otros tejidos de los sujetos pigmentados, los que por exposición al
sol, se transformarían en un compuesto purpúreo. Este mismo proceso ocurriría
también en condiciones aparentemente fisiológicas "in vitro". En segundo lugar
que su presencia los haría responsables del aumento de la actividad tirosinásica
y de la producción de melanina. El color purpúreo de la piel pigmentada sugeriría
que un metabolite purpureo de la cloropromacina se añadiría a la melanina o que
se formaría por una polimerización de un derivado quinoide nuclear de la fenotiacina, una seudomelanina de color diferente a la melanina.

Con respecto a las opacidades de la córnea y las cataratas centrales y estrelladas
que ocasionalmente pueden observarse en algunos pacientes pigmentados, se
encontraría una explicación si se las relacionase con la sensibilidad a los rayos
ultravioletas que demostraron estas drogas a través de sus metabolitos, en especial
el 7-hidroxiclorpromacina susceptible de transformarse en otro derivado.

El informe de las biopsias practicadas a estos pacientes hiperpigmentados
demostraron: una hiperqueratosis laminar discreta; conservación de la capa
granulosa; hiperacantosis de los brotes intercapilares, alargados e irregulares y en-
sanchados. En los espacios intercelulares; células emigrantes; degeneración vacuolar en el cuerpo mucoso. En la capa basal: abundantes gránulos de melanina y
algunos en las filas inferiores de las células epiteliales; infiltrados perivasculares;
extensión variable en la dermis superficial, formado por linfocitos, abundantes
histiocitos, eosinófilos y fibroblastos; gránulos de pigmento amarillo-obscuros en
los fibroblastos e histiocitos y extracelulares.

Interpretación patogénica de esta discromía

Quienes se ocuparon de los accidentes cutáneos producidos por este grupo y
con preferencia por los originados por la cloropromacina, los interpretaron como
una consecuencia de los depósitos de melanina en la epidermis y en la dermis. La
afinidad de este pigmento con los producidos por la fenotiacina o sus productos,
fue motivo para considerar como la causa del tinte purpureo de las áreas hiperpig-
mentadas descubiertas. El incremento de la melanina en estos se debería a la
acción de la luz ultravioleta sobre esa droga fotosensibilizante, la que reaccionaría
de maneras diferentes; como fotoalérgica, originando urticaria, erupciones
maculopapulosas, reacciones eccematosas, alteraciones cosméticas desagradables,
etc. despues de un periódo de incubación variable, en aquellos pacientes a los que
se les administra pequeñas dosis de este psicofármaco; o como expresión de una
curiosa discromia consecutiva a una reacción fototóxica, cuando las dosis son
masivas y prolongadas, teniendo en cuenta una concentración adecuada del fotosensibilizante en las células vivas de la epidermis.

Comprobaciones obtenidas en el H. N.

Prescindiendo de las reacciones fotoalérgicas mencionadas en nuestra comunicación anterior, nos referiremos exclusivamente a las discromías de las zonas
cutáneas descubiertas, observadas en un grupo de alienados, sometidos a tratamiento prolongado con dosis elevadas de cloropromacina. La lectura de trabajos

extranjeros nos indujo a buscar esta nueva dermatosis en nuestro medio, en el Hospital Nacional de Neuropsiquiatría de Varones, de la Capital Federal. Para realizar nuestra investigación nos dedicamos al examen de esta población de recluidos. No nos sorprendió encontrar una incidencia elevada de esta discromía, justificada en parte por la gran densidad de población de enfermos a los que se les administraba cloropromacina; de los 3550 recluídos, 2435 estaban sometidos a esta droga, a dosis y tiempo variable. Las circunstancias de funcionar el hospital en una área de amplios jardines, en pabellones bien orientados, provisto de grandes ventanales, sirvió para que la exposición a la luz jugase un papel importante en la mayor frecuencia de esta discromia. En aquellos pabellones mal orientados, en los cuales el sol penetra con dificultad, el número de afectados por la máscara pigmentaria fue muy inferior a la de los ubicados en los pisos altos. La conveniencia técnica de administrar cloropromacina con resultados favorables y aún superiores en algunos casos a los obtenidos por los tratamientos clásicos, vino a reemplazarlos en parte, a partir de 1958, con el advenimiento de los psicofármacos, facilitando su control y administración, y a reducir el personal encargado de su aplicación. Por otra parte también su uso permitió el abaratamiento de los costos de los tratamientos, de vital importancia en el presupuesto de los hospitales del estado. Estas circunstancias y otras de menor importancia resultaron favorables para el hallazo de esta nueva dermatosis pigmentaria. De los 3550 psicópatas recluídos a 1097 no se les administraba esta droga. Los restantes 2435, sin excepción estaban sometidos a ella, pero su dosificación y tiempo de administración era variable, en concordancia con el control de su proceso demencial. De estos últimos pacientes, solamente 700 presentaron la máscara pigmentaria y eran los que recibían dosis elevadas de cloropromacina desde hacía más de 12 meses. En el cuadro N° 1 hacemos un resumen de estos datos.

Cuadro 1

A. Enfermos que no recibían cloropromacina:	1097
B. Enfermos que recibian la droga y no se pigmentaron	1753
C. Enfermos que recibian la droga y se pigmentaron	700
D. Total de enfermos examinados	3550

Los primeros pacientes de este cuadro que no se medicaron con cloropromacina nos sirvieron de control para las conclusiones de si esta droga era o no causa de discromía. Los del segundo grupo a los que se les administró el medicamento en pequeñas dosis y no se pigmentaron (el 71,47% de los medicamentos). También nos sirvieron como testigos de las consecuencias de la administración del medicamento en grandes o pequeñas cantidades. Los del tercer grupo de 700 pacientes con máscaras (el 28,53% restante) confirmaron las opiniones de los autores extranjeros sobre esta discromia.

En el cuadro N° 2 resumimos el tiempo y la posología que estuvieron sometidos los 2453 pacientes a los que se les administró cloropromacina de los cuales 700 solamente presentaron la máscara pigmentaria. Total de psicopatas examinados 3550; pacientes a los que se les administró la droga 2435. N° de pacientes con meses de Posología. Máscara administración de la droga. Mg. día.

Cuadro 2

2453	423	25 m	93 m[a]	300	1500
2453	127	19 m	84 m	150	1200
2453	68	17 m	72 m	100	900
2453	52	15 m	53 m	50	800
2453	30	12 m	46 m	25	800[b]
T. 2453	700		[a] meses		[b] Inicial y de sosten

De los enfermos psicópatas que usaron la droga y no se pigmentaron, sus historias clínicas demostraron que el tiempo de administración de la cloropromacina era relativamente breve y en ninguna oportunidad superó el año calendario. Fácilmente controlables a dicha posología, estos pacientes se volvieron tranquilos y sociables; debemos añadir que en el grupo de 1753 pacientes no pigmentados están incluidos 123 recluidos de los pabellones MELENDEZ y CHARUGA a quienes también se les administraba la droga, en dosis superiores a los 800 mg diarios y por lapsos variables nunca inferiores a 15 meses, siendo el motivo de no presentar la pigmentación de sus áreas descubiertas el estar privados de luz solar, por su condición de alienados peligrosos. Tampoco encontramos máscaras pigmentarias en algunos gotosos y enfermos que permanecían en el lecho por afecciones clínicas o quirúrgicas, que les impedía la deambulación. El grupo de psicópatas con discromías, reducido a 700 en total eran hombres adultos, cuyas edades oscilaban entre los 20 y los 50 años. Un hecho a destacar es que los mas pigmentados procedían de servicios bien iluminados, con amplios ventanales y ocupaban los pisos mas altos de los pabellones y que por ser alienados cuyo control se había logrado eficientemente con dosis altas y prolongadas, les estaba permitido ausentarse de sus salas de internación para desempeñar ciertas tareas al aire libre, tales como las de jardineros, mensajeros, acompañantes de otros recluídos, etc. El cuadro clínico dermatológico pigmentario fué muy variado en sus matices y comprometía la casi totalidad de las superficies expuestas a la luz. Su extensión nos hizo compararlos con la escafandra de los trajes de los buzos. Pocos fueron los pacientes parcialmente pigmentados, remedando manchas cloasmáticas localizadas en las áreas de piel normal. No encontramos ningún caso de melanosis generalizada, ni alteraciones oculares ni de las faneras. El Dr. PLATER, oftalmólogo del hospital no logró constatar complicaciones oculares en los pacientes que le enviamos.

A dos de los pacientes bajo nuestro control después de elevarle las dosis de clorpromacina aprovechando que las anteriormente indicadas eran insuficientes, los expusimos en el mes de enero del año en curso a baños de sol consiguiendo la aparición de una discromía con los caracteres clínicos observadas en los demas enfermos pigmentados. Las primeras manifestaciones consistieron en un eritema activo, que en uno de ellos llegó a producirle flictenas, obligándonos a suspender los baños de luz, y a tratar su dermatosis, sin necesidad de disminuir la posología a la que estaba sometido.

Superada la crisis, con toda precausión lo expusimos nuevamente al sol, logrando broncearlo. Este paciente fue biopsiado, encontrándose pigmentos en su dermis y epidermis, completamos el estudio de los demas estudios pigmentados, con pruebas de laboratorio y biopsias que tomamos de la cara o del cuello. Para tal fin escogimos aquellos que no ofrecían dudas, al menos clínicas, de su cuadro discrómico. Las pruebas de laboratorio que solicitamos consistieron en análisis completo de orina, hemograma, eritrosedimentación y hepatograma. En las pruebas de orina, las bandas de Kimmig variaron entre EH: 0,03 y 0,07. El resultado de las biopsias, fue el signiente:

Con la hematoxilina-eosina se comprobaron la presencia de abundantes depósitos de un pigmento amarillo castaño en las células adyacentes a los capilares de la dermis superficial y en menor cantidad en la capa basal de la epidermis. Con la coloración de Masson-Fontana para la melanina, en esos sitios se observó un depósito de gránulos finos y negruzcos. La actividad tirosinásica fué particularmente intensa en la capa basal y en menor grado en los depósitos pigmentarios dérmicos. Con la técnica del hierro de lillie se lograron los mismos resultados que con la coloración de Masson-Fontana. La reacción de Perl, del azul de prusia los resultados fueron negativos, demostrando la ausencia de hierro, descartando así la hemosiderina. Histológicamente el pigmento fue indistinguible de la melanina, de acuerdo a las reacciones consideradas como específicas. Los depósitos pigmentarios parecen hallarse localizados en los macrófagos adyacentes a los capilares y en la capa basal.

Referencias. 1. CASALA, A., y S. WAINFELD: Arch. argent. Derm. **7**, 297 (1957). — 2. CASALA A., y D. MENDOZA: Arch. argent. Derm. **9**, 47 (1959). — 3. CORDERO, A. A.: Orientación méd. **VII**, 330 (1959). — 4. MOLINA LEGUIZAMÓN: Trabajo de adscripción Cloropromacine como causa de enfermedad profesional. Bs. As. 1958. — 5. PERROT, et BOURIALA: Bull. Soc. franç. Derm. Syph. **69**, 631 (1962). — 6. ZELICKSON, A.S., and H.C. ZELLER: J. Amer. med. Ass. **188**, 394 (1964). — 7. GREINER, AC., and BERRY: Canad. med. Ass. J. **90**, 663 (1964). — 8. A New Chlorpromazine lick affect. Lancet, Annotations, N° 7344, 1206 (1964). — 9. PERRY, TL., and C. F. A. CULLING: Science **146**, 81 (1964). — 10. SATANOVE, A.: J. Amer. med. Ass. **191**, 4 (1965). — 11. MARGOLIS, H., and JL. GOBLE: J. Amer. med. Ass. **193**, 7 (1965). — 12. KELLUM, R. E.: Arch. Derm. **91**, 670 (1965). — 13. HASHIMOTO, K.: J. invest. Derm. **47** 296 (1966).

Necrolisis Epidermica Toxica
Observaciones sobre 12 Casos

A. CORTÉS CORTÉS y V. CÁRDENAS JARAMILLO, Facultad de Medicina de la Universidad de Antioquia, Medellin (Colombia)

Introducción. El objeto de esta comunicación es simplemente el de presentar una breve descripción de la necrolisis epidérmica tóxica y luego nuestros comentarios sobre doce casos que hemos tenido la oportunidad de observar.

Definición. Dermatosis de aparición súbita y curso agudo, caracterizada por eritema mas o menos generalizado, el cual al cabo de horas, sigue un desprendimiento de la piel en colgajos que dejan áreas de piel denudadas con tendencia a la rápida cicatrización. En la fase de desprendimiento cutáneo se aprecian, con frecuencia, ampollas fláccidas y hay signo de Nikolsky positivo.

Sinonimia: Rara erupción ampollosa (LANG, WALKER, 1956); Necrolisis epidermica toxica (LYELL, 1956); Epidermolisis necroticans combustiformis (SOLTERMANN, 1959); Epidermolisis acuta toxica (KORTING, HOLZMANN, 1960); Epidermonecrolisis ampollosa (VÁNKOS, BORZA, 1962); Sindrome de Brocq, Lyell (MACORELA, RUIZ, 1963); Necroepidermolisis (LADA, JAGAS, KOLACZKOWSKI, 1965).

Etiología: 1. Intolerancia a drogas, 2. infecciones bacterianas, virales etc., 3. asociación de las anteriores, 4. autoinmunidad.

Considerada inicialmente por LYELL [1] como una necrosis epidérmica secundaria a una toxina circulante, podemos decir hoy que la necrolisis epidérmica tóxica es un síndrome polietiológico en el cual la intolerancia a las drogas juega un papel desencadenante en la mayoría de los casos. Las infecciones, especialmente las de la región faríngea también se encuentran frecuentemente en los antecedentes inmediatos de estos pacientes, por lo cual algunos autores han pensado que pueden éstas actuar como factor predisponente. Igualmente han considerado algunos la posibilidad de una infección viral [2]. Hay inclusive quien considere los fenómenos autoinmunes como responsables de esta afección [3].

Cuadro clínico. Se caracteriza por la aparición subita de eritema más o menos generalizado, que afecta frecuentemente las mucosas, el cual es seguido al cabo de 12 a 24 h por desprendimiento epidérmico con ampollas fláccidas, con signo de Nikolsky generalmente positivo, después de cual quedan grandes áreas de piel denudada. Hay con frecuencia dolor a la presión e hipertermia. Llama la atención que a pesar del extenso compromiso no se advierten los signos del "shock".

Histopatología. Se aprecia al microscopio necrosis más o menos marcada de las células epidérmicas, la cual lleva a la pérdida de cohesión y a la formación de vesículas intraepidérmicas que cuando llegan a ser muy grandes y localizadas en la parte inferior de la epidermis llegan a dar el aspecto de ser subepidérmicas. Llama la atención la escasa, casi nula, reacción dérmica.

Diagnostico diferencial. La necrolisis epidérmica tóxica se diferencia del Pénfigo Verdadero porque éste es de curso crónico, no se instala con tanta rapidez y sus ampollas asientan en general sin que haya una base eritematosa tan amplia y extensa, como sucede en la necrolisis epidérmica tóxica. En el eritema exudativo multiforme predominan los elementos pápuloedematosos con su morfología en iris. En el síndrome de Stevens-Johnson se notarán igualmente lesiones de tipo eritema multiforme; faltará el desprendimiento epidérmico en grandes áreas y la denudación subsiguiente. Finalmente desde el punto de vista histológico se apreciarán los cambios dérmicos del Eritema multiforme. La Patomimia o dermatitis facticia debe ser considerada sobretodo en las formas localizadas y este diagnóstico sólo es posible descartarlo después de larga observación. Las quemaduras son consideradas a primer golpe de vista en estos pacientes pero el interrogatorio nos descarta esta posibilidad.

Tratamiento. La pérdida de líquidos y electrolitos debe ser vigilada estrechamente y de acuerdo a esto se debe hacer una administración muy cuidadosa de los mismos. Igualmente los cuidados de enfermería deben ser estrictos: cambios de posición, asepsia hasta donde sea posible para evitar la infección secundaria etc. Los corticoesteroides son usados por la mayoría de los autores dado el dramatismo de la afección con el objeto de minimizar la reacción inflamatoria. Los antibióticos de amplio espectro también son usados profilácticamente dada la extensión de las áreas denudadas. Ultimamente MACOTELA-RUIZ y col. en vista de sus hallazgos de autopsia — fenómenos tromboembolíticos — recomiendan el uso de anticoagulantes.

Resumen y conclusiones

1. Se presentan 12 casos de N.E.T. (3 de forma localizada y 9 de forma generalizada).

2. En 6 casos se encontró relación con la ingestión de drogas. En 4 de éstos había además una infección asociada (3 amigdalitis y 1 gonococcia).

3. De los 12 pacientes 2 terminaron fatalmente. Estos 2 tenían compromiso extensísimo y su tratamiento fue iniciado después del 50. día de comienzo de la dermatosis.

4. Consideramos que la N.E.T. es una dermatosis reaccional de etiología multiple muy cercana del E.M. ampolloso pero con características clinicas e histológicas tan definidas que justifican su autonomía clínica.

Pronóstico. Los factores que han sido considerados de valor para el pronóstico de la necrolisis epidérmica tóxica son la edad, la extensión del proceso, la rapidez de iniciación del tratamiento y en especial la aplicación rápida de cuidados generales. De acuerdo a lo visto en nuestros casos será más grave el curso mientras más extenso sea el compromiso cutáneomucoso y mientras más se demore la iniciación de los cuidados al estado general: hidratación, administración de antibióticos de amplio espectro y corticoesteroides.

Dermatosis por anovulatorios

Y. Ortiz, Centro Dermatológico Pascua, México, D. F. (México)

Los Cinco Jinetes de la Apocalipsis dermatológica son en la actualidad insuficientes para englobar las numerosas afecciones cutáneas provocadas por las drogas. *Los años de los cincuentas fueron de los corticoesteroides, los años de los sesentas son de los anovulatorios.*

En todos los sectores de la población se habla del tema de moda "Control de la Natalidad" y "Planeación de la Familia", debido a la gran propaganda que se les ha hecho a los Anticonceptivos por vía oral, llamados corrientemente "*La píldora*". Esto ha llegado a ser un tema de interés en los Concilios Ecuménicos. Los Antiovulatorios contienen un progestágeno y un estrógeno, pertenecen a un grupo caracterizado por la presencia de un anillo del ciclo-pentano-per-hidro-fenantreno, con la particularidad de inhibir la secreción hipofisiaria de gonado-tropina, impidiendo la maduración folicular y la ovulación. La fase proliferativa del ciclo menstrual con estos medicamentos dura 3 días, luego aparece la fase secretoria temprana que es únicamente de 6 días y los 14 restantes del ciclo son la Fase Pseudodecidual. Esto equivaldría a un Pseudoembarazo. Los medicamentos se derivan de cuatro categorías químicas: 1. de la 19-Nortestosterona, 2. de la 3 dexosi de la 19-Nortestosterona, 3. de la 17 Hidroxiprogesterona y 4. de la Retro-progesterona. No solo se emplean como Anticonceptivos, aunque sea esta su principal indicación, también se utilizan en Amenorrea secundaria, Dismenorrea, Esterilidad funcional y otras indicaciones, así como en la Normalización del ciclo menstrual. Más de 10 millones de mujeres en el mundo los toman por prescripción médica. Pensamos que un número elevado lo hace por automedicación, sobre todo en México, en donde este porcentaje alcanza cifras altas.

En lo que respecta a los efectos secundarios de estas drogas se ha encontrado; Mareos naúseas, vómitos, mastalgia, cefalea, cloasma, edema, aumento de peso, dolor abdominal, hemorragias intermedias, acné, tromboflebitis, ictericia, nerviosismo e irritabilidad y algunas otras como alteraciones oculares. Se mencionó en 1965 que en Inglaterra 27 mujeres fallecieron por el uso de estas drogas. Tres de cada 100,000 mueren en la actualidad por las píldoras.

El interés dermatológico de estos medicamentos reside en que algunos autores como Wansker, Palitz, Milberg, Kantor, Strauss y Pochi en Estados Unidos y Ahumada en México los han utilizado en el tratamiento del Acné.

Por el contrario, en forma aislada se ha hecho mención de los efectos secundarios en la piel (Goldzieher, Rock, Tiller, Cook, Satterthwaite) reportan la presencia de Cloasma. Rice-Wray en México observó Cloasma, Acné y Urticaria. Netz menciona Cloasma, Exacerbación de dermatosis preexistentes (Neuro-dermatitis, Psoriasis). Ijzerman, Dukes y Kopera encontraron edema de la cara, urticaria, caída del cabello, pelo grasoso, telangiectasias, edema angioneurótico, pigmentación de la areola y del pezón y acné. También se ha reportado: Hirsutismo, Eritema polimorfo, Eritema nudoso, Púrpura, Lupus eritematoso, Erupción papulosa, Prurito y Leucodermia.

De las publicaciones dermatológicas en 1963, Esoda menciona el Cloasma por el uso de Anticonceptivos orales y comunica un caso. En 1965 en una comunicación preliminar de las dermatosis por el uso de estos medicamentos mencionamos 20 casos y a fines de ese mismo año comunicamos 50 casos.

En 1966 Rice-Wray y Ferrer hablan del Cloasma relacionado con Proges-tágenos. Resnik reune en 1967, 15 casos de Cloasma y aporta datos sobre ellos, afirma que de un grupo de 212 pacientes con tratamiento por Anticonceptivos orales el Cloasma se presentó en 61 (29%), como resultado directo de la droga. SIDI, BOURGEOIS-SPINASE y AROUETE en el actual Congreso, mencionan entre las causas de Alopecia en la mujer a las Píldoras Anticonceptivas.

En México hay más de 20 marcas comerciales de estas drogas, la mayoría de ellas pertenecen al grupo I y al III. Las del Io. contienen Noretindrona y Mestranol. Las del IIIo. Clormadinona y Mestranol. Las dosis en los últimos tres años han disminuído en forma considerable, en especial del progestágeno. Se administran en forma clásica, consistentes en que por 20, 21 o 22 días se toma el medicamento y las tabletas contienen un progestágeno y un estrógeno. Otro método es la Terapia Secuencial, que se afirma es más fisiológico y superior al anterior, se administran en los primeros 15 o 16 días el estrógeno y los cinco restantes el progestágeno y el estrógeno juntos.

Material. Nuestra casuística consta de 100 casos observados en tres años en la consulta en el Centro Dermatológico Pascua de la Ciudad de México, las dermatosis aparecidas por el empleo de los Anovulatorios. En la tabla se observan los datos.

	casos
Cloasma	63
Dermatitis medicamentosa	5
Dermatitis medicamentosa tipo Eritema pigmentario fijo	5
Dermatitis medicamentosa tipo Eritema polimorfo	4
Melanosis facial	5
Cloasma y Acné	4
Agravación de dermatosis preexistentes (Neurodermatitis y D. solar)	4
Acné	3
Alopecia difusa	3
Rosácea	2
Urticaria	2

El mayor número de las pacientes estaban entre la 3a. y la 4a. década de la vida (84 casos). El Anovlar fue el medicamento causante en 58 casos, Ortho-Novum en 7, Prolestín 6, Enavid 5 casos, Seqüens 5, Gynovlar 4 casos, Lindiol 4, Ovulen 3, Provestral 3 casos, Ovral 2 casos, Noraciclina 1 caso, Norace 1 caso y Orlest 1 caso. Las Dermatitis medicamentosas se presentaron en forma brusca, las otras dermatosis en forma lenta y progresivamente. Solo fue necesario en 11 de los casos suspender el medicamento durante un ciclo o dos, en dos de ellos la suspensión fue definitiva porque presentó el mismo cuadro con tres diferentes anticonceptivos. La terapéutica es difícil o fácil en razón de que el diagnóstico sea adecuado y oportuno. Las Dermatitis medicamentosas, el Acné, la Urticaria y la Alopecia difusa son regresivas al suspender por una temporada el medicamento causante. Al contrario la Rosácea y el Cloasma son rebeldes, debido a que se presentan después del 3er. ciclo de administración o meses o hasta un año después. Cuando se continúa con la administración del medicamento la dermatosis puede acentuarse, como sucede con el Cloasma, en el que es evidente la hiperpigmentación de un tono café con leche en las regiones de la parte central de la frente, regiones superciliares, maseterinas, al grado de que cuando se ve a una persona con esta morfología se le puede preguntar de inmediato. *Desde cuando toma el Anovlar?*

El interrogatorio debe ser cauto por los problemas sociales que esto entraña en nuestros países con influencia religiosa arraigada. Prejuicios existentes que encierra el uso de estos medicamentos, por ser un tabú el tema del Control de la Natalidad. El problema del Cloasma es estético, consultan con el objeto de que se les indique algo para mejorar la pigmentación, sin que se pretenda quitar el medicamento que las provoca. En la terapéutica se han utilizado: Cloroquinas, cremas despigmentantes y un colerético, colepoyético y espasmolítico, no obteniendo resultados satisfactorios con ninguno de ellos por el uso continuo del Anovulatorio. Estamos en el XII año de estudio y empleo de estos medicamentos, su uso se encuentra extendido, ya sea por prescripción médica o por automedicación, lo que nos da la oportunidad de observar una nueva etapa en el gran capítulo de la *Dermatología Iatrogénica* y nos permite estar alertas en los problemas sociales de la población, para un manejo adecuado de las pacientes en cuanto a la orientación, comprensión del problema socio cultural y religioso, que representa el uso de los *Anovulatorios*.

A pesar de todos estos problemas seguimos optimistas y pensamos que lo mejor de la vida continua siendo el amor.

Bibliografía. AHUMADA, P. M.: Tratamiento del acné juvenil. Efecto terapeútico de la combinación de clormadinona y mestranol. Reporte preliminar. Rev. Fac. Med., Méx. **6**, 715 (1964). – COOK, H. H., C. J. GAMBLE, and A. P. SATTERTHWAITE: Oral contraception by norethynodrel. A three year field study. Amer. J. Obstet. Gynec. **82**, 437 (1961). – ESODA, E. C. J.: Chloasma from progestational oral contraceptives. Arch. Derm. **87**, 486 (1963). – GOLDZIEHER, J. W.: Newer drugs in oral contraception. Med. Clin. N. Amer. **48**, 529 (1964). – IJZERMAN, G. L., M. N. G. DUKES und H. KOPERA: Klinische Ergebnisse der Fertilitätskontrolle nach cyclischer Anwendung von Lynestrenol in Kombination mit einem Oestrogen. Arzneimittel-Forsch. (Drug Res.). **13**, 507 (1963). – ORTIZ, Y.: Anovulatorios. Un nuevo factor patógeno en dermatología. Comunicación preliminar en 20 casos. Dermatología (Méx.) **9**, 63 (1965). – PALITZ, L. L., I. L. MILBERG, and I. KANTOR: Enovid for acne in the female. Skin **1964**, 243. – RESNIK, S.: Melasma induced by oral contraceptives drugs. J. Amer. med. Ass. **199**, 601 (1967). – RICE-WRAY, E., y A. DE S. FERRER: El cloasma relacionado con progestágenos. Sem. méd. Méx. **50**, 322 (1966). – ROCK, J., C. R. GARCIA, and G. PINCUS: Synthetic progestins in the normal human menstrual cycle. Recent Progr. Hormone Res. **13**, 323 (1957). – SATTERTHWAITE, A. P., and C. J. GAMBLE: Conception control with norethynodrel: Progress report of a four-year field study at Humacao, Puerto Rico. J. Amer. med. Ass. **17**, 797 (1962). – SIDI, E., J. BOURGEOIS-SPINASSE et J. AROUETE: Causes actuelles des alopécies féminines diffuses. XIII Congress. Internat. Derm., München, 1967. Berlin-Heidelberg-New York: Springer 1968. – STRAUSS, J. S., and P. E. POCHI: Effect cyclic progestin-estrogen therapy on sebum and acne in women. J. Amer. med. Ass. **190**, 815 (1964). – TYLER, E. T., H. J. OLSON, F. WOLF, S. FILKELSTEIN, J. THAYER, N. KAPLAN, J. LEVIN, and J. WEINTRAUB: An oral contraceptive. A year study of norethindrone. Obstet. Gynec. **18**, 363 (1961). – WANSKER, B. A.: Norethynodrel with mestranol in the treatment of acne. Sth. med. J. (Bgham. Ala.) **57**, 917 (1964).

Case Presentations and Fundamentals on Film

Représentation cinématographique de démonstrations de cas et de principes fondamentaux

Representación cinematográfia de demonstraciones de casos y de principos fundamentales

Falldemonstrationen und Grundlagenforschung im Film

Organizers

M. B. SULZBERGER, USA

R. Z. SULZBERGER, USA

Delegates of the Organization Committee

H. TH. SCHREUS, Germany

A. WIEDMANN, Austria

Second International Film Presentation of the Institute for Dermatologic Communication and Education

President: MARION B. SULZBERGER
Executive Secretary: ROBERTA Z. SULZBERGER
Treasurer: HERMAN BEERMAN
Board of Directors: ALFRED W. KOPF, Vice President,
REES B. REES, B. MATHIEU ROOS

On Friday afternoon, August 4, 1967, in the Bayernhalle, the Institute presented a première of its newly produced educational motion pictures. The films were in color with sound and with simultaneous translations in the four official languages of the Congress. The large auditorium was filled by an attentive audience throughout the $3^1/_2$ h program. The following films, emanating from nine different countries, were presented:

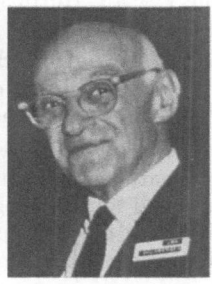

1. Keratosis Follicularis (Darier's Disease)

Presented by N. KARLTORP, Umeå Universitet, Umeå (Sweden) and St. FLODERUS, Kungälv (Sweden)

This film shows Darier's disease appearing in a family which could trace the disease back through several generations. The small farming community and sparsely inhabited area permits the precise demonstration of the family tree and the genetic transmission. The cardinal clinical and histologic features are discussed in detail and several aberrant forms are shown as well as typical ones.

2. Congenital Ichthyosiform Erythroderma

Presented by K. REHTIJÄRVI, with the assistance of K. KUOKKANEN and P. KARMA, University of Oulu (Finland)

Five different forms of the disease are presented and the differential diagnosis from other forms of Ichthyosis including Ichthyosis vulgaris is stressed. The findings and histology coincide with those described by VAN SCOTT and FROST under the title "Epidermolytic Hyperkeratosis" and pictures are shown comparing the presenters' cases and those of the American authors. The film is particularly instructive because it demonstrates not only the full-blown extensive and severe cases of this geno-dermatosis but also the rudimentary and abortive forms. In these latter, the disease can appear as simply palmar or plantar hyperkeratosis or even present only the picture of a typical linear nevus.

3. Xeroderma Pigmentosum

Presented by H. EL-HEFNAWI, Kasr-el-Aini University, Cairo (Egypt)

A very great number of cases of this severe and disfiguring and eventually cancerous and fatal dermatosis are presented with emphasis upon the consanguinity of the marriages, and the rôle of sunlight. The various forms are shown, ranging from the most benign which permit survival into middle life and even old age and those which are so malignant that they kill rapidly within the first years of life. The large case material permits the presentation of all the various stages and all the cardinal manifestations of the disease both of the skin and the eye.

37*

4. Metastasizing Basal Cell Carcinoma

Presented by C. CH. THOMAS, Woman's Medical College of Pennsylvania, Philadelphia (USA)

This most unusual case emphasizes the absolute need for histologic examination in the endeavor to make a precise microscopic diagnosis of every obstinate ulcer, no matter where situated. In the present instance, before being seen by the presenter the ulcer of the lower leg was misdiagnosed as an ordinary stasis ulcer until it was too late. The patient is shown in his downhill course until he died of metastases not only to various parts of the skin but to practically every one of the viscera. Autopsy and histologic findings are included.

5. The Nevoid Basal Cell Carcinoma Syndrome

A report by J. B. HOWELL and D. E. ANDERSON, University of Texas, and M. D. Anderson Hospital and Tumor Institute, Texas (USA)

This genetically determined and most unusual type of cancerous nevus is presented in a father and son. The presenters demonstrate the skin cancers, the unusual and pathognomonic pits of the palms, the X-ray findings including the cysts in the jaw bones, the skeletal anomalies and the intra-cranial calcifications. There is a detailed discussion of the course, prognosis and management.

6. Gold Leaf Treatment of Cutaneous Ulcers

Presented by N. M. KANOF, Georgetown University Medical School, Washington, D.C. (USA)

On a series of patients the presenter demonstrates the technique she has developed, describes the rationale of the treatment and shows the rapid healing which is brought about in torpid ulcers of the skin from a great variety of causes. The indications and the causes of failures are also discussed.

7. Diagnosis of Latent Psoriasis

Presented by G. HOLTI, University of Newcastle-upon-Tyne (England)

This film is an exception since it was presented not in color but black and white. By capillary microscopy, HOLTI demonstrates direct motion picture photography showing the form, calibre and circulation of the capillaries, stressing the typical changes which are present in the capillaries even in the normal skin of psoriatics when viewed with the capillary microscope. In this way, latent psoriasis can be diagnosed and perhaps even the psoriatic trait in members of the family not affected by the clinical disease.

8. Surgical Treatment of Benign Acanthosis Nigricans

Presented by H. OLLENDORFF CURTH, Department of Dermatology, College of Physicians and Surgeons, Columbia University, New York (USA)

Dr. CURTH, together with Dr. CRICKELAIR, plastic surgeon, demonstrate the procedure of dermabrasion and show the rehabilitation and excellent results which can be obtained by encouragement, careful selection of dermabrasion and surgical techniques for removal of the pigmented acanthotic lesions in the benign form of acanthosis nigricans. Differential diagnostic criteria which distinguish this benign form from other forms of acanthosis nigricans are presented, as a confirmation of the presenter's suggestion for classification. At the close, one sees the graduation picture of the young man who has been so successfully rehabilitated that he is now able to face life and plans to study medicine, whereas before he was completely incapacitated by his skin disease.

9. Pellagra and other Avitaminoses in the Bantu

Presented by M. ROSE, Transvaal Provincial Hospitals, Johannesburg (South Africa)

In an extraordinarily beautiful series of photographs, Pellagra and other forms of avitaminoses in the Bantu natives of South Africa are shown. Unfortunately, the presenter of this photographically and medically excellent film died before he was able to view it at its premiere showing. The pictures are most unusual and instructive and the differential and characteristic features of the skin changes in various forms of avitaminoses are illustrated, together with some demonstrations and comments as to proper treatment.

10. Lupus Erythematosus

Presented by D. L. TUFFANELLI, University of California, School of Medicine, San Francisco, and W. B. REED, University of California, School of Medicine, Los Angeles (USA)

The origin of the name with CAZENAVE, the various important steps and publications which have enlarged the concept and led to the modern classification and knowledge of Lupus erythematosus are shown in historical sequence and perspective. A great number of patients with different varieties of this most protean disease are presented, ranging from patients with severe systematic forms, which rapidly ended fatally in the pre-corticosteroid era, to the benign discoid forms and the exceedingly rare Lupus erythematosus profundus. The immunologic features and other laboratory findings are included.

11. Lipoid Proteinosis

Presented by R. M. CAPLAN, The University of Iowa, Iowa City (USA)

This relatively rare malady is shown, with examples demonstrating the characteristic deposits not only in the clinically affected skin but in apparently normal skin areas. Furthermore, it is shown that these deposits occur in practically every one of the viscera. The clinical features of the disease are clearly demonstrated in a series of patients. The remarkably characteristic deposits on the vocal cords are shown together with the evidence of the ensuing hoarseness and at times even airway obstruction. In one of the cases, tracheotomy was required. The characteristic hoarseness is beautifully brought to the attention of the audience by actual sound recordings of the patients' voices.

12. Acrodermatitis Chronica Atrophicans (Herxheimer)

Presented by F. HERRMANN and O. SCHULTKA, Univ.-Hautklinik, Frankfurt a. M. (Germany)

Perhaps the most autoritative presentation of this condition is embodied in this film, since it emanates from the University Clinic at which KARL HERXHEIMER first described the disease and where Prof. HERRMANN is now Director. The statistical data are authoritative since they include not only the presenter's own figures but also the figures of his predecessor, Prof. OSCAR GANS. The regional geographic occurrence is emphasized as an excellent illustration of geographic pathology. An historical review of the origin of the concept, the confirmation of the original findings, and both the classic and unusual features of the disease are included in this film which has been photographed in superb fashion by SCHULTKA.

13. Granulomatous Dermo-Hypodermitis with Progressive Atrophy

Presented by J. CONVIT, Division of Sanitary Dermatology, FR. KERDEL-VEGAS, Vargas Hospital and Central University of Venezuela (Caracas), with the assistance of M. F. ALLENDE, University of California School of Medicine, San Francisco (USA)

The case presented, while it resembles von Recklinghausen's disease, with the tremendous flaps of redundant skin which literally hang down in elephantine folds, is demonstrated not to be a neurofibromatosis but a most unusual and rare form of skin atrophy following a granulomatous infiltrate. While laboratory evidence is not able to substantiate the hypothesis, it is considered possible that auto-sensitivity on the part of the patient to elastic tissue of his own skin may have led to its destruction through a granulomatous process.

Report of the Institute for Dermatologic Communication and Education to the International Committee of Dermatology

Munich, Germany, 30. August, 1967

After the XII International Congress of Dermatology in Washington in 1962, the Institute for Dermatologic Communication and Education was incorporated as a non-profit, tax-exempt educational institute under the laws of the District of Columbia, U.S.A.

This was done according to the wishes of the International Committee of Dermatology, in order to assume continuing responsibility for the motion pictures which had been produced and to continue the production and dissemination of educational motion pictures and materials on an international basis.

Since its incorporation early in 1963, the Institute for Dermatologic Communication and Education (hereinafter called "the Institute") has produced 46, 16 mm, sound and color educational motion pictures, with timed scripts in four languages (English, French, German and Spanish). In addition it has acquired the rights to three more pictures and has translated these.

31 of these motion pictures have been produced in 8 mm format in English, French and Spanish in cartridges for use in Fairchild Automatic projectors. This was done in collaboration with the Audiovisual Facility of the U.S. Public Health Service. The dissemination of these pictures is done by the Institute in 16 mm and 8 mm and by the U.S. Public Health Service in 8 mm.

The funds for the production and sound recording of the films; securing duplicate inter-negatives for making copies; translation into the four languages; the maintenance of the circulating library; the maintenance of an office; legal fees; accounting, etc. during 7 years were supplied from the following sources in the approximate amounts listed:

	approximately
Dome Chemicals	$ 100,000.00
Marion B. Sulzberger Foundation:	
— Direct grants to the Institute	33,000.00
— Grants to the University of California, Continuing Education in Health Sciences (used in major part for work on writing, production and translation of Institute films)	30,000.00
U.S. Public Health Service	14,000.00
E. R. Squibb & Sons	10,000.00
Schering Corporation	5,500.00
Westwood Pharmaceuticals	5,000.00
Montefiore Hospital (Victor Riesenfeld Memorial)	3,000.00
Revlon Research Laboratories	3,000.00
Duke Laboratories	1,000.00
Edgar Stern Foundation	1,000.00
Marion B. Sulzberger (for prizes)	1,000.00
Total (approx.)	$ 206,500.00[1]

[1] A few contributions under $ 1,000.00 have not been listed.

For this expenditure the Institute owns the 46 (plus 3) films having a running time of approximately 480 min. The usual cost of production of films of this kind is estimated by experts to be no less than $ 1,000.00 to $ 1,500.00 per min, which gives the Institute's property in 16 mm films a book value of $ 500,000.00 to $ 720,000.00.

This estimate does *not* include the value of the translated scripts, the 31 pictures in 8mm format in three languages, nor the value of the services rendered in circulating the films for dermatologic education and the organization and production of film showings at numerous meetings and congresses during the past 6 years.

The above services to dermatologic education include the following:

1. Selected films loaned and/or supplied to almost all the departments of dermatology in major medical schools in the U.S.A.

2. Complete sets of films purchased by the following, or donated by the Institute to the following for circulation:

a) The U.S. Army Pictorial Service,
b) Armstrong Laboratories (for Latin America),
c) Japanese Laboratories (for Japan),
d) Rockefeller Fund (for India),
e) National Medical Library of the U.S. Public Health Service,
f) Copies of films supplied to each presenter (his own).

3. Regular showings annually by the Institute at the following meetings: American Academy of Dermatology, Pacific Dermatologic Association, U.S. Army meetings, Europe.

4. Special showings at meetings in several countries of Europe and South America including Israel, Germany, Switzerland, France, Venezuela, England, Japan and other countries.

The work of the Institute to date has been performed with the approval of the Board of Trustees and carried out and/or supervised by the President and Executive Secretary with part-time secretarial help and regular inspection of bank accounts by the Treasurer. The work has included: fund raising; final writing and production of films; distribution of films; securing and checking translations; preparing reports to trustees; legal and tax reports; accounting; arranging projection for showings; demonstrations of films in 8 mm; cooperation with U.S. Public Health Service, etc.

In order to proceed and to develop the Institute's work, additional help will be required; and this necessitates more firm and broader support.

The International Committee of Dermatology can best help the Institute's work by enlarging its international effectiveness through the establishment of branches and affiliates in various countries. These affiliates of the Institute will be able to acquire copies of films or, better still, printing materials to make copies of all the films in the Institute's library.

To purchase the internegatives for making prints at actual laboratory cost for all 46 films and to maintain and circulate these prints would require an estimated sum of $ 10,000.00. Such a fund could start a circulating library which could disseminate, in the language concerned, films having a total value of $ 500,000.00 to $ 750,000.00 and would represent a fine contribution to international dermatologic education. Steps to start such affiliates are already under way in England, France and Germany.

At the present XIII International Congress, the film showings prepared by the Institute at the request of the International Committee will include 22 motion pictures running a total of 5 h and 9 min. 9 of these 22 films have been previously shown, and will, through the kindness of Dozent Dr. KLAUS BOSSE, be included in the daily motion picture program. The remaining 13 motion pictures have never been shown before and will be premiered at the Institute's program on Friday afternoon in the Bayernhalle.

Dr. SULZBERGER recently received an award of $ 1,000.00 (the first Stephen Rothman Memorial award) from the Society for Investigative Dermatology, U.S.A. In memory of his friend and great teacher, Dr. SULZBERGER is contributing this money for prizes being awarded by the Institute for the best films made especially for this Congress. The awards are given with the advice of a committee of Institute trustees. We now ask the approval of the International Committee for the presentations to be made by the Institute's Executive Secretary during the film program on Friday afternoon.

Awards are based on the standards published: Scientific validity, world-wide interest, technical motion picture quality.

They are as follows:

For the best complete film, to

Diagnosis of Latent Psoriasis — HOLTI	$ 250.00
Le Cyto Diagnostic — SIDI †, MAWAS and MEIGNANT	250.00

For the best raw materials to

Lipoid Proteinosis — CAPLAN	250.00
Nevoid Basal Cell Carcinoma Syndrome — HOWELL and ANDERSON	250.00
Total	$ 1,000.00

Citations of Merit for constant and continued support to

1. EDWIN SIDI †, JEAN AROUETE and JACQUELINE BOURGEOIS-SPINASSE, Paris (France);
2. FRANZ HERRMANN and OTTO SCHULTKA, Frankfurt/Main (Germany);
3. JACINTO CONVIT and FRANCISCO KERDEL-VEGAS, Caracas (Venezuela);
4. ALFRED W. KOPF, New York (U.S.A.);
5. H. E. KLEINE-NATROP, Dresden (Germany);
6. STEN FLODERUS, Kungälv (Sweden), and NILS KARLTORP, Umeå (Sweden);
7. MAX ROSE, Johannisburg (South Africa);
8. ERIC M. DONALDSON, Stoke-on-Trent (Great Britain).

Scientific Exhibition

Exposition scientifique

Exposición científica

Wissenschaftliche Ausstellung

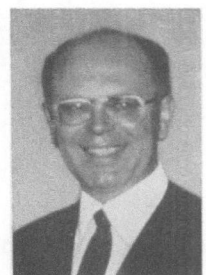

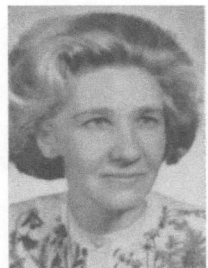

Organizers

H.-J. BANDMANN, Germany

L. KREMPL-LAMPRECHT, Germany

The Scientific Exhibition has been demonstrated in three sections:

    1. section: Clinical Dermatology

    2 section: Experimental Dermatology

    3. section: Mycology

In connexion with the Scientific Exhibition a botanical show of sensibilizing plants — according to an idea of H.-J. BANDMANN — has been performed by L. KREMPL-LAMPRECHT and by F. SCHÖTZ, Director of the Botanic Garden, Munich.

Clinical Dermatology

Die spontane Heilungsquote der Blutschwämme und die daraus zu ziehenden Schlüsse für die Prognose und Therapie

G. F. KLOSTERMANN, Universitäts-Hautklinik Göttingen (Deutschland)

Tabellarische Darlegung eigener *Verlaufsbeobachtungen unbehandelter Blutschwämme* an 377 Kontrollbefunden belegt mit 70% Spontanheilungen und weiteren 30% gut zurückgebildeten Herden im Alter von 6 bis 10 Jahren die grundsätzliche Rückbildungsneigung dieser Gebilde [Einzelheiten bei KLOSTERMANN u. JUST, Strahlentherapie 125, 10 (1964)].

Nachkontrolle bestrahlter Hämangiome ergibt wahrnehmbare Röntgenspätfolgen in einem meist höheren Prozentsatz als gewöhnlich angenommen. Die Ergebnisse an 202 mit Strahlenqualitäten einer GHWT von 3 bis 4 mm bestrahlten Blutschwämmen wurden tabellarisch aufgeschlüsselt. Ohne sichtbare Röntgenfolgen sind bei einer Gesamtdosis bis 1000 R nur 41,5%, bei einer Gesamtdosis von > 1000 bis 2000 R nur 13,7% (Einzelheiten bei KLOSTERMANN, Strahlentherapie 130, 205 (1966)].

Folgende *Empfehlungen für das derzeitige Vorgehen* werden aus den Ergebnissen abgeleitet:

1. Im Regelfall Spontanremission abwarten. Keine Therapie.

2. Behandlungsindikationen:

a) absolut: Raumverdrängende Blutschwämme mit Druck auf lebenswichtige Organe (eigenes Beispiel: tiefreichendes Hämangiom des Halses mit Druck auf Atemwege). Kasabach-Merritt-Syndrom.

b) relativ: Erhebliche Wachstumstendenz des Hämangioms (soweit keine Einschränkungen gemäß 3.).

3. Kontraindikation der Strahlenbehandlung (absolut im Hinblick auf die Spontanremission): Hämangiome im Bereich von Knochenwachstumszonen, Gonadennähe (Rippenbogen bis Knie), Mammazone, Fontanellen.

Spontanverlauf der Säuglingshämangiome

A. PROPPE und H. HAUSS, Universitäts-Hautklinik Kiel (Deutschland)

An der Hautklinik Kiel ist der Verlauf von 532 unbehandelt gebliebenen Säuglingshämangiomen fotografisch dokumentiert worden. G. GROTHUSEN hat die gesammelten Befunde ausgewertet. In einem Diagramm ist der Zeitplan der unbeeinflußten Verlaufsweise dargestellt. 50% der Blutschwämme hatten sich bis zum 5. bis 6. Lebensjahr, 70% bis zum 7. bis 8. Lebensjahr, 80% bis zum 10. Lebensjahr vollständig zurückgebildet. Vom 14. Lebensjahr ab sind fast in keinem Fall mehr Blutschwammreste nachweisbar. Bleiben die Säuglingshämangiome unangetastet, so verschwinden sie in 70% der Fälle spurlos. In den übrigen 30% finden sich Residuen in Form von epidermalen Unebenheiten, Narben und gelegentlich auch ungenügend zurückgebildeten Hautsäcken. Sie sind in der Regel unscheinbarer als Folgezustände nach therapeutischen Eingriffen.

Die Bilddemonstration zeigt Beispiele von unberührt belassenen Säuglings-hämangiomen, darunter große, die das Gesicht, die Schläfenregion oder den Unter-arm in Anspruch genommen haben, und auch solche, die eine Zeitlang durch vor-übergehende Vergrößerung ausgezeichnet sind. Neben den Ausgangsbildern werden die Endstadien gezeigt, wie sie 4 bis 11 Jahre später gefunden wurden.

Das Behandlungsrisiko ist vergleichsweise an Beispielen von Bestrahlungs-folgen (ausgebliebenes Wachstum der Brust im Alter von 12 Jahren, Skelettschäden) sowie an kosmetisch belastenden Narben durch chirurgische und elektrokaustische Verfahren ausgewiesen.

Die Zuverlässigkeit der Spontanheilung ist ein wesentliches Argument für die These der Autoren über die Pathogenese der Säuglingshämangiome. Sie sehen in ihnen passagere Blutgefäßschlingenbildungen ähnlich solchen in entzündlichen Gewebsveränderungen. Der Zusammenhang mit dem Feldzerfall der primären Haarkeimanlage im Moment der hormonell in Gang gesetzten Beihaarentwicklung erscheint u. a. in Übereinstimmung mit der These des Gefällesystems morphogene-tischer Potentiale von DALCQ sowie der Vormustertheorie STERNS (1954) gut begründet. Auch die in einem weiteren Diagramm dargestellte verschiedenartige topographische Verteilung der Blutschwämme bei den Geschlechtern zählt zu den Argumenten für diese These. Die verspätete Reifung der passager derangierten Hautregion hat nicht zuletzt zur Folge, daß sich die unpassenden Blutgefäß-konvolute wieder zurückbilden. Das demonstriert am eindrucksvollsten die Bild-serie über einen großen Blutschwamm, in dessen Zentrum sich ursprünglich eine mißgestaltete Ohrmuschel befunden hat. Mit dem Verschwinden der Gefäß-konvolute hat auch die Ohrmuschel völlig normale Gestalt angenommen; sie ist jetzt im Vergleich zur anderen Ohrmuschel nur größer proportioniert.

Literatur. GROTHUSEN, G.: Aesthet Med. 17, 27, 47 (1968). — PROPPE, A., u. H. HAUSS: Arch. klin. exp. Derm. **216**, 194 (1963).

Laser Surgery of Angiomas with Special Reference to Port-Wine Angiomas*

L. GOLDMAN, E. J. RITTER, R. J. ROCKWELL jr., R. MEYER, B. HENDERSON and K. WM. KITZMILLER, Laser Laboratory, The Childrens Hospital, University of Cincinnati, Medical Center, Cincinnati, Ohio (USA)

The exhibit shows the progressive steps in the development of the use of the laser for investigative studies in angioma. First, there are charts and pictures of various types of lasers which have been used in these experiments. These lasers include the pulsed ruby laser, pulsed neodymium laser und the continuous wave argon laser. The continuous wave carbon dioxide laser was used only in animal experiments. The characteristics of the ruby, neodymium and argon lasers may be correlated with color absorption of angiomas. The absorption curves of hemo-globin, however, primarily would refer to the 5145 Å of the argon laser. To provide for animal test model systems, tattooed skin of the rabbit, the miniature pig, the rabbit ear, and the comb and wattle of the chicken were used. Because of the morphology and the dynamics of the vascular system of the comb and wattle of

* Supported by a grant from The John A. Hartford Foundation, and Division of Pediatric Surgery, The Children's Hospital, University of Cincinnati, Medical Center, Cincinnati, Ohio (USA).

chicken, this was preferred. Tattooed animal skin gave only artificial pigment masses, static in tissue. The rabbit ear provided some value in the study of a few vascular channels in response to laser impact, but it did not give mass areas necessary for investigative studies of various forms of angiomas in man.

Investigative studies over the past 4 years have included the following types of vascular lesions: the resistant port-wine lesion of all types, cavernous angiomas, spider angiomas, so-called "senile" angiomas, the glomus tumor, and, of the malignant lesions, Kaposi's hemorrhagic sarcoma and angiosarcoma.

The results in the clinical series were shown in a series of colored pictures illustrating the results of the laser treatment and the follow-up studies. It was shown that the laser did have value in the treatment of resistant port-wine lesions and angiomas with the production of small areas of lightening, approximately 1.76 cm². The small size is one of the practical difficulties of current laser research. The mechanism of the lightening effect was studied in repeated biopsies of patients. These biopsies revealed nonspecific scarring with decreased vascularity and changes in the connective tissue and disappearance of the elastic tissue. There was relative resistance of the pilosebaceous unit. This may explain some of the good cosmetic results after laser impact. The adverse reactions which were uncommon included a pitted type of scarring, increased redness which was also temporary, and the revascularization of previously whitened areas. The optical quality of the angioma was changed by previous tattooing. Therapeutic results were poor in previously tattooed areas and in patients with very light type of port-wine lesions. The most significant improvement occurred in patients with the mixed cavernous port-wine type of lesion. In several patients tattooing with titanium dioxide and zinc oxide pigment after laser impact showed improvement in the treated areas.

Table 1. *Laser surgery of 73 patients*

	Total number	Improved[a]	Not improved
Port-wine lesions	57	39	18
Cavernous angiomas	4	4	
Senile angiomas	4	4	
Spider angiomas	2	2	
Maffuci's syndrome	1	1	
Lymphangioma	1		1
Kaposi hemorrhagic sarcoma	3	3 (For small lesions biopsies negative)	
Angiosarcoma	1	1	

[a] Improvement: Persistent lightening in color of treated areas.

Table 2. *Laser surgery. Reactions of treated areas of Port-Wine Lesions in 57 patients*

Superficial scarring	3
Revascularization of some areas	4
Telangiectasia	2

Through the courtesy of the Siemens Company, a helium-neon gas laser was used to illustrate the value of medical holography to provide third-dimensional pictures. The comb of the chicken was dried and mounted in acrylic plastic. Then, holograms were taken of this. The laser was used to reconstruct these holograms. Reconstruction showed a third-dimensional red picture.

Conclusions. Studies over the past 4 years, then, have shown that the laser can be used as a safe but limited form of investigative surgery for many types of benign and malignant vascular lesions, especially the incurable port-wine lesion. Scarring and telangiectasia are minimal and the treatment is safe. These initial results warrant continued controlled studies. The laser is recommended as a research tool, not for conventional therapy. Additional research with the laser is in the direction of the development of precise, safe, so-called bloodless surgery instrumentation.

Therapie hypercholesterinämischer Xanthomatosen

N. Zöllner, M. Gudenzi und G. Wolfram, Medizinische Poliklinik der Universität München (Deutschland)

Zahlreiche Medikamente sind zur Behandlung hypercholesterinämischer Xanthomatosen angewendet worden — D-Thyroxin, Heparinoide, Phosphatide, Linolsäure —, aber ohne sicheren Erfolg. Erst die Nicotinsäure führte in vielen Fällen zur völligen Rückbildung der Xanthome. Beta-Pyridylcarbinol, ein Nicotinsäurederivat,

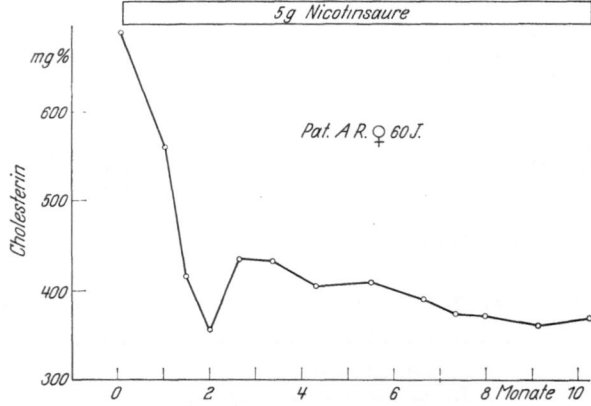

übt die gleiche Wirkung aus. Wird es in einer retard-Form (Ronicol retard) verabreicht, so liegen die notwendigen Dosen deutlich niedriger und Nebenerscheinungen sind seltener.

Abb. 1. Frau A. R. hatte eine ausgeprägte Hypercholesterinämie, die auf 5 g Nicotinsäure/Tag gut ansprach. Unter dieser Behandlung wurden auch die Xanthome an Händen und Ellenbogen deutlich kleiner

Bei etwa 12% unserer Patienten mit Hypercholesterinämie (1) beobachteten wir Haut- und/oder Sehnenxanthome. Eine medikamentöse Senkung des Cholesterins im Serum mit Nicotinsäure oder Beta-Pyridylcarbinol führte in fast allen

Fällen auch zu einer Rückbildung der Xanthome (Abb. 1, 2). Die Wirkung der Nicotinsäure bzw. des Beta-Pyridylcarbinol hängt von der Grundkrankheit ab. Besonders zuverlässig ist ein Erfolg bei der familiären Hypercholesterinämie (Abb. 3), biochemisch regelmäßig ausgewiesen durch normale Triglyceridspiegel,

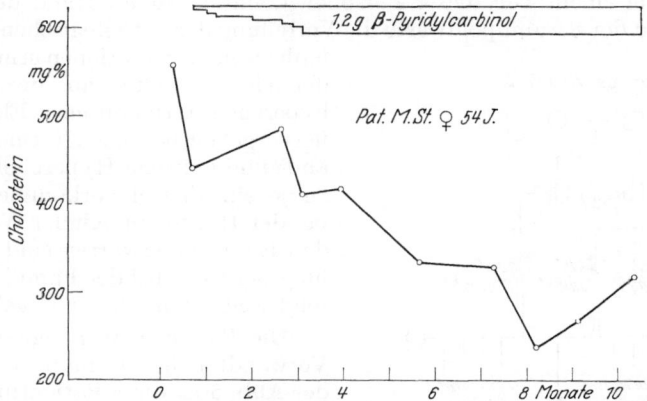

Abb. 2. Frau M. St. hatte Xanthome der Haut an beiden Ellenbogen und Knien. Unter Beta-Pyridylcarbinol kam es zu einer Normalisierung des Cholesterinspiegels, die Xanthome waren nach einem Jahr vollständig zurückgebildet

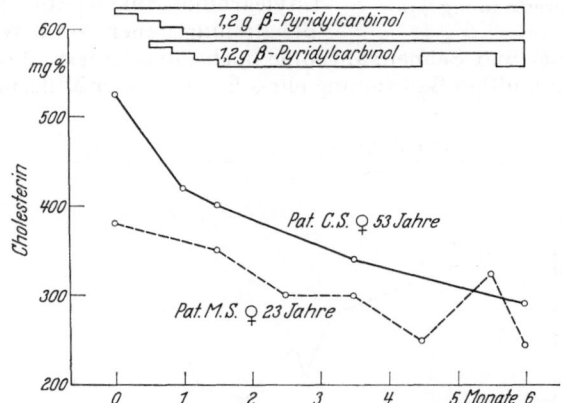

Abb. 3. Die Pat. C. S. und M. S., Mutter und Tochter, hatten Sehnenxanthome am Handrücken, die unter der Behandlung mit Beta-Pyridylcarbinol deutlich kleiner wurden

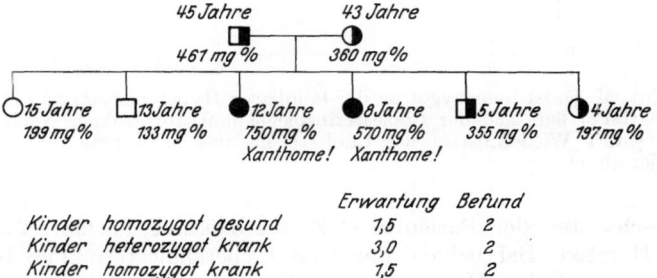

Abb. 4. Stammbaum der Familie A (Gesamtcholesterinwerte in mg-%)

während von der Hypercholesterinämie mit Neutralfettvermehrung nur ein Teil der Fälle befriedigend behandelt werden kann.

Unter den Therapieversagern bei der familiären Hypercholesterinämie fanden sich vorwiegend homozygot an der familiären Hypercholesterinämie erkrankte Patienten. Bei einem Teil dieser Personen konnten wir an Hand der Familienanamnese und der Serumlipoidwerte die Verteilung der pathologischen Gene innerhalb zweier Generationen ermitteln. Nach der Theorie sollten aus der Ehe zweier hypercholesterinämischer Eltern Kinder hervorgehen, bei denen Normocholesterinämie und extreme Hypercholesterinämie zu je ein Viertel vorkommen, während bei der Hälfte der Kinder Werte wie bei den Eltern zu erwarten sind. Die Verteilung der Gene bei der Familie A (Abb. 4) folgt weitgehend dieser Regel.

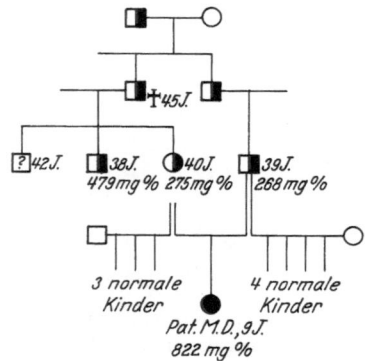

Stammbaum der Familie D.

Abb. 5. Stammbaum der Familie D (Gesamtcholesterinwerte in mg-%)

Die Patientin M. D. entstammt einer Verwandtenehe. Gemäß dem Erbgang der Abb. 5 ist diese Patientin homozygot an der familiären Hypercholesterinämie erkrankt. Trotzdem ließ sich der Cholesterinspiegel des Serums durch Beta-Pyridylcarbinol senken (Abb. 6). Nach einer Behandlungsdauer von 8 Wochen waren die zahlreichen Haut- und Sehnenxanthome noch unverändert; dieser Zeitraum ist jedoch für eine endgültige Beurteilung eines Erfolges oder Mißerfolges zu kurz.

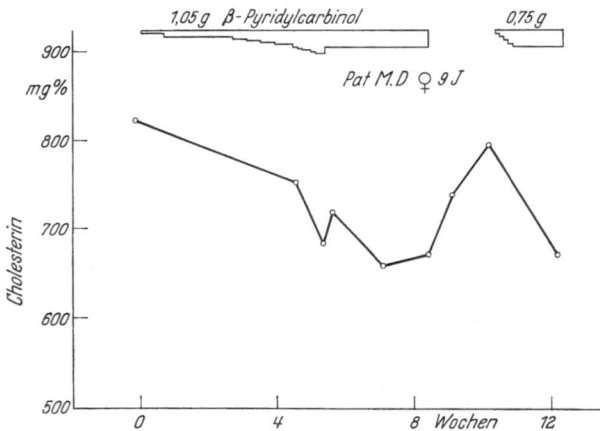

Abb. 6. Die Pat. M. D. ist homozygot an der familiären Hypercholesterinämie erkrankt. Mit Beta-Pyridylcarbinol ließ sich der Cholesterinspiegel langsam senken. Nach Absetzen des Medikaments sofort Wiederanstieg des Cholesterins, das nach erneuter medikamentöser Therapie wieder abfiel

Zwei Geschwister der Patientin C. Z. starben mit 17 bzw. 22 Jahren am plötzlichen Herztod. Bei beiden war eine Hypercholesterinämie bekannt. Die Hautxanthome am linken Handgelenk der Patientin C. Z. bildeten sich unter der Behandlung mit bis zu 1,8 g Beta-Pyridylcarbinol pro Tag vollständig zurück, nach Unterbrechung der Therapie vergrößerten sich die Xanthome am Hand-rücken.

Die günstige Wirkung von Beta-Pyridylcarbinol auf den Serumcholesterin-spiegel und die Hautxanthome wird durch die Auslaßversuche bei den Patien-tinnen M. D. und C. Z. eindrucksvoll belegt.

Literatur: ZÖLLNER, N., u. M. GUDENZI: Med. Klin. **61**, 1996 (1966).

Proteolytic Enzyme Treatment of Skin Ulcers

M. C. SPENCER, Danville (USA)

Chemosurgery for the Microscopically Controlled Excision of Skin Cancer

F. E. MOHS, University Hospital, Madison, Wisconsin (USA)

The chemosurgical technique by which complete microscopic control of the excision of cancer of the skin is attained was illustrated by photographs of patients in all stages of treatment. The treatment of an early but troublesome basal cell carcinoma and of a more advanced recurrent neoplasm was described and illus-trated. Photos taken before, during and after chemosurgical excision depicted some of the indications. Besides skin cancers, carcinoma of the lip and melanoma

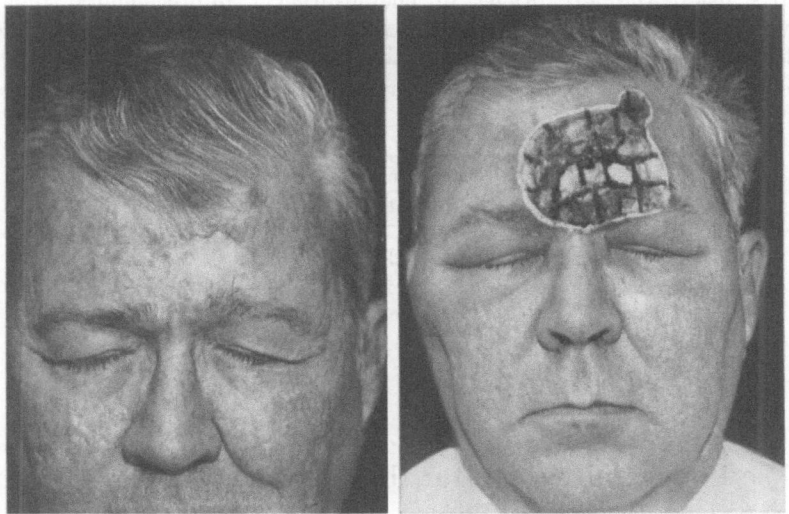

1   2

Fig. 1. Basal cell carcinoma, morphea-like type, duration 22 years. The cancer had persisted despite electrodesiccation and curettage on three occasions

Fig. 2. Lesion after chemosurgical excision, showing the final layer of fixed tissue with mark-ings to show the sites from which the specimens were removed. Frozen sections were cut through the undersurface of each specimen. The sections were scanned systematically to provide complete microscopic control of excision. Most of the "silent extension" of this cancer was in the dermis at the periphery

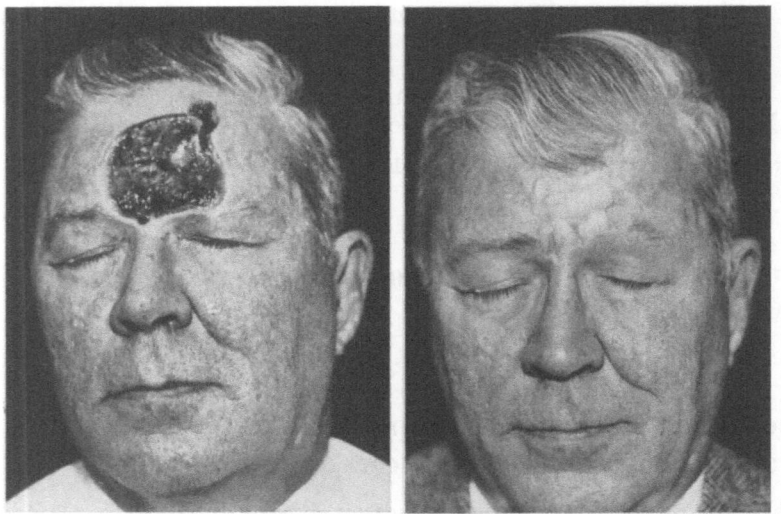

3   4

Fig. 3. Granulation tissue after separation of final layer of fixed tissue 11 days later. Epithelization already is under way

Fig. 4. Healed lesions 5 months later. The wound healed with better cosmetic result then would have been obtained with grafts

were illustrated. The illustrations here depict a patient in various stages of treatment.

Charts listed the advantages of chemosurgery: unprecedented reliability, conservatism, low operative mortality, excellent healing and extension of operability to patients with cancers too extensive for hope of cure with other methods.

The reliability of chemosurgical treatment is evidenced by the 5-year end results:

	Number of cases		5-year rate of cure (%)
	Total	Determinate	
Basal cell carcinoma, skin	5423	4159	99.1
Squamous cell carcinoma, skin	1912	1330	92.3
Squamous cell carcinoma, lips	1009	798	92.5
Melanoma, skin	68	61	45.9

Multiple Punch Autografts for the Alopecias

D. B. STOUGH, Hot Springs (USA)

Evaluation of Parental Methotrexate for Intractable Psoriasis

CH. P. DEFEO, B. ALLYN and S. EISENBERG, New York (USA)

Zur Wirkung des hochalpinen Klimas bei der atopischen konstitutionellen Neurodermitis

S. Borelli, gemeinsam mit H. Brenn, St. Chlebarov, C. Ene-Popescu, H. Gehrken, B. Kopecka, P. Michailov und H. Vossieck, Dermatologische Klinik der Universität München (Deutschland) und Klinik für Dermatologie und Allergie (Hochgebirgs-Sanatorium Valbella) Davos (Schweiz)

Basierend auf den Veröffentlichungen von Turban, Spengler, Campbell u. a. Autoren über therapeutische Erfolge durch Hochgebirgs-Klimakuren bei Kranken mit Asthma bronchiale, sammelte Marchionini seine ersten Erfahrungen mit der Hochgebirgsklimatherapie bei atopischer konstitutioneller Neurodermitis während seines Aufenthaltes in der Türkei, indem er die Kranken auf den bitynischen

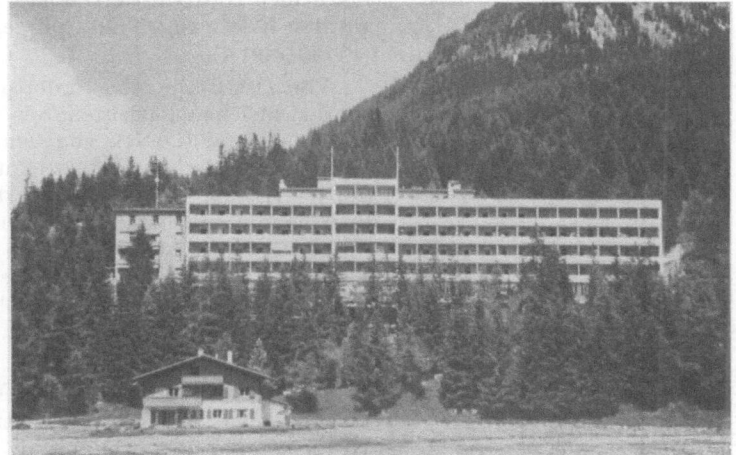

Abb. 1. Hochgebirgs-Sanatorium Valbella (Davos-Dorf/Schweiz) Sommer

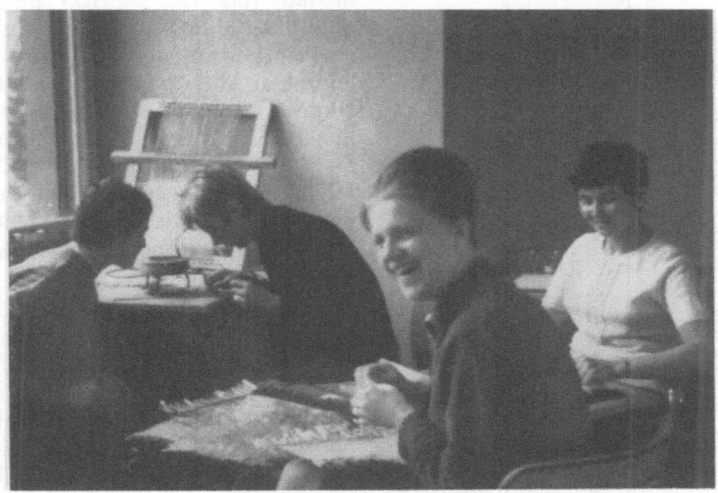

Abb. 2. Pat. mit atopischer Neurodermitis bei der Beschäftigungstherapie mit Holz-, Schnitz-, Web- und Flechtarbeiten

88*

Absetzung der Cortisonmedikation
Zeitraum: vom 1. April 1961 bis 31. März 1967

Nach Davos eingewiesene Kranke, die unter Cortisonmedikation stehen		Cortison bei Aufnahme	sofort abgesetzt	Woche der Absetzung										vorübergehend abgesetzt	nicht abgesetzt	Cortison insgesamt abgesetzt Summe
				1	2	3	4	5	6	7	8	9	10			
Cortison innerlich 31,11%	absolute Zahl	1020	748	33	49	54	35	18	21	1	2	1	2	53	53	964
	%	100	73,33	3,24	4,80	5,29	3,43	1,76	2,06	0,10	0,20	0,10	0,20	0,29	5,20	94,51
äußerlich Cortisonsalben 68,89%	absolute Zahl	2462	516	61	102	145	125	90	48	18	9	8	8	306	1026	1130
	%	100	20,95	2,48	4,14	5,89	5,08	3,66	1,95	0,73	0,36	0,33	0,33	12,43	41,67	45,90

Olymp (Uludag) zur Kur schickte. Auf Veranlassung von MARCHIONINI wurden nach seiner Rückkehr nach Deutschland (1948) systematisch Beobachtungen über die Wirkung des einfachen Milieuwechsels sowie des Klimawechsels in das Mittelgebirge, das Hochgebirge und an der Nordsee oder Ostsee gesammelt.

In den darauf folgenden Jahren erstand an der Nordsee (Norderney) eine klimatherapeutische Abteilung (PÜRSCHEL) seitens der Hautklinik Hannover-Linden (HARTUNG) zur Ausnutzung des maritimen Nordsee-Reizklimas. Zugleich wurden Erfahrungen auf Sylt gesammelt (PFLEIDERER).

Von Ost-Berlin aus förderte LINSER für den gleichen Patientenkreis aus Mitteldeutschland (DDR), von dem infolge der innerdeutschen Grenzziehung und der politischen Gegebenheiten die westdeutschen Möglichkeiten leider nicht genutzt werden können, in den an sich weniger geeigneten Klimazonen der Ostsee und des Mittelgebirges klimatherapeutische Abteilungen (Kap Arkona, Fichtelberg).

Im *Hochgebirge* liefen von München aus Versuche auf der Zugspitze, dem Kreuzeck und dem Wendelstein bei Garmisch, Bayern/Deutschland, sowie in Samedan (bei St. Moritz) im Engadin/Schweiz, die im Anfang des Jahres 1961 zur Einrichtung der Deutschen Dermatologischen Abteilung in dem im Besitz der Bundesrepublik Deutschland befindlichen Sanatorium Valbella in Davos-Dorf in Graubünden/Schweiz (1560 m Höhe) durch die zuständigen Organe und den Bundesminister für Arbeit und Sozialordnung, Bonn, auf Anregung des Referenten, führte.

Die *Deutsche Dermatologische Abteilung** im Sanatorium Valbella*, Davos-Dorf, Schweiz (100 Betten), befindet sich unter der ärztlichen Leitung des Referenten (BORELLI) und steht insofern in personellem Zusammenhang mit der Dermatologischen Klinik und Poliklinik der

---

* Inzwischen: Klinik für Dermatologie und Allergie.

Universität München*. Es werden Kranke mit atopischer Neurodermitis aus der gesamten Bundesrepublik Deutschland, d. h. Kranke sämtlicher Krankenkassen und Rentenversicherungsträger ebenso wie Selbstzahler, dort aufgenommen. Die Dermatologische Abteilung steht darüber hinaus selbstverständlich Kranken mit atopischer Neurodermitis aus sämtlichen Ländern zur Verfügung.

Diese wissenschaftliche Ausstellung kennzeichnete in 36 tabellarischen Übersichten die Ergebnisse der in den sechs vergangenen Jahren an mehr als 3000 behandelten Neurodermitiskranken gewonnenen Erfahrungen im Sinne eines kurz gefaßten Überblicks. Zugleich vermittelten 10 Abbildungen einen Eindruck von der Deutschen Dermatologischen Abteilung im Sanatorium Valbella in Davos-Dorf.

* Inzwischen: Der Fakultät für Medizin der TH München.

Klimatherapie von Hautkrankheiten an der Nordsee

W. PÜRSCHEL, Allergie- und Hautklinik Norderney der Gesellschaft für Klimabehandlung e. V. Hannover (Deutschland)

Klimatherapie von Hautkrankheiten an der Nordsee ist die umfassendste Art der physikalischen Therapie (PFLEIDERER), da sie den gesamten gesunden wie kranken Organismus erfaßt, wenn auch, wie z. B. bei der Heliotherapie von Hautkrankheiten, die heilende Wirkung direkt am Hautorgan erfolgt. Als Träger der günstigen Nordseeklimawirkung konnten von uns insbesondere die maritimen Luftkörper mit cyclonalem Westwettergeschehen erkannt werden. Als Reiz- bzw. Umstimmungstherapie führt die Klimatherapie zur Regulierung des vegetativen Nervensystems und des Nebennierenrinden-Hypophysensystems bei vielen Dermatosen. Neben der allgemeinen Klimawirkung ist die direkte Einwirkung bestimmter meteorologischer Elemente und Elementkomplexe auf das Hautorgan von hervorragender Bedeutung. Auf Grund der intensiven Sonnen- und Himmelsstrahlung befindet sich in der sog. Strandzone das natürliche Solarium, die hier herrschende maximale Abkühlungsgröße am Tage führt zum Training der terminalen Strombahn, die größte Konzentration des maritimen Kernaerosols in der Brandungszone bedingt die Allergenkarenz. Unter diesen günstigen Klimagegebenheiten werden, je nach Krankheitsfall durch schuldermatologische und balneologische Maßnahmen unterstützt, optimale Behandlungsergebnisse erzielt.

Zehn Aufnahmen und Darstellungen sollen zum Verständnis dieser Ausführung über die Klimatherapie von Hautkrankheiten an der Nordsee beitragen.

1. Luftbild der Nordseeinsel Norderney in West-Ostrichtung (Abb. 1).

2. Aufnahme der Allergie- und Hautklinik Norderney (Abb. 2).

3. Darstellung der eindeutigen Rückbildung des Pruritus bei ,,chronischen Ekzematikern", besonders bei Kranken mit konstitutionellem Ekzem (Synonyma: Neurodermitis, endogenes Ekzem, atopic dermatitis u. a.) mit/ohne Asthma bronchiale (Abb. 3). Nach PAHL, O. u. W. PÜRSCHEL: Hautarzt 7, 27 (1956).

4. Darstellung des Gangs meteorologischer Größen in der Umgebung von für die Klimatherapie an der Nordsee sich günstig auswirkenden biotropen Tagen mit starker Umstimmungswirkung. Luftdruck am Boden, Mitteltemperatur Boden/500 mb, relative Luftfeuchtigkeit 800/500 mb, Labilität der Luftschicht Boden/600 mb und Windrichtung und -stärke in 700 mb sind an diesen Tagen abrupten

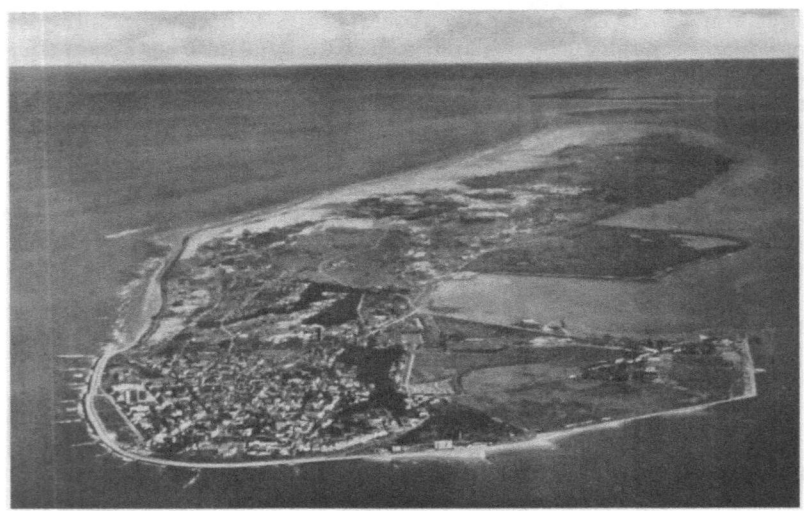

Abb. 1

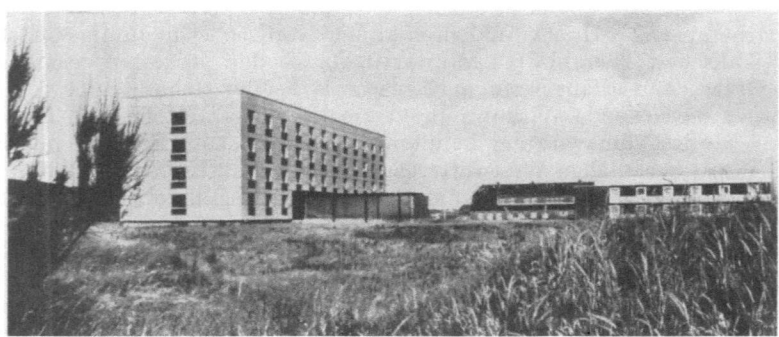

Abb. 2

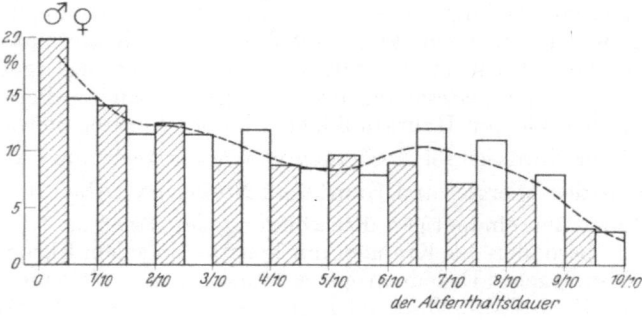

Abb. 3

Änderungen unterworfen und sind Ausdruck für das cyclonale Westwettergeschehen, das auf der Nordseeinsel Norderney volle Reizwirkung zeigt (Abb. 4).
Nach PAHL, O. u. W. PÜRSCHEL: Hautarzt 7, 27 (1956).

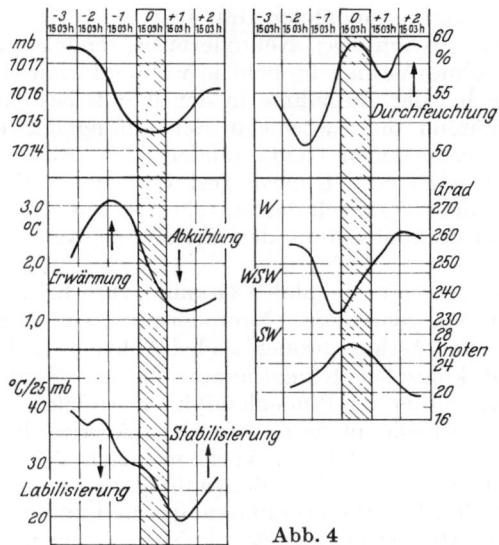

Abb. 4

5. Darstellung der Windverteilung in den Monaten Juli und August zweier Jahre mit verschiedenem Witterungscharakter. Zu beachten ist die überwiegende Anströmung aus dem West-Nord-Halbraum mit maritimen Luftkörpern und die geringe Anströmung aus dem Süd-Ost-Halbraum mit kontinentalen Luftkörpern. Nach PAHL, O. u. W. PÜRSCHEL: Z. Haut- u. Geschl.-Kr. 20, 253 (1956).

6. Häufigkeitsverteilung der Äquivalenttemperatur in den Monaten Juli bis August zweier Jahre (1954 und 1955) mit verschiedenem Witterungscharakter. 1954 zeigte gute Umstimmung von vegetativem Nervensystem und endokrinem System (NNR-Hypophyse) durch die vorherrschenden polar-maritimen Luftmassen. 1955 zeigte besonders einen therapeutischen Effekt der Heliotherapie bei Ichthyosis vulgaris, Psoriasis vulgaris, Acne vulgaris/conglobata, Parapsoriasis, Mykosis fungoides und vielen anderen bedingt durch stärkere Beteiligung kontinentaler Luftmassen höheren Wärme- und Strahlungsinhaltes. Nach PAHL, O. u. W. PÜRSCHEL: Z. Haut- u. Geschl.-Kr. 20, 253 (1956).

7. Die Kurven stellen den mittleren Jahresgang der Lufttemperatur auf Norderney in Form von gewogenen Pentadenmitteln dar, wobei sich eine Kurve auf solche Pentaden bezieht, in denen die Luftzufuhr aus dem Westhalbraum, die andere auf solche mit vorherrschender Zufuhr aus dem Osthalbraum bezieht. Sie zeigen in erster Näherung die Unterschiede des „maritimen" und des „kontinentalen" Klimaanteiles, wobei ersichtlich ist, daß der so definierte „maritime" Klimaanteil in ganz überwiegendem Maße dominiert. Der Jahresgang der Lufttemperatur zeigt für den „maritimen" Klimaanteil eine wesentlich geringere Amplitude — im Sommerhalbjahr kühler, im Winterhalbjahr milder (annähernd +/— 5 °C).

8. Die Kurven stellen den mittleren Jahresgang der Sonnenscheindauer auf Norderney in Form von gewogenen Pentadenmitteln dar, wiederum getrennt für den „maritimen" und „kontinentalen" Klimaanteil. Die größere Sonnenscheindauer ist an die Luftzufuhr aus dem Osthalbraum gebunden, wobei besonders die Monate Mai bis August durch Sonnenscheinreichtum hervortreten. Nach O. PAHL, Dipl.-Met., Norderney.

9. Verlauf der absoluten eosinophilen Granulocyten bei 26 Patienten mit konstitutionellem Ekzem (Synonyma: Neurodermitis, endogenes Ekzem, atopic dermatitis u. a.) mit/ohne Asthma bronchiale während klinischer Klimatherapie an der Nordsee. Die bei der Aufnahme in der Klinik bestehende Eosinophilie normalisiert sich während der 8wöchigen Behandlungszeit bei gleichzeitigem Abklingen der neurodermitischen Hautveränderungen. Absicherung der Ergebnisse erfolgte nach dem R- oder Duncan-Test bzw. der F-Verteilung mit 95% Aussagesicherheit bei dem Vergleich der Mittelwerte und 99% Aussagesicherheit bei dem Vergleich der Streuungen um den Mittelwert. Nach W. PÜRSCHEL u. O. PAHL, Norderney.

10. Verlauf der absoluten eosinophilen Granulocyten bei zwölf Patienten mit konstitutionellem Ekzem (Synonyma: Neurodermitis, endogenes Ekzem, atopic dermatitis u. a.) mit/ohne Asthma bronchiale bei Abbau einer Langzeit-Corticoidbehandlung während klinischer Klimatherapie an der Nordsee. Absetzen der Corticoidtherapie war vorher im Binnenlandklima erfolglos. Bei der Aufnahme in die Klinik war keine Eosinophilie nachweisbar. Anstieg der Eosinophilen bei und nach Corticoidabbau in der 2. bis 3. Woche mit nachfolgender Normalisierung der Eosinophilenzahl nach 7 Wochen Behandlungszeit und gleichzeitigem Abklingen der neurodermitischen Hautveränderungen und unerwünschten Corticoid-Nebenwirkungen. Die Absicherung der Ergebnisse erfolgte wie bei Darstellung 9 mit gleicher Aussagesicherheit von 95% bzw. 99% für Mittelwert bzw. Streuungsberechnung. Nach W. PÜRSCHEL u. O. PAHL, Norderney.

Die Verbrennung — ein dermatologisches Problem
Komplikationen, Therapie und Prophylaxe

G. WEBER und H. JURSCH, Hautklinik der Städtischen Krankenanstalten Nürnberg (Deutschland)

Während die Behandlung Verbrennungskranker vor dem II. Weltkrieg ein der Dermatologie zugehöriges, da sachverwandtes Gebiet war, wurde diese Aufgabe danach im wesentlichen von der Chirurgie übernommen. Nur einzelne dermatologische Kliniken führen heute diese Aufgabe weiter. Die Berechtigung hierzu leitet sich nicht nur aus den fachlichen Kenntnissen des Dermatologen von den physiologischen und pathologischen Stoffwechselvorgängen am Hautorgan ab, sondern auch aus der Entwicklung neuer Medikamente und therapeutischer Maßnahmen, die eine chirurgische Intervention, abgesehen bei begleitenden Unfallverletzungen, in den meisten Fällen erübrigen.

Die Versorgung und Behandlung des Verbrennungskranken wird von uns nach folgenden Gesichtspunkten durchgeführt, wobei eine Schematisierung dieser Maßnahmen wegen der beträchtlichen Variabilität des Krankheitsverlaufs nur begrenzt möglich ist.

Die *Allgemeinbehandlung* richtet sich auf die Therapie des Schockzustandes, dessen Auftreten nicht zwangsläufig von der Ausdehnung oder dem Schweregrad der Verbrennung abhängt, sondern zumeist von der Dauer der Schmerzeinwirkung bis zum Behandlungsbeginn sowie der Schmerztoleranz des Patienten. Deren Bedeutung wird ersichtlich einerseits am Beispiel zweit- bis drittgradiger Verbrennungen zwischen 50 und 70% und Ausbleiben eines Schocks und andererseits an zweitgradigen Verbrennungen von 15% der Körperoberfläche und tiefen

Schockzuständen. Zwischen beiden Extremen findet sich ein fließender Übergang, so daß die Prognose eines Schockeintritts oftmals schwierig. wird. Gelingt es, den Zeitpunkt zwischen Verbrennung und Beginn der ärztlichen Behandlung zu kürzen, so nimmt das Risiko eines Schocks (abgesehen von schwersten Verbrennungen) beträchtlich ab. Seine Behebung erfolgt durch Rückverschiebung des Blutvolumens aus dem Abdominalbereich in die minderdurchblutete Peripherie, wofür sich die Applikation von Effortil und Elektrolytgemischen stets bewährte. Von den sog. Plasmaexpandern sehen wir keinen Vorteil, Adrenalinabkömmlinge vom Typ des Novadral, Akrinor und Hypertensin sind wegen ihrer peripher vasoconstrictorischen Wirkung nicht indiziert.

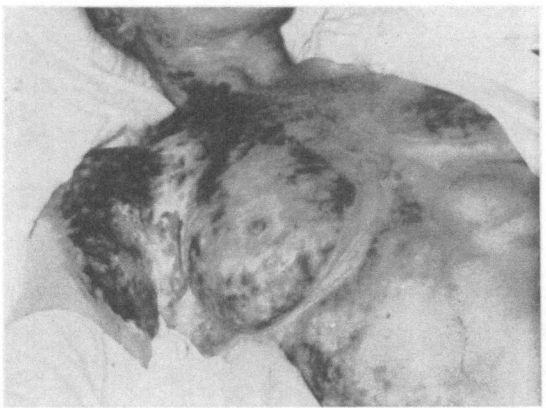

Abb. 1. Verbrennung III. Grades mit beginnender Spontandemarkation

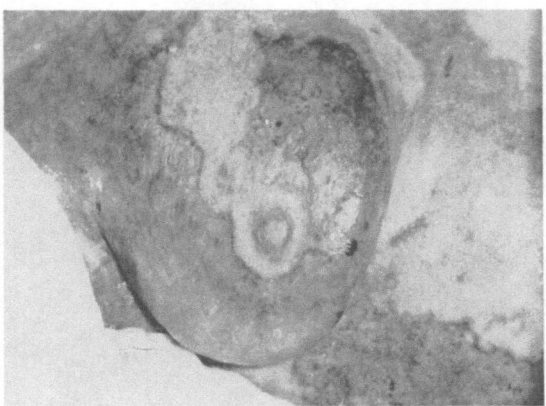

Abb. 2. Zustand nach chemisch-enzymatischem Debridment

Die *primäre Lokalbehandlung* besteht in der sofortigen Beseitigung spontandemarkierten, d. h. blasig abgehobenen Epithels, während bei drittgradig verbranntem Gewebe bis zum Einsetzen der spontanen Demarkation abgewartet und diese dann durch ein chemisch-enzymatisches Debridment unterstützt wird (Abb. 1, 2, 3). Von einer chirurgischen Abtragung sehen wir ab, um nicht unnötige Gewebsverluste in Kauf nehmen zu müssen. Zwar wird damit die Gefahr einer, jeder Demarkierung vorausgehenden, Entzündung riskiert; wir schätzen

letztere aber nicht allzu hoch ein, da durch eine hohe parenterale Corticosteroid-
applikation in den ersten Behandlungstagen die Entzündung in ihrer Stärke und
im zeitlichen Ablauf abgebremst wird.

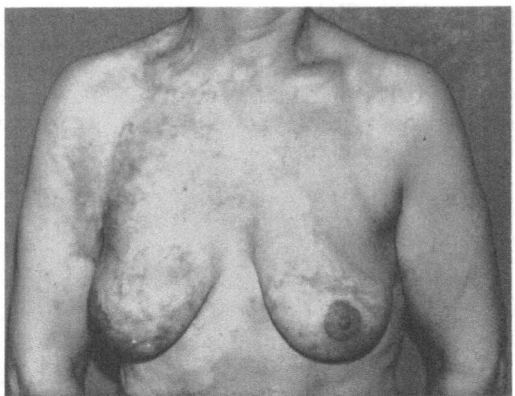

Abb. 3. nach Abheilung

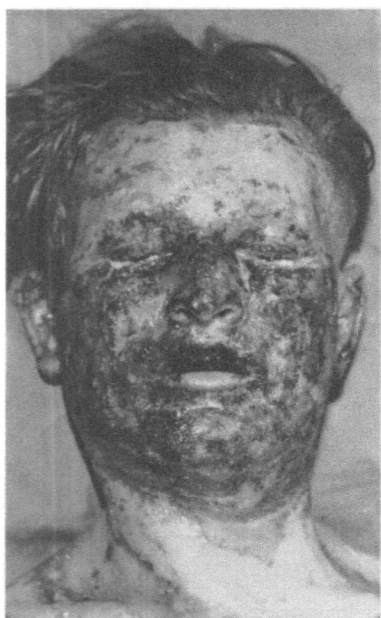

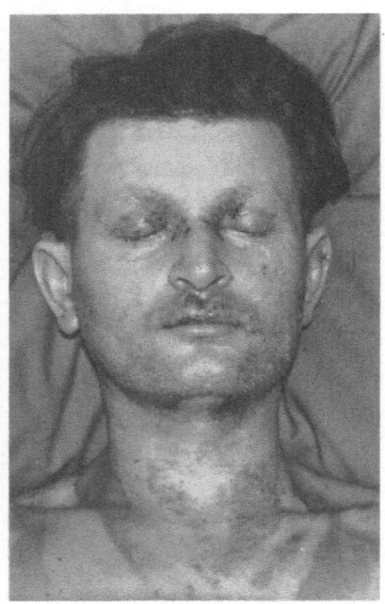

Abb. 4. Zweitgradige Verbrennung   Abb. 5. nach Ödemeliminierung
mit Ödematisation

Auch auf die Applikation der üblicherweise schon initial verabreichten hohen
Antibioticamengen verzichten wir bis etwa zum 7. Tag, dem Zeitpunkt der fortgeschrittenen Demarkation, da in diesem Zeitraum einsetzendes Fieber durch
Antibiotica nicht zu beherrschen und demzufolge nicht auf eine Bakterieninvasion,
sondern auf die Resorption toxisch wirkenden Gewebsdetritus zurückzuführen ist.

Eine weitere Maßnahme ist die Behandlung des *Verbrennungsödems* (Abb. 4, 5). Unabhängig von der Tiefe und Ausdehnung der Verbrennung, vom Schock oder einer Organmitbeteiligung kommt es beim Überleben der ersten 24 Std zu einem Ödem im Verbrennungsbereich, aber auch in verbrennungsfernen Bezirken als Hirn- oder Glottisödem. Ganz abgesehen von der akuten Bedrohung des Patienten,

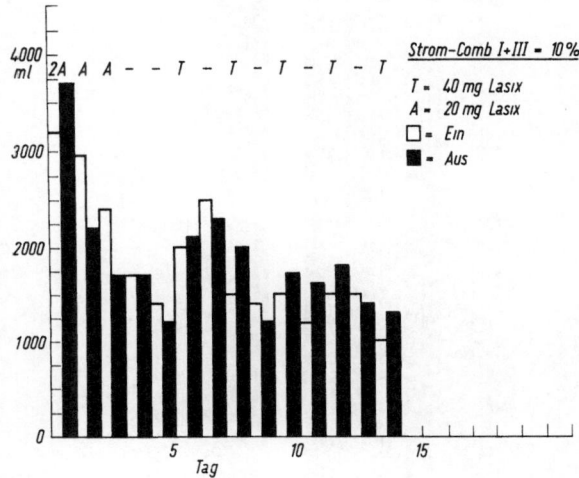

Abb. 6. Intakte Diurese nach Verbrennung unter sofort einsetzender Furosemid-Behandlung

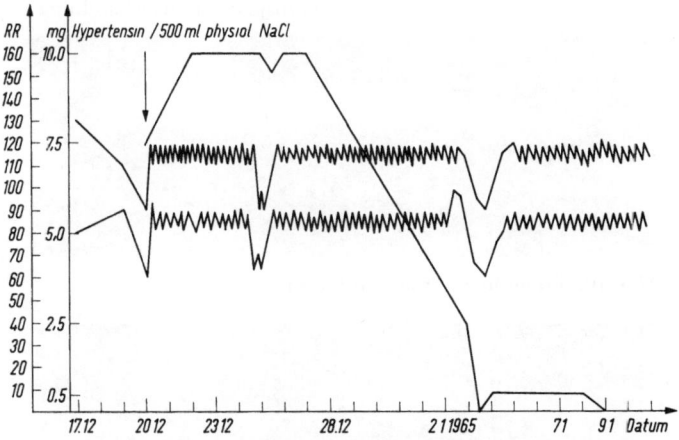

Abb. 7. Sekundäres Kreislaufversagen bei 70% zumeist drittgradiger Verbrennung

liefert das Ödem im Wundbereich eine wichtige Voraussetzung für das Zustande-kommen der Sepsis. Das oftmals zu monströsen Schwellungen führende Verbren-nungsödem wird durch Furosemid praktisch mit Sicherheit ausgeschwemmt, was eine Verminderung der Infektausbreitung zur Folge hat und darüber hinaus die Nierenfunktion intakt hält. Es zeigte sich, daß die gefürchtete oligurische bis anurische Phase (Abb. 6) abgeschwächt verlief bzw. ausblieb (WEBER und VOGEL).

In einem routinemäßigen Prüfverfahren werden, tabellarisch aufgezeichnet,
außer kliniküblichen Messungen (Temperatur, Puls, RR usw.) zunächst täglich,
dann nach Erfordernis, die folgenden Regulationen überwacht: Hämatokrit,

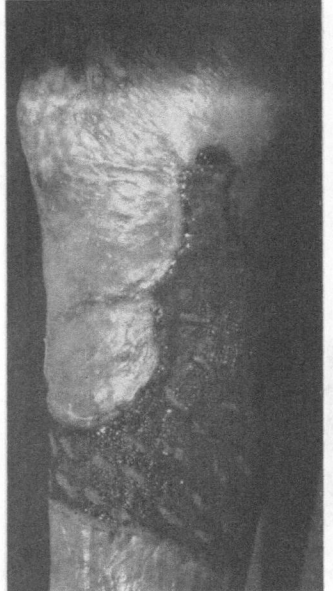 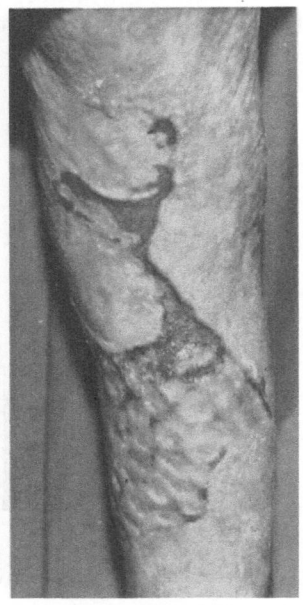

Abb. 8. Reverdin   Abb. 9. Zustand nach Reverdin-
                                    Transplantationsbehandlung

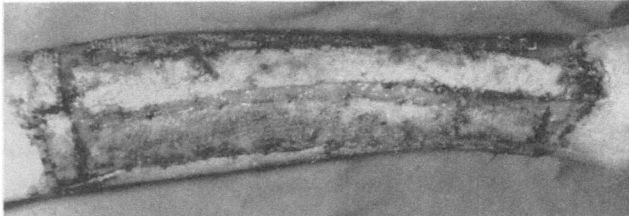

Abb. 10. Fremdhaut-Transplantation

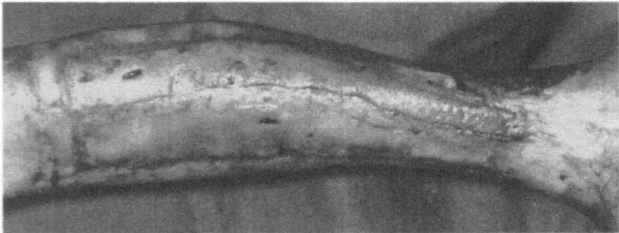

Abb. 11. Zustand nach 4 Wochen

Hämoglobin, Blutbild, BSG, Elektrolyte, Gesamteiweiß, Albumin/Globulin-
quotient, Einfuhr — Ausfuhr, Harnstoff, Transaminasen, Bilirubin i.S., Urobilin
und Urobilinogen.

Während Hämatokrit und Hämoglobin zunächst bei starker Exsudation rasch ansteigen, fallen Erythrocyten, Hämoglobin und wenige Tage später die Serumeiweiße, unter diesen das Albumin stärker, ab. Gleichzeitig oder anschließend kann es zum Elektrolytverlust kommen. Um den 10. Tag beginnen die Transaminasen, das Bilirubin und die ohnehin beschleunigte Senkung anzusteigen, Urobilin und Urobilinogen werden im Harn positiv. Die Temperaturen erreichen vom 7. Tag Werte um über 39°, der Blutdruck sinkt bei steigender Herzfrequenz langsam ab.

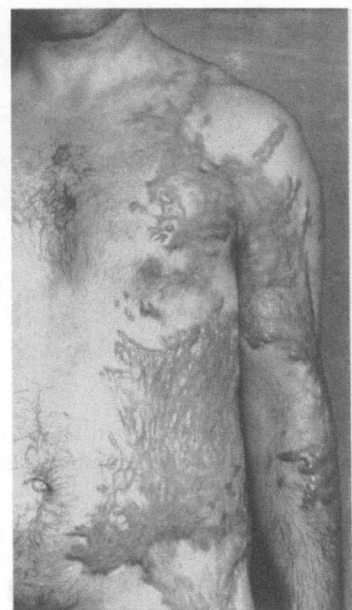

Aus diesem fast als gesetzmäßig zu bezeichnenden Verlauf können sekundäres, peripheres Kreislaufversagen (Abb. 7), Sepsis, Ödeme und Hepatitis resultieren. Daher wird die Therapie auf die Substitution der jeweiligen Mangelzustände und die Prophylaxe der zu erwartenden *Komplikationen* ausgerichtet. Diese lassen sich in folgende Abschnitte gliedern: Normalisierung des Hämatokrits durch Infusion von Elektrolyt- und Aminosäuregemischen. Bei Absinken der Serumeiweiße, besonders des Albumins, werden Albuminlösungen infundiert, oral anabole Steroide und Nahrungseiweiße appliziert; vor der Gewebsdemarkation auftretende Temperaturen durch Antipyretica, später durch Tetracycline behandelt. Die sich um den 8. bis 10. Krankheitstag einstellende Anämie wird durch Bluttransfusionen, die krankheitsbedingte Elektrolytverarmung durch parenterale und orale Elektrolytgaben behandelt. Vom 9. Tag an werden die meist über

Abb. 12. Ausgedehnte Verbrennungskeloide (familiär)

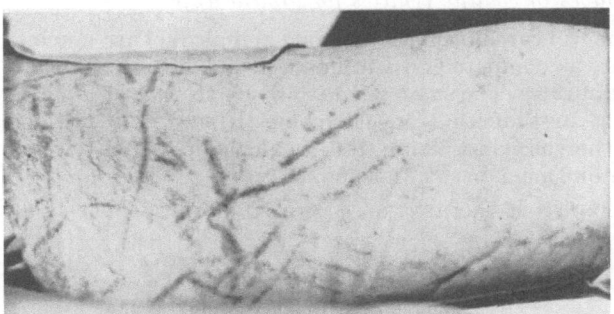

Abb. 13. Hautblutungen 10 Tage nach Verbrennungsschock

einen Kavakatheter laufenden Dauerinfusionen durch eine auf KALK zurückgehende Leberschutztherapie abgelöst.

Zum frühest möglichen Zeitpunkt, d. h. bei intakter Herz-Kreislauffunktion und bei Abstoßung nekrotischen Gewebes, beginnen Reinigung und Bewegungsübungen, je nach Ausdehnung der Verbrennungen im Teil-, Voll- oder

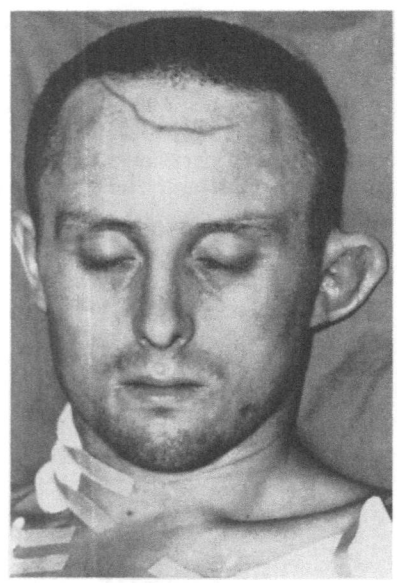

Abb. 14. Perichondritis

Schmetterlingsbad. Die Wundbehandlung besteht ferner in der Hemmung überschießender Granulationen (durch Touchieren oder Umschläge mit Argentum nitricum oder durch Corticoidemulsionen unter Occlusivverbänden). Eine verlangsamte Wundepithelisierung verlangt die plastische Deckung nach RE-VERDIN (Abb. 8, 9) bzw. THIERSCH mit Eigen- oder Fremdhauttransplantaten (Abb. 10, 11). Diese Maßnahmen verringern die besonders im Kindesalter beträchtliche Gefahr der Keloidbildung. Bei konstitutioneller bzw. familiärer Keloidneigung sind diese Behandlungsformen allerdings weitgehend wirkungslos (Abb. 12). Die Nachbehandlung mit der Thioharnstoff-Iontophorese führt gelegentlich zu einer Besserung.

Zu den weiteren *Komplikationen* zählen die ab der 2. Krankheitswoche auftretenden Haut- (Abb. 13) und Intestinalblutungen, die Perichondritis (Abb. 14), Thrombosen sowie erneut Herz- und Kreislaufversagen. Deren Behandlung ist symptomatisch und bei rechtzeitiger Erkennung zumeist reparabel.

A New Principle in Topical Corticosteroid Treatment

G. HAGERMAN, Department of Dermatology of the University Lund (Sweden)

General advantages of volatile vehicles for topical application

In experimental carcinogenesis, acetone and alcohol are much superior vehicles for benzpyrene, as compared to vaseline and polyethylene glycol, which tend to retain it at the surface. The same seems to apply to several topically applied, toxic substances, e. g. urethane, nitrocyclohexane (RISKA, SCHÜTZ), and also to sexual hormones. In the vasoconstriction test, an alcoholic corticosteroid vehicle appears superior to an ointment base (VICKERS).

In topical corticoid therapy, an entirely volatile vehicle has proved to have several advantages:

Formula used in this investigation:

Triamcinolone acetonide Squibb	0.2%
Salicylic acid	2%
Benzalkonium chloride	0.05%
Alcohol	70 to 100%

1. Cosmetically superior, leaving no greasy, smearing residue.

2. Maximum utilization of the applied amount of corticoid, as no part of it can be retained in vehicle residues.

3. The efficacy may be further increased through repeated (double or triple) application of the corticoid tincture, allowing a couple of minutes evaporation between each application. This does not apply to non-volatile vehicles (see figure).

4. *Combination treatment*. After evaporation of the volatile vehicle, the corticosteroid effect may be *combined* with that of other topical remedies suitable in the individual case, as the corticoid layer on the surface does not impede the penetration of the other formula applied afterwards. An ointment containing *e.g.* corticoids, tar or antibiotics may then add its activity to that of the primary corticoid deposit, on which the ointment layer may also have an occlusive, penetration-increasing action.

The dermatologist, using this combination principle, may individualize the treatment according to the needs of each patient more freely than when he is bound to the fixed drug combinations available.

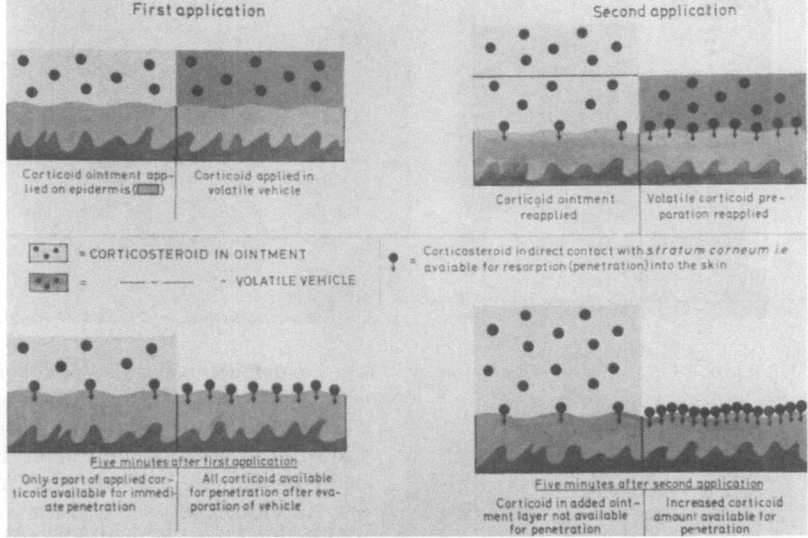

Fig. Possibilities for increasing the effect through repeated application.

Several pictorial examples of the efficacy of Kenalog Tincture, used alone or in combination treatment, were given in the exhibition.

In psoriasis of the scalp (particularly in visible border areas), the tincture is applied in the evening under occlusive bandaging. Thus, very good results may be obtained without the cosmetical inconveniences inherent to the use of ointments, creams or non-volatile lotions.

In lupus erythematodes or psoriasis of the face, where occlusive bandaging is difficult or non-feasible, Kenalog Tincture under corticoid cintment during the night and tincture only during the day, has proved a cosmetically very acceptable and therapeutically effective treatment. The same pertains to the hands, greasy, smearing applications are impossible in many working conditions.

In non-psoriatic *otitis externa*, the low surface tension of the tincture makes it „explode" into all crevices of the auditory channel, assuring maximum anti-inflammatory and drying activity (has been used with excellent results in several hundred cases in the E.N.T.-Department).

Casus rari muco-cutanei

A. GREITHER und O. HORNSTEIN, Universitäts-Hautklinik Düsseldorf und
Universitäts-Hautklinik Erlangen (Deutschland)

1. Pareiitis plasmacellularis bullosa et Balanitis plasmacellularis Zoon. 71jäh-
riger Mann mit blasigen Erscheinungen und Infiltraten an der Wangenschleimhaut und auf der Eichel. Histologisch in beiden Lokalisationen kennzeichnende
plasmocelluläre-lymphocytäre Infiltrate, zum Teil mit lymphfollikulären Reak-
tionszentren. Besserung bzw. Abheilung durch Steroide.

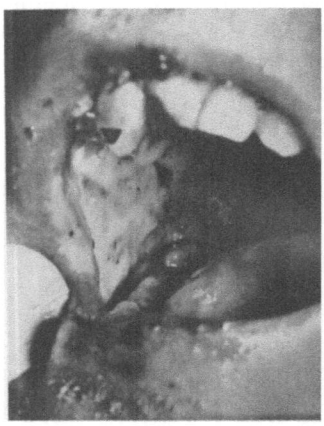

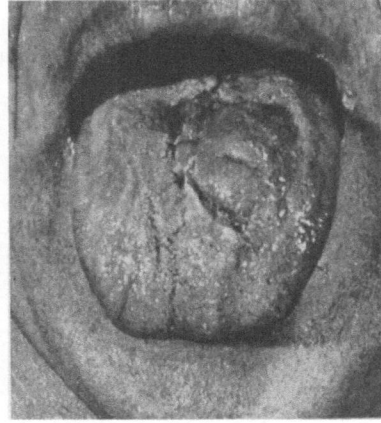

Abb. 1   Abb. 2

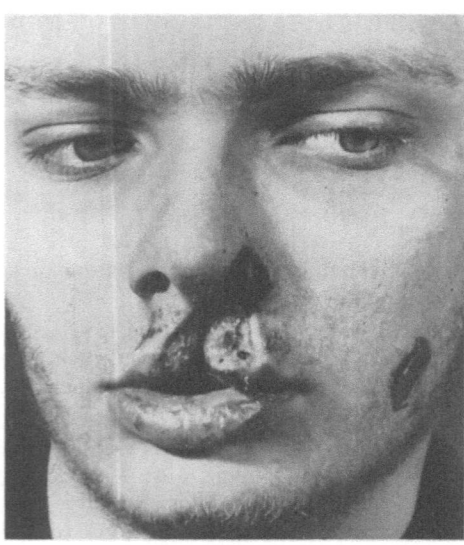

Abb. 3

*2. Combustiones I.—III.° faciei,
oris, labii, naris ex aluminio liquido.*
27jähriger Mann, dem am 31. Januar
1966 durch einen technischen Fehler
beim Gießen heißes Aluminium aus
der Maschine geflossen und ins Gesicht
und in den Mund gespritzt ist (Abb. 1).

3. Lupus vulgaris labii superioris.
63jährige Frau, in der Vorgeschichte
Leukämie. Seit 4 Jahren lupöse Infiltrate der Ober- und Unterlippe, am
harten Gaumen und an der Nasen-
schleimhaut. Langsame Abheilung un-
unter Tuberkulostatika (Abb. 2).

*4. Tuberculosis granulomatosa lin-
guae.* 44 Jahre alter Mann, Erscheinungen seit 4 Jahren, 1966 Probeexcision: Tuberkulose vom proliferie-
rend-verkäsenden Typ. Unter Tuberkulostatika nur langsame Rückbildung.

5. Combustio (et scissio) labii superioris et nasi e currente electrico. 20jähriger
Mann, der am 24. Oktober 1966 während der Reparatur eines Durchlauferhitzers,
der unter einem Spülstein montiert war, mit einem Stromkreis von 380 Volt in

Kontakt kam und das Bewußtsein verlor. Er fiel dann mit dem Gesicht auf den stromführenden Leiter und wurde in dieser Stellung von einem mitarbeitenden Kollegen gefunden, der den Stromkreislauf sofort unterbrach. Stromeintrittsmarke am rechten Daumengrundglied. Durch direkten Kontakt mit dem Stromleiter entstand eine völlige Spaltung der Oberlippe und eine Verletzung des linken Nasenflügels. Durch Sekundärnaht und inzwischen erfolgten plastischen Aufbau des linken Nasenflügels ist bereits eine wesentliche Annäherung an den früheren Zustand erzielt worden (Abb. 3).

6. *Angulus infectiosus et tumores e leukaemia.* 54jähriger Mann mit Knoten am Mons pubis, aus denen histologisch (an auswärtiger Stelle) die Diagnose eines angeblichen Stachelzellcarcinoms gestellt wurde. Die Tumoren wurden mit Bestrahlung behandelt. Erst später wurde eine Leukämie entdeckt, die Tumoren wurden jedoch nicht darauf bezogen. Bei der ersten Untersuchung (am 14. Februar 1967) fanden sich auch leukämische Infiltrate an den Mundwinkeln (Perlèche), die durch Erhöhung der Leukerandosis innerhalb weniger Wochen abheilten, ebenso wie sich die leukämischen Tumoren am Genitale zurückbildeten.

Visualization in Dermatology

K. K Mustakallio, Helsinki (Finnland)

Examen radiographique des tissus cutanés et sous-cutanés normaux et pathologiques

Ch. Gros, A. Basset, S. Schraub, J. Maleville, E. Grosshans et E. Heid, Service Central de Radiologie et Clinique Dermatologique, Strasbourg (France)

L'examen radiologique de la peau ou dermoradiographie permet une étude intéressante du revêtement cutané in vivo.

D'abord réalisée sans préparation, la radiographie de la peau a bénéficié des travaux d'Aleu Saldanha de Lisbonne qui, injectant un produit de contraste dans le tissu cellulaire sous-cutané, a introduit une technique d'exploration particulière et a décrit une sémiologie radiologique nouvelle.

Nous nous sommes inspirés de A. Saldanha et avons étudié les tissus cutanés et sous-cutanés sans préparation et après injection de substance opaque en suivant la résorption de celle-ci.

Le technique radiologique employée est celle des parties molles: rayonnement de bas voltage (25 à 30 kV), intensité élevée, film sans écran à haute définition, compression modérée de la peau et cône localisateur pour éviter la diffusion, source de flou. Des améliorations de l'image peuvent être obtenues par des procédés électroniques (logétron).

Les régions explorées dépendent des localisations pathologiques. Ont été essentiellement étudiés, les membres supérieurs et inférieurs, le revêtement cutané de l'abdomen et du cou. Après avoir pratiqué un cliché sans préparation, on procède à l'injection de 1 millilitre d'un produit iodé hydrosoluble rendu isotonique par adjonction d'eau distillée. La quantité injectée en sous-cutané ne distend pas les tissus et n'entraîne aucune réaction locale ni générale.

Il est difficile de dégager une sémiologie radiologique simple de la peau normale ; il existe en effet plusieurs aspects normaux selon l'âge et chaque individu. L'épiderme est bien visible, néanmoins ses variations d'épaisseurs sur le cliché doivent être appréciées avec circonspection ; en effet, la projection tangentielle de l'épiderme sur le film peut entraîner une image radiologique d'épaississement ne correspondant pas à une augmentation réelle d'épaisseur du tissu épidermique. Le tissu sous-cutané est plus ou moins développé selon l'âge et le sexe du sujet, ainsi chez la femme l'espace sous-épidermique est plus important que chez l'homme. Les tractus fibreux, notamment le fascia superficialis sont parfois bien visibles ; il existe une transition progressive entre l'épaississement normal et pathologique

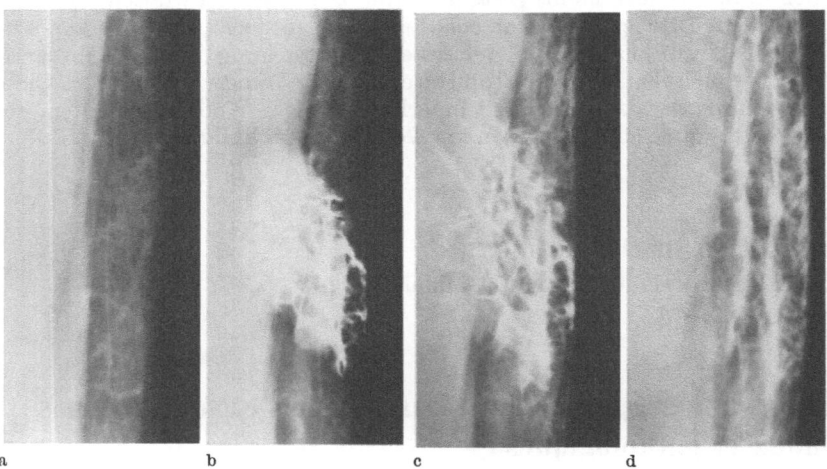

a   b   c   d

Fig. 1. Peau normale : a Sans préparation. On reconnait l'épiderme, le derme avec le facia superficialis, des veinules, le muscle et son aponévrose. b 1 min après injection du produit de contraste. c 5 min après injection du produit de contraste. Celui-ci diffuse dans le tissu sous-cutané. d 30 min après injection : le produit diffuse le long des tractus fibreux et selon deux réseaux longitudinaux, le plus profond étant situé au voisinage immédiat du facia superficialis

de ces éléments fibreux. Les veines du tissu sous-cutané sont nettement reconnaissables, l'aponévrose et les muscles se distinguent très facilement sur les clichés radiologiques.

Après injection d'un produit iodé hydrosoluble, isotonique, il existe une résorption progressive de celui-ci que l'on suit facilement sur les clichés pratiqués 5 min, 15 min, 30 min et 1 h après l'injection. La résorption se fait d'une façon homogène après diffusion du produit le long des tractus fibreux — alors bien délimités — perpendiculaires à la peau, et le long d'un ou des fascias parallèles à la surface épidermique. Il y a formation d'un réticule (SALDANHA), puis les traits opaques diminuent progressivement d'intensité et disparaissent en 40 min.

Les différents états pathologiques étudiés ont permis des remarques intéressantes. Dans la lipomatose, le tissu adipeux refoule l'architecture fibreuse habituelle, avec notamment distention des logettes.

Les varices apparaissent nettement sur les clichés radiologiques sans préparation sous forme de gros pelotons veineux dont les parois sont plus ou moins épaissies.

Dans la sclérodermie ,il existe une nette diminution d'épaisseur du tissu sous-cutané avec un aspect lamellaire fibreux particulier.

Les œdèmes déterminent une augmentation importante de l'espace sous-cutané avec épaississement des tractus fibreux surtout en cas d'œdème chronique, et distention des logettes. Dans les états d'œdèmes inflammatoires (érysipèle par exemple), l'épiderme est épaissi et le tissu sous-cutané est distendu, les tractus fibreux ont perdu leur finesse habituelle. Le produit iodé injecté, diffuse plus largement aussi bien en épaisseur qu'en surface, sa résorption est assez rapide.

Les œdèmes chroniques présentent un aspect analogue, cependant la résorption se fait lentement.

Le myxœdème prétibial entraîne dans la région intéressée un épaississement de l'espace sous-cutané avec un aspect arachnéen des tractus fibreux mieux dessinés après injection du produit de contraste.

Dans la cellulite, outre l'épaississement net du tissu sous-cutané, on note une

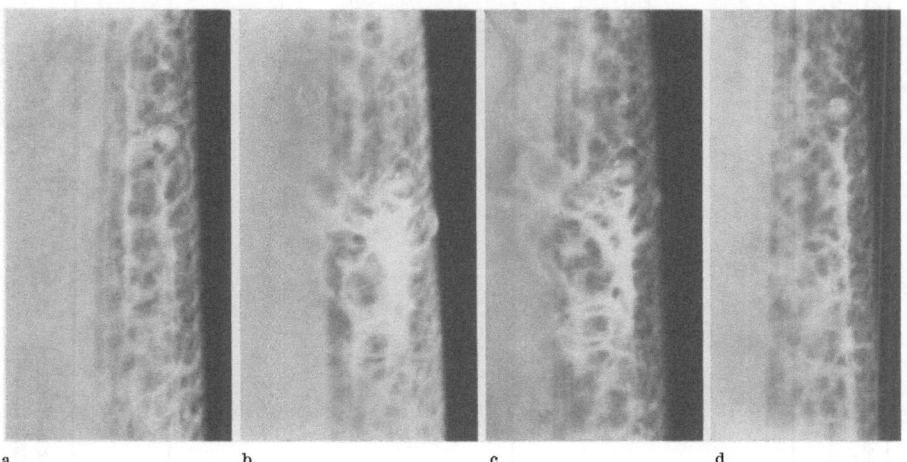

a   b   c   d

Fig. 2. Oedème chronique (état inflammatoire local chronique). a Sans préparation: épaississement de la peau, nette accentuation des tractus fibreux qui sont plus épais et plus nombreux. b 1 min après injection du produit de contraste. c 5 min après injection du produit opaque. d Dès la 30ème min le produit qui a diffusé le long des tractus s'est résorbé

altération des tractus fibreux qui peuvent prendre un aspect grossier, flou et diffus. Le produit injecté diffuse peu, sa résorption est lente.

Telles sont les premières conclusions que nous avons pu tirer de notre étude radiologique des tissus cutanés et sous-cutanés. Cette méthode récente nous semble apporter des éléments intéressants dans le diagnostic et dans la compréhension physio-pathogénique de certaines affections.

Bibliographie. SALDANHA ALEU: Contribution radiologique à l'étude du tissu cellulaire sous-cutané. Leçon de concours de professeur titulaire de la chaire de Séméiotique Radiologique. Lisbonne 1964; — Etude radiologique de la circulation plasmo-tissulaire.

Klassifizierung der Ichthyosen

U. W. SCHNYDER, Universitäts-Hautklinik Heidelberg (Deutschland) und B. KONRÁD, Brünn (Tschechoslowakei)

Die Autoren schlagen auf Grund der heutigen Kenntnisse folgende Klassifizierung der Ichthyosen vor (s. Tab. S. 1412):

Tabelle. *Klinisch-genetische Klassifizierung der Ichthyosen*

	Klinischer Typ der Ichthyose				P.P.K	Erbgang		Kon-genital
	I. vulg.	I. cong.	I. hy.	Ü. Formen		ges.	fragl.	
I. Autosomal-dominante Ichthyosen:								
1. Ichthyosis vulg. simplex	+					+		—
↕ nitida	+					+		—
↕ serpentina	+					+		—
2. Erythrodermie cong. ichth. bull. (BROCQ)	++				(+)	+		+
3. Ichthyosis vulg. localisata (HERMANN)	++				(+)	+		—
4. Ichthyosis vulg. bullosa (SIEMENS)			+			++		—
5. Ichthyosis hystrix gravior (LAMBERT)	+		+				+	+
6. Ichthyosis vulg. mit Kryptorchismus (SONNECK)	+						+	—
II. Autosomal-recessive Ichthyosen:								
1. Ichthyosis cong. gravis (RIECKE I)		+			(+)	+	+	+
↕ mitis (RIECKE II)		+			(+)			+
↕ tarda (RIECKE III)		++			(+)	+	+	—
2. Sjögren-Larsson-Syndrom		+			(+)	+		+
3. Rud-Syndrom	++				(+)	++		+
4. Refsum-Syndrom	++							—
5. Ichthyosis vulg. (SPINDLER)	++							?
6. Maleformatio ectodermalis generalisata			+				++	+
↕ „Porcupine Man" (BÄFVERSTEDT)							+	+
7. Jung-Vogel-Syndrom	+				+		+	?
III. x-chromosomal-recessive Ichthyosen:								
1. Ichthyosis „vulgaris" (WELLS u. KERB)		?		+	(+)	++		+/—
2. Ichthyosis mit Hypogenitalismus (LYNCH et al.)					?	++		+

I. vulg. = Ichthyosis vulgaris
I. cong. = Ichthyosis congenita
I. hy. = Ichthyosis hystrix

Ü. Formen = Übergangsformen
P.P.K. = Palmoplantarkeratose
ges. = gesichert

fragl. = fraglich
(+) = fakultativ
↕ = nosologische Beziehungen unklar

Andrologie in Klinik und Praxis

C. Scherren und H. Grell, Universitäts-Hautklinik Hamburg (Deutschland)

Auf einer 4 × 2 m großen Demonstrationstafel werden die einzelnen Untersuchungsmöglichkeiten im Bereich der Andrologie unter spezieller Abtrennung praktischer Belange und ausschließlich klinischer Möglichkeiten dargestellt. Während für die Praxis die Untersuchung des Patienten, die Erhebung der Anamnese mit allen Kautelen sowie morphologische, biochemische und physikalische Untersuchung des Spermas einschließlich der Fructosebestimmung in Betracht kommen, sind die Möglichkeiten der klinischen Diagnostik sehr viel weiter gefaßt. In einer klinischen andrologischen Spezialabteilung kommen die Patienten zur Untersuchung und eingehenden Beratung, wenn die Untersuchung in der Praxis zu keiner verbindlichen Diagnosestellung gelangen kann. Für den Bereich der andrologischen Spezialabteilung kommen an Untersuchungsmethoden in Betracht: Geschlechtschromatinbestimmung, Hormonanalysen, Hodenbiopsien sowie weitergehende endokrinologische Spezialuntersuchungen. Zu diesen einzelnen Gesichtspunkten erfolgt eine ausgiebige Bilddemonstration.

Papulonecrotic and Acneiform Tuberculids

C. E. Sonck, Department of Dermatology, University of Turku (Finland)

This demonstration of 8 cases of papulonecrotic or acneiform tuberculids comprised 40 colour pictures in all. Six of the cases are shortly described below.

Case 1: K. R. Business man, born 1921.

Brother had Tbc. Pat. heavily exposed to TB: lived together with a tuberculotic, without getting clinical manifestations. Only some calcified foci found in the pulmonary roentgenogram.

Chronic otitis media since the age of 7, cured 1955. Numerous furuncles and septic fever ad 40 °C, Nov. 1941, duration 5 m. SR 128 mm/1 h. Erythema induratum-like lesions appeared in 1948 on the distal parts of his legs, recurring every winter, often several croups pro year, less frequently after 1960. Spontaneous healing without ulceration. First onset of papulo-necrotic lesions on penis in 1954. They were at that time insignificant and recurred very seldom. Inflammation of the left eye, in 1958, after exposure to bright sun. Dg. Chorioiditis, "probably of tuberculous origin". New chorioideal foci continued to occur year after year, accompanied by attacks of episcleritis, scleritis and iridocyclitis.

In May 1964 papulo-necrotic lesions re-appeared on glans penis, this time with great violence, numerous recurrences, subfebrile temperatures. Some of the lesions were fairly deep-sited, causing severe destruction of the glans penis. The occupation of penis, however, seemed to have a favourable influence on the eye.

General condition very good. Almost an athletic habitus, body weight ad 107 kg. Tuberculin R. (Mantoux) strongly positive. No reactions after stich with needles. No aphthae. Disappearance of all active lesions in short time following antituberculous treatment (SM + INH + PAS), which was started in Dec. 1965.

Case 2: R. S. Female Farmaceutist, born 1925.

Onset of disease in 1953 to 1954 with long periods of "atypical rheumatic fever" ad 39 °C., followed by erythematous lesions on arms and legs, some conjunctivitis, and swelling of left wrist and right ankle. SR ad 117 mm/1 h. WIDAL-, WEIL-FELIX —. No tuberculous foci. No angina. No other bacterial foci found. Several blood cultures negative. No LE-cells. Normal values for AST and ASTa.

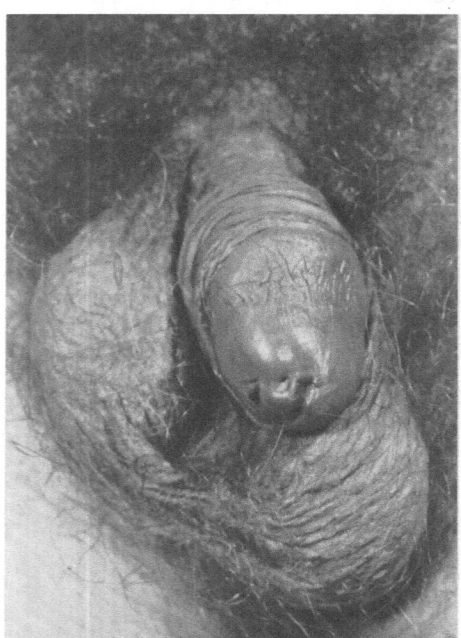

Fig. 1. Case 1. Papulonecrotic lesions on the penis (July 1964)

Later no joint troubles. Last febrile period with temp. ad 39 °C, in 1958. Subfebrile temp. ad 37,2 °C still occur.

Since 1956 to 1957 quite an amazing combination of recurring dermatological phenomena have been observed year after year up to 1967:

1. Erythematous non-suppurating lesions on legs and arms, resembling a mild erythema induratum.

2. Papulo-necrotic lesions, especially on the nose, finger-tips and toes, leaving pitted scars behind.

3. Aphthous lesions on the oral mucosa and in vulva.

4. Hidradenitis axillae et labii majoris pudendi (less frequently).

5. Herpes simplex (only occasionally).

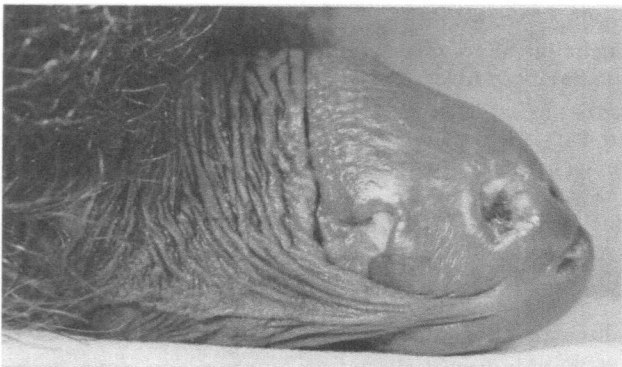

Fig. 2. Case 1. Papulonecrotic lesions on the penis

Tuberculin test (MANTOUX) very strongly positive both with Alt-Tuberculin 1:1.000.000, and 1:100.000, as well as with Danish Purified Tuberculin (1 TU/ 0,1ml).

No reaction to intracut. inj. of physiol. saline or on stich with needles. Only slight redness without infiltrate after intracut. inj. of Frei's antigen. No isomorphic

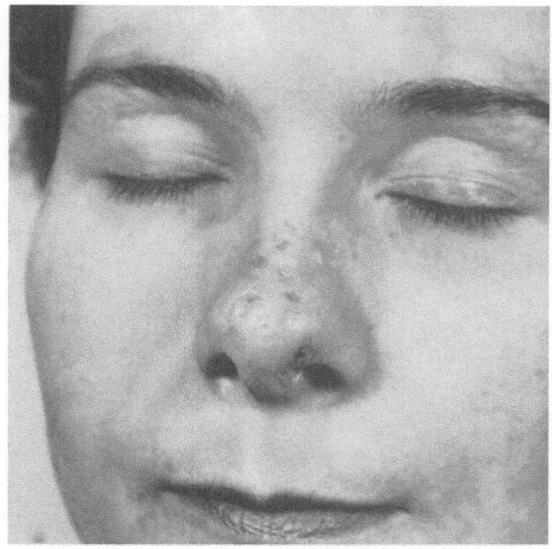

Fig. 3. Case 2. A recent lesion and numerous pitted scars on the nose

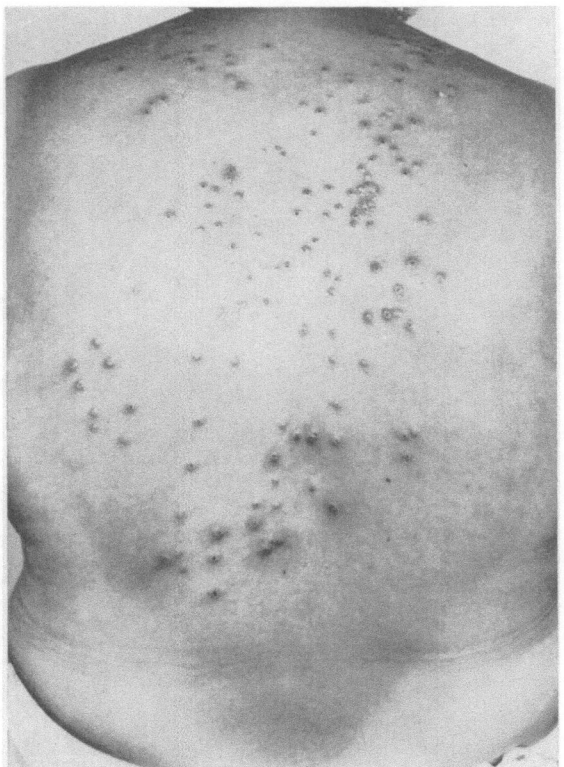

Fig. 4. Case 5. Acneiform lesions on the back

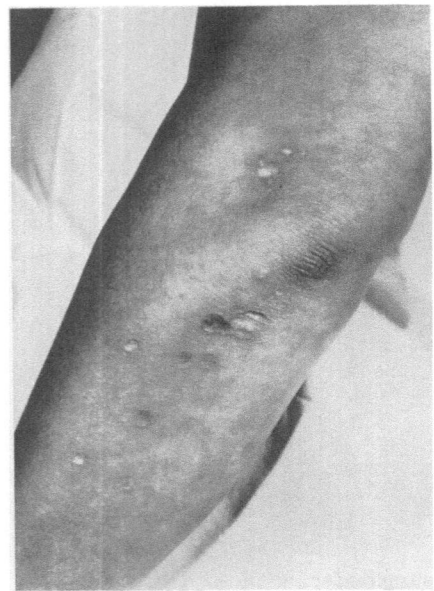

Fig. 5. Case 5. Typical scars on
the elbow

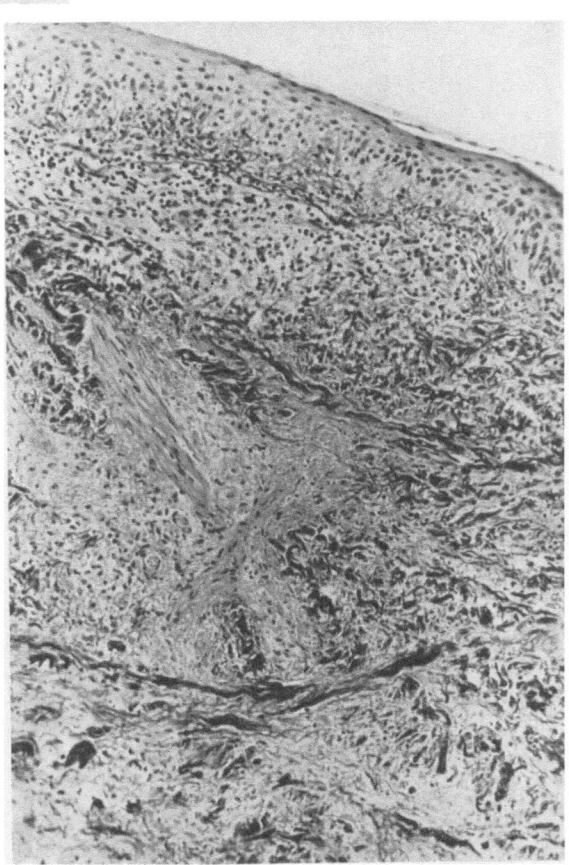

Fig. 6. Case 6. Biopsy showing
a necrotic focus

reactions (OLLENDORFF-CURTH) have been observed. Herpes simplex complement fix. reaction + (1:128).

Case 3: M. H. Carpenter, born 1902.

Tuberculous lymph nodes on the neck at the age of five. His brother had it, too. His wife died in pulmonary tuberculosis in 1931. Two papulonecrotic lesions on the glans penis about 1947, leaving pitted scars. Recurring papulonecrotic lesions on the penis, Febr. to June 1957. When examined, June 6th 1957, six papulonecrotic lesions and seven scars were seen. Biopsy showed granulomatous structures and necroses.

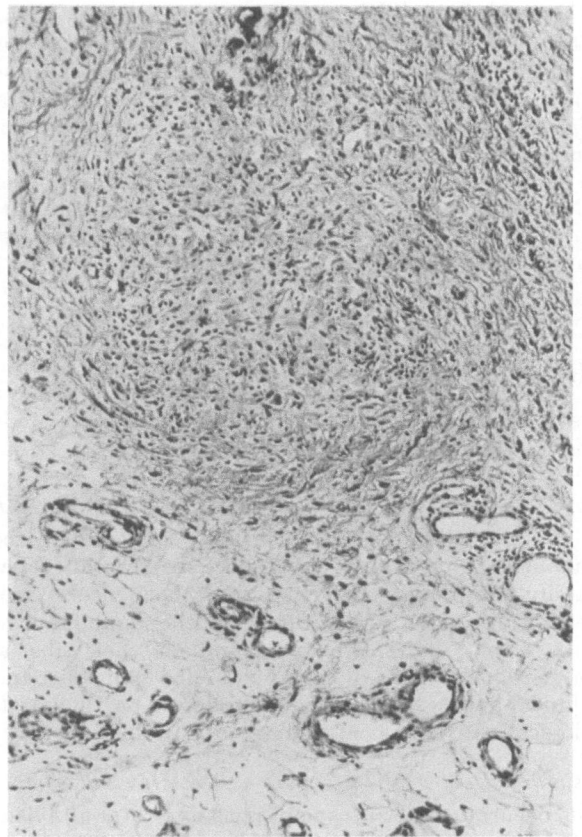

Fig. 7. Case 6. Granulomatous reaction in the lower corium

Case 4: K. V. Business man's wife, born 1931.

Phlyctaenular keratoconjunctivitis o. a. at the age of 17, followed by several recurrences. *Tub. pulm. 1. dx.* at the age of 19. Th.: Pneumothorax. Three years later empyema pleurae. Three thoracoplastic operations with resection of costae. Periapical processes in several teeth.

Sudden outbreak, in 1955, of acneiform, pustular lesions on the forehead and the neck, followed by new crops symmetrically on the medial and ventral surfaces of her thighs, and in the sternal region. After their healing very small (1 to 2 mm) pitted scars remained. Simultaneously with the acneiform lesions the patient suffered from Keratoconjunctivitis phlyctaenulosa o. dx. Aphthous lesions have appeared on the oral mucosa. In January 1958 there was a severe exacerbation of the acneiform lesions, this time accompanied by Hidradenitis axillaris et genitalis l. a. Mantoux test was strongly positive (1:1.000.000) and caused an exacerbation of the eruption. — No skin lesions after 1959.

Case 5: E. S. female, aged 41.

Mother died in pulmonary tuberculosis. Pat. has calcified hilar nodes. Acneiform and papulonecrotic tuberculids (TB culture positive).

Case 6: K. H. Foreman, born 1926.

Recurring tonsillitis with abscessus peritonsillaris at the age of 15 to 18. *Tub. pulm.* l. a. 1947. Hospitalized several times. Th.: Pneumothorax. Erythema nodosum with arthralgies in Dec. 1954. Pulmonary roentgenogram in 1955 still showed signs of active tuberculosis. Recurring papulonecrotic lesions during many years, on legs and arms, on the feet and fingers and on the buttocks. When seen in Febr. 1967, the patient still had a circinate group of papulonecrotic lesions on his left elbow. Numerous pitted scars on the extremities and buttocks. Mantoux test with Alt-Tuberculin 1:1.000.000 very strongly positive (infiltrate 20 × 20 mm, halo 60 × 50 mm). Controls with saline etc. negative.

Exhibit on Genodermatoses

L. ZIPRKOWSKI, University Department of Dermatology, Medical School, Tel Hashomer Government Hospital, Tel Aviv (Israel)

1. Partial Albinism and Congenital Deafness due to a Recessive sex Linked Gene

14 patients affected by partial albinism and congenital perceptive deafness, all male descendants of one family, are reported. A detailed pedigree has been given of the family comprising six generations. Evidence is presented that the pathological gene is recessive and located on the nonhomologous part of the X-chromosome. 5 of the 7 living affected members, their sibs, and descendants as well as 3 carrier mothers have been examined clinically and by laboratory methods. The clinical findings are presented in detail, particulary the dermatological, ophthalmological and otological findings.

2. Total Albinism and Deaf-Mutism Due to a Recessive Autosomal Gene

Simultaneous occurrence of autosomal recessive total albinism and congenital perceptive deafness is presented in 4 children belonging to 2 related consanguineous Jewish-Moroccan sibships. In 1 of these sibships 3 other sisters are affected with congenital deafness only. The clinical findings are presented, particulary the dermatological and the ophthalmological findings, and the genetical interpretations is discussed.

3. Hereditary Porphyria Cutanea Tarda

Three generations of a family with an inherited abnormality of porphyrin metabolism are described. The propositus took sleeping drugs (barbiturates) for a long time. He had an overt, scleroderma — like porphyria cutanea tarda and signs of only mild liver damage. His son was symptomless but excreted considerable quantities of porphyrins in urine and feces. Somewhat elevated fecal coproporphyrin excretion was observed in a grandson. Only the laboratory investigations of the family disclosed the genetic nature of the disease as both family history and clinical examinations were negative.

4. Basal Cell Nevus Syndrome

A 40 year old Jewish male, of Polish extraction began to develop from the age of 32 multiple basal cell epitheliomata, which appeared on the skin even in non light exposed areas. The family history was non-contributory. Clinical, radiological and other laboratory examinations revealed the following abnormalities listed by systems:

a) Skin-multiple basaliomata, plantar porokeratosis of Manthoux, milia and comedones of face and a lipoma.

b) Bones — bifid rib, multiple deformities of spine, multiple stigmata of Marfan's syndrome, abnormal dentition and a supernumerary finger.

c) Ligaments — hyperelastic.

d) The E.E.G. showed nonspecific changes.

e) Calcium-phosphor metabolism — calcification of falx cerebri, costal cartilage and intra-abdominal calcifications.

f) Chromosomal studies on leukocytes cultures showed an anomaly of the E-17 pair.

5. Maffucci's Syndrome
(Osteo-Chondro-Dysplasia and Haem and Lymphangiomatosis)

A 53 year old woman, of Iraqi origin with multiple skeletal and vascular changes is presented. The family history was not-contributory. From birth till the age of 8 years she was apparently well. At the age of 8 she sustained a pathological fracture of the left forearm, which brought attention to the existence of bony defects. She is of short stature, height 146 cm, in good general condition. Clinical and radiological examinations revealed the following defects: Bony skeleton — The left upper and lower extremeties are shorter than the right upper and lower extremities. The bones of the left forearm are bowed. There are many exostoses of the thorax, scapula fingers and toes. Skin — The skin changes show manifestations of vascular changes. In the left calf and foot there is elephantiasis and tumors consisting of distended vessels. The skin is atrophic with brown pigmentation. In certain areas of the body cavernous haemangiomata are found. In other parts of the body superficial lymphangiomata, each the size of a pin head, are found.

6. Epidermolysis Bullosa Dystrophica

A 18 year old male, born in Roumania, developed vesicles on hand and feet a short time after his birth. It was noticed in the same time that his fingernails were absent. There are no similar cases within his family. His grandfathers were brothers. Later, severe deformities of the hands and feet developed with spontaneous amputations of the distal phalanges. Most of his teeth fell out, and it became difficult for him to swallow. Radiological examinations show a stricture of the oesophagus and changes in the bones of the hands and feet. The histology of one of the vesicles showed subepidermal bullous formation.

7. Multiple Trichoepithelioma

Three cases of trichoepithelioma (mother, daughter and son) are described. Four generations of this Yemenite family were affected. The transmission was dominant. The typical lesions of trichoepithelioma began to appear at the age of 15 and were found on the face, neck and upper trunk and extremities. In one of the cases (the mother) developed a baso-squamous cell carcinoma, which is rarely recorded in the world literature. The histology of one of the benign tumors and that of the baso-squamous tumor is presented.

A Case of Congenital Erythropoietic Porphyria

K. YAMAMOTO, Department of Dermatology, National Children's Hospital, Tokyo (Japan)

Among the various forms of inherited diseases of porphyrin metabolism, congenital erythropoietic porphyria stands out as a well-defined and very rare disorder. So far, a total of 13 proved cases have been reported in Japan. The metabolic defect is found in the maturing erythroid cells of the bone marrow and leads to overproduction of porphyrins of type I isomer. We recently had an opportunity to observe and investigate a patient with clinical manifestations of this type.

Report of a Case. A 5-year-old Japanese girl was first seen at our clinic on May 21, 1966, with cutaneous lesions of the face and back of the hands, and an excretion of dark reddish brown urine of 4 years duration. Family history elicited nothing of significance.

Examination revealed vesicular or bullous eruption containing serous fluid and mild pigmentation with several depressed scars on the face, the back of the hands, and other exposed parts of the body. Moreover, these parts of the skin showed the abnormal mechanical fragility. Fine dark hair resembling lanugo covered markedly the face and extremities. Deciduous teeth showed a brownish discoloration (erythrodontia), and under ultraviolet light exhibited red fluorescence.

Splenomegaly at the time of study was absent. Hypertension and abdominal or neurologic symptoms were not found.

Laboratory studies; liver function tests were all within normal limit, and liver biopsy showed no particular change.

Table. *Urinary Porphyrin Excretion* (μg/100 ml)

	PBG	PROTO	COPRO	URO
June 10, 1966	0	0	231	521
June 11, 1966	0	0	218	480

Note: PBG, PROTO, COPRO, URO = porphobilinogen, protoporphyrin, coproporphyrin, uroporphyrin, respectively.

Hematologic examination; hemoglobin concentration 12.4 gm-%; red blood cell count 3.74 million; white blood cell count 6,300; reticulocytes $8^0/_{00}$. A decreased erythrocyte life span was demonstrated by the ^{51}Cr method. Bone marrow showed erythroid hyperplasia, and studies of unstained bone marrow preparations in the fluorescence microscope revealed intense porphyrin fluorescence in nucleated red cells, particularly in the nucleus. Many fluorescing normoblasts exhibited morphologic abnormalities in nuclear structure, consisting of PAS (—) inclusion. Protoporphyrin concentration of circulating red blood cell was 22.0 $\mu g/100$ ml.

Chemical examination; porphyrin determinations in urine are given in the table. The amounts of uroporphyrin excreted were always increased. In addition, the urine contained large amounts of coproporphyrin, but the concentration was less than that of uroporphyrin. Smaller amounts of porphyrins with six and five carboxyl groups were also demonstrated. These urinary porphyrins were identified as the type I isomer. Porphobilinogen and protoporphyrin were consistently absent from the urine.

Contact Allergy in Scandinavia

B. MAGNUSSON, Gothenburg (Sweden), S.-G. BLOHM, Stockholm (Sweden), S. FREGERT, Lund (Sweden), N. HJORTH, Copenhagen (Denmark), G. HØVDING, Bergen (Norway), V. PIRILÄ, Helsinki (Finland), E. SKOG, Stockholm (Sweden)

Since 1962 a Scandinavian Committee has been working on standardization of patch testing. The aims were: 1. Standardization of methods; 2. Selection of substances for a standard patch test series; 3. Study of the incidence of contact allergy [2, 3, 4].

In Scandinavia, balsam of Peru is one of the most common causes of positive reactions to standard patch tests. The balsam is a common denominator of a large number of allergens. Any of these may be the primary sensitizer, but the positive reaction to balsam of Peru may help to trace it. All allergens can initially sensitize a person to a wide range of immuno-chemically related allergens, and these in turn can cause a chronic recurrent dermatitis, despite continued later avoidance of the primary sensitizer.

A positive reaction to balsam of Peru may be a symptom of dermatitis from any of the products shown.

Sensitivity to balsam of Peru occurs also in countries where the substance as such is little used.

Fig. 1

1. Standardization of Methods for Patch Testing

Several factors influence the patch test response for example choice of patch test, dosage of the allergen, choice of test site, choice of adhesive tape for fixation.

Choice of patch test. The test patches should be standardized in regard to size as well as quality. Furthermore the patch itself and the material separating it from the tape should be as free as possible from allergen. Filter paper, which is standardized in quality, readily available and inert, has been satisfactorily employed as carrier material. The size of the absorbent patch should be adjusted to the amount of allergen to be applied. In large scale patch testing it is advisable to take advantage of ready-made tests units. Test patches with aluminium foil as insulating material have for example been designed by S. FREGERT.

Dosage and storing of test agents. The allergen — whether an ointment or in solution — should be applied to the test patches so that the dose will be the same each time it is administered. Storing patch test agents in hypodermic syringes as designed by HJORTH and TROLLE-LASSEN [7] saves labour by reducing by as much as 75% the time necessary to apply test substances to the tape. It eliminates or

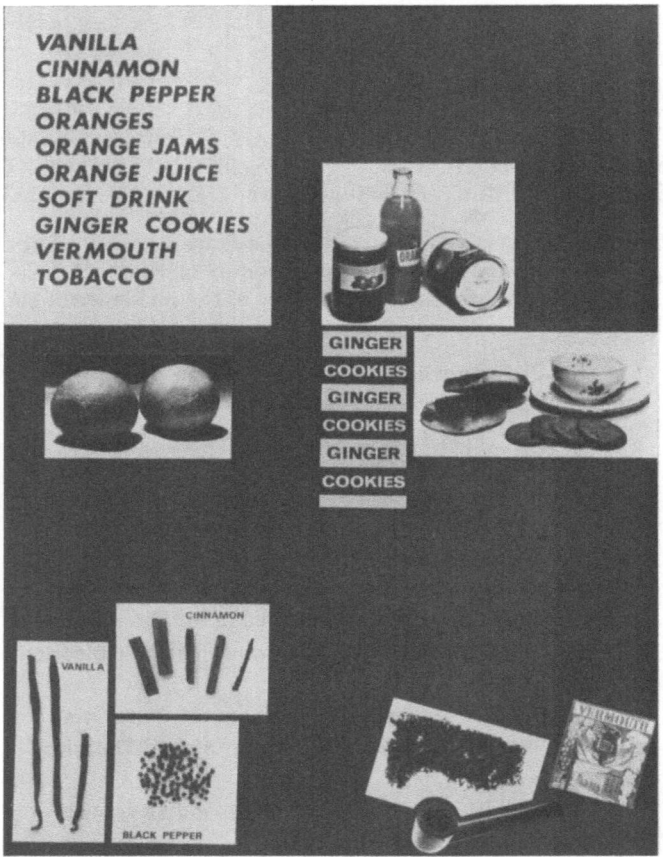

Fig. 2

greatly reduces the problems raised by oxidation and evaporation and obviates possible contamination with rubber. Dose-pipette flasks entirely made of glass have been constructed by BLOHM and by PIRILÄ. When the capillary tube which is melted to the stopper is held against the test patch it delivers a constant quantity of the allergen solution.

Application site of test patches. Skin regions usually employed for patch testing are the back, thigh and arms. Dermatological handbooks present varying and superficial information on which of these areas is the most suitable. According to MAGNUSSON and HERSLE [5] the test responses on the upper and lower back are significantly stronger than those on the arm or thigh. That means that one can obtain clearly positive results on the back, but with the same method a negative response can be obtained on the arms or thighs. In order to ensure comparable and reproducible results one must therefore confine the patch testing to the same region.

Influence of adhesive tape on test-response. Skin irritation and discomfort from adhesive tape are not unusual complications from patch testing. In recent years,

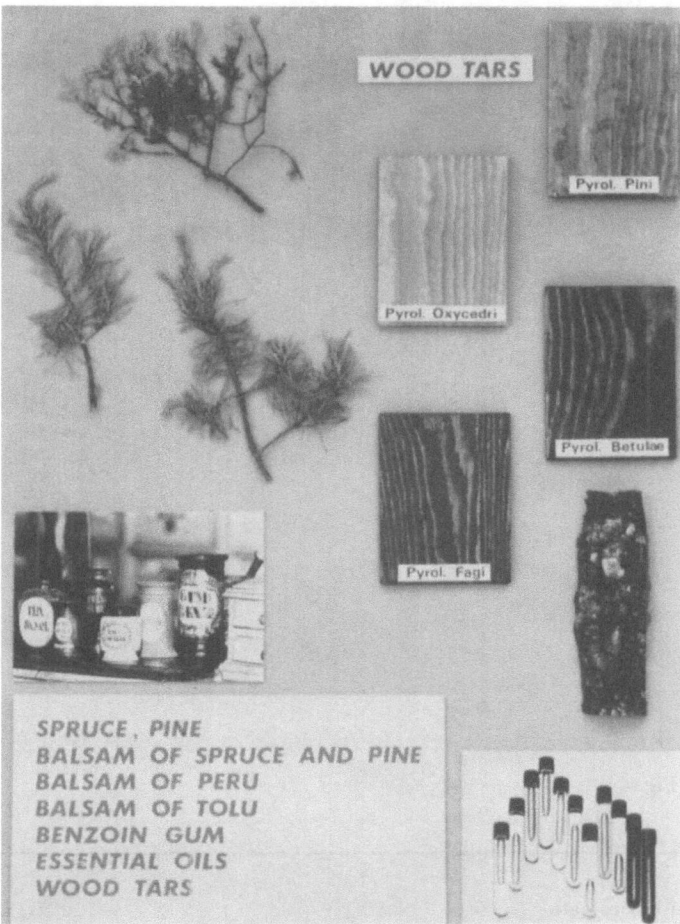

Fig. 3

new types of adhesive tapes, composed of synthetic material with allegedly low irritation and high adhesive capacities have been introduced and recommended especially in connection with patch testing. When using these types which were both of occlusive and non-occlusive types, it was found by MAGNUSSON and HERSLE [6] that some patients with known sensitivity showed false negative responses even when the patch was properly fixed for 48 h. When water was used as vehicle and fixation was performed with non-occlusive tapes, the skin responses were significantly weaker then with occlusive tapes. Almost 50% negative responses were obtained. This difference was not observed when petrolatum was used as vehicle.

When non-occlusive tapes are employed for fixation of test patches it is therefore recommended that petrolatum is used as vehicle of test substances to avoid false negative test responses.

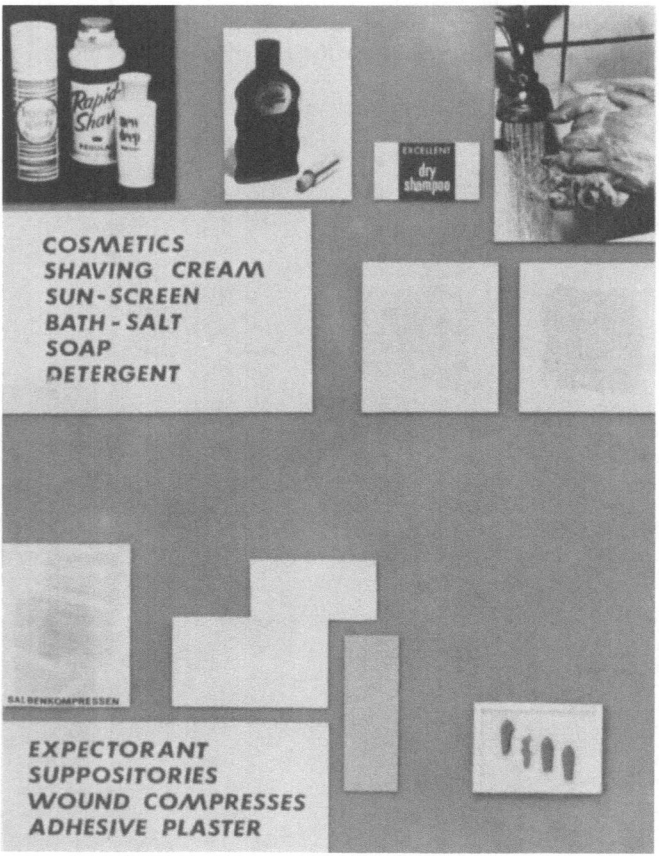

COSMETICS
SHAVING CREAM
SUN-SCREEN
BATH-SALT
SOAP
DETERGENT

EXPECTORANT
SUPPOSITORIES
WOUND COMPRESSES
ADHESIVE PLASTER

Fig. 4

Table 1

Metals	
Potassium bichromate	0.5% in petrolatum
Nickel sulfate	5.0% in petrolatum
Cobalt chloride	2.0% in petrolatum
Mercuric chloride	0.05% in water
Rubber chemicals	
N-Phenyl-N^1-cyclohexyl-p-phenylenediamine (PCPPD)	2.0% in petrolatum
N.N^1-diphenyl-p-phenylenediamine (DPPD)	2.0% in petrolatum
Tetrametylthiuramdisulfide (TMTD)	2.0% in petrolatum
Mercaptobenzthiazole (MBT)	2.0% in petrolatum
Medicaments	
Neomycin	20.0% in petrolatum
Vioform	5.0% in petrolatum
Sterosan	5.0% in petrolatum
Benzocaine	5.0% in petrolatum

Other contactans

p-Phenylenediamine (PPD)	1.0% in petrolatum
Formaldehyde	2.0% in water
Lanolin	30.0% in petrolatum
Turpentine	10.0% in olive oil
Colophony	20.0% in petrolatum
Balsam of Peru	25.0% in petrolatum
Wood tars	25.0% in petrolatum
Coal tar	5.0% in petrolatum
Primula obconica	as is

2. Selection of substances for a standard patch test series

All patients suspected of contact dermatitis were patch tested with the substances shown in Tab. 1. The investigation was performed at the same time at six Scandinavian skin clinics.

Table 2

Chromate	7.4	PCPPD	2.8
Balsam of Peru	6.9	TMTD	2.5
Nickel	5.9	Hydroxychinolines	2.4
Cobalt	5.0	Mercuric chloride	2.3
Neomycin	4.5	Colophony	2.3
PPD	4.5	Primula	2.3
Wood tars	3.8	Benzocaine	2.1
Turpentine	3.3	MBT	1.9
Coal tar	3.1	DPPD	1.9
Formaldehyde	2.8	Lanolin	1.5

3. Incidence of contact allergy

The study comprised 5588 consecutive patients. The frequency of positive reactions is shown in Tab. 2. The two most important allergens were chromate and balsam of Peru, but there were considerable sex differences and differences between the clinics. Balsam of Peru sensitivity was frequent in all clinics except in Helsinki and was the only rate which was high and similar for both sexes. In the exhibit is exemplified how one can get in touch with the different allergens included in balsam of Peru.

References. 1. MAGNUSSON, B., S.-G. BLOHM, S. FREGERT, N. HJORTH, G. HØVDING, V. PIRILÄ, and E. SKOG: Proc. North. Dermat. Soc. 1962, p. 126. — 2. MAGNUSSON, B., S.-G. BLOHM, S. FREGERT, N. HJORTH, G. HØVDING, V. PIRILÄ, and E. SKOG: Acta derm.-venereol. (Stockh.) 46, 153 (1966). — 3. MAGNUSSON, B., S.-G. BLOHM, S. FREGERT, N. HJORTH, G. HØVDING, V. PIRILÄ, and E. SKOG: Acta derm.-venereol. (Stockh.) 46, 396 (1966). — 4. MAG-NUSSON, B., S.-G. BLOHM, S. FREGERT, N. HJORTH, G. HØVDING, V. PIRILÄ, and E. SKOG: Acta derm.-venereol. (Stockh.) 48, 110 (1968). — 5. MAGNUSSON, B., and K. HERSLE: Acta derm.-venereol. (Stockh.) 45, 257 (1965). — 6. MAGNUSSON, B., and K. HERSLE: Acta derm.-venereol. (Stockh.) 46, 275 (1966). — 7. HJORTH, N., and C. TROLLE-LASSEN: Acta derm.-venereol. (Stockh.) 43, 324 (1963).

Klinische Pharmakologie des neuen Histaminblockers Tavegil

L. KERP und H. KASEMIR, Freiburg (Deutschland)

Hautveränderungen und Antikörper-Mangelsyndrome

G. Brehm, Universitäts-Hautklinik Mainz (Deutschland)

Gezeigt wurden zwei Tabellen mit einer Aufstellung über die wichtigsten Formen der Antikörper-Mangelsyndrome (Tab. 1) und die bei diesen vorkommenden Hautveränderungen (Tab. 2).

Tabelle 1	Tabelle 2
## Antikörpermangelsyndrome	## Dermatosen bei AMS

Tabelle 1 — Antikörpermangelsyndrome

I. Idiopathische, isolierte AMS
  1. Kongenitale AMS der Knaben (Bruton)
  2. mit Lymphopenie (Schweizer Form)
  3. mit Leukopenie
  4. mit lymphatischer Hyperplasie
  5. ohne lymphoreticuläre Dysplasie
  6. Dys-γ-Globulinämie Typ II
  7. erworbene AMS

II. Symptomatische (Begleit) AMS
  Bei: chron. lymphatischer Leukämie, Plasmocytom, Makroglobulinämie Waldenström, Thymom, M. Hodgkin Proteinverlust-Syndromen, Vaccinia progressiva, Amyloidose, Louis–Bar-Syndrom, Pyoderma gangränosum, Wiskott-Aldrich-Syndrom, idiopath.-fam. Dysproteinaemie, Perniziöse Anämie.

III. frühkindliche, transitorische AMS

Tabelle 2 — Dermatosen bei AMS

Pyodermien
Pyoderma gangraenosum
Bakterielle Ekzeme
Suppurative Lymphadenitis
Erythrodermie
Soor-Mykose der Haut-u. Schleimhäute
Therapie-resistente Tinea
Endogenes Ekzem (Milchschorf)
Herpes zoster
Vaccinia progressiva
Eccema herpeticatum
Exantheme verschiedener Morphe
Petechiale Blutungen
Uhrglasnägel und Trommelschlegelfinger
Teleangiektasien (LOUIS-BAR-Syndrom)
Lupus erythematodes
Progressive Sklerodermie, Dermatomyositis
Erythema nodosum
Urticaria, Strophulus
Jchthyosis vulgaris

Als Beispiel für Antikörper-Mangelzustände wurden vier Abbildungen gebracht, wobei den immunelektrophoretischen Befunden die Hautveränderungen gegenübergestellt wurden. Es handelt sich im einzelnen um eine kongenitale AMS der Knaben mit Ichthyosis vulgaris (Abb. 1), eine psoriatische Erythrodermie mit Gamma-A-Mangel (Abb. 2), ein Gamma-G-Plasmocytom mit Furunkel (Abb. 3) und ein Franceschetti-Zwahlen-Syndrom mit Gamma-M-Mangel (Abb. 4).

Diese Ausstellung bildet die Ergänzung zu dem Vortrag des Ausstellers im Symposium 11, Seite 1149.

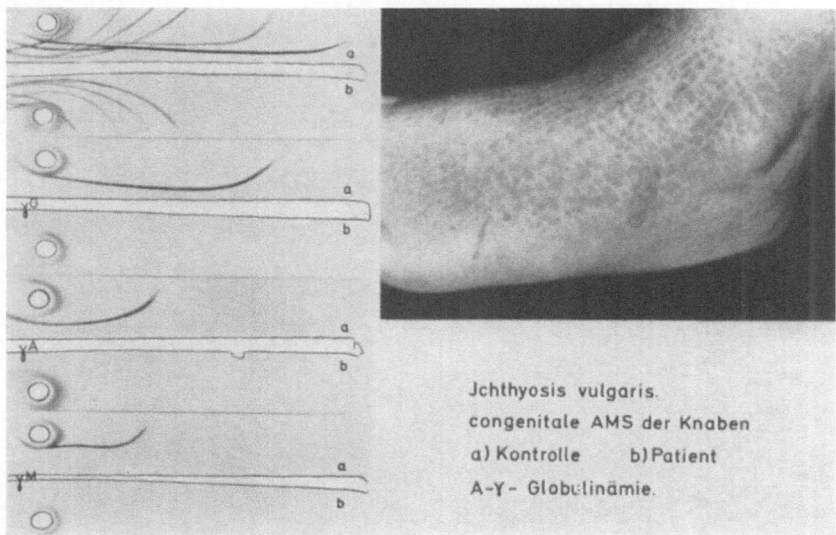

Jchthyosis vulgaris.
congenitale AMS der Knaben
a) Kontrolle   b) Patient
A-γ- Globulinämie.

Abb. 1

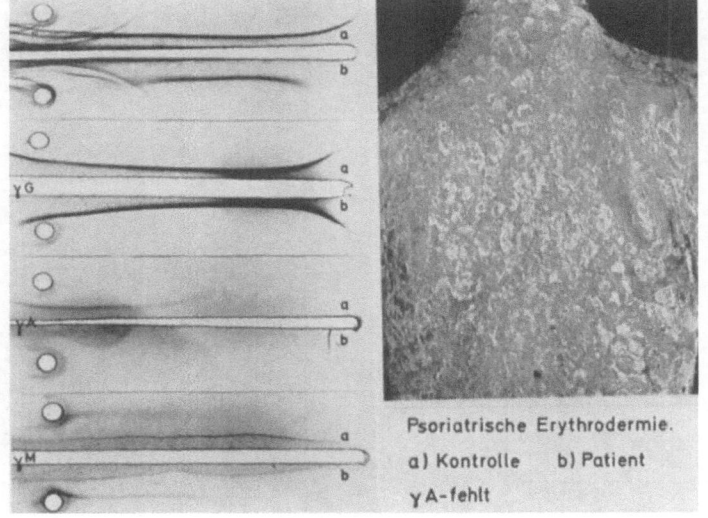

Psoriatrische Erythrodermie.
a) Kontrolle   b) Patient
γA-fehlt

Abb. 2

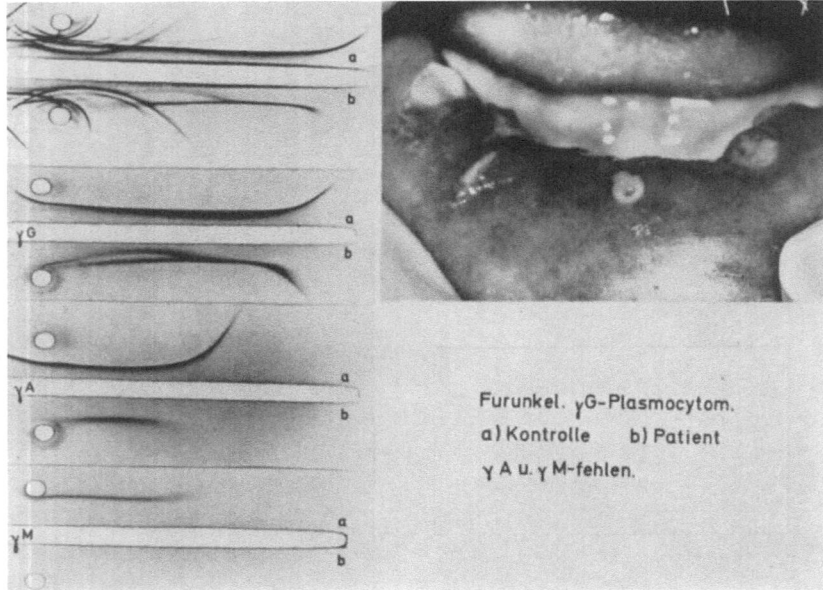

Furunkel. γG-Plasmocytom.
a) Kontrolle   b) Patient
γ A u. γ M-fehlen.

Abb. 3

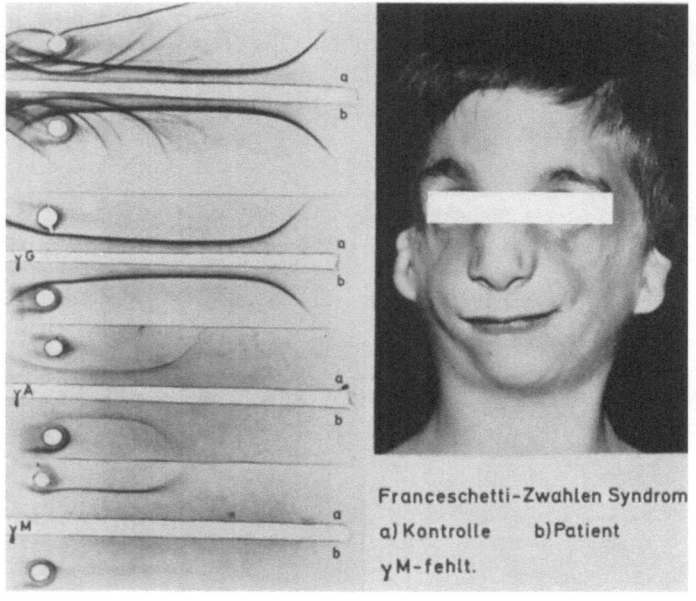

Franceschetti-Zwahlen Syndrom
a) Kontrolle   b) Patient
γ M-fehlt.

Abb. 4

L'allergie de contact

J. FOUSSEREAU, Service d'Allergologie de la Clinique Dermatologique, Strasbourg (France)

Divers documents présentés ont trait à quelques allergènes d'actualité en dermato-allergologie. Il s'agit d'allergènes médicamenteux (laurier noble, baume du Pérou) et professionnels (Frullania, Piperazine).
— le laurier noble représente à Strasbourg la majorité des allergies médicamenteuses. Ce réactogène végétal entre dans la composition de certaines pommades sous forme d'huile de laurier. La sensibilisation à cette substance a donné lieu à une recherche d'identification chimique de l'allergène menée de front par les chimistes (CL. BENEZRA et G. OURISSON) et les allergistes (J. FOUSSEREAU).

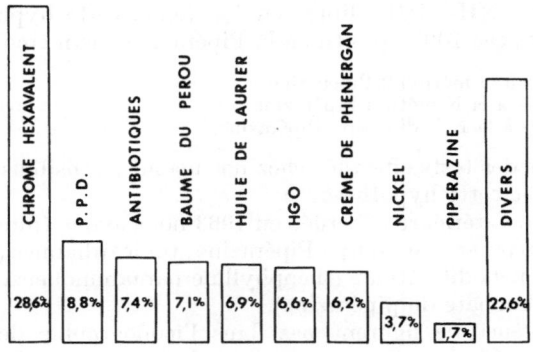

1962-1966 = 688 CAS D'ALLERGIE

TESTS CHEZ 6 ALLERGIQUES A LA PIPERAZINE

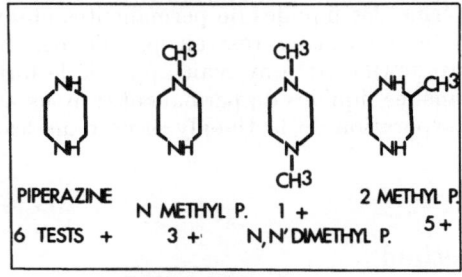

LA METHYLATION DE LA P
SUR LES NH SUPPRIME L'ALLERGIE

Cette étude montre que l'allergène a une fonction cétone, une double liaison époxydable et ne possède pas de fonction alcool facilement estérifiable. D'autres travaux sont en cours.

— le baume du Pérou vient en deuxième position dans le cadre des allergies médicamenteuses. Pour HJORTH l'allergène responsable est le benzoate de coniféryle et le test à ce produit est généralement positif chez les sujets sensibilisés au baume du Pérou. Dans tous les cas d'allergie à cette substance les tests effectués à notre clinique ont montré une positivité pour le benzoate de coniféryle.

— le Frullania est un allergène végétal de connaissance plus récente et moins bien connu. Cette muscinée hépatique est un réactogène puissant responsable de dermites chez les bûcherons, gardes forestiers, agriculteurs, etc. L'allergie de contact à Frullania est bien connue depuis les travaux de l'Ecole bordelaise de LE COULANT (1956). Cet auteur relève 73 cas d'allergie de contact à Frullania pour plus de 1700 dermites par sensibilisation soit près de 4%. Le Frullania est très répandu sur les écorces de certains arbres (chênes, peupliers, hêtres, acacias, chataigniers, etc.) et aussi sur les pierres, les rochers ou les talus. En ce qui concerne les bois du pays, les allergènes parasylvestres nous paraissent au moins tout aussi importants que les allergènes sylvestres. Deux grandes catégories d'allergènes parasylvestres sont à connaître: d'une part les muscinées hépatiques (Frullania) et d'autre part les lichens du type Parmélia (TENCHIO).

— la Pipérazine: une étude effectuée en collaboration avec. Cl. BENEZRA a montré que l'intolérance à la pipérazine est étroitement liée à la présence simultanée des groupes —NH —NH— libres en 1,4. Selon cette hypothèse on devrait s'attendre pour des cas 100% positifs à la Pipérazine elle-même:

à 100% de cas + à la méthyl 2 Pipérazine,
à 50% des cas + à la N méthyl Pipérazine,
à   0% de cas + à la N,N'diméthyl Pipérazine.

Or les résultats des tests effectués chez nos malades sensibilisés à la pipérazine sont en accord avec cette hypothèse:

Dans une étude antérieure effectuée en 1963 nous avons énuméré les différents médicaments appartenant au groupe Pipérazine: tonicardiaques (camphosulfonate de pipérazine), bronchodilatateurs (théophylline-paraaminobenzoate de pipérazine et théophylline éthanoate de pipérazine).

D'autres allergènes ne figurent pas dans l'iconographie de la Consultation d'Allergologie de la Clinique Dermatologique de Strasbourg. Il s'agit de réactogènes médicamenteux (triéthanolamine des pommades à la prométhazine et d'autres crèmes) et cosmétologiques. Un cas de sensibilisation à l'égard de la thioglycérine des crèmes à épiler a été observé tout récemment et rejoint les allergies à la thioglycérine des liquides de permanentes observées il y a quelques années en Allemagne et en Suisse. Instruit par l'expérience de nos confrères étrangers (BORELLI, BURCKHARDT) qui avait apprécié le fort pouvoir réactogène de la thioglycérine dans les liquides de permanentes, nous avons mis en garde le fabricant contre l'incorporation de la thioglycérine dans les crèmes dépilatoires.

Chamber Test Method

V. PIRILÄ and L. FÖRSTRÖM, Institute of Occupational Health, Helsinki (Finland)

ROKSTAD, in connection with his investigations on skin reactions caused by oil of turpentine, observed that the customary patch test "failed on non-hypersensitive individuals where the point was to determine the toxic effect of the substances". A new method was therefore devised by him. This method, from its principle, was called the adhesion chamber method or briefly the chamber method. A circular patch stamped out of boiled linen absorbed the test substance, and for the impermeable layer a celluloid chamber was used (Fig. 1). PIRILÄ agreed with ROKSTAD and used the chamber method slightly modified. The method gave reproducible results in patients sensitized to oil of turpentine and even proved suitable for determining the threshold concentrations of toxic reactions to solvents.

In testing with other substances such as neomycin and bacitracin it has also given more reliable results than the ordinary patch test method. We have recently used radioisotopes (^{60}Co) and chemical methods to compare absorption of various test substances into the skin from the ordinary patch test and the chamber test. The results indicate that the amounts of test substances absorbed from the chamber test clearly exceed and

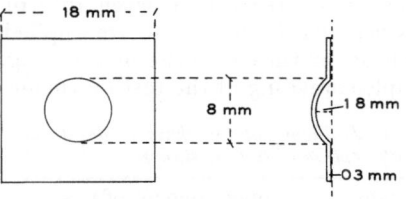

Fig. 1. Original adhesive chamber of ROKSTAD. Prepared of celluloid

are more uniform than those absorbed from the customary patch test.

Description of the method

As material for the latest model of the chamber cellulose acetate has been used. The form and dimensions are seen in Fig. 2. In order to obtain a uniform distribution of the test substance the roof of the chamber was made flat. The inner border of the brim is slightly elevated towards the skin to prevent the spread

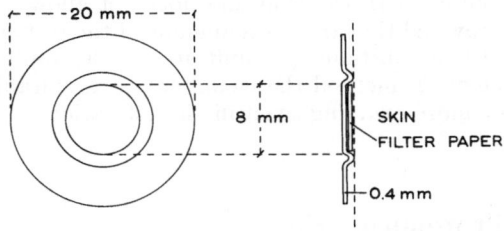

Fig. 2. Modified chamber. Prepared of cellulose acetate. Depth of the chamber: 0.35 or 0.5 mm. Filter paper: Whatman GF/A 0.25 mm or 3 MM 0.4 mm, in tests with ointments no patch disc is necessary

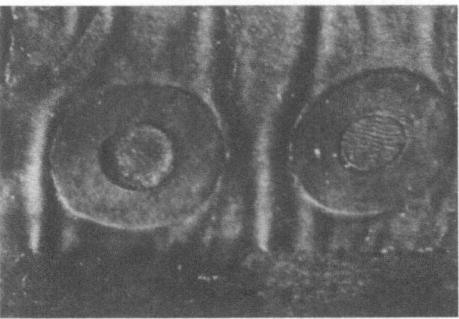

Fig. 3. Successful negative tests immediately after removal of the chambers. Left with solution, right with ointment

of the test solution under the brim. After removal of the chamber the success of the test is indicated by a ring-formed depression around the site of the patch (Fig. 3). As patch for test solutions a disc 8 mm in diameter, 0.5 sq cm, of Whatman filter paper No 3 MM was chosen. This patch absorbs 15 μl test solution. As our observations, however, suggested that this cellulose filter paper and other materials customarily used reduce a high proportion of Cr^{VI} to Cr^{III} within a few hours, more recently a patch disc of glass fibre paper (Whatman paper GF/A) has been used. Ointments are applied, without using the patch disc, by stroking them across the cup of the chamber e.g. from Blohm's standard tubes. A subsequent simple spreading of the test ointment over the cup area, before placing the chamber, possibly followed by slight pressure on the roof of the chamber at its place on the skin, seems to be sufficient for even distribution of the test substance.

Table. *Influence of the chamber depth on the absorption of test substances*

Chamber depth	Average amount of test substance disappeared from the patch	
	Chromate %	Cobalt %
0.85 mm	20	5
0.35 mm	47	12

Test solutions: Potassium dichromate 0.5%, cobalt chloride 2%. Exposure: 24 h.

The influence of the depth of the chamber cup has recently been investigated by us (table). On the basis of the results, by using Whatman filter paper GF/A, 0.25 mm thick, a chamber depth of appr. 0.4 mm (0.35 mm as absolute minimum) can be recommended. With thicker patch discs correspondingly deeper chambers have to be used.

The chamber test is handy and inexpensive. It holds the tightly covered test substance in close contact with the skin and does not allow it to spread outside the test area. Thus provided that the total amount of the test substance applied is equal, the amount of test substance per unit area is also uniform. As a practical and at the same time exact method the chamber test is suitable both for routine patch testing and for more exacting scientific investigations.

Erythropoietic Protoporphyria

R. M. Fusaro, W. J. Runge, E. S. Peterka, M. O. Jaffe, E. W. Goltz and C. J. Watson, Department of Dermatology, University of Minnesota, Minneapolis, Minn. (USA)

The exhibit demonstrates a review of the clinical and laboratory findings of the disease along with the results of our research.

1. History and Symptoms: (A) Begins in the first decade of life and occurs on all exposed areas (usually face and hands), (B) In northern latitudes (Minnesota, USA) from spring to fall on exposure to sunlight (even through window glass) the following symptoms can occur: burning, itching, and prickling sensation.

2. Physical Findings: One or more of the following can be present: erythema, edema, purpura, eczematization, leather-like thickening of skin and sometimes absence of physical findings (only symptoms).

3. Pertinent Laboratory Findings: Erythrocyte protoporphyrin level is elevated while urine protoporphyrin is absent.

4. Results of our Research: (A) Fluorescence Microscopy: Recording microfluorospectrometric measurements of a single red cell and recording histofluorescence spectrometry of frozen skin tissue sections showed the presence of only free protoporphyrins. (B) Sunlight Protection: Patient treated with a mixture of 3% dihydroxyacetone and 0.13% lawsone in an experimental non UV absorbing cream or in 50% isopropyl alcohol-water solution once a day. Patient received 10 h/day sunligth protection with the cream and 2 h/day protection with the

alcohol-water solution. It is necessary to prevent leakage of light through fissures in the stratum corneum therefore the integrity of the keratin appears to be important. (C) Infrared Sensitivity: Radiation at 26,000 A caused immediate urticaria (within minutes) and a bullous lesion several hours later. The above sunscreen mixture gave protection against infrared radiation at 26,000 A.

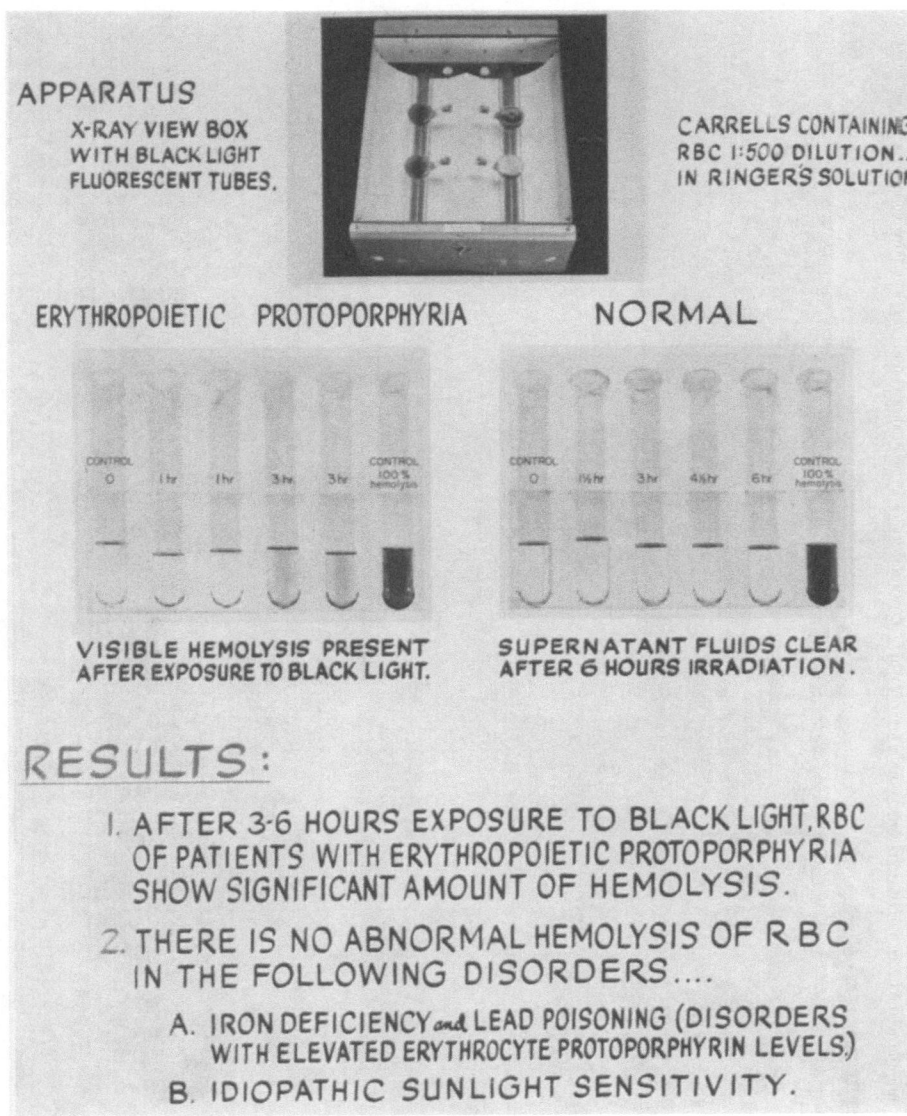

Fig. 1

I METHOD

  A. ANY ERUPTION IS FIRST CLEARED BY STEROID THERAPY + AVOIDANCE of LIGHT.
  B. TECHNIQUE OF SUNLIGHT PROTECTION.
    1. MIXTURE
       3% DIHYDROXYACETONE & 0.13% LAWSONE IN A 50% SOLUTION OF ISOPROPYL ALCOHOL
       AND DISTILLED WATER.
    2. USE OF MIXTURE
       (1) INITIAL: 6 TO 8 APPLICATIONS IN FIRST 48 HOURS.
       (2) MAINTENANCE: ONE TO FOUR APPLICATIONS (SPRAYINGS) PER DAY.
    3. SKIN MUST BE KEPT INTACT & SOFT WITH A TOPICAL CREAM OR OINTMENT WHICH
       DOES NOT DESTROY THE SUNSCREEN FILTER IN THE STRATUM CORNEUM. PATIENT MUST
       NOT APPLY OINTMENT OR WASH WITHIN ONE HOUR AFTER APPLICATION OF MIXTURE.

II RESULTS

  A. TOTAL PROTECTION WITH USE OF SUFFICIENT AMOUNTS OF TOPICAL MIXTURE.

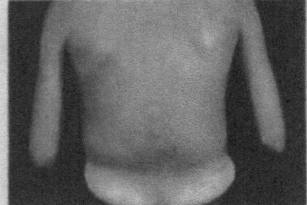

  IN SUMMER OF 1964 PATIENT ACQUIRED A
  NORMAL TAN THROUGH THE SUN FILTER IN THE
  STRATUM CORNEUM. PATIENT PARTICIPATED IN
  NORMAL OUTDOOR ACTIVITIES INCLUDING SWIM-
  MING. PRIOR TO PROTECTION HE COULD TOLERATE
  LESS THAN ONE HOUR SUNLIGHT.

  B. SYMPTOMS OCCUR IF INSUFFICIENT AMOUNTS OF TOPICAL MIXTURE ARE USED OR IF
     THE AMOUNT OF EXPOSURE EXCEEDS THE PROTECTION WHICH CAN BE INDUCED INTO THE
     PARTICULAR PATIENT'S STRATUM CORNEUM.

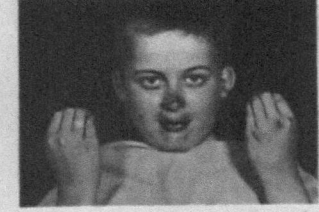

  SAME PATIENT IN SUMMER 1965 RECEIVED 8 to 10
  HOURS OF DIRECT SUNLIGHT IN AN OPEN FIELD
  AND EXCEEDED HIS PROTECTION. HE WAS USING
  TOPICAL MIXTURE ONLY ONE OR TWO TIMES
  A DAY.

  C. PREVENTION OF BULLOUS REACTION PRODUCED EXPERIMENTALLY WITH INFRARED RADIATION (26,000 A).

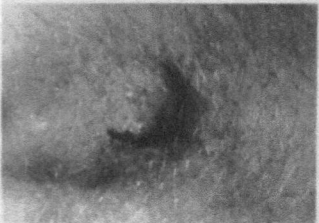
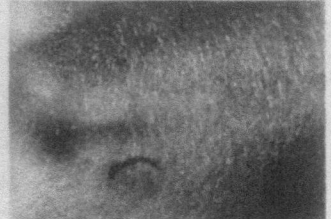

BULLA ON UNTREATED AREA AFTER EXPOSURE TO   AFTER PROTECTION OF SKIN WITH SUNSCREEN
26,000 A FOR 2 MINUTES (NOTE BLISTER NEXT to   MIXTURE, EXPOSURE TO 26,000 A FOR 2 MIN-
RED MARKING PENCIL). NORMAL PERSON SHOWS   UTES CAUSES ONLY TRANSIENT ERYTHEMA.
NO REACTION, NOT EVEN ERYTHEMA.   (NOTE ABSENCE OF BLISTER NEXT TO RED...
                                                 MARKING PENCIL). IN THIS EXPERIMENT...
                                                 JUGLONE WAS USED INSTEAD of LAWSONE.

Fig. 2

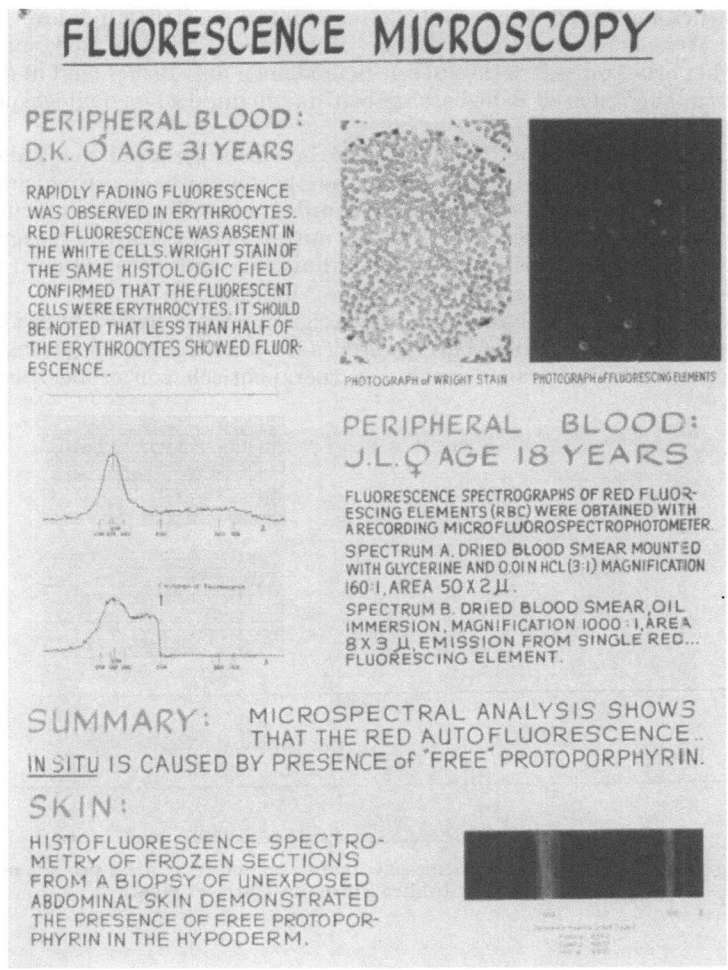

Fig. 3

Gegenüberstellung von Angiomatosis Kaposi (Sarcoma idiopathicum haemorrhagicum multiplex) und Stewart-Treves-Syndrom (Sarcoma angioplasticum in elephantiasi)

H. TELLER und H. KRÜGER, Dermatologische Abteilung des Städt. Krankenhauses Berlin-Britz (Deutschland)

Das 1948 erstmals von STEWART und TREVES als ,,Lymphangiosarcoma in Postmastectomy Lymphedema" beschriebene Krankheitsbild ist charakterisiert durch das Aufschießen einer symptomatischen Sarkomatose vom Typ Kaposi auf dem Boden chronischer Extremitätenlymphödeme.

Es tritt in einer Häufigkeit von 0,5% nach durchschnittlich 9 Jahren bei post-operativen Armödemen infolge radikaler Mastektomie und in 1,5% nach etwa 20 Jahren bei primären oder sekundären Beinödemen auf. Bisher sind in der Welt-literatur ungefähr 70 bis 80 Fälle beschrieben, davon nur drei im deutschsprachigen Schrifttum.

Dieser Umstand und die Tatsache, daß in einem Großteil der Fälle zuerst klinisch und/oder histologisch ein Sarcoma idiopathicum haemorrhagicum multi-plex (Angiomatosis Kaposi) diagnostiziert wurde, gaben Veranlassung zur Gegen-überstellung dieser beiden Krankheitsbilder mittels einer Serie von fotografischen Abbildungen und einer Tabelle, welche die klinischen und histologischen Gemein-samkeiten und Unterschiede aufzeigen (siehe Abbildungen).

Die besonders im Anfangsstadium schwierige, im Knötchenstadium aber mög-liche differentialdiagnostische Abgrenzung des Stewart-Treves-Syndroms von der Angiomatosis Kaposi ist prognostisch und therapeutisch von großer Bedeutung.

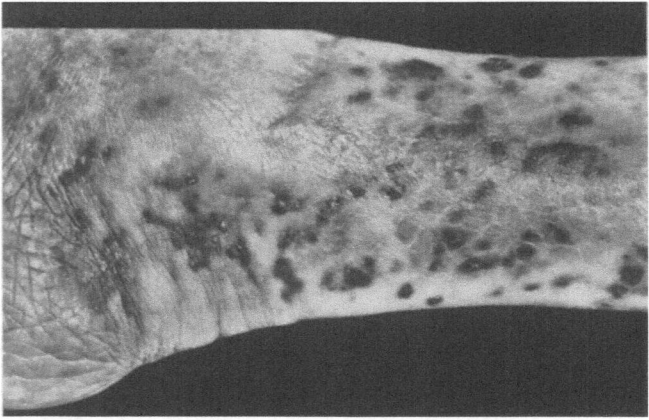

Abb. 1. Angiomatosis Kaposi. Dichte Aussaat livid-bräunlichroter, flach prominenter Knöt-chen und kleinflächiger, gleichfarbiger Infiltrationen am Unterschenkel

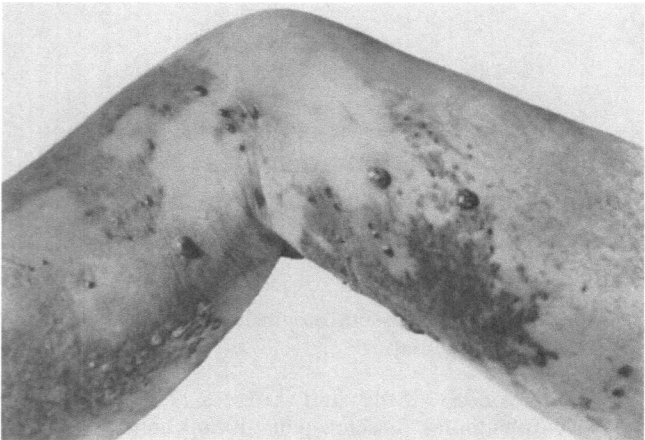

Abb. 2. Angiomatosis Kaposi. Großflächige hämorrhagische Infiltrate an Unter- und Ober-schenkel mit einzelnen, bis haselnußgroßen, blauroten, kugeligen Tumoren

Tabelle. *(In Anlehnung an die Tabelle von* U. BRUNNER*)*

	Angiomatosis Kaposi	Stewart-Treves-Syndrom
Klinik der Haut-veränderungen	Oft symmetrisches Auftreten braunroter Infiltrate und derber Knoten an den Extremitäten. Später kompaktere Tumoren und elephantiastisches Lymph-ödem. Ulceröser Zerfall und spontane Rückbildung möglich. Hämorrhagien und Pigmenta-tionen.	Hämorrhagische Induration und Aufschießen bläulich-schwarzer cutaner Papeln an lymphödematöser Extremität. Ulceröser Zerfall und spontane Rückbildung der Efflorescen-zen möglich. Später kontinuier-liche Eruptionen von braun- bis blauroten großknotigen Tumo-ren, auf die benachbarten An-teile des Stammes übergreifend.
Histologisches Bild	Gefäßgeschwulst mit angioma-tösen und fibroblastischen Tu-morbezirken, Geschwulstzell-bild nur geringgradig polymorph und mitosearm. Erythrocyten-extravasate, Hämosiderinabla-gerungen.	Angioplastisches Sarkom mit angiomatösen und fibroblasti-schen Tumorbezirken. Ge-schwulstzellbild polymorph und mitosereich. Erythrocyten-extravasate und Hämosiderin-ablagerungen.
Geschlecht	vorwiegend Männer	vorwiegend Frauen
Lebensalter bei Erstmanifestationen	alle Altersstufen, vorwiegend 6. bis 7. Dekade	5. bis 7. Dekade bei Lymph-ödem nach Mammaradikalope-ration, 2. bis 7. Dekade bei an-deren Lymphödemen.
Rassische Bevorzugung und geographische Verbreitung	umstritten	keine
Prädilektionsstellen	Extremitäten bilateral, symme-metrisch	Extremitäten unilateral, auf Lymphödem
Lymphödem	gelegentlich vorbestehend, oft Späterscheinung	immer vorbestehend
Organbefall	Magen-Darm-Trakt, äußeres Genitale, retroperitoneale Lymphknoten, Leber, Lunge (eher systematisierter Prozeß)	paraortale Lymphknoten, Lunge, Leber, Milz (metasta-sierende Sarkomatose)
Prognose	unsicher, Überlebensdauer wenige Monate bis Jahrzehnte	infaust, stürmischer Verlauf, Überlebensdauer 5 Monate bis 4 Jahre, durchschnittlich $1^1/_2$ Jahre
Therapie	Methode der Wahl: Röntgen-bestrahlung	Methode der Wahl: radikale Exartikulation

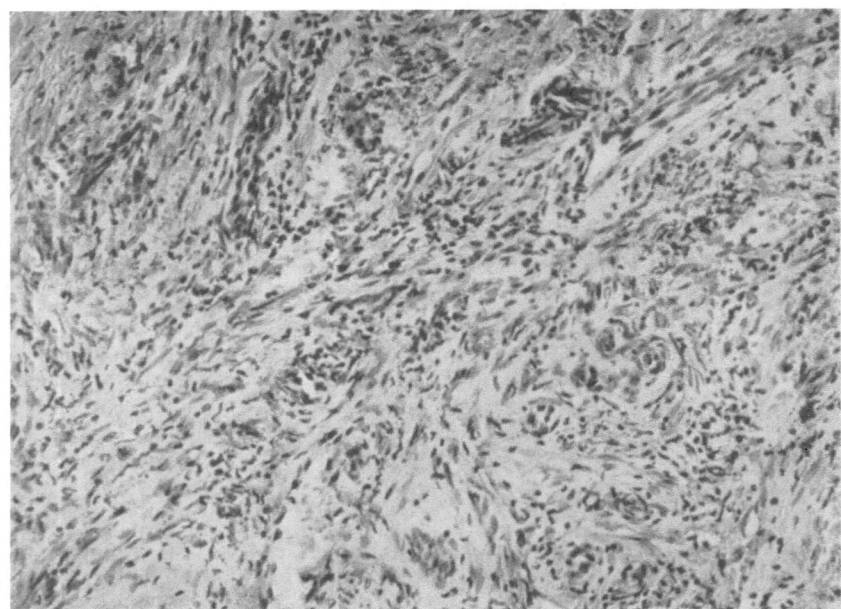

Abb. 3. Angiomatosis Kaposi. Proliferation und Ektasie von Blutcapillaren, strangförmige Wucherung fusiformer Zellen, Hämosideringranula, lympho-plasmacelluläres Infiltrat. HE.-Färbung, Abbildungsmaßstab 900:1

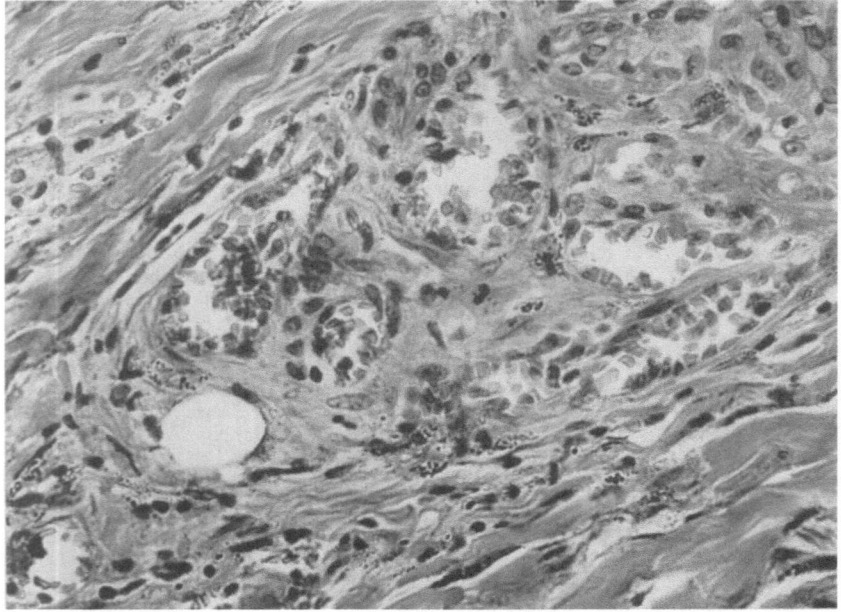

Abb. 4. Angiomatosis Kaposi. Ektatische Blutcapillaren mit großkernigen Endothelzellen, Hämosideringranula. Hämangiomatöser Bezirk, HE.-Färbung, Abbildungsmaßstab 1850:1

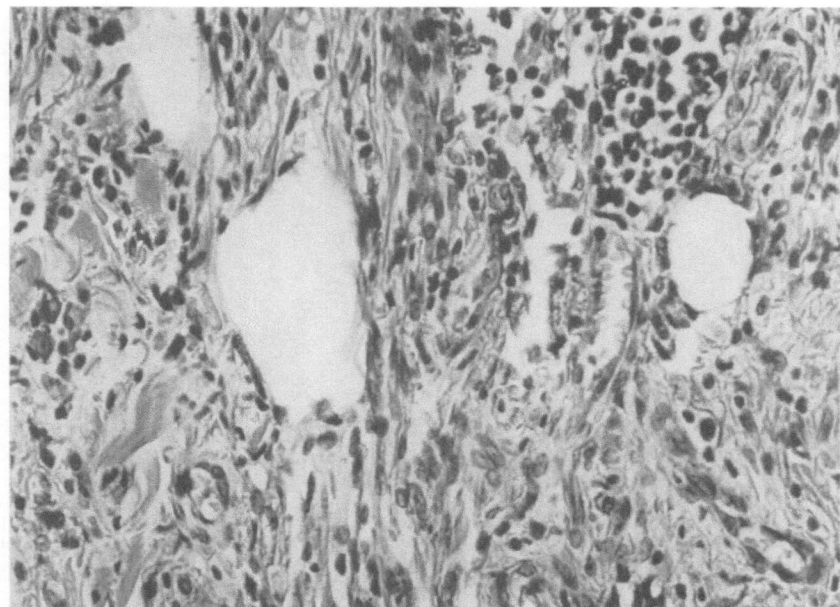

Abb. 5. Angiomatosis Kaposi. Ektatische Lymphcapillaren, Endothel- und Perithelzellen geringgradig polymorph, herdförmig lympho-plasmacelluläres Infiltrat. Lymphangiomatöser Bezirk, HE.-Färbung, Abbildungsmaßstab 1 750:1

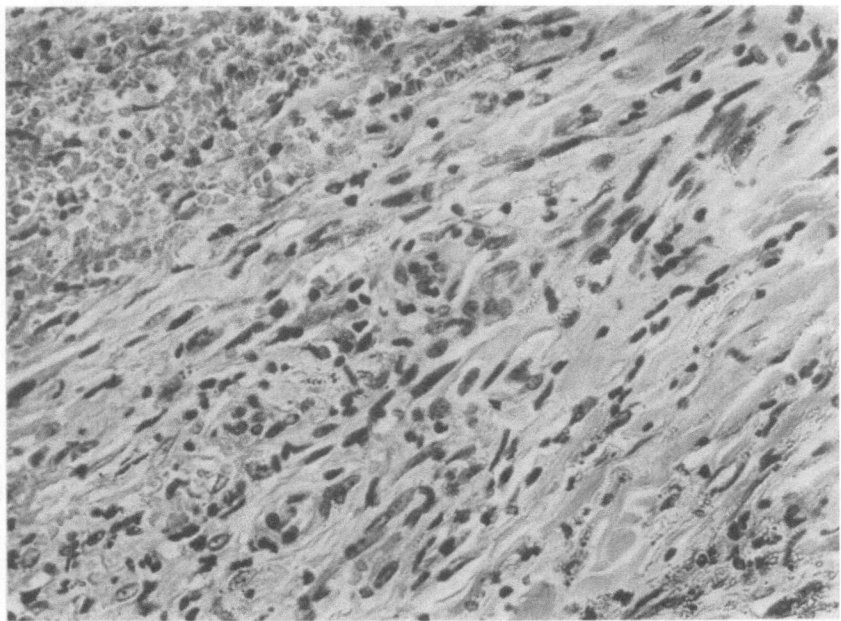

Abb. 6. Angiomatosis Kaposi. Spindlige und blaßkernige Zellen in strangförmiger Lagerung, Blutextravasate und Hämosideringranula. Fibroblastischer Bezirk, HE.-Färbung, Abbildungsmaßstab 1 800:1

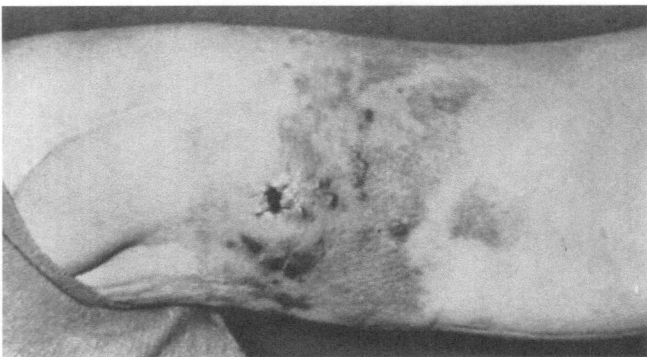

Abb. 7. Stewart-Treves-Syndrom. Bandförmige, livid-hämorrhagische Induration am lymph-
ödematösen Oberarm mit einzelnen, bis erbsgroßen, livid-schwärzlichen, flach-prominenten
Knötchen, 10 Jahre nach Ablatio mammae aufgetreten

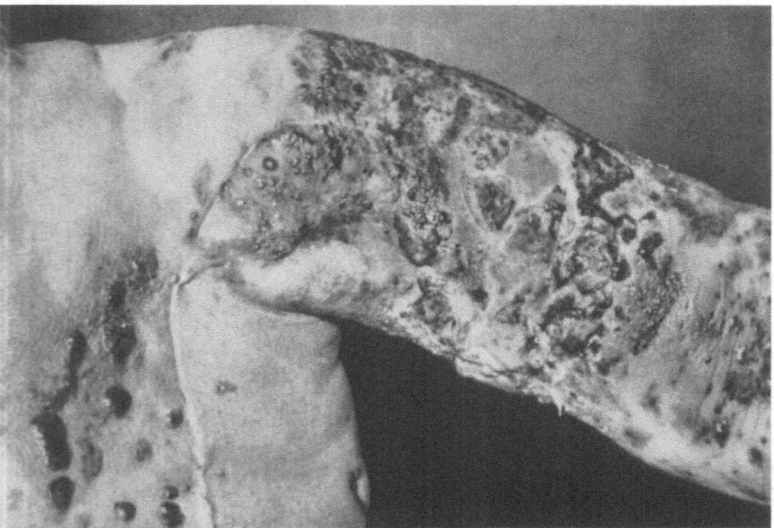

Abb. 8. Stewart-Treves-Syndrom. Metastatische Ausbreitung bräunlichroter, knotiger und
ulcerierender Tumoren am Unter- und Oberarm sowie den angrenzenden Thoraxabschnitten,
6 Monate nach Erstmanifestation

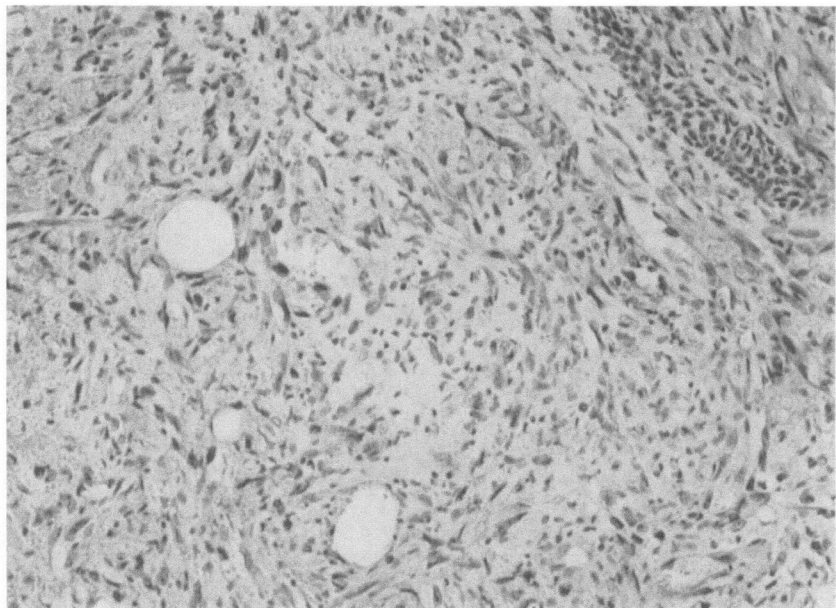

Abb. 9. Stewart-Treves-Syndrom. Proliferation und Ektasie von Blut- und Lymphgefäßen, Zellpolymorphie, Blutextravasate, lymphoidzellige Infiltration. HE.-Färbung, Abbildungsmaßstab 850:1

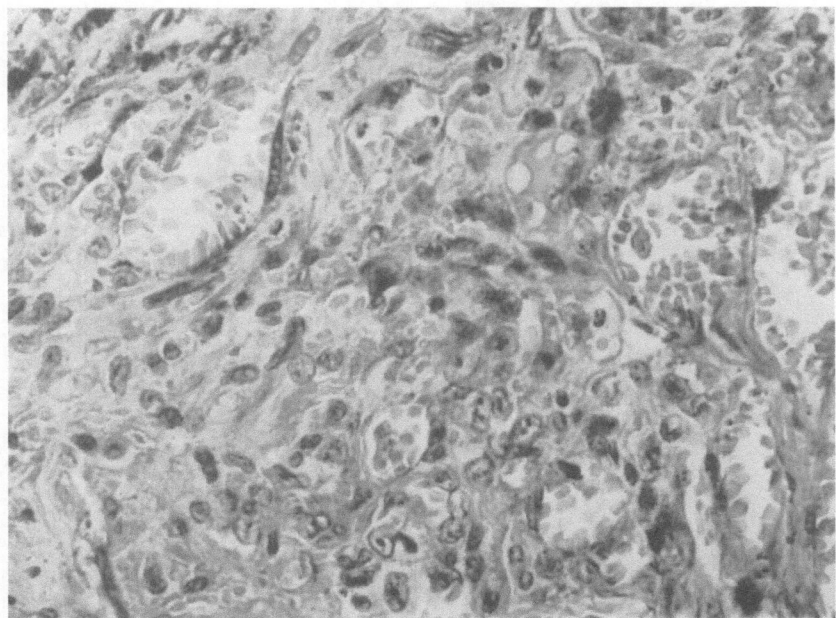

Abb. 10. Stewart-Treves-Syndrom. Ektatische Blutcapillaren mit atypischen Endothelzellen, perivasale Geschwulstzellinfiltration mit starker Kernpolymorphie. Hämangioplastischer Bezirk, HE.-Färbung, Abbildungsmaßstab 2200:1

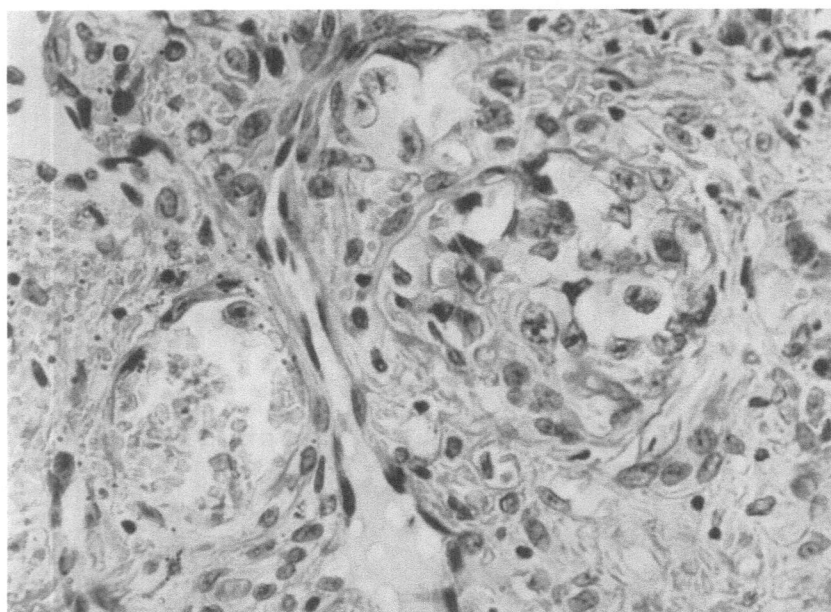

Abb. 11. Stewart-Treves-Syndrom. Polymorphe Tumorzellen mit meist ovoiden, blassen oder vesiculösen Kernen in einem Capillarlumen und perivasal. Tumorzellembolus, HE.-Färbung, Abbildungsmaßstab 2200:1

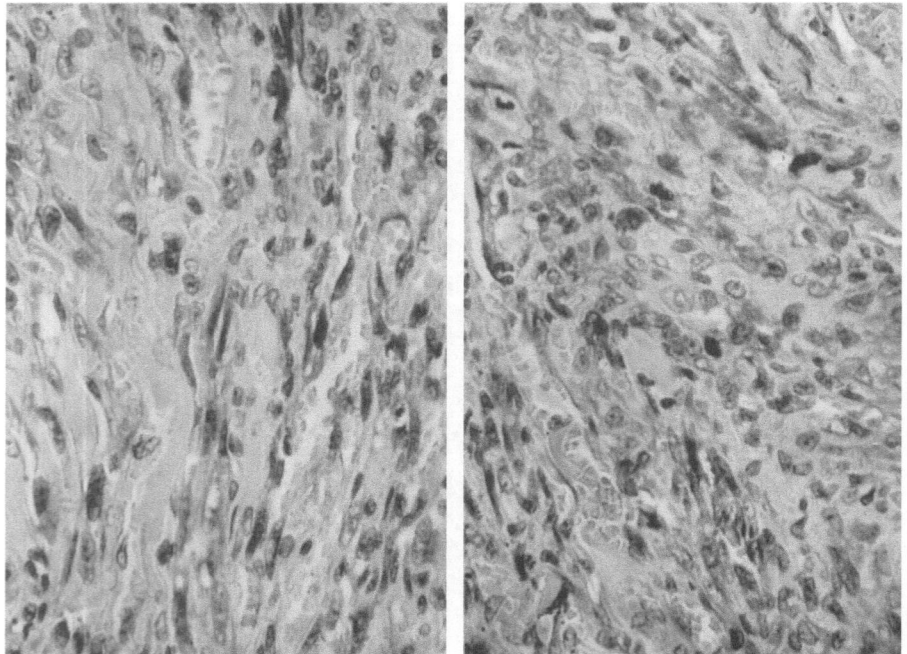

Abb. 12. Stewart-Treves-Syndrom. Linke Bildhälfte: Fusiforme, in Strängen gelagerte, fibro-blastenähnliche Zellen. Rechte Bildhälfte: Polymorphe, vorwiegend ovoide Zellen, gehäuft Mitosen. Zellbild aus Tumorzentrum, HE.-Färbung, Abbildungsmaßstab 350:1

Une affection liée au sexe: la gérodermie ostéodysplasique

D. Klein, F. Bamatter, A. Franceschetti, G. Boreux, J. E. W. Brocher, Genève (Suisse) et P. Holenstein, Bâle (Suisse)

Les auteurs présentent une étude génétique, clinique et radiologique d'une famille valaisanne, suivie depuis près de 20 ans.

Dans une branche de la famille, un homme de 35 ans (le probant) présentait depuis sa naissance une peau plissée sur toute la surface du corps. Il eut de nombreuses fractures osseuses, la première à l'âge de 8 mois. A 6 ans, sa démarche devint dandinante. Entre 8 et 10 ans, il fut traité orthopédiquement pour une luxation de la hanche. A 13 ans, il cessa de grandir.

Il présente actuellement un nanisme disproportionné avec troubles osseux: déformation des têtes et des condyles fémoraux, coxa valga, corps vertébraux biconcaves et aplatis; les plateaux vertébraux concaves présentent des lignes multiples, pareilles aux anneaux de croissance d'un arbre. Il y a ostéoporose généralisée. On note une hyperlaxité ligamentaire, extrêmement marquée aux pouces, des pieds plats, un équino-valgus, et une hypotrophie des muscles de la jambe (jambes d'oiseau).

La peau, qui manque de turgescence, apparaît flétrie et sénile, particulièrement sur le dos des mains et des pieds, où les veines superficielles sont très saillantes.

Le visage a un aspect sénile et grincheux que l'on a comparé aux figures des nains de Walt Disney. Il y a ptose palpébrale, avec «hochstehender Blick», un léger degré de microcornée et une myopie.

Le maxillaire supérieur est hypoplasique, le palais ogival, avec mauvaise implantation des dents, et il y a prognathisme inférieur.

On a trouvé une forte augmentation de l'élimination des 17-OH corticostéroïdes urinaires.

La sœur aînée du probant, née en 1922, est apparemment normale, mais elle a deux enfants atteints de gérodermie ostéodysplasique héréditaire:

Une fille, née en 1948, chez laquelle le diagnostic a été posé déjà à l'âge de 3 mois: expression sénile du visage et peau des mains ridée. Actuellement, la peau est lâche, flétrie, spécialement sur le dos des mains et des pieds, et le visage apparaît comme celui d'une personne beaucoup plus âgée. Il y a aussi une ptose palpébrale. Le palais est ogival, avec mauvaise implantation des dents; les incisives médianes supérieures sont très grandes. On note la présence de scapulae alatae et d'une scoliose dorsale.

Le fils, né en 1954, est cliniquement superposable à son oncle. Il a une taille courte, une démarche dandinante avec luxation bilatérale marquée des hanches, une hypotrophie des muscles des jambes (jambes d'oiseau), des pieds plats et des scapulae alatae. Les os sont de transparence anormale. Les vertèbres présentent des lignes transverses multiples parallèles aux plateaux. On remarque un enfoncement du plateau vertébral supérieur de L 4.

La peau est fine, ridée, particulièrement sur le dos des mains et des pieds, où le réseau veineux est très apparent. Les joues sont tombantes, et le visage est d'aspect grincheux. Il y a rétrognathie supérieure. Le palais est ogival, avec un raphé médian profond, et les dents ont une mauvaise implantation. Les incisives médianes supérieures sont aussi très grandes, comme chez la sœur.

Dans une autre branche de la famille, un homme né en 1920 présente les caractéristiques suivantes: il a eu aussi de nombreuses fractures — la première à l'âge de 6 ans — peu douloureuses et se consolidant facilement. La taille est normale. Par contre, les hanches sont larges et les fémurs allongés. Il y a une coxa valga, une ostéodystrophie articulaire des hanches et des genoux, et des pieds plats; cet homme présente également une ostéoporose généralisée. Le palais est ogival, avec mauvaise implantation des dents, et la région nasale paraît enfoncée. Comme ses cousins, le patient a un «hochstehender Blick» et un léger degré de microcornée. Les joues sont tombantes, les sillons du visage très marqués, ce qui confère à cet homme un aspect beaucoup plus âgé. Les mains et les pieds sont également gérodermiques. On note en outre un daltonisme.

Une sœur, née en 1931, a aussi un aspect gérodermique avec joues tombantes, sourcils hauts, narines larges et physionomie grincheuse. A 17 ans, elle en paraissait au moins 35. Comme chez son frère, on remarque une ptose palpébrale avec «hochstehender Blick» et légère microcornée. La peau du dos des mains est aussi très ridée. Les dents sont mal implantées. On note la présence d'omoplates saillantes, de genua valga, et de pieds affaissés. Il y a une laxité ligamentaire des doigts et des orteils.

Dans une troisième branche de la famille, deux filles issues d'un mariage consanguin, nées respectivement en 1914 et en 1915, ont une microphthalmie, une opacité cornéenne congénitale, une buphtalmie et actuellement une cécité complète.

Bien qu'il existe des analogies avec la progérie de HUTCHINSON-GILFORD et avec l'acrogérie de GOTTRON, il semble que nous sommes en présence, ici, d'une entité clinique encore non décrite, se transmettant de façon liée au sexe.*

---

* Le travail original paraîtra dans le Journal de Génétique Humaine.

Elektronenmikroskopische, histochemische und polarisations-optische Untersuchungen bei Pemphigus familiaris benignus (Hailey und Hailey)

F. NÜRNBERGER und G. MÜLLER, Mainz (Deutschland)

Pemphigus Benignus Chronicus and Keratosis Palmo-plantaris in a Finnish Family

C. E. SONCK, Department of Dermatology, University of Turku (Finland)

In a family, with 27 members, originating from Pyhäjärvi O. l., two different genodermatoses with dominant inheritance have been demonstrated in four successive generations.

Fig. 1 shows the pedigree in which 8 of the 27 members are affected with benign chronic pemphigus Hailey-Hailey. (4 of the children are so far too young to show manifestations of this disorder). The lower (black) square indicates Hailey and Hailey's disease. The birth year of each person is listed underneath the individual symbol. There is in the same family, however, another skin disorder with dominant inheritance, keratosis palmo-plantaris, which in the family pedigree is indicated by the upper (striped) square. This skin affection originates from the grandfather, and is present in 14 members out of 27. In all affected members the hyperkeratosis ist most prominent on the plantar surface of their heals, which in addition to the keratosis show numerous fissures. All cases show this same type of diffuse hyperkeratosis on the heals. The palmae are involved, too, although somewhat lesser. The palmar keratosis has appeared in two varieties. Some members have shown a diffuse keratosis with fissures over the whole palmar surface, while other members of the same family have had an insular type of keratosis. *Biopsies* taken from the hyperkeratotic and fissurated soles show no clefts in the epidermis and no signs of acantholysis.

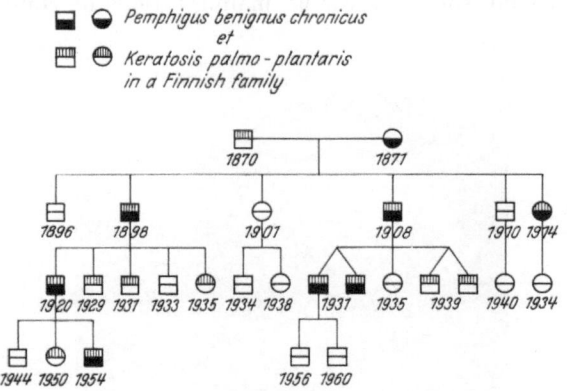

Fig. 1. Family pedigree showing two different genodermatoses in four successive generations

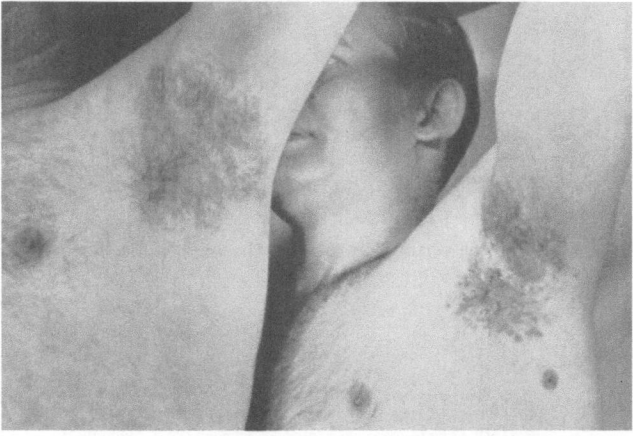

Fig. 2. Father (born 1908), and son (born 1931) with Hailey and Hailey's disease

Two dizygotic male twin pairs can be seen in the pedigree. Two of the twins are affected with benign chronic pemphigus; all four show keratosis palmo-plantaris.

Besides the typical symptoms of familial benign chronic pemphigus (Hailey-Hailey) and the keratosis palmo-plantaris there are some other features common to several members in this family:

1. Most of the members with Hailey and Hailey's manifestations are, with few exceptions, of rather pycnic constitution and stout. In this they are like their grandmother, born 1871, who suffered from benign chronic pemphigus, while their grandfather (born 1870), who suffered from keratosis palmo-plantaris is said to have been of a taller and lanker type.

2. Many of the members are troubled by hyperhidrosis, having moist hands and feet.

3. The eyelids of several members of the family show a blepharitis-like redness, due to numerous and large capillaries in the free margins of the eyelids. In one branch of the family this blepharitis with redness and some scaling is very pronounced in both grand-father, father, and all three children, two of whom (born 1944 and 1950) so far show no visible manifestations of Hailey and Hailey's disease.

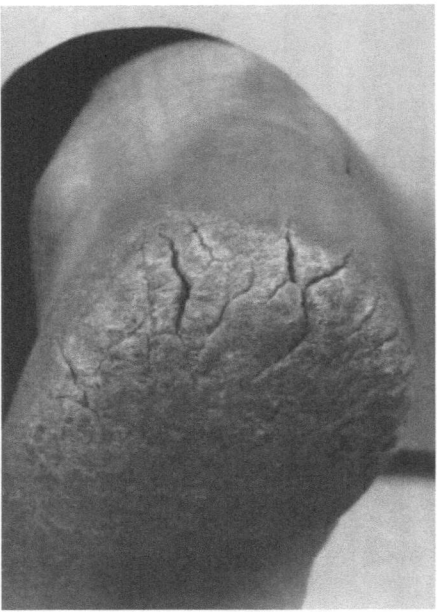

Fig. 3. Plantar keratosis on the heal (male, born 1908)

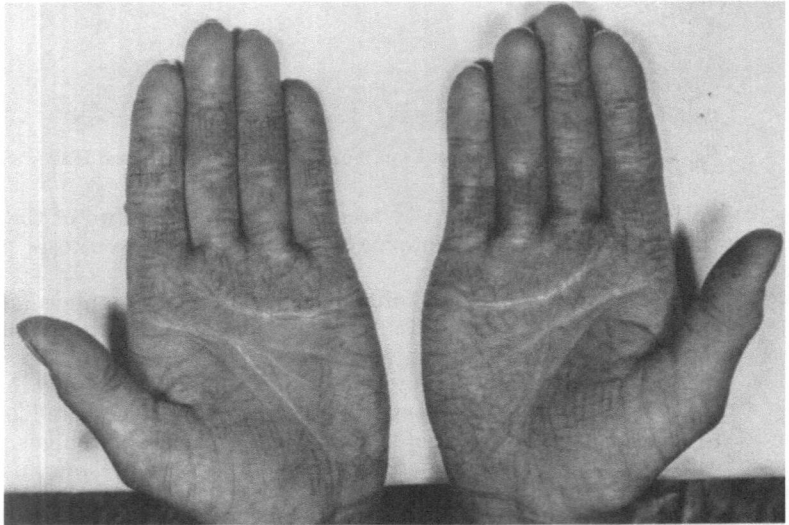

Fig. 4. Palmar keratosis (female, born 1935)

Shibi-Gatchaki-Syndrome

Y. KATABIRA, Department of Dermatology, University School of Medicine, Hirosaki (Japan)

Shibi-gatchaki syndrome is an endemic disease in the Tsugaru District (latitude about 41 °N) of Aomori Prefecture in Japan. It is a kind of undernutrition defined as a syndrome accompanied by itching and pain in the anogenital region, of which clinical manifestations mainly correspond with those of ariboflavinosis and pellegra.

Symptoms. 1. Angular stomatitis, cheilitis and glossitis. 2. Cutaneous thickening, pigmentation, roughness, rhagades and erosions in the backs of the hands and feet

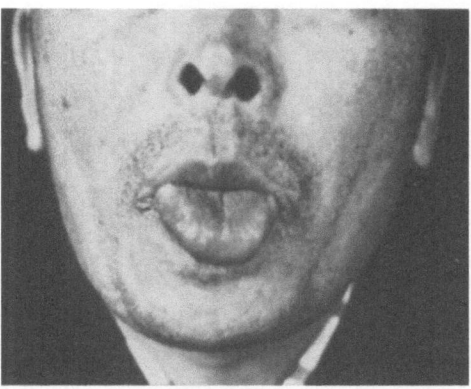

Fig. 1. A man aged 42. Angular stomatitis. Cheilitis. Edematous, swollen tongue. Eczematous eruptions around the anus also present

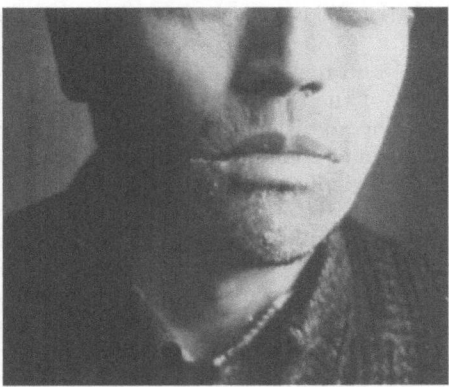

Fig. 2. A man aged 41. Angular stomatitis. Thickened and scaly perioral skin. Magenta tongue also present

as well as the anogenital region. 3. Angular blepharitis, Hyperemia, vascularization and pigmentation of the corneal margin. 4. Subjective symptoms consisting of itching and pain of the affected areas, headache and general fatigability. (As the initial symptoms, glossal pain and genital pruritus are common.)

Clinical course. The onset is in infancy and the course is chromic. The symptoms are usually manifested or aggravated from May to June and from September to October.

Laboratory data. Serum levels of vitamin B_2, nicotinic acid or vitamin C is decreased; reduction of all these vitamins was seen in 50% of the cases. Other abnormal data include insufficiency of the liver and adrenal body functions, macrocytic anemia, myocardosis, and hypoalbuminemia with hyperglobulinemia.

Histopathology. Slight acanthosis, increase of melanin in the basal layer, increase of dermal melanophages and slight cell infiltration in the upper dermis are usual findings.

Etiology. The principal cause is the disturbance in the utilization of vitamin B_2 due to a hepatic disorder (histologically, vacuolar degeneration and edema of the hepatic cells, stenosis of the intrahepatic bile ducts, etc)., which resulted from

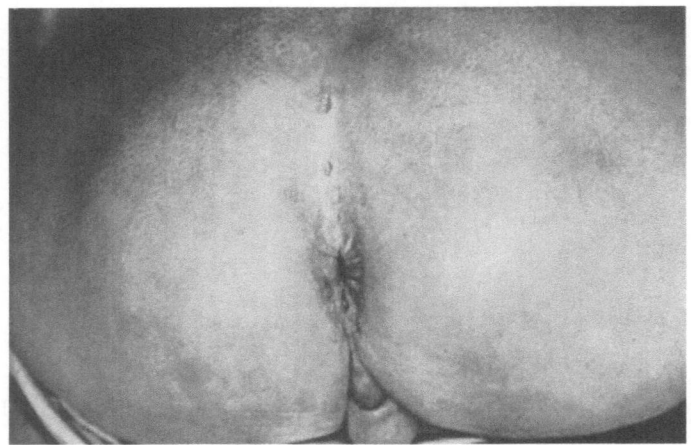

Fig. 3. Same case (Fig. 2). Perianal skin is thickened, reddened, fissured and scratched

overeating of polished rice and inadequate intake of protein. The above condition is aggravated by daily use of the well water in this district, which shows a rather high concentration of Mn. The predisposition to angular stomatitis may be explained by the fact that degeneration of the mucosal epithelia due to lysozyme activity in the saliva is exacerbated by riboflavin deficiency.

Statistical data. Both sexes are equally affected. The age is evenly distributed from young to old. A mass examination performed 15 years ago in the villages where the disease occurs frequently revealed morbidity rates of 70% in children and 62% in farmers. In the group in which vitamin-enriched soy containing 75 mg of B_1 75 mg of B_2 and 750 mg of nicotinic acid per 2 L was used for a year, clinical improvement and increase of serum level of ester-form B_2 were observed compared with the group using usual soy. A statistical study of incidence of patients of the recent 20 years (1947 to 1966) in Hirosaki University revealed a peak of 0.11% in 1953 followed by a decreasing tendency in the subsequent period. However, the statistical data of the recent 10 years (1957 to 1966) made in Dermatological Clinic of the City Hospital of Goshogawara City, the center of the prevalent area, disclosed the incidence of patients of 0.91 to 0.85%; therefore, a decreasing tendency is not obvious, although severe cases are rarely seen.

Cas Cliniques

A. BASSET, Strasbourg (France)

Gnathostomiasis Cutis. Yangtze Edema in China and Similar Migrating Intermittent Swellings of the Skin in Japan, Both Due to Gnathostoma Spinigerum Owen, 1836

K. Kitamura, Teishin Hospital, Tokyo (Japan)

During the past years *Yangtze edema* has occasionally occurred among Japanese people who lived in the Yangtze Kiang Valley in China. It was first interpreted as Quincke's acute circumscribed edema because of the migrating intermittent swellings of the skin. Later it was regarded as a food allergy, for it occurs usually in people who have eaten *Ophicephalus argus Cantor* and other fresh-water fishes uncooked.

In Yangtze edema, the presence of superficial indurated areas and progressively extending linear eruptions are noteworthy. Moreover, the swellings are more compact, brighter red and more inflammatory than the edematous, rather pale swellings of Quincke's edema. The swellings migrate as those of Quincke's edema do, but as a rule remain localized several days or more, while swellings of Quincke's edema appear and disappear more quickly.

The skin lesions of Yangtze edema were examined histologically and larvae morphologically identical with those of *Gnathostoma spinigerum* Owen, *1836* were found in the skin showing marked tissue eosinophilia. In Shanghai, it was discovered that Ophicephalus argus and other fresh-water fishes have encysted larvae of Gnathostoma spinigerum in their

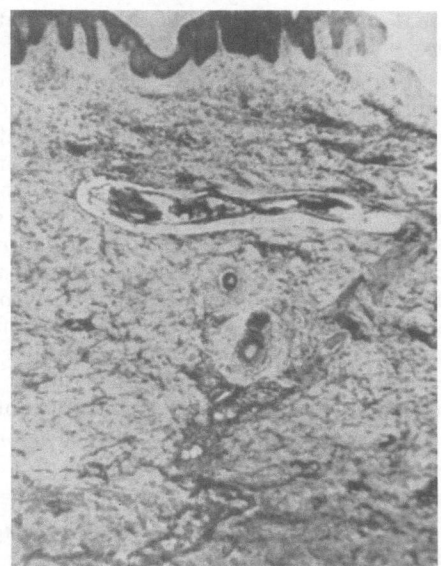

Larva of Gnathostoma spinigerum in the skin lesion of Yangtze edema

muscles and livers and cats and dogs have its adult worms in the digestive tract.

Later in Japan also, the infection of Ophicephalus argus and other fresh-water fishes with Gnathostoma spinigerum was confirmed. And in cases of Yangtze edema-like swellings of the skin developing after the eating of Ophicephalus argus larvae of this worm were found histologically in the skin lesions or extirpated from them.

So it became clear that Yangtze edema in China and similar swellings of the skin occurring in Japan after the eating of Ophicephalus argus are both *Gnathostomiasis cutis* like *Tua Chid*, an endemic disease in Thailand, which has skin lesions resembling those of Yangtze edema. Tua Chid is caused by the eating of *Ophicephalus striatus Bloch* and other fresh-water fishes, which also were found to have larvae or Gnathostoma spinigerum.

Clinical pictures of Yangtze edema and similar swellings of the skin occurring in Japan after the eating of Ophicephalus argus, histological pictures of both diseases showing larvae of Gnathostoma spinigerum in the skin, pictures of Ophicephalus argus and encysted larvae of Gnathostoma spinigerum are presented.

Plusieurs dermatoses

G. SAKELLARIOU, Clinique des Maladies Cutanées et Syphilitiques
de la Faculté de Médecine Thessaloniki (Grèce)

1. Toxidermie par Dramamine (Sel de 2-diphénylométhoxy-éthylo-diméthyl-amine de la 8-chlorothéophylline). Apparition de lésions disséminées érythémato-urticariennes prurigineuses avec œdème du visage chaque fois que la malade (jeune fille de 19 ans) prenait une dragée de Dramamine préventivement avant de voyager. Les lésions en regressant prennent un aspect de lichénification et une coloration brune foncée ou brunâtre; elles diparaissent lentement (plus d'un mois) après une désquamation.

2. Erythème polymorphe (forme bulleuse). Localisation insolite, presque seulement sur les jambes. Lesions érythémato-bulleuses énormes. Récidives. Amygdalite et bronchocèle.

3. Pemphigus vulgaire et corticothérapie. Dans nombreux cas de pemphigus traités par les corticoïdes, on observe diverses manifestations, absentes ou rares avant la corticothérapie, dont l'explication est difficile ou impossible. Dans notre Clinique Dermatologique de Thessaloniki nous avons observé, en dehors des symptômes habituels (Œdème du visage, des extrémités, d'une seule région articulaire; hypertrichoses étendues surtout chez les jeunes filles, innombrables cystes milliaires, vergetures...) et des myopathies, artérites, lymphangites, thrombophlébites, attaques cardiaques, rhinorragie, encéphalite. De plus, différenciations des images histologiques et du cytodiagnostic de Tzanck. Chez les photos exposées, il s'agit d'une jeune fille qui présente: faciès lunéaire, innombrables cystes milliaires, hyperpigmentations et taches achromiques, hypertrichose étendue, zona thoracique et certains nodules hémangiomateux qui montrent histologiquement une image approchante d'angiomatose de Kaposi.

4. Epidermolyse bulleuse dystrophique. Deux nourrissons: bulles énormes et érosions extensives; NIKOLSKY $+++$ (pseudo-Nikolsky); Cystes milliaires innombrables. La mère d'un: hémiplégie, altérations des articulations, bronchocèle.

5. Aplasies cutanées circonscrites congénitales. Nouveau-né prématuré, portant d'aplasies absolument symétriques et étendues sur les régions abdominales et costales, où on distingue de nombreux réseaux vasculaires. Mort par bronchopneumonie 15 jours après la naissance. (Malade de la Clinique Gynécologique et Obstétrique de l'Univ. de Thessaloniki. Dir.: Prof. P. PANAYOTOU).

6. Erythema gyratum perstans de Colcott-Fox. Très rare génodermatose érythémato-vésiculeuse, serpigineuse et desquamative chez un homme de 36 ans, souffrant dès l'âge de 11 ans. Diagnostic différentiel très difficile: «génodermatose en cocarde» de DEGOS; «érythème perstans» de WENDE (Ier cas); «éruption circinée papulo-squameuse» de DARIER; «psoriasis et psoriasis pustuleux à type d'érythème annulaire centrifuge» de LAPIÈRE, de HURIEZ, de DEGOS même de BASEX et coll.; «familial annular erythema» etc. Pas d'image histologique spéciale, pas de cancer interne, pas de signe de psoriasis, pas un facteur sûr étiologique ou influent à l'évolution de la maladie.

7. Naevus hyperkératosique généralisé sous forme d'ichtyose hystrix. Homme de 20 ans atteint dès la 2ème mois après la naissance. Histologiquement: hyperkératose orthokératosique; hypergranulation; hypéracanthose. Papilles et prolongements interpapillaires augmentés. Glandes sudoripares hyperplasiques.

8. Maladie de Jadassohn-Lewandowsky. ♀ 16 ans souffrant dès la naissance. Papules kératosiques péripillaires partout du corps. Hyperkératoses diffuses plantaires et palmaires. Plaques hyperkératosiques de la langue. Pachyonychie. Chevelure frisée. Hyperthyroïdisme.

9. Naevus comédonien. ♀ 22 ans. Comédons énormes, nodules inflammatoires et purulents, atrophies cicatricielles localisés à disposition zoniforme sur la fesse gauche. Quelques comédons disséminés sur le tronc. Histologiquement: hyperkératose très accentuée; prolongations des papilles; immersions pseudocystiques de l'épiderme contenant en abondance de lames kératinisées.

10. Hémangiomes et lymphangiomes multiples de la langue chez une fille de 19 ans. Apparition à l'âge de 14 ans. Périodes d'aggravation, durant un mois environ, et périodes de régressions. Tendance d'effacement des lésions et de la douleur vers le soir. Histologiquement: kératinisation; hyperplasie d'épithélium; accentuation de vaisseaux avec hyperhémie et infiltrations hémorrhagiques étendues. Pas de crase sanguine.

11. Cystes épidermiques du scrotum.

12. Epithélioma baso-cellulaire du visage.

13. Epithélioma spinocellulaire sur la nuque avec multiples lésions kératosiques disséminées et une corne sur le nez chez un homme de 56 ans.

14. Epithélioma spinocellulaire balanoprépucial d'aspect vermiculures.

15. Epithélioma métastatique à la région inguinale gauche, 18 mois après la « guérison » d'un épithélioma spinocellulaire — sans tuméfaction des ganglions inguinals-balanoprépucial et de la glande. Le plus intéressant: c'est la fluorescence orangée sur le même point de la glande, avant et après la métastase, et rouge vif sur la tumeur métastatique. Mort du malade 8 mois après l'apparition de la métastase.

16. Epithéliomas métastatiques, chez un homme de 71 ans souffrant d'un cancer pulmonaire. Apparition de lésions vésiculo-bulleuses, très douloureuses, en disposition zoniforme bilatéralement sur la nuque, le visage, les oreilles; aussi sur les mains. Cytodiagnostic: cellules épithéliales un peu volumineuses en groupes avec kératinisation en début du protoplasme et un noyau volumineux forcement coloré. Histologiquement: image d'épithélioma spino-cellulaire?

17. Syphilides papuleuses géantes (condylomes plats). Sur la glande d'un homme syphilitique (Sy secondaire).

Seltene Hautkrankheiten

G. HARGITA, Dermatologische Abteilung des Bezirkskrankenhauses in Szombathely (Ungarn)

Keratosis palmo-plantaris in cutem penetrans hereditaria mit dominantem Erbgang. Typ: Unna-Thost.

Feldarbeiter, 68 Jahre alt. Er wurde 1966 und 1967 in unserer Abteilung *wegen Pemphigus vulgaris* behandelt. Die Keratose trat schon bei seinem Vater und bei einem seiner drei Brüder im 30. Lebensjahr in Erscheinung. Unter seinen drei Töchtern traten bei einer, die jetzt 32 Jahre alt ist, vor einigen Jahren dieselben Hautveränderungen in Erscheinung, und zwar ebenfalls an den Handflächen und Fußsohlen. Unser Kranker hat noch einen 20jährigen Sohn, der taubstumm und schwachsinnig ist. *Hautbefund:* an beiden Hand- und Fußflächen

dichtstehende, inselförmig eingelassene, teilweise stachelähnliche Hyperkeratosen.
Stammbaum: 1. unser Kranker, 2. sein Sohn.

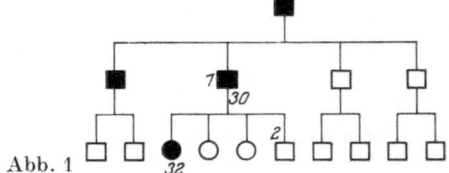

Abb. 1

Keratosis palmo-plantaris hereditaria. Typ: Unna-Thost.

67 Jahre alt, Rentner, dessen Hautveränderung seit Kindheit besteht. Es sind
kegelartige, tief in die Haut der Handinnenflächen und Füße eingelassene Verhornungen. Allgemeinbefund ohne Besonderheiten. Untersuchung der Angehörigen
war nicht möglich. Sein Vater hatte ebensolche derben Hände.

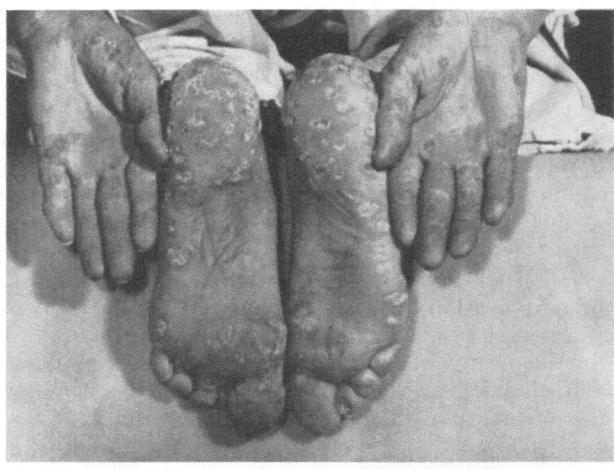

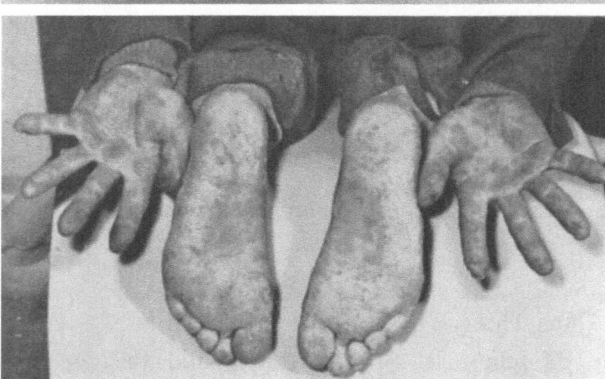

Abb. 2

*Naevus pigmentosus systematisatus partim verrucosus congen. Megaloureter et
calculus renis* lateris sinistri.

34jähriger Landarbeiter. Er führt seine Hautveränderung darauf zurück, daß
seine Mutter, als sie mit ihm schwanger war — bei einer großen Feuersbrunst im

Dorfe, in ihrem Schrecken —, ihre Hand zu ihrer linken Hüftengegend drückte. Beim Patienten ist die Hautveränderung an derselben Hautfläche. Seine Hautveränderung besteht seit seiner Geburt, sie wuchs mit ihm in Ausdehnung, verdickte

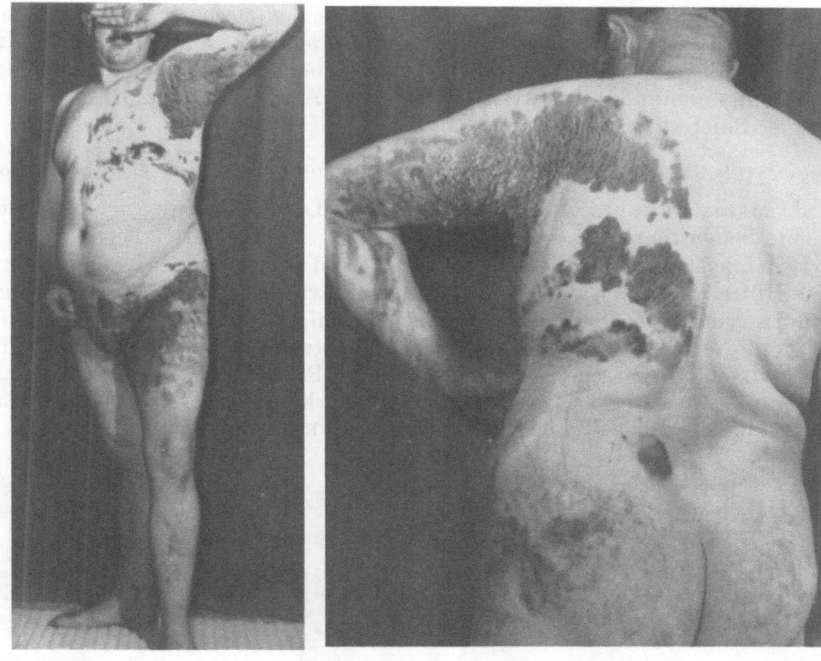

Abb. 3   Abb. 4

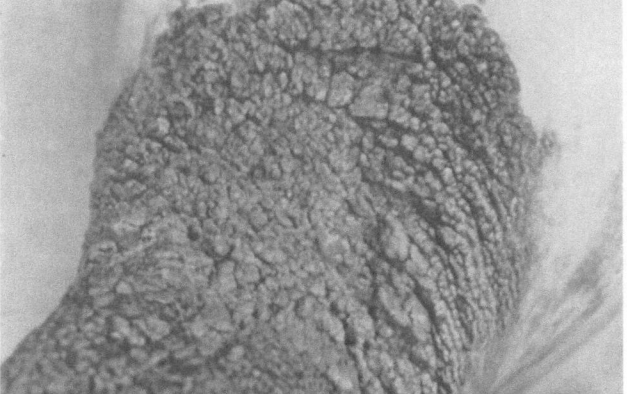

Abb. 5

sich und stellenweise, in der Achselgrube und in der inguinalen Gegend, verdickte sie sich stärker und wurde warzenartig. Der Patient ist weder in seiner Arbeit noch im sexuellen Leben behindert.

Sklerodermia generalisata exulcerans.

45jährige Kranke, ihr gegenwärtiger Zustand entwickelte sich in 4 Monaten. Am Anfang schwoll ihr linker Fußknöchel an und von hier verbreitete sich die Hautveränderung. Gegenwärtig ist die Haut fast der ganzen linken Körperfläche und des linken unteren Fußgliedes glatt, glänzend, abgezehrt, fast gar nicht zu runzeln, gelblich weiß. Ähnlich ist der Zustand der Haut auf der rechten Hüfte, fast bis zur Kniebeuge. Auf dem linken inneren Knöchel anfängliche Exulceration. Labor-Roentgenbefunde: negativ, auch der Augenhintergrund ist normal. Histologie: Skleroderma diffusum.

Angiokeratoma des Skrotum, Elephantiasis femoris sinistri et Hydro-Varicocele.

H. J., Mann, 24 Jahre alt. Bis zu seinem 5. Lebensjahr war er gesund ohne irgendeine bemerkbare Veränderung am Körper. Mit 5 Jahren begann sich sein linkes Bein langsam, stufenweise zu verdicken, und zwar in seinem ganzen Umfang von der Hüfte bis zu den Zehen. Mit 18 Jahren wurde bei ihm durch plastischen Eingriff Fettgewebe entfernt und Sympathektomie vorgenommen. An der linken Skrotumseite entwickelten sich multiple, etwa stecknadelkopf- und linsengroße, juckende, nachher nässende und schuppende Papeln. *Histologisch:* Deutliche Hyperkeratose. Das verdünnte Epithel faßt mehrkammerige, mit dünnem Endothel ausgekleidete Blutlakunen ein. *Diagnose:* Lymphangioma cavernosum.

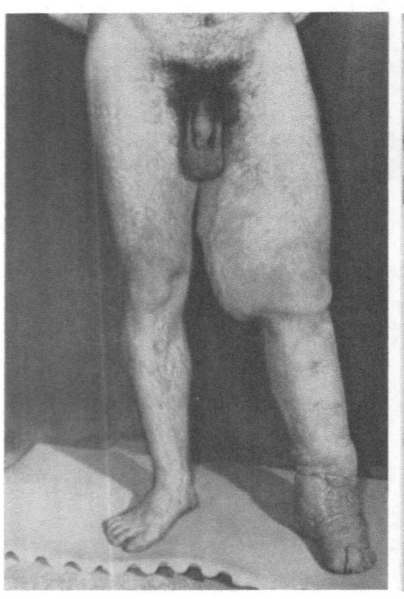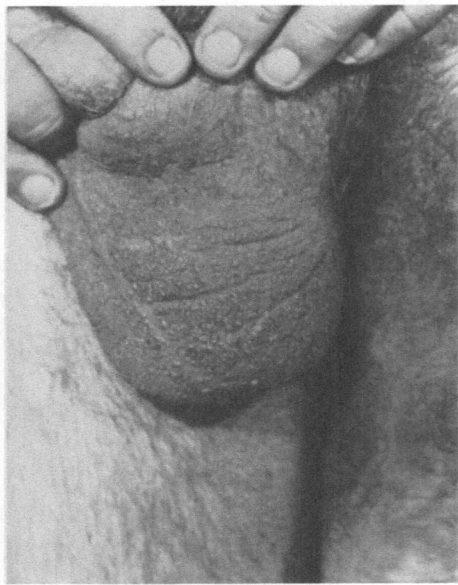

Abb. 6

Auf unserer Tabelle berichten wir über Resultate, die wir durch Bekämpfung von Infektionen gewisser Eingeweideparasiten, bei Patienten der Dermatologischen Abteilung im Laufe von 8 Jahren, erlangten. Unserer Bewertung gemäß fanden wir bei vielen Kranken mannigfaltige, wechselungsreiche und nicht selten mehrfache Infektionen. Bei gleichzeitiger Fach- und antiparasitärer Behandlung hatten wir in mehreren Fällen günstige Erfahrungen. Ein ausführlicherer Bericht ist in der Derm. Wschr. im H. 36/1967 erschienen.

Tabelle. *Über die parasitären Infektionen in der dermatologischen Abteilung des Bezirkskrankenhauses in Szombathely/Ungarn*

	Jahr 1958	1959	1960	1961	1962	1963	1964	1965	Insgesamt
Zahl der Untersuchungen	855	826	621	804	679	691	555	514	5545
Einfache Infektion	322	372	195	214	160	161	105	77	1606
Zweifache Infektion	55	41	23	11	14	11	13	2	170
Dreifache Infektion	6	10	—	—	1	—	—	2	19
Vierfache Infektion	4	—	—	—	1	—	—	—	5
Gesamtzahl der Infektionen	387	423	218	225	176	172	118	81	1800

Infektion	Jahr 1958	1959	1960	1961	1962	1963	1964	1965	Insgesamt
Zweifache									
Entam. hist. + Trich. trichiura	29	25	10	7	6	6	7	2	92
Entam. hist. + Ascaris lumbric.	2	2	3	—	1	—	—	—	8
Entam. hist. + Giardia lamblia	5	5	7	3	2	1	2	—	25
Entam. hist. + Chilom. mesnili	1	—	—	—	—	—	—	—	1
Entam. hist. + Enterob. vermic.	8	2	2	—	2	1	—	—	15
Entam. hist. + Strong. steror.	—	1	1	—	—	—	—	—	2
Trich. trichiura + Giardia lamblia	4	3	—	—	3	—	—	—	10
Trich. trichiura + Ascaris lumbric.	5	3	—	1	—	3	4	—	16
Ascaris lumbric. + Trichom. hom.	1	—	—	—	—	—	—	—	1
Insgesamt	55	41	23	11	14	11	93	2	170
Dreifache									
Entam. hist. + Ascaris lumbric. + Trich. trichiura	2	3	—	—	1	—	—	1	7
Entam. hist. + Enterob. vermic. + Trich. trichiura	2	2	—	—	—	—	—	—	4
Giard. lamblia + Ascaris lumbric. + Trich. trichiura	1	1	—	—	—	—	—	1	3
Giard. lamblie + Trichom. hom. + Trich. trichiura	1	1	—	—	—	—	—	—	2
Giardia lamblia + Entam. hist. + Trich. trichiura	—	3	—	—	—	—	—	—	3
Insgesamt	6	10	—	—	1	—	—	2	19
Vierfache									
Entam. hist. + Giardia lamblia + Enterob. vermic. + Trich. trichiura	1	—	—	—	1	—	—	—	2
Entam. hist. + Giardia lamblia + Enterob. vermic. + Trich. trichiura	3	—	—	—	—	—	—	—	3
Insgesamt	4	—	—	—	1	—	—	—	5

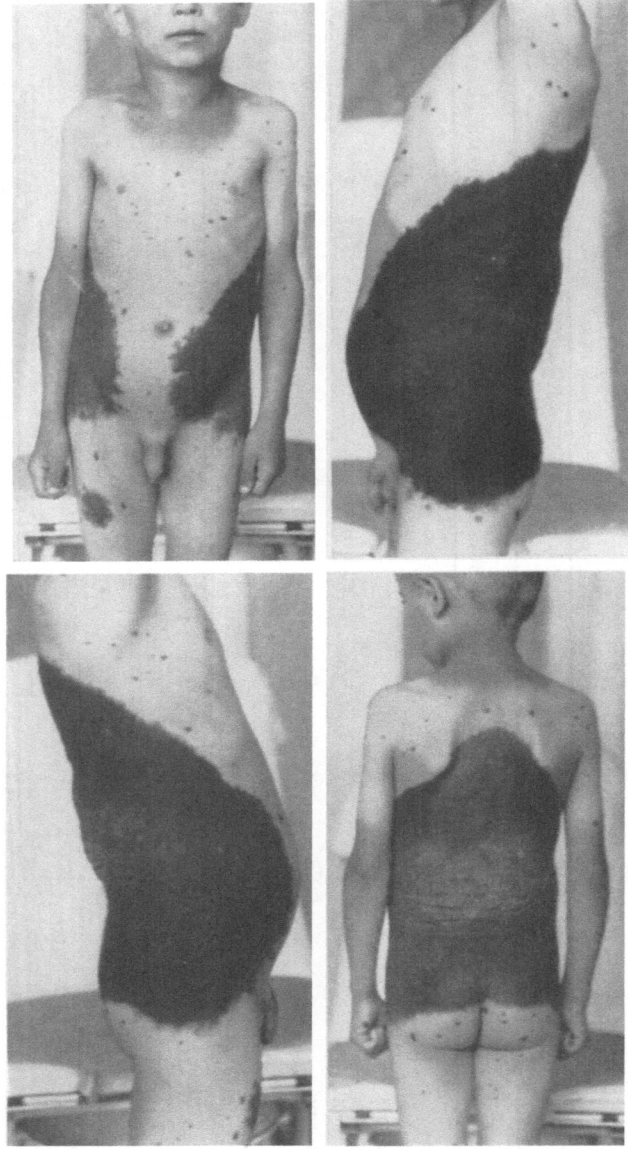

Abb. 7

Naevus pigmentosus spilosus (Tierfellnaevus).

36jähriger Maschinenschlosser. Er wurde als 8jähriges Kind im Jahre 1939 durch seine Mutter in unsere Abteilung gebracht. Nach Aussage der Mutter war bei seiner Geburt die ganze Körperfläche behaart.

Auf der sacralen Gegend und auf den beiden Rumpfseiten war die Haut ohne bemerkbaren Farbenunterschied. Die Mutter erklärte die Hautveränderung ihres Sohnes folgendermaßen: als sie im 2. Monat ihrer Schwangerschaft mit diesem

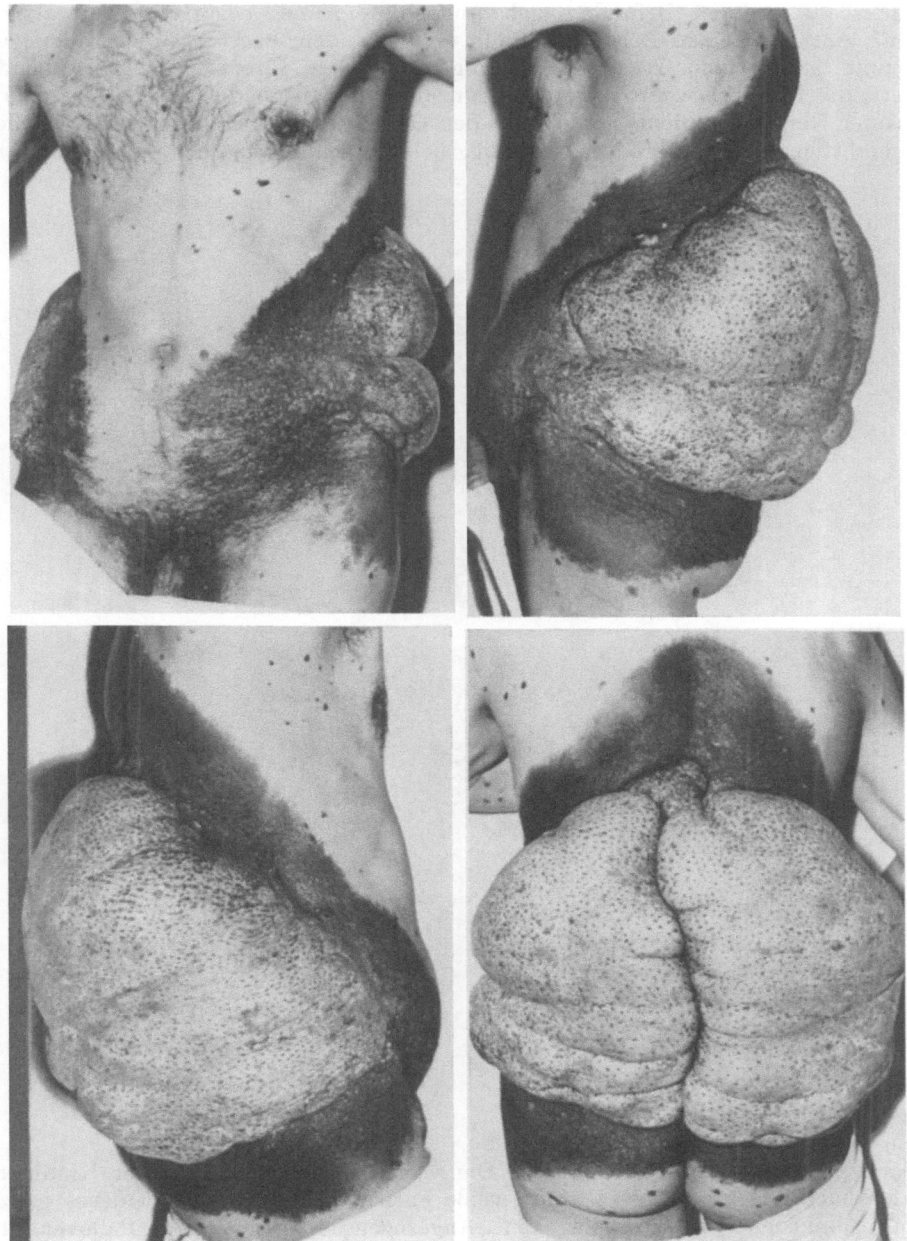

Abb. 8

Kinde war, führte sie an der Hand einen älteren Sohn, den ein schwarzer Hund
beißen wollte. Sie bekam einen großen Schrecken.

Im Jahre 1939: Der histologische Befund eines solitären Herdes: Naevus
pigmentosus. Das Hautexcindat aus dem Rücken: Melanoma malignum. Damals

waren alle anderen Befunde, auch Augenhintergrund, negativ. Gegenwärtig, 1967, sind auf beiden Beckenschaufeln und über dem Sacrum voneinander getrennte, große tumorartige Veränderungen zu sehen. Ihre Oberfläche ist nicht glatt, die Haut ist weiß bestreut mit unzählbaren stecknadelkopf-linsenartigen, aus der Hautfläche nicht heraustehenden Gebilden. Bei Betastung scheinen die tumorartigen Gebilde bindegewebsartig, sie sind schmerzlos und beweglich. Ihr

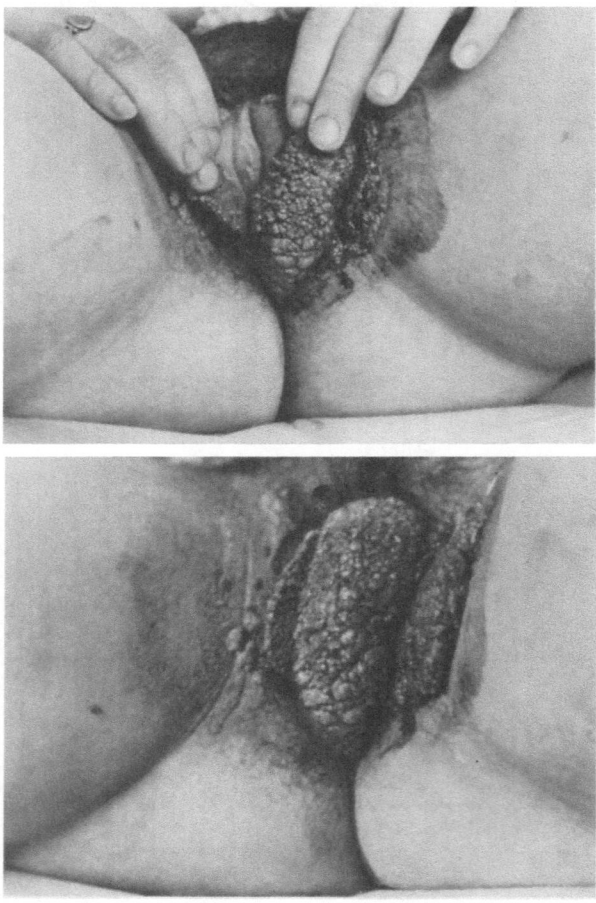

Abb. 9

Wachsen ging stufenweise vor sich. Die schwarze, dicke Haut seiner Kindheit nahm nach und nach diese schwarz-weiße Farbe an, gleichzeitig mit dieser ganz ungewöhnlichen Verdickung der Haut. Angezogen immer mit einem Pullover, ist er in der Hüftgegend sehr breit. Er wiegt 80 kg, die tumorartigen Gewebshypertrophien wiegen schätzungsweise 10 kg. Der Mann hat ein hübsches Gesicht, ist 1,70 m groß und lebt in glücklicher Ehe. Seine beiden lebenden Kinder, seine Eltern und seine Geschwister sind gesund und haben keinerlei Hautveränderungen. Ein drittes Kind, zwischen den beiden Gesunden geboren, kam mit Hydrocephalus auf die Welt und starb mit $4^1/_2$ Jahren. Von einer Operation wollten die Beteiligten nichts hören.

Condyloma acuminatum labii utriusque et regions inguinalis bilateralis ohne Gonorrhoe

Mädchen, 17jährig, führte Geschlechtsleben während eines Monats. Die Hautveränderung entwickelte sich während dieser Zeit in 3 Wochen. Nur chirurgisches Eingreifen konnte helfen.

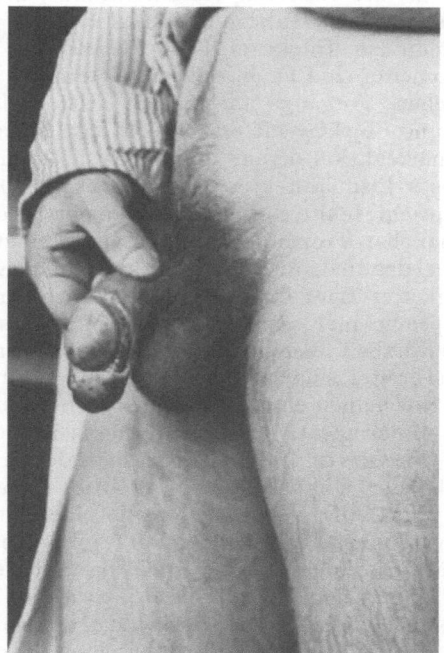

Abb. 10

Ulcus mixtum destructivum.

Mann, 24 Jahre alt. WR: $++++/++++/++++$. Der fehlende Teil des Präputium wurde während der Behandlung abgestoßen, der zurückgebliebene Hautrest mußte durch Operation entfernt werden.

Angiokeratoma corporis diffusum Fabry

R. DENK, Universitäts-Hautklinik Mainz (Deutschland)

Die primäre Hautreaktion nach infektiösem Tsetsefliegenstich bei der afrikanischen Schlafkrankheit

H. E. KRAMPITZ, Institut für Infektions- und Tropenmedizin der Universität München (Deutschland)

Aus mehreren Gründen war die Existenz einer spezifischen Intoleranzreaktion des menschlichen Hautorgans an der Eintrittsstelle der Schlafkrankheits-Trypanosomen jahrelang etwas *umstritten*. In der letzten Zeit wurde zunehmend bekannt, daß die Ausbildung einer Primärreaktion bei dieser Blutparasitose entscheidend abhängt von der wechselnden Zahl und vor allem der in weiten Grenzen variierenden Virulenz der durch die Fliege beim Saugakt mit dem Speichel verimpften Trypanosomen. Lokale entzündliche Reaktionen als Resultanten der Wechselwirkung zwischen Wirt und Parasit lassen sich im *Experiment* nur unter bestimmten Voraussetzungen an der rasierten Kaninchenhaut, nicht aber bei anderen Laboratoriumsnagern oder bei Huftieren rekonstruieren, wobei es weitgehend gleichgültig ist, ob man zur Infektion Tsetsefliegen oder die Injektionsspritze benutzt. Wichtige Momente sind auch, daß die tiefdunkle Haut dem ungeübten Auge alle entzündlichen Vorgänge tarnt und ernste allgemeine Krankheitssymptome subjektiv und objektiv oft erst in späteren Phasen der Infektion auftreten, wenn die Primärreaktion bereits erloschen ist. Auch nach der klassischen Erstbeschreibung dieses Primäraffektes durch GRAF (1929), seit der man vom Grafschen Schanker spricht, fehlte es weitgehend an entsprechenden Abbildungen.

Die Abneigung mancher Tropenmediziner gegen eine strikte *Dreiteilung* des Krankheitsverlaufes bei der afrikanischen Schlafkrankheit (KRAMPITZ u. DE RAADT 1967) etwa in Analogie zur Lues ist daher verständlich und bei der *Variationsfreudigkeit* aller Symptome hier auch bis zu einem gewissen Grade berechtigt. Neuere Beobachtungen haben aber besonders dort, wo virulente Trypanosomenstämme endemisch verbreitet sind, also vor allem in Ostafrika, die Tatsache bestätigt, daß mit dem Erscheinen einer initialen Lokalreaktion bei 50 bis 70% der frischen, d. h. noch liquornegativen Trypanosomiasisfälle an Patienten aller Rassen zu rechnen ist (KRAMPITZ, 1967). Damit erhält der Grafsche Schanker trotz mancher noch bestehender Unklarheiten in funktionell-parasitologischer Sicht für den Kliniker den Wert eines *Frühsymptoms* in einer therapeutisch günstigen Phase des Infektionsverlaufes. Für die Therapie ergibt sich damit aber auch die Notwendigkeit, Primärsensationen anderer infektiöser Ätiologie, wie sie bei Lues, den Leishmaniasen, bei manchen Rickettsiosen, sowie bei Tularämie oder Milzbrand auftreten, differentialdiagnostisch sicher abzugrenzen.

Übereinstimmend wird angegeben, und wir haben es durch vielfache auch sehr persönliche Erfahrungen mit Tsetsestichen in Uganda bestätigt gefunden, daß ein nichtinfektiöser Stich dieser Blutsauger zwar sehr schmerzhaft sein kann, aber sonst keine persistierenden Sensationen am Hautorgan zu hinterlassen pflegt. Nach GRAFS Worten (1937) erzeugt die Trypanosomeneinimpfung jedoch „eine furunkelähnliche empfindliche Schwellung der Haut des Menschen, die bald nach dem infektiösen Glossinenstich auftritt und ohne zu vereitern bald wieder vergeht." Zweifellos ist der Primäraffekt auch hier Ausdruck einer intensiven lokalen *Vermehrung der Erreger* in der Umgebung der Eintrittspforte in den Körper, während der oft noch keine Parasitämie nachgewiesen werden kann. Die ersten deutlichen Hautreaktionen treten gewöhnlich innerhalb 4 bis 9 Tage nach dem Stich auf, sie lassen aber manchmal aus den eingangs genannten Gründen auch 15 und mehr Tage auf sich warten. Infektionsexperimente an menschlichen Freiwilligen haben viel zur Aufklärung dieser Verhältnisse beigetragen.

Histologisch ist in den Frühstadien eine allmählich zunehmende, vorwiegend lymphocytäre Infiltration und umschriebene ödematöse Durchtränkung der Stichregion zu bemerken. Die Trypanosomen vermehren sich bevorzugt in den obersten Schichten des cutanen Fettgewebes, treten aber regelmäßig auch in Punktaten der Gewebsflüssigkeit des Schankerbereichs auf. Zunächst palpiert man einen etwa Fünfmarkstück-großen, verhältnismäßig scharf umgrenzten, leicht indurierten und *entzündlich geröteten Bezirk*, der sich rasch deutlich über das Hautniveau erhebt. Das Faltenmuster ist dann immer vergröbert und schließlich besonders im Zentrum gestört (Abb. 1). Dort wird oft auch für kurze Zeit ein

Bläschen wahrgenommen, das sich später zum Zentrum der sehr *typischen Des-quamation* entwickelt. Diese schreitet zusammen mit dem Abklingen der akuten Entzündung kontinuierlich konzentrisch und zentrifugal fort und ist im Gegensatz zur Entzündungsrötung auf der dunklen Haut besonders gut zu sehen (Abb. 2). Diese Schuppung pflegt, auch ohne daß bereits eine spezifische Therapie eingeleitet wird, nach etwa 3 Wochen beendet zu sein und kann einen hyperpigmentierten Fleck hinterlassen, dessen Genese jetzt allerdings ohne Kenntnis der Vorgeschichte kaum mehr zu deuten ist. Zu eitrigen Einschmelzungen oder Ulcerationen kommt es nur bei Schankern, die im ödematösen Stadium durch Kratzen superinfiziert wurden. Es scheint dies allerdings nach unseren Beobachtungen trotz regelmäßiger lokaler Mißempfindungen verhältnismäßig selten vorzukommen. Die *erhaltene Epitheldecke* ist vielmehr von differentialdiagnostischer Wichtigkeit. Bei der oft

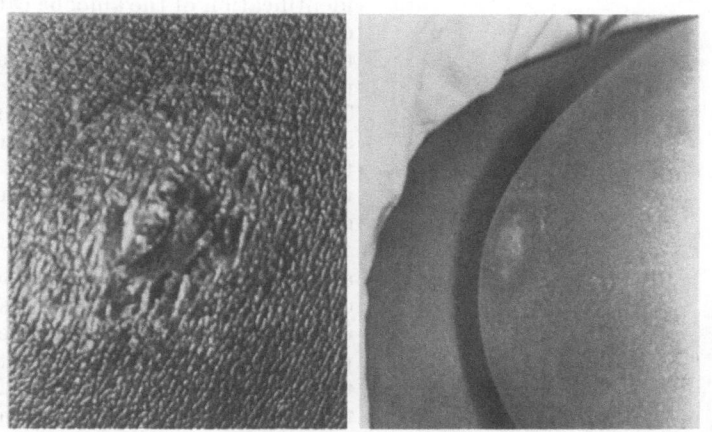

1   2

Abb. 1. Typischer Grafscher Schanker im entzündlichen Stadium an der Haut eines Afrikaners bei dem die Infektion nicht länger als höchstens 10 Tage zurückliegt

Abb. 2. Älterer, bereits desquamierender Schanker am Gesäß im früher febrilen Stadium (nach KRAMPITZ u. DE RAADT, 1967)

recht stürmisch verlaufenden ostafrikanischen Lokalvariante der Schlafkrankheit können sich die einzelnen Stadien weitgehend *ineinanderschieben* und sowohl Parasitämie wie Liquoreinbruch der Trypanosomen bereits nachweisbar sein, wenn noch Schankerreste zu sehen sind.

Da Glossinen auch gern durch dünne, eng anliegende Kleidung stechen, sind Schanker *an allen Körperstellen*, einschließlich des behaarten Kopfes, möglich, die unbedeckten Hautpartien werden aber zum Saugakt bevorzugt angeflogen. Im Rahmen der Schlafkrankheitstherapie bedarf der Schanker in der Regel keiner besonderen *Lokalbehandlung*. Sie kann aber bei bakterieller Superinfektion notwendig werden, besonders dann, wenn der Allgemeinzustand des Patienten bereits zu wünschen übrig läßt.

Literatur. GRAF, H.: Arch. Schiffs- u. Tropenhyg. **41**, 214 (1937). — KRAMPITZ, H. E., u. P. DE RAADT: Münch. med. Wschr. **109**, 441 (1967); — Z. Tropenmed. Parasit. **18**, 273 (1967).

Amoebiasis Skin Manifestations

TH. DOXIADES and J. CAPETANAKIS, Athen (Greece)

The exhibited photographs show the significance of cutaneous manifestations in chronic amoebiasis. As it is well-known, the protozoon Entamoeba histolytica invades the wall of the large bowel causing acute dysentery with many daily blood-stained stools. Stool examination may easily reveal the amoeba. In the chronic form the symptoms are milder, with constipation alternating with bouts of diarrhoea. Sometimes the liver is involved either in the form of chronic non-suppurative hepatomegaly (chronic hepatitis) or by the formation of a true amoebic abscess. In the chronic form, identification of the amoeba can be easily obtained after repeated stool examinations and/or colon biopsy or even more rarely by means of positive liver biopsy. The value of the stool examination is the same as the value in the sputum examination for baccilus Koch, in that the negative result does not exclude the presence of E. histolytica.

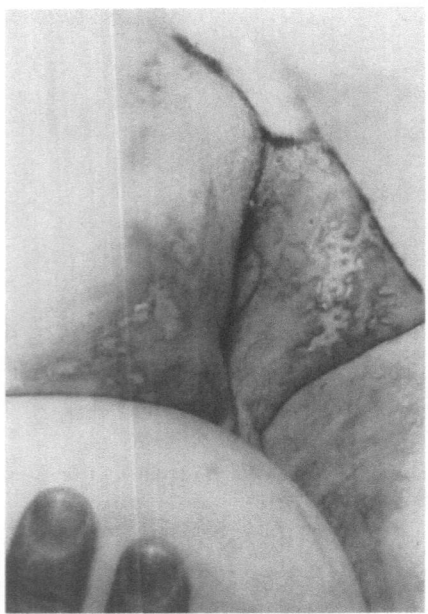

Fig. 1. Ulcers of the perianal region

In Greece there is the same incidence as in other mediterranean countries of dysentery or chronic amoebiasis with liver involvement. The same incidence could probably be found in many other countries if the repeatedly performed examinations were carried out in each case and doctors considered the possibility of the presence of amoeba. Anyway, statistically the incidence of amoebiasis is geographically universal. Many individuals who are considered as being "healthy" carriers eventually, as a result of the dermatological picture, make the adjective "healthy" appear obsolete.

During many years study of clinical material, we have witnessed a great improvement and in many cases a complete disappearance of many of the intractable well-known dermatological entities occuring in patients with chronic amoebiasis after anti-amoebic treatment (emetine, chloroquine, contractamebicides) had been instituted without any special treatment for the dermatosis itself.

We have studied the skin manifestations of chronic amoebiasis and we have come to the following conclusions as regards the classification of this disease:

1. The "true" skin manifestation, where the Entamoeba histolytica can be found in the skin lesions.

Such lesions can be caused as follows: by spreading mainly in the perianal region or along the drainage area after incision of an hepatic abscess or amoebic granuloma. The most often seen ulcers are those of the perianal region.

E. histolytica enters the skin through a fissure or sinus or through a post-operative ulcer. Amoebic lesions have been described in the genitalia of men and women in the form of balanitis, ulcero-vegetating lesions on the glans penis, vaginitis and cervicitis. There have also been described ulcers of the skin after

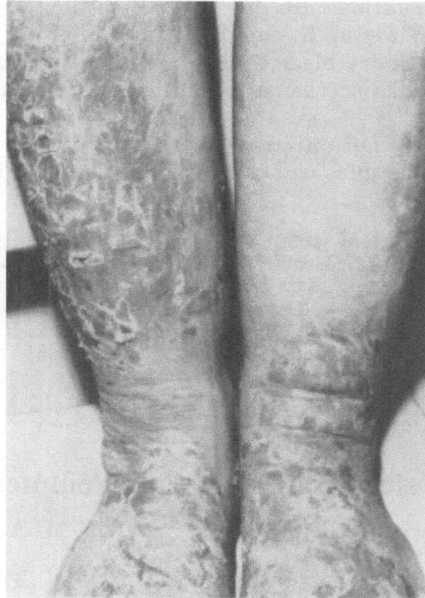 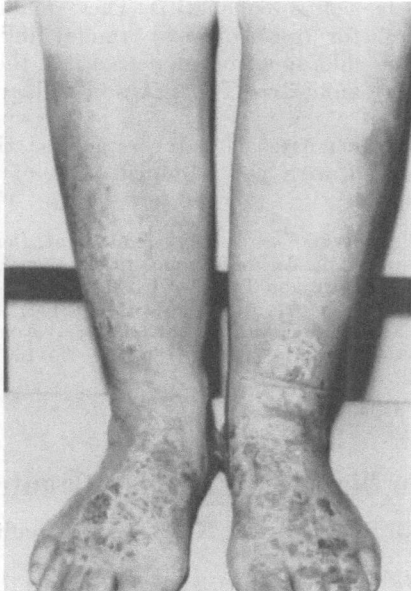

Fig. 2a. Eczema of the legs due to   Fig. 2b. The same after treatment
chronic Amoebiasis (before treatment)

appendicectomy. Clinically we find ulcer-vegetating and granulomatous lesions, which show a tendency to "phagedenic" spreading (Fig. 1).

2. The "allergic" manifestations.

We consider as allergic the skin manifestations where the parasite cannot be detected in the dermatological lesion, but where the skin manifestations are due to a sensitivity as a result of the toxins. The amoeba is present in the body but not in the region of the skin lesion. Eczema (Fig. 2a and 2b), urticaria, angineurotic oedema of Quinque, ano-genital pruritus, pruritus vulvae, Schönlein-Henoch's allergic purpura, eczematid-like purpura may show up as clear allergic reactions. We may include in the same group of skin manifestations as being allergic reactions other skin diseases, such as erythrodermia, psoriasis, acne rosacea, acne necrotica, dermatitis herpetiformis etc.

3. The manifestations due to "nutritional deficiency" or "avitaminosis".

The above manifestations are probably due to inadequate absorption from the gastro-intestinal tract following chronic

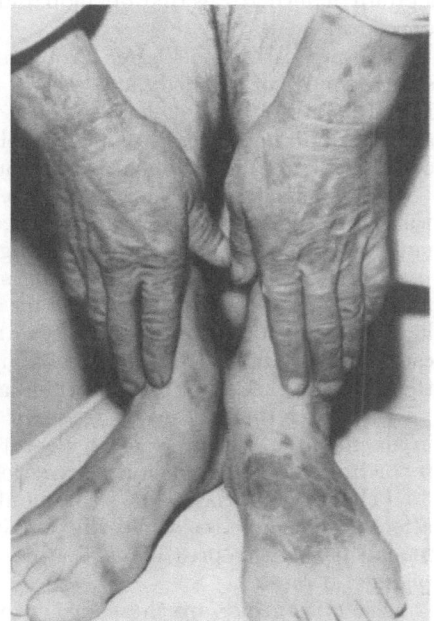

Fig. 3. Pellagra-like erythema due to chronic Amoebiasis

amoebic colitis or hepatitis. These manifestations are due to a deficiency of the
P.P. factor (nicotinic-acid amide) and Vitamin B. complex. In this group we
include chloasma, melanodermatitis, the "hairy black tongue" and glossitis marginata exfoliativa. Pellagra and pellagra-like erythema (Fig. 3) are more characteristic.

In such cases it is recommended that the anti-amoebic therapy should be
combined with the administration of nicotinic acid and vitamin B. complex
injections.

References. CASALA, A.: Arch. argent. Derm. 2, 181 (1952). — DOXIADES, TH.: Hautveränderungen bei der Amöbenhepatitis (Leber, Haut und Skelet), S. 40. Stuttgart: Thieme 1963;
— Prophylaxe und Therapie 1, 23 (1962). — DOXIADES, TH., N. CANDREVIOTIS, Z. YIOTSAS,
and F. SMYRNIOTIS: Arch. intern. Med. 111, 219 (1963). — DOXIADES, TH., and J. CAPETANA-
KIS: Nosokom. Chron. 26, 481 (1964); — Amer. J. Proctol. 17, 58 (1966). — ROLLIER, R., u.
P. BRU: Hautarzt 15, 493 (1964). — TOURAINE, A., et B. DUPERRAT: Presse méd. 54, 1087
(1939).

Skin Diseases in Arabian Countries: Certain Notes and Comments

M. EL ZAWAHRY, Kasr-el-Aini Faculty of Medicine, Cairo University (U.A.R.)

In Arabian countries skin diseases fall into three categories.

The vast majority are more or less the same as those frequently met with
elsewhere with no or minor differences that do not reflect any special importance
on this *first* category of the dermatoses in the Arabic area.

The *second* group are those dermatoses that show an appreciable difference
that materially alter their aetiology and hence their management. To this belongs
a group of dermatoses that develop under the influence of light and after undue sun
exposure.

The first is Lichen Planus Tropicus which is a form of L.P. that occurs on the
exposed parts of the body and mostly during summer and subsides during winter.
It is itchy and itching is more intense with light exposure. The lesions are usually
annular and have persistent post-lichen pigmentation. Lichen planus tropicus
constitutes 40% of ordinary L.P. in our area.

Vitiligo may follow sun burn on exposed parts of body. Such cases increase
with ultra violet rays and may be successfully treated by administration of antimalarial drugs and protection from light.

Psoriasis constitutes 3% of our skin disorders. Certain clinical varieties of
psoriasis may be itchy and occur on exposed parts of body and endangered by
light and subside during winter. The mucous membranes may be site of election
especially the lips, while the hands and feet involvement constitutes 26% of all
the psoriasis cases and most of them are not pustular.

Lupus erythematosus is frequent and no drop in its incidence opposite to
lupus vulgaris. We rarely meet ulcerated discoid lupus erythematosus or even the
seborrhoeic and telangiectatic varieties.

Pellagra is nowadys less commonly seen and constitutes 0.2% of all the skin
affections in our area while the nutritional deficiencies come to 1.25%. Pellagra
in our patients represents a double border, that of scaleness and another of
pigmentation.

The *third* group are those dermatoses which are either endemic in our area or
characteristic to the Arabian zone. Schistosomal granuloma of the skin, the so
called bilharzioma, is met with in some of our patients infected with schistosom-

iasis, and the bilharzia ova and even the worms could be demonstrated in the skin and subcutaneous tissue.

Amoebiasis cutis is also met with and commonly it complicates surgical operations.

Elephantiasis Arabum is a próblem in some regions of our area and huge sizes of leg or scrotal involvement may be seen and sheathed microfilaria bancrofti could be demonstrated in the peripheral blood in a higher percentage than usual. The mosquito is culex pipiens.

Leprosy is endemic in our area and child leprosy, meaning infection from a family member, is occasionally seen. Erythema nodosum leprosum is not rare.

Oriental sore is endemic in certain Arabian countries especially Iraq, Syria and U.A.R. Multiplicity of the lesions to huge numbers was reported especially from patients coming from Yemen and the Arabia Sauedi. The vector is the sand fly (phlebotomus papatasii) and the parasite is leishmania tropica. The incidence of Oriental sore is on the whole less nowadays than before.

Statistical reports and illustration of the cases are to be demonstrated in the exhibit.

Die Tumormetastasierung von der Haut und in die Haut

H. Drepper und F. Ehring, Haus Hornheide, Klinik für Geschwülste und Tuberkulose der Haut und Mundhöhle, Handorf ü. Münster (Westf.) (Deutschland)

Die verschiedenen an der Haut beobachteten Arten maligner Tumoren verhalten sich nach Häufigkeit, Geschwindigkeit und Ausbreitung der Metastasen sehr unterschiedlich. Dies ist gemeinsam mit dem Lokal- und Allgemeinbefund im Therapieplan zu berücksichtigen. Denn auch der regionär metastasierte Hautkrebs bietet eine echte Heilungschance. Die dargestellten Erfolge wurden erzielt, nachdem alle modernen Behandlungsmethoden in einer Klinik zusammengefaßt und so individuell kombiniert werden konnten. Hierzu gehören vor allem die Operation, weiche und ultraharte Strahlen (Cobaltron II, Ehring), Schnellschnitthistologie auch zur Kontrolle der vollständigen Tumorexcision (Drepper), Chemotherapie und Wiederherstellung durch Plastik und Epithese.

Das *Plattenepithelcarcinom* metastasiert häufiger als früher angenommen, nachdem man das Keratoakanthom und andere Pseudocancerosen von ihm zu trennen weiß. Die Metastasen bleiben aber oft regionär und so radikaler Behandlung zugänglich. Von vier demonstrierten Kranken wies der folgende eine besonders große Metastase auf:

68jähriger Rentner. Durch Bestrahlung geheiltes Plattenepithelcarcinom am linken Mundwinkel. 2 Jahre später Metastasen. Rö.-Bestrahlung a. a. O. erfolglos (Abb. 1). Excision mit neck-dissection, Rotationsplastik. Nachbestrahlung mit Cobaltron II (22 × 250 r). Seit 2 Jahren rezidivfrei (Abb. 2).

Das *Basalzellcarcinom* metastasiert nicht. Auch im fortgeschrittenen Stadium bedeutet die Beseitigung des Tumors Heilung, wie an zwei sehr fortgeschrittenen Tumoren demonstriert wird (s. Drepper-Ehring). Beim Cylindrom der Haut, dem Basalzellcarcinom verwandt, sind jedoch Metastasen mehrfach beobachtet worden.

Hausfrau, 62 Jahre. Seit 20 Jahren Cylindrom der Haut an der linken Fußsohle. Nach „Ätzungen" begann es vor 2 Jahren zu wuchern. Dazu Metastasen in der Haut des linken Beines, des Rückens, in Lymphknoten der linken Leiste, der rechten Halsseite und rechten

Wange und in den Knochen des Beckens und der Wirbelsäule, welche zum Tode führten (Inaug. Diss. SCHULTE-STRATHAUS, Münster 1965).

Das *maligne Melanom* metastasiert früh und weit streuend. Isolierter Befall der regionären Lymphknoten ist jedoch nicht ganz selten. Radikale Behandlung bietet auch hier eine Heilungschance. Hierzu werden u. a. drei Kranke demonstriert, bei welchen nach Entfernung und Nachbestrahlung von regionären Metastasen bisher eine 5-Jahres-Heilung erzielt wurde. Bei folgenden Kranken blieb der Primärtumor unbekannt:

Kaufmann, Xeroderma pigmentosum. Mit 19 Jahren Plattenepithelcarcinom. Excision. Mit 21 Jahren erneut Plattenepithelcarcinom, Excision. Zwischenzeitlich Excision kleiner Hauttumoren ohne histologische Untersuchung beim Hautarzt. Mit 22 Jahren 3,5 cm große Metastase eines malignen Melanoms. Neck-dissection. Seit $2^{1}/_{2}$ Jahren rezidivfrei. Mit 25 Jahren Keratoakanthom. Excision.

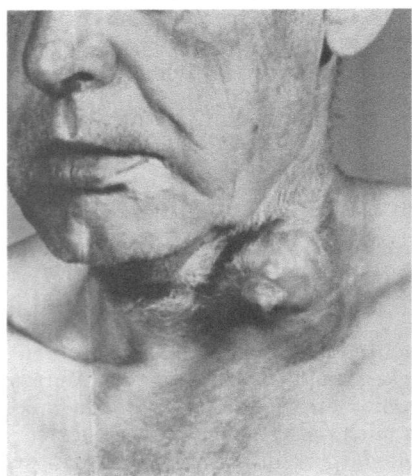

Abb. 1. Metastasen nach Unterlippen-carcinom, die mit den tiefen Gefäßen fest verwachsen waren

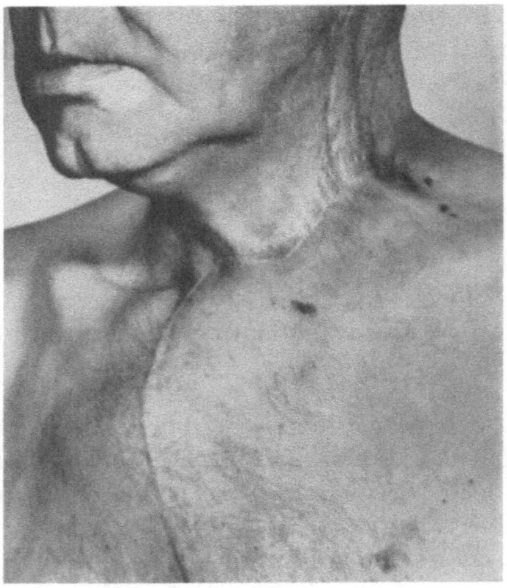

Abb. 2. Nach Operation und ^{60}Co-Bestrahlung seit 2 Jahren rezidivfrei

Auch bei *Sarkomen* gibt es solche, welche nie — und solche, welche nur regionär metastasieren. Sie sind daher nicht selten radikaler Behandlung zugänglich, während die generalisierten zum Teil vorübergehend cytostatisch zu beeinflussen sind. Auch hierfür wurden Beispiele gezeigt, z. B. ein Reticulosarkom an der Schulter von 10 cm Durchmesser mit Metastasen in der Achselhöhle. Es wurde der rechte Schultergürtel amputiert und mit dem Cobaltron II nachbestrahlt. Bis zum Tod durch Unfall war die Kranke 3 Jahre rezidivfrei.

Hautmetastasen maligner Geschwülste anderer Organe sind nach Mammacarcinomen häufig — sonst selten. Sie fallen oft durch bei primären Hauttumoren ungewöhnliche Lokalisation auf. Bei ihrer Erkennung ist das Grundleiden meist schon inkurabel. Hierzu werden demonstriert ein Plattenepithelcarcinom des Daumens mit Abdominalcarcinom, Hautmetastasen an der Brust nach Kehlkopfcarcinom, eine Hypernephrom-Metastase hinter dem rechten Ohr und Metastasen eines Ovarialcarcinoms in einem Radioderm am Rücken (s. DREPPER-EHRING).

Literatur. DREPPER, H.: Hautarzt **14**, 420 (1963). — EHRING, F.: Arch. Derm. **219**, 504 (1964). — EHRING, F., u. H. DREPPER: Krebsforschung und Krebsbekämpfung, Bd. VI, S. 269. München: Urban & Schwarzenberg 1967.

Zur Pathologie cutaner Lymphgefäße

J. Tappeiner und L. Pfleger, I. Universitäts-Hautklinik Wien (Österreich)

Bei Beurteilung von Zirkulationsstörungen der cutanen Lymphgefäße wird die röntgenologische Darstellung derselben — die bei totaler Gefäßobliteration nicht gelingt — durch histologische Untersuchungen von Lymphgefäß- und Hautbiopsien ergänzt. Außerdem wird auch das Verhalten des zur Markierung der Lymphgefäße injizierten Farbstoffes berücksichtigt.

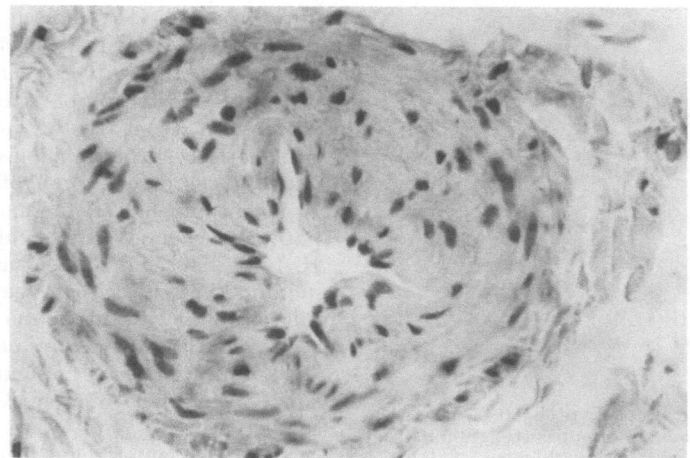

Abb. 1. Normales Lymphgefäß mit sternförmigem Lumen und dreischichtiger Gefäßwand. HE-Färbung 500×

Bei normalen Lymphgefäßen sind nach i.c. Injektion von Patentblauviolett einige präfasciale Lymphbahnen am Fußrücken sichtbar. Nach Freilegung eines derartigen Gefäßes wird das Kontrastmittel injiziert. Röntgenologisch findet man, bei Darstellung des vorderen Lymphgefäßbündels, an der Medialseite der unteren Extremität bis zum Lymphknoten ziehend, eine größere Zahl nahezu parallel verlaufender, wenig geschlängelter Bahnen von einem durch die Klappen bedingten perlschnurartigem Aussehen. Die Lymphabflußbahnen haben, wie der histologische Befund ergibt, eine dreischichtige Wand: die Intima besteht aus dicht angeordneten, längsverlaufenden kollagenen Fasern, die Media aus sich durchkreuzenden Muskelbündeln und die Adventitia aus lockerem kollagenen Gewebe (Abb. 1).

Bestehen manifeste Lymphgefäßläsionen, so entwickeln sich als Folge von Lymphkreislaufstörungen Lymphödeme. Beim idiopathischen Lymphoedema praecox kommt es nach Farbinjektion zur diffusen oder netzförmigen Anfärbung eines etwa handtellergroßen Areals im Injektionsbereich. Röntgenologisch findet man nur eine einzige fadendünne Abflußbahn, welche histologisch entzündliche oder degenerative Wandveränderungen und eine hochgradige Einengung des Lumens aufweisen kann. Als Kriterium des Lymphödems besteht in der Haut eine Verquellung und Homogenisierung des kernarmen kollagenen Gewebes.

Beim symptomatischen Lymphödem, das sich am häufigsten nach rezidivierendem Erysipel entwickelt, kommt es im Bereich des vom Rotlauf befallenen Gebietes zu einer diffusen Verfärbung durch den injizierten Farbstoff. Röntgenologisch ist das Phänomen des „dermal backflow" nachweisbar, das ist die Darstellung eines zarten, bis an die Oberfläche reichenden capillaren Netzwerkes. Histologisch findet man organisierte Lymphthromben (Abb. 2) oder fibrös veränderte Gefäßstränge.

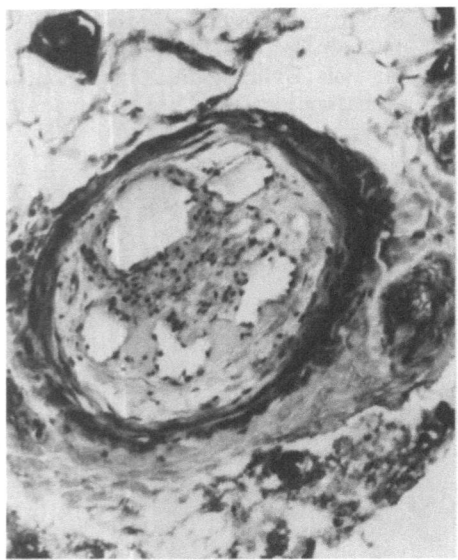

Abb. 2. Obliteriertes Lymphgefäß, dessen Lumen durch einen organisierten, rekanalisierten Lymphthrombus verschlossen ist. HE-Färbung 125×

Beim Ulcus cruris kann es zu profusem Farbaustritt aus dem Ulcus oder zur rückläufigen Anfärbung einer im Ulcus stehengebliebenen Hautinsel kommen. Im Lymphangiogramm sind die Lymphbahnen im Ulcusbereich unterbrochen. Histologisch sind die Lymphgefäße zwar hochgradig dilatiert, sonst aber unverändert.

Beim postthrombotischen Syndrom wird der Farbstoff normal abtransportiert. Röntgenologisch findet man entlang dem Lymphgefäßverlauf Kontrastmittelaustritte als Zeichen pathologischer Wanddurchlässigkeit. Histologisch sind die Lymphgefäße maximal erweitert, die vasa vasorum dilatiert und gestaut. In der Haut besteht ein Stauungsödem, das ist eine Ansammlung freier Flüssigkeit, insbesonders in den oberen Coriumabschnitten.

Bei den entstellenden elephantiastischen Schwellungen sind röntgenologisch häufig Lymphvaricen in Form unregelmäßig erweiterter, elongierter und mäanderartig geschlängelter Lymphbahnen nachweisbar. Histologisch sind die Lymphgefäße ektatisch, die Gefäßwand

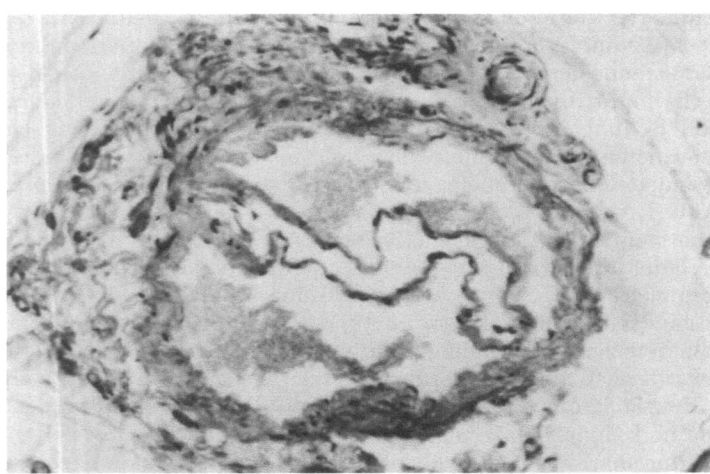

Abb. 3. Ektatisches Lymphgefäß mit atrophischer Gefäßwand und gedehnten Klappen. Im Lumen Fibringerinnsel. HE-Färbung 125×

infolge des Muskelschwundes der Media atrophisch. Die gedehnten Klappen sind insuffizient (Abb. 3). In der Haut besteht eine ausgeprägte Fibrose des Corium. Das subcutane Fettgewebe ist durch neugebildetes kollagenes Gewebe ersetzt. Vielfach finden sich Lymphgefäße und Lymphcapillaren mit wandständigen Thromben.

Neuere Aspekte zur Histopathologie der Alopecia areata

W. Thies und Ch. Fischer, Hautklinik der Freien Universität Berlin im Rudolf Virchow-Krankenhaus (Deutschland)

Der Ausstellung liegen histologische Serienschnitte von 53 Alopecia areata (A. a.)-Patienten zugrunde. 40 Excisate stammten aus erkrankten Bezirken, bei 13 Kranken handelte es sich um Biopsien aus klinisch unauffälligen Kopfhautpartien. Außerdem wurde bei 46 A. a.-Patienten das Verhalten der Haarwurzeln an Hand einzeitig epilierter Haarbüschel (Methode nach van Scott) geprüft, davon bei 33 Patienten der Haarwurzelstatus vom Herdrand mit klinisch gesunden Bezirken verglichen. Eine Mitbeteiligung der übrigen Kopfhaut fand sich bei 70%.

Bei den histologischen Untersuchungen findet sich als wesentliches und in allen aktiven Herden übereinstimmendes Kennzeichen neben den allgemein bekannten peribulbären und intrapapillären lympho-histiocytären Infiltraten an den Proliferationshaaren eine mehr oder minder ausgeprägte Degeneration von Matrixzellen in der oberen Bulbushälfte, vornehmlich oberhalb der Papillenspitze, in Form dissoziierter, homogen eosinophil tingierter Zellkomplexe mit pyknotischen oder nicht mehr anfärbbaren Kernen, offenbar bedingt durch eine vermehrte inter- und intracelluläre Flüssigkeitsansammlung ähnlich der trüben Schwellung. In besonders foudroyant verlaufenden A. a.-Fällen kommt es zur Nekrobiose der Matrixzellen. Weiterhin sieht man zwischen die Matrixzellen eingestreut eingewanderte Lymphocyten (Abb. 1a—c u. 2).

Bemerkenswert ist das Fehlen morphologischer Besonderheiten in der unteren Bulbushälfte, d. h. unterhalb des durch den größten Papillendurchmesser gedachten „critical level". Die degenerativen Veränderungen im Bulbus beschränken sich ausschließlich auf jene Bezirke, in denen bereits eine beginnende Differenzierung der Matrixzellen in Richtung innere Wurzelscheide und Haarcortex zu erkennen ist. Außerdem beherbergt dieser Bulbusabschnitt die Melanocyten. Weiterhin resultiert daraus eine Abnahme der Mitoserate in derartig geschädigten Haarbulbi, sie sind atrophisch und gehen vorzeitig in das Katagenstadium über (Abb. 3). Außerdem kommt es zu unvollständiger Haarschaftbildung. Offenbar bedingt die Degeneration der Haarmatrixzellen auch eine Störung der Melaninaufnahme in den suprapapillären Bulbusabschnitten, statt dessen wird vermehrt Melanin an die Haarpapille bzw. an den Haarstengel abgegeben (Abb. 4). In älteren A. a.-Herden überwiegen die vorzeitig hochgestiegenen dystrophischen Haarfollikel (Miniaturfollikel).

In makroskopisch nicht sichtbar erkrankten Kopfhautarealen finden sich zum Teil recht massive perivasculäre und perifolliculäre lymphocytäre Infiltrate mit in die äußere und innere Wurzelscheide eingedrungenen Rundzellen, auch im Bereich von Kolbenhaaren, deren prozentualer Anteil angestiegen ist, während eine Degeneration der Haarmatrixzellen, wie sie für die erkrankten Kopfhautpartien beschrieben wurden, vermißt wird.

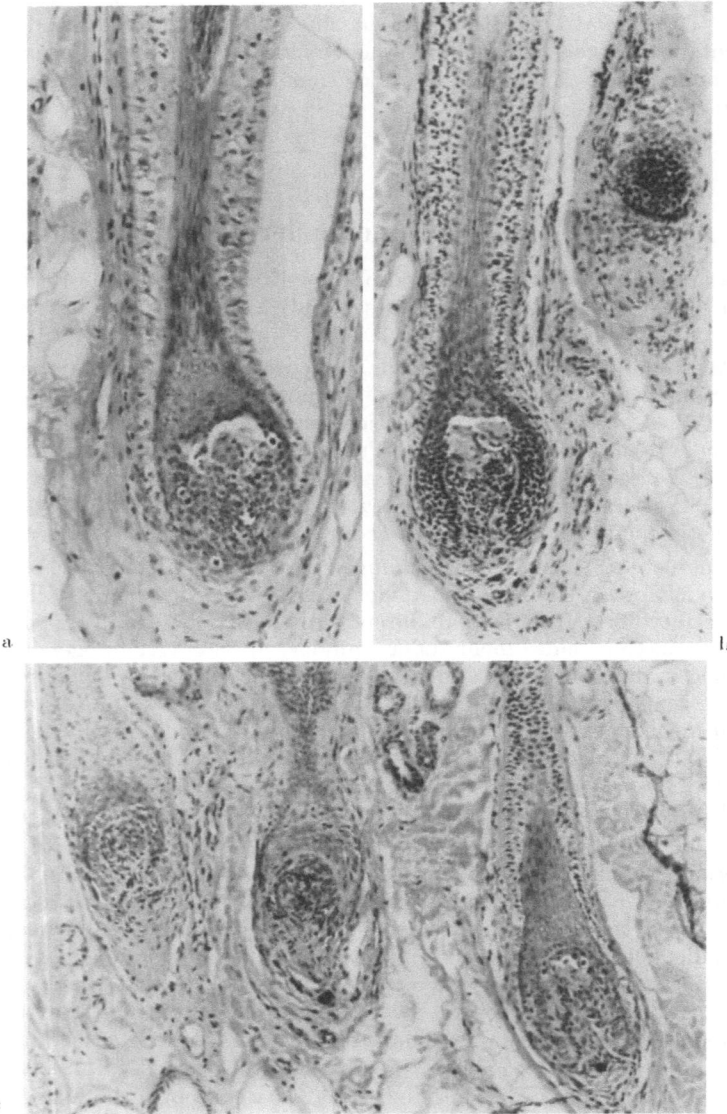

Abb. 1 a—c. Alopecia areata. 17jähriger Pat. Beginn von 10 Jahren. Vor 7 Jahren Alopecia totalis. Nach Vitamin D$_2$ und Corticosteroiden erneut Haarwachstum. Seit einem Jahr nach Absetzen der Corticosteroide Verschlimmerung. Schlanker anagener Haarbulbus mit Dissoziation und Degeneration der Haarmatrixzellen und eingewanderten Rundzellen. H.-E. Num. Ap. 0,32

Abb. 1 b. Proliferationshaar mit atrophischem Haarbulbus und degenerierten Haarmatrixzellen, intrapapillären und peripulbären lympho-histiocytären Infiltraten. Pigmentschollen unterhalb der Papille. H.-E. Num. Ap. 0,32

Abb. 1 c. Atrophische hochgestiegene Haarbulbi mit unterschiedlicher Degeneration der Haarmatrixzellen bzw. der inneren Wurzelscheidenzellen. Lympho-histiocytäre Infiltrate mit Melanophagen und Pigment in den Haarpapillen und subpapillär. H.-E. Num. Ap. 0,32

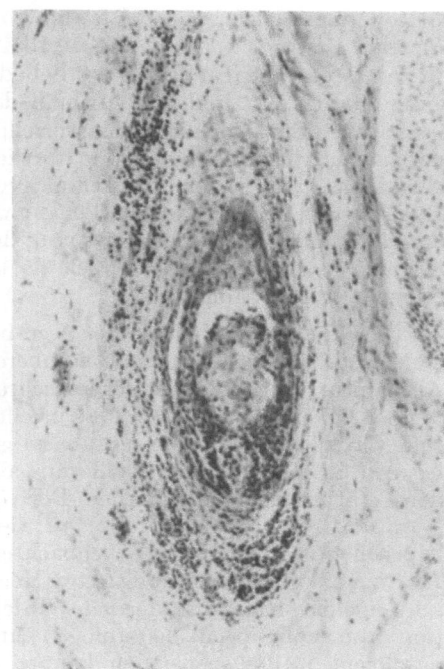

Abb. 2. Alopecia areata maligna. 23jähriger Pat. Beginn vor 2 Monaten mit einzelnen Herden, in kurzer Zeit zum Verlust sämtlicher Kopfhaare führend. Hochgradige Atrophie des Haarbulbus und der Haarpapille. Degeneration und Dissoziation der inneren Wurzelscheidenzellen, durchsetzt von eingewanderten Lymphocyten. Massive peribulbäre lymphocytäre Infiltrate. H.-E. Num. Ap. 0,32

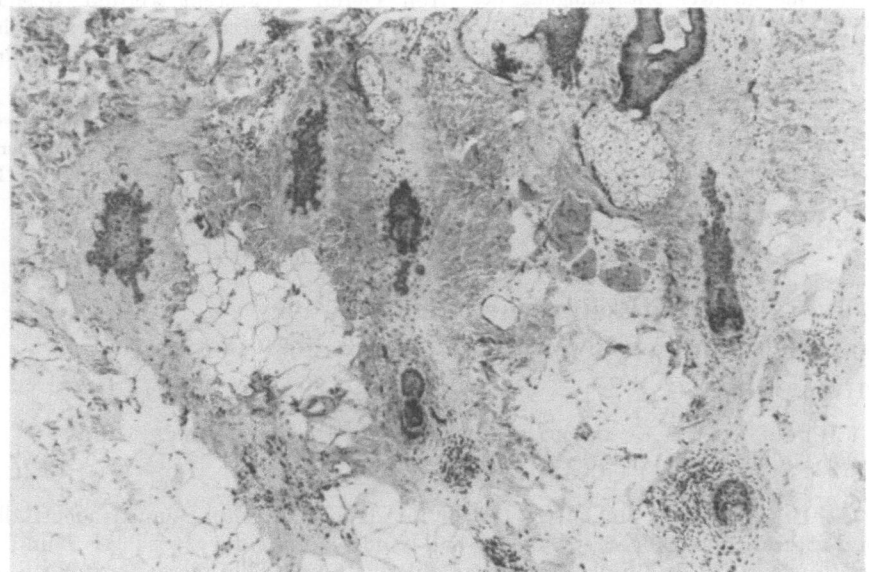

Abb. 3. Alopecia areata. 70jähriger Pat. Seit 3 Monaten mehrere Herde am Hinterkopf. Excisat vom Herdrand. Hochgestiegene Mikrofollikel, zum Teil im Katagenstadium. Peribulbäres Infiltrat um atrophischen anagenen Haarbulbus (unten rechts). H.-E. Num. Ap. 0,32

Die histopathologischen Befunde bestätigen, daß es sich bei der A. a. um eine diffuse Erkrankung der Haarfollikel handelt (BRAUN-FALCO u. ZAUN, 1962), wobei Dauer und Intensität der Schädigung für die Art und das Ausmaß der pathogenen Reaktion an den Matrixzellen der anagenen Haarfollikel verantwortlich sind. Dysenzymosis der mitotisch-aktiven Haarmatrix (BRAUN-FALCO u. THIANPRASIT, 1963) im Sinne einer Hemmung des Atmungs- und Energiestoffwechsels ist offenbar erst die Folge.

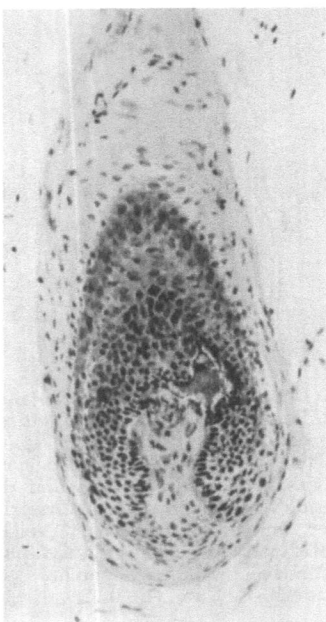

Über die Ätiopathologie der A. a. besteht noch keine Einigkeit. Die oberen Abschnitte des Bulbus mit der fortschreitenden Differenzierung der Matrixzellen sind vergleichbar mit den suprabasal gelegenen Stachelzellen der Epidermis, die der Keratinisation anheimfallen. Der von WILHELMJ u. Mitarb. (1962) in tierexperimentellen Studien beobachtete Haarausfall bei autosensibilisierten Meerschweinchen nach intradermaler Injektion von homologen, heterologen und autologen Hautsuspensionen konnte in eigenen orientierenden, recht eingreifenden Sensibilisierungsstudien (gem. mit KLASCHKA, unveröffentlicht) bei mehreren Tieren festgestellt werden, weshalb bei der A. a. an einen allergischen Mechanismus vom Typ der Spätreaktivität ähnlich dem Ekzem zu denken wäre.

Abb. 4. Alopecia areata. Seit 10 Wochen einzelne Herde. Trichogramm: Gemischte Alopecie mit geringer Mitbeteiligung des gesamten Capillitiums. Excisat aus klinisch unauffälligerKopfhaut. Auffallend geblähte pigmentreiche Melanocyten in oberer Bulbushälfte. H.-E. Num. Ap. 0,32

Literatur. BRAUN-FALCO, O., u. H. ZAUN: Hautarzt 13, 342 (1962). — BRAUN-FALCO, O., e.M. THIANPRASIT: Atti Soc. ital. Derm. Sif. 1963, 252. — THIES, W.: Arch. klin. exp. Derm. 227, 541 (1966). — WILHELMJ, CH. M., R. R. KIERLAND, and CH. A. OWEN: Arch. Derm. Syph. (Chigago) 86, 161 (1962).

Befund Langerhans-ähnlicher Zellen in den Hauterscheinungen der Reticuloendotheliose von Letterer-Siwe

V. PUCCINELLI, F. GIANOTTI und R. CAPUTO, Dermatologische Klinik der Universität Mailand (Italien)

Die Untersuchung der Ultrastruktur der Hauterscheinungen von vier Fällen von Letterer-Siwescher Erkrankung bei Kindern im Alter zwischen 8 und 18 Monaten zeigte in drei Fällen ein reticulohistiocytäres Zellinfiltrat, bestehend aus voluminösen polimorphen Zellen verschiedener Größe mit gelapptem Kern und Vacuolen unterschiedlichen Durchmessers und schwach osmophylen Inhaltes im Cytoplasma, gut entwickeltem Reticulum, Lisosomen, Phagosomen, Myelin-

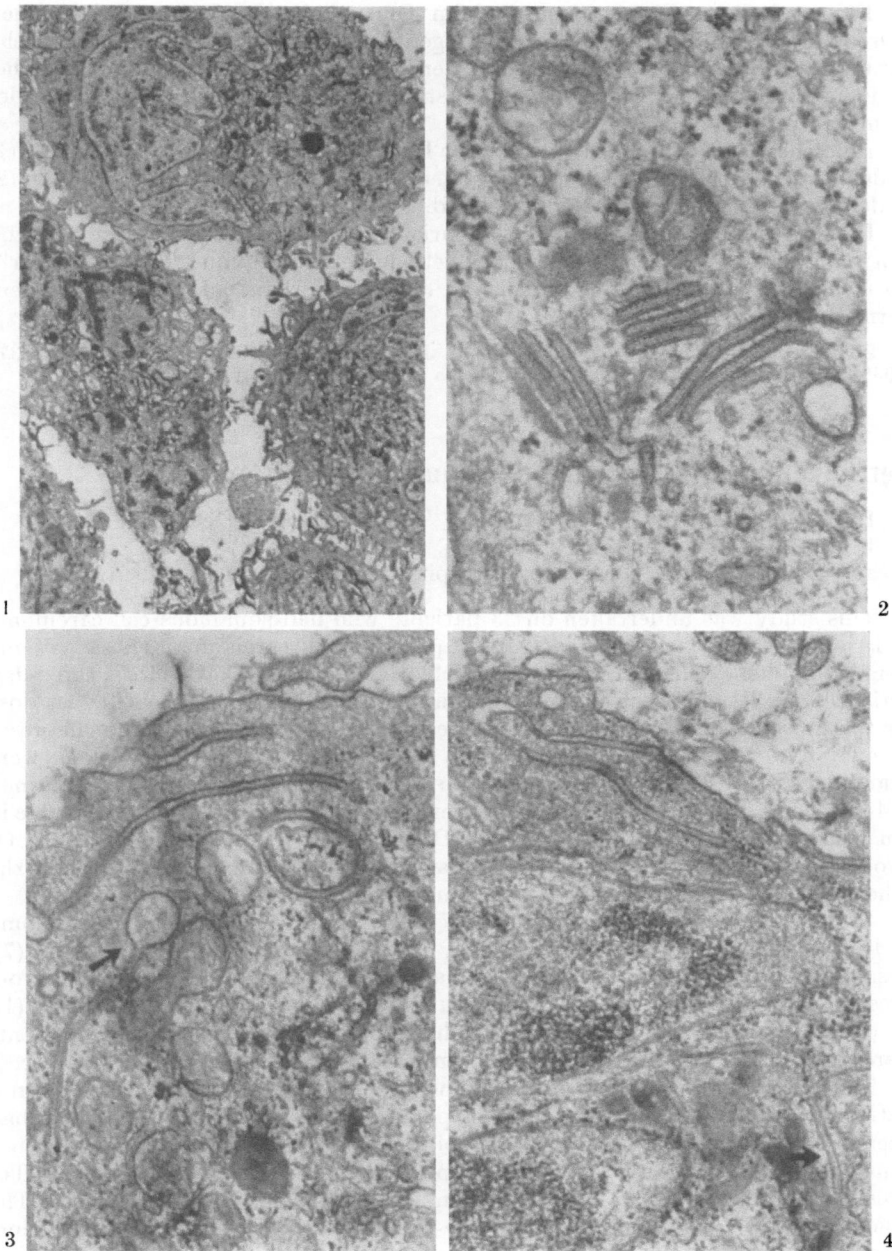

1 2 3 4

formationen und Glykogenkörnern. Beim 8 Monate alten Kind war das reticulo-histiocytäre Infiltrat fast monomorph (Abb. 1) und bestand aus Langerhans-ähnlichen Zellen, deren Cytoplasma eine große Menge durch eine doppelte Membran abgegrenzte tubuläre Formationen verschiedener Länge mit abgerundeten Polen enthielt (Abb. 2); die „Tennisschläger"-Form trat selten auf (Abb. 3).

Diese tubulären Formationen sind im Querschnitt ringförmig, haben einen Durchmesser von 300 bis 400 Å und zeigen nur selten eine interne periodische Struktur (Abb. 4). Sie sind in der Nähe der Zellmembran länger als in Kernnähe, und man hat oft den Eindruck, als entstünden sie durch eine Einstülpung der Membran (Abb. 3 und 4).

Ähnliche Befunde beschrieben bei der Histiocytosis-X BASSET und TURIAF (1) in den Lungen- und Knochenveränderungen von 15 Fällen und DE BEUKELAAR (2) in den Hauterscheinungen bei einem Kind.

Die von uns beobachteten und beschriebenen Zellen unterscheiden sich von den Langerhansschen Zellen durch das seltene Auftreten von „Tennisschläger"-Formen, das Fehlen von Melaninkörnern und das Vorhandensein von Glykogenkörnern.

Bibliographie. 1. BASSET, F., et J. TURIAF: Bull. Mem. Soc. Méd. Hôp. (Paris) **117**, 373 (1966). — 2. DE BEUKELAAR, L.: Dermatologica (Basel) **134**, 337 (1967).

Tetracycline Fluorescence in Squamous Cell Carcinoma

H. J. DONSKY, University of Toronto, Toronto General Hospital, Department of Dermatology, Toronto, Ontario (Canada) and G. R. MIKHAIL, Henry Ford Hospital, Detroit (USA)

This study was undertaken on 33 patients who had squamous cell carcinoma or lesions suspected clinically of being squamous cell carcinoma. These patients were given tetracycline (TC) or demethylchlortetracycline (DMCT) for a three-day period. Their lesions were examined under Wood's light 48 h after the last dose for the presence of a canary-yellow fluorescence. Lesions which did not fluoresce or exhibited a dull yellow colour were considered negative. All lesions were examined histologically. The presence of squamous cell carcinoma was confirmed in 14 patients. Eleven of these patients were given TC with positive fluorescence in ten instances. All three patients given DMCT showed positive fluorescence. Of two patients with Bowen's disease, one lesion failed to fluoresce with TC, while the other showed a "leopard spot" type of fluorescence with DMCT.

17 patients who were clinically suspected of having squamous cell carcinoma had the following diagnoses on biopsy examination: chronic ulceration (7), basal cell epthelioma (4), keratoanthoma (1), metastatic adenocarcinoma from breast (1), syringocystadenoma papilliferum (1), ulcerated periarteritis nodosa (1), thermal burn ulceration (1), lymphatic hyperplasia (1). Seven of these patients were given DMCT and none fluoresced. Ten were given TC, and only one fluoresced.

The only false negative result was encountered with TC. This occurred in a patient who had a scaling erythematous papule on the side of his neck which had been present for 10 months. The pathology report in this case was „Grade I squamous cell carcinoma". The only false positive result was also observed with TC. This patient had a chronic ulceration in the pretibial region for 5 years. The lesion had been enlarging over the one-and-a-half year period before testing. Histology showed "pseudoepitheliomatous hyperplasia".

Fluorescence, when present, was mainly restricted to the necrotic or granulomatous portions of tumours. The intensity of fluorescence was evenly distributed in the lesion except in the case of Bowen's disease which showed a "leopard spot" arrangement.

One of the patients was first given a course of TC without eliciting fluorescence. At that time he had a granulomatous mass which had gradually developed in the periana region for 3 years. The pathology reports in the first seven biopsy examinations were "pseudoepitheliomatous hyperplasia". The report on the eighth biopsy specimen was "grade II squamous cell carcinoma". By this time the lesion had become necrotic and ulcerative. The lesion then showed positive fluorescence with DMCT. This was the only lesion which demonstrated the "live coal" fluorescence described by RONCHESE. The entire skin was exposed to Wood's light in all patients, and in no instance was fluorescence observed in any of the following lesions: nevi, seborrheic and actinic keratoses, psoriasis, seborrhoids, and xanthelasma palpebrarum.

Many lesions have been reported that fluorescence with ultra violet light. MARGAROT and DEVEZE, in 1929, were the first to report fluorescence in naturally occurring cancers. RONCHESE later found that of the various types of skin carcinomata, only the squamous or epidermoid cell variety is naturally fluorescent. The fluorescence is restricted to the necrotic ulcerated areas of these lesions. PHILIPS and his group observed that a thin layer of normal tissue may obscure the fluorescence of an underlying malignant growth.

RALL and his co-workers induced fluorescence in necrotic animal tumours by administering tetracycline. DUBUY and SHOWACRE demonstrated that tetracycline combined specifically with mitochondria of animal cells. These mitochondria were found to have decreased oxidative phosphorylation, but their oxygen uptake remained normal.

Conclusion: These findings confirm the affinity tetracyclines have for tumour tissue. Their value as an ancillary procedure in the diagnosis of squamous cell carcinoma remains limited by the fact that the tumour must be superficially located in the skin in order to demonstrate positive fluorescence. Demethylchlortetracycline was found to fluoresce more intensely than tetracycline.

Concept of the Molecular Cause of Albinism

G. F. WILGRAM, Dermatologic Genetics Laboratory, New England Center Hospital, Boston, Mass. (USA)

In a mutation of the S 91 mouse melanoma, an albino tyrosinase is extractable and a few melanosomes are detectable with electron microscopy. The ultrastructure of these few albino melanosomes is different from that of the abundant melanosomes in the wild pigmented strain. Tyrosinase activity can be demonstrated in vitro after the inhibitor is removed by cell fractionation. Both the RNP-bound and the freely soluble forms of this albino enzyme are susceptible in vitro to the normally present inhibitor. It is proposed that through mutation a small change took place in the protein carrier of albino tyrosinase, as detected by refined electrophoresis. The active center of the mutant enzyme does not seem to be altered since the Michaelis constant is almost identical to that of the wild enzyme. In the wild pigmented strain, tyrosinase apparently "aggregates" itself into melanosomes where the enzyme is protected from its inhibitor. Therefore, despite the presence of an inhibitor, tyrosinase activity can be shown in the whole tumor as well as in whole homogenates. In the Type B albino mutant the small change in the protein carrier of the enzyme does not allow the "aggregation" of albino tyrosinase into melanosomes. As a result, the albino tyrosinase does not reach its stable form in the melanosome where it would be protected from its inhibitor. Thus, melanosome formation and melanin production cannot take place in vivo, although albino tyrosinase with a fully functioning active center is present.

The application of these findings in mouse and hamster tumors to cutaneous albinism in man is not easy, but there are indications that in human albino hair bulbs a few malformed melanosomes are present and that traces of tyrosinase are demonstrable with histiochemistry under favorable substrate conditions. It seems like that the tyrosinase inhibitor is washed out during histochemical procedures.

CONCEPT OF THE "MOLECULAR CAUSE" OF ALBINISM

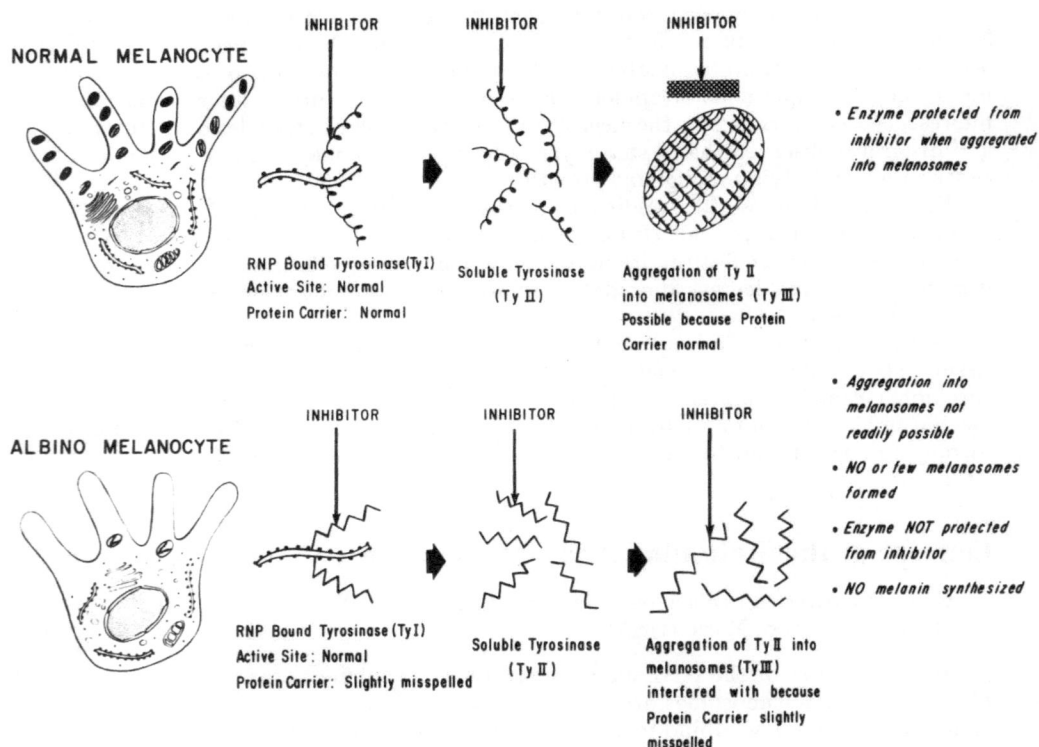

Since RNP-bound tyrosinase and tyrosinase "aggregated" into a few melanosomes remain in the histologic tissue section, a positive dopa reaction may be obtained under these circumstances. Thus it appears that the Type B mutation in the S 91 albino melanoma may be an experimental model of the conditions as they prevail in albinism in man.

Xeroderma pigmentosum

H. El Hefnawi, Dept. of Dermatology of the University of Cairo (U.A.R.)

Skin Tuberculosis, Leprosy, Cutaneous Leishmanosis, Favus

M. A. Maleki, Dept. of Dermatology, Razi Univ. Hospital, Teheran (Iran)

Experimental Dermatology

A Cutaneous Rôle in the Regulation of the Body's Carbohydrate Milieu

R. M. FUSARO and J. A. JOHNSON, Department of Dermatology, University of Minnesota, Minneapolis, Minn. (USA)

The exhibit demonstrates the results of our research with a new method of doing the cutaneous glucose tolerance test; that is, the dextrose was given intravenously rather than orally. In this manner, the kinetics of the dermal extracellular compartment with respect to the disappearance of glucose were defined. After a rapid i. v. dextrose load, the concentration of dermal glucose reached a peak concentration in approximately 30 min and fell as a first order decay expression. Assuming the skin mass to be 10% of body weight, knowing the i.v. dextrose dose (35 to 45 Gm) and using the 30 min dermal glucose value, it was shown that 20% of the i.v. dose was absorbed by the skin and a major part of the absorbed glucose was released back to the blood over a four hour period. In contrast, the blood glucose levels had returned to normal prefasting values within $1^1/_2$ h. The cutaneous lymphatics glucose levels also took approximately four hours to return to prefasting levels and had the same glucose disappearance rate constant as glucose in the dermal extracellular compartment.

Results

Blood and Skin

A. Blood:

Glucose disappears from the blood in a first order decay manner and can be expressed as a single constant, k in % of glucose cleared per min.

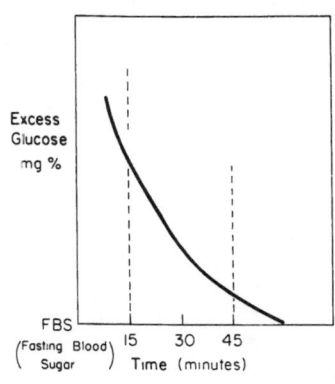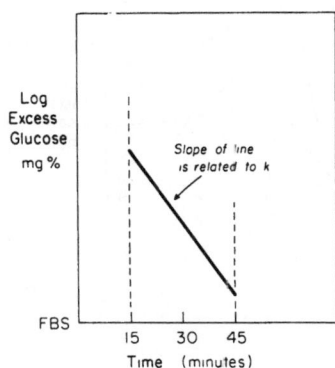

B. Skin:

Glucose disappears from the extracellular compartment of the skin and can be expressed by the first order decay expression:

$$S_t = S_0 e^{-k't}$$

where

S_t = the glucose excess in mg per 100 gm of whole skin (wet weight) at time (t) between the time interval of 35 to 65 min;

S_0 = the glucose excess in mg per 100 gm of whole skin extrapolated to time zero;

and k' = the rate of disappearance of glucose from the skin (expressed in % per min).

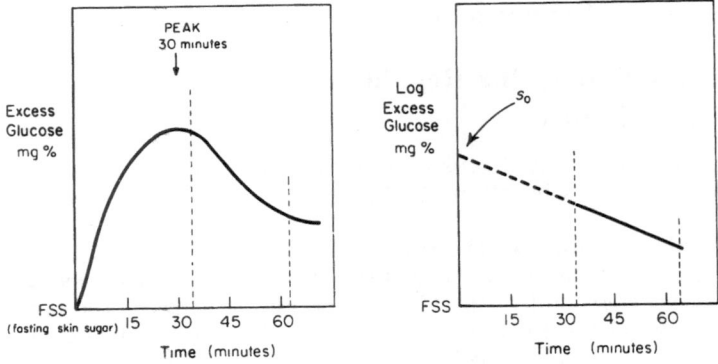

Results
Lymph and Skin

Experimental Conditions:

In a patient with lymphectasia of the leg, 35 g of dextrose was given i.v. (antecubital) within 4 min. Glucose concentrations were followed for $1\frac{1}{2}$ h in the blood, lymph, and skin.

1. Blood glucose levels returned to fasting concentration in approximately $1\frac{1}{2}$ h, while skin and lymph glucose levels remained significantly elevated at $1\frac{1}{2}$ h.

2. Both lymph and skin glucose values peaked simultaneously (at approximately 35 min) indicating that the extracellular compartment of the skin and the lymphatic vascular system were in equilibrium.

3. Skin is a temporary reservoir for excess blood glucose and the lymphatic system is a route for the drainage of the excess glucose from the extracellular compartment of the skin

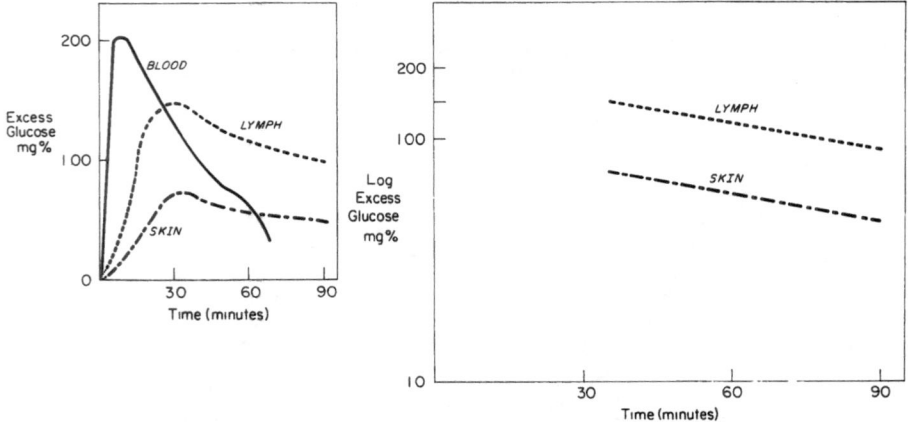

Results
Amount of Glucose Absorbed by Normal Skin

Experimental Conditions:

Ten normal young men were given the cutaneous glucose tolerance test three times in 3 months. Each was given the following dose of intravenous dextrose:

$$
\begin{aligned}
&\text{Test 1} \quad 35 \text{ g}\\
&\text{Test 2} \quad 40 \text{ g}\\
&\text{Test 3} \quad 45 \text{ g}
\end{aligned}
$$

Since glucose concentration reaches its peak in the skin at 30 min this value along with estimated weight of the skin was used to calculate the percentage of the i.v. dose which was found in the extracellular compartment of the skin.

Dosage

Subject	35 g %	40 g %	45 g %
1	24.8	19.4	25.0
2	21.9	22.0	21.5
3	30.2	23.5	19.3
4	23.3	21.8	17.4
5	18.2	18.0	23.4
6	16.4	29.8	25.7
7	22.7	21.3	21.7
8	17.5	14.9	20.4
9	18.2	26.9	25.6
10	29.2	13.6	26.5
average	22.2	21.1	22.6
S.D.	±4.9	±5.0	±3.1
S.E.	±1.6	±1.6	±1.0

The Relationship of the Skin to the Whole Body

Excess glucose deposited in the skin takes the following routes:

1. Diffuse into the blood,
2. Flow via the lymphatic system into the blood,
3. Enter the epithelial compartment to follow metabolic pathways.

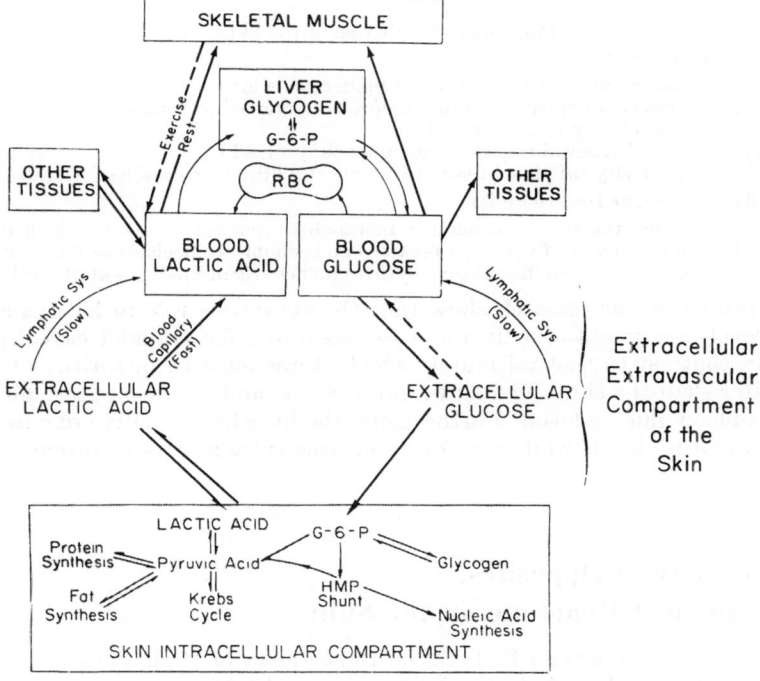

Since the skin needs large quantities of ATP for epithelial regenerations and Krebs cycle activity in the epidermis is low (as demonstrated by high *in vivo* skin lactate levels and low *in vitro* radioactive glucose incorporation into the Krebs cycle), we propose that the skin has a continous Cori cycle with the liver, in order to provide sufficient ATP (for epithelial regeneration) by an otherwise inefficient glycolytic sequence (anaerobic glycolysis — EMBDEN-MEYERHOF PATHWAY). In addition, this cycle provides the skin with another mechanism for the control of blood carbohydrate levels; that is, the conversion of lactate from the skin into glucose and glycogen by the liver.

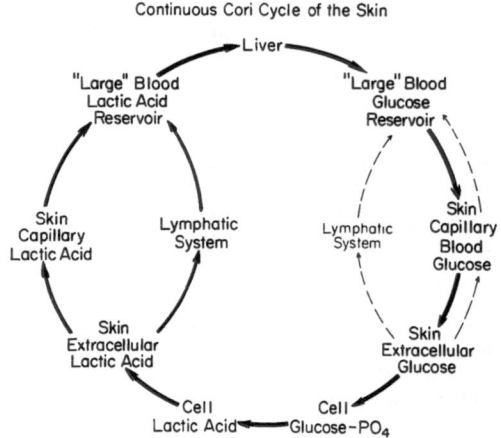

Continuous Cori Cycle of the Skin

Consideration of these facts —

1. Oxygen consumption and tension of the epidermis is low.
2. The major portion of glucose utilized *in vitro* is converted to lactate.
3. Lactate diffuses freely back to blood.
4. Rapid epidermal renewal requires large quantities of ATP.
5. Krebs cycle activity supplies a limited amount of ATP via oxidation of NADH (DPNH).

— suggests the concept that there is:

a Cori Cycle in which the skin continuously metabolizes glucose to lactate which in turn is reconverted to glucose by the liver. This provides an economical mechanism for ATP production by way of an otherwise inefficient glycolytic sequence (EMBDEN-MEYERHOF Pathway).

The results of our research show that the cutaneous rôle in balancing blood glucose levels is second to the liver as a storage center for available carbohydrates. This is in contrast to skeletal muscle which stores massive quantities of glucose (far greater than the skin) for its own internal use and can not release glucose to maintain blood glucose levels. Furthermore, the liver has an active rôle in balancing blood glucose levels while the cutaneous role is by passive diffusion.

The Interplay of Opposites.
Immunological Reactions in the Skin

TH. M. INDERBITZIN and P. J. GROB, Department of Dermatology, Tufts University School of Medicine, Boston, Mass. (USA)

The term immunology comprises two phenomena, namely immunity, meaning protection, and hypersensitivity, meaning disease. The ability of an organism to react towards an aggression with immunity or with hypersensitivity is acquired through previous exposures to antigens.

Antigenic stimuli may induce the production of immunoglobulins (antibodies) and may enable certain cells to recognize and to react with an antigen. Accordingly, immune and hypersensitivity reactions are the result of an interplay of opposites, namely of the antigen either with immunoglobulins, or with immunologically competent cells, or with both.

The exhibit illustrated the pathways following stimulations with antigens and also illustrated some hypersensitivity reactions in the skin.

The urticarial wheal, the Arthus type lesion and the acantholysis in pemphigus were shown as examples of hypersensitivity reactions mediated by immuno-globulins.

The happenings at sites of hypersensitivity reactions mediated by cells, the so called delayed type hypersensitivity reactions, were illustrated with the allergic contact dermatitis.

Finally, a "dual hypersensitivity reaction" mediated by both, cells and immunoglobulins was demonstrated.

Autoradiographic Studies on Psoriatic Epidermis

S. Sotomatsu, Y. Igarashi and Y. Ooshima, Kyoto Prefectural University of Medicine, Kyoto (Japan)

The cytodynamics and amino acids-metabolism in the epidermis of psoriasis vulgaris were studied autoradiographically giving ^{3}H-compounds in vivo or in vitro.

Materials and Methods

The skin of the extensor aspect of upper arm of psoriatic and normal young adults (controls) was used. Physiological saline solution containing a ^{3}H-compound (^{3}H-thymidine $25 \mu c/0.1$ ml or ^{3}H-uridine $50 \mu c/0.1$ ml) was injected intracutaneously at the area to be examined, then the injected area were biopsied at various times after injection of the tracer, or biopsied materials were incubated in vitro for 2 to 6 h in Eagle's medium containing a ^{3}H-compound (^{3}H-glycine $50 \mu c/ml$ or ^{3}H-tyrosine $35 \mu c/ml$). These specimens were fixed in 10% formalin solution, dehydrated and embedded in paraffin. They were cut 4μ and mounted on slides. Autoradiographs were prepared with FUJI ET-2E stripping films and developed with ED 111 after 3 weeks of exposure at 4 °C. The specimens were stained hematoxylin and eosin after the development.

Results

1. In the specimens from psoriatic lesions, labeled in vivo for 1 h, not only basal cells but also cells of a few layers above the basal layer were labeled with ^{3}H-thymidine. The labeling index was 35% (Fig. 1).

2. In the specimens from normal subjects, labeled in vivo for 1 h, only the basal cells were labeled with ^{3}H-thymidine. The labeling index was 7 %.

3. In the specimens from psoriatic lesions, labeled cells had migrated into the superficial layer of spinous cells on the 3rd day after intracutaneous injection of ^{3}H-thymidine.

4. In the specimens from normal subjects, labeled cells had migrated to the granular cell layer on the 14th day after intracutaneous injection of ^{3}H-thymidine.

5. In the specimens from psoriatic lesions, all the epidermal cells were labeled at 40 min after intracutaneous injection of ^{3}H-uridine (Fig. 2).

6. In the specimens from normal subjects, ^{3}H-uridine was incorporated in all the epidermal cells at 40 min after intracutaneous injection.

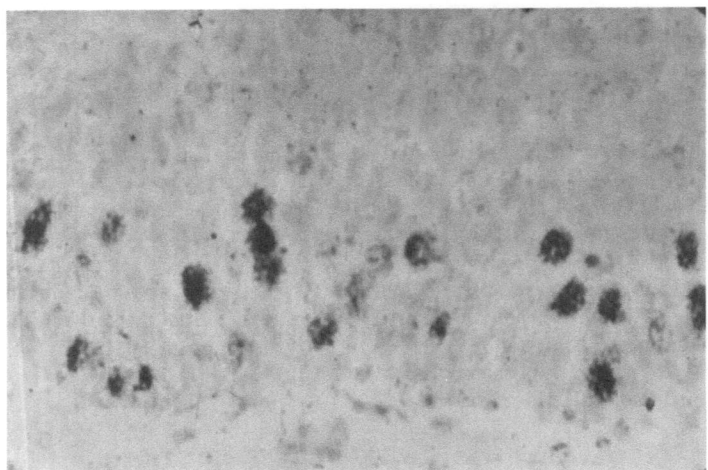

Fig. 1

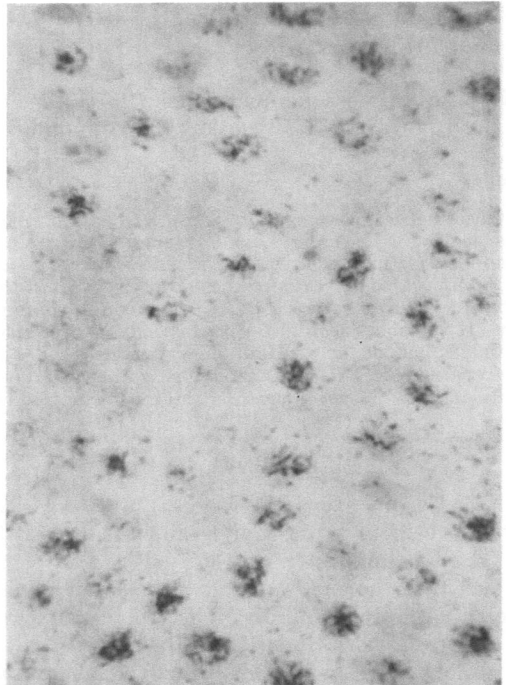

Fig. 2

7. In the specimens from psoriatic lesions, incubated in vitro with ^{3}H-tyrosine for 2 h, silver grains predominated over the cells in the upper spinous layer.

8. In the specimens from normal subjects, incubated in vitro with ^{3}H-tyrosine for 2 h, silver grains were found over the lower spinous layer.

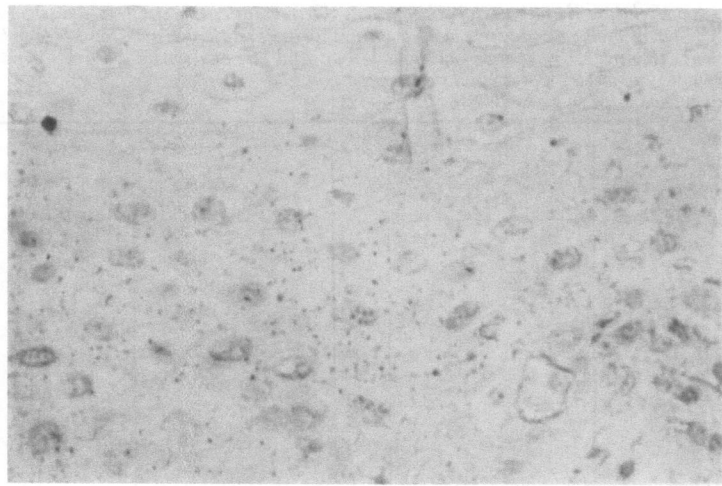

Fig. 3

9. In the specimens from psoriatic lesions, incubated in vitro for 4 h, labeling of ³H-glycine was seen over the cells of all layers (Fig. 3).
10. In the specimens from normal subjects, incubated in vitro for 4 h, ³H-glycine was mainly incorporated in the upper spinous and basal layers.

Die Mastzelle*

A. SCHAUER, Pathologisches Institut der Universität München (Deutschland)

Es wird über histochemische und biochemische Untersuchungen an normalen und Mastocytomzellen berichtet. Ein zum Teil gemeinsam mit EDER bearbeiteter Fragenkomplex ist der Nachweis proteolytischer, esterolytischer und Phosphat-spaltender Enzyme in den Mastzellen verschiedener Species sowie ihrer Bedeutung und Aktivitätsänderung unter physiologischen und pathologischen Zuständen, insbesondere bei der akuten Entzündung.

Dabei wurde gefunden, daß bei allen untersuchten Species und beim Menschen in den Mastzellen eine Aminopeptidase vorkommt, deren Aktivität an die Mast-zellgranula gebunden ist (Abb. 1). Dies ergibt sich aus dem Aktivitätsnachweis an den nach akuter Entgranulierung mit der Substanz 48/80 frei vorliegenden Mastzellgranula. Ein weiterer Beweis ist darin zu sehen, daß an fetalen Ratten-mastzellen die Enzymaktivität mit der Entwicklung und Reifung der Mastzell-granula (Tab. 1), die zunächst einzeln auftreten, an diesen nachweisbar wird (Abb. 2).

Bei der akuten Kreislaufstörung kommt es wie beim akuten Entzündungsab-lauf zum weitgehenden Verlust der Aminopeptidasereaktion (Abb. 3). Die Amino-peptidase vermag verschiedene künstliche Substrate, bei denen Aminosäuren mit Beta-Naphthylamid verbunden sind, zu spalten. Von besonderem Interesse ist in diesem Zusammenhang, daß auch Histidin-Beta-Naphthylamid hydrolysiert wird,

* Mit Unterstützung durch die Deutsche Forschungsgemeinschaft und der Stiftung Volks-wagenwerk. Elektronenoptische Abbildungen von Prof. Dr. F. MILLER.

Tabelle 1. a—d *Relative Zunahme toluidinblau-färbbarer Rattenmastzellen, bei abgestuftem pH in verschiedenen Entwicklungsstadien, a Ergebnisse an frühfetalen Mastzellen, b Ergebnisse kurz vor und nach der Geburt, c Ergebnisse zwischen dem 5. und 20. Lebenstag, d Färbbarkeit der Zellen des P-815 Mastocytoms mit Toluidinblaulösungen von abgestuftem pH,*
[aus Virchows Arch. path. Anat. **335**, 72 (1962)]

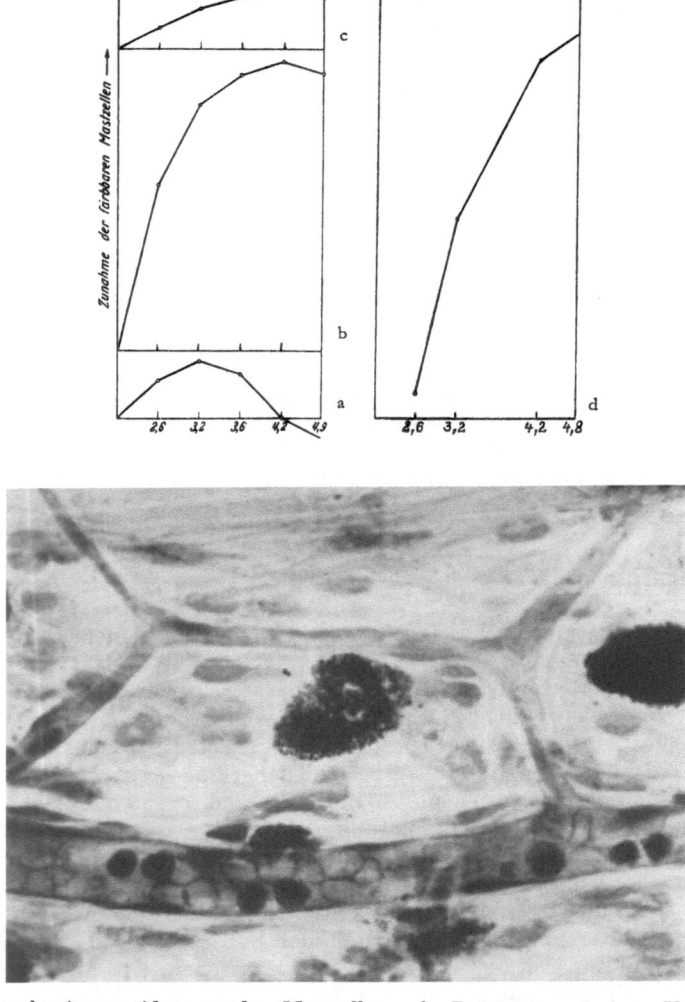

Abb. 1. Leuzylaminopeptidase an den Mastzellgranula, Rattenmesenterium. Vergr. 800fach
[aus Beitr. path. Anat. **124**, 251 (1961)]

wobei Histidin frei wird, das sekundär decarboxyliert werden kann, ein Befund, der für die Biochemie der akuten Entzündung bedeutungsvoll erscheint.

Eine Glutamylpeptidase oder Glutamyltranspeptidase wurde nicht nachgewiesen (Tab. 2).

Ganz besonderes Interesse gewinnt ein beim Menschen und beim Hund nachweisbares Trypsin-artiges Enzym, das durch die bekannten Trypsininhibitoren

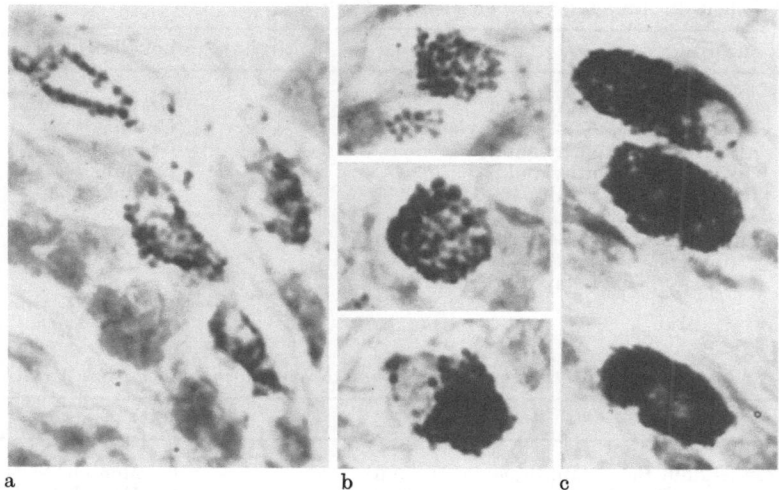

a   b   c

Abb. 2a—c. Aminopeptidasereaktion bei verschiedenen Entwicklungsstufen der Mastzellen. Stetige Zunahme des Reaktionsniederschlages an den Granula. Vergr. 1500fach. a 19 Tage alter Fet, b 2 Tage alte Ratte, c 9 Tage alte Ratte [aus Virchows Arch. path. Anat. **335**, 72 (1962)]

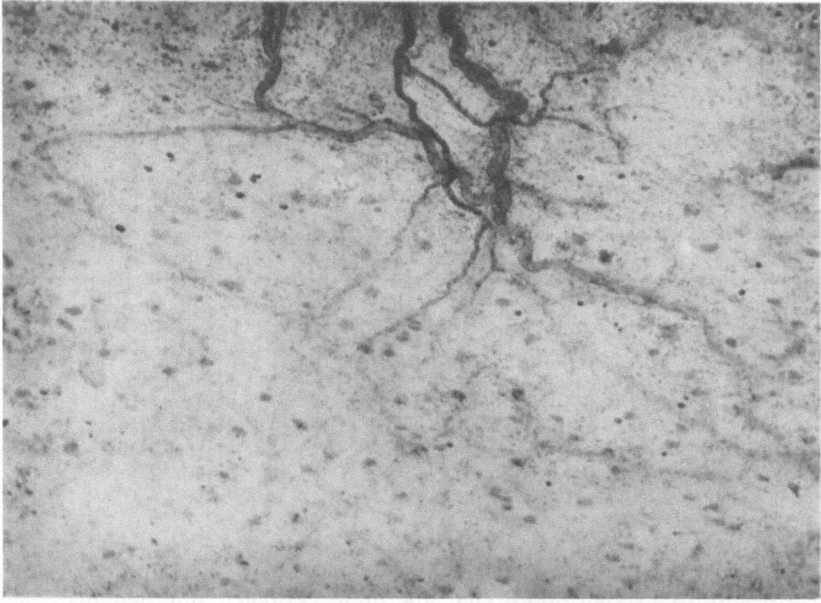

Abb. 3. Akute Zirkulationsstörung am Rattenmesenterium nach Gefäßunterbindung. Starke Abnahme der Leuzylaminopeptidasereaktion an den meisten Mastzellen. Vergr. 30fach [aus Beitr. path. Anat. **124**, 251 (1961)]

nicht hemmbar ist, das jedoch durch den Esteraseblocker Diisopropylfluorophosphat gehemmt wird (Tab. 3).

Auch andere von uns in den Mastzellen histochemisch nachgewiesene Enzyme, wie saure Phosphatase und ATP-ase, sind an die Mastzellgranula gebunden und werden mit der Entwicklung der Mastzellen an den Granula nachweisbar (Abb. 4).

Tabelle 2. *Aminopeptidasenachweis an Mastzellen*

Substrat	Aktivität	Lokalisation
Leuzyl-Beta-Naphthylamid	+++	Granula
Leuzyl-4-Methoxy-2-Naphthylamid	+++	Granula
Alanyl-Beta-Naphthylamid	+++	Granula
Glycil-Beta-Naphthylamid	++	Granula
Histidin-Beta-Naphthylamid	+	Granula
Alpha-Glutamyl-Beta-Naphthylamid	—	
Gamma-Glutamyl-Beta-Naphthylamid (transpeptidaseartiges Enzym)	—	
L-Cystin-di-Beta-Naphthylamid	—	

Tabelle 3.
Amidase- und esterolytische Aktivität mit Trypsin-ähnlichen Eigenschaften beim Menschen

Substrat	Aktivität
DL-Benzoyl-Arginin-Beta-Naphthylamid (BANA)	+++ Mensch +, Hund +
DL-Benzoyl-Lysin-Beta-Naphthylamid (BLyNA)	+++ Mensch +, Hund —
L-Tosyl-L-Arginin-Beta-Naphthylamid (TANA)	—
D-Benzoyl-Arginin-Beta-Naphthylamid	— kompetitiver HK
Epsilon-Aminocaproyl-Beta-Naphthylamid (ε-ACA-NA)	— kompetitiver HK
Trypsininhibitoren	
BANA + Sojabohneninhibitor	+++
BANA + Ovomucoid	+++
BANA + Trasylol	+++
BANA + DFP	—

Tabelle 4. *Esteraseaktivitäten an den Mastzellen verschiedener Species und des Menschen. Nachweis mit synthetischen Substraten*

Substrat	Aktivität	Species
Alpha-Naphthylacetat	— (+)	Ratte —, Mensch (+)
Naphthol-ASD-Acetat	+	Ratte
Naphthol-AS-Cl-Acetat	+++	Mensch, Hund
Naphthol-ASD-Cl-Acetat	+++	Mensch, Ratte
Naphthol-AS-Beta-Alanyl-Glycinat	+++	Mensch, Hund
Naphthol-AS-Epsilon-Aminocaproat	+++	Mensch, Hund
Naphthol-AS-D-Epsilon-Aminocaproat	+++	Mensch, Hund
Thioessigsäure	—	Ratte
5-Bromindoxylacetat	—	Ratte

Beim Nachweis esterolytischer Aktivitäten wurden zahlreiche künstliche Substrate geprüft. Dabei ergab sich aus dem Vergleich mit den histochemisch nachweisbaren Esterasen des tubulären Systems der Niere und verschiedener Organe, daß die Mastzellen mehrere Esterasen besitzen (Tab. 4).

Zum Vergleich esterolytischer Aktivitäten in Blut- und Bindegewebszellen mit Enzymaktivitäten an Mastzellen wurden die Ergebnisse anderer Autoren und die eigenen tabellarisch zusammengefaßt (Tab. 5).

Während die Bedeutung der Proteolyse bis zur Peptidspaltung beim Entzündungsgeschehen leicht verständlich ist, ist die esterolytischer Aktivitäten wesentlich schwieriger zu beurteilen.

Auch Beta-Glucuronidase war an den Mastzellen besonders des Meerschweinchens nachweisbar (Abb. 5).

Elektronenoptisch stellen die Mastzellgranula dichte Partikel dar, deren
Struktur deutliche Speciesunterschiede aufweist (Abb. 6 bis 8). Während sie bei der
Ratte weitgehend homogen erscheinen, ergibt sich beim Meerschweinchen ein
stoffartiges, wie gewebt aussehendes Muster. Für die menschlichen Mastzellgranula typisch sind wirbelartige Strukturen, die wie Fingerabdrücke erscheinen.

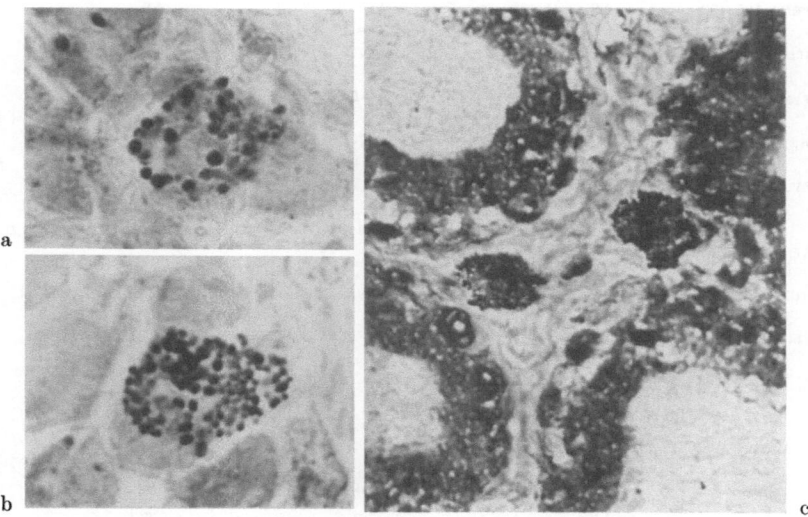

Abb. 4a—c. Saure Phosphatasereaktion. a Enzymreaktion an den Granula bei einem 20 Tage
alten Feten, b Reaktion bei 2 Tage alter Ratte, c Reaktion beim erwachsenen Tier. Vergr.
a und b 1800fach, c 800fach [aus Virchows Arch. path. Anat. **335**, 72 (1962)]

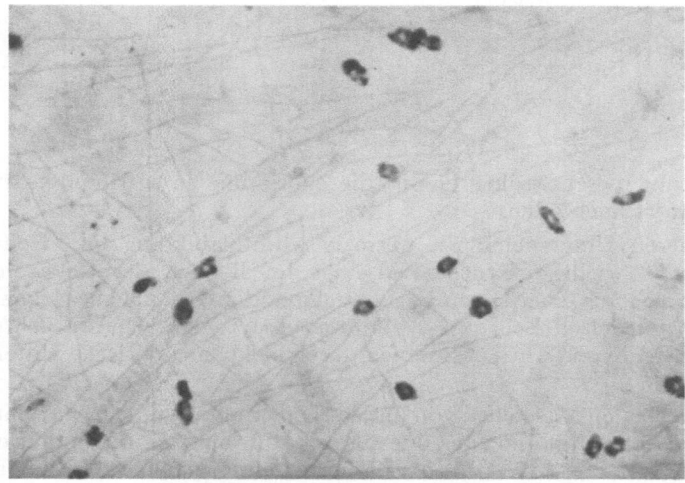

Abb. 5. β-Glucuronidasereaktion an den Mastzellen des Meerschweinchenmesenteriums. Vergr.
180fach [aus Beitr. path. Anat. **124**, 251 (1961)]

Tabelle 5. *Esteraseaktivitäten in Blut- und Bindegewebszellen.*
Nachweis mit verschiedenen synthetischen Substraten.

| Autor | Blut | | | | | | | | |
| | Lymphocyten | | | Monocyten | | | Neutrophile | | |
	N	N-Cl	Br-J	N	N-Cl	Br-J	N	N-Cl	Br-J
GOMORI, 1953	AS-Cl ∅			AS-D (+)	AS-Cl ∅			AS-Cl ∅-+	
BENDITT, 1956									
WACHSTEIN, 1958/59	AS (+)			AS ++			AS ++		
BRAUNSTEIN, 1958/59	α-N (+)			α-N +			∅		
ACKERMAN, 1959/60	x+ß-N AS ∅		(+)	α+ß-N AS ∅		(+)	NAS ∅ ASD (+)		(+)
LÖFFLER, 1959/61	α-N-AS (+)		(+)	α-N-AS +++			α-NAS +		+
MOLONEY, 1960		ASDCl ∅			ASDCl ∅		AS, ASD ∅	AS-Cl ASDCl +++	
LENNERT, LÖFFLER, 1960									
SCHÜMMELFEDER, 1961				AS +				ASDCl +	
LAMBERS, 1962							ASD +++		
KELLER, 1962									
KELLER, 1963									
BAKALOS, 1963	AS (+)			AS +++			AS ++		
HOPSU, 1963									
LEDER, 1963	AS +	ASDCl ∅		AS +++	ASDCl (+)			ASDCl +++	
LENNERT, 1963	α-N-AS ASD (+)								
LÖFFLER, 1963	AS +			AS +++	ASDCl (+)		AS +	ASDCl +	
Eigene Befunde				AS +++	ASDCl ∅	∅	AS ∅	ASDCl +++	∅

Die Bedeutung dieser Strukturen und die Zuordnung zu bestimmten Inhaltstoffen der Granula ist noch offen.

In früheren Untersuchungen über die Granulabildung und Reifung wurde gefunden, daß wichtige Synthesevorgänge im Bereich der Golgizone erfolgen. Dies ergibt sich aus einer engen Lagebeziehung der Granula zur Golgizone, besonders an abgesiedelten Zellen von Mäusemastocytomen. Unsere lichtoptisch gewonnenen Ergebnisse wurden kürzlich durch elektronenoptische Untersuchungen bestätigt.

Die in normalen Mastzellen von uns erstmals wahrscheinlich gemachte Histidindecarboxylaseaktivität und von SCHAYER mit Hilfe einer Isotopendilutionsmethode sicher nachgewiesene Aktivität, die an normalen Mastzellen sehr niedrig ist, aber an Mastocytomen außerordentlich hoch sein kann (Tab. 6), ist nicht an die Granula gebunden, sondern es handelt sich um ein cytoplasmatisches Lyoenzym.

N = jeweiliges Naphthylacetat (Naphthylacetat Naphthol AS-Acetat Naphthol AS-D-Acetat)
NCl = Naphthol AS-D-Chloracetat   BrJ = 5-Bromindoxylacetat

Blut						Gewebe								
Eosinophile			Basophile			Mastzellen			Makroph. Histiocyten			Reticulumzellen		
N	N-Cl	Br-J	N	N-Cl	Br-J	N	N-Cl	Br-J	N	N-Cl	Br-J	N	N-Cl	Br-J
	AS-Cl ∅						+++							
?									α-N +++					
α-ß-N AS ∅ α-NAS (+)	ASDCl ∅	(+)	α-ß-N AS ∅ AS ++	ASDCl ∅					α-NAS +	ASDCl +++				
ASD ∅			ASD ∅			AS +++ α-N +	ASDCl ∅ ASCl +++	+++						
AS (+)			?			α-N, AS ∅	+							
?	ASDCl ∅					α-NAS +	ASDCl +++		AS +++	ASDCl (+)		α-N ++ ASD +		
AS +		∅	AS +		∅	AS ++ α-N, + ASD	ASDCl + ASDCl	+++						

Tabelle 6. *Histidindecarboxylaseaktivität an Mäusemastocytomen*
Enzymquelle: Überstand nach Zentrifugierung des Tumorhomogenates bei 150000 (g)

Tumor I: erzeugt durch Methylcholanthren	Tumor I (DUNN u. POTTER P 815 Mastocytom)		Tumor II (FURTH u. Mitarb.)	
	γ/g Gewebe			
Tumor II: erzeugt durch Röntgenstrahlen	Histamin im Leeransatz	Bildung bei Zusatz von Pyrid.-5' Ph.	Histamin im Leeransatz	Bildung bei Zusatz von Pyrid.-5' Ph.
niedrigster Wert	380	0	200	360
höchster Wert	1680	1920	720	2100
Mittelwert aus 7 Messungen	720	390	540	1200

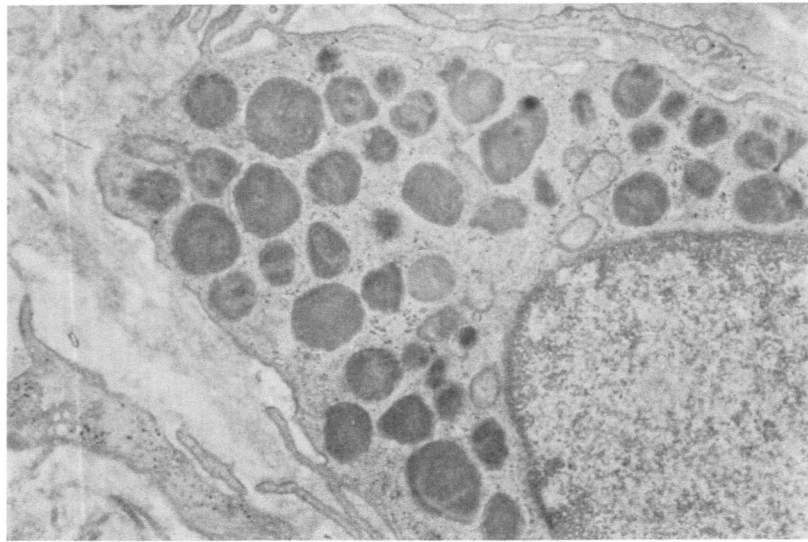

Abb. 6. Mastzelle aus der Haut des Menschen. Zellkern rechts unten. Vergr. 105000fach

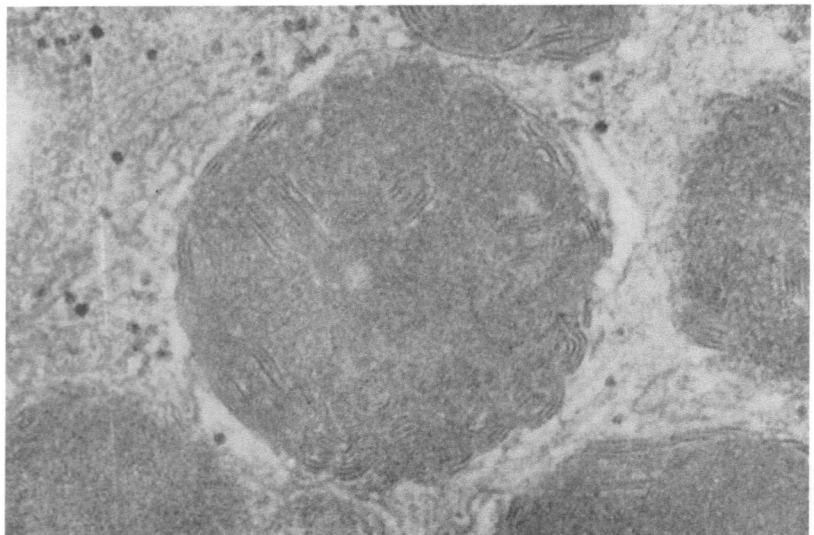

Abb. 7. Feinstruktur der Mastzellgranula des Menschen. Vergr. 660000fach

Ein zweites nicht mastzellgebundenes histidindecarboxylierendes Enzym ist wahrscheinlich an das Capillarmesenchym gebunden. Dies ergibt sich aus Untersuchungen SCHAYERs und eigenen Versuchen über die Aktivitätssteigerung der Histidindecarboxylase im Endotoxinschock, die durch Glucocorticoide zu verhindern ist (Tab. 7 bis 10).

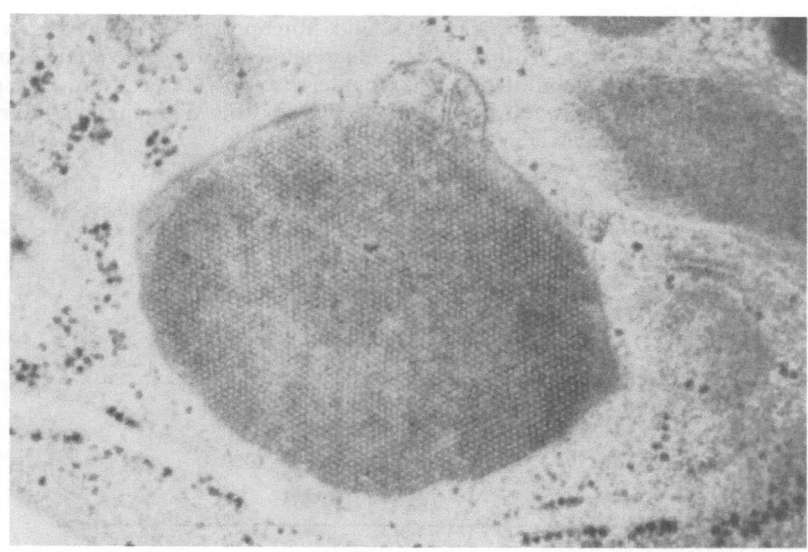

Abb. 8. Feinstruktur eines Mastzellgranulums des Meerschweinchens. Vergr. 480000fach

Tabelle 7. *Isotopendilutionsmethode zur Bestimmung der Histidindecarboxylaseaktivität in Anlehnung an* Schayer

Inkubat:		*Trennungsschritte:*
Gewebsextrakt, Pyridoxalphosphat $5 \cdot 10^{-4}$ m Ring-2-C^{14}-Histidin 5 γ Aminoguanidin 10^{-4} Tetracyclin 10/ml	37 °C, 3 Std, N_2-Atmosphäre $\longrightarrow$ Inaktivierung mit 2n $HClO_4$ Eindampfen	Histidin-Histamin-Trennung durch Butanolextraktion mit Carriersubstanzen, Überführung in HCl
Kristallisation:		*Messung:*
Histamin + Benzolsulfochlorid $\rightarrow$ Benzolsulfonylhistamin (Sulfonamidreaktion), Kristallreinigung	Trocknen der Kristalle $\longrightarrow$	Auflösung der Kristalle in Szintillatorflüssigkeit und Impulsmessung im Szintillationszähler

Tabelle 8. *Erhöhung der Histidindecarboxylaseaktivität der Rattenlunge nach Endotoxingabe und Hemmung dieses Effektes durch Glucocorticoide*

	Kontrollen	Verabreichung von Endotoxin	Verabreichung von Endotoxin und Glucocorticoid
	900	3900	500
	0	8000	0
	1100	3200	0
	1500	1400	1300
	0	3800	0
	1400	2500	0
	900	5500	
	2000	3700	
	4700	(3000—5000)	
Mittelwerte:	1388	4000	300

Ergebnisse in Impulse/min/100 mg BSH.

Außer den bekannten Aminwirkungen und Mucopolysaccharidwirkungen ist somit noch eine dritte Stoffgruppe in den Mastzellen aktuell geworden, nämlich die meist an die Granula gebundenen Enzyme der Proteo-, Estero- und Phosphat-hydrolyse (Tab. 11), wobei sich die Diskussion über die Wertung der Mastzell-granula als eine Sonderform von Lysosomen aufdrängt.

Tabelle 9. *Die Histidindecarboxylaseaktivität in der Mäuselunge im Endotoxinschock. Änderung des Effektes nach Glucocorticoid-behandlung*

	Kontrollen	Verabreichung von Endotoxin	Verabreichung von Endotoxin und Gluco-corticoid
	0	15500	3700
	0	18300	3000
	0	17000	4680
	0	17500	
		18580	
Mittelwerte:	0	17378	3793

Impulse/min/100 mg BSH.

Tabelle 10. *Zeitlicher Ablauf der Enzyminduktion und Verhalten der Corticosteronkonzentration im Blutplasma*

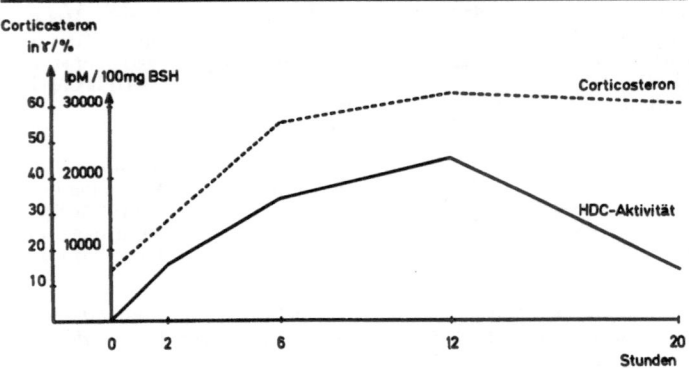

Tabelle 11. *Effects of substances and enzymes of mastcells*

1. *Biogenous amines:* a) Histamine: vasodilatation, increase of permeability, stimulation of phagocytosis; b) 5-hydroxytryptamine (rat, mouse): increase of permeability, pain-pro-ducing substance.

2. *Heparin and other Mucopolysaccharides:* decrease of blood coagulation (dog), poly-electrolyte-effect: inhibition of different enzymes.

3. *Proteolytic enzymes:* a) Aminopeptidase: liberation of different amino-acids, f.i. histidine of dipeptides; b) chymase (chymotrypsin-like enzyme); c) tryptase (trypsin-like enzyme) (man and dog).

4. *Esterolytic enzymes:* splitting of different synthetic substrates.

5. *Phosphate-hydrolysis:* unspecific acid phosphatase and ATPase.

6. *Splitting of glucuronide* (guinea pig).

7. *Amino acid-decarboxylases* (Histidine- and 5-Hydroxytryptophan-decarboxylase.)

Electronmicroscopy of Merkel's Tastzelle

K. K. Mustakallio and U. Kiistala, Univ. Centr. Hosp., Dept. of Dermatology, Helsinki (Finland)

Bilddemonstration zur mikroskopischen Anatomie des Haarfollikels im Verlauf des Haarcyclus

H.-J. Bandmann und K. Bosse, Dermatologische Klinik und Poliklinik der Universität München (Deutschland)

An insgesamt 13 Abbildungen wird die Gestalt des menschlichen Follikels in seinen verschiedenen Wachstumsphasen gezeigt*.

Während das Kolben(= Telogen)-Haar in seinem Bulbusbereich völlig verhornt in der äußeren Wurzelscheide ruht oder bereits gänzlich abgestoßen ist, wächst aus der Matrix ein Epithelstrang der Papille entgegen. Die Abbildung zeigt, daß ein solcher Strang mehrfingerig ausgebildet sein kann.

Die Oberflächenhäutchen (= Cuticulae) des Haares und der inneren Wurzelscheide weisen in ihrem proximalen Bereich eine feine ineinandergreifende Zähnelung auf, welche beim Anagenhaar der Extraktion entgegenwirkt.

Der Übergang vom Bulbus(Anagen)-Haar zum Kolben(Telogen)-Haar wird über das Katagenhaar vollzogen. Die Abbildung zeigt ein Haar von diesem Typ im Tangentialschnitt mit Beginn der Wurzelverhornung.

Bei Fluorchromierung mit Akridinorange (1:200 bei pH 4,79) lassen sich die morphologischen Unterschiede des extrahierten Anagen- und Telogenhaars besonders deutlich demonstrieren.

Der total verhornte Telogenhaarbulbus leuchtet hellgrün in einem orangefarbenen Epithelsäckchen (äußere Wurzelscheide), während sich bei Anagenhaaren die gelbgrüne innere Wurzelscheide deutlich von der orangefarbenen äußeren Wurzelscheide abhebt.

Die Stratigraphie eines Anagenhaares wird an einem medianen Sagittalschnitt demonstriert. Von den nur unregelmäßig anzutreffenden Bestandteilen ist hier eine nah distal reichende Marksäule zu beobachten.

In einem paramedianen Sagittalschnitt eines Anagenhaares wird der Übergang vom Matrixepithel zum verhornten Schaft demonstriert.

Ein dicker Schnitt zeigt an einem mit Gallocyanin gefärbten Präparat die Stratigraphie der verschiedenen Schichten und deren Verhornungszonen (Anagenhaar).

Die Henlesche Schicht mit ihren eigenartigen Verhornungen ist im Gegensatz zu den anderen Schichten des Anagenhaares peroxydasehaltig. Sie kann deshalb mit Benzidin oder 1-Naphtol dargestellt werden.

Auch durch den Verlust der inneren Wurzelscheiden kann das Telogenhaar charakterisiert werden, wie an Transversalschnitten von Anagen- und Telogenhaaren demonstriert wird.

---

* Die Abbildungen sind als Serie mit 12 Kleinbild-Dias gesondert erschienen. Rückfragen bei: Literarische Abteilung der Firma Carl Zeiss, 7082 Oberkochen/Württ., Deutschland.

Zur Ultrastruktur des menschlichen Haarfollikels

V. Puccinelli und R. Caputo, Dermat. Klinik der Universität Mailand
(Italien)

In der Entwicklung des Reifungsprozesses des Follikels zeigen die Ultralängsschnitte, wie von der Zone der undifferenzierten Zellen verschiedene Zellstränge

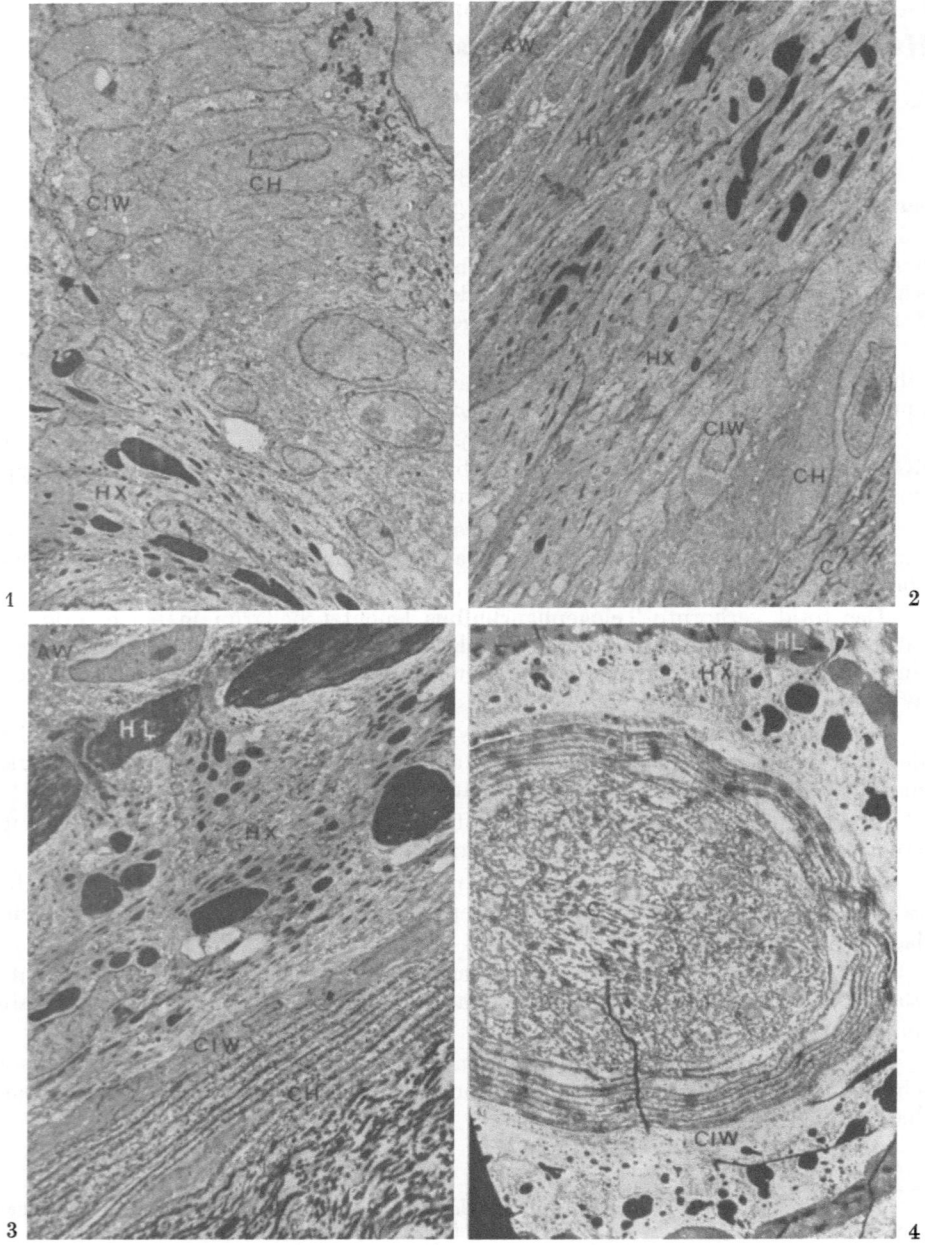

ausgehen, die einen gut differenzierten Charakter haben und sich von der Peripherie zur Haarachse hin zusammensetzen aus: 1. äußerer Wurzelscheide; 2. innerer Wurzelscheide, bestehend aus a) der Henleschen, b) der Huxleyschen Scheide und c) der Cuticula der inneren Wurzelscheide; 3. Cuticula des Haares; 4. Cortex des Haares.

Abb. 1 zeigt im Längsschnitt im untersten Abschnitt des Follikels, wie die Cuticula des Haares und diejenige der inneren Wurzelscheide aus zwei Zellsträngen bestehen, deren cylindrische Zellen zur Haarachse im rechten Winkel stehen.

Aus Abb. 2 und 3 ersieht man sowohl die progressive Reifung der Zellen der Scheiden von HENLE und HUXLEY, gekennzeichnet durch das Vorhandensein von Trichohyalinkörnern, als auch die typische Entwicklung der Zellen der beiden Cuticulae, die sich verlängern und nach und nach parallel zur Haarachse zu liegen kommen.

Die Zellen der Henleschen Scheide vervollkommnen den Prozeß der Keratogenese vor denen der Huxleyschen Scheide (Abb. 3).

Abb. 4 gibt im Querschnitt einen panoramischen Überblick über alle Lagen des Follikels und veranschaulicht, wie unterschiedlich in ihnen der keratogenetische Vorgang abläuft.

C Cortex, CH Cuticula des Haares, CIW Cuticula der inneren Wurzelscheide, HX Huxleysche Scheide, HL Henlesche Scheide, AW Äußere Wurzelscheide.

Zur licht- und elektronenoptischen Struktur der Nerven am Haar

E. HAGEN, Abteilung für Experimentelle Biologie im Anatomischen Institut der Universität Bonn (Deutschland), und
G. NIEBAUER, II. Universitäts-Hautklinik Wien (Österreich)

Während eines Zeitraumes von mehr als 50 Jahren waren die morphologischen Studien von v. FREY (1895) für die Sinnesphysiologie der Haut maßgebend. Heute kann seine Lehre von der Spezifität der Endkörperchen nach vergleichenden, neurohistologischen Ergebnissen in ihrer ursprünglichen Konzeption nicht mehr vertreten werden; denn nur die *unbehaarte* Haut zeichnet sich durch eine formenreiche und mit verschiedenen Sinnesqualitäten identifizierte Endigungsweise cerebrospinaler Fasern aus. Derartige nervöse Endkörperchen fehlen in der *behaarten*, nicht krankhaft veränderten Haut bis auf vereinzelt vorkommende Lamellenkörperchen fast gänzlich. Regelmäßig läßt sich jedoch eine spezialisierte Nervenformation im Bereich der Haarfollikel nachweisen (Abb. 1). Die sog. ,,nervöse Haarmanschette'' stellt in ihrer Funktion ein sensibles Receptororgan dar. Eine dichte vegetative Nervenfaserhülle ergänzt die Innervation des Haares (Abb. 2). Das anatomische Prinzip der Innervation des Haares zeigt beim Menschen keine Unterschiede zwischen den kleinen Terminalhaaren und den Borsten- und Langhaaren. Die Differenzen liegen in der Quantität und im Kaliber der Fasern.

Die Nervenmanschette um das Haar, die hauptsächlich aus sensiblen Fasern aufgebaut ist, liegt an der oberen Einschnürung des Follikels zwischen der Einmündung der Talgdrüse und dem Ansatz des Haarmuskels. Wahrscheinlich kommt dieser Lagerung der nervösen Hülse bei den Vorgängen des Haarcyclus besondere Bedeutung zu (NIEBAUER, 1966).

Die Nervenmanschette des Haares wird aus zwei gitterförmig übereinander gelagerten Formationen von Nervenfasern gebildet. Sie liegt hülsenartig der

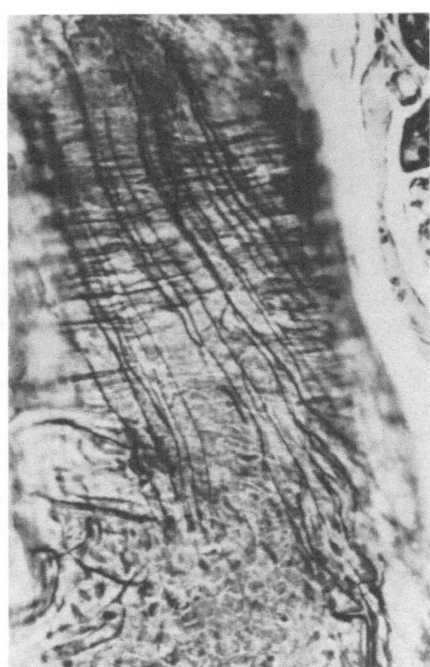

Abb. 1. Nervengitterbildung an der Haarwurzelscheide, Hund, Palisadenfasern, Ringfasern. Richardson-Newton-Methode. Präp.: G. TROSSMANN. Neg.-Vergr.: 64×

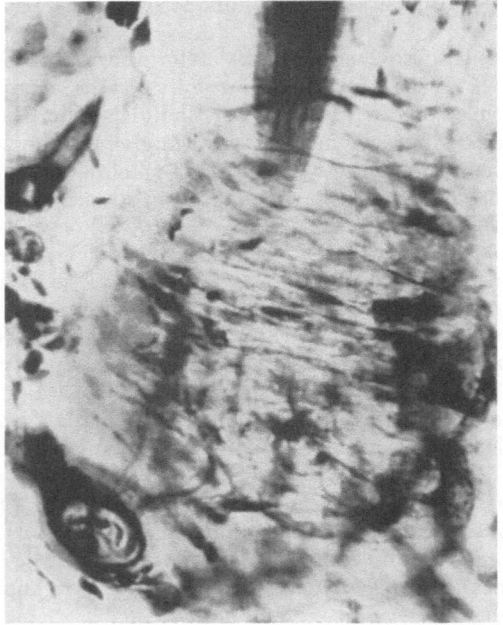

Abb. 2. Bindegewebiger Haarbalg mit Spiraltouren vegetativer Nervenfasern. Behaarte Haut, Mensch. Bielschowsky-Gross-Methode. Neg.-Vergr.: 160×

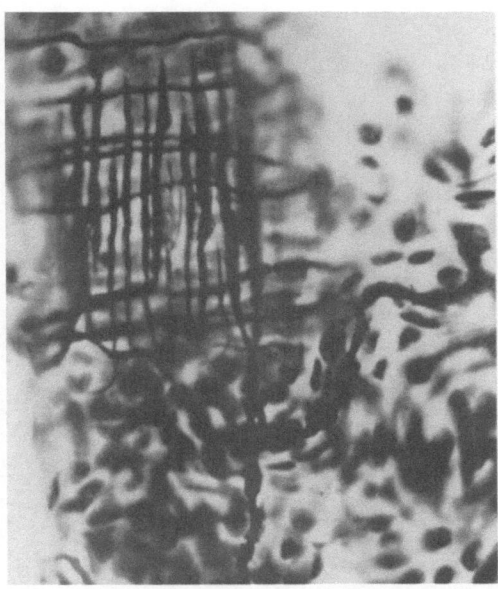

Abb. 3. Nervengitterbildung (Manschette) an der Haarwurzelscheide mit zuführender mark-
haltiger Nervenfaser in der Haarpapille. Behaarte Haut, Mensch. Bielschowsky-Gross-Methode.
Neg.-Vergr.: 325 ×

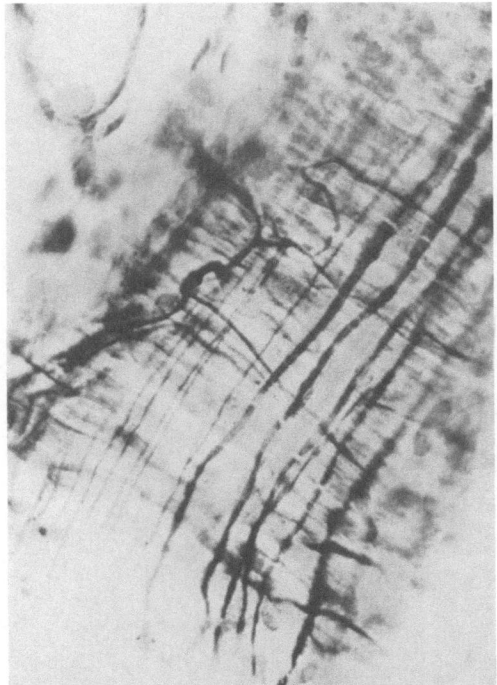

Abb. 4. Aufteilung einer Nervenringfaser an der äußeren Haarwurzelscheide, sowie pali-
sadenförmig angeordnete Nervenfasern. Richardson-Newton-Methode. Präp.: G. TROSSMANN.
Neg.-Vergr.: 160 ×

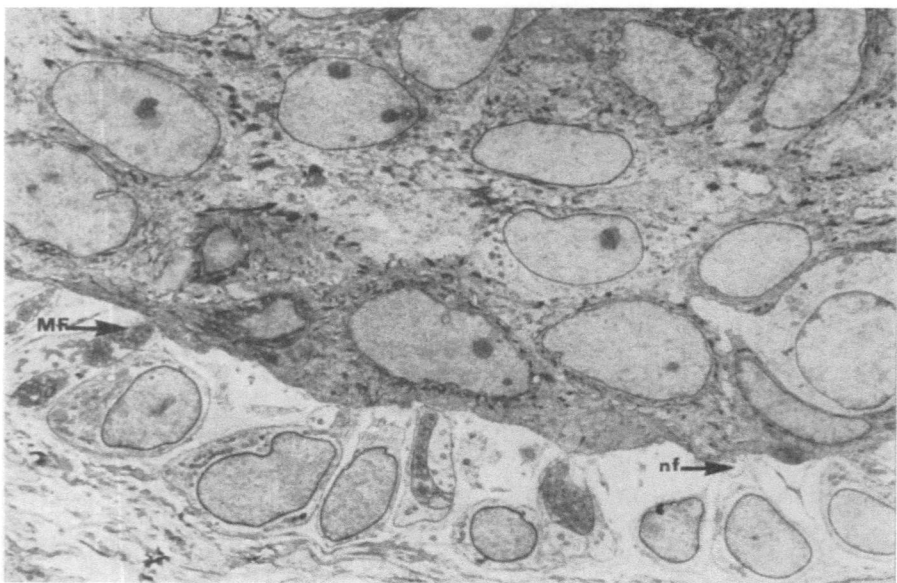

Abb. 5. Mitochondrienreiche große Axone (MF) und strukturarme kleinere Axone (nf) an der äußeren Wurzelscheide des Haares, Mensch. Schwannsche Zellen, Epithelzellen der äußeren Wurzelscheide. Neg.-Vergr.: 1700 ×

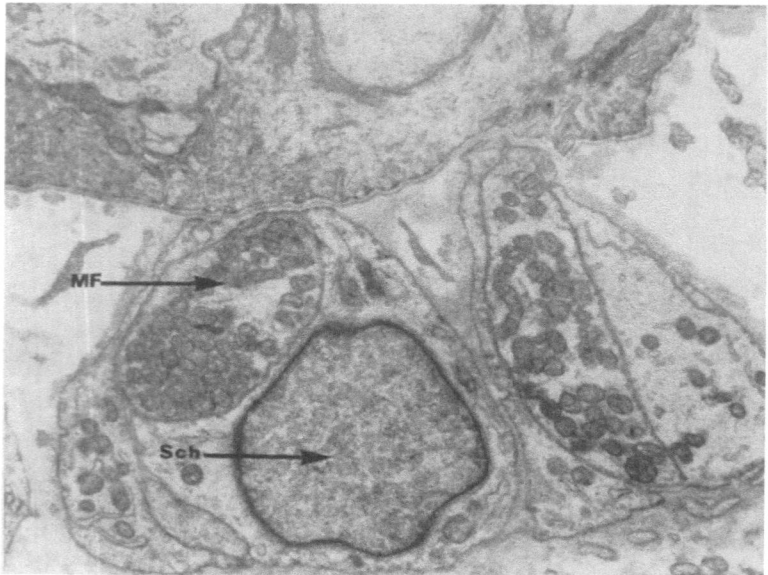

Abb. 6. Große, mitochondrienreiche Nervenfasern (MF) (cerebrospinale Nerven) mit Schwannscher Zelle. Schwannscher Nucleus (Sch). Haarwurzelscheide, Mensch. Neg.-Vergr.: 7000 ×

epidermalen Wurzelscheide unmittelbar auf. Die Nervenformationen ziehen mit ihren Nervenfasern parallel zur Haarwurzelachse aufwärts. Sie teilen sich gabelartig in dickere und dünnere Äste und bilden schließlich auf Höhe des Haarwurzelhalses eine palisadenartige Endformation (Abb. 3). Nach KADANOFF lassen sich etwa 30 bis 50 derartige Nervenendigungen kranzförmig um das Epithel der äußeren Wurzelscheide angeordnet nachweisen. Distal von dieser Formation liegt ein zweites System ringförmig verlaufender Nervenfasern (sog. ,,Nervenring") (Abb. 4). Palisaden und Ringgeflecht lassen die als nervöse Hüllschicht des Haares charakteristischen Gitterstrukturen entstehen. Es ist bisher nicht gelungen, eine Beteiligung der palisadenartigen Endigungen am Aufbau der Ringgeflechte zu beobachten.

Im bindegewebigen Haarbalg verlaufen dichte Spiraltouren vegetativer Nervenfasern. Auch in der bindegewebigen Papille lassen sich zahlreiche vegetative Nervenfasern nachweisen. Ihre Hauptmasse begleitet die Blutgefäße. Die zur Wurzelscheide ziehenden cerebrospinalen Nerven zeigen im bindegewebigen Bereich des Haares meist eine deutliche Markscheide (Abb. 3).

Zwei besondere morphologische Typen von Nervenfasern sind elektronenmikroskopisch an der äußeren Wurzelscheide des menschlichen Haares zu unterscheiden. Ein auffälliger Reichtum an Mitochondrien charakterisiert eine Anzahl von Axonen, die in Schwannsches Cytoplasma eingebettet der Basalmembran der äußeren Epithelzellen der Wurzelscheide eng anliegen (Abb. 5). Ein Teil kleinkalibriger Nervenfasern zeigt nur wenig Binnenstruktur, und die Axone entbehren ebenso wie die mitochondrienreichen Nervenfasern stellenweise zur Basalmembran der Wurzelscheide hin einer Schwannschen Cytoplasmahülle (Abb. 6). Das beträchtliche Kaliber und die Fülle der Mitochondrien sowie lichtmikroskopische Kontrollschnitte sprechen für die cerebrospinale Abkunft und die Identität der Nerven mit den Palisadenfasern, während die kleinen Axone wahrscheinlich als vegetative Nerven zu deuten sind.

Literatur. v. FREY, M.: 3. Ber. Sächs. Ges. Wiss. Leipzig **23**, 166 (1895). — HAGEN, E.: Nervensystem der Haut. In: J. JADASSOHNS. Hdb. der Haut u. Geschlechtskrankheiten, Erg.-Werk. Bd. I, 1. Berlin-Heidelberg-New York: Springer 1968. — KADANOFF, D.: Acta neuroveg. (Wien) 18, 159 (1958). — NIEBAUER, G.: Arch. klin. exp. Derm. **227**, 409 (1966).

Neuere Entwicklung der dermatologischen Virusforschung

TH. NASEMANN, Dermatologische Klinik und Poliklinik der Universität München (Deutschland)

Durch eine Auswahl elektronenmikroskopischer Abbildungen folgender fünf dermotroper Virusarten:

1. Molluscum contagiosum-Virus,
2. Paravaccinevirus (Melkerknoten),
3. Zostervirus,
4. Herpes simplex-Virus,
5. Warzenvirus,

sollte der Vortrag über neuere Entwicklung der dermatologischen Virusforschung anschaulicher gemacht werden (s. S. 301). Hier können nur drei Bilder wiedergegeben werden:

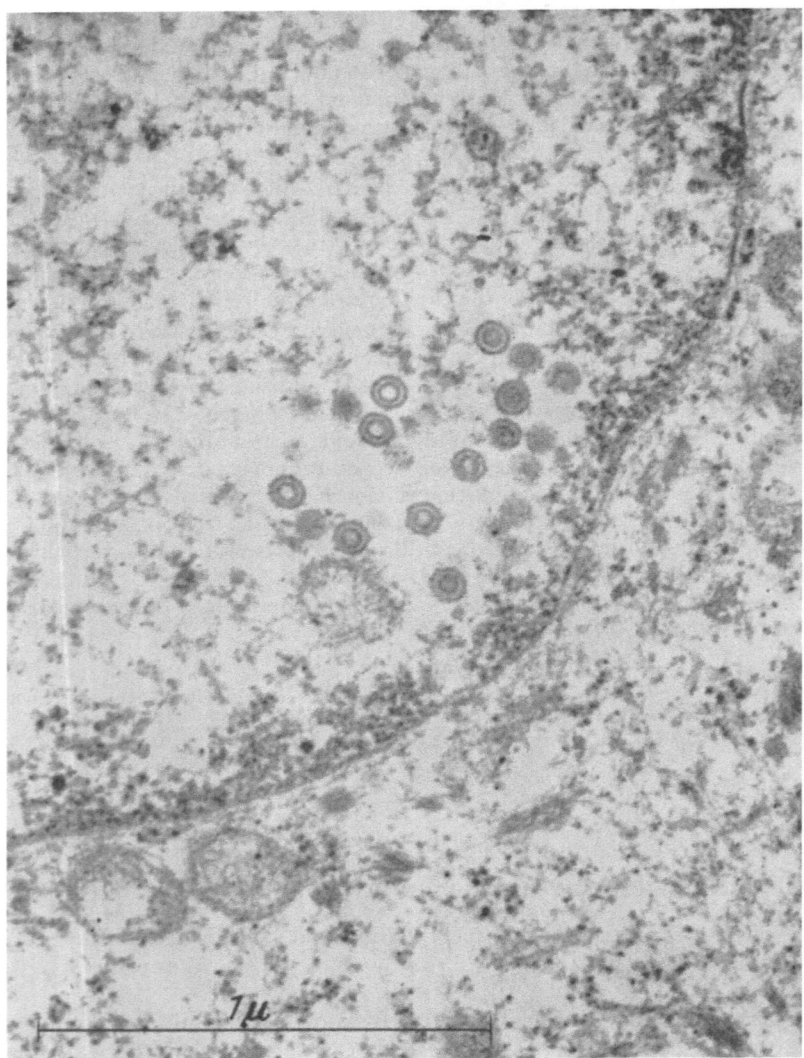

Abb. 1. Zostervirus. Ultraschnitt von Epidermis. Elementarkörper im Zellkern.
Vergr.: 60 000×

2 b   2 a

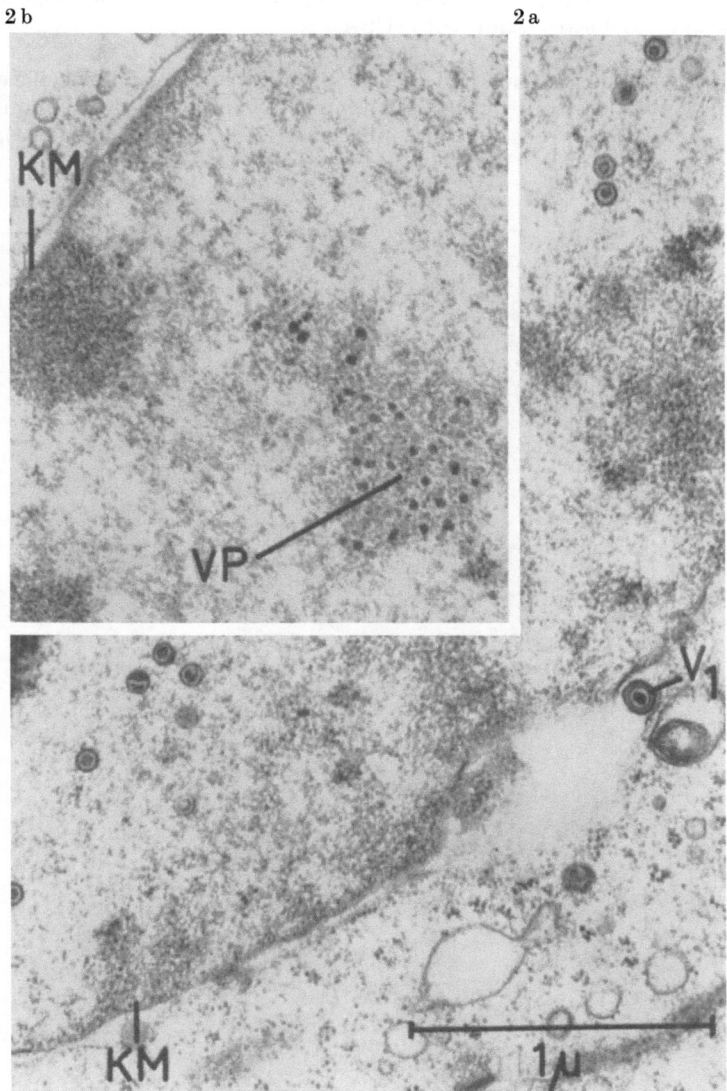

Abb. 2a: Herpes simplex-Virus. Ultraschnitt von HeLa-Zelle. Elementarkörper im Zellkern. V_1 aus dem Kernplasma in das Cytoplasma ausgeschleuster Elementarkörper. Beim Verlassen des Kernes wird aus der Kernwand die zweite Virusmembran aufgezogen. KM Kernmembran

Abb. 2b: wie Abb. 2a. Kernausschnitt aus frisch infizierter HeLa-Zelle. Noch keine reifen Elementarkörper vorhanden. Bildung des Herpesvirus in früher Phase, DNS-Verdichtungen als kleine Kugeln im Viroplasma (VP) sichtbar. Vergr.: 40000 ×

Recent Observations on Langerhans Cells

K. Wolff, R. K. Winkelmann and K. Holubar, I. Dermat. Clinic,
University of Vienna, and Section of Dermatology, Mayo Clinic and Mayo
Foundation, Rochester, Minnesota (USA)

1. These intraepidermal dendritic cells contain several species specific enzymes
which are probably controlled by genetic factors: In man, the rhesus monkey and
guinea pig Langerhans cells contain nucleoside phosphatases (Fig. 1a), in the

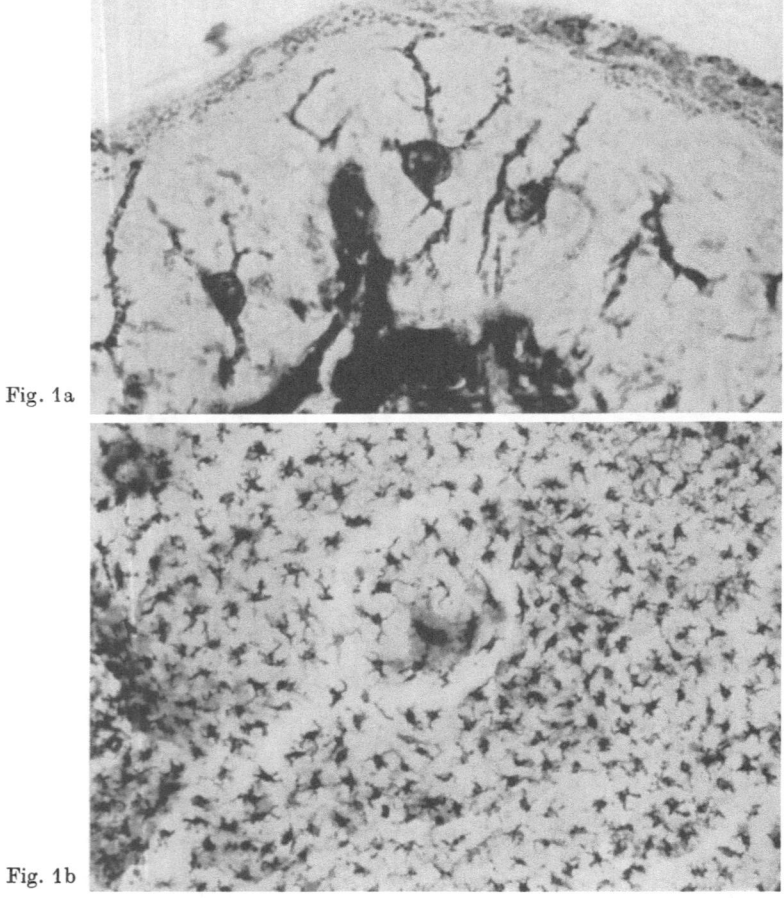

Fig. 1a

Fig. 1b

guinea pig also aminopeptidase, in Lorisidae alkaline phosphatase, in the sheep
and bat cholinesterase and in the mouse and rat aliesterase. Presumably, these
enzymes represent a hydrolytic capacity inherent in Langerhans cells.

2. Electronmicroscopically, Langerhans cells are characterized by a relatively
clear cytoplasm, a lobulated nucleus, a well developed Golgi zone, mitochondria,
endoplasmatic reticulum and lysosomes (Fig. 2). They produce peculiar disc-

shaped granules which appear as rod- or tennis racket-like profiles in cross-sections (Fig. 3) or as plate-like structures if cut face on. These organelles contain four sheets of particles which are spaced regularly at 60 Å and form   a three-dimensional lattice.

3. Quantitatively, Langerhans cells of the guinea pig constitute a constant intraepidermal cell population of approximately 920 cells per square millimeter

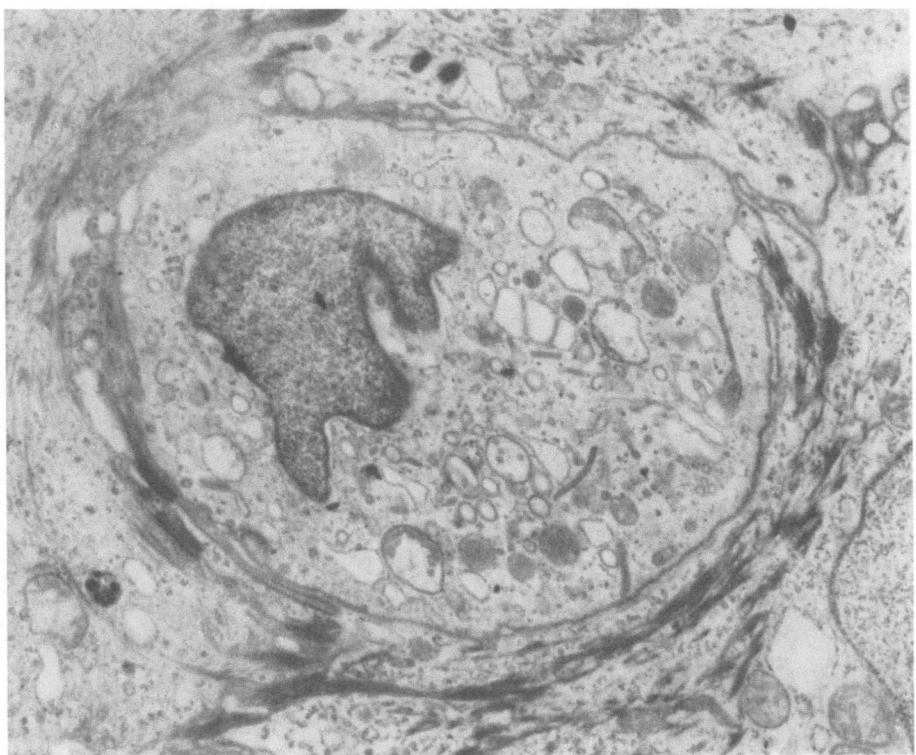

Fig. 2

of skin surface (Fig. 1 b). There are no significant differences between Langerhans cell counts in different animals of the same pigmentary strain, in pigmented and albino guinea pigs and in the pigmented and white spots of recessively spotted animals. In addition, the Langerhans cell population does not exhibit regional variations contrasting the pattern of distribution of melanocytes. There is no constant numerical relationship between the two cell types.

4. Ultraviolet light which induces considerable changes in melanocytes fails to elicit qualitative or quantitative changes in Langerhans cells which indicates that alterations of one dendritic cell population leaves the other completely unaffected.

5. After complete removal of the horny layers of the epidermis by the keratin-stripping technique almost the entire Langerhans cell population is trapped within a massive parakeratotic sheet of the epithelium and subsequently shed with it. The regenerating epidermis is initially almost devoid of but is gradually repopulated by Langerhans cells. So far, there is no proof for an immigration of these cells from the dermis but this process appears probable.

6. Langerhans cells are unique intraepidermal dendritic cells which differ from melanocytes in many respects: in their ultrastructural features, in their definitely different capacity for melanin production, in their different enzymatic properties, in their localization within the epidermis, their quantitative behaviour, regional distribution and in their dissimilar response to experimental stimuli. These data indicate that they *represent two distinct, independent and self maintaining cell populations.*

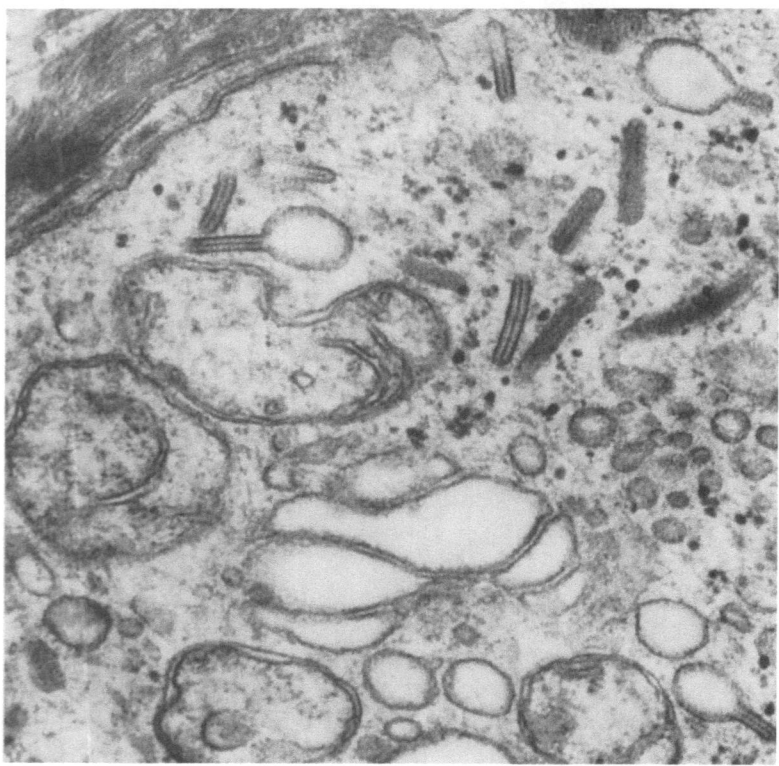

Fig. 3

Recent observations of "Langerhans cell granules" in histiocytic cells of histiocytosis X suggest that there may be a relationship of these cells and the intraepidermal dendrocytes. The structural identity of Langerhans cells and histiocytosis X-cells, their enzymes which are typical for mesenchymal tissues, their phagocytic ability and the possibility of their migration from the dermis into the epidermis may be considered suggestive of their mesenchymal nature.

Malignant Melanomas: Subcellular Differentiation of Nevocytic and Melanocytic Ontogeny*

Y. Mishima, Departments of Dermatology, Wayne State University, School of Medicine, Detroit General Hospital, Detroit, Michigan, and Veterans Administration Hospital, Dearborn, Michigan (USA)

Two biologically and clinically distinct entities of malignant melanoma have been found in man [1]. In contrast to malignant melanoma (malignant nevocytoma) developing from junction nevus, melanoma (malignant melanocytoma) arising from melanosis circumscripta praecancerosa (Dubreuilh) shows slower growth, delayed metastasis, and radiosensitivity [2, 3]. Furthermore, nevus cells of junction nevi are infrequently transformed to malignant melanoma cells and

Table. *Ontogenesis of melanotic tumors. Benign juvenile melanoma is considered a variant of nevus cell nevi and similarly has junctional, compound, and intradermal forms*

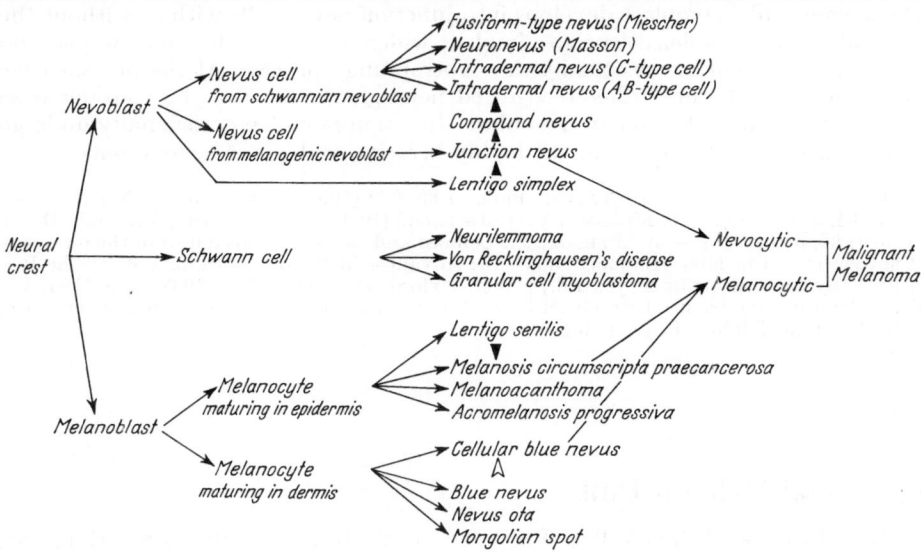

generally become intradermal nevus cells by the "dropping off" process, losing their ability for active melanin synthesis [4]. On the other hand, the neoplastic melanocytes of Dubreuilh's precancerous melanosis usually develop in exposed areas after middle age and are frequently transformed to malignant melanoma cells, acquiring intense melanin biosynthesis. It was further found that Dubreuilh's precancerous melanosis and precancerous junction nevus differ in their melanosome fine structure as well as other subcellular and cellular characteristics: enzymic activities of tyrosinase, cholinesterase and acid phosphatase; pigment transfer; mode of genesis; and mode and rate of malignant transformation [5]. The differences in malignancy, radiosensitivity, and prognosis, together with differences in

* This investigation was supported by Public Health Service Research Grant No. CA-05580-06 and CA-08891-01 from the National Cancer Institute, No. AM-07981-04 from the National Institute of Arthritis and Metabolic Diseases.

biological behaviour, may be explained by the separate ontogenies of these two malignant melanomas.

Our working hypothesis for the origin and pathogenesis of all "melanotic tumors" [6] is summarized in the table. The neural crest differentiates to melanoblasts and further into melanocytes which can undergo initial neoplastic changes and result in lentigo senilis. Lentigo senilis can further assume premalignant changes becoming Dubreuilh's precancerous melanosis which generally assumes malignant changes leading to malignant melanocytoma. Neoplasms of the adult junctional melanocyte can also occur as melanoacanthoma and acromelanosis progressiva. The dermal melanocyte tumors such as Mongolian spot, nevus Ota, blue nevus, and cellular blue nevus are developed from melanoblasts maturing in the dermis. The cellular blue nevus may also develop from blue nevus and can undergo malignant change. The neural crest also differentiates to the Schwann cell whose neoplasms are found in the center of the table. The nevus cell nevi can be thought of as derived from the "nevoblast", a bipotential cell which can differentiate in two directions, melanogenic nevoblast and Schwannian nevoblast, just as melanocytes and Schwann cells are differentiated from the neural crest cell [4]. The melanogenic nevoblast develops into junction nevus cells with or without the stage of nevus incipiens, lentigo simplex, which may then become A-type and B-type intradermal nevus cells by the "abtropfung" process. At the present time C-type nevus cells, like other recognized neurogenic nevi may be considered as deriving from the Schwannian nevoblast. Junction nevi can occasionally undergo malignant changes resulting in the highly invasive malignant nevocytoma.

References. 1. MISHIMA, Y.: Cancer (Philad.) 20, 632 (1967). — 2. MISHIMA, Y.: J. invest. Derm. 34, 361 (1960). — 3. MISHIMA, Y.: Cutis 2, 588 (1966). — 4. MISHIMA, Y.: Arch. Derm. 91, 519; 92, 393 (1965). — 5. MISHIMA, Y.: Cellular and subcellular activities in the ontogeny of nevocytic and melanocytic melanomas. In: Advances in Biology of Skin, Vol. 8: The Pigmentary System. MONTAGNA, W., Ed., p. 509. Oxford: Pergamon Press 1967. — 6. MISHIMA, Y.: Melanotic tumors, in: Ultrastructure of Normal and Abnormal Skin, p. 612. ZELICKSON, A. S., Ed. Philadelphia: Lea & Febiger 1967.

Epidermal Melanin Unit

M. A. PATHAK, G. SZABÓ, T. B. FITZPATRICK, Y. HORI, S. S. BLEEHEN, E. FRENK and M. MIYAMOTO, Harvard University (U.S.A.);
M. SEIJI, Tokyo Medical and Dental University (Japan) and
A. BREATHNACH, London University (Great Britain)

Normal melanin pigmentation of the skin is related to the number and distribution of *melanosomes*, the subcellular units (organelles) of melanin formation. These specialized organelles are the product of melanocytes, which are specialized exocrine glands in the skin and hair bulb that arise from the neural crest. The melanocytes transfer melanosomes to malpighian cells, and these organelles are thus distributed throughout the epidermis. Melanosomes contain a basic protein framework (matrix) and a large, extremely dense polymer, melanin. This polymer is formed by the enzymatic action of a copper-containing aerobic oxidase, *tyrosinase*, on the naturally occurring amino acid, tyrosine. The process of melanin pigmentation involves the production, transfer, and distribution of melanosomes. The number of melanosomes produced and the rate of their transfer to malpighian cells are regulated by hormones and ultraviolet radiation, but primarily by genetic factors. Genes control the morphology of melanocytes and melanosomes and also the color (yellow-red; brown and black) of the melanin polymer.

A close integration of melanocytes and malpighian cells in pigmentation in vertebrates has been proposed in the concept of the "epidermal melanin unit" (EMU). The EMU may be defined as a melanocyte with an associated pool of malpighian cells, the size of which is variable. The concept of the EMU presupposes close interaction between epidermal melanocytes and malpighian cells during the synthesis and distribution of melanosomes. To illustrate this interaction, two examples have been selected. One deals with suntanning or melanogenesis after solar radiation, and the other deals with depigmentation of the skin by chemical agents (see Fig. 1—9 pag. 1507—1513).

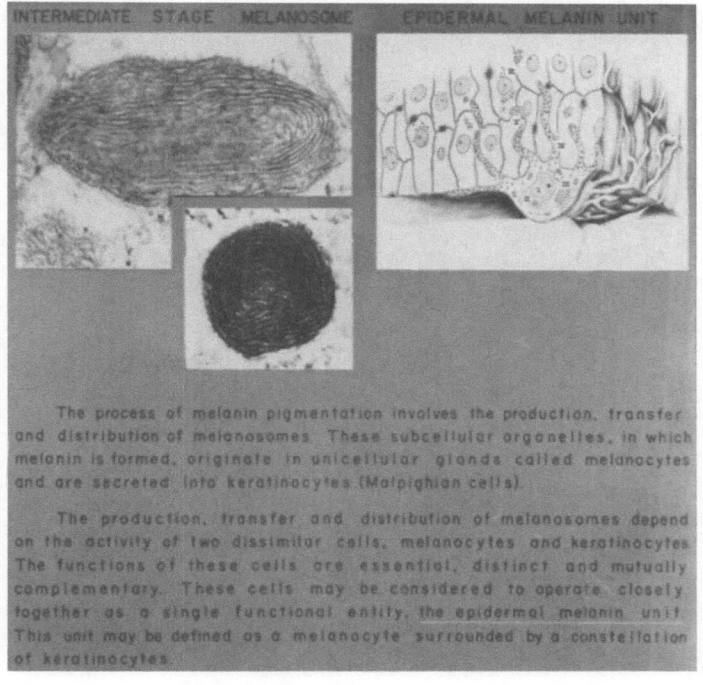

The process of melanin pigmentation involves the production, transfer and distribution of melanosomes. These subcellular organelles, in which melanin is formed, originate in unicellular glands called melanocytes and are secreted into keratinocytes (Malpighian cells).

The production, transfer and distribution of melanosomes depend on the activity of two dissimilar cells, melanocytes and keratinocytes. The functions of these cells are essential, distinct and mutually complementary. These cells may be considered to operate closely together as a single functional entity, the epidermal melanin unit. This unit may be defined as a melanocyte surrounded by a constellation of keratinocytes.

Fig. 1

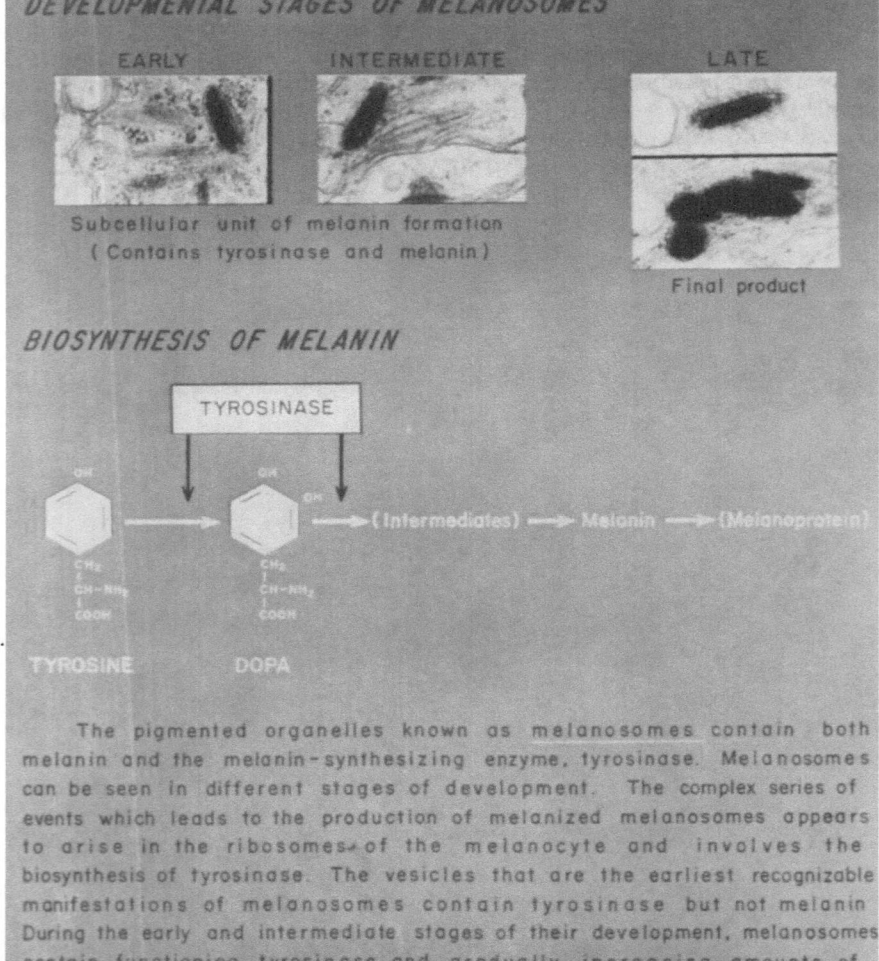

Fig. 2

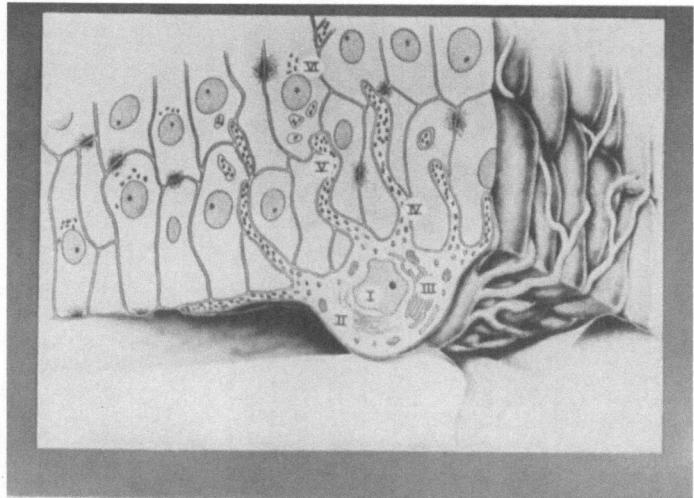

The population of epidermal melanocytes and the melanocyte : keratinocyte ratio are constant and characteristic for each body region. Racial differences in skin color are not due to differences in the number and distribution of melanocytes, but appear to result from differences in the degree of melanization of melanosomes and in the total number and distribution of melanosomes within the epidermal melanin unit. Genetic endowment in some way determines ability to produce melanin. Differences in skin color are due, therefore, to characteristic differences in the rate at which melanosomes are produced by melanocytes and transferred and distributed in keratinocytes.

Fig. 3

BIOLOGICAL CONTROL OF MELANIN PIGMENTATION AT VARIOUS LEVELS OF ORGANIZATION OF THE MELANOCYTE

LEVEL I   Melanocyte distribution

LEVEL II   Melanosome production

LEVEL III   Tyrosinase biosynthesis

LEVEL IV   Tyrosine – melanin biosynthesis

LEVEL V   Transfer of melanosomes to keratinocytes

LEVEL VI   Oxidative darkening of early, intermediate and late melanosomes

REGIONAL DIFFERENCES IN MELANOCYTE DISTRIBUTION		
MELANOCYTES/mm^2	REGION	KERATINOCYTES:MELANOCYTE
2120 ±90	face	4.5:1
1160 ±40	arm	10.0:1
890 ± 70	trunk	13.0:1
1130 ±60	leg	10.0:1

Fig. 4

MELANOGENESIS FOLLOWING SOLAR RADIATION

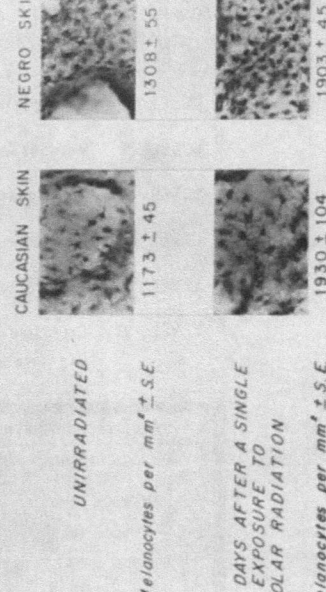

- LEVEL II   An increased number of melanosomes due to increased synthesis.

MELANOCYTE   KERATINOCYTE

UNIRRADIATED SKIN

AFTER SOLAR RADIATION

notice increased number of melanosomes.

Other factors that can play a role at various levels in the melanogenesis induced by ultraviolet radiation.

- LEVEL III   An increase in tyrosinase activity due to the synthesis of new tyrosinase in proliferating melanocytes.
- LEVEL IV   Activation of tyrosinase; increased tyrosine-melanin formation.
- LEVEL V   An increase in the transfer of melanosomes as the result of increased turnover of keratinocytes.
- LEVEL VI   Oxidative darkening of early, intermediate and late melanosomes.

Fig. 6

MELANOGENESIS FOLLOWING SOLAR RADIATION

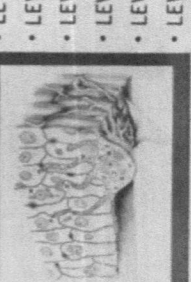

- LEVEL I   Increased melanocyte numbers.
- LEVEL II   Increased melanosome production.
- LEVEL III   Increased tyrosinase biosynthesis.
- LEVEL IV   Increased tyrosine-melanin formation.
- LEVEL V   Increased melanosome transfer.
- LEVEL VI   Oxidative darkening of melanosome stages.

The cutaneous pigmentation stimulated in mammals by solar radiation involves an increase in the formation of melanosomes within melanocytes and in their transfer and distribution in keratinocytes. This augmentation of melanin pigmentation appears to occur at the following levels

- LEVEL I   An increase in the number of functional melanocytes as the result of proliferation and/or activation of melanocytes. Hypertrophy of melanocytes and increased arborization of melanocytic dendrites may accompany this increase.

	CAUCASIAN SKIN	NEGRO SKIN
UNIRRADIATED		
Melanocytes per mm² ± S.E.	1173 ± 45	1308 ± 55
FIVE DAYS AFTER A SINGLE EXPOSURE TO SOLAR RADIATION		
Melanocytes per mm² ± S.E	1930 ± 104	1903 ± 45

Fig. 5

CUTANEOUS DEPIGMENTATION BY CHEMICAL AGENTS

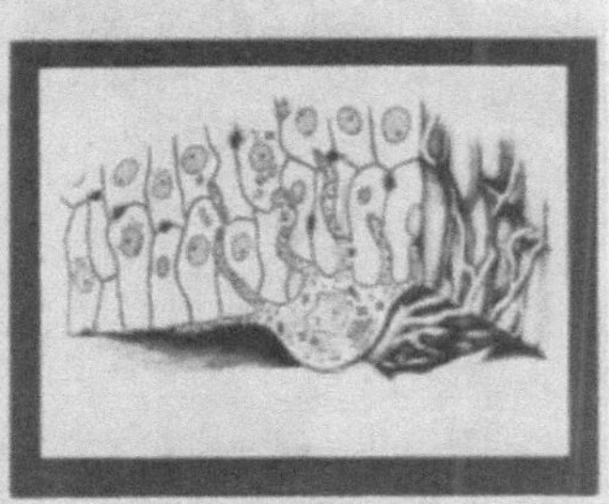

- LEVEL I   Loss of melanocytes.
- LEVEL II   Inhibition of melanosome formation or structural alteration of melanosomes.
- LEVEL III   Inhibition of tyrosinase biosynthesis or inactivation of tyrosinase.
- LEVEL IV   Inhibition of tyrosine–melanin formation.
- LEVEL V   Interference with the transfer of melanosomes.
- LEVEL VI   Chemical reduction of melanin in melanosomes.

The close functional relationship between epidermal melanocytes and keratinocytes is affected by chemical agents that induce cutaneous depigmentation. The depigmenting agent may selectively act on the melanocytes, which synthesize melanosomes, and thus cause loss or disappearance of melanocytes and a decrease in the production and transfer of melanosomes. An epidermis devoid of melanosomes appears depigmented.

Monobenzyl ether of hydroquinone (MBH)
Monomethyl ether of hydroquinone (MMH)
Hydroquinone (HQ)
Sulfanilic acid
Guanofuracin
2-Mercaptoethylamine hydrochloride (MEA)
N(2-mercaptoethyl) dimethylamine hydrochloride (MEDA)
Catechol and several catechol derivatives
4-Isopropyl catechol (4-IPC)

CHEMICAL AGENTS KNOWN TO INDUCE
CUTANEOUS DEPIGMENTATION

Experiments with various topically applied compounds have demonstrated that MEDA and 4-IPC are very potent agents that cause depigmentation in treated areas only, 4-IPC being the most effective. When applied to the skin of black guinea pigs, both MEDA and 4-IPC inhibited melanogenesis, acted selectively on melanocytes, decreased melanocyte distribution significantly and rendered the melanocytes degenerative.

Fig. 7

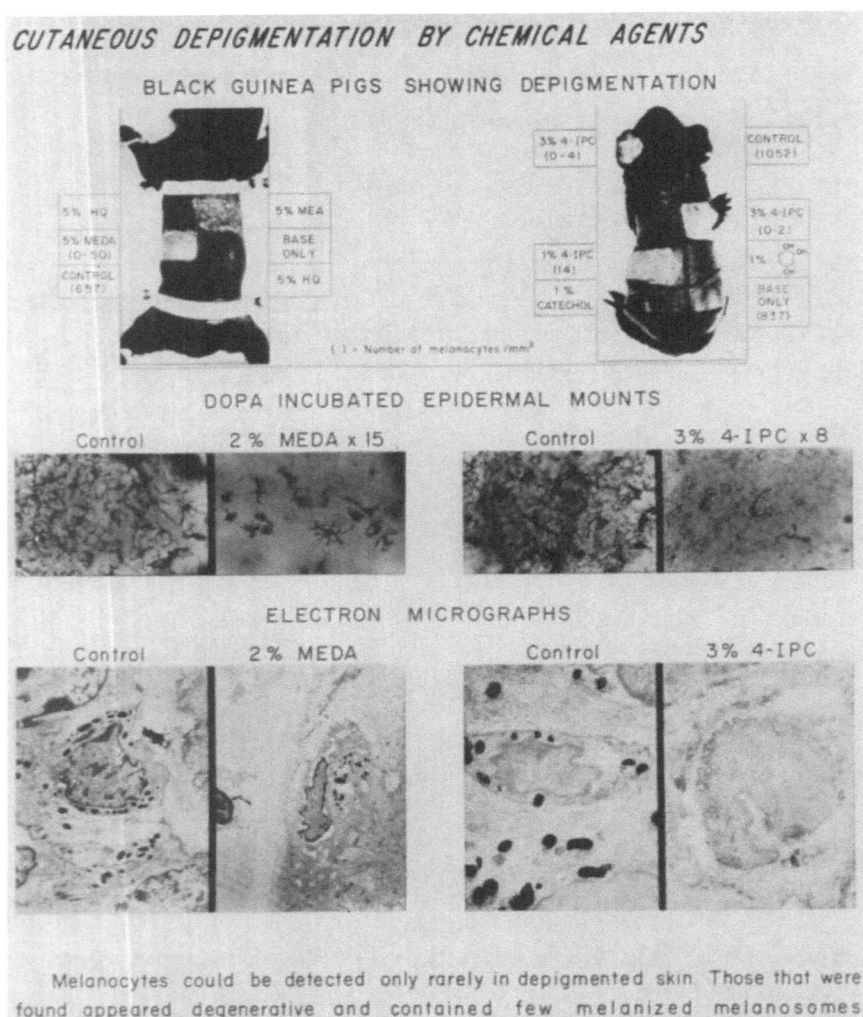

Fig. 8

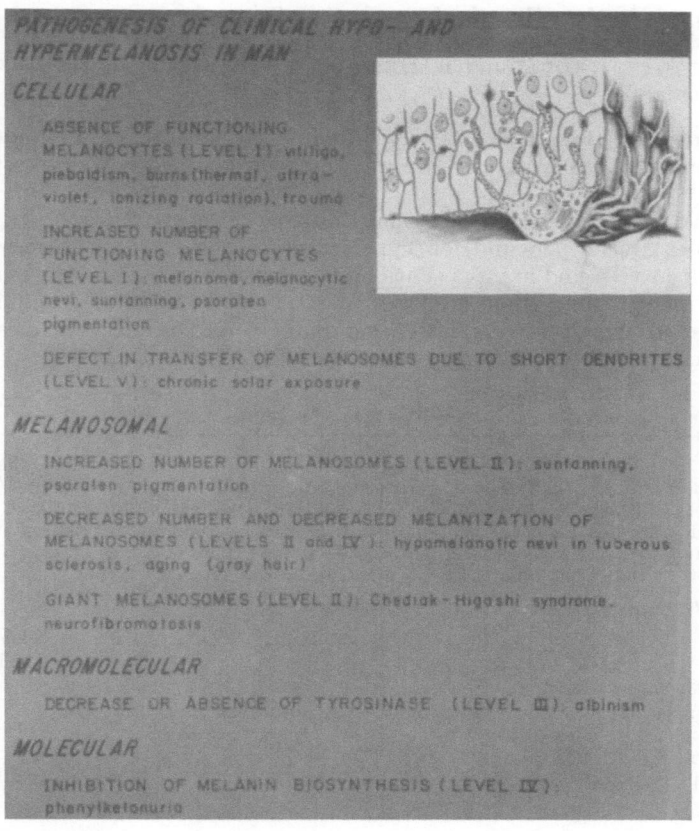

Fig. 9

Dermo-Epidermal Separation by Suction

N. KIISTALA and K. K. MUSTAKALLIO, Univ. Centr. Hosp.,
Dept. of Dermat., Helsinki (Finland)

Comparative Study with the Akantholysis in Pemphigus. Experimental Investigations on the Akantholysis Induced by the Staphylococcus pyogenes

B. ZILBERBERG, Sao Paolo (Brazil)

Pathophysiologie allergischer Dermatosen*

G. Stüttgen, I. Gigli und F. Herrmann, Univ.-Hautklinik Frankfurt a. M. (Deutschland)

An klinischen Beispielen mit zugehörigen experimentellen Befunden werden verschiedene pathogenetische Wege zu allergisch bedingten Hautveränderungen gezeigt.

Das Bild einer allergischen Dermatose wird weitgehend durch die Natur des Antigens, des Antikörpers und den Typ der Antikörperreaktion bestimmt. Letztere läßt sich oft in vivo und in vitro (Patient, Tierversuch) erfassen. Am Beispiel eines Patienten mit „Dermographia haemorrhagica" bei Penicillinüberempfindlichkeit (Abb.) werden Resultate von Antikörperanalysen im Hinblick auf ihre mutmaßliche pathogenetische Bedeutung aufgeführt (Tab. 1).

Tab. 1. *Hämorrhagischer Dermographismus nach Penicillin*

Pat. C. C., 53 Jahre, Arzt. Seit 4 Jahren Schwächeanfälle und Kreislaufstörungen. Schmerzhafte dermographische Ekchymosen. Zahlreiche Konsultationen in Amerika und Europa.

    Anamnese: Früher Beschäftigung mit Produktion von Penicillinpräparaten. Vor einigen Jahren, zu Beginn des Hautleidens, Anfall von Bewußtlosigkeit im Betriebsgelände, gefolgt von Ödemen. Untersuchungen Frankfurt a. M., Sommer 1966.

    Hauttteste: Prick-Test, Pen. G (neg.), intracutane Injektion, PPL (neg.).

Zirkulierende Antikörper gegen Penicillin (bei Pat. C. C.)

In vitro		Mutmaßliche Antikörper
Passive Hämagglutination		
Serum agglutiniert Hammelerythrocyten, Pen. G überzogen		
Titer	1:10240	
nach Erwärmen	1:320	IgM reichlich
nach Mercaptoathanol	1:240	IgG spärlich
Imunadhärenz		
Nach R. A. Nelson		
Titer	1:3200	IgA reichlich (?)
Hämolytische Antikörper		
Hammelerythrocyten überzogen mit Pen. G. hämolysiert in Gegenwart von		
Komplement durch Pat.-Serum		
Titer 1:200		IgG spärlich

In vivo

Passiv ausgelöste Reaktionen bei Tieren
Passive cutane Anaphylaxie (PCA) Meerschweinchen: PPL konjugiert mit menschlichem Gamma-Globulin

Systematische Anaphylaxie
Meerschweinchen: Intraperitoneale Vorbehandlung mit Pen. G; nach 24 Std i.v. Injektion von Pat.-Serum

Arthus-Phänomen (pass.)
Kaninchen: Pat.-Serum i.c., PPL konjugiert mit menschlichem Gamma-Globulin i.m.

Passiver Transfer
Affe: Pat.-Serum i.c., PPL konjugiert mit menschlichem Gamma-Globulin i.v.

Antigene: Pen. Proteinkonjugat $\longrightarrow$ Auto (Z) $\begin{cases} \text{Endothel-Pen.} \\ \text{Erythrocyten-Pen.} \end{cases}$

---

* Ermöglicht durch Unterstützung der August-Scheidel-Stiftung Frankfurt a. M.

In einer weiteren Übersicht weisen Analysen der Komplementfaktoren bei allergischen Arzneimittelexanthemen Unterschiede zu den Faktoren bei angioneurotischem Ödem (Anaphylaxie) auf. Bei letzterem fällt insbesondere die Abwesenheit des Inhibitors der Komplementesterase C'1 auf, die eine Gefäßwandpermeationserhöhende Wirkung hat (Tab. 2).

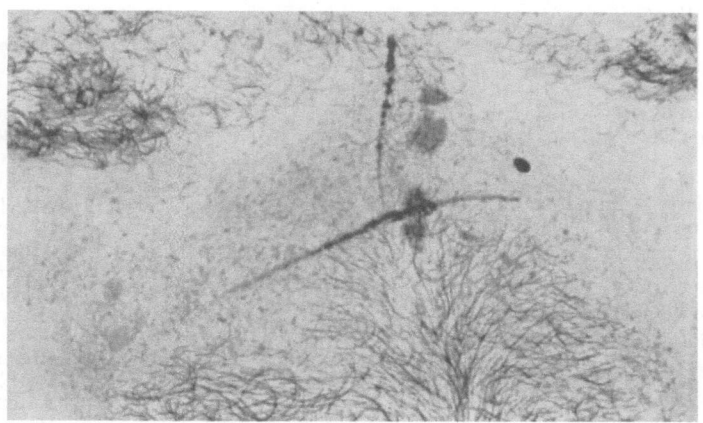

Abb. Hämorrhagischer Dermographismus. Entstehung einige Sekunden nach dem Strichreiz

Tab. 2. *Anaphylaktische Dermatosen und Komplementsystem (C')*

Inhibitoren im Serum
Komplementfaktoren
Sequenz ⟶

$$\begin{array}{ccccccccc} & \downarrow^{+} & & \downarrow^{+} & & ^{(+)}\downarrow & & & \\ C'1 & 4 & 2 & 3 & 5 & 6 & 7 & 8 \end{array}$$

Esterase
notwendig für
Phagocytose

alle zusammen integrierend für
cytotoxische Antigen-
Antikörper-Reaktion

	Gesunde Probanden	Arzneimittel-exantheme	Angioneuro-tisches Ödem
Gesamtkomplement C'	140	200	50
C'-Faktoren:			
C'1	52000	67000	107000
C'4	100000	550000	7000
C'2	10000	20000	6000
C'3	3200		2400
C'5	3200		4000
C'6	96000		100000
C'7	16000		14000
C'8	32000		32000
C'9	24000		20000
C'1-Inhibitor:			
Erfassung: enzymatisch	20	27	0
hämolytisch	12000	16000	0
C'3-Inhibitor	1200	1200	1200

Die Haut als Bildungsort sowie Speicherorgan gewebs-, insbesondere gefäß-
aktiver Substanzen, deren Kenntnis mittels pharmakologischer, insbesondere
chemischer Methoden erweitert werden konnte, gibt bei allergischen Reaktionen
wie auch nach anderen Reizen verschiedener Genese sekundär ein unspezifisches
Spektrum derartiger Wirkstoffe ab (Abb. 2).

Abb. 2. *Die Haut als*

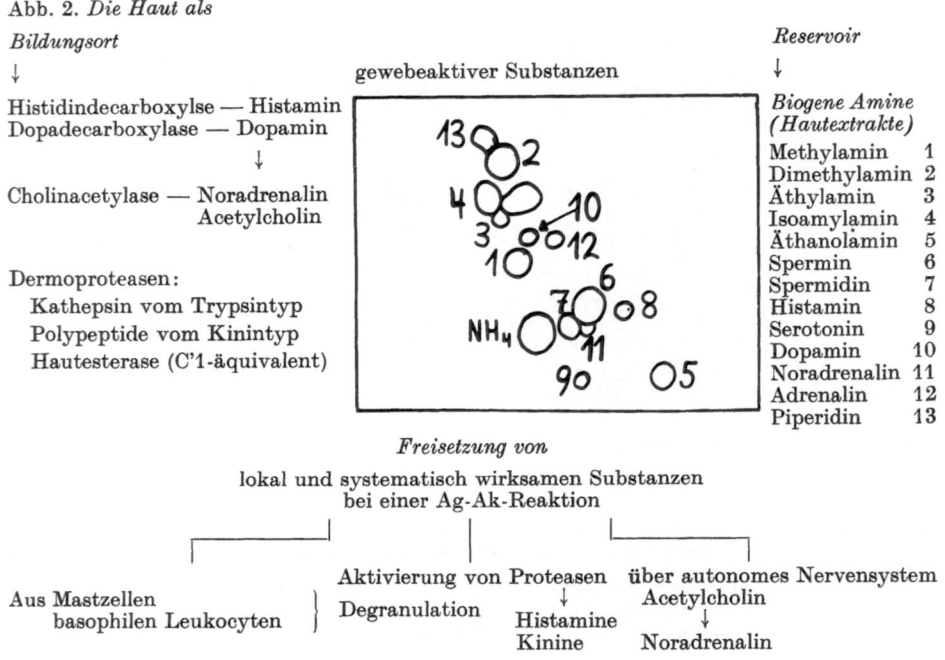

Bildungsort   *Reservoir*
↓   gewebeaktiver Substanzen   ↓

Histidindecarboxylse — Histamin   *Biogene Amine*
Dopadecarboxylase — Dopamin   *(Hautextrakte)*
                                                                          Methylamin   1
                                                                          Dimethylamin   2
Cholinacetylase — Noradrenalin   Äthylamin   3
            Acetylcholin   Isoamylamin   4
                                                                          Äthanolamin   5
                                                                          Spermin   6
Dermoproteasen: Spermidin   7
    Kathepsin vom Trypsintyp   Histamin   8
    Polypeptide vom Kinintyp   Serotonin   9
    Hautesterase (C'1-äquivalent)   Dopamin   10
                                                                          Noradrenalin 11
                                                                          Adrenalin   12
                                                                          Piperidin   13

Freisetzung von
lokal und systematisch wirksamen Substanzen
bei einer Ag-Ak-Reaktion

                              Aktivierung von Proteasen   über autonomes Nervensystem
                                      ↓   Acetylcholin
Aus Mastzellen   ⎫   Degranulation   Histamine   ↓
    basophilen Leukocyten ⎭   Kinine   Noradrenalin

Das mikrobielle Ekzem

H. Röckl, F. Schröpl, E. Müller und G. Peter, Dermatol. Klinik und Poliklinik der Universität Würzburg (Deutschland)

An Hand von ausgewählten Farbaufnahmen wird das klinische Bild des
mikrobiellen Ekzems und mikrobieller Streuphänomene demonstriert. Die massive
Besiedelung dieser Ekzemherde mit Staphylococcus aureus im Vergleich zur umgebenden und zur gesunden Haut wird dokumentiert. Ferner werden klinische
und histologische Bilder von Testreaktionen mit Cellophankulturfiltrat von
Staphylococcus aureus (CKF) gezeigt, deren Morphologie mit der des klassischen
Kontaktekzems übereinstimmt. Die Möglichkeiten der analytischen Auftrennung
von CKF wird an Hand der folgenden schematischen Darstellung deutlich gemacht. Durch die Bestimmung der hydrolytischen Spaltprodukte wird gezeigt,
daß es sich bei einem der zwei vorhandenen Ekzematogene um das Polysaccharid
A handelt, während die Natur des zweiten Ekzematogens, das möglicherweise
einen Eiweißkörper darstellt, noch nicht geklärt ist.

Isolierung der Staphylokokkenekzematogene aus Cellophankulturfiltrat (CKF)

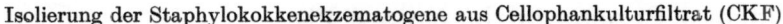

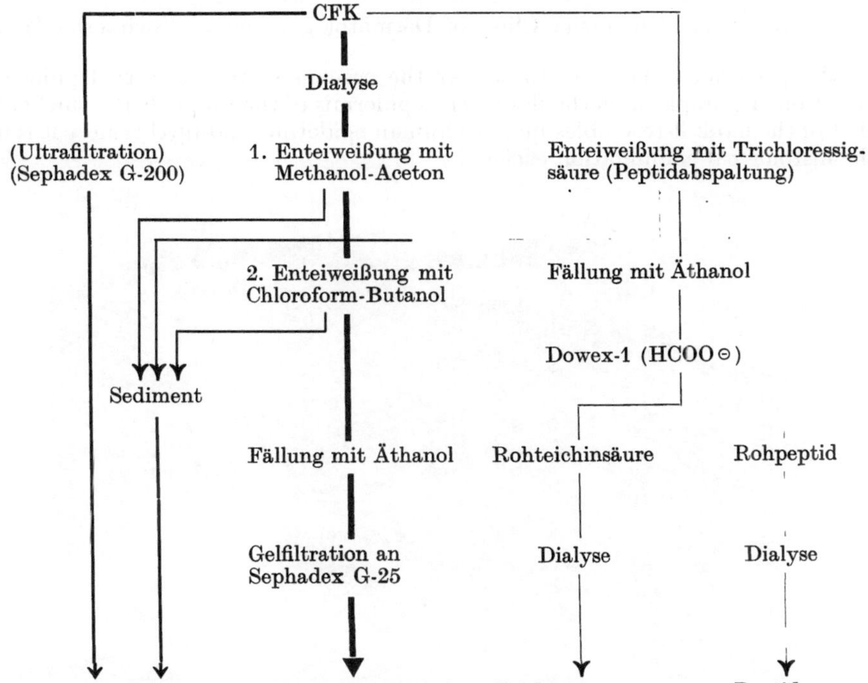

CFK

Dialyse

(Ultrafiltration)   1. Enteiweißung mit   Enteiweißung mit Trichloressig-
(Sephadex G-200)   Methanol-Aceton   säure (Peptidabspaltung)

                           2. Enteiweißung mit   Fällung mit Äthanol
                              Chloroform-Butanol

                                                        Dowex-1 (HCOO⊖)

        Sediment

                           Fällung mit Äthanol   Rohteichinsäure   Rohpeptid

                           Gelfiltration an   Dialyse   Dialyse
                           Sephadex G-25

		Teichinsäure-Peptid-	Teichinsäure	Peptid
hochmolekulares		Komplex=Poly-		
Ekzematogen		saccharid A		
Chemische	Protein?	Ala, Gly, Lys, Glu,	Glucosamin, Ribitol,	Ala, Gly,
Zusammen-		Glucosamin, Ribitol,	Anhydroribitol,	Lys, Glu
setzung		Anhydroribitol,	Phosphat, Alanin,	
		Phosphat, Muramin-	Muraminsäure	
		säure		
Im Epicutan-	schwach	wirksam	schwach wirksam	unwirksam
test	wirksam			

Schematische Darstellung der analytischen Auftrennung von CKF, der Wirksamkeit der gewonnenen Fraktionen und ihrer Zusammensetzung. Da bei den verwendeten Hydrolyse-bedingungen die Acetylgruppe abgespalten wird, ist bei den Spaltprodukten das zu erwartende N-Acetylglucosamin nicht vorhanden

Literatur. MÜLLER, E.: Arch. klin. exp. Derm. **219**, 874, 876 (1964). — MÜLLER, E., F. SCHRÖPL und H. RÖCKL: Arch. klin. exp. Derm. **218**. 298 (1964). — PETER, G., F. SCHRÖPL und G. CAMPHAUSEN: Arch. klin. exp. Derm. **231**, 111, (1968). — RÖCKL, H.:Hautarzt **6**, 532 (1955); **7**, 14, 70, 113, 248, 304 (1956); — Arch. klin. exp. Derm. **219**, 830 (1964); — Z. Haut-u. Geschl.-Kr. **42**, 475 (1967). — RÖCKL, H., u. F. SCHRÖPL: Arch. klin. exp. Derm. **219**, 862 (1964). — SCHRÖPL, F.: Arch. klin. exp. Derm. **219**, 877 (1964); **226**, 383 (1966); **229**, 411 (1967); **230**, 48, 111, 402, 413 (1967). — Z. Haut- u. Geschl.-Kr. **42**, 497 (1967). — SCHRÖPL, F., E. MÜLLER und H. RÖCKL: Arch. klin. exp. Derm. **215**, 523 (1963); **218**, 91, 312 (1964).

Experimental Eczema of the Guinea Pig

N. Hunziker, University Clinic of Dermatology, Geneva (Switzerland)

We performed the tests to trigger the eczema in the sensitized guinea pig, either on the nipple or on the flank. The epidermis of the nipple being thicker than that of the flank it resembles more to human epidermis and furthermore it renders the histological examination easier.

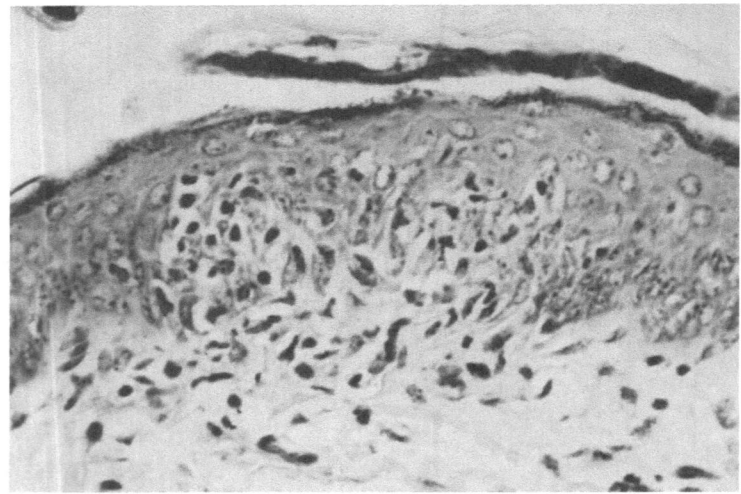

Fig. 1. Guinea pig sensitized with dinitrochlorobenzene. Nipple 14 h after one application of 0,1% dinitrochlorobenzene in acetone: spongiosis

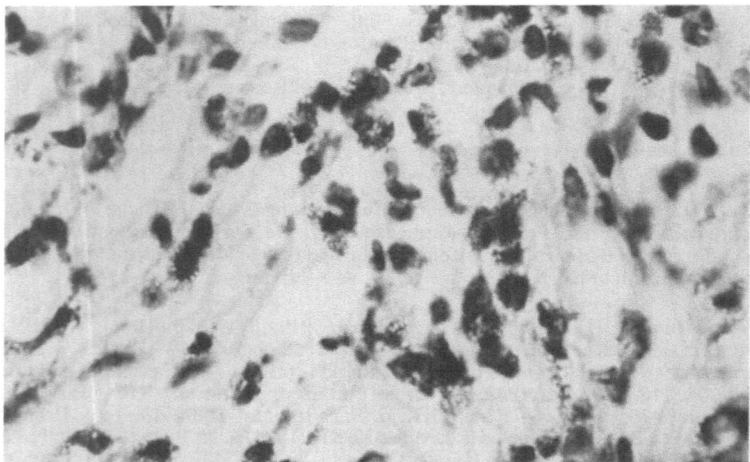

Fig. 2. Guinea pig sensitized with citraconic anhydride. Nipple 14 h after one application of 25% citraconic anhydride in dioxane: numerous eosinophils in the infiltrate

Among the results obtained we will only summarize some.

1. Eczema of the guinea pig caused by dinitrochlorobenzene closely resembles, from the histological point of view (especially on the nipple and on the flank made

acanthotic) to contact eczema of man: more or less wide spread spongioses, intra-epidermal vesicles, infiltrate, composed mostly of small round cells which invade the epidermis (Fig. 1).

2. Eczema of the guinea pig's flank due to paranitrosodimethylaniline is manifested in several ways in the histological examination, according to the group

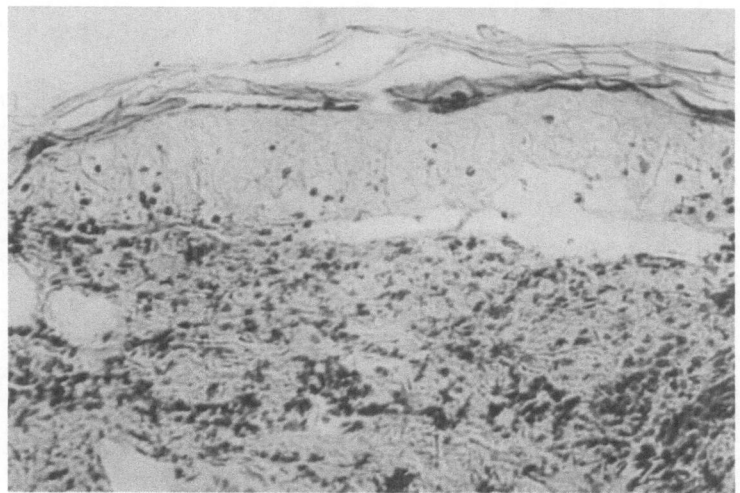

Fig. 3. Guinea pig sensitized with propionic anhydride. Flank 14 h after one application of 25% propionic anhydride in dioxane: necrosis of the epidermis

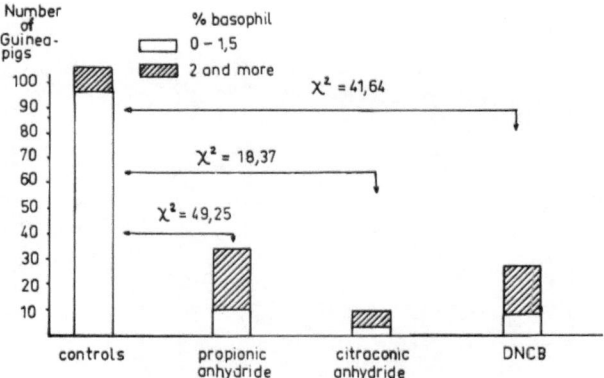

Fig. 4. Basophilia in control guinea pigs (non sensitized) and in treated guinea pigs (towards the end of sensitization treatment)

of animals, even though the sensitization technique has always been the same. We observed either spongioses, either acanthosis, accompanied or not by an infiltrate which is very abundant in eosinophils.

3. Eczema of the guinea pig caused by citraconic anhydride is preceeded by an urticarial reaction. The urticarial reaction is progressively transformed to a delayed reaction. In the histological examination of the two reactions we observed an infiltrate very rich in eosinophils (Fig. 2).

4. Eczema on the guinea pig's flank due to propionic anhydride can resemble from the histological point of view to toxic epidermal necrolysis (Lyell's disease): necrosis of the epidermis. Whereas, the lesions on the nipple do not show a necrosis but only spongiosis (Fig. 3).

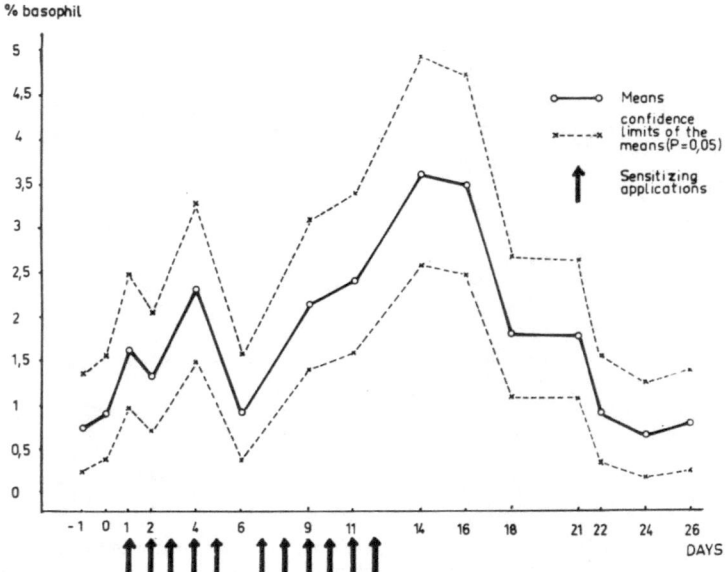

Fig. 5. Evolution of basophilia during the sensitization with propionic anhydride

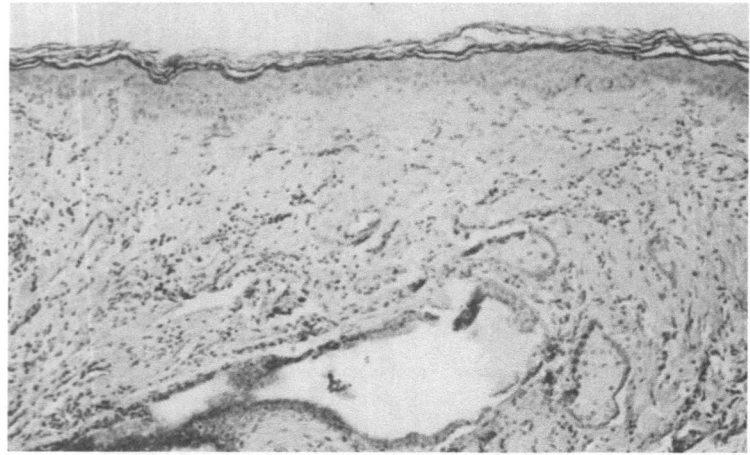

Fig. 6. Guinea pig sensitized with dinitrochlorobenzene. Daily applications of 0.1% dinitrochlorobenzen in acetone on the left nipple for 100 days. Right nipple after one application of 0.1% dinitrochlorobenzene in acetone: no lesions

5. In the course of sensitization with simple chemical compounds (dinitrochlorobenzene, propionic anhydride and citraconic anhydride) a blood basophilia is observed. In guinea pigs sensitized to dinitrochlorobenzene we found at the end

of sensitization 3.9% basophils (mean of 28 guinea pigs), at the end of sensitization with propionic anhydride 4.05% (mean of 34 guinea pigs), and at the end of the sensitization with citraconic anhydride 3.0% (mean of 9 guinea pigs).

In normal guinea pigs we found 0.6% basophils (mean of 107 animals).

The animals of each group (controls, and guinea pigs sensitized with dinitrochlorobenzene, citraconic anhydride and propionic anhydride) are separated in two classes: animals having 0 to 1.5% blood basophilia, and animals having a blood basophilia of 2% or more. The difference between the control group and the three groups of sensitized guinea pigs is highly significant (χ^2 method) (Fig. 4).

This basophilia appears towards the end of sensitization* (10 to 16 days after beginning of treatment) and is transient (Fig. 5).

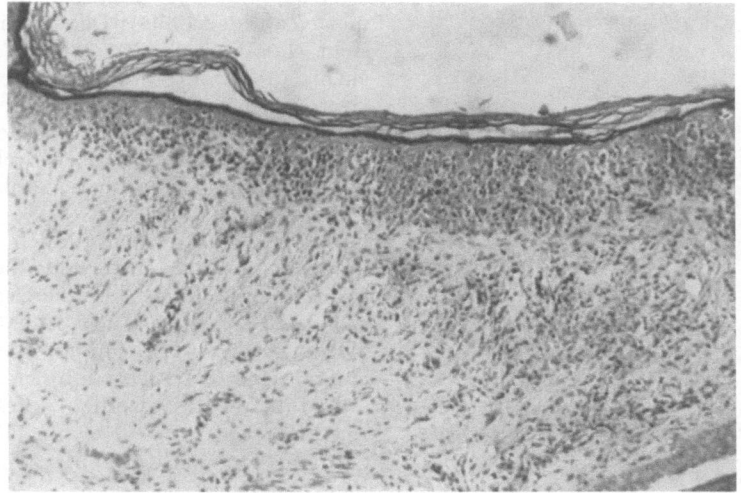

Fig. 7. Guinea pig sensitized with dinitrochlorobenzene. No treatment for 100 days. Nipple after one application of 0.1% dinitrochlorobenzene in acetone: spongioses

6. In the experimental eczema of the guinea pig it is possible to obtain a general desensitization by repeated applications of a primary non toxic solution of the eczematogen upon a small surface (nipple).

a) After 100 to 150 daily applications of dinitrochlorobenzene on guinea pigs sensitized to this substance, we observe after a patch test, practically no macroscopic or microscopic reaction (Fig. 6); whereas the sensitized guinea pigs without desensitization treatment, show still a strong eczema: spongiosis and infiltrate composed mostly of small round cells (Fig. 7).

b) After 57 daily applications of paranitrosodimethylaniline on a group of guinea pigs sensitized to this substance, we observe after a patch test no macroscopic or microscopic reaction; whereas, the sensitized guinea pigs of the same group but without desensitization treatment, show epidermal lesions and an important infiltrate which is rich in eosinophils.

---

* Sensitization by epicutaneous applications only, for dinitrochlorobenzene; by epicutaneous applications combined with injections for citraconic anhydride and propionic anhydride.

Terpentinöl-Intoxikation bei Arbeitern einer Schuhcreme-Fabrik, verursacht durch d-Alpha-Pinen

F. Nürnberger, Hautklinik der Universität Mainz (Deutschland)

Sechs Arbeiter einer Schuhcremefabrik, die alle in einer Abteilung tätig und dabei Dämpfen terpentinhaltiger Schuhcreme ausgesetzt waren, klagten im Winter 1965/66 hauptsächlich bei kalter Witterung unterschiedlich und zeitweise über folgende *Beschwerden:* 1. Schwindel- und Trunkenheitsgefühl, vor allem morgens bei Arbeitsbeginn, 2. brennende Hautrötung im Gesicht-Hals-Bereich, 3. Juckreiz und Brennen im Analbereich, 4. schmerzhafte Defäkation und hauptsächlich über 5. Pollakisurie mit Makrohämaturie.

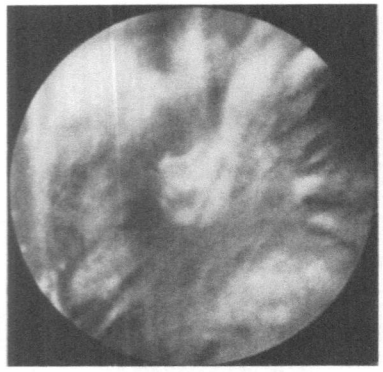

Abb. 1. Massive ödematös-hämorrhagische Cystitis mit einem linsengroßen Ulcus vesicae der Hinterwand (Diagnose und Photo: Dr. Rapp, Urolog. Abt. der Chirurg. Univ.-Klinik Mainz)

Untersuchungsergebnisse (in Klammern Zahl der Fälle): Dermatitis im Gesicht-Hals-Bereich (3), subakutes Analekzem (3), Proktitis (2), hämorrhagische Cystourethritis (3) mit zusätzlichem Ulcus vesicae (2) (Abb. 1), toxische Nierenreizung (1), toxische Milzschwellung (1, szintigraphisch errechnetes Milzgewicht 400 g). Der Urin der sechs Arbeiter hatte „Veilchengeruch", auch die Nylander-Probe war unterschiedlich stark positiv (s. Abb. 2). Anamnestisch ergab sich, daß zumindest seit 1962/63 jeden Winter von ca. November bis Februar einige Arbeiter der Abteilung an den oben aufgeführten Beschwerden erkrankt waren. Bei warmer Witterung (Frühjahr, Sommer, Herbst) waren die Arbeiter immer beschwerdefrei.

Eine *Arbeitsplatzuntersuchung* ergab, daß in der Abteilung keine Be- und Entlüftungsanlage eingebaut war. Die Entlüftung erfolgte nur durch große Fenster,

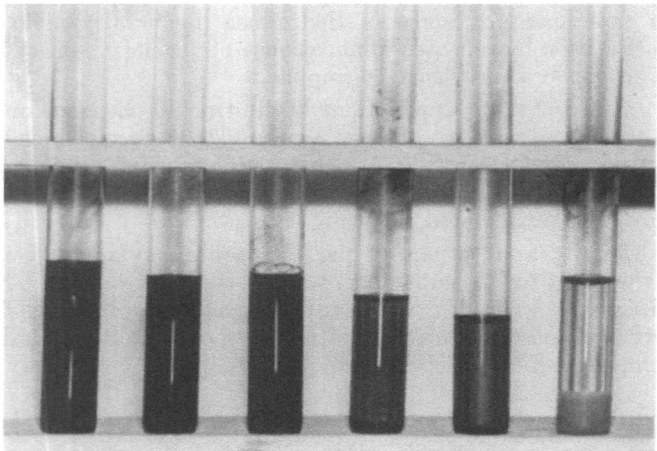

Abb. 2. Unterschiedlicher Reaktionsausfall der Nylander-Probe im Urin von sechs Arbeitern durch vermehrte Ausscheidung „gepaarter Glucuronsäuren"

die bei warmem Wetter weit geöffnet wurden, aber im Winter wegen der Kälte
weitgehend geschlossen blieben. Dadurch kam es zu einer Ansammlung terpentinhaltiger Dämpfe im Raum, zu vermehrter Inhalation und damit zur Intoxikation.

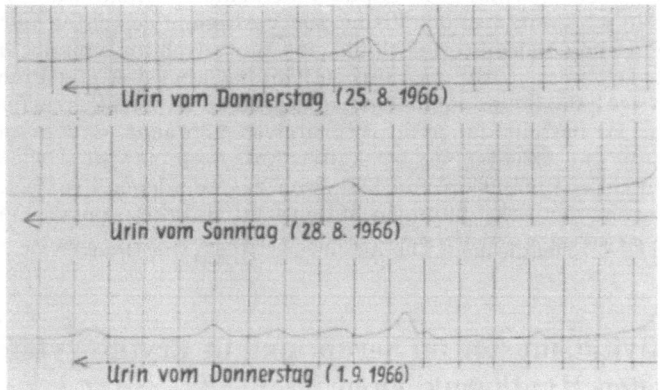

Urin vom Donnerstag (25. 8. 1966)

Urin vom Sonntag (28. 8. 1966)

Urin vom Donnerstag (1. 9. 1966)

Abb. 3. Gaschromatographische Urinuntersuchungen bei einem Arbeiter: Eingeatmete
Schuhcremedämpfe werden zum Teil im Urin ausgeschieden. Am arbeitsfreien Sonntag ist nur
noch eine kleine Bande vorhanden

Gaschromatographisch ließen sich im Urin der Arbeiter
Lösungsmittel nachweisen (Abb. 3), wahrscheinlich
hauptsächlich Terpentinöl (Veilchengeruch der Urine!).
Durch Glucuronsäurebestimmungen wurde bewiesen,
daß der unterschiedlich positive Reaktionsausfall der
Nylander-Probe im Urin auf eine mehr oder weniger
vermehrte Ausscheidung von Glucuronsäure zurückzuführen ist. Im *Selbstversuch* und bei einem besonders
exponierten Arbeiter wurde festgestellt, daß am Ende
eines achtstündigen Arbeitstages nach intensiver Inhalation von Dämpfen terpentinhaltiger Schuhcreme
eine Methämoglobinämie von 7% bzw. 8,3% auftrat
(Normalwert bis 2,2%), die am nächsten Morgen wieder
verschwunden war. Das Methämoglobin wurde also
über Nacht wieder abgebaut. Methämoglobinbestim-
mungen, die bei den Arbeitern am Vormittag durchgeführt wurden, ergaben deshalb immer normale Werte.
Bei dem gleichen Selbstversuch konnte auch gezeigt
werden, daß nach mehrstündigem Aufenthalt in dem
terpentinreichen Milieu der Abteilung beim Verfasser
im Urin eine starke Positivität der Nylander-Probe
nachweisbar war. Am nächsten Morgen war die Nylander-Probe wieder negativ (Abb. 4). Der Urin hatte
jedoch noch ca. 2 bis 3 Tage einen typischen „Veilchengeruch".

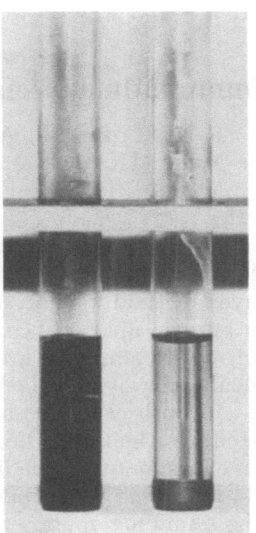

Abb. 4.
Selbstversuch (s.Text): links:
Nylander-positiver Urin am
Abend des 3.3.1966; rechts:
Nylander-negativer Urin
am nächsten Morgen

   Die von der Firma hergestellte Schuhcreme hat im
wesentlichen folgende Zusammensetzung: Terpentinöl (bzw. Alpha-Pinen) 65 bis
70%, Testbenzin 7%, Wachskomposition 23 bis 24%, Diphenylamin 0,4%, Farben
0,8%. Obwohl die Firma schon seit Jahrzehnten Schuhcreme herstellt, sind früher
bei den Arbeitern angeblich niemals Beschwerden aufgetreten. Während der letzten

Jahre wurde aber an Stelle von Terpentinöl verschiedener Provenienz immer mehr konzentriertes amerikanisches Alpha-Pinen verwendet, weil es konstanter ist in seiner Zusammensetzung und besser riecht. Nach unseren polarimetrischen Messungen hatte dieses amerikanische Alpha-Pinen eine Rechtsdrehung von 41°, während die beiden anderen, von der Firma zur Verfügung gestellten portugiesischen und österreichischen Balsamterpentinöle eine Linksdrehung von 58° bzw. 50° aufwiesen. Nach DANBOLT u. BURCKHARDT (1935) hat aber d-Alpha-Pinen mehr eine toxische und l-Alpha-Pinen mehr eine allergisierende, ekzemerregende Wirkung auf die Haut. Es besteht daher der begründete Verdacht, daß mangelhafte Be- und Entlüftung am Arbeitsplatz bei kalter Außentemperatur sowie die dadurch bedingte vermehrte Inhalation von Dämpfen des vorwiegend toxischen d-Alpha-Pinen als Ursache der Erkrankungen in den letzten Jahren anzusehen sind.

[Ausführliche Veröffentlichung: Zbl. Arbeitsmed. (1967) (Im Druck).]

Enzymaktivitätsmuster im Serum und in Erythrozyten bei verschiedenen Hautkrankheiten

H. HOLZMANN, B. MORSCHES, G. W. KORTING und R. DENK, Univ.-Hautklinik Mainz (Deutschland)

Immunofluorescence Studies of the Skin

R. H. CORMANE, Amsterdam, E. H. BAART DE LA FAILLE, J. B. VAN DER MEER, Utrecht, and A. A. W. TEN HAVE-OPBROEK, W. W. MUIJS VAN DE MOER, Leiden (Netherlands)

Antigens as well as antigen-antibody complexes present in tissues can be detected by means of immunofluorescent (I.F.) staining. In the direct or single layer method a fluorescein-labelled antibody interacts directly with the antigen or antigen-antibody complex. In the indirect or double layer method the antigen-antibody complexes are incubated previously with unlabelled antibodies and then incubated with labelled antibodies directed against the antibodies first used.

In both cases the result is that in the fluorescence microscope the U.V. light excitates the fluorochrome components of the labelled antibodies which results in an emission of visible light.

In *Lupus erythematosus* (L.E.) with cryostate sections and the direct method the immunoglobulins (Ig) can be detected in the region of the dermal-epidermal junction of skin lesions while in normal skin or skin lesions of other dermatoses (with the exception of pemphigoid) no fluorescence can be seen.

Specificity tests (unrelated antibodies, blocking method, neutralizing method) are necessary to exclude false positive results. With the same procedure (cryostate sections and direct I.F. method) human complement can be detected in the region of the dermal-epidermal junction in the skin of L.E. skin lesions. The Ig and the complement appear to be concomitantly bound which can be proved by previous incubation with unconjugated anti-human Ig (resp. complement) and subsequent staining with labelled anti-human complement (resp. anti-human Ig).

The anti-Heavy and the anti-Light chains antisera used have been shown to be capable of detecting the different major classes (IgG, IgA, IgM) and types ($\varkappa$ and

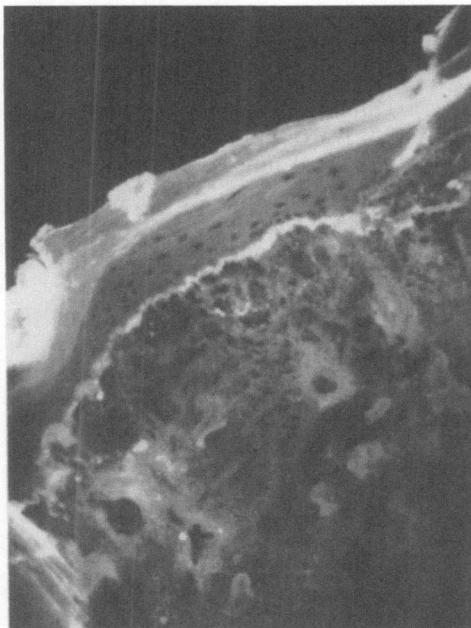

Fig. 1. Lupus Erythematosus. Fluorescence of the region of the dermal-epidermal junction

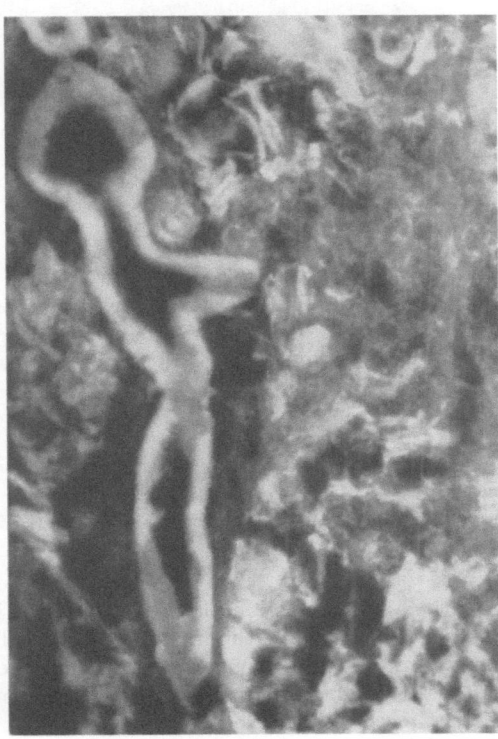

Fig. 2. Lupus Erythematosus.
Uninvolved skin.
Fluorescence of the vessels

λ) of Ig in the dermal-epidermal junction in discoid and systemic L.E. IgG appear to be consistently located in the region in question in contrast to IgM and IgA. Data obtained in L.E. studies:

L.E. and lymphocytic infiltration (JESSNER). The I.F. method is a valuable aid for the differential diagnosis between L.E. and L.I. Jessner. In L.I. Jessner no Ig can be detected in the region of the dermal-epidermal junction.

L.E. and pemphigus and other bullous dermatoses. In Pemphigus the pattern of I.F. is of another type: circulating antibodies are capable of staining the inter-cellular spaces of the cells of the stratum spinosum. In pemphigoid there are circu-lating antibodies directed against the basement membrane of the skin.

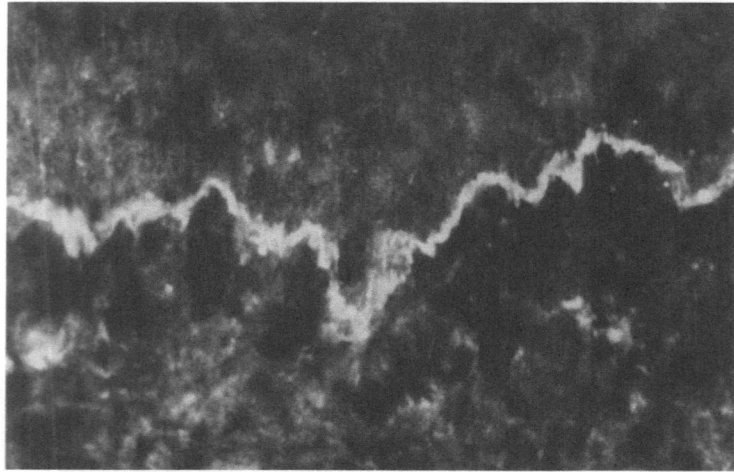

Fig. 3. Pemphigoid. Stained by the direct I.F. method. Note the presence of Ig in the region of the dermal-epidermal junction

Immunofluorescent Methods

Direct = single layer method

Antigen-antibody complexes present in tissues can be detected after a single incubation with fluorescein-labelled antibodies directed against antibodies (human immunoglobulins) of these complexes.

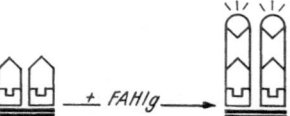

Indirect = double layer method

Antigen-antibody complexes present in tissues can also be detected after a previous incubation with unlabelled antibodies directed against the antibodies (human immunoglobulins) of these complexes and subsequent incubation with fluorescein-labelled antibodies directed against the unlabelled antibodies used for the first incubation.

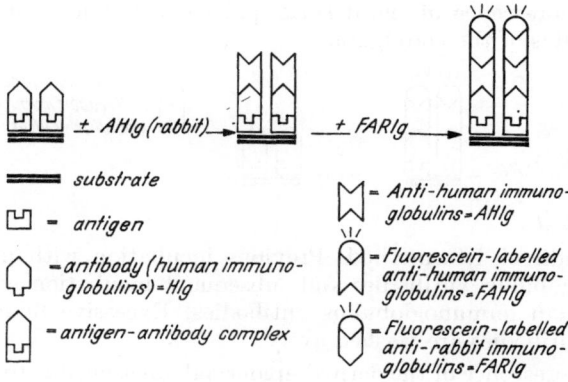

Detection of Immunoglobulins in the Region of the Dermal-Epidermal Junction

Lupus Erythematosus

Substrate: Cryostate sections of L.E. skin lesions.

Procedure: Direct I.F. method. Incubation with fluorescein-labelled anti-human immunoglobulins antibodies (conjugate).

Result: Fluorescence of the dermal-epidermal junction, due to the presence of human immunoglobulins.

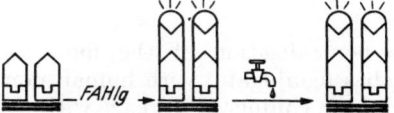

Controls

Substrate: Cryostate sections of normal skin or skin lesions of various other dermatoses (with the exception of pemphigoid and dermatitis herpetiformis).

Procedure: As above.

Result: No fluorescence of the dermal-epidermal junction, due to the absence of human immunoglobulins.

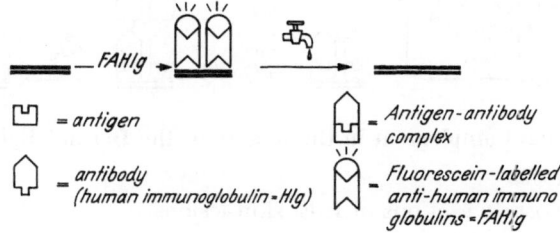

Specificity Tests I

Substrate: Cryostate sections of L.E. skin lesions.

I. Unrelated antibodies

Procedure: Direct I.F. method. Incubation with fluorescein-labelled unrelated antibodies (conjugate). Excessive conjugate is washed away.

Result: No fluorescence of the dermal-epidermal junction, due to absence of specific binding sites of the conjugate.

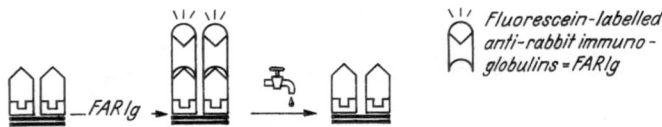

II. Blocking method

Procedure: Indirect I.F. method. Previous incubation with unlabelled anti-human immunoglobulins antibodies and subsequent incubation with fluorescein-labelled anti-human immunoglobulins antibodies. Excessive fluorescein-labelled and unlabelled antibodies are washed away.

Result: No fluorescence of the dermal-epidermal junction, due to blocking of the human immunoglobulins.

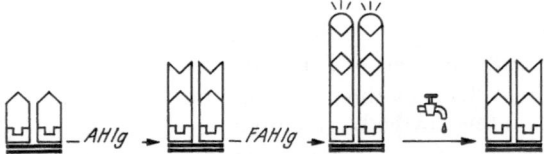

Specificity Tests II

Neutralizing Method

Procedure: Previous neutralization of the fluorescein-labelled anti-human immunoglobulins antibodies (conjugate) with human non-labelled immunoglobulins removes the ability of the conjugate to react with the human immunoglobulins in the dermal-epidermal junction.

Result: No fluorescence of the dermal-epidermal junction, due to neutralizing of the conjugate with the human immunoglobulins.

Specificity tests are necessary to exclude false positive results

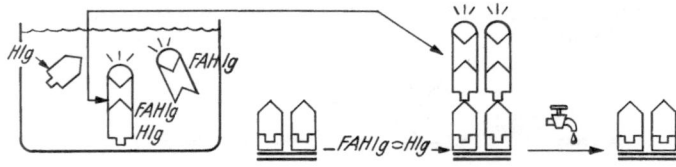

Detection of Human Complement in the Region of the Dermal-Epidermal Junction

Lupus Erythematosus

Substrate: Cryostate sections of L.E. skin lesions.

Procedure: Direct I.F. method. Incubation with fluorescein-labelled anti-human complement (conjugate). Excessive complement is washed away.

Result: Fluorescence of the dermal-epidermal junction, due to the presence of human-complement.

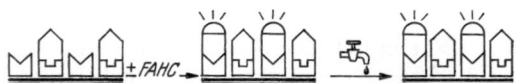

Controls

Substrate: Cryostate sections of normal skin or skin lesions of various other dermatoses (with the exception of pemphigoid and dermatitis herpetiformis).

Procedure: As above.

Result: No fluorescence of the dermal-epidermal junction, due to the absence of human complement.

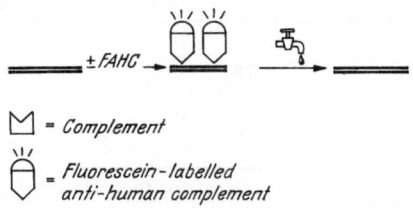

$\sqcap$ = *Complement*

$\overset{\sqcup}{\ominus}$ = *Fluorescein-labelled anti-human complement*

Immunoglobulins and Complement

Immunoglobulins and complement appear to be concomitantly bound in the region of the dermal-epidermal junction.

Substrate: Cryostate sections of L.E. skin lesions.

Procedure: Previous incubation with unconjugated anti-human immuno-globulins and subsequent staining with fluorescein-labelled anti-human complement.

Result: Fluorescence of the dermal-epidermal junction, due to the presence of human complement.

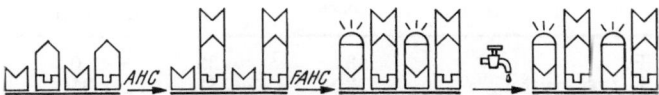

Procedure: Previous incubation with unconjugated anti-human complement and subsequent staining with fluorescein-labelled anti-human immunoglobulins.

Results: Fluorescence of the dermal-epidermal junction due to the presence of human immunoglobulins.

This means that immunoglobulins and complement are concomitantly bound to the region of the dermal-epidermal junction. Apparently the conjugates possess different binding sites on their molecules for the region of the dermal-epidermal junction.

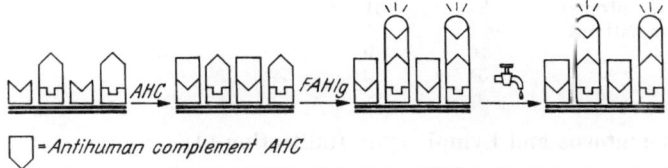

$\bigsqcup$ =*Antihuman complement AHC*

Classification of the Immunoglobulins

Three classes of immunoglobulins are studied: IgG, IgA, IgM. Differences between these Ig are determined by the structure of the H(eavy) chains, which also confer immunological specificity.

All classes of Ig have structural units in common: L(ight) chains. Based on the similarity to the corresponding types of Bence-Jones proteins, the L-chains are classified as belonging to either of two immunological types, $\varkappa$ or λ.

Diagnosis	No of Patients	Classes of Ig in Dermo-Epidermal Junction				
		H-chains			L-chains	
		IgG	IgA	IgM	type $\varkappa$	type λ
C.D.L.E. lesions	12	12	1	2	12	12
Systemic L.E. lesions	3	3	0	2	3	3
uninvolved skin	2	2	1	0	2	2

Diagnosis	No of Patients	Classes of Ig in Dermo-Epidermal Junction		
		IgG	IgA	IgM
C.D.L.E.	5	4	0	5
S.L.E.	5	4	0	5

Result: The fluorescein-labelled anti-Heavy and anti-Light chains antisera have been shown to be capable of detecting major classes and their subsequent types of Ig in the dermal-epidermal junction in discoid and systemic L.E.

Results

Lupus Erythematosus

Diagnosis	No. of cases	Dermal-Epidermal junction	
		skin lesion	uninv. skin
C.D.L.E.	133	133	0
C.D.L.E. ("transistory")	31	31	31
C.D.L.E. (syst. inv.)[1]	17	17	17
S.L.E. (probable possible)[1]	40		40
S.L.E. (definite)[1]	26		26

[1] Classification of L.E. according to DUBOIS.

Diagnosis	Skin lesion			Uninvolved skin		
	No. of patients	positive	negative	No. of patients	positive	negative
C.D.L.E. (with or without suggestive symptoms)	35	31	4	15	1	14
S.L.E. (with or without skin lesions)	10	9	1	16	9	7
Controls	54	0	54	—	—	—

Lupus Erythematosus and Lymphocytic Infiltration (JESSNER)

Diagnosis	No of Patients	I.F. Dermal-Epidermal Junction			
		anti-human Ig		anti-human complement	
		pos.	neg.	pos.	neg.
L.E.	11	10	0	6	0
L.I.	4	0	4	1	3

Differences in the immunofluorescence pattern support the view that chronic discoid lupus erythematosus and infiltratio cutis lymphocytica Jessner are different diseases.

Fluorescense microscopy is a valuable aid for the differential diagnosis between the two diseases.

Comparative Immunofluorescent Results[1] in L.E. and Bullous Dermatoses

| Diagnosis | Direct method | | Indirect method (serum antibodies) | |
| | Skin lesions | | Skin of normal controls | |
	Dermal-epidermal junction	Epidermis (intercell. spaces)	Dermal-epidermal junction	Epidermis (intercell. spaces)
Lupus erythematosus	+	—	—	—
Pemphigus	—	+	—	+
Pemphigoid	+	—	+	—
Dermatitis herpetiformis	—	—	—	—

[1] Data obtained from literature and own investigations.

Herkunft der mononucleären Entzündungszellen (Makrophagen) bei der unspezifischen Entzündung (Untersuchungen am Rebuck'schen Hautfenster bei der Ratte)

M. BEGEMANN, München (Deutschland)

Unspezifische und spezifische Wirkstoffe bei allergischen Reaktionen der Cutis

G. STÜTTGEN, J. GIGLI und F. HERRMANN, Univ.-Hautklinik Frankfurt (Main)

Allergens of Quinone Structure

K. H. SCHULZ, P. SCHMIDT and H. GRELL, Dermatological Clinic of the University, Hamburg (Deutschland)

During the past years it has been possible to isolate and to identify allergens of low molecular weight from plants and tropical woods. These sensitizers are chemically characterized by a quinone nucleus to which an aliphatic or a cyclic side chain is attached.

I. Teak wood (Tectona grandis)

In patch test studies performed with several constituents of Teak in sensitized patients we found allergic reactions only to Desoxylapachol and to Lapachol (both derivatives of naphthoquinone). Desoxylapachol, isolated by SANDERMANN and SIMATUPANG [1], was about 100 times more effective than Lapachol (minimal threshold concentration of Desoxylapachol 0.0001% to 0.0005%) [2]. Experiments on guinea pigs confirmed the strong sensitizing capacity of Desoxylapachol which must be regarded as the primary sensitizer of Teak. Lapachol was only capable to elicit contact reactions in animals previously sensitized to Desoxy-lapachol.

Desoxylapachol (sensitizer and elicitor)   Lapachol (elicitor)

II. Dalbergia species

The valuable woods of the Dalbergia family, called Rio-Palisander, s. Jacarandá (Dalbergia nigra), Indian Palisander (Dalbergia latifolia), Cocobolo (Dalbergia retusa) contain 3 or 4 compounds of quinone structure, called Dalbergiones.

In patients with contact dermatitis due to these woods allergic patch test reactions to Dalbergiones, especially to 4-Methoxydalbergion, were obtained (minimal treshold concentration 0.01% to 0.05% [3]. Chemically the Dalbergiones are derivatives of p-benzoquinone [4].

4-Methoxydalbergion

III. Mansonia (Mansonia altissima)

The sensitizing factor of Mansonia wood is also a derivative of benzoquinone, called Mansonon A. In patch test studies concentrations of 0.01% to 0.1% were still effective. The sensitizing effect of Mansonon A could also be proved in experiments on guinea pigs. The chemical structure is the following [5]:

Mansonon A

IV. Iroko (Kambala)-wood (Chlorophora excelsa)

Epicutaneous tests in patients sensitized by this wood showed positive results to Chlorophorin, a 4 times oxidized derivative of stilbene, isolated by KING and GRUNDON [6]). The chemical structure shows some similarity to pentadecyl-catechol, the sensitizing agent of poison ivy. Chlorophorin is itself not a quinone compound, but it may be converted into a compound of quinone structure (quinone-methid) within the organism.

Chlorophorin

V. Primrose (Primula obconica)

The chemical structure of Primin, the allergen of Primula obconica, has re-recently been clarified by SCHILDKNECHT and co-workers [7]. The molecule consists of a benzoquinone nucleus which is connected with an aliphatic side chain.

$$\text{H}_3\text{CO} \overset{\text{O}}{\underset{\text{O}}{\bigcirc}} \text{CH}_2-\text{CH}_2-\text{CH}_2-\text{CH}_2-\text{CH}_3$$

Primin

VI. A quite similar quinone has been isolated from *Phagnalon saxitale*, a shrub-like plant which is growing on the coasts of the Mediterranian [8].

$$\overset{\text{O}}{\underset{\text{O}}{\bigcirc}} -\text{CH}_2-\text{CH}=\text{C}\overset{\text{CH}_3}{\underset{\text{CH}_3}{\diagup}}$$

Quinone from Phagnalon saxitale Cass

For future research in this field it may be useful to direct attention towards compounds of quinone structure.

References. 1. SANDERMANN, W., u. M. H. SIMATUPANG: Chem. Ber. **96**, 2182 (1963). — 2. SCHULZ, K. H.: Z. Haut- u. Geschl.-Kr. **42**, 499 (1967). — 3. SCHULZ, K. H., u. H. H. DIETRICHS: Allergie u. Asthma 8, 125 (1962). — 4. EYTON, W. B., W. D. OLLIS, J. O. SUTHERLAND, L. M. JACKMAN, O. R. GOTTLIEB, and M. TAVEIRA MAGALHAES: Proc. Chem. Soc. **1962**, 301. — 5. TANAKA, N., M. JASUE, and H. IMAMURA: Tetrahydron Letters **1966**, 2767. — 6. KING, F. E., and F. M. GRUNDON: J. chem. Soc. **1949**, 3348; **1950**, 3547. — 7. SCHILDKNECHT, H.: Angew. Chemie **76** (1964), blaue Beilage S. 177. — SCHILDKNECHT, H., J. BAYER und H. SCHMIDT: Z. Naturforsch. **22 b**, 36 (1967). — 8. BOLLMANN, F., u. K. M. KLEINE: Chem. Ber. **99**, 885 (1966).

Methode zur Hornschichtdickenmessung in vivo

F. KLASCHKA und R. A. KRAUSE, Hautklinik der Freien Universität Berlin (Deutschland)

Methodische Grundlagen: Die trockene Hornschicht (HS) mit einem Wassergehalt von $\leq 10\%$ besitzt gegenüber dem lebenden Epidermis- bzw. Körpergewebe (Feuchtigkeitsgehalt $> 60\%$) eine herabgesetzte elektrische Leitfähigkeit. Wird in einem definierten Stromsystem eine Nadelelektrode mechanisch regulierbar durch die zwischen Innenkörper und Außenwelt isolierende HS geführt, so zeigt der kontinuierlich aufgezeichnete elektrische Wechselstromwiderstand beim Erreichen der vermutlich filmartig dünnen Übergangszone vom toten zum lebenden Epidermisepithel einen abrupten Abfall. Aus dem Weg-Zeit-Verhältnis zwischen Nadelvorschub und Stromkurve resultiert der Abstand vom initialen Oberflächenkontakt (Abfall des Wechselstromwiderstandes von ∞ auf $50 \sim \text{M}\Omega$) bis zum Erreichen der nichtverhornten Epidermis. Diese Entfernung kann nach Umrechnung an der Stromkurve nachgemessen werden und entspricht annähernd der HS-Dicke.

Methodische Ausführung: Der Meßkopf, hergestellt aus Plexiglas und Injektionsspritzen, fixiert mittels Unterdruck (Wasserstrahlpumpe) die zu prüfende

Hautregion (Abb. 1). Durch eine motorgetriebene und exakt steuerbare Hydraulik wird die im Meßkopf bewegliche Nadelelektrode aus Wolfram mit einem Spitzenkrümmungsradius von $\leq 2\,\mu$ durch die Hornschicht geführt, wobei die gegen eine indifferente Flächenelektrode abgeleitete Stromkurve simultan aufgezeichnet

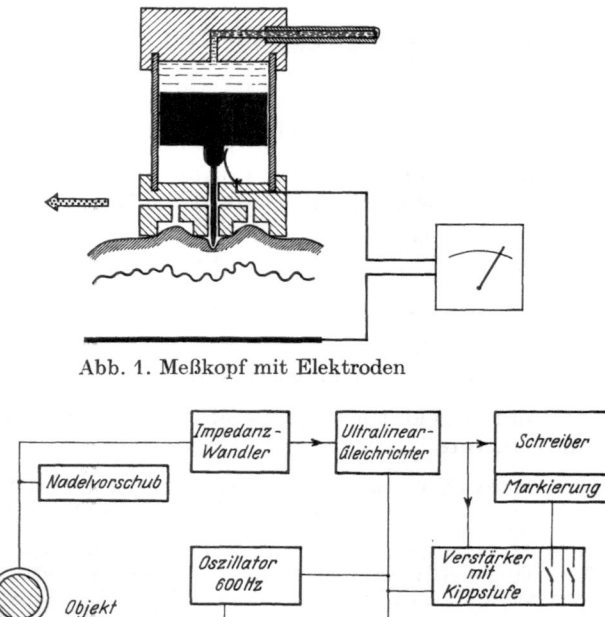

Abb. 1. Meßkopf mit Elektroden

Abb. 2. Blockschaltbild zum Hornschichtdicken-Meßgerät

wird. Ein Oszillator erzeugt eine Wechselspannung von 600 Hz, die an der Flächenelektrode 0,7 V — gegen Erde — beträgt. Der während der HS-Passage von der Nadelelektrode abgeleitete Wechselstrom wird einem Impedanzwandler zugeführt, von einem Ultralineargleichrichter in Gleichspannung umgewandelt und vom Linienschreiber aufgezeichnet (Abb. 2). Die Gleichspannung erreicht über einen Verstärker eine Kippstufe, die beim Auftreffen der Nadelelektrode auf das lebende Epidermisepithel ein Relais zum Ansprechen bringt und gleichzeitig eine Markierung im Schreiber betätigt. Nadel- und Papiervorschub haben einen wahlweise verstellbaren Synchronmotorantrieb. Aus dem Verlauf der Stromkurve vom ersten Nadel-Hautkontakt bis zum Erreichen des lebenden Epidermisepithels ergibt sich eine der Hornschichtdicke entsprechende Strecke.

Literatur. Document II. Sympos. Dermat. S. 261, Brno (1965).

Dermatological and Immunological Aspects of Cryoglobulinaemia

K. K. Mustakallio and O. Wagner, Univ. Centr. Hosp., Dept. of Dermat., Helsinki (Finland)

R.U.V., X-Ray and Alpha-particles Micrography of the Skin

A. Tosti, Department of Experimental Dermatology,
University of Palermo (Italy)

The absorption image by superimposition

If a tissue section is put in contact with a photographic plate and the whole is exposed, an "absorption image" of the same size as the section will be obtained.

By observing the plate with a lens or a microscope, it will be found that the various structures of the tissue are reproduced according to the grade of their

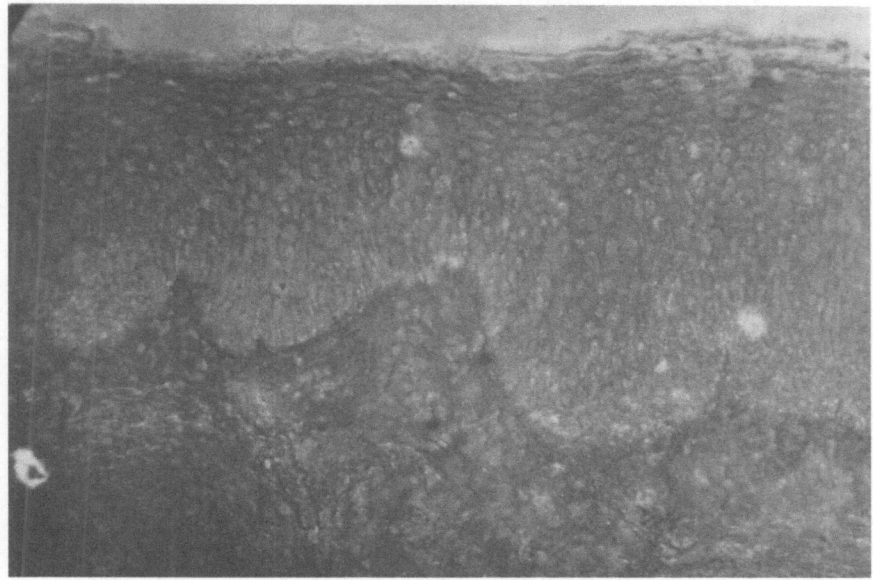

Fig. 1. Human epidermis (Ultraviolet, λ 2520 Å)

absorbing ability. Under correct photographic conditions there is a linear relation between "blackening" of the plate and light absorption of the specimen, so that the more a given structure is absorptive, the lower will be the blackening (or photographic density) of its reproduced image.

The method represent an useful tool, therefore, for the morphologic and absorptiometric exploration of tissue samples at micrological level.

The kind of information given by the absorption images depend on the source of energy used for the exposure, the most interesting sources being the ones of invisible "light", to which the photographic emulsion, however, are sensitive.

Technical steps

1. Floating sections (deparaffined or from criostat) are carried down to distilled water.

2. The sections are picked up on extremely fine grained photographic plates, and allowed to dry (dark room).

3. The plates carrying the sections are exposed.

4. The sections are removed from the photographic plates in a water bath (dark room), and eventually stained and mounted.

5. The photographic plates are developed, examined under microscope and analyzed by microdensitometry.

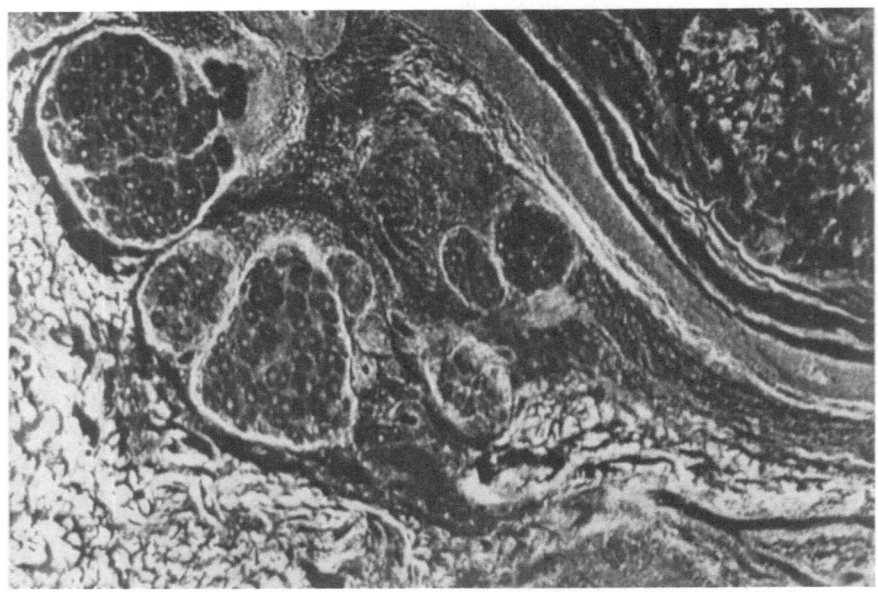

Fig. 2. Favre-Racouchot elastoidosis (Soft X-rays, 1.5 kV)

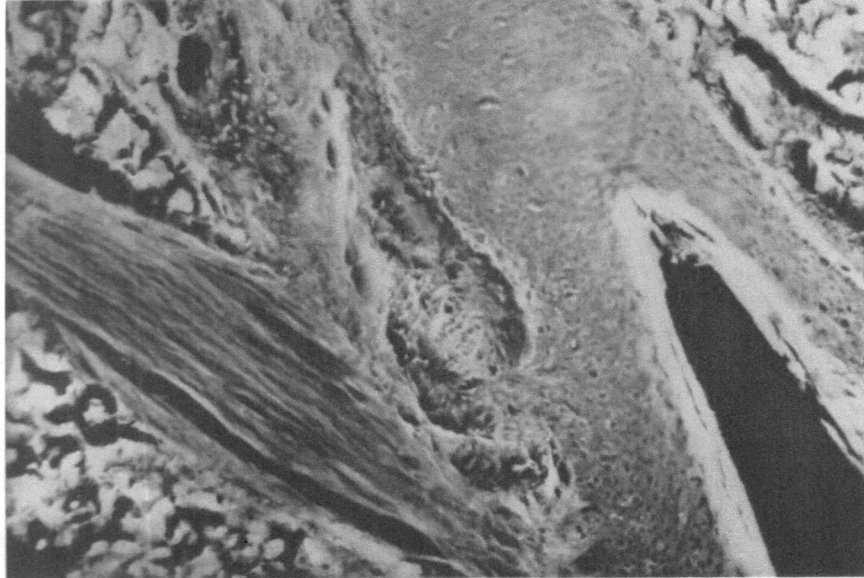

Fig. 3. Hair follicle with arrector pili muscle (Soft X-rays, 1.2 kV)

Exposure

Visible light, monochromatic (λ 5450 Å, interference filter).

Ultraviolet, monochromatic (various wavelengths) as well as wood light (Mx.s.d. 3660 Å).

X-rays

Soft X-rays. Sealed off X-ray tube with Be window (Philips) operating at tension between 1.1 and 5 kV.

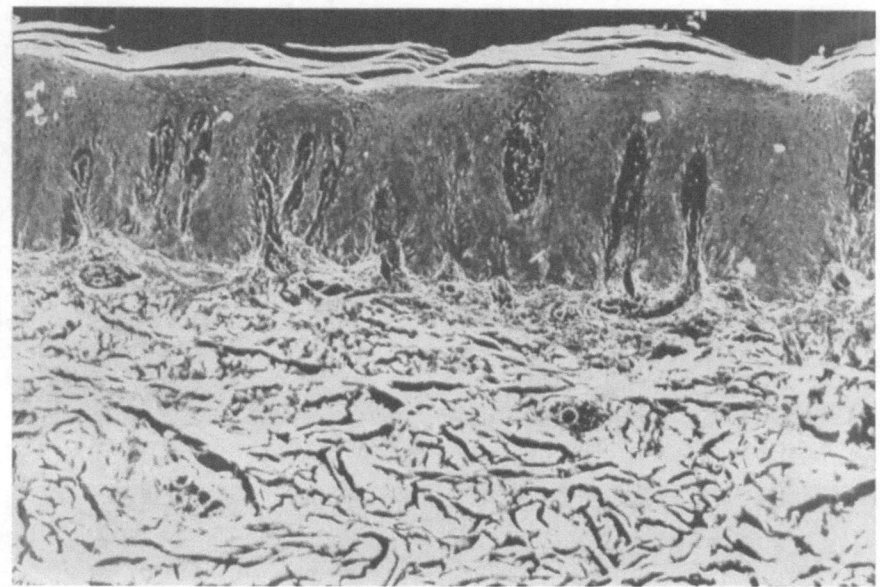

Fig. 4. Neurodermatitis (Ultrasoft X-rays, 0.8 kV)

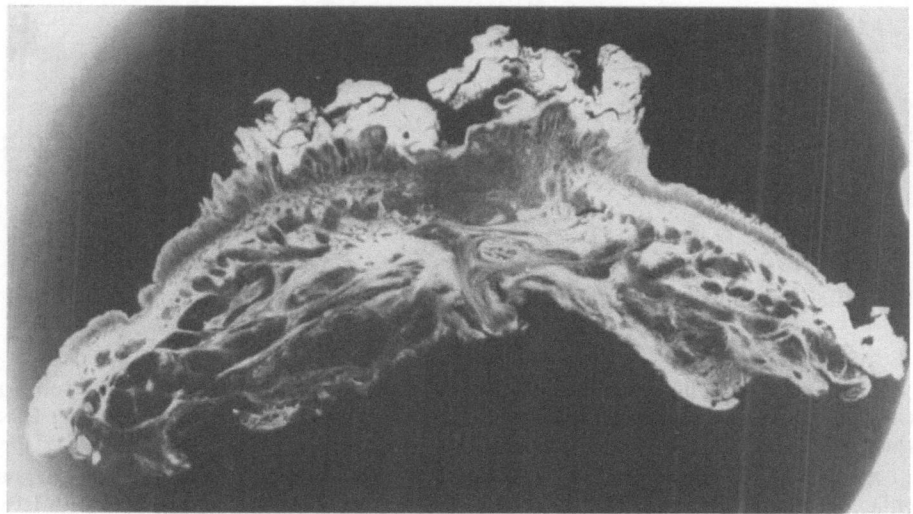

Fig. 5. Angiokeratoma (200 μ thick section, 3.5 kV tension)

Ultrasoft X-rays. Open X-ray tube devised by the author and realized in the Raytheon Laboratories in Palermo. The tube makes possible the exposition to a quite unfiltered and light free ultrasoft X-ray beam, required for the highest resolution and contrast.

X-ray images of thick sections. 200 to 3000 μ sections; tensions ranging from 4 to 10 kV.

Alpha-particles: Alpha-emitting [110]Po source.

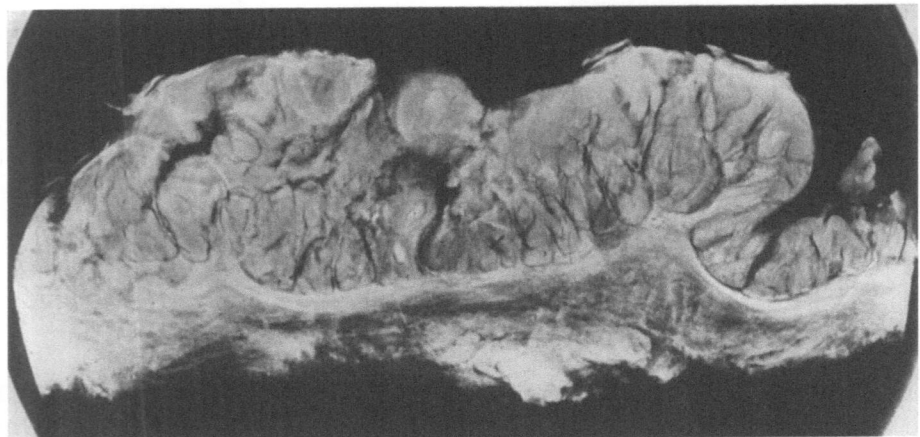

Fig. 6. Basal cell epithelioma (300 μ thick section, 4 kV tension)

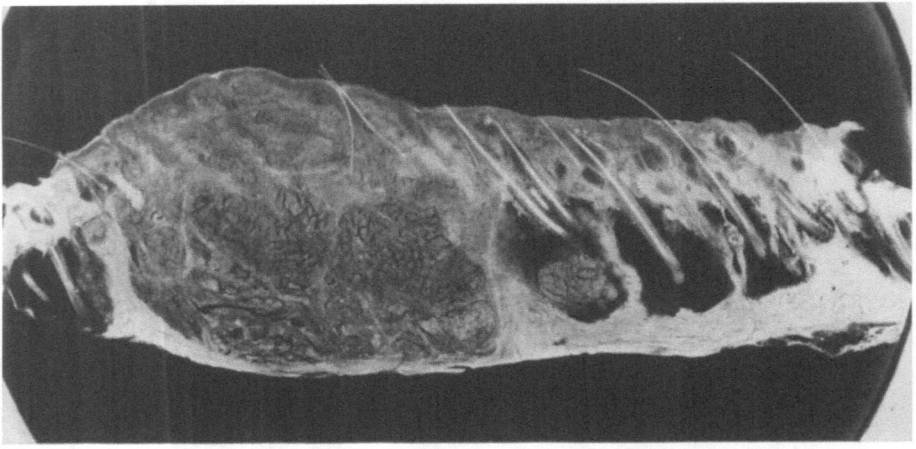

Fig. 7. Hairy skin, basal cell epithelioma (200 μ thick section, 3.5 kV tension)

Advantages of the method

1. From a morphological viewpoint the absorption images represent a tool for the microanatomic investigation of the skin structures at energy regions other than the visible light.

2. Turning to the biological problem of the penetration of radiant and corpuscular energy in the skin, the method is helpful, as it reveals the pattern and the intensities of the absorptions at micrological level.

3. The absorption images are also apt for investigation of histophysical order, in force of the relation between the chemistry of the structures and their absorbing ability. When the X-rays are used the absorptions may be converted, under proper conditions, in term of concentration of dry mass (and dry weight). The same is expected to occur when alpha-particles are used.

4. Further, the X-ray images of thick sections are suitable for the architectural and istometric analysis of the tissue.

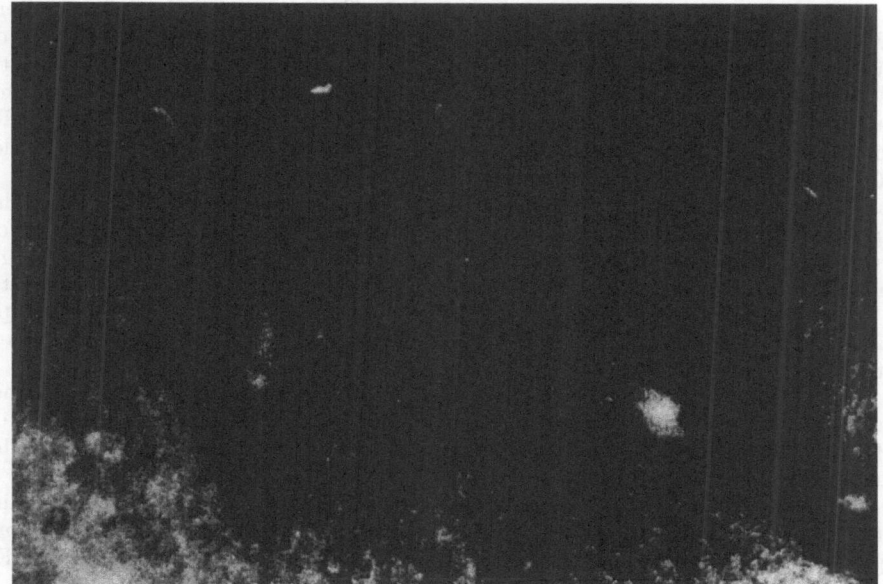

Fig. 8. Epidermoid carcinoma (alpha-emitting ^{110}Po source)

References. Tosti, A., e M. L. Fazzini: Ann. ital. Derm. Sif. **15**, 53 (1960); — **16**, 1, 185 (1962); — Contact microradiographs and contact photomicrographs of human skin in several pathological condition. Proc. XII Int. Congr. of Dermatology Washington, September 1962, p. 1623; — Riv. Istoch. norm. pat. **9**, 2 (1963); — Arch. Derm. **89**, 131 (1964). — Tosti, A., M. L. Fazzini, and J. Záhejský: Čs. Derm. **39**, 73 (1964). — Tosti, A.: Microradiografia da contatto della cute umana. Ind. Graf. Naz. (Palermo) 1964. — Tosti, A., M. L. Fazzini e M. Aricò: Ann. ital. Derm. Sif. **19**, 125 (1965). — Tosti, A.: G. ital. Derm. **107**, 1339 (1966). — Tosti, A., e G. Brancato: Ann. ital. Derm. Sif. **20**, 1 (1966). — Tosti, A., G. Brancato e C. Cappadona: Atti Accad. Sci. Med. (Palermo) 1967.

L'Exploration thermographique en dermatologie

Ch. Gros et C. Vrousos, Service Central de Radiologie;
J. Alt et A. Basset, Clinique Dermatologique; Strasbourg (France)

La thermographie vient de faire son entrée sur la scène des explorations biophysiques médicales. Depuis de nombreuses années, pendant lesquelles des perfectionnements ont été apportés, la thermographie est restée dans l'ombre et dans le secret des applications militaires et astronautiques. Les premiers résultats cliniques de la thermographie obtenus dans certains centres des Etats-Unis et de l'Europe sont plus qu'encourageants. Les principales indications semblent se dégager mais de nombreux secteurs de la pathologie dans lesquels la thermographie peut apporter de précieux renseignements, restent encore à explorer.

Tout corps dont la température dépasse le zéro absolu (— 273 °C) est une source d'émission infra-rouge. Nous vivons donc dans un véritable «bain» de rayonnement I.R. invisible. Chaque objet émet, absorbe et re-émet un rayonnement I.R. jusqu'à ce qu'un équilibre thermique s'établisse.

Le corps humain n'échappe pas à cette règle. Il est la source d'un rayonnement I.R., c'est-à-dire d'ondes électro-magnétiques dont la longueur d'onde s'étend de 3 à 20 μ avec maximum d'énergie de 10 μ. Si l'œil humain percevait cette partie du spectre électromagnétique, il verrait des plages brillantes alternant avec d'autres beaucoup plus sombres, correspondant à des niveaux de chaleur différents. Ceci serait dû au fait que la température cutanée varie largement selon les endroits alors que la température centrale reste remarquablement stable.

L'œil humain était cependant incapable de saisir ce spectre infra-rouge, des appareils très sensibles: les thermographes permettent de capter cette information infra-rouge, de la transformer en énergie électrique proportionelle à l'énergie émise. Ce courant est amplifié et alimente un tube à décharge qui, lui, par la suite, va impressionner une plaque photographique. On obtient ainsi une image qui est une véritable carte géographique de la distribution thermique de la surface cutanée.

La thermographie ainsi obtenue comporte des plages noires (froides) et des zones blanches (chaudes). Pour passer du noir au blanc, il faut une différence de l'ordre de 1 °C, les appareils actuels étant sensibles pour des variations des gris à des différences de température cutanée de l'ordre de 0,1 °C.

On conçoit aisément que tout processus pathologique qui modifie la température dont l'émission I. R. altère l'image thermographique. Non seulement les lésions superficielles sont perceptibles, mais également celles situées en profondeur. En effet, un foyer chaud situé en profondeur modifie la température superficielle car par un mécanisme de conduction, celle-ci «projette» à la superficie.

Le thermographe (BARNES, USA) utilise un détecteur thermique ou bolomètre qui capte tout le spectre I. R. et permet un enregistrement de 60.000 points sur 200 lignes en 4 min.

La thermographie voit s'ouvrir devant elle un domaine d'applications aussi vastes que celui de la radiologie.

L'intérêt de la thermographie en Dermatologie, peut ne pas paraître évident a priori. En effet, les lésions sont superficielles, visibles à l'œil nu et directement accessible à un prélèvement biopsique.

Cependant, l'étude d'un certain nombre de cas (Colloque international de Thermographie médicale, à Strasbourg, en mars 1966) a démontré que cette technique ouvre des perspectives nouvelles vers le diagnostic des affections cutanées.

Il est par exemple possible de détecter l'extension d'un angiome sous-cutané et de guider ainsi l'acte thérapeutique. De même, il sera possible de déceler une infiltration cutanée à un stade infra-clinique, et de diriger la biopsie.

Mais c'est surtout dans l'exploration des tumeurs cutanées pigmentées que la méthode donne des résultats encourageants. Elle permet de détecter précocément la dégénérescence des lésions naeviques et de visualiser les métastases infra-cliniques. Une étude récente (Bulletin de la Société Française de Dermatologie 73, 1966, 5 bis pp 726—729 — Journées Nationales de Besançon 3 à 5 juin 1966) portant sur 23 lésions pigmentées examinées au point de vue anatomo-clinique et thermographique a permis les conclusions suivantes: les naevi banaux se traduisent du point de vue thermographique par des zones froides ou par des zones isothermiques par rapport aux régions cutanées avoisinantes. Les mélanomes malins, par contre, se caractérisent par une zone d'hyperthermie nette, débordant largement la lésion anatomique. La thermographie permet, par ailleurs, la détection des métastases ganglionnaires ou viscérales de ces tumeurs.

Les données thermographiques doivent cependant être interprétées en fonction du contexte clinique.

Toute hyperthermie au niveau d'un naevus ne signifie pas forcément une dégénérescence maligne. Un naevus pigmentaire surinfecté par exemple, se manifeste également par une zone d'hyperthermie pouvant simuler un mélanome malin. Dans ces cas, la répétition des examens thermographiques dans le temps permettra de suivre l'évolution de cette anomalie de la thermogénèse et conclure en faveur de la surinfection ou de la dégénérescence.

Dans le premier cas, l'hyperthermie régressera avec disparition de l'infection alors que dans la deuxième éventualité la zone chaude persistera.

Il est évidemment prématuré de conclure que cette méthode nouvelle d'appréciation du relief thermique permet toujours de différencier d'une façon absolue le naevus thermographiquement froid, du mélanome malin, thermographiquement chaud. Il est permis de penser que dans l'avenir, avec les améliorations techniques et la meilleure connaissance des aspects thermographiques, cette investigation deviendra un examen d'orientation précis dans le dépistage des tumeurs pigmentées.

Mais dès maintenant, elle peut apporter une contribution importante au diagnostic et au pronostic des tumeurs pigmentées et présente avec la lymphographie et la scintigraphie, une méthode d'appoint appréciable surtout par son innocuité totale.

The History of the Dermatological Section of the Royal Society of Medicine

This exhibit briefly records and illustrates the history of the Dermatological Section of the Royal Society of Medicine and the buildings in which its activities take place. Its monthly meetings, the publication of its monthly Proceedings and its fine library are the product of a long tradition.

Capillary Microscopy

T. J. RYAN, St. John's Hospital for Diseases of the Skin, London

This exhibit illustrates the concept that the patterns of the microcirculation in the skin are manifestations of growth. There is a spectrum of capillary shape ranging from atrophy to hypertrophy which can be correlated with similar changes of atrophy and hypertrophy in the tissue supplied. The vessels supplying the epidermis grow towards the epidermis and this growth is influenced by the products of epidermal cells, by nerve endings, by cells of the reticulo-endothelial system, as well as by factors of blood flow within the vessel (RYAN, 1966a, 1967a).

A new technique is described which by dispersing tissue fluid enables quick and easy exposure of the papillary vessels and subpapillary plexus (RYAN, 1965, 1967b). By use a of code and the wild M 5 microscope with drawing tube attachment the spectrum of vessel growth can be recorded and presented as a graph.

Since the chief function of the papillary vessel is to supply the epidermis, a further guide to vessel behaviour is the state of nourishment and orientation of the epidermal cell (Ryan, 1966 b, 1967 c).

Because growth influences vascular patterns the physiology of blood flow in the skin can be altered by changes towards atrophy or hypertrophy in the papillary system (Ryan, 1967 d).

Bibliography. Ryan, T. J.: J. roy. micr. Soc. **84**, 230 (1965); — Geront. clin. (Basel) **8**, 327 (1966 a); — Brit. J. Derm. **78**, 403 (1966 b); — **1**, 79 (1967 a); — Biorheology (1967 b) (In press); — Histiophysiologic study of living animals. Bourne, G. H., Ed. Baltimore: Williams & Wilkins Co (1967 c) (In press); — Variations on the morphological pattern of the microcirculation of the skin and how they may influence the interpretation of studies of blood flow. (1967 d) (In press).

Unusual Dermatophytes

Y. M. Clayton, St. John's Hospital, London

In the Department of Medical Mycology, St. John's Hospital for Diseases of the Skin, London, over 2,700 patients were seen during 1966 and material from another 3,000 patients were received from hospitals and institutions in London and other parts of England. Approximately 35% of these patients yielded positive cultures for either ringworm fungi or *Candida albicans*. The most common fungi isolated were *Trichophyton rubrum* (40% of all positive cultures), *C. albicans* (27%), *T. mentagrophytes* var. *interdigitale* (15%) and *Epidermophyton floccosum* (9%). Other fungi grown included *Microsporum audouinii*, *M. canis*, *T. mentagrophytes*, *T. verrusocum*, *T. sulphureum* and *T. violaceum*. In addition, a variant of *T. mentagrophytes* (*T. mentagrophytes* var. *erinacei*) parasitic on the hedgehog (*Erinaceus europaeus*) was isolated and four species indigenous to Africa, *T. soudanense*, *T. gourvilüi*, *T. yaoundei* and *M. audouinii* var. *rivalierii* were grown.

The cultures were all grown on Sabouraud's dextrose agar containing chloramphenicol and actidione and the temperature of incubation was 26 °C.

The isolation of *T. mentagrophytes* var. *erinacei* from hedgehogs was first reported from New Zealand in 1960 and since then has been recovered from hedgehogs in the British Isles. Human infections contracted from hedgehogs have been reported but the fungus has also been isolated from cases where no direct contact could be established. The case illustrated is one such example. The girl had numerous pet animals and attended a riding school but it was not possible to trace the source of infection.

The variant is distinguished from *T. mentagrophytes* by the production of a bright yellow pigment on the reverse of the colony, by its ability to grow at a higher temperature (optimum temperature 35 °C) and the fact that growth is inhibited at pH 4.

The three Trichophyton African species all produce endothrix scalp infection and *T. soudanense* and *T. gourvilii* can also give rise to skin and nail infections.

During 1966, seven patients with *T. soudanense* infections were seen, two of whom were children of West Indian parents but had been born in Britain. The child illustrated, although African, had been born in England and had not visited Africa although she was in contact with relatives recently arrived from Ghana. A younger brother also had scalp and skin lesions. The scalp lesions produced by *T. soudanense* are often minimal and sometimes difficult to detect; there is no fluorescence under Wood's light.

The colony is very distinctive and has no special growth requirements.

Trichophyton gourvilii was isolated from one patient in 1966 and only one other case has been seen at St. John's Hospital. Both cases were in African subjects. The lesions produced by this fungus resemble those of *T. violaceum* or *T. rubrum*.

Colony morphology is diagnostic; there are no specific growth requirements.

Trichophyton yaoundei was originally reported from the French Cameroons and is a common cause of scalp ringworm in Equatorial Africa. The case illustrated was in a white girl recently arrived from Rhodesia with a rash in the scalp which was reported to have been present for 18 months and which had not responded to local treatment.

The white, slowly growing glabrous colony could at first be confused with that of *T. verrucosum* but the colony soon darkens to deep tan or brown with the pigment diffusing into the medium. Also, unlike *T. verrucosum*, growth is not enhanced at 37 °C and there is no specific requirement for thiamin.

Microsporum audouinii var. *rivalierii*, also an African species, produces small-spored fluorescing scalp ringworm. It was first isolated from the Congo in 1963 but in 1965 19 cases of tinea capitis were reported in negro children in Florida. The case illustrated is the first recorded in Britain. The child was born in London but his parents were from Jamaica.

The rapidly growing colony is characterised by the development of many folds and microscopically the presence of abundant pectinate hyphae is diagnostic of the species.

Acknowledgement is made to the Clinicians of St. John's Hospital for Diseases of the Skin, to Dr. K. V. SANDERSON of St. George's Hospital, London, for the case of *T. gourvilii* infection, and to the Department of Medical Illustration, Institute of Dermatology.

Hyalinosis Cutis et Mucosae: Demonstration of Abnormal Metabolism of Mucopolysaccharides in the Epidermis

E. J. MOYNAHAN, London, and J. F. KENNEDY, Birmingham

It is now well established that the hyaline changes seen in connective tissue are not confined to the skin and mucosae, but are found in other organs where perivascular infiltrates may be found — e.g. brain, but despite much investigation the chemical nature of the hyaline material has not yet been determined. However, chemical studies of the mucopolysaccharides of the skin, using an isotope incorporation micromethod, in two cases, has revealed a striking increase in the keratan (keratosulphate) content of the epidermis. This may be secondary to the changes in the underlying dermis or represent the pleiotropic action of the gene. These findings were presented to the Section of Dermatology in March, 1966 [MOYNAHAN, E. J.: Proc. roy. Soc. Med. 59, 1125 (1966); KENNEDY, J. F.: Proc. roy. Soc. Med. 59, 1126 (1966)] and will be published *in extenso* elsewhere.

Progressive Profuse Lentiginosis, Progressive Cardiomyopathy, Short Stature with Delayed Puberty, Mental Retardation or Psychic Infantilism, and other Developmental Anomalies: A new Familial Syndrome

E. J. MOYNAHAN and P. POLANI, London

This striking familial syndrome, which appears to be transmitted by an autosomal gene with complete penetrance, but variable expressivity, is characterised by a progressive profuse, symmetrical lentiginosis, usually associated with a progressive cardiomyopathy. Growth is retarded, leading to short stature, puberty is delayed. Mental retardation may be present, but other patients display psychic infantilism (their behaviour is more in conformity with their stature than their intellectual capacities), other developmental anomalies include hypospadias, and cryptorchidism (Case 2) and absence of one ovary and ovarian cysts in (Case 1). Representative E.C.G.s., phonocardiographs, chest x-ray films as well as angiocardiographs illustrate the cardiomyopathy which like the lentiginosis is progressive, and may be extremely severe (Case 3), whose angiocardiograms show marked hypertrophy of muscle in all chambers of the heart and the muscular part of the septum.

Case 1 was first shown to the Clinical Section in 1960, and the first male case (2) was shown to the Section of Dermatology early in 1962 [MOYNAHAN, E. J.: Proc. roy. Soc. Med. **55,** 959 (1963)]. The disorder is not a *forme fruste* of von Recklinghausen's neurofibromatosis, as there is no evidence of neurofibromata in any patient or near relative. Similar, but clinically and genetically distinct, syndromes have recently been recorded including 'Pulmonary Stenosis, Café-au-lait spots, and Dull Intelligence' [WATSON, G. H.: Arch. Dis. Childh. **42,** 303 (1967)] and 'Electrocardiographic abnormalities in a family with generalised lentigo' [R. J. WALTHER, B. PLANSKY, and I. A. GROTS: New Engl. J. Med. **275,** 1220 (1966)]. Other familial cases with profuse lentiginosis, normal stature, bizarre E. C. G. and congenital deafness (again a separate gene) were seen at Prof. Victor McKusick's clinic at Johns Hopkins Hospital, Baltimore, USA. It is probable that the gene concerned in this new syndrome is one which interferes with the development of neural crest elements, leading to hyperactivity of melanocytes in skin (lentiginosis) and of the beta-adrenergic effectors in cardiac muscle, thus accounting for the gross abnormalities in the electrocardiograms and the marked muscular hypertrophy demonstrated. It is known that melanocytes play a part in the development of the male genital tract (Hypospadias, and ? cryptorchidism). It is also possible that some disturbance of pigmentary metabolism inside the brain, associated with dopamine and other catechol amines may lead to the delay in growth and sexual maturation. The syndrome accounts satisfactorily for the origin in some patients of so called sub-aortic valvular stenosis. The full series will be reported in detail, in the Quarterly Journal of Medicine.

Acrodermatitis Enteropathica: Evidence in Favour of Inherited Enzyme Defect (Intestinal Oligopeptidase)

E. J. MOYNAHAN, Guy's Hospital and the Hosp. for sick Children, London

Acrodermatitis enteropathica is a recessively inherited disorder, characterised by malabsorption of fats, revealed by pale, bulky, foaming, stinking stools, which is confirmed by fat balance studies, in some cases the absorption of carbohydrates is interfered with, clinically recognisable by the profuse watery, foul smelling, acid stools, glucose and galactose intolerance, and lactosuria [(MOYNAHAN, E. J.: Proc. roy. Soc. Med. **59,** 445 (1966)]. The striking resemblance of some of the cutaneous manifestations to those seen in a recently recognised nutritional deficiency state in infants on synthetic diets (MANN, T. P., E. M. WILSON, and B. E. CLAYTON: Arch. Dis. Childh. **40,** 364) suggests that the absorption of some of the vitamins of B complex (biotin, inositol, choline, pantothenic acid and pyridoxine) is interfered with. The disorder is one of weaning suggesting that the noxious agent is produced by incomplete breakdown of some substance in the infants diet, probably a protein, the incomplete hydrolysis of which yields a small peptide which has toxic properties. The enzyme-histochemical and ultrastructural studies displayed provide evidence which points towards a defective or absent oligo-peptidase. Current views on the localisation of enzymes in the intestinal villus cell were illustrated and evidence presented to show that the toxic peptide may depress, some of the enzymes located in or on the cell membrane of the microvillus (leucine aminopeptidase): depression of mitochondrial enzymes was revealed by the weak succinic dehydrogenase reaction in biopsy specimens. No evidence of interference with lysosomal enzymes was obtained, in contrast to enzyme histochemical findings in coeliac disease. Fat absorption may be interfered with by the presence of the toxic peptide in or at the surface of the cell membrane, and further evidence of this interference is well shown in the electron micrograph in which marked pinocytotic activity, as well as dilatation of the intercellular spaces and the golgi apparatus is seen. In Case 2, secondary lactose intolerance was demonstrated by jejunal biopsy, which revealed that lactase was present but the reaction was weak. Lactase is found deep in the microvillus and not at its surface. Clinical evidence of glucose and galactose intolerance in the same patient indicated that transport of these monosaccharides was being interfered with. The absorption of the toxic peptide into blood, probably interferes with the synthesis of hard keratin (alopecia, and loss of nails). Psychic depression and apathy could result from the toxic action of the peptide itself, or might be the consequence of the vitamin deficiency state. Tryptophane loading does not aggravate this disorder, thus excluding a possible defect in tryptophane metabolism. The therapeutic action of both hydroxyquinolone derivatives and penicillamine is accounted for by their chelation of the oligo-peptide itself which may well contain a cystyl residue. The evidence presented overall points to absence of or defect in an oligopeptidase as the cause of acrodermatitis enteropathica.

The Photodermatoses

L. A. MAGNUS, Institute of Dermatology, London

This exhibit illustrates the investigation, classification and treatment of the photodermatoses. Using a monochromator light testing apparatus it is possible to find causative wavelengths and to reproduce lesions as well as to identify abnormal photosensitising substances in the skin.

People with certain diseases, notably porphyria or those exposed to some industrial hazards e.g. pitch, show photosensitivity. This can be reproduced experimentally by placing porphyrins or anthracene on the skin and illuminating at the wavelength of maximum absorption of these compounds (400 m. for porphyrins and 360 m for anthracene). Within 10 min a painful weal develops. This does not happen if the skin is deprived of oxygen during the illumination.

Some of these compounds, such as porphyrins and anthracene tend to be stored in intra-cellular bodies known as lysosomes. These contain powerful hydrolytic enzymes, which, when released into the cell, will cause its disruption and death.

If lysosomes in the skin containing porphyrins etc., are illuminated with an appropriate wavelength in the presence of oxygen, they rupture releasing their hydrolytic enzymes. It is suggested that this mechanism may be the basis of the skin lesion in photosensitivity.

Zellphysiologische Aspekte der Psoriasis vulgaris

O. Braun-Falco, E. Christophers, S. Marghescu, D. Petzoldt, G. Rassner und M. Rupec, Dermatol. Univ.-Klinik Marburg/Lahn (Deutschland)

Die statisch-morphologische Betrachtung der Hautveränderungen bei Psoriasis vulgaris hat bereits Ansatzpunkte für die Analyse von Ätiologie und Pathogenese dieser Erkrankung geliefert. Weitere interessante Aspekte hat die Anwendung neuerer Untersuchungsmethoden (Histochemie, Biochemie, Autoradiographie, Immunologie, Elektronenmikroskopie) ergeben. Die Ausstellung demonstriert einige entsprechende Ergebnisse unseres Arbeitskreises.

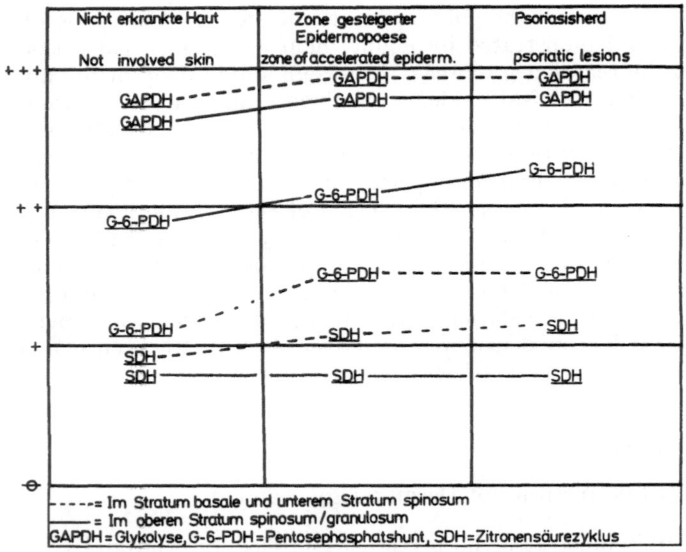

Abb. 1. Histochem. Enzymaktivitätsmuster in der Epidermis von Psoriasispatienten

Histochemische Untersuchungen: Mit histochemischer Methodik wurden Enzyme des energieliefernden Stoffwechsels untersucht. Um zur Dynamik der psoriatischen Hautveränderungen eine Aussage machen zu können, erfolgten die Untersuchungen im Psoriasisherd, in der Zone gesteigerter Epidermopoese und in herdnaher, klinisch und histologisch normaler Epidermis (Abb. 1). Es wurde gezeigt, daß in herdnaher, klinisch und histologisch normaler Epidermis die Aktivitätsmuster der geprüften Enzyme genau die gleichen sind wie in der Epidermis von hautgesunden Kontrollpersonen.

In der Zone gesteigerter Epidermopoese steigen die Aktivitäten einiger glykolytischer und NADP-spezifischer Enzyme in der Epidermis stark an. Der Aktivitätsanstieg der Enzyme des Citronensäurecyclus und der Atmungskette ist vergleichsweise weniger stark und auf die coriumnahen Epidermislagen begrenzt. In der Epidermis des Psoriasisherdes setzt sich der Anstieg der Enzymaktivitäten nur noch geringfügig fort. Lediglich die geprüften Enzyme des Pentosephosphatcyclus zeigen im oberen Stratum spinosum und Stratum granulosum des Psoriasisherdes deutlich stärkere Aktivitäten als in den entsprechenden Schichten der Zone gesteigerter Epidermopoese.

Es wird festgestellt, daß der epidermale energieliefernde Stoffwechsel in der Zone gesteigerter Epidermopoese und im Psoriasisherd gegenüber normaler Epidermis qualitativ nicht verändert, sondern nur durch eine Änderung des Verhältnisses von oxydativem zu glykolytischem Stoffwechsel zugunsten des letzteren gekennzeichnet ist. Die erhöhten Aktivitäten von Enzymen der Glykolyse und NADP-spezifischer Dehydrogenasen lassen auf einen gesteigerten energieliefernden Stoffwechsel im Bereich der Glykolyse und eine vermehrte Bereitstellung von Wasserstoff für reduktive Biosynthesen schließen (Ausführliche Veröffentlichung erfolgt im Arch. klin. exp. Derm.).

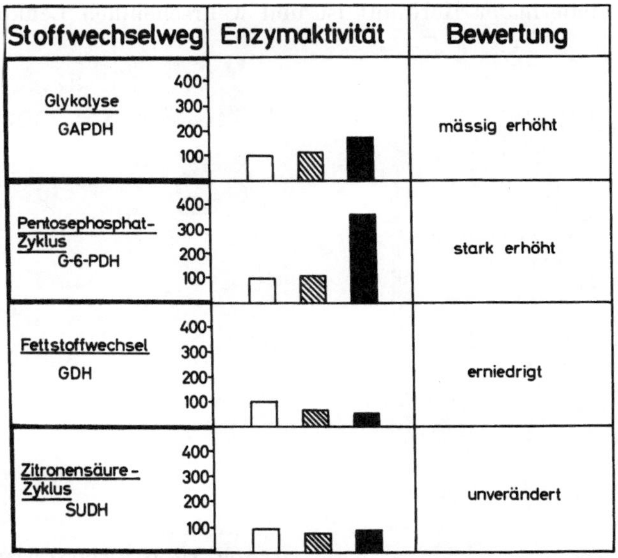

Stoffwechselweg	Enzymaktivität	Bewertung
Glykolyse GAPDH		mässig erhöht
Pentosephosphat- Zyklus G-6-PDH		stark erhöht
Fettstoffwechsel GDH		erniedrigt
Zitronensäure- Zyklus SUDH		unverändert

Abb. 2. Prozentuale Aktivitätsveränderung von jeweils einem Enzym der untersuchten Stoffwechselwege. Epidermis: Normal, Enzymaktivität ▭; Psoriasis vulgaris: klinisch unveränderte Haut, Enzymaktivität ▨; Psorisais vulgaris: Herdbereich, Enzymaktivität ▬

Biochemische Untersuchungen: In der Epidermis von Normalpersonen, in der Epidermis klinisch nicht befallener Bezirke bei Patienten mit Psoriasis vulgaris und der Epidermis des Psoriasisherdes wurden 15 bzw. 18 Enzyme der Glykolyse, des Pentosephosphatcyclus, des Citronensäurecyclus und angeschlossener Reaktionen quantitativ-biochemisch bestimmt. In nicht erkrankter Epidermis von Patienten mit Psoriasis vulgaris war die Aktivität fast aller untersuchter Enzyme geringgradig, aber nicht signifikant erhöht. Lediglich die Aktivität des Enzyms Glycerin-1-Phosphat-Dehydrogenase war vermindert (nicht signifikant). In der Epidermis des Psoriasisherdes fanden sich vorwiegend ausgeprägte Enzymaktivitätserhöhungen, die im Bereich der Glykolyse ca. 75%, bei den NADPH-liefernden Dehydrogenasen ca. 200% betrugen. Eine Aktivitätsverminderung fand sich lediglich bei den Enzymen GDH und GPT (Abb. 2).

Die sehr starke Aktivitätserhöhung NADPH-liefernder Dehydrogenasen wird mit einem erhöhten Bedarf der Epidermiszellen an NADPH für reduktive Biosynthesen im Rahmen einer stark beschleunigten Zellreifung gesehen. Die Erhöhung der Enzymaktivitäten glykolytischer Enzyme bei gleichbleibender Enzymaktivität im Bereich des Citronensäurecyclus deutet auf eine Steigerung der sauerstoffunabhängigen, energieliefernden Reaktionen hin. Die Aktivitäts-verminderung der Enzyme GDH (→ Fettstoffwechsel) und GPT (→ Eiweißstoff-wechsel) ist funktionell noch nicht sicher erklärbar.

Immunologische und enzymelektrophoretische Untersuchungen: Die Fraktio-nierung wasserlöslicher Psoriasis-Schuppenextrakte mit Hilfe der diskontinuier-lichen Polyacrylamidgel-Elektrophorese (PAA-El.) ergab zahlreiche Proteinbanden (Abb. 3). Eine Aufschlüsselung der Proteinfraktionen nach ihrer Herkunft mittels PAA-El. von isolierten Leukocyten und von Homogenaten normaler Epidermis sowie durch Immunoelektrophorese der Extrakte gegen Antihumanserum von Kaninchen zeigte, daß ein Teil der Proteine in den Extrakten psoriatischer Horn-schicht nicht epidermaler Herkunft ist und wahrscheinlich Leukocytenproteine

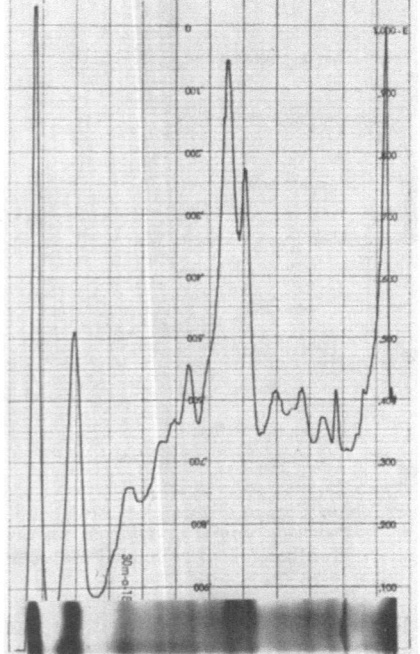

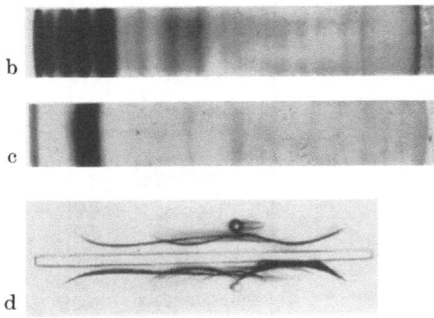

Abb. 3a—d. a Polyacrylamidgel-Elektro-phorese wasserlöslicher Psoriasis-Schuppenextrakte. b Polyacrylamidgel-Elektrophorese isolierter Leucocyten. c Polyacrylamidgel-Elektrophorese nor-maler Epidermis. d Immunoelektro-phorese wasserlöslicher Psoriasis-Schuppenextrakte

(Munro-Absceß) und Serumproteine (Exoserose) darstellt (Abb. 3). Aus diesen Untersuchungen geht hervor, daß der wasserlösliche Gesamtextrakt psoriatischer Hornschicht ein inhomogenes Antigen ist und als solches für immunologische Zwecke ungeeignet erscheint.

Die *enzymelektrophoretische* Untersuchung von Homogenaten psoriatischer Epidermis auf Lactatdehydrogenase(LDH)-Aktivität diente der Klärung der Stoffwechsellage. Das Homogenat normaler Epidermis enthielt nur LDH_4 als ein-ziges Isozym. Dieses Muster ist typisch für eine vorwiegend anaerobe Stoffwechsel-situation eines Organs. Das LDH-Cymogramm psoriatischer Epidermis zeigte das gleiche LDH_4-Isozym, nur stark vermehrt. Eine zusätzliche schwache LDH_3-Bande kann auf die Exoserose und/oder auf die Leukocyten der Munro-Abscesse zurückgeführt werden. Es ergibt sich daraus auch für die psoriatische Epidermis eine vorwiegend anaerobe Stoffwechsellage bei stark erhöhter Enzymaktivität.

Autoradiographische Untersuchungen: Nach autoradiographischer Darstellung

[3]H-Thymidin-markierter DNS-synthetisierender Epidermiszellen fand sich an der klinisch normalen Haut von Patienten mit Psoriasis vulgaris eine im Vergleich zu Normalpersonen signifikant erhöhte Zahl dieser prämitotischen Zellen. Nach Hornschichtabriß wurde der Anstieg ^{3}H-Thymidin-markierter Kerne in Abhängig-

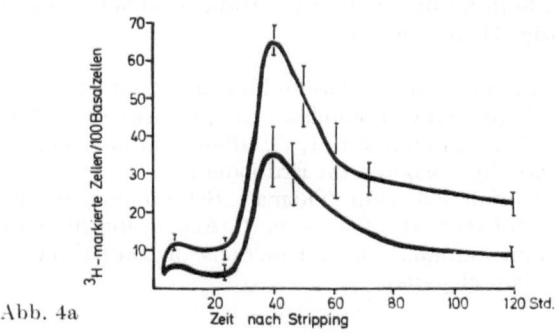

Abb. 4a

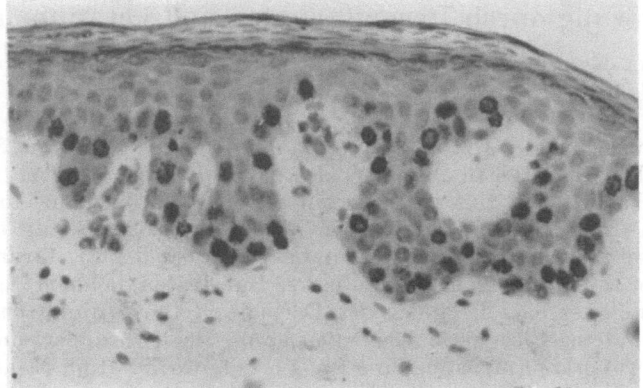

Abb. 4b

keit von der Zeit verfolgt. Es konnte auch hier eine überschießende Reizbeantwortung durch Zunahme DNS-synthetisierender Zellen beobachtet werden (Abb. 4).

Inkubation von Excisaten psoriatischer Haut mit RNS- und Aminosäurevorläufern ergab eine stärkere Silberkornschwärzung der angefertigten Autoradiogramme als Hinweis gesteigerter Syntheseleistungen der psoriatischen Epidermis (Abb. 5).

Elektronenmikroskopische Untersuchungen: Es wird gezeigt, daß die saure Phosphatase in der normalen, unveränderten Epidermis und der psoriatischen Epidermis folgendermaßen verteilt ist:

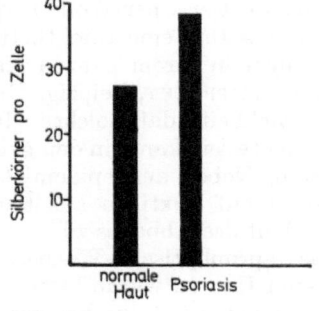

Abb. 5

1. Intracellulär, und zwar als freie, nicht strukturgebundene, an Keratohyalingranula gebundene und lysosomale saure Phosphatase.

2. Extracellulär im Intercellularraum der ortho- und parakeratotischen Hornschicht.

Mycology

Mikroskopische Demonstration von Fadenpilzen und Hefen

H. Braun und C. Schönborn, Klinik für Hautkrankheiten der Karl Marx-
Universität Leipzig (Deutschland)

1. Farbaufnahmen zum Thema ,,Anwendungsmöglichkeiten der Fluorescenzmikroskopie bei mykologischen Untersuchungen" (Nachweis von Pilzelementen im
KOH-Präparat und in Hautfrischmaterial; Vitalfluorochromierung von Hefezellen;
Nachweis von Dermatophytensporen im Erdboden).
2. Schwarz-weiß-Aufnahmen zum Thema ,,Schimmelpilze aus Krankheits-
erscheinungen — Saprophyten oder Parasiten?" (Aspergillus nidulans; Penicillium
claviforme; Verticillium cinnabarinum; Rhizopus oryzae; Chrysosporium keratinophilum; Thamnidium elegans).

Faserzerstörung durch Dermatophyten und keratinophile Pilze

L. Krempl-Lamprecht, Dermatologische Universitätsklinik München
(Deutschland)

Der Lebenscyclus der Dermatophyten kann entweder nach dem Schema einer
kontinuierlichen Infektkette ablaufen, also einer ununterbrochenen Übertragung
von einem lebenden Wirt zum anderen (mit anderen Worten: einer fortwährenden
parasitischen Entwicklung), oder einer diskontinuierlichen Infektkette, d. h.
einem Wechsel zwischen parasitischer und saprophytischer Ernährung.

Unter den saprophytisch besiedelbaren Substraten nehmen Skleroproteine
eine Sonderstellung ein, da außer der Dermatophytenverwandtschaft nur eine
kleine Zahl anderer Pilze sie aufschließen kann. Beide Gruppen sind gegenüber
anderen Nahrungskonkurrenten dort im Vorteil, wo keratinhaltige Substanzen
vorliegen. In der freien Natur stellt z. B. der Erdboden mit seinem stellenweise
gehäuften Anfall tierischer Skleroproteine (Federn, Haare, Hufe, Horn, Stacheln...)
ein solches Auslesesubstrat dar. Daneben erfüllen aber — bei entsprechender
Feuchtigkeit — auch Gegenstände des täglichen Bedarfs diese Voraussetzungen,
etwa die aus tierischer Wolle hergestellten Garne und Textilien, Filz usw. Es gelingt zwar selten, eine Infektkette mit langdauerndem saprophytischen Stadium
in Textilien in ihrem ganzen Entwicklungsverlauf zu verfolgen (Vgl. Vortrag
Krempl-Lamprecht, Leipzig, Mai 1966). In der Praxis berücksichtigt man aber
die Möglichkeit, daß solches Material Zwischenträger und Reservoir lebender
Pilzelemente sein kann, in den bekannten hygienischen Empfehlungen an Mykose-
patienten. Neben den epidemiologisch bedeutsamen Folgerungen läßt das Pilz-
wachstum auf Textilien aus tierischen Fasern auch interessante Aussagen über
den Verlauf des Abbaues zu.

Das saprophytische Wachstum der Dermatophyten auf natürlichen, unver-
arbeiteten Haaren wurde bisher schon von verschiedener Seite beschrieben, teils
bei Untersuchungen zur Ermittlung der keratinolytischen Potenz, teils mit dem
Ziel, aus unterschiedlichen Befallsformen artdiagnostische Merkmale abzuleiten.
Zusammengefaßt ergibt sich aus diesen Beobachtungen, daß Dermatophyten beim
Aufschluß der Skleroproteine praktisch eine eigene Wuchsform entwickeln, bei
der mechanische und enzymatische Komponenten vereinigt sind. Angaben über

den Haarangriff durch Nichtdermatophyten sind dagegen spärlich und teilweise widersprüchlich.

In meiner Demonstration habe ich versucht, in 16 Abbildungen (hier eine Auswahl von 8 Abbildungen), die wesentlichen Unterschiede der Wuchsformen beider Pilzgruppen darzustellen, wie sie auf verarbeiteter Wolle auftreten.

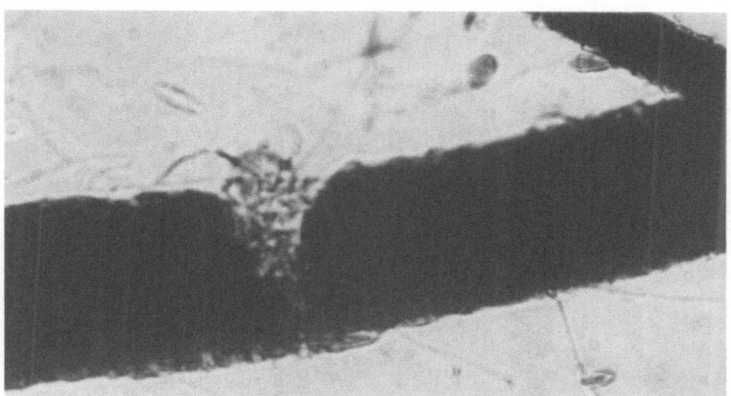

Abb. 1. Perforation der Wollfaser durch Microsporum gypseum

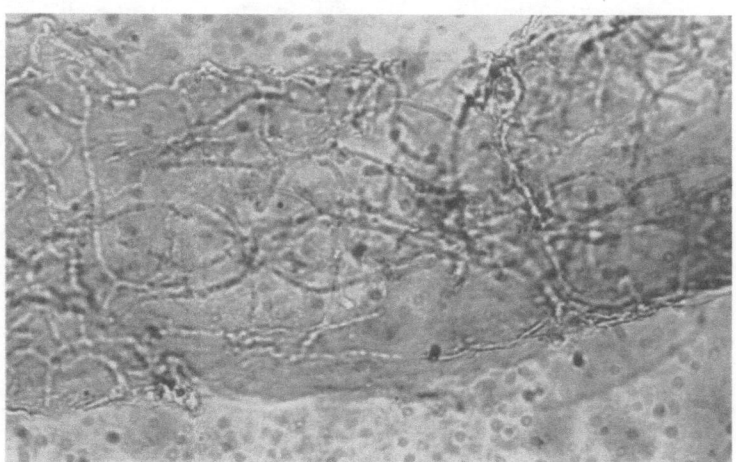

Abb. 2. Trichophyton terrestre, Erosionsmycel vor der Bildung der Perforation

Mit Ausnahme von *Trichophyton mentagrophytes*, der aus einer Kamelhaardecke isoliert worden war, stammten sämtliche Pilze von Fangproben aus Schafwollstoffen, die im Rahmen anderer Untersuchungen im Boden vergraben und anschließend in feuchter Kammer gehalten wurden. Es handelte sich um Stoffstücke 1. aus reiner Merinowolle, 2. Wolle mit Naturseide (tierische Faser), 3. Wolle mit Baumwolle (pflanzl. Faser), 4. Wolle mit sog. Zellwolle (synthet. Faser). Von den dabei isolierten Pilzen wurden als Demonstrationsbeispiele ausgewählt:

a) die beiden geophilen Dermatophyten *Trichophyton terrestre* und *Microsporum gypseum*,

b) die auf allen Fangproben regelmäßig auftretenden *Schimmelpilze* aus den Gattungen *Scopulariopsis, Chrysosporium* und *Chaetomium*.

Obwohl damit gerechnet wurde, daß mit den verschiedenartigen chemischen Einflüssen bei der Textilherstellung eine Veränderung der Wollfaser einhergeht, die sich eventuell in einem veränderten Pilzangriff äußert, ließen sich doch bei den

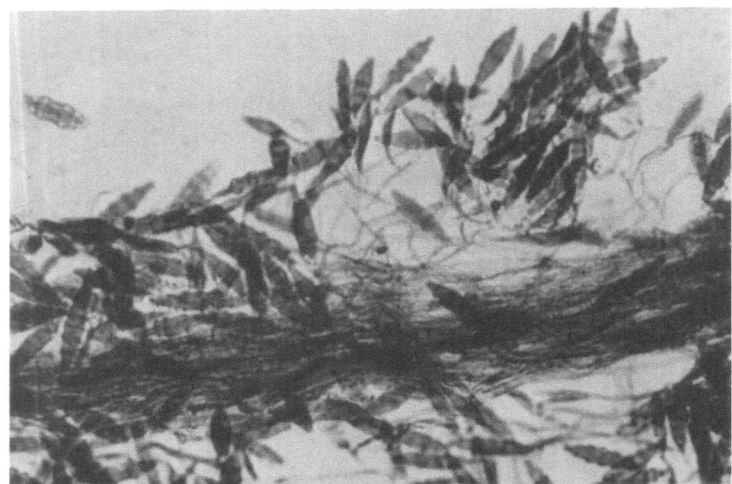

Abb. 3. Endstadium des Abbaus durch Microsporum gypseum

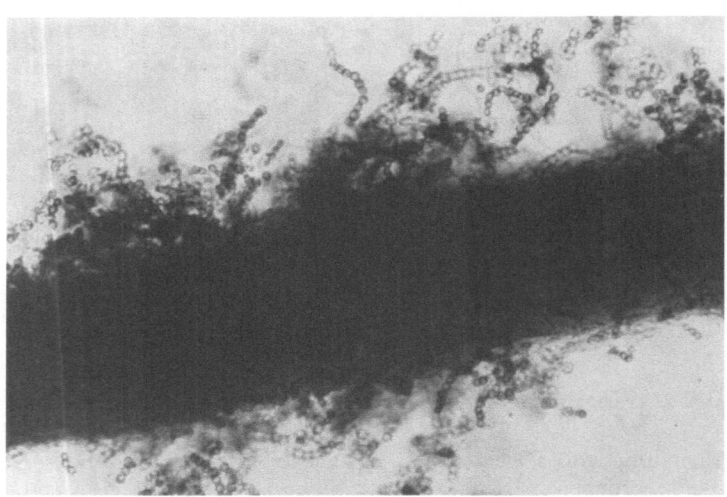

Abb. 4. Scopulariopsis sphaerospora auf Wollfaser

drei Arten aus der Dermatophytenverwandtschaft die für sie typischen Befallsformen nachweisen:

1. *Anhebung der Cuticularschuppen*, wenn kurze Seitenhyphen des ursprünglich längs der Haaroberfläche verlaufenden Mycels unter diese eindringen.

2. *Abbauerscheinungen der Rindenschicht* (Kortex): Hier herrschte der *diffuse Haarabbau* vor, es konnten aber auch — wenn auch erheblich seltener als auf

natürlichen Schafhaaren — bei allen drei Stämmen relativ schmale *Perforationen* beobachtet werden. Dabei fiel auf, daß hier die enzymatisch bedingte Erweiterung zur breiten Trogform fehlte. Der ganze Einbruchskeil war von Lufthyphen erfüllt, die fast unmittelbar nach der Ausbildung der dick- und kurzzelligen Perforations-hyphe an deren Basis entstanden (Abb. 1).

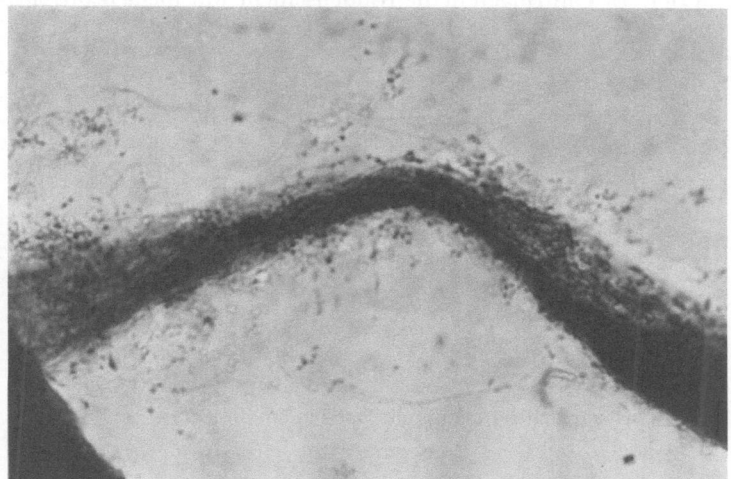

Abb. 5. Diffuser Faserabbau durch Chryososporium pannorum (beachte die sehr kleinen, fast dreieckigen Conidien!)

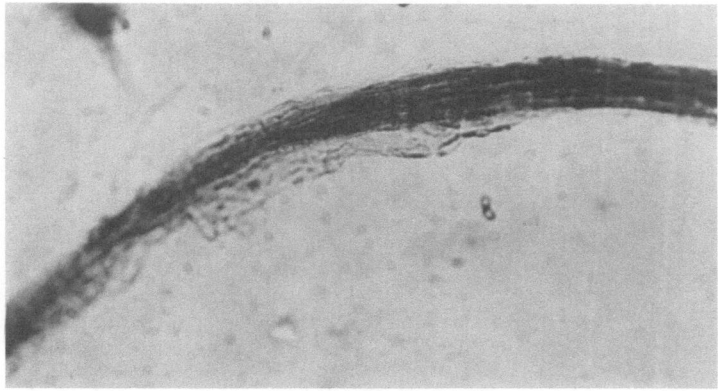

Abb. 6. Cuticulaablösung durch Chaetomium indicum

3. Bei Trichophyton terrestre konnten in künstlich aufgehellten Präparaten auch die vom Erosionsmycel ausgehenden *Mycelstrukturen in Farnwedel-* oder Palmetten*form* erkannt werden, von denen später die Perforationsorgane ihren Ausgang nehmen (Abb. 2).

Das Endstadium des Abbaus ließ sich mit Microsporum gypseum bei den Mischtextilien besonders deutlich darstellen: Selektiv waren neben unversehrten Baumwollfasern die Wollfasern praktisch aufgelöst („Geisterhaare"). An ihrer Stelle markierten lebhaft makrokondienbildende Hyphenbüschel ihren ehemaligen Verlauf (Abb. 3).

Schimmelpilze

Scopulariopsis brevicaulis und sphaerospora (Abb. 4). Auf eine dichte Umhüllung der Wollfasern mit Luftmycel folgte ein dermatophytenähnliches *Ein-
wachsen seitlicher Hyphenverzweigungen unter die Cuticularschuppen*, an das sich
eine reichliche Konidienbildung nach außen hin anschloß. Damit war der Angriff
beendet, ein tieferes Vordringen in die Rindenschicht war nicht beobachtbar, auch

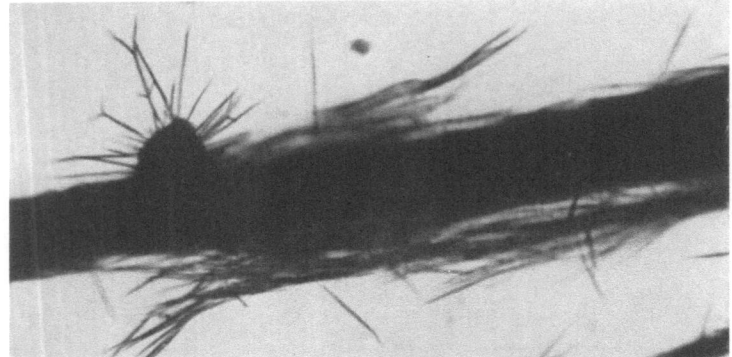

Abb. 7. Cortexaufsplitterung durch Chaetomium indicum

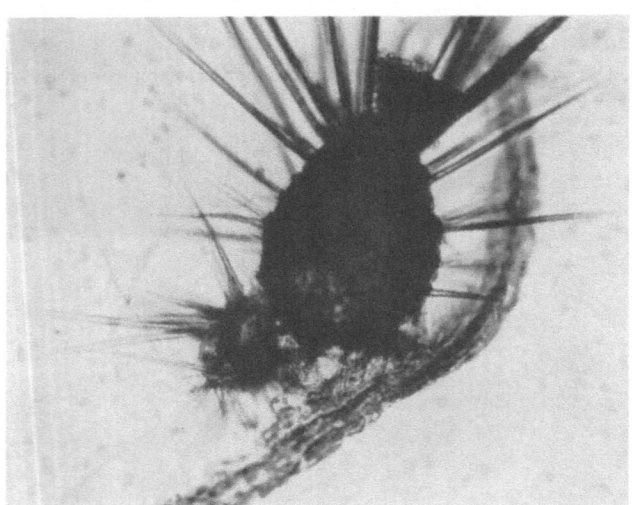

Abb. 8. Bohr- bzw. Hafthyphen, von der Basis des Ascocarps von
Chaetomium indicum ausgehend

nicht in künstlich aufgehellten und gequollenen Fasern, die mit ihren hochgedrück-
ten Schuppen, unter denen Mycel lag, an ausgetrocknete Coniferenzapfen erinnerten.

Chrysosporium pannorum (Abb. 5). Dieser nicht selten von der Haut isolierte
Schimmelpilz zeigte beachtliche Ähnlichkeit mit der Angriffsform der Dermatophyten. Vorherrschend war eine *Lockerung der Cuticula*, gepaart mit einer Mycel-
umhüllung der Wollfaser. Nach einiger Zeit traten Schwunderscheinungen auf,
die der *großflächigen, diffusen Haarverdauung* der Dermatophyten gleichen. Echte
Perforationshyphen fehlten, vereinzelt drangen Hyphenäste senkrecht in die
Rindenschicht ein.

Chaetomium indicum (Abb. 6, 7, 8). Obwohl sich diese Pilzgattung vor allem durch cellulolytische Fähigkeiten auszeichnet, war der Abbau tierischer Fasern weitgehender als erwartet. Schmale *Hyphen* etwa vom Durchmesser der Lufthyphen *durchbohrten* besonders an den Schuppenrändern *die Cuticula* und drangen senkrecht in die Rinde ein. Dort kam es zu teils rechtwinkeligen Verzweigungen, wobei sukzessive *spindelförmige Zellen aus der Rindenschicht abgestoßen wurden.* Im Stadium der Ascocarpbildung drangen von deren Basis zusätzliche dunkle Bohrhyphen wie Haftorgane in die Faser ein. Echte Perforationen fehlten auch hier ebenso wie Erscheinungen enzymatischen Abbaus.

Die Gegenüberstellung des Faserabbaus in schafwollhaltigen Textilien bestätigte somit, daß die Angriffsform der Dermatophyten Ausdruck ihrer echten Keratinophilie ist, während die Wuchsformen der — nur selten als Parasiten auftretenden — Schimmelpilze dafür sprechen, daß sie vor allem von den Kittsubstanzen leben, die die keratinisierten Zellen zusammenhalten.

Dermatophyten und ihre Hauptfruchtformen

G. A. DE VRIES, Centraalbureau voor Schimmelcultures, Baarn (Niederlande), und L. KREMPL-LAMPRECHT, Dermatologische Universitätsklinik München (Deutschland)

Im Verlauf des letzten Jahrzehnts hat die Systematik der Dermatophyten eine beachtliche Erweiterung erfahren, vor allem durch die Beschreibung einer Reihe der zugehörigen perfekten Formen. Um den mykologisch interessierten Dermatologen aus aller Welt Gelegenheit zu geben, nicht nur diejenigen Pilze, die tagtäglich in Klinik und Praxis vorkommen, in ihrer saprophytären Wuchsform zu sehen, sondern auch seltene oder erst kürzlich beschriebene Arten, hat das Centraalbureau voor Schimmelcultures (DE VRIES) eine Reihe von Teststämmen zur Verfügung gestellt, von denen im Mykologischen Laboratorium der Dermatologischen Universitätsklinik München (KREMPL-LAMPRECHT) in Petri-Schalen sog. Riesenkolonien auf Czapek-Dox-Agar + 1% Pepton angelegt wurden.

Selbst wenn man die bei Dermatophyten besonders ausgeprägte Nährbodenvarianz in Rechnung zieht, dürften für einen Großteil der Betrachter diese Kulturen der lebenden Pilze mit ihrer Farb- und Formcharakteristik anschaulichere Demonstrationsobjekte darstellen als fotografische Aufnahmen.

Perfektes Stadium	*zugehöriges imperfektes Stadium*
1. Nannizzia incurvata Nannizzia gypsea Nannizzia fulva	Microsporum gypseum
2. Nannizzia cajetana	Microsporum cookei
3. Nannizzia obtusa	Microsporum nanum
4. Nannizzia grubyia	Microsporum vanbreuseghemi
5. —	Microsporum canis
6. —	Microsporum distortum
7. —	Microsporum audouini
8. —	Microsporum ferrugineum
9. Arthroderma quadrifidum	Trichophyton terrestre

Seltene, bzw. kürzlich beschriebene Arten:
Trichophyton yaoundei
Trichophyton indicum
Trichophyton evolceanui

Serological Relationship of the Dermatophytes of Emmons-Conant-System

H. PALDROK and K. R. SUNDSTRÖM, Stockholm (Sweden)

Adaptationsphasen der Dermatophyten in Zusammenhang mit ihrer Klassifikation

V. A. BALABANOFF, Dermatologische Universitätsklinik Sofia (Bulgarien)

Bei ihrem Übergang vom Saprophytismus zum Parasitismus haben die primitiven Dermatophyten neue Eigenschaften zum Vorschein gebracht. Sie lassen sich bereits wie pathogene Arten von anderen Gesetzen leiten. Deshalb muß man bei ihrer Klassifizierung, im Vergleich mit den saprophytären Arten, andere Kriterien anwenden.

Die Studien über den Polymorphismus und die Variabilität der Dermatophyten (1955) haben uns die einzelnen Stufen ihrer biologischen Differenzierung gezeigt. Die vergleichenden Untersuchungen über die Bodendermatophyten aus Kontrast-biotopen (1963) — Höhlen und Tierställen — mit verschiedenem Gehalt an organischen Resten sowie aus pflanzlichen Resten durch eine von uns modifizierte Haarködermethode (1965) haben einerseits ihre Ökologie in Zusammenhang mit den Adaptationsphasen gezeigt und andererseits unsere Vorstellungen über ihre Phylogenie erweitert. Bei Kultivierung von *A. quadrifidum*, *N. cajetana*, *N. incurvata* und des perfekten anascogenen Stadiums von *T. mentagrophytes* auf Dextrose-agar nach SABOURAUD (24 °C) sind drei Entwicklungsphasen des perfekten und des imperfekten Stadiums zu beobachten: 1. wollig-noduläre Phase des perfekten ascogenen Stadiums, 2. granulöse Phase des perfekten anascogenen Stadiums und 3. gipsartige, asteroide oder flaumige Phase des imperfekten makroconidialen Stadiums. Diese Phasen gehen parallel mit ausgeprägter morphologischer Reduktion ihrer Fruchtkörper.

Für die Bestimmung einer pathogenen Dermatophytenart, die gegenüber einer vergleichbaren saprophytären Art völlig abweichende Merkmale aufweist, muß nicht nur der Wert der rein botanischen, sondern auch der sog. „sekundären" und „phylogenetischen" (BALABANOFF, 1955) (s. Tab. 1) Merkmale hervorgehoben werden. Von den genannten phylogenetischen Merkmalen zeigt sich in den Grenzen ein- und derselben Dermatophytenart, bei Bodenisolaten mit vollständiger Fruktifikation, ein schnelleres Wachstum (Diametermessung und Durchwachsen von Agarsäulchen nach HRUSZEK, 1934) und eine geringfügigere Pigmentierung im Gegensatz zu verlangsamtem Wachstum sowie stärkerer Pigmentierung bei Isolaten von pathologischen Läsionen mit reduzierter Morphologie des imperfekten Stadiums. Gleichlaufend geht der Übergang von wollig-nodulären Kulturen in granulös-gipsartige oder flaumige vor sich. Dieser Übergang kann mit einer Erhöhung der Pathogenität einhergehen. Durch CO_2-Einwirkung war es uns möglich (1963), ähnliche Erscheinungen hervorzurufen.

Die geschilderten Adaptationsphasen, die sich schon früh bei den saprophytären Formen äußern, sind der Ausgangspunkt gewesen für eine erweiterte Gradierung der Dermatophyten in eine wollig-granulöse saprophytäre Phase des perfekten Stadiums, eine gipsartig-granulöse oder asteroide Übergangsphase und

Tabelle 1

Degree of parasitic adaptation	Cultures of dextrose agar of SABOURAUD (24 /C)	Micromorphology	Physiology	Parasitology	Ecology (habitat)
1. Perfect state grade I Type Arthroderma quadrifidum Nannizzia cajetana Nannizzia incurvata	Downy-nodular or granular	Ascigerous, cleistothecial state	Rapid growth as a mold, rich enzyme and antibiotic activity. Perforating organs are regular observed. Relative resistance to fungistatic drugs.	Saprophytism	Soil or organic wast matter of plant origin (BALABANOFF, 1965), rodents or other mamalian pels.
2. Perfect state grade II Type A. quadrifidum	Granular or downy-nodular	Anascigerous cleistothecial state	Rapid growth as a mold, rich enzyme and antibiotic activity. Perforating organs are regular observed. Relative resistance to fungistatic drugs. Slower growth	Saprophytism or rarely atypical parasitism (soil or plant trauma), tendency toward spontaneus cure, positive trichophytine tests.	Soil or organic wast matter of plant origin (BALABANOFF, 1965), rodents or other mamalian pels.
3. Imperfect state grade I Type T. terrestre T. cookei M. gypseum	Granular, asteroid or fluffy	Macroconidial, abortiv-cleistothecial state	Slower growth More marked pigment production	Saprophytism or rarely atypical parasitism (soil or plant trauma), tendency toward spontaneus cure, positive trichophytine tests.	Rare infections of animals and humans
4. Imperfect state grade II Type T. mentagrophytes M. canis	granular, asteroid or fluffy	Macroconidial (with reduced number of macroconidia) pseudocleistothecial, rarely abortive-cleistothecial state	More marked pigment production	Inflammatory mycoses with tendency toward spontaneus cure, positive trichophytine tests and inoculation to experimental animals.	Heteroreceptive, zooantropophilic infections
5. Imperfect state grade III Type T.(A.) quinckeanum T. rubrum M. audouini	Fluffy or velvety "withe species" ingrowing into the agar	Microconidial state (relyadaptive forms of macroconidia)	More marked pigment production.	Balanced parasitism, transition from ecto- to endothrixy-epidermphytosis, superficial pilomycosis resistent to treatment.	Monoreceptive zoophilic or antropophilic infections—school infections, chronic trichophytosis of the adult, epidermophytosis of bath in swimmers, occupational contact in medical personal, farmers etc.
6. Imperfect state grade IV Type T. violaceum T. tonsurans M. ferrugineum-withe varieties	Cerebriform or waxy-faviform with disappearing air mycelium, or finegranular with cerebriform or crateriform center, slow pleomorphism	Microconidial state with marked morphological reduction.	Physiological specialisation and reduction (BALABANOFF, 1960) as regards the utilisation of vitamine (vitamin-deficient species), aminoacids and lipids, and growth rate. Perforating organs are hardly to obtain or lacking. Hyperpigmented species.	Balanced parasitism, transition from ecto- to endothrixy-epidermphytosis, superficial pilomycosis resistent to treatment.	Monoreceptive zoophilic or antropophilic infections—school infections, chronic trichophytosis of the adult, epidermophytosis of bath in swimmers, occupational contact in medical personal, farmers etc.
7. Imperfect state grade V Type T. concentricum M. ferrugineum var. aureum	Cerebriform or waxy-faviform	Mycelial or chlamidosporial state with complete morphological reduction.	Physiological specialization and reduction (BALABANOFF, 1960) as regards the utilisation of vitamine (vitamin-deficient species), aminoacids and lipids, and growth rate. Perforating organs are hardly to obtain or lacking. Hyperpigmented species.	Balanced parasitism, transition from ecto- to endothrixy-epidermphytosis, superficial pilomycosis resistent to treatment.	Monoreceptive zoophilic or antropophilic infections—school infections, chronic trichophytosis of the adult, epidermophytosis of bath in swimmers, occupational contact in medical personal, farmers etc.

eine flaumig-samtige oder cerebriformfaviforme pathogene Phase (BALABANOFF, 1965; Abb. 1, 2, 3).

Tabelle 2. *Dermatophytes*

A. Perfect state "Gymnoascaceae"
(ascigerous and anascigerous state)

1. Arthroderma
A. quadrifidum, DAWSON and GENTLES, 1961
A. uncinatum, DAWSON and GENTLES, 1961
A. gertleri BÖHME, 1967
A. benhamiae AJELLO and CHEN, 1967

2. Nannizzia
N. cajetana AJELLO, 1961
N. incurvata, STOCKDALE, 1961
N. grubyia, GEORG and al., 1962
N. obtusa DAWSON and GENTLES, 1961

B. Imperfect State "Fungi imperfecti"
(I, II, III, IV and V grade)

1. Vanbreuseghemia
Grade I
    K. ajelloi VANBREUSEGHEM, 1952

2. Matruchotia
Grade I
    T. terrestre, DURIE and FREY, 1957
    T. vanbreuseghemii RIOUX and al., 1964
Grade II
    T. mentagrophytes ROBIN, 1853
    T. interdigitale PRISTLEY, 1917
Grade III
    T. cerebriforme SABOURAUD, 1909
Grade IV
    T. tonsurans, MALMSTEN, 1845

3. Sabouraudia
Grade 1
    M. cookei AJELLO, 1959
    M. gypseum (BODIN), GUIART et GRIGORAKIS, 1928
    M. vanbreuseghemii GEORG and al. 1962
    M. nanum FUNTES, 1956
Grade II
    M. canis BODIN, 1902
Grade III
    M. audouini GRUBY, 1843

Grade IV
    M. ferrugineum OTA, 1922
Grade V
    T. concentricum BLANCHARD, 1896?

4. Harzia
Grade III
    E. floccosum (HARZ), LANGERON et MILOCHEVIC, 1930

5. Bodinia
Grade III
    T. quinckeanum (ZOPF), MACLEOD et MUENDE, 1940
    T. gallinae (MÉGNIN), SILVA et BENHAM, 1952
    T. equinum (MATRUCHOT et DASSON-VILLE) GOEDELST, 1902
    T. mégnini BLANCHARD, 1890
    T. rubrum (CASTELLAN), SABOURAUD, 1911
Grade IV
    T. verrucosum BODIN, 1902
    T. schönleinii (LEBERT, 1845) LANGERON et MILOCHEVIC, 1930
    T. violaceum BODIN, 1902

6. Langeronia
Grade III
    T. soudanense JOYEUX. 1912

Arthroderma Berkely und *Nannizzia Stockdale* der *Gymnoascaceae Baranetzky*, von denen die echten Dermatophyten stammen, zeigen jedoch gewisse Unterschiede bei ihrer biologischen Differenzierung. Die Arthroderma-Arten behalten nämlich länger ihre granulöse Struktur mit Abortiven- und Pseudocleistothecien (ohne Gemsenhörner) — die sog. „Gypseum-Gruppe" (Matruchotia Balabanoff, 1964). Jedoch verläuft die Phylogenie der Nannizza-Arten in ihrem imperfekten Stadium (Sabouraudia oder Mikrosporum) mit wollig-flaumiger Struktur ohne abortive Cleistothecien — M. Nanum, M. canis. Unsere Studien mit STRASCHILOVA (1966) über den Vitaminbedarf der Dermatophyten in Zusammenhang mit den Adaptationsphasen stützen die Hypothese vom „Gesetz der physiologischen Reduktion beim Parasitismus" (1960).

Mit Hilfe von sieben bei Arthroderma, Nannizia und ihren imperfekten Formen erkennbaren Adaptationsphasen (Tab. 1) gelingt es uns, eine phylogenetisch geordnete Klassifizierung der Dermatophyten und der ihnen verwandten Formen der Gymoascaceen durchzuführen. In der letzten Redaktion dieser

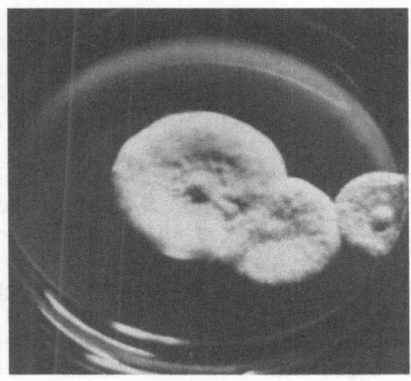

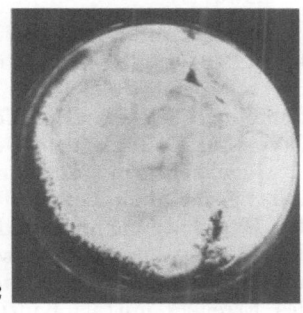

2

1

Abb. 1. Wollig-noduläre (phylogenetisch primitivste) Adaptationsphase — Microsporum gypseum (Bodenursprung)

Abb. 2. Granulöse, abortiv-cleistotheticale Adaptationsphase — Trichophyton mentagrophytes var. granulosum

Abb. 3. Faviforme, wachsartige parasitäre Adaptationsphase mit verlangsamtem Wachstum und stark reduzierter Morphologie — T. (A.) schönleinii

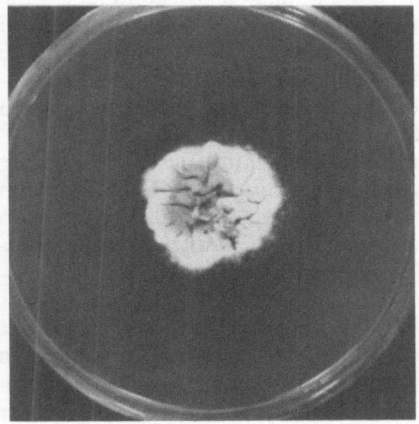

3

Kulturen auf Standardnährboden mit Dextrose nach SABOURAUD (24 °C).

Klassifikation (Tab. 2) ist die Gruppe Vanbreuseghemia (Keratinomyces Vanbreuseghem, 1952), phylogenetisch eine der jüngsten, an den Anfang des imperfekten Stadiums gestellt. T. (A.) gallinae hat seinen richtigen Platz als höher differenzierte zoophile Art im Vergleich mit T. (A.) quinckeanum in der Gruppe Bodinia gefunden. Die von uns im Erdboden Bulgariens beobachteten T. vanbreuseghemii und ihre perfekte Form — A. gertleri Böhme, — haben ihre entsprechenden Plätze eingenommen.

Damit wurden die Regeln des Internationalen Code der Systematik der Mikroorganismen vom 1. Januar 1930, was die Einteilung des imperfekten Stadiums der Dermatophyten in Vanbreuseghemia, Matruchotia, Sabouraudia, Harzia, Bodinia und Langeronia anbetrifft, befolgt.

Literatur. BALABANOFF, V. A.: Mycopathologia (Den Haag) **25**. 323 (1965).

Epidemiologische Analyse des Vorkommens von Dermatophyten in der Slowakei

L. Chmel, Hautklinik der medizin. Fakultät der Univ., Bratislava (Tschechoslowakei)

Die Erkrankungen an Dermatomykosen nehmen in der Slowakei seit dem Jahre 1940 ständig zu. Auf diese Tatsache verweisen die Tabellen und graphischen Darstellungen, welche eine kurze Übersicht der langjährigen Verfolgung der epidemiologischen Situation des Vorkommens von Trichophytien, Mikrosporien und Favus auf slowakischem Gebiete darstellen.

Gleichzeitig mit der zunehmenden Anzahl dieser mykotischen Erkrankungen änderte sich auch die qualitative Zusammensetzung der Mykoflore. Die Grundlage der Einschätzung der epidemiologischen Situation wurde vor allem durch die Einführung der obligatorischen Meldung von Dermatomykosen (Trichophytien, Mikrosporien und Favus) im Gebiete der CSSR sowie auch durch die Feststellung des Erregers mittels Kultivierung gebildet. Die Übersichten der Kultivationsergebnisse für die Periode der Jahre 1953 bis 1961 zeigten, daß in der globalen Gesamtheit der Erreger von Dermatomykosen zoophile Stämme vorherrschen und daß unter den Erkrankungen Trichophytien am häufigsten vorkommen. Eine detaillierte Analyse zeigte, daß die Haupterreger der zoophilen Dermatomykosen eindeutig das Trichophyton gypseum und das Trichophyton faviforme in beinahe gleichem Maße sind und daß bei der verhältnismäßig niedrigen Anzahl der anthropophilen Dermatomykosen das Trichophyton violaceum und das Microsporon audouini relativ am häufigsten vertreten sind.

Die Analyse der Erkrankungen an Dermatomykosen laut der Beschäftigung zeigte, daß die durch zoophile Dermatophyten hervorgerufenen Erkrankungen sich ausdrucksvoll in der Landwirtschaft konzentrieren. Von 621 evidierten kranken landwirtschaftlichen Angestellten mit positivem Kultivationsergebnis wurde die Erkrankung in 614 Fällen durch Trichophyton gypseum und Trichophyton faviforme verursacht.

In den tiefliegenden südlichen Gebieten der Slowakei herrscht als Erreger das Trichophyton faviforme vor, während in den Gebirgsgegenden das Trichophyton gypseum das häufigste ist. Die auf die Art der Bewirtschaftung gerichtete eingehendere Analyse zeigte, daß in den Großwirtschaften, die sich vorwiegend in der Südslowakei befinden, sich günstigere Vorbedingungen für die Verbreitung von durch Trichophyton faviforme hervorgerufene Trichophytien bilden. Demgegenüber ist in den Gebirgsgegenden, wo der Typ von Kleinwirtschaften vorherrscht, die Verbreitung von Infektionen durch Trichophyton gypseum, ermöglicht durch das leichtere Vordringen der Hauptwirte des Dermatophytes (kleine Nagetiere) in die Wirtschaftseinrichtungen, ausdrucksvoller. Dem Kontakt des Menschen mit der Infektionsquelle unter verschiedenen Bedingungen der Wirtschaftsführung entspricht auch die Saisonmäßigkeit des Vorkommens von zoophilen Trichophytien.

Einige biochemische Eigenschaften der Isothiocyanate

A. Bojanovská, Bratislava (Tschechoslowakei)

Isocyanate, welche als natürliche pflanzliche Substanzen entdeckt wurden, sind wegen ihrer biologischen Eigenschaften in manchen Studien tiefer verfolgt als die Isothiocyanate. Ihre antimikrobielle Wirksamkeit liegt gerade in ihrem Eingriff in den energetischen Metabolismus. Bei den Experimenten mit den Gewebszellen und mit den Zellen von Tumoren zeigte es sich, daß die Isothiocyanate die Aktivität der Hexokinase, 3-P-Glyceraldehyd-, Alkoholdehydrogenase inhibieren (Studien aus der Slovakischen Technischen Hochschule, Lehrstuhl für Mikrobiologie und Biochemie, Nemec, Drobnica). Weiter sah man, daß der Mechanismus der Inhibition in der Bindung der Isothiocyanate und SH-Gruppen der Proteine liegt. Die Entzündung der Haut, welche durch die Applikation von p-bromphenylisothiocyanat (PBFI) hervorgerufen wurde, war in ihrem Verlauf charakteristisch und wurde deshalb zum Anlaß unserer Studien über die Aktivität der Dehydrogenasen unter dem Einfluß von PBFI.

Wir haben die Wirksamkeit des 0,1%-PBFI auf die Aktivität der Glycerophosphat-, Lactat-, Glutamat- und Succinatdehydrogenase in Kryostatschnitten bei der Verwendung von Nitro-BT verfolgt. Das Verschwinden der Formazangranulen nach der zweistündigen Präinkubation der Kryostatschnitte der menschlichen Haut mit PBFI signalisierte das Absinken der Aktivität der Dehydrogenasen. Eine kleinere Inhibition wurde bei der Verwendung von Natriumsuccinat und Natriumlactat als Substrate bemerkt. Wir nehmen an, das die Inaktivation als Folge der Reaktion von PBFI mit SH-Gruppen der verfolgten Enzyme kam.

Trichofytocid Spofa® (5% p-bromphenylisothiocyanat) bei der Behandlung von Trichophytosis

L. CHMEL, M. VALENTOVÁ und J. BUCHVALD, Bratislava (Tschechoslowakei)

Trichofytocid ung. Spofa ist ein Antimykotikum, dessen wirksame Komponenten aus p-bromphenylisothiocyanat C_7H_4NSBr in einer Menge von 50 mg in 1 g Vaselin-Lanolin-Salbenbasis bestehen. Der Mechanismus der Wirksamkeit des Heilmittels wird durch die Inhibition der Prozesse des energetischen Metabolismus der Mikroorganismen erklärt, welche in der Blockierung der Enzyme und in der Bindung der SH-Gruppen besteht. Durch die Einwirkung des Trichofytocids auf die menschliche Haut entsteht eine Entzündungsreaktion, verbunden mit der Bildung von sich abschälenden Hautschuppen. Dieser Effekt, zusammen mit der antimykotischen Wirkung des Heilmittels, stellt einen zweiseitigen äthiotrophen Eingriff in den Krankheitsprozeß dar. Nach der Applikation der Salbe für 24 bzw. 48 Std entsteht bei schnellem Rückgang der Entzündungsreaktion in dem trichophytischen Herd im Zeitraum von 7 bis 9 Tagen eine Abschälung der Hautschuppen, Krusten; es empfiehlt sich, die Haare und Härchen, soweit sie nicht eliminiert wurden, nach der Entfernung des Heilmittels mechanisch zu epilieren. Nach der Heilung verbleiben keine Hautveränderungen.

Indikationen: Trichophytis superficialis cutis glabrae, Trichophytia profunda cutis glabrae, Trichophytia profunda capilitii et barbae.

Durch die neue Heilmethode werden die Dauer der Heilung sowie die Dauer der Arbeitsunfähigkeit wesentlich verkürzt.

Histopathomorphologische Befunde der Haut nach der Applikation von Trichofytocid

L. CHMEL und A. BOJANOVSKÁ, Bratislava (Tschechoslowakei)

Die bedeutenden therapeutischen Erfolge mit dem Trichofytocid (5%-p-bromphenylisothiocyanat-PBFI) haben uns zum Studium des Pathomechanismus der Wirksamkeit von PBFI auf die Haut geführt. Die sterile Entzündung, welche nach der Applikation von PBFI entsteht, potenziert als organotroper Faktor die antimikrobielle Wirksamkeit des PBFI. Strukturelle cytologische Änderungen, welche durch den Eingriff von PBFI in metabolische Prozesse entstehen, präsentieren ein gewisses Modell der Entzündungsreaktion. Neben dem pathomorphologischen Bild ist auch die Zellendifferentiation des Mesenchyms, welche als Antwort des Makroorganismus auf den irritierenden Stoff entsteht, interessant. Die initialen Veränderungen der Lysis der intercellulären Verbindungen Strati spinosi sind morphologisch sehr ähnlich jenen Befunden, welche nach der Applikation von Cantharidin, Lewisit und Yperit entstehen. Diese Ähnlichkeit liegt in dem Eingriff identischer enzymatischer Prozesse. In der Zellendifferentiation des Coriums liegt ein gewisser Zusammenhang zwischen der Intensität des wirkenden Stoffes (PBFI) und der Transformation der Zellen. Nach der lymphocytären und monocytären Antwort vermehren sich die neutrophilen und eosinophilen Granulocyten, welche aber der monocytären Reaktion abgetreten sind. In 4 Tagen hat sich eine parakeratotische Lamelle gebildet, welche mit Granulocyten, Lymphocyten und zerronnenem Fibrin ausgefüllt war.

Das schnelle Abklingen der Entzündung erklären wir mit der Inhibition der Proteinasen, welche für Aufhälter der entzündlichen Reaktion gehalten wurden. Früher haben wir die Inhibition unter dem Einfluß von PBFI experimentell überprüft. Das Studium der Dehydrogenasesysteme unter dem Einfluß von PBFI sowie auch das Verfolgen der Aktivität der Proteinasen geben uns eine gewisse Vorstellung über den Pathomechanismus der Entzündungsreaktion nach PBFI. Einerseits beschleunigt die Inhibition einiger Dehydrogenasen durch den Einfluß von PBFI die Entwicklung der Entzündungsreaktion. Anderseits kommt es mit dem Verhindern der Wirkung der Proteinasen zum schnellen Abnehmen der Inflammation. Diese zweiseitige Beeinflussung gibt uns eine umfangreichere therapeutische Möglichkeit.

Chromomycosis Caused by a New Species Chmelia slovaca

L. CHMEL, I. KOCHOVÁ and A. BOJANOVSKÁ, Bratislava (Czechoslovakia)

Thorough taxonomic study of the strain BYS/61 isolated from the lesions on the human skin led to the identification of a new pathogenic agent of chromomycosis: Chmelia slovaca, SVOBODOVÁ. By classification it is a new genus with one species listed in the artificial group Deuteromycetes, order Moniliales, family Dematiaceae, tribus Torulae. Cultivation: on Sabouraud-glucose agar the colony is at the beginning cream coloured, later brown, the reverse of the culture is of black colour. The mature colony is quite black, of felt-like character. The mycelium has partly grown into the soil. The young hyphae are thin septated, the more mature ones septated, expressively thick walled. The width of hyphae varies between 2,6 to 3,5 μ. From the micromorphological aspect Chmelia slovaca is characteristic for the formation of chlamydospores of four types, for the formation of spirally hyphae and a sporadic formation of blastospores. Most characteristically in the histological section from the affected human skin are the chlamydospores which form with their microstructure a much varied picture. They appear as cells of 12 to 15 μ with a double wall with a hyalinic, foamy, granular protoplasma. They sometimes obtain a yellow-brown pigment. They are usually of a round shape, sometimes divided. The hyphae overgrow the whole corium, they are either thin-walled, not septated with terminal chlamydospores of a brown colour, or thickwalled, septated, often coiled into spiral forms. The fumagoid cells are only sporadically present. The tissue reaction of the host is greatly manifested.

The Third Case of Chromomycosis in the Territory of Czechoslovakia

L. CHMEL, I. KOCHOVÁ, A. BOJANOVSKÁ and B. KONRÁD, Bratislava
(Czechoslovakia)

For 10 years the patient A. Ch. was treated as lupus vulgaris. Because the antituberculotic therapy was without result the diagnosis was corrected. Immediately after repeated biopsy the process on the affected skin spread (trauma!). The histopathological findings indicated deep mycoses. From the lesions of the affected skin has been isolated the pathogenic agent: Phialophora pedrosoi.

Pilzerkrankungen innerer Organe

T. WEGMANN, Medizinische Klinik des Kantonspitals St. Gallen (Schweiz)

Klinische Einteilung:

Primär (exogen)	Nordamerikanische Blastomykose	
	Südamerikanische Blastomykose	
	Chromomykose	außereuropäische Mykosen
	Histoplasmose	
	Coccidiomykose	
	Nokardia	
	Sporotrichen	
Sekundär (endogen)	Candida	
	Actinomyces[a]	
	Geotrichum	einheimische Mykosen
Exogen und endogen	Cryptokokken	
	Aspergillus	
	Penicillium	
	Mucoraceen	

[a] Keine Pilze (Mykobakterien).

Klinisches Bild: Meistens unspezifisch, so daß die Diagnose nur per exclusionem gestellt werden kann. Der Pilznachweis ist lediglich für die primär-exogenen Erkrankungen, also vornehmlich für die außereuropäischen oder tropischen Mykosen signifikant, während er für einheimische Methoden nur von untergeordneter Bedeutung ist.

Es werden folgende eigene Beobachtungen dargestellt:

A. Einheimische Mykosen

1. *Soorpneumonien* primär und sekundär nach antibiotischer, cytostatischer und Corticosteroidbehandlung, histologische Präparate.

2. *Aspergillosen* mit typischen Aspergillomen, ferner ein Fall von miliarer Aspergillose mit entsprechenden histologischen Präparaten.

3. *Geotrichose* mit doppelseitigem Befall der Lunge und Spontanpneumothorax.

4. *Actinomykose* mit Rippenperiostitis (Rippencaries), ferner miliare Form sowie Form mit apikalem Rundschatten, einen Lungentumor vortäuschend.

B. Außereuropäische Mykosen

- 5. *Südamerikanische Blastomykose* bei einem Schweizer Schreiner, der tropische Hölzer verarbeitete, mit Ulcus an der Gingiva und Lungenveränderungen, die weitgehend einer doppelseitigen Oberfeldtuberkulose entsprachen. Nachweis der

Pilze im Biopsiematerial. Heilung durch Amphotericin B-Behandlung. Histologische Präparate.

6. *Nordamerikanische Blastomykose* bei einer Schweizer Tabakarbeiterin, die beim Tabaksortieren Blastomyces dermatitidis inhaliert hat. Uncharakteristisches Lungenbild, eine Lungentuberkulose vortäuschend.

7. *Histoplasmose* bei einem jungen Mann, der die Krankheit in Südamerika aquirierte. Initialsyndrom Erythema nodosum beider Unterschenkel, dann Lungenbefund, der während Jahre als Lungentuberkulose interpretiert wurde.

Survey of Mycoses in U.A.R.

M. El Zawahry, Kasr el Aini University, Dept. of Dermatology, Cairo (U.A.R.)

Clinical Diagnosis of Onychotrichophytosis

J. Alkiewicz and W. Sowinski, Institute of Medical Mycology,
Medical Academy, Poznan (Poland)

The investigations carried out by Alkiewicz and Sowinski have shown the following development of the process of the Trichophyton growth in the nail plate: At the beginning the fungus penetrates into the intercellular spaces and therein

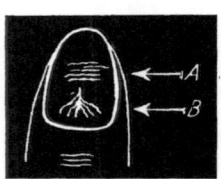

Fig. 1. Onychomycosis.
Scheme of the transverse *A* and spriggy *B* network

it develops in two directions: a) transversely to the axis of the nail and b) towards the nail root. It is only later that it affects the very nail cell. This latter process verified by histological investigations which reveal the corrosion of the cytoplasm. At that later stage the nail keratin is being destroyed by fungus enzymes. The released gases fill long tunnelshaped cavities resulting from the process of corrosion. The tunnels whose diameter is about 20 μ, form a double network: 1. The transverse network, observable through an ordinary magnifying glass after greasing the surface of the plate with cedar oil (see Fig. 1, *A*, and 2) and 2. the spriggy network which is formed in a similar way, but wherein the tunnels, in the shape of sprigs, are centripetally directed, i.e. towards the nail root (see Fig. 1, *B*, and 3). The second variant is a consequence of the infection having penetrated under the eponychium (Sowinski).

The two kinds of network are those manifestations of fungous infection of the nail which can be observed only in clinical examination.

During the miscroscopic examination of the ablated nailplate a broad net of fungi is visible. This stage is the initial phase of the fungus growth in the nail plate, i.e. before the gas tunnels are produced.

Mummy Nails

Microscopic investigations of a nail taken from an Egyptian mummy 1500 B.C. (XVIIIth dynasty) have revealed that the nail plate cells have well preserved their shape and structure.

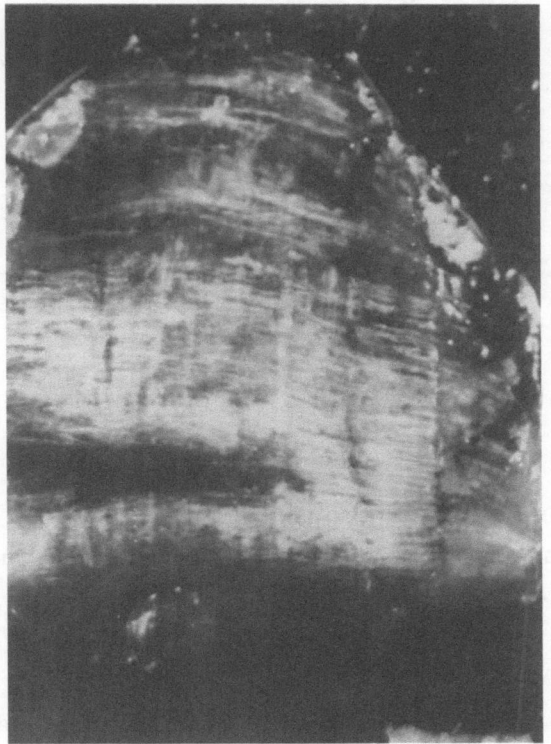

Fig. 2. ALKIEWICZ: Onychomycosis, transverse network

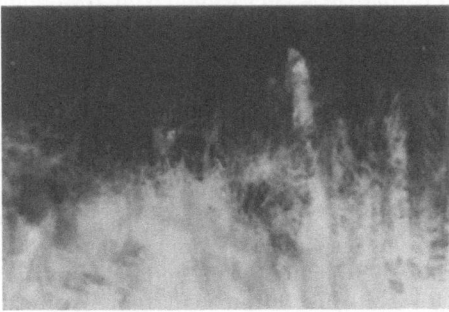

Fig. 3. SOWINSKI: Onychomycosis, spriggy network

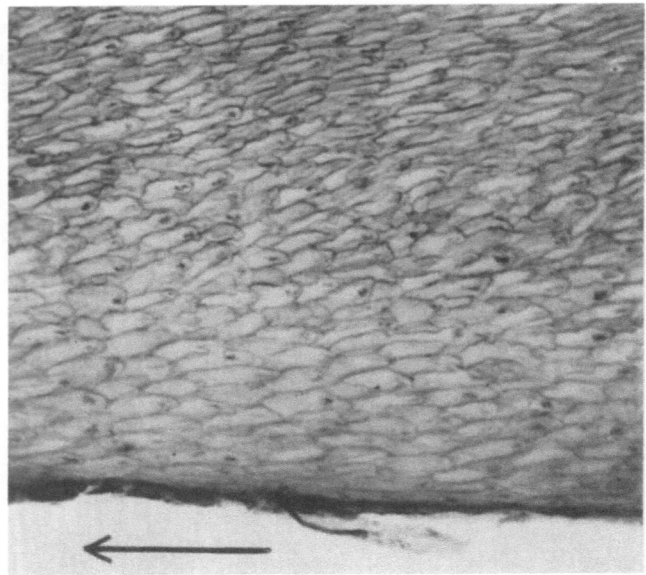

Fig. 4. ALKIEWICZ: Egyptian mummy nail, XVIII dynasty. Longitudinal section

Favic Infections in the Surroundings of Göttingen

M. KIRSCH-NIETZKI, Universitäts-Hautklinik Göttingen (Deutschland)

Pilzinfektionen im Bereich des Auges

D. H. HOFFMANN, Univ.-Augenklinik Hamburg (Deutschland)

Die Zunahme mykotischer Erkrankungen am und im Auge läßt sich als Phänomen aus der Literatur eindeutig belegen. Als Erreger sind Hefen, Schimmel, Dermatophyten und Aktinomyceten anzutreffen. In den verschiedenen Abschnitten des Auges überwiegt jeweils eine dieser Hauptgruppen humanpathogener Pilze.

So werden die *Tränenröhrchen* vorwiegend von *Aktinomyceten* befallen, in der Mehrzahl der Fälle durch den anaeroben Actinomyces Israelii. Es kommt zur Bildung von Konkrementen, die sich aus dem erkrankten Canalicus ausdrücken lassen.

An den *Lidern* trifft man hingegen vorzugsweise *Dermatophyten* an. Trichophytie- und Favus-ähnliche Bilder sowie Lidrandentzündungen mit Verlust der Wimpern sind typisch. Auch Mykide werden beschrieben.

Bei den in Europa noch selten zu beobachtenden Mykosen der *Orbita* sind häufig *Schimmelpilze* wie Phykomyceten und Aspergillusarten zu finden. Die Mucormykose der Orbita befällt komatöse oder präkomatöse Diabetiker. Über die Nasennebenhöhlen dringt der schnell wachsende Pilz in die Augenhöhle ein, wodurch das Bild des Orbitaspitzensyndroms entsteht. Weitere Infiltrationen führen zur Meningoencephalitis.

Klinisch besonders wichtig sind die *Pilzinfektionen der Cornea*. Hier überwiewiegen *Schimmel und Hefen*, Dermatophyten und Aktinomyceten sind Seltenheiten. Charakteristisch für die mykotische Ätiologie eines Ulcus serpens cornea sind rosenkranzartig angeordnete Infiltrate, die man als Satellitenphänomen be-

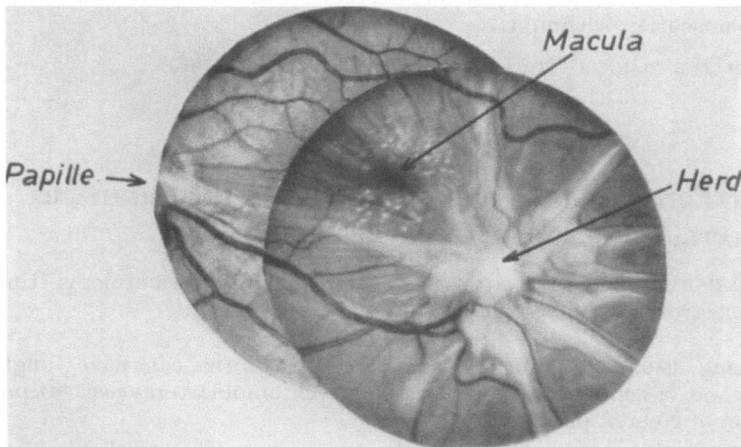

Abb. 1. Metastatischer Candida albicans-Herd am linken Augenhintergrund eines 13jährigen Mädchens. Blutkultur mehrfach positiv. Abheilung durch Langzeitbehandlung mit i.v. Amphotericin B-Infusionen. Zur Verminderung der Keimzahl im Darm wurde zusätzlich Moronal p.o. gegeben

zeichnet. Durch vorsichtiges Abschaben befallener Hornhautstellen kann man Material für Direktpräparat und Kultur gewinnen. Keratomykosen durch Hefen sprechen gut auf lokale Nystatintherapie an. Amphotericin B (Augensalbe, Augentropfen, subconjunctivale Injektion) ist bei Schimmelpilzen zu empfehlen. Auch Pimaricin erscheint geeignet. Bei weit fortgeschrittenen Mykosen der Cornea muß der erkrankte, von Mycel durchsetzte Hornhautbezirk excidiert und durch ein gleich großes Stück Spenderhornhaut ersetzt werden (Keratoplastik).

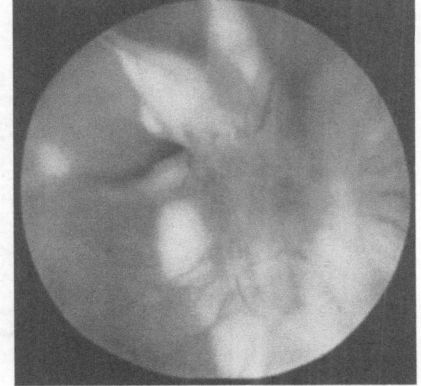

Abb. 2. Rechtes, schwerer befallenes Auge derselben Pat.

Mykosen des Augeninnern können auf *exogenem* Wege, d. h. nach perforierenden Verletzungen, Durchbruch eines Hornhautulcus oder bulbuseröffnenden Operationen auftreten. Der Verlauf einer derartigen Pilzendophthalmitis ist schleichend. *Schimmel und Hefen* überwiegen.

Endogene intraoculare Pilzinfektionen beginnen am Augenhintergrund, wo das Aufschießen der Herde mit dem Augenspiegel zu verfolgen ist. Die Pilze werden bei generalisierten Mykosen oder bei Mykosen der Lunge auf dem Blutweg metastatisch in das Auge verschleppt (Abb. 1 u. 2).

Intraoculare Mykosen exogenen oder endogenen Ursprungs sind nur durch i.v.-Amphotericin B-Infusionen zu behandeln.

Beim Kaninchen lassen sich durch i.v. Applikation einer geeigneten Menge von Candida albicans-Blastosporen regelmäßig Kolonien am Augenhintergrund erzeugen, die über Wochen mit dem Ophthalmoskop zu beobachten sind. Das histologische Bild gibt im Verein mit den Rückzüchtungsergebnissen Aufschluß über das jeweilige Stadium der Auseinandersetzung zwischen Wirt und Erreger zu jedem gewünschten Zeitpunkt.

Literatur. HOFFMANN, D. H.: Fortschr. Augenheilk. **16**, 63 (1965).

Parasitic Forms of the Causative Fungi in the Cutaneous and Visceral Lesions of Chromoblastomycosis

R. FUKUSHIRO and S. KAGAWA, Departments of Dermatology, University of Kanazawa and University of Tokyo (Japan)

Following usual and unusual parasitic forms of the causative fungi in the cutaneous and visceral lesions in seven cases of chromoblastomycosis are presented in the form of colored photomicrographs:

1. *Hormodendrum pedrosoi:* a) Dark brown, septate bodies in fresh preparation of pus from a lesion on the leg and b) germinating sclerotic cells in PAS stained smear of the same material. Case 1: A 26-year-old carpenter with cutaneous chromoblastomycosis with femoral lymph node involvement.

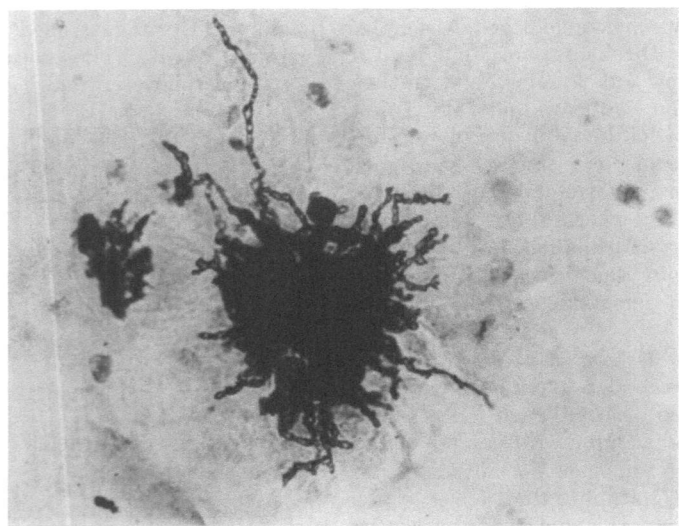

Fig. 1. *Hormodendrum pedrosoi.* Germinating sclerotic cells in smear of pus. PAS, 400 ×

2. *H. pedrosoi:* a) Sclerotic cells and hyphae in the horny layer and b) budding sclerotic cells within a giant cell in the epidermis. Sections from a lesion on the finger in a 3-year-old girl of disseminated cutaneous chromoblastomycosis with axillary lymph nodes involvement.

3. *H. pedrosoi:* Dark brown round bodies within a giant cell in the cutis. Section from a solitary lesion on the right breast in a 56-year-old farmer with cutaneous chromoblastomycosis.

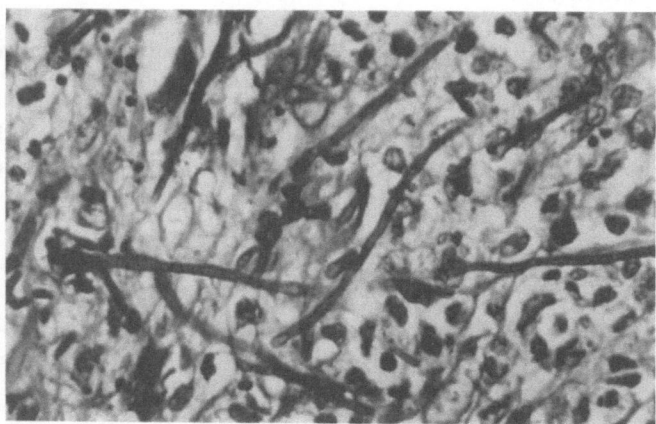

Fig. 2. *Phialophora verrucosa:* Mycelial elements in a granulomatous lesion in the dermis. PAS, 500×

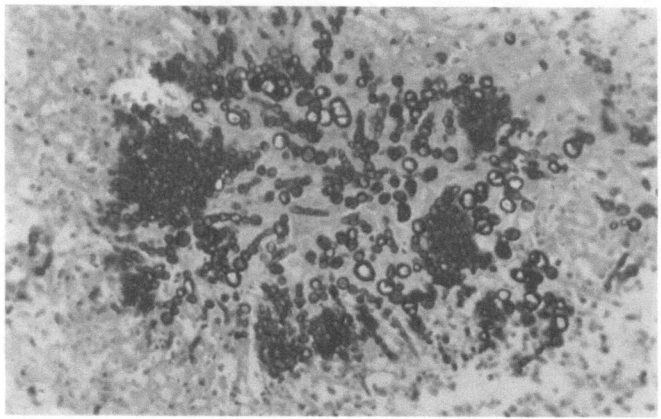

Fig. 3. *Hormodendrum dermatitidis:* Sclerotic cells and clusters of small round fungal cells in granuloma in the brain. PAS, 200×

4. *Phialophora verrucosa:* a) Chiefly mycelial elements in the granulomatous lesion in the dermis and b) those in a nodule of the axillary lymph node. Sections from a 21-year-old woman with a cutaneous lesion on the back of chromoblastomycosis and axillary lymph nodes involvement.

5. *H. pedrosoi:* A cluster of dark brown cells in the necrotic area of a nodule in the femoral lymph node in case 1.

6. *H. dermatitidis:* a) Predominantly mycelial growth of the fungus in a nodule on the surface of the cerebral basis, b) mass of small round brown cells in a different area of the same nodule and c) large brown septate bodies and chains of small round or ovoid fungal cells in a necrotic area of a granuloma in the brain. Sections from

an autopsy case, a 30-year-old housewife, of the brain abscess due to *H. dermatitidis.*

7. *H. pedrosoi:* Exclusively hyphal growth of the fungus in a granulomatous lesion of the brain. Section from a 8-year-old girl of cutaneous chromoblastomycosis with metastases to the brain.

8. Fungal elements in the lesions of the liver: a) Chains of brown round bodies in a nodule and b) mycelial forms of the organism in another area of the nodule. Sections from a fatal case, a 3-year-old boy, of systemic chromoblastomycosis without cutaneous lesions. No cultures. (Courtesy of Dr. SASANO et al.)

9. *H. pedrosoi:* a) A cluster of sclerotic cells with radiate formations in an intraperitoneal nodule in the inoculated rat and b) budding brown cells in a nodule of another rat.

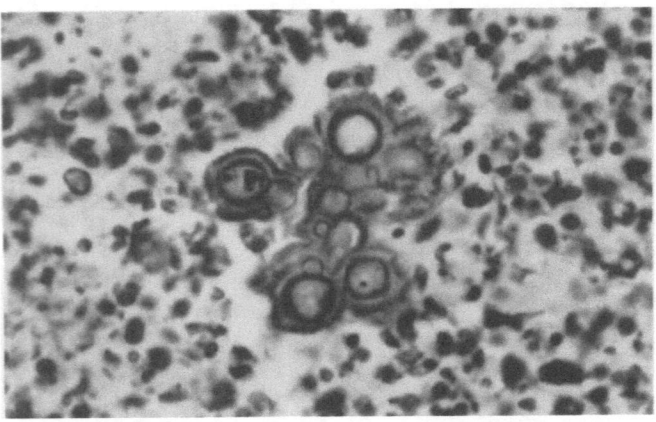

Fig. 4. *Hormodendrum pedrosoi:* Cluster of sclerotic cells with radiate formations in an intraperitoneal nodule of the inoculated rat. H & E, 800 ×

Chromomycosis (in the World and in Finland)

T. PUTKONEN, Univ. Centr. Hosp., Dept. of Dermatology, Helsinki (Finland)

Relations entre formes cliniques et espèces mycologiques

A. BASSET et M. BASSET, Clinique Dermatologique de Strasbourg (France)

Dermatomykosen bei Säugetieren

H. KRAFT, Medizinische Tierklinik der Universität München (Deutschland)

Die Abbildungen sollen einen Ausschnitt der bei Säugetieren vorkommenden Dermatomykosen zeigen. Es gibt praktisch keine Tierart, die nicht von Dermatophyten befallen werden kann. Die klinischen Symptome sind mannigfaltig und durch die starke Behaarung des ganzen Körpers oft erst im fortgeschrittenen Stadium zu erkennen. Die auf Bildern gezeigten Veränderungen durch Trichophyton mentagrophytes und Microsporum canis demonstrieren die Vielfalt der klinischen Erscheinungen. Bei einem abgebildeten Pferd waren kleine, etwa pfenniggroße, haarlose Stellen mit Schuppenbildung in der „oberen Halsgegend" und linsengroße ähnliche Stellen in der Nackengegend verdächtig für eine Dermatomykose. Die kulturelle Untersuchung auf Sabouraud-Agar des entnommenen Materials ergab einen Befall mit Trichophyton mentagrophytes.

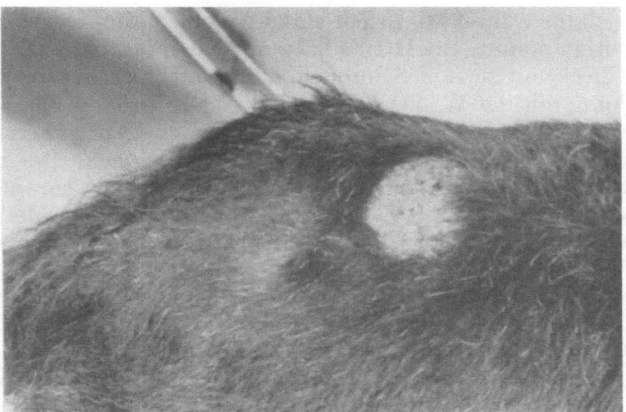

Abb. 1. Microsporum canis am Rücken eines Scotch-Terriers

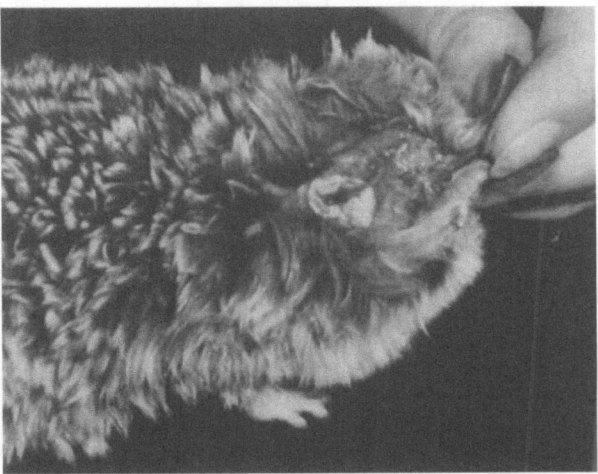

Abb. 2. Trichophyton mentagrophytes beim Chinchilla velligera

Bei einem Rind fielen spritzerartig verteilte haarlose, kreisrunde Stellen verschiedener Größe am Hals und auf den Hinterschenkeln auf. Schuppenbildung fehlte bei diesen Veränderungen. Auch hier ergab die kulturelle Untersuchung einen Befall mit Trichophyton mentagrophytes. In beiden Fällen — sowohl beim Pferd als auch beim Rind — brachte eine mehrmalige äußerliche Behandlung mit einem antimykotisch wirkenden Waschmittel (Herpetren = Pentachlorpgenol) rasche Heilung.

99*

Obgleich vom selben Erreger verursacht, waren die Erscheinungen bei einem Schäferhund ganz anders. Hier sah man runde haarlose Stellen mit wallartiger Begrenzung der entzündlich veränderten Haut an der Innenseite der Schenkel-innenfläche. Das Auftreten der typischen Makroconidien und von Spiralhyphen in der Kultur ergab die Diagnose: Dermatomykose verursacht durch Trichophyton mentagrophytes. Auch hier führte die äußerliche Behandlung zu einer raschen Heilung. (Die Besitzerin des Hundes hatte ebenfalls typische Veränderungen an ihren Armen.)

Die beiden dargestellten Mikrosporiefälle bei einem Mops bzw. Scotch-Terrier wurden frühzeitig erkannt. Die Hunde hatten je einen fünfmarkstückgroßen haar-losen runden Fleck mit starker Schuppenbildung am Ellbogen bzw. Rücken. Bei der Untersuchung mit der Woodschen Lampe trat bei beiden Patienten deutliche Fluorescenz auf, und an ausgerissenen fluorescierenden Haaren konnte man schon makroskopisch eine deutliche Sporenmanschette erkennen. Die innerliche Be-handlung mit Griseofulvin und eine gleichzeitige äußerliche Therapie brachten die Veränderungen innerhalb von 8 Wochen zur Abheilung, und wiederholte Kontrol-len mit Woodscher Lampe und Kultur bewiesen die Pilzfreiheit der Haut der Patienten (Abb. 1).

Bei den beiden Abbildungen vom Chinchilla handelt es sich um ein und das-selbe Tier. Es fällt eine deutliche Rötung der Haut mit Haarausfall in der Um-gebung der Ohren, im Nacken und am Hals auf. Außerdem sieht man am Hals ein ca. markstückgroßes gelbes Scutulum. Die Kultur zeigte starkes Wachstum von Trichophyton mentagrophytes. Nach Entfernen der Schuppen und Ausreißen der Haare in der Umgebung der Veränderungen konnte durch äußerliche Behandlung innerhalb 3 Wochen Heilung erzielt werden (Abb. 2).

Mit dieser Demonstration könnte der Eindruck entstehen, daß bei Säugetieren nur Microsporum canis und Trichophyton mentagrophytes vorkommen. Das ist nicht der Fall. Microsporum gypseum, Trichophyton verrucosum, T. equinum und Epidermophyton floccosum wurden ebenfalls beobachtet.

Mykosen bei Tieren (Befall durch Aspergillus, verschiedene Dermatophyten und Alternaria)

H. KRAFT, Medizinische Tierklinik der Universität München (Deutschland)

Besondere Sorge bereiten dem Tierarzt Luftsackmykosen bei verschiedenen Vogelarten. Vor allem Wassergeflügel wie Enten, Gänse und Pinguine leiden an Aspergillose. Aber auch Papageienvögel zeigen nicht selten starke Atemnot, deren Ursache ein Aspergillusbefall in den Luftsäcken ist, wie die Abbildung zeigt. Man erkennt im aufgeschnittenen Luftsack mit schwartig verdickter Wand deutliche Pilzrasen. Die Züchtung auf Sabouraud-Agar ergab: *Aspergillus fumigatus*. Die Ausschnittaufnahme aus der Kultur zeigt die typischen Aspergillus-Conidienträger.

In der zweiten Reihe der Abbildungen sind Makroconidien von *Trichophyton vanbreuseghemi* dargestellt, die einer Primärkultur aus den Mähnenhaaren eines Pferdes entnommen wurden. Deutliche klinische Veränderungen lagen in diesem Falle nicht vor; dem Besitzer fiel lediglich auf, daß das Tier sich am Mähnenansatz immer stark schabte und Haarausfall bestand. Erst nach dem Scheren der Haare konnten haarlose, mit Schuppen bedeckte Flecken gefunden werden.

Ab und zu kommt *Trichophyton equinum* beim Pferd vor und bewirkt eben-falls besonders am Mähnenansatz Haarausfall und geringgradige Schuppenbildung.

Die im nächsten Bild dargestellten Makroconidien sind einer Primärkultur vom Pferd entnommen.

Als drittes Bild in dieser Reihe der Demonstration sieht man schließlich zahlreiche Makroconidien von *Alternaria* (Kultur auf Sabouraud-Agar), wie man sie bei Hunden mit Seborrhoea squamosa fast immer findet. Vermutlich handelt es sich hier um eine spezifische Sekundärinfektion. Neben der üblichen Behandlung der Seborrhoe nehmen wir deshalb in solchen Fällen eine ein- bis zweimalige Waschung mit Antimykotika vor. Die Heilungserfolge sind ausgezeichnet.

In der untersten Reihe ist im ersten Bild die ektotriche Anordnung von Sporen von Microsporum canis dargestellt. Eine Makroconidie ist ebenfalls zu erkennen. Deutlich erscheint die Abschilferung der Haarcuticula durch die Sporen. Es handelt sich um eine Phasenkontrastaufnahme eines Haares aus einer Primärkultur.

Im zweiten Bild der gleichen Reihe sind endotriche Sporenketten von Microsporum canis im mit Kalilauge aufgehellten Nativpräparat photographiert. Auch hier handelt es sich um eine Phasenkontrastaufnahme.

Das dritte Bild stellt die Chlamydosporenbildung von Epidermophyton floccosum dar. Das Material stammt aus einer Primärkultur vom Rind. Deutliche fleckenhafte Veränderungen bei diesem Tier ließen die Verdachtsdiagnose einer Dermatomykose zu. Bevor jedoch die Diagnose durch die kulturelle Untersuchung gesichert werden konnte, hatten bereits zwei Leute des Pflegepersonals heftige Veränderungen an ihren Armen. Gleichzeitig wurden noch andere Kühe im gleichen Bestand durch das Putzzeug oder durch die Pfleger infiziert. Bei den Kühen reichte eine 14tägige äußerliche Behandlung mit Antimykoticis aus, um diese bei Tieren relativ seltene Dermatomykose zum Abheilen zu bringen.

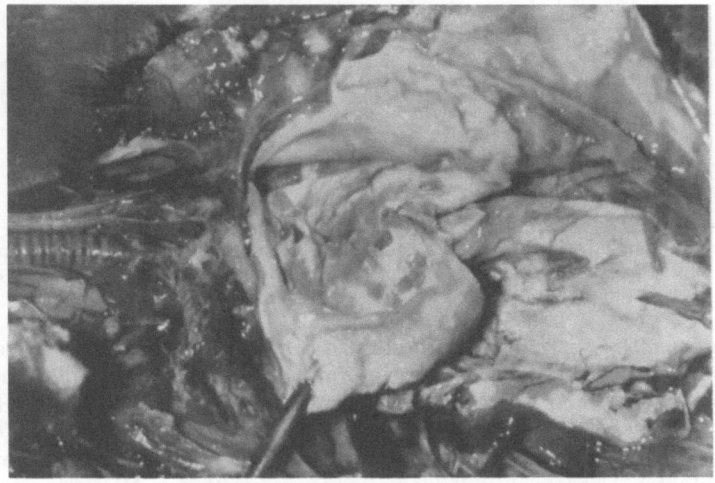

Abb. Befall der Luftsäcke eines Papageien mit Aspergillus fumigatus

Maduromykose beim Pferd

B. Schiefer und B. Gedek, Inst. für Tierpathologie der Univ. München (Deutschland)

Beitrag zur Mykologie der Systemmykosen:
Histoplasmose und Kryptokokkose

H. Karuga, Tuberkulose- und Varia-Abteilung an der Staatl. Bakteriologischen Untersuchungsanstalt München (Deutschland)

Unter Systemmykosen versteht man generalisierte Pilzinfektionen, die — von einer Eintrittspforte ausgehend — den ganzen Körper befallen. Vorzugsweise werden dabei die inneren Organe, wie Lunge, Leber, Milz, Drüsen, Nebenniere, Gehirn und Hirnhäute, ergriffen. Daneben kommt es auch zum Befall zahlreicher anderer Organe, vor allem der Haut. Bei den hier gezeigten Erregern (Mikrophotos 1 bis 5) handelt es sich um 1. *Histoplasma capsulatum*, den Erreger der Histoplasmose, und 2. *Cryptococcus neoformans*, den Erreger der Kryptokokkose.

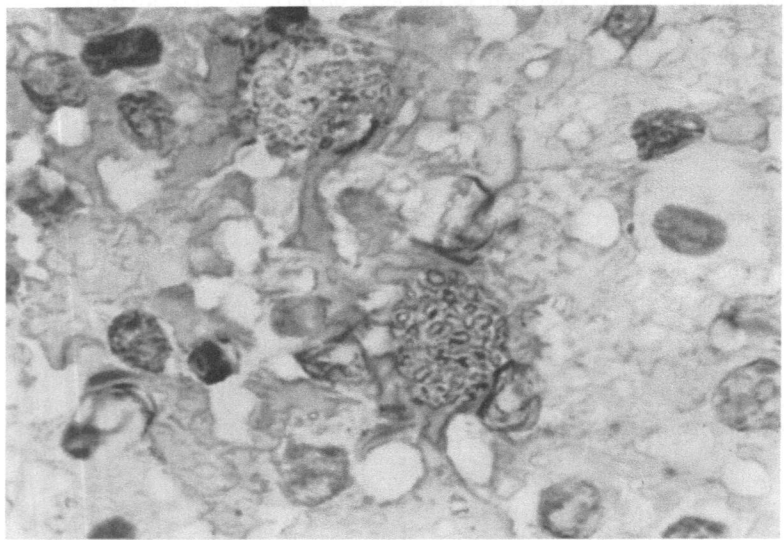

Abb. 1. *Histoplasma capsulatum:* Experimentelle Histoplasmose beim Goldhamster, Knochenmarkausstrich (Giemsafärbung). Der Erreger befindet sich in der Hefephase. Neben Knochenmarkzellen sind die Erreger in zwei größeren Ansammlungen in Form kleiner ovaler, bis zu 5 μ großen Körperchen sichtbar

Die Histoplasmose ist eine hochinfektiöse Inhalationsmykose, die in verschiedenen Stadien auftritt: in der akuten, primären Lungenform und in der chronischen, progressiven, bösartigen Form der Systemmykose, dazwischen liegen Übergänge. Der Erreger, Histoplasma capsulatum, ist ein ovales Körperchen von 1 bis 5 μ ⌀ und befällt primär das RES. Er lebt saprophytär im Boden, vor allem in den Endemiegebieten. Das größte Endemiegebiet umfaßt das Mississippibecken der USA, ferner wurde der Erreger auch in Mexiko, Mittelamerika, Zentralafrika, Philippinen, Java und England beobachtet, hingegen nicht in Mitteleuropa. Der Erreger kommt auch enzootisch und epizootisch vor. Auf Grund von Intracutanreaktionen nimmt man an, daß 90% der Primärinfektionen asymptomatisch verlaufen. In Endemiegebieten ist die Infektion im Alter bis zu 18 Jahren achtmal so häufig wie eine Tuberkulose. Die meisten Formen heilen im Stadium des pulmonalen Primärinfektes unter entsprechender Verkalkung aus. Die klinischen Symptome sind dabei gering. Prognostisch gelten die gleichen Überlegungen wie für die

Tuberkulose. Tiere kommen nur als Reservoir für den Erreger, aber nicht als direkte Überträger in Betracht.

Der Nachweis des Erregers ist nur im gefärbten Präparat möglich. Das Untersuchungsmaterial aus Sputum, Eiter, Hautgeschabsel, Gewebsstückchen, Knochenmark oder Liquor wird am besten nach Giemsa oder PAS gefärbt; Betrachtung bei

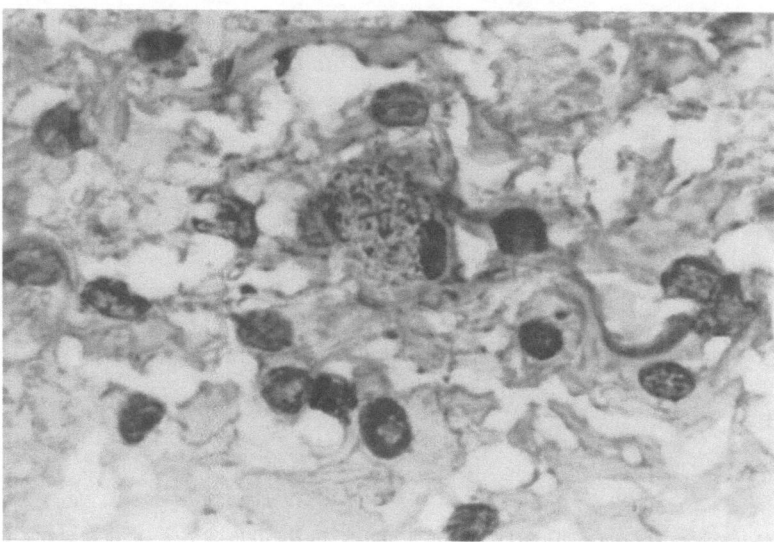

Abb. 2. *Histoplasma capsulatum:* Experimentelle Histoplasmose beim Goldhamster, Knochenmarkausstrich (Giemsafärbung). Der Erreger befindet sich in der Hefephase; eine größere Ansammlung in der Mitte der Abbildung

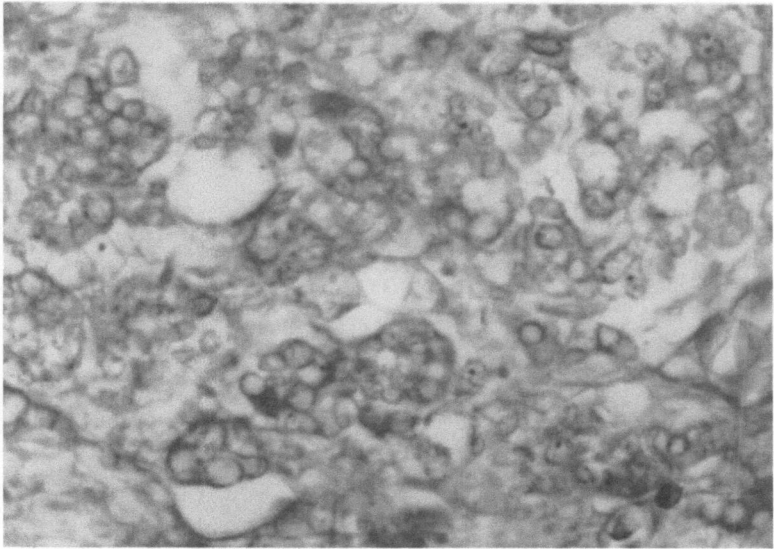

Abb. 3. *Histoplasma capsulatum:* Experimentelle Histoplasmose beim Goldhamster. Schnitt vom lymphatischen Gewebe des Intestinaltraktes (PAS). Der Erreger ist massenhaft in lymphatischen Elementen eingebettet

Ölimmersion. Dabei wird die Hefephase intracellulär in Form ovaler Körperchen gefunden; meist in Monocyten und Reticulumzellen. Kulturell zeigt der Erreger einen Dimorphismus, d. h. er wächst bei Zimmertemperatur z. B. auf Sabouraud-Agar in der Mycelform, während die Hefephase sich vor allem bei Züchtung auf

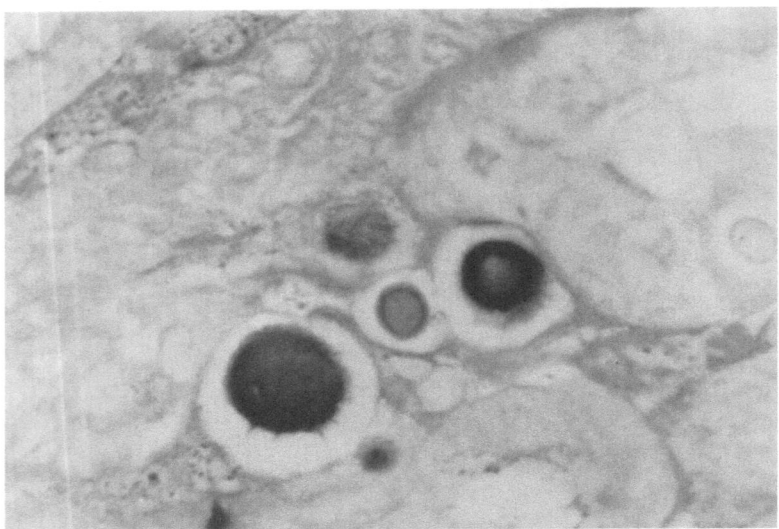

Abb. 4. *Cryptococcus neoformans:* Experimentelle Kryptokokkose der weißen Maus. Gewebs-schnitt der Niere (PAS). Der Erreger findet sich im Bindegewebe in Form mehrerer kugeliger Gebilde, die dunkel tingiert und von einer dicken hellen Schleimkapsel umgeben sind, da-neben sind die Querschnitte mehrerer Tubuli erkennbar

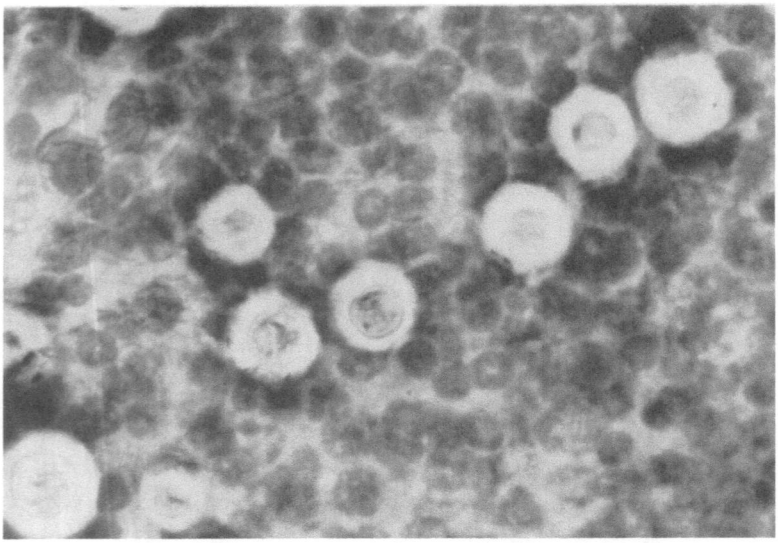

Abb. 5. *Cryptococcus neoformans:* Experimentelle Kryptokokkose der weißen Maus. Milz-ausstrich (Toluidinblaufärbung). Der Erreger ist in Form mehrerer kugeliger, z. T. doppelt konturierter Gebilde, die von einer deutlichen Schleimkapsel umgeben sind, zwischen Lympho-cyten und Reticulumzellen eingebettet

Blut-Cystin-Agar unter verminderter O_2-Spannung bei 37 °C entwickelt. Bei der Mycelphase sind die kleinen birnenförmigen Conidien und die großen dickwandigen Chlamydosporen mit handschuhartigen Fortsätzen auffällig. Versuchstiere sind Goldhamster und weiße Mäuse.

Die Kryptokokkose, häufig auch Torulose oder europäische Blastomykose genannt, ist eine weltweit verbreitete Infektionskrankheit, die durch Cryptococcus neoformans verursacht wird. Der Erreger lebt saprophytär im Boden und wurde vielfach aus Vogelmist isoliert. Durch Inhalation kommt es beim Menschen zunächst zu einer Lungenmykose, oft zur Entwicklung mächtiger Granulome, Absceß- und Fistelbildung, oberflächlicher und tiefer Ulcerationen, papillomatösen und tumorartigen Veränderungen z. B. der Haut und Knochen durch hämatogene Aussaat. Am gefährlichsten ist die Infektion der Hirnhaut. Die Cryptococcus-Meningitis verläuft chronisch protrahiert und ist fast immer tödlich. Cryptococcus neoformans ist auch tierpathogen und als Ursache einer sporadischen bzw. epizootischen Mastitis beim Milchvieh bekannt. Von 1954 bis 1957 waren in Deutschland etwa zehn Fälle beim Menschen bekannt geworden. Wahrscheinlich ist die Krankheit noch viel häufiger. In der gesamten Literatur sind bisher nur ca. 500 Fälle beschrieben. Die Häufigkeit der durch Cryptococcus neoformans hervorgerufenen Hirnmykosen ist auffallend, die cutane Kryptokokkose tritt demgegenüber zurück. Eine Übertragung von Mensch zu Mensch oder vom Tier auf den Menschen hat man bisher nicht nachgewiesen.

Der Nachweis des Erregers gelingt im Nativpräparat mit stark abgeblendetem Trockensystem, im Tuschepräparat und im gefärbten Präparat mit Toluidinblau oder PAS. Untersuchungsmaterial: Eiter von Hautläsionen und subcutanen Granulomen, Sputum, Liquor und Gewebsmaterial. Die Kultur gelingt auf Sabouraud- oder Grütz-Agar bei 30 °C, ferner auf Hirn-Herz-Infusions- und Blut-Agar bei 37 °C. Das Wachstum ist glasig-schleimig oder creme-weiß, später bräunlich. Abzugrenzen sind apathogene Kryptokokkusarten, die nicht mäusepathogen sind. Im Tierversuch an der weißen Maus sind die Erreger gut im Peritonealexsudat nachweisbar. Die oft in beträchtlicher Dicke vorhandene Schleimkapsel läßt sich am einfachsten im Tuschepräparat sichtbar machen. Die apathogenen Verwandten gedeihen bei Körperwärme nicht oder nur sehr schlecht. Cycloheximid (Actidion) verhindert das Wachstum von Cryptococcus neoformans.

Literatur. HAZEN, and REED: Laboratory identification of pathogenic fungi simplified. Springfield: Ch. C. Thomas 1960. — Moss, and MC QUOWN: Atlas of medical mycology. Baltimore: Williams & Wilkins 1960. — POLEMANN: Klinik und Therapie der Pilzkrankheiten. Stuttgart: Thieme 1961. — SEELIGER: Leitfaden zur mykologischen Diagnostik, Scriptum. Bonn 1957. — WIEBECKE, u. STAIB: Münch. med. Wschr. **107**, 361 (1965).

Vorkommen von Dermatophyten im Boden und bei Tieren als mögliche Infektionsquellen

D. JANKE, Fulda (Deutschland)

An Hand von stilisierten Zeichnungen werden Vorkommen und Häufigkeit verschiedener Dermatophyten im Erdboden, Spontanbefall bei Haus- und Wildtieren sowie mögliche Infektionswege dieser Pilze demonstriert.

Auf Abb. 1 werden die mit Hilfe der Haarködermethode aus unterschiedlichen Bodenarten (Wiese, Feld, Laubwald, Gartenerde, Blumenerde, Seesand) kulturell nachgewiesenen keratinophilen Dermatophyten aufgeführt. Als häufigster Fundort erwies sich Garten- und Großstadterde — als seltenster der sandige Meeresstrand. Der Zusammenstellung von Tieren mit spontanem Dermatophytenbefall auf Abb. 1 sind die diesbezüglichen Mitteilungen von GÖTZ [2] im Ergänzungswerk

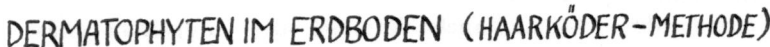

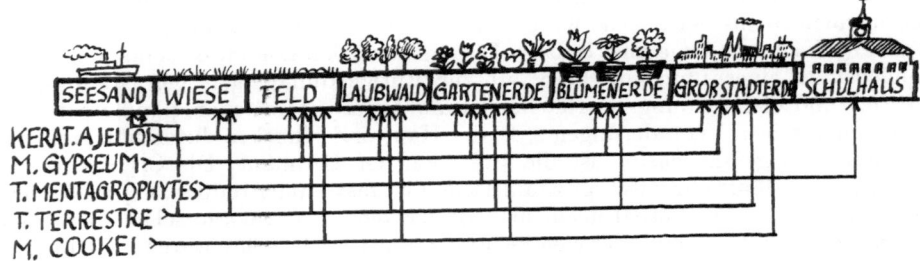

Abb. 1

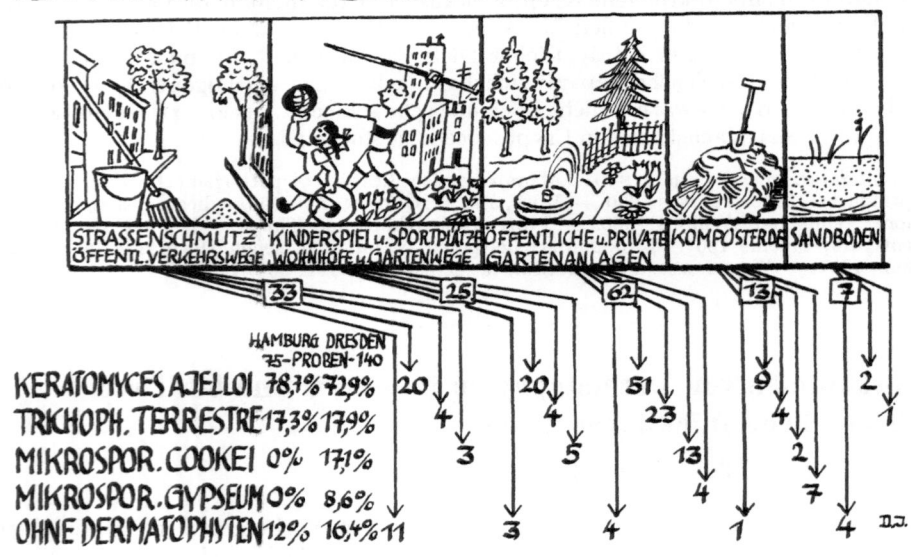

Abb. 2

zu J. JADASSOHNs Handbuch der Haut- und Geschlechtskrankheiten zugrundegelegt. Spontanbefall mit T. mentagrophytes, T. rubrum und T. verrucosum wird bei Haustieren beobachtet; T. mentagrophytes auch bei Wildtieren, die mit Haustieren in Berührung kommen. Das Vorkommen von T. rubrum bei Tieren gilt als Seltenheit.

Die unterschiedliche Verteilung von keratinophilen Dermatophyten in Bodenproben verschiedenartiger Lokalitäten der Großstadt wird in Abb. 2 dargestellt, wobei Kulturergebnisse von BLASCHKE-HELMESSEN [1] aus Dresden und von MEINHOF, THIANPRASIT u. RIETH [4] aus Hamburg zugrundeliegen. Zahlenmäßig am häufigsten wurden diese Pilze aus Bodenproben von Gartenanlagen und aus Straßenschmutz öffentlicher Verkehrswege isoliert.

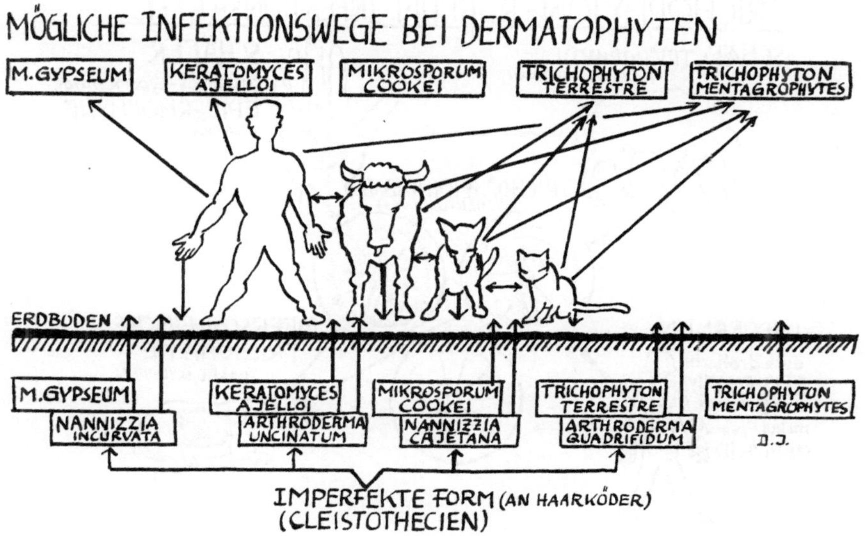

Abb. 3

Bei Demonstration möglicher Infektionswege der Dermatophyten auf Abb. 3 werden die keratinophilen Dermatophyten mit ihren speziell benannten im Erdboden vorkommenden und an Haarködern nachgewiesenen imperfekten Formen aufgeführt. Eine imperfekte Form mit Ausbildung sog. Cleistothecien wurde bei keratinophilen Dermatophyten gefunden, die bisher nur in seltenen Fällen als Krankheitserreger bei Mensch und Tier nachweisbar sind (Keratinomyces ajelloi, Microsporum cookei, Trichophyton terrestre), weiterhin von Microsporum gypseum, aber noch nicht in überzeugender Weise von T. mentagrophytes als häufigstem Dermatomykoseerreger bei Mensch und Tier.

Die Frage nach Herkunft der Dermatophyten bleibt bis heute noch offen. Bereits 1936 vertrat SZATMARY [5] die Ansicht, daß sich die Dermatophyten im perfekten Stadium als Saprophyten in der Natur in einer Urform finden, aus welcher sich erst später auf dem Umweg über das Tier die uns bekannten Arten entwickeln. WILLIAMS [6] züchtete 1934 pleomorphe Kulturen von T. mentagrophytes und E. floccosum aus Geschabsel von Fußböden, Matten und Turngeräten einer Schule und glaubte, daß es sich um die gesuchte Urform handeln könnte. Hingegen muß man jedoch annehmen, daß die in der Umgebung von Menschen und Haustieren isolierten Dermatophyten durch Verstreuung kleiner Epidermisteilchen in die nahe Umgebung gelangt sind.

Abb. 4 veranschaulicht die wohl einmalige Beobachtung einer Trichophyton rubrum-Infektionskette [ausführliche Publikation: JANKE, D.: Z. Haut- u.

Geschl.-Kr. **33**, 151 (1962)]. Es handelt sich um Übertragung des T. rubrum vom Schaf auf einen Schäfer und weiterhin auf die mit den isolierten T. rubrum-Stämmen hantierende Laborantin. Zuerst wurde die Trichophyton rubrum-Infektion an den Klauen bei 10 von 52 Schafen einer monatelang auf Wiesengelände weidenden Herde beobachtet, später als hyperkeratotische Epidermophytie der Hohlhände beim Schäfer, nachdem er die erkrankten Tiere ohne Handschutz behandelt hatte. Bei Laboratoriumsarbeiten mit den von Schafen und Schäfer gezüchteten T. rubrum-Stämmen kam es zu einer Infektion bei einer

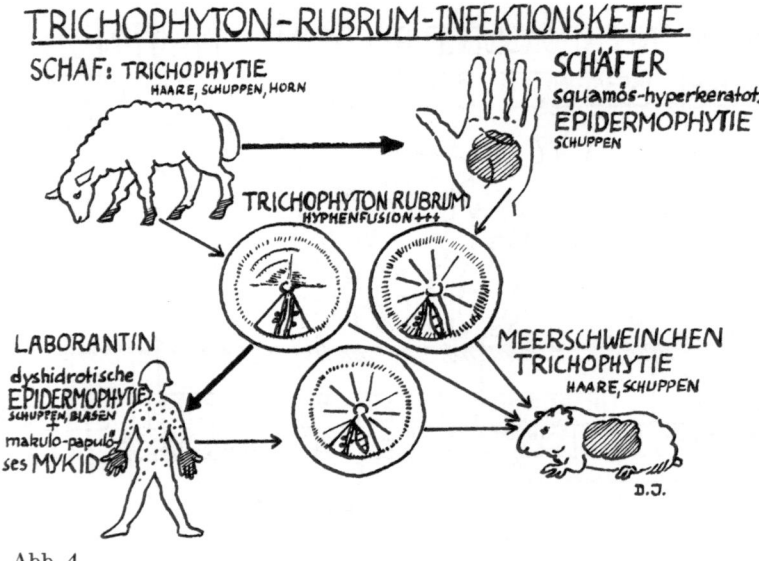

Abb. 4

Laborantin mit Erscheinungen einer dyshidrotischen Epidermophytie der Hände und späterem fieberhaften generalisierten maculo-papulösen Mykid. Bei vergleichenden mykologischen Untersuchungen zeigten die von Schafen, Schäfer und Laborantin isolierten T. rubrum-Stämme geringgradige morphologische Unterschiede, jedoch untereinander Hyphenfusion, und verursachten in gleicher Weise eine experimentelle Trichophytie bei Meerschweinchen.

Literatur. 1. BLASCHKE-HELLMESSEN, R.: Z. Haut- u. Geschl.-Kr. **36**, 169 (1964). — 2. GÖTZ, H.: Erg.-Werk zu J. Jadassohns Handbuch der Haut- und Geschlechtskrankheiten, Bd. IV/3, S. 107. Berlin-Göttingen-Heidelberg: Springer 1962. — 3. JANKE, D.: Z. Haut- u. Geschl.-Kr. **33**, 151 (1962). — 4. MEINHOF, W., M. THIANPRASIT und H. RIETH: Arch. klin. exp. Derm. **212**, 30 (1960). — 5. SZATHMARY, S.: Magy. orv. Arch. **37**, 394 (1936). — 6. WILLIAMS, J. W.: Proc. Soc. exp. Biol. (N.Y.) **31**, 984 (1934).

Trichophytie und Blastomykose

Zs. HERPAY, Debrezen (Ungarn)

Ultrastructure of Dermatophytes

W. MEINHOF, Dermatologische Klinik und Poliklinik der Universität München,
W. VOGELL, Institut für Physikalische Biologie und Elektronenmikroskopie
der Universität Marburg a. d. Lahn (Deutschland)

The dermatophyte *cell wall* and septa are composed of fibrillar material. The outer layer (lamina densa) consists of electron-dense material and has a rough surface. The lamina densa may be absent, especially in glabrous fungi (T. Schön-leinii, T. verrucosum). The fibrillar structure of the electron-transparent lamina

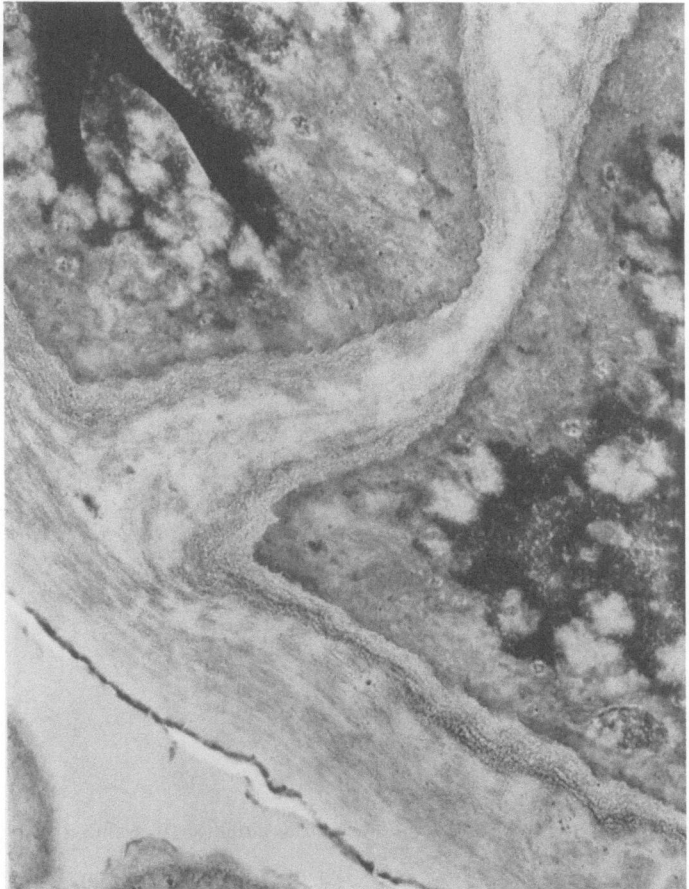

Fig. 1. Keratinomyces Ajelloi. Structure of cell wall and septum in macroconidium. 30 000 × (¹/₄ reduced)

lucida is more distinct than it is in the lamina densa. The inner layers of the lamina lucida take part in the formation of septa. The septa are usually tapering towards the centre of the hyphal lumen. Often a *central pore* can be demonstrated. Central pore plugs (Woronin bodies) are frequently found, either in contact with the septal pore or in it's close vicinity.

A *cytoplasmic membrane*, which appears to be double-layered in some preparations, covers the inner face of the cell wall and both sides of the septa. The continuity of the cytoplasmic membrane is not interrupted by the septal pore. In some instances the cytoplasmic membrane appears to be broken into small, curved fragments. In other mycelia there are found numerous vesicular structures at the site of the cytoplasmic membrane. This applies especially to the hyphal tips of vegetative mycelia.

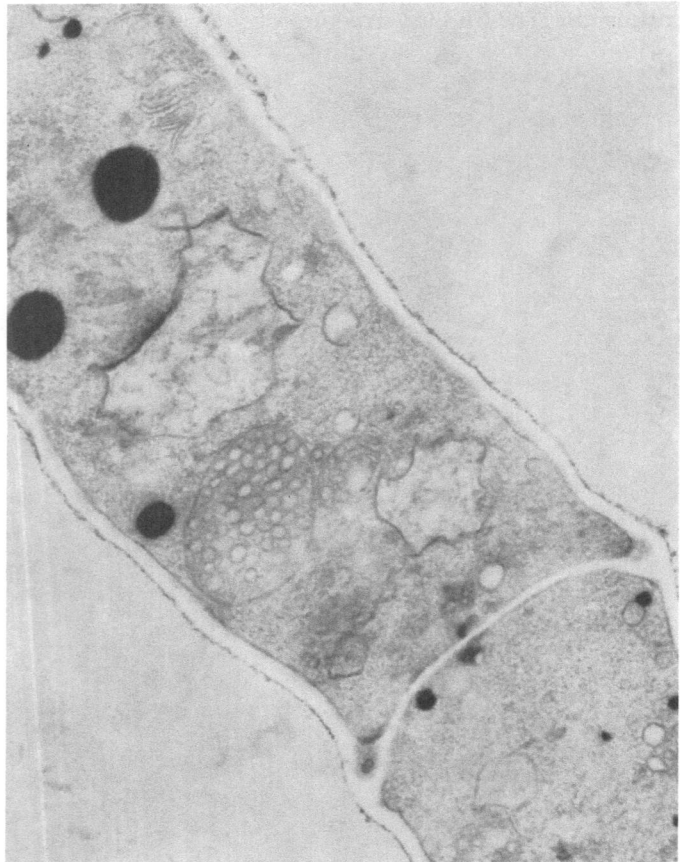

Fig. 2. Microsporum gypseum. Tubular mitochondria. 30000× (¹/₄ reduced)

Nuclei are rarely seen as irregular shaped, electron-transparent organells with a double-layered nuclear membrane which is perforated by nuclear pores. Nucleoli could not be detected. The number of *mitochondria* varies greatly in different sections of mycelia and conidia. The cristate type is predominant and was found in all dermatophytes that were investigated (K. Ajelloi, M. gypseum, T. Schönleinii, T. verrucosum). Within the mycelia of M. gypseum, however, tubular mitochondria could be demonstrated together with cristate mitochondria, sometimes, even in the same hyphal section. Dumb-bell shaped cristate mitochondria in M. gypseum suggest a process of division of these organells. Mitochondria in close contact with large vacuoles or even protruding into the lumen of the vacuole seemed to have lost their characteristic structure and contained droplets of opaque material. *Ribosomes* were observed in all sections but only rarely in connection with a cytoplasmic reticulum. In older mycelia and in the macroconidia of K. Ajelloi large amounts of glycogen are found as particulate, electron-dense inclusions. Dark osmiophilic droplets, which may represent lipid material, where seen in some preparations.

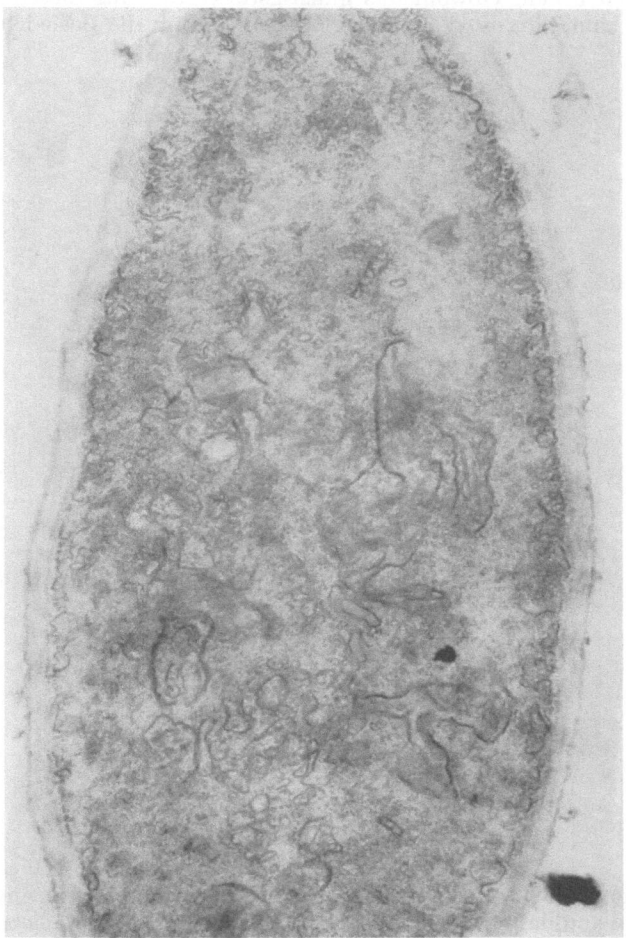

Fig. 3. Microsporum gypseum. Lamellate mitochondria, vesicular structures at the site of the cytoplasmic membrane. $30\,000 \times$ ($^{1}/_{4}$ reduced)

Exposure of M. gypseum mycelia in submersed culture to small Aerosil particles resulted in *phagocytosis* of these particles, which were found after a certain period of time, within the fungal cytoplasma.

References. W. MEINHOF: Arch. klin. exp. Derm. **226**, 33 (1966); **228**, 111, 122, 265 (1967).

Infektionen durch Candida albicans

J. THURNER, II. Universitäts-Hautklinik Wien (Österreich)

In den letzten Jahren wird Candida albicans häufiger als Erreger von Dermatomykosen kultiviert. Die Ursache für das Ansteigen der Candidainfektionen könnte
aber auch lediglich in der höheren Frequenz der durchgeführten Laboratoriumsuntersuchungen liegen. Obwohl das günstigste Terrain für diesen Sproßpilz die
Schleimhäute sind, gibt es oft einfache Erklärungen für die Besiedelung der Cutis.

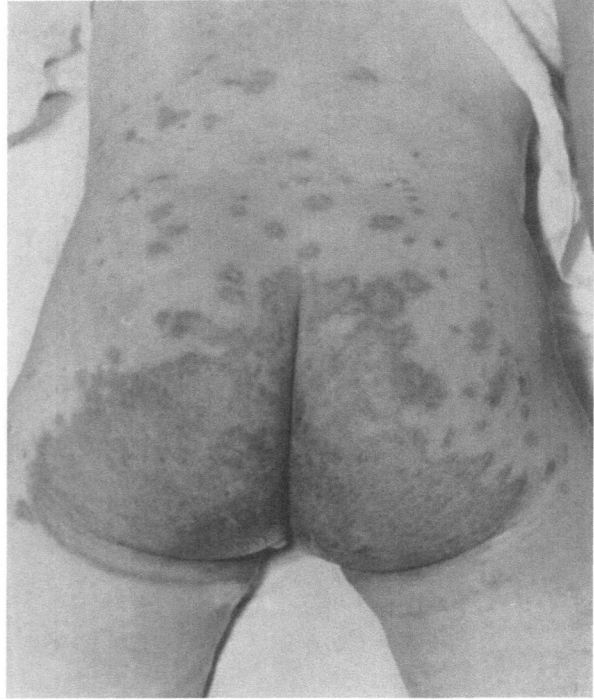

Abb. 1. Candidamycosis cutis eines Säuglings

Fast ausschließlich leiden Hausfrauen und Geschirrwäscher an einer Paronychia
und Onychia candidamycetica, weil sie infolge des vielen Waschens dem Pilz die
besten Wachstumsbedingungen schaffen. Beim Säugling dürfte als primäre
Ursache der Infektion die Candida-besiedelte Vagina der Mutter anzusehen sein.
Beim Kind sind Mundhöhle und Intestinaltrakt besiedelt, und von dort aus kann,
ebenso wie beim Erwachsenen, eine Infektion der Rima ani die Folge sein, die sich
unter dem Bereich der Windelhose rasch ausbreitet. Durch Fingerlutschen werden
sowohl Infektionsmöglichkeit als auch günstiges Milieu für den Sproßpilz bei den
Fingernägeln geschaffen.

In allen Fällen ist neben der Lokaltherapie die Beseitigung der Infektionsmöglichkeit zu beachten, und der Patient müßte jene Faktoren meiden, die dem
Pilz Möglichkeit zur Ansiedlung geben.

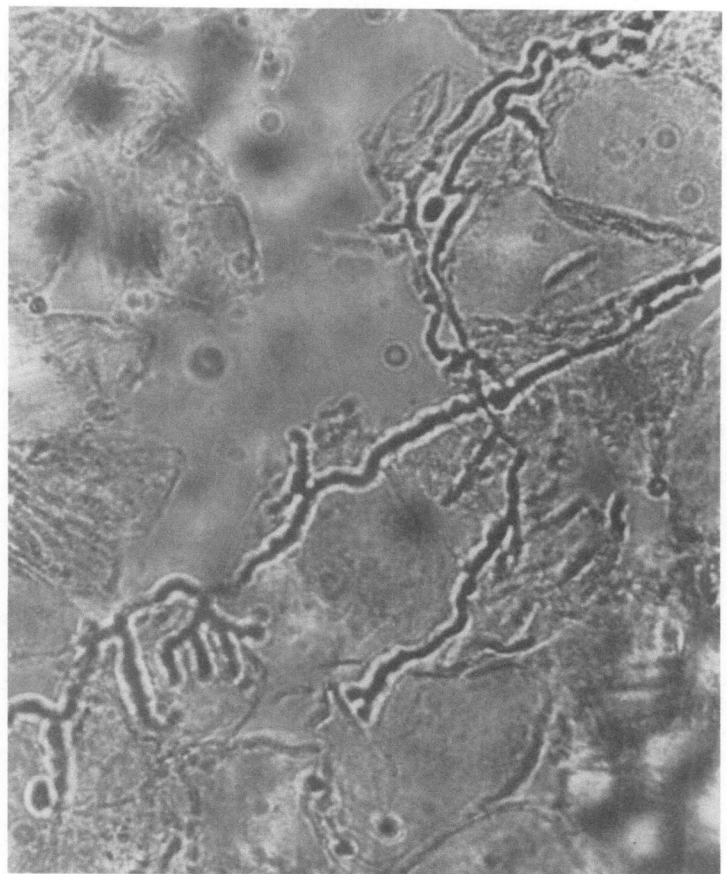

Abb. 2. Nativpräparat zu Abb. 1 (hauptsächlich Pseudomycel)

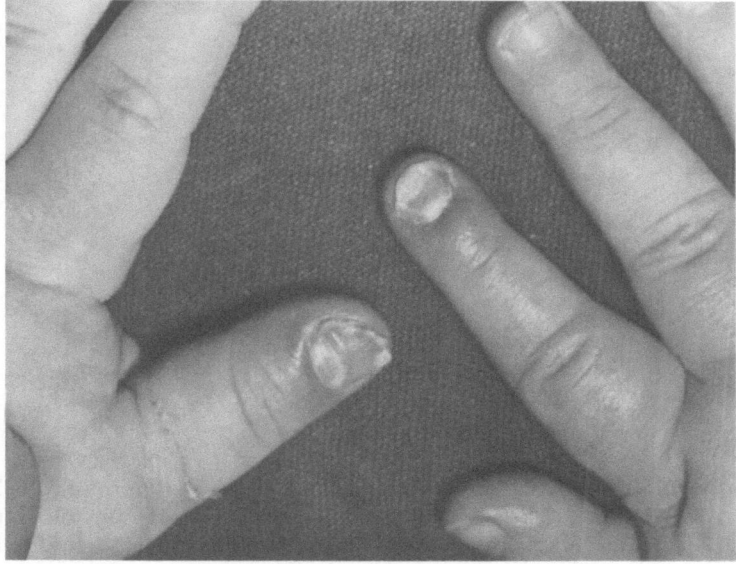

Abb. 3. Paronychia und Onychia candidamycetica eines Säuglings

Die Nativuntersuchung gelingt mühelos, wenn im Präparat Ansammlungen von Blastospren zu sehen sind. Scheint im Präparat nur Pseudomycel auf, ist eine Verwechslungsmöglichkeit mit echtem Mycel, also Dermatophytenhyphen, gegeben. In diesem Fall ist einzig die Kultur entscheidend.

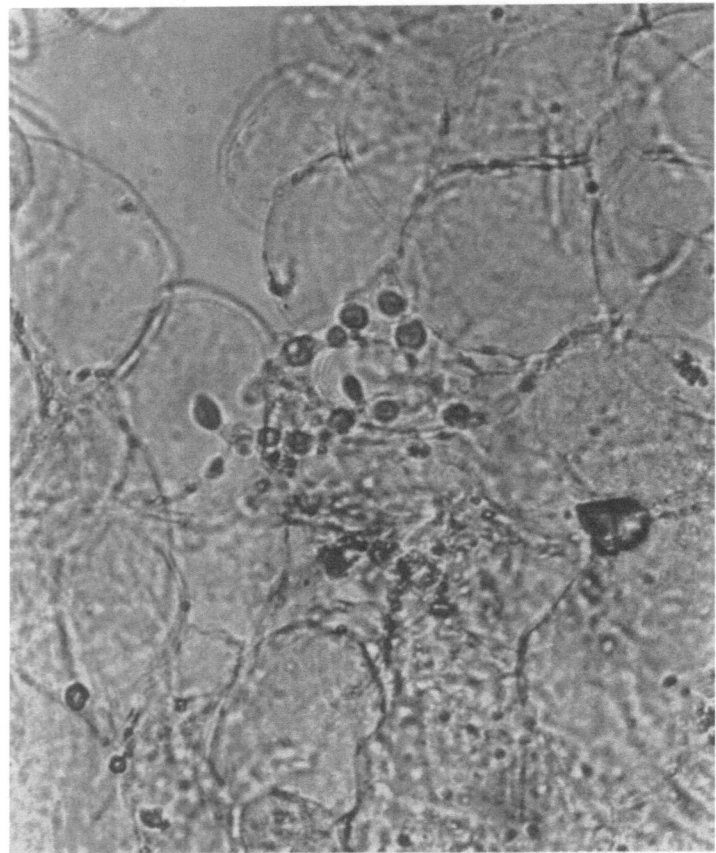

Abb. 4. Nativpräparat zu Abb. 3 (vereinzelt Blastosporen)

Quantitative Methoden der Antimykotikaprüfung

W. DITTMAR, Farbwerke Hoechst AG., Frankfurt (Main)-Höchst (Deutschland)

I. Einführung

Laboratoriumsmethoden zur Wirksamkeitsprüfung von antimikrobiellen Substanzen, z. B. von Antimykotika, sollen gut abgestufte Werte für die Hemmwirksamkeit ergeben und mit gebräuchlichen Laboratoriumsapparaturen durchführbar sein. Von grundlegender Wichtigkeit für die Gewinnung der Versuchsergebnisse ist, daß generell die Relationen zwischen den einzelnen Meßwerten eines Experimentes besser reproduzierbar sind als die Absolutwerte der einzelnen Messungen. Bei Vornahme von Konzentrationsbestimmungen in einem Untersuchungsmaterial (Serum, Gewebe) von Mensch oder Tier ist der meßbare Grad an Hemmaktivität im unverdünnten Versuchsmaterial von größerer Bedeutung als die Totalkonzentration der Substanz, da diese keinen Schluß auf die aktuelle Aktivität zuläßt. Bei Spiegelbestimmungen sollte darum neben den Gesamtkonzentrationen auch die therapeutisch wichtigere Hemmaktivität der nicht an Körpersubstanzen gebundenen Präparatmenge erfaßt werden. Für die Beurteilung von Behandlungserfolgen bei experimentellen Mykosen stehen bisher nur zum Teil befriedigende Meßmethoden zur Verfügung, auf die hier nicht eingegangen werden kann.

II. Versuchstechnik (in vitro)

Die sicherste Bestimmung der in vitro-Hemmwirkung eines Präparates gegenüber Mikroorganismen erfolgt an Hand von Wachstumsphasen mit konstanter Vermehrungsrate. Mittels Zeit-Wachstumskurven wird zunächst festgestellt, ob und in welchem Kulturabschnitt mit einer Hemmsubstanz und einem bestimmten Testkeim solche Phasen auftreten.

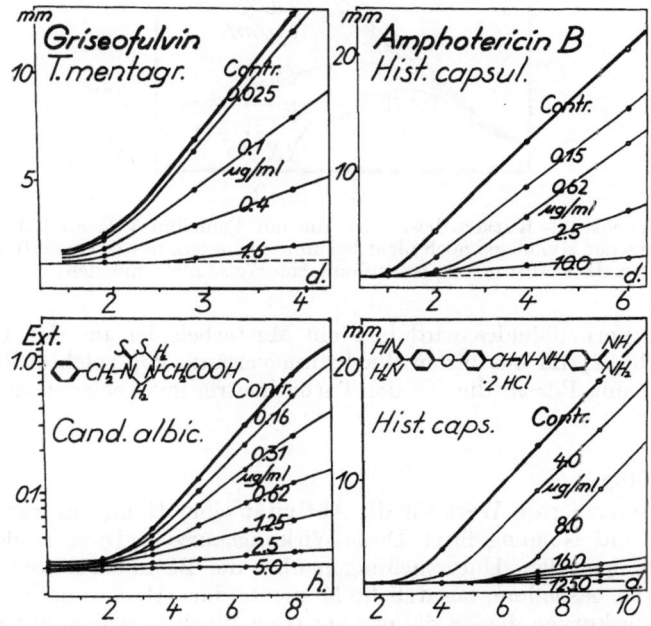

Abb. 1. Zeit-Wachstums-Kurven von vier antifungalen Verbindungen nach Mycelwuchs- bzw. Turbidimetrieversuchen. Im Fall der Kurve rechts unten wird der Wachstumsbeginn durch geringere Hemmstoffkonzentrationen (4 μg/ml) beeinflußt als das nachfolgende Mycelwachstum (16 μg/ml)

Techniken (je nach Wachstumsweise der Testkeime):

(M) *Mycelwachstumstechnik* für Hyphomyceten und Mycelphasen von Sproßpilzen:

Die mehrfach während des Versuches ermittelten Mycellängen bzw. die radialen Größen der wachsenden Kolonien ergeben die Ordinatenwerte der Zeit-Wachstumskurven.

(T) *Turbidimetrietechnik* für Hefen (und analog für Bakterien):

Die laufend photometrisch gemessenen Extinktionswerte für die Keimmasse in Schüttelkulturen ergeben, auf logarithmisch unterteilter Ordinate aufgetragen, die Zeit-Wachstumskurven (angenäherte Proportionalwerte für die Keimmasse).

In vielen Fällen wird der Beginn der exponentiellen Wachstumsphase bereits durch niedrigere Hemmstoffkonzentrationen verzögert als das nachfolgende Keimwachstum (Abb. 1, rechts unten), so daß vor Auswertung der Meßwerte eine Differenzierung in Wirkung auf Auskeimung und folgendes Wachstum nötig wird.

In einzelnen Fällen, wie beim Griseofulvin, wird dagegen das spätere Keimwachstum stärker gehemmt als das beginnende. Wegen seines besonders ein-

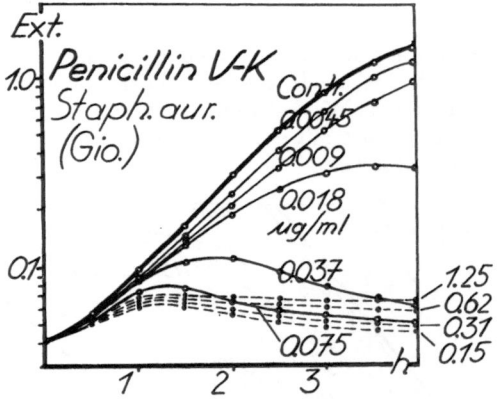

Abb. 2. Zeit-Wachstums-Kurven dieser Art, die mit Penicillin V-K an Bakterien erhalten wurden, sind aus der Mykologie noch nicht bekannt geworden, mit ihrem Auftreten muß aber gerechnet werden. Ihre Auswertung ist auf einfache Weise nicht möglich

drucksvollen Verlaufsbildes wird hier ein Musterbeispiel aus der Bakteriologie angeführt (Abb. 2), da uns bisher Wachstumsverläufe von solch auffallender Art in Versuchen mit Pilzen, die für die Turbidimetrie gut geeignet sind, nicht begegnet sind.

III. Auswertung

Einen differenzierten Wert für die Aktivität einer Hemmsubstanz liefern uns die Position und Neigung ihrer Dosis-Wirkungskurven. Diese stellen die beste Basis für alle speziellen Untersuchungen über die Beeinflußbarkeit der Hemmaktivität durch besondere, zusätzliche Momente dar. Als Ordinatenwerte für die Dosis-Wirkungskurven dienen die prozentualen Wachstumshemmungen, die über den entsprechenden Hemmstoffkonzentrationen (Abszisse, logar. Teilg.) aufgetragen werden.

Die Prozentwerte werden aus linearen Abschnitten der Zeit-Wachstumskurven ohne und mit Hemmstoffeinwirkung ermittelt. In der *Theorie* wird die Differenz zwischen den Wachstumskonstanten der Kontrollen und der einzelnen Hemmstoffkonzentrationen in Prozent der Kontrollkonstanten ausgedrückt und ergibt die prozentuale Hemmwirkung der einzelnen Präparatkonzentrationen.

Im *praktischen* Fall kann das ganze Rechenverfahren erspart werden, indem mittels eines geeigneten, graduierten Rechtecklineals (Abb. 3) aus den Zeit-Wachstumskurven direkt die Prozentwerte abgelesen werden.

Die Nachweisempfindlichkeit solcher Verfahren, mit denen noch kleine Teil-hemmwirkungen graduell erfaßt werden können, ist bis zu 100fach höher als die-jenige von üblichen Verdünnungs- und Diffusionsmethoden.

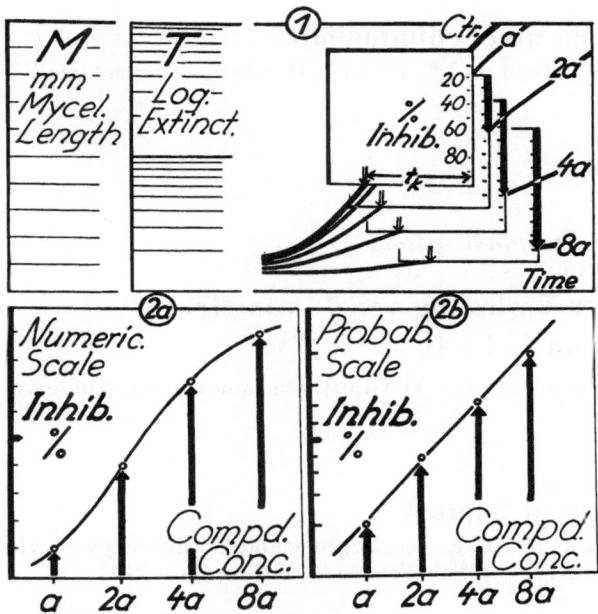

Abb. 3. Zur schnellen Ermittlung der % Wachstumshemmung aus Zeit-Wachstums-Kurven kann eine Schablone verwendet werden. Durch Anlegen derselben an der Kontrollkurve wird ein Zeitabschnitt t_k ermittelt, der an alle anderen Kurven angelegt wird. Auf dem vertikalen Rand der Schablone kann sodann der % Hemmwert abgelesen werden

IV. Anwendungsgebiete

1. Differenzierte und graduelle Messung der Hemmwirksamkeit gegenüber Sporenauskeimung, sich teilenden Zellen und wachsenden Mycelien.

2. Wirksamkeitsvergleiche.

3. Haltbarkeitsprüfungen.

4. Einflüsse auf die Präparataktivität (biochem. Antagonismus, Eiweißbin-dung, etc.).

5. Fungizidie (Messung der Auskeimungsverzögerung nach Inkubation mit Hemmstoff und anschließender Auswaschung desselben).

6. Mikrobiologischer Nachweis von antifungalen Substanzen und Aktivitäten in Untersuchungsflüssigkeiten (kompliziert in eiweißhaltigem Körpermaterial).

a) *Standard*verfahren auf Agarmedium, besonders für Serumspiegelunter-suchungen, mit Verdünnung des Materials. (Unsicherheitsfaktor: mögliche Metabolisierung des Präparates und Änderung seiner Eigenschaften).

b) *Mikro*testverfahren, besonders zum Nachweis der Hemmfähigkeit von nicht eiweißgebundenem (dialysablem) Hemmstoff im unverdünnten Versuchsmaterial.

Enzymhistochemische Untersuchungen an Dermatophyten

K. HOLUBAR und O. MALE, I. Univ.-Hautklinik Wien (Österreich)

Dermatophyten und Schimmelpilze

B. BRAUN, H. RIETH und C. FINGER, Hamburg (Deutschland)

Additional Demonstrations

Kollegheft der Vorlesung von F. von Hebra, geschrieben von F. Curti

zur Verfügung gestellt von O. GRUMBACH unter Vermittlung von O. GANS (Schweiz)

Histopathology of Leprosy

M. L. BRUBAKER and P. FASAL, Leprosy and Dermatology Service, U. S. Public Health Service Hosp.), San Francisco, California (USA)

Antibiotics and the Placebo Reaction in Acne

R. C. SAVIN and MARIA CHANCO-TURNER, Section of Dermatology, Department of Medicine, Yale University School of Medicine, New Haven, Connecticut (USA)

Tetracycline has been widely accepted as a highly effective and reliable agent in the treatment of Acne Vulgaris. Only four controlled studies as to pharmacologic effectiveness of this have been reported and the results are divided. We undertook this double-blind study to determine the effectiveness of antibiotics in the treatment of Acne and to delineate the percentage of placebo reactors.

Materials and Methods

42 outpatients with papulopustular and cystic Acne cooperated in a short term double blind study. The active medication was a combination of tetracycline hydrochloride 250 mg and novobiocin sodium 125 mg. Prior to and during the study, subjects were kept on a simple topical program employing a nonabrasive soap, one percent salicyclic acid in ethyl alcohol, and a sulfur-resorcin lotion.

All patients were given four capsules per day of active drug and placebo for a period of 2 weeks. If improvement was noted, the dose was decreased.

Results

42 patients completed their course of therapy. 23 patients received the tetracycline-novobiocin combination; 18 showed improvement. 19 patients were treated with placebo with nine showing improvement (Table).

Table

	Number of patients	Improved	No improvement
Tetracycline-novobiocin	23	18 (78%)	5 (22%)
Placebo	19	9 (47%)	10 (53%)

Statistical analysis of the data in the table shows that it is significant at the 4% level of probability. Fisher's exact test gives a "one tailed" probability of 0.03925 (P = 0.04).

Discussion

The evidence to support the effectiveness of antibiotics in Acne is based on only few controlled clinical studies.

HICKS [1] and STEWART [2] have published double-blind studies supporting the effectiveness of tetracyclines.

SMITH [3] published a double-blind study of 60 patients treated with demethylchlortetracycline, phenethicillin, and placebos; no significant difference was found among the three groups. Recently, CROUNSE [4] reported a double-blind study of 45 Acne patients treated with demethylchlortetracycline, tetracycline, and a placebo in a sequential cross-over manner. He found that neither antibiotic was superior to the placebo.

Neither SMITH nor CROUNSE used concomitant topical therapy in contrast to those investigators who found antibiotics more effective. Thus it would appear that continued topical therapy is important in the antibiotic therapy of Acne.

Clinical evaluation of new drugs is subject to bias; the placebo effect is but one of its many facets. The placebo reaction is a function of suggestion brought about by the high value our culture places on drug therapy [5]. The information derived from uncontrolled clinical trials, in which there are no fixed end points or inherent controls, is impossible to evaluate without knowledge of the percentage of placebo reactors to the same illness and mode of therapy. BEECHER [6] has shown that 15 to 58% of patients show significant improvement with placebo therapy; the mean was 35.2 ± 2.2%.

Studies of placebo reactors to tetracycline therapy in Acne do not yield the same consistency of results: HICKS [1] found 31% placebo reactors, STEWART [2] 56%, SMITH [3] 19%, CROUNSE [4] 24%. The Upjohn Company [7] 50%, and BECKER [8] 50%. We found 47% placebo reactors. These findings suggest that in the therapy of Acne a placebo reaction rate of 45 to 50% should be expected.

Most physicians would be satisfied with a 50% rate of clinical improvement and patient satisfaction in a chronic, embarrassing disease that is difficult to control and impossible to cure. Yet, the above data demonstrate that this rate is to be expected from the placebo effect alone. Therefore, in the clinical evaluation of Acne medication, the nonplacebo controlled clinical trial adds little to our knowledge of drug efficacy. The double-blind study stands out as an important method in the clinical evaluation of medication for Acne.

The high percentage of placebo reactors does not detract from the evidence that tetracyclines and the tetracycline-novobiocin combination are pharmacologically beneficial drugs in the treatment of Acne but rather emphasizes the fallacy of relying on uncontrolled clinical trials to evaluate pharmacologic benefits.

References. 1. HICKS, J. H.: Sth. med. J. (Bgham, Ala.) **55**, 357 (1962). — 2. STEWART, J. D.: Canad. med. Ass. J. **89**, 1096 (1963). — 3. SMITH, W. A., P. M. WATERWORTH, and M. P. CURWEN: Brit. J. Derm. **74**, 86 (1962). — 4. CROUNSE, R. G.: J. Amer. med. Ass. **193**, 906 (1965). — 5. BEECHER, H. K.: J. Amer. med. Ass. **176**, 1102 (1961). — 6. BEECHER, H. K.: J. Amer. med. Ass. **159**, 1602 (1955). — 7. The Upjohn Company. Pers. communication. Unpublished data. — 8. Becker, F. T.: Arch. Derm. **91**, 155 (1965).

Authors Index

Abdel Gawad, M. S. 654
Abeliuk, S. 267
Abulafia, J. 58
Achten, G. 46, 828
Adam, A. 562
Adam, W. 884
Adari, S. 575
Afifi, A. K. 79
Agache, P. 276
Agius, J. R. G. 1241
Agrup, G. 273
Ahumada, M. 615
Aiuti, F. 1189
Akano, A. 84
Alessi, E. 1033
Aliaga, A. 581, 968
Alkiewicz, J. 1564
Allegra, F. 521
Allegrini, J. 886
Allende, M. F. 1381
Allyn, A. 1394
Alt, J. 1539
Alteras, I. 830, 859
Amor, F. 377
Anderson, D. E. 587, 1380
Anderson, T. E. 1153
Andrade, G. O. 1159
Andrade, L. M. C. de 858, 1328
Andrade, R. 936
Angyal, J. 333
Andreassi, L. 693
Antonescu, S. 892
Antoniades, H. N. 158
Anzai, T. 509
Aono, K. 370
Araki, H. 1357
Argenziano, G. 700
Armengaud, M. 316
Arouète, J. 771
Asboe-Hansen, G. 133
Aschheim, E. 458
Ashurst, P. J. 644
Aso, K. 184
Astore, I. 783
Avila, J. J. 373
Avram, A. 881
Azevedo Carneiro, J. de 858
Azulay, R. 731
Azulay, R. D. 858, 1328

Baart de la Faille, E. H. 1524
Baccaredda-Boy, A. 1212
Bădăniou, Al. 192
Baer, R. L. 226, 1144
Bajdekov, B. 1063
Baker, H. 1017
Balabanoff, V. 879
Balabanoff, V. A. 1556
Balabanov, K. 119
Balevska, N. 1110
Baliña, L. M. 373, 1334

Balosu, P. 895
Bamatter, F. 1443
Bandmann, H.-J. 665, 1493
Barman, J. M. 783
Barriere, H. 49, 747
Barták, P. 478
Basset, A. 316, 1359, 1409, 1448, 1539, 1570
Basset, M. 1570
Bastide, J.-M. 886
Bastide, M. 886
Bazex, A. 565, 1197
Bechelli, L. M. 1323
Beck, J. S. 1153
Beerman, H. 381
Begemann, M. 1531
Belaïch, S. 153
Belisario, J. C. 99
Bell, M. 521
Bellone, A. G. 1285
Bellringer, H. E. 289
Benedetto, A. 1047
Beninson, J. 452
Benjamin, B. 481
Benne, M. 1162
Berdichesky, R. 1234
Berger, D. 1112
Berger, H. 53, 522
Bergoend, H. 1359
Bermont, A. 1352
Bernstein, I. A. 1008
Berowa, N. 1191
de Bersaques, J. 37, 1103
Bertchev, K. 1063
Betetto, M. 1096
Bettinelli, C. A. 1222
Beukelaar, L. de 176
Beurey, J. 1156, 1352
Bianchi, C. 1060, 1283
Bianchi, O. 1060, 1283
Bichis, M. 87
Bielický, T. 282, 1170
Bignami, A. 728
Bihari, Ö. 973, 975
Binazzi, M. 791
Bismuth, V. 750
Björnberg, A. 207, 340
Bleehen, S. S. 941, 1506
Blohm, S.-G. 1421
Blois, M. S. 976
Bloom, D. 529
Böszörményi, J. 611
Bogdaszewska-Czabanowska, J. 73
Bojanovská, A. 1560, 1561, 1562, 1563
Bojkov, B. 1063
Bolgert, M. 645, 1317
Bologa, E. I. 583
Bolubasz, J. 44
Boncinelli, U. 419
Bonelli, M. 1033

Bonneau, H. 741
Boraud, P. 1264
Borelli, S. 238, 1185, 1395
Boreux, G. 1443
Born, W. 1101
Borota, A. 474
Bosco, I. 13
Bosse, Kl. 70, 1493
Bottyan, E. 333
Botzov, P. 205
Boulle, St. 1217
Bourdon, R. 750, 752
Bourgeois-Spinasse, J. 771
Bourlond, A. 626
Boutet, B. 413
Bowden, L. 918
Brauer, E. W. 761
Braun, B. 1590
Braun, H. 1550
Braun, W. 31
Braun-Falco, O. 1546
Breathnach, A. 1506
Brehm, G. 1149, 1426
Brehmer-Andersson, E. 735
Brenn, H. 1395
Brničević, M. 893
Brocher, J. E. W. 1443
Brown, S. 1016
Brown, W. J. 360
Brubaker, M. L. 1590
Brun, R. 755
Brunk, U. 735
Bubola, D. 310, 329
Buchvald, J. 851, 1561
Burckhardt, W. 224
Bureau, B. 747
Bureau, Y. 49
Burnett, J. B. 943

Cabré, J. 1083
Cabrera, H. N. 373
Cabrini, R. L. 714
Čajkovac, V. 166
Calabresi, P. 739
Calap, J. 81, 968
Calas, E. 741
Calnan, C. D. 229
Cantwell, A. R. 1320
van Caneghem, P. 1069
Capetanakis, J. 1462
Capilla, A. J. 117
Caplan, R. M. 1381
Căpusan, I. 895, 1222
Caputo, G. 1285
Caputo, R. 1472, 1494
Cardama, J. E. 373, 1334
Cárdenas Jaramillo, V. 1371
Carniol, M. 861
Carslaw, R. W. 209
Carton, F.-X. 286
Casalá, A. 1060, 1283
Casper, W. A. 1249

Castermans, A. 501
Catterall, M. 1215
Catterall, R. D. 372
Cavalieri, R. 534
Ceppellini, R. 514
Cerimele, D. 43
Cernea, R. 673
Cerutti, P. 698
Cesarini, J. P. 741
Chanco-Turner, M. 1590
Chernosky, M. E. 587
Chiappino, G. 326
Chieregato, G. C. 410
Chisleag, G. 461
Chlebarov, St. 652, 1395
Chmel, L. 851, 1560, 1561, 1562, 1563
Chorzelski, T. 1135
Christiansen, J. V. 1319
Christol, B. 565, 1197
Christophers, E. 1546
Ciarrocchi, L. 415
Cipriani, C. 765
Civatte, J. 61
Clarke, G. H. V. 644
Clayton, Y. M. 1542
Clodi, P. H. 574
Coburn, J. G. 257
Cojocaru, I. 830, 859
Collart, P. 400
Comaish, J. S. 1179
Constantine, V. S. 831
de Conti, R. C. 739
Contreras, M. A. 1094
Convit, J. 1314, 1381
Corbett, M. B. 334
Cordero, A. A. 1363
Cormane, R. H. 1146, 1524
Cortés, A. C. 835
Cortés Cortés, A. 1371
Cortese jr., Th. A. 1273, 1288
Coser, A. 1248
Costea, V. 861
Cottenot, F. 1305, 1326
le Coulant, P. 338, 1264
Cox, A. J. 171
Cozza, G. 249
Craggs, E. 1320
Cristofolini, M. 685
Crosti, A. 310, 330
Crovato, F. 765, 1212
Cruickshank, C. N. D. 156
Curth, W. 369
Curti, F. 1590
Curtis, A. C. 140

Dabrowa, N. 813
Daguet, G. L. 359
Dajani, A. S. 612
Dana, M. 750, 752
Danbolt, N. 1202
Davies, R. E. 24, 1112
Defeo, Ch. P. 1394
Degiovanni, G. 501

Degos, R. 17, 75, 363
Delacrétaz, J. 863
Delaire, P. L. 1317
Denk, R. 1459, 1524
Desmons, F. 444
Desprez-Curely, J. P. 750
Díaz, J. 1234
Didisheim, P. 1208
Dillaha, C. J. 128
Dimitrescu, Al. 86
Dittmar, W. 1586
Dlabalová, H. 468
Dobson, R. L. 1024
Dodica, C. 702
Dogo, G. 496
Dohi, J. 370
Domonkos, A. N. 1347
Donald, G. F. 1296
Donaldson, A. D. 569
Donaldson, E. M. 569
Donsky, H. J. 74, 1474
Dorfman, M. 1314, 1329
Doxiades, Th. 1462
Drepper, H. 125, 1465
Dufourmentel, C. 946, 954
Duheille, J. 1156
Dulamită, L. 859
Dulanto, F. de 118, 520
Dumas, K. J. 179
Dumitriu, R. 1248
Duncan, W. C. 595
Dunoyer, F. 400
Dunoyer, M. 400
Duperrat, B. 92, 917
Dupont, Ad. 626
Dupré, A. 565, 1197
Dutu, R. 78

Eberhartinger, Chr. 1229
Ehlers, G. 38
Ehring, F. 125, 1308, 1465
Ehrmann, G. 419
Eisenberg, S. 1394
Ejmont-Skrzypczyk, B. 613
El-Hefnawi, H. 524, 654, 1379, 1476
Eliasson, R. 659
El Komy, H. M. 908
Ellena, V. 510
Ellickson, B. E. 481
El Mofty, A. M. 908, 1224
El Zawahry, K. 847
El Zawahry, M. 847, 1107, 1464, 1564
Ene-Popescu, C. 1064, 1395
Epstein, J. 1045
Epstein, J. H. 566, 939
Epstein, W. L. 939, 1148
Esteller, J. 581
Evdos, P. 755
Even-Paz, Z. 729
Everett, M. A. 988, 1056

Faerman, J. 1234
Faldarini, G. 410

Farah, F. S. 79, 612, 1090, 1176
Farber, E. M. 171, 458
Fasal, P. 1337, 1590
Fegeler, F. 385, 903
Feinstein, A. 562
Feiwel, M. 194, 202
Fejér, E. 864
Feldmann, R. J. 186
Fellner, M. J. 226, 1144
Fenster, M. L. 813
Fettich, J. 244
Fiedler, H. P. 1022
Filkov, T. 879
Finger, C. 1590
Fischer, Ch. 1469
Fischer, H. 1252
Fitzpatrick, T. B. 913, 941, 1506
Fixa, B. 1294
Fjelde, A. 1185
Flarer, F. 389
Fleisher, T. L. 1124
Floderus, St. 1379
Földvári, F. 145
Förström, L. 1430
Follmann, E. 1363
Forck, G. 270, 948
Forsbeck, M. 268
Fortea, J. M. 81
Fournet, M. 153
Foussereau, J. 1429
Fraga, S. 831
Franceschetti, A. 553, 1443
Freedberg, I. M. 776
Freeman, R. G. 466, 587
Fregert, S. 1421
Frenk, E. 941, 1506
Friederich, H. C. 503
Friedman-Kien, A. E. 505
Fry, L. 1301
Fujita, H. 724
Fukushiro, R. 1568
Fukuyama, K. 1288
Furtado, T. A. 1159
Fusaro, R. M. 1048, 1332, 1432, 1477

Gabino, G. 1306
Galloway, J. M. D. 441
Gans, O. 1590
Gardenghi, G. 181
Garretts, M. 1061
Gartmann, H. 958
Gatti, J. C. 373, 1334
Gavrilescu, M. 518
Gay Prieto, J. 77, 107, 1306
Gedda, L. 534
Gedek, B. 1573
Gehrken, H. 1395
Geniaux, M. 338
Georgiadis, Chr. 854
Giacometti, G. 327
Giacometti, L. 521
Giannetti, A. 1003, 1050

Giannotti, B. 265
Gianotti, F. 310, 330, 1472
Gigli, I. 1514
Gigli, J. 1531
Gimenez Camarasa, J. M. 262
Gimferrer, E. 581
Girdwood Fergusson, A. 163
Glicenstein, J. 946, 954
Glickman, F. S. 1335
Goddard, A. R. 110
Goetschel, G. E. 951
Götz, H. 807
Gokhale, B. B. 833
Goldberg, H. C. 866
Goldman, L. 1084, 1388
Goldschmidt, H. 105
Goldstein, N. 283
Goltz, E. W. 1432
Gómez Orbaneja, D. J. 1262
González Ochoa, A. 819
Goppel, A. 19
Governa, M. 330
Gózony, M. 611
Graciansky, P. de 628
Graham, J. H. 89, 470
Granelli, U. 728
Grant Peterkin, G. A. 1214
Gray, H. R. 470
Greaves, M. W. 1176
Gregorczyk, K. 393
Gregory, P. B. 1097
Greither, A. 1408
Grell, H. 1413, 1531
Griem, M. L. 1099
Griffin, T. B. 1273
Grigoriou, D. 863
Grinspan, D. 1234
Grob, P. J. 1154, 1158, 1480
de Groot, W. P. 559
Gros, Ch. 1409, 1539
Grosshans, E. 1409
Grots, I. A. 72, 578
Grütz, O. 960
Grumbach, O. 1590
Grupper, Ch. 1349
Gudenzi, M. 1390
Guigon, M. 44
Guilaine, J. 1217
Gulati, O. D. 1053
Gulbert, A. 957, 973
Guthe, T. 345

Hadida, E. 551, 748
Haeger, K. 450
Haenen-Severyns, A. M. 501
Hagen, E. 1495
Hagerman, G. 1406
Hahn, E. 310, 327
Haisuc, M. 1248
Hamada, Y. 588
Hargita, G. 1451
Hasegawa, T. 375
Haserick, J. R. 1204
Hashimoto, K. 3, 1278
Hasselmann, C. M. 1224

Hauser, W. 650
Hauss, H. 1387
ten Have-Opbroek, A. A. W.
    1524
Hearst, B. R. 1251
Hebra, F. von 1590
Hegyi, E. 294
Heid, E. 1409
Heitmann, H. J. 1174
Hellerström, S. 102, 103, 104,
    105
Hellgren, L. 207, 340
Hellinga, G. 679
Helwig, E. B. 89
Henderson, B. 1388
Herpay, Zs. 1580
Herrmann, F. 995, 1381,
    1514, 1531
Herrmann, R. 668
Herrmann, W. P. 663
Herzberg, J. J. 933
Hewitt, J. 44
Heyns, W. 660
Higoumenakis, C. G. 378
Higuchi, K. 639
Higuchi, M. 1171
Hjorth, N. 275, 1421
Hodgson, G. 29
Hoffmann, D. H. 1566
Hofmann, M. F. 685, 1285
Holenstein, P. 1443
Hollander, A. 72
Holti, G. 1380
Holubar, K. 1502, 1590
Holzmann, H. 572, 1524
Honeycutt, W. M. 128
Hontaru, M. 1248
Horáček, J. 999
Horáková, M. 168, 204
Hori, Y. 941, 1506
Hornstein, O. 1408
Hornstein, O. P. 672
Høvding, G. 1421
Howell, J. B. 1380
Hundeiker, M. 53
Hunter, G. A. 1296
Hunziker, N. 755, 1518
Hurel, G. 645
Huriez, Cl. 276, 444

Iacob, P. 87
Iacovacci, G. 1189
Idsøe, O. 345
Igarashi, Y. 561, 1481
Ikeda, S. 915
Ilca, St. 702
Ilea, R. 589
Ilies, M. 861
Illig, L. 258, 1187
Inderbitzin, Th. M. 1154,
    1158, 1480
Indianer, L. 872
Inglesini, C. 1283
Ioanovici, Z. 702
Ippen, H. 1218

Isaac, Z. 580
Ishibashi, Y. 1325
Ishiwara, K. 1171
Ishizu, S. 915
Ismirov, I. 1063
Ito, K. 380
Iwashita, K. 335, 561, 1012

Jablonska, S. 17
Jackson, R. 949
Jadassohn, W. 23, 59, 76
Jänner, M. 1232
Jaffe, M. O. 1432
James, V. H. T. 194, 202
Janke, D. 1577
Janoušek, B. 468
Jansen, G. T. 128
Jaqueti, G. 107
Jaramillo, V. C. 835
Jeandidier, P. 1352
Jeffries, C. D. 908
Joel, Ch. A. 676
Johnson, A. 76
Johnson, F. R. 1301
Johnson, J. A. 1048, 1477
Johnson, M.-L. T. 1097
Johnson, W. C. 470
Jones, F. T. 786
Jordan, P. 948
Jovović, D. 291
Jowev, S. 1110
Józefczyk, Z. 609
Juhlin, L. 198
Juon, M. 793
Jursch, H. 1400

Kaden, R. 686
Kästner, H. 948
Kagawa, S. 1568
Kahn, D. S. 75
Kalkoff, K. W. 53
Kaminsky, A. 58, 630
Kaminsky, A. R. de 58
Kaminsky, C. A. 58
Kanitakis, C. 854
Kanof, N. M. 1380
Karasek, M. A. 513
Karlić, D. 166
Karltorp, N. 1379
Karma, P. 1379
Kárpáti, Gy. 973
Karuga, H. 1574
Kasemir, H. 1425
Kass, G. 758
Katabira, Y. 1447
Katzenellenbogen, J. 321
Kawamura, T. 915, 1325
Keddie, F. M. 867
Kennedy, J. F. 1543
Kerdel-Vegas, F. 775, 1381
Kerp, L. 1425
Kiffe, M. 385
Kiistala, N. 1513
Kiistala, U. 1493
Kikuchi, Y. 84

Kimmig, J. 1139
Kinmont, P. D. C. 97, 1237
Kint, A. 542, 1103
Kirsch-Nietzki, M. 1566
Kitamura, K. 1316, 1449
Kitzmiller, K. Wm. 1388
Klaschka, F. 232, 1151, 1533
Klein, D. 1443
Klostermann, G. F. 928, 1387
Klüken, N. 476
Knoth, W. 668, 712
Knox, J. M. 466, 595, 1126
Knudsen, E. A. 1038
Koblenzer, P. J. 1298
Kobori, T. 788, 1357
Kochová, I. 1562, 1563
Kocsard, E. 607
Kogoj, Fr. 244
Kojima, T. 370
Komárková, O. 1294
Konrád, B. 1411, 1563
Konstantinović, S. 423
Kooji, R. 1322
Kopecká, B. 1185, 1395
Kopf, A. W. 54
Korossy, S. 611
Korting,   G.   W.   72,   623,
  1524
Kostanecki, W. 780
Kotter, L. 22
Kraft, H. 1570, 1572
Krampitz, H. E. 1459
Krause, R. A. 1533
Krempl-Lamprecht, L. 1550,
  1555
Krepsz, I. 974
Kreysel, H. W. 1232
Krizek, H. 1016
Krstitsch, A. 288
Krüger, H. 1435
Kukita, A. 188
Kunick, I. 1187
Kuokkanen, K. 1379
Kurban, A. K. 79, 612, 1090,
  1176
Kúta, A. 67

Lachapelle, J. M. 1362
Lacková, E. 168, 204
Lagerholm, B. 500
Lalević, B. 725
Lamberg, S. I. 517
Lambergeon, S. 640, 795
Lańcucki, J. 609
Landau, J. W. 813, 872
Lane Brown, M. 970, 978
Langhof, H. 803
Langner, A. 17
Lanzl, L. H. 796
Lapeyre, J. 413
Lapière, Ch. M. 986
Lapiere, S. 531
Latourelle, Ph. 1162
Laugier, P. 510
Lazăr, M. 861

Lebeuf, M. 1162
Leclercq, R. 1238
Ledoux-Corbusier, M. 1093
Leigheb, G. 398, 514
Lejeune, G. 501
Lejman, K. 73
Lempriere, W. W. 159
Lesińska, W. 411
Lesiński, J. 387, 411
Lever, W. F. 3
Levi, L. 1222
Levy, L. 1337
Lewis, M. B. 1297
Lima, A. O. 1159
Lipkin, G. 1029
Lisbôa Miranda, J. 831
Litoux, P. 747
Löwy, G. 900
Logan, J. C. P. 163
Londoño, F. 1122
Longhin, C. 78
Longhin, S. 135
Lorincz, A. L. 1016
Lortat-Jacob, E. 353
Lowney, E. D. 247
de Luca, M. 688, 698
Ludwig, G. 160
Lutzner, M. A. 720
Lyell, A. 1346

Mach, K. W. 721
Magnin, P. H. 714
Magnus, I. A. 1195, 1545
Magnusson, B. 1421
Maibach, H. I. 186, 602
Maier, N. 895
Majcan, D. 725
Male, O. 852, 1590
Maleki, M. A. 1476
Maleville, J. 1359, 1409
Malina, L. 1170
Malkinson, F. D. 796, 1099
Malmquist, J. 1006
Mammen, A. 580
Mantellassi, G. 1087, 1088
Manuel, Y. 1289
Many, P. 413
Marcel, G. A. C. 1349
Marcelou-Kinti, U. 854, 856
March, C. 576
Marchand, J. P. 1162
Marghescu, S. 1546
Marill, F. G. 551, 748
Markuch, T. 421
Marples, M. J. 602
Marques, A. S. 470
Martin, P. 276
Martin-Scott, I. 781
Martina, G. 143, 1168
Mascaro, J.-M. 61, 917
Masszi, J. 145
Matanić, V. 120
Matěja, F. 1294
Mathai, R. 580
Matoltsy, A. G. 1014

Matsuzawa, T. 188
Mavor, G. E. 441
McBride, M. E. 595
McCallum, D. I. 97, 1237
McDonald, Ch. J. 739
Meenan, F. O. 197
van der Meer, J. B. 1524
Meerts, P. 367
Mehareb, R. 908
Mehregan, A. H. 68
Meinhof, W. 876, 1581
Melczer, N. 925
Memmesheimer, A. 32
Meneghini, C. L. 249, 1222
Mennecier, M. 276
Merello, A. 211
Merklen, F.-P. 1305, 1326
Meyer, R. 1084, 1388
Meyer-Rohn, J. 600
Meyhöfer, W. 666, 668
Michailov, P. 1191, 1395
Midana, A. 143, 1168
Middleton, J. D. 1010
Miguens, M. P. 896
Mikhail, G. R. 74, 1474
Mikol, Cl. 1180, 1190
Milton, G. W. 970, 978
Miranda, R. N. 898
Mishima, Y. 961, 1505
Misson, E. 413
Miura, Y. 84
Miyamoto, M. 1506
Miyazawa, T. 479
Mochizuki, H. 370
Möller, H. 1355
Mohs, F. E. 122, 1393
Molina Leguizamón, E. B. 1363
Mom, A. M. 165
Monacelli, M. 331
Montagnani, A. 688
Montes, L. F. 831
Montet, Y. 1156
Montgomery, H. 707
Moor, P. de 660
Moreno, A. R. 835
Moretti, G. 765
Morgenfeld, M. C. 714
Moriame, G. 367
Morohashi, M. 1028
Morsches, B. 572, 1524
Moulin, G. 1289
Moulton, J. E. 607
Mouly, R. 946, 954
Moynahan, E. J. 208, 1543,
  1544
Müller, E. 1036, 1516
Müller, G. 1444
Muijs van de Moer, W. W.
  1524
Mullins, J. F. 877
Munro, D. D. 194, 202
Munteanu, M. 803
Mustakallio, K. K. 1409,
  1493, 1513, 1534
Mustakov, G. 1110

Nagashima, T. 907
Nakagawa, T. 84
Nakai, T. 939
Nakajima, T. 915
Nakashima, K. 907
Nannelli, M. 1088
Nasemann, Th. *39, 46, 48, 50,*
  301, 1499
Nastase, G. 461
Nazzaro, P. 331, 728
Negulescu, V. N. 259
Nékám, L. 1243
Nelson, C. T. 1270
Németh, Gy. 973
Neumann, L. 615
Newcomer, V. D. 813, 872
Nicholas, L. 381
Nicolau, R. 87
Nicolau, St. G. 325
Nicolson, J. M. 209
Niebauer, G. 35, 1495
Nielsen, H. A. 357
Niepel, G. 1246
Niermann, H. 696
Nikolowski, W. 682
Nishiyama, Sh. 1240
Noaghea, G. 325
Noda, S. 915
Noel, J. 645
Noguchi, Y. 1171
Nolting, S. 385
Nordquist, J. 1056
Nordquist, R. 1056
Noury, J. Y. 92
Novák, M. 282
Nürnberger, F. 1444, 1522

Oancea, C. C. 296
Oates, J. A. 1006
Ocampo, F. A. 841
Ocaña, J. 91
Ocaña Sierra, J. 117
Oehlschlaegel, G. 745
Ofner, F. 607
Ohara, K. 212
Okamura, K. 1012
Oleffe, J. 252
Olitzki, A. L. 1329
Ollendorff Curth, H. 557, 1380
Olson, R. L. 988, 1056
Ooshima, Y. 1481
Opplt, J. 1170
Orentreich, N. 497
Orfanos, C. 798
Ortega, E. 615
Ortiz, Y. 1373
Osbourn, R. A. 481
Ottolenghi, F. 405, 406

Pace, N. 576
Padhye, A. A. 833
Padilha-Gonçalves, A. 824,
  839
Pages, F. 413
Pagnes, P. 408

Paldrok, H. 1556
Palese, D. 1234
Panconesi, E. 255, 261
Panti, A. 404
Parejo, P. 91
Pascalev, T. 205
Pathak, M. A. 941, 1506
Paupe, J. 1190
Pavel, M. 589
Pecoraro, V. 783
Pegum, J. S. 279
Pelfini, C. 43
Pentschev, P. 119
Perdrup, A. 463
Perez, R. T. 841
Perišić, S. 291, 423
Pernis, B. 330
Perry, H. O. 1208
Peryassú, D. 900
Peter, G. 1516
Peterka, E. S. 1432
Petkov, J. 1110
Petrarca de Mesquita, A. 731
Pettinger, W. 1006
Petzoldt, D. 1546
Pfleger, L. 1467
Piccinini, S. 1033
Pichot, P. 640
Piérard, J. 37, 542
Pierquin, B. 1081
Pietschmann, H. 1293
Pinetti, P. 826
Pinkus, H. 8.
Piñol Aguadé, J. 455, 581
Piret, J. M. 645
Pirilä, V. 236, 1421, 1430
Pizano, I. R. 835
Pochi, P. E. 762
Poggi, G. 400
Polani, P. 1543
Polano, M. K. 176
Polansky, B. 578
Poligny, O. de 628
Polychronopoulou, A. 856
Popchristov, P. 605, 879
Pospišil, L. 395
Pozzo, G. 685
Price, V. H. 786
Proppe, A. 1070, 1387
Prose, Ph. H. 505
Prutkin, L. 57
Puccinelli, V. 1472, 1494
Puccinelli, V. A. 1228
Pürschel, W. 169, 1397
Puhvel, S. M. 1136
Puissant, A. 1238
Putkonen, T. 1570

Quiroga, M. I. 1343

Raab, W. 901, 1293
Rabbiosi, G. 1003, 1050
Rabito, C. 389
Race, R. R. 562
Rádl, J. 168

Rahim, G. F. 837
Rahmann-Esser, M. 903
Rajka, E. 611
Rajka, G. 1187
Ramos-Silva, J. 839
Rampini, E. 765
Rantuccio, F. 249
Rasiewicz, W. 460
Rassner, G. 876, 1546
Rausch, N. G. 366
Rauschkolb, E. W. 1126
Raven, R. W. 926
Rebora, A. 765
Reed, W. B. 646, 1381
Rehák, A. 11
Rehtijärvi, K. 1379
Reich, H. 1214
Reid, J. 257
Reisner, R. M. 1136
Reiter, L. 1248
Renoux, M. 1180
Ribuffo, A. 21
Rieth, H. 1590
Rimbaud, P. 886
Rimington, C. 569
Risold, J. C. 510
Ritter, E. J. 1388
Riveiro, C. 377
Robinson, H. M. 634
Rocha, G. L. 731
Rockwell jr., R. J. 1084,
  1388
Rodermund, O.-E. 1091
Roe, D. A. 1231
Röckl, H. 1244, 1516
Rohde, B. 938
Rollier, R. 421
Ronchi, E. 326
Rook, A. J. 993
Roqué, O. 1060
Rorsman, H. 942
Rose, M. 1381
Ross, C. M. 636
Rostenberg, A. 758
Rothenstein, J. 1106
Rothfield, N. 576
Rovenský, J. 1020
Rowell, N. R. 1131, 1153
Rozsívalová, V. 468, 1294
Rueda, L. A. 955
Runge, W. J. 1432
Rupec, M. 1546
Ryan, T. J. 727, 1541

Sabra, F. A. 79
Sagher, F. 729, 1314, 1329
Saitoh, M. 788
Sakamoto, M. 788
Sakellariou, G. 1450
Samii, R. 1339
Samman, P. D. 733
Samos, J. 609
Sánchez-Muros, J. 118, 520
Sandru, G. 78
Sanger, R. 562

Santler, R. 469
Santoianni, P. 700
Santori, G. 690
Santos, F. 731
Sartoris, S. 397, 398
Sasai, Y. 479
Sato, Y. 1028
Sauter, L. S. 1235
Savin, R. C. 1590
Sayag, J. 551, 748
Sberna, P. 883
Scarpa, C. 280
Schauer, A. 1483
Schiefer, B. 1573
Schirren, C. 660, 662, 1413
Schirren, C. G. 27, 78
Schmalbruch, H. 672
Schmid, P. 224
Schmid, R. 224
Schmidt, P. 1531
Schneider, W. 56, 59, 429
Schneiderman, J. 1234
Schnyder, U. W. 539, 1411
Schönborn, C. 1550
Schöpf, E. 254
Scholtz, J. R. 179
Schraub, S. 1409
Schröpl, F. 246, 1516
Schultka, O. 1381
Schulz, K. H. 254, 1181, 1531
Schuppli, R. 769
Schutter, K. 1041
Schwarz, E. 1043
Schwarz, K. 1106
Schwarz-Speck, M. 1106, 1183
Schwarzwald, M. 33
Scolari, E. G. 1078
Seabra, O. 1159
Seiji, M. 1506
Seiler, H. 943
Semmola, L. 694
van Senden, K. G. 1025
Serri, F. 43, 763
Sertoli, A. 261, 265
Sertoli, P. 1291
Shelley, W. B. 1143
Sheskin, J. 1314, 1329
Shinoda, R. 375
Siage, J. 691
Sidell, Ch. M. 334
Sidi, E. 771
Silva, D. 842
Silvers, S. H. 1335
Simon, N. 1312
Simonart, J. M. 944
Simpson, J. R. 549
Sitay, Z. 1246
Skog, E. 268, 1267, 1421
Sneddon, I. B. 1061
Söltz-Szöts, J. 425
Sofronić, A. 291
Sonck, C. E. 65, 1413, 1444
Soo Duk Lim 1332
Sorkin, E. 1185

Sotman, S. 158
Sotomatsu, S. 1481
Soule, M. 645
Sowinski, W. 1564
Spagnoli, U. 405, 406
Spangler, A. S. 158
Spencer, M. C. 1393
Spier, H. W. 232
Spinelli-Ressi, F. 1222
Spiridon, M. 78
Spirov, G. 205
Stanowska, E. 609
Stava, Z. 1230
Steeno, O. 660
Steigleder, G. K. 983
Stein, G. 112
Stene, J. 463, 464
Sternberg, T. H. 1136
Stevanović, D. 725
Stevanović, D. V. 51
Stoian, M. 881
Stoker, G. L. 140
Storck, H. 438
Stough, D. B. 1394
Strani, G. F. 397, 398
Strauss, J. S. 1031
Strauss, W. G. 602
Strehler, E. 438
Stringa, S. 1060, 1283
Strozzi, F. 326
Stüttgen, G. 306, 1514, 1531
Sturde, H.-C. 670
Sugár, J. 83
Sulzberger, M. B. 32, 1273, 1382
Sundström, K. R. 1556
Surdan, C. 325
Suskind, R. R. 217
Suurmond, D. 200
Swatek, F. 1320
Sweet, R. D. 339
Sylvester, E. 267
Szabó, G. 941, 1506
Szita, J. 611
Szodoray, L. 16
Szymczyk, B. 460

Takenouchi, K. 184
Tamisier, J. M. 338
Tanabe, Y. 184
Taplin, D. 593
Tappeiner, J. 1257, 1467
Tarquini, B. 181
Taura, T. 1097
Teillard, J. 413
Teller, H. 1435
Temime, P. 1162
Teodorescu, St. 192
Texier, L. 338, 1264
Thibaut, D. 113
Thiele, F. A. J. 1025
Thiers, H. 1002
Thies, W. 63, 1469
Thirumalachar, M. J. 833
Thivolet, J. 1134

Thomas, C. Ch. 1380
Thomas, R. S. 786
Thurner, J. 1584
Tîrlea, P. 1222
Todorov, A. 605
Tomasini, C. 1033
Tomášková, J. 801
Tomov, G. 1110
Tosti, A. 490, 1535
Tóth, F. 1243
Touraine, R. 153
Towpik, J. 416
Trichopoulos, D. 856
Trinh Thi Kim Don 1326
Tritsch, H. 48
Tronnier, H. 172
Tsuyuki, Sh. 1240
Tuffanelli, D. L. 391, 1381

Ueda, K. 335, 561, 1012
Ujváry, E. 974
Ulbrich, A. P. 292
Ulivi, S. 404
Ungari, S. 1189
Urabe, H. 907
Urbach, F. 24, 1112
Usunov, P. 879
Uzuka, M. 788

Valentová, M. 851, 1561
Vallecchi, C. 1087
Vanbremeersch, F. 92, 1238
Vanbreuseghem, R. 817
Vavruska, G. W. 75
Vélez, G. C. 835
Veltman, G. 575, 642
Venkei, T. 973, 975
Verhagen, A. R. H. B. 1118
Verma, B. S. 1053
Véron, M. 510
Vértes, B. 145
Vezekenyi-Nagy, Cl. 16
Victoria, R. V. 841
Viglioglia, P. A. 213
Vignale, R. A. 377
Villapol, L. O. 1234
Visetti, M. 514
Viziam, C. B. 580
Vlček, F. 1246
Vogel, H.-J. 19
Vogell, W. 1581
Vossieck, H. 1395
de Vries, G. A. 1555
Vrousos, C. 1539

Wachsmann, F. 1074
Waddington, E. 314, 336
Wagner, O. 1534
Wakasugi, M. 335
Wallace, H. J. 1207
Walther, R. J. 578
Wanet, J. 46
Warin, R. 314
Warin, R. P. 336
Watson, C. J. 1432

van Waveren Hogervorst,
  J. W. 1322
Weber, G. 1400
Wegmann, T. 1563
Weitgasser, H. 474
Weitz, R. 642
Wells, G. C. 1200
Welton, W. A. 19
Wheatley, V. R. 1029
Whimster, I. W. 487
Whiteley, H. J. 29
Wiedmann, A. *22, 29*, 355
Wilgram, G. F. 571, 1475
Wilkinson, D. S. 1266
Willcox, R. R. 345
Willis, C. J. 877
Wilson, J. W. 1320
Wilson-Jones, E. 70

Winer, L. H. 1259
Winkelmann, R. K. 707,
  1045, 1502
Winkler, K. 187
Wiskemann, A. 1125
Wisniewska, C. 387
Wittels, W. 515
Witten, V. H. 149
Woeber, Kh. 960
Wohlstein, E. 1219
Wolff, K. 1045, 1502
Wolfram, G. 1390
Wright, E. T. 1259
Wuepper, K. D. 391, 566

Yamamoto, K. 1420
Yasuda, T. 1240
Yoshida, S. 1171

Ytterborn, K. 268

Zacarian, S. A. 126
Zachariae, H. 1006
Zackheim, H. S. 22, 458
Záhejský, J. 1020
Zaias, N. 593
Zajac, W. 387, 411
Zajfen, M. 613
Zbojanova, M. 1246
Ziegler, G. 570
Zilberberg, B. 1275, 1513
Zimmerman, M. 334
Zina, G. 143, 1047
Ziprkowski, L. 562, 1418
Zivkovitch, V. 288
Zlatkov, N. 1110
Zöllner, N. 1390